EIGHTEENTH EDITION

Maternity Nursing

FAMILY, NEWBORN, AND WOMEN'S HEALTH CARE

Sharon J. Reeder
RN, PhD, FAAN

Professor Emeritus of Nursing and Former Chair,
   Primary Care Section
School of Nursing
University of California
Los Angeles, California

Leonide L. Martin
RN, MS, DrPH

Professor Emeritus, Department of Nursing
Sonoma State University
Rohnert Park, California
Family Nurse Practitioner
Sierra Family Medical Clinic
Nevada City, California

Deborah Koniak-Griffin
RN, EdD, FAAN

Professor
Women's Health Care Nurse Practitioner
School of Nursing
University of California
Los Angeles, California

EIGHTEENTH EDITION

Maternity Nursing

FAMILY, NEWBORN, AND WOMEN'S HEALTH CARE

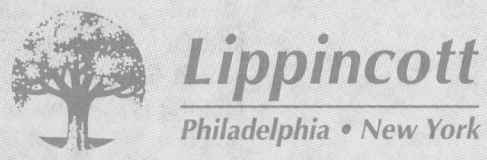
Lippincott
Philadelphia • New York

Acquisitions Editor: Jennifer Brogan
Developmental Editor: Sarah Andrus
Coordinating Editorial Assistant: Danielle DiPalma
Project Editor: Susan Deitch
Production Manager: Helen Ewan
Production Coordinator: Nannette Winski
Design Coordinator: Kathy Kelley-Luedtke

18th Edition

Library of Congress Cataloging in Publications Data

Reeder, Sharon J.
    Maternity nursing : family, newborn, and women's health care /
Sharon J. Reeder, Leonide L. Martin, Deborah Koniak-Griffin. — 18th ed.
        p.   cm
    Includes bibliographical references and index.
    ISBN 0-397-55166-5
    1. Marternity nursing.   I. Martin, Leonide L.   II. Koniak,
Deborah.   III. Title.
    [DNLM: 1. Maternal-Child Nursing.   2. Women's Health.   WY 157.3
R325m 1997]
    RG951.R44   1997
    618.2 — dc20
    DNLM/DLC   96-15970
    for Library of Congress   CIP

Care has been taken to confirm the accuracy of the information presented and to describe generally accepted practices. However, the authors, editors, and publisher are not responsible for errors or omissions or for any consequences from application of the information in this book and make no warranty, express or implied, with respect to the contents of the publication.

The authors, editors and publisher have exerted every effort to ensure that drug selection and dosage set forth in this text are in accordance with current recommendations and practice at the time of publication. However, in view of ongoing research, changes in government regulations, and the constant flow of information relating to drug therapy and drug reactions, the reader is urged to check the package insert for each drug for any change in indications and dosage and for added warnings and precautions. This is particularly important when the recommended agent is a new or infrequently employed drug.

Some drugs and medical devices presented in this publication have Food and Drug Administration (FDA) clearance for limited use in restricted research settings. It is the responsibility of the health care provider to ascertain the FDA status of each drug or device planned for use in their clinical practice.

9 8 7 6 5 4 3 2 1

Contributors

Ida Stanley Bird, RN, MN
Assistant Clinical Professor
UCLA School of Nursing
UCLA Center for the Health Sciences
Childbirth Educator in Private Practice
Los Angeles, California
*Chapter 19: Education for Pregnancy and
Parenthood, Coauthor Chapter 23: Pain Management
During Childbirth, and Appendix C: Prenatal
and Postpartum Exercises*

Judith Bunten, BSN, MSN, RNC
Administrative Nurse II, Perinatal Unit
UCLA Medical Center
Los Angeles, California
Chapter 38: Postpartum Complications

Roberta J. Gerds, RN, MN
Associate Professor, Department of Nursing
California State University, Bakersfield
Bakersfield, California
*Chapter 18: Nutritional Care in Pregnancy, Chapter
24: Immediate Care of the Newborn, Chapter 28:
Assessment of the Newborn, Chapter 29: Nursing Care
and Sensory Enrichment of the Normal Newborn,
and Chapter 30: Nutritional Care of the Newborn*

Judith N. Halle, RNC, PhD
Perinatal Clinical Nurse Specialist
Postdoctoral Fellow
Division of Maternal-Fetal Medicine
UCLA School of Medicine
Los Angeles, California
*Chapter 22: Management of Normal Labor, Chapter
31: Gestational Related Complications, Chapter 36:
Complications of Labor, and Chapter 37: Operative
Obstetrics*

Jane McAteer, RN, MN
Associate Professor of Nursing
College of San Mateo
San Mateo, California
*Chapter 41: The High-Risk Newborn: Disorders
of Gestational Age and Birth Weight, Chapter 42:
The High-Risk Newborn: Developmental Disorders,
and Chapter 43: The High-Risk Newborn: Acquired
Disorders*

Catherine Walla, RN, MA, MN
Assistant Clinical Professor
School of Nursing, Los Angeles
Research Coordinator
Department of Obstetrics and Gynecology
Cedars-Sinai Medical Center
Los Angeles, California
*Chapter 39: Fetal Diagnosis and Treatment (Nursing
Care Plan provided by Alison Keller, RN, MN)
and Chapter 40: Intrapartum Fetal Monitoring and Care*

Wynne Waugaman, CRNA, PhD
Director, USC and UCLA Programs of Nurse
    Anesthesia
Associate Professor of Nursing, University of Southern
    California
Professor of Clinical Anesthesiology, University
    of California, Los Angeles
Los Angeles, California
*Coauthor Chapter 23: Pain Management During
Childbirth*

Wendy Wetzel, RN, MSN, FNP
Private Practice
"A Woman's Place"
Flagstaff, Arizona
*Chapter 13: Management of Infertility, Chapter 14:
Genetic Counseling and Diagnosis During Pregnancy,
and Chapter 15: Biophysical Aspects of Normal
Pregnancy*

Reviewers

Lynne Hutnik Conrad, RNC, MSN, BSN
Program Director, ObGyn
Elkins Park Hospital
Elkins Park, Pennsylvania

Laurie Kaudewitz, BSN, MSN, RNC
Assistant Professor of Nursing
East Tennessee State University
Johnson City, Tennessee

Celesta Kirk, RN, CS, MA, MSN, FNP
Assistant Professor
Department of Family-Community Nursing
East Tennessee State University
Johnson City, Tennessee

Cecilia Tiller, RN, DSN
Associate Professor
Medical College of Georgia
Augusta, Georgia

Katherine Carnaghan-Scherrard, RN, BN, MSC(A)
Faculty Leader, School of Nursing
McGill University
Consultant, Montreal Children's Hospital
Montreal, Quebec, CANADA

Greta Wiener Fox, RNC, FNP, BSN, MSN
Family Nurse Practitioner
Mount Auburn Women's Health Association
Watertown, Massachusetts
Gynacare Clinic
Boston, Massachusetts

Preface

Maternity Nursing: Family, Newborn, and Women's Health Care has been extensively revised and updated to reflect many of the changes evident in today's society, family, and healthcare system.

One very exciting change is the growing health promotion focus in healthcare, with clients wanting to take a more active and informed role. For example, many women are taking an active role in choosing the birthing experience with which they feel most comfortable—whether that be with a physician, nurse-midwife, or practitioner in the hospital, home, or alternative birthing center. Cultural diversity among healthcare recipients and providers is increasing, bringing new ideas, practices, and challenges into family, maternal, and newborn care.

Family structures are continuing to change and evolve. There are many more single mothers and fathers, and many women are continuing to work while raising children. The healthcare system itself is undergoing evolution. Many community hospitals are being closed, insurance policies are cutting the amount and types of procedures they will cover, and there is tremendous growth in the home and community care practices. One example of the impact insurance policies are having on maternal-newborn care is seen in the decreased length of hospital stay for vaginal and cesarean births.

New health discoveries, for example in the field of infertility treatment, are changing the scope of healthcare and providing hope for many people. Health problems in today's society are having a devastating impact on the family, women, and newborns. For example, HIV/AIDS is now the third most common cause of death in the 25- to 44-year-old male and female population.

These changes have had a profound impact on maternal-perinatal healthcare. The traditional role of the maternal-perinatal nurse must expand to meet the challenges these new changes are posing. This starts with an awareness and acknowledgment of these changes and a willingness to evolve along with them. These current issues and their impact on the maternal-perinatal specialty are examined in depth to enable students to understand their importance. The intent of the authors is that today's students take this knowledge and incorporate it into the care they provide.

Organization

The 18th edition of *Maternity Nursing* has been reorganized into eight units. All chapters within the units have been revised and updated to reflect current standards of practice, technology, and nursing care:

Unit I: Nursing, Family Health, and Reproduction includes five chapters: Philosophy of Contemporary Maternity Care, Critical Thinking in the Nursing Process, The Family and Nursing Practice, Sociocultural Considerations, and Ethical and Legal Considerations.

Unit II: Biophysical Aspects of Human Reproduction includes two chapters: Sexual and Reproductive Anatomy and Physiology and Conception and Development of the Embryo and Fetus.

Unit III: Assessment and Management of Women's Health includes seven chapters: Women's Health Promotion, Sexual Health and Family Planning, Common Problems in Women's Health, Infectious Diseases, Clinical Interruption of Pregnancy, Management of Infertility, and Genetic Counseling and Diagnosis During Pregnancy.

Unit IV: Assessment and Management in the Antepartum Period includes five chapters: Biophysical Aspects of Normal Pregnancy, Psychosocial Aspects of Pregnancy, Nursing Care in the Prenatal Period, Nutritional Care in Pregnancy, and Education for Pregnancy and Parenthood.

the Passageway and Passenger, The Process of Labor and Birth, Management of Normal Labor, Pain Management During Childbirth, and Immediate Care of the Newborn.

Unit VI: Assessment and Management in the Postpartum Period includes six chapters: Biophysical Aspects of the Postpartum Period, Psychosocial Aspects of the Postpartum Period, Nursing Care in the Postpartum Period, Assessment of the Newborn, Nursing Care and Sensory Enrichment of the Normal Newborn, and Nutritional Care of the Newborn.

Unit VII: Assessment and Management of High-Risk Maternal Conditions includes eight chapters: Gestational Related Complications, Concurrent Medical Complications of Pregnancy, Violence Toward Women in the Childbearing Years, Addictive Disorders in Pregnancy, Adolescent Sexuality, Pregnancy, and Childrearing, Complications of Labor, Operative Obstetrics, and Postpartum Complications.

Unit VIII: Assessment and Management of High-Risk Perinatal Conditions includes five chapters: Fetal Diagnosis and Treatment, Intrapartum Fetal Monitoring and Care, The High-Risk Newborn: Disorders of Gestational Age and Birth Weight, The High-Risk Newborn: Developmental Disorders, and The High-Risk Newborn: Acquired Disorders.

New Features for This Edition

Color A vibrant four-color design has been implemented for this edition to highlight all displays, charts, boxes, tables, illustrations, and photographs.

New **Chapters** have been added to address the concepts and changes discussed earlier in the preface. These include:

Chapter 2: Critical Thinking in the Nursing Process

Chapter 8: Women's Health Promotion

Chapter 10: Common Problems in Women's Health

Chapter 33: Violence Toward Women in the Childbearing Years

In addition several chapters were combined to tighten the focus of the material:

Chapter 23: Pain Management During Childbirth (Formerly, *The Nurse's Contribution to Pain Relief During Labor and Analgesia and Anesthesia During Childbirth*).

Chapter 29: Nursing Care and Sensory Enrichment of the Normal Newborn (Formerly, *Nursing Care of the Normal Newborn and Sensory Enrichment with the Newborn*).

Sociocultural Sensitivity

Sociocultural sensitivity is an important aspect of maternal-perinatal care. It is important for the student to understand sociocultural differences in order to provide the best possible, nonbiased care for each individual client.

Chapter Four: Sociocultural Considerations focuses on these issues and examines social, economic, and cultural diversity and the changing relationship between the client and the healthcare provider. In addition, the critical thinking exercises at the end of each unit emphasize the diversity of our society, and the photographs throughout the text were chosen to depict culturally diverse clients and healthcare providers.

Critical Thinking

Critical thinking skills are an important component of nursing care, especially with the more independent role that nurses are taking in healthcare today. Students should begin to practice these skills early in their education. The text provides several ways for the student to develop and practice these essential skills.

Chapter 2: Critical Thinking in the Nursing Process explains what critical thinking is and how the nurse can use these skills when providing client care. The chapter also explains how critical thinking relates to the nursing process and nursing care.

Critical Thinking Exercises are provided after each unit. These exercises contain material covered in each chapter of the unit. The student is challenged to use critical thinking skills to discuss the issues that are presented in each exercise.

Learning Tools

Chapter Outlines are presented at the beginning of each chapter and contain the major topics covered in the chapter.

Chapter Objectives (*new to this edition*) are presented at the beginning of each chapter and provide guidelines that enable the student to focus on the most important material in that particular chapter.

Key Terms (*new to this edition*) are presented at the beginning of each chapter. The key terms are defined in the glossary at the back of the textbook.

Nursing Process provides a unifying conceptual basis for the nursing care throughout the book. Nursing diagnoses have been revised according to the current NANDA recommendations. All nursing care plans and clinical chapters reflect the nursing process.

Bulleted Lists (*new to this edition*) are presented throughout the chapters to highlight important information in an easy-to-read format.

Summary Points (*new to this edition*) appear at the end of every chapter to highlight the most important information within the chapter.

Assessment Tools appear throughout the text and contain either questions or step-by-step assessment criteria for a specific situation.

Research Highlights appear in a majority of chapters. These displays contain current research pertaining to a topic discussed in the particular chapter. Each Research Highlight includes a critique of the reseach study.

Assessment Guidelines (*new to this edition*) appear throughout the text and contain general information that the nurse can use to assess and evaluate the client.

Nursing Guidelines recur throughout the text and contain nursing care guidelines for specific problems that the nurse can refer to when performing care for the clients.

Client Teaching Guidelines appear throughout the text. These boxes provide information for the nurse on what should be addressed with a client concerning a certain topic.

Client Education boxes appear throughout the text and provide information directed to the client about what to expect with a specific condition or how-to information on performing self-care activities.

Numbered Procedures (*new to this edition*) appear throughout the text in a two-column format. These how-to displays provide the student with specific nursing actions and rationales.

Critical Pathways (*new to this edition*) can be found in several chapters and provide the student with visual examples of these relatively new, insurance or hospital cost-cutting driven tools used to plan care for a particular procedure or problem.

Nursing Care Plans are included in the majority of chapters. New to this edition are rationale statements added to the new Intervention/Rationale column.

Tables, Boxes, and Charts appear throughout the text to highlight information and provide examples of information discussed in the chapter.

References and Selected Readings have been updated with current professional literature and are located at the end of each chapter.

Conference Material

The conference material at the end of each unit has been completely revised in order to better prepare the student for examinations and clinical practice. The conference material is arranged in three separate sections: *Critical Thinking Exercises, Study Questions, and NCLEX-Style Multiple Choice Questions.*

Each critical thinking exercise consists of a brief case study related to material covered within a specific chapter in the unit. A question is asked at the end of the case study that requires the student to think critically in order to determine possible answers to the question.

Study questions are provided for each chapter within the unit. The student may be asked to list several items, fill in the blank, name a particular disorder or treatment, or state the specific plan of care. The answers to the study questions are found in the Instructor's Manual.

NCLEX-style multiple choice questions are provided for each chapter within the unit to help the student become familiar with answering questions for the board exam. Each multiple choice question has only one possible correct answer. In addition, each question has been categorized according to the components of the NCLEX. The Cognitive Level, Client Need, and Phase of the Nursing Process for each question are found in the Instructor's Manual, just after the correct answer and rationale for that question.

Self-Study Computer Disk

A free Interactive Self-Study Computer Disk is stored on the inside back cover of each book. Over 250 multiple choice NCLEX-style questions challenge the student's comprehension and application of important material. Feedback is provided for each answer.

For the Instructor

(*The following items are available free to the instructor upon adoption of the text.*)

- **Computerized Testbank**—IBM-formatted disks contain 1000 new NCLEX-style multiple choice questions. A sophisticated ParTEST program allows the instructor to edit the questions in the testbank or add new questions if desired.
- **Printed Testbank**—A printed copy of the questions in the computerized testbank is provided to enable the instructor to see the questions that are in each chapter or unit at a glance.
- **Instructor's Manual**—The instructor's manual contains 43 chapters that correspond to each chapter in the text. Each chapter in the manual includes:

Chapter Overview: A summary of the content covered in each chapter.

Chapter Outline: A listing of the topical headings and subheadings of the chapter.

Key Terms: A list of key terms associated with the material presented in the chapter.

Teaching/Learning Activities: Classroom activities, clinical experiences, discussion questions, and written activities.

- **Student Review Sheets**—Review questions and activities for students to use in place of a Study Guide. The Student Review Sheets are printed on perforated pages so they can be copied and distributed to the students.
- **Transparencies**—*Fifty* full-color transparencies are included, enabling instructors to provide visual examples of what is being taught.

Acknowledgments

We wish to acknowledge our contributors to the 18th edition of *Maternity Nursing: Family, Newborn, and Women's Health Care* who have brought a wealth of expertise to this edition. Again, in this edition, all of the contributors are nurses with a wide range of clinical skills and knowledge, who have continued to deepen and broaden the book's content and orientation.

We also wish to express our thanks for the help and encouragement of all of our colleagues who have played such an important part in the revision of this edition. In particular, Kathy DeMattis provided invaluable help in the revision of several of the care plans, and Carmen Mathenge played a key role by providing help with literature searches, computer support, general assistance, and expert editorial services. In addition, Marian Heller helped out with literature searches and general assistance, and Nancy Siris Rauls, Juan Tan, and Jim Kimmick provided staunch and creative computer-related support.

We would like to acknowledge all of the publishers, colleagues, and the various organizations for use of their assessment tools, illustrations, and other displays that are found in the text. We are also indebted to the parents, children, nurses, and students who graciously agreed to be photographed for this edition.

Last but certainly not least, we wish to express our sincerest thanks and appreciation to the staff of Lippincott-Raven Publishers for their crucial support and suggestions throughout the production of this edition. We are indebted to Donna Hilton, Vice President and Publisher, Nursing and Allied Health Editorial and to Diana Intenzo, formerly with Lippincott, who was with us for the start of this revision and has been helpful in many past editions. We wish to thank particularly those with whom we have worked so closely in this revision: Jennifer Brogan, Acquisitions Editor, Mary Ann Foley, Developmental Editor, Sarah Andrus, Developmental Editor, Susan Deitch, Production Editor and Danielle DiPalma, Editorial Assistant for their steadfast patience and assistance to the authors and contributors in the preparation of this edition.

Finally, we salute our families, who have provided staunch support during production deadlines, computer glitches, misplaced manuscript, and all the other traumas that often beset revisions.

Contents

UNIT II
Biophysical Aspects of Human Reproduction   91

UNIT III

Assessment and Management of Women's Health   159

CHAPTER 10
Common Problems in Women's Health   227

CHAPTER 11
Infectious Diseases   267

CHAPTER 12
Clinical Interruption of Pregnancy   301

CHAPTER 13
Management of Infertility   *319*

CHAPTER 14
Genetic Counseling and Diagnosis During Pregnancy   *341*

UNIT IV
Assessment and Management in the Antepartum Period   *363*

CHAPTER 15
Biophysical Aspects of Normal Pregnancy   *365*

UNIT V

Assessment and Management in the Intrapartum Period   501

CHAPTER 20
Assessment of the Passageway and Passenger   503

CHAPTER 21
The Process of Labor and Birth   519

CHAPTER 22
Management of Normal Labor   537

CHAPTER 23
Pain Management During Childbirth   573

CHAPTER 24
Immediate Care of the Newborn   617

UNIT VI
Assessment and Management in the Postpartum Period   633

CHAPTER 25
Biophysical Aspects of the Postpartum Period   635

CHAPTER 29
Nursing Care and Sensory Enrichment of the Normal Newborn   727

CHAPTER 30
Nutritional Care of the Newborn   761

UNIT VII
Assessment and Management of High-Risk Maternal Conditions   801

CHAPTER 31
Gestational Related Complications   803

CHAPTER 32
Concurrent Medical Complications of Pregnancy   849

CHAPTER 33
Violence Toward Women in the Childbearing Years   889

CHAPTER 34
Addictive Disorders in Pregnancy   905

CHAPTER 35
Adolescent Sexuality, Pregnancy, and Childrearing   931

CHAPTER 36
Complications of Labor   955

CHAPTER 37
Operative Obstetrics   1009

CHAPTER 38
Postpartum Complications   1027

UNIT VIII

Assessment and Management of High-Risk Perinatal Conditions   1055

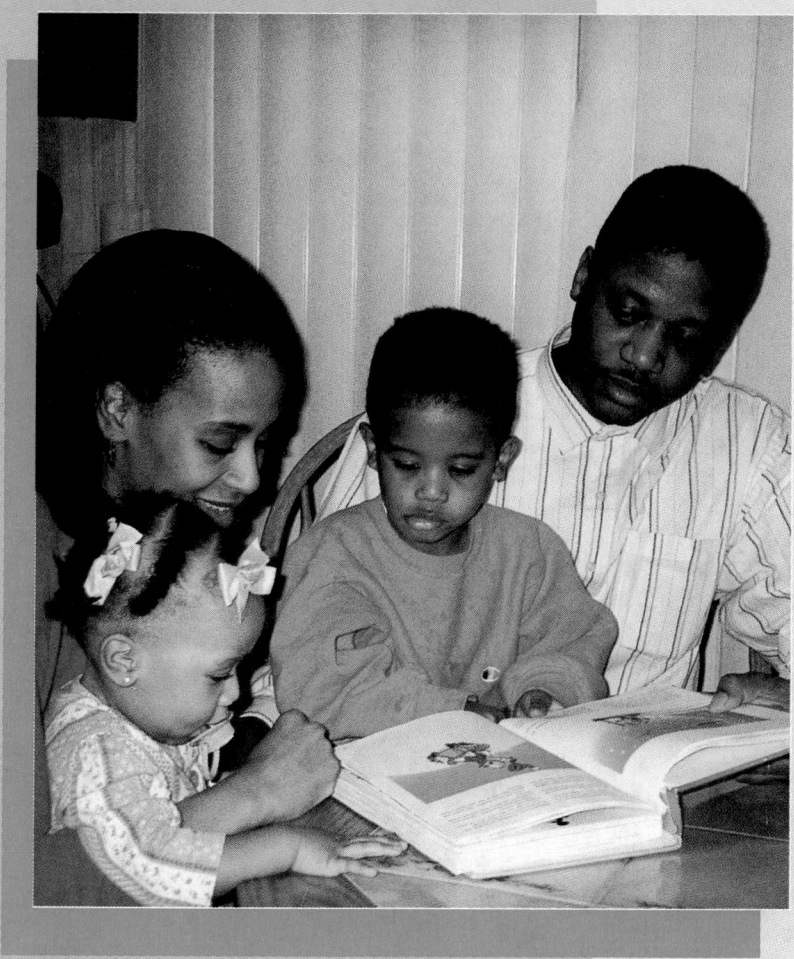

Nursing, Family Health, and Reproduction

1

Philosophy of Contemporary Maternity Care

Objectives

- Describe the philosophy and assumptions underlying family-centered maternity-perinatal nursing.
- Develop an understanding of the various aspects of family-centered maternity care.
- Compare and contrast the various nursing advanced practice roles in maternity-perinatal care.
- Summarize the relevance of vital statistics for perinatal care.
- Describe and discuss the development and trends in maternity-perinatal nursing.
- Describe the innovations in institutional and community or home health settings in maternity-perinatal care.

Key Terms

Fetal death	Obstetrics
Level I hospitals	Perinatal
Level II hospitals	Perinatal care
Level III hospitals	Perinatal mortality
Maternal-child health	Puerperal infection
Maternal mortality	Tertiary care
Neonatal mortality	

The l990s have been called the decade of women's health; reproduction has been given prime importance. Legislation and policy efforts have focused attention on women as recipients and providers of healthcare. The increasing numbers of women and children living in poverty, the epidemic of adolescent pregnancy, the number of women in the work force, the increasing numbers of women with acquired immunodeficiency syndrome, the effect of immigration and population shifts, and continued advances in reproductive technology all impact the childbearing family and create enormous pressures for critical problem solving (Quimby, l994). These complexities of current societal trends impose a challenge to the providers of maternal-child healthcare. Professionals from the social sciences and health sciences, policy makers, and providers of healthcare services are combining their efforts to develop useful strategies for the 21st century.

Birth is a family affair, and the reproductive health of the total family is the cornerstone of a healthy society. Thus, the study of obstetrics and nursing care of women and their families during childbearing includes the study of anatomic and physiologic adaptations to human reproduction, human growth and development, and the many complex, interdependent relationships to society.

Knowledge of the anatomy and physiology of the reproductive organs and of the development of the fetus from conception to birth is required by everyone who participates in maternity care. The physiologic mechanism by which conception takes place and the new human being that develops have far-reaching implications for the family. The health, well-being, and safety of each mother, father, and newborn must be protected, and the highest level of wellness possible for ever─ childbearing family must be achieved in the ─t sense of physical, emotional, and social well- ─ is important to understand the extent to which ─ture and function of the family as it relates to ─fluence the reproductive behavior and health

of the childbearing family, particularly in these highly complex, technological times.

This chapter introduces many of these issues in an effort to orient the student to maternity nursing. The philosophy and assumptions underlying care for the family during reproduction are given, and basic concepts of care are examined. In the remainder of the unit, information and concepts relating to childbearing families and how they mesh with society are explored (Box 1-1).

Development of Maternity Care

All definitions and modes of healthcare have a history. Maternity care is no exception. The following paragraphs introduce some key terms and concepts of care that have become associated with them.

Obstetrics

Obstetrics is defined as the branch of medicine that deals with parturition, its antecedents, and its sequelae. Thus, obstetrics is concerned principally with the phenomena and management of pregnancy, labor, and the puerperium under normal and abnormal circumstances (Cunningham et al., l993).

The word obstetrics is derived from *obstetricia* or *obstetrix*, meaning midwife. The Latin verb *obsto* means to stand by. In England and the United States, this branch of medicine was called *midwifery* until the latter part of the 19th century when the term obstetrics came to the forefront.

After World War II, the terminology changed to *maternity care* as the focus came to be on the recipient of care rather than on the provider of care. Maternity care now implies a broader meaning of care to mother, newborn, and other members of the family. It emphasizes the importance of interpersonal relationships that are significant in the family and takes into consideration the factors that are crucial in promoting the general health and well-being of the expanding family group.

The term **maternal-child health** has been used for more than 70 years when speaking of the health needs and delivery of care to the mother and newborn. In 1912, the U.S. Children's Bureau was created by an act of Congress to promote maternal and child health "among all classes of people." Until its reorganization into the National Institutes of Health, the Children's Bureau continued to make significant contributions to the promotion of maternal-child health in this country.

BOX 1–1
Characteristics of Maternity Care and the Emergence of Maternity Nursing

Maternity Care

Birth considered a family and community event, integrated into everyday life

⬇

Development of scientific medicine and physician participation in childbirth

⬇

Increasing understanding of asepsis and increased technology in obstetrics

⬇

Growing emphasis on hospital deliveries rather than on home births

⬇

Increasing numbers of women delivering in the hospital

⬇

Necessity for efficient, organized aseptic care in hospitals, due to organizational structure

⬇

Borrowing of time-saving approaches and work-efficient procedures from industry

⬇

"Assembly line care" in hospitals

⬇

Ritualistic practices, rigid adherence to rules and procedures

⬇

Impersonal, routine care

⬇

Resurgence of family and participant focus in childbearing through natural childbirth and consumer movements

⬇

Pressure for change in hospital routines and procedures, alternative birth approaches

⬇

Development of family-centered maternity care, participant childbirth, rooming-in, alternate birth centers

Maternity Nursing

Midwives usual birth attendants, precursors to maternity nurse

⬇

Gradual replacement of midwives by physicians as birth attendants

⬇

Nursing as women's occupation, paralleling growth of scientific medicine

⬇

Nurses in obstetrics taught by medical (pathologic) model

⬇

Nursing students focused on technical competence and physical care of clients in hospitals

⬇

Nursing students service provided to hospitals where trained

⬇

Nursing orientation toward efficient care of a number of clients, without in-depth nursing therapy (no theoretical foundation)

⬇

Institution-oriented nurses, physician's "right arm"

Development of the humanistic-supportive nursing model as distinct from the pathologic-intervention medical model

⬇

Expansion of the maternity nurse's role to include personalized care, parent education, counseling and psychosocial support, advocacy, alternative-care services to childbearing families

⬇

Emergence of new roles (nurse practitioner, clinical specialist) and resurgence of nurse-midwifery

Perinatal Care

During the last decade, as knowledge and technology have continued to burgeon, an effort has been made to provide a conceptual umbrella to encompass maternal-fetal healthcare as a unit. Consequently, the term **perinatal care** has evolved. By definition, the word **perinatal** means the 6 weeks preceding and following birth; however, in actual use, the connotation is much more encompassing. All of the definitions imply that an obstetric and pediatric orientation are involved. Hence, perinatal care is a method of healthcare delivery that decreases the segmentation and fragmentation of care for the mother and newborn (Fig. 1-1).

Perinatal care also has become associated with the high-risk mother and newborn in hospitals designated as **tertiary care**, or **level III hospitals.** These hospi-

tals have the resources and expertise to manage any complication of pregnancy or that the newborn may experience. The personnel in level III institutions provide care for normal clients and for all types of maternal-fetal and neonatal illnesses and abnormalities. By contrast, **level I hospitals** provide for management of uncomplicated maternal and neonatal clients. In these institutions, there should be a strong component of preventive services and early detection of existing or potential problems, which then may be referred to the level III institutions. **Level II hospitals** provide the same services as level I hospitals; however, they can provide for some high-risk obstetric problems and certain types of neonatal illnesses that do not require the wide array of expertise and technology found in the level III hospitals (Box 1-2 and Table 1-1; DeVane, 1991; Andersen et al., 1993; Chiu et al., 1993).

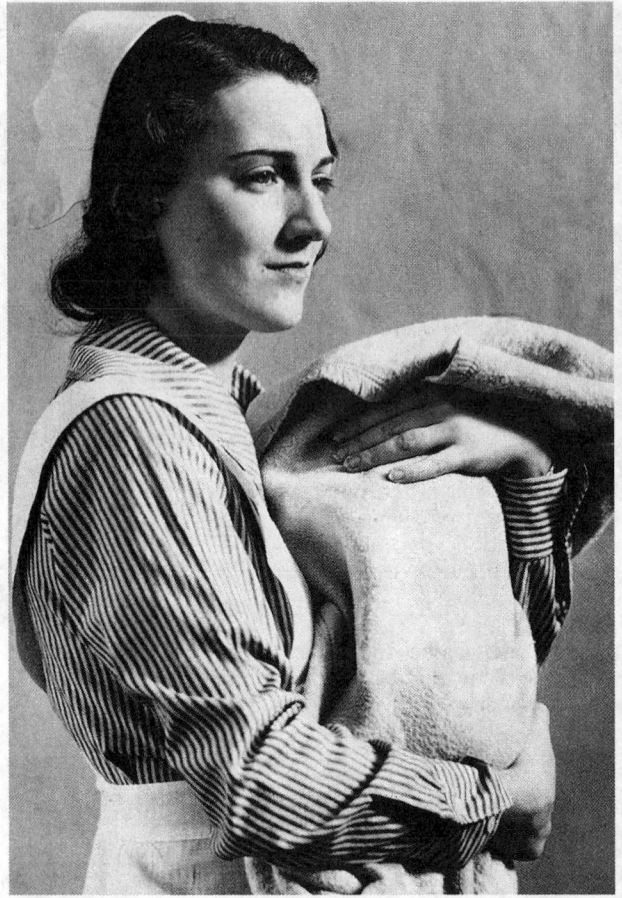
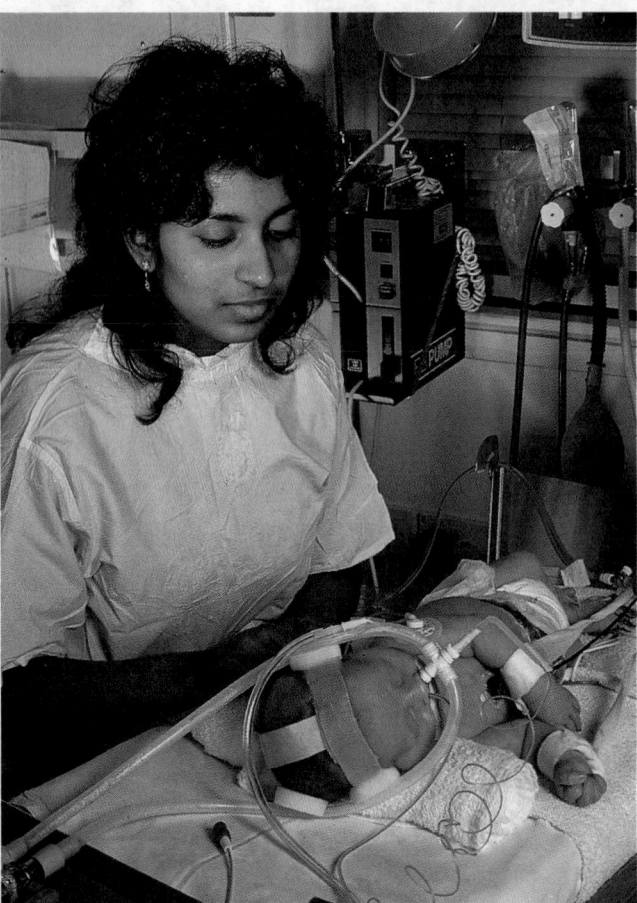

A   B

FIGURE 1–1 The concept of obstetrics, which focused primarily on the physician and nurse as providers of care during labor and delivery, has expanded to become a concept entitled perinatal care. This is a shift in focus that encompasses the mother's health, fetal health, and care of the normal or high-risk newborn.

Philosophy of Maternity Care

When responding to their clients' health maintenance and illness management needs, health providers must take into consideration current attitudinal, social, and cultural changes. Healthcare is not delivered in a vacuum; it takes place in a larger social context and is greatly influenced by current thinking and change manifested by the host society. Philosophies of care evolve from this thinking and change.

We believe maternity care to be a philosophy of client care, rather than a special area of medical services or nursing. As previously stated, having children is a family affair; thus, the medical and nursing care of maternity clients is a family-centered activity.

In almost no other normal physiologic process does one find such individual extremes of reactions within a normal context. For the woman and her partner, reactions to becoming parents may be based on events

from childhood, adolescence, or adulthood. Certainly, they are influenced by the immediate home environments from which the mother and father come. In addition, the expectant parents' level of satisfaction and the level of contentment of the postpartum mother and newborn are modified by the interpersonal relationships of those most significant to them in the healthcare environment.

Assumptions About Maternity Care

Underlying the philosophy about maternity care are the following assumptions:

- All individuals have the right to be born healthy, and to ensure this right, every pregnant woman and fetus has the right to quality healthcare.
- The sexuality of individuals is inextricably bound to reproduction but not subordinate to it; changing societal attitudes toward sexuality, role relationships, and childbearing, together with technological ad-

experience will be influenced by his or her cultural heritage.

Maternity-Perinatal Nursing and Family-Centered Care

The following paragraphs address important terminology associated with the concepts and delivery of maternity-perinatal nursing care. Some of the terms are used interchangeably, but each has a slightly different nuance; thus, it is important to use the term appropriate to the phenomenon under discussion.

Definition

Maternity-perinatal nursing is the delivery of professional quality healthcare that recognizes, focuses on, and adapts to the physical and psychosocial needs of the childbearing woman, family, and newborn. Implicit in this definition is the notion of a family-centered approach that assumes the family to be the basic unit in society whose important functions are childbearing, childrearing, and mutual support of its members.

BOX 1-2
Services Provided in Level I, II, and III Hospitals

Level I

- Surveillance and care of all clients admitted to the obstetric service, with an established triage system for identifying high-risk mothers who should be transferred to a level II or III facility prior to delivery
- Proper detection and supportive care of unanticipated maternal-fetal problems that occur during labor and delivery
- Performance of cesarean delivery
- Care of postpartum conditions
- Resuscitation of all newborns in their delivery facilities
- Stabilization of unexpected small or sick newborns before transfer to a level II or III facility
- Evaluation of the condition of healthy newborns and continuing care of these newborns until their discharge

Level II

- Performance of level I services
- Management of high-risk mothers and newborns admitted and transferred

Level III

- Provision of perinatal service for all mothers and newborns
- Research support
- Compilation, analysis, and evaluation of regional data

---

vances in fertility control, have made parenthood an increasingly voluntary state.

- Reproduction is not experienced alone; whatever the circumstances, it involves one or more additional individuals.
- Reproduction is a normal psychophysiologic process and can be physically and emotionally rewarding for those involved.
- The childbearing experience is a developmental opportunity; it can be a situational crisis during which family members benefit from the solidarity of the family unit.
- The profound physiologic changes and adjustment that the mother and her offspring experience during the childbearing process make them particularly vulnerable to changeable and noxious environments and situations that would ordinarily not prove hazardous.
- Each individual's attitudes, values, and health behavior are influenced by the culture and society from which he or she comes; thus, each individual's reproductive outcomes and childbearing

---

TABLE 1-1
Recommended Nurse–Client Ratios for Perinatal Services

Nurse–Client Ratio	Care Provided
1:2	Prenatal testing
1:2	Laboring clients
1:1	Clients in second stage of labor
1:1	Ill clients with complications
1:2	Oxytocin induction or augmentation of labor
1:1	Coverage of epidural anesthesia
1:1	Circulation for cesarean delivery
1:6	Prenatal or postpartum clients without complications
1:2	Postoperative recovery
1:3	Clients with complications but in stable condition
1:4	Recently born newborns and those needing close observation
1:6	Newborns needing only routine care
1:3	Mother–newborn care
1:1	Newborns requiring multisystem support
1:3–4	Newborns requiring intermediate care
1:1–2	Newborns needing intensive care

"Family" does not necessarily mean the traditional nuclear family composed of a married couple and their children. In Chapter 3, the various definitions and emerging family forms are examined.

Implementation

Maternity-perinatal nursing involves direct, personal care to the childbearing woman and her newborn and the related activities of teaching, counseling, and supervising during the various phases of the childbearing experience. A cornerstone of care is client education with respect to health maintenance and reproductive health. This is unique in that the nurse must attend, educate, and counsel all age groups, because the childbearing unit may span many stages in the life cycle.

The nurse will intervene to relieve or reduce problems caused by physiologic, psychological, or social stress. In addition, the nurse must make clients aware of the principles of health maintenance so that they may incorporate these into their preventive health behavior patterns.

A significant aspect of maternity-perinatal nursing on the professional level is that the nursing care involves purposeful, sustained interaction during which the nurse makes an assessment of the client's problems and resources and then takes action to relieve the problem and support the strengths. If the condition requires additional services from the other members of the health team, referral or consultation is given.

The successful implementation of family-centered nursing care includes recognition that the provision of high-caliber care requires a team effort by the woman and her family, the healthcare providers, and the community. The composition of the team may vary from setting to setting and includes obstetricians, pediatricians, family physicians, certified nurse-midwives (CNM), nurse practitioners, and perinatal clinical nurse specialists. Although physicians are responsible for providing direction for medical management, other team members share appropriately in managing the healthcare of the family, and each team member must be individually accountable for the performance of his or her facet of care. The team concept includes the cooperative inter-relationships of hospitals, providers, and the community in an organized care system to provide for the total spectrum of maternity-newborn care.

Advanced Practice Roles in Maternity Nursing Care

As the healthcare system evolves, so too does the scope of practice for the maternity-perinatal nurse. In the 1970s, the concept of *expanded role* was introduced into nursing. The connotation was that the functions of nurses needed to be expanded so that they could assume more responsibility in primary care, acute care, and long-term care. In the 1980s, the term *advanced nursing practice* came into use. Advanced nursing practice has been defined as the deliberate diagnosis and treatment of the full range of human responses to actual and potential health problems. The definition also includes the application of a broad range of theories and a broad set of postgraduate nursing skills (Calkin, 1984; California Nurses' Association, 1984). It is generally accepted that preparation for the advanced practice role occurs at the graduate level and incorporates the components of theory, clinical practice, consultation, education, and research. Thus, Frik et al. (1994) offer a revised definition of advanced practice: specialists in various areas of nursing practice who have been prepared through theory-based education and supervised clinical practice at the graduate level.

These advanced practice roles developed in two directions. The nurse practitioner role focuses on primary ambulatory care, and the nurse clinical specialist role focuses on secondary and tertiary hospital care. The CNM combines antepartum, intrapartum, and postpartum management. The practitioner and clinical specialist roles require graduate study at the master's level. The CNM can be achieved by a certification program, although the preparation is more frequently at the master's level.

The Obstetrician-Gynecologist Nurse Practitioner

The obstetrician-gynecologist (OB-GYN) nurse practitioner, provides prenatal care for uncomplicated pregnancies in conjunction with a physician consultant. The nurse takes a health and pregnancy history, performs the physical and obstetric examination, orders and interprets laboratory and other diagnostic studies, plans for necessary treatments and medications in conjunction with the physician, and assesses family relationships and psychosocial needs.

Throughout the pregnancy, the OB-GYN nurse practitioner sees the woman on prenatal visits, sometimes alternating with the physician; evaluates the progress of the pregnancy; and manages minor physical problems. Information and counseling related to pregnancy and childbirth and assessment of the couple's adjustments and family problems are part of the nurse practitioner's role. Referrals to community agencies, prepared childbirth classes, and other medical specialties also may be made. Most maternity-nurse practitioners are skilled in provision of family planning counseling and can select and teach about appropriate methods for the client, including natural methods for pregnancy spacing, oral contraceptives, intrauterine devices, and diaphragms.

The Family Nurse Practitioner

Family nurse practitioners also can provide care during pregnancy. These nurses are generalists who care for all family members similarly to family practice physicians. In addition to the functions described for maternity-nurse practitioners, family nurse practitioners provide postdelivery care for the baby as it grows, thus providing continuity throughout the reproductive process except during the intrapartum phase.

The Maternity-Perinatal Clinical Specialist

Maternity-perinatal clinical specialists undergo advanced study of maternity nursing at the graduate level and are able to provide in-depth intervention for many of the adaptational and physiologic problems encountered in maternity care. Frequently, clinical specialists have an area of expertise within the specialty field, such as the care of pregnant diabetics, breast-feeding mothers, parents experiencing neonatal death or abnormalities, or Rh-sensitized mothers. These nurses with master's degrees also are consultants to other maternity nursing staff, assisting them to plan care for difficult problems or special situations encountered in the unit. Although clinical specialists also may be involved in staff education, their primary function is direct client services that require a high degree of knowledge, skill, and competence in their area of specialty.

Critical Care Obstetrics

This subspecialty is only recently emerging and relates primarily to high-risk deliveries and postpartum critical care. As yet there are no "specialists," and there has

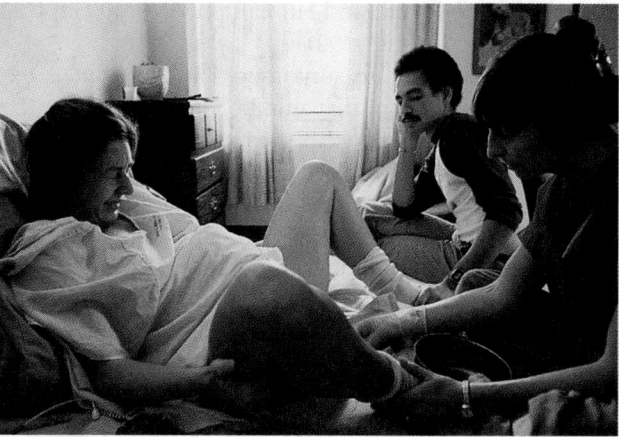

FIGURE 1–2 The certified nurse-midwife can administer care to the mother during labor and delivery in the home, birthing center, or hospital as long as the mother's progress is considered normal and uncomplicated.

been little in the literature regarding this type of practice. However, with the increasing number of high-risk clients and the implementation of technical equipment, it is expected that this specialty will become prominent (Andersen, 1993).

Nurse-Midwife

The "expanded" role known as nurse-midwife has been around for centuries. Modern practice requires certification and special education. CNMs are registered nurses who have completed a specific program of study and have clinical experience recognized by the American College of Nurse Midwives. They also must pass a certification test before beginning practice. They are qualified to take complete health histories and perform complete physical examinations for their clients. They can provide complete prenatal care, including teaching and counseling. They are qualified to give comprehensive care during the intrapartum period, including delivery of the newborn (Fig. 1-2). They are able to deliver care to the mother and newborn in the postpartum period, including family planning information and devices. Thus, they attend the mother and newborn throughout the maternity cycle, including the delivery, as long as the woman's progress is considered normal and uncomplicated (Box 1-3).

Social Context of Maternity Nursing Care

Maternity care is practiced in the context of the total society and as such, is influenced by the values, attitudes, and practices of that society. Lately, society has adopted a new stance, particularly with regard to attitudes toward the roles of men and women. The maelstrom of social change this country has experienced, particularly in the last 25 years, has greatly expanded options for behavior.

Social Change and Personal Choice

Women in particular expect more choices of lifestyle. Increasingly, they are demanding a large decision-making role regarding economic and social policies that affect their lives and the larger society in which they live. At one time, women had to make a choice between a family or a career. Now, women are increasingly combining the two. Moreover, many types of occupations and professions formerly closed to women are becoming more accessible. Federal legislation supports equal treatment of working women, and more mechanisms to challenge discrimination and unfair em-

BOX 1–3
Nurse-Midwifery

What Is a Certified Nurse-Midwife?

A certified nurse-midwife (CNM) is an individual educated in the two disciplines of nursing and midwifery, who possesses evidence of certification according to the requirements of the American College of Nurse-Midwives.

What Is Nurse-Midwifery Practice?

Nurse-midwifery is the independent management of care of essentially normal newborns and women, antepartally, intrapartally, postpartally, or gynecologically, occurring within a healthcare system that provides for medical consultation, collaborative management, or referral. This is in accord with the *Functions, Standards, and Qualifications for Nurse-Midwifery Practice* as defined by the American College of Nurse-Midwives.

The nurse-midwife provides care for the normal mother during pregnancy and stays with her during labor, providing continuous physical and emotional support. She evaluates progress and manages the labor and delivery. She evaluates and provides immediate care for the normal newborn. She helps the mother to care for herself and her newborn, to adjust the home situation to the newborn, and to lay a healthful foundation for future pregnancies through family planning and gynecologic services. The nurse-midwife is prepared to teach, interpret, and provide support as an integral part of her services.

AJN (1990) 90(12)

ployment practices against women are being developed at the state level. Antidiscrimination laws in effect until recently have had an impact on educational institutions. This has forced a gradual change in the social biases toward a male privilege, perpetuated through values taught in primary and secondary schools and culminating in the sex-linked admission practices and career choices fostered by colleges and universities.

Women who rear families today spend significantly less of their lifetime in childbearing and childrearing than women did years ago. This fact has a direct impact on the structure and function of the family. Today's families are smaller, and for those who start childbearing early, the last child is often born when the mother is in her middle to late 20s or early 30s. The high degree of technology in many American households has freed the woman from hours of household chores; thus, homemaking does not provide the full-time occupation that it once did. With her life span lengthened and her health improved, the 35- to 40-year-old woman can be healthy and vigorous and can look ahead to at least another 25 years of productivity in a sphere outside the home.

More egalitarian relationships are slowly developing between the two sexes. Increasingly, men are assuming more responsibility in childrearing and running the household as their partners are continuing with careers or occupations. When both parties are pursuing a career, household management, chores, and child-related activities tend to be shared. Thus, social power is slowly being equalized, and sex-linked exploitation is gradually being diminished. However, there is still a long way to go before true equality can be achieved.

Statistics

Statistical profiles are useful because they summarize a large amount of data about various populations and therefore supply healthcare providers and policy makers with a valuable overview of needs and gaps in care in a particular social context. In the United States, these *vital statistics reports* are published officially by the U.S. Public Health Service, National Center for Health Statistics, Vital Statistics Division (Box 1-4). Mortality and morbidity terminology are classified according to the World Health Organization's *Manual of International Classification of Diseases, Injuries, and Causes of Death.*

Birthrates

The increase in the number of births is the result of the increase in the number of women in the childbearing ages of 15 to 44 years. These childbearing women were born as a result of the "baby boom" of the post-World War II era. In 1992, the provisional fertility rate was 69.2, higher than it was through most of the 1970s and 1980s. The average number of lifetime births expected for women 18 to 34 years in 1992 was 2.1 (U.S. Department of Health and Human Services, 1993b; U.S. Bureau of the Census, 1992).

In 1989, the birthrate surpassed 4 million but is expected to drop below that number in the 1990s as the baby boom generation finishes its childbearing. By 2007, an upswing is expected, and by 2050, the number may pass 5 million (U.S. Department of Health and Human Services, 1993a; U.S. Bureau of the Census, 1992). Thus, an important consideration that influences the number of children being born annually is the size and age composition of the female population of childbearing age. Although the fertility rate is computed on the basis of births per 1,000 women between 15 and 44 years, most of the childbearing continues to be concentrated among women in their 20s. There has been a slight rise in the rate of marriages since 1968. However, many married couples are electing not to have

BOX 1–4
Definitions Pertaining to Vital Statistics

Birthrate. The number of births per 1,000 population; also known as the crude birthrate

Marriage rate. The number of marriages per 1,000 total population

Fertility rate. The number of births per 1,000 women aged 15 through 44 years

Neonatal. The period from birth through the 28th day of life

Neonatal death rate. The number of neonatal deaths per 1,000 live births

Stillbirth or fetal death. A death in which the fetus of 20 weeks or more gestational age dies *in utero* prior to birth

Perinatal mortality. All stillborn infants whose gestational age is 28 weeks or more, plus all neonatal deaths under 7 days per 1,000 births.* The 1979 revision of the ICD, however, uses birth weight rather than gestational age as a criterion. It also recommends two different categories of reporting. (For national data collection, the recommendation is that 500 g be used as the minimum weight of stillborn and live-newborns. For international comparisons, however, the weight should be 1,000 g or more. When weight is unknown, either gestational age [28 weeks] or body length corresponding to 1,000 g may be used.) Obviously, these different criteria will make comparisons with previous data impossible and will make national and international statistical comparisons difficult. There is current debate as to the efficacy of using the newly developed criteria.

Infant mortality rate. The number of deaths before the first birthday per 1,000 live births

Maternal mortality rate. The number of maternal deaths resulting from the reproductive process per 100,000 live births

Race and color. Births in the United States are classified for vital statistics according to the race of the parents in the categories of white, African American, American Indian, Chinese, Japanese, Aleut and Eskimo combined, Hawaiian and part-Hawaiian combined, and "other nonwhite." In most tables, a less detailed classification of "white" and "nonwhite" is used. The white category includes births to parents classified as white, Mexican, Puerto Rican, or "not stated."

*Current definition approved by the World Health Organization.

children, and more children are born from social contract and other nonlegal unions.

The Birth Certificate. All 50 states and the District of Columbia demand that a birth certificate be filled out on every birth and that the certificate be submitted promptly to the local registrar. After the birth has been registered, the local registrar sends a notification to the parents of the child. Also, a complete report is forwarded from the local registrar to the state authorities and then to the National Office of Vital Statistics in Washington.

Complete and accurate registration of births is a legal responsibility (Fig. 1-3). The birth certificate gives evidence of age, citizenship, and family relationships and is often required for military service, for passports, and to collect benefits on retirement and insurance.

A revision of the U.S. Standard Certificate of Live Birth was adopted by all but three states in the early 1990s. Form and content have been changed significantly. Check boxes will be used to obtain detailed medical, health, and lifestyle information and obstetric procedures, medical conditions of the newborn, birth attendant, and place of birth (Fig. 1-4). When these data are combined with other socioeconomic and health data, it is anticipated that a wealth of new information can be accumulated relevant to the etiology of neonatal health problems and adverse pregnancy outcomes (Taffel et al., 1989).

Mortality Rates

These statistics are valuable in providing policy makers and health professionals with necessary data to plan and implement research and programs that address diseases and conditions endangering the population.

Maternal Mortality. **Maternal mortality** refers to deaths that result from childbearing; that is, the underlying cause of the woman's death is the result of complications of pregnancy, childbirth, or the puerperium. The reduction in maternal mortality rates has been consistent since 1951. The dramatic decline in these rates began about the mid-1930s and continued until 1956. Since then, the decline has been slow but steady, culminating in a 7.6 rate per 1,000 births in 1990 and a 7.3 rate in 1992 (Maternal Child Health Bureau, 1994). Rates are projected to continue to fall for white women. Unfortunately, the nonwhite woman in the United States does not fare well in comparison. A nonwhite woman in the United States has a threefold greater incidence of death related to childbearing than her white counterpart. This is unfortunate, especially in the richest country in the world. The mortality rate for nonwhite women is equivalent to that of white women *30 years ago.*

The risk of maternal death for all women is lowest between ages 20 to 24 years. It is slightly higher in women younger than 20 years and in those 25 years and older. Increasing age is associated with a steep rise in maternal mortality. At 40 to 44 years, the mortality rate is six times greater than at 20 to 24 years. At the

H105.142 Rev. 5-78

COMMONWEALTH OF PENNSYLVANIA
DEPARTMENT OF HEALTH
VITAL STATISTICS

CERTIFICATE OF LIVE BIRTH

TYPE OR PRINT IN PERMANENT INK

PRIMARY DIST. NO.____________ STATE FILE NO.

A.____________
B.____________
C.____________
D.____________
E.____________
F.____________
G.____________
H.____________
I.____________

CHILD–NAME 1.	FIRST	MIDDLE	LAST	SEX 2.	DATE OF BIRTH (Mo. Day Year) 3a.	HOUR 3b. ______ AM ______ PM
HOSPITAL NAME (If not in Hospital, Give Street and Number) 4a.		City, Boro, or Twp. of Birth 4b.			COUNTY OF BIRTH 4c.	
I CERTIFY THAT THE STATED INFORMATION CONCERNING THIS CHILD IS TRUE TO THE BEST OF MY KNOWLEDGE AND BELIEF 5a. (Signature)		DATE SIGNED (Mo, Day, Year) 5b.	CERTIFIER–NAME AND TITLE (Type or Print) 5c.			
Name and Title of Attendant at Birth if other than Certifier (Type or Print) 5d.		CERTIFIER'S MAILING ADDRESS (Street or R.F.D. No., City or Town, State, Zip) 5e.				
MOTHER–MAIDEN NAME 6a.	FIRST	MIDDLE	LAST	AGE (At time of this Birth) 6b.	STATE OF BIRTH (If not in U.S.A., Name Country) 6c.	
MAILING ADDRESS 7.	STREET AND NUMBER		CITY AND STATE		ZIP CODE	
WHERE DOES MOTHER ACTUALLY LIVE? 8.	STATE		COUNTY		CITY, BORO, TWP. (Specify)	
FATHER–NAME 9a.	FIRST	MIDDLE	LAST	AGE (At time of this Birth) 9b.	STATE OF BIRTH (If not in U.S.A., Name Country) 9c.	
INFORMANT 10a.		Relation to Child 10b.	REGISTRAR'S SIGNATURE AND DATE RECEIVED 11.			

Death Under One Year Of Age – Number of Death Certificate For This Child

Multiple Births Enter State File Number for Mate(s)

Live Birth(s)

Fetal Death(s)

CONFIDENTIAL INFORMATION FOR MEDICAL AND HEALTH USE ONLY

RACE–MOTHER (e.g., White, Black, American Indian, etc. – Specify) 12.		RACE–FATHER (e.g., White, Black, American Indian, etc. – Specify) 13.		EDUCATION–MOTHER (Specify only highest grade completed) ELEMENTARY OR SECONDARY (0-12) | COLLEGE (1-4 or 5+) 14.		EDUCATION–FATHER (Specify only highest grade completed) ELEMENTARY OR SECONDARY (0-12) | COLLEGE (1-4 or 5+) 15.	IS MOTHER MARRIED TO FATHER? ☐ Yes ☐ No 16.
PREGNANCY HISTORY (Complete each section)							
LIVE BIRTHS (Do not include this child)		OTHER TERMINATIONS (Spontaneous and Induced)		Date Last Normal Menses Began (Mo. Day, Year) 18.	Month of Pregnancy Pre-Natal Care Began (1st, 2nd, etc.) (Specify) 19a.	Pre-Natal Visits – Total (If none, so state) 19b.	Length of Pregnancy in weeks. 20.
17a. Now living Number___ None ☐	17b. Now dead Number___ None ☐	17d. Before 16 wks. Number___ None ☐	17e. After 16 wks. Number___ None ☐	BIRTH WEIGHT 21.	THIS BIRTH–Single, Twin, Triplet, etc. (Specify) 22a.	If NOT Single Birth – Born First, Second, Third etc. (Specify) 22b.	APGAR SCORE 1 Min. 23a. 5 Min. 23b.
17c. Date of Last Live Birth (Mo. Year)		17f. Date of Last Other Termination (Mo. Year)		Method of Delivery 24.	COMPLICATIONS OF PREGNANCY (Describe or write "none") 25.		
CONCURRENT ILLNESSES OR CONDITIONS AFFECTING THE PREGNANCY (Describe or write "none") 26.					COMPLICATIONS OF LABOR AND/OR DELIVERY (Describe or write "none") 27.		
BIRTH INJURIES OF CHILD (Describe or write "none") 28.					CONGENITAL MALFORMATIONS OR ANOMALIES OF CHILD (Describe or write "none") 29.		

FIGURE 1–3 Certificate of live birth used by Pennsylvania Department of Health. Similar forms are used by other cities and states.

oldest age in the reproductive age span, 45 years or older, the mortality is about 12 times greater than the lowest figure (U.S. Department of Health and Human Services, 1993b).

Causes of Maternal Mortality. The major causes of maternal mortality are illustrated in Fig. 1-5. The reduction in maternal mortality from hemorrhagic disorders of pregnancy and childbirth was the largest single factor responsible for the reduction in the total maternal mortality rate. The hypertensive disorders and sepsis (other than abortions) were next in importance as conditions affecting the mortality rate (see Fig. 1-5). These three conditions are discussed in subsequent chapters in more detail. These conditions, and especially deaths from these conditions, are preventable.

Hemorrhage, though no longer the primary cause of maternal death, remains an important factor in the morbidity of mothers and in the underlying cause of death. According to the official classification, only the direct cause of death is considered, although predisposing causes may be just as important factors. For example, a mother may have a massive hemorrhage, and in her weakened condition, she may develop a puerperal infection that eventually causes her death. The death, however, is classified as a result of puerperal infection. Hemorrhage is often a predisposing factor, and its toll in maternal mortality should not be underestimated.

Puerperal infection is a wound infection of the birth canal after childbirth, which sometimes extends to cause phlebitis or peritonitis. The nurse can play an important role in helping to prevent such infections by maintaining flawless technique in performing nursing procedures.

The hypertensive disorders of pregnancy are certain disturbances peculiar to gravid women, characterized

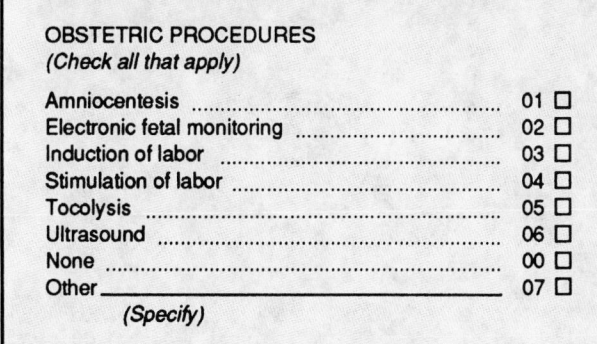

MEDICAL RISK FACTORS FOR THIS PREGNANCY
(Check all that apply)

Anemia (Hct. < 30/Hgb. < 10)	01 ☐
Cardiac disease	02 ☐
Acute or chronic lung disease	03 ☐
Diabetes	04 ☐
Genital herpes	05 ☐
Hydramnios/Oligohydramnios	06 ☐
Hemoglobinopathy	07 ☐
Hypertension, chronic	08 ☐
Hypertension, pregnancy-associated	09 ☐
Eclampsia	10 ☐
Incompetent cervix	11 ☐
Previous infant 4000+ grams	12 ☐
Previous preterm or small-for-gestational-age infant	13 ☐
Renal disease	14 ☐
Rh sensitization	15 ☐
Uterine bleeding	16 ☐
None	00 ☐
Other _____	17 ☐
(Specify)	

OTHER RISK FACTORS FOR THIS PREGNANCY
(Complete all items)

Tobacco use during pregnancy .... Yes ☐ No ☐
    Average number cigarettes per day _____
Alcohol use during pregnancy .... Yes ☐ No ☐
    Average number drinks per week _____
Weight gained during pregnancy _____ lbs.

OBSTETRIC PROCEDURES
(Check all that apply)

Amniocentesis	01 ☐
Electronic fetal monitoring	02 ☐
Induction of labor	03 ☐
Stimulation of labor	04 ☐
Tocolysis	05 ☐
Ultrasound	06 ☐
None	00 ☐
Other _____	07 ☐
(Specify)	

FIGURE 1–4 Medical risk factors, other risk factors, and obstetric procedures for the pregnancy, are listed on the new U.S. Standard Certificate of Live Birth that will help give new information and statistics regarding the etiology of neonatal health problems and adverse pregnancy outcomes. (Reproduced from 1989 U.S. Standard Certificate of Live Birth.)

mainly by hypertensive edema and albuminuria and in some severe cases, by convulsions and coma. Prenatal care is an important part of prevention or early detection of symptoms, and with suitable treatment, the disturbance often can be allayed.

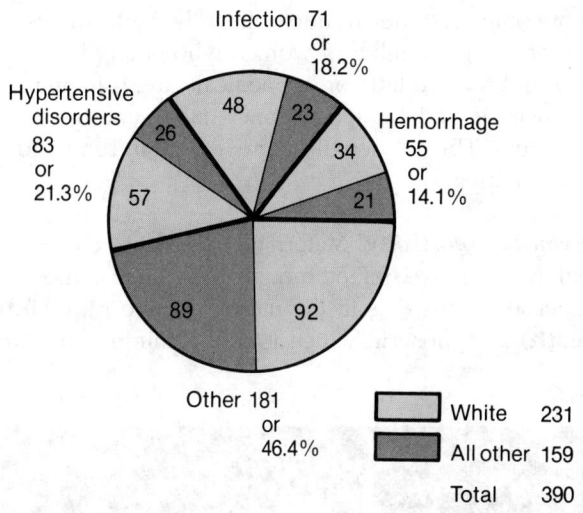

FIGURE 1–5 Annual summary of births, deaths, marriages, and divorces. ([1989]. United States, 1988 DHHS Pub. No. (PHS) 110–111. *Monthly Vital Statistics Report, 37,* 59.)

Reduction in Maternal Mortality. The following factors are mainly responsible for achieving the overall reduction in maternal mortality in this country during the last 25 years:

- Medical management has improved. The widespread use of intravenous products and monitoring of fluid and electrolyte balance, antibiotics, and sophisticated anesthesia management have contributed to the reduction. Legal access to abortion also has helped reduce the number of maternal deaths associated with illegal abortion.
- The development of widespread training and education programs in obstetrics and maternity care has provided better qualified specialists, professional nurses, and other caregivers. This has been a critical factor in the effort to reduce the maternal mortality rate.
- Better hospital facilities and the development of alternative hospital facilities to meet consumer demands for a more homelike setting for parturition is proving to be a helpful factor.
- The distinct change in attitudes of physicians, nurses, and parents has contributed. The orientation has shifted from curing the problem and a helpless "cope as best as we can" attitude to prevention and encouraging a state of preparedness.
- Prenatal care has been an important achievement in maternity care during this century. When used, pregnancy outcomes improve. However, many economically disadvantaged women still underuse prenatal care (Robert Woods Johnson Foundation, 1993).
- The development of maternal child health programs by state departments of public health and the work

of community health nurses have helped. Nurses visit a large number of women who otherwise would receive little or no medical care, bringing much-needed aid in pregnancy, labor, and the puerperium. This service fills a great need in rural and urban areas.

Perinatal Mortality. Maternity nursing is concerned mainly with two infant mortality problems: those in which the fetus dies in the uterus prior to birth (**fetal death**) and those in which it dies within a short time after birth (neonatal death). The term **perinatal mortality** is used to designate deaths in these two categories.

The perinatal death rate has fallen almost 50% in the last 25 years (Table 1-2). There are about 180 perinatal deaths for every maternal death. Because the maternal death rate is low, the perinatal loss rate is a better indicator of the level of obstetric care. Several factors are believed to have affected this decline, including a declining fertility rate, better contraceptive practices, the availability of safe clinical abortions, and a higher stan-

TABLE 1–2
Infant Mortality Rates, Fetal Death Rates, and Perinatal Mortality Rates According to Race: United States, 1950–1993

Year (all races)	Neonatal Mortality Rate* (Deaths per 1,000 Live Births)				Fetal death rate†	Late fetal death rate‡	Perinatal mortality rate§
	TOTAL	UNDER 28 DAYS	UNDER 7 DAYS	POST-NEONATAL			
1950"	29.2	20.5	17.8	8.7	18.4	14.9	32.5
1960"	26.0	18.7	16.7	7.3	15.8	12.1	28.6
1970	20.0	15.1	13.6	4.9	14.0	9.5	23.0
1980	12.6	8.5	7.1	4.1	9.1	6.2	13.2
1981	11.9	8.0	6.7	3.9	8.9	5.9	12.6
1982	11.5	7.7	6.4	3.8	8.8	5.9	12.3
1983	11.2	7.3	6.1	3.9	8.4	5.4	11.5
1984	10.8	7.0	5.9	3.8	8.1	5.2	11.0
1985	10.6	7.0	5.8	3.7	7.8	4.9	10.7
1986	10.4	6.7	5.6	3.8	7.7	4.7	10.3
1987	10.1	6.5	5.4	3.6	7.6	4.6	10.0
1988	10.0	6.3	5.2	3.6	7.5	4.5	9.7
1989	9.8	6.2	5.1	3.6	7.5	4.5	9.6
1990	9.2	5.8	4.8	3.4	7.5	4.3	9.1
1991	8.9	5.6	4.6	3.4	7.3	4.1	8.7
1992	8.5	5.4	4.4	3.1	7.4	4.1	8.5
Provisional data							
1992	8.5	5.4	—	3.1	—	—	—
1993	8.3	5.4	—	2.9	—	—	—

*Rates are infant (younger than 1 y), neonatal (less than 28 d), early neonatal (less than 7 d), and postneonatal (28–365 d) deaths per 1,000 live births in specified group.
†Number of fetal deaths of 20 wk or more gestation per 1,000 live births plus fetal deaths.
‡Number of fetal deaths of 28 wk or more gestation per 1,000 live births plus late fetal deaths.
§Number of late fetal deaths plus infant deaths within 7 days of birth per 1,000 live births plus late fetal deaths.
"This includes births and deaths of nonresidents of the United States.
"Infant deaths and fetal deaths are tabulated by race of decedent; live births are tabulated by race of child.
¶Infant deaths are tabulated by race of decedent; fetal deaths and live births are tabulated by race of mother.
(Sources: Centers for Disease Control and Prevention, National Center for Health Statistics: Vital Statistics of the United States, Vol. II, Mortality, Part A, for data years 1950–1992 Public Health Service. Washington. U.S. Government Printing Office. Annual summary of births, marriages, divorces, and deaths: United States, 1992 and 1993. *Monthly Vital Statistics Report, 41,* 42 (13), Hyattsville, Md.: Public Health Service, 1993 and 1994; Advance report of final mortality statistics, 1992. *Monthly Vital Statistics Report, 43* (6. Suppl.) Hyattsville, Md.: Public Health Service, 1994. Data computed by the Division of Health and Utilization Analysis from data compiled by the Division of Vital Statistics.)

dard of living in the general population. However, it has been shown that these national statistics do not accurately reflect trends in large urban areas and southern states, where the decline has been much less (Cunningham et al., 1993).

Many factors are responsible for **neonatal mortality.** The leading causes are low birth weight, congenital malformations, injury to the central nervous system (including hypoxia in utero), traumatic injury to the brain during labor and delivery, and respiratory distress syndrome. The recent national statistics also reflect a startling increase in the category of newborns affected by maternal complications, showing an increase from 3.4 per 100,000 births in 1982 to 36.7 per 100,000 births in 1987. These maternal complications often relate to the mother's lifestyle or habits, including substance abuse, smoking, or poor prenatal care. This category has now become a major cause of perinatal mortality (Cunningham et al., 1993).

The welfare of approximately 3,500,000 newborns annually in the United States is a legitimate concern of perinatal nurses and obstetricians. The goals of care include reducing the enormous loss of newborn lives, protecting the fetus and newborn, and laying a solid foundation for the newborn's health throughout life.

Reproductive Wastage

About 10% of all pregnancies terminate in spontaneous abortion due to such factors as faulty genetic development, unsatisfactory environmental conditions, and hormonal and many other unknown etiologic causes (Cunningham et al., 1993). The term *reproductive wastage* is used to describe the loss of the products of conception.

The concern for the United States, stemming from the overall problem of reproductive wastage, reflects a symptom of far-reaching social change. The current major concern is that a large segment of the American population does not receive maternity care. This is particularly true for many disadvantaged, low-income families and foreign immigrants, who have concentrated in the major cities. With the increased cost of health services in general and the cost of hospital care in particular, these low-income families are straining the local resources of the communities in which they reside. However, the most serious problem is that many of these women receive poor, or often no, prenatal care; this is in part because of limited access or dissatisfaction with the kind of care provided.

Not only the very poor are affected by the increasing costs of healthcare. With the recent economic fluctuations, middle class couples are feeling the impact of being unable to afford adequate healthcare. They are not considered poor enough for welfare coverage yet are not affluent enough to afford appropriate care.

Difficulty in providing adequate care is due to an artificial shortage of professional personnel in the maternity field. The rapid growth of the population in certain sections, such as rural and inner city areas, has not been accompanied by a proportionate increase in the number of physicians and nurses willing to staff these underserved areas.

Trends in Perinatal Care

There are several major current trends in society that influence the healthcare industry. These trends will have direct and indirect effects on perinatal care, particularly perinatal nursing. The settings in which healthcare is delivered, the practitioners who deliver care, and the manner in which reimbursement is provided will all be transformed by economic, demographic, social, and health status changes (Klerman, 1994; Haller, 1994).

The collision of societal trends, changing client needs, and consequent changes in the provider role can lead to confusion about practice standards for maternity-perinatal nursing. To clarify basic standards of practice, The Association of Women's Health, Obstetrics and Neonatal Nurses (formerly the Nurses' Association of the American College of Obstetricians and Gynecologists [NAACOG]) has developed standards for obstetric, gynecologic, and neonatal nursing. These standards are not meant to limit innovation in nursing care but should be viewed as part of an ongoing process being constantly revised as the need arises. Students are advised to familiarize themselves with these important standards of practice and the Pregnant Patient's Bill of Rights (see Appendix A and Box 1-5; NAACOG, 1991).

Demographic Trends

Several trends in the population have already had a major impact on the healthcare delivery system and will continue to do so. These include the birthrate, marital status, and age distribution, particularly of the chilbearing and aging populations.

Birth Rate. As described in the discussion of vital statistics, the number of births has increased in the last 10 years. Although the number of births is expected to drop in the 1990s, by 2007, the number should total 4 million and should continue to increase (U.S. Bureau of the Census, 1992).

Age Distribution. The age range of 20 to 35 years is still the most popular time for childbearing, but there is a trend toward beginning a family when the woman is in her late 30s and early 40s. The risks of childbear-

---

BOX 1–5
Recommendations for Perinatal Nurses Regarding Trends

- Become knowledgeable and active in the political arena; use national health policy fellowships, Robert Wood Johnson fellowships, and so forth to prepare to contribute.
- Voice support for continued resources for perinatal services.
- Stand in the forefront to maintain a balance between technology and humanized care.
- Conduct market surveys to determine need for services, and tailor services accordingly. Conduct clinical nursing research to determine relevant problems in the healthcare of women and their fetuses and infants and the relationship of these problems to clinical nursing practice.
- Expand the leadership and practice roles to nontraditional practice settings, such as ambulatory care settings, and the home. The perinatal home care aspect will become increasingly important.

---

ing for this group in the 1990s are less than for the older childbearers in the past because these women are generally well educated, healthy, and start families after establishing their careers. The needs of these pregnant women may be different from those of younger pregnant women.

The trend in childbearing among girls younger than 18 years is uncertain. The increased use of contraceptives and the availability of abortion may account for the decline of births in this group through 1986. However, since that time, the teenage birth rate has increased. Until the economy and the educational system improve, teenage parents probably will not consciously balance the benefits and burdens of childbearing and childrearing against the benefits and burdens of preventing pregnancies (Klerman, 1994).

The *"graying of America"* may be one of most important trends affecting the healthcare delivery system between 2010 and 2030, when the baby boomers are expected to reach 65 years. Perinatal nursing professionals will feel the impact of the growing number of elderly people (21% of the population will be older than 65 years by 2040) in the form of decreased resources for infants and women in their childbearing years. Elderly people are expected to continue to use a disproportionate share of health resources, and healthcare will become increasingly focused on the long-term care and rehabilitation of older clients. Moreover, it is anticipated that the growing number of older people, with the use of their economic and political power, will wield considerable influence in tailoring healthcare policy, services, and resources to the

needs of the elderly (Andreoli et al., 1986; Klerman, 1994).

Marital Status. Childbearing outside of marriage has increased during the last few decades in all western industrialized countries (see Chap. 3). More older women and teenagers are bearing children outside of marriage, although they may be living with a male partner. The stigma attached to such birth is lessening for all ethnic groups and will probably continue to do so, especially for women who can afford to care for a child without becoming dependent on public funds (Klerman, 1994).

Demographic Changes and Reproductive Health. If the trends enumerated previously continue as predicted, reproductive healthcare will be affected. If the birthrate stays at 4 million per year, the high demand will continue for obstetricians and advanced practiced maternity-perinatal nurses, including midwives, nurse practitioners, and clinical specialists. Hospital facilities and maternity centers will be needed to accommodate these clients and healthcare practitioners. The organization of care will need to change to accommodate the working mother and those who have differing amounts of education. This will be necessary in the prenatal education and care areas and in clinics. Different types of advanced practice nurses (nurse-midwives and nurse practitioners) will be needed for the various ages and types of maternity populations.

The current movement in public policy is to restrict Aid to Families with Dependent Children to prevent additional births among welfare recipients, particularly those who are unmarried. In addition, there are plans to enforce the Family Support Act of 1988 to compel absent fathers to support their families. These are strategies aimed at reducing federal and state costs for the support of childbearing (Klerman, 1994).

Healthcare Reform

Since the mid-1970s, efforts have been made in the various levels of government to reduce the costs of healthcare and improve the access to medical care. These efforts are known collectively as "healthcare reform." However, to date, no serious uniform measures have been passed. Thus, large segments of the population have no health insurance at all or have severely limited access to services.

- Healthcare measures. As a result of the escalating cost of healthcare, the United States spends approximately $1 billion a day on healthcare, which is about 10.8% of the gross national product, and this proportion is expected to keep rising. Several "healthcare packages" have been proposed that have created a great deal of controversy. The content of the benefit packages and how services will be financed and delivered are yet to be determined. It is anticipated that no pregnant woman who is an American citizen will experience financial barriers to prenatal care, labor, and delivery services or a postpartum checkup. Family planning services, contraceptives for adolescents without parental knowledge, and unrestricted abortion services continue to be areas of debate and controversy (Klerman, 1994; Mundinger, 1994).

- Medicaid. It is still unclear if Medicaid will be maintained under healthcare and welfare reform. Many perinatal healthcare advocates would like to see it terminated to provide more equality across socioeconomic groups. Proponents of Medicaid fear that the benefits will not be as comprehensive as those now available. The required and optional services now included under Title XIX (Medicaid) legislation make a wide variety of case management, home visits, and other services, many of which are in the purview of nursing, available to the childbearing family. Economically disadvantaged women would suffer if services were abolished and the total perinatal package was "lean." One proposed solution is to find public health departments to provide these supportive health services, even if traditional prenatal and infant care is obtained in private offices or health maintenance organizations.

- Perinatal and family planning. Other aspects of healthcare reform will affect perinatal and family planning services by impinging on other factors besides the financial one. There is a shortage of qualified physicians and midlevel advanced practice nurses in the inner city and rural areas. These areas are seen as less desirable because of lack of current facilities, lower income production, lack of professional and social colleagues for self and family, and personal danger. Incentives, such as educational support in return for a limited time of practice in these settings, are being considered in the reform measures. Unless planning for the underserved is included, these practitioners, especially the advanced practice nurses, such as CNMs and nurse practitioners, will be absorbed into current hospital and office practices (Klerman, 1994).

- Home visiting. Home visiting is another strategy to cut costs. Public health nurses and institutionally based nurses skilled in home healthcare can increase compliance with medical regimens and recommendations during the prenatal and postpartum periods, especially if the mother or infant is sick. Even if the infant suffers only from low birth weight, the nurse can provide counseling, education, support, and help with adjustments in the household (Klerman, 1994; Styles, 1990). See the

section entitled, "Emergence of Perinatal Home Healthcare" later in this chapter.

Biomedical Research

Technological improvements that can reduce preterm delivery, infertility, and unintended pregnancy should lead to fewer compromised fetuses, fewer childless families, and smaller completed family size, all of which should reduce the costs of perinatal care (Klerman, 1994; Hoffman, 1993). Scientific improvements, especially in the area of contraception, will have an impact on reproductive health. The development of new and improved contraceptives, including those designed for male use and those that can be used reliably by adolescents, would limit health costs significantly. RU486 will probably receive approval from the Food and Drug Administration within the next 5 years. Its availability would reduce the need for abortion clinics and would replace the combination estrogen-progesterone combination pills as "the morning after pill." Women who want an abortion would seek care from primary care providers and return home to await the expulsion of the fetus (Hoffman, 1993).

Health Status

The high incidence of low–birth-weight newborns in the United States and the increasing rate of sexually transmitted diseases are health trends that have implications for perinatal practice. The high proportion of low–birth-weight newborns is largely responsible for the slowing in the decline of the national infant mortality rate. Most low–birth-weight newborns are premature, and this condition accounts for two-thirds of the yearly 39,000 infant deaths nationally. A variety of risk factors contribute to low birth weight and prematurity. These are discussed in detail in other chapters. However, the other factors mentioned previously, particularly the changing healthcare economics, will contribute to the incidence of these conditions (U.S. Department of Health and Human Services, 1991).

Healthcare Preferences

- Perinatal care preferences. Increasing numbers of women, particularly those who are more affluent and better educated, are making their perinatal care preferences known. Less technological and more family-centered birth experiences are frequently sought and requested. Hospitals who want to keep their clientele and increase their number of deliveries are redesigning their units to ensure profitability.

- Labor and delivery environment. Single rooms that can accommodate labor, delivery, and recovery are in demand. Nurse-midwives are often requested as the practitioner of choice. Tensions often develop between physicians with a highly technological orientation to birth and its management and the desire of many women for a more natural, family-centered approach to the reproductive process. The outcome of this tension is uncertain (Young, 1992; Klerman, 1994).

Future Directions in Maternity-Perinatal Care Settings

In current nursing practice, there has been a shift from institution-based nursing services to two other areas: home healthcare and community-based healthcare. The latter is not a new phenomenon in maternity care; public health nursing has always had its roots in the delivery of care to mothers and their children with home visits, well baby clinics, and immunization clinics.

Emergence of Perinatal Home Healthcare

Home care is a growing phenomenon in present day healthcare. The U.S. Department of Commerce has called it one of the fastest growing sectors in the healthcare field (Weinstein, 1993). Home health visits, once centered on maternal-child care, chronic care, and health promotion must meet the newer demands of many populations with a variety of medical problems, some of which are acute and require intensive care.

Community and home healthcare differ from institutional care in that the setting, the home, is exclusively in the domain of the client. Basic to the meaning of home are various elements of ownership, control, security, family development, independence, comfort, and protection. The nurse is invited into the home, and control belongs to the client. Family issues become more prominent. The nurse's practice is solitary, and accountability looms large; thus, the nurse must be able to think and act autonomously without the presence of medical supervision (Stulginsky, 1993a, 1993b).

Home health nurses are no longer exclusively generalists. Advanced practice nurses are needed to address the increasing complexity and acuity in the home (Stulginsky, 1993). Predictions for 2000 indicate that home health will need 8,000 more registered nurses than employed in 1990 to keep pace with the growing demand (U.S. Department of Health and Human Services, 1991; Box 1-6).

BOX 1–6
Factors in the Growth of Home Healthcare

- One-half of home care recipients are older than 65 years.
- Diagnostic-related groups (DRGs) for third-party payment have resulted in clients being discharged "quicker and sicker" from the hospitals, including mothers and newborns.
- Third-party payer focus on cost effectiveness allows technical interventions in the home.
- Consumers prefer the home over institutional healthcare.

(Lindman, 1992)

Innovations in the Delivery of Perinatal Care Services

Given the problems of access, retention, and relevant prenatal content, supplements to existing programs for healthcare delivery during pregnancy and after birth are necessary. *Healthy People 2000* states that prenatal care is a priority on the nation's health agenda and suggests exploring alternative models of care to decrease or eliminate several of the undesirable perinatal outcomes that plague society. These include uneven rates of low–birth-weight newborns among culturally diverse groups and increasing rates of women who do not seek or are slow to seek prenatal care (Affonso et al., 1993).

Various plans have been developed to evaluate innovative interventions for prenatal care services. The *Community Health Nursing Prenatal Care Program* was designed to complement standard obstetric services with specific nursing services and community outreach interventions targeted to be culturally sensitive and congruent with the lifestyles of ethnic women in Hawaii (Affonso et al., 1993). Public health nurses with special expertise in maternal-child health are the main providers of care.

Similarly, home care for the client at risk for preterm labor involves home uterine monitoring. When care is performed in the home and the providers are perinatal nurses, the focus is on the client, and health maintenance is the goal rather than the goal of "cure" with technology. In 1989, the Kaiser Permanente of Ohio and Professional Nurse Associates, Inc. collaborated to provide a home-centered postpartum recovery program to meet postdelivery needs of the mother, newborn, and families after shortened hospital stays. Outcomes were uniformly good, and the authors recommend establishing postpartum home nursing care as a recognized standard of care for postpartum child-bearing families (Williams et al., 1993). Other authors have researched feasibility and outcomes during the prenatal and postpartum periods. Some studies have used public health nurses; others have used perinatal clinical specialists and practitioners. All have found positive health outcome and a heightened level of health maintenance (Dineen et al., 1992; Olds, 1992; Starn, 1992; Bradley et al., 1993).

Summary Points

✔ Maternity care has evolved from a provider orientation to a recipient orientation, and various terms have been used to describe the concepts of care. In contemporary times, there has been a great increase in high technology and increasing specialization in the care of mothers and infants. To decrease the fragmentation and segmentation of care and provide a conceptual umbrella to encompass maternal-fetal care as a unit, the term perinatal has come into current usage.

✔ The use of statistics enables health policy makers and healthcare providers to discern trends and events in the health arena; thus, they are able to predict and plan to minimize or control health outcomes.

✔ Major trends in society and the healthcare industry today have direct and indirect effects on perinatal care:
  ▪ Demographic trends in the population, particularly marital status and the age distribution, affect the birthrate.
  ▪ Healthcare reform includes controversial "healthcare reform packages" aimed at improving access for all and cost reduction but may impact negatively on many perinatal services.
  ▪ Biomedical research includes new discoveries, technological improvements, and research and development, resulting in scientific applications to improve perinatal outcomes.
  ▪ Women's preferences are focused on community and home care rather than institutional care and less technological interference in the birth process.

✔ Advanced practice nursing roles in perinatal care are becoming increasingly needed as perinatal care moves from the hospital to the community and home settings. Innovative programs and creative methods of care delivery are being developed to provide better access and cost reduction and provide summaries of national and international trends. They are valuable in planning programs of care.

REFERENCES

Editorial. (1993). *Access to health care: Key indicators for policy* (pp. 1–98). Princeton: Robert Wood Johnson Foundation.

Andersen, H. F., & Genesen, L. B. (1993). Partnership in perinatal care. *Journal of Perinatology, 13*(4), 259–260.

Andreoli, K. G, & Musser, L. A. (1986). Major trends shaping the future of perinatal nursing. *Journal of Perinatology, 6*(2), 325–330.

Affonso, D. D., Mayberry, L. J., Graham, K., Shibuya, J., & Kunimoto, J. (1993). Prenatal and postpartum care in Hawaii: A community based approach. *Journal of Obstetric, Gynecologic, and Neonatal Nursing, 22*(4), 320–325.

Bradley, J., & Mawn, B. (1993). Standards of care for high-risk prenatal clients: The community nurse case management approach. *Public Health Nursing, 10*(2), 78–88.

California Nurses' Association (1984). *Position statement on specialization in nursing practice.* San Francisco: Author.

Calkin, J. D. (1984). A model for advanced nursing practice. *Journal of Nurse Administration, 14*, 24–30.

Chiu, H. S., Jogt, J. F., Chan, L. S., & Rother, C. E. (1993). Regionalization of infant transports: The southern California experience and its implications. 1: Referral patterns. *Journal of Perinatology, 13*(4), 289–296.

Cunningham, F. G., McDonald, P. C., Gant, N. F., Leveno, K. J., & Gilstrap, L. C. (1993). *Williams' obstetrics* (19th ed.). Norwalk, CT: Appleton & Lange.

DeVane, D. M. (1991). *The crises in perinatal care in Los Angeles county* (pp. 25). Burbank, CA: March of Dimes.

Dineen, K., Keller, L., Lia-Hoagberg, B., & Rossi, M. (1992). Antepartum homecare services for high-risk women. *Journal of Obstetric, Gynecologic, and Neonatal Nursing, 21*(2), 121–125.

Frik, S. M., & Pollock, S. E. (1994). Preparation for advanced nursing practice. *Nursing and Health Care, 14*(4), 190–195.

Haller, K. B. (1994). Agenda for 1994-2000. *Journal of Obstetric, Gynecologic, and Neonatal Nursing, 23*(1), 10.

Hoffman, J. (1993). The morning after pill. *The New York Times Magazine*, 12–16, 30–32.

Klerman, L. C. (1994). Perinatal health care policy: How it will affect the family in the 21st century. *Journal of Obstetric, Gynecologic, and Neonatal Nursing, 23*(2), 124–128.

Lindeman, C. (1992). Nursing and technology, moving into the 21st century. *Caring Magazine, 11*(9), 5–10.

Maternal Child Health Bureau (1994). Maternal mortality rates for complications of pregnancy, childbirth, and the puerperium, according to race and age: United States, selected years 1950-92. Vital Statistics of the U.S., Vol. II. *Mortality.*

Mundinger, M. O. (1994). Health care reform: Will nursing respond? *Nursing and Health Care, 15*(1), 28–33.

Nurses' Association of the American College of Obstetricians and Gynecologists (1991). *Standards for obstetric, gynecologic, and neonatal nursing* (4th ed.). Washington, DC: Author.

Nurses' Association of the American College of Obstetricians and Gynecologists (1988). *Nursing practice resource: Considerations for professional nurse staffing in perinatal units.* Washington, DC: Author.

Olds, D. L. (1992). Home visitation for pregnant women and parents of young children. *American Journal of Diseases of Children, 146*(6), 704–708.

Quimby, C. H. (1994). Women and the family of the future. *Journal of Obstetrics, Gynecologic, and Neonatal Nursing, 23*(3), 113–121.

Starn, J. R. (1992). Community health nursing visits for at-risk womn and infants. *Journal of Community Health Nursing, 9*(2), 103–110.

Stulginsky, M. M. (1993a). Nurses' home health experience: Part I: The practice setting. *Nursing and Health Care, 14*(8), 402–407.

Stulginsky, M. M. (1993b). Nurses' home health experience: Part II: The unique demands of home visits. *Nursing and Health Care, 14*(9), 476–485.

Styles, M. M. (1990). Challenges for nursing in this new decade. *MCN: American Journal of Maternal Child Nursing, 13*(6), 347ff.

Taffel, S. M., Ventura, S. J., & Gay, G. A. (1989). Revised U.S. certificate of birth: New opportunities for research on birth outcomes. *Birth, 16*(4), 188–193.

U.S. Department of Health and Human Services, Health, Education, Welfare (1991). *Healthy people 2000.* Washington, DC: U.S. Government Printing Office.

U.S. Department of Health and Human Services (1991). *Health personnel in the U.S., eighth report to congress* (DHHS no. HRS-P-00-92-1). Rockville, MD: U.S. Government Printing Office.

U.S. Bureau of the Census (1992). *Population projections of the United States by age, sex, race and Hispanic origin 1992-2050. Current population reports* (P20-470). Washington, D.C.: U.S. Department of Commerce.

U.S. Department of Health and Human Services, National Center for Health Statistics (1993a). Advance report of official natality statistics, 1991. *Monthly Vital Statistics Report, 42*(Suppl.).

U.S. Department of Health and Human Services, National Center for Health Statistics (1993b). Annual summary of births, marriages, divorces and deaths: United States, 1992. *Monthly Vital Statistics Report1, 41*(13).

Weinstein, S. (1993). A coordinated approach to home infusion care. *Home Health Care Nurse, 11*(1), 15–20.

Williams, L. R., & Cooper, M. K. (1993). Nurse-managed postpartum home care. *Journal of Obstetric, Gynecologic, and Neonatal Nursing, 22*(1), 25–31.

Young, D. (1992). Family centered maternity care: Is the central nursery obsolete? *Birth, 19*(4), 183–184.

SUGGESTED READINGS

Ernst, E. K (1994). Health care reform as an ongoing process. *Journal of Obstetric, Gynecologic, and Neonatal Nursing, 23*(2), 129–137.

Wood, S. H. et al. (1994). The 1990s: A decade for change in women's health care policy. *Journal of Obstetric, Gynecologic, and Neonatal Nursing, 23*(2), 139–152.

Taffel, S. M., Placek, P. J., & Kosary, C. L. (1992). U.S. cesarean rates 1990: An update. *Birth, 19*(1), 21–23.

2

Critical Thinking in the Nursing Process

Objectives

- Explain the relationships among critical thinking, clinical judgments, problem solving, decision making, the nursing process, and the research process.
- Identify three methods for problem solving. Describe the five steps of the nursing process.
- Explain how critical thinking and the nursing process are essential to nursing practice.
- Describe how nursing research can be successfully integrated into nursing practice.

Key Terms

Assessment	Inferences
Critical thinking	Integrity
Decision making	Nursing process
Deductive reasoning	Nursing diagnosis
Defining characteristics	Problem solving
Human responses	Research utilization
Humility	Scientific method
Implementation	Trial and error
Inductive reasoning	

In the current environment of healthcare delivery, nurses constantly are faced with rapidly expanding technology and changing situations. They are required to make crucial decisions about a client's well-being, possibly even about a client's survival. Calm, fact-finding, and judicious deliberation become increasingly difficult. Conflicts between principle and expediency arise. These conflicts carry even more significance for maternity and perinatal nurses, because two clients, the woman and fetus, are involved.

Today, nursing practice requires organized, purposeful, and disciplined thinking. The contemporary nurse must constantly solve problems; establish priorities; assess, plan, and implement treatment options; evaluate outcomes; and reassess. To perform these complex processes swiftly and accurately, the nurse must develop the ability to think critically, using a systematic approach. This systematic approach allows the nurse to move quickly through the myriad of data and options available and make clinical judgments and decisions resulting in effective treatment plans and desired outcomes.

Maternity and perinatal nurses must use critical thinking in all aspects of their nursing practice to ensure the best possible outcome. Beginning with the knowledge base obtained as a student and expanding to include the application of research findings and nursing standards of care, maternal and perinatal nurses continually use critical thinking skills to analyze data and make decisions about the woman and fetus.

This chapter explores the concepts of critical thinking, problem solving, the nursing process, and the research process. The elements essential to each are presented, and the inter-relationship among the concepts is described.

Critical Thinking

Critical thinking is a method of problem analysis. It involves the examination of assumptions, beliefs, pro-

spectives, and the meaning and uses of words, statements, and arguments related to a problem (Bandman, et al., 1994).

In nursing, critical thinking is evidenced when the nurse performs the following functions:

- Discriminates among the uses and misuses of language in nursing
- Identifies and formulates nursing problems
- Analyzes meanings of terms in relation to their indication, their cause or purpose, and their significance
- Analyzes arguments and issues into premises and conclusions
- Examines nursing assumptions
- Reports data and clues accurately
- Makes and checks **inferences** based on data, making sure that the inferences are, at least, plausible
- Formulates and clarifies beliefs
- Verifies, corroborates, and justifies claims, beliefs, conclusions, decisions, and actions
- Gives relevant reasons for beliefs and conclusions
- Formulates and clarifies value judgments
- Seeks reasons, criteria, and principles that effectively justify value judgments
- Evaluates the soundness of conclusions (Bandman, et al., 1994)

Three components are essential to critical thinking. They include a solid knowledge base, ability to react to change and adapt, and ability to make decisions. For more information about these three components, see Table 2-1.

Characteristics of Critical Thinking

Evaluating and integrating information are essential steps in the critical thinking process. As a result of critical thinking, facts can be separated from opinions; prejudices, stereotypes, biases, and preconceptions can be identified; new or different ideas can be explored; and new conclusion, solutions, or ideas can be developed. All of these results aid the nurse in **decision making.**

Critical thinking is reasonable, rational, and reflective; it promotes an attitude of inquiry; and involves autonomous, creative, fair thinking with a focus on believing and doing. For a description of these characteristics and examples, see Table 2-2.

Attitudes and Cognitive Skills

Creative thinking involves affective (emotional) attitudes and cognitive skill. To think critically, a person must possess the skills and be motivated to use them.

RESEARCH HIGHLIGHT

Relationship Between Professionalism and Critical Thinking Abilities

This descriptive study was undertaken to investigate the relationship between professionalism and critical thinking abilities in senior nursing students in four different types of National League for Nursing (NLN) accredited nursing education programs (ie, generic baccalaureate, associate degree, diploma, and the RN completion [upper division baccalaureate]). Fifty students from each type of program were selected by means of convenience sampling during the same spring semester before graduation. The instruments used were the Health Care Professional Attitude Inventory, which measured professionalism, and the Watson-Glaser Critical Thinking Appraisal, which measured critical thinking. Demographic data were analyzed by percentage distributions and ANOVA to determine the characteristics of the sample and to see if they differed significantly from national samples compiled by the NLN. They were not significantly different, and in general, the sample groups' data were comparable to national data. The Pearson Product Moment Correlation and ANOVA were used to analyze relationships between professionalism and critical thinking among the students in the programs.

For individual programs, low to moderate correlations ranging from $r=0.263$ (diploma) to 0.516 (RN completion) were found between critical thinking and professionalism. There was a significant but low positive correlation between critical thinking and professionalism across all programs. The RN completion students showed significant low to moderate positive correlations for age with critical thinking ($r=0.487$) and professionalism ($r=0.327$), which were not observed in the other groups of students. The RN completion students scored highest in professionalism when scores were compared across programs, and the diploma students showed the lowest level of professionalism. Professionalism scores for generic baccalaureate students and associate degree students were not significantly different. When critical thinking abilities were compared, both the generic baccalaureate and the RN completion students showed significantly higher levels than those from the associate degree and diploma programs.

Critique: In general this is a well-written and timely article. The authors set out their rationale for the study (ie, the scarcity of research literature that addresses the relationship between professionalism and critical thinking skills *across the four types of nursing curricula from which students must choose*). They document their rationale with a concise literature review that speaks to the importance of these skills and the responsibility that nursing education has in developing these skills for nurses in modern healthcare. The research questions are clear and address what the authors intend to do.

However, when describing their sampling methods, the authors do not say *how many* programs were actually contacted to supply the 50 students from each type of program, nor do they say how they selected the *programs*. This discussion would have strengthened the paper. They give an appropriate rationale for the convenience sampling of the *students* but not the *programs*; therefore, the reader is unclear, for instance, if the group of 50 baccalaureate students came from several programs in southeastern Pennsylvania or just one; the same is true for the other groups. Thus, the unit of analysis (program or students) is unclear.

They analyze the demographic data and ascertain that their student data are comparable to other national data on several important demographic characteristics. The statistics used are appropriate, and the issues of the validity and reliability of their instruments are clearly addressed. They do not mention the problem with low correlations and significance; that is, even if significance is reached in a low correlation, one cannot have real confidence in the significance of the relationship. The authors are careful to caution against making any generalizations from the data, citing the convenience sampling and the small numbers in the groups. This is an article worth reading because it illustrates the difficulty in trying to measure these "slippery" constructs. The section on limitations and recommendations is particularly useful, because the authors point out the direction that subsequent research should take to compensate for the limitations in their study.

Brooks, K. L., and Shepherd, J. M. (1992). Professionalism verses general critical thinking abilities of nursing students in four types of nursing curricula. *Journal of Professional Nursing, 8*(2), 87–95.

Attitudes

Attitudes involved with critical thinking are interrelated and integrated. They are not used in isolation. Some critical thinking attitudes include the following:

- Thinking independently
- Humility (awareness of own knowledge limits)
- Courage
- Integrity (challenging own knowledge beliefs in the same fashion as one would challenge others)
- Perseverance
- Empathy
- Fair mindedness
- Exploring thoughts and feelings (Paul, 1993)

Cognitive Skills

Complex thinking skills are necessary for critical thinking. These skills involve the logical process of reasoning. The four types of reasoning include deductive, inductive, informal (or everyday), and practical.

TABLE 2-1
Components of Critical Thinking

Component	Description
Solid knowledge base	▪ Requisite studies in the biologic and social sciences and humanities ▪ Foundational courses in nursing concepts, theories, and models ▪ Required courses in clinical nursing skills ▪ Continuing education and certification ▪ Standards of care
Ability to react to change and adapt	▪ Stressful care environments with constant changes in client condition and areas, such as technology, treatments, and medications ▪ Recognition and analysis of cues, information, and quick response ▪ Application of knowledge base with adjustments to specific situations based on analysis of cues and information
Decision making	▪ Use of sound judgment based on analysis of situation and knowledge base ▪ Determination of important versus unimportant information ▪ Follow through with actions

Deductive reasoning involves arriving at a conclusion that is certain. The conclusion is unmistakable. There is complete evidence that supports the conclusion. With deductive reasoning, if the information is true, the conclusion also is true. Use of deductive reasoning reduces dependence on forces of unreason to settle the deepest issues of life (Bandman, et al., 1994). For example, involution of the uterus is substantiated by cessation of lochia and progressive diminution in size of uterus during the postpartum period.

Inductive reasoning involves the use of generalizations formed from a set of facts or observations. When viewed together, certain information appears to promote a certain interpretation. There is some evidence for the conclusion. However, the information is not sufficient enough to assure, ensure, or guarantee the truth of the conclusion. With inductive reasoning, even if the information is believed to be true, the conclusion still may be false. The conclusion is at most probable or likely and implies the need for further verification and corroboration. Inductive reasoning may be used to make differential **assessments** relating to attachment and bonding behaviors between mother and child.

Informal reasoning involves the use of knowledge about everyday events, activities, and practices to arrive at a conclusion. **Practical reasoning** involves the use of experiences related to one's participation or role in events, activities, and so forth to formulate a conclusion. These types of reasonings rely on experience with a variety of parents in childbirth situations.

Relationship of Critical Thinking to Clinical Judgment

Critical thinking is key to making accurate clinical judgments and using the nursing process. Critical thinking involves fact finding, sorting pertinent information, making decisions, and applying solutions to problems. In nursing practice, the nurse gathers data from a variety of sources—records, observation, interviews, and questioning—and then organizes these data into a meaningful unit by asking the following questions: What are the appropriate groupings, what is extraneous, what seems "intuitively" right, what is missing, and what does experience tell? The nurse then begins making decisions based on these findings and experience, subsequently developing a plan of care that includes evaluation (Reeder, 1994).

Nursing practice, particularly in acute care settings, has grown so complex that it is no longer possible to standardize all that nurses must do to provide safe, effective care. Moreover, expanding knowledge about **human responses** to health problems constantly affects the relevance of nurses' interventions (Box 2-1). In today's practice settings, regardless of clinical assignments, nurses must be able to perform technical, interpersonal, and critical thinking skills in a simultaneously integrated, thoughtful process to arrive at accurate, appropriate clinical judgments (del Bueno, 1990).

The art and science of making clinical judgments is a complex skill involving several cognitive phases and integrative processes. It is perhaps the most important dimension of nurses' work. The development of such competence, however, is time consuming, difficult, and complex for the new nurse and the employer. Research indicates that baccalaureate nurses have stated that it takes about 8 months of clinical experience before feeling confident about the accuracy of clinical judgments (del Bueno, 1990). Thus, well prepared, independent, hands-on experience is necessary to bring all of the elements together in a cohesive whole.

Problem Solving

Problem solving refers to a process by which an individual obtains information related to a problem or situ-

TABLE 2–2
Characteristics of Critical Thinking

Characteristic	Description	Examples
Reasonable and rational	▪ Based on reason and logic rather than prejudice, preferences, or self-interest	A nurse chooses to work in labor and delivery after consulting with a nurse recruiter and other staff members about job opportunities rather than on the desire to work in an area that is usually less stressful.
Reflective	▪ Time taken to collect data, weigh facts and evidence, and think things through	During an inservice program prepared by a company introducing a new and better Doppler fetoscope, a nurse questions the company representative about what makes this device better and asks for information to support this claim.
Attitude of inquiry	▪ Examination of existing claims and statements to determine the truth and validity rather than blindly accepting them ▪ Constructive criticism and questioning with "why" and "how"	A nurse caring for a client with pregnancy-induced hypertension wants to know why the body responds the way it does and how magnesium sulfate works to control seizures.
Autonomous thinking	▪ Self-thinking ▪ Analysis of issues with decisions about what information is credible ▪ Not easily manipulated ▪ Acceptance of beliefs based on rational reasons and rejection of beliefs held for incorrect reasons	After reviewing the reasons for and against, a nurse working in labor and delivery decides to work 12-hour shifts, even though coworkers try to convince the nurse otherwise.
Creative thinking	▪ Development of original ideas by establishing relationships and connections among thoughts and concepts ▪ Ability to transfer concept to a new setting or apply it in a different way	A nurse uses relaxation and imagery with a client who is having trouble sleeping after a difficult delivery.
Fair thinking	▪ Removal of own biases and recognition of others' biases in thinking and accepted standards ▪ Questioning of suppositions and practices based on prejudice or bias	The nurse manager of the postpartum unit responds positively to a nurse's holiday request to be off, only after determining that staffing was adequate for that day.
Focus on believing and doing	▪ Argument evaluation and conclusions ▪ Communication of new ideas or alternative courses of action ▪ Reliable observations leading to sound conclusions and problem solving ▪ Use of accepted standards to examine own views and those of others	In all examples above, each nurse decided on a course of action.

Adapted from Kozier, B., et al. (1995). *Fundamentals of nursing* (5th ed.). Addison-Wesley.

ation and then, based on that information, develops possible solutions. Critical thinking helps the nurse identify a variety of potential solutions, limit the number of solutions by identifying possible stereotypes and biases, and then choose the best possible solution. Thus, problem solving represents the careful examination of the information obtained through critical thinking (Grant, 1994). Closely related to problem solving are the nursing process and research process.

Once the best solution is implemented, the nurse continues to monitor the situation to evaluate its effectiveness. Other solutions identified previously, but not chosen, are not discarded but held in reserve in case the solution chosen was not effective or it becomes ineffective. In other instances, a different client's situation or problem is similar to a previous one. In this case, the nurse may find that one of the alternative solutions would be more effective for this client. Thus,

BOX 2–1
Human Responses to Health and Illness

Definition: Human responses are actions, reactions, and at times, lack of actions that individuals may use when faced with the pressures from illness or in an attempt to remain in a state of wellness. They are phenomena that may be viewed from multiple perspectives: **behavioral**–actions or lack of action that a person uses (ie, eating a well-balanced diet during pregnancy or not attending pre-natal care); **experiential**–experiences in the past or present that a client may have (ie, finding a pleasant compatible obstetrician or experiencing bleeding); **physiologic**–a body's normal physiologic response (ie, progressing normally through pregnancy); and **pathophysiologic**–untoward negative physiologic response (ie, development of pernicious anemia or vomiting in pregnancy).

Rationales for studying human responses include the following:

- To explain and understand the range of responses in individuals to the demands of healthy living and illness from at least the four perspectives mentioned
- To understand the inter-relationships of those responses with the social, cultural, and environmental context in which they occur
- To predict the potential for change in health status when nursing therapies are applied to specific human responses
- To measure the effectiveness of nursing therapies in promoting health responses and in preventing, modifying, or eliminating health-damaging responses.

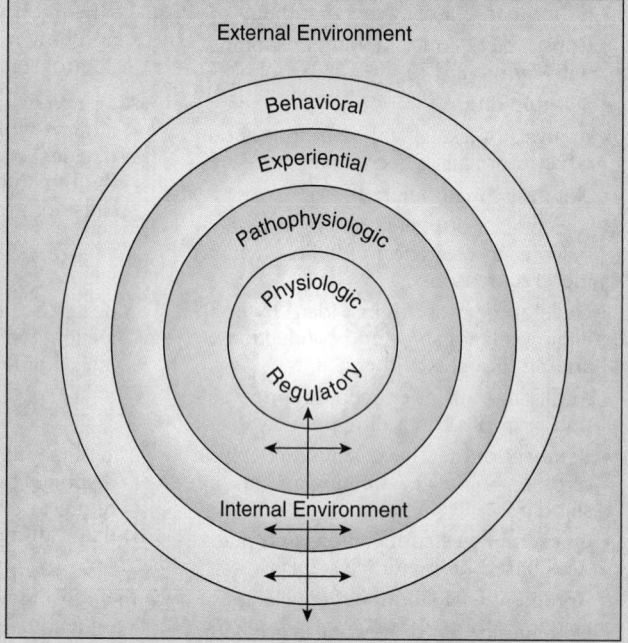

Relationship of perspectives on human responses to the internal and external environment. (Adapted from Mitchell et al. 1991.)

Adapted from Mitchell, et. al. (1991)

the nurse's initial knowledge base expands, thereby contributing to the overall knowledge base from which to draw in the future.

Steps

The problem-solving process consists of a series of specific steps, which correspond to the components in the nursing process:

- Assessing and accumulating data
- Defining the problem
- Determining the options
- Taking actions
- Evaluating outcomes

The nursing process and the research process are closely related to the problem-solving process with some distinct differences. (See the sections "Nursing Process" and "Research Process" later in this chapter.)

Methods

Various approaches, such as **trial and error, intuition,** and the **scientific method,** may be used for problem solving. Different approaches can lead to different results, some of which may be more effective than others. Regardless of the method chosen, critical thinking is essential.

Trial and Error

Trial and error, as its name suggests, involves the use of a variety of different approaches. Each approach is tried until a solution is found. Because the alternatives are randomly selected, it is difficult to ascertain exactly why one approach works. Using trial and error to solve nursing problems is considered dangerous because client harm may result from an inappropriate approach.

Intuition

Intuition is often viewed as a form of guessing. Controversy exists as to whether intuition is an appropriate method for solving nursing problems. Opponents argue that clinical judgments should be based on scientific data alone in an attempt to establish nursing as a scientific discipline. Proponents argue that intuition is an essential component of clinical judgment obtained through knowledge and experience with similar situations.

Intuition is based on experience and knowledge. The nurse first must have the knowledge base necessary to practice in the clinical area, then use that knowledge in clinical practice. Clinical experience allows the nurse to recognize cues and patterns and begin to make appropriate decisions (Kozier, et al., 1995)

Scientific Method

The *scientific method* is a formalized, logical, systematic approach to solving problems. Usually the researcher, under a controlled situation, isolates a single aspect of a problem to be studied. The study may last from a few weeks to a few years.

The scientific method is used in nursing research. However, clinical problem solving differs in some re-

---

TABLE 2–3
Comparing the Scientific Method With the Nursing Process of Clinical Problem Solving

Scientific Method	Clinical Problem Solving (Nursing Process)
1. Recognize general problem area: Survey pertinent information (literature, past expeience, observation). Construct data base (organize, select). Develop "hunches."	1. Collect data (subjective, objective): Gather information on the physical, social, and psychological aspects of the health status of the individual and family. Construct data base by observation, interview, history taking, physical examination, and role taking. Develop impressions.
2. Define specific problem: Make decisions about relevance. Review related information (research already done, theoretical formulations).	2. Define the problem: Make decisions regarding deficits or potential deficits in health status of the individual and family. Make nursing diagnoses based on clinical judgment and inference, and review related information, that is, theoretical formulations and research.
3. Propose hypotheses.	3. Plan the intervention: Make decisions regarding the actions believed to be appropriate to effect a solution of defined problems. Decisions include goal setting, priority setting, and nursing prescriptions.
4. Test hypotheses. Establish baseline data. State criteria for acceptance or rejection. Collect data.	4. Implement the intervention. Execute a nursing regimen by administering a prescribed medication or treatment, executing a medical regimen, providing comfort measures and physical care, providing counseling, providing referral services, coordinating services for the patient, and providing health education.
5. Analyze data, and interpret results.	5. Evaluate the intervention. This in turn may lead to further reassessments: Determine the degree of effectiveness of the actions taken to solve the defined problems by observation, interview of patient status and conditions, physical examination, and reading of current records. Predict future nursing action and patient potential for change.
6. Terminate or modify study: Make recommendations and predictions for future research.	6. Terminate or modify relationship.

TABLE 2–4
Decision-Making Elements

Element	Description	Example
Cue	▪ A piece of data or information	Contractions increasing in intensity, length, and frequency
Hypothesis	▪ Projected or proposed possibility; may include what is wrong with the client; what nurse, doctor, or client might do, think, or feel; or what orders or policies may be used ▪ Often introduced by subjects with words, such as probably, might, if, could be, maybe, perhaps, sounds like, or looks like	Probable active phase of first stage of labor
Knowledge base	▪ Correct and incorrect information; used as rationale or support for statements made by subject	Knowledge of phases and stages of labor
Nursing intervention	▪ Any proposed nursing action, such as assessment, physical care, teaching, communication, or collaboration	Monitor maternal and fetal vital signs closely; explain what is happening.
Search	▪ Indication of desire for additional or supplemental information about the client or situation	Observe fetal monitor. Observe mother's behavioral and verbal cues. Adjust behavior accordingly.
Assumption	▪ Conclusion verbalized for which there is insufficient information given; may lead to a search	Contractions continue to increase in intensity, frequency, and duration and woman feels uncontrollable urge to push, evidence indicates that labor is progressing and transition has been accomplished.

Adapted from Tschikota, S. (1993). *The clinical decision making process of student nurses. Journal of Nursing Education, 32* (9), 393.

spects from this formal research. Often, the nurse's time frame is much shorter, requiring an immediate solution to a client's problem. The clinical environment also does not allow for strict scientific control. In most situations, the nurse must deal with multiple, complex problems at one time, rather than one isolated aspect of a problem. As a result, clinical problem solving involves a modified scientific approach (Table 2-3).

Decision Making

Decision making refers to the process of determining the best solution to a situation or problem. It occurs during the problem-solving process as a result of critical thinking. Strader defines decision making as the process of establishing criteria by which alternative courses of action are developed or selected.

Decisions are made whenever mutually exclusive choices exist. Nurses make decisions about themselves and for their clients, and they assist clients in making decisions. When faced with more than one personal or client need, the nurse must decide which needs take priority by using critical thinking. When helping clients with decision making, the nurse also may need to supply the clients with information or resources to aid them in making the decision.

In a research study, Tschikota (1993) identified six elements for clinical decision making. These six elements include cue, hypothesis, knowledge base, nursing intervention, search, and assumption. Nurses use a variety of these elements in combination as part of their critical thinking process for decision making (Table 2-4).

The Nursing Process

Implicit in the delivery of effective, professional nursing care is the ability to use a method that helps the nurse think critically and arrive at informed judgments about clients based on sound data. With the data base and appropriate clinical judgments, nursing care can be planned and implemented to enable clients to maintain, return to, or reach a higher state of high-level wellness.

In an effort to describe a lucid, organized, scientifically based problem-solving approach to professional nursing practice, this method has been conceptualized as the *nursing process* by a variety of authors (Carpenito, 1995; Avant, 1990; Maas, et al., 1990; Jenny, 1989; Turkoski, 1988).

Nursing process is the organizing conceptual framework used throughout this text to help the student learn to make clinical nursing judgments appropriate to nursing care. It supplies a mechanism that enables the nurse to arrive at a responsible, valid judgment about clients from which to assess, diagnose, plan, implement, and evaluate nursing care that is responsive to the client's varied needs.

Components of the Nursing Process

The purpose of the nursing process is twofold: to provide a method for critical thinking that becomes second nature for quick but appropriate nursing decisions and conclusions and to provide a scientific approach to problem solving, which is essential to any profession.

The nursing process also can help the student understand how nursing practice can be made operational. The various operations have been classified under stages, headings, or steps. These have been derived by nurse theorists, practitioners, and researchers (Carpenito, 1995). These stages are not mutually exclusive and do not stand alone. Rather, there are constant feedback loops in the process.

With time, the nursing process has come to be composed of five stages: assessment, **nursing diagnosis,** planning, intervention (or **implementation**), and evaluation. Various authors have conceptualized the process using different terminology, including assessment, problem identification, diagnostic phase, validation, action, and evaluation (McClosky, 1994; Turkoski, 1988). New conceptualizations and terminology have evolved over the years. As nursing science develops, other terminology no doubt will be used.

Although the components may be described in slightly different ways by various authors, it is generally agreed that the process is as follows: In *assessment,* data are gathered on the state of the client's health, and *nursing diagnoses* are made from these data. Following the construction of the diagnoses, the nurse develops a *plan* using scientific rationale for intervention, based on assessment data and diagnoses. After *planning,* the nurse implements *interventions.* Throughout the process and as the client's condition changes, *evaluations* are made of the outcomes of the interventions. Additional assessments, diagnoses, plans, and interventions are made as indicated by evaluating the outcomes. Thus, a continuous feedback loop is in operation (Fig. 2-1).

For clarity and ease, a four-step format for nursing process and care plans is used in this book: assessment, nursing diagnosis, planning and intervention, and evaluation.

Assessment

Assessment is the act of reviewing a human situation based on information from the client and a variety of other sources. The information gathered forms a crucial data base. Assessing affirms the degree of client wellness or illness and to diagnose potential problems. The assessment phase incorporates a variety of data-gathering efforts and activities, which are illustrated in Box 2-2.

If these gathering activities are approached logically and systematically, they will provide the information to make valid nursing judgments and diagnoses. Thus, the purpose of the assessment phase is to identify and obtain data about the client's needs that enable the nurse, client, and family to assess the degree of wellness, recognize actual and potential problems, and plan care that will ensure that the client and family will arrive at appropriate solutions.

During assessment, the nurse must consider the inter-relationships of such factors as the client's age, sex, education, stage of growth and development, culture, and socioeconomic status. These factors are discussed more fully in Chapter 4.

Specific data can be obtained by interviewing the client and performing a health examination. Using a systematic format, such as an assessment tool or form, the interview and examination incorporate physical and psychosocial dimensions. Previous records and charts should be considered to ensure that information is complete; this avoids fragmentation, which could impact on the continuity of care.

Throughout the data collection process, cues and emerging patterns will become evident. Often, these cues will be related in clusters or groups. The nurse uses knowledge and experience to perceive the cues and understand their meanings. From this, the nurse begins to make *inferences,* defined as the movement of thought that proceeds from something given, a cue or data, to a conclusion as to what those data mean or suggest (Bandman, et al., 1994).

While the nurse collects data, inferences are validated to ensure accuracy in interpretation. When the existence of a problem, condition, or situation is inferred from the accumulated facts, it is confirmed with the client. The client then has the opportunity to confirm or deny the perceptions or diagnosis.

Carpenito (1995) has pointed out that after the data are gathered and examined, alternative explanations need to be tested and ruled out. At this time, the nurse will have reached one of four conclusions illustrated in Table 2-5.

Nursing Diagnosis

As data are collected, the existence and extent of a problem become evident: Generally, a problem exists when there is a goal to be obtained (ie, a healthy pregnancy), but the client sees no well-defined, well-established means of attaining it. For instance, she may be

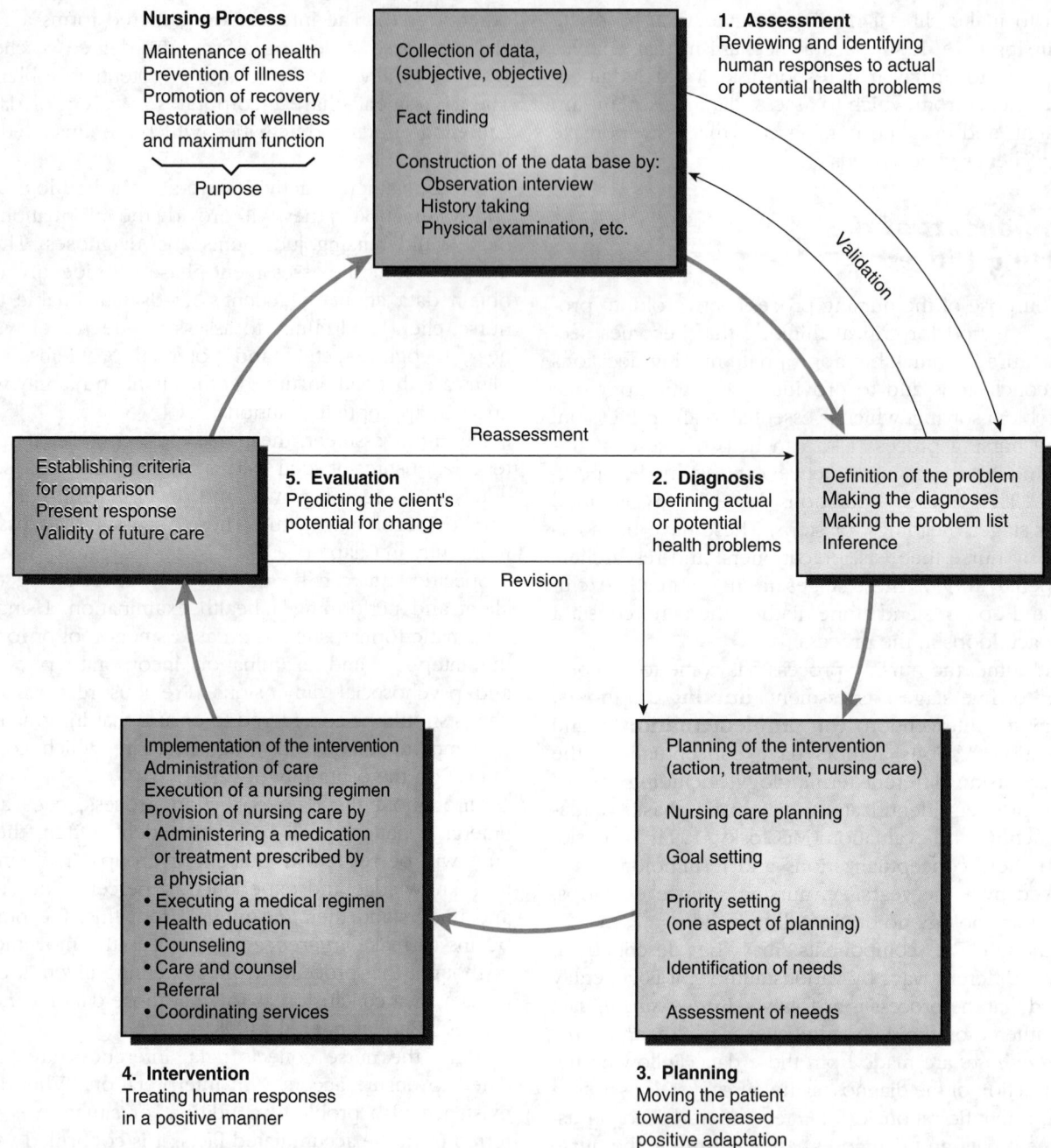

Nursing Process

Maintenance of health
Prevention of illness
Promotion of recovery
Restoration of wellness
and maximum function

Purpose

Collection of data,
(subjective, objective)

Fact finding

Construction of the data base by:
    Observation interview
    History taking
    Physical examination, etc.

1. Assessment
Reviewing and identifying
human responses to actual
or potential health problems

Validation

Reassessment

Establishing criteria
for comparison
Present response
Validity of future care

5. Evaluation
Predicting the client's
potential for change

2. Diagnosis
Defining actual
or potential
health problems

Definition of the problem
Making the diagnoses
Making the problem list
Inference

Revision

Implementation of the intervention
Administration of care
Execution of a nursing regimen
Provision of nursing care by
• Administering a medication
  or treatment prescribed by
  a physician
• Executing a medical regimen
• Health education
• Counseling
• Care and counsel
• Referral
• Coordinating services

Planning of the intervention
(action, treatment, nursing care)

Nursing care planning

Goal setting

Priority setting
(one aspect of planning)

Identification of needs

Assessment of needs

4. Intervention
Treating human responses
in a positive manner

3. Planning
Moving the patient
toward increased
positive adaptation

FIGURE 2–1 Conceptualization of nursing care using the nursing process.

too ill or too weak to help herself. Again, the goal (ie, a "healthy diet") may be so vaguely defined or unclear that the client cannot determine relevant means of achieving it. Thus, she may not understand or know how to accept conditions and instruction for achieving the goal of health.

A decision about the existence and extent of the problem or need initiates a diagnosis (Carpenito, 1995). Through the years, various definitions of nursing diangosis have been offered (Box 2-3).

A review of the literature reveals that the term *nursing diagnosis* has taken on two somewhat different meanings. (Turkoski, 1988; Carpenito, 1995). In some

situations, the term describes the process of problem solving. In other situations, it means an actual statement of the problem. This dual use has created a good deal of confusion. When the term is used to define the process of analyzing data and identifying a problem, the outcome of this process can be the delineation of medical, nursing, or other problems. The former must be referred to the physician, and the nurse may participate in the implementation of the medical regimen. Nursing problems, on the other hand, can be treated by the nurse, because they are within the nurse's legal and educational purview (Carpenito, 1995; McClosky, 1994).

BOX 2–2
Data Gathering Activities for Assessment

- Taking a nursing history including client and family history
- Using previous health records
- Performing a physical assessment
- Using a variety of data-gathering tools, such as thermometer, sphygmomanometer, stethoscope, and diagnostic tests
- Using the techniques of physical examination: inspection, palpation, auscultation, and percussion

BOX 2–3
Definitions of Nursing Diagnosis

- The actual or potential health problems that nurses, by virtue of their education and experience, are capable and licensed to treat
- The judgment or conclusion that occurs as a result of nursing assessment
- A clinical judgment about an individual, family, or community that is derived through a systematic process of data collection and analysis and that provides the basis for prescription for definitive therapy for which the nurse is accountable. The diagnosis is expressed concisely and includes the etiology when known.
- A statement that describes the human response (health state or actual/potential altered interaction pattern) of an individual or group that the nurse can legally identify and for which the nurse can order the definitive interventions to maintain the health state or to reduce, eliminate, or prevent alterations
- A clinical judgment about individual, family, or community responses to actual or potential health problems or life processes. Nursing diagnoses provide the basis for selection of nursing interventions to achieve outcomes for which the nurse is accountable.

Adapted from Carpenito 1995 and NANDA 1994

In this book, a nursing diagnosis is defined as a statement that describes the human response (which may be a health state or actual or potential altered interaction pattern) of an individual or group that the nurse can legally identify and for which the nurse can order the definitive interventions to maintain the health state or to reduce, eliminate, or prevent alterations (Carpenito, 1995).

For nursing diagnoses in this text, the North American Nursing Diagnosis Association (NANDA) classification taxonomy is used. NANDA classifies nursing diagnoses as actual, risk, or wellness. See Box 2-4 for a description of each. NANDA is a group that evolved from a series of national conferences (the first conference was held in 1973) on nursing diagnosis. It is made up of representatives from all areas of the nursing profession: clinical practice, education, and research.

The work of NANDA, considered extremely important by most members of the profession, is viewed as a major advancement toward nursing professionalism. Some controversy about the practicality of using a method such as nursing diagnosis in contrast to a more holistic approach to patient care has existed within the nursing profession. Some nurses have suggested alternatives to the extant classification taxonomies, such as NANDA's (McClosky, 1994). Whatever the concerns of those who have conflicting opinions and whatever the data show, it is crucial that this discussion and alternatives be aired. It is only through such informed discussion and debate that the profession advances.

Carpenito (1995) advises that a nursing diagnosis be a two- or three-part statement. In a two-part statement,

TABLE 2–5
Conclusions in Assessment

Conclusion	Example for Maternity and Perinatal Nursing
No problem is evident at present; hence, no health promotion or intervention is indicated.	All physiologic signs are normal for stage of pregnancy; patient is keeping all regular appointments.
No problem is evident, but health-promotion activities are indicated to ensure and maintain the present level of wellness and to prevent health alterations.	Patient is not eating healthy diet—go over rationale for diet during prenatal visits.
Actual or potential clinical problems are evident, requiring medical referral or implementation of the medical regimen by the nurse.	Blood pressure is slightly elevated; diet contains excess fat and salt—refer to dietitian or physician.
Actual or potential nursing problems are apparent that are within the legal and educational domain of the nurse and that require nursing orders.	Patient does not know components of healthy diet—nurse provides counseling.

BOX 2-4
Classification of Nursing Diagnoses

Actual nursing diagnosis	Human responses to health conditions or life processes that exist in an individual, family, or community	Knowledge deficit related to physiologic changes of pregnancy
	Supported by defining characteristics that cluster in patterns of related cues and inferences	
Risk nursing diagnosis	Human responses to health conditions or life processes that may develop in a vulnerable individual, family, or community	Risk for infection related to prolonged rupture of membranes
	Supported by risk factors that contribute to increased vulnerability	
Wellness nursing diagnosis	Human responses to levels of wellness in an individual, family, or community that have a potential for enhancement to a higher state	Effective breastfeeding related to appropriate infant weight gain patterns

Source: NANDA Nursing Diagnosis and Classification 1995–1996, page 102

the first part is a diagnostic label or statement, followed by a statement about the contributing factors associated with the problem. "Body image disturbance related to physiologic and psychosocial changes of pregnancy" is an example of a two part statement. A three-part statement includes the diagnostic label, contributing factors, followed by the **defining characteristics** (signs and symptoms) of the diagnosis. "Anxiety related to prolonged, painful labor as evidenced by client statements about not being able to deliver her baby" is an example of a three-part nursing diagnosis. Critical thinking is essential to identifying the contributing factors and defining characteristics and to determining their relationship to the problem. The relationship also provides evidence to support the problem.

Carpenito (1995) cautions about the importance of not linking the statements with words that imply cause and effect, because such a relationship can result in legal and professional difficulty for the nurse. The phrase *related to* rather than *caused by* or *due to* eliminates this problem. Thus, additional potential diagnoses that the nurse might make while attending a maternity patient might be "Anxiety related to uncertainty of labor process" or "Risk for altered body temperature related to inadequate hydration."

Sometimes it is impossible to ascertain any related factors despite a complete assessment. In this instance, the following diagnosis might be appropriate: "Fear of caring for the newborn related to unknown factors." Moreover, there may be several diagnoses relating to a constellation of inter-related problems. The diagnoses

given previously could conceivably apply to one client at any time. Therefore, it is essential for the nurse to use critical thinking to prioritize the nursing diagnoses and plan and intervene based on these priorities.

Finally, the same nursing diagnosis can have different related factors. In the case of a newly delivered infant, for instance, the diagnosis might be "Impaired gas exchange related to a possible congenital heart defect" or "Impaired gas exchange related to immature lungs associated with prematurity." The nurse needs to evaluate critically the related factors and use them to guide any actions.

Planning

Following the assessment and nursing diagnosis stages, the next component of the nursing process involves developing a plan. The skills involved with planning include establishing priorities, establishing client goals (expressed in behavioral, measurable terms) and outcome criteria, and determining nursing interventions. Using all of the information available to the nurse from the previous two stages, coupled with the solid knowledge base and experience, the nurse uses critical thinking and decision making to arrive at the plan. This plan provides a framework for action for the next stage.

Implementation

Implementation is the action stage of the nursing process, requiring the use of intellectual, interpersonal,

BOX 2–5
Example of Nursing Orders and Interventions in a Given Situation

Nursing Prescriptions or Orders	*Nursing Intervention*
Increase fluids to at least 2,400 mL/24 h	Increase fluid intake.
1,000 mL 7–3	
700 mL 3–11	
100 mL 11–7	
Allow all juices and carbonated beverages (client likes).	
Do not count coffee or tea in above amount.	
Tell client to nurse infant on each breast at each feeding.	Ensure that breasts are emptied.
Allow time on each breast as tolerated.	
Nurse q2h or on demand; do not allow longer intervals than q4h between feedings.	Ensure that breasts are stimulated frequently.
Allow client to nurse sitting or lying down.	

Adapted from Carpenito, 1995

and technical skills. Analysis, integration, and synthesis occur. It is the actual initiation of the plan, evaluation of the response to the plan, and recording of nursing activities and the client's response to these activities. These activities may encompass everything from the administration of comfort measures to counseling and health education. These activities are directed at moving the client toward increased positive adaptation to the environment and high-level wellness.

Nursing prescriptions or orders are given here. These are required to prevent, reduce, or eliminate the alteration in the client's health–illness continuum based on scientific rationale. It has been suggested that nursing orders should be composed of the following:

- The date when written
- A directive verb
- What, when, how often, how long, and where the order is to be executed
- The signature of the nurse who wrote the order (Carnevali, 1983; Carpenito, 1995)

The objective of the nursing prescription or order is to direct individualized care to the client. Orders differ from nursing actions. Nursing actions are broad interventions that can apply to any number of people sharing a similar problem or health alteration. Examples of nursing orders and interventions for a mother who is recovering from dehydration and is having some difficulty establishing breast-feeding are given in Box 2-5 (Carpenito, 1995).

The implementation phase is fluid because it is based on a diagnosis or diagnoses that may be reassessed at any point in the process. Additionally, as care is provided, the client's condition will be expected to change, which, on evaluation, will necessitate modifying care and possibly changing or adding new diagnoses. Therefore, continuous feedback loops are built into the process. For example, placing a woman on her side may help the fetal heart rate to improve, thus changing the diagnosis of fetal distress and the evaluation status.

During this stage, the nurse has the responsibility to communicate his or her plan of care to medical and nursing colleagues so that comprehensive care for the client can be attained. This can be done by means of the Kardex, verbal reporting, charting, critical pathways, clinical guidelines, and nursing care plans. Most hospitals have instituted some kind of care-plan format, and they provide a thorough but brief summary of pertinent client data together with space to write and record nursing prescriptions, interventions, evaluations, and client response to care.

Evaluation

The last component of the nursing process includes evaluation and prediction aspects. A worthwhile evalu-

BOX 2–6
Components of Evaluation

- Establishing observable and measurable criteria
- Assessing the present response for evidence of achievement
- Comparing the response to the established criteria
- Revising or modifying the current plan

TABLE 2-6
Primary Knowledge and Skills Needed to Implement the Nursing Process

Critical Thinking	Theoretical Knowledge	Communication Skills	Technical Skills	Therapeutic Use of Self
Discrimination or differentiation	Basic science	Interviewing	Organization	Goal setting for self and others
Analysis	General physiology	Mutual sharing	Use of equipment	Ability to use past experiences and role take
Synthesis	General pathophysiology	Writing	Knowledge of general and specific:	Ability to appreciate others' value systems
Formulation	Nursing research	Nonverbal	Techniques	Ability to recognize limitations in self and others
Clarification	Social science	Listening	Safety	
Reason	Ethical or religious		Physics	
Logic	Family systems		Asepsis	
Reflection	Reproductive:			
Inquiry	Physiology			
Self-thinking	Pathophysiology			
Creativity	Psychosocial			
Fairness	Pharmacology			
Verification	Nutrition:			
Validation	Basic			
	Relating to reproduction			

ation includes an estimation of the results of past nursing care activities. In addition, evaluation may help to predict the validity of future care. Critical thinking plays an important role. Objectivity, self-corrective feedback, objective standards, and verification are crucial to evaluation. The components of an accurate evaluation are illustrated in Box 2-6.

Evaluation, although a separate and distinct stage, is an ongoing and continuous process performed throughout all stages of the nursing process. Many different skills are required for evaluation. These include knowledge of the standards of care, knowledge of normal client responses, knowledge of conceptual models and theories, ability to monitor effectiveness of nursing interventions, and awareness of clinical research.

Any statement about the effectiveness and reliability of actions is best made with qualifications indicating the degree or amount of effectiveness and the reliability claimed:

- What is the present state of the client?
- Were all symptoms relieved?
- What was the extent of the results?
- What is the evidence (observation of self, others, verbal response, cessation of symptoms)?
- Who was involved (nurse, client, others)?

TABLE 2-7
Secondary Knowledge and Skills Needed to Implement the Nursing Process

Assessment	Nursing Diagnosis	Planning and Implementation	Evaluation
Ability to	Ability to	Ability to	Knowledge of
- Differentiate cues and inferences	- Differentiate nursing problems from medical clinical problems	- Identify goals	- Process criteria
- Observe systematically		- Identify interventions	- Outcome criteria
- Perform a nursing health assessment	- Identify and test alternatives	- Write nursing orders	
- Identify patterns of problems	- Recognize patterns of problems	Management skills	
- Validate impressions	- Correctly label patterns	Communication skills	
		Teaching skills	
		Ability to implement change theory	

Adapted from Carpenito (1995) and NANDA (1994).

■ In what context did this occur (what else was happening when the action was performed)?

When these points are established, effective nursing actions are identified; in the future, under certain circumstances, for certain patients, given certain conditions, the nurse may use this information again. Nurses are then in a better position to predict the client's potential for change toward stability or a wellness condition.

Knowledge and Skills Necessary to Implement the Nursing Process

There are certain basic knowledge and skills that the nurse must have to implement the nursing process. Tables 2-6 and 2-7 provide a quick reference listing of the knowledge and skills needed as the nursing process is used with the maternity client and her family. With in-

TABLE 2–8
Comparing the Research Process, Nursing Process, and Problem-Solving Process

Problem-Solving Process	Nursing Process	Research Process
Assessing and accumulating data	Assessment: Collect data (subjective, objective). a. Gather information on the physical, social, and psychological aspects of the health status of the individual and family. b. Construct the data base by observation, interview, history taking, physical examination, and role taking. c. Develop impressions.	Recognize general problem area. a. Survey pertinent information (past experience, observation). b. Construct data base (organize, select). c. Develop "hunches"—research question.
Defining the problem	Nursing diagnosis: Define the problem. a. Make decisions regarding deficits or potential deficits in health status of the individual and family assigning resources. b. Make nursing diagnoses based on clinical judgment and inference and review of related information, that is, theoretical formulations and research.	Define specific problem. a. Make decisions about relevance. b. Review related information, literature review (research already done, theoretical formulations).
Determining the options	Planning: Plan the intervention. a. Make decisions regarding the actions believed to be appropriate to effect a solution of defined problems. b. Decisions include goal setting, priority setting, and nursing prescriptions.	Propose hypotheses. a. Define variables. b. Select test method. c. Select population, sample, and setting.
Taking actions	Implementation: Implement the intervention. a. Execute a nursing regimen by administering a prescribed medication or treatment, executing a medical regimen, providing comfort measures and physical care, providing counseling, providing referral services, coordinating services for the patient, and providing health education.	Test hypotheses. a. Establish baseline data. b. State criteria for acceptance or rejection. c. Collect data.
Evaluating outcomes	Evaluation: Evaluate the intervention. This in turn may lead to further reassessments. a. Determine the degree of effectiveness of the actions taken to solve the defined problems by observation, interview of patient status and conditions, physical examination, and reading of current records. b. Predict future nursing action and patient potential for change.	Analyze data, and interpret results.
Terminate or modify process	Terminate or modify relationship.	Communicate conclusions and implications. Terminate or modify study. a. Make recommendations and predictions for future research.

creased expertise, increasing proficiency in using the nursing process, relationships with clients will develop more quickly, be on a greater empathetic level, and ultimately be more effective.

Nursing Research

The research process, or the scientific method as it is sometimes called, is used for problem solving. It also is used as a basis from which to formulate additional research that will expand the theoretical base of the discipline. Because nursing also has the concern of expanding its theoretical knowledge to provide a sound basis for its practice, the nursing process must be scientifically grounded (Table 2-8).

Research and Practice

As Wilkerson-Faulk and Smith (1994) have pointed out, an understanding of the research process is critical to all healthcare professionals because of the new emphasis placed on quality improvement by the Joint Commission on Accreditation of Healthcare Organizations. Research not only provides the basis for building new nursing knowledge, but also it is a way to attain the highest quality of care in practice. Unfortunately, practicing staff nurses often see research as something the nurse does not understand and therefore cannot do. In addition, the nurse often is compelled to participate in the research activities, adding to an already packed client care assignment.

Research Utilization

The term currently used for incorporating or applying research findings in the delivery of patient care is **research utilization.** Research utilization has been defined as a complex activity involving planned change, the transfer of specific research-based knowledge into practice, and the activity of client problem solving. It can be conceptualized as the translation of practice-based research findings into research-based nursing practice (Keefe, 1994).

Although there is still much to be done, the progress made, particularly in the last 20 years, has been impressive. In the 1950s, research in maternity nursing and the critical reading of literature was not even an ideal. In the 1960s, an acceptance of the importance of research began to be considered but was not implemented consistently in nursing curricula. In the maternity nursing field, for example, some clinicians were aware that rooming in resulted in a positive expense for the mother and did not increase her anxiety. This finding was the result of pioneer research. By the 1970s, research began to be a consistent theme but

only a vague ideal in education. During the last 20 years, professional nursing practice has been based on research. As May (1991) points out, we have more nurses with graduate degrees prepared to conduct research; more expert clinicians throughout the country are becoming involved in nursing research programs (not just intermittent studies). Moreover, and nursing is now a bona fide research institute within the National Institutes of Health. However, nurses continue to grapple with the problem of irrelevancy; that is, much of the research has little applicability to the reality of practice. Many pressing clinical problems, such as nursing interventions specifically designed to promote better prenatal care in recovering substance abusers or reexamination with large samples of the attachment process are receiving inadequate attention because they do not fit into nurse researchers' "program" of research; they are not viewed by promotion committees, peer reviewers, and prestigious journals as "impressive" enough to study, or the researcher simply does not realize what the salient problems in the clinical area are.

May (1991) argues that there is great potential for the practicing clinician to assume a leadership role in identifying priorities for clinical investigation. Although the clinician cannot do this alone, it is imperative that the working clinician and the working researcher or scientist collaborate to bring their different but necessary perspectives to bear on setting research priorities. This perspective is becoming increasingly recommended by a variety of clinicians and researchers (Young, 1994; Wilkerson-Faulk & Smith, 1994; Keefe, 1994).

Methods to Enhance Research Integration

Wilkerson-Faulk and Smith (1994) and Keefe (1993) offer several strategies to enhance collaboration and integra-

---

BOX 2-7
Steps in Integrating Clinical Nurses Into Research

- Identify a common problem.
- Validate the problem with the staff.
- Simplify the data collection process.
- Encourage staff input.
- Use staff suggestions.
- Encourage and support staff participation in the research process.
- Keep the staff updated throughout the study.
- Discuss how findings can be applied to practice with the staff.

Wilkerson-Faulk D., & Smith, A. (1994). Involving staff nurses in research: A practical approach. MCN, 19(4), 194–196.

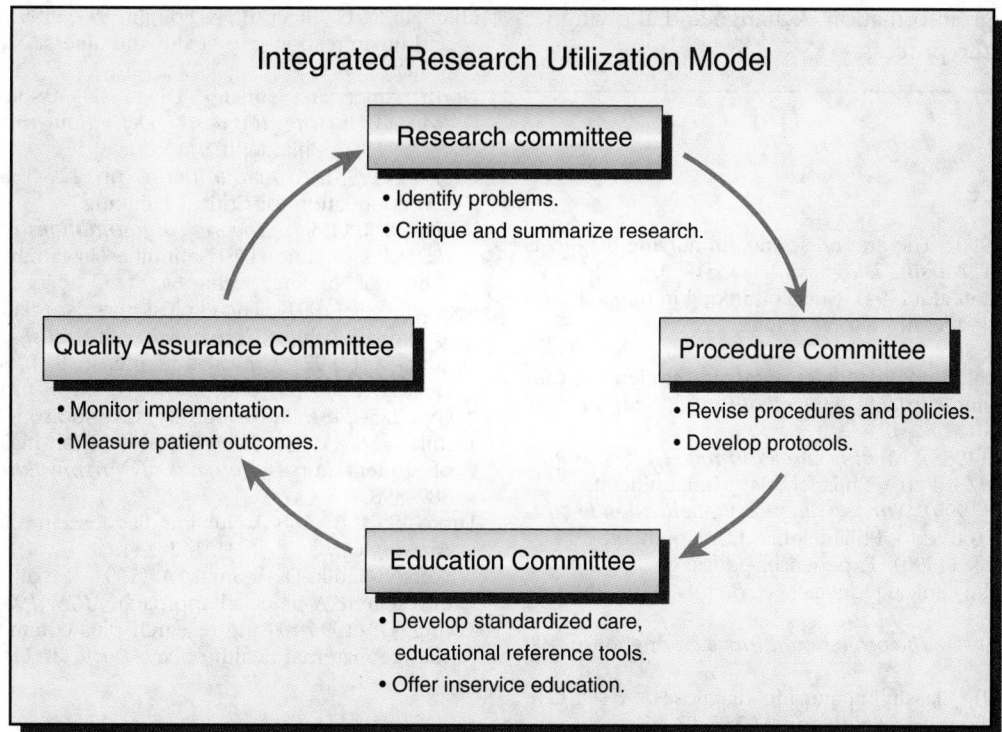

FIGURE 2-2 An integrated model illustrating an approach to integrating research findings into clinical practice. Adapted from Keefe, 1994.

tion of research into practice. Wilkerson-Faulk and Smith (1994) suggest eight steps to enhance the involvement of the clinical nurse in research participation and utilization. Box 2-7 illustrates these steps. As can be seen, the focus is on the staff and their needs, input, and decisions. This kind of decision making and input empowers the staff and makes them an integral part of the research team.

Keefe (1994) offers a model for integrating research at the institutional level (Fig. 2-2). This model emphasizes getting support from administrative and institutional committee sources and the various activities that each committee can perform to ensure integration. Because the committees are often made up in part of staff clinicians, service on these committees can empower as well.

Critical thinking, accurate clinical judgments, problem-solving, decision making, the nursing process, and research are the crucial foundations on which our contemporary nursing practice is built.

Summary Points

✔ Critical thinking is a basic component in making accurate clinical judgments, problem solving, decision making, and using the nursing process. It involves fact finding, sorting information, making decisions, and applying solutions to client health problems.

✔ Problem solving refers to a process by which an individual obtains information related to a problem or situation and then based on that information, develops possible solutions. Various methods can be used in problem solving, including trial and error, intuition, and the scientific method.

✔ Decision making occurs during the problem-solving process as a result of critical thinking to determine the best possible solution to a situation or problem.

✔ Nursing diagnoses are statements that describe the human rresponse of an individual or group that the nurse can legally identify and for which the nurse can order definitive interventions to maintain the health state or to reduce, eliminate, or prevent alterations.

✔ The nursing process is a five-step process that involves assessment, nursing diagnosis, planning, implementation, and evaluation. It is a continuous feedback loop.

✔ Although research is the basis of quality nursing practice, integrating the practicing clinician into ongoing research studies has been difficult because much of the nursing research in the past had little relevance for clinical problems. Staff felt exploited and burdened if they did participate. Strategies to improve integration include making the clinician a participating member of the research team by defining mutual clinical problems and empowering staff through information exchange and allowing input into the process.

REFERENCES

Avant, K. C. (1990). The art and science in nursing diagnosis development. *Nursing Diagnosis, 1*(2), 51–56.

Bandman, E. L., et al. (1994). Critical thinking in nursing (2nd ed.). Norwalk, CT: Appleton & Lange.

Brooks, K. L., & Shepherd J. M. (1992). Professionalism verses general critical thinking abilities of nursing students in four types of nursing curricula. *Journal of Professional Nursing, 8*(2), 87–95.

Carnevali D. L. (1983). *Nursing care Planning: Diagnosis and management* (3rd ed.). Philadelphia: J.B. Lippincott.

Carpenito L. J. (1995). *Nursing diagnosis: Application to clinical practice* (6th ed.). Philadelphia: J.B. Lippincott.

del Bueno, D. J. (1990). Experience, education and nurses' ability to make clinical judgements. *Nursing & Health Care, 11*(6), 290–294.

Grant, A. B. (1994). *The professional nurse*. Springhouse, PA: Springhouse.

Jenny, J. (1989). Classifying nursing diagnoses: A self-care approach. *Nursing & Health Care, 10*(2), 83–88.

Keefe, M. R. (1994). An integrated approach to incorporating research findings into practice. *MCN, 18*(2), 65–70.

Kozier, B., et. al. (1995). *Fundamentals of nursing. Concepts, processes and practice* (5th ed.). Redwood City, CA: Addison-Wesley.

Maas, J., Hardy, M., & Craft, M. (1990). Some methodological considerations in nursing diagnoses. *Nursing Research, 1*(1), 24–30.

May, K. A. (1991). The leader in nursing research. *MCN, 16*(1) 30–31.

McClosky, J. C. (1994). Standardizing the language for nursing treatments: An overview of the issues. *Nursing Outlook, 42*(2), 56–63.

Meleis, A. (1991). *Theoretical nursing: Development and progress* (2nd ed.). Philadelphia: J.B. Lippincott.

Mitchell, P., Gallucci, B., & Fought, S.G. (1991). Perspectives on human response to health and illness. *Nursing Outlook, 39*(4).

North American Nursing Diagnosis Association (1994). *NANDA nursing diagnosis—Definition and classification 1995–1996*. Philadephia: Author.

Paul, R. (1993). *Critical thinking* (pp. 129–130). Santa Rosa, CA: Foundation for Critical Thinking.

Reeder, S. J. (1994). *Theoretical foundations in care of families*. Class lecture: Discontinuities in family health. UCLA School of Nursing, Spring.

Sparacino, P. (1991). The clinical nurse specialist—case manager relationship. *Clinical Nurse Specialist, 5,* 180.

Strader, M. (1992). Critical thinking. In E. J. Sullivan & P. J. Decker (Eds.), *Effective management in nursing* (3rd ed.) (pp. 225–248). Redwood City, CA: Addison-Wesley.

Tschikota, S. (1993). The clinical decision making processes of student nurses. *Journal of Nursing Education, 32*(9), 389–398.

Turkoski, B. B. (1988). Nursing diagnosis in print, 1950–1985. *Nursing Outlook, 36*(3), 142–144.

Wilkerson-Faulk, D., & Smith, A. (1994). Involving staff nurses in research: A practical approach. *MCN, 19*(4), 194–196.

Young, D. (1994). Using research plus community action to change maternal health policy. *Birth, 21*(1), 2–3.

SUGGESTED READING

Connelly, J. M., Keele, B. S., Kleinbeck, S. V., Schniederr, J. K., & Cobb, A. K. (1993). A place to be yourself: Empowerment from the client's perspective. *Image, 25*(3), 297–303.

Korbert L., & Folan M. (1990). Coming of age in nursing: Rethinking the philosophies behind holism and nursing process. *Nursing Health Care, 11*(6), 308–312.

Levin R. F., Blake, E. R., & Dunn, S. A. (1989). Diagnostic content validity of nursing diagnoses. *Image, 21*(1), 40–44.

Reynolds, A. (1994). Patho. flow diagramming: A strategy for critical thinking and clinical decision making. *Journal of Nursing Education, 33*(7), 333–336.

Vincent K. G., & Coler M. S. (1990). A unified nursing diagnostic model. *Image, 22*(2), 93–95.

3

The Family and Nursing Practice

Objectives

- Develop knowledge and understanding of the structure and function of the modern American family.
- Acquire knowledge of the various theoretical frameworks used in family study and their relationship to nursing practice.
- Develop knowledge and understanding of the cultural and societal changes that are impacting the modern family.
- Develop an understanding of the implications that these changes have for family functioning, particularly in the areas of childbearing and the use of health services.
- Acquire knowledge about and develop expertise in delivering quality nursing care to today's evolving families.

What Is the Family?

Most people know intuitively what is meant by the phrase "the family." They have known families throughout their lives, and intuitive definitions are sufficient for everyday conversation and action. However, when defining what constitutes a family, analyzing the unit as a social institution, or attempting to deliver comprehensive care to its members, personal, intuitive definitions are inappropriate. The characteristics of families of one segment of society often do not fit those of families of other segments or cultures.

The family has been defined in a variety of ways. For instance, the U.S. Census Bureau defines the family as a group of two or more people who are related by blood, marriage, or adoption and who reside together (U.S. Bureau of the Census, 1994). The concept of residing together is important for purposes of census enumeration, but there are times and situations in which family members do not share the same household. Other authors have defined the family as a system of roles or as a unit of interacting personalities who may not necessarily be sanctioned by law but have some commitment to each other (Feetham et al., 1993; Gilliss et al., 1989; Quimby, 1994). Generally, family can be defined as a group of kin united by blood, marriage, or adoption who share a common residence for some part of their lives, assume reciprocal rights and obligations with regard to one another, and are the principal source of socialization of its members (Eshelman et al., 1990).

Common to all these definitions is the fact that the members relate to each other in some way. They interact with specified patterns of behavior and in so doing, differentiate and structure roles for themselves; thus, they provide valuable functions for the unit and for society.

The Changing American Family

American society is living through a period of historic change that is impacting greatly on the American family. Various forms of the American family are continuing to evolve rapidly: single-parent families, unmarried couples with and without children, gay and lesbian parents, mothers working while fathers keep house, both parents working, grandparents parenting, and second- and third-marriage blending of families (Fig. 3-1).

As late as the 1950s, the family was thought to have an "ideal" form. Often it was religiously sanctioned and based on an ideal set of values. This was the **traditional nuclear family** of husband, wife, and children who lived together in their separate residence, with the father as breadwinner and mother as homemaker. Forms that varied from this traditional definition were viewed as deviant. Research in the 1950s and 1960s on single-parent families, working mothers, or dual-working families was primarily focused on the harmful effects that absent spouses or working mothers had on the children. The implication was that the woman should be in the home, and if a spouse was alone for any reason, he or she had the obligation to remarry (not just live with someone) as soon as possible (Thornton, 1989; Whall et al., 1991).

Today, people often ask, "What has happened to the family?" The problems are many: Children are having babies; adolescents refuse to grow up and leave home and often return home in their 20s and 30s; drugs and drug use are rampant among parents and children; and some parents seem to care more about making money and being affluent than they do for their children's

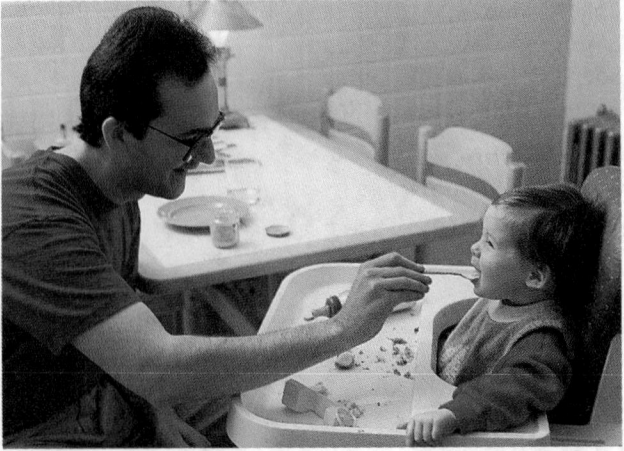

FIGURE 3-1 In some American families the traditional roles are being reversed. This father stays at home to care for the child while the mother works outside the home.

welfare. Marriage is tenuous at best, and divorce seems to be an easy and handy solution. For some, the family just does not exist anymore (Newsweek, 1990; Feetham et al., 1993).

Is the Family Simply Changing, or Is it in Decline?

The structure and function of the American family have changed remarkably in the past quarter of a century. Among the most notable of the changes, documented through an analysis of census data and research on the composition of the American family, is the near tripling of one-parent and one-person households and the more than quadrupling of households composed of unmarried couples. These shifts are the result of profound demographic and social changes in America. Other social indicators suggest that the rapid changes in the roles of men and women, begun in the 1960s and continuing today, are of primary importance in effecting change in the American family (U.S. Bureau of the Census, 1994; Popenoe, 1993a; Glenn, 1993; Cowan, 1993; DeMaris et al., 1993; Glick, 1988).

The changes in women's roles in particular have been caused primarily by three inter-related factors (Quimby, 1994; Thornton, 1989; DeMaris et al., 1993; Popenoe, 1993a):

■ Changes in the economy affecting labor force participation
■ Changes in the age structure of our society due to the baby boom of the 1950s and the subsequent lowering of the birthrate (Fig. 3-2)
■ Changes in values

These role and value changes have been intimately tied to what has been called the *contraceptive revolution* of the 1960s, and the continuing effective use of these products has allowed women to regulate their childbearing effectively. More younger women are delaying marriage or choosing not to have children. Similarly, women are increasingly working outside the home (and more frequently in professions); they choose to do so to actualize themselves as individuals and to earn a needed second income (Fig. 3-3). There continues to be a restructuring of values and roles within the home toward a more egalitarian or democratic orientation, and the power base is gradually shifting from a strong patriarchal orientation to a more egalitarian orientation, particularly among the upper middle class. However, there is a notion that in these egalitarian roles, the partners are supposed to be dutiful parents, dual wage earners, fascinating lovers, and providers of unqualified emotional support for all concerned. Obviously, the goals of this type of relation-

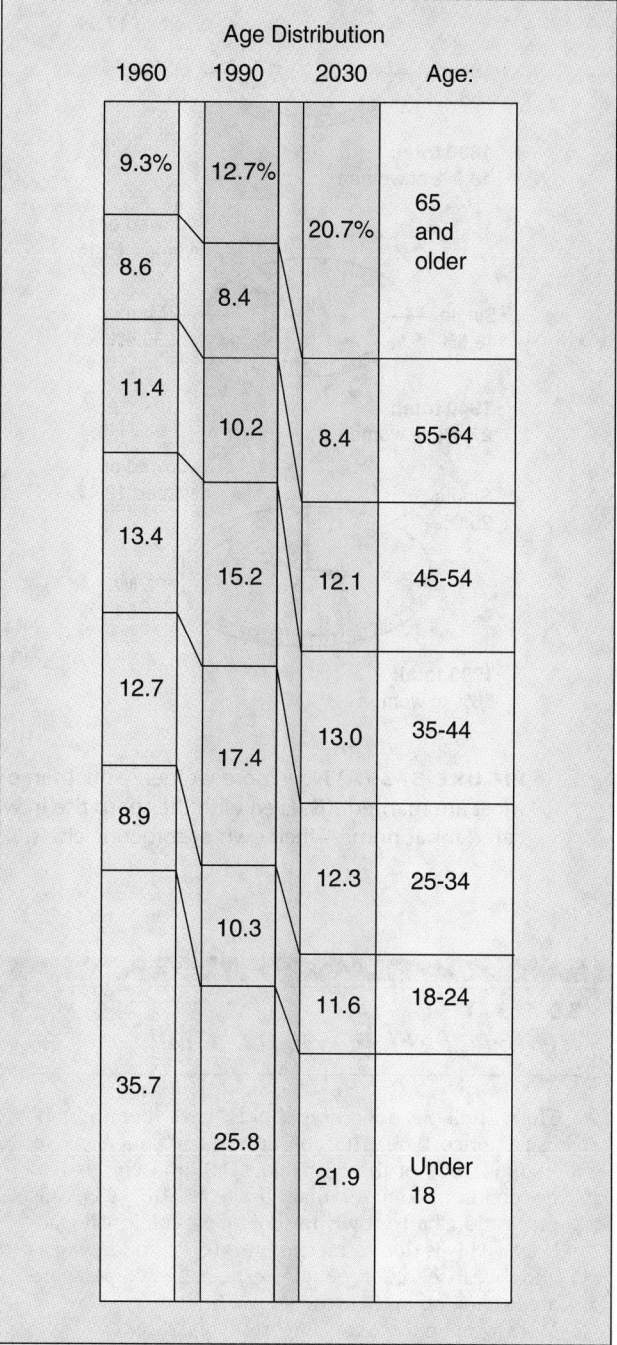

FIGURE 3–2 As the old get older, the percentage of young gets dramatically smaller.

ship are incredibly demanding, and a highly flexible divorce system has arisen in response. With divorce and remarriage, partners may shift, but the monogamous ideal remains (Newsweek, 1990; Friedman, 1992). Some startling changes in the family are highlighted in Box 3-1.

Among scholars of the family, however, a controversy rages. Popenoe (1993b) and Thorton (1989) refer

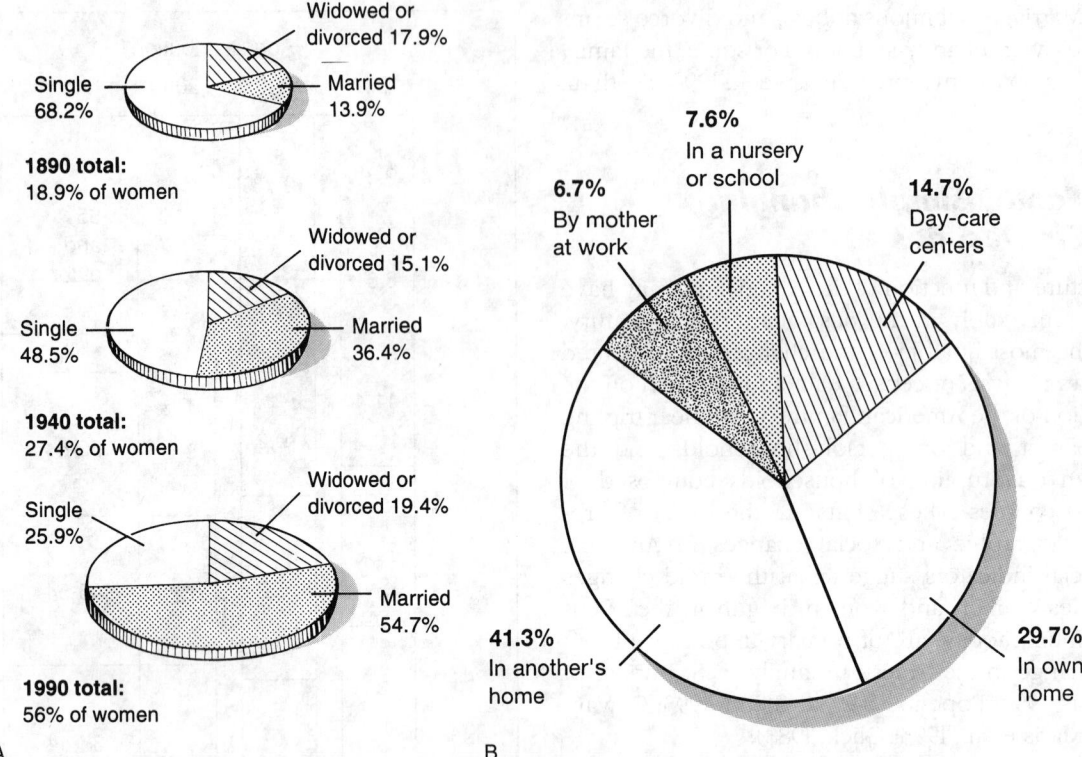

FIGURE 3–3 (A) Now more women work than do not, and of the women who do work, most are married. **(B)** Even with the sharp rise in working mothers, most children are still cared for at home—their own or someone else's.

BOX 3–1
Historical Changes in the Family

- Thirty million new households have been established since 1960. This constitutes a 58% increase.
- In 1960, 52% of the 53 million U.S. households had no children younger than 18 years. By 1983, this proportion had grown to 63% of 84 million households. This is due to increasing rates of childlessness and because older people, especially women, are able to maintain their own households.
- More women are expecting to be childless.
- Since 1960, the overall rate of married-couple households has increased slowly; in 1983, they accounted for 6 in 10 households. Cohabitation, on the other hand, has skyrocketed, primarily since 1970, increasing by 331%!
- There has been a 175% increase in one-parent households compared with a 26% increase in married families. This rise was most accelerated during the 1970s, when divorce rates greatly increased and the number of out-of-wedlock births also was greatest.
- Nearly one-half of all marriages in the 1980s ended in divorce; one in every three marriages is a remarriage.

to this dialectic as the "national family wars." Popenoe (1993a) contends that the American family is declining, not just changing. He maintains that since the 1960s, this decline has been extraordinarily steep and the social consequences serious, especially for children. Drawing on a variety of sources, he argues that families have lost their function, power, and authority; familism as a cultural value has diminished; and people have become less willing to invest time, money, and energy into family life, preferring to invest in themselves. The recent decline in the last decade is more serious than any in the past because the fundamental unit of society, the nuclear family, is breaking up. It is stripped of relatives and left with two crucial functions that cannot be performed better elsewhere: childbearing and provision to its members of affection and companionship.

Cowan (1993) and Glenn (1993, 1991), take different perspectives, arguing that the "decline," if there is one, is finishing for the family, and the family has emerged more "streamlined" and more adaptable to contemporary issues. Some of the authors feel that Popenoe's interpretations of his source data are in error and his predictions too dire. Thus, the debate promises to continue.

Structure of the Modern Family

There will always be different conceptualizations of the family as a unit of society and what the "appropriate" functions ought to be. The nurse should be well informed about the various contemporary issues regarding the family, including the changes in the structure of the American family.

Traditional Structures

Although it may seem that the traditional family structure is on the wane, many traditional family forms are still common. The most prominent among these are the following:

- Single adult: An adult lives alone.
- Nuclear family: Husband, wife, and children live in a household. Continuous or interrupted career is pursued by wife as children are born (Fig. 3-4).
- Nuclear dyad: Husband and wife live alone, either childless or with children leaving home. Dual careers may be present.
- Single-parent family: One head is present as a result of death, divorce, or abandonment. Children are usually present. When financial aid is not available from the absent spouse, a career or occupation is pursued.
- Extended family or kin network: Nuclear household with close kin or unmarried members live in the household or in close proximity with an exchange of reciprocal services (Duvall et al., 1990).

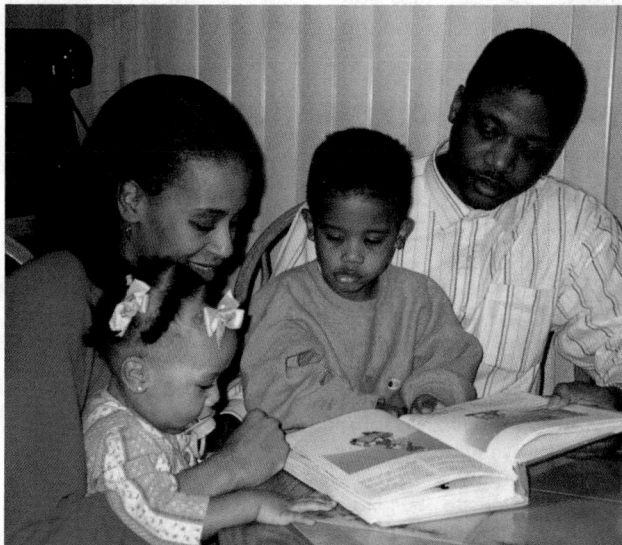

FIGURE 3–4 The nuclear family is an important and prominent type of family structure in American society. This nuclear family enjoys reading together after dinner.

Each of these may have its problems and resources with respect to health needs and use of services. Generally, society favors traditional households because they are considered stable and provide a legitimate anchor for the family's children (DeMaris et al., 1993; Quimby, 1994).

It has been said that nuclear families suffer from isolation and cannot cope with illness, repeated pregnancy, or reproductive wastage (eg, abortion, stillbirths); hence, they must turn to professionals for sustenance and care. However, research indicates that the nuclear family probably has less isolation and better coping ability than formerly was thought. This is because there appears to be great role adaptability and flexibility in times of stress and a greater use of kin and other social networks for advice and sustenance during childbearing and other health conditions (Quimby, 1994; Feetham et al., 1993; Antonovsky, 1989).

It is apparent that extended family forms can counter isolation and provide help during periods of stress. However, kin and friends also can deter family members from appropriately identifying themselves as being in need of care and can prohibit or deter them from prompt and continued use of health services.

Single-Parent Families

This type of traditional family structure deserves particular mention because it is one of the fastest growing types of families. As shown in Figure 3-5, the proportion of children living with one parent nearly tripled from 1970 to 1990. Census Bureau statistics for 1990 indicate that single parents headed 37.9% of the families with children younger than 18 years. It is anticipated that this percentage will continue to rise. As many as one-fourth of all now-married mothers and fathers with children will be single parenting by the end of the decade (U.S. Bureau of the Census, 1994). The intact, conventional family accounts for only 45% of American households, whereas 55% of households are represented by single parents, childless couples, or reconstituted families (remarried couples with or without children; Glick, 1988; Glenn, 1991).

The quality of the single-parent experience depends on the circumstances that occur in this type of household. In the case of widows and widowers, for instance, if there is adequate insurance coverage or the remaining spouse has a lucrative occupation, there may not be the economic hardship or social stigma that occur when divorce is the cause of single parenting.

Single-Mother Households. The one common characteristic shared by almost all female-headed, single-parent families is poverty or at best, reduced economic circumstances. Even with supplemental insurance and

Nuclear Family vs. One-parent Family

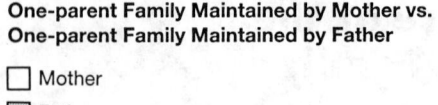

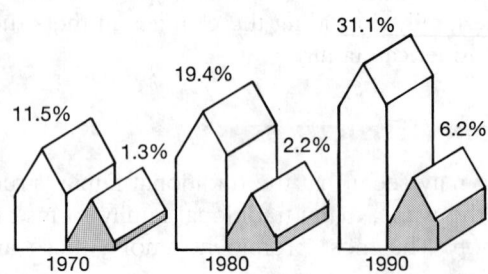

One-parent Family Maintained by Mother vs.
One-parent Family Maintained by Father

FIGURE 3–5 The changing American family.

child support payments, the economic situation is often grim. Even in today's "enlightened" society, mothers are still awarded custody of the children in more than 90% of all divorces and must bear most of the financial burden of childbearing and household management, regardless of whether the husband contributes financially (Glick, 1988). Child support and alimony supplements are often inadequate to keep the divorced mother and her children from a poverty subsistence level. Unfortunately, society still tends to view many single-parent families as deviant and pathologic, especially when headed by a woman in stringent economic circumstances. Rather than looking for ways to assist these families and assessing their strengths, health professionals in particular often view them negatively and emphasize their alleged weaknesses. This has led to biased governmental, employment, and social policies that have been detrimental to these families. To make matters worse, many separated and divorced women have incorporated these negative images into their self-concepts. Thus, they have another obstacle to overcome in their readjustment to new circumstances (Bank et al., 1993).

Several types of personal and community supports are available to single mothers. These women should be given a variety of options because of their different support needs. Most importantly, a mother must enlarge her social-support networks if she is to become economically independent and socially involved. Box 3-2 illustrates some of these supports.

Single-Father Households. Myer et al. (1993) maintain that although father-only families still constitute a small fraction of all families with children (4%), the percentage of these types of families has been increasing dramatically. Between 1960 and 1990, the number of father-only families has increased by almost 300%,

compared with a 200% increase in mother-only families.

Father-headed households include group living arrangements and living alone with the child. Because the man's economic status is generally better than the woman's, he has more options for child care and living quarters. Thus, caretakers in the home are found more frequently, although ample use is made of child care centers and children's programs (Pruett, 1993). Parents should take special care when choosing day care facilities to ensure the safety and well-being of their children (see Client Education).

The beginning of the breakdown in parental roles has begun to have some effect on custodial outcomes. Hence, after divorce, more fathers are now requesting and getting joint and sole custody of their children. In Gersick's (1979) pioneering study of fathers and custody,

---

BOX 3–2
Resources for Single Parents

- Group living homes—individual apartments per family or communal residences where food preparation, child care, and general living quarters are shared. Sleeping arrangements are private. These are useful first residences, particularly for people with little or no economic resources. Advantages include peer-group interaction for the children, shared child care responsibilities, and lower cost.
- Community and organizational support—programs that facilitate the parent's return to school or work and have community-sponsored child care facilities. Community support groups, such as Parents Without Partners, the Momma League, or La Leche League, can help women, in particular, build stronger personal social networks.

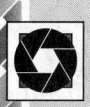

CLIENT EDUCATION
Questions to Consider When Selecting a Day Care Center

- *What are the educational and training backgrounds of staff?*
- *What is the child-staff ratio for each age group?* Recommended: no more than 4:1 for infants; 5:1 for 18 months to 2 years; 8:1 for 2 to 3 years; 10:1 for 3 to 4 years; and 15:1 for 5 to 6 years.
- *What are the disciplinary policies and procedures?*
- *May the parents visit any time?*
- *Are the facilities clean and well cared for?*
- *Are safety precautions observed? What are the procedures for reporting accidents and notifying parents?*
- *Are staff members careful about their own and the children's hygiene?* It is important to wash hands between diaper changes to avoid cross-contamination; changing tables should be kept clean.
- *Are facilities and staff for caring for sick children available?*
- *Is there adequate indoor and outdoor play space for the children?*
- *Do the children look happy and cared for?*

four interacting variables appear to determine whether fathers consider assuming custody of their children:

- The father's own family relationships: Many want to overcome, in their relationships with their children, the problems and emotional detachment they experienced with their parents.
- Feelings toward the ex-wife: When the father believes that the wife has betrayed him in some way, he is motivated to seek custody by a combination of a desire to punish his wife and a concern for the well-being of the children.
- The wife's pretrial consent: A court battle was not necessary, and the father could assume custody with a minimum of conflict.
- The attorney's attitudes: If the attorney is reluctant to press for custody, the father tends to let the wife have the children.

Although Greif (1985a) did not examine the determinants of seeking custody, he did find that the fathers in his study who wanted custody "very much" felt they shared in the marital breakup; were better prepared for assuming custody, having participated a great deal in rearing the children and doing household chores; and were generally more satisfied with their relationship with their children. Greif notes, however, that most of the custodial fathers "ended their marriages in an uncomfortable state."

As with the voluntary single-male parent, research indicates that divorced fathers generally have sufficient material resources to provide at least an adequate lifestyle for their children (Meyer et al., 1993). Research shows that many of the difficulties that men experience are the same as those of the single-parent women. Economic circumstances become more stringent (but not as dire as for women), and arranging child care becomes a problem. In Greif's study, visits from the wife were anticipated with anxiety, and for many of the men, the strain of the divorce coupled with the new demands of total responsibility for the children made readjustment to the single lifestyle difficult. However, none of the fathers studied regretted their decision to assume custody of their children (Grief, l985a; l985b; Meyer et al., l993; Feetham et al., l993).

The student is referred to *Fatherhood U.S.A.* in the Suggested Readings list for excellent resources for the single parent, particularly the father.

Evolving Family Structures

The creation of a communal alternative to the nuclear family is not new in this country. Communes of the past varied according to the cause of their members' dissent and their organizational structure. Some were based on religious conviction, some on economic idealism, and some on rebellion against authority.

Communal Living Groups

Today, communes remain varied in terms of membership type, organizational structure, general purpose, and size, which varies from less than 12 people to hundreds of people. A significant number of communes are based on religious commitment, common interests, or a unifying goal. Eastern philosophy is often a guiding force in many. In others, the "Jesus movement" is central, with a search for a new way to live out the traditional Judeo-Christian convictions (Thornton, l989). The following are the most frequently seen communal arrangements:

- Several monogamous couples with children share a single household: Common facilities are shared and socialization of the children is a common responsibility.
- Several nonmonogamous couples with children share a household: Individuals are "married" to each other, and all parent the children. A charismatic leader is often present, and a status system exists. Cultism is often involved.
- Unmarried parent and child live together: A voluntary situation where marriage for the mother is not desirable or possible. Children are natural or adopted.

■ Unmarried couple and child live together: A *social contract* situation exists with an ideologic commitment to a union not sanctioned by law. Parents are committed to their relationship, and the father is heavily involved in parenting. Another situation involves a *common law* union with possible problems or constraints associated with legal marriage. Children may be born to the partners or informally adopted.

Functions of the Modern Family

It has been said that the modern family has lost many of its former socialization functions. Protective services are now provided by law enforcement, the fire department, child protective services, and the like. Education and religious training are now entrusted to schools and churches. Even the production, preservation, and preparation of food have become largely the domain of industry. Duvall and Miller (1990) state that at least six basic functions are left to the family: *Generating Affection, Ensuring Continuity of Companionship, Providing Personal Security and Acceptance, Giving Satisfaction and a Sense of Purpose, Providing Social Placement and Socialization,* and *Inculcating Controls and a Sense of What Is Right.* These functions, described in detail in Box 3-3, are crucial for producing competent persons who must survive in a complex, ever-changing world.

It is no wonder that those who are concerned with the "decline" of the family also are concerned with the loss of family functions. The kinds of rewards and punishments that the child experiences influence his or her sense of right and wrong, and these carry into adulthood as moral values. Thus, the family becomes the primary source of transmitting human values that radiate into the society as a whole.

BOX 3–3
Functions of the Modern Family

Generating Affection

This is a phenomenon that occurs between all members of the unit, as well as among members of the different generations. Love is generated through family living. In western societies, couples generally marry for love and have children as an expression of that love. In the ideal situation, both parents and children grow in a climate of mutual affection that contributes to a healthy development of all concerned. In actuality, we know that the ideal is often not achieved.

Ensuring Continuity of Companionship

In today's highly mobile world, often only family associations endure. One's friends, colleagues, neighbors, and acquaintances enter and leave one's social network; jobs change, neighborhoods expand and contract, and social mobility continues. The family unit provides a continuing presence of sympathetic companions who encourage family members to share both disappointments and successes.

Providing Personal Security and Acceptance

Most persons look to their family for the security and acceptance they need to make their lives dignified and worthwhile. It is within the family's protective security that the members can make mistakes, learn from them, and form complementary rather than competitive relationships. These relationships allow the members to develop naturally and at their own pace.

Giving Satisfaction and a Sense of Purpose

The family, at its best, can give its members a basic sense of satisfaction and worth that the other arenas in a person's life often do not fulfill. Family rituals, celebrations, gatherings, and the like serve to act as cohesive factors to dilute the frustrations and problems found in the larger society.

Providing Social Placement and Socialization

Every society demands that individuals learn what is expected of them and where they fit in the larger social hierarchy. At birth, the child automatically acquires a rich heritage by virtue of his or her family's attributes and position in society, including such things as genetic, physical, national, ethnic, cultural, economic, political, religious, and educational attributes. The individual will change some of these over time; others remain immutable. Families also act as the transmitter of their personal as well as societal values, goals, and sentiments to the child. Thus, the child becomes socialized to the expectations of both the family and society.

Inculcating Controls and a Sense of What Is Right

Within the family unit, the child first learns the rules, obligations, responsibilities, rights, and privileges of the larger society to which he or she belongs. In the socialization process, family members criticize, correct, order, praise, blame, coerce, entice, reward, and punish in ways that would be unthinkable elsewhere. In this way, the family becomes the agent of the larger society. If it fails to perform its socialization tasks adequately, the goals of the larger society may not be attained. It is no wonder that those who are concerned with the "decline" of the family also are concerned with the loss of family functions.

Theoretical Approaches to the Study of the Family

In an attempt to study systematically and delineate patterns of interaction in the family, scholars of the family, both psychologists and sociologists, have developed several interpretive approaches to variations in family life. Each approach generates a unique understanding about family organization, while emphasizing a different aspect. These variations in emphasis result in slightly modified definitions of the family in each approach.

In the early 1960s, Hill and Hanson (1960) wrote an original article describing the five major conceptual frameworks then in existence for family study. It remains a source for family scholars. Recent analyses of the use of these frameworks indicate that the interactionist, systems, exchange, and developmental theories are the major theories in use today. These frameworks are summarized below to help the student understand the relationship between these important frameworks and practice (Gilliss et al., 1989; Friedman, 1992; Duvall et al., 1990; Whall et al., 1991).

Conceptual Frameworks in Family Study and Practice

- *The symbolic interaction approach* views the family as a unit of interacting personalities. Each person has a position in the family in which he or she perceives the norms or role expectations held by the other individuals (or by the family as a whole) as the basis for attitudes and behaviors. Individuals will define their role expectations primarily in light of their source and self-conception. The family is studied through analyzing the interactions and communication patterns of the role-playing members. The primary focus is on the internal structure of the family; this framework, however, neglects the family's relation to the community. The central theme is that actions, behaviors, and objects have a symbolic meaning and acquire shared meaning with time as a result of interaction between individuals; hence, socialization is a key concept, because it is the mechanism of transmitting values, goals, sentiments, and meaning to the family members.
- *Systems approaches* are used across various disciplines, including the natural and social sciences and engineering. The family is viewed as an open system composed of interdependent subsystems that work toward common goals. Systems theory emphasizes sets of objects, their relationships, and their boundaries; the system as a whole experiences inputs and outputs from its own subsystems and from society as a whole and responds to feedback with control mechanisms. Family assessment depends on analysis of the interdependent parts, communication patterns, and the family's adaptation patterns.
- The *exchange approach*, although relatively new, is gaining in popularity. This perspective holds that all human interactions, including those in the family, can be viewed as social "exchanges." Individuals weigh rewards and costs in their interactions, and if the exchange is perceived as unequal, one person will be at a disadvantage, and the other will control the relationship. The goal is to minimize costs and maximize rewards. Important concepts in this approach are rewards, costs, profits, and a normative context of reciprocity and equity. The ability to choose is central to this formulation. Although no analysis has been done, some authors say that this approach has relevance at institutional and individual levels. To date, only family assessment has been at the interpersonal level of analysis.
- The *developmental approach* focuses on the family as it evolves. It holds that families have a predictable life cycle with changing developmental tasks and role expectations associated with each phase of the cycle. Family assessment is based on analysis of task fulfillment at each stage, with consideration given to physical and emotional maturation, the development of personality and values, and the impact of social and cultural factors. It is an eclectic approach in that it borrows concepts from many disciplines. For instance, sociology contributes the concepts of social class, social change, cultural influences, and the generational sweep of the life cycle; psychology contributes learning theory concepts and interaction processes; and home economics contributes the themes of home management, housing, and family practices.

Any of these frameworks can be used, depending on the problem under study. These frameworks are helpful tools and are not to be considered "right" or "wrong." When choosing a framework, an individual must consider the assumptions he or she makes about human behavior, how he or she views people in relation to the environment, and the problem that he or she is trying to solve. Only one framework should be used for any one problem under study—when frameworks are mixed, the assumptions underlying each framework tend to become confused, and the conclusions will be deceptive.

Symbolic Interaction Approach

One of the most useful of the previous frameworks for those who must deal with the family as a unit is the interactional framework. This conceptual scheme provides a system for viewing the personal relationships between the man and woman and between parents and children and for viewing the impact of various health conditions on the family unit. The family is viewed as a unit of interacting personalities and as a living, changing, growing thing. This conceptualization does not view the family in a legalistic way or in a family contract sense, but as it exists by virtue of the interaction of its members. Thus, a single parent with a child is a family unit, as is an unmarried couple with or without children.

Within the family, each member occupies a position or positions to which a number of roles are assigned or allocated. Through socialization and role differentiation (structuring a role), the individual perceives certain norms (rules) or role expectations that the other members of the family have set for his or her behavior in role performance. The responses of the others in the family reinforce or challenge this conception that the individual is developing. Thus, people define their role expectations in a situation in terms of a reference group (others who are important to them) and by means of their own self-concept.

Implicit in this formulation is the fact that humans interpret or define one another's actions instead of merely reacting to them. For instance, a woman does not respond to her mate merely on the basis of his actions; it also depends on the meaning that both partners attach to such actions. Thus, the family members act and react by using symbols. The key concept involved in the use of symbols is communication.

Interpersonal relations based on communication among family members is one of the major distinguishing aspects of the interactional approach. The emphasis in this framework is on the development of competence in interpersonal relations, and as such, it describes a process rather than a state (Gilliss et al., 1989; Friedman, 1992; Feetham et al., 1993).

Family Interaction and Stress

Several problems for investigation have grown out of these concerns and emphases on family unity, communication, and interpersonal competence. The one that is particularly important for health practitioners is the study of discontinuities in family life, particularly family crises or stresses. This includes the impact of the reproductive process and parenthood on the family, stress created by acute or chronic illness of various family members at any time during the life cycle, and the crisis brought about by death of a family member, particularly during the reproductive years.

Using a family interaction perspective, the nurse can look inside the family group, observe interaction among members, and analyze how the family is coping. Each family member, therefore, can be viewed as a developing member in a changing group. This approach can be particularly useful to the helping professions not only because it provides a practical way of assessing the family, but also because it allows the professional to isolate and specify the potential sources of difficulty as family members relate to one another and to their society (Gilliss et al., 1989; Friedman, 1992; Whall et al., 1991).

Role Theory and Implications for Nursing Practice

As a background for understanding the family, another concept permeates lay and professional language today. That concept is role, and it is an integral part of the structure and function of the family.

As with the concept of family, people have an intuitive sense of what a "role" is, but when systematically studying the concept, a broad latitude in definitions and understandings of it exists. Personality develops within a social system, which in American culture is the family. Roles, which are crucial to personality development, may be viewed from a psychosocial viewpoint, which focuses on the individual and how he or she integrates role relationships, and from a sociologic viewpoint, which focuses on group or social relationships, primarily those within the family. The self can be viewed as a unit of personality, a person's status, position in a unit of society, or a role enacted in the culture (Eishelman, 1990; Gilliss et al., 1989; Feetham et al., 1993).

Roles and Status

It is important to distinguish between the terms "role" and "status." **Status,** or position, generally refers to a person's location in a system of interaction. On the other hand, **role** applies to behavior that reflects the goals, values, and sentiments operating in a certain situation.

From an interactionist frame of reference, role is more than a series of "dos" and "don'ts" (the structuralist position) for the behavior expected of a person occupying a position. Rather, it is a collection of behaviors that emerges from interactions between the self and others that constitute a meaningful unit and an expression of the values, goals, or sentiments that provide direction for that interaction. These collections of behaviors become patterned with time, and the actors proceed as if there were prescriptions for performance (Friedman, 1992). The interactionist interpretation allows for innovative, individualistic designing of a person's role performance on the basis of assigning some sentiment or goal to the behavior of relevant others.

This conception of role is particularly important for nursing practice because it allows for a broader interpretation of the behavior of all actors than do more traditional concepts. Moreover, it does not prescribe the interpretation of the behavior or the nurse's response to the behavior. Hence, it permits creativity and innovation in interaction with clients.

Role Socialization and Role Models

Roles are learned through the process of **socialization.** As stated previously, individuals learn the ways of social groups so that they can function within these groups. Socialization takes place through intentional and incidental instruction. Specific instruction regarding a certain facet of behavior is given, and examples of desired behavior are provided. This is called role modeling. Various socialization agencies, the family in the beginning and later the church and schools, teach the child certain role behaviors through intentional programs of learning and study. Operating conjointly may be incidental learning in which the child adopts the ways of others through play acting, peer group relations, and observations of adult and peer role models.

Thus, significant people in the child's world teach him or her by defining the world and by serving as **models** for attitudes and behavior. The child learns through a system of rewards and punishment. If the child behaves as the significant others desire, he or she receives positive attention and invitations to continue participation and interaction. If the child behaves otherwise, he or she is refused attention, reprimanded, or punished.

Much of the role learning that takes place in the family is indirect. The child learns by observing and participating in the interpersonal relationship patterns established by the family, the examples set by the other family members, and the role that the child develops within the family. As a result, the child learns and adopts basic role skills from family members and concurrently adapts to the roles of the other family members (Gilliss et al., 1989; Eshelman, 1990; Feetham et al., 1993).

There are many techniques of socialization, and evidence indicates that no one technique is better than another. Rather, parents must choose and modify what is best for them. This will depend on the many factors to which we have referred previously.

Emotional Basis of Learning

Learning for adults and children is not merely a cognitive process. It is associated with multiple emotional or affective ties that the individual makes with others. These attachments begin with the mother and gradu-

RESEARCH HIGHLIGHT

How Publications Transmit Current Knowledge of Child Development

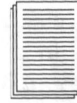 Magazines that give advice to parents about infant care are full of information from experts. Two widely read publications were studied to find out how they transmit current knowledge about child development.

Articles from 1955 through 1984 were reviewed and categorized by topic. Topical content analysis found that 53% of the articles dealt with daily infant care and common childhood illnesses, whereas 47% addressed and provided advice in child development. Themes included mother-infant attachment, day care for working mothers, fathers, breast versus bottle-feeding, infant cognition, temperament, and language development. Excluding articles on infant language, Young found that articles on child development accurately revealed the most current knowledge. However, advice given in the articles more often reflected social norms rather than research findings. These results render concrete evidence on the strengths and weaknesses of these publications for new parents.

Critique: This article reflects a well-designed and rigorous content analysis of publications that are frequently read by parents. The length of time the articles were reviewed, 1954 to 1984, strengthens the analysis. The authors are careful with their interpretations and do not overreach in their conclusions.

Nurses who typically distribute publications to assist in teaching parents about child care should be aware of the bias of these articles and carefully screen the written materials to ascertain the philosophy being presented. By selecting materials that agree with the clinician's philosophy, the nurse can avoid giving conflicting advice. Parents also would benefit from being taught how to evaluate critically the infant-care publications that they may read.

Young, K. (1990). American conceptions of infant development from 1955 to 1984: What the experts are telling parents. *Child Development, 61,* 17–28.

ally include increasing numbers of people with whom the child interacts and comes to identify. As these attachments grow, children develop a sense of self. They can take a position from the outside and view their own thoughts, feelings, and actions. In this way, the expected behavior is gradually internalized as they figuratively stand back and look at themselves. Children judge, reflect on, and guide their own behavior according to their perception of others' expectations for their behavior.

Although individuals learn role behavior in much the same way, there are differences in respective role performances. This differential role performance may be due to differences in the ways people respond in interpersonal situations, their knowledge of the role in general, their motivation to perform specific roles, their attitude toward themselves, and their response to the behavior of other people in the interaction (Gilliss et al., 1989; Quimby, 1994). Tension and discontinuities in role relations also must be considered when considering the concept of role. Many terms have been used to illustrate the idea of tension or interruptions in a smooth process of interaction. Terms such as *role conflict, role strain, role change,* and *role transition* have been used to convey the various aspects of tension that can occur in a role system.

As stated previously, role interaction is dynamic. When theories of the development of human nature change, so do socialization patterns. As socialization patterns change, variant family life systems evolve that redefine reciprocal role relationships. Tensions and disruptions in smooth and rewarding role interaction may occur at any point (Friedman, 1992). The major determinants of the degree of adjustment a person makes to a role are summarized in Box 3-4. When there is a high degree of adjustment, the enactment of a person's set of roles can be rewarding in that they define a self-concept anchor and a sense of belongingness and purpose. They provide social recognition and support, which allow individuals to buy or earn desired conditions or things in the world and to view themselves as worthwhile, contributing members of society (Friedman, 1990).

Social Power in the Family

As roles become differentiated (structured) and allocated (who gets what role), the element of social power comes into play. Various authors have defined this dynamic concept as the ability to influence a decision, influence the emotions and behavior of others, or

---

BOX 3–4
Determinants of Role Adjustment

- The clarity with which a specific role and its complementarity are defined and demonstrated
- The clarity or definiteness of the transitional procedures in the acquisition of a new role
- How well the role is learned and enacted; partly dependent on the first two determinants and the strength of the socialization process to the new role
- The consistency of the responses a role evokes
- A role's compatibility with the other roles in the person's set of roles
- A role's congruity with the emotional needs of the person
- The degree of complementarity that exists between reciprocal roles
- The bases and use of social power in the family

BOX 3–5
Bases of Social Power

- *Legitimate power.* The shared belief that one person in the family system has the right to make decisions for others in the system. The basis for such power is traditional; thus, parents exert legitimate power over their children. In some families, it is the father's traditional prerogative to make most of the decisions. When role relationships are egalitarian, legitimate power is a more shared phenomenon.
- *Expert power.* The perception that a family member or group has particular knowledge or skills. Thus, nurses are often seen by their clients as having expert knowledge to effect a change in behavior.
- *Referent power.* The influence of one person over another. This occurs through positive identification with the more powerful person, and one person adopts the behaviors, values, and attitudes of the powerful person. Role modeling is an example.
- *Reward power.* The expectation that the person has the resources to reward others. Parents are invested with this type of power. The hierarchical structure of nursing also carries this power.
- *Coercive power.* The expectation that punishment will occur if certain things are done or not done, certain behavior is exhibited or not exhibited, or certain expectations are met or not met. Examples include abuse in the family or denying a child access to school if not immunized.
- *Informational power.* Conveying a message that change is necessary. The media is an example. Families use this power when providing instruction to the members; often used in conjunction with expert power.

---

achieve intended outcomes or goals. Decision making is one indicator of social power or dominance in the family. Several bases of power have been delineated (Box 3-5). Families tend to use one type of power predominantly, although each may be used at different times, and several may be used simultaneously.

Decision making reflects how the family meets its members' needs, including health needs. In addition, it has implications for family cohesiveness (Gilliss et al., 1989; Feetham et al., 1993; Friedman, 1992). Several areas can be assessed to give the nurse vital information in this area (see Assessment Guidelines).

Aspects of the Nurse's Role

A discussion of the client's role would not be complete without a reference to the complementary nurse's role. As with any role, multiple facets or aspects must be considered (Fig. 3-6).

First, the nurse is a *practitioner*—the nursing process is used to assess, prescribe, and implement nursing regimens for clients and to assist the physician in im-

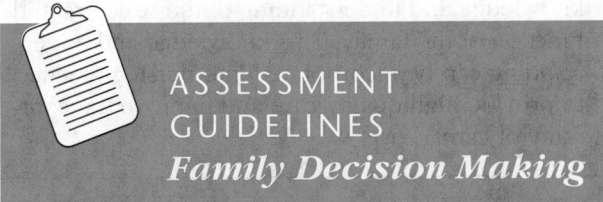

ASSESSMENT GUIDELINES
Family Decision Making

The following are several questions for the nurse to keep in mind as family decision making is assessed:

- Who usually instigates a decision-making process?
- Who decides who will be involved in the decision?
- Who actually is involved, and how did this come about?
- What processes are used in making decisions? For instance, are control, negotiation, persuasion, or authoritativeness modes used, and how frequently?
- Who seems to exert the most power during decision making?
- Who makes the final decision?
- How is it implemented?
- What is the significance of the decision for the family, and what are the effects on family interaction?

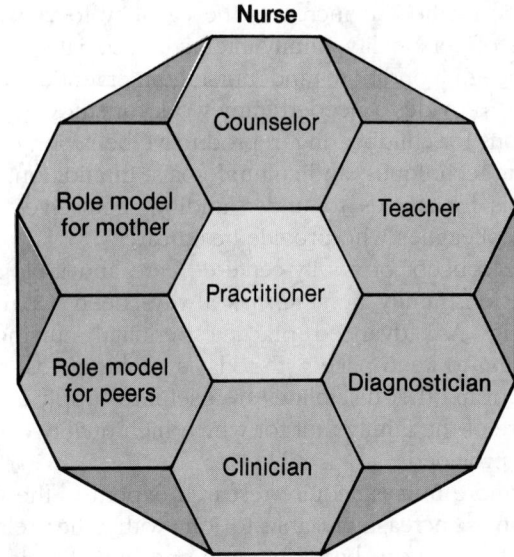

FIGURE 3–6 Maternity nursing is a multifaceted role.

plementing the medical regimen for these clients. The nurse's role also includes being a *role model*. Maternity and perinatal nurses and community health nurses commonly are role models for new mothers who are inexperienced or who exhibit maladaptive behavior in childrearing and child care. In a sense, the nurse acts as a surrogate mother by meeting the dependency needs of the young mother, thus allowing her to devote time and effort to mothering her own children. The nurse also may be a role model for peers and other professional colleagues by demonstrating an interest in high quality care while initiating newcomers into the institutional or agency routines and practices.

An additional aspect of the nurse's roles is that of *teacher and counselor*. Nurses are becoming increasingly involved in all levels of parent education to socialize groups of parents efficiently. The role of counselor is often required, particularly with family planning, child health services, and abortion and genetic counseling.

Finally, in the *advanced practice role,* the nurse also may provide physical diagnosis and clinician skills. In many instances, nurses working in an ambulatory care setting provide the link between the family in the community and acute care institutions to which they must go occasionally for more severe conditions.

The potential for developing these multiple facets of the nursing role is unlimited and will be fully realized only when nursing recognizes its own unique, independent contribution to healthcare.

When delivering care to individuals and families, nurses will observe and analyze the role behaviors of all people involved, including their own. They will analyze various dimensions of the roles, behaviors, values, expectations, and attitudes of the actors and their underlying motivations and emotions. Role conflict and perceptions of inadequacy in role performance have the potential to undermine emotional and physical well-being in the client and the nurse. In contrast, satisfactory role performance enhances self-concept and can promote growth and emotional well-being.

Relationship of Family Theory to Nursing Practice

The structure and function of the family help determine their use of health services. As discussed previously, all members of the healthcare team need to be aware of the variety of theories regarding human behavior and how families develop their various patterns of behavior. This necessitates using knowledge from other specific disciplines when appropriate.

In addition, an understanding of the populations that will be served gives some anchorage to nursing's therapeutic method. It increases the capacity to view the forces of personality, family interaction, social systems, the health condition, and nursing intervention as a unit. It provides a needed framework for studying motivations for childbearing, reproductive behavior, child-rearing techniques, and cultural goals. In addition, it is a basis for nurses to understanding themselves and their colleagues who provide healthcare.

The concept of family-centered care and its logical extension, family nursing, has always been a part of nursing. As advanced practice perinatal nursing is evolving to keep pace with today's health needs, concepts from other disciplines are useful to supply a total picture of the family unit for which high quality care is to be provided.

As more nurses acquire research expertise, the profession is increasingly able to join with other related disciplines whose basic interests and expertise in the family may some day ensure team approaches to research in clinical matters, multidisciplinary educational programs, and most important, family care.

Summary Points

✔ The family remains the basic unit of society. In today's rapidly changing world, many cultural and societal changes are impacting the family. These changes are resulting in dramatic changes in the traditional structure and function of the family. New family forms are evolving, being tested and retained or discarded.

✔ Some students of the family are fearful that the nontraditional structures that are evolving are not suitable for the appropriate socialization of children or the support and mentoring of the adult members. Moreover, there is additional concern that the functions of the family (ie, socializing child and adult members, generating affection, ensuring continuity in companionship, providing personal security and acceptance, giving satisfaction and a sense of purpose to members, providing social placement, and inculcating controls and a sense of what is right) are being stripped away from the family unit and not being adequately assumed by other institutions.

✔ Other researchers hold a more optimistic view, concluding that the "decline in the family" is almost finished and that the experimentation with alternate family forms and functions has resulted in a unit that is more adequately prepared to cope with society's changes. The "national family wars" controversy continues to rage, however.

✔ A variety of theoretical perspectives regarding family study are available to nurses to improve their

knowledge and understanding of the structure and function of the family. This knowledge and understanding can be incorporated into nursing practice to provide high quality care and improve the continuity of care.

REFERENCES

Antonovsky, A. (1987). *Unraveling the mystery of health: How people manage stress and stay well.* San Francisco: Jossey-Bass.

Bank, L., Forgatch, M. S., Patterson, G. R., & Fetrow, R. A. (1993). Parenting practices of single mothers: Mediators of negative contextual factors. *Journal of Marriage and the Family, 55*(2), 371–384.

Cowan, N. D. (1993). The sky is falling, but Popenoe's analysis won't help us do anything about it. *Journal of Marriage and the Family, 55*(3), 548–552.

DeMaris, A., & MacDonald, W. (1993). Premarital cohabitation and marital instability: A test of the unconventionality hypothesis. *Journal of Marriage and the Family, 55*(3), 399–407.

Duvall, E. M., & Miller, B. C. (1990). *Marriage and family development.* New York: Harper & Row.

Eshelman, J. R., & Cashion, B. G. (1990). Sociology: An introduction. Boston: Little, Brown.

Feetham, S. L., Meister, S. B., Bell, J. M., & Gilliss, C. L. (Eds.) (1993). *The nursing of families: Theory/research/education/practice.* Newbury Park, CA: Sage Publications.

Friedman, M. M. (1992). *Family nursing: Theory and practice* (3rd ed.). Norwalk, CT: Appleton & Lange.

Gersick, K. E. (1979). Fathers by choice: Divorced men who received custody of their children. In G. Levinger, O. C. Moles (Eds.), *Divorce and separation: Context, causes and consequences* (pp. 303–323). New York: Basic Books.

Gilliss, C. L., Highley, B. L., Roberts, B. M., & Martinson, I. M. (1989). *Toward a science of family nursing.* New York: Addison-Wesley.

Glenn, N. D. (1993). A plea for objective assessment of the notion of family decline. *Journal of Marriage and the Family, 55*(3), 542–544.

Glenn, N. D. (1991). The recent trend in marital success in the United States. *Journal of Marriage and the Family, 53*(3), 261–270.

Glick, P. C. (1988). Fifty years of family demography: A record of social change. *Journal of Marriage and the Family, 50*(4), 861–873.

Greif, G. L. (1985a). Single fathers rearing children. *Journal of Marriage and the Family, 47*(1), 185–191.

Greif, G. L. (1985b). *Single fathers.* Lexington, MA: Lexington Books.

Grief, G. (1987). A longitudinal examination of single custodial fathers: Implications for treatment. *The American Journal of Family Therapy, 15*(3), 253–260.

Grief, G. (1990). *The daddy track and the single father.* Lexington, MA: Lexington Books.

Hill, R., & Hanson D. A. (1960). The identification of conceptual frameworks utilized in family study. *Marriage and Family Living, 22*(4), 308–320.

Myer, D. R., & Garasky, S. (1993). Custodial fathers: Myths, realities, and child support policy. *Journal of Marriage and the Family, 55*(1), 73–89.

Popenoe, D. (1993a). American family decline: 1960-1990. *Journal of Marriage and the Family, 55*(3), 527–541.

Popenoe, D. (1993b). The national family wars. *Journal of Marriage and the Family, 55*(3), 553–556.

Pruett, K. D. (1993). The paternal presence. *Families in Society, 71*(1), 46–51.

Quimby, C. H. (1994). Women and the family of the future. *Journal of Obstetric, Gynecologic, and Neonatal Nursing, 23*(3), 113–121.

(1990). The 21st century family [Special issue]. *Newsweek, Winter/Spring,* 3–108.

Thornton, A. (1989). Changing attitudes toward family issues in the United States. *Journal of Marriage and the Family, 51,* 873–893.

U.S. Bureau of the Census (1994). *Household and family characteristics: March 1994. Current Population Reports Series* (No 428). Washington, DC: Department of Commerce.

Whall, A. L., & Fawcett, J. (1991). *Family theory development in nursing: State of the science and art.* Philadelphia: F.A. Davis.

SUGGESTED READINGS

Carlson, G. E. (1993). When grandmothers take care of their grandchildren. *MCN: American Journal of Maternal Child Nursing, 18*(4), 206–207

Collins, C., & Tiedje, L. B. (1987). A program for women returning to work after childbirth. *Journal of Obstetric, Gynecologic, and Neonatal Nursing, 17*(4), 246–253.

DeJoseph, J. F. (1994). Redefining women's work during pregnancy: Toward a more comprehensive approach. *Birth, 20*(2), 86–93.

Klinman, D. G., & Kohl R. (1984). *Fatherhood USA.* New York: Garland Publishing.

Quimby, C. H. (1994). Women and the family of the future. *Journal of Obstetric, Gynecologic, and Neonatal Nursing, 23*(3), 113–123.

4

Sociocultural Considerations

Objectives

- Identify the sociocultural factors that influence motivations for childbearing and the use of health services.
- Discuss the current societal trends affecting childbearing motivations and the impact these trends have on maternity and perinatal services.
- Relate the influence that ethnicity and cultural belief systems have on the childbearing cycle.
- Explain the influence of sociodemographic, social, and behavioral risk factors on reproductive outcomes.
- Discuss the changing relationships between clients and providers and basic principles regarding nursing care of today's families.

Social and Cultural Meaning of Childbearing

As discussed in Chapter 1, pregnancy needs to be considered in terms of the social context in which it occurs, namely, the family and the larger society. Pregnancy and childbearing generally have different meanings in various societies and even within any given society, depending on a person's position in society and socioeconomic status.

Childbearing Motivations

No biologic event has greater significance for society than reproduction and its outcome. It is important in family and population dynamics and therefore has a

Values, roles that shape a person's attitudes, beliefs, and behaviors, are formed and conditioned by social groups formed in early childhood. Consequently, there are different orientations to health and healthcare, reflecting memberships in differing ethnic, racial, religious, and social class groups. These varying health orientations become manifest in the behavior of individuals and in the institutions that are organized to deliver health services.

In recent years, there has been a heightened awareness of the importance of social and cultural factors in health status, specifically maternity care. Although Americans are accustomed to thinking of their health status as being the best in the world, their healthcare is still far short of its potential. Large segments of the population either do not have access to adequate medical care or are deprived of quality care in the services that they do receive. There has been a great stimulus to improve the prenatal care system to improve reproductive outcomes. There has been some expansion and elaboration of the existing system of maternity and perinatal services. Whether this will have the desired effects depends on a variety of factors, which are discussed in Chapter 1.

This chapter focuses on the forces in society that influence the field of maternity and perinatal services and reproductive outcomes. The social and cultural meanings of pregnancy, including the current social, cultural, and economic forces that influence motivations for childbearing, are examined. Some of the critical issues in the use of maternity services, including the influence of race and **ethnicity** on health beliefs, the use of healthcare services, and the risks factors associated with reproductive outcomes, are discussed. Implications of these variables for nursing also are discussed.

BOX 4–1
Belief Systems Surrounding Childbearing

Antepartum

Who may have a child?

At what age?

By whom may one have a child?

How many children can one have?

Can one space pregnancies?

What should be the behavior during pregnancy?

Are there restrictions on the father?

Are there any restrictions on sexual activity?

Who may see and touch certain body parts?

How is a fetus formed?

What are the beliefs regarding conception?

Intrapartum

What causes labor?

How does one behave during labor?

How should one respond to pain?

Should one take medication?

Where should labor take place?

Postpartum

What general behavior is expected?

What behavior is expected of the father and others?

Are there restrictions on food or activity?

Care of the Newborn

When is he or she recognized?

What are the rules for his or her care?

Who cares for him or her?

(Adapted from Kavanagh, K. H., & Kennedy, P. H. [1992]. Promoting cultural diversity: Strategies for health care professionals. Newbury Park: Sage Publications.)

heavy impact on individual and national welfare. Women begin their preparation for childbearing early in life. From birth, women are affected by the cultural values of their family, which influence how they see themselves and their approach to situations, such as healthcare.

As mentioned previously, society is organized primarily for families with children, and the argument for having children can be very persuasive. Even in this era of voluntary childbearing, couples without children can still be made to feel "out of place." Research has indicated that the value of having children remains generally accepted by the majority of Americans (Feetham et al., 1993; Whall et al., 1991; Friedman, 1992). Theoretically, the availability of contraceptive methods should permit childbearing to result from motivated human action rather than mere biologic happenstance. However, when pregnancies occur, whether they were planned, the number of children that a couple has, and the time at which they have

them are a function of the couple's childbearing motivations to a large extent. These, in turn, are influenced by **culture,** the system of goals, beliefs, attitudes, and roles shared by a group of people. The questions listed in Box 4-1 focus on culturally important areas the nurse can assess to help plan interventions for clients.

Present Societal Trends Affecting Childbearing Motivations

Fertility Control. Improvement in the number and reliability of contraceptive methods has resulted in a more effective means of fertility control. Previously, women could not confidently plan the prevention of unwanted pregnancies. Thus, the role expectations of women were structured around motherhood and became rationalizations for the inevitable (Patterson et al., 1990). The ability to control fertility has resulted in an apparent change in how decisions about childbearing are made. It has become a voluntary endeavor.

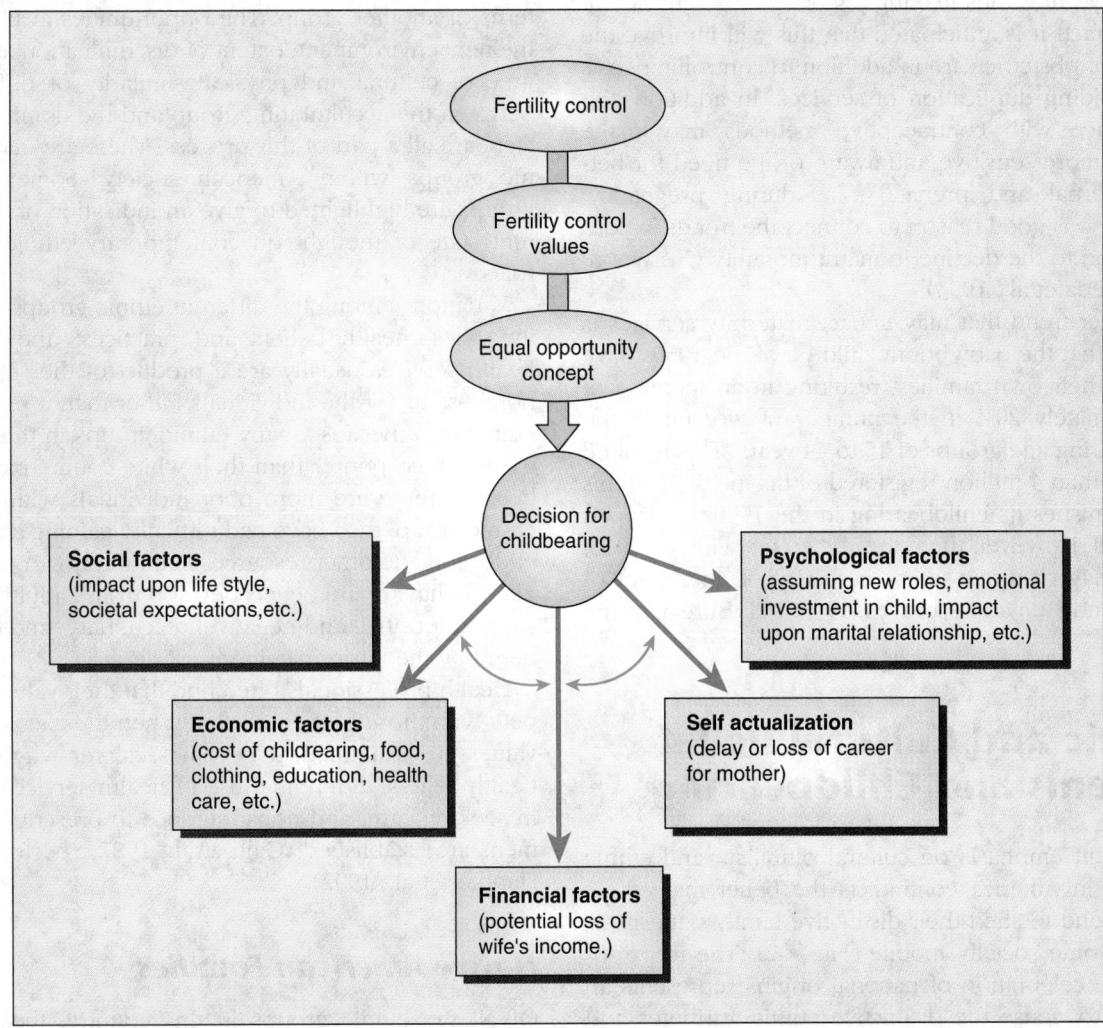

FIGURE 4–1 Fertility control has made childbearing a matter of choice. This illustration shows some of the factors that may be included in the decision for childbearing.

Competing Social Roles. The changes associated with contraception have given support to the equal opportunity concept by making nonfamilial roles a realistic and viable option for women. One of the consequences has been to place motherhood more directly in competition with alternative, socially desirable career roles. When there is choice for childbearing, emphasis is placed on planning. Factors that are considered include the direct social, psychological, and economic costs of having children; the financial factor, including the loss of the wife's earnings; and the need for self-actualization, including the intrinsic satisfaction with the mother's occupation and the effect of the delay or loss of the career (Fig. 4-1; Patterson et al., 1990).

Impact of Trends on Maternity Services

Societal trends also are affecting the delivery of maternity care. Some hospitals are closing or merging their maternity units, thus making regionalization an accomplished fact. It is anticipated that this will improve the quality of obstetric care in addition to controlling costs and avoiding duplication of services. In addition, the experience with contraceptive methods may make women more sensitive and aware of the need for better maternal and prenatal care during pregnancy. There also is good reason to connect the trends in contraception to the decline in infant mortality (Norwood, 1994; Freda et al., 1993).

Another trend that may impact maternity services is the fact that the baby boom children of the 1950s have formed their own families, resulting in an increase of approximately 20% in the number of women in the childbearing age groups of 15 to 44 years. This resulted in more than 4 million registered births in 1989. As this group finishes its childbearing in the 1990s, a drop is expected. However, there may be an upswing by 2010, which may continue to increase (U.S. Department of Health and Human Resources, 1993; U.S. Bureau of the Census).

Ethnic and Cultural Belief Systems and Childbearing

The recent emphasis on cultural pluralism and ethnic heritage in America contradicts the belief that ethnic groups tend to shed their distinctive family patterns as they become socially mobile (Fig. 4-2). The move toward the celebration of national origins represents an attempt to praise the distinctive ethnic attributes and artifacts to promote a positive identity and ancestral pride in those who have had little of either (see the Research Highlights).

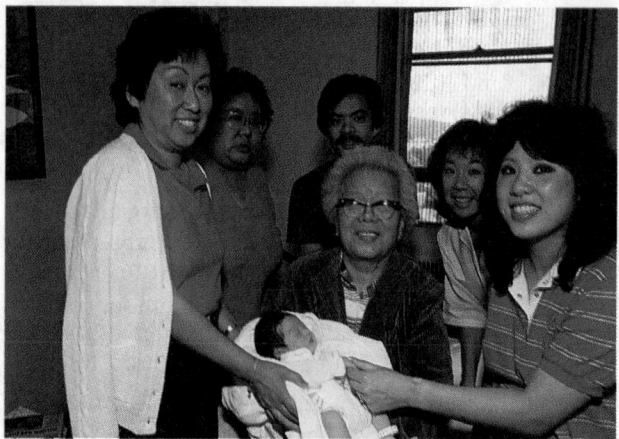

FIGURE 4–2 Families with rich ethnic and cultural heritages are a vital part of American society.

The contemporary family roles of various ethnic groups undergo a process called **acculturation,** which consists of adopting the cultural traits or social patterns of another group. The opportunities available in the new environment, extent of discrimination, and degree of cultural and physical similarity or difference between the acculturating group and the dominant society are all a part of this process. There are many ethnic groups within American society. Some of the groups are highlighted to give an indication of the current state of thought on contemporary ethnic family roles.

Variations among the different ethnic groups in family styles, health beliefs and practices, and use of health services usually are a product of the socioeconomic status of the individuals rather than a particular ethnic bias. Because many ethnic groups in this country are often poorer than their white counterparts and because there are more poor individuals within each ethnic group, they have had difficulty gaining access to education and other resources that money can provide. Their behavior and beliefs develop from a multitude of sources: positive and negative, reactionary, and engendered by the intrinsic culture.

Health professionals often find that their values compete with those of their clients. When the client's basic values are examined, it becomes clearer why certain health beliefs, differential use of health services, delay in seeking care, and nonadherence to prescribed regimens are established (Galli et al., 1987; Spector, 1991; Handler et al., 1992).

Native American Families

Of all the ethnic groups in this country, the Native American has perhaps the most remarkable history, which reflects severe exploitation, astounding endurance, and incredible capability for adaptation. The

RESEARCH HIGHLIGHT

Relationships Among Immigration, Ethnic Identity, and Faith

The relationships among immigration, ethnic identity, and health were investigated in people who emigrated from the Middle East to the United States. Immigrants from Egypt, Yemen, Iran, Armenia, and other Arab countries (Iraq, Syria, Palestine-Israel, and Lebanon) were interviewed to determine the relationship among ethnic group, strength of ethnic identity, and mental and physical health. Findings showed significant differences among the five groups on cultural attitudes, social attitudes, family orientation, the number of physical symptoms and psychological symptoms, perceived health status, and positive morale. There were more physical symptoms and less positive morale among those who perceived themselves to be more traditionally ethnic. Ethnic group accounted for a significant percentage of variance in positive morale and perceived health status. Ethnic identity accounted for a significant proportion of variance in physical symptoms. The author concludes that ethnic identity and country of origin should be considered when providing care for clients.

Critique: The study was well designed and timely, although the sample size was small. Eighty-eight subjects responded to a solicitation through Middle Eastern churches, cultural clubs, gatherings, and a "snowball" sampling technique of referral. There were 14 to 24 subjects in each ethnic group. Hence, generalizations cannot be made to all Middle Eastern clients. Because of the complexity of the health and ethnic identity constructs, the authors used multiple indicators of the variables, thus adding rigor to the design and data. The authors are careful not to overstep their findings. In the discussion, the authors outline the implications of the findings not only for the health practitioner, but also for researchers and policy makers. The article is well written and easy to follow.

Native American's history has been marred by disease, starvation, deliberate attempts at genocide, and blatantly inconsistent treatment by governmental agencies. Even today there is not a single accepted definition of Native American. Governmental agencies and the Census Bureau rely on individuals to identify themselves as Native American; some require proof of at least one-fourth Native American blood. It is clear that identification of the number of individuals and tribes is difficult (Lamarine, 1989; Spector, 1991; Bell, 1994).

It is estimated that approximately one-half of the Native American population lives on reservations whose development was a result of governmental policy of exclusion. Life on the reservation today is fraught with the twin plagues of poverty and substandard housing, which give rise to myriad health problems (Bell, 1994; Hsu et al., 1991; Spector, 1991).

An urban resettlement program attempted in 1952 was supposed to aid the assimilation of the Native American into the mainstream American culture. The program is generally regarded as a failure because of bureaucratic red tape, disinterest, and the inadequacy of financial and other aid (Lamarine, 1989; Boyle et al., 1989; Spector, 1991).

The cultural background of the Native American varies according to tribal affiliation. Thus, generalizations about the Native American family must be made with caution. In the main, family life is influenced by tribal beliefs. There is a great deal of variation among the tribes with respect to holding to traditional values and customs. The variability occurs in the reservation and urban Native American communities.

In spite of the fact that most Native American women deliver in hospitals, their maternal mortality rate is nearly 2% higher than the overall maternal mortality rate in the United States. This results from a variety of factors, including poverty, general health, nutrition, and social risk factors. Progress has been made in the last 3 decades with respect to childbearing, which has been marked by an 82% decline in infant mortality and an 89% decline in maternal mortality. Alcoholism, tuberculosis, other infectious diseases, and suicide remain the main killers of Native Americans (Bell, 1994; Hsu et al., 1991; Spector, 1991).

African American Families

One of the most significant factors affecting the family roles of the African American population of the United States and other groups from the Caribbean and West Indies has been the concentration of most of these families at income levels that are grossly inadequate. This has largely been caused by discrimination, which is more severe for African Americans than for other, less visible groups. New opportunities have opened up for the African American community in recent years. However, these have mainly benefited upper working-class and middle-class families. The poorest strata have not gained proportionally (Spector, 1991). Also, among this group there are wide variations in languages, religious and cultural practices and beliefs, and economics and culture.

Hispanic Families

There are approximately 15 million people of Latino or Spanish ethnic origin living in the United States. There are several ethnicities represented: Puerto Rican, Cuban, Central and South American, and Mexican Americans. Of these, Mexican Americans constitute the largest majority, approaching 9 million, and are concentrated in Texas, New Mexico, Colorado, Arizona, and California. To that number, 1 million or so undocumented immigrants should be added. Hence, Mexican Americans have become the fastest growing and largest minority ethnic group in the United States (Spector, 1991; Enderlein et al., 1994).

In the last 2 decades, many Hispanic families have become less isolated as new perspectives and opportunities have had an impact of family life. Neighborhood enclaves (barrios) still exist, and middle-class Mexican American and Hispanic people reside in some small rural or isolated urban areas. The great influx of illegal and legal immigrants into the country in the 1980s has led to a persistence of barrios among the poor (Higgenbotham et al., 1990; Aponte, 1993). Traditional values and certain folk beliefs persist, particularly if the family tends to isolate in the barrio; this isolation can make the acquisition of modern health knowledge and practice difficult (Spector, 1991).

Asian Families

Asian families have been a part of the American scene for generations. As with the Native American families, one should not make sweeping generalizations about these families because the cultural prescriptions and preferences can be distinct. However, especially among the older generations, family roles tend to be more clearly defined and differentiated than is the case elsewhere.

Japanese American Families

The largest concentration of Japanese Americans is in California. This segment of the population has the highest median levels of income and education of any minority group. Japanese Americans also have very low rates of crime and delinquency, which indicate the greater persistence of traditional values of obedience and conformity to parental values and norms. The generational pattern of increasing acculturation is clearly illustrated in the contemporary Japanese American community, because other factors, such as urban-rural residence, do not vary significantly (Spector, 1991; Morris, 1990).

Southeast Asian Families

Since 1975, approximately 850,000 Southeast Asian refugees have emigrated to the United States, according to the Refugee Resettlement Program (U.S. Department of Health and Human Services, 1988). The immigrants settled in all of the states, but the highest concentration is found in California. The first wave of refugees arrived in the early 1970s before the collapse of the Vietnamese government. These immigrants were middle class by American standards. They had secondary-school education and were largely multilingual

in French, English, and their native tongue. About 23% held university degrees. The second great wave arrived after the government's collapse. These immigrants had less fortunate circumstances. Many were penniless and poorly educated, with little or no command of English. In general, they were less likely to be exposed to western culture. In addition, the majority were in poor health, with such diseases and health conditions as malaria, tuberculosis, intestinal parasites, anemia, and malnutrition. These conditions, combined with cultural diversity, multiple languages and dialects, and different health belief systems, present a continuing challenge to the American healthcare system. Most of the available data about the homeland culture and mores and recent adjustment endeavors are experiential and anecdotal and derive from interviews with families as they make their varying adjustments (U.S. Department of Health and Human Services, 1988; Poss, 1989).

More recently, there has been an influx of Hmong, Cambodians, and Laotians. Each of these groups brings with it specific talents, such as organization, willingness to learn new languages and ways of life, and extensive cultural beliefs surrounding childbearing and childrearing (Judkins et al., 1992; Mattson et al., 1992). Many of these groups suffered terrible hardships trying to gain freedom from repressive regimes. The physical and sexual abuse suffered by many of the women may impact on their response to pregnancy and childbearing.

More is known of the Vietnamese than the other Asian groups. Vietnamese social concerns and problems, including health needs, are not significantly different from those of many Americans, especially those who live in reduced circumstances. Economic opportunities may be limited for the unskilled. For the educated former urban dweller, economic opportunities may not be commensurate with the Vietnamese's considerable skill and expertise. Culture shock and language barriers also may be troublesome. Moreover, waiting for news or the arrival of loved ones from their old home has serious economic and emotional impact on the lifestyle of these people (Poss, 1989; Mattson et al., 1992).

Community agencies and research programs have been developed to assist southeast Asian families in adjusting to American culture and to provide information about available health services. The Southeast Asian Health Project's aim is to provide information for immigrants on health practices, use of healthcare, and satisfaction with services, particularly those associated with childbearing. Social support systems, including friend and family networks, also have eased the transition to the American culture (Judkins et al., 1992; Mattson et al., 1992; Faller, 1992).

The Vietnamese family is not averse to using the existing American healthcare delivery system, including hospital care during parturition, if the providers are sensitive to the family structure and try to use family members as resources for the care of the child in an extended-family manner. Telephone outreach programs based in the maternity ward and a well-monitored referral system to public health agencies have been beneficial in the delivery of health services (Mattson et al., 1992; Faller, 1992).

There are several culture-based customs that have relevance for those providing maternity care to these clients. As a sign of respect, the client may not look the provider in the eye when speaking and may often answer "yes" to a direct question when "no" is more appropriate, again out of deference and fear of giving offense. Direct questions, loud conversation, getting on a first-name basis, touching, pointing, and other accepted western behaviors are considered inappropriate by the southeast Asian. There also is a belief that touching the baby's head can make the spirit fly out. Thus, using questions that do not require a negative answer, making indirect rather than blunt requests, and maintaining a formal, respectful attitude will increase the family's comfort and therefore the effectiveness of the nurse's care (Faller, 1992; Table 4-1).

Sociocultural Factors and the Use of Maternity Services

Specific predictor variables influence all types of human behavior, including those relating to health and use of healthcare. this group of variables deals with personal sociodemographic factors, such as education, marital status, gender, and socioeconomic status, and societal organizational factors, such as the organization of healthcare, institutional social supports, and economic supports. These groups, although similar, differ in certain aspects.

Socioeconomic Status

Socioeconomic status is a complex concept referring to a theoretical formulation of relationships between subgroups in our society. It is a term frequently used by sociologists and epidemiologists in medical research to subdivide populations into a few descriptive categories that differ in a variety of social and economic characteristics, background, and behavior (Collins, 1990; Feetham et al., 1993). Socioeconomic status is an important determinant of maternal reproductive behavior and use of services. Socioeconomic status, or social class as it is sometimes called, has a pervasive influence on health and healthcare.

To determine socioeconomic status, the usual procedure is to select one or several characteristics as indicators of social difference. Each characteristic is closely related to income, education, occupation, housing and place of residence, social values, and the general lifestyle of population subgroups. By far, the most widely used indicator of socioeconomic status is occupation. It is the best indicator of a person's income, education, standard of living, and social values.

However, not all social differences stem from socioeconomic status. Dividing a population along one social dimension does not automatically provide categories that are socially meaningful in other respects. Such social variables as age, geographic region, height, parity, and ethnicity each contribute independently to the total picture of social variation in pregnancy outcome. The same may be said of other more complex social influences (Feetham et al., 1993).

It is generally accepted that adequate medical care during pregnancy, particularly in the early stages, reduces the incidence of neonatal and maternal mortality, congenital malformations or other birth defects, and prematurity. The relationship between low socioeconomic status and failure to receive adequate antenatal care has been well documented. The data appear to be similar in the United States, Great Britain, and various other western nations. Not only do women of lower socioeconomic status typically comprise the highest proportion of those who have not received antenatal care, but they contribute to the highest proportion of underusers of antenatal care (Norbeck et al., 1989; Patterson et al., 1990).

As a result, socioeconomic status may have more impact on maternity visits than ethnicity. However, nonwhite mothers typically are in a lower socioeconomic group compared with white mothers. On average, women living in families below the poverty level make 9.3 visits for medical care, while women from middle-income families average 13.7 visits. Most lower income women attend clinics or hospitals for their care, in contrast to the higher income women who have a private physician (Patterson et al., 1990; Enderlein et al., 1994).

Healthcare Organization

Many features about the organization of healthcare hinder some clients from receiving appropriate care. The major issues correlated with underuse are discussed below.

Inadequate Outreach Program

In the 1970s, there was a national commitment to equality of healthcare for all citizens. This led to a variety of important legislative acts with an aim to extend and improve the system of health organization so that care could be offered more efficiently to the poor and

TABLE 4–1
Ethnic and Cultural Belief Systems

Group	Family	Beliefs and Health Providers
Native Americans	<ul><li>Family as basic structural unit</li><li>Extended family included</li><li>Children valued and admired</li><li>All members participate in childrearing</li><li>Matriarchal lineage</li><li>Child automatically member of mother's clan at birth</li><li>Women influential in tribal affairs; held in esteem because of childbearing ability</li><li>Children considered assets</li><li>Elderly held in high regard</li></ul>	<ul><li>Vary with tribal identity</li><li>Religion as a powerful force for guiding childbearing, birth, and childrearing</li><li>Pregnancy part of normal cycle of life and death</li><li>Harmonious stress-free prenatal period crucial</li><li>Prenatal care and hospital delivery with obstetricians, other physicians, and tribal midwives</li><li>Tribal medicine man to provide special items to increase strength, prevent illness, and aid in healthy delivery</li></ul>
African Americans	<ul><li>Persistent myth of lack of strong patriarchal tradition</li><li>Mother seen as head of household and provider</li><li>Father seen as absent, powerless parent</li><li>Research showing no significant differences (from white people) regarding role differentiation, values, and orientations</li><li>More use of extended household among middle and lower socioeconomic strata*</li></ul>	<ul><li>Traditional value system, including strong sense of family, superstition, religion, and fatalism (lower socioeconomic strata)</li><li>Middle class urban value system, including rationalism, pragmatism, individualism, egalitarianism, secularism, and achievement</li><li>Health services used promptly if family is middle class with attendant economic resources</li><li>Possible delay and underuse of services if family is poor†</li></ul>
Hispanic or Mexican Americans	<ul><li>Familism strong with patriarchism and "machismo"</li><li>Masculinity equating maleness with sexual prowess</li><li>Women subordinate to husbands</li><li>Childbearing confers high status on male involvement</li><li>Religious (Catholicism/Christian)</li><li>Children valued; trust that Creator will provide</li></ul>	<ul><li>Artificial contraception frowned on</li><li>Life in barrios with own set of beliefs about illness and treatment, usually handed down from generation to generation</li><li>Two categories of illness: emotional origin and magical origin</li><li>Folk healers (*Curanderas* [women] or *Curanderos* [men]) used; often important with respected standing in community</li><li>Many illnesses viewed as result of evil forces, spells, or punishment —Mal aire (bad air entering body) —Mal ojo (evil eye causing nonspecific but often serious symptoms) —Susto (nervousness and loss of appetite and sleep caused by fright) —Mollera calda (fallen fontanel causing diarrhea, sunken eyes, and vomiting)</li></ul>
Japanese Americans	<ul><li>Woman married to serve husband and often his mother and others in household</li><li>Extended family important</li><li>Elderly and children valued and respected</li><li>Grandparents often the decision makers, advisors, and supervisors of children's upbringing</li><li>Filial respect</li><li>Service orientation</li><li>Harmony, patience, modesty, gentleness, and reserve important</li><li>Confrontation avoided</li></ul>	<ul><li>Few hold beliefs</li><li>Scientific medicine accepted generally</li><li>Preventive medicine solicited</li><li>Health and medical regimens usually followed</li><li>Some reliance on herbal medicine</li><li>Interest in acupuncture</li></ul>

(continued)

TABLE 4–1 *(Continued)*
Ethnic and Cultural Belief Systems

Group	Family	Beliefs and Health Providers
Southeast Asians	<ul><li>Traditional values, with diversity within each tribe and ethnicity</li><li>Children and elderly generally respected</li><li>Strong sense of familism</li><li>Strong belief in male authority</li><li>Grandfather considered head of family; authority carried down to oldest son</li><li>Extended family highly valued</li></ul>	<ul><li>Commitment to stoicism and strong belief in fate and enduring pain</li><li>Folk traditions with herbal medicines; family members and elders initial source of healthcare</li><li>Modesty important</li><li>Surgery viewed as mutilation and loss of spirit</li><li>Possible activity restrictions for 40 to 60 days after delivery with other women assuming household and child care duties</li><li>Body heat conservation during childbirth and postpartum</li><li>Bathing after childbirth considered risky</li><li>Possible embarrassment with breast-feeding in front of others</li></ul>

*Dawkins (1989) McAdoo (1993), Alexander et al (1993)
†Ahijevych, (1994)

economically disadvantaged. For example, the federally subsidized maternal and infant care (MIC) projects were instituted to help reduce infant and maternal mortality and reduce the incidence of mental retardation and other handicapping conditions caused by complications associated with childbearing. They emphasized early, comprehensive prenatal care for all clients in the geographic area served. However, the results have been only partially successful. With the current era of economic austerity in governmental subsidies, it remains to be seen whether there will continue to be a national commitment to quality health services for all strata of society (Patterson et al., 1990).

Size of the Organization

The massiveness of most medical organizations can be intimidating. Most lower income women tend to visit medical facilities, such as hospitals and clinics, which are often large, complex, specialized, and often impersonal. Poorly educated clients are ill equipped to cope with these complexities. In addition, they often feel that they are not receiving the best care possible. They realize that two kinds of care exist: one for those who can pay and another for those who cannot.

Providing adequate health services for everyone requires a restructuring of present national priorities and an escalation of the public's social consciousness. Most health professionals agree that any worthwhile program should provide financial support while maintaining the mother's dignity. The concept of comprehensive health planning by states and localities, including area health education centers, community clinics, and innovative programs in hospital clinics, has attempted to provide a higher caliber of care for all segments of society (Handler et al., 1992; Enderlein et al., 1994).

Within the last 10 years, the focus of service in many outpatient departments and clinics has changed from dispensing first aid to giving ambulatory care with a dynamic, change-oriented focus. In these settings, nurses function in more independent and expanded roles, educating clients, providing supportive guidance, and making observations. The professional nurse becomes primarily responsible for maintaining continuity of healthcare for a specific client population. Increasingly, expanded nursing roles provide routine prenatal care in outpatient, ambulatory settings (Handler et al., 1992).

Skills and Education Needed to Cope With Professionalization in Healthcare

Professionalization in healthcare demands that the client is able to communicate, understand, and comply with appointment schedules and prescribed regimens. Many ordered regimens are impossible for low-income clients to follow. The simple order to take medication "with each meal" may be difficult for many lower income families who eat irregularly or who cannot afford to eat three meals a day. Lower income people may be less skilled in obtaining information and explanations from professionals about their care. Higher income clients have greater assertive, interactional skills and can cope more effectively with the professional's failure to communicate (Boyle et al., 1989; Handler et al., 1992).

Middle-Class Bias

Another characteristic of medical organization that influences the quality of medical care is the middle-class bias of most professional health workers. There may be a distinct bias expressed against lower income clients, based honestly on professional conceptions. Typically, staff members do not understand the perspectives, attitudes, customs, and lifestyles of lower income clients, especially if they come from another culture. **Ethnocentrism,** the practice of judging cultural beliefs or practices by standards from another culture, is common. Healthcare workers often take for granted that their clients have the same attitudes about health as they do. Therefore, they tend to issue orders that are not understood or cannot be followed easily. In addition, healthcare workers may tend to think of lower income people in stereotypical terms. For example, they cannot keep appointments, or they have little sense of time or responsibility. Lower income clients may perceive these class biases, which can affect use of services. The many hours of waiting, the impersonal routines of institutional care in large hospitals or clinics (particularly in the municipal and county hospitals), and the real or imagined perceptions of racial and class bias all tend to maximize dissatisfactions of lower income clients, thereby reducing use.

Facility Location

The distances that clients must travel to the facilities and the cost of transportation are realistic concerns. Customarily, poorer people organize their lives so they do not have to go far for the necessities of living. This is one of the reasons for the relative success of the MIC program and the neighborhood health centers that have reached into the lower income communities and brought clinic facilities into the neighborhood (Kavanagh et al., 1992; Boyle et al., 1989).

Maldistribution of Health Personnel and Manpower

Rural and geographically isolated communities and the inner cities have traditionally experienced difficulties obtaining adequate healthcare because professional socialization and economic considerations promote practice in desirable metropolitan areas. Lack of coordination and overlap in agencies also add to this problem. For example, there may be several community health nursing services in one area, such as the health department, a voluntary nursing agency, and school nursing services. They may all serve one family, but they seldom communicate with one another. Similarly, some hospitals may be overcrowded, while others have empty beds.

Future Trends

It is believed that quality maternity care in the future will be provided by a closely integrated team of physicians, professional nurses, nurse-midwives or nurse practitioners, laboratory technicians, social workers, nutritionists, health educators, and homemakers. The development of expanded roles for nurses is proving to be a viable effort to deliver quality care. Research has indicated that when nurses are used in advanced practice, in expanded roles, and as integral members of the healthcare team, there are considerably fewer broken antepartum appointments, better postpartum clinic attendance, better use of family-planning services and techniques, and reduced infant mortality (Pettitti, Coleman et al., 1990; Finlay et al., 1990).

Government programs have been developed to encourage health professionals to enter practice in medically underserved rural or inner-city urban areas. Efforts such as the following are steps toward ensuring greater availability and appropriate distribution of health personnel: National Health Service Corps, which supports team practices between physicians and nurse practitioners in rural communities; Medicare reimbursement of nurse practitioners and physicians' assistants in rural clinics; scholarships and educational subsidies for primary care providers; and program grants for primary care to schools of nursing and medicine (Finlay et al., 1990).

Training indigenous community members through decentralized educational programs also has has been an effective method of providing quality care to underserved populations. Their familiarity with the lifestyles of childbearing families, knowledge of the socioeconomic factors to be considered, and willingness to provide whatever service is needed are important factors in their success.

Innovations have been developed in an attempt by the healthcare system to respond to consumer needs. Examples of these innovations include community clinics and alternative birth centers. Community clinics are initiated and organized by the indigenous population and are staffed largely by local people. Supported largely by federal and state funds, which are in increasingly short supply, community clinics can be effective in responding to specific healthcare needs.

Health Insurance Coverage

The national goals for healthcare include ensuring quality, access, and control of costs. However, methods of financing these services continue to support disparities among population groups. The chief protection for the health needs of most young parents lies in voluntary and commercial prepayment insurance. Maternity benefits traditionally have been distressingly low. Young low-income families are frequently saddled with large medical and hospital bills at a time when they can least afford to pay. Many professionals feel that maternity care should be entirely covered, but the insurance providers believe that the rates for this kind of coverage would be prohibitive. However, insurance companies have had this opinion about other forms of coverage and under public pressure have increased benefits. Many community health leaders believe that the resources of this country are so vast that full coverage is feasible if there is a public mandate to provide it (Pettitti et al., 1990; Patterson et al., 1990).

Various bills for national health insurance have been introduced in the U.S. Congress, but conflicting goals continue to make it difficult for legislators to develop a comprehensive, widely acceptable plan. Figure 4-3 depicts the necessary requirements for quality maternity

and perinatal care. The involvement of concerned nurses in governmental processes can help promote an equitable healthcare system.

Risk Factors and Reproductive Outcomes

Certain risk factors may jeopardize the health of the maternity client. Some of these factors, such as age, may be beyond the client's control; others, however, such as behavioral risk factors, life events, and stress, are capable of being changed. Box 4-2 lists the factors that place the mother or fetus at risk.

Sociodemographic Risk Factors

Sociodemographic risk factors are a subset of sociocultural risk factors that involve society and culture. They include maternal age, parity, socioeconomic status,

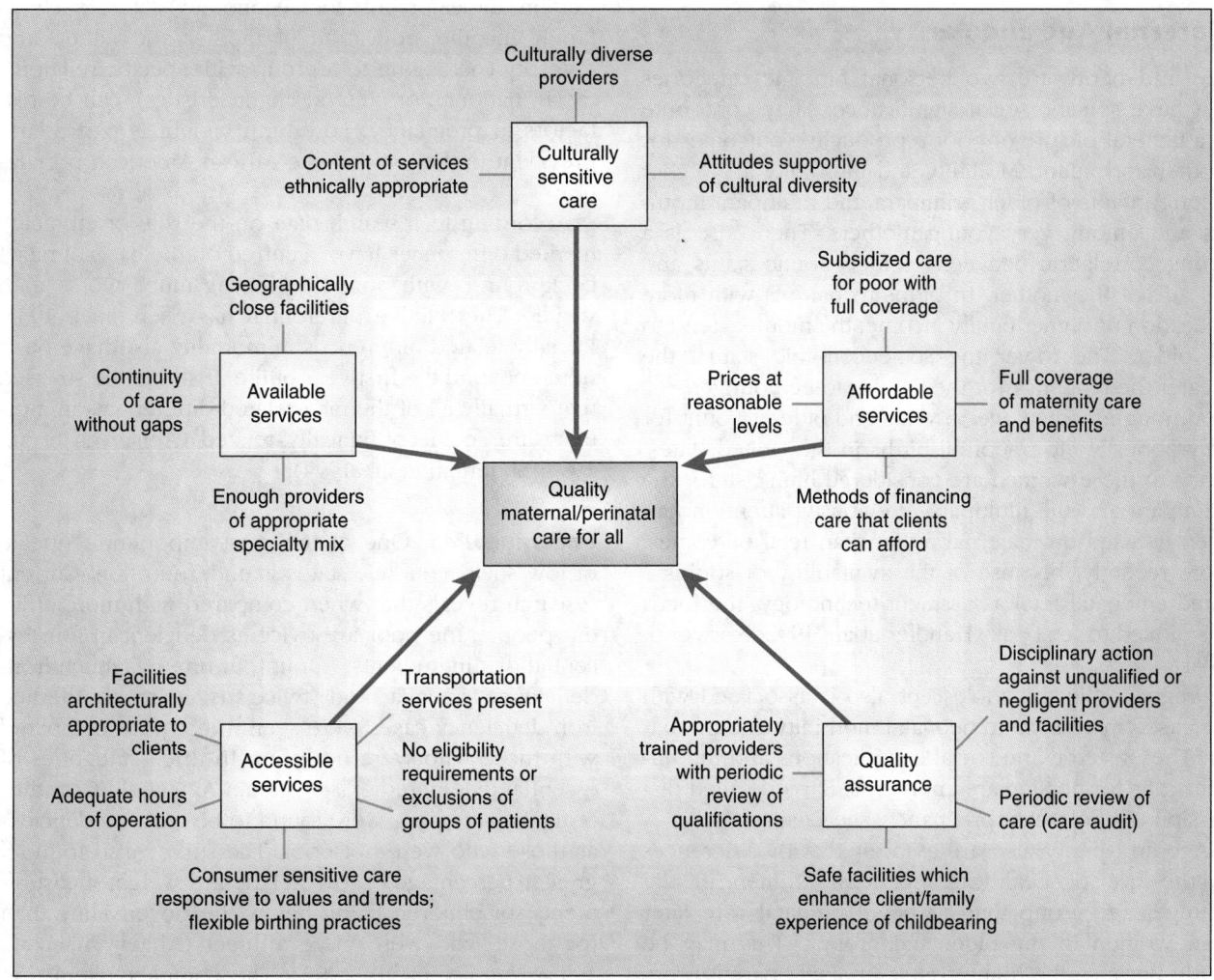

FIGURE 4–3 Healthcare system requirements for providing quality maternity and perinatal care for all.

BOX 4–2
Factors Placing Woman or Fetus at Risk

- Sociodemographic risk factors
  - Older than 35 years
  - Adolescence
- Socioeconomic and ethnic factors
  - Education of parent
  - Ethnicity
  - Family income
  - Undernutrition
- Behavioral risk factors
  - Addictive habits: smoking, alcohol, drugs
  - Teratogenic foods and additives
- Life events and life stress
  - High life stress and low social support
  - Attitudes and emotions

---

ethnicity, and geographic area. These factors are not easily controlled by the client.

Maternal Age and Parity

Age and parity are two personal biologic categories that have specific social significance. They contribute to a general picture of poor reproductive outcomes for mother and infant. Mortality and morbidity are higher among infants of older primipara and multipara mothers and among very young mothers. There also is a strong correlation between socioeconomic status and the age of the mother. In births to parents with more education or higher family income, the mothers tend to be older. The lower the socioeconomic status, the greater the tendency for the mother to be younger.

Although women age 35 years and older account for only about 5% to 6% of all births in the United states, births to these women are considered high risk for the primipara and the multipara. Previously, attention had been focused on maternal rather than fetal outcomes. More recently, because of the availability of sophisticated antenatal fetal assessment technology, the focus has moved to fetal risk (Handler et al., 1992; Norwood, 1994).

Pregnancy in the adolescent also is associated with increased maternal and neonatal morbidity and mortality. The obstetric and social complications and the implications for nursing are enormous. For a detailed discussion of adolescent pregnancy, see Chapter 35.

Age and parity also are associated with differences in the use of healthcare services. Women in the younger age group tend to begin prenatal care later than women in the older age groups. This may be partly because the highest rates of single-parent pregnancies are in the youngest age groups. Multiparas who have had little trouble with previous pregnancies

also tend to come later and be more lax in keeping appointments (Norwood, 1994).

Nursing Implications. The role of the maternity nurse becomes particularly important in counseling women whose age or parity places them at risk for problems with their pregnancies and with some of the prenatal diagnostic techniques. The mother and father need to be appraised of the limitations associated with these tests. The tests are not a panacea for a safe pregnancy outcome. They are useful because they can determine if some fetal defects exist, allowing the parents to consider their options. The also can give a good indication of the age and well-being of the fetus, which helps if early delivery is indicated. Thus, these parents need meticulous prenatal care, particularly from the nurse, beginning as early as possible in the pregnancy.

Socioeconomic Ethnic and Geographic Risk Factors

Certain indicators of socioeconomic status, such as family income, education of mother and father, and ethnicity (belonging to a group with specific religious, racial, national, or cultural characteristics), can be risk factors in pregnancy. Low birth weight is particularly prevalent in the low-income African American population.

According to research data on the role of ethnicity, marked differences have occurred on the basis of racial background, with nonwhites faring much worse than whites. The relative differential has risen since 1935. Racially related differences in mortality also have been noted beyond the first year of life. It should be stressed that virtually all of the race-related differentials in mortality are socioeconomically related (Ahijevych et al., 1994; Enderlein et al., 1994).

Undernutrition. One of the most important sequelae of low socioeconomic status is undernutrition. Current research reveals that when compared with more affluent people, the poor are twice as deficient in four essential diet ingredients. About four times as much iron-deficiency anemia and twice as many borderline iron-deficiency cases were seen in the poor compared with those who were not poor. In three categories of essential diet ingredients—vitamin A, vitamin C, and riboflavin—the poor were found to be twice as deficient as those who were not poor. The survey also found a greater percentage of low height and weight measurements for children living below the poverty line than for those who were more affluent (Ahijevych et al., 1994; Handler et al., 1992). The complex interaction between undernutrition, poverty, and other environmental and genetic factors is apparent.

Effects on Fetal Brain Development. Studies also have found that deficiencies in the diet of a pregnant woman can have profound effects on a number of pregnancy outcomes. For some of these effects, see Figure 4-4.

It is estimated that 10% of the children born today are seriously affected as a consequence of maternal malnutrition. Research at the National Institutes of Health suggests that there is a correlation between the level of the amino acids in the blood of a pregnant woman and the subsequent intelligence of her baby (Super et al., 1990; Norwood, 1994).

Low Birth Weight. Maternal undernutrition has been identified as one of the causes of low–birth-weight infants born to poor urban mothers. The relationship between low birth weight and malnourished populations may have a more complex explanation than simple nutrition. It may reflect long-term maternal undernutrition and social deprivation from the early childhood of the woman (Super et al., 1990).

Hypertensive Disorders. There is some evidence that the incidence of hypertensive conditions can be modified by environmental changes, either situational or behavioral. During World War II in Great Britain, pregnant nursing mothers were given preferential treatment in food rationing during the evacuation. Therefore, women of lower socioeconomic groups were fed as well as other population groups. The result was a dramatic fall in the mortality rate from pregnancy-induced hypertensive disorders (Ahijevych et al., 1994; Handler et al., 1992).

Nursing Implications. The nurse can be a force in the community and in ambulatory care settings to help improve preventive services to those at highest risk because of situational factors. Health education, including clear nutritional counseling and information about environmental risk factors and their solutions, needs to be incorporated into all prenatal counseling. Moreover, the nurse can be a positive force in the community to exert influence on other institutions, such as schools, health departments, government agencies, and voluntary agencies, to provide preventive services to the population at greatest risk.

Behavioral and Lifestyle Risk Factors

Certain behavioral factors can result in lifestyles that are detrimental to a pregnancy. These behaviors should be changed. Concepts of healthy living and stress management should be encouraged during pregnancy.

Addictive Disorders

Various substances, such as alcohol, drugs, and tobacco, have been found to be addictive and harmful to the user's health, particularly during pregnancy. The harmful effects to the woman and fetus have been

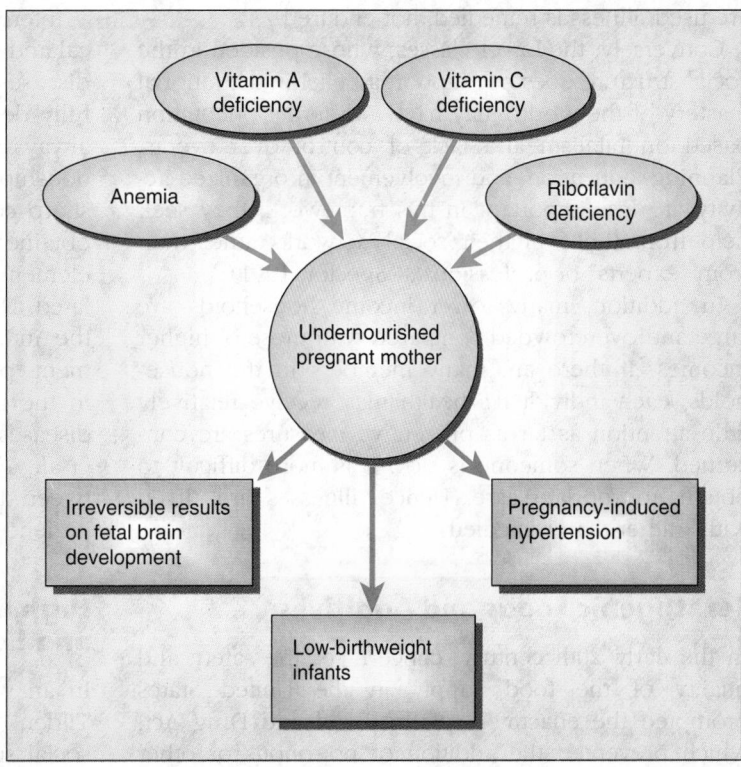

FIGURE 4–4 Some of the effects of undernutrition on pregnancy outcomes.

much publicized. Clients with addictive disorders who are pregnant need thorough education, counseling, and follow-up. A referral to treatment programs may be necessary if the pregnancy is to result in a positive outcome. A detailed discussion of this topic is found in Chapter 34.

Lifestyles

Lifestyle refers to a way of living that can have implications for health. It is important to take into account the characteristic lifestyles of clients, particularly those of the economically disadvantaged. The experiences of the lower income person and his or her world is distinctive for its problems and crisis-dominated character. Health concerns are minor to those who feel they confront much more pressing troubles; health problems are just one crisis among many with which they must try to cope. Therefore, maternal and child health services need to be comprehensive and multidisciplinary to assess and address the client's needs in the perceived priority as much as possible.

In general, middle class people value specific orientations. They are activistic in their attitudes about actions in interpersonal relationships and demonstrate **rational mastery** (power and technology to solve all problems) over the natural or supernatural environment. They also value **future time,** planning for the future, being on time, saving time, and placing importance on novelty and youth. These orientations tend to result in a specific outlook on life that is reflected in health beliefs and behavior. Preventive health practices are used; illness is remedied, not endured.

Conversely, the lower classes, whose position in the social structure does not support a belief in the rational mastery of the world, may have a different orientation based on fatalism and lack of control over events. Planning, education, and involvement in organized activity are less important in this framework; they seek help from those in their social network rather than from "experts" or professionals (Spector, 1991).

In addition, many lower income households are large and overcrowded compared with those of higher incomes. If there are many members in the households, each individual's health may receive relatively little attention as far as preventive measures are concerned. When someone is sick, it is more difficult to obtain appropriate care. Hence, illnesses are "lived with" rather than remedied.

Teratogenic Foods and Additives

In the early 20th century, concern for the safety and quality of the food supply in the United States prompted the enactment of the Food and Drug Act, which prevented the addition of poisonous or other deleterious ingredients to foods. With advanced technology and increased sophistication of food production, processing, and advertising, concern has mounted about the safety of foods and additives. It has been found that many unsuspected substances, both naturally occurring and artificially added, are **mutagens, teratogens,** or **embryotoxins.** Mutagens change the inherited chromosomal structure of cells; teratogens produce congenitally malformed infants; and embryotoxins kill or alter the embryo (Wilson, 1987; Thomson et al., 1992).

Problems associated with the study of teratogens revolve around the choice, dosage, and amount of experimental substance; the choice of subject animals (humans cannot be used for experimentation); the difficulty in isolating variables and hence measuring results; the difficulty in determining preconditioning factors; and the need for multigenerational studies. Therefore, definitive data are lacking. It is particularly important that the pregnant woman be made aware of the potential hazards, because ingesting large quantities of these substances may be harmful to her fetus (Wilson, 1987; Thomson et al., 1992). The groups of foods and additives are summarized in Box 4-3.

Life Events and Life Stress as Risks

Life events and **life stress** refer to the effects on the pregnancy of divorce, illness, assault, eviction, death of a close family member or friend, and job loss. Appropriate intervention by nursing staff can be especially effective in meeting the needs and reducing the risks associated with such life stress.

Interest in the relationship between the psychological and social world of individual human disorders and diseases has a long history. Even the findings of carefully designed and conducted investigations have not always yielded clear-cut results concerning this relationship (Walker, 1989; Di Leonardi, 1993). This is in sharp contrast to the dramatic results that have been obtained with animal experiments in which the various elements in the social environment have been correlated. Nevertheless, there is accumulating evidence of the intimate interaction between the social environment, physiologic reactions, and pathologic outcome in the individual. This is particularly true of chronic diseases, such as heart disease and cancer (Alexander et al., 1993). However, studies on the relationship between disorders of pregnancy and life changes and experiences that may be stressful are relatively few.

High Life Stress and Low Social Support

In an well-designed prospective study, Norbeck and Tilden (1983) looked at the relationship of life stress, social support, and emotional disequilibrium to complications in pregnancy outcomes. They found that

BOX 4–3
Potential Hazards of Foods and Additives

Nitrosamines (N-nitroso Compounds)

These compounds are potent carcinogens in all tested species, including amphibians, birds, fish, and mammals. Although nitrosamines are rarely found in foods, their precursors, nitrites (which combine with other nitrogen-containing compounds) are common. Sodium nitrite and sodium nitrate are added to most smoked and cured meat and fish to act as an antioxidant to ensure preserving the food. Nitrate, which may break down to nitrite, is found in soybean oil and naturally in leafy vegetables, such as cauliflower, broccoli, lettuce, cabbage, and beets, especially when high levels of nitrate fertilizers are used. Drinking water in areas experiencing fertilizer runoff also may contain high levels. Ascorbic acid (vitamin C) can be used in place of nitrites as an antioxidant.

Aflatoxins

These substances are related to mycotoxins and are produced by fungal growths on a wide range of food. Contamination is usually caused by excessive moisture before harvest or during storage. Aflatoxins are toxic to humans. For instance, the mycotoxin ergotism of rye can induce abortion, gangrene, and other ills of the vascular system. Peanuts are particularly susceptible to infection, as are cereal grains, legumes, cocoa, cassava, sweet potatoes, improperly fermented foods and alcoholic beverages, and dairy products from animals fed contaminated feed. These toxins are not destroyed by home cooking or freezing, but milling is effective because the infected outer shells are removed. Regulation of harvest, storage, and marketing protects the consumer to a great extent.

U.S.-Certified Food Colorings

These are the "azo" dyes, which include red #2 (amaranth), red #4, yellow #6 (tartrazine), green (ferrous gluconate), and some others. Red #2 was found to be embryotoxic to rats and to cause small litters in the same species; it has been banned since 1976. There is no clear-cut carcinogenic or teratogenic evidence regarding the other dyes; hence, Public Law 86–618 provides for setting "safe limits" for these and other food substances.

Artificial Sweeteners

Again there is no clear evidence of a carcinogenic or teratogenic effect with sodium cyclamate, saccharin, mannitol, and xylitol. Researchers have found that mothers who had taken cyclamates during pregnancy had children who suffered from hyperactivity and learning disabilities.[30] At present, research is continuing on these products, because the studies suffer from the methodologic problems mentioned previously.

Caffeine

This substance is of concern because of its chemical structure, purine, one of the constituent groups of DNA. Moreover, it crosses the human placenta and penetrates the pre-implantation blastocyte in mammals. In addition, it causes chromosomal rearrangements in the sperm of mice. The data on human populations are not conclusive, and conflicting evidence is given. A recent large study in Finland, the country that leads the world in coffee consumption, did not produce any definitive data or recommendations.[32]

Thus, although there is reason for caution in using caffeine during pregnancy (and excessively in general), there is insufficient evidence to implicate it as a teratogen.

Trace Elements and Metallic and Chemical Contaminants

Such trace elements and metallic contaminants as lead, selenium, arsenic, cadmium, mercury, and methylmercury occur in the ground; in fish and crustaceans, especially when they come from contaminated waters; and in some fruits, cheeses, cereals, and other food. When taken in large quantities they are teratogenic, producing a variety of symptoms from congenital malformations to central nervous system problems.

Similarly, chemical contaminants, including pesticides, space sprays (DDVP, dichloros, vapona), herbicides, and fungicides are embryotoxic, mutagenic, and teratogenic in mammals. The pesticide DVCP has been banned because of the occurrence of sterility in farm workers who used the substance in their work. Ingestion of these in pregnancy should be avoided.

---

high life stress and low social support were significantly related to high emotional disequilibrium, although social support and life stress were not significantly related to each other. They also found a relationship between high life stress, social support, and gestational and infant complications. Social support appeared to play a mediating role. In a separate study, Tilden (1983) documented a significant relationship of life stress and social support to emotional disequilibrium during pregnancy. What contribution the pregnancy itself might have made to the overall relationship was not measurable.

Additional research is needed, but data of Norbeck and Tilden (1983) help to explain some of the discrepant results in the literature (Walker, 1989). In short, the research and the approach cast serious doubt on the usefulness of specificity (as far as current clinical syndromes are concerned) in research concerned with psychosocial factors in disease etiology.

Attitudes and Emotions

A great deal of research on the role of emotional and attitudinal factors, psychological stress during pregnancy, and pregnancy outcomes has been done. The evidence is inconclusive. Much of it is based on poorly designed research and on inadequate samples of the population at risk. Despite this, there is a general consensus in medical science that psychological factors are in some way associated with various aspects of the maternity cycle. Some investigators have asserted that early psychological assessment of pregnant women holds promise of being predictive of the course and outcome of pregnancy. Most of the literature attempts to measure the attitudes of the women toward her pregnancy, her perception of herself as a mother, and other psychosocial factors, because these may influence the outcome (Walker, 1989). There are clearly attitudinal differences among women toward their individual pregnancies, and there may be an intimate interaction between the psychosocial stress experienced by the person, the buffering effects of social supports, and psychological reactions. Complications of pregnancy, labor, and delivery can be obscured by this interaction. Thus, physiologic changes and discomfort may trigger psychologically negative attitudes toward the pregnancy, and conversely, life stress may precipitate somatic problems (Norbeck et al., 1983, 1989; Walker, 1989).

Nursing Implications. Many women experience some psychological stress during pregnancy. However, nursing and medical literature tend to assume that some of these conditions are psychosomatic or emotional. As researchers have pointed out, there should be continued criticism of the cloudy thinking that has characterized such conditions as menstrual pain, nausea of pregnancy, and pain in labor as caused or aggravated by psychogenic factors. They suggest sexual prejudice as the basis for such thinking. Scientific evidence clearly suggests organic causes for these conditions (Norbeck et al., 1989; Walker, 1989; Kavanagh et al., 1992; Spector, 1991).

Nurses must avoid accepting long-established attitudes that are rooted in prejudice rather than in scientific evidence. Stereotypical thinking is poor in scientific terms and tends to influence the course and quality of treatment of female clients. Nurses must play an important role in assisting the pregnant woman to use her psychosocial assets to cope with the fears, anxieties, somatic complaints, and other problems associated with pregnancy in the prenatal and intrapartum periods. Emotional and social support during and following the pregnancy can be a comfort to the client and may assist in reducing problematic outcomes.

Changing Relationships Between Clients and Providers

Changes affecting the healthcare system have affected the way clients and providers interact. Clients are demanding satisfaction and changing the ways they communicate with their providers.

Consumer Satisfaction

Consumer satisfaction refers to the attitudes toward the healthcare system of those who have experienced contact with the system. It is concerned with the satisfaction of the client with the quantity or quality of care received and relates to several dimensions (see Box 4-4).

Consumers complain that it is more difficult to find a primary care physician who will give them the personal attention they want. Regardless of the socioeconomic status of the woman, it is difficult for her to receive continuity of care from maternity care providers. Group practices sometimes disrupt the relationship between client and physician, and hospital structure requires nursing personnel shift changes. Clients often have difficulty determining the status of the person in the medical office to whom they are speaking on the telephone. Clients feel that obstetricians seem to relinquish their responsibility for the neonate during the postpartum period. Similarly, in this period, pediatricians (from the mother's perspective) do not appear to be centrally involved with the needs of the mother. These features of the medical care system are reflected in the concept of fragmented healthcare and consumer dissatisfaction (Finlay et al., 1990; Patterson et al., 1990).

Communication

One important transaction that occurs in the provider–client relationship is effective communication from the provider to the client concerning the nature of her condition and the actions to be taken. The degree to which she has understands the physician and nurse and can verbalize the advice and instructions given depends on the quality of the relationship. Similarly, good healthcare results in communication from the client to the providers. In particular, the degree to which the woman's concerns, worries, and fears about her condition have been perceived by the provider is equally important.

BOX 4-4
Dimensions of Consumer Satisfaction

- Accessibility and convenience of services: convenience of care and emergency care
- Availability: family physicians, hospitals, specialists
- Continuity: regular family physician, same physician
- Physician conduct: consideration of feelings, explanations
- Financial aspects: cost of services, insurance coverage, payment mechanisms

Commentators on the physician–client relationship frequently have discussed the social-class and value differences between providers and clients as one barrier to communication and ultimately, to use of health services. Numerous studies indicate that middle-class clients tend to obtain most of their information about illness by asking their physicians and nurses direct questions. In contrast, working-class clients receive their information from a passive process in which they are given information without asking; they also tend to receive less information (Handler et al., 1992; Ahijevych et al., 1994; Norwood, 1994). Despite their reluctance to request information, working-class maternity clients are not much different from upper-class clients in their desire for information. Although upper-class clients may desire more technical details regarding their health condition, there is no general social-class difference in clients' desires for as much information as possible presented in nontechnical language (Handler et al., 1992).

Part of the issue of better communication between provider and client results from a reflection of a general social-class difference in language use. Working-class clients sense a social distance between themselves and their physician and feel that they are not expected to ask questions. Even middle-class clients hesitate to communicate freely with their physician about troublesome problems or symptoms because they perceive their physician as busy and hard-working.

The Nurse as Communicator

The maternity nurse plays a crucial role in communication. Generally, the nurse in not perceived by the client in the same manner as the physician. Several studies have indicated that the nurse can more effectively perform roles involving the giving and receiving of information to clients. Thus, the nurse has an opportunity to fill a much-needed role by seizing the initiative and asking the client about any concerns and questions about the pregnancy. This helps to close the communication gap in the client–provider relationship. Because communication problems have a significant effect on the appropriate use of services, the nurse's contribution to communication is crucial (Freda et al., 1993; Norwood, 1994).

Nursing Care of Today's Families

There are several principles to remember when the nurse is assessing, diagnosing, planning, implementing, and evaluating care for families today. Although each family must be assessed with care tailored to their needs, some basic principles remain. Families today may assume a more questioning attitude. Rationales for treatment plans are questioned, and prognoses and alternatives are requested. This may prove disconcerting to some health providers, but clients' questions should be answered, and options must be discussed. The nurse also plays a key role in assessing the client for social and obstetric risk factors. Specific risk factors are listed in the Assessment Guidelines.

Evaluating Health Information

Health professionals often expect clients to accept information as true because it is drawn from a scientific body of knowledge. However, some clients may question information before accepting it.

Expectant parents will have many questions. When the nurse responds to their inquiries, parents may then relate information that they have gathered from other sources. It becomes important to discuss this information seriously and with respect because it is valuable to the parent. Health teaching that is documented with rational explanation is much more readily accepted. The advice and teaching must be practical, especially if there are others in the family to consider. Similarly, ethnic variables, such as food preferences and preparation, no matter how repugnant to the nurse, must be taken into consideration.

Families today also expect a fuller and more complete explanation, particularly if they are well educated. If a mother prefers a vegetarian diet and wants to know the food values of the items she wishes to include in her diet, she may not be satisfied with only a suggested menu. Exchanges and equivalents must be discussed. Similarly, it is not sufficient to tell a mother in a prenatal clinic to return in so many weeks for another blood test without telling her the reason for returning and the purpose of the procedure. If clients reject some advice, this must be treated with respect.

Choosing Reproductive Services

Certain factors influence the choice of prenatal services. These include experience with health personnel, geographic location, economics, feelings about the pregnancy, the influence of significant others, and the patents' physical condition. These areas need a complete assessment.

Increasingly, selection of services is made on the basis of client consultation with friends, referrals from professionals, and experience with health providers. In general, couples are taking a more active role in the planning and execution of their care. They tend to seek out health professionals who allow them this right. This is particularly true for immigrant families, who tend to select professionals who are sensitive to

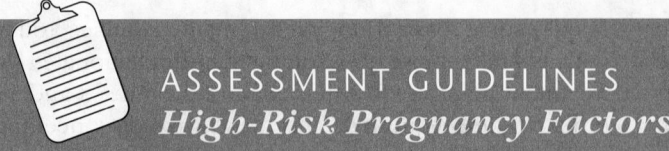

ASSESSMENT GUIDELINES
High-Risk Pregnancy Factors

Use the following as a guide to help identify potential risk factors that may affect the outcome of the pregnancy.

Prenatal Factors

1. Maternal disease
   a. Diabetes mellitus
   b. Preeclampsia and eclampsia
   c. Hypertension
   d. Cardiopulmonary disease
   e. Renal disease
   f. Infection: syphilis, rubella, tuberculosis
   g. Drug addiction
   h. Alcoholism
   i. Endocrinopathy
   j. Severe anemia and blood dyscrasias
   k. Malnutrition
   l. Malignancy during pregnancy
2. Maternal practices
   a. Taking medications associated with adverse fetal effects
   b. Smoking, drugs, alcohol
   c. Excessive exposure to radiation
   d. Less than three prenatal visits; general use of health services
3. Age: <16 years and >35 years
4. Short maternal stature
5. Severe isoimmunization (Rh or other)
6. Multiple gestation (eg, particularly second of twins, third of triplets)
7. Premature rupture of the membranes (PROM): >37–38 weeks (not considered here as a high-risk factor because all preterm infants are PROM)
8. Prolonged rupture of membranes: >18–24 h (predisposes to neonatal sepsis, intrauterine pneumonia, and infections)

9. Polyhydramnios, oligohydramnios
10. Evidence of intrauterine growth retardation
11. Previous perinatal and neonatal deaths, preterm or low–birth-weight deliveries
12. Lower socioeconomic status
13. Previous or current abuse (physical, sexual, emotional)
14. Geographic location: rural, urban, inner city, barrio
15. Life stress and social supports

Previous Labor and Delivery Factors

1. Placental accident or hemorrhage
   a. Abruptio placentae
   b. Placenta previa
2. Cesarean section
3. Mechanical factors
   a. Abnormal presentation (ie, breech, transverse)
   b. Anatomy of the birth canal: cephalopelvic disproportion
4. Fetal distress
5. Prolonged or obstructed labor that leads to fetal asphyxia (>24 h for primigravidas; >18 h for multigravidas)
6. Prolonged second stage of labor
7. Prolapsed, knotted, or entangled umbilical cord leading to fetal asphyxia
8. Maternal fever
9. Depressant drugs given to mother near delivery (eg, meperidine [Demerol])

(Modified from Trotter, C. W., Chang, P.-N., & Thompson, T. [1982]. Appendix: High-risk pregnancy factors. Journal of Obstetric, Gynecologic, and Neonatal Nursing, 11, 90.)

---

their cultural needs. It then becomes important in planning care with the client to be sure that the couple is duly informed about the nature of their care, including their right to sign themselves out of the hospital. This information, together with a genuine regard for the couple, is usually sufficient to lessen apprehension about the particular service.

Selecting a hospital or choosing between a hospital or home delivery involves many of the same factors as those considered by the client when selecting prenatal

services. For most couples today, childbirth is regarded as a natural process; thus, alternative birth centers may be sought. Modern equipment and technologic expertise may be much less important than an environment that simulates the home.

The need for control over one's own life also may be a strong motivating factor when choosing a home delivery. However, having a baby at home is a controversial decision. Safety of the mother and infant continues to be a grave concern for health professionals, and

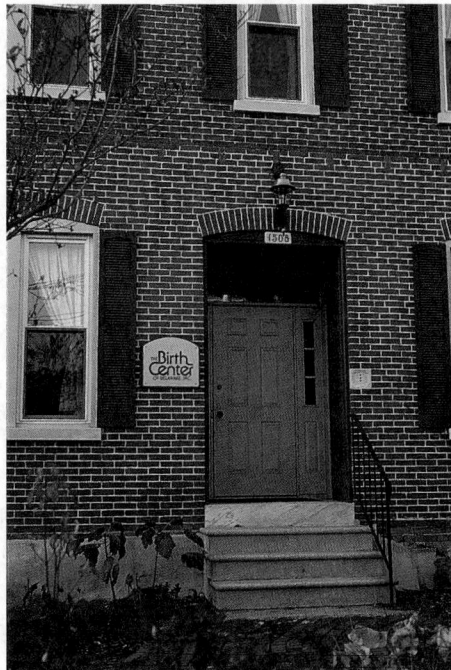

FIGURE 4–5 Many hospitals institute birth centers in the surrounding communities to provide a homelike alternative to the traditional hospital setting.

data indicate that this concern is well founded. Birth carries a strong symbolic meaning, however, and the home typifies this meaning. The traditional hospital setting is seen by many couples as a sterile place with little room for intimacy and family integration. Many hospitals have instituted birthing rooms or birth centers that simulate a homelike atmosphere free from many of the restrictions and rigidities imposed by traditional delivery suites (Fig. 4-5). Couples enjoy and use these services, and data indicate that the risk to the infant and mother is minimal during low-risk deliveries.

Today, parents generally come to their deliveries with more knowledge than in previous years. This is partly due to the large variety of books now available that deal with nutrition during pregnancy and the physiology of pregnancy, labor, and delivery. There are even "how to" books on home delivery. Parents, therefore, expect their requests to be considered. Hospitals that have the reputation for having a great deal of restrictions usually are avoided.

Summary Points

✔ Several trends in society affect the motivation for childbearing. These include availability of contraceptive methods and competing social roles, both of which give women options for a variety of roles besides motherhood. These trends impact on maternity and perinatal services as fertility and birth rates rise and fall.

✔ Examining the contemporary family roles of various ethnic groups shows that the process of transition into the American culture has been accelerated or delayed by several factors: opportunities available for employment in the new environment, the extent of discrimination, and the cultural and physical differences and similarities between the acculturating group and the dominant society.

✔ Socioeconomic status is one of the most powerful predictors in the use of health services, including maternity services. It is as important as race and ethnicity. However, problems in the organization of healthcare impinge negatively on the appropriate use of maternity and perinatal services, irrespective of socioeconomic status and ethnicity.

✔ Several groups of risk factors impact negatively on reproductive outcomes. Some are sociodemographic risk factors, such as age, parity, ethnicity, socioeconomic status, undernutrition, and geographic area. Some of these are beyond the client's control. Behavioral risk factors, such as substance abuse, lifestyle, use of teratogenic foods and additives, life events and life stress risk factors (such as attitudes and emotional stress management), and the use of social support systems, are generally within the client's control.

✔ The modern American family is changing its relationships with health providers. Paramount among its criteria for quality care is satisfaction with provider relations, access to care, and continuity of care. Positive communication patterns also are important. There must be time and opportunity to converse freely with the provider, be informed of options, and participate in planning care. There must be a sense of mutual respect on both sides.

REFERENCES

Ahijevych, K., & Bernhard, L. (1994). Health-promoting behaviors of African American women. *Nursing Research, 43*(2), 86–89.

Alexander, G. R., Baruff, G., Mor, J. M. Keiffer, E. C., & Hulsey, T. C. (1993). Multiethnic variations in pregnancy outcomes of military dependents. *American Journal of Public Health, 83*(12), 1721–1725.

Aponte, R. (1993). Hispanic families in poverty: Diversity, context, and interpretation, Families in society. *The Journal of Contemporary Human Services, 74*(9), 527–537.

Bell, R. (1994). Prominence of women in Navajo health beliefs and values. *Nursing and Health Care, 15*(5), 232–241.

Boyle, J. S., & Andrews, J. M. (1989). Trancultural concepts in nursing care. Boston: Scott, Foresman/Little Brown College Division.

Collins, J. W., & David, R. J. (1990). The differential effect of traditional risk factors on infant birthweight among blacks and whites in Chicago. *American Journal of Public Health, 80*(1), 679–686.

Dawkins, C., Ervin, N., Wiessfeld, L., & Yan, A. (1988). Health orientations, beliefs and use of health services among minority, high-risk expectant mothers. *Public Health Nursing, 5,* 7–11.

Di Leonardi, J. W. (1993). Families in poverty and chronic neglect of children, families in society. *The Journal of Contemporary Human Services, 74*(9), 557–562.

Draper, E. D. (1992). Parabola: The oral tradition. *Focus, 17*(3), 2–3.

Enderlein, M. C., Stephenson, P. A., Holt, L., & Hikok, D. (1994). Health status and timing of onset of prenatal care: Is there an association among low-income women? *BIRTH, 21*(2), 71–75.

Faller, H. S. (1992). Hmong women: Characteristics and birth outcomes, 1990. *BIRTH, 19*(3), 144–148.

Finlay, W., Mutran, E. S., Zeitler, R. R., & Randall, C. S. (1990). Queues and care: How medical residents organize their work in a busy clinic. *Journal of Health Social Behavior, 31*(2), 292–305.

Freda, M. C., Andersen, H. F., Damus, D., & Merkatz, I. R. (1993). What pregnant women want to know: A comparison of client and provider perception, *Journal of Obstetric, Gynecologic, and Neonatal Nursing, 22*(3), 237–244.

Friedman, M. (1992). *Family nursing, theory and practice.* Norwalk, CT: Appleton & Lange.

Feetham, S. L., Meister, S. B., Bell, J. M., & Gilliss, C. (1993). *The nursing of families: Theory/research, education/practice.* Newbury Park, CA: Sage Publications.

Galli, N., Greenbert, J. S., & Tobin, F. (1987). Health education and sensitivity to cultural religious and ethnic beliefs. *Journal of School Health, 57*(6), 177–180.

Gunn, P. (1991). *Grandmothers of the light.* Boston: Beacon Press.

Handler, A., & Rosenbert, D. (1992). Improving pregnancy outcomes: Public versus private care for urban, low-income women. *BIRTH, 19*(3), 123–130.

Higgenbotham, J. C., Trevino, F. M., & Ray, L. A. (1990). Utilization of curanderos by Mexican-Americans: Prevalence and predictors; finding from HANES, 1982–84. *American Journal of Public Health, 80*(Suppl.), 32–35.

Hsu, J. S., & Williams, S. D. (1991). Injury prevention awareness in an urban Native-American population. *American Journal of Public Health, 81*(11), 1466–1471.

Judkins, R. A., & Judkins, A. B. (1992). Commentary: Cultural dimensions of Hmong birth. *Birth, 19*(3), 148–150.

Kavanagh, K. H., & Kennedy, P. H. (1992). *Promoting cultural diversity: Strategies for health care professionals.* Newbury Park, CA: Sage Publications.

Lamarine, R. (1989). The dilemma of Native-American health. *Health Education, 20*(2), 15–18.

Leninger, M. (1990). Ethomethods: The philosophic and epistemic bases to explicate transcultural nursing knowledge. *Journal of Transcultural Nursing, 1*(2), 40–51.

Mattson, S., & Lew, L. (1992). Culturally sensitive prenatal care Southeast Asians. *Journal of Obstetric, Gynecologic, and Neonatal Nursing, 21*(1), 48–54.

Morris, T. M. (1990). Culturally sensitive family assessment: An evaluation of the family assessment device used with Hawaiian-American and Japanese-American families. *Family Process, 29*(6), 105–116.

Norbeck, J. S., & Tilden, V. P. (1983). Life stress, social support and emotional disequilibrium during pregnancy: A prospective, multivariate study. *Journal of Health and Social Behavior, 24*(6), 30–46.

Norbeck, J. S., & Anderson, N. J. (1989). Psychosocial predictors of pregnancy outcomes in low-income Black, Hispanic and white women. *Nursing Research, 38*(4), 204–209.

Norwood, S. L. (1994). First steps: participants and outcomes of a maternity services support system. *Journal of Obstetrics, Gynecologic and Neonatal Nursing, 23*(6), 467–476.

Patterson, E. T., Freese, M. P., & Goldenberg, R. L. (1990). Seeking safe passage: Utilizing health care during pregnancy. *Image, 22*(4), 27–31.

Pettitti, D., Coleman, C., Binsacca, D., & Allen, B. (1990). Early prenatal care in urban Black and white women. *BIRTH, 17*(1), 1–5.

Poss, J. E. (1989). Providing health care for Southeast Asian refugees. *Journal of New York State Nurses Association, 20*(4), 4–6.

Solis, J. M., Marks, G., Garcia, M., & Shelton, D. (1990). Acculturation, access to care, and use of preventive services by Hispanics: findings from HANES, 1982–84. *American Journal of Public Health, 80*(Suppl.), 11–19.

Spector, R. E. (1991). Cultural diversity in health and illness. Norwalk, CT/San Mateo, CA: Appleton & Lange.

Super, C., Herrara, M., & Mora, J. (1990). Long term effects of food supplement and psychosocial intervention on the physical growth of Colombian infants at risk for malnutrition. *Child Development, 61*(4), 29–49.

Thomson, E. J., & Cordero, J. F. (1992). The new teratogen: Accutane and other Vitamin A analogs. *MCN, 14*(4), 244–248.

Tilden, V. P. (1983). The relation of life stress and social support to emotional disequilibrium during pregnancy. *Research in Nursing and Health, 6*(4), 167–173.

U.S. Department of Health and Human Services, National Center for Health Statistics (1993). Advance report of official natality statistics, 1991. *Monthly Vital Statistics Report, 42*(Suppl.).

U.S. Department of Health and Human Services, Social Security Administration (1988). *Refugee resettlement program: Report to Congress* (pp. 1–56). Washington, DC: Author.

Walker, L. (1989). Longitudinal analysis of stress process among mothers and infants. *Nursing Research, 38*(6), 339–343.

Whall, A. L., & Fawcett, J. (1991). *Family theory development in nursing: State of the science and art.* Philadelphia: F.A. Davis.

Wilson, T. (Ed.) (1987). Handbook of teratology. New York: Plenum Press.

SUGGESTED READINGS

Marchione, J., & Stearns, S. J. (1990). Ethnic power perspectives for nursing. *Nursing and Health Care, 11*(6), 296–301.

McAdoo, J. (1993). The roles of African-American fathers: An ecological Perspective. *Families in society, 74*(1), 28–35.

Moore, R. (1991). Awakening the hidden storyteller. Boston: Shambhala. *Navajo Treaty.* (1868) Library of Congress number 68-29989.

Morris, T. M. (1990). Culturally sensitive family assessment: An evaluation of the family assessment device used with Hawaiian-American and Japanese-American families. *Family Process, 29*(6), 105–116.

Patterson, E. T., Freese, M. P., & Goldenberg, R. L. (1990). Seeking safe passage: Utilizing health care during pregnancy. *Image, 22*(4), 27–31.

Pruett, K. D. (1993). The paternal presence, families in society. *The Journal of Contemporary Human Services, 74*(1), 45–50.

5

Ethical and Legal Considerations

Objectives

- Develop an understanding of the ethical choices that must be made in maternity-perinatal care.
- Define ethics.
- List the three ethical principles underlying ethical decision making.
- Identify the characteristics that make ethical problems unique.
- Compare and contrast ethics and law.
- Develop an ability to differentiate between ethical and legal decisions.
- Discuss the nurse's role regarding accountability, particularly with respect to breach of duty and negligence.
- Describe the critical ethical and legal considerations for the client prior to conception, including those relating to abortion.
- Discuss the critical ethical, and legal considerations for the client during the childbearing cycle, including considerations regarding the mother, her fetus, and the newborn.

Key Terms

Artificial insemination	Justice
Autonomy	Laws
Beneficence	Malpractice
Ethical dilemma	Natural law
Ethics	Scope of practice
Gamete intrafallopian	Standards of care
transfer	Surrogate
In vitro fertilization	motherhood
and embryo transfer	

Maternity and perinatal nursing care often present more ethical and legal questions to the nurse than any other area of nursing care. Maternity and perinatal nurses provide a wide range of services and care for clients in a variety of different practice settings. These nurses are faced with the issues surrounding birth, life, death, and the ability to create life on a daily basis. Critical to these issues is the involvement of two clients, the mother and the fetus or newborn.

This chapter discusses the ethical and legal considerations involved with maternity and perinatal nursing care. As a foundation of this discussion, an overview of ethics, law, and nursing accountability is presented. Specific information surrounding the ethical and legal issues prior to conception, abortion, and care of the fetus, sick neonate, and mother is provided.

Overview of Ethics and Law

Before beginning the discussion about the complex area of ethical and legal considerations in reproduction, the terms used must be defined and clarified. There are distinct differences and similarities between ethics and laws.

Ethics

Ethics are the principles of conduct governing one's relationships with others. They are basic beliefs about values of right and wrong that provide a framework for decisions and actions. For example, ethics provide the basis for deciding whether or not to go to work in the morning. There are no rules in such a situation, so a personal decision must be made to do what is right. A person could pretend to be sick and stay home; however, colleagues, friends, and the community would agree that to feign illness is inappropriate behavior.

Moreover, an employer would have the right to dismiss an individual if this were a continuing occurrence. Sometimes situations arise in which a decision needs to be made, but no one solution seems completely satisfactory. An **ethical dilemma** exists. More than one solution may exist; however, they may be in opposition to each other. Any or all possible solutions may be unfavorable. Ethical decisions have consequences for oneself and others (Ellis et al., 1995).

Moral philosophers have identified three ethical principles that underlie moral judgments and ethical decision making. These are **beneficence,** respect for **autonomy,** and **justice** (Goode et al., 1993; Box 5-1). The nurse needs to weigh these principles when making ethical decisions about the welfare of her clients.

Laws

Laws are rules of conduct or action recognized as binding or enforced by a controlling authority, such as the local, state, or national government. They are designed to prevent the actions of one party from infringing of the rights of another party. All law is ultimately derived from **natural law,** the innate human tendency to do good and avoid evil. The U.S. federal government and the states hold constitutional authority to create and enforce laws. The legal system sets guidelines rather than rigid rules for practice. All laws, regardless of origin, are subject to change and interpretation. Ellis et al. (1995) make the point that ethics and the law may go hand in hand and support each other. If, for example, an individual chooses to steal money from an employer, the behavior is not only unethical but also illegal. Many laws are written to provide a basis for enforcing ethical principles that are deemed necessary for the well-being of the majority of the people.

Relationship Between Ethics and Law

Ethics may address different questions than does the law. The example of coming to work as expected is not governed by laws, although most people would have similar views in the situation. At times, though, individuals find that the law and their ethical beliefs diverge. An example might be a soldier required to kill enemy soldiers during a war. Whole countries consider this to be a legal act, but some people have ethical reservations and stipulate a conscientious objection when required to serve in the armed services. These individuals are often given noncombat assignments, although they may be in combat zones. A nursing example would be a nurse who objects to assisting with abortions, feeling that it is unethical to take the life of the fetus. The nurse could be assigned other duties in

---

BOX 5–1
*Ethical Principles Underlying
Moral Judgments*

- *Principle of beneficence:* The promotion of the welfare of others (a positive aspect) and doing no harm to others (a negative aspect)
- *Respect for autonomy:* The acknowledgement of the individual's freedom to be in control and make decisions
- *Principle of justice:* The governing of the distribution of benefit and harm and the addressing of who is included or excluded; fair and equal treatment of all

---

which personal ethics are not in conflict with the current law or practice.

Authors writing in the field of ethics make the point that not all choices or problems are ethical ones (Ellis et al., 1995; Reilly, 1989; Bushy et al., 1989). They outline several characteristics that make ethical problems unique:

- The problem cannot be resolved entirely from empirical data; for example, should a healthy person be forced to donate an organ to someone who would otherwise die without the donor organ? Clearly, any of the sciences cannot answer this question definitely. The various sciences and humanities can contribute information, but the answer lies beyond the competence of the scientific disciplines.
- The problem is inherently perplexing. There are conflicts of values and uncertainties about the amount or type of information needed to make a decision. If a newborn has repairable multiple congenital anomalies but has a chromosomal aberration that will eventually cause death at an early age, should aggressive efforts be made to keep the newborn alive as long as possible, even if these efforts may cause pain and suffering for the parents and the newborn?
- The answer to the ethical problem will have profound relevance for several areas of human concern. The decision will have far-reaching effects on one's perception of fellow human beings, the relationships among human beings, their relationship to society, and the relationship of various societies to the world at large. If, for example, the decision is made to force a person to donate a body part to a family member, the decision is based on several premises and assumptions (which may not be held by all societies): A person's right to bodily integrity may be violated if someone else can benefit by it; a person's right to life includes the right to require another to undergo painful surgery with the result of permanent loss of body part and damage to general

body integrity; and health professionals and others in authority can force or otherwise coerce a person to sacrifice body integrity for the well-being of another. This choice involves the concepts of human rights, the limits of benevolence, and the power of those in authority. Although the previous example is dramatic, other issues, such as a woman's right to take drugs and alcohol during pregnancy or how long to prolong the life of an irreparably damaged newborn, are less clear-cut. The nurse should apply the previous characteristics when determining whether or not a decision involves an ethical problem.

Legal Aspects of Maternity and Perinatal Care

The maternity and perinatal field has become especially high risk for **malpractice and professional negligence suits,** for several reasons. Some hospitals are facing financial crises, causing them to implement inadequate staffing patterns that can be dangerous for the client and nurse. In addition, advancements in technology for monitoring the mother and fetus preconceptually, conceptually, and postconceptually and the many techniques and procedures performed carry with them the risk of producing iatrogenic effects that can damage the mother, fetus, or both, sometimes irreversibly. Perhaps most importantly, there are potentially two claimants in any instance of mother-baby damage, thus doubling the risk to the nurse and other health providers (Ellis et al., 1995; Lederman, 1991).

Nursing Practice and Accountability

Nursing practice today is legislated by each state in the form of nurse practice acts. Nurse practice acts define the **scope of practice,** stating what the nurse is and is not allowed to do by establishing certain requirements for education, licensure, and standards of care. Because these requirements vary among the states, it is the nurse's responsibility to be familiar with the nurse practice act of the states in which he or she practices.

Standards of care describe the level of care that can be expected for practitioners. They are derived from the definition of nursing practice established by the nurse practice acts. Standards of care are developed by the hospitals or other institutions that employ the nurse and by professional organizations, such as the Association of Women's Health, Obstetric and Neonatal Nurses, formerly known as the Nurses Association of the American College of Obstetricians and Gynecologists. Nurses are held accountable to these standards. It is important for nurses to know and implement the accepted standards of care in their community, because failure do so would result in a *breach of duty* or a charge of *negligence* (Ellis et al., 1995). Certain facts are necessary to establish that a nurse has failed to conform to the standards of care; Box 5-2 lists these facts.

In nursing practice today, nurses are accountable for their clients' care not only morally and ethically, but legally as well. In the past, before healthcare became so complex and nurses expanded their roles, institutions and physicians were considered primarily responsible. However, with the increased independence in nursing came the responsibility to be accountable to the client for nursing care and to some degree, accountable for the client's well-being.

Accountability also extends beyond the nurse's individual sphere of care. If the nurse knows that the care given by other members of the health team is inappropriate or inferior, he or she also has the legal and ethical obligation to report such care to the appropriate authorities (Ellis et al., 1995; Purcell, 1988; Reilly, 1989). Legal action can be brought against a nurse for breach of duty or negligence. Personal liability insurance is a preventive measure to protect nurses from incurring large losses that may result from legal action against them. Every nurse should carry professional liability insurance. This is in addition to any insurance provided by the institution that employs the nurse. Institutional insurance generally covers the nurse only for the hours that he or she is on duty at the institution, not at other times when he or she might practice. The legal costs of a lawsuit and possible settlements or judgments can be devastating. Moreover, it is becoming more common for an institution to sue the nurse involved if the institution loses a malpractice suit (Ellis et al., 1995; Lederman, 1991). Because adequate coverage usually can be purchased at a reasonable price, it is a worthwhile investment for the nurse's personal protection.

Ethical and Legal Considerations Prior to Conception

Often a couple will have difficulty conceiving. The National Center for Health Statistics estimates that almost half of currently married women 15 to 44 years old suffer from some degree of infertility, and 10% of married couples fail to conceive after 1 year of no contraceptive use (Goode et al., 1993).

In the last 15 years, advances in medical engineering have resulted in methods of reproduction without intercourse, including artificial insemination and in vitro fertilization with embryo transfer (IVF/ET). As with contraception, artificial reproduction is defended by its proponents as life affirming while denounced by its detractors as unnatural. In addition, there has arisen what one author called a "hucksterism," or hype, surrounding much of the technology, particularly that of IVF/ET. Some see this hype as an exploitation of the infertile couple, especially when accompanied by the publicity about success rates that some centers use. Those professionals urging caution point out that the incidence of live births (not pregnancy) is still low with these techniques (Goode et al., 1993; Macklin, 1991; Shearer, 1988).

Artificial Insemination

Artificial insemination, the depositing of sperm at the cervical os or in the uterus by mechanical means, can be accomplished by two methods. In artificial insemination from the husband (AIH), sperm from the client's husband is deposited within her reproductive tract. This is perhaps the least controversial of all of the assisted reproductive methods, because it is clear who the genetic and sociologic parents are. Some religious denominations object to masturbation as a means of sperm collection, but this method generally is without grave ethical or legal questions.

The second method, artificial insemination from a donor (AID), is more problematic. With AID, the woman is inseminated with the sperm from an anonymous donor. This method separates the sociologic parent (the woman's husband) from taking part in his offspring's conception. AID has become the preferred treatment when the husband has an absence or

---

BOX 5-2
Facts to Establish Proof of Breach of Duty or Guilt of Negligence

Breach of Duty	Negligence
The nurse performs an unauthorized act.	The nurse had a responsibility to the client.
The nurse fails to act.	The nurse failed to carry out the responsibility.
The nurse carries out an authorized act improperly.	Injury was sustained by the client.
	A causal relationship existed between the client's injury and the nurse's breach of duty.

If the nurse is found guilty of a breach of duty, he or she may lose his or her license or be a defendant in a malpractice lawsuit. (Ellis, J. R., & Hartley, C. L. [1995]. Nursing in today's world [5th ed.]. Philadelphia: J. B. Lippincott.)

marked decrease in the amount of sperm. AID also is used when the husband suffers from a genetic defect or is Rh sensitized. This procedure has decreased in recent years because of the possibility of human immunodeficiency virus (HIV) transmission. Currently, all donors and each specimen are screened for HIV. As long as the husband of the woman consents, the donor is not considered the legal father of the child. Thus, the husband replaces the genetic father as the legal father of the child. As can be seen, this therapeutic model places contracts among the parties ahead of genetic or "bloodline" considerations. This model has been suggested as a model for embryonic transfer, but there is question as to whether it fits (Holmes, 1988; Macklin, 1991; Goode et al., 1993).

Legal obligations are satisfied by written, informed consent by all parties—wife, husband, and donor. Anonymity of all parties is recommended. It also is recommended that the physician be given the right to select the donor. This recommendation raises questions about the limits of authority for the professional, especially because there has been some scandal in recent years when the physician is given this right; the consent usually includes a clause removing liability from the health professionals if the child is born with abnormalities. The question of the child's legitimacy can be resolved by adoption (Goode, 1993; Bonnicksen, 1988).

In Vitro Fertilization and Embryo Transfer

In vitro fertilization and embryo transfer is a procedure in which an egg or eggs are removed from a woman's ovary, fertilized by sperm in a laboratory dish, cultured, and then transferred back into the woman's uterus when the embryo has reached the four- to six-cell stage. IVF is the only method of reproduction available for women whose fallopian tubes are damaged or missing. It also can be used for wives whose husbands have low sperm counts, women whose cervical mucus is nonreceptive to sperm, and women with infertility of unknown causes (Holmes, 1988; Ellis et al., 1995; Prattke et al., 1993).

A variety of ethical and legal questions have been raised regarding IVF/ET. The first live birth using IVF occurred in 1978, and by January 1984, more than 200 children had been born in the United States and abroad following IVF/ET.

In 1984, **gamete intrafallopian transfer** (GIFT) was developed; this procedure involves retrieving eggs from the woman and then transferring the eggs along with sperm into the ampullary portion of the fallopian tubes, usually using laparoscopy. It is the procedure of choice when there is at least one functional fallopian tube. Data suggest that the *pregnancy rate* is better with GIFT than with IVF/ET alone, perhaps due to the timing of implantation (Pace-Owens, 1989; Macklin, 1991; Goode et al., 1993).

The demand for these procedures continues to grow. According to the American Fertility Society, at least 46 centers in the United States have or are planning to have IVF clinics. Practically every major city where western medicine is practiced has at least one IVF/ET clinic. There have been five World Congresses devoted to this topic (Holmes 1988; Pace-Owens, 1989).

While these procedures move ahead clinically, there has been no federally funded research in humans since 1975 because of a de facto moratorium. Congress first imposed a temporary moratorium on fetal research on July 12, 1974 (Public law 93-348). This was lifted technically on August 8, 1975, when regulations were issued by what was then the Department of Health, Education, and Welfare. These regulations required all proposals dealing with IVF and fetal research to be reviewed by a national Ethics Advisory Board (EAB) in addition to the usual review by peer and Institutional Review Board for scientific merit. The EAB was duly but slowly constructed. It examined the topic of IVF thoroughly, concluding that although the controversy was legitimate, IVF/ET was acceptable from an ethical standpoint (Holmes, 1988; *Medical Ethics Advisor*, 1994). The major conclusions of the EAB are listed in Box 5-3. However, at subsequent public hearings and presentations to Congress, the response was overwhelmingly negative, so a de facto moratorium set in.

Over the years, the ethical and legal concerns have changed. The current concerns regarding IVF/ET can be summarized as follows:

- *The moral status of the fetus.* The human embryo is entitled to profound respect, but this respect does not necessarily encompass the full array of legal and moral rights attributed to a person. Mainstream ethicists and theologians generally concur that IVF/ET is not problematic as long as the EAB's guidelines are followed. Conservative theologians, however, believe that any tampering with the procreative process is unnatural and should not be attempted. Thus, the use of human embryos for research remains a problem (Raymond, 1990; Annas, 1988a).
- *Safety and efficacy.* During the late 1970s, there was only limited understanding about the risks involved with this procedure. As data have been collected, there is a good (but not conclusive) indication that there are no patterns of abnormality or short-term risks either in laboratory research with animals or in clinical experience with humans. Until further research is conducted, however, this concern will remain (*Medical Ethics Advisor*, 1994).

1. The department should consider support of carefully designed research involving in vitro fertilization and embryo transfer in animals, including nonhuman primates, to obtain a better understanding of the process of fertilization, implantation, and embryo development; to assess the risks to woman and offspring associated with such procedures; and to improve the efficacy of the procedure.
2. Research involving human in vitro fertilization and embryo transfer is ethically acceptable provided that if the research involves human in vitro fertilization without embryo transfer, these conditions must be satisfied:
   a. The research complies with the regulations governing research with human subjects.
   b. The research is designed to establish the safety and efficacy of embryo transfer and to obtain important scientific information not reasonably attainable by other means.
   c. Informed consent is obtained.
   d. No embryos will be sustained in vitro beyond the stage normally associated with the completion of implantation (14 days after fertilization).
   e. The public is advised of possible risk.

In addition, if the research involves embryo transfer following human in vitro fertilization, embryo transfer will be attempted only with gametes obtained from lawfully married couples.

(Adapted from Abramowitz, S [1984]. The stalemate on (test-tube) baby research. Part I. Test-tube. Hastings Center Report, 14(7).)

- *"The slippery slope."* This concern relates to the fear that research procedures performed on nonhuman mammalian species might be performed on human embryos with the results possibly leading to undesirable clinical applications. Some ethicists are concerned about extending the procedure to unmarried people, such as surrogate mothers and third-party donors. They see the basic relationship between husband and wife and the institution of marriage as being threatened. These were the same concerns that artificial insemination generated decades ago (Macklin, 1991; Schneider, 1994).
- *Funding and cost.* There is general acknowledgment that the procedure is costly. Although some believe that it is ethical to federally fund research projects relating to IVF, it should have a low national priority, because there are many other national health problems that are far more pressing. Those who oppose the procedure say that efforts would be better spent finding and preventing the causes of infertility and tubal obstruction (*Medical Ethics Advisor*, 1994).

Surrogate Motherhood

Surrogate motherhood involves the contractual hiring of a woman to bear another couple's child. The father's sperm may be used to impregnate the surrogate, or, in surrogate embryo transfer, the surrogate is implanted with the genetic parent's embryo. When the fetus is born, the surrogate mother relinquishes her rights to the newborn to the couple as per the terms of a contract.

Some people view this as another instance of collaborative reproduction, such as AID and IVF, saying these methods are no different ethically and legally from adoption, which separates conception and gestation from childrearing (Snowdon, 1994). However, ethical and legal issues remain.

There is the issue of "hiring" the surrogate mother. The mother typically receives a fee for carrying the child. Although this may seem fair for the surrogate mother's efforts, some find the idea of payment for producing a child repugnant and morally offensive. Children are reduced to commodities to be bought and sold. Some have suggested that mothers who need money may "sell" themselves as surrogates to keep their own families together. There also is the stress of the complex relationship involving a stranger in such an intimate context, which may be entangling and disturbing to the parties. For example, the surrogate may experience depression when giving up the child, or the couple may continue the relationship with the mother out of misplaced feelings of indebtedness. Third, the lineage of the children may become confused, and the fabric of the marriage may be damaged. However, it has been argued that although these concerns are legitimate, they must be balanced against the deep desires of the infertile couple to have children (Annas, 1988b; Raymond, 1990).

Legal concerns surround the contractual arrangements. It had been maintained that a well-drawn contract would obviate some of the difficulties in the three-way relationship. However, this was not true for the Baby C case litigated in California in 1990, wherein the surrogate mother abrogated the well-drawn contract with the parents by charging them with neglect during pregnancy and bonding to the newborn she carried. The surrogate mother is suing for shared custody of the child (Gerwertz 1990a; Gerwertz, 1990b). In the Baby C case and in the famed Baby M case, it is evident that well-drawn contracts can be contested, causing a great deal of stress for all parties, including the infant (Gerwertz, 1990a). Some critics also are concerned about cases in which neither party wants a child born with impairments or in which the surrogate is reluctant to surrender the newborn. The legality of such contracts remains a controversial issue, because the courts are still battling the extent to which these contracts are binding.

The amount of control the couple can exert over the surrogate also is a difficult issue. Certainly the couple wishes to ensure the best possible "environment" for the fetus and may want to regulate the surrogate's nutrition and lifestyle. Issues of the surrogate mother's right to privacy and freedom of choice come into play. Because of these and other complexities, Great Britain has made it a criminal offense for third parties to benefit from commercial surrogacy. However, voluntary surrogacy is still legal. Because of the legal climate and hostile public and medical sentiment surrounding surrogacy, the method is essentially banned in that country (Brahams, 1987; Annas, 1988b). Researchers caution that the use of a surrogate mother, even for a short time; the inconvenience of synchronizing the donor and recipient menstrual cycles; and the medical risks to the donor make this method less appealing to many (Prattke et al., 1993: Goode et al., 1993).

Amniocentesis

Amniocentesis has been available for more than a decade and is discussed fully in Chapter 13. Ethical and legal issues surrounding this procedure involve errors of omission or commission. For example, if a woman who is a candidate for the test because of age (older than 35 years) produces a child with a chromosomal anomaly or has a history of genetic disease and is not made aware of the test, the healthcare professional may be liable if she produces a defective newborn. Risks and benefits of the tests also must be explained to the client, and an informed consent must be obtained. If the mother has the test, is told that her fetus is normal, and then subsequently produces a defective newborn, the healthcare professional and laboratory performing the test could be held accountable. If the healthcare professional has personal beliefs about the efficacy of the test, opinions about whether the woman should abort if the test shows a defective fetus, or moral, ethical, or religious objections to the test, the healthcare professional nevertheless has the obligation to inform the client about the test and refer her elsewhere (Stern, 1988; Freda, 1994).

Ethical and Legal Considerations in Abortion

The current conflict between the prochoice and the prolife groups has rekindled the fires that have raged around the topic of abortion. Nurses must understand their own ethical position on this matter if they are to render quality care to their clients. Because the nurse is involved in counseling clients about abortions from a variety of standpoints, a brief review of the ethical and legal considerations is given in the following sections.

Ethical Considerations

The ethics involved in the abortion issue revolve around terminating the life of a fetus by removing it from its life support system. It has been argued that given a choice, humans would choose health and lack of suffering for themselves. Furthermore, the argument continues, humans do not have the right to inflict the tragic consequences of detectable diseases on a fetus. By aborting a defective fetus, "nothingness" results rather than the pain of living with an abnormality. The damaged fetus can be replaced with a normal one in a subsequent pregnancy. Although this line of reasoning supports aborting damaged fetuses, it does not address the ethics of aborting healthy (or unplanned) products of conception. It also raises the issue of who determines what is normal or healthy (Cohen, 1990; Overall, 1990; Freda, 1994).

Prochoice advocates take the position that the mother has the ultimate responsibility and freedom of choice about what happens to her body. Prochoice is not proabortion. Prochoice advocates stress using abortion only as a last resort. They uphold responsible use of contraception, amniocentesis to determine fetal defects, and adoption whenever possible. Prolife advocates believe that the fetus is human from the time of conception and that to destroy human life is murder and, hence, indefensible morally.

Legal Considerations

In 1973, in the historic Roe versus Wade case, the U.S. Supreme Court declared that abortion was legal anywhere in the United States. The decision rendered existing state laws prohibiting abortion as unconstitutional on the grounds that such laws invaded the mother's privacy (Annas, 1986a). The decision also stipulated several other points:

- A state *could not* prevent a woman from obtaining an abortion from a licensed physician any time during the first trimester.
- The state *could* regulate the performance of an abortion to protect the woman's health during the second trimester.
- The state *could* regulate and even prohibit abortions in the third trimester, except when the mother's life or health might be jeopardized.
- The state had the right to impose safeguards for the fetus in the last trimester.

BOX 5–4
Legal Status of Abortion

In 1973, the United States Supreme Court ruled that abortion was legal. A summary of the decision follows:

- The abortion decision and its implementation must be left to the judgment of the woman and her physician when pregnancy is in the first trimester.
- After the first trimester and before the end of the second trimester, the state, in promoting its interest in the health of the pregnant woman, may choose to regulate abortions in ways that are reasonably related to health.
- After pregnancy has reached the time of viability (defined as 24 to 26 weeks' gestation), the state, in promoting its interest in the potentiality of human life, may, if it chooses, regulate and even proscribe abortion, except when it is necessary, in medical judgment, to preserve the life or health of the pregnant woman.

In 1976, the Supreme Court further ruled that the state cannot impose the requirement of consent by a third party on the woman's right to abortion; thus, abortion cannot be denied if a spouse or parent objects.

In 1983, the Supreme Court struck down state restrictions that impose waiting periods for first-trimester abortions, that require specific informed consents, and that require hospitalization for second-trimester abortions.

Although states can implement requirements for parental notification of abortion services to pregnant minors, this can be waived by a state court or administrative agency if the minor is judged mature enough to give informed consent.

Implications of Roe Versus Wade

The decision did not provide "abortion on demand." It was the intent that physicians would still use their clinical judgment when clients requested abortion.

The law also did not consider pregnant minors. Some states allow pregnant minors to have an abortion without parental consent. A precedent of sorts was set in 1981 when the Supreme Court upheld the constitutionality of a Utah law that required physicians to inform parents of a minor's request for abortion (Annas, 1986a; Annas, 1989; Overall, 1990).

A major problem with the ruling is that there was no decision as to when life begins. The Court felt that because no other scholars or scientist were able to reach a consensus opinion on this matter, it would be presumptuous for the Court to do so. They did decide that the fetus was not a "person" for the purposes of the 14th amendment and that neither the father of the fetus nor the woman's husband had the right to interfere in or prevent the abortion (Annas, 1989; Overall, 1990; Freda, 1994). The issue of when life actually begins

and when the fetus becomes a person continues to be debated.

In many states, there are laws that include "conscience clauses," which allow institutions, health providers, and others to refuse to assist in abortions without risk of reprisal if participation is against their moral, ethical, or religious beliefs. However, public hospitals must allow the use of their facilities for abortion because they are supported by public funds (Box 5-4).

Reaffirmation of Women's Rights. At the center of the debate about abortion is the issue of women's rights. Ethicists point out that abortion must remain a moral decision for the mother unless sexual inequality is to be governmentally institutionalized. The Roe versus Wade decision is somewhat of a technological decision, because it still relies on medical technology and expertise to ascertain the viability of the fetus and to determine at what stage of pregnancy abortion is safer for the woman. However, there are positive and negative sides to decisions based solely on available technology. For example, if advances in drug technology produce a safe method of allowing all women to self-induce early abortion by way of medication, then abortion decisions will be automatically removed from governmental interference. However, such methods will confuse the distinction between methods of contraception and methods of abortion, allowing women to find the whole issue less morally troubling (Annas, 1986a; Annas, 1989; Cohen, 1990).

Abortion Opponents Continue to Seek Legislation

Abortion opponents continue to seek laws and regulations that discourage or restrict abortions. See Box 5-5 for some of the tactics used to try and restrict abor-

BOX 5–5
Tactics to Restrict Abortion

- State laws that require physicians to take the same degree of care in aborting a possibly viable fetus as they would take in delivery of a live birth
- Requiring physicians to use the abortion method most likely to result in fetal survival, unless this significantly increases risk to the woman; impacts on second-trimester abortions and often involves fetuses with diagnosed genetic abnormalities
- Increasing the burden to providers and the woman through reporting or lengthy information requirements, including filing the reports, which contain personal and social data, with state health departments.

Cohen (1990); Freda (1994).

tions. The constitutionality of such proposed regulations usually is tested before the Supreme Court by such advocates of legalized abortion as Planned Parenthood, the National Organization for Women, and the American Public Health Association. The Supreme Court has, in the past, upheld the principle that a woman's right to choose may not be burdened with excessive or discouraging regulations. However, the changing political composition of the Court is a crucial factor and leaves open the possibility of more conservative and restrictive interpretations (Cohen, 1990; Freda, 1994).

Ethical and Legal Considerations for the Fetus, Sick Newborn, and Mother

Perhaps the area in perinatology and neonatology that is most fraught with dissension, discussion, debate, and ethical and legal dilemmas is the areas of neonatal intensive care and fetal research and treatment. Ironically, many of the problems in this area are a result of the technological advances developed in the field of neonatology and perinatology. Fetuses that would have naturally aborted or been stillborn 5 years ago now often can be sustained in utero until they are almost full term. Infants who had no chance of survival a decade ago now may look forward to a relatively healthy and productive life. What, then, is the cause for debate?

As technology and expertise continue to increase, there will be more attempts to save fetuses at earlier and earlier stages, even those with severe conditions. In many of these cases, the "saved" newborn may be severely physically or mentally handicapped. Heroic efforts are made by health professionals to prolong life, when it is questionable whether it is in the best interest of the newborn or family. Health providers and parents are often faced with these ethical and moral dilemmas because of federal regulations and guidelines (Cunningham et al., 1990; Penticuff, 1994).

The Fetus

The fetus has rights from the time of conception and can be a beneficiary of a trust and inherit property. Although not legally considered a person until born, the rights of the fetus have been upheld in courts. For example, a woman was ordered to have a cesarean section by the courts because of fetal distress. The woman had refused the procedure and was adamant about leaving the hospital. After conferring with her, the legal staff of the hospital procured a court order for the woman to undergo the cesarean section. This was the first time a woman had been legally coerced into surgery. In another case, the courts ordered a mother who was a Jehovah's Witness to have a blood transfusion to save the life of her fetus (Nelson et al., 1988; Mattingly, 1992).

Fetal Research

Although federal funding for fetal research remains a controversial issue, many advocates believe the research has great potential for preventing costly diseases. However, many states have made fetal research illegal, especially when the fetus is an abortus or is still in utero. The ethics of fetal tissue transplants are hotly debated. Several difficult questions have been raised regarding the rights of the mother versus the rights of the fetus:

- Does the woman have the right to determine what will be done with fetal remains?
- Does a woman who plans an abortion have the right to allow experimentation in utero?
- Can an aborted fetus be kept alive for experimental purposes?

Federal guidelines require that fetal research be designed to meet the needs of the fetus, be of minimal risk, and have the potential to develop important medical knowledge. These global guidelines allow for wide interpretation. Experts agree that we are on the threshold of great discoveries. However, with this progress will come even more difficult decisions for expectant parents and those who care for them (Stotland, 1990; Ryan, 1990; Robertson, 1994; McCormick, 1994).

Fetal Therapy

Advances in technology have resulted in the ability to drain spinal fluid from the brain of a fetus (cephalocentesis), catheterize the fetus in utero, remove its lower body from the uterus to repair a urinary tract obstruction, transfuse the fetus in utero, repair gastroschisis, and surgically repair skeletal defects. Although these are certainly milestones in the area of therapy, investigators generally advise caution and note the experimental nature of many of the treatments (McCormick, 1994; Grodin, 1990; Evans et al., 1990). Those who take a more conservative approach state that the only anatomic malformations that warrant consideration are those that interfere with fetal organ development and that if alleviated, would allow normal fetal development to proceed.

The Committee on Bioethics of the American Academy of Pediatrics (1990) points out that the woman and her fetus are being viewed more often as two treatable entities. They caution, however, that while some fetal diagnostic procedures and treatments in utero, such as amniocentesis and intrauterine transfusion of the fetus, have become standard practices of proven efficacy, other fetal interventions, such as shunt diversions for hydrocephalus or obstructive uropathy, are considered research procedures and are not standard medical practice. Thus, their use is equivocal at this time. In their opinion, these interventions should be registered with the international registry that has been established to record experience with these experimental interventions. In general, this opinion is held by a majority of practitioners in the field, but others want to push the frontiers of research in the interest of future "common good" (Grodin, 1990; Stotland, 1990; Robertson, 1994).

Ethical and legal questions and possible conflicts can emerge as these treatments are used more frequently. What happens if a physician feels he or she can help a fetus, but the mother refuses consent, or the surgical consent is ambiguous? If a court orders the mother to submit to fetal treatment, does this invade her right to privacy and her own body integrity? Could she be charged with fetal abuse if she refuses treatment? Is the risk-to-benefit ratio favorable enough to cause this costly therapy to be a national priority? Finally, who will be required to pay for these experimental procedures? Health insurance often refuses coverage in "experimental" conditions (Grodin, 1990; Ryan, 1990). Answers to these questions are not easy, and solutions are becoming more difficult as technology improves.

The Sick Newborn

Ethical and legal questions and conflicts also emerge for the sick newborn. How much should a newborn have to suffer for the sake of life? More importantly, which should be regarded more highly—the sanctity of life or the quality of life? Doctors, nurses, and parents will continue to face these dilemmas as infant mortality rates continue to decline. Of the approximately 3.5 million newborns delivered in the United States each year, about 250,000 are born with significant defects or experience a birth injury. Clearly, medicine is advancing in its effort to save lives, but the long-range outcomes may be questionable.

Effects of Invasive Procedures

Some of the procedures deemed necessary for a sick newborn can have an iatrogenic effect, resulting in another disease or defect. For example, prolonged use of ventilators can scar respiratory passages. Oxygen therapy, if it is give at too high a concentration, can cause varying degrees of vision impairment. Newborns are subjected to numerous needle punctures, tubes down their throats, and catheters into their hearts, bladders, and other orifices. Healthcare providers often view the newborn's suffering as justifiable, something that must be endured to make the newborn better in the long term. Although this point of view enables them to practice with less guilt and is often required by current legal regulations, it may be dismal from the newborn's point of view. The newborn clearly has no choice, unlike adults who have the option of refusing treatment. Therefore, the decision about what is reasonable treatment for newborns is more difficult (Mattingly, 1992; Cunningham et al., 1990).

There is a growing consensus among providers and ethicists that society must come to terms with several difficult questions in the next few years:

- Should the lives of certain newborns be saved only to have them lead lives of pain, disability, and deprivation?
- Should the newborn who would not otherwise survive without major intervention be left to die? If so, who makes the decision?
- What is the family's role in these decision? How much power should the family have in decision making?
- What kind of care does one deny or give a newborn to allow death with comfort and dignity?

Baby Doe Regulations

Some of the questions listed previously have received partial, although ambiguous, answers in the controversial "Baby Doe" regulations (Carter, 1993; Gates, 1990; Evans et al., 1990). In March 1983, the first Baby Doe regulation was issued by the Secretary of the Department of Health and Human Services (DHHS). This was in response to a report that an infant with Down's syndrome had died in an Indiana hospital because her esophageal atresia was left uncorrected. The main thrust of the regulation was the threat to remove federal funding from hospitals that did not comply with a notice to be posted stating that failure to feed or care for handicapped infants was against federal law. In addition, a Baby Doe hotline was established to allow reporting of suspected hospital failures to comply. Some alleged failures were reported, and "Baby Doe squads" were dispatched to suspected hospitals. This resulted in major disruptions at all levels, including actual medical and nursing care. Charts were confiscated, providers were interrogated, and time was taken from care. It was eventually proved that the hospitals in question were entirely blameless.

The American Academy of Pediatrics and others sought an injunction against the regulation. This was denied. However, a waiting period was granted in which public comment was to be solicited. Debate was heated. Healthcare professionals felt the judicial system was interfering with decision making that was in the purview of the healthcare providers and the parents and was insidiously labeling the parties "child abusers." In September 1983, the regulation was reissued with only little change. One of the changes was the posting of hotline notices only in nurses' stations, presumedly to encourage nurses to report "abuse," because they often were "afraid of reprisal" otherwise. Nurses, neonatologists, and ethicists have stated that this was a demeaning rationalization for nurses, because it infers that nurses are not intelligent, participating members of the health team (Hastings Center Report, 1986; Baggs, 1993; Carter, 1993).

On October 11, 1983, a newborn was born in Port Jefferson, New York, with multiple neural tube defects. After consulting with physicians and their Roman Catholic priest, the parents chose conservative medical rather than surgical treatment to reduce the chance of infection rather than correct the defects. A lawyer in Vermont, unrelated to any of the participants, managed to get a court order to appoint a guardian *ad latem* for the child (depriving the parents of their parental authority) to have the surgery performed. The trial court's ruling was struck down eventually by New York's State Court of Appeals. The court commented on the often "offensive activities of those who sought to displace parental responsibility for management of her medical care." Nevertheless, fears were aroused once more about the possibility of further interference in the provider–client relationship (Carter, 1993).

In January 1984, what were thought to be the final regulations pertaining to handicapped infants were issued by the Secretary of DHHS. They were entitled, "Nondiscrimination on the Basis of Handicap, 1984." Legal rights of handicapped infants were required to be posted. State protective services were to develop procedures for protecting infants from medical neglect. The regulations did not require neonatal intensive care units to provide futile efforts to prolong the act of dying. Hospitals were encouraged (but not required) to set up infant care review committees (ICRC) to review all cases of infants who might be deprived of care because of their health conditions(s). The American Academy of Pediatrics has developed guidelines for the composition and duties of such a committee, regarding them as viable alternatives to hotlines and squads of investigators (Carter, 1993).

On May 15, 1985, the latest Baby Doe regulation went into effect as the Child Abuse Amendments of 1985 to Public Law 98-457—the Child Abuse Prevention and Treatment Act (Murray, 1985). Included in this amendment are the following definitions:

- **Medical neglect:** withholding of medically indicated treatment from a disabled infant with a life-threatening condition.

- **Withholding medically indicated treatment:** failure to respond to the infant's life-threatening conditions by providing treatment (including appropriate nutrition, hydration, and medication) which, in the treating physician's (or physicians') reasonable medical judgement, will be most likely to be effective in ameliorating or correcting all such conditions.

- **Withholding medical treatment is not neglect under three conditions:**

    The infant is chronically and irreversibly comatose.

    The provision of such treatment would merely prolong dying, not be effective in ameliorating or correcting all of the infant's life-threatening conditions, or otherwise be futile in terms of the survival of the infant.

    The provision of such treatment would be virtually futile in terms of the survival of the infant and the treatment itself under such circumstances would be inhumane.

- **Reasonable medical judgement:** medical judgement that would be made by a reasonably prudent physician knowledgeable about the case and the treatment possibilities with respect to the medical treatment involved.

However, the amendment has had minimal impact on medical and ethical decision making, because the trend is toward aggressive treatment of nonlethal conditions and the narrowing of parents' and physicians' discretion on treatment decisions (the "best interest of the infant" standard). Moreover, although encouraging hospitals to form ICRCs, DHHS was careful to maintain that these are only guidelines. DHHS does not offer sanctions or rewards for their establishment. Confusion remains about the language, particularly the "chronically and irreversibly comatose" phrase, which is interpreted in narrow and broader senses depending on the judge and attorneys (Hasting Center Report, 1986; Carter, 1993).

Carter (1993) has pointed out that these regulations have not changed decision making or care practices by neonatologists in the sample he studied. Comfort care, limited care, and withdrawal of support when appropriate was noted. Thus, exceptional measures and invasion of the mother's and infant's body integrity were not found (see Research Highlight). This aspect of care, however, continues to be fraught with ethical and legal issues.

The Mother

One controversial legal and ethical issue surrounding the mother is whether pregnant women should be compelled by law to receive medical or surgical treat-

RESEARCH HIGHLIGHT

Use of Hospital Ethics Committees

The use of hospital ethics committees or infant care review committees has been recommended for difficult decisions regarding federal regulations that have become known as "The Baby Doe Regulations." The author surveyed both military and civilian neonatologists and found that ethics committees had been established in 27 of their 28 hospitals, however, fewer than 50% had infant care review committees. The data were obtained from a mailing to all neonatologists in the Army, Air Force, Navy, and Public Health Service stationed at 18 medical centers in the U.S., Europe, and the Philippines (*n*=46). Additional mailings were sent to all practicing civilian neonatologists in Colorado at 10 different NICUs (*n*=46). A second mailing or telephone follow-up was made to non-respondents. Thirty four (74%) neonatologists responded from the military, and 23 (62%) civilian neonatologists responded. This response rate is adequate for the descriptive analysis that was done, although 62% borders on marginal.

Despite the frequency of potential cases for committee review, the committees were seldom consulted. The educational background of the neonatologists indicated that at least 62% had received ethics education during their professional careers. The majority made difficult decisions in conjunction with parents or used a multidisciplinary patient care conference. Use of the conferences antedated any federal regulations. Sixty-seven percent indicated that the Baby Doe Regulation had affected neither their thinking about ethical issues nor their practice. In 13 hypothetical cases in delivery room, intensive care nursery, and long-term care settings, the provision of comfort care, limited care, or withdrawal of support was noted by a sizable percentage of neonatologists, except in the case of meningomyelocele and trisomy 21, which tended to receive maximal support. The aggressive support for these conditions has become the standard of practice in most communities. The author concludes that the need for an ethics committee input for neonates is questionable, but the value of multidisciplinary deliberations and parental input in the difficult cases is obvious. He feels that the resultant process of decision making continues to reflect the maturation of both the healthcare professional team and the contemporary society that is served by them.

Critique: The study is timely and, in general, well done. However, the small sample size does not lend itself to generalizability. The description of the questionnaire in the materials and methods section is brief but may be a function of the particular requirements of the journal, which favors brevity. Tables are concise and easy to read, and the discussion is clearly written. The conclusions the author draws are consistent with the data presented, and he concludes with a well-defined point that there is a continued need to address these ethical issues even though the federal regulations advise a different type of input than that which has become the standard of care.

Carter, B. S. (1993). Neonatologists and bioethics after Baby Doe. *Journal of Perinatology, 13*(2), 144–150.

ment for benefit of the fetus. Several cases of unusual circumstances have focused on these issues. In one case, the ethical question revolved around the appropriateness of using life support systems on the mother for a short period to improve substantially the outcome of the fetus. It has been noted that the use of the mother's body to serve the interest of her fetus would be permissible if the mother had given prior consent or signed an anatomic donation card. Without the mother's consent, permission must be obtained from next of kin (Annas, 1986b). Such cases inevitably create controversy and conflicting opinions between relatives and the healthcare providers. They raise questions about the limits of benevolence, authority, and the right of the client to bodily integrity. In the present climate, this opinion would not be held by the majority of clients, health personnel, and ethicists.

In April 1990, the District of Columbia court of Appeals issued its opinion in *Re A. C.*, the much publicized case involving a court-ordered cesarean section performed on a dying woman in June 1987. The court's decision holding that "in virtually all cases the question of what is to be done is to be decided by the client— the pregnant woman—on behalf of herself and the fetus," is a precedent-setting reaffirmation of a pregnant woman's autonomy in making her own healthcare decisions (Allen, 1990). The student can read the details of this precedent-setting ruling from the sources listed in the suggested readings list.

In its commentary, the court emphasized the importance of the client's bodily integrity and reaffirmed that this belongs to *competent and incompetent* people. Its decision also recognized judicially the autonomous decision-making authority of the pregnant woman, further stating that the court should not even engage in a balancing of maternal and fetal interests. This opinion is consistent with the American College of Obstetricians and Gynecologists (ACOG) Committee Opinion on Maternal-Fetal Conflict. With the decision rendered in *A. C.*, it is hoped that health providers will avoid resorting to the courts (Allen, 1990). Unlike the extreme case noted previously, there is still question regarding just how far laws should extend to compel women to accept even routine medical or surgical treatment for the benefit of the fetus during pregnancy. Such treatments could include attending frequent medical appointments, submitting to various tests and treatments, or even complying with medical recommendations to refrain from sexual intercourse, taking drugs, consuming alcohol, or exercise. In the eyes of some, if the mother refuses to comply with the suggested regimen, she should be liable to criminal prosecution. Most ethicist and physicians believe, however (as reaffirmed in *A. C.*), that no legal, ethical, or moral basis justifies requesting the courts to order a woman to undergo a medical or surgical procedure for the benefit of the fetus, particularly when the pregnant woman objects to the proscription, treatment, or procedure (Nelson et al., 1988; Annas, 1986b; Ryan, 1990; Gates, 1990).

Nurse's Responsibility

The nurse working in maternal and perinatal care has a responsibility to the woman and fetus or newborn. An understanding of one's own values and beliefs together with knowledge of the standards of care, scope of practice, and legal regulations aid in effective decision making.

The nurse has certain obligations to the woman. He or she must have the knowledge and expertise to use the equipment necessary for the woman's care, particularly fetal monitors. He or she should be familiar with the guidelines for monitoring developed by ACOG. The nurse must be proficient in reading the monitor accurately, making appropriate notations, and reporting complications to the physician immediately. Monitoring tapes should be appropriately stored, because often they are important evidence in the event of a medical malpractice suit.

The importance of the nurse recording promptly and accurately his or her observations, treatments, procedures, medicines, and any other appropriate information cannot be stressed enough. Many weak malpractice cases come to court because of errors or omissions in charting and recording (see the suggested readings list).

Another important area of responsibility is to observe the newborn and mother carefully after delivery and report and record any signs of a complication or problem. Nurses can be held liable in the event of maternal or newborn complications. It is extremely important that they are knowledgeable regarding their appropriate responsibilities and care.

Summary Points

✔ Ethics and laws are similar, but they also have distinct differences. Not all problems or choices the nurse must make are ethical ones.

✔ An ethical problem is unique because 1) the problem cannot be resolved entirely from empirical data; 2) the problem is inherently perplexing; and 3) the answer to the ethical problem will have profound relevance for several areas of human concern.

✔ Nurses are accountable for their actions based on standards of care. To establish guilt or negligence of the nurse in her practice, the following must be proven: 1) The nurse had a responsibility to the client. 2) The nurse failed to carry out that responsibility. 3) Injury was sustained by the client. 4) There was a causal relationship between the

client's injury and the nurse's breach of duty. A breach of duty occurs when the nurse fails to act, performs an unauthorized act, or carries out an authorized act improperly.

✔ A variety of ethical and legal concerns have arisen for the client prior to conception relating to the medical engineering developed to combat infertility. These include concerns in the area of artificial insemination, IVF/ET, and surrogate motherhood. Of these, IVF/ET and surrogate motherhood are the most controversial.

✔ Concerns about IVF/ET include the moral state of the fetus, which entitles it to profound respect but not necessarily the full array of human rights attributed to a person who has been born; safety and efficiency of the procedures, which have yet to be proven to be free of long-term risks; the "slippery slope," which relates to the fear that experiments performed on nonhuman mammalian species might be performed on human embryos and result in undesirable clinical applications; and funding and expenditures for these highly technical procedures, which are costly, and the concern about the deployment of limited research funds for such endeavors.

✔ Baby Doe regulations are still in force, but research indicates that they do appear to have influenced the thinking or care that health providers render.

✔ The rendering of the decision of *A. C.* set a precedent that reaffirmed the right of the mother to her bodily integrity; that is, she cannot be ordered by healthcare professionals or the court or otherwise coerced to undergo a treatment, procedure, or medical regimen that she does not want, even if the well-being of the fetus is at stake. This decision coincides with the recommendations of ACOG.

✔ Nurses working in maternity and perinatal care have obligations to the woman and the fetus or newborn. A thorough knowledge base, careful observation and monitoring, and accurate recording and reporting are essential.

REFERENCES

Allen, A. E. (1990). In re A. C.—An affirmation of ACOG committee opinion number 55: Maternal-fetal conflict. *Women's Health Issues, !*(1), 37–40.

Annas, G. J. (1986a). Roe vs. Wade reaffirmed, again. *Hastings Center Report, 16*(3), 26–27.

Annas, G. J. (1986b). Pregnant women as fetal containers. *Hastings Center Report, 16*(6), 13–14.

Annas, G. J. (1988a). *Redefining parenthood and protecting embryos, in Judging Medicine.* Clifton, NJ: Humana Press.

Annas, G. J. (1988b). Death without dignity for commercial surrogacy; The case of Baby M. *Hastings Center Report, 16*(3), 21–24.

Annas, G. J. (1989) Webster and the politics of abortion. *Hastings Center Report, 19*(6), 36–38.

(1994). The future of human embryo research: NIH guidelines raise concerns about public education. *Medical Ethics Advisor, 10*(8), 103–104.

Baggs, J. G. (1993). Collaborative interdisciplinary bioethical decision making in intensive care units. *Nursing Outlook, 41*(3), 108–112.

Bonnicksen, A. (1988). Some consumer aspects of in vitro fertilization. *Birth, 15*(3), 145–147.

Brahams, D. (1987). The hasty British ban on commercial surrogacy. *Hasting Center Report, 17*(3), 16–19.

Bushy, A., Randall, R., & Matt, B. F. (1989). Ethical principles; Applications to an obstetric case. *Journal of Obstetric, Gynecologic, and Neonatal Nursing, 18*(3), 7–212.

Carter, B. S. (1993). Neonatologists and bioethics after Baby Doe. *Journal of Perinatiology, 13*(2), 144–150.

Cohen, S. S. (1990). Health care policy and abortion: A comparison. *Nursing Outlook, 38*(1), 20–25.

Committee on Bioethics of the American Academy of Pediatrics (1990). Fetal therapy: Ethical considerations. *Women's Health Issues, 1*(1), 16–17.

Committee on Ethics of the American College of Obstetricians and Gynecologists (1990). Patient choice: Maternal-fetal conflict. *Women's Health Issues, 1*(1), 13–15.

Confusion over the language of the Baby Doe regulations (1986). *Hastings Center Report, 162*(2), 1–2.

Cunningham, S. H. (1990). Myths in health care ethics. *Image, 23*(4), 235–238.

Elkins, T. E. (1990). The case for a middle ground. *Women's Health Issues, !*(1), 34–36.

Ellis, J. R., & Hartley, C. L. (1995). *Nursing in today's world* (5th ed.). Philadelphia: J. B. Lippincott.

Evans, M. I., Johnson, M. P., & Holzgrove, W. (1990). Fetal therapy: The next generation. *Women's Health Issues, 1*(1), 31–33.

Freda, M. C. (1994). Childbearing, reproductive control, aging women, and health care: The projected ethical debates. *Journal of Obstetric, Gynecologic, and Neonatal Nursing, 23*(2), 144–152.

Gates, E. A. (1990). Maternal choice: Will it work both ways? *Women's Health Issues, 1*(1), 25–27.

Gewertz, C. (1990a). Genetic parents given sole custody of child,. *Los Angeles Times, October 23,* A1, A23.

Gewertz, C. (1990b). Surrogate-born baby now with genetic parents. *Los Angeles Times, September 23,* A1, A28.

Goode, C. J., & Hahn, J. F. (1993). Oocyte donation and in vitro fertilization: The nurses role with ethical and legal issues *Journal of Obstetric, Gynecologic, and Neonatal Nursing, 22*(2), 106–111.

Grodin, M. A. (1990). Patient choice and fetal therapy. *Women's Health Issues, 1*(1), 18–20.

Hardwig, J. (1990). What about the family? *Hastings Center Report, 20*(2), 5–10.

Holmes, H. B. (1988). In vitro fertilization: Reflections on the state of the art. *Birth, 15*(3), 134–145.

Lederman, R. P. (1991). Professional liability and obstetrical health care delivery. *Nursing Outlook, 39*(1), 14–21.

Macklin, R. (1991). Maternal-fetal conflict: An ethical analysis. *Women's Health Issues, 1*(1), 28–30.

Mattingly, S. S. (1992). The maternal-fetal diad: Exploring the two-patient obstetric model. *Birth, 22*(1), 13–18.

McCormick, R. A. (1994). Blastomere separation. *Hastings Center Report, 24*(2), 14–16.

Murray, T. H. (1985). The final anticlimactic rule on Baby Doe. *Hastings Center Report, 15*(3), 5–7.

Nelson, L. J., & Milliken, N. (1988). Compelled medical treatment of pregnant women: Life, liberty and law in conflict. *Journal of the American Medical Association, 259*(5), 1060.

Overall, C. (1990). Selective termination of pregnancy and women's reproductive autonomy. *Hastings Center Report, 20*(3), 6–11.

Pace-Owens, S. (1989). Gamite intrafallopian transfer (GIFT). *Journal of Obstetric, Gynecologic, and Neonatal Nursing, 18*(2), 93–97.

Pearse, W. H. (1990). Maternal-fetal conflict. *Women's Health Issues, 1*(1), 12–13.

Penticuff, J. (1994). Ethical issues in genetic therapy. *Journal of Obstetrics, Gynecologic, and Neonatal Nursing, 23*(6), 498–501.

Prattke, T. W., & Gass-Sternas, K. A. (1993). Appraisal, coping and emotional health of Infertile couples undergoing donor artificial insemination. *Journal of Obstetric, Gynecologic, and Neonatal Nursing, 22*(3), 516–527.

Purcell, G. (1988), Quality assurance/utilization management and risk management; Deterrents to professional liability. *Clinical Obstetrics and Gynecology, 31*(1), 162–168.

Raymond, J. G. (1990). Reproductive gifts and gift giving: The altruistic woman. *Hastings Center Report I, 20*(6), 7–11.

Reilly, D. E. (1989). Ethics and values in nursing: Are we opening Pandora's box? *Nursing and Health Care, 10*(2), 91–95.

Robertson, J. A. (1994). The question of human cloning. *Hastings Center Report, 24*(2), 6–14.

Ryan, K. J. (1990). Erosion of the rights of pregnant women: In the interest of fetal well-being. *Women's Health Issues, 1*(1), 21–24.

Schneider, C. E. (1994). Bioethics in the language of the law. *Hastings Center Report, 24*(4), 16–22.

Schneider, C. E. (1988). Rights discourse and neonatal euthanasia. *California Law Review, 76,* 151–176.

Shearer, B. H. (1988). Some effects of assisted reproduction on Perinatal care. *Birth, 15*(3), 131–133.

Snowden, C. (1994). What makes a mother? Interviews with women involved in egg donation and surrogacy. *Birth, 21*(2), 77–84.

Stern, L. (1988). On ethics, difficult choices and the responsibility of physicians. *Journal of Perinatology, 1, 8*(3), 81.

Stotland, N. L. (1990). Social change and women's reproductive health care, *Women's Health Issues, 1*(1), 4–11.

Williams, L. S. (1988). It's going to work for me: Responses to failures of IVF. *Birth, 15*(3), 154–156.

SUGGESTED READINGS

Allen, A. E. (1990). In re A. C.—An Affirmation of ACOG Committee Opinion Number 55: Maternal-Fetal Conflict. *Women's Health Issues, 1*(1), 37–40.

Baggs, J. G. (1993). Collaborative interdisciplinary bioethical decision making in intensive care units. *Nursing Outlook, 41*(3), 108–112.

Schifrin, B. S. (1990). Polemics in perinatology: The abortion thing. *Journal of Perinatology, 10*(3), 81–83.

Smith, J. B. (1989). Ethical issues raised by new treatment options. *MCN, 14*(3), 183–187.

Snowdon, C. (1994). What makes a mother? Interviews with women involved in egg donation and surrogacy. *Birth, 21*(2), 77–84.

Ward, C. J. (1991). Analysis of 500 obstetric and gynecologic malpractice claims: Causes and prevention. *American Journal of Obstetrics and Gynecology, 165*(6), 298–306.

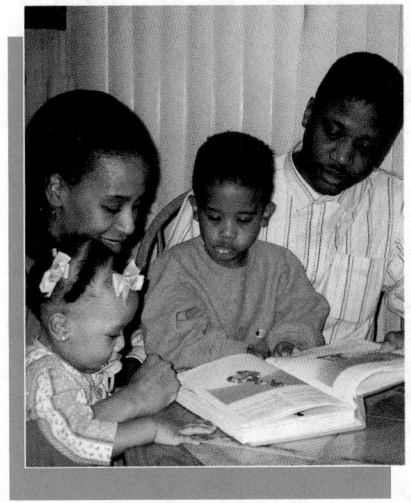

Nursing, Family Health, and Reproduction

Critical Thinking Exercises

1. Jennifer Chin, age 28, has come to the women's health clinic associated with a Level III perinatal healthcare facility suspecting that she is pregnant for the first time. History and physical examination reveal that she is 9 weeks pregnant. Jennifer is married and has a supportive family nearby. She states, "I'm so excited. I can't wait to tell my husband. He'll be thrilled!"

    You begin discussing the options available for perinatal care with Jennifer. She states, "One of my friends used a midwife and another one had a nurse practitioner. They both used natural childbirth and were fine. My sister used a doctor for both of her pregnancies. She planned for natural childbirth but she had problems. The babies were premature and had to be sent to another hospital because they couldn't take care of them. I'm so confused. I don't know what to do."

    When preparing to address Jennifer's concerns, what issues should be addressed and how would you address them?

2. The Shock family consists of the following members: Jeffrey, age 35; Brenda, age 33; and their 5 children—John, age 12; Mary, age 10; Jason, age 7; Karen, age 3; and Kyle, age 1. They live next door to Jeffrey's parents who are in their sixties. His parents play an active role in watching the children. Jeffrey has two younger siblings, both of whom live out of state and visit infrequently. Brenda's parents live about 60 miles away and visit at least once a month. Brenda has no brothers or sisters.

    Using each of the four conceptual frameworks presented in the text, evaluate this family's interactional patterns.

3. Maria Gonzalez, a 24-year-old woman, is brought to the clinic by her husband, Jose, age 28 for a prenatal check-up. Maria has two other children, ages 1 and 3. The family lives with Jose's older parents and elderly grandmother. Maria speaks very little English, so her husband acts as the translator. She does not work outside the home, but spends her time caring for the members of the household. Jose is an auto mechanic and does odd jobs to earn extra money. They do not own a car but use public transportation.

    When planning appropriate care for Maria, what socioeconomic aspects and ethnic and cultural beliefs about the family and healthcare providers must you address and how can you address them without stereotyping the client?

4. As part of a seminar course, you and a group of your fellow classmates are asked to debate the issue of surrogacy, addressing the specific ethical and legal concerns associated with it. You will be assigned to argue either for or against the issue just prior to the class.

    In preparing for the seminar, what issues would you address and how would you support your position for each side of the argument?

Multiple Choice Questions

1. A nurse is preparing a class presentation about the advanced practice roles in maternity nursing for a group of senior nursing students. When describing the maternity/perinatal clinical specialist role, the nurse explains that this advanced practice role:

    A. Focuses on primary ambulatory care
    B. Requires passing a certification examination
    C. Focuses on secondary and tertiary hospital care
    D. Manages labor and delivery independently

2. When developing a prenatal health promotion program for a group of first time mothers, the nurse reviews the statistics for maternal mortality, noting that the risk of maternal mortality is lowest for the age group:

A. Between ages 20 and 24
B. Below age 20
C. Between ages 30 and 35
D. Over age 40

3. The nurse is teaching a group of students about the trends occurring in perinatal care. When reviewing the demographic changes, the statement that accurately illustrates the nurse's understanding of these trends is:

   A. "Over the last 10 years, the number of births has increased."
   B. "More women are beginning a family in their late 30's and early 40's."
   C. "Childbearing outside the marriage has decreased during the last few decades."
   D. "Since 1986, the teen birth rate has decreased."

4. While assessing a postpartum client, the nurse notes a firm fundus, 1 fingerbreath below the umbilicus, moderate lochia rubra, and vital signs within normal limits. The nurse determines that the client is stable and experiencing a normal postpartum period. To arrive at this conclusion, the nurse uses:

   A. Inductive reasoning
   B. Deductive reasoning
   C. Informal reasoning
   D. Practical reasoning

5. The nurse documents the following on a client's chart: Fatigue related to physiologic demands of early pregnancy. This statement is an example of:

   A. Objective data
   B. Subjective data
   C. Nursing diagnosis
   D. Client outcome

6. The nurse makes a follow-up home visit to a client recently discharged early from the hospital after delivery. While talking with the client, the nurse learns that the client, husband, and three children live in the house. The client's and husband's parents live out of the state. The nurse identifies this family type as:

   A. Nuclear
   B. Extended/kin network
   C. Nuclear dyad
   D. Dual adult

7. When interviewing a client and her family during the prenatal period, the nurse asks questions that relate to specific accomplishments of tasks, such as education, career, and family. Based on the nurse's knowledge of conceptual frameworks used in family study, the nurse is most likely using the:

   A. Symbolic interaction approach
   B. Systems approach
   C. Exchange approach
   D. Developmental approach

8. The parents of a newborn are planning to take the baby home. They ask the nurse if they can take the baby to a family reunion scheduled in a few weeks. Based on the nurse's knowledge of family functions, the nurse interprets this question as a means to fulfill:

   A. Giving satisfaction and a sense of purpose
   B. Providing social placement and socialization
   C. Inculcating controls and a sense of what is right
   D. Ensuring continuity of companionship

9. When caring for the client of Vietnamese descent, the nurse notices that the client does not maintain eye contact when the nurse speaks to her and she responds. The nurse interprets this as:

   A. Disgust with the healthcare system
   B. A sign of respect
   C. Noncompliance
   D. Inappropriate

10. When the nurse acknowledges the client's choice to decide whether to have an abortion, the nurse is using the ethical principle of:

    A. Negligence
    B. Beneficence
    C. Respect for autonomy
    D. Justice

Study Questions

1. Define what is meant by the term "maternity care."

2. Name the three major causes of maternal mortality.

3. What are the leading causes of neonatal mortality?

4. List the three components essential to critical thinking.

5. Identify the components of a two-part nursing diagnosis statement.

6. What skills are involved with the planning stage of the nursing process?

7. Which family structure has been identified as one of the fastest growing types of families?

8. List the six functions of the modern family.

9. Define acculturation.

10. What are the three ethical principles underlying moral judgment?

11. What facts are necessary to establish negligence by a nurse?

12. List four ethical and legal concerns that currently surround in vitro fertilization and embryo transfer.

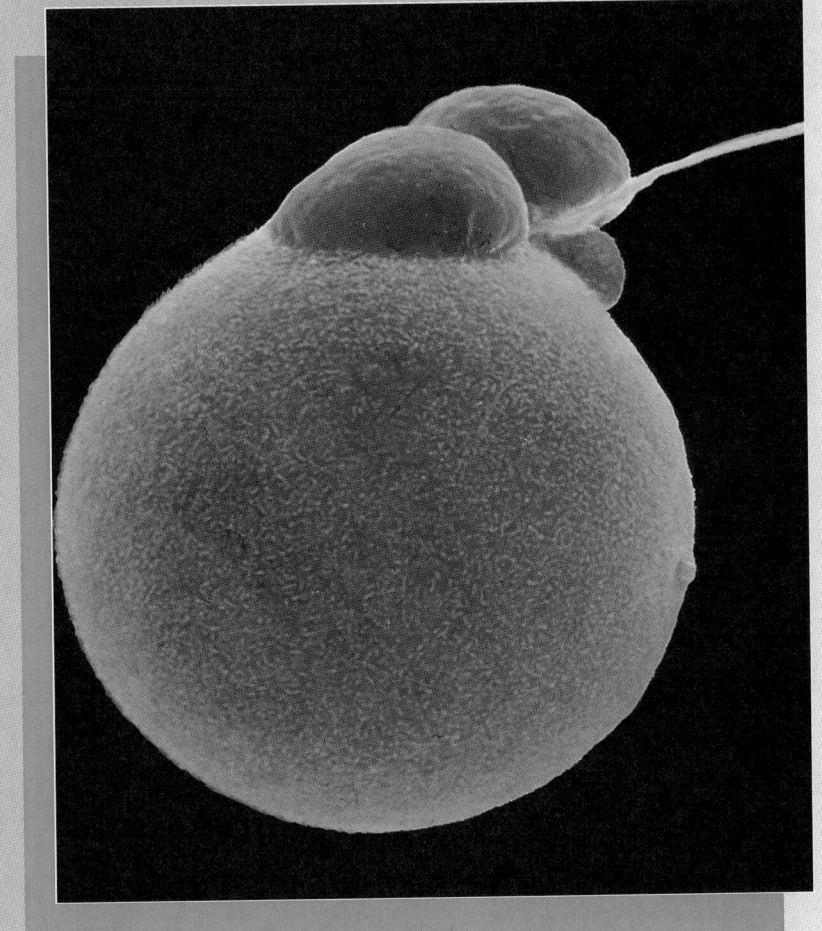

*Biophysical Aspects of
Human Reproduction*

6

Sexual and Reproductive Anatomy and Physiology

Objectives

- Identify the anatomic features of male and female reproductive structures and organs.
- Explain the major physiologic functions of the male and female reproductive structures and organs.
- Explain the anatomic features and functions of the mammary glands.
- Outline the major processes involved in male and female sexual maturation.
- Discuss endocrine influences on male and female reproductive functioning.
- Summarize the ovarian and menstrual cycles.
- Describe the physiology of menopause and perimenopause.

Key Terms

Cervix
Corpus luteum
Corpus
Endometrium
Fallopian tubes
False pelvis
Female reproductive
    cycle
Fundus
Graafian follicle
Menarche
Menopause
Menstrual phase
Menstruation
Mittelschmerz
Mons veneris

Ovaries
Perimenopause
Perineum
Primordial follicle
Progesterone
Proliferative phase
Puberty
Secretory phase
Seminiferous tubules
Spermatogenesis
Testosterone
True pelvis
Uterus
Vagina
Vulva

Although women and men share many similarities in the structure and function of their reproductive systems, many unique characteristics differentiate each sex. Most notably, women have a limited reproductive life span that begins soon after the first menstrual period, declines somewhat in the late reproductive years, and terminates at menopause. No more than 500 eggs or ova may be released during the course of reproductive life. In the man, sperm production is initiated at the time of puberty and continues well into old age. Mature spermatozoa produced by the testes during this long interval number in the billions.

Another important difference is that in the man, the capacity to reproduce is associated with sexual excitement, erection of the penis, and ejaculation. However, the capacity of the female to reproduce may be disassociated from sexual excitement and receptivity; conception can occur by mechanical placement of the ejaculate through artificial insemination. The capacity of the woman for sexual pleasure, however, is extremely important. The physical aspects of a relationship may play a critical role in the communication process that brings a couple closer together.

Anatomy and physiology of the reproductive organs and human sexual response are discussed in this chapter; ovum and sperm development and fertilization are discussed in Chapter 7.

Male Organs of Reproduction

The male reproductive system consists of the *external genitals* (the penis and scrotum) and the *internal geni-*

tals (the testes and an excretory duct system) with their accessory structures (Fig. 6-1). The main function of the male reproductive system is to produce and transport sperm from the male reproductive organs out to female reproductive organs. The specific functions of individual structures are summarized in Box 6-1 and discussed below.

Penis

The penis is the male sex organ and consists of a body, which contains two lateral columns (*corpora cavernosa*) and a central core of erectile tissue (*corpus spongiosum*), and the glans *penis*, an extension of the corpus spongiosum. The glans contains the external opening of the urethra. It is covered by a fold of retractable skin called the *foreskin*, or prepuce, often removed by circumcision. The two corpora cavernosa are covered by a thick fibrous connective tissue and are closely connected along their course. The columns separate at their base into two *crura*, strong tapering fibrous processes firmly attached to the pubic bone.

The corpora cavernosa receive their blood supply from branches of the dorsal artery of the penis. These divide further and terminate in a capillary network, the branches of which open directly into the cavernous spaces. These spaces are usually empty, and the organ is flaccid. Filling of the cavernous spaces with blood causes the penis to become turgid (an *erection*). The flow of blood, controlled by the autonomic nervous system (vasodilator fibers), varies with sexual arousal. When the erect penis is intensely stimulated, impulses from the autonomic nervous system trigger pulsatile release of semen along the urethra (an *ejaculation*). The size of the penis may vary considerably in the flaccid state; however, there is less size variation in an erect penis.

Scrotum

The scrotum, a saclike structure suspended between the penis and the anus, is composed of fascial connective tissue containing smooth muscle fibers (dartos fascia) with overlying corrugated skin. The skin of the scrotum is pigmented with scattered hairs and sebaceous glands. Its wrinkled appearance is produced by the underlying dartos fascia. The muscle contained in the dartos fascia responds to cold by contracting, accentuating the wrinkled appearance as the scrotum is drawn closer to the body wall.

Inside the scrotum lie two compartments separated by a medial septum, which is an extension of the dartos fascia. Each compartment contains one testis and its related structures. A ridge on the external surface of the scrotum at midline marks the position of the me-

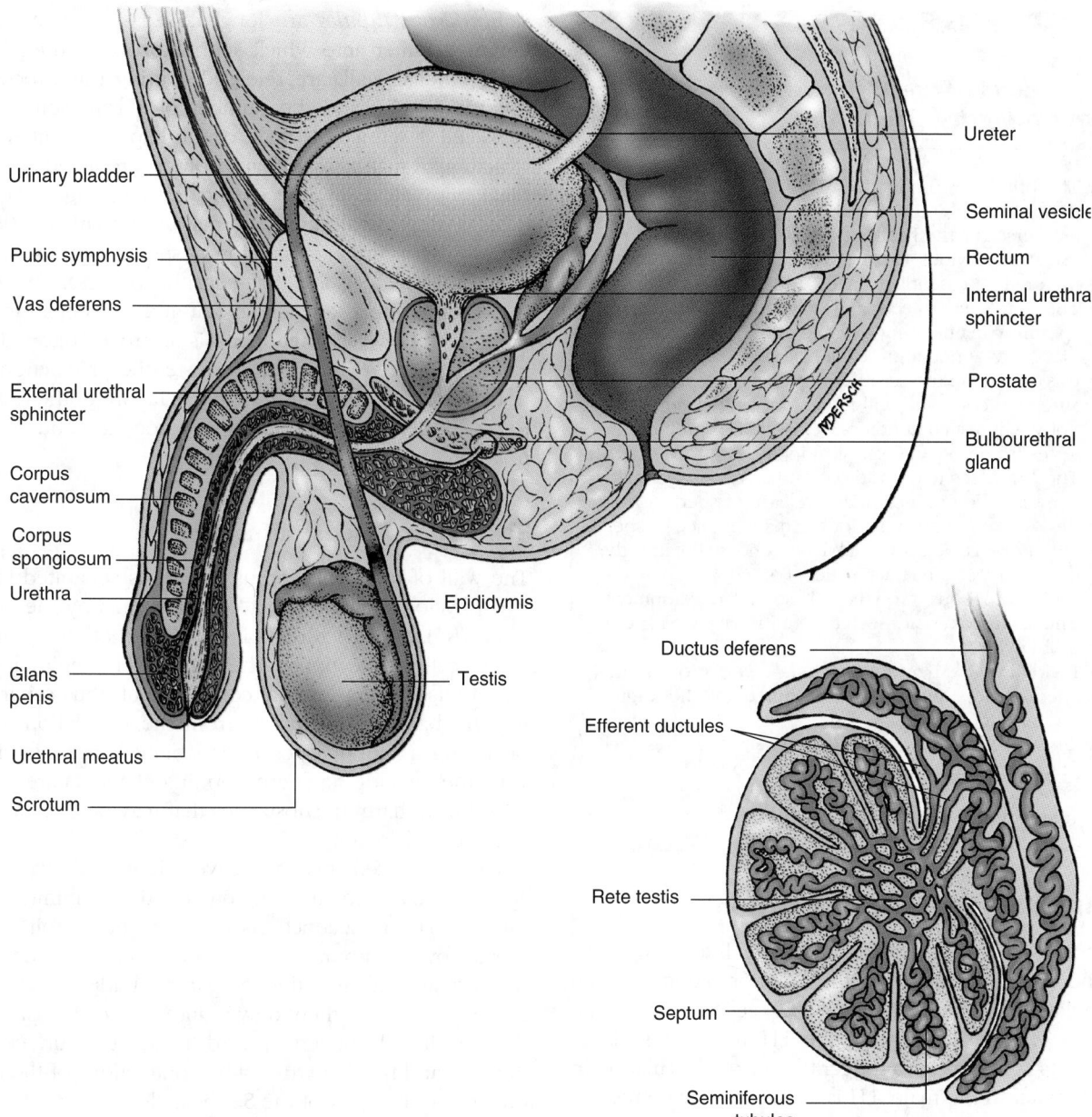

FIGURE 6–1 Organs of the male reproductive system.

dial septum. The scrotum maintains a temperature that is 2°F to 3°F lower than that of normal body temperature, which allows spermatogenesis to take place (see below).

Testes

The testes are a pair of oval, glandular organs located outside the abdominal cavity in the scrotum. They play a principal role in controlling male reproductive function. Approximately 5 cm long, the testes are contained in a fibrous protective covering, the *tunica albuginea*, which subdivides them into lobules (see Fig. 6-1). Each lobule contains **seminiferous tubules**, coiled ducts; spermatogenesis occurs in the walls of these tubules.

The testes also contain testosterone-producing cells, the *interstitial cells of Leydig*, and larger supporting *Sertoli cells*, important for sperm transport within the seminiferous tubules.

During early fetal life, the testes are abdominal; as the fetus develops, they move downward and enter the scrotum through the inguinal canal shortly before birth.

The testes depend on an interplay between the brain, the hypothalamus, and the pituitary gland. Their two functions are secretion of **testosterone** (the male hormone) and **spermatogenesis** (the production and release of spermatozoa). Both are initiated at about the time of puberty and under normal circumstances, continue well into senescence.

BOX 6–1
Functions of the Male Reproductive Organs

- The primary reproductive function of the *penis* is to deposit sperm in the female vagina during sexual intercourse for the fertilization of the ovum. (The penis also provides for the passage of urine through the urethra, essential to male urinary function.)
- The *scrotum* protects and supports the testes and sperm by maintaining a temperature lower than normal body temperature (thus, allowing spermatogenesis). Because the scrotum is sensitive to pain, pressure, and cold, and will retract, moving closer to the body when such conditions exist, it also protects the testes from potential physical injury.
- The *testes* secrete testosterone and carry out spermatogenesis—the production and release of spermatozoa.
- *Testosterone* is essential for the maintenance of spermatogenesis; it also establishes and maintains the secondary sex characteristic of the man and contributes to body growth and general development.
- The *seminal vesicles* secrete a fluid that helps sperm mobility.
- Fluid produced by the *prostate gland* protects the sperm from the acidic environment of the vagina and urethra.
- *Bulbourethral (Cowper's) glands* secrete a substance that lubricates the tip of the penis to aid in vaginal penetration and helps to neutralize the acidic environment of the vagina.

Testicular Hormone Production

Testosterone is produced when the luteinizing hormone (LH) released from the anterior pituitary gland stimulates the interstitial (*Leydig*) cells of the adult testes. This is identical to the LH released in large amounts at midcycle to trigger the onset of ovulation in the female. In the male, LH is sometimes called the *interstitial cell stimulating hormone*. Its release is controlled by hormones from the brain and hypothalamus; there is a reciprocal relationship between LH release and testosterone production.

Testosterone establishes and maintains the secondary sex characteristics of the male, such as development and maturation of the external genitalia, prostate, and seminal vesicles; growth of body and facial hair; and maturation of the larynx. It also contributes to body growth and general development.

The principal role of testosterone in terms of reproduction is maintenance of spermatogenesis. If this hormone is not present in normal amounts, fertility is impaired.

Spermatogenesis

Production of spermatozoa is initiated and maintained in the seminiferous tubules of the testes (Fig. 6-2). The *seminiferous tubules* are long, coiled structures containing a lumen into which spermatozoa, produced in the epithelial wall, are released. During this process, meiosis occurs, and the number of chromosomes in each cell is reduced to half, or the haploid number. A structurally mature spermatozoon is produced, complete with head, midpiece, and tail (see Fig. 7-3). It takes 60 days for a human spermatozoon to mature (see Chapter 7 for further discussion of spermatogenesis).

Spermatogenesis is a heat-sensitive process. The 2°F to 3°F difference between scrotal and abdominal temperatures allows spermatogenesis to proceed normally in the cooler environment. Testosterone production is not affected by temperature; hence, failure of the testes to descend severely impairs spermatogenesis but does not affect testosterone production.

Testicular Release of Sperm

The wall of the seminiferous tubules is separated into two physiologically distinct compartments by the *Sertoli cells*, large structures joined to each other by firm cell-to-cell connections. They divide the epithelium into a basal and a luminal compartment, thus separating the basal compartment from the circulation and providing a blood–testes permeability barrier. In this way, the developing sperm-forming elements are protected from harmful substances that may be circulating in the bloodstream.

The Sertoli cells play an active role in the release of spermatozoa into the lumen of the seminiferous tubules. The tight junctions between the Sertoli cells break down temporarily to permit upward movement of spermatocytes into the compartment adjacent to the lumen. They are then drawn into the cytoplasm of the Sertoli cell, moved upward toward the surface of the cell, and finally extruded by contractions of the cytoplasm at the apex of the Sertoli cells (Fig 6-3). These spermatozoa possess tails but are not yet capable of motility.

Duct System

Leading from the testes are the transporting and storage ducts of the male reproductive tract, which include the following:

- The *epididymis* is a duct about 6 m (20 ft) long that is adjacent to the testis (see Fig. 6-1) and is a reservoir where sperm can survive for extended periods. It is divided into a head portion (caput) and a tail (cauda). The seminiferous tubules coalesce at the rete testis (see Fig. 6-1) and enter the epididymis. Spermatozoa acquire motility and become fertile as they pass along the epididymis.
- The *vas deferens*, also known as the ductus deferens, is the transporting passage along which sper-

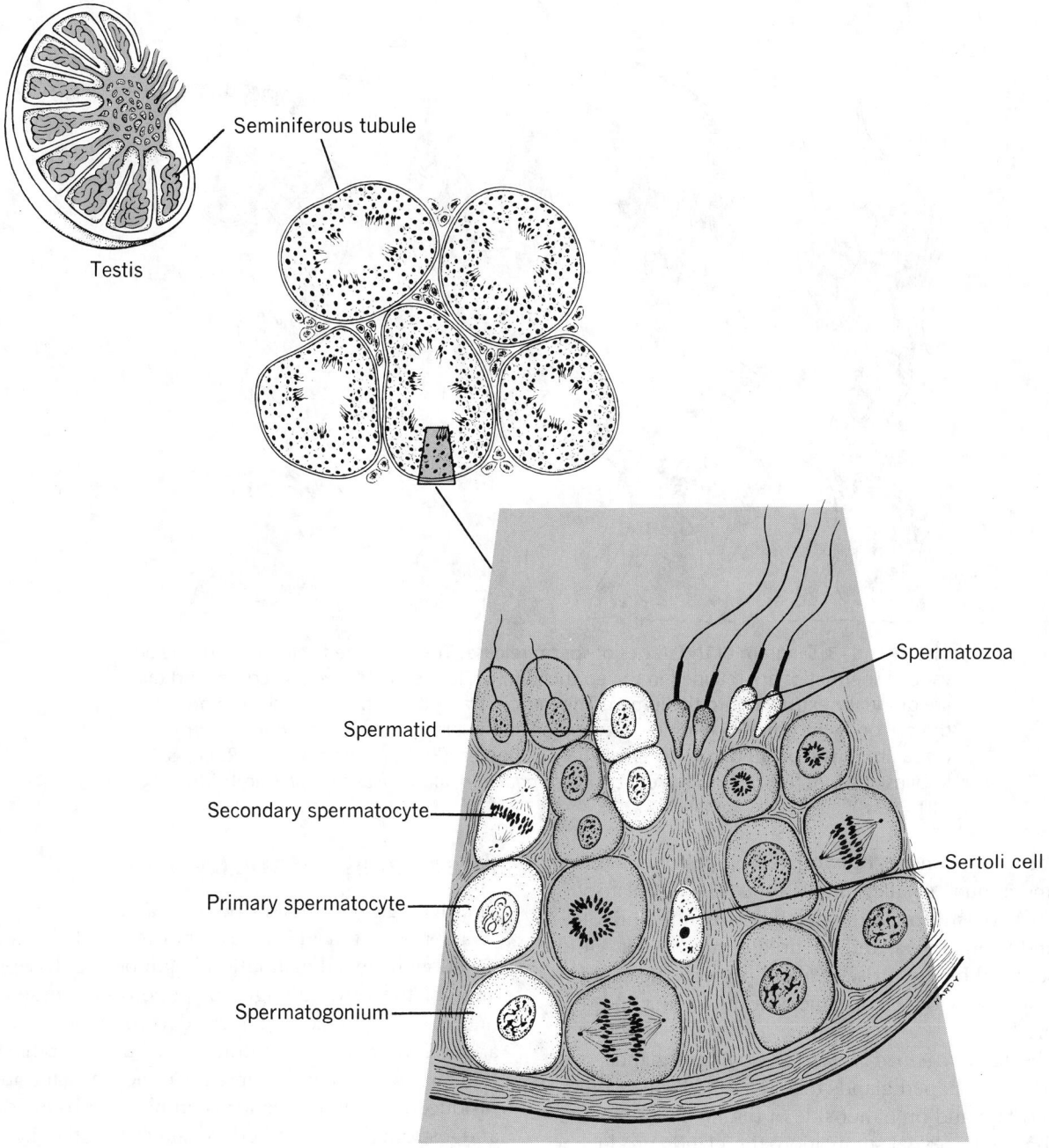

FIGURE 6–2 Section of a seminiferous tubule, showing various stages of spermatogenesis.

matozoa traverse after release from the epididymis (see Fig. 6-1). The ductus deferens has contractile power to propel the spermatozoa upward to the ejaculatory duct and through the urethra to the base of the penis.

Accessory Structures

The accessory structures, which consist of the *seminal vesicles*, the *prostate gland*, and the *bulbourethral glands*, aid in ejaculation and safe delivery of the sperm to the site of fertilization (see Fig. 6-1). The secretions of all of these structures facilitate transporta-

tion of spermatozoa along the urethra during the ejaculatory process and provide a temporary milieu where spermatozoa can survive. Testosterone is essential to their functioning. Each of these structures is described briefly:

■ The *seminal vesicles* are sacculated structures located behind the bladder and in front of the rectum at the base of the prostate. They produce prostaglandins (PGs) and a viscous secretion abundant in fructose that mixes with sperm in the ejaculatory ducts during ejaculation and helps sperm mobility.

■ The *prostate gland* surrounds the base of the urethra and the ejaculatory duct and rests on the

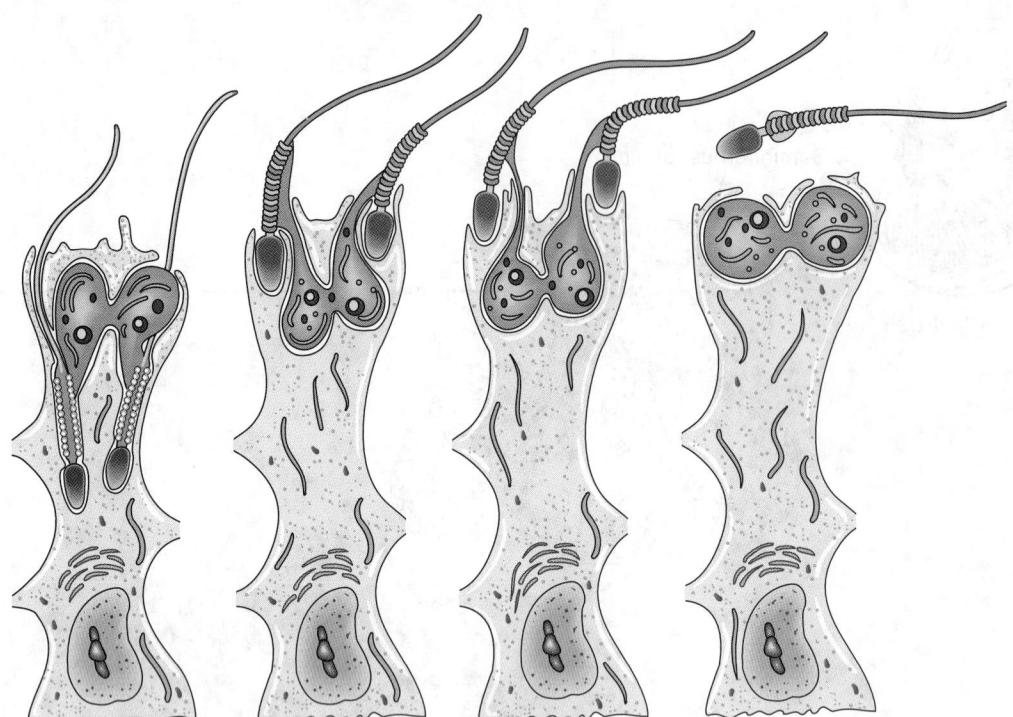

FIGURE 6-3 Diagram of the stages of sperm release. The conjoined cell bodies of the advanced spermatids are retained in the epithelium, while the nucleus, neck region, and tail are gradually extruded into the lumen. The narrow stalk connecting the neck region with the cell body becomes increasingly attenuated and finally gives way. Individual spermatozoa are thus separated from the syncytial cell bodies. (Redrawn from Greep, R. O., & Koblinsky, M. A. [Eds.] [1977]. *Frontiers in reproduction and fertility control.* Cambridge: MIT Press.)

rectum. It consists of two lateral lobes of equal size and a much smaller middle lobe. The ejaculatory ducts pass through the gland between the middle and lateral lobes, and the urethra traverses it. Fluid secreted by the prostate gland protects the sperm from the acidic environment of the vagina and the urethra.

■ The *bulbourethral glands*, or Cowper's glands, are two pea-shaped glands that lie at the base of the prostate and on either side of the membranous urethra. With sexual stimulation, the glands produce a viscous mucus that becomes part of the semen and lubricates the penile urethra in preparation for intercourse. This secretion also aids in neutralizing the pH environment.

During ejaculation, the secretions contributed by the seminal vesicles and the prostate gland join the semen so that the ejaculate is made up of spermatozoa contained in seminal vesicular and prostatic secretions, with a small contribution from the Cowper's glands. On intravaginal ejaculation, some spermatozoa leave the ejaculate almost immediately and begin to traverse the cervical mucus. Within minutes, some spermatozoa are on their way to the site of fertilization.

Male Sexual Maturity

The average man enters puberty at 11.6 years of age (Wasserman et al., 1981). The hormonal changes associated with sexual maturation begin before the appearance of the physical signs of puberty. Increased production of adrenal sex steroids (adrenarche) occurs about 2 years before maturation of the hypothalamic-pituitary-gonadal axis. Three major adrenal steroids are produced: dehydroepiandrosterone, androstenedione, and estrone. A decreased sensitivity to the negative feedback system between the central nervous system and the testes is believed to cause the hypothalamus and pituitary gland to begin secreting increased amounts of gonadotropin-releasing hormone (GnRH), follicle-stimulating hormone (FSH), and LH.

With increased secretion of pituitary hormones, testosterone levels rise progressively during maturation. On the average, changes associated with puberty in the man occur 1 year later than in the woman and span approximately 4 years. These include development of axillary, pubic, and body hair and maturation and growth of the testes and penis; these occur over 2 to 3 years and are accompanied by a growth spurt and general muscular development. Development of the internal accessory glands (prostate, bulbourethral,

TABLE 6–1
Tanner Staging in Boys

Stage	Testes	Penis	Pubic Hair	Other*	Range in Years
I	No change, testes 2.5 cm or less	Prepubertal	None		Birth–15
II	Enlargement of testes, increased stippling and pigmentation of scrotal sac	Minimal or no enlargement	Long, downy, slightly pigmented hair often occurring several months after testicular growth; chiefly at base of penis		10–15
III	Further enlargement of testes and scrotum	Significant penile enlargement, especially in length	Increase in amount; now darker, coarser, and curled at and lateral to the base of the penis	Peak growth spurt begins.	10½–16½
IV	Further enlargement, increased pigmentation of scrotum	Further enlargement, especially in diameter	Adult type but not distribution, limited to pubic region	Axillary hair and some facial hair develop.	Variable 12–17
V	Adult size and shape	Adult size and shape	Adult distribution and quality (medial aspects of thighs)	20% have peak height velocity; body hair development and increase in musculature may continue for several months to years.	13–18

seminal vesicles) occurs synchronously with penile and testicular growth. Ejaculation of fluid with penile erection may occur within 1 year after the beginning of growth of the penis, even before it is of mature size. Approximately 25% of adult height and 50% of adult weight occurs during puberty (Oski et al., 1994). The peak growth spurt occurs about 2 years after the onset of genital enlargement. Circulating testosterone affects muscle development by increasing lean body mass (a percentage of body weight) from 80% to 85% to 90%.

Tanner's staging system for describing and categorizing secondary sex characteristics in boys (sexual maturity ratings) is summarized in Table 6-1. Although adolescents pass through a sequential series of pubertal events as they mature, the age at onset of events and the time interval between one event and the next is variable (Oski et al., 1994).

Female Structures and Organs of Reproduction

The female reproductive system includes external and internal organs. The internal reproductive organs are housed inside the pelvis, which also contains the canal through which the fetus passes during birth. Following puberty, the primary purpose of the female reproductive system is to produce and release a mature female sex cell (ovum) each month and to transport it to the structure where fertilization can occur. The specific functions of the female reproductive structures and organs are summarized in Box 6-2.

Female Pelvis

The *pelvis*, named for its resemblance to a basin, is a bony ring interposed between the trunk and the thighs. The vertebral column, or backbone, passes into the pelvis from above and transmits the weight of the upper part of the body to it. The pelvis, in turn, transmits weight to the lower limbs. The pelvic cavity contains the generative organs and is the canal through which the fetus must pass during birth.

Bony Structure

The pelvis is made up of four connected bones: the two hipbones (*os coxae*, or innominate), situated laterally and in front, and the *sacrum* and *coccyx*, situated behind (Fig. 6-4).

BOX 6-2
Functions of the Female Reproductive Structures and Organs

- The *pelvis* is a bony structure that supports and protects the lower abdominal and internal reproductive organs. During pregnancy, the pelvis provides support for the growing fetus and an essential passageway for birth.
- The *external reproductive organs* (mons veneris, labia majora, labia minora, clitoris, vaginal vestibule, and perineum) serve a variety of functions, such as providing protection and support for the structures beneath or adjacent to them and playing a role in sexual arousal and coitus.
- The primary functions of the *ovaries,* or female gonads, include ovulation and production of estrogen, progesterone, and androgens.
- The *fallopian tubes* capture and transport the ovum from the ovaries to the uterus and provide a supportive site for fertilization.
- Functions of the *uterus* include providing a safe and nourishing environment for the developing fetus, contracting rhythmically during labor to facilitate birth, and preparing for pregnancy on a monthly basis from puberty until menopause.
- The *vagina* functions as the birth canal and the organ for sexual intercourse (coitus).

Anatomically, the hipbones are divided into three parts: the *ilium,* the *ischium,* and the *pubis.* These bones become firmly joined into one by the time the growth of the body is completed (between the ages of 20 and 25 years) so that when the pelvis is examined, no trace of the original edges or divisions of these

three bones can be discovered. Each of these bones is briefly described below:

- The *ilium,* the largest portion of the bones, forms the upper and back part of the pelvis. Its upper flaring border forms the prominence of the hip, or crest of the ilium (hipbone).
- The *ischium* is the lower part below the hip joint, and from it projects the tuberosity of the ischium, on which the body rests when in a sitting position.
- The *pubis* forms the anterior part of the hipbone. It extends from the hip joint to the joint in front between the two hipbones (the *symphysis pubis*) and then turns down toward the ischial tuberosity; it thus forms, with the bone of the opposite side, the arch below the symphysis, the *pubic* or *subpubic arch.* This articulation of the two pubic bones encloses the pelvic cavity anteriorly.
- The *sacrum* and the *coccyx* form the lowest portions of the spinal column. The sacrum is a triangular wedge-shaped bone consisting of five vertebrae fused together. It is the back part of the pelvis. The coccyx forms a tail end to the spine. In the child, the coccyx consists of four or five small, separate vertebrae; in the adult, these bones are fused into one. The coccyx is usually movable at the point of attachment to the sacrum, the sacrococcygeal joint, and may become pressed back during labor to allow more room for the passage of the fetal head.
- The *sacral promontory* is the marked projection formed by the junction of the last lumbar vertebra with the sacrum. This is one of the most important landmarks in obstetric anatomy.

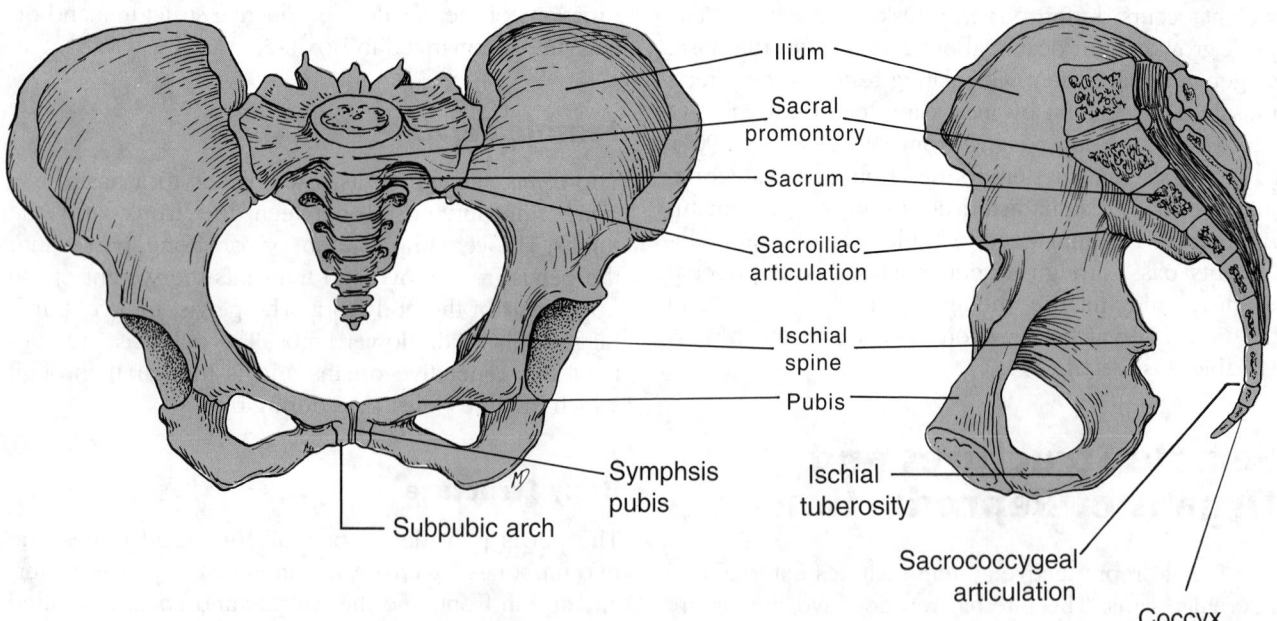

FIGURE 6-4 Front and lateral views of the pelvis, showing major bones and articulations.

Articulation and Surfaces

Four *articulations*, or joints of the pelvis, are important in obstetric care:

- Two *sacroiliac articulations*—posterior, located between the sacrum and the ilia on either side
- *Symphysis pubis articulation*—anterior, between the two pubic bones
- *Sacrococcygeal articulation*—between the sacrum and the coccyx

All of these articular surfaces are lined with fibrocartilage, which becomes thickened and softened during pregnancy; likewise, the ligaments that bind the pelvic joints together become softened, and as a result, greater mobility of the pelvic bones develops. A certain definite, although very limited, motion in the joints is desirable for normal labor; however, there is no change in the actual size of the pelvis. The increased mobility of pelvic joints in pregnancy results in a slight "wobbliness" in the pelvis and puts greater strain on the surrounding muscles and ligaments. This accounts for much of the backache and leg ache in the later months of pregnancy.

The pelvis is lined with muscular tissue, providing a smooth, somewhat cushioned surface for the fetus to pass over during labor. These muscles also help support the abdominal contents.

True and False Pelves

The pelvis is divided into two parts by a natural line of division, the *inlet* or *brim* (see Fig. 20-1). The **false pelvis**, or upper flaring part, supports the uterus during late pregnancy and directs the fetus into the true pelvis at the proper time. The **true pelvis**, or lower part, forms the bony canal through which the fetus must pass during parturition. For descriptive purposes, it is divided into three parts: an inlet or brim, a cavity, and an outlet. The importance of these parts and the various ways of assessing them during pregnancy and labor are discussed in Chapter 20.

External Organs

The external female reproductive organs, called the **vulva**, consist of everything visible externally from the lower margin of the pubis to the perineum (Fig. 6-5) and are listed in Box 6-3. They include the mons veneris, labia majora, labia minora, clitoris, vaginal vestibule (the vaginal opening or *introitus*, the ducts of Bartholin's glands, the ducts of Skene's glands, and the hymen), urethral meatus, and perineum.

Mons Veneris

The **mons veneris**, or *mons pubis*, is a firm, cushion-like formation of subcutaneous fatty tissue and loose connective tissue over the symphysis pubis. It is covered with pubic hair, varying in texture among ethnic or racial groups from thick, coarse, and curly among African American women to sparse and fine among Asian women. The mons veneris protects the pelvic bones during sexual intercourse.

Labia Majora

The *labia majora* are two prominent longitudinal folds of adipose tissue covered with skin, extending downward and backward from the mons veneris and disappearing to form the anterior border of the perineal body. These two thick folds of skin, covered with hair

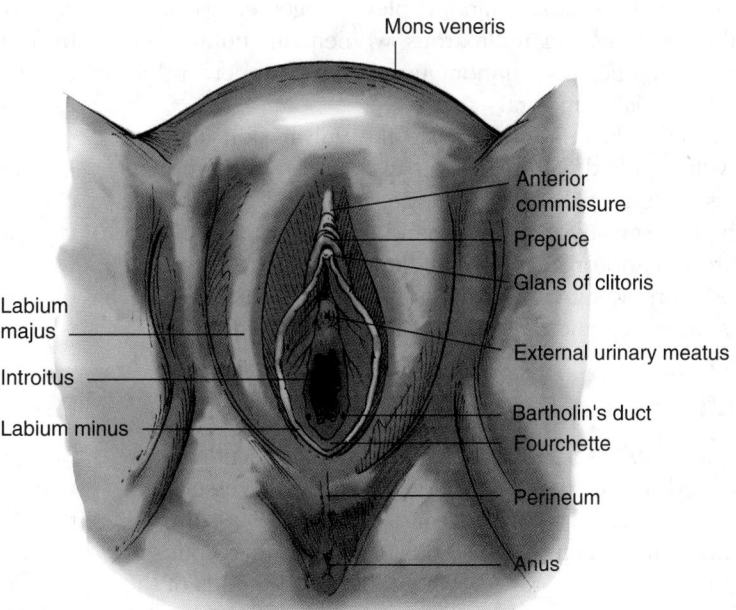

FIGURE 6–5 External genitalia of the female.

BOX 6–3
Female Organs of Reproduction

External	Internal
Vulva	Ovaries
Mons veneris	Fallopian tubes
Labia majora	Uterus
Labia minora	Corpus (body)
Clitoris	Cervix (neck)
Vaginal vestibule	
Perineum	

on their outer surfaces after puberty, are smooth and moist on their inner surfaces. At the bottom, they fade away into the perineum posteriorly, joining together to form a transverse fold, the posterior commissure, directly in front of the fourchette. This fatty tissue is supplied with an abundant plexus of veins that may rupture as the result of injury sustained during labor and give rise to an extravasation of blood, or hematoma. The labia majora protect the structures lying between them.

Labia Minora

The *labia minora* are two thin folds entirely covered with thin membrane, situated between the labia majora. Their outer surfaces join with the inner surfaces of the labia majora. The labia minora extend from the clitoris downward and backward on either side of the opening of the vagina. In the upper extremity, each labium minus separates into two branches, which, when united with those of the opposite side, enclose the clitoris. The upper fold forms the *prepuce*, and the lower fold forms the *frenum of the clitoris*. At the bottom, the labia minora blend together to form the *fourchette* in nulliparous women; in multiparous women, the labia minora usually pass imperceptibly into the labia majora.

The labia minora lubricate the vulvar skin and are well supplied with blood vessels, nerves, and lymphatics. Often called the "sex skin," the labia minora are highly sensitive to touch and play a major role in arousal and orgasm through their draping over the clitoris, providing continual clitoral stimulation as tension is increased and decreased with penile thrusting.

Clitoris

The *clitoris* is a small, highly sensitive projection, composed of erectile tissue, nerves, and blood vessels and covered with a thin epidermis. The organ is a complex anatomic structure with both external and cryptic, or partially hidden, parts between the anterior ends of the labia minora. It is comparable to the penis and is re-

garded as the chief area of female sexual pleasure. There are four parts to the clitoris: the glans, shaft, crus, and vestibular bulbs. The glans and shaft are the most external and smallest portions and are largely hidden under the prepuce. The clitoral glans is the most sensitive female erogenous area. The cryptic structures of the clitoris include the crus and vestibular bulbs. The clitoral crus is homologous to the corpus cavernosum in the man, which becomes the crus of the penis. A cheeselike fatty substance with a distinctive odor, known as *smegma*, is secreted by the sebaceous glands of the clitoris.

Vaginal Vestibule

The *vestibule* is the almond-shaped area enclosed by the labia minora, extending from the clitoris to the fourchette. It is perforated by four openings: the urethra, the vaginal opening or *introitus*, the ducts of Bartholin's glands, and the ducts of Skene's glands. Bartholin's glands (*vulvovaginal glands*) are two small glands situated beneath the vestibule on either side of the vaginal opening. They secrete a clear and viscous mucus that increases the viability and motility of sperm in the vestibule. Skene's glands (*paraurethral glands*) are tubular structures opening on the vestibule on either side of the urethra. They produce mucous secretions that lubricate the vaginal vestibule, facilitating sexual intercourse.

The *hymen* marks the division between the internal and the external organs. It is a thin sheath of mucous membrane situated at the introitus. It may be entirely absent, or it may form a complete septum across the lower end of the vagina. The hymen changes in shape and consistency throughout the life cycle. In the newborn, it projects beyond the surrounding parts. In adult virgins, it is a membrane of varying thickness with a circular or crescent shaped opening that varies in size from a small slit to a larger space that readily admits one or even two fingers. The hymen may be torn during strenuous physical work or exercise, masturbation, or use of tampons without the initiation of intercourse. In rare instances, the hymen may be imperforate and cause retention of menstrual discharge if it occludes the vaginal orifice completely.

The *urethral meatus* is located about 2.5 cm below the clitoris in the midline of the vestibule. The opening is pink or reddened and may vary in shape.

Perineum

The **perineum** consists of muscles and fascia situated between the thighs and extending from the vaginal introitus to the anus. The muscles of the perineum are illustrated in Figure 6-6. One of the most important muscles in terms of pelvic support is the *pubococcygeus muscle*, immediately adjacent to the urethra, vagina,

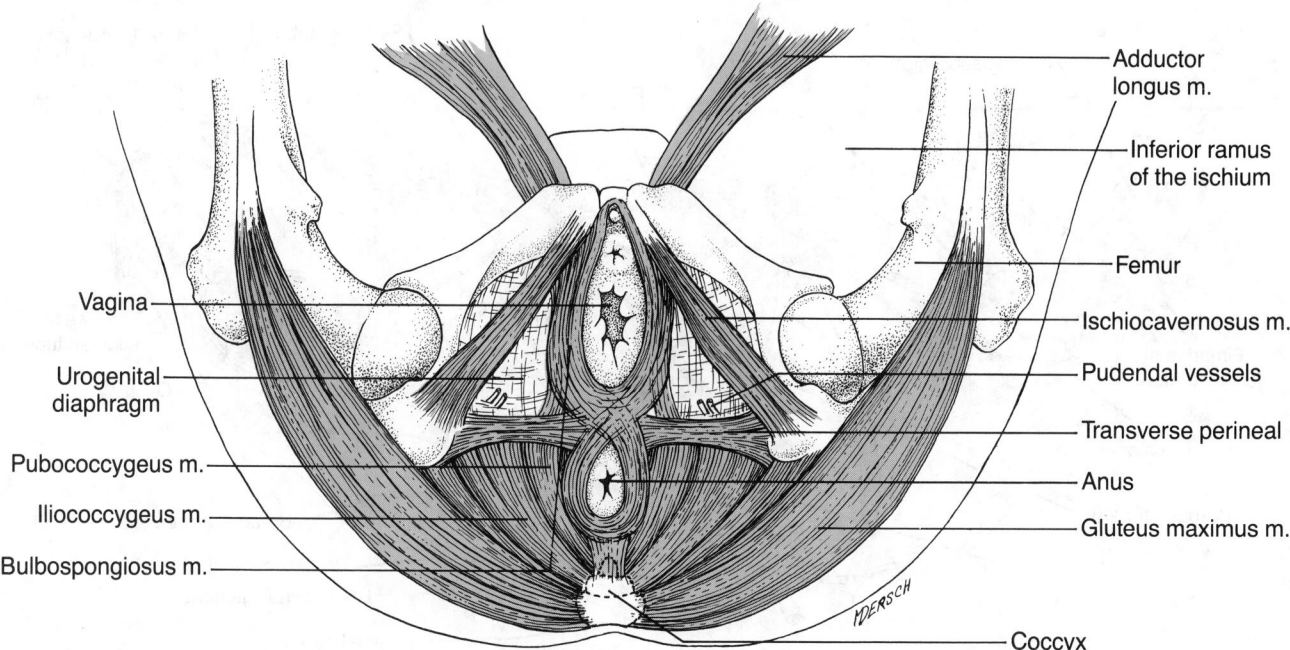

FIGURE 6–6 Muscles of the pelvic floor (female perineum).

and rectum. If this muscle becomes attenuated as a result of childbirth, the support of these structures is altered, with possible herniation of the bladder (cystocele) and rectum (rectocele) and descent into the vagina of the cervix and uterus.

Internal Organs

The internal organs of reproduction (see Figs. 6-7 and 6-8 and Box 6-3) include ovaries, fallopian tubes, uterus (including the corpus [body] and cervix), and vagina.

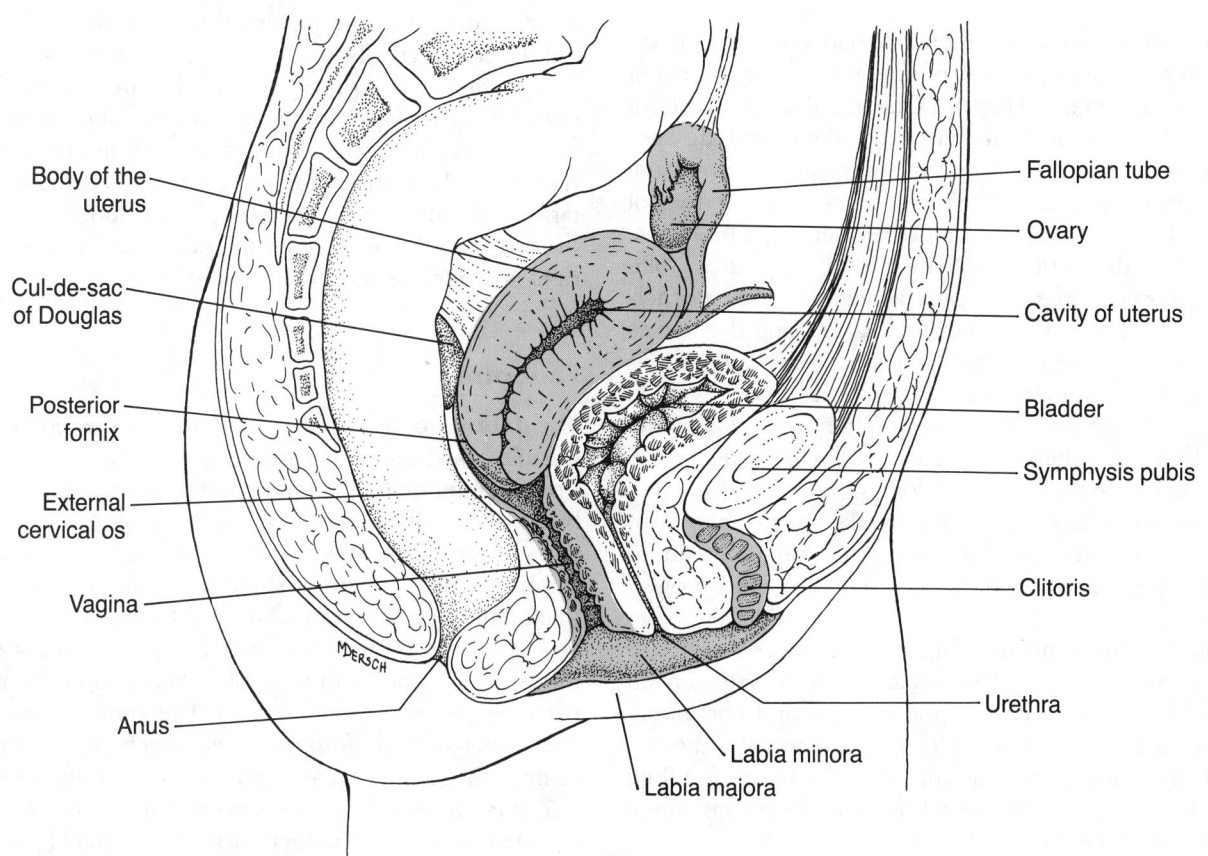

FIGURE 6–7 Female reproductive organs as seen in sagittal section.

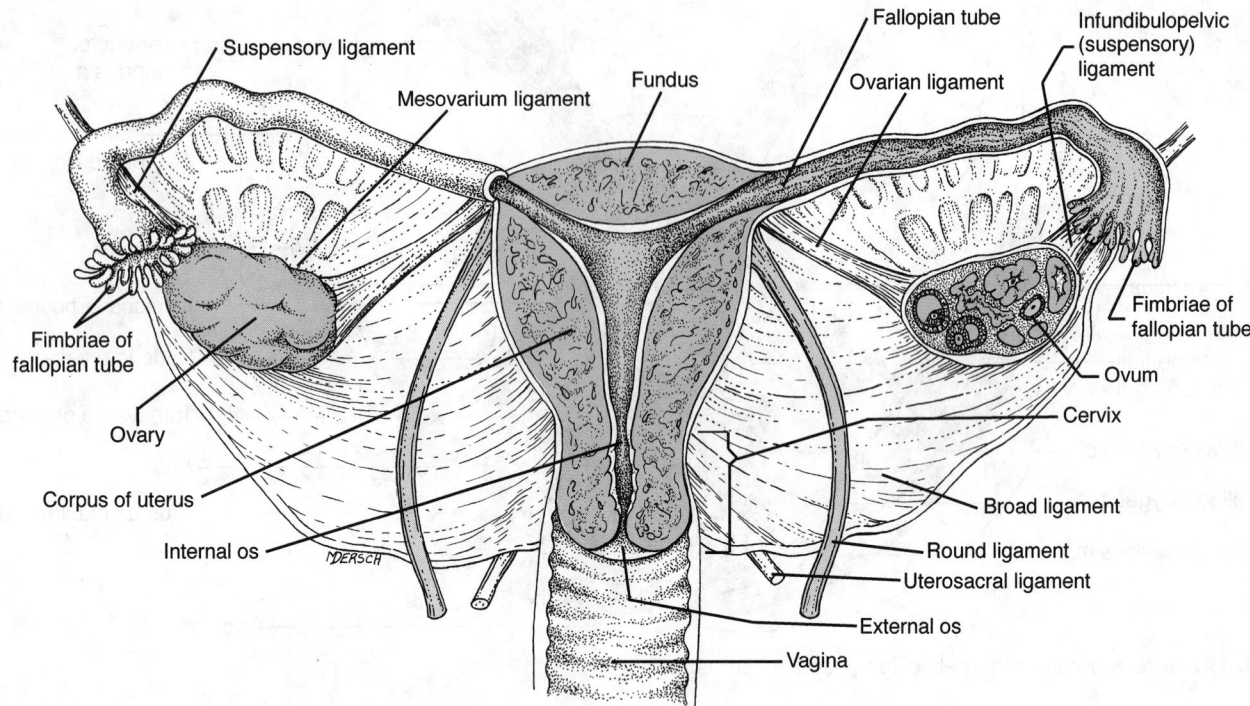

FIGURE 6–8 Anterior view of the uterus and related structures.

Ovaries

The **ovaries** are two almond-shaped glandular organs located in the upper part of the pelvic cavity on either side of the uterus. They are embedded in the posterior fold of the broad ligament of the uterus and are supported by the suspensory, ovarian, and mesovarium ligaments (see Fig. 6-8). The ovaries are composed of three layers: the *tunica albuginea*, serving a protective function; the *cortex*, containing the ova, graafian follicles, corpora lutea, corpora albicantia, and degenerated follicles; and the *medulla*, containing the nerves and the blood and lymphatic vessels. Although there is some variation in the size of the ovaries among women and according to the phase of the menstrual cycle, each organ weighs approximately 6 to 19 g and is 1.5 to 3 cm wide and 2 to 5 cm long.

The chief functions of the ovaries include development and expulsion of ova and provision of certain internal secretions, or hormones (estrogen and progesterone).

Each ovary contains a large number of germ cells, or primordial ova, in its substance at birth, sufficient in number for life. Beginning at puberty and continuing to menopause, one of the follicles that contains the ova enlarges each month and ruptures. The ovum and fluid content of the follicle are released from the ovary, then swept into the tube.

There is no peritoneal covering on the ovaries. This assists eruption of the mature ovum but allows easier spread of malignant cells from cancer of the ovaries.

The arteries that supply the ovaries are four or five branches that arise from the anastomosis of the ovarian artery with the ovarian branch of the uterine artery (Fig. 6-9). The veins that drain the ovary become tributaries to the uterine and ovarian plexus. Superiorly, the ovarian vein drains into the inferior vena cava on the right and into the renal vein on the left.

Fallopian Tubes

The **fallopian tubes** are two trumpet-shaped, thin, flexible, muscular tubes about 12 cm long, extending from the uterine cornua along the upper margin of the broad ligaments to the ovaries. Each tube has three parts: the isthmus, the ampulla, and the infundibulum (fimbria). The *isthmus* is straight and narrow, with a thick, muscular wall and a lumen 2 to 3 mm in diameter. The curved *ampulla*, containing the outer two-thirds of the tube, is the site of fertilization of the primary oocyte by a spermatozoon. The ampulla ends in the funnel-shaped *infundibulum*, which is composed of many finger-like projections known as *fimbriae*.

The fallopian tubes have two openings, one into the uterine cavity and the other into the abdominal cavity.

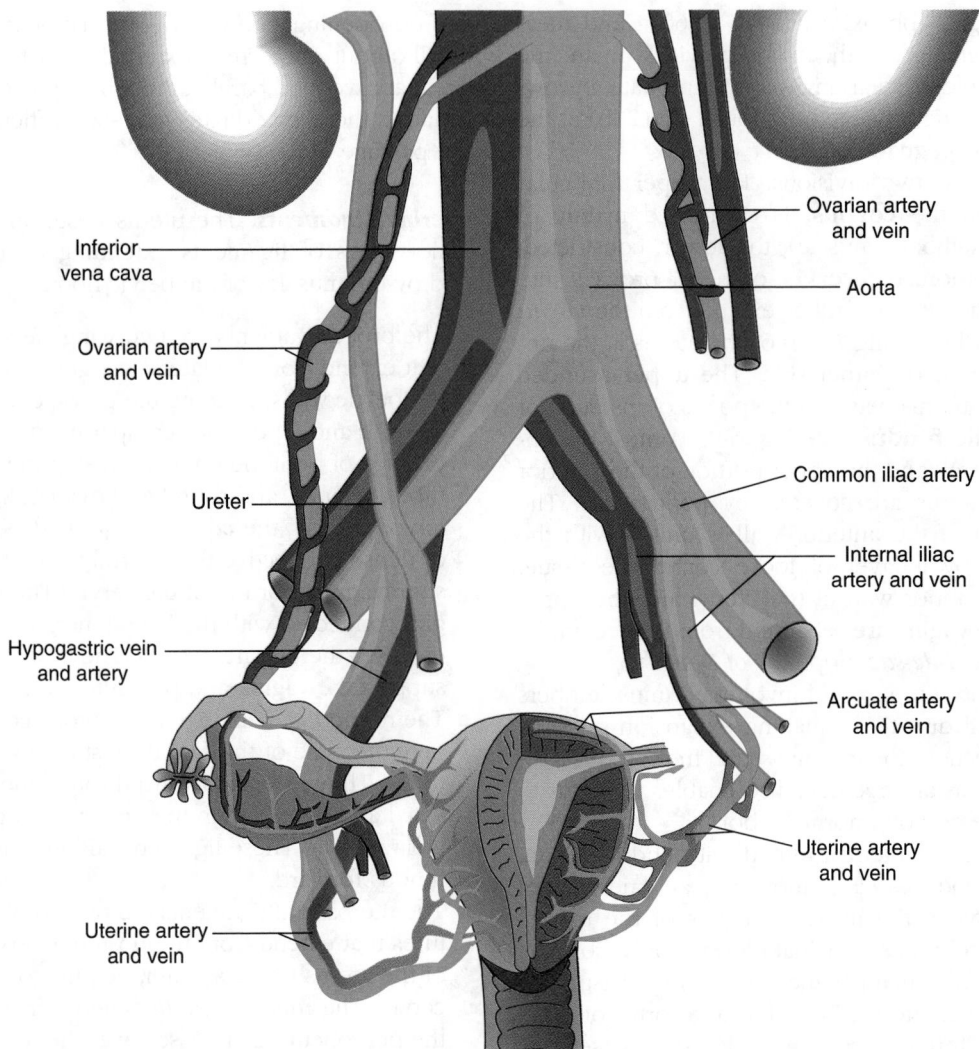

FIGURE 6-9 Blood supply of the uterus and the adnexa.

The opening into the uterine cavity is 1 mm in diameter. The larger abdominal opening is surrounded by many fimbriae. The cilia on the fimbriated end of the tube create a current in the layer of fluid that surrounds the various pelvic organs, allowing the ovum to enter the tube. Ciliary action and peristalsis propel the ovum from the tube to the cavity of the uterus.

The fallopian tubes are lined with mucous membrane that contains ciliated and secretory epithelium. The muscular layer is made up of longitudinal and circular fibers that provide peristaltic action. The serous membrane covering the tubes is a continuation of the *peritoneum*, a membrane that lines the whole abdominal cavity.

The fallopian tubes receive their blood supply from the ovarian and the uterine arteries (see Fig. 6-9). The veins of the tubes follow the course of these arteries, emptying into the uterine and ovarian trunks. The tubes are innervated by parasympathetic and sympa-thetic motor and sensory nerves from the pelvic plexus and ovarian plexus.

Uterus

The **uterus**, or womb, is a hollow, thick-walled, muscular organ (see Fig. 6-8) situated in the cavity of the true pelvis of the nonpregnant woman, behind the bladder and in front of the rectum. The uterus is the organ of menstruation. In addition, during pregnancy, the uterus serves several other important functions:

- Receiving the fertilized ovum and retaining and nourishing it until birth
- Protecting the fetus from injury
- Contracting during labor

Generally pear shaped, the size and shape of the uterus vary according to the woman's age and whether or not she has borne children. The uterus of the adult nullipara weighs approximately 40 to 60 g and measures 6 to 8 cm in length. In the gravid woman, the uterus is capable of enlarging to accommodate a growing fetus, reaching a weight of about 1 kg (2 lb) at the termination of pregnancy.

The uterus has two divisions. The upper triangular portion, called the **corpus,** is composed mainly of myometrium (smooth muscle); the lower, constricted, cylindrical portion, the **cervix** or neck, projects into the vagina. The fallopian tubes extend from the *cornu* (the Latin word meaning *horn*) of the uterus at the upper outer margin on either side. The upper rounded portion of the uterus between the points of insertion of the tubes is the **fundus** (see Fig. 6-8). Almost the entire posterior wall and the upper portion of the anterior wall of the uterus are covered by peritoneum. The lower portion of the anterior wall is united with the bladder wall by a layer of loose connective tissue. The lower posterior wall of the uterus and the upper portion of the vagina are separated from the rectum by the *Douglas' cul-de-sac,* or *pouch of Douglas.*

The uterus is composed of involuntary muscle fibers arranged in all directions, making expansion possible in every direction to accommodate the products of conception. This arrangement also enables the fetus to be born at the end of a normal labor.

The body of the uterus is lined with endometrium. Numerous blood vessels, lymphatics, and nerves are arranged between the muscular layers of the uterus. The uterus receives its principal blood supply from the uterine artery, the main branch of the hypogastric artery. The ovarian artery, a branch of the aorta, joins the uterine artery, further increasing blood supply (see Fig. 6-9). The uterovaginal plexus returns the blood from the uterus and the vagina to the venous circulation.

The nerve supply of the uterus is provided principally by the sympathetic nervous system and partly by the cerebrospinal and parasympathetic systems. Both the sympathetic and the parasympathetic nerve supplies contain motor and a few sensory fibers. These two systems are mostly antagonistic (ie, they work against each other): The sympathetic system causes muscular contraction and vasoconstriction, while the parasympathetic system inhibits contraction and leads to vasodilatation.

Cervix. Less movable than the body of the uterus, the cervix is composed mainly of fibrous connective tissue with some muscle fibers and elastic tissue. Its muscular wall is not as thick, and its lining is different from the uterine body in that it is folded and contains glands that produce mucus; these are the chief source of the mucous secretion during the menstrual cycle and in pregnancy. The cervix has an upper opening, the *internal os,* leading from the cavity of the uterine body into the cervical canal, and a lower opening, the *exter-*

nal os, opening into the vagina. The cervical canal is small (about 2–2.5 cm in external diameter) in the nonpregnant woman, barely admitting a probe. At the time of labor, the cervix dilates to a size sufficient to permit the passage of the fetus.

Uterine Ligaments. The uterus is supported by three major types of ligaments extending from either side and by the muscles of the pelvic floor:

- The broad ligaments are two winglike structures that extend from the lateral margins of the uterus to the pelvic walls, dividing the pelvic cavity into an anterior and a posterior compartment. Each consists of folds of peritoneum that envelop the fallopian tubes, ovaries, and round and ovarian ligaments. A lower portion, the *cardinal ligament,* is composed of dense connective tissue firmly joined to the supravaginal portion of the cervix. The median margin, connected with the lateral margin of the uterus, encloses the uterine vessels. The broad ligaments support the vagina and prevent uterine prolapse.
- The round ligaments are two fibrous cords attached on either side of the fundus, just below the fallopian tubes. They extend forward through the inguinal canal and terminate in the upper portion of the labia majora. These ligaments aid in holding the fundus forward.
- The uterosacral ligaments are two cordlike structures that extend from the posterior cervical portion of the uterus to the sacrum, helping to support the cervix. The *uterovesical ligament* is merely a fold of the peritoneum that passes over the fundus and extends over the bladder. The *rectovaginal ligament* is a fold of the peritoneum that passes over the posterior surface of the uterus and is reflected on the rectum.

Position of Uterus. Because the uterus is a freely movable organ suspended in the pelvic cavity, its position may be influenced by physiologic conditions, such as a full bladder or rectum. The uterus can be pushed backward or forward. Its position also changes when the woman stands, lies flat, or turns on her side. The uterus is usually inclined somewhat anterior and forward (anteflexion); however, variations in position may occur, including retroversion, in which the fundus is tipped far backward, and prolapse, which occurs when the muscles of the pelvic floor and the uterine ligaments are attenuated (Fig. 6-10).

Vagina

The **vagina** is a dilatable, mucous membrane-lined passage between the bladder and the rectum (see Fig. 6-7). The vaginal opening occupies the lower portion

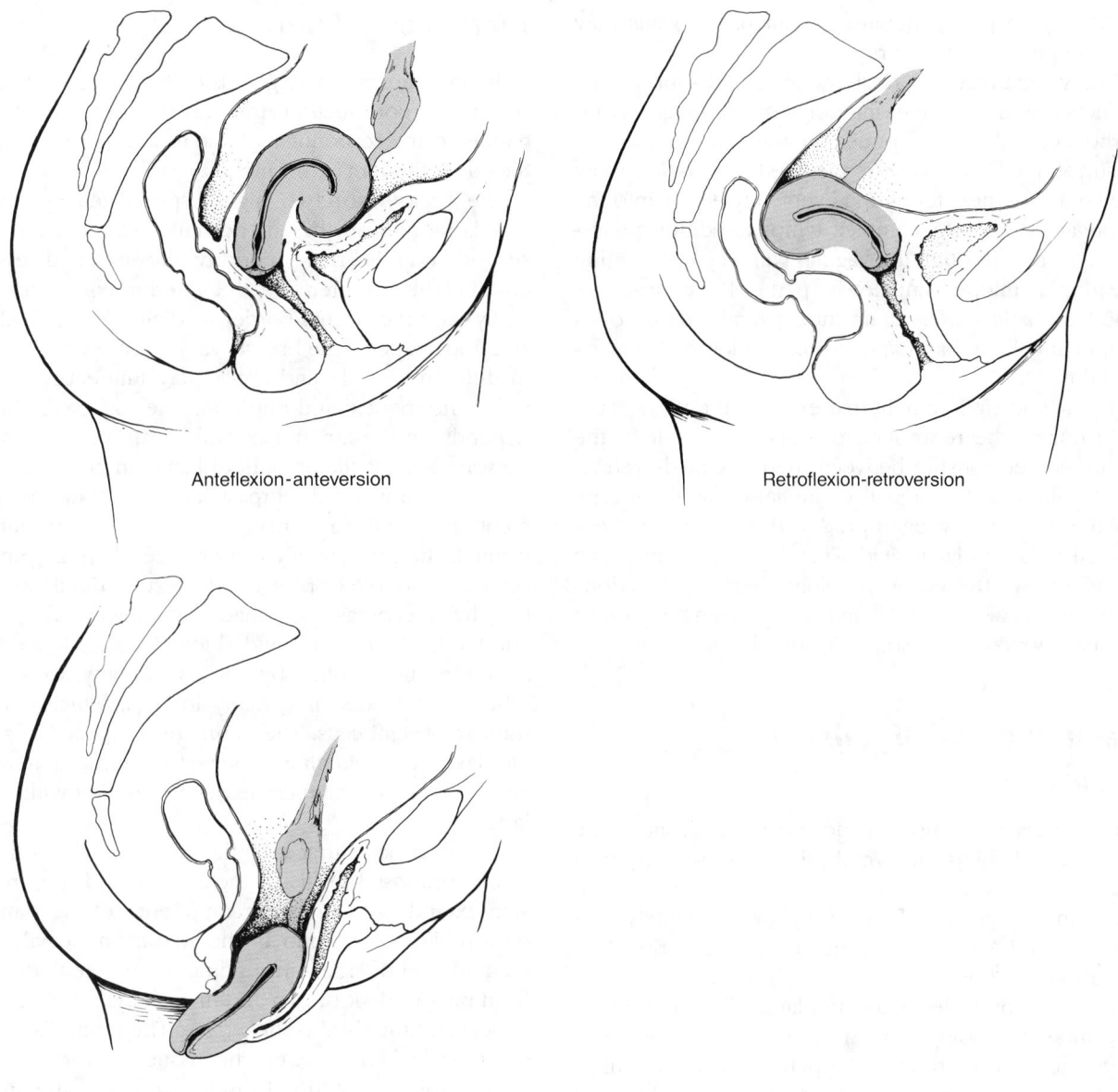

Anteflexion-anteversion

Retroflexion-retroversion

Complete prolapse

FIGURE 6-10 Positions of the uterus, showing anteflexion–anteversion, retroflexion–retroversion, and complete prolapse.

of the vestibule. The vagina is 8 to 12 cm long. In the upper end of the vagina, the *blind vault*, there is a recess into which the lower portion of the cervix projects. This area is commonly called the *fornix*.

The fornix is divided into four parts: the *lateral fornices*, or the spaces between the vaginal wall on either side and the cervix; the *anterior fornix*, between the anterior vaginal wall and the cervix; and the *posterior fornix*, between the posterior vaginal wall and the cervix. The posterior fornix is considerably deeper than the anterior fornix, because the vagina is attached higher up on the posterior than the anterior wall of the cervix. The fornices are important for two reasons: They provide space for semen to collect after inter-

course, thereby improving the chances of conception, and their thin walls allow the examiner to palpate the internal pelvic organs, including the uterus, ovaries, appendix, cecum, colon, and ureters.

The vagina serves three important functions:

- It represents the excretory duct of the uterus through which secretion and menstrual flow escape.
- It is the female organ of copulation.
- It forms part of the birth canal during labor.

The walls of the vagina are pinkish with *rugae*, ridgelike structures caused by folding of the mucous membranes. These are capable of stretching to allow marked distention of the passage in the process of childbirth. In postmenopausal women, the walls may be pale pink with fewer rugae.

The vagina receives an abundant blood supply from branches of the uterine, inferior vesical, median hemorrhoidal, and internal pudendal arteries. The passage is surrounded by a venous plexus; the vessels follow the course of the arteries and eventually empty into the hypogastric veins. A complex lymphatic drainage system channels through the vagina, with vessels draining the upper, middle, and lower parts of the structure. The lymphatic vessels drain into several lymph nodes (eg, inguinal, lumbar, hypogastric, and internal and external iliac).

The acidic environment that exists in the vagina (pH 4–5) during the reproductive years is a result of the symbiotic relationship between the lactic acid-producing bacilli and the vaginal epithelial cells. The bacilli break down the glycogen produced by the vaginal epithelial cells into lactic acid. This delicate balance may be adversely affected by antibiotic therapy, alterations in the levels of ovarian hormones, douching, or use of vaginal suppositories, sprays, or deodorants.

Related Pelvic Organs

Bladder

The bladder is a muscular sac situated in front of the uterus and behind the symphysis pubis (see Fig. 6-7) that is a reservoir for urine. The bladder remains entirely in the pelvis when empty or moderately distended, but if it becomes greatly distended, it rises into the abdomen.

Urine is conducted into the bladder by the ureters, two tubes extending down from the basin of the kidneys and over the brim of the pelvis beneath the uterine vessels to open into the bladder at about the level of the cervix. The bladder is emptied through the urethra, a short tube that terminates in the urethral meatus. Lying on either side of the urethra and almost parallel with it are the two small *Skene's glands*. Their ducts empty into the urethra just above the meatus. Often in cases of gonorrhea, Skene's glands and ducts are involved.

Anus

The anus lies close to the field of delivery, so it is considered in any discussion of the organs of reproduction. The *anus* is the entrance to the rectal canal. The rectal canal is surrounded at the anus by its sphincter muscle, which binds it to the coccyx behind and to the perineum in front. It is supported by the muscles passing into it; these muscles help to support the pelvic floor (see Fig. 6-7).

Mammary Glands

Although the mammary glands or *breasts* are not actual organs of reproduction, they are important accessory glands to the reproductive system and are directly affected by the female hormones.

The breasts are two highly specialized cutaneous glands located on the anterior chest wall between the second and third ribs superiorly, the sixth and seventh costal cartilages inferiorly, the anterior axillary line laterally, and the sternal border medially (Fig. 6-11). The size and shape of the breasts vary at different ages and in different people and are largely influenced by heredity, hormones, and nutrition. The size of the breast depends on the amount of fatty tissue present and in no way denotes the amount of lactation possible.

The functions of the breasts are to provide nourishment and protective maternal antibodies to infants through the process of lactation (see Chap. 25) and to serve as a source of pleasurable sexual stimulation. Internally, the breasts are made up of glandular tissue and fat. Each organ is divided into 15 or 20 lobes, separated from each other by fibrous and fatty walls. Each lobe is subdivided into many lobules, which contain numerous acini cells. The *acini* are composed of a single layer of epithelium, beneath which is a small amount of connective tissue richly supplied with capillaries.

The external surface of the breast is divided into three portions: The first is the smooth and soft area of skin extending from the circumference of the gland to the areola; the second is the *areola*, a heavily pigmented area of skin surrounding the nipple that varies from pink to dark brown and may change during pregnancy; and the third is the *nipple*. The nipple is largely composed of sensitive, erectile tissue and forms a large conic papilla projecting from the center of the areola; its summit is at the openings of the milk ducts. There are 3 to 20 milk duct openings. Small papillae, called *Montgomery glands*, roughen the surface of the nipple and areola. These enlarged sebaceous glands and the areola darken during pregnancy.

The internal mammary and intercostal arteries supply the breast glands, and the mammary veins follow these arteries. Many cutaneous veins become dilated during lactation. The lymphatics are abundant, especially toward the axilla. These breast glands are present in the male but exist only in the rudimentary state.

Nerves abundantly supply the breasts, which contain tissue that responds to hormones. Breast development at puberty and lactation is a result of endocrine influences. Estrogenic hormones stimulate the growth and development of the ductal epithelium. Progesterone, in combination with estrogen, is responsible for the acinar and lobular development during the luteal phase of menstruation.

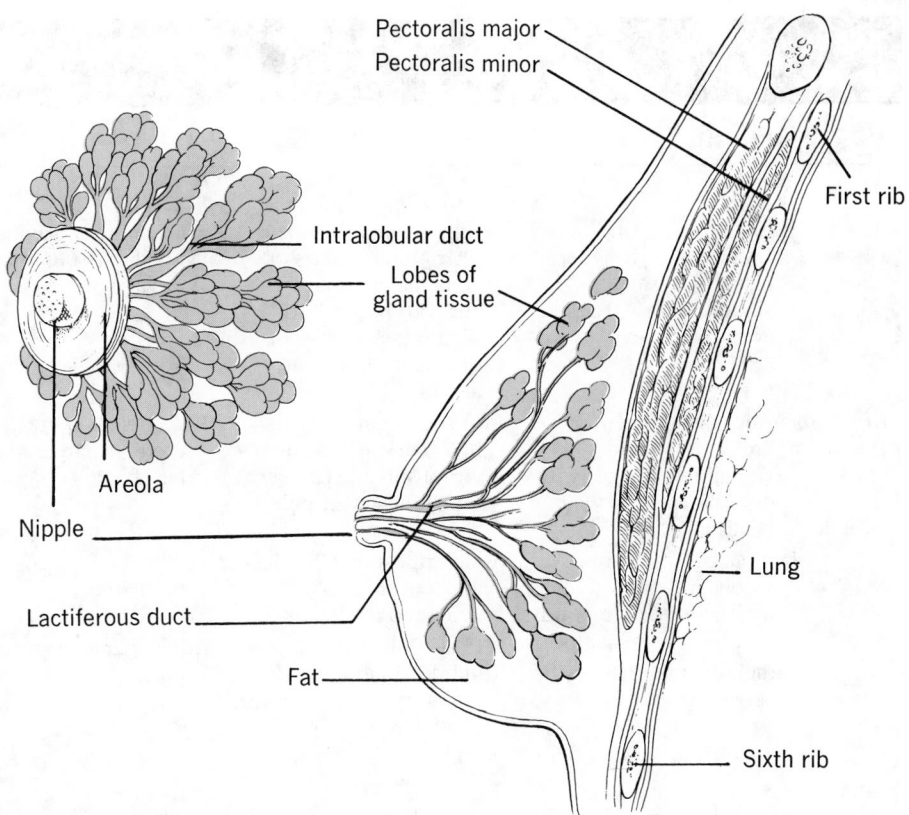

FIGURE 6-11 Glandular tissue and ducts of the mammary gland.

Female Sexual Maturity

Sexual maturity in the female begins at puberty, with the onset of dramatic bodily changes. The first sign of pubertal development is the onset of breast budding (*thelarche*), which occurs at about 10 years, with a range from approximately 8 to 13 years (Oski et al., 1994). The process of puberty spans about 3 years. Early in the course of puberty, axillary and pubic hair appears. Shortly thereafter, the contour of the labia gradually change. The peak growth spurt in girls occurs approximately 1 year after the onset of puberty, and growth is largely completed when menstruation begins, **menarche**. Establishment of the menstrual cycle is the most clearly identifiable sign of puberty and is an indication that the internal sex organs are approaching maturity. These physical changes are accompanied by emotional changes.

With maturation, fat deposition in girls increases, and their lean body mass decreases from 80% to 75%. The increase in body fat to a critical level of about 17% is believed by some to stimulate the onset of menses (Oski et al., 1994). This theory, if correct, would explain the trend for earlier onset of menarche evident in western countries since 1840, based on better nutrition among adolescents (Oski et al., 1994).

Tanner's stages for the development of female secondary sex characteristics are displayed in Table 6-2. Girls are assigned a sexual maturity rating based on pubic hair and breast development. The time sequence of changes culminating in the attainment of reproductive potential varies considerably from person to person. Bodily manifestations of puberty precede the actual onset of menstruation.

The interplay of physiologic and sociocultural forces acting on girls throughout puberty often raises many questions and concerns among prepubescent girls and their mothers. Frequently, the nurse must explain the bodily and psychological changes of puberty to mothers and their daughters. There is often anxiety about the onset of pubertal changes that are thought to be occurring too early or too late. Therefore, it is important to recognize the wide variability from one young woman to the next.

The Female Reproductive Cycle

Menstruation is the periodic discharge of blood, mucus, and epithelial cells from the uterus. It usually occurs at monthly intervals throughout the reproductive period, except during pregnancy and lactation, when it is usually suppressed. Menstruation is part of the menstrual cycle, a vital component of the **female reproductive cycle** (FRC). The FRC also includes the ovarian cycle; combined, these two cycles make child-

TABLE 6-2
Tanner Staging in Girls

Stage	Breasts	Pubic Hair	Other*	Range in Years
I	None	None		Birth–15
II	Breast budding (the-larche): areolar hyper-plasia with small amount of breast tissue, erect papillae	Long, downy pubic hair over mons veneris or labia majora; may oc-cur with breast bud-ding or several weeks or months later (pub-arche)	Thickening of vaginal ep-ithelial tissue, lowering of vaginal pH occurs.	8½–15
III	Further enlargement of breast tissue and widening of areola with no separation of their contours	Increase in amount of hair (dark, coarse, and curly) spread sparsely over junction of pubes	Peak height spurt begins; uterus enlarges; axillary hair begins to appear.	10–15
IV	Double contour form: areola and papillae form secondary mound on top of breast tissue	Adult appearance but less area covered, no spread to medial as-pects of thighs	Axillary hair present; uterus enlarges; vaginal discharge.	10–17
V	Larger, mature breast with single contour form	Adult distribution and quantity with spread to medial aspects of thighs	Adult characteristics present.	12½–18

*Criteria not included in original Tanner stages.
(Adapted from Wasserman, G., & Gromisch, D. S. [1981]. *Survey of clinical pediatrics* [7th ed.]. New York: McGraw-Hill; Tanner, J. M. [1969]. *Growth at adolescence* [2nd ed.]. Oxford: Blackwell Scientific Publications; and Marshall, W. A. & Tanner, J. M. [1969]. Variations in pattern of pubertal changes in girls. *Archives of Diseases in Children, 44,* 291–303.)

bearing possible and influence the unique qualities and lives of women. In general, a woman who men-struates is able to conceive naturally, whereas one who does not is probably infertile. The processes of ovula-tion and menstruation are closely interlinked and play a vital role in childbearing.

Menarche

Puberty refers to the entire transitional period be-tween childhood and sexual maturity. Menarche is one sign of puberty, usually occurring between 9 and 16 years. In the majority of girls, menarche begins during breast development (Tanner stage 3 or 4), but in some, it will not occur until the breasts are fully mature (Scott et al., 1994). Heredity, race, state of nutrition, climate, and environment may influence the onset of menar-che. For example, maturity tends to occur earlier in warm climates and later in cold regions. The age of menarche has declined steadily; this decline has now ceased in the United States. The mean age of American girls at menarche is 12.3 to 12.8 years (Scott et al., 1994). The reproductive period spans about 35 years, from some point after the beginning of menstruation until its cessation during menopause.

Throughout childhood, the *gonadotropins*, hor-mones produced by the pituitary gland to stimulate the ovaries, appear in low concentrations. Estrogen, pro-duced by the ovaries in the adult, remains unde-tectable. Puberty begins with a rise in the release of gonadotropins from the pituitary gland. These stimu-late the ovary to secrete increasing amounts of *estro-gen*, the hormone responsible for many of the bodily changes of puberty.

An orderly sequence of endocrinologic events result-ing in ovulation may not occur initially. The first few FRCs (commonly called menstrual cycles) following menarche may not be associated with ovulation and are often irregular. However, once menstruation has occurred, it must be assumed that ovulation is present, signifying fertility and the potential for pregnancy.

The Ovarian Cycle and Ovulation

The ovarian cycle refers to the process in which a hu-man ovum is matured and expelled into the fallopian tube, while maturation of another ovum is restrained until the next cycle. Each month, with considerable regularity, a blister-like structure about 1 cm in diame-ter develops on the surface of one of the ovaries.

Within this bubble, almost lost in the fluid and cells around it, lies a tiny speck called the *human ovum,* scarcely visible to the unaided eye (a thimble would hold 3 million of these specks). This ovum not only has the potential to develop into a human being, but it also embodies the mental and physical traits of the woman and her ancestry.

In the process of ovulation, one blister on one ovary ruptures at a given time each month and discharges an ovum. The precise day on which ovulation occurs is a matter of no small significance. For instance, because the ovum can be fertilized (impregnated by the spermatozoon, or male germ cell) only within 24 hours after its escape from the ovary, the day after ovulation a woman is no longer fertile. However, a woman is potentially fertile for a number of days preceding the actual time of ovulation, because spermatozoa can survive in the female reproductive tract for 24 to 72 hours, awaiting the arrival of the ovum.

In a given cycle, the time of ovulation is unpredictable. Even the woman who has regular menstrual periods could experience a delayed or early ovulation in any cycle. This possibility of irregularity, combined with the potential for fertility just before ovulation, makes it difficult to identify precisely the fertile phase of a given cycle.

The only really infertile interval is after ovulation has occurred. The time between ovulation and menstruation is relatively constant (14 ± 2 days); the time between menstruation and ovulation is variable enough that ovulation cannot be accurately predicted from one cycle to the next.

Graafian Follicle

At birth, each ovary contains a huge number of undeveloped ova, probably more than 400,000. These are rather large, round cells with clear cytoplasm and a good-sized nucleus occupying the center. Each ovum is surrounded by a layer of a few small, flattened or spindle-shaped cells. The whole structure, ovum and surrounding cells, is a *follicle,* but in its underdeveloped state at birth, it is a **primordial follicle**.

The formation of primordial follicles ceases at birth or shortly thereafter, and the large number contained in the ovaries of the newborn represents a lifetime supply. The majority have disappeared before puberty, at which time there are approximately 30,000 left. This disintegration of follicles continues throughout reproductive life until menopause when none are usually found.

Meanwhile, from birth to menopause, a few of these primordial follicles show signs of development. The surrounding granular layers of cells begin to multiply rapidly until they are several layers deep; at the same time, they become cuboid in shape. As this proliferation of cells continues, an important fluid called the *follicular fluid* develops between them.

After puberty, the cells within the developing follicles produce *estrogenic hormones,* which, in turn, act on the reproductive organs and bring about cyclic bodily changes. During each FRC, several follicles develop further; however, usually only one of these is selected for complete maturation and ovulation.

Follicular fluid accumulates in such quantities that the multiplying follicle cells are pushed toward the margin; the ovum itself is almost surrounded by fluid and is suspended from the periphery of the follicle by only a small neck of cells. The structure is now known as the **graafian follicle**.

As it increases enormously in size, the graafian follicle naturally pushes aside other follicles that form each month, and a noticeable, blister-like projection appears on the surface of the ovary. At one point, the follicular capsule becomes thin, and as the ovum reaches full maturity, it breaks free from the few cells attaching it to the periphery and floats in the follicular fluid. The thinned area of the capsule now ruptures, and the ovum is expelled from the ovary in the process of ovulation (Fig. 6-12).

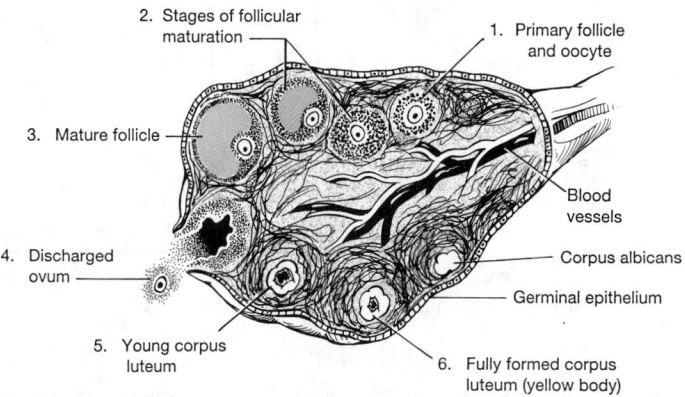

FIGURE 6-12 Ovarian follicle development.

Changes in the Corpus Luteum

After the discharge of the ovum, the ruptured follicle undergoes a change. It becomes filled with large cells containing a special yellow matter. The follicle then is known as the **corpus luteum,** or yellow body. If pregnancy does not occur, the corpus luteum reaches full development in about 8 days, then retrogresses and is gradually replaced by fibrous tissue, the *corpus albicans.*

If pregnancy occurs, the corpus luteum enlarges somewhat and persists throughout gestation, reaching its maximum size about the fourth or fifth month and retrogressing slowly thereafter. The corpus luteum secretes an extremely important substance, progesterone, which is discussed later in this chapter.

In the absence of pregnancy, the corpus luteum remains active for about 2 weeks. The corpus luteum produces progesterone for the standard duration of the postovulatory phase of the menstrual cycle.

The Menstrual Cycle

If the **endometrium,** the lining membrane of the uterus, was observed daily, some remarkable alterations would be noted (Fig. 6-13). These changes have only one purpose, to provide a suitable bed for the fertilized ovum to secure nourishment and grow. If an ovum is not fertilized, these alterations serve no useful function.

The menstrual cycle is broken into three phases: proliferative, secretory, and ischemic. The menstrual cycle is related directly to the ovarian cycle, and both are under hormonal influences, as described in the following section.

Proliferative Phase

Immediately following menstruation, the endometrium is very thin. During the subsequent week or so, it proliferates markedly. The cells on the surface become taller, while the glands that dip into the endometrium become longer and wider. As a result of these changes, the thickness of the endometrium increases sixfold or eightfold. Its glands become more active and secrete a rich, nutritive substance.

Each month during this phase of the menstrual cycle (from approximately the fifth to the 14th day), a graafian follicle is approaching its greatest development and is manufacturing increasing amounts of follicular fluid. This fluid contains the estrogenic hormone *estrogen.* Because estrogen causes the endometrium to grow or proliferate, this phase of the menstrual cycle is called the **proliferative phase.** Sometimes it is called the *follicular* or *estrogenic phase.*

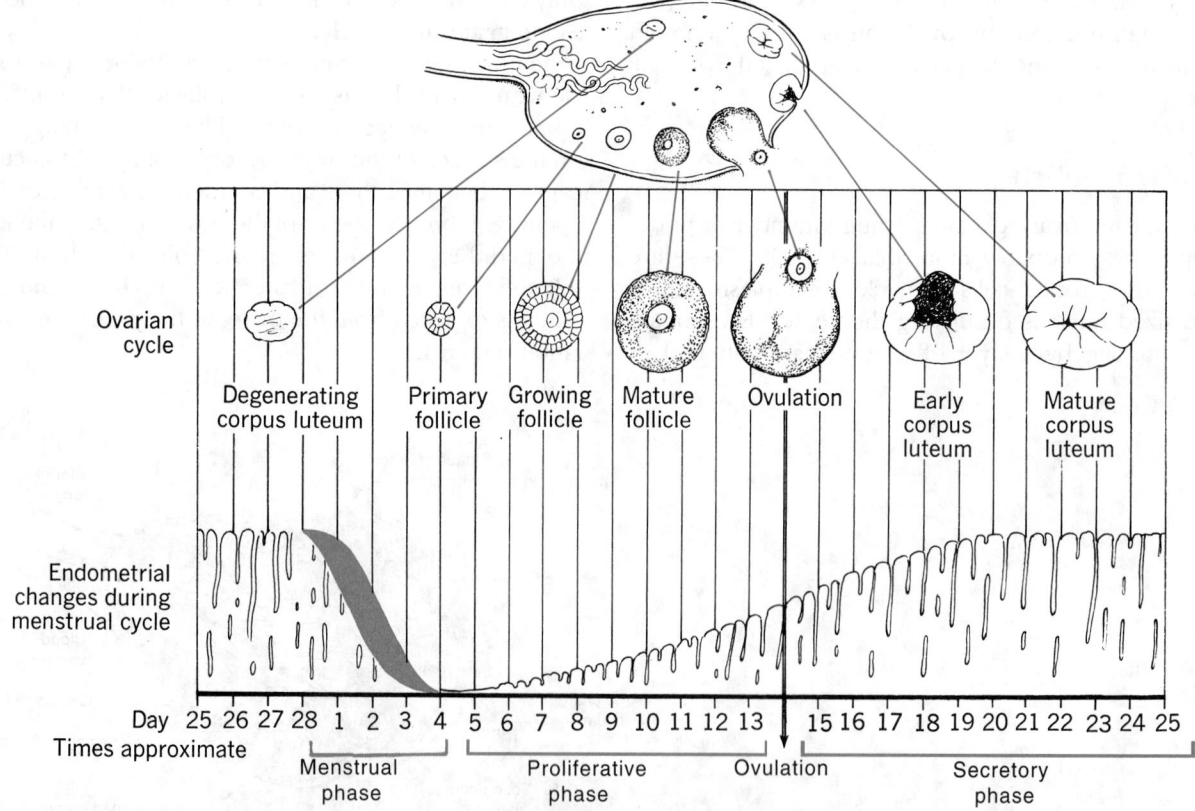

FIGURE 6-13 Schematic representation of one ovarian cycle and the corresponding changes in thickness of the endometrium. It is thickest just before the onset of menstruation and thinnest just as it ceases.

Secretory Phase

Following the release of the ovum from the graafian follicle (ovulation), the cells that form the corpus luteum begin to secrete another important hormone, **progesterone**, in addition to estrogen. This supplements the action of estrogen on the endometrium in such a way that the glands become tortuous, and the lumens are greatly dilated and filled with secretion.

Meanwhile, the blood supply of the endometrium is increased, and it becomes vascular and succulent. The spiral arteries continue to extend into the superficial layer of the endometrium and become convoluted. These effects are directed at providing a bed for the fertilized ovum. This phase of the cycle occupies the last 14 ± 2 days and is called the **secretory phase**; it is also sometimes called the *progestational, luteal,* or *premenstrual phase.*

Menstrual Phase

Unless the ovum is fertilized, the corpus luteum regresses, secretion of progesterone and estrogen declines, and the endometrium undergoes involution. As the endometrium degenerates, countless small blood vessels rupture with innumerable minute hemorrhages. The disintegrated endometrium and blood and glandular secretions escape into the uterine cavity, pass through the cervix, and flow out through the vagina, carrying the tiny unfertilized ovum with them. Thus, menstruation represents the abrupt termination of a process designed to prepare lodging for a fertilized ovum. Its purpose is to clear away the old bed so that a new and fresh one may be created the next month. This phase of the cycle (from approximately the first to the fifth day) is called the **menstrual phase**.

Hormonal Control of the Cycles

The FRC is regulated primarily through the highly coordinated function of the brain, hypothalamus, pituitary, ovaries, and uterus (Fig. 6-14). The whole sequence represents the harmonious, integrated reactions of several processes within the human organism, all of which are necessary to maintain proper relationships in the FRC. For synchronized function of this system, each component must know what the other is doing and must at times be able to stimulate or suppress one of the other elements.

Role of the Pituitary Gland

The anterior lobe of the pituitary releases the gonadotropins to stimulate the ovary and other hormones. These hormones produce the ovarian alterations associated with ovulation. The two principal gonadotropins are the FSH and LH. FSH stimulates the development

of the follicle. LH is principally active during ovulation and the luteal phase of the cycle.

The *hypothalamus,* a specialized structure within the brain located just above the pituitary, regulates the release of the gonadotropic hormones by the pituitary. The hypothalamus has a vascular connection to the pituitary gland and nerve connections to the central nervous system. Its function can be modified by influences within the central nervous system.

The cyclic release of gonadotropin by the pituitary gland is controlled by a hormonal agent released by the hypothalamus. This is called GnRH or LH- and FSH-releasing hormone because it triggers the release of FSH and LH from the pituitary gland. Prostaglandins (PGs) influence gonadotropin secretion by acting on the hypothalamus. These hormones play a major role in the FRC.

Cyclic Pattern

Sensitive laboratory methods now allow accurate measurement of day-to-day changes in circulating pituitary

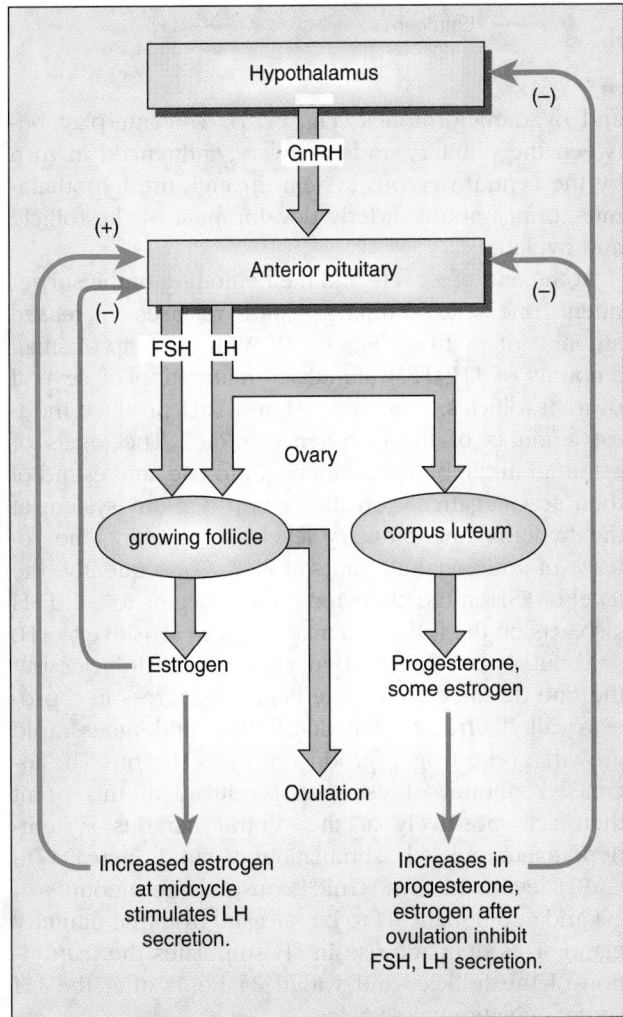

FIGURE 6–14 Feedback loops among the hypothalamus, anterior pituitary, and ovaries during the female reproductive (menstrual) cycle.

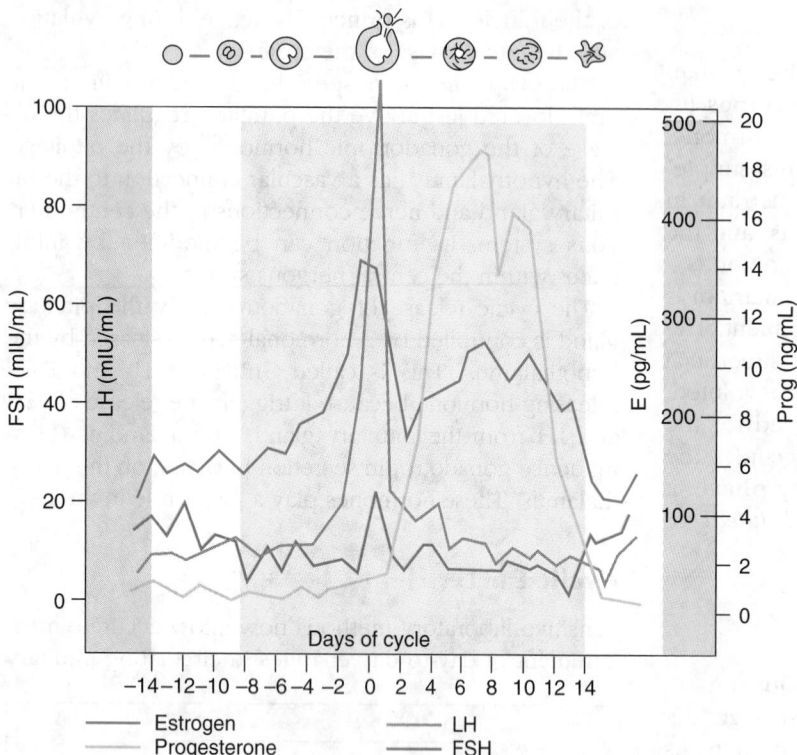

FIGURE 6-15 Plasma hormones in the normal female reproductive cycle.

and ovarian hormones (Fig. 6-15). The interplay between the pituitary and the ovary, influenced in turn by the central nervous system through the hypothalamus, brings about orderly development of the follicle and ovulation.

At the end of a cycle and the beginning of the subsequent one, the pituitary gland releases increased amounts of FSH (see Fig. 6-15). With the help of small amounts of LH, FSH stimulates maturation of several ovarian follicles. Together, LH and FSH produce modest amounts of the estrogen estradiol. The levels of estradiol in the bloodstream begin to rise, and estradiol then acts negatively on the central nervous system at the hypothalamic-pituitary level by inhibiting the release of additional amounts of FSH. Consequently, the level of FSH in the circulating blood begins to fall. FSH also acts on the follicle to make it more sensitive to LH.

About 2 days before ovulation, all the follicles but the one destined to ovulate begin to regress in a process called *atresia.* That one follicle undergoes rapid growth, and estrogen production rises sharply. The increased amount of estrogen produced at this point then acts positively at the central nervous system-hypothalamic level, stimulating a rapid increase in GnRH levels. In turn, GnRH causes large amounts of LH and additional FSH to be released from the pituitary gland. This dramatic rise in LH stimulates the maturation of the follicle, and within 24 hours after the LH surge, ovulation takes place.

The increased levels of preovulatory estrogen prepare the genital tract for sperm migration. The secretions of the cervix, scanty and viscous early in the cy-

cle, become thin and watery and more receptive to spermatozoa. The vaginal wall also reflects the effects of estrogen. A vaginal smear taken at this time reveals a large percentage of mature, or "cornified," cells. The endometrium displays maximal proliferation (see Fig. 6-13).

Following ovulation, the cyclic pattern continues. The ruptured follicle is transformed into a corpus luteum. The second function of LH is to maintain the corpus luteum. These endocrine events are associated with further modifications in the cervical mucus, vagina, and endometrium. The mucus becomes thick, sticky, and viscous and is no longer as receptive to spermatozoa. The vaginal smear reflects the influence of progesterone with a decreasing "maturation index." The endometrium takes on secretory changes to prepare for implantation.

Progesterone secretion by the corpus luteum reaches its maximum about 5 to 7 days after ovulation (see Fig. 6-15). This is the time when the fertilized egg, now a *blastocyst,* is ready to implant. If pregnancy has occurred, another hormone, *human chorionic gonadotropin,* appears within 2 to 3 days of implantation. This hormone, produced by the conceptus, acts on the corpus luteum to maintain its progesterone-providing function and transforms it into a corpus luteum of pregnancy. If pregnancy has not intervened, the corpus luteum begins its demise at this time. Approximately 10 to 11 days after ovulation, progesterone levels decline precipitously, and on about the 14th postovulatory day, no longer receiving hormones, the endometrium begins to shed in the process of menstruation.

Other Functions of Estrogen and Progesterone

In addition to their role in controlling menstruation, estrogen and progesterone serve other important functions:

- Estrogen is responsible for the development of the secondary sex characteristics (eg, the growth of the breasts at puberty, the distribution of body fat, the size of the larynx, and the resulting influence on the quality of the voice).
- Progesterone helps to relax the uterine muscle, in addition to its action on the endometrium. It plays an important role in preserving the life of the embryo in early pregnancy by preventing its expulsion from the uterus and by preparing the endometrium to receive and nourish it.

Prostaglandins

As biologically active lipids, PGs have many functions in reproduction. They are not classified as true hormones, because they are synthesized at or near their site of action rather than transported through the blood to another site. PGs can arise from nearly all tissues of the body, but they are present in high concentrations in the male and female reproductive tracts. There are many different forms of PGs; the subscript refers to the number of double bonds, and the letter refers to the type of PG (eg, A, B, C, D, E, F) according to chemical structure. Particular effects of the PGs are determined by the tissue, the specific PG, and its concentration. PGs can cause smooth muscle contraction or relaxation, tachycardia, hypotension, nausea, vomiting, diarrhea, and bronchial changes. In the man, PGs have been isolated from semen and are believed to play a role in sperm motility and transport. PGs may act as central nervous system transmitters, mediating the effects of hypothalamic-releasing hormones on the pituitary gland (Scott et al., 1994). PGE_2 increases pituitary content of LH in animals, and evidence suggests that $PGF_{2\alpha}$ is involved in ovulation (Scott et al., 1994).

The synthesis of PGs in the uterus occurs predominantly in the endometrium and is related to the phase of the menstrual cycle, rising toward the end of the luteal phase. Progesterone withdrawal in the absence of pregnancy is thought to be related to $PGF_{2\alpha}$. PGs are believed to play a major role in cervical ripening and the initiation and control of labor. PGE_1, PGE_2, and $PGF_{2\alpha}$ cause contraction of the uterus and vasodilation. Certain PGs have been related to dysmenorrhea and premanifestations of preeclampsia (see Chap. 31). Administration of PGE_2 or $PGF_{2\alpha}$ induces labor or abortion at any point in gestation. Certain medications, such as aspirin and indomethacin, may inhibit the production or activity of PGs.

Variations in Cycles

Although the interval of the FRC or menstrual cycle, counting from the beginning of one period to the onset of the next, averages 28 days, there are wide variations even in the same woman. It is rare for a woman to menstruate exactly every 28 or 30 days. Several studies on normal young women show that the majority (almost 60%) experience variations of at least 5 days in the length of their cycles; differences in the same woman of even 10 days are not uncommon and may occur without explanation or apparent detriment to health (Barlow et al., 1988).

The degree and intensity of the outward manifestations of the ovulatory cycle vary from one woman to the next. Some women consistently experience pelvic discomfort during ovulation, or **mittelschmerz**, so named because it typically appears in the middle of a 28-day menstrual cycle. Slight staining or occasional bleeding may occur in association with ovulation. In the postovulatory interval, there may be breast tenderness and fullness, typically reaching a peak just before menstruation.

A variety of clinical syndromes may cause women to experience tension and other affective and somatic symptoms premenstrually. Chief among these is *premenstrual syndrome* (PMS), with symptoms that occur in repetitive fashion prior to menses (eg, irritability, depression, and somatic complaints). A detailed discussion of PMS and other clinical variations in the menstrual cycle, such as dysmenorrhea and amenorrhea, is found in Chapter 10.

Determinants of Phases of Cycles

Not all menstrual cycles are 28 days, and ovulation cannot be determined by counting 14 days from the last menstrual period. Therefore, other means of establishing phases of ovulation have been determined. Two useful means of determining ovulation are observing daily variations in cervical mucus and checking basal body temperature. Both are used in infertility clinics and as natural methods of contraception (see Chaps. 9 and 13). Ultrasound also is being used to observe follicular development and to determine time of ovulation, particularly in infertility clients.

Variations in Cervical Mucus

Under the influence of rapidly rising preovulatory levels of estrogen (see Fig. 6-15), the cervical mucus, scant and sticky early in the cycle, becomes copious and clear. It is most abundant on the day preceding ovulation and is most receptive to spermatozoa at that time. Following ovulation, under the influence of progesterone, the mucus becomes scant, thick, and sticky once again.

BASAL BODY TEMPERATURE RECORD

NAME: _____

AGE: _____

↓ COITUS

■ MENSES

AUGUST / SEPTEMBER

DAYS OF CYCLE ▶	1	2	3	4	5	6	7	8	9	10	11	12	13	14	15	16	17	18	19	20	21	22	23	24	25	26	27	28	29	30	31	32	33	34	35	36	37	38	39	40	41	42
DATE OF MONTH ▶	11	12	13	14	15	16	17	18	19	20	21	22	23	24	25	26	27	28	29	30	31	1	2	3	4	5	6	7	8	9	10	11	12	13	14	15	16	17	18	19	20	21

Temperature scale: 99.0° .8 .6 .4 .2 98.0° .8 .6 .4 .2 97.0°

August Period — *Best Chance Missed* — *15 Days* — *Menses*

SEPTEMBER / OCTOBER

DAYS OF CYCLE ▶	1	2	3	4	5	6	7	8	9	10	11	12	13	14	15	16	17	18	19	20	21	22	23	24	25	26	27	28	29	30	31	32	33	34	35	36	37	38	39	40	41	42
DATE OF MONTH ▶	8	9	10	11	12	13	14	15	16	17	18	19	20	21	22	23	24	25	26	27	28	29	30	1	2	3	4	5	6	7	8	9	10	11	12	13	14	15	16	17	18	19

September Period — *Patient Pregnant*

Intercourse Evening Of Temperature Drop

AUGUST / SEPTEMBER

DAYS OF CYCLE ▶	1	2	3	4	5	6	7	8	9	10	11	12	13	14	15	16	17	18	19	20	21	22	23	24	25	26	27	28	29	30	31	32	33	34	35	36	37	38	39	40	41	42
DATE OF MONTH ▶	11	12	13	14	15	16	17	18	19	20	21	22	23	24	25	26	27	28	29	30	31	1	2	3	4	5	6	7	8	9	10	11	12	13	14	15	16	17	18	19	20	21

August Period — *Menses*

—— *Rectal Temperature*

----- *Mouth Temperature*

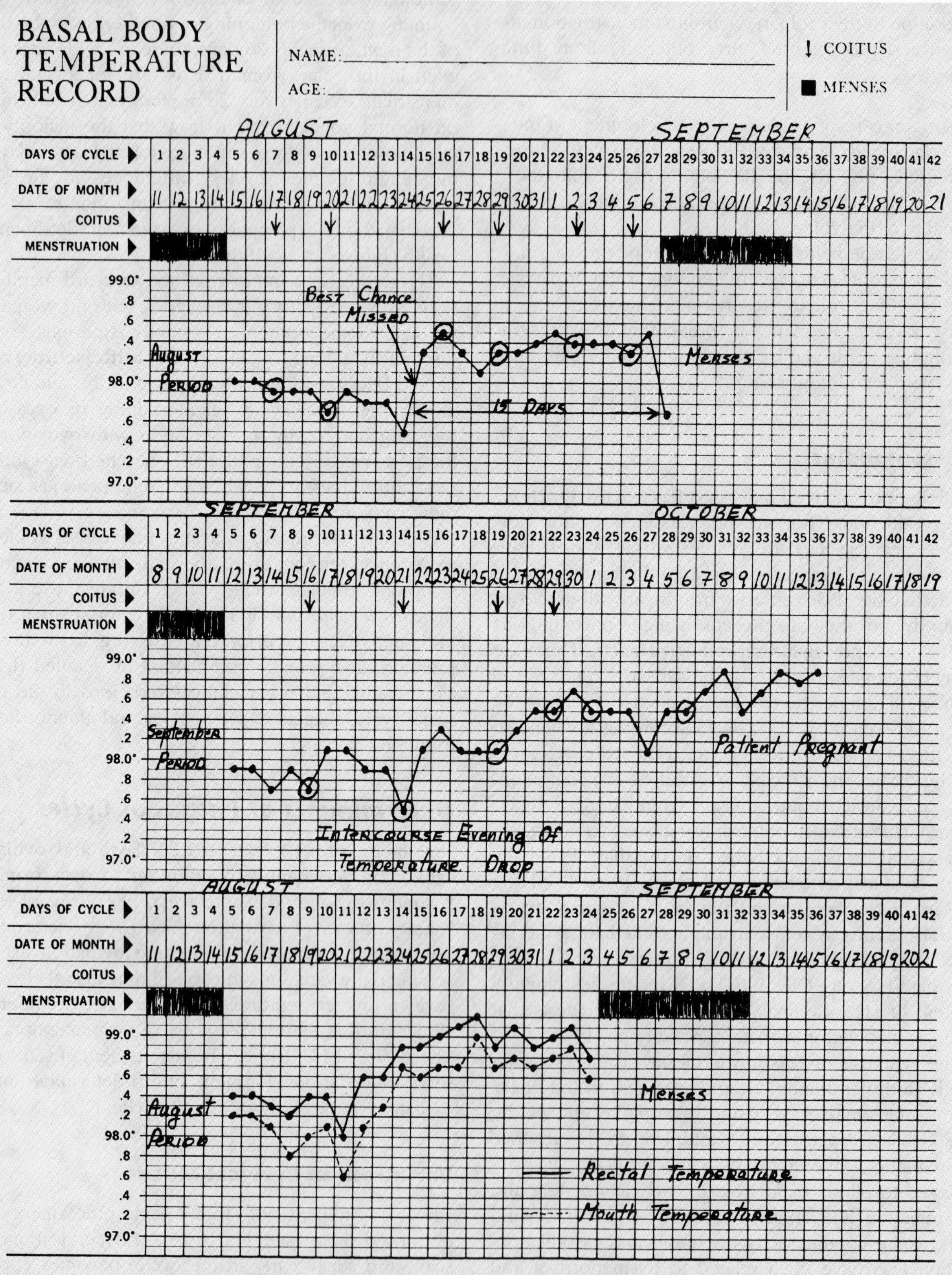

Samples of basal temperature charts indicating menstrual cycles and daily temperature readings. Temperature drops are clearly indicated on all charts, with optimal time for fertilization. Phases of the cycles are determined by these charts. Charts may be used in family planning or in management of infertility. The bottom chart contrasts oral and rectal temperatures. Directions for using this chart are given on the facng page.

(Published by Merrill-National Laboratories, Div. of Richardson-Merrill, Inc., Cincinnati, Ohio 45215.)

These cyclic changes in the quality of the cervical mucus are often easily detected by the normally menstruating woman once she is aware of them. In some cases, a clear, translucent, stretchable (*spinnbarkeit*) mucus appears at the labia or may be wiped from the cervix to provide suggestive evidence of impending ovulation. In the postovulatory phase of the cycle, the sticky and less abundant mucus is not as easily detected. Daily observations of cervical mucus have been suggested as a useful parameter when using the rhythm method of contraception, also referred to as the *symptothermal approach.*

If the cervical mucus is aspirated from the cervical os, spread on a glass slide, allowed to air dry for a few minutes, and examined microscopically, characteristic patterns can be visualized that depend on the stage of the ovarian cycle and the presence or absence of pregnancy. From about the 7th day of the menstrual cycle to about the 18th day, a *fernlike* pattern of dried cervical mucus is seen. The crystallization of the mucus, which is necessary for the production of the fern, depends on the concentration of electrolytes, mainly sodium chloride, in the secretion (Cunningham et al., 1993). After approximately the 21st day of the cycle, this fernlike pattern is not evident; a different pattern forms that has a beaded or cellular appearance. This beaded pattern usually also is observed during pregnancy.

Basal Body Temperature

Slight daily variations in body temperature normally occur in all human beings. These temperature variations are relative to the time of day and the nature of the circumstances surrounding the person. For example, the body temperature is lowest in the morning before breakfast, after a good night's rest, and before activity. After a day of normal activity, the body temperature is usually highest toward afternoon and early evening. The fact that physiologic variations in basal body temperature also occur in relation to the menstrual cycle is important, because it can be useful for estimating the time of ovulation. Such an index becomes extremely important in studies of fertility and sterility.

In the woman who is ovulating, normally a rhythmic variation in the basal body temperature curve occurs during the menstrual cycle (see the Assessment Tool). The basal temperature is lower during the first part of the menstrual cycle, the proliferative phase. It may drop slightly before ovulation and then rise approximately 0.2° to 0.4°C (0.4°–0.8°F) in association with ovulation. During the luteal phase of the cycle, the temperature remains relatively higher as a result of the influence of progesterone produced by the corpus luteum following ovulation. Progesterone causes this thermogenic effect through its influence on the central nervous system.

If pregnancy occurs, the progesterone level is maintained, and under its influence, the basal temperature remains high past the expected time of the period. In the absence of pregnancy, the basal temperature usually drops a day or so before the menstrual period.

The Use of the Basal Temperature Graph. The basal body temperature is one of the most practical means of diagnosing ovulation. The relative difference in basal body temperature during the course of the cycle is the important diagnostic criterion for ovulation. It is only useful in the timing of ovulation retrospectively. Thus, when there is infertility, efforts to time intercourse to coincide with changes in the temperature chart may not be helpful. In fact, such regulation of coital habits is seldom recommended. However, for the diagnosis of ovulation, the temperature chart is valuable. The temperature chart also may be useful as an adjunct to the rhythm method of family planning (see Chap. 9). Women require specific instructions on how to obtain and record their basal temperature accurately (see Client Teaching Guidelines).

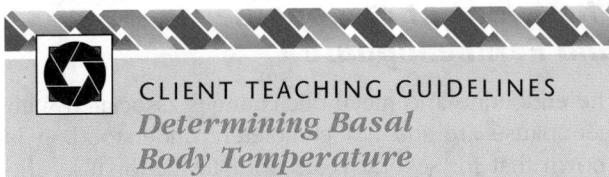

CLIENT TEACHING GUIDELINES
Determining Basal Body Temperature

- Discuss the relationship between basal body temperature (BBT) and ovulation.
  Biphasic pattern of BBT: Temperature is lower during first half of the cycle (<98°F or <36.7°C) than during the second half of the cycle (>98°F or >36.7°C). BBT sometimes drops 12-24 hours before ovulation; this change does not occur in all women.
  At ovulation, the temperature will rise 0.4–0.8°F (0.2°–0.4°C) above preovulatory baseline.
  The first day of menses is considered to be day 1 of the cycle.
- Instruct client to record duration of menstrual flow, beginning on cycle day 1 (see graph). The date of onset of flow is recorded, and each subsequent date is recorded in the spaces provided.
- Demonstrate BBT thermometer and chart.
- Instruct client to perform the following procedures: Take temperature (oral, rectal, BBT thermometer) for 5 minutes immediately after waking and before getting out of bed, eating, drinking, or smoking and at the same time each day. The thermometer is read within 0.1°. Record BBT immediately after obtaining the reading by entering a dot for the recorded temperature each day and connecting the series of dots.
  Shake the thermometer down after each use.
  Record the occurrence of sexual intercourse with a circle around the BBT recording the following morning.
  Note other occurrences that can affect BBT, for example, illness, inadequate sleep, travel, alcohol consumption the evening before, use of an electric blanket or a heated waterbed, and emotional upset.
  Record observable signs of ovulation, such as mittelschmerz or clear preovulatory vaginal discharge.

Menopause and Perimenopause

Menopause refers to the time in a woman's life when she has her last menses. **Perimenopause** begins prior to the last menstruation and includes the year after the permanent cessation. Menopause occurs because of a marked decrease in estrogen; it usually occurs between 50 and 55 years of age in most women, with an average of 51 years (Wren, 1992). Although the word *climacteric* is often used synonymously with menopause, the term refers to the total syndrome of endocrine, somatic, and psychic changes associated with declining fertility in an aging woman. Menopause rarely occurs as a sudden loss of ovarian function. However, ovulation may occur sporadically or may cease abruptly. Hence, periods may end suddenly, become scanty or irregular, or be intermittently heavy before ceasing altogether.

Physiology of Menopause and Perimenopause

The endocrine and metabolic changes associated with menopause are still not completely understood. It is known that for several years prior to menopause, the ovaries begin to exhaust the supply of oocytes and surrounding cellular structures that produce most of the estrogen available during the reproductive years. The loss of functioning ovarian follicles and the resulting decrease in circulating estrogen also cause a change in the sex hormone output of the hypothalamus, pituitary gland, and adrenal glands (Scharbo-DeHaan et al., 1991). For example, the decreasing production of estradiol and progesterone allows release of increased amounts of gonadotropins from the pituitary, resulting in higher circulating levels of FSH and LH. The hypothalamus secretes increasing amounts of GnRH into the portal circulation in a pulsating fashion, which is believed to be responsible for inducing the hot flashes that often accompany menopause (Wren, 1992). With estrogen withdrawal, neurotransmitters decrease opioid endorphin activity and modify dopamine and serotonin metabolism (Rinehart et al., 1985). These fluctuations in hormone levels contribute to emotional changes.

The physiologic impact of perimenopause may cause a woman to experience a variety of symptoms. Changes in the vaginal mucosa vary among perimenopausal women. Even minimal changes may result in painful intercourse (dyspareunia). Thinning of the vaginal lining and the decrease in lubrication can be corrected with estrogen administered orally or locally with vaginal suppositories or cream. Dyspareunia is a common symptom that should not be overlooked in the management of the postmenopausal woman.

Each woman reacts somewhat differently to the changes in menopausal endocrine function. These reactions are unpredictable and depend to some extent on a woman's emotional history, her support systems within the family, and the fact that the menopausal reproductive-endocrine system may be quite labile during this interval, which may last as long as 8 or 9 years (Ravnikar, 1990; Ferguson et al., 1989).

Some of the difficulties of perimenopause can be subdued through education about aging, menopause, and related concerns (Cook, 1993). It is particularly important for women to be counseled about the increased risk of adverse changes associated with estrogen deprivation (eg, osteoporosis, atherosclerosis, myocardial infarction, stroke, and cancer) and methods to promote health during the aging process.

Human Sexuality

Human sexuality encompasses multiple dimensions, which include physiologic development of the reproductive systems and self-identity, sexual expression, and the need for love and personal fulfillment. All people are sexual beings and are aware of and react to their own femaleness or maleness. Sexuality is holistic, integrating biologic, psychological, and cultural factors into a whole that is greater than the sum of its parts. Each person has a unique style of sexuality, even those who limit sexual expression in celibacy. Human sexuality extends from before birth in early embryonic development, throughout life, and until death. It is a fundamental and pervasive characteristic of human activity and interaction.

Sexual response in men and women is a complex process with both psychological and physiologic components that canot really be separated. These components are intricately inter-related and create numerous feedback loops that can enhance or inhibit sexual response. The changes in bodily function and the perceptions and emotions that precede or accompany these are closely related to physiologic processes. The psychogenic stimuli that affect sexual response work largely through the relatively simple process of conditioning by association, or conditioned response. However, sexual meanings can be attached to stimuli through more complex psychological processes. The mental state in which people are likely to initiate or respond to sexual advances is created by a complex interplay of many factors. Human emotions and thoughts are complicated, so it is not surprising that sexual responsiveness varies greatly among different people and in the same person at different times. Sex can be considered one of the basic human drives; however, it is much more malleable in expression than food or sleep, for example. Although a nearly universal behavior among humans, sex can be postponed for long periods, or in some instances, never activated, without adverse effects. Although cultural expression leads to a wide variety of sex-related behaviors, the biologic foundations of sexual interaction lead to more underlying similarities than differences among people.

Differences have been identified between male and female sexuality across the life span, which may be culturally based. Men seem to have an intense, genitally focused sexuality as teenagers. Approaching 30 years, men are still highly interested in sex but without such urgency and are satisfied with fewer orgasms. With increasing age, men's sexual experience becomes more sensuously diffuse and has a greater emotional component. In contrast, women have an early awareness of the sensuous and emotional aspects of sex, but their orgasmic response is slow and inconsistent while in their teens and early 20s. By 30 to 35 years, women's sexual response becomes quicker and more intense, with more consistent orgasms. Sexuality for the adolescent girl is person centered, emphasizing the relationships and emotions between two people. It becomes more body centered, emphasizing physical pleasure later in midadulthood (Hyde, 1990).

Physiology of Sexual Response

Research on human sexuality has found that male and female sexual responses and behavior are more alike than different. The basic similarities of physiologic sexual responses between both sexes have been stressed by such researchers as Kinsey, Masters, and Johnson. Aside from the obvious anatomic differences, men and women are homogeneous in their physiologic responses to sexual stimuli. There are direct parallels in male and female anatomic responses to effective sexual stimulation, and the same underlying physiologic mechanisms are involved: vasocongestion and myotonia. For example, vaginal lubrication in the woman parallels penile erection in the man; both responses occur as a result of vasocongestion. Increases in muscle tension (*myotonia*) and changes in heart rate, blood pressure, and respiration are common to men and women during sexual excitement. The reflexive contractions of orgasm are virtually identical in both sexes, although there are variations in the results that these contractions produce. Furthermore, there is a considerable overlap in the subjective experience of orgasm. In a study comparing women's and men's written descriptions of orgasms, in which the sex of the person writing the description could not be identified, professional judges could not distinguish the writer's sex by the way orgasms were described. The study concluded that the experience of orgasm, as described by this college-age population, was essentially the same (Denney et al., 1992).

The systems of sexual anatomy and physiology, organized around the clitoris in women and the penis in men, are exact homologues of each other. Each part in one sex has its counterpart in the other. These counterparts, structurally the same in women and men, may be modified to perform the same function in a different way or may perform a different function. The sexual response cycle progresses through identical phases with corresponding changes in genital and other body organs in women and men. There are certain differences in timing and patterns that are characteristic of both sexes within this common physiologic process.

The sexual organs receive messages from the sympathetic and parasympathetic systems, as do most other body organs. Penile erection and vaginal lubrication are caused by the effects of the parasympathetic system, which produce vasodilation. As arousal progresses, the sympathetic system plays a larger role, causing increases in heart rate and blood pressure. The sympathetic system may take over completely at orgasm, with ejaculation and vaginal spasms set off by a sudden discharge of adrenaline. The release of acetylcholine from the parasympathetic system quickly compensates for the autonomic imbalance produced by this sudden release of adrenaline. This parasympathetic rebound phenomenon, with its vasodilation, contributes to the subjective feelings of warmth and relaxation that many people feel after orgasm.

The sexual response cycle in men and women can be divided into several stages. An orderly sequence of psychophysiologic events takes place, bringing about marked changes in the shape and function of the genital organs. Regardless of whether sexual stimulation is reflexogenic or psychogenic, the reactions in the neurologic, vascular, muscular, and hormonal systems affect many parts of the body.

Sexual Response Theories

The most popular sexual response model was introduced by Masters and Johnson (1966) in *Human Sexual Response*. Their four-stage model proposed that human sexual response progresses from excitement to plateau, orgasm, and finally resolution. Each stage is accompanied by anatomic and physiologic reactions (Table 6-3). The *excitement stage* begins with the onset of erotic feelings and sensations, producing an immediate and intense vasocongestion and increased myotonia if stimulation is effective. As excitement progresses, the *plateau stage* is reached; this is the stage immediately preceding orgasm. The *stage of orgasm* is reached when vasocongestion passes a critical point, and a reflex stretch mechanism is set off in the pelvic muscles of both sexes. The muscles contract vigorously, pressing on distended structures and expelling blood trapped in tissues and vessels, which creates the sensation of orgasm. Ejaculation occurs in the man, with spurts of semen from the urethral meatus and contractions of the penis and urethra. In the woman,

TABLE 6-3
Summary of Physiologic Changes in Four-Stage Sexual Response Cycle

General Description	Physiologic Changes in Women	Physiologic Changes in Men
Excitement stage begins with onset of arousal from physical or psychic stimuli. This produces an immediate and intense vasocongestion and increased myotonia (contraction of muscles) if stimulation is effective. Other responses include elevated pulse, blood pressure, and respiratory rate and flushing of the skin on abdomen and over chest.	External genitalia: *labia majora*—spread flat and elongate anterioposteriorly; changes more exaggerated in multiparous women. *Labia minora*—deepen in color, engorge, and extend outward. *Clitoris*—glans and shaft engorge, shaft elongates two to three times, vestibular bulbs distend. Internal genitalia: *vagina*—upper two-thirds widen and lengthen, upper vagina balloons out, rugae become smooth, droplets of clear fluid (transudate) appear on walls within 10–30 sec of stimulation, coalesce and produce lubrication. *Uterus*—enlarges and pulls upward, away from vagina. *Cervix*—moves upward and backward posteriorly. Related structures: *Breasts*—enlarge and areola engorges, nipples erect and increase in size. *Pelvic muscles*—engorge and contract.	*Penis*—engorges, lengthens, and rapidly develops erection; penile bulb distends; glans enlarges to almost twice its normal size. *Scrotum*—skin thickens and wrinkles; scrotal sac elevates and flattens against body; spermatic cord contracts. *Testes*—increase in size and partially elevate with scrotum. *Urethral meatus*—dilates and moistens with mucus. *Cowper's glands*—may secrete fluid. *Breasts:* Nipples may become erect.
Plateau stage is the period preceding orgasm that is characterized by heightened sexual arousal of the entire body. Physiologic responses reach a maximum level (eg, continued vasocongestion and myotonia, elevated pulse, blood pressure, respiratory rate).	External genitalia: *Labia minora*—distends maximally and turns bright to deep red. *Clitoris*—glans completely retracts under the prepuce, enlarges, and completes upward arc; vestibular bulbs distend maximally; may be very sensitive. *Bartholin glands*—secrete 1 to 3 drops. Internal genitalia: *Vagina*—distends maximally; "orgasmic platform" (thickened area of congested tissue producing gripping effect) builds up in outer third of vagina; upper vagina widely balloons. *Uterus*—ascends from true pelvis. *Cervix*—fully elevated. Related structures: *Breasts*—enlarge, and areola fully engorges.	*Penis*—fully distends and erects to maximum size; glans becomes purplish. *Testes*—increase in size (up to 50%) and fully elevate closely against perineum, rotate anteriorly. *Urethral meatus*—contains drops of fluid from the Cowper's glands (may contain sperm). *Prostatic urethra*—collects seminal fluid, producing feeling of imminent ejaculation.
Orgasm stage is the phase of maximum sexual (physical, psychological, or both) arousal in which there is a release from muscle tension and blood engorgement. Men and women show a decrease in voluntary muscle control demonstrated by muscle spasm throughout the body (eg, facial twitching, contractions of muscles of neck, limbs, abdomen). Physiologic responses include greater elevation in pulse, blood pressure, and respiratory rate; marked sex flush occurs.	External genitalia: *Labia minora*—change in color. *Clitoris*—contracts rhythmically. *Urinary meatus*—dilates in some women. Internal genitalia: *Vagina*—Contractions of orgasmic platform occur 3–15 times; intensity may vary from mild to strong. *Uterus*—contracts rhythmically from fundus to cervix. *Cervix*—os opens slightly immediately after orgasm. Related structures: *Breasts*—enlarge and areola swell; nipples become erect and increase in size. *Rectal sphincter*—contracts. *Pelvic muscles*—engorge and contract.	*Penis*—expulsive contractions of entire penile urethra, starting at 0.8-second intervals; after the first three or four contractions, they decrease in frequency and intensity. *Urethra*—semen ejects with force as bulb contracts. *Vas deferens*—contract. *Seminal vesicles, prostate,* and *Cowper's glands*—contract, expelling semen and fluid into urethra. *Breasts*—nipples may become erect. *Internal sphincter of bladder*—contracts.

(continued)

TABLE 6–3 *(Continued)*
Summary of Physiologic Changes in Four-Stage Sexual Response Cycle

General Description	Physiologic Changes in Women	Physiologic Changes in Men
Resolution stage is the final phase of the sexual response cycle when man or woman returns to an unexcited state. This is the period of involuntary relaxation when changes in genitals and other organs are reversed as the congested blood is released back into the general circulation. Physiologic responses, such as pulse, blood pressure, and respiratory rate, return to normal; sex flush fades slowly. The duration of this stage varies proportionately with length of excitement and plateau stage.	External genitalia: *Labia majora*—return to normal size, color, and midline. *Labia minora*—return slowly to normal size and position; lose color. *Clitoris*—returns to normal size and position (5–10 sec), no refractory period; multiple orgasms may be experienced. Internal genitalia: *Vagina*—outer ⅓ returns quickly to normal; inner ⅔ returns to normal more slowly. *Uterus*—slowly returns to normal position. *Cervix*—drops into seminal pool, os closes in 20–30 minutes. Related structures: *Breasts and nipples*—decrease in size.	*Penis*—decreases rapidly in size to 50% larger than unstimulated state; refractory period needed. *Urethra*—minor contractions continue for short period after semen is released. *Scrotum*—thins and folds return. *Testes*—decrease in size and descend. *Breasts and nipples*—decrease in size.

contractions occur at the same time interval (0.8 second) as blood and fluid move out of distended pelvic tissues and veins; the main sites of orgasmic sensation involve the clitoris and lower part of the vagina.

Female ejaculation, the expulsion of fluid during orgasm by women, has been reported by women in a number of investigations (Bullough et al., 1984; Masters and Johnson, 1985; Ladas et al., 1982; Zaviacic et al., 1993). Researchers propose the existence of a rudimentary female prostate gland in the urethral wall near the bladder that produces a gush of fluid from the urethra during orgasm. This has been associated with the *Grafenberg spot*, a sensitive area on the anterior wall of the vagina, which may be very erotic and promote orgasm for some women (see Research Highlight). The paraurethral (Skene's) glands are another possible source of female orgasmic fluid. Studies have found that some women expel a fluid similar to urine from the urethra during sexual response, while others expel a fluid different from urine (Zaviacic et al., 1993).

During *resolution*, the final stage of the sexual response cycle, the changes in genitals and other organs and structures are reversed. The term *refractory period* refers to the time necessary to complete the sexual response cycle again. This period varies with age and physical and emotional health.

If orgasm does not occur, resolution follows the same physiologic processes but takes considerably longer. Muscle tension and vasocongestion recede more gradually, and the pelvic area may remain congested for several hours. Response to sexual experiences without orgasm vary by occasion and individual. In some instances, it may be desirable to avoid orgasmic release, and even if not deliberate, nonorgasm on occasion is usually accepted. Consistent absence of or-

RESEARCH HIGHLIGHT

Female Prostate Gland

Despite previous contradictory claims, some researchers have recently reported a possible homologous female prostate gland, potentially involved in female ejaculation at the moment of orgasm. Physicians have speculated that the fluid being expelled is urine. This descriptive study was undertaken to examine a series of variables thought to be associated with female ejaculation and its relationship, if any, to a sensitive anatomic area known as the Grafenberg spot. An anonymous questionnaire was developed for this study and distributed by mail to 2,350 professional women in the United States and Canada with a subsequent 55% return rate. Of these respondents, 40% reported having a fluid release (ejaculation) at the moment of orgasm. Further, 82% of the women who reported the sensitive area also reported ejaculation with their orgasms. Several variables were found to be associated with the perceived existence of female ejaculation; examples include the experience of multiple orgasms during sexual intercourse and orgasms of longer duration.

Critique: The generalizability of findings is limited because the sample was self-selected and included subjects with high educational backgrounds. Furthermore, a number of participants had read about the possibility of female ejaculation and discussed the topic with friends or relatives prior to participation. All data were collected through self-report, and direct observations were not performed. It is possible that some of the women's confusion about the anatomy and physiology of their sexual organs made them mistake their vaginal lubrication or urinary incontinence for an ejaculation.

Darlin, C. A., Davidson, J. K., & Conway-Welch, C. (1990). Female ejaculation: Perceived origins, the Grafenberg spot/area, and sexual responsiveness. *Archives of Sexual Behavior, 19*, 29–47.

gasm, however, often leads to frustration, resentment, feelings of inadequacy, and unhappiness. There are cultural differences between male and female responses to nonorgasm: A man generally is not satisfied with sex unless he has ejaculated, whereas women do not find it unusual to have some percentage of nonorgasmic sexual encounters. However, a long-term, high proportion of encounters without orgasm in women gradually can lead to less interest in sex (Kaplan, 1974).

Other models of sexual response patterns have been proposed. Based on her work as a sex therapist, Helen Kaplan (1974, 1979) has described a *triphasic model* of sexual response. Instead of the previously described four sequential stages, she conceptualizes three relatively independent phases; two are physiologic (vasocongestion, reflex muscular contractions), and one is psychological (desire). The phase of vasocongestion is comparable to the excitement and plateau phases of Masters and Johnson and is controlled by the parasympathetic nervous system. The phase of reflex muscular contractions compares with orgasm in Masters' and Johnson's model and is controlled by the sympathetic nervous system. The phase of sexual desire involves psychological and cognitive factors. Because different systems are involved (perceptive, neuromuscular, and vascular), difficulties can develop in one phase relatively independently of another.

A *five-component model* proposed by Zilbergeld and Ellison (1980) takes psychological and subjective aspects of human sexual response into account. These five components are related to each other but also are independent. The components are interest or desire; arousal; physiologic readiness, including vasocongestion of reproductive structures, erection, and vaginal lubrication; orgasm; and satisfaction, the subjective feeling of the sexual experience. This model includes more focus on cognitive and subjective aspects, stressing the importance of perception and evaluation of sexual events.

Male Sexual Patterns

There appears to be less variability in the man's pattern of sexual response than the woman's:

- Excitement usually progresses continuously in the man, unless prolonged by deliberate use of delaying tactics, until the plateau stage is reached.
- Plateau lasts for a relatively short time, then peaks in one definitive, usually strong orgasm.
- Resolution occurs rapidly, with a supposed refractory period during which restimulation of the penis is not possible.
- The refractory period is much shorter in younger men, who may have another erection in a few min-

utes. Some have questioned the concept of a time during which the man cannot respond to sexual stimuli (Fig. 6-16).
- Men report experiencing orgasms of different intensity.

Female Sexual Patterns

There are three basic types of sexual response patterns in women (Masters et al., 1966):

- Pattern one resembles the male pattern, in that excitement builds rapidly to plateau, with some peaks and dips along the way, leading to one intense orgasm and a rapid resolution stage (see pattern C, Fig. 6-16).
- Pattern two involves a slower progression of excitement and a longer plateau stage. An intense and definite orgasm is then experienced, followed by a slower resolution stage. Instead, after orgasm, the woman may return to plateau for a while, then have another orgasm that may be either more or less intense. Some women can have multiple orgasms while rising and falling into plateau levels of arousal, followed by slower resolution (see pattern A, Fig. 6-16).
- In pattern three, excitement progresses more slowly until plateau is reached, then there are minor surges toward orgasm, causing repeated and prolonged pleasurable and tingly sensations without a definite orgasm. Resolution tends to be longest with this pattern (see pattern B, Fig. 6-16).

A few other differences between male and female sexual response warrant discussion. Erection is attained within 3 to 5 seconds, while vaginal lubrication takes about 30 seconds. It takes longer for the woman to fill the much larger structures in her pelvic area, and greater amounts of vasocongestion and edema are required. The man has three erectile bodies to fill (two corpora cavernosa and one corpus spongiosum with its bulb), while the woman has five bodies to fill (two corpora cavernosa, two vestibular bulbs, and a large circumvaginal plexus). With all the bulbs and venous plexi maximally distended, the blood volume that a woman has to remove during orgasm is considerably greater than that of a man. Women need longer pelvic muscles to do this because the female pelvic outlet is greater in diameter. In the man, the greatest strength of muscle contractions occurs in the first three to four orgasmic contractions. This strong, concentrated muscular activity assures deposition of semen deep within the vaginal barrel, resulting in a short, intense orgasm that enhances conception. The woman's orgasmic contractions generally last twice as long as the man's, and their strength is not as markedly concentrated in the first few contractions. These types of contractions re-

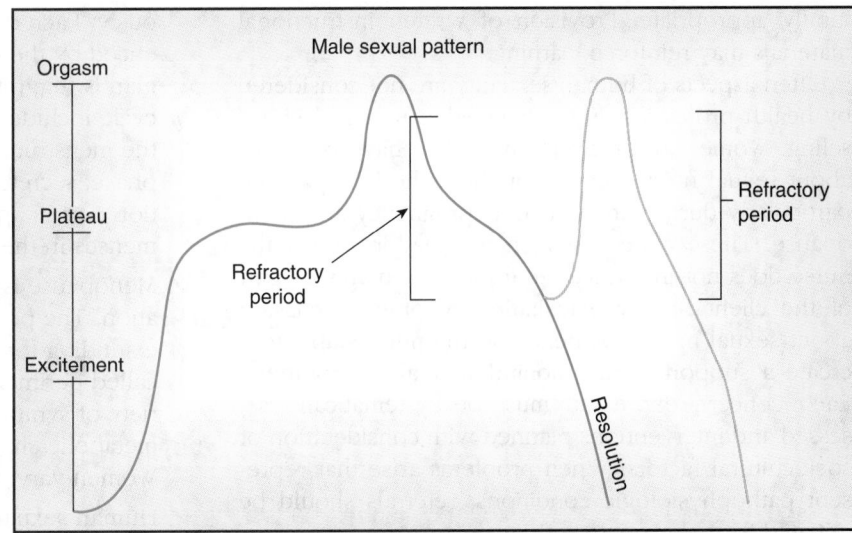

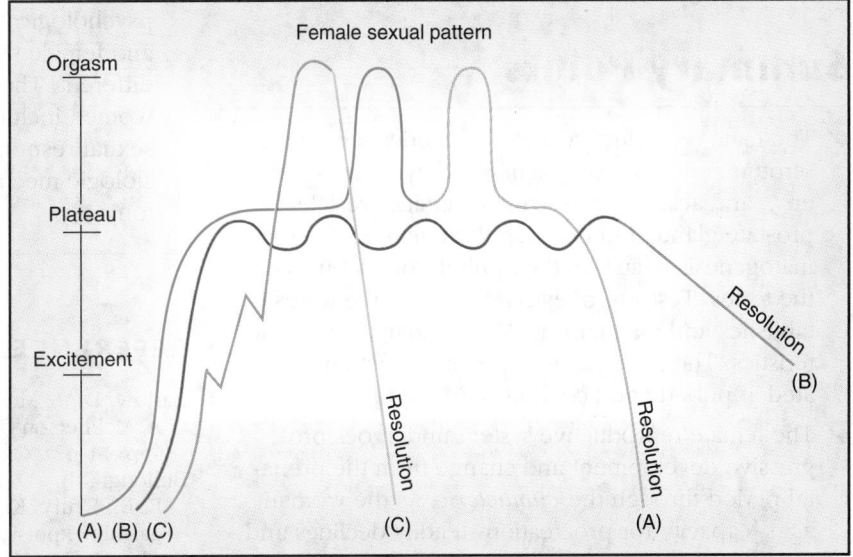

FIGURE 6–16 Male and female sexual response patterns. Female sexual patterns: (A) Steady progression to plateau stage is followed by intense orgasm; subsequent orgasms may occur; resolution is slower. (B) Slower progression to plateau stage is followed by minor surges toward orgasm, causing prolonged pleasurable feelings without definitive orgasm; resolution is slowest. (C) Rapid progression to plateau stage with some peaks and dips; one intense orgasm follows with rapid resolution. This most closely resembles the male pattern.

move a greater amount of the woman's more widespread pelvic congestion. However, there is wide variation in a woman's orgasmic response, with a generally greater range in intensity and duration than a man's.

Nursing Process

Basic knowledge of the male and female reproductive systems and human sexuality is necessary for the nurse to understand the process of conception and human development. The nurse needs to be familiar with the anatomic features of the man and woman to perform physical assessments and health histories. Psychological factors influencing sexual behaviors and preferences constitute another important component of the comprehensive nursing evaluation related to the reproductive system. This area of inquiry must be considered with the utmost confidentiality and respect. The data obtained are used to formulate nursing diagnoses

and develop care plans that consider the unique features of each individual.

Information about sexual and reproductive anatomy and physiology should be incorporated into client education to promote health from childhood through aging. Knowledge about reproductive functioning provides a basis for self-care, fertility control, and sexual decision making. Adolescents and young adults often lack information about how their body functions (eg, menstrual cycle, sexual response patterns), which may contribute to risk-taking behaviors. Pregnancy and childbirth provide an opportune time for instructing women and their partners about changing reproductive anatomy and alterations in function associated with gestation. As menopause approaches, numerous questions may arise concerning methods for alleviating symptoms. These should be anticipated and routinely addressed in client education. The nurse should provide anticipatory guidance and instruction in language that is clearly understandable by the client and is culturally appropriate. Provision of written instructional materials may reinforce learning.

Often aspects of human sexuality are not considered by health professionals in client education and counseling. Women and their partners may have concerns about sexual functioning throughout the life span but particularly during times such as pregnancy and menopause. These concerns often go unaddressed if the nurse does not introduce the topic of sexuality as part of the client history. Facilitation of open discussion about sexual matters depends on the nurse's ability to create a supportive and nonjudgmental environment. Each concern expressed must be systematically assessed and interventions planned with consideration of sociocultural factors. When problems arise that represent pathophysiologic conditions, referrals should be initiated for appropriate assistance.

Summary Points

✔ The male reproductive system includes the penis, scrotum, testes, duct system (epididymis, vas deferens), and accessory structures (seminal vesicle, prostate gland, and bulbourethral glands). Spermatogenesis occurs in the seminiferous tubules of the testes. Testosterone secretion from the testes establishes and maintains male secondary sex characteristics. The male capacity for reproduction is initiated at puberty and continues into old age.

✔ The female reproductive system undergoes progressive development and change from the prenatal period through the *climacteric*. As the woman ages, capacity for procreation steadily declines and finally ends with menopause. A lifetime supply of primordial follicles (germ cells) is present at birth. The development and maturation of these follicles containing the ova continue from puberty to menopause.

✔ The female reproductive system includes external organs (mons veneris, labia majora, labia minora, clitoris, vaginal vestibule, and perineum) and internal organs (ovaries, fallopian tubes, uterus, and vagina). The ovaries are the site for development and expulsion of the ova, and they secrete hormones (estrogen and progesterone) that play a central role in the FRC. The fallopian tubes transport the ova to the uterus and are the site of fertilization of the primary oocyte. The uterus is the implantation site for the fertilized ovum and protects the fetus until birth; its lining is shed during menstruation. The vagina is the organ of copulation; it also provides an avenue for escape of menstrual flow and forms part of the birth canal.

✔ The FRC has two components, the ovarian cycle and the menstrual cycle, which occur simultaneously. Each of these cycles includes phases influenced by the central nervous system and endocrine glands (eg, pituitary, hypothalamus). The ovarian cycle includes the follicular phase and luteal phase; the menstrual cycle consists of the proliferative phase, secretory phase, and ischemic phase. Ovulation occurs approximately 14 days before each menses in the normally occurring FRC.

✔ Menopause is the point of a woman's last menstruation. The period preceding the last menses and extending for 1 year after permanent cessation is called perimenopause and is characterized by a variety of symptoms attributed to endocrine and metabolic changes (eg, estrogen deprivation). Women vary widely in response to these changes.

✔ Human sexual behavior is influenced by complex inter-relations between physiologic development, psychological factors, culture, and emotions. Male and female sexual behavior is more alike than different. The reproductive systems of men and women include homologous sex organs. The sexual response cycle includes two basic physiologic mechanisms: vasocongestion and myotonia.

REFERENCES

Barlow, D., & McPherson, A. (1988). Menstrual problems. In A. McPherson (Ed.), *Women's problems in general practice* (pp. 14–42). Oxford: Oxford University Press.

Bullough, B., David, M., Whipple, B., Dixon, J., Allgeier, E. B., Drury, K. C. (1984). Subjective reports of female orgasmic expulsion of fluid. *Nurse Practitioner, 9*(3), 55–59.

Cook, M. J. (1993). Perimenopause: An opportunity for health promotion. *Journal of Obstetric, Gynecologic, and Neonatal Nursing, 22*, 223–228.

Cunningham, F. G., PacDonald, P. C., Gant, N. F., Leveno, K. J., & Gilstrap, L. C. (1993). *Williams obstetrics* (19th ed.). Norwalk, CT: Appleton & Lange.

Denney, N. W., & Quadagno, D. (1992). *Human sexuality.* St. Louis: C.V. Mosby.

Ferguson, K. J., Hoegh, C., & Johnson, S. (1989). Estrogen replacement therapy: A survey of women's knowledge and attitudes. *Archives of Internal Medicine, 149*(1), 133–136.

Hyde, J. S. (1990). *Understanding human sexuality* (4th ed.). New York: McGraw-Hill.

Kaplan, H. S. (1974). *The new sex therapy.* New York: Brunner/Mazel.

Kaplan, H. S. (1979). *Disorders of sexual desire.* New York: Simon & Schuster.

Ladas, A., Whipple, B., & Perry, J. (1982). *The G spot and other recent discoveries about human sexuality.* New York: Holt Rinehart & Winston.

Masters, W., & Johnson, V. E. (1966). *Human sexual response.* Boston: Little, Brown.

Oski, F. A., Feigin, R. D., & DeAngelis et al. (Eds.) (1994). *Principles and Practice of Pediatrics.* Philadelphia: J.B. Lippincott.

Ravnikar, V. (1990). Physiology and treatment of hot flushes. *Obstetrics and Gynecology, 75*(Suppl. 4), 3S–8S.

Rinehart, J., & Schiff, I. (1985). Menopause. In D. H. Nichol (Ed.), *Ambulatory gynecology* (pp. 399–425). Philadelphia: Harper & Row.

Scharbo-DeHaan, M., & Brucker, M. C. (1991). The perimenopausal period. *Journal of Nurse-Midwifery, 36,* 9–15.

Scott, J. R., DiSaia, P. J., Hammond, C. B., Spellacy, W. N. (Eds.) (1994). *Danforth's obstetrics and gynecology.* Philadelphia: J.B. Lippincott.

Wasserman, E., & Gromisch, D. (1981). *Survey of clinical pediatrics* (7th ed.). New York: McGraw-Hill.

Wren, B. G. (1992). The menopause. In N. F. Hacker & J. G. Moore (Eds.), *Essentials of obstetrics and gynecology* (pp. 543–550). Philadelphia: W. B. Saunders.

Zaviacic, M., & Whipple B. (1993). Update on the female prostate and the phenomenon of female ejaculation. *The Journal of Sex Research, 30*(2), 148–151.

Zilbergeld, B., & Ellison, C. R. (1980). Desire discrepancies and arousal problems in sex therapy. In S. R. Leiblum & L. A. Pervin (Eds.), *Principles and practice of sex therapy.* New York: Guilford Press.

SUGGESTED READING

Flint, M., Kronenberg, F., & Utian, W. (Eds) (1990). *Multidisciplinary perspectives on menopause* (Vol. 592). New York: New York Academy of Sciences.

Gray, S. (Ed) (1994). *Gray's anatomy.* New York: Vintage Books.

Haas, A., & Haas, K. (1990). *Understanding sexuality.* St. Louis: Times Mirror/Mosby College Publishing.

Hammond, C. B., Haseltine, F. P., & Schiff, I. (Eds) (1989). *Progress in clinical and biological research: Menopause: Evaluation, treatment and health concerns* (Vol. 320). New York: Alan R Liss.

Marshall, W. A., & Tanner, J. M. (1969). Variations in pattern of pubertal changes in girls. *Archives of Disease in Childhood, 44,* 291–303.

Masters. W., Johnson, V., & Kolodny, R. (1985). *Human sexuality* (2nd ed.). Boston: Little, Brown.

Mastroianni, L., & Coutifaris, C. (1990). *Reproductive physiology* (ed.). Park Ridge, NJ: Parthenon Pub Group.

Speroff, L., Glass, R. H., & Kase, N. G. (Eds) (1994). *Clinical gynecologic endocrinology and infertility* (5th ed.). Baltimore: Williams & Wilkins.

Tanner, J. M. (1962). *Growth at adolescence* (2nd ed.). Oxford: Blackwell Scientific Publications.

Tanner, J. M., & Preece, N. A. (Eds) (1989). *The physiology of human growth, Society for the Study of Human Biology Symposium series 29.* New York: Cambridge Press.

Williams, P. L., Warwick, R., Dyson, M., & Bannister, L. H. (Eds) (1989). *Gray's anatomy of the human body* (37th ed.). New York: Churchill Livingstone.

Yen, S. S., & Jaffe, R. B. (1991). *Reproductive endocrinology: Physiology, pathophysiology and clinical management* (3rd ed.). Philadelphia: W. B. Saunders.

7

Conception and Development of the Embryo and Fetus

Objectives

- Describe the structure of the human sperm and ovum.
- Explain the process of fertilization and implantation.
- Describe how multifetal pregnancy can occur.
- Identify and describe the three developmental stages.
- Explain the process of prenatal sex differentiation.
- Identify the major milestones in prenatal development from conception through birth.
- Describe the structure and function of the placenta and factors influencing uteroplacental blood flow.
- Compare fetal and neonatal circulation, identifying differences in anatomy and physiology.

Key Terms

Amnion	Genes
Amniotic cavity	Genetics
Autosomes	Growth
Blastocyst	Heterozygous
Brown fat	Homologous
Capacitation	Meiosis
Chorion	Mitosis
Chromosomes	Morphogenesis
Cleavage	Oogenesis
Decidua	Placenta
Differentiation	Sex chromosomes
Embryo	Spermatogenesis
Estimated date of birth	Trophoblast
Gametes	Viability
Gametogenesis	Zygote

In all of the universe, there is no process more wondrous and no mechanism more fantastic than the one by which a tiny speck of tissue, the human egg, develops into a fully devloped baby. Primitive people considered this phenomenon so miraculous that they frequently ascribed it to superhuman intervention and overlooked the fact that sexual intercourse was a necessary precursor. Throughout the ages, primitive human ancestors doubtless held similar beliefs, but it is now known that pregnancy comes about in only one way: from the union of a female germ cell, the egg, or ovum, with a male germ cell, the spermatozoon. These two germ cells, or **gametes**, become fused into one cell, or **zygote**, which contains the characteristics of the woman and the man. Subsequent human development may be divided into three essential phases:

- **Growth**: increase in size, involving cell division and elaboration of cell products
- **Morphogenesis**: development of form, including mass cell movement that allows cells to interact with each other during the formation of tissues and organs
- **Differentiation**: maturation of physiologic processes, resulting in the organs being able to perform specialized functions (Moore et al., 1993)

This chapter describes these phases of human development, including fertilization, implantation, prenatal development (pre-embryonic, embryonic, and fetal), and physiology of the embryo, fetus, and placenta.

Genetics

Genetics, the science of heredity, explains the influence of the **genes**, the functional units of heredity, on human development. Genes are responsible for the transmission of particular biologic and behavioral characteristics from one generation to the next. The genes wield their influence at the cellular level, dictating which proteins are found in a cell and how the proteins determine the form and function of a particular cell (Bullock, 1996). They consist of a particular sequence of nucleotides found in the deoxyribonucleic acid (DNA) of **chromosomes**, which are present in the nucleus of every body cell. Each chromosome contains a sequence of thousands of genes; each of these genes is believed to have a specific location on a particular chromosome. In the last decade, more than 2,000 human genes have been localized to specific chromosomes, and approximately 5,500 human genes have been cataloged so far (Scott et al., 1994).

Chromosomes

There are normally 46 chromosomes in every body cell; the only exception are the mature sex cells (sperm and egg cells), which have 23 chromosomes each.

Chromosomal Structure

The individual chromosomes differ in form and size, ranging from small, spheric masses to long rods (see Fig. 14-1 in Chap. 14). Normally, the chromosomes within each somatic cell are paired. Each cell contains 22 pairs of **autosomes** (*auto,* self) and one pair of **sex chromosomes**. The chromosomes are composed of strands of deoxyribonucleic acid (DNA) and protein. The genes are located in linear order on the DNA of cell nuclei. Pairs of autosomes that carry similar genes are called **homologous**; those with dissimilar genes are called **heterozygous.** The genes located on the 44 autosomes are involved, with few exceptions, in aspects of development and physiology that do not relate to sex determination (Cunningham et al., 1993).

Chromosomes contain two longitudinal halves called *chromatids,* which are visible under a microscope. The chromatids are united at a point called the *centromere.* Chromosomes are classified according to their length and position on their centromere.

The two sex-determined chromosomes in each cell consist of two X chromosomes in normal girls and one X and one Y chromosome in normal boys. The Y chromosomes predominantly contain genes for maleness, whereas X chromosomes carry several genes, in addition to those for sexual traits. The sex chromosome of the mature ovum is always of the X type. The mature spermatozoon may have either an X chromosome or a Y chromosome (Fig. 7-1). When fertilization occurs with a spermatozoon containing the X chromosome, a girl is produced. When an ovum is fertilized by a spermatozoon containing a Y chromosome, a boy is produced. Thus, the sex is determined at the time of fertilization by the spermatozoon, not by the ovum.

Cell Reproduction

Cell reproduction is achieved by two different but related processes. **Mitosis** is the process by which body (somatic) cells replicate to produce two new identical cells with the same genetic makeup. The cells created have the same *diploid* number (n = 46) of chromosomes as the parent cell. Mitosis is divided into five stages: *interphase, prophase, metaphase, anaphase,* and *telophase* (Fig. 7-2). **Meiosis** is the process by which specialized male and female germ cells (gametes) are produced. The gametes have a haploid number (n = 23) of chromosomes. Meiosis is essential

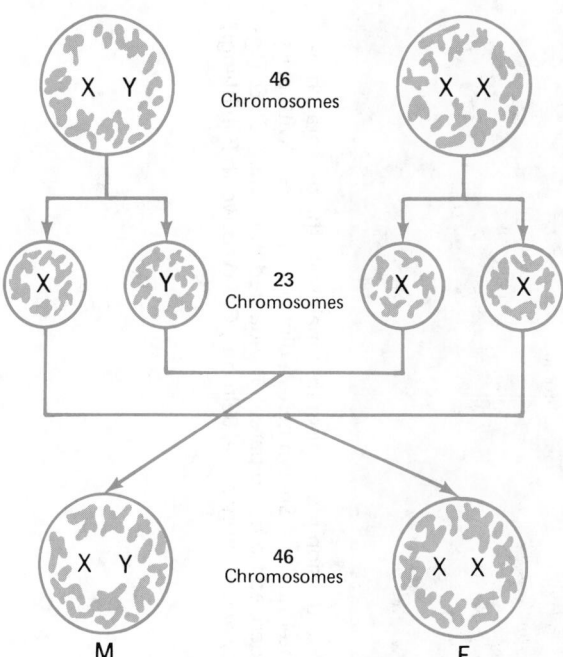

FIGURE 7–1 The sex of the offspring is determined at the time of fertilization by the combination of the sex chromosomes of the spermatozoon (either X or Y) and the ovum (X). The ovum fertilized by a sperm cell containing the X chromosome produces a female (44 regular chromosomes + 2 X chromosomes). If it is fertilized by a spermatozoon containing the Y chromosome, the union produces a boy (44 regular chromosomes + X + Y). Note that the structures depicted as chromosomes are diagrammatic only. In this illustration, it is not possible to include the total correct number.

for sexual reproduction. The term **gametogenesis** refers to the process of formation and development of the specialized male (spermatozoon) and female (ovum) gametes for fertilization. This maturation process is called **spermatogenesis** in men and **oogenesis** in women (Fig. 7-3).

Maturation of Ovum and Sperm Cells

The oogonia enlarge to form primary oocytes during early fetal life. No primary oocytes form after birth. Although the first meiotic division of primary oocytes begins before birth, the completion of prophase does not occur until after puberty. The ovum remains in a resting stage of development until about 2 days before ovulation. Its nucleus is large and round and has been described as vesicular because it resembles a vesicle. The ovum completes the first *meiotic division* while still in the follicle. Through meiosis, the ovum matures, and its genetic material prepares for fertilization. The second meiotic division begins at ovulation; however, it is arrested until a sperm penetrates the secondary oocyte (see Fig. 7-3).

The cells that eventually produce mature spermatozoa within the seminiferous tubules of the testes are called *spermatogonia*. These are located at the periphery of the seminiferous tubules (see Fig. 7-3). The spermatogonia begin to increase in number at puberty. After several mitotic divisions, the spermatogonia grow and undergo gradual changes that transform them into primary spermatocytes. Before they leave the testis, the primary spermatocytes subsequently undergo meiotic processes, producing spermatozoa in preparation for fertilization. Spermatogenesis requires about 74 days. The spermatozoon is fully matured when it is discharged in the ejaculate.

The primary oocyte and primary spermatocyte replicate their DNA just before the first meiotic division. Thus, at the beginning of the maturation divisions, the *germ cells* (primary spermatocyte and primary oocyte) contain double the normal amount of DNA, and each of the 46 chromosomes is a double structure. During this reduction process, the cytoplasm divides, but the chromosomes do not split; they are divided between two new cells. The *daughter cell* (secondary spermatocytes and secondary oocyte) contains one member of each chromosome pair (22 regular chromosomes, or *autosomes,* and an X chromosome) and thus has 23 double-structured chromosomes. The amount of DNA in each secondary cell equals that of a normal somatic cell.

Immediately after the first meiotic division, the cell begins its second maturation division, in which each

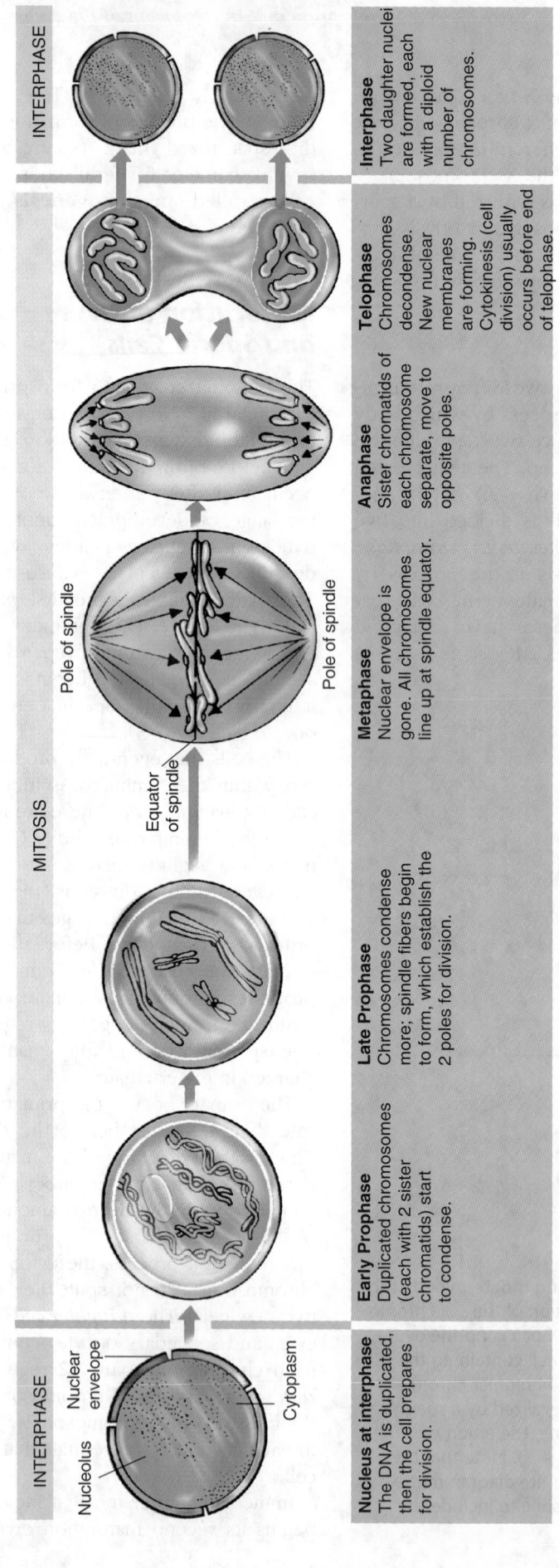

FIGURE 7-2 Mitosis: the nuclear division mechanism that maintains the parental chromosome number in each daughter nucleus. Shown here, a diploid animal cell (with pairs of homologous chromosomes, derived from two parents). (Adapted from Starr, C., & Taggart, R. [1989]. *Biology: The unity and diversity of life*. Belmont, CA: Wadsworth Publishing.)

INTERPHASE

MITOSIS

INTERPHASE

Nucleolus

Nuclear envelope

Cytoplasm

Pole of spindle

Equator of spindle

Pole of spindle

Nucleus at interphase
The DNA is duplicated, then the cell prepares for division.

Early Prophase
Duplicated chromosomes (each with 2 sister chromatids) start to condense.

Late Prophase
Chromosomes condense more; spindle fibers begin to form, which establish the 2 poles for division.

Metaphase
Nuclear envelope is gone. All chromosomes line up at spindle equator.

Anaphase
Sister chromatids of each chromosome separate, move to opposite poles.

Telophase
Chromosomes decondense. New nuclear membranes are forming. Cytokinesis (cell division) usually occurs before end of telophase.

Interphase
Two daughter nuclei are formed, each with a diploid number of chromosomes.

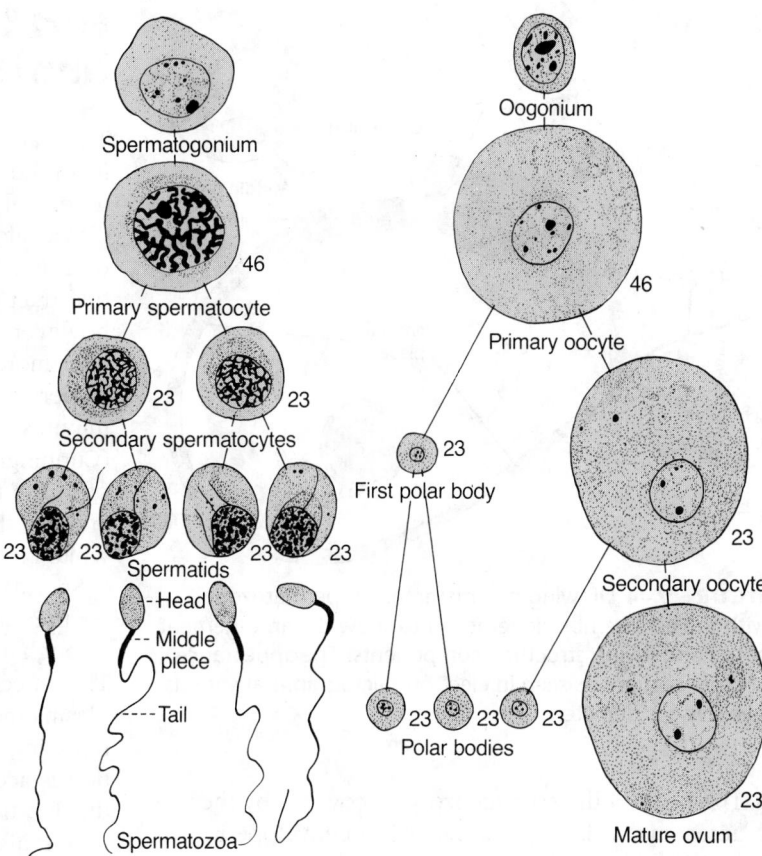

FIGURE 7-3 Diagram of gametogenesis. The various stages of spermatogenesis are indicated on the left; one spermatogonium gives rise to four spermatozoa. On the right, oogenesis is indicated; from each oogonium, one mature ovum and three abortive cells are produced. The chromosomes are reduced to one-half the number characteristic for the general body cells of the species. In humans, the number in the body cells is 46, and that in the mature spermatozoon and secondary oocyte is 23.

gamete normally receives only one chromosome of each pair and half the amount of DNA of a normal somatic cell. Thus, each mature spermatozoon has 23 chromosomes in its nucleus, and each mature ovum also contains 23 chromosomes, the haploid number.

As a result of the meiotic division, one primary oocyte produces four daughter cells, each with 22 + 1 X chromosomes. Only one of these daughter cells develops into a mature gamete, the oocyte; the other three, known as *polar bodies,* have little cytoplasm and eventually degenerate. The primary spermatocyte also gives rise to four *spermatids:* two with 22 + 1 X chromosomes and two with 22 + 1 Y chromosomes. Each spermatid develops a tail and eventually becomes a mature spermatozoon.

The importance of meiosis is that it provides for constancy of the chromosome number from generation to generation by producing haploid germ cells, and it allows random assortment of maternal and paternal chromosomes among the gametes (Moore et al., 1993).

Ovum

As described in Chapter 6, one ovum per month is normally discharged from the human ovary. Under the influence of the gonadotropins, the graafian follicle, which is destined to release an ovum, has matured.

The ovum has been pushed to one side of the fluid-filled cavity of the follicle. It is surrounded by a translucent coat, the *zona pellucida.* Immediately adjacent and connected to the zona pellucida is a layer of follicular cells, the *corona radiata,* which are arranged in a radial pattern. The *cumulus oophorus* is a more loosely structured layer of cells peripheral to the corona radiata. The ovum, surrounded by this entourage of cells and having matured through release of its first polar body, is released through the process of ovulation. The ovum, within its sticky cumulus mass, is rapidly and efficiently transported into the fallopian tube, the site of fertilization. The ovum is about 0.2 mm (⅛ of an inch) in diameter and is barely visible to the naked eye.

Spermatozoa

Spermatozoa resemble microscopic tadpoles, with oval heads and long, lashing tails about 10 times the length of the head. They are much smaller than ova; their overall length measures about one-quarter the diameter of the egg, and it has been estimated that the heads of 2 billion of them could be placed, with room to spare, in the hull of a grain of rice.

The human spermatozoon consists of three parts: the head, the middle piece (neck), and the tail (Fig. 7-4).

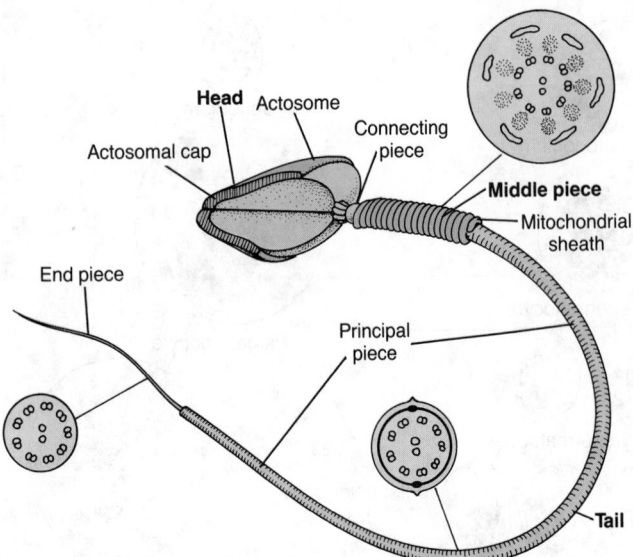

FIGURE 7–4 Drawing of a mammalian spermatozoon with the cell membrane removed to show the arrangement of the underlying structural components. The appearance of cross-sections as seen in electron micrographs at various levels also is depicted.

- The head of the spermatozoon is covered by the acrosome. This *acrosomal cap* is an envelope in which enzymes that play an important role in sperm penetration are contained. The nucleus, and consequently the chromatin material, is in the head.
- The middle (neck) of the sperm supplies energy for the tail's wriggling motions.
- The tail is a propeller allowing spermatozoa to swim with a quick vibratory motion, as fast as 3 mm/min.

To ascend the uterus and the fallopian tube, spermatozoa must swim against the same currents that pull the ovum downward; they are assisted by uterine contractions induced by prostaglandins in the seminal fluid, which propel them upward in the direction of the tube. Spermatozoa have been observed in the fallopian tube within minutes of insemination.

At each ejaculation during intercourse, approximately 300 million spermatozoa are discharged into the vagina. Of the millions of spermatozoa deposited in the vagina during coitus, many are expelled immediately; some remain in the vagina and are later extruded. Those retained in the vagina lose their motility in about 1 hour because of the acidic environment provided by the vagina.

Some spermatozoa reach the cervix almost immediately after ejaculation. Those transferred into the secretions of the cervix find a more favorable environment and may remain motile for as long as several days, especially in the preovulatory phase of the cycle.

Fertilization and Implantation

Thousands of spermatozoa find their way into the cavity of the uterus; fewer reach the lumen of the fallopian tube. Only one is given the opportunity to continue biologic life through fertilization, and this occurs only occasionally. The spermatozoa in the female reproductive tract may retain their motility for hours or days; however, few spermatozoa are capable of fertilization after more than 24 hours. Fertilization of the ovum by a spermatozoan occurs in the fallopian tubes within 2 minutes or no more than a few hours after ovulation (Cunningham et al., 1993). Spermatozoa are disposed of in the reproductive tract or in the peritoneal cavity, and as they degenerate, they are phagocytized by white blood cells.

Spermatozoa are conditioned to fertilize an ovum after they are exposed to the female reproductive tract through a physiologic change known as **capacitation**. This mechanism involves removal of the overlying plasma membrane and the outer acrosomal membrane, releasing an enzyme called *hyaluronidase*. Capacitation is accomplished in the fluids of the female reproductive tract and is an essential requisite to fertilization. It also is possible for human sperm to acquire the ability to fertilize after a short incubation in defined media without entering the female reproductive tract. This capacity makes in vitro fertilization possible.

Transport Through the Fallopian Tubes

The fallopian tube is an important structure that is crucial to fertilization and eventual implantation of the ovum (Fig. 7-5). First, it is responsible for transporting the ovum from the rupturing follicle into its lumen where it provides a temporary environment for the ovum and the spermatozoon. Second, fertilization occurs in the fallopian tube, as does cell division of the fertilized ovum during the early stages of human life. Third, the fallopian tube transports the fertilized, cleaving ovum into the uterus.

The fallopian tube is uniquely designed for its various functions: It contains *fimbriae* and *cilia*, which facilitate ovum transport (see Fig. 6-8 and 7-6). The structure of the fimbriated end of the tube is important in ovum pickup mechanisms. A separate strand of fimbriae, the *fimbria ovarica*, extends from the tube to the ovary to which it is attached. This contains a separate bundle of smooth muscle. During ovulation, this muscle contracts and pulls the ovary in the direction of the tubal opening. The remainder of the fimbriae are

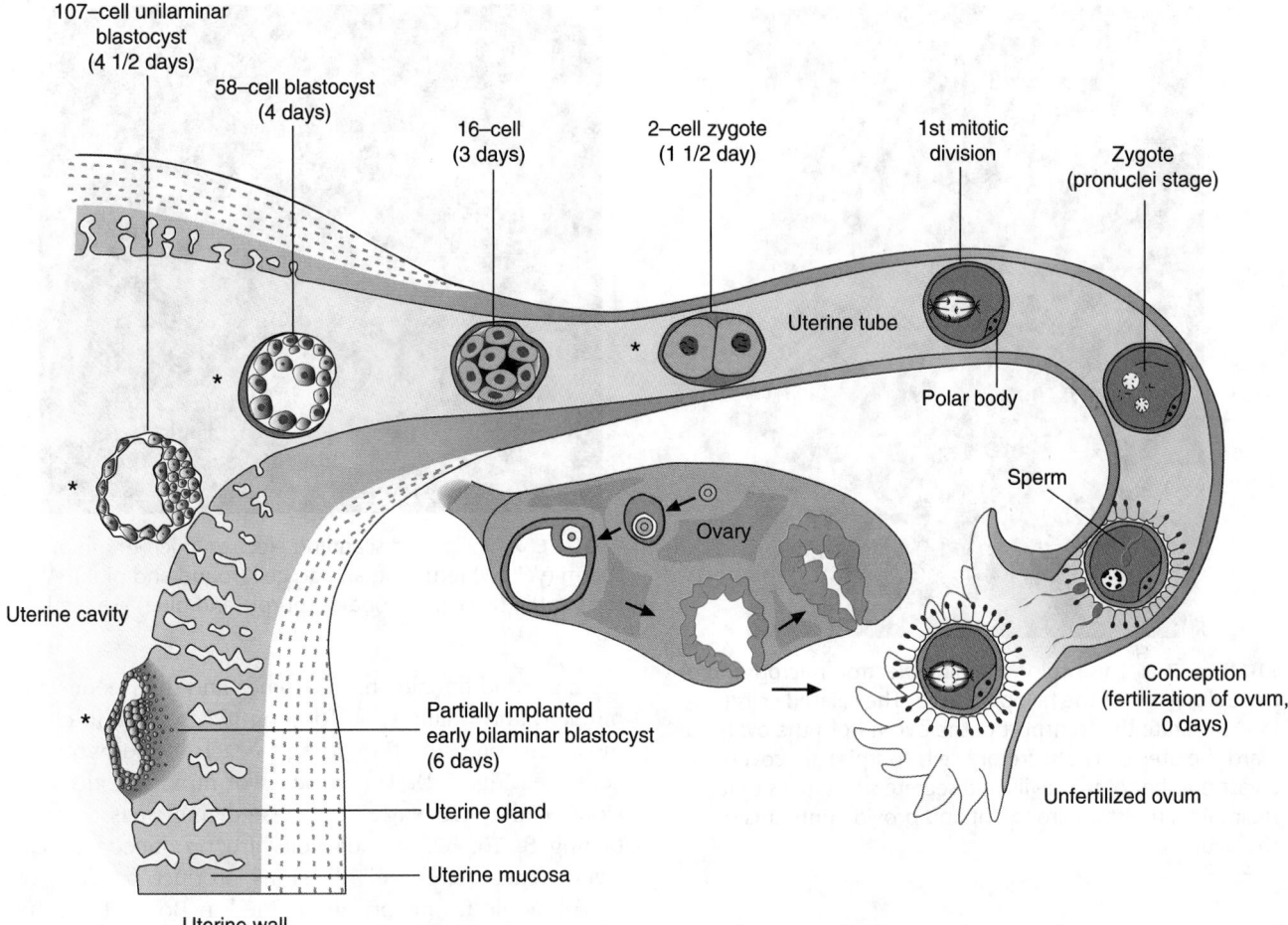

107–cell unilaminar
blastocyst
(4 1/2 days)

58–cell blastocyst
(4 days)

16–cell
(3 days)

2–cell zygote
(1 1/2 day)

1st mitotic
division

Zygote
(pronuclei stage)

Uterine tube

Polar body

Sperm

Ovary

Uterine cavity

Conception
(fertilization of ovum,
0 days)

Partially implanted
early bilaminar blastocyst
(6 days)

Unfertilized ovum

Uterine gland

Uterine mucosa

Uterine wall

FIGURE 7–5 Transport of the ovum into the fallopian tube and fertilization within the tube followed by cleavage (cell division) to the 8- to 16-cell stage. The product, now referred to as a morula, is delivered into the uterus where it develops into a blastocyst and implants in the endometrium on the sixth to seventh postfertilization day. (Modified from Gasser, R. F. [1975]. *Atlas of human embryos.* Hagerstown: Harper & Row.)

thought to embrace the ovary near or over the point of ovulation. They exercise muscular movement that moves them over the rupturing follicle. Thus, the cilia lining the fimbriae soon come into contact with the cumulus oophorus surrounding the ovum, and as they beat in the direction of the tubal lumen, they carry the sticky cumulus mass past the tubal ostium to a point well within the fallopian tube. An efficient process of ovum transfer is arranged through these mechanisms, and ovum pickup is practically ensured, despite the fact that the ovum is minuscule.

Once the ovum is safely past the tubal ostium, it is rapidly transported to the ampulla of the fallopian tube where fertilization occurs. After fertilization, the ovum passes through several cell divisions, during which it is retained in the fallopian tube for approximately 3 days. The mechanism by which the human ovum is retained in the tube is not well understood. Premature expulsion of the ovum from the tube could result in failure of implantation. Prolonged retention could result in ec-topic pregnancy, causing tubal rupture and hemorrhage (see Chap. 31).

Fertilization and Changes After Fertilization

After the ovum is well within the fallopian tube, the cells surrounding the ovum (cumulus oophorus) disperse. These cells begin to separate, partly as a result of the influence of the enzyme hyaluronidase contained in the acrosome surrounding the head of the spermatozoon. The spermatozoon makes its way through this peripheral layer of cells; meanwhile, the densely packed corona radiata (outer layer of ovum) has undergone certain changes. These cells become looser under the influence of tubal fluid, and the spermatozoon finds its way through this layer to the zona pellucida. Sperm connect firmly to the surface of the zona pellucida at specific binding or "receptor" sites

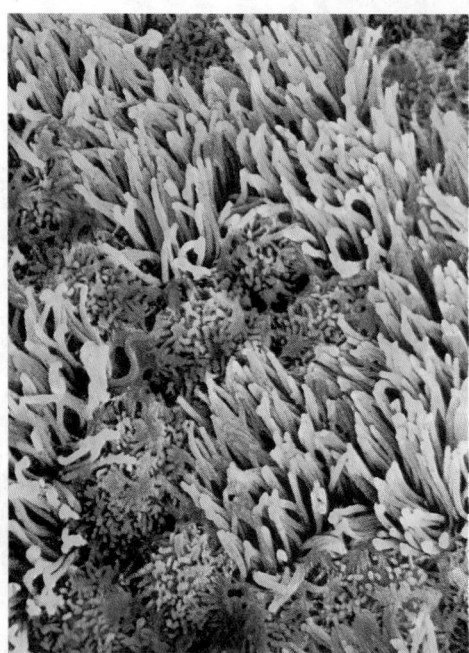

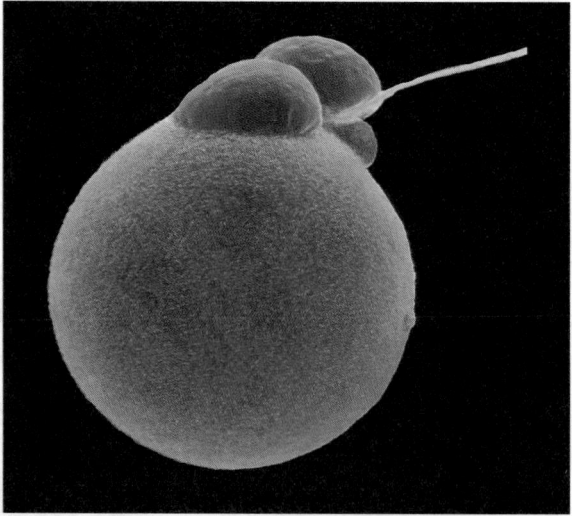

FIGURE 7-7 Colored scanning electron micrograph of sperm (yellow) fertilizing an egg cell (round and pink). At top center, three polar bodies (purple and blue) are seen.

FIGURE 7-6 False color scanning electron micrograph of the epithelium of the fallopian tube. The ciliated cells (yellow) facilitate the transport of the ovum from the ovary toward the uterus. The secretory cells (purple) are covered by a vast number of microvilli and secrete substances that maintain a moist environment and provide nutrients to the ovum.

(Scott et al., 1994). It is thought that the zona pellucida is penetrated by the spermatozoon because of a trypsin-like enzyme (*acrosin*) present in the spermatozoon's acrosome. Before penetration, openings are created in the outer membrane of the acrosome through which the enzyme-rich contents of the acrosome escape. This process, called the *acrosome reaction*, leads to a loss of the membrane over the anterior half of the sperm's head. The spermatozoon makes a channel through the zona pellucida as the acrosin dissolves the protein-containing zona with which it comes into contact. After the spermatozoon traverses the zona pellucida, it is in a position to penetrate the membrane of the ovum. As the spermatozoon penetrates the ovum, it brings its tail with it. (Fig. 7-7)

Once penetration is complete, a physiologic barrier occurs, and penetration of the ovum by other spermatozoa is prevented. Soon after penetration, the nucleus of the spermatozoon and the nucleus of the ovum undergo characteristic changes. They become *pronuclei*: distinct, clearly identifiable bodies of chromatin, each contained in a membrane. The male and female pronucleus fuse to form the fertilized ovum, or zygote. The new cell possesses the full complement of chromosomes (46—23 from the spermatozoon and 23 from the ovum). Soon thereafter, the single-celled zygote undergoes first cell division through mitosis. In this process,

the male and female chromosomes and their genes are mingled and finally split, forming two sets of 46 chromosomes, one set of 46 going to each of the two new cells (see Fig. 7-2). This process of rapid mitotic divisions, called **cleavage**, is repeated until masses containing 8, 16, 32, and 64 cells are produced successively. These early cell divisions produce a series of morphologic formations as defined in Box 7-1. At the 8- to 16-cell stage, the dividing ovum is delivered into the uterus. The fertilized ovum spends about 4 days in the uterine cavity developing further into a blastocyst before actual embedding takes place. Thus, a total interval of about 7 days elapses between ovulation and implantation. When the ovum remains unattached in the uterine cavity, it lies in a lake of endometrial secretion that is rich in glycogen and provides nourishment.

Meanwhile, several important changes are occurring in the internal structure of the fertilized ovum. Fluid appears in the center of the mulberry-like mass that pushes cells to the periphery of the sphere. At the

BOX 7-1
Early Morphologic Formations

- Zygote: The cell that results from the fertilization of the ovum by a spermatozoan
- Blastomere: The cells that result from mitotic division of the zygote (cleavage)
- Morula: The solid ball of cells formed by 16 or so blastomeres
- Blastocyst: The inner cell mass, formed from further differentiation of the morula, that develops into the embryo and embryonic membranes

same time, it becomes apparent that this external envelope of cells is made up of two different layers, an inner and an outer layer (Fig. 7-8). The inner solid mass of cells is called the **blastocyst** and develops into the embryo and an embryonic membrane (the **amnion**). The outer layer is a sort of foraging unit called the **trophoblast**, which means feeding layer; the principal function of these cells is to secure food for the embryo. The trophoblast eventually develops into one of the embryonic membranes known as the chorion.

While the ovum is undergoing these changes, the lining of the uterus is preparing for its reception. Considering that ovulation takes place on the 14th day of the menstrual cycle and that the tubal journey and the uterine sojourn require 7 days, 21 days of the cycle have passed before the ovum develops its trophoblastic layer of cells. This is when the lining of the uterus reaches its greatest thickness and succulence.

Implantation of the Ovum

The trophoblast is responsible for embedding the ovum, usually in the upper part of the posterior uterine wall. This process is carried out by means of enzymes. These cells not only burrow into the endometrium and eat out a nest for the ovum, but they also can digest the walls of the many small blood vessels that they encounter beneath the surface. The woman's bloodstream is tapped, and the ovum is deeply sunk in the lining epithelium of the uterus, surrounded by tiny pools of blood. Finger-like projections, or *chorionic villi*, develop out of the trophoblastic layer and extend into the blood-filled spaces. Another name for the trophoblast, and one more commonly used as pregnancy progresses, is the **chorion**. These chorionic villi contain blood vessels that are connected to the fetus and are extremely important because they are the sole means by which oxygen and nourishment are received

from the woman. The entire ovum becomes covered with villi, which grow out radially and convert the chorion into a shaggy sac.

The cells of the chorionic villi begin to secrete *human chorionic gonadotropin* (hCG), the hormone that maintains progesterone production by the corpus luteum. In turn, progesterone stimulates and supports endometrial growth by providing a suitable environment for continued development of the conceptus. Thus, the newly formed pregnancy is essentially self-sufficient and is in control of its own environment.

Throughout the 2-week interval after fertilization, there is a substantial incidence of pregnancy loss, associated with abnormal development of the fertilized ova. Such a pregnancy loss is not surprising considering the complicated series of events that culminate in a successfully implanted pregnancy. For surviving ova, the third week of gestation marks the beginning of the embryo stage of prenatal development, in which development occurs relatively rapidly.

Multifetal Pregnancy

Twins are the most frequent type of multifetal pregnancy, with an incidence of approximately 12 per 1,000 in the United States. There are two types of twins: *Dizygotic* or fraternal twins originate from two zygotes, and *monozygotic* or identical twins develop from one zygote. The frequency of identical twins is relatively constant throughout the world at about 1 set in every 250 pregnancies. The occurrence of identical twins also is largely independent of race, heredity, maternal age, parity, infertility drugs, and environmental factors. The incidence of fraternal twins, however, is influenced by these factors. The frequency of dizygotic birth increases until about age 40; it also increases with parity, independent of maternal age. The incidence of fraternal twins in white people is about 1 set in 95, and

FIGURE 7-8 Early stages of development. (*Top, left and center*) The cells are separated into a peripheral layer and an inner cell mass. The peripheral layer is called the trophoblast, or trophectoderm; the entire structure is called a blastodermic vesicle. (*Top, right*) The formation of the amniotic cavity and yolk sac is indicated. The former is lined with ectoderm, the latter with entoderm. (*Bottom, left*) The location of the embryonic disk and the three germ layers is shown, together with the beginning of the chorionic villi. (*Bottom, right*) The external appearance of the developing mass is shown; the chorionic villi are abundant.

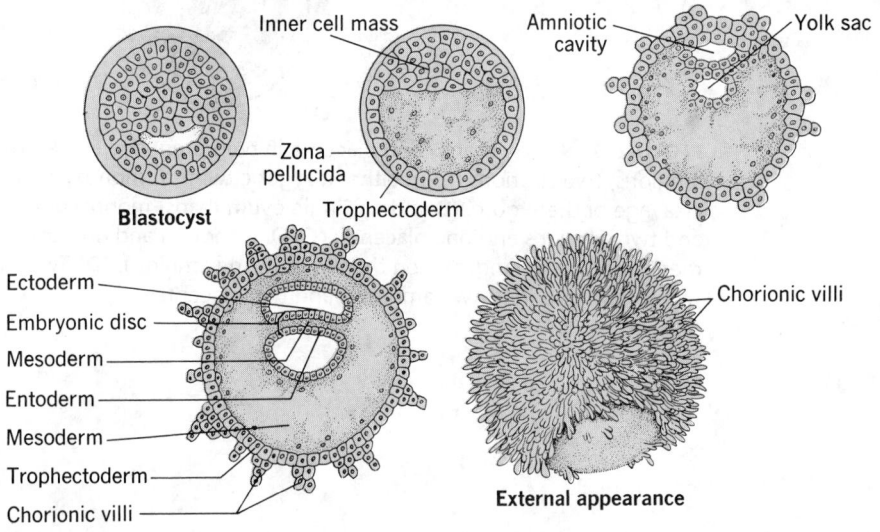

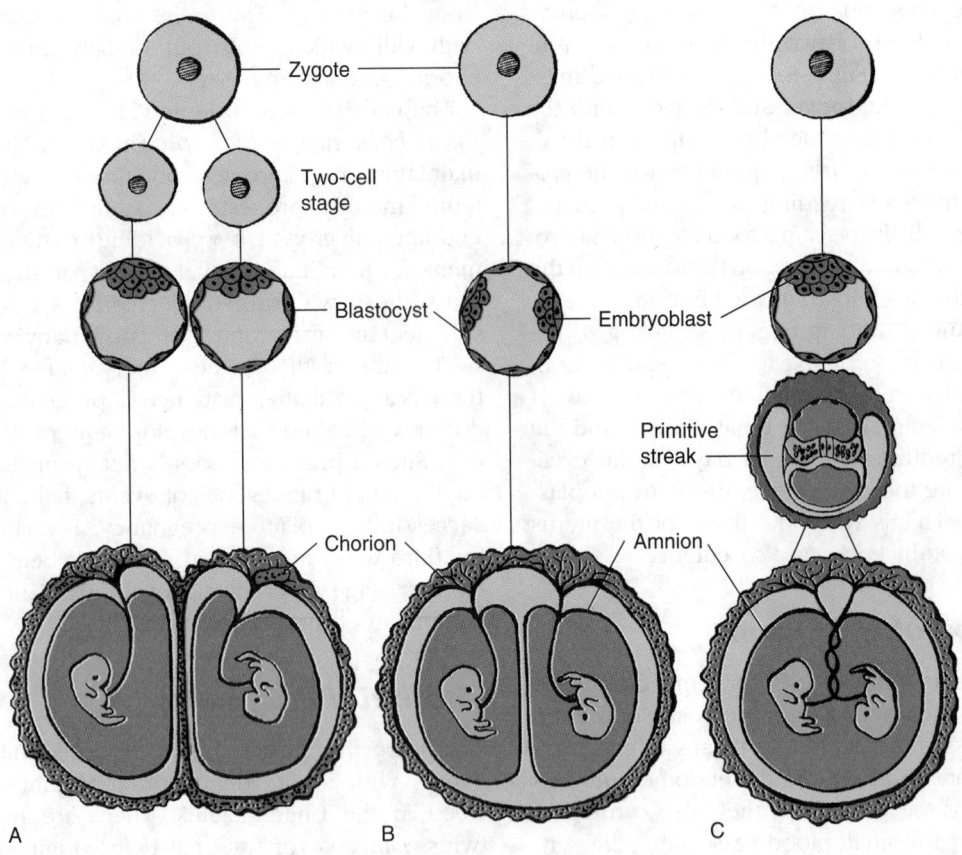

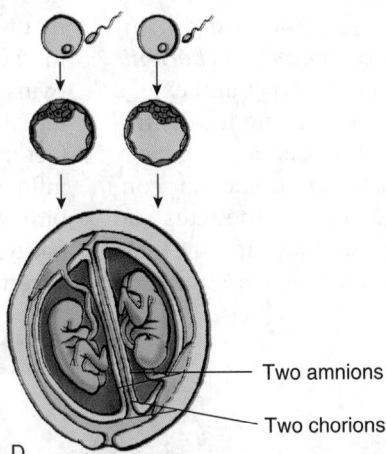

FIGURE 7–9 Membranes and placenta in twin pregnancies. (**A**) Two placentas, two amnions, two chorions (from either dizygotic twins or monozygotic twins) with early cleavage of the zygote. (**B and C**) Single ovum twins (monozygotic). (**B**) One chorion and two amnions and one placenta. (**C**) One chorion and one amnion (note entanglement of cords, a danger when there is only one amnion). (**D**) Two ovum (dizygotic twins), two chorions, two amnions, and two placentas.

in African Americans, it is 1 set in 78. Twins among Asians are less common (Cunningham et al., 1993).

About two-thirds of twins are dizygotic, and dizygotic twins tend to repeat in families. Because they develop from the fertilization of two separate ova by two different sperms, dizygotic twins are genetically distinct and may be of the same sex or different sexes. In contrast, monozygotic twins are genetically identical and are of the same sex. Monozygotic twins arise from the fertilization of a single ovum. At the blastocyst stage, division of the inner cell mass creates two embryonic primordia. Research findings suggest that monozygotic twins are not only more genetically similar, but also may experience more similar environments than dizygotic twins (Brennen et al., 1993). An interesting feature of twinning is that although dizygotic twins are not genetically identical, if they are of the same sex, they often resemble each other as closely at birth as a pair of monozygotic twins. The process of the division of one fertilized zygote into two does not always result in an equal sharing of the protoplasm; thus, the growth of monozygotic twins may be dramatically discordant (Cunningham et al., 1993).

Two types of placentas exist in twins, those with monochorial (one chorion) and those with dichorial (two chorions) membranes. Also, the placenta may be fused, separate, or a single disk, and there may be one or two amnions. However, each fetus usually has its own umbilical cord. The possible combinations include the following (Fig. 7-9):

- Monozygotic (identical)
    Diamniotic dichorionic (two amnions, two chorions), second most common
    Diamniotic monochorionic (two amnions, one chorion), most common
    Monoamniotic monochorionic (one amnion, one chorion), rare
- Dizygotic (fraternal or nonidentical)
    Diamniotic dichorionic (two amnions, two chorions)

The number of triplets and higher order births rose dramatically (113%) in the United States between 1972 and 1989, particularly among white women 30 through 39 years old being treated for infertility (Cunningham et al., 1993). Triplets can be produced from one to three zygotes and may be identical or fraternal. Quadruplets have similar possible origins, arising from one to four zygotes. Multifetal pregnancy has become increasingly common as a consequence of infertility therapies that involve administration of human gonadotropins (eg, Pergonal or clomiphene citrate) to women with ovulatory failure. In vitro fertilization and embryo transfer have further increased the incidence of multifetal pregnancy. Evidence suggests that in vitro fertilization pregnancies may yield a multiple pregnancy rate as high as 22% (Kurachi et al., 1985; Australian In-

Vitro Fertilization Collaborative Group, 1988). A discussion of multifetal pregnancies is found in Chapter 36.

Stages and Duration of Pregnancy

Development Stages: Ovum, Embryo, and Fetus

Fertilization initiates the process of human development. Prenatal development is divided into three periods, as summarized in Box 7-2.

Although each of the these stages is important, the embryonic period is most critical because all the main organ systems are differentiating and are vulnerable to environmental influences (eg, teratogens such as drugs, viruses, radiation, infections). The adequacy of the woman's diet also is important to the developing embryo and fetus. Nutritional deficiencies during pregnancy may contribute to intrauterine growth retardation when the needs of the rapidly growing fetus are not being met.

Duration of Pregnancy

The length of pregnancy may be divided into days, weeks, or lunar months (Table 7-1); however, misunderstandings may arise if it is not clearly stated whether the age is calculated from date of onset of the last menstrual period (LMP) or the estimated day of fertilization (conception). **Estimated date of birth** is usually calculated from LMP. Length of gestation may vary and is under hormonal control. Some fetuses require a longer time, while others require a shorter time in the uterus for full development. The frequency of postdate pregnancies (>42 weeks) has been reported between 3% and 12% (Scott et al., 1994).

Viability

The length of gestation is important because it affects the unborn child's chances of survival after birth. **Via-**

BOX 7-2
Periods of Prenatal Development

Preembryonic (ovum): Fertilization through the first 2 weeks of prenatal life (includes formation of the morula, blastocyst, primary villi, and implantation)

Embryonic: From the third to the eighth week of gestation, during which all essential structures are developing and a definite form is being assumed

Fetal: From the eighth week to the time of birth, a period of growth and maturation of existing structures

TABLE 7–1
Comparison of Gestational Time Units

Reference Point	Days	Weeks	Calendar Months	Lunar Months
Fertilization	266	38	8¾	9½
LMP	280	40	9¼	10

LMP = last menstrual period.

bility refers to the capability of the fetus to live outside the uterus at the earliest gestational age. It was believed that a fetus was viable at a weight of 1,000 g (about 28 weeks' gestation). The age at which a fetus reaches viability has declined in recent years as a result of improvements in maternal and neonatal care. Fetal viability has been reported as early as 22 weeks (Moore et al., 1993), but the chances of survival are poor until several weeks later, mainly because the respiratory and central nervous systems are not completely differentiated.

Physiology of the Embryo

Decidua

The **decidua** is the structure of thickened endometrium that develops after conception. It is a direct continuation, in exaggerated form, of the already modified premenstrual endometrium. For descriptive purposes, the decidua is divided into three portions (Fig. 7-10):

- *Decidua basalis*: the part lying directly under the embedded ovum that forms the maternal component of the placenta
- *Decidua capsularis*: the portion that overlies the ovum and separates it from the rest of the uterine cavity
- *Decidua vera* (sometimes called *decidua parietalis*): the remaining portion that is not in immediate contact with the ovum

As pregnancy advances, the decidua capsularis expands rapidly over the growing embryo and at about the fourth month, lies in intimate contact with the decidua vera.

Amnion

Even before the previously noted structures become evident, a fluid-filled space develops around the embryo. This space, the **amniotic cavity**, is lined with a smooth, slippery, glistening membrane, the amnion (see Fig. 7-10). The amnion originates from the ectoderm, a primary germ layer. It has an important role in prostaglandin (PGE$_2$) formation, particularly after labor commences.

Because the amniotic cavity is filled with fluid, it is often called the bag of waters; the fetus floats and moves within this space. The amniotic fluid is composed of water (98%) and organic and inorganic solids (1%–2%). It serves a number of important functions for the embryo and fetus:

- Helping to maintain even body temperature
- Providing a cushion against possible injury
- Permitting symmetric external growth
- Preventing adherence of the amnion
- Providing space for free movement

The amniotic cavity enlarges throughout gestation; at the end of the fourth month of pregnancy, it is the size of a large orange and with the fetus, occupies the entire interior of the uterus. By full term, this cavity normally contains 500 to 1,000 mL of liquor amnii, or the "waters." The amniotic fluid contains albumin, urea, uric acid, creatinine, lecithin, sphingomyelin, bilirubin, fat, fructose, leukocytes, proteins, epithelial cells, enzymes, vernix, and fetal hair (lanugo). The fetus contributes to the amniotic fluid volume by the passage of urine. Amniotic fluid volume and composition are controlled by a complex system of fluid exchange between the maternal and fetal fluid compartments. The amniotic fluid index at term is an important determinant of fetal well-being that is used to diagnose an abnormally small quantity of fluid (*oligohydramnios*) or an excessive amount of fluid (*polydramnios* or *hydramnios*; see Chap. 39).

Chorion

The shaggy chorionic villi that originally cover the ovum and invade the decidua basalis enlarge and multiply rapidly to form the *chorion frondosum* (leafy chorion). This structure becomes the fetal component of the placenta. The chorionic villi covering the decidua capsularis degenerate and almost disappear, leaving only a slightly roughened membrane, the *chorion laeve* (bald chorion). The chorion laeve lies separated from the amnion by the exocoelomic cavity until near the end of the third month, after which they establish close contact. The chorion laeve and amnion form an avascular *amniochorion,* an important site of transfer and metabolic activity (Cunningham et al.,

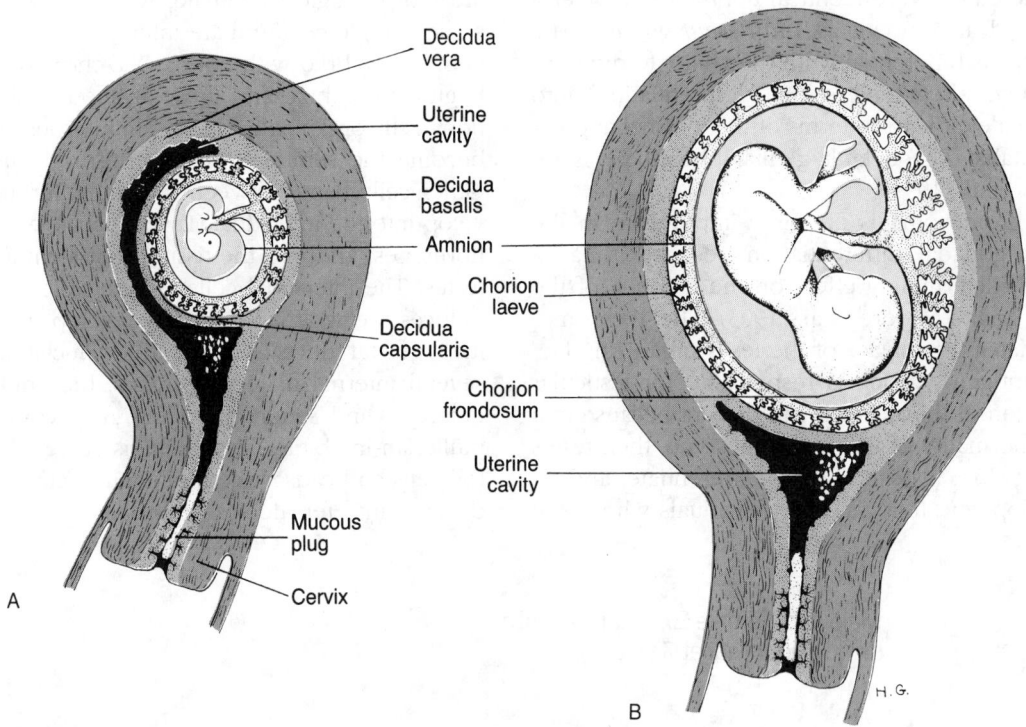

FIGURE 7-10 Enlargement of the chorionic vesicle and progressive obliteration of the uterine cavity. (**A**) At 6 weeks after fertilization. (**B**) At 16 weeks after fertilization. (Modified from Cunningham, F. G., MacDonald, P. C., & Gant, N. F. [1993]. *Williams obstetrics* [18th ed.]. Norwalk, CT: Appleton & Lange.)

1993). The fetus is thus surrounded by two membranes, the amnion and the chorion.

Yolk Sac

The small yolk sac develops as a cavity in the blastocyst about 8 or 9 days after fertilization. It serves many functions in embryonic development, such as helping to transfer nutrients to the embryo during the second and third weeks while uteroplacental circulation is being established and forming early blood cells until hematopoietic activity begins in the liver during the sixth week. The dorsal section of the yolk sac becomes part of the primitive gut. The yolk sac detaches from the midgut loop by the end of the sixth week and shrinks as gestation advances.

Three Germ Layers

The three germ layers that arise from the inner mass of blastocyst cells during the third week grow rapidly with adequate nutrition and give rise to all the tissues and organs of the embryo. At first, they all look alike, but soon after embedding, certain groups of cells assume distinctive characteristics and differentiate into three main groups: an outer covering layer (ectoderm), a middle layer (mesoderm), and an internal layer (endoderm). These are described in more detail in Box 7-3.

Sex Differentiation

Sex is established at the time of fertilization based on whether an X- or a Y-bearing sperm fertilizes the X-bearing ovum. The XX or XY combination of sex chromosomes passes the sexual program to the primordial gonad of the embryo. The primitive genital

---

BOX 7-3
Three Germ Layers

Ectoderm: The epithelium of the skin, hair, nails, sebaceous glands, sweat glands, and nasal and oral passages; the salivary glands and mucous membranes of the mouth and nose; the enamel of the teeth; the mammary glands; the central nervous system (brain and spinal cord) and the peripheral nervous system

Mesoderm: Muscles, bone, cartilage, the dentin of the teeth, ligaments, tendons, areolar tissue, striated and smooth muscles, kidneys, spleen, ureters, ovaries, testes, heart, blood, lymph and blood vessels, and the lining of the pericardial, pleural, and peritoneal cavities

Endoderm: Epithelium of the digestive tract and respiratory tract (except the nose), thymus, liver, pancreas, bladder, urethra, thyroid, and tympanic antrum and auditory tube

ducts of the embryo are identical until about 6 weeks' gestation and are known as *indifferent gonads.* The early embryo is bipotential, with the ability to differentiate sexually (phenotypic sexual differentiation) into male or female, at least in terms of the internal and external genitalia. The default genital phenotype is female (Scott et al., 1994).

The Y chromosome is of prime importance in the process of gonadal differentiation because it has a strong testis-determining effect on the medulla of the indifferent gonad (Moore et al., 1993). The Y chromosome regulates the release of the testis-organizing factor (H-Y antigen), which is responsible for testicular differentiation. If this factor is not present because of a genetic abnormality of the Y chromosome, then testes will not develop; instead, ovaries differentiate, and female development follows. The individuals who result

are morphologically female, with an XY sex chromosome complement and are infertile.

In the embryo with normal XY chromosomes, testes begin to organize and grow at about 7 weeks' gestation. Cells organize into the seminiferous cords, which become the seminiferous (sperm-producing) tubules. Other cells lying between the seminiferous cords develop into the interstitial (Leydig) cells, which produce hormones, and into the tissues that form and hold the testes. The interstitial cells secrete testosterone, which induces the wolffian ducts to develop from the primitive genital ducts. The wolffian ducts develop into several internal male sex organs: the epididymis, vas deferens, and seminal vesicles. A glycoprotein called müllerian-inhibiting substance, is secreted by the Sertoli cells and causes the müllerian ducts (which would develop into female sex organs) to regress and disap-

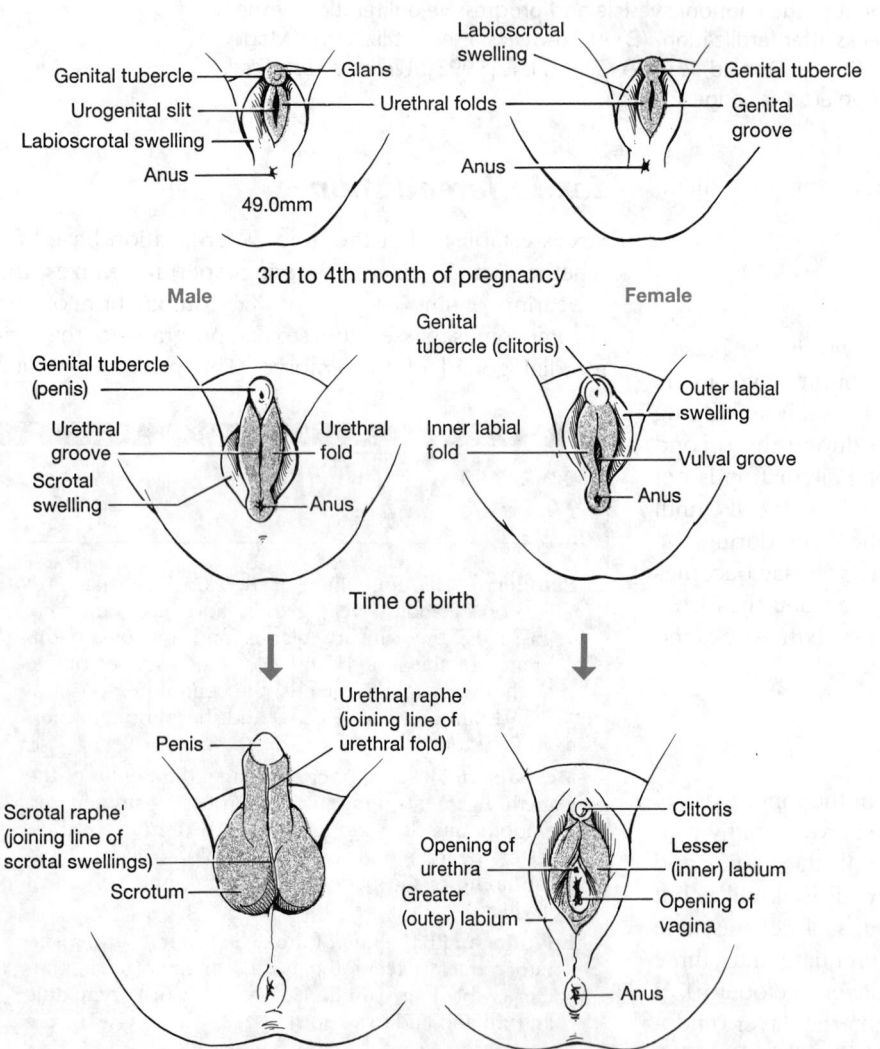

FIGURE 7–11 (A) Male and female external genitalia are identical at 7 weeks, but changes occur after the third month, and genital differentiation continues until birth. **(B)** Differentiation of internal male and female sex organs.

(A)

pear. Differentiation proceeds from the internal reproductive structures and is completed with the differentiation of the external genitals as male or female (Money et al., 1975). Dihydrotestosterone (peripherally metabolized from testosterone) produces normal masculinization of the external genitalia (Scott et al, 1994).

In an embryo with normal XX chromosomes, the process is somewhat slower, with ovaries beginning to develop at about 11 to 12 weeks' gestation. Cells form small clusters and become follicles of the ovaries, giving rise to oocytes (immature ova) by the 16th week. Other cells that produce hormones develop in the follicles, and still others form tissues around the ovarian follicles. Although the initial formation of the ovaries requires the absence of a Y chromosome, continued development depends on the presence of two X chromosomes. If only one X chromosome is present,

ovaries do not fully develop, and the woman is infertile. Female sexual differentiation in the fetus does not depend on hormones; it happens even if the ovaries are absent (Money et al., 1973). The lack of testosterone and müllerian-inhibiting substance causes the wolffian ducts to regress and disappear in the female embryo. The müllerian ducts continue to develop in the female embryo and give rise to the fallopian tubes, uterus, cervix, and possibly the upper vagina. There seems to be a built-in propensity for primitive genital structures to develop in the female pattern. Androgens must be present to produce male sexual differentiation, whereas their absence leads to female differentiation. If embryonic gonads do not secrete hormones (either testosterone or estrogens) and even if embryonic reproductive tracts (without gonads) are removed in experimental animals who are kept alive, the genital

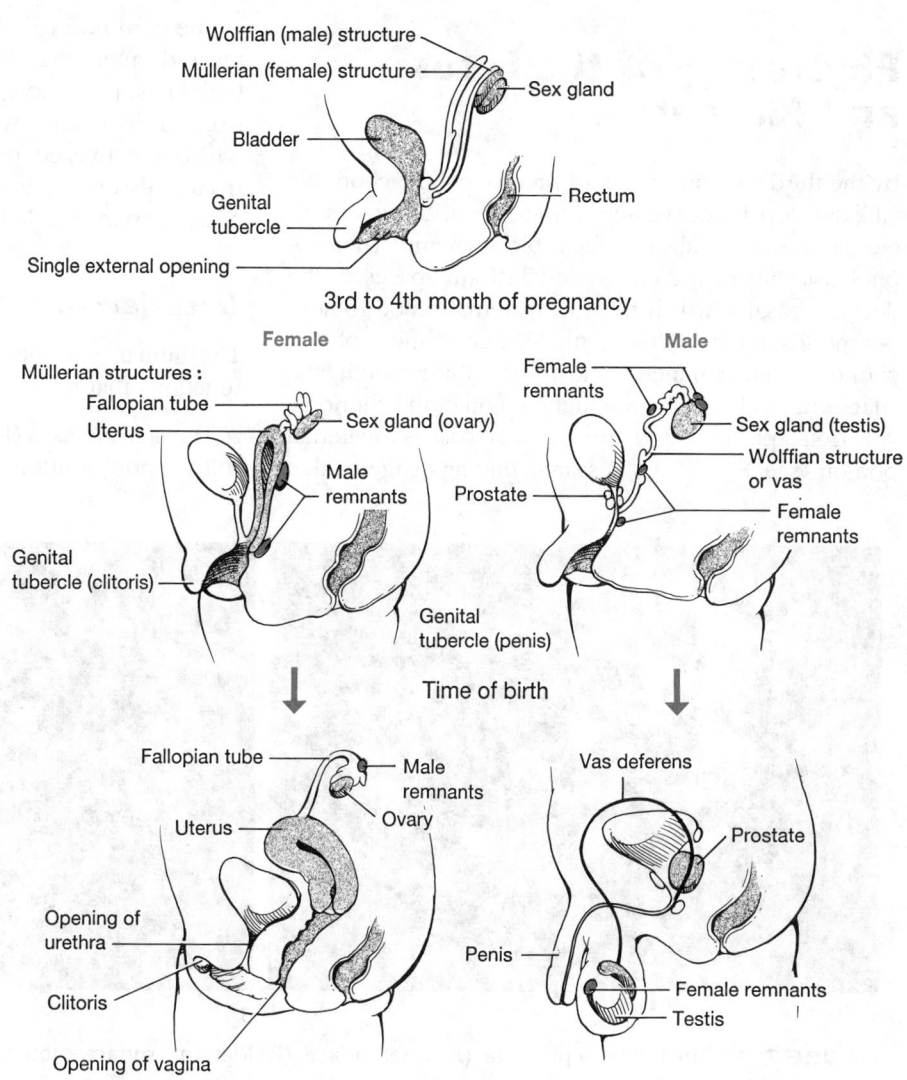

Male and Female Internal Sexual Organs
(identical at 2nd to 3rd month of pregnancy)

Wolffian (male) structure
Müllerian (female) structure
Sex gland
Bladder
Genital tubercle
Rectum
Single external opening

3rd to 4th month of pregnancy

Female

Müllerian structures :
Fallopian tube
Uterus
Sex gland (ovary)
Male remnants
Genital tubercle (clitoris)

Male

Female remnants
Sex gland (testis)
Wolffian structure or vas
Female remnants
Prostate
Genital tubercle (penis)

Time of birth

Fallopian tube
Male remnants
Ovary
Uterus
Opening of urethra
Clitoris
Opening of vagina

Vas deferens
Prostate
Penis
Female remnants
Testis

(B)

Figure 7-11B (continued)

structures continue to develop the female pattern (Johnson et al., 1988; Sherfey, 1972).

The external female and male genitals develop from the same embryonic tissues. These folds and swellings of embryonic tissue develop into the *homologous* or corresponding male and female structures and structures common to both, such as the bladder and urethra. The embryonic glands and genital tubercle develop into the clitoral system in the female embryo and the penis in the male embryo. The labioscrotal swelling becomes the female labia or male scrotum, and the urogenital slit and urethral folds form the different male and female urethral systems. The other homologous sex organs (male and female, respectively) are (1) the prostate gland and Skene's glands and (2) the Cowper's glands and Bartholin's glands (Fig. 7-11).

The development of ambiguous genitalia is attributed to abnormal androgenic representation in utero (Cunningham et al., 1993). In other words, an embryo that was destined to be female received too much androgen, or an embryo that was destined to be male received too little androgen.

Physiology of the Fetus and Placenta

By the third or fourth week of pregnancy, the chorionic villi develop blood vessels within them; these vessels are connected with the fetal bloodstream. The trophoblast cells of the chorionic villi form spaces in the decidua basalis, which fill with maternal blood to supply nourishment to the fetus. Differentiation of the chorionic villi continues, and by the third month, the **placenta** has formed through the union of the chorionic villi (fetal portion) and the decidua basalis (maternal portion; see Fig. 7-10). Research findings suggest that smoking during the first months of pregnancy may induce morphologic changes in the trophoblast that may explain biologic disturbances observed during early gestation and later in pregnancy (Jauniaux et al., 1992).

During pregnancy, the placenta's weight and mass increase in proportion to that of the fetus. The normal fetal-placental weight ratio at term is 6:1. The placenta grows to about 20 cm in diameter and 2 cm in thickness late in pregnancy. It appears to be a fleshy, disk-like organ that at term, weighs about 500 g and covers about one-quarter of the uterine wall. The structure of the placenta includes the following components (Fig. 7-12):

- The *fetal surface*, which is smooth and glistening and is covered by amnion. Beneath this membrane, a number of large blood vessels may be seen.
- The *maternal surface*, which is red and fleshlike and is divided into 15 to 20 segments, or *cotyledons*, about 2.5 cm in diameter
- The *umbilical cord*, which connects the placenta to the fetus and is usually about 55 cm in length and about 1 to 2.5 cm in diameter

The cord normally leaves the placenta near the center and enters the abdominal wall of the fetus at the umbilicus, just below the middle of the median line in front. It contains two arteries and one large vein, which are twisted on each other and are protected from pressure by a transparent, bluish white, gelatinous substance called *Wharton's jelly*.

Overview of Placental Function

The human placenta is a versatile organ. It has many functions that are similar to organs and body systems:

- Transfer of gases (lung)
- Transport of nutrients (gastrointestinal tract)

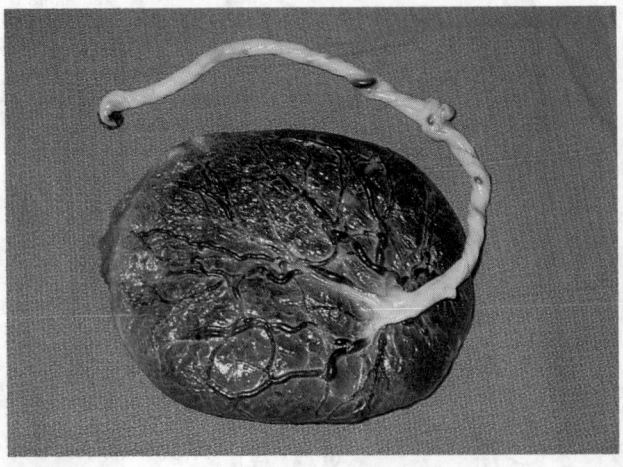
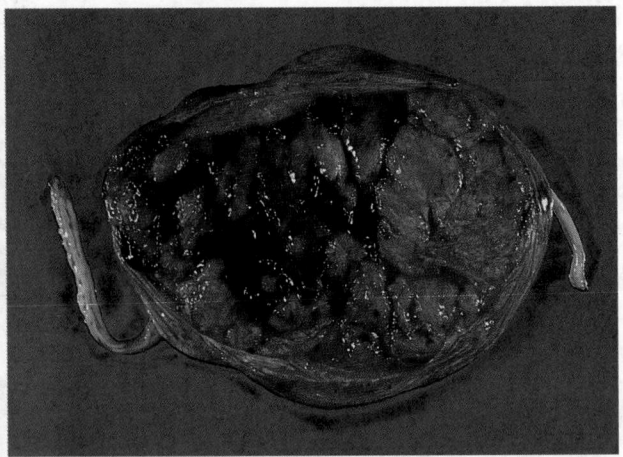

A

B

FIGURE 7-12 The full-term placenta. **(A)** Fetal surface. **(B)** Maternal surface. Note the presence of two umbilical cords indicating twins.

- Excretion of wastes (kidney)
- Transfer of heat (skin)
- Conjugation of drugs and hormones (liver)
- Production of various protein and steroid hormones (endocrine gland)

These important activities are able to be accomplished because of the unique human type of placentation (ie, hemochorioendothelial). The "heme" refers to maternal blood, which bathes the syncytiotrophoblasts (chorio) directly and is separated from the fetal blood by the endothelium of the fetal capillaries in the intravillous space (Cunningham et al., 1993). The maternal blood entering the intervillous space from the spiral arterioles is rich in nutrients and is well oxygenated. The fetal blood contained within finger-like villi extending into the intervillous space is deoxygenated and depleted of nutrients (Fig. 7-13); it is delivered there from the umbilical arteries. The transfer of oxygen and a great variety of nutrients from the woman to the fetus and conversely, the transfer of carbon dioxide and other metabolic wastes from the fetus to the woman occur across the chorionic membrane (chorial), which constitutes the outer surface of the villi. The newly restored blood is returned to the fetus along the veins contained within the villi, which converge into the umbilical vein. The inflowing maternal arterial blood drives venous blood into the endometrial veins, which are located over the surface of the decidua basalis.

Fetoplacental Oxygen Exchange

The partial pressure of oxygen (pO$_2$) in the intervillous space is approximately 35 to 40 mm Hg. This is the highest oxygen tension to which the fetal circulation is exposed. Despite this relatively low pO$_2$, the fetus normally does not suffer from hypoxia because of several adaptive mechanisms, including a greater cardiac output per unit of body weight than the adult, increased oxygen-carrying capacity of fetal blood, and higher hemoglobin concentration than in adults. Fetal hemoglobin can carry 20% to 30% more oxygen than adult hemoglobin. At any time, the oxygen in the intervillous space is capable of satisfying fetal oxygen consumption for about 1½ minutes. On their way to the intervillous space, the spiral arteries cross the muscular wall of the myometrium. The spiral arteries are compressed by the myometrium, and blood flow through these vessels is interrupted with each uterine contraction. Thus, delivery of oxygen to the intervillous space is interrupted. The normal fetus can tolerate this brief period of oxygen deprivation without damage. In certain cases of abnormal labor, when the contractions are unusually prolonged, the resulting anoxia could cause fetal damage.

The umbilical cord is the other vulnerable link in the system for maternal–fetal exchange of oxygen. Under certain conditions of labor, the umbilical cord can be compressed, for example, between the fetal head and the pelvis or entangled above the fetus. Prolonged interference with cord circulation can seriously affect fetal oxygenation.

Gross examination of the maternal side of the placenta reveals approximately 20 cotyledons or lobes. These are further divided into approximately 200 lobules, each of which is a circulatory unit containing a single spiral artery. When a spiral artery becomes obstructed, as when there has been a thrombosis or development of a clot within its lumen, the blood supply to that circulatory unit is disrupted, resulting in tissue destruction or infarction of the area. Many full-term placentas contain an area of infarction. Fortunately, the placenta is endowed with a substantial reserve. It can withstand loss of an estimated 30% of the functioning villous tissue surface by fibrin deposition or 50% due to thrombotic obliterations of fetal stem vessels without fetal compromise (Scott et al., 1994).

At the microscopic level, three layers of tissue separate the fetal circulation from the maternal blood. A molecule passing from the fetus to the woman must cross these tissues:

- The fetal trophoblast is the outermost layer, which contains an outer *syncytiotrophoblast* and inner *cytotrophoblast.*
- A connective tissue layer is immediately beneath the trophoblast.
- The endothelial layer of the fetal capillary is the innermost layer.

As pregnancy progresses, the fetal capillaries are brought closer to the surface of the villi, and exchange is facilitated.

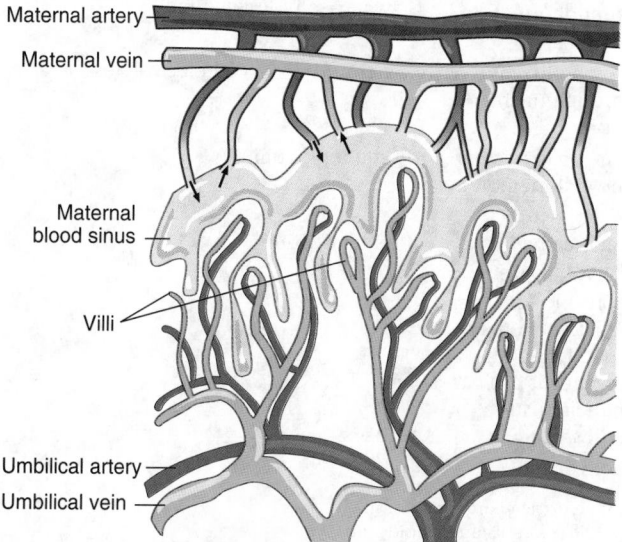

Maternal artery
Maternal vein
Maternal blood sinus
Villi
Umbilical artery
Umbilical vein

FIGURE 7–13 Diagram of placental circulation. Note that maternal and fetal circulations are completely separate.

Placental Transmission of Nutrition

The six mechanisms for the transport of nutrients from the woman to the fetus are diffusion, facilitated diffusion, active transport, bulk flow, pinocytosis, and defects in placental membrane. These transport methods are described in Table 7-2.

Placental Permeability

Diffusion is the most important mechanism regulating the transfer of substances between woman and fetus. Thus, impaired diffusion is often the cause of clinically evident placental dysfunction. Diffusion depends on the characteristics of the placental membrane. It is purely a physical process and requires no energy. The process is governed by certain principles, which, in combination, are described in *Fick's law*. Fick's law states that the rate of transfer of materials is directly proportional to the thickness of the membrane. This means that the more permeable the membrane and the greater the area presented by the membrane, the greater the rate of transfer. Conversely, the thicker the membrane, the slower the rate of transfer.

Other determinants of permeability for any molecule include the size of the molecule and its molecular charge and lipid-solubility properties. In general, mole-

TABLE 7–2
Mechanisms of Placental Transport

Mechanism for Transport*	Description	Examples of Substances Exchanged
Diffusion	<ul><li>A substance passes from one area to another on the basis of its concentration gradient.</li><li>Transport of gases depends on their partial pressures.</li></ul>	Respiratory gases, oxygen, and carbon dioxide; the electrolytes, sodium, and chloride; and some lipid-soluble vitamins
Facilitated diffusion	<ul><li>Passage along a concentration gradient occurs when the concentration of material on the maternal side is greater than that on the fetal side.</li><li>This occurs without the use of energy, but at a faster rate than can be explained on the basis of the concentration gradient alone.</li><li>It is carrier mediated (ie, it is transferred by cellular elements that carry it into and through the membrane).</li></ul>	Glucose
Active transport	<ul><li>Substances pass from one area to another against a concentration gradient.</li><li>This requires the expenditure of energy by the cells.</li></ul>	Amino acids (2:1 concentration gradient from mother to fetus); iron, calcium, phosphorus, iodine, and water-soluble vitamins
Bulk flow	<ul><li>Substances transfer by hydrostatic or osmotic gradients through micropores in the membrane.</li></ul>	Water and dissolved electrolytes
Pinocytosis	<ul><li>Materials contained in small vessels located at or near the cell membrane transfer across a cell.</li></ul>	Immunoglobulins
Defects in the membrane	<ul><li>Tears in the membrane can allow the transfer of large materials.</li><li>This process is responsible for sensitization of the Rh-negative woman carrying an Rh-positive fetus. Rh-positive fetal red blood cells are carried into the maternal circulation and produce antibodies.</li><li>This may occur at delivery.</li></ul>	Red blood cells

*Placental transfer may be affected by molecular size and concentration, electric charge, rate of maternal blood flow through intervillous space, area available for exchange, diffusion distance, lipid solubility, specific binding, or carrier protein in fetal or maternal circulation.

cules with a molecular weight greater than 1,000 do not cross the placental membrane. For example, the anticoagulant heparin is a large molecule that because of its size, does not traverse the placental membrane; hence, heparin treatment can be used safely in pregnancy. In contrast, the anticoagulant dicumarol is a much smaller molecule that readily crosses the placenta and when used in pregnancy, may affect the fetus. Other more common drugs, such as caffeine, alcohol, and nicotine, and many viruses (eg, rubella, chickenpox, measles, cytomegalovirus) may cross the placenta and adversely influence the fetus.

Lipid solubility is an extremely important characteristic in the transport of drugs from woman to fetus, as is the electrostatic charge of the molecules. Many of the narcotic agents and analgesics used in labor and delivery are designed to reach the maternal brain quickly to provide rapid pain relief. The characteristics that allow this rapid transport to the brain also allow them to cross the placental membrane rapidly, and they can equally quickly affect the fetal central nervous system.

Factors Influencing Placental Exchange

Blood Flow to Uteroplacental Circulation

In general, impaired exchange of carbon dioxide and oxygen is not usually related to problems of diffusion. There is little, if any, resistance to the diffusion of these molecules. Their transfer is most often affected by interference with blood flow into the intervillous space and back to the fetus. Oxygen is brought to the intervillous space by the maternal uterine circulation. Uterine blood flow is approximately 600 to 700 mL/min, representing 10% of the total maternal cardiac output at term. Almost 90% of the total uterine blood flow goes into the intervillous space; 10% supplies the myometrium. The amount of blood that flows into the intervillous space is directly affected by the perfusion pressure within the uterine arteries. Uteroplacental circulation is widely dilated at rest and therefore has little capacity to expand further. This circulation is capable of marked vasoconstriction, however, which occurs through hormonal or neural mechanisms. Hence, uterine blood flow during pregnancy can be increased significantly by only one mechanism, maternal bed rest. At rest, blood flow to other organs and tissues, such as muscle and fat, is diminished, and the supply of blood to the placenta and fetus is enhanced.

Blood flow to the uteroplacental circulation may be diminished due to a number of causes:

- *Uterine contractions* interrupt the supply of blood into the intervillous space. A contraction that lasts 45 seconds stops the blood flow for approximately 30 seconds. This is normally well tolerated by the healthy fetus who can exist on stored nutrients or on those present in the stagnant blood of the intervillous space.
- *Abnormal labor pattern* (eg, prolonged uterine contractions or increased frequency of uterine contractions) can greatly diminish blood flow to the uteroplacental circulation and cause hypoxia.
- *Compression of the inferior vena cava* interferes with the return of blood to the right heart. Decreased cardiac output diminishes delivery of blood to the uteroplacental unit. A large full-term uterus may cause this condition.
- *Maternal hypertension and pregnancy-induced hypertension* involve vasospasm and thereby reduce uteroplacental circulation.
- *Various pharmacologic agents, such as vasopressors,* may cause constriction of the vessels.
- *Vigorous maternal exercise* increases blood flow to the muscles and may divert blood from the uteroplacental circulation.

Fetal Blood, Fetal Hemoglobin, Bohr Effect

Several other important determinants of oxygen transfer from woman to fetus should be considered. These include the affinity of fetal blood for oxygen, the concentration of fetal hemoglobin within the fetal blood, and the Bohr effect.

Fetal hemoglobin, because of its special characteristics, has a greater affinity for oxygen than does maternal blood. By virtue of certain biochemical constituents, maternal hemoglobin has a greater capacity to unload oxygen, whereas fetal hemoglobin is endowed with a greater ability to accept oxygen. The actual concentration of hemoglobin in fetal blood also is greater than in maternal blood. At midpregnancy, fetal blood contains 15 g of hemoglobin/dL, and at term, it is somewhat higher, about 18 g/dL (Cunningham et al., 1993). Because hemoglobin is the agent that actually carries the oxygen and because the fetus has more hemoglobin, a unit of fetal blood can carry much more oxygen than can maternal blood.

The *Bohr effect* is the effect of pH on the ability of hemoglobin to accept or unload oxygen. A more acidic pH is associated with an increased ability of hemoglobin to unload oxygen; a more alkaline pH increases the ability to accept oxygen. Blood returning from the fetal circulation in the umbilical artery is more acidic and has a greater capacity to unload oxygen. It reaches the intervillous space, where it gives up its hydrogen ions and carbon dioxide, and its pH rises. Concomitantly, these hydrogen ions and carbon dioxide are accepted by the maternal circulation, and the pH of the maternal blood decreases. The increased fetal pH results in a greater capacity to accept oxygen, and the decreased maternal blood pH results in a greater capacity to deliver oxygen.

Adjustments in Fetal Blood Flow

Fetal blood flow is redistributed during periods of oxygen deprivation. Increased amounts of blood are supplied to the fetal brain and heart; blood flow to the fetal gastrointestinal tract is diminished. This helps to ensure survival of the most vital fetal organs during temporary oxygen lack. Nature has endowed the fetoplacental unit with a unique system of checks and balances to preserve fetal well-being throughout pregnancy.

The Placenta as an Endocrine Organ

From early pregnancy, the cells that eventually form the placenta are hormonally active. Even before the skipped menstrual period, the trophoblastic cells that have been responsible for allowing the embryo to invade into the endometrium have begun to secrete hCG.

Human Chorionic Gonadotropin

Produced by the syncytial cells of the trophoblast, hCG is a glycoprotein with a large molecular weight of 36,000 to 40,000. hCG is similar to pituitary luteinizing hormone in structure and activity, but it differs physiologically in that its levels are maintained in the circulation for longer periods of time. It is composed of two subunits, an alpha and a beta subunit, which are important for pregnancy testing (see Chap. 15). hCG levels increase steadily in early pregnancy, reaching a maximum in 60 to 90 days, and then the levels in the blood begin to fall. Little hCG is secreted into the fetal compartment compared with the large quantities that are released in the maternal circulation.

Human Placental Lactogen or Human Chorionic Somatomammotropin

The placenta produces a second protein hormone, human placental lactogen (HPL), also called human chorionic somatomammotropin. This hormone also is formed in syncytial cells within the trophoblast of the placenta. Its production increases progressively during pregnancy, with a marked increase after the 20th week. Very little HPL reaches fetal circulation. There is a distinct correlation between HPL levels and placental weight. For example, maternal HPL levels are higher in multiple gestations. This hormone has an action similar to human growth hormone:

- HPL regulates maternal metabolism to maintain a supply of nutrients for the fetus by facilitating transport of glucose across the placenta by facilitated diffusion.
- HPL has a mammotropic effect.

Progesterone and Estrogen

The placenta also produces the steroid hormones progesterone and estrogen. Throughout pregnancy, there is a steady increase in *progesterone* levels, which reach a maximum just before delivery. This progesterone maintains the endometrium and endometrial blood supply, brings about uterine growth, inhibits the activity of the uterine muscle, and stimulates alveolar development in the maternal breast. It also has significant effects on the woman's metabolism.

The *estrogens*, estriol 17β-estradiol, and estrone are products of the placenta. Estriol is biologically the weakest of the three major estrogens, but it is produced in greatest quantity. Its production by the placenta involves a unique interplay among the fetal adrenals, fetal liver, and placenta. Estriol is produced by a weak androgen, dehydroepiandrosterone (DHA) sulfate, which comes from the fetal adrenal gland. Ninety percent of all the estriol seen in pregnancy is derived from fetal adrenal DHA sulfate. The fetal liver further modifies DHA sulfate and converts it to a hormone the placenta can use in estriol production. Thus, the prerequisites for the placenta to produce significant quantities of estriol are an intact fetal adrenal gland and a normally functioning fetal liver.

The placenta converts the modified DHA sulfate into estriol. The estriol levels in the blood rise steadily during pregnancy as the fetus gains weight and the placenta increases in size. The levels of the other two hormones, estradiol and estrone, parallel the estriol levels in maternal blood.

Functions. The physiologic functions of the estrogens during pregnancy are multifold:

- They stimulate the growth of the uterus and uterine placental blood flow.
- They stimulate contractile activity of the myometrium.
- They stimulate growth of mammary tissue.
- They have significant effects on maternal metabolism.

In the past, measurement of estriol level was considered useful corroborative evidence of fetal death; however, current evidence indicates there is no clinical utility of these tests in the selection of management options for the high-risk pregnancy (Cunningham et al., 1993). A wide range of variation exists in the amount of urinary estriol excreted in the plasma or urine among different normal pregnant women. Factors un-related to the fetoplacental unit may be associated with decreased urinary estriol levels (eg, administration of potent glucocorticosteroids or certain antibiotics to the woman or maternal pyelonephritis).

Effects on the Newborn. Maternal estrogen is transmit-ted to the fetus and produces striking effects on the newborn. As a result of the action of this hormone, the breasts of male and female newborns may become markedly enlarged during the first few days of life and even secrete milk. In addition, the endometrium of the female fetus hypertrophies as it does in an adult woman. When estrogen is suddenly withdrawn after birth, the endometrium breaks down and bleeding sometimes occurs. This is a normal occurrence mani-fested by a little spotting on the diaper during the first week of life.

Size and Development of the Fetus

Size of the Fetus at Various Months

Length is generally considered a more accurate crite-rion of the age of the fetus than weight. *Hasse's rule* suggests that for clinical purposes, the length of the embryo in centimeters may be approximated during

the first 5 months by squaring the number of the month of pregnancy; in the second half of pregnancy, the month may be multiplied by five to estimate the length of the fetus. Conversely, the approximate age of the fetus may be obtained by taking the square root of its length in centimeters during the first 5 months and thereafter by dividing its length in centimeters by five. For example, a fetus that is 16 cm long is about 4 months old; a fetus that is 35 cm long is about 7 months old.

Highlights of Embryonic and Fetal Development

Conception does not take place until ovulation, 14 days after the onset of menstruation in a 28-day cycle, and an embryo is not 1 month old until about 2 weeks after the first missed period (assuming a 28-day cycle). Its "birthday" by months regularly falls about 2 weeks after any numerically specified missed period (Fig. 7-14). If the cycle is longer than 28 days or if ovulation was delayed in the conceptive cycle, the duration of actual pregnancy relative to the last menstrual period is shorter. This should be considered when evaluating the month-by-month development of the fetus.

Although no formal system of staging prenatal de-velopment has been developed, it is useful to con-sider the distinctive changes that occur in periods of 4 to 5 weeks. In Box 7-4 and in the discussion that follows, time periods for major development of the

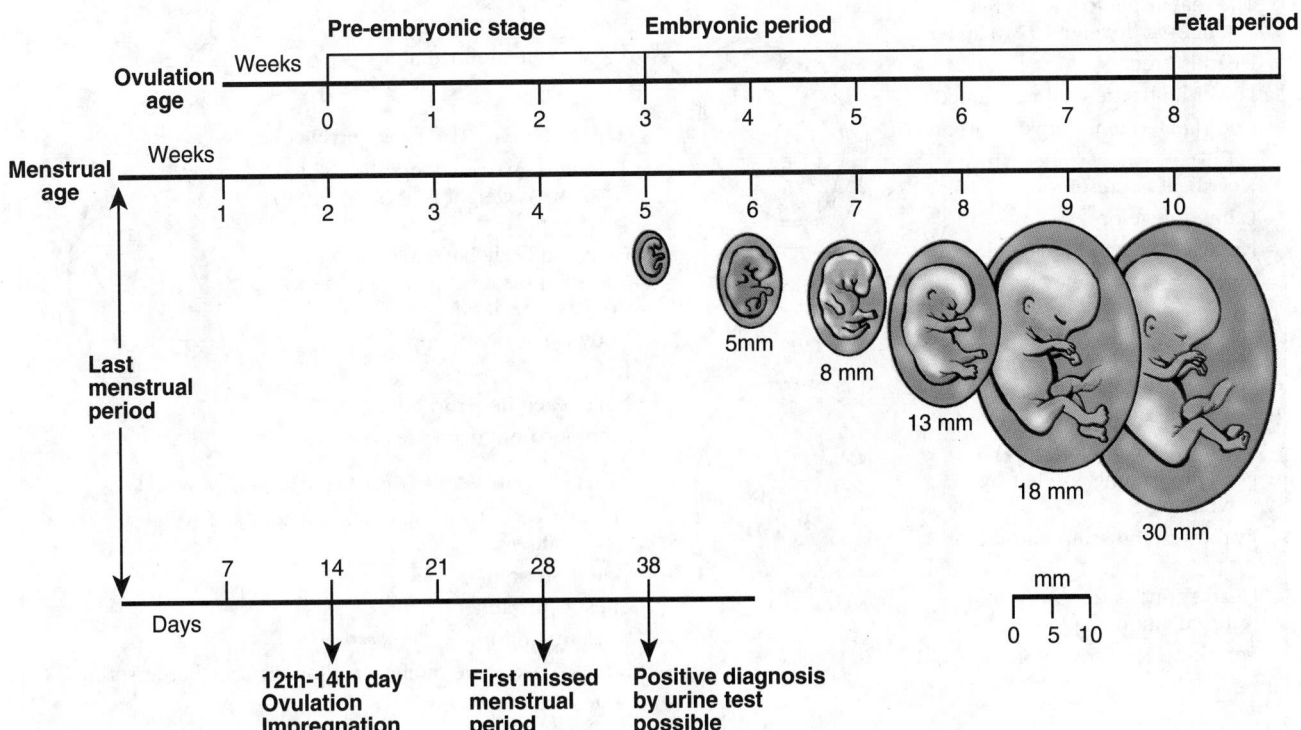

FIGURE 7-14 Growth of the ovum, embryo, and fetus during the early weeks of preg-nancy.

BOX 7–4
Fetal Development*

Four Weeks

The embryo is 4 to 5 mm in length.

Trophoblasts embed in decidua.

Chorionic villi form.

Foundations for nervous system, genitourinary system, skin, bones, and lungs are formed.

Buds of arms and legs begin to form.

Rudiments of eyes, ears, and nose appear.

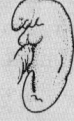

4 weeks

Five to Eight Weeks

The fetus is 27 to 31 mm in length and weighs 2 to 4 g.

Fetus is markedly bent.

Head is disproportionately large as a result of brain development.

Sex differentiation begins.

Centers of bone begin to ossify.

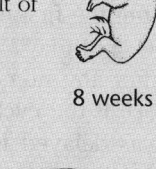

8 weeks

Nine to Twelve Weeks

The fetus average length is 50 to 87 mm and weight is 45 g.

Fingers and toes are distinct.

Placenta is complete.

Rudimentary kidneys secrete urine.

Fetal circulation is complete.

External genitalia show definite characteristics.

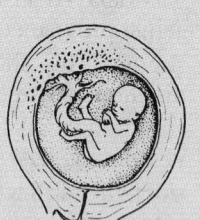

12 weeks

Thirteen to Sixteen Weeks

The fetus is 94 to 140 mm in length and weighs 97 to 200 g.

Head is erect.

Lower limbs are well developed.

Coordinated limb movements are present.

Heartbeat is present.

Lanugo develops.

Nasal septum and palate close.

Fingerprints are set.

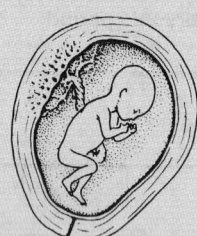

16 weeks

Seventeen to Twenty Weeks

The fetus is 150 to 190 mm in length and weighs approximately 260 to 460 g.

Lanugo covers entire body.

Fetal movements are felt by woman.

Eyebrows and scalp hair are present.

Heart sounds are perceptible by auscultation.

Vernix caseosa covers skin.

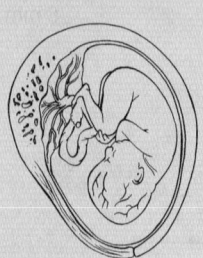

20 weeks

Twenty-one to Twenty-Five Weeks

The fetus is about 200 to 240 mm in length and weighs 495 to 910 g.

Skin appears wrinkled and pink to red.

REM begins.

Eyebrows and fingernails develop.

Sustained weight gain occurs.

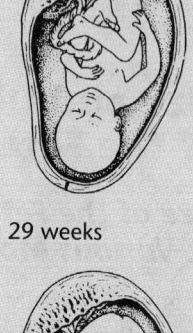

25 weeks

Twenty-Six to Twenty-Nine Weeks

The fetus is 250 to 275 mm in length and weighs about 910 to 1,500 g.

Skin is red.

Rhythmic breathing movements occur.

Pupillary membrane disappears from eyes.

The fetus often survives if born prematurely.

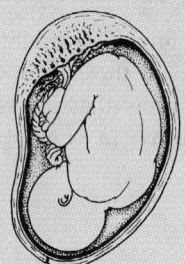

29 weeks

Thirty to Thirty-Four Weeks

The fetus is 280 to 320 mm in length and weighs 1,700 to 2,500 g.

Toenails become visible.

Eyelids open.

Steady weight gain occurs.

Vigorous fetal movement occurs.

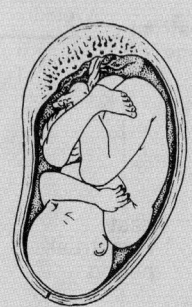

34 weeks

Thirty-Five to Thirty-Seven Weeks

The fetus' average length is 330 to 360 mm; weight is about 2,700 to 3,400 g.

Face and body have a loose wrinkled appearance because of subcutaneous fat deposit.

Body is usually plump.

Lanugo disappears.

Nails reach fingertip edge.

Amniotic fluid decreases.

37 weeks

Thirty-Eight Weeks (Full Term)

The average fetus is 360 mm in length and weighs 3,400 to 3,600 g.

Skin is smooth.

Chest is prominent.

Eyes are uniformly slate colored.

Bones of skull are ossified and nearly together at sutures.

Testes are in scrotum.

*All lengths given are crown to rump.

As pregnancy progresses, the fetus becomes capable of increasingly complex behaviors, which may be detected in utero by sonographic techniques. By the eighth week, movements of the trunk can be observed; the limbs begin to move 1 week later. Hiccuping is a common occurrence that may be perceived by the mother beginning around the ninth week. By the 11th week, there is movement of the fetal chest, and soon thereafter, the fetus becomes capable of moving amniotic fluid in and out of the respiratory tract—intrauterine fetal "breathing." The fetus actually swallows amniotic fluid and, because the taste buds are already developed, can actually react to substances injected into the amniotic fluid, which are swallowed by the 7th month. The internal and middle ear are well developed by mid-pregnancy, and the fetus is capable of reacting to sudden noise with active movement at about the 24th week.

croscopic arteries. The beginnings of the future digestive tract also are discernible. A long, slender tube leading from the mouth to an expansion becomes the stomach; connected with the latter, the beginnings of the intestines may be seen. Foundations for the nervous system, genitourinary system, skin, bones, and lungs are formed. The backbone is apparent but is so bent on itself that the head almost touches the tip of the tail. The head is extremely prominent, representing almost one-third of the entire embryo. The head is large in proportion to the body throughout intrauterine life. This is still true at birth but to a lesser degree.

The embryo is susceptible to the effects of teratogens, which may cause major congenital defects during this period.

Five to Eight Weeks

The fetus begins to assume human form during this period (Fig. 7-16). As the brain develops, the head becomes disproportionately large (constituting about one-half of the embryo), so the nose, mouth, and ears become relatively less prominent. It has an unmistakably human face and arms, legs, fingers, toes, elbows, and knees (Fig. 7-17). In the seventh week, a fetal heartbeat can be detected with real-time sonography. Early in the eighth week, the eyes are open, but toward the end of the eighth week, the eyelids often begin to unite by epithelial fusion (Moore et al., 1993). By the end of the eighth week, all of the regions of the limbs are apparent, and the digits have lengthened and are separated. Purposeful limb movements begin, and centers of the bones start to ossify. The external genitalia have become apparent, but it is difficult to distinguish accurately between male and female fetuses. During the last 4 weeks, the embryo has quadrupled in length and measures about 27 to 31 mm from head to buttocks. Weight ranges from 2 to 4 g.

embryo and fetus are presented using *postconception age* as a reference point. Box 7-5 summarizes in utero fetal behavior

Four Weeks

At 4 weeks, the embryo is about 4 to 6 mm long if measured in a straight line from crown to rump. Recognizable traces of all organs are differentiated. The rudiments of the eyes, ears, and nose make their appearance (Fig. 7-15). The incipient arms and legs resemble buds. The tube that eventually forms the heart has been formed, producing a large, rounded bulge on the body wall; even at this early age, this structure is pulsating regularly and propelling blood through mi-

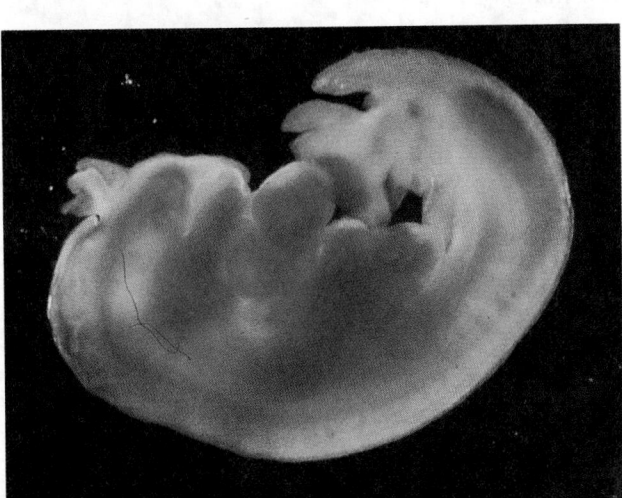

FIGURE 7-15 Embryo at 4 weeks.

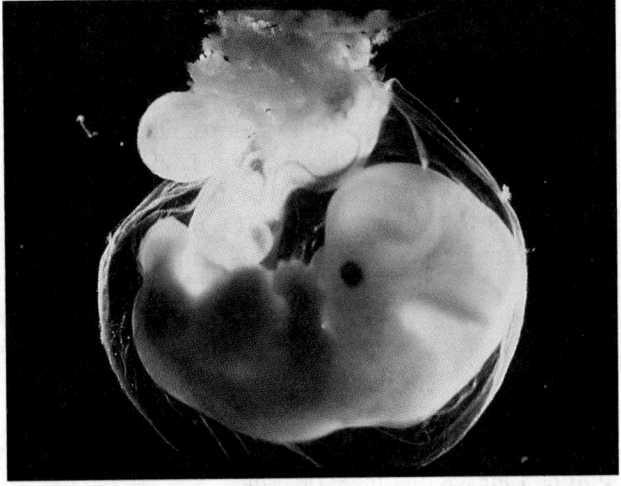

FIGURE 7-16 Fetus at 5½ weeks.

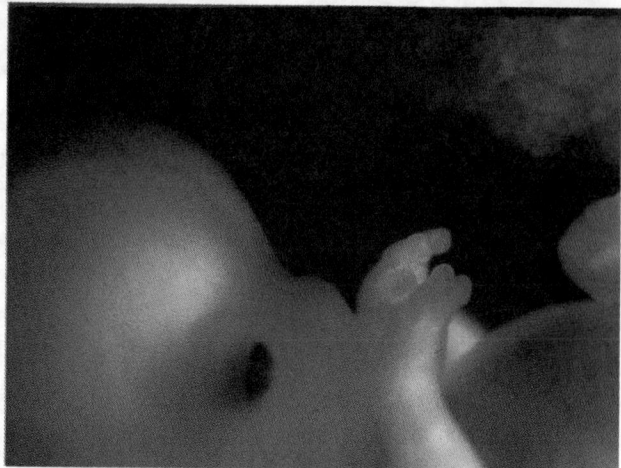

FIGURE 7-17 Fetus at 8 weeks.

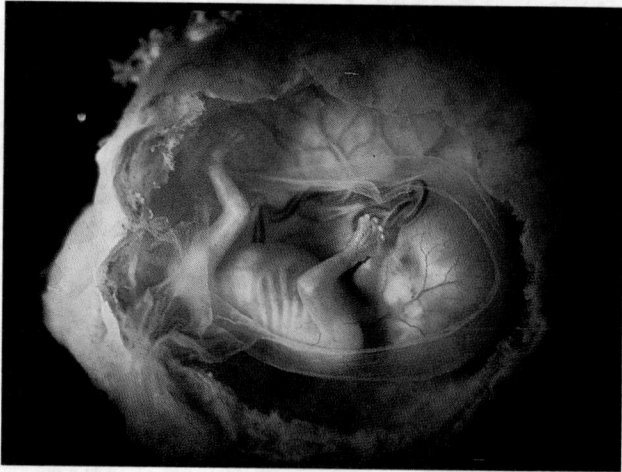

FIGURE 7-18 Fetus at 16 weeks.

Nine to Twelve Weeks

During this period, the fetus is 50 to 87 mm long and weighs 45 g. The sex can be distinguished because the external genitalia are beginning to show definite characteristics. Early in this period, buds for all the temporary "baby" teeth are present, and sockets for these develop in the jawbone. Rudimentary kidneys have formed and secrete small amounts of urine into the bladder, which escape later into the amniotic fluid. Movements of the fetus occur at this time, but they are too weak to be felt by the woman. By the end of 12 weeks, primary ossification centers appear in the skeleton, especially in the skull and long bones. The upper limbs have almost reached their final relative lengths, but the lower limbs are not as well developed and are slightly shorter than their final relative lengths. The fingernails and toenails appear as fine membranes. Fetal circulation is complete, and the **placenta** is fully formed.

Thirteen to Sixteen Weeks

During this period, rapid fetal growth occurs. Length extends between 94 and 140 mm and weight ranges from 97 to 200 g (Fig. 7-18). The sex, as evidenced by the external genital organs, is obvious. Fingerprints are set, and ossification of the skeleton is active. Coordinated limb movements are present by the 14th week but are still too slight to be felt by the woman. Slow eye movement occurs. The fetus can stretch, move around, and swallow amniotic fluid. The nasal septum and palate close. *Lanugo*, fine, downy hair, begins to develop. Blood vessels are visible under the transparent fetal skin. The head is relatively small compared with that of the 12-week fetus. In the female fetus, the ovaries are differentiated by 16 weeks and contain primordial follicles that have oogonia.

Seventeen to Twenty Weeks

The crown-to-rump length extends between 150 to 190 mm, and the fetal weight ranges from 260 to 460 g. Lanugo appears on the skin over the entire body. **Brown fat**, the source of heat production, forms during this period. By 18 weeks, the uterus is developed, and canalization of the vagina has begun in the female fetus. In the male fetus, the testes are at the inguinal ring at about 20 weeks. Eyebrows and scalp hair are present at the end of the 20th week (Dimmick et al., 1992). The skin is now covered with a greasy, cheese-like material known as *vernix caseosa* (Moore et al., 1993). Usually, the woman becomes conscious of slight fluttering movements in her abdomen as a result of fetal movement. Their first appearance is called *quickening,* or the perception of life. Fetal heart tones can easily be detected by auscultation at 20 weeks. If a fetus is born now, it may make a few efforts to breathe, but its lungs are insufficiently developed to cope with conditions outside the uterus, and it invariably dies within a few hours.

Twenty-One to Twenty-Five Weeks

The length of the fetus from crown to rump extends from 200 to 240 mm, and its weight ranges from 495 to 910 g. The skin appears wrinkled, translucent, and is pink to red because blood is visible in the capillaries beneath it. Rapid eye movements begin at 21 weeks. Blink-startle responses have been reported at 22 to 23 weeks. Fingernails and eyelashes are present by 24 weeks. The secretory epithelial cells in the interalveolar walls of the lungs have begun to secrete surfactant, a surface-active lipid that maintains the patency of the alveoli of the lungs (Moore et al., 1993). Sustained weight gain occurs during this period.

Twenty-Six to Twenty-Nine Weeks

The fetus measures between 250 and 275 cm in length from crown to rump and weighs from 910 to 1,500 g during this period. The pupillary membrane has just disappeared from the eyes, allowing the eyes to reopen at 26 weeks (Moore et al., 1993). The fetal spleen is now an important site of hematopoiesis. Lanugo and head hair are well developed, and toenails become visible. In the male fetus, scrotum descent may begin as early as the 28th week. During this period, a fetus often survives if born prematurely and given intensive care because the fetal lungs are capable of breathing air (Dimmick et al., 1992). Furthermore, the central nervous system has matured to the stage where it can direct rhythmic breathing movements and control body temperature.

Thirty to Thirty-Four Weeks

The fetus measures between 280 to 320 mm from crown to rump and weighs approximately 1,700 to 2,500 g. Its skin is still red and wrinkled, and vernix caseosa and lanugo are present. Vigorous fetal movements are present. Pain pathways to the brain stem and thalamus are completely myelinated by 30 weeks (Anand et al., 1987), and the pupillary light reflex of the eyes can be elicited. Fetuses 32 weeks and older usually survive with proper incubator and good nursing care. At this stage, the quantity of white fat (adipose tissue) is about 8% of body weight.

Thirty-Five to Thirty-Eight Weeks

For all practical purposes, the fetus is a mature infant at 35 to 38 weeks' gestation. It measures about 330 to 360 mm from crown to rump and weighs between 2,700 and 3,400 g. Because of the deposition of subcutaneous fat, the body has become more rotund, and the skin is less wrinkled and red. Lanugo hair is beginning to disappear, and the nails reach the edge of the fingertip. The fetus at 35 weeks has a firm grasp and exhibits a spontaneous orientation to light. By 36 weeks, circumference of head and chest are approximately equal. During this period, the fetus gains about 220 g/wk. Its chances of survival are as good as though it were born at full term. Most fetuses during this "finishing period" are plump. As term approaches (37–38 weeks), the nervous system is sufficiently mature to carry out some integrative functions, and the amount of white fat is about 16% of body weight. A fetus adds about 14 g of fat during these last weeks of gestation (Moore et al., 1993).

Thirty-Eight Weeks (Full Term)

By this point, full term has been reached (38 weeks after fertilization or 40 weeks after LMP), and the fetus

weighs, on an average, 3,400 to 3,600 g and is about 360 mm long from crown to rump. Male fetuses usually weigh more than female fetuses. Skin is smooth and normally bluish-pink and thickly coated with the cheesy vernix in body creases and skin folds. The fine, downy hair that previously covered its body has largely disappeared except on the upper arms and shoulders. The fingernails are firm and protrude beyond the end of the fingers. Eyes are uniformly slate colored, and the bones of the skull are ossified and nearly together at sutures. The chest is prominent, and the breasts protrude slightly in both sexes. Testes are in the scrotum, and labia majora are well developed.

Fetal Circulation

Fetal circulation differs from extrauterine blood flow in several ways. The fetus receives oxygen and excretes carbon dioxide through the placenta because its lungs do not function as organs of gas exchange in utero. The fetal circulation contains certain special vessels ("bypasses" or "detours") that shunt the blood around the lungs, with only a small amount circulating through them for nutrition.

The oxygenated blood flows up the cord through the umbilical vein and passes into the inferior vena cava; on the way to the inferior vena cava, part of the oxygenated blood goes through the liver, but most of it passes through a special fetal structure, the *ductus venosus,* which connects the umbilical vein and the inferior vena cava. The liver is proportionately large in a newborn because it receives a considerable supply of freshly vitalized blood directly from the umbilical vein. Blood flow in the umbilical circulation has been estimated at approximately 125 mL/kg of body weight or approximately 500 mL/min in the average fetus at term (Scott et al., 1994).

From the inferior vena cava, the current flows into the right auricle and goes directly to the left auricle through a special fetal structure, the *foramen ovale*. It then flows into the left ventricle and out through the aorta. The blood that circulates up the arms and the head returns through the superior vena cava to the right auricle again, but instead of passing through the foramen ovale as before, the current is deflected downward into the right ventricle and through the pulmonary arteries. Part of it goes to the lungs (for purposes of nutrition only), but most of it goes into the descending aorta through the *ductus arteriosus*.

The blood in the aorta, with the exception of that which goes to the head and upper extremities, passes downward to supply the trunk and lower extremities (Fig. 7-19). Most of this blood finds its way through the internal iliac, or hypogastric, arteries and back through

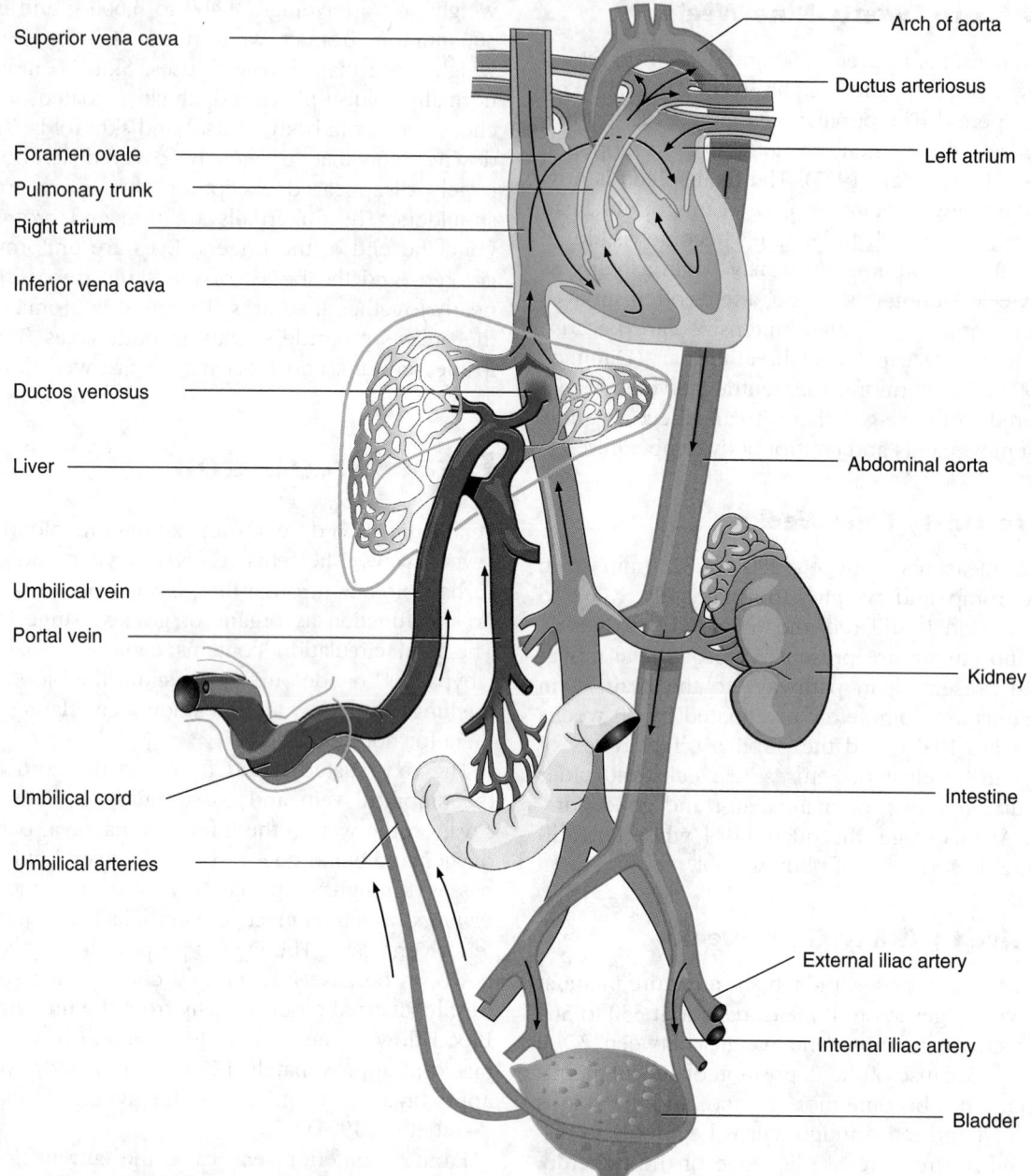

FIGURE 7–19 Diagram of the fetal circulation shortly before birth. The course of blood is indicated by arrows.

the umbilical arteries to the placenta, where it is again oxygenated; however, a small amount passes back into the ascending vena cava to mingle with fresh blood from the umbilical vein and again makes the circuit of the entire body.

Change in Circulation at Birth

The fetal circulation is arranged so that the passage of blood to the placenta through the umbilical arteries and back through the umbilical vein is possible up to the time of birth, but it ceases entirely the moment the baby breathes and begins to take oxygen directly from its own lungs. During intrauterine life, the circulation of blood through the lungs is for the nourishment of the lungs and not for the purpose of securing oxygen.

In the transition to extrauterine life, the newborn circulatory pathway becomes comparable to that of the adult. Venous blood circulates from the two venae cavae into the right auricle of the heart, to the right ventricle, and through the pulmonary arteries to the lungs, where it gives up its waste products and takes up a fresh supply of oxygen. After oxygenation, the arterial blood flows from the lungs, through the pulmonary veins to the left auricle, to the left ventricle, and out through the aorta; it is then distributed through the capillaries to all parts of the body and eventually collected as venous blood in the venae cavae and recirculated into the right auricle.

Circulation Path After Birth

The primary changes in the circulation at birth are, first, loss of the large blood flow through the placenta, which approximately doubles the systemic vascular resistance at birth (Guyton, 1991). This increases the aortic pressure and the pressures in the left ventricle and left atrium. Second, the pulmonary vascular resistance greatly decreases, as a result of lung expansion. These changes alter the character of the blood in many vessels and make many of these vessels useless. The umbilical arteries within the baby's body become filled with clotted blood and are ultimately converted into fibrous cords. After occlusion of the vessel, the umbilical vein within the body becomes the round ligament of the liver. After the umbilical cord is tied and separated, the large amount of blood returned to the heart and the lungs, which are functioning, causes equal pressure in both of the auricles. This pressure causes the foramen ovale to close. The foramen ovale remains closed and eventually disappears, and the ductus arteriosus and the ductus venosus shrivel up and are converted into fibrous cords or ligaments in 2 or 3 months. The instantaneous closure of the foramen ovale changes the entire course of the blood current and converts the fetal circulation into the adult type.

The changes in the fetal circulation after birth are shown in Table 7-3.

The Nursing Process

Nurses caring for childbearing families and prospective parents have an ideal opportunity to provide teaching and counseling regarding genetics, conception, and prenatal development. Because couples are generally eager to have a healthy baby, they are motivated and receptive to learning about their unborn child and influences on the intrauterine environment. Basic concepts of embryology can be introduced, highlighting important milestones during gestation (see Client Teaching Guidelines). Information needs to be presented in simple terms, using language appropriate for the client(s). Use of childbirth graphics (eg, pictures and videos) may further reinforce client education and feelings of identification with the fetus.

Anticipatory guidance should be provided about ultrasonography, if indicated. The procedure should be explained as an effective method for dating pregnancy, detecting gross fetal abnormalities, and monitoring fetal well-being. Use of ultrasound techniques is often a routine part of early prenatal care.

Assessment for potential environmental hazards is another important component of the comprehensive prenatal evaluation of all clients (see Chap. 17). Referrals for genetic counseling should be initiated for couples at risk for congenital or genetic disorders and chromosomal anomalies (see Chap. 14). Ideally, preconception counseling will have been performed in many of these situations.

TABLE 7-3
Changes in Fetal Circulation After Birth

Structure	Before Birth	After Birth
Umbilical vein	Brings arterial blood to liver and heart	Obliterated; becomes round ligament of liver
Umbilical arteries	Brings arteriovenous blood to placenta	Obliterated; become vesicle ligaments on anterior abdominal wall
Ductus venosus	Shunts arterial blood into inferior vena cava	Obliterated; becomes ligamentum venosum
Ductus arteriosus	Shunts arterial and some venous blood from pulmonary artery to aorta	Obliterated; becomes ligamentum arteriosum
Foramen ovale	Connects right and left auricles (atria)	Obliterated usually; at times open
Lungs	Contain no air and very little blood	Filled with air and well supplied with blood
Pulmonary arteries	Bring little blood to lungs	Bring much blood to lungs
Aorta	Receives blood from both ventricles	Receives blood only from left ventricle
Inferior vena cava	Brings venous blood from body and arterial blood from placenta	Brings venous blood only to right auricle

(Guyton, A. C. [1986]. *Medical physiology* [7th ed.]. Philadelphia: W. B. Saunders.)

CLIENT TEACHING GUIDELINES
Development of the Embryo and Fetus

■ Instruct the client about development of the embryo and fetus
  - Weeks 4–8 are critical for cell differentiation and organ development; the embryo is most vulnerable to developmental or environmental influences that may cause malformations. (Avoid individuals with infectious diseases, such as rubella; avoid exposure to potential teratogenic substances, such as high-dose ionizing radiation, organic mercury compounds, lead, polybrominate biphenyls, organic solvents).
  - Body organs are formed by 8–12 weeks; remaining weeks of gestation are for maturation and growth.
  - Sex of baby is evident.
  - Oxygen transferred from mother to baby through the placenta; factors influence uteroplacental blood flow (eg, smoking).
  - Fetal heart beat is audible by Doppler at 8–12 weeks and by fetoscope at 20 weeks.
  - Fetal movements are felt by woman around 20 weeks (quickening).
  - During week 24–26, the fetus is capable of survival if born prematurely.
■ Explain how ultrasound examination may provide important information during early pregnancy (see Chap. 37 for further details).
  - 5–6 weeks: formation of gestational sac
  - 6–7 weeks: embryonic outline
  - 6–7 weeks: heart activity
  - 8–9 weeks: early placenta
■ Caution against environmental hazards.
  - Sauna or hot tub use may cause maternal hyperthermia, which has been associated with central nervous system defects.
  - Substance use can cause a variety of problems that relate to the type of chemical ingested, quantity, and duration of use (see Chap. 33 for further details).
■ Counsel regarding maternal nutrition to promote optimum intrauterine environment (see Chap. 18 for further details).

Summary Points

✔ Mitosis is the major process by which somatic cells containing 46 chromosomes (diploid) are produced. Gametes (germ cells) with 23 unpaired chromosomes (haploid) are created through the process of meiosis.

✔ Oogenesis is the process by which female gametes are produced; the process by which male gametes are produced is known as spermatogenesis. The ovaries begin to develop early in the female fetus. Meiosis begins in all oocytes during the prenatal period and stops before the first division is complete until puberty. During puberty, the first meiotic division is completed in the primary oocyte.

✔ The male can produce sperm from puberty through old age. Both capacitation and acrosomal reaction must occur for the sperm to fertilize the ovum.

✔ The zygote (46 chromosomes) forms from union of the sperm and ovum. Fertilization is followed by rapid mitotic divisions (cleavage), which produce a series of morphologic formations (eg, blastomeres, morula, blastocyst).

✔ Sex is determined at the time of fertilization by the spermatozoon not by the ovum. A female embryo is produced when the spermatozoon contains the X chromosome, whereas a male embryo is produced by a spermatozoon containing a Y chromosome. Until approximtately 7 weeks, the genital ducts are undifferentiated. Hormones play an essential role in male sex differentiation; however, female sexual differentiation does not depend on hormones.

✔ Multifetal pregnancy may result from the fertilization of one or more ovum. Twinning is the most frequent type of multifetal pregnancy. Twins may be monzygotic (identical) or dizygotic (fraternal). The birth of dizygotic twins is more prevalent and is affected by fertility drugs, maternal race, age, and parity. Dizygotic twins result from two separate ova that have been fertilized by two different spermatozoa.

✔ The first 8 weeks of development represent the most critical period because all of the major organ systems are developing. Exposure to teratogens and environmental hazards at this time may lead to morphologic defects.

✔ The three primary germ layers known as the ectoderm, endoderm, and mesoderm give rise to all tissues, organs, and organ systems.

✔ Major prenatal developmental milestones include pulsating heart (4 weeks), completion of organ systems (8–12 weeks), visible external genitals (16 weeks), audible heart beat by ausculation and perceivable fetal movements (20 weeks), viability (24–26 weeks), eyes reopening (26 weeks), and fingernails reaching end of fingers (35–37 weeks).

✔ The placenta is a major organ for gaseous exchange (oxygenation), nutrient transport, excretion of wastes, and production of hormones. Exchange of substances from woman to fetus occurs across the intervillious space. Most substances in the maternal blood may be transferred to the fetus by one of the following processes: diffusion, facilitated diffusion, active transport, bulk flow, or pinocytosis. Defects in the placental membranes may cause leakage of substances.

✔ Hormones produced by the placenta play a major role in pregnancy. Progesterone maintains the endometrium and endometrial blood supply, brings about uterine growth, and stimulates developmental of breast tissue. Estrogens stimulate growth of the uterus and uterine blood flow, enhance contractility of the myometrium, and affect growth of mammary tissue. Other hormones produced by the placenta include HPL and hCG.

✔ Embryonic membranes include the chorion and amnion. The chorion encloses the amnion, embryo, and yolk sac. The amnion is the membrane adjacent to the embryo. Amniotic fluid contained within the amniotic cavity protects the fetus from injury, maintains even intrauterine temperature, permits symmetric external growth, and provides space for free movement. The quantity of amniotic fluid provides an index of fetal well-being.

✔ Uteroplacental blood flow may be influenced by a number of factors, such as uterine contractions, cord compression, maternal blood flow, and hypertension.

✔ The one umbilical vein carries oxygen and nutrients from the placenta to the fetus; the two umbilical arteries carry deoxygenated blood and waste products to the placenta. Wharton's jelly provides a protective covering over the umbilical cord.

✔ Three major shunts exist in the fetal circulation. Blood is shifted from the right atrium to the left atrium through the *foramen ovale*. The *ductus venosus* allows blood to bypass the fetal liver partially. The *ductus arteriosus* allows blood to bypass the lungs and enter the descending aorta. These structures functionally close shortly after birth.

REFERENCES

Anand, K. J. S., Phil, D., & Hickey, P. R. (1987). Pain and its effects in the human neonate and fetus. *The New England Journal of Medicine, 317*(21), 1321–3127.

Australian In-Vitro Fertilization Collaborative Group (1988). In-vitro fertilization pregnancies in Australia and New Zealand. *Medical Journal of Australia, 148,* 429.

Brennan, P. A., & Mednick, S. A. (1993). Genetic perspectives on crime. *Acta Psychiatric Scandinavia,* Supplementum 370, 19–26.

Bullock, B. (1996). *Pathophysiology* (pp. 65–67) (4th ed.). Philadelphia: Lippincott-Raven Publishers.

Cunningham, F. G., MacDonald, P. C., & Gant, N. F. (1993). *Williams obstetrics* (19th ed.). Norwalk, CT: Appleton & Lange.

Dimmick, J. E., & Kalousek, D. K. (1992). *Developmental pathology of the embryo and fetus.* Philadelphia: J.B. Lippincott.

Guyton, A. C. (1991). *Medical physiology* (8th ed.). Philadelphia: W.B. Saunders.

Jauniaux, E., & Burton, G. J. (1992). The effect of smoking in pregnancy on early placental morphology. *Obstetrics and Gynecology, 79*(5), 645–648.

Johnson, M. H., & Everett, B. J. (1988). *Essential reproduction.* Boston: Blackwell Scientific.

Kurachi, K., Aono, T., Susuki, M. et al. (1985). *Results of HMG (Hurregon)-hCG therapy in 6,096 treatment cycles of 2,166 Japanese women with anovulatory infertility. European Journal of Obstetrics, Gynecology & Reproductive Biology, 19*(1), 43–51.

Money, J., & Ehrhardt, A. A. (1973). *Man and woman: Boy and girl.* Baltimore: Johns Hopkins University Press.

Money, J., & Tucker, P. (1975). *Sexual signatures: On being a man or a woman.* Boston: Little, Brown.

Moore, K. L., & Persaud, T. V. N. (1993). *The developing human* (5th ed.). Philadelphia: W.B. Saunders.

Scott, J. R., DiSaia, P. J., Hammond, C. B. (Eds.) (1994). *Danforth's obstetrics and gynecology* (16th ed.). Philadelphia: J.B. Lippincott.

Sherfey, M. J. (1972). *The nature and evolution of female sexuality.* New York: Random House.

Swaab, D. F., Hofman, M. A., Lucassen, P. J., Purba, J. S., Raadsheer, F. C., & Van de Nes, J. A. P. (1993). Functional neuroanatomy and neuropathology of the human hypothalamus. *Anatomy and Embryology, 187,* 317–330.

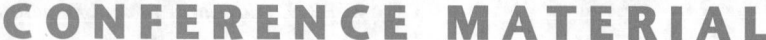
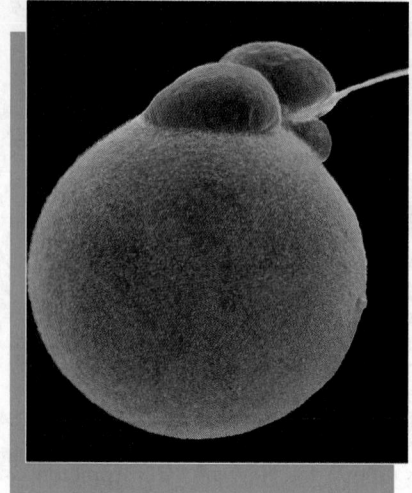

II

Biophysical Aspects of Human Reproduction

Critical Thinking Exercises

1. You are the school nurse at a local middle school. The health teacher asks you to teach a class of 10- to 13-year-old girls about the female reproductive system, including the menstrual cycle. As the school nurse, you know that the class is at various stages of sexual maturity development.

    How would you approach this task? Include any ideas for possible audiovisual aids to enhance your teaching plan.

2. M.K., a 23-year-old married woman, comes to the woman's clinic for a routine check up. She reports that she and her husband are planning to have a child. She is concerned that she might have trouble getting pregnant. She states, "My periods are somewhat irregular, and I have a hard time knowing when I'm ovulating." After further discussion, M.K. decides to use the cervical mucus method and basal body temperature to determine ovulation.

    When developing your teaching plan, what areas should you address and, specifically, how will you address them?

3. A group of couples, all in the early second trimester of pregnancy are attending childbirth education classes. Many of the participants are asking about the changes occurring with the fetus at this time. You are hearing questions like: "When will we be able to hear the baby's heartbeat?"; "When can we tell if its a boy or a girl?"; "Can the baby hear us talking?"; "How big is the baby now?". You plan to focus the next class on fetal growth and development.

    How would you meet the needs of this group and what aspects would your teaching plan address?

Multiple Choice Questions

1. A client with small breasts in her first pregnancy is worried about her ability to breast-feed her baby. The most correct response by the nurse would be:

    A. "You probably will be unable to breast-feed your baby."
    B. "The size of the breasts will not influence the amount of lactation possible."
    C. "Mothers with small breasts usually have less difficulty feeding their babies."
    D. "Your baby would be fed better by means of formula feeding."

2. During a teaching session, a client asks "When does ovulation generally occur?" The nurse responds correctly when stating that it generally occurs:

    A. 14 days after the last day of the menstrual cycle
    B. 14 days before the end of the menstrual cycle
    C. 5 days after the last day of the menstrual cycle
    D. 5 days before the end of menstruation

3. When performing a pelvic exam, the nurse would expect that normally the uterus is:

    A. Attached anteriorly to the bladder wall
    B. Suspended and freely movable in the pelvic cavity
    C. Posterior to the rectum
    D. Attached posteriorly to the anterior wall of the sacrum

4. When determining the stage of sexual maturity for a female client, the nurse understands that the time sequence of changes that occur at puberty in the female is:

A. Appearance of axillary and pubic hair, breast development, menarche
B. Menarche, breast development, appearance of axillary and pubic hair
C. Breast development, menarche, appearance of axillary and pubic hair
D. Breast development, appearance of axillary and pubic hair, menarche

5. When developing a teaching plan for a client using basal body temperature, the nurse keeps in mind that the hormone that brings about the postovulatory increase in basal body temperature is:

A. Gonadotropins
B. Estrogen
C. Progesterone
D. GnRH

6. A client delivered a 600-g fetus. The nurse would determine that the approximate age of the fetus is:

A. 13 to 16 weeks
B. 17 to 20 weeks
C. 21 to 25 weeks
D. 26 to 29 weeks

7. When teaching a pregnant client about fetal development, the nurse emphasizes that the most critical period of physical development for the fetus occurs from:

A. 2 to 8 weeks
B. 16 to 20 weeks
C. 20 to 28 weeks
D. 28 to 40 weeks

8. For an embryo to differentiate as a male, what hormonal event must occur?

A. Maternal estrogen secretion
B. Fetal gonadal secretion of androgen
C. Fetal gonadal secretion of estrogen
D. Maternal androgen secretion

9. A pregnant woman of 6 weeks' gestation asks how early can the baby's heart beat be detected? The nurse correctly replies:

A. "The heartbeat can be easily heard by 8 weeks."
B. "We can do an ultrasound now to show you the fetal heart."
C. "The fetal heart beat can be heard now."
D. "The fetal heart beat can be easily heard by 28 weeks."

10. During a teaching session, the nurse describes the umbilical cord as consisting of:

A. Two arteries and one vein
B. One artery and two veins
C. Two arteries and two veins
D. One artery and one vein

STUDY QUESTIONS

1. Name the core of erectile tissue found in the penis.

2. Why is the temperature of the scrotum 2 to 3 degrees lower than that of body temperature?

3. List the two functions of the testes.

4. List the two parts of the female pelvis.

5. Identify the chief function of the ovaries.

6. What type of environment exists in the vagina?

7. What breast structure is composed of highly sensitive erectile tissue?

8. Define menarche.

9. Name the hormone that appears within 2 to 3 days of implantation if pregnancy has occurred.

10. Define mittelschmerz.

11. What change in cervical mucus suggests impending ovulation?

12. List the stages of the four-stage sexual response cycle.

13. Define mitosis.

14. Identify the three germ layers of the embryo.

15. List the six mechanisms for transporting nutrients through the placenta.

16. During which stage of fetal development does the head constitute about half the size of the fetus?

17. When does quickening occur?

18. Identify the three fetal structures that differentiate fetal circulation from extrauterine circulation.

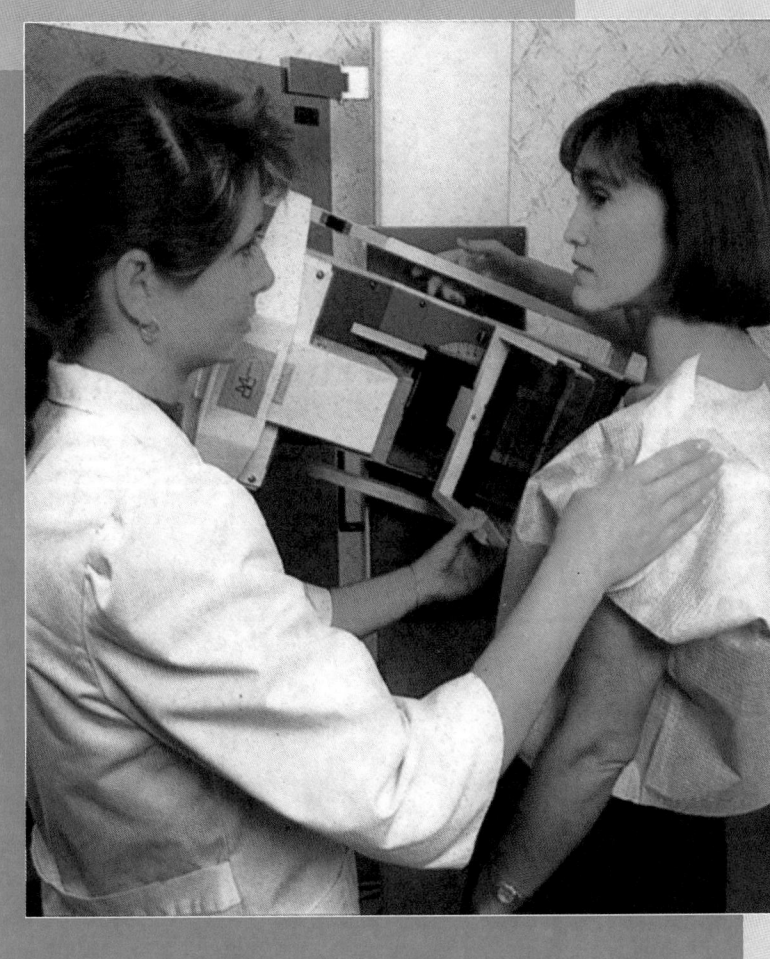

Assessment and Management of Women's Health

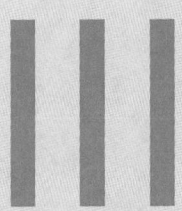

8

Women's Health Promotion

Objectives

- Describe periodic screening procedures for women's health promotion.
- Identify personal and cultural factors that affect women's health promotion and screening behaviors.
- Describe variations in common menstrual patterns.
- Discuss the effects of cigarette smoking on women's health.
- Describe the procedures for taking a Pap smear and performing breast examinations.
- Discuss the impact of stress on women's health.
- Describe physiologic and psychological characteristics of menopause.
- Identify risk factors for cancer, depression, substance abuse, osteoporosis, and heart disease in women.
- Develop nursing care plans for promoting women's health and reducing risk of disease.

Key Terms

Breast cancer
  screening
Cervical cancer
  screening
Depression

Hormone replacement
  therapy
Menopause
Osteopenia
Osteoporosis

BOX 8-1
Health Promotion:
Personal Responsibility

Health promotion requires first and foremost that individuals (including the nurse) take responsibility for their own personal health habits. "Improving personal health can count among the most potent means to prevent disease and promote health. . . . Each person must choose to make these changes a personal priority"

U.S. Department of Health and Human Services. (1992). Healthy people 2000: national health promotion and disease prevention objectives. Washington, DC: DHHS.

Nurses who provide women's healthcare have the opportunity to promote wellness and reduce the risk of illness. In hospital and community settings, nurses may respond to healthcare needs that include teaching health-enhancing practices, identifying risk factors, screening for and early detection of illness, counseling clients about issues related to growth and development (including the life stages of adolescence and menopause), and caring for women with common health problems, such as menstrual or breast disorders, genital infections, depression, abuse, neoplasia, and reproductive surgery. Techniques and skills for assessing and managing women's healthcare are adapted for different cultural perspectives, ages, and disabilities.

Wellness Care of Women in the Community

Health promotion for women often takes place in a community-based setting, such as a family planning clinic, community clinic, office practice, ambulatory care facility, or prenatal clinic. *Nursing's Agenda for Health Care Reform* (Executive Summary, 1992) supports delivery of primary healthcare in community-based settings to ensure access and quality services at affordable costs. Such settings provide essential services for women and children (Capan, 1993). Nurse-managed centers that are directed by nurses and staffed by nurse practitioners focus on wellness care. While such centers are not yet common throughout the country, data show that clients of nurse-managed centers are highly satisfied with their care, have excellent compliance and outcomes, and experience substantial cost savings (Lundeen, 1985; McGrath, 1990).

Healthy People 2000

The Department of Health and Human Services (DHHS) has established goals toward helping the nation achieve better health. The central purpose of *Healthy People 2000* is to increase the number of Americans who live long and healthy lives (DHHS, 1992). Priorities for

health promotion include increasing physical fitness; improving nutrition; decreasing alcohol, tobacco, and drug use; promoting family planning and mental health; and preventing violent and abusive behavior. Priorities for illness prevention include reducing the incidence of heart disease and stroke, cancer, diabetes, human immunodeficiency virus infection, sexually transmitted diseases (STDs), and infectious diseases. Women's healthcare is concerned with most of these areas; emphasis will vary according to individual characteristics and stage of life.

The best health promotion strategies include those related to individual lifestyle (Box 8-1). The personal choices people make in a social context have a significant influence on their health status. Nurses play an important role in promoting health through teaching and counseling that assists clients to make and implement healthy choices in their daily lives. For example, studies have demonstrated that teaching and counseling by health professionals is effective in helping people change dietary and smoking behaviors (Burns, 1994). Taking responsibility for personal health behavior also must be a priority for the nurse.

Nursing Assessment

Women's Health History

Assessment begins with a general health history, paying particular attention to the reproductive system and special risk areas for women. The history includes identifying data, occupation, family structure, menstrual history, obstetric history, significant illnesses (with emphasis on gynecologic problems), immunizations, lifestyle and behavior history, sexual history, and family health history. A review of symptoms related to each body system provides data on current health status.

Periodic screening procedures are reviewed for early detection of breast and cervical cancer. The woman is asked about her performance of breast self-examination (BSE) and about her most recent mammogram and Papanicolaou (Pap) smear and the results. Particular risks suggested by the history are further explored. For example, women with multiple sexual partners are at higher risk for STDs, and those with rectal bleeding are at greater risk for polyps or cancer of the colon. Smokers have greater risk of lung cancer and cardiovascular disease. Occupational hazards and high stress levels that increase risk also can be identified and explored.

See the Assessment Tool: Women's Health History for details.

Physical Examination

The nurse performs or assists with the physical examination. The format closely follows that described in Chapter 17. Age, individual health history, cultural factors, and risk status of clients direct the examination to emphasize certain systems or parts.

ASSESSMENT TOOL
Women's Health History

Personal Data

Age, marital or relationship status
Education and occupation
Cultural or ethnic group
Children or people living in home
Religion
Support systems

Menstrual History

Menarche or menopause
Menstrual cycle characteristics
    Length of cycle
    Days of flow
    Character of flow
    Premenstrual symptoms
    Degree of discomfort
    Medications or remedies used
Date and results of last Pap smear
If menopausal, any vaginal bleeding or other symptoms
If menstruating, any irregular bleeding

Pregnancy History

Age at first pregnancy
Total number of pregnancies and outcomes
Pregnancy complications

Contraceptive History

Current contraceptive (if any)
Other contraceptives used
Satisfaction and problems with contraceptive methods
Future fertility plans

Major Illnesses or Health Problem

Date and type of illness or health problem
Date and type of operations, procedures,
or hospitalizations
Current medical treatment and medications

Family Health History

Type of illness or health problems of relatives
    Heart attack
    Stroke
    Cancer
    Diabetes
    High blood pressure
    Blood clots (lungs, legs)
    Mental illness
    Obesity

Current Health Status

Client's definition of state of health
Concerns about symptoms or possible problems
Self-care activities
Last physical, gynecologic, and dental examination

Lifestyle and Habits

Nutrition and eating patterns
Sleep and rest
Exercise and recreation
Elimination (bladder, bowel, skin)
Sexual patterns
Stress and stress management
Leisure activities
Environment at home (satisfactions, concerns, physical or emotional abuse, see Chap. 33)
Environment at work (job satisfaction, hazards, sexual harassment, or discrimination)
Smoking
Alcohol use
Drug use (prescription, over-the-counter, recreational)

For the adolescent, particular attention is paid to the progress of sexual development by noting stage of the secondary sex characteristics (see Table 6-2, Chap 6). Examination for scoliosis also is important for adolescents. The pelvic examination and health history provide data concerning common health problems of adolescent girls, such as dysmenorrhea, irregular menses, vaginitis, and contraception. The first pelvic examination must be conducted gently and with sensitivity. The nurse's attitudes and actions can positively affect the adolescent's emerging sexual identity.

Women in young and middle adulthood have health needs related to contraception, pregnancy, menstrual problems, vaginal and urinary infections, and neoplasms of the breasts or reproductive organs. Examinations focus on the breast and reproductive systems. In older adulthood, menopausal concerns become important, and the physical examination can focus on physiologic changes expected with declining hormonal function. Cancers of the breast, reproductive organs, and colon become a greater risk and are carefully assessed during examination.

Periodic Screening

Women are more susceptible to certain diseases at different ages. Periodic screening procedures have been recommended according to an age-related schedule. The most critical screening procedures for women include the following:

- Breast examination by health professional
- Mammography
- Pelvic examination
- Pap smear
- Hematocrit and hemoglobin

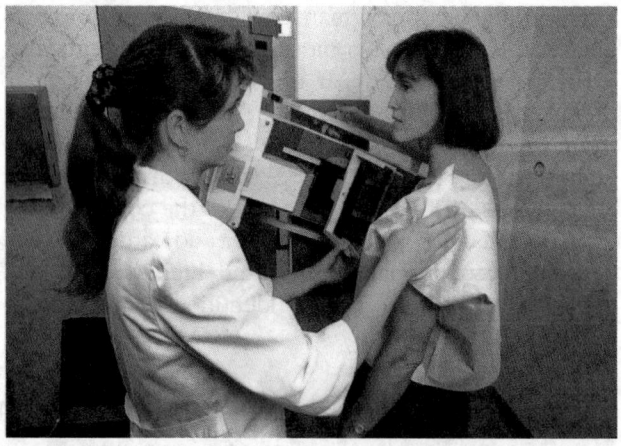

FIGURE 8–1 Women should receive periodic mammographies on an age-related schedule. Nurses can perform mammographies in the hospital, clinic, or physician's office.

- Rectal examination and stool guaiac
- Height and weight
- Lipid profile
- Blood pressure

The nurse can perform many of these procedures in the hospital, clinic, or physician's office (Fig. 8-1). Table 8-1 provides a schedule for screening tests and examinations.

Effects of Cultural Factors on Screening

Cultural values often shape definitions of health and illness. The perception of need for screening procedures is affected by culture. Specific beliefs related to sexual and reproductive behavior are powerful determinants

TABLE 8–1
Schedule for Periodic Screening for Women

Screening Test or Examination	Age of Woman (Years)			
	12 TO 19	**20 TO 49**	**50 TO 59**	**60 AND ABOVE**
Breast examination	Annual	Annual	Annual	Annual
Mammogram	*	*	Annual	Annual
Pelvic examination/Pap smear	Annual if sexually active	Annual	Annual	Annual or every 2 y
Hematocrit/hemoglobin	Every 2 y	Every 2 y	Every 5 y	Every 5 y
Rectal examination	*	*	Annual	Annual
Stool guaiac	*	*	Annual	Annual
Height and weight	Annual	Annual	Annual	Annual
Blood pressure	Every 2 y	Every 2 y	Annual	Annual
Urinalysis	*	Every 5 y	Every 5 y	Annual
Lipid panel	*	Every 2–5 y	Annual	Annual

*Not indicated unless increased risks or symptoms are present.

of acceptable screening procedures. When premarital virginity is culturally prescribed, pelvic examinations and Pap smears may be avoided due to concern about maintaining an intact hymen. Among cultures where the woman's body must remain covered, breast and pelvic examinations may be unacceptable.

Researchers have found that older women, especially African American women, do not perform BSE regularly and have lower rates of professional breast examination and mammography. Barriers to BSE include lack of confidence, embarrassment, and lack of knowledge; barriers to mammography and professional examination include lack of knowledge, cost, inconvenience, lack of symptoms, and social influences (Champion, 1991). Strategies to increase screening participation include reducing cost and increasing accessibility. Breast health education with ethnic and cultural sensitivity can increase women's knowledge. Health practitioners need to recommend **breast cancer screening** to all their clients, explaining the procedures involved and their importance. Community networks (family, friends, churches, clubs, leaders) are important in distributing information (Brown et al., 1994).

Nursing Diagnoses

Data from the assessment process provide the basis for nursing diagnoses. Common diagnoses in the area of women's healthcare might include the following:

- Altered Health Maintenance related to unhealthy lifestyle
- Knowledge Deficit about periodic screening recommendations related to lack of access to information sources
- Anxiety related to
    Cost of screening procedures
    Discomfort and dangers of screening procedures
    Fear of cancer
    Uncertainty about health conditions
- Ineffective coping related to
    Lack of knowledge
    Poor learning skills
    Inadequate support systems
    Poor self-esteem
- Health-seeking behaviors related to interest in maintaining high-level wellness

Nursing Planning and Intervention

Plans for health promotion depend on age and health needs. However, teaching and counseling in the following areas are appropriate for women of all ages (DHHS, 1992):

- Nutrition: low sodium, low fat, high complex carbohydrates, high fiber, caloric intake balanced with activity
- Activity: regular physical activity
- Substance use: alcohol in moderation (no more than two drinks per day, 3 d/wk), no smoking, no drug use, no prescription drug abuse
- Sexual practices: contraception, STD prevention
- Injury prevention: seat belts, smoke detectors, violence prevention
- Skin protection: sun screens, limited ultraviolet light exposure
- Immunizations: tetanus and diphtheria booster every 10 years
- Dental health: regular brushing and flossing, periodic dental examinations

The following teaching relates to adults 40 to 64 years old:

- Hormone replacement: prevention of osteoporosis, coronary artery disease

The following teaching relates to adults older than 65 years:

- Injury prevention: preventing falls, burns
- Immunizations: annual influenza vaccine, one-time pneumococcal vaccine

Promoting Menstrual Health

The nurse assists women to understand menstrual processes and develop healthy attitudes regarding menstruation. Women need information about normal patterns and variations, preparation for changes in menstrual patterns, support for positive attitude formation, and counseling on self-care and adaptations to special conditions.

Variations in Menstrual Patterns

Normal menstrual patterns vary greatly (Box 8-2). The menstrual cycle ranges from 24 to 35 days in women with normal hormone profiles. At either extreme, only about 1% of women have very short or very long cycles (Scott et al., 1994). Other characteristics include the following:

- Mean length of first half of the menstrual cycle (from menstruation to ovulation) is 14.8 days; the range is 9 to 23 days.
- Mean length of second half of the cycle (from ovulation to onset of menses) is 13.3 days; the range is 9 to 20 days.
- Average menstrual phase (menstrual bleeding) lasts 5 to 6 days; the range is 2 to 9 days.
- Amount of menstrual blood loss averages 50 mL; the range is 30 to 100 mL per menses.

BOX 8-2
Menstrual Patterns

Hypomenorrhea is a regular pattern of menstrual bleeding with decreased amount of flow.

Hypermenorrhea is a regular pattern of menstrual bleeding with increased amount of flow.

Dysmenorrhea is pain or discomfort experienced during menstrual flow.

Amenorrhea is absence of menstruation.

Oligomenorrhea is infrequent menstrual periods.

Polymenorrhea is too frequent menstrual periods.

- Average amount of iron lost during menses is 0.5 to 1 mg daily.

The menstrual cycle is controlled by multiple complex interactions between the endocrine, nervous, and humoral systems. These interactions involve the hypothalamic-pituitary axis, the ovaries, and the uterus and are mediated by gonadotropic neurohormones (see Chap. 6). Virtually all body cells have receptors for estradiol and progesterone (secreted by the ovaries). Widespread effects of these gonadotropins are felt in many tissues.

The immunoglobulin (Ig) content of cervical mucus and vaginal fluid varies during the menstrual cycle. Cervical mucus IgG levels are lowest at the time of ovulation, while vaginal fluid IgG levels are low from ovulation through the luteal phase. Vaginal fluid IgG is relatively high in the postmenstrual and early proliferative phases, and IgA levels are lowest in the luteal phase (Scott et al., 1994). Decreased Ig activity around ovulation may facilitate sperm survival and support conception.

Many other metabolic changes occur in association with the menstrual cycle. The basal metabolic rate (BMR) is lowest about 1 week before ovulation; it then increases 8% to 16% during the luteal phase. This produces the subtle temperature changes useful in predicting and detecting ovulation (see Chaps. 9 and 13). Plasma electrolytes (sodium, magnesium) are lower around ovulation, and colloid osmotic pressure in the plasma and interstitial fluid is significantly lower during the luteal phase. These may contribute to tissue fluid retention premenstrually.

Numerous psychocognitive changes are associated with various phases of the menstrual cycle. Information processing seems faster during the periovulatory phase (Woods et al., 1995). Women tend to have food cravings and increased eating during the luteal phase, probably as a consequence of increased BMR. A slight but significant increase in body weight occurs during the luteal phase, probably due to fluid retention. Variations in mood and feeling state are reported by many women in the late luteal or premenstrual phase. Most common are a decrease in positive affect, more reactivity, depression, lower frustration tolerance, and increased irritability.

Effects of Cigarette Smoking. Women who smoke cigarettes are relatively estrogen deficient. Smoking affects the hypothalamus, pituitary and adrenal glands, ovaries, and other glands controlling steroid production and metabolism. Nicotine decreases luteinizing hormone release directly, increases circulating cortisol levels, and inhibits adrenal enzymes. Carbon monoxide or polycyclic aromatic hydrocarbons in smoke may affect activity of enzymes involved in gonadotropin hormone metabolism and may be directly toxic to ovarian follicles (Baron et al., 1990). Serum levels of estrogen and estradiol in smokers are 50% lower than in nonsmokers. Cigarettes may decrease production of estrogens, alter estrogen metabolism, and increase circulating androgens.

Women who smoke have more symptoms related to estrogen deficiency, such as irregular menses, menopausal symptoms, and hirsutism. Infertility is more common among smokers, probably due to fallopian tube dysfunction. Smokers generally have menopause 1 to 1.5 years earlier than nonsmokers, with an apparent dose-effect relationship (earlier menopause in heavier smokers). Smokers also have an increased incidence of osteoporotic fractures, especially of the hip and spine. Bone mass decreases at a higher rate in smokers, and postmenopausal women who smoke have lower bone mineral content.

Because of the antiestrogenic effects of smoking, there are beneficial effects on some diseases caused by estrogen excess. Smokers have a decreased risk of endometrial hyperplasia and half the risk for endometrial cancer of nonsmokers. Smokers have fewer uterine fibroids, less endometriosis, and less benign breast disease. Smoking does not appear to affect risk of breast cancer (Baron et al., 1990; Yeh et al., 1989).

Menstrual Counseling

In the following ways, nurses can promote healthy adaptation to the menstrual experience:

- Providing accurate information about menstruation and menarche
- Correcting misunderstandings, myths, and exaggerations
- Acknowledging stress, fear, or embarrassment about menstruation
- Helping adolescents develop effective coping with practical needs, menstrual self-care, and feelings

- Encouraging positive attitudes toward menstruation as an expression of feminine identity and a normal, healthy process
- Validating the adolescent's realistic concerns about hassles, messiness, interference with activities, and discomforts associated with menstruation (see Client Education: Menstrual Self-Care).

Breast Cancer Screening

Breast Self-examination

Women should perform BSE for early detection of minimal breast lesions. Every nurse should be well versed in teaching BSE. This is a professional service nurses can offer clients in a variety of settings. BSE is usually taught initially at an adolescent health examination and should be reviewed and reinforced every 2 to 3 years. It is recommended that women perform BSE every month about 1 week after their menses. Many women practice BSE less often or avoid it due to fear, confusion about technique, or embarrassment. The nurse can encourage BSE practice by reviewing examination technique, using breast models and return demonstration, and reinforcing the woman's confidence in her BSE ability. Positive attitudes, social influences, and stated intention to perform BSE have been found to correlate well with actual BSE performance (Lierman et al., 1990).

The American Cancer Society's approach to teaching BSE is shown in the Client Education: Breast Self-Examination Technique.

Mammography

Mammography is an important screening and diagnostic procedure for breast conditions. More than 90% of breast cancers can be detected by mammography; of these lesions, between 20% and 50% can be found only by mammography. Breast examination by health professionals can detect about one-third of minimal cancers; mammography finds smaller cancers earlier with less metastases to lymph nodes (Cooper, 1989).

The American Cancer Society recommends annual mammograms for all women older than 50 years, combined with annual breast examination by a health professional and monthly BSE (American Cancer Society, 1994). Women with risk factors for breast cancer (Box 8-3) should have mammograms more frequently.

Baseline mammography for women 30 to 49 years old has not been found to save lives. Although evidence is clear that mammograms in women older than 50 years save lives, it appears that women in their 40s do not benefit from regular mammograms in terms of prolongation of life. This may be because younger breasts are denser, making mammograms less accurate.

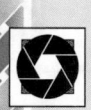

CLIENT EDUCATION
Menstrual Self-Care

Tampons and Pads

Absorbent tampons of many sizes and shapes are available. Most have disposable applicators for ease of insertion. Tampons with higher absorbency should be worn during heavy flow days. When flow is light, thinner or less absorbent tampons or minipads are better. Superabsorbent tampons worn during light flow can absorb too much vaginal moisture, leaving the walls dry and more susceptible to injury. Tampons are too absorbent if they are difficult to pull out or shred when being removed. When leakage is a concern, tampons that expand in width are helpful. Tampons with deodorants should be avoided because they can cause rashes or allergic reactions.

Pads (sanitary napkins) come with adhesive strips and in various shapes, lengths, and thicknesses (minipads to maxipads). Some women prefer pads throughout menstruation; others use them when flow is light. For extremely heavy flow, women may use a tampon and pad together. Wearing tampons during the day and pads at night reduces the risk of vaginal irritation. When the woman is concerned about toxic shock syndrome, pads are preferable. Deodorized pads are available, but they may cause skin irritation, a rash, or allergies.

Douches and Vaginal Sprays

Many products are available for "feminine hygiene" that encourage women to control odor and promote cleanliness. Others are to enhance sexual pleasure. Menstrual fluid usually has very little odor until it contacts bacteria on the skin or in the air. Daily bathing or showering is adequate to control this odor. Douching is unnecessary because the vagina cleans itself unless infection is present. Douches wash off normal mucus and vaginal flora that are protective, making the vagina more susceptible to infection. Perfumed or deodorized douches can cause irritation and allergic reactions. Douching is especially risky during menstruation, when the cervical os is slightly more open and there is danger of introducing foreign matter and bacteria into the endometrial cavity.

Vaginal sprays can cause irritation, burning, itching, rashes, infections, allergic reactions, and increased vaginal discharge. Unless part of sexual enhancement, there is little reason to use them. Normal bathing or showering keeps the vulva and vagina clean and free of problematic odor.

Breast cancer in younger women usually is more aggressive, contributing to lower survival statistics. Mammograms in women younger than 50 years are more likely to result in false-positives, leading to unnecessary biopsies, expense, and emotional upset (UC Berkeley Wellness Letter, 1994).

CLIENT EDUCATION
Breast Self-Examination Technique

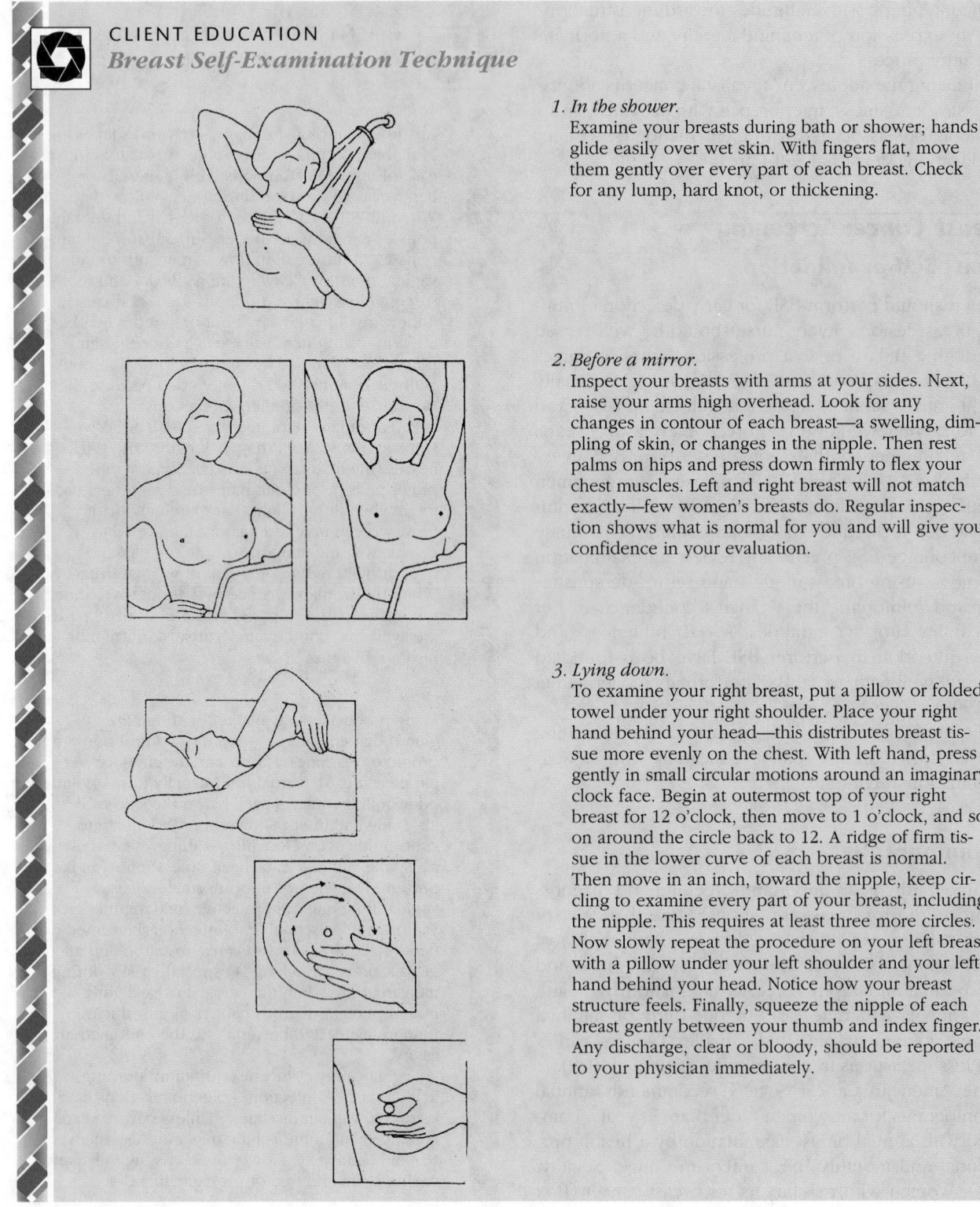

1. *In the shower.*
Examine your breasts during bath or shower; hands glide easily over wet skin. With fingers flat, move them gently over every part of each breast. Check for any lump, hard knot, or thickening.

2. *Before a mirror.*
Inspect your breasts with arms at your sides. Next, raise your arms high overhead. Look for any changes in contour of each breast—a swelling, dimpling of skin, or changes in the nipple. Then rest palms on hips and press down firmly to flex your chest muscles. Left and right breast will not match exactly—few women's breasts do. Regular inspection shows what is normal for you and will give you confidence in your evaluation.

3. *Lying down.*
To examine your right breast, put a pillow or folded towel under your right shoulder. Place your right hand behind your head—this distributes breast tissue more evenly on the chest. With left hand, press gently in small circular motions around an imaginary clock face. Begin at outermost top of your right breast for 12 o'clock, then move to 1 o'clock, and so on around the circle back to 12. A ridge of firm tissue in the lower curve of each breast is normal. Then move in an inch, toward the nipple, keep circling to examine every part of your breast, including the nipple. This requires at least three more circles. Now slowly repeat the procedure on your left breast with a pillow under your left shoulder and your left hand behind your head. Notice how your breast structure feels. Finally, squeeze the nipple of each breast gently between your thumb and index finger. Any discharge, clear or bloody, should be reported to your physician immediately.

Breast Examination by a Health Professional

An annual professional breast examination is usually included when women have their annual Pap smear. Not all breast lesions can be detected by mammography, and the nurse can assess the presence of suspi-

cious tissue. Although professional breast examinations are clearly necessary beginning at 40 years when the risk of breast cancer starts to increase, most women benefit from these examinations during their 20s and 30s. The health professional can reinforce BSE practice, review technique, reassure women who are confused about breast findings, and detect lesions that

BOX 8-3
Risk Factors for Gynecologic Cancer

Breast Cancer

Older than 40 years

White

Living in cold climate, western hemisphere

Unmarried

Higher socioeconomic status

Nulliparous or first pregnancy after 35 years

Family history of breast cancer (grandmother, mother, sister, daughter)

Previous breast cancer or fibrocystic breast disease

Early menarche (before age 12)

Late menopause (more than 30 years after menarche or after age 50)

Diet high in fat and protein, low in selenium (possible risk)

Other malignancies, lowered immunocompetency

Cervical Cancer

Multiple sexual partners

Beginning sexual contact before age 20

First pregnancy at an early age

High parity

Intercourse with men who have had venereal disease or prostatic cancer

History of sexually transmitted disease (herpes, trichomoniasis, chlamydia, genital warts, syphilis)

Ovarian Cancer

Delayed onset of childbearing

Low parity

Infertility

Nulliparity

Several spontaneous abortions

Family history of ovarian cancer

White of European or North American origin

Endometrial Cancer

White, middle class

Irregular menses

Infertility

Late menopause

Obesity, hypertension, and diabetes mellitus

Personal or family history of other cancers

History of atypical endometrial hyperplasia

Postmenopausal bleeding

---

need further diagnostic testing (see Client Teaching Guidelines: Common Questions About Mammograms).

Cervical Cancer Screening

Women of all ages are concerned about cervical cancer. It is the second most frequent cancer in women (after breast cancer); about 2% of women will develop cervical cancer before they are 80 years old. The death rate from cervical cancer has fallen steadily in the last 40 years, with most cases diagnosed as carcinoma in situ (CIS) because of **cervical cancer screening** through the Pap smear. The average age at diagnosis of CIS is 35 years; for invasive disease, it is 45 years. Women in their teens and early 20s are increasingly diagnosed in both stages of disease. Cervical cancer is progressive, with most untreated clients developing invasive disease within 5 to 9 years after CIS.

Women are at increased risk for cervical cancer in the following situations:

- They have multiple sexual partners.
- They begin sexual activity before 20 years.
- They have their first pregnancy at an early age.
- They have high parity.

- They have male partners with venereal disease or prostatic cancer.
- They have STDs.

All types of cervical dysplasia, from moderate to CIS, may be considered part of the same process called cervical intraepithelial neoplasia (CIN). Histologically, the changes in tissue involve the same processes but are a matter of degree. When normal squamous metaplasia proceeds to atypical changes, the cervical epithelium may then develop varying degrees of dysplasia (Berman, 1985).

Papanicolaou Smear Screening

The American College of Obstetricians and Gynecologists and the American Cancer Society recommend Pap smear screening intervals of 1 to 3 years (American College of Obstetricians and Gynecologists, 1989). There is greater risk for invasive cervical cancer when Pap smear screening intervals are 3 to 4 years or greater. Women who have Pap smears every 3 years are at three times the risk of developing squamous cell cervical cancer than those who have Pap smears every 1 to 2 years. Having four or more lifetime sexual part-

CLIENT TEACHING GUIDELINES
Common Questions About Mammograms

- *Does breast cancer run in families?*
  Heredity is not a factor in the majority of breast cancers. Probably only 5% to 10% of breast cancers can be linked to family history. The main risk for breast cancer is simply growing old. Most women who develop breast cancer have no identifiable risk factors except their age.
- *Is there a gene for breast cancer?*
  A gene has been discovered that may transmit susceptibility to breast and ovarian cancer in some families. Inherited breast cancer is a rare disease. It will be years before there is a reliable test for this susceptibility.
- *Are x-rays for mammograms dangerous?*
  Very low doses of radiation are delivered by the new, dedicated mammography machines (0.7–0.22 rad). Radiology centers are required to meet the Mammography Quality Standards Act for minimal radiation exposure. The possibility that mammograms could promote breast cancer is very remote.
- *Are mammograms painful?*
  You may feel pressure or pinching during a mammogram, because the breast must be compressed between plates for the x-ray. Most women report temporary discomfort. If your breasts are tender before your period, schedule the mammogram for just afterward.
- *Are mammograms really necessary after a few negative ones?*
  The older you are, the greater your risk for breast cancer. Data from studies show that annual mammograms for women older than 50 years save lives. Putting mammograms off could delay discovery of breast cancer, allowing the disease to progress. The earlier a malignancy is discovered, the better your chances to overcome it.

ners also puts women at greater risk (Shy et al., 1989; Boyce et al., 1990).

About 50% of women receive an annual Pap smear, and 30% have Paps at 3-year intervals or greater. Women may over-report their last screening interval, because obtaining Pap smears is socially acceptable and expected behavior. Recommending a 3-year interval for Pap screening appears to increase the woman's risk for more advanced cervical cancer. Pap smear screening should occur every 1 to 2 years, unless risk factors are present.

The risk of cervical cancer is increased in lower socioeconomic groups, African Americans, elderly women who have not been screened, and more sexually active women. Women exposed to diethylstilbestrol in utero also have increased risk and should have a Pap smear every 6 months (Clay, 1990).

Nursing Responsibilities

Nurses must be able to identify women at increased risk for cervical cancer. Many nurses have the skills to perform vaginal examinations and Pap smears. Women often have no symptoms associated with CIN, and the condition usually is detected with a routine Pap smear. Vaginal infections or cervicitis may alter cell characteristics due to inflammation. Usually the infection is treated and the Pap smear repeated in 3 months.

A complete pelvic examination is done, including speculum examination, bimanual examination, and collection of specimens. Before taking the Pap smear, the cervix is inspected and its condition noted. Findings may include nabothian cysts, ectropion, erosion, cervicitis, polyps, leukoplakia, or neoplasia (Fig. 8-2).

Nurses have increasing responsibility for Pap smear screening, especially nurse practitioners and clinical specialists (see Nursing Procedure 8-1: Taking a Pap

PROCEDURE 8–1
Taking a Pap Smear

The Pap smear is taken using a cotton-tipped applicator or cytobrush and a spatula (wooden or plastic). The cervix is wiped gently only if there is excessive mucus. Lubricating jelly should not be used because it distorts the cell sample; water is used to aid speculum insertion. Samples are taken from the endocervical canal with the cotton-tipped applicator, which may be saturated with saline, or the cytobrush. The applicator is placed high in the cervix, rotated a few times, then withdrawn and applied to a slide by gentle rolling. The spatula, with the long tip placed into the cervical os, is used to scrape the ectocervix. The material is spread thinly on a slide. Slides are sprayed or immersed im-

mediately in a fixative; air drying can distort cells. The presence of inflammation, infection, or other conditions (such as hormone therapy) should be noted on the Pap request form.

Vaginal pool specimens are recommended for women older than 50 years to screen for endometrial cancer. Specimens may be taken for microscopic examination by saline or potassium hydrochloride mounts or cultures done for *Chlamydia* or gonorrhea as indicated. With exposure to diethylstilbestrol, samples are obtained with a spatula by scraping the vaginal walls, placing on a slide, and fixing as above.

Pap smear classifications are shown in Box 8-4.

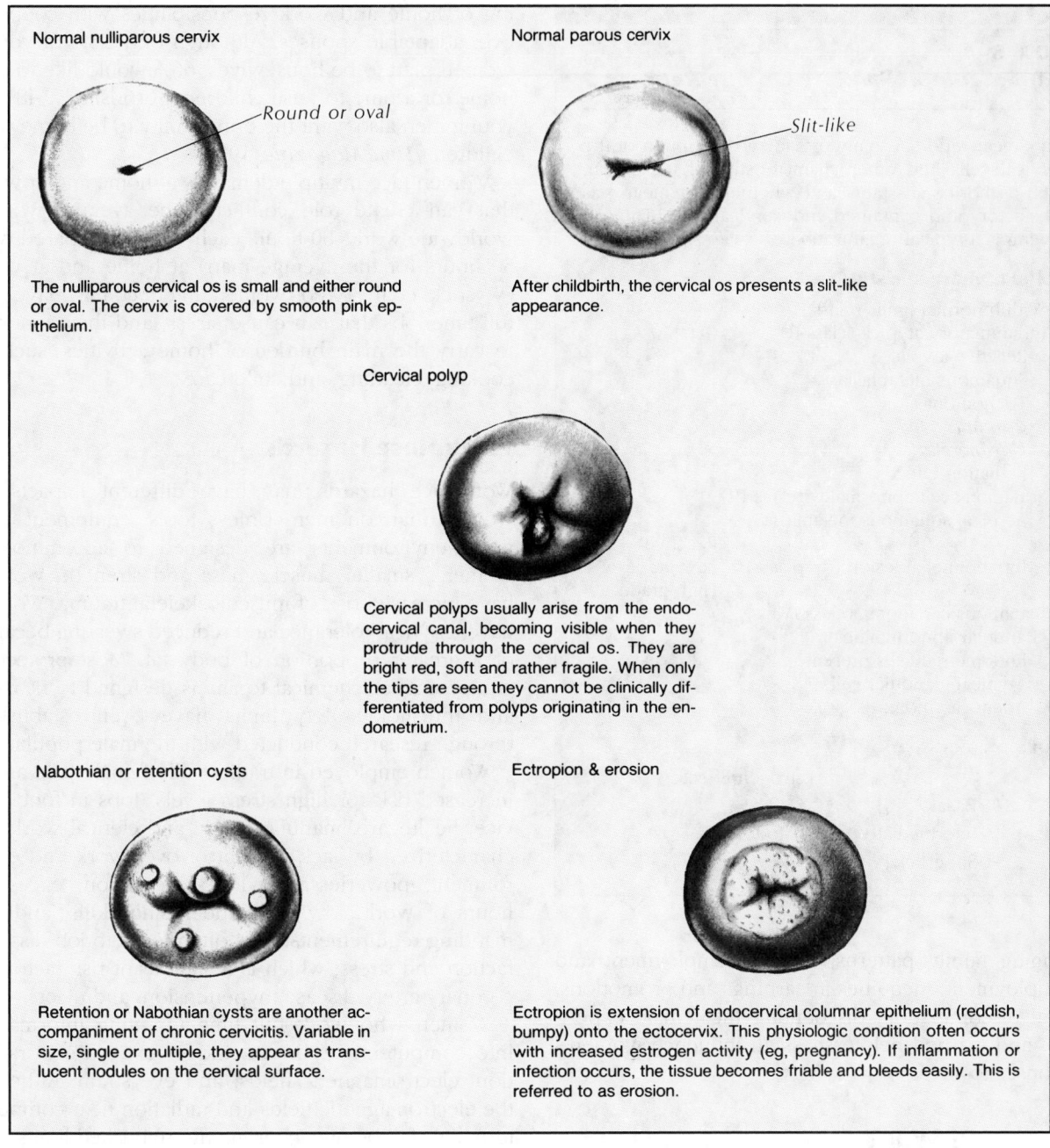

Normal nulliparous cervix

Round or oval

The nulliparous cervical os is small and either round or oval. The cervix is covered by smooth pink epithelium.

Normal parous cervix

Slit-like

After childbirth, the cervical os presents a slit-like appearance.

Cervical polyp

Cervical polyps usually arise from the endocervical canal, becoming visible when they protrude through the cervical os. They are bright red, soft and rather fragile. When only the tips are seen they cannot be clinically differentiated from polyps originating in the endometrium.

Nabothian or retention cysts

Retention or Nabothian cysts are another accompaniment of chronic cervicitis. Variable in size, single or multiple, they appear as translucent nodules on the cervical surface.

Ectropion & erosion

Ectropion is extension of endocervical columnar epithelium (reddish, bumpy) onto the ectocervix. This physiologic condition often occurs with increased estrogen activity (eg, pregnancy). If inflammation or infection occurs, the tissue becomes friable and bleeds easily. This is referred to as erosion.

FIGURE 8–2 Common cervical conditions.

Smear). Box 8-4 gives an example of a typical Pap smear report.

Women and Stress

Stress is an unavoidable part of life. The body's response to stress includes physical, mental, emotional, and chemical reactions. Events that frighten, excite, confuse, endanger, or irritate can create stress. A certain amount of stress is natural and probably necessary for life, but continuous stress at a sufficiently high level can have adverse effects on health.

Biologic factors lead to characteristic patterns and rates of illness, longevity, and causes of death. Although women are more resistant to infectious and degenerative disease and to major illness (eg, cancer, heart disease), they do have more acute, limited conditions than men. Women seek care earlier, more often, and for less serious problems than do men.

Research indicates that higher levels of symptoms are experienced by people with oppressive life conditions, such as financial insecurity, abusive families, unemployment, and social isolation. Women, minorities, and the poor with these conditions have more physical and emotional health problems (Hafner et al., 1992).

BOX 8-4
Papanicolaou Smear Cytology Reports

Pap smear reports usually provide a description of the cervical cells and other characteristics of the smear, such as hormonal status and whether the smear was satisfactory and contained endocervical cells. The following is a typical organization of a Pap smear report:

Cellular characteristics

- Within normal limits (class I)
- Inflammatory atypica (class II)
  Reactive atypia
  Squamous metaplasia
  Trichomonas
  Candida
  Gardnerella
  Radiation effect
- Squamous cell abnormality (class III)
  Atypical squamous metaplasia

		Reactive
Intraepithelial lesion (dysplasia)		Low grade
		High grade

- Squamous carcinoma (class IV)
- Glandular abnormalities
  Endometrial cells present
  Atypical glandular cells
  Adenocarcinoma

Hormonal evaluation

	Estrogen Effect
_____ % Basal	High
_____ % Intermediate	Moderate
_____ % Superficial	Low

Changing family patterns, divorce, employment and unemployment, inequities in earnings and promotions, sexual discrimination, discounting the female experience, and learned helplessness all influence women's responses to stress.

Stress and Work

The number of women in the work force has increased dramatically. Nearly one-half of all workers are women, and more than 90% of women work for at least some period during their lives. Women workers earn less than men with the same education, although about half are responsible for financially maintaining their families.

While the composition of the labor force continues to change (with women and minority men and immigrants accounting for a large portion of new or returning workers), the needs, work styles, and career goals of this labor force also have changed. Young women now beginning careers want recognition of family and parenting needs, flexible work patterns, the ability to advance without "workaholism," and successful blend-

ing of home and work responsibilities with cooperative, adaptable spouses. Although only 25% of young women plan to be housewives, 66% would like to stay home for a time to raise children. Surprisingly, 48% of young men also want the opportunity to be home with children (*Time Magazine*, 1990).

Women face multiple demands at home and at work that can create role conflicts. The average woman worldwide works 80 hours each week (compared with 50 hours for the average man) at home and at work (Wysocki et al., 1983). Women, in effect, may have two full-time jobs that can cause stress, and they continue to carry the main burden of home activities, such as cooking, cleaning, and child care.

Workplace Hazards

Workplace hazards may have different impacts on women than on men. Unless tools, equipment, and work environments are designed to accommodate women's smaller muscle mass and strength, women have increased risk of musculoskeletal trauma. Women have less heat tolerance and reduced sweating because of a greater proportion of body fat. Most protective equipment for chemical toxins is designed to fit men, and threshold safety limits have been established through research conducted with the male population.

Women employed in traditionally female jobs are at increased risk for high stress levels. Jobs in food service, healthcare, manufacturing, and clerical work are characterized by lack of control over work and environment, powerlessness, less recognition, excessive hours of work, low pay, underusing skills, and demanding requirements. This often leads to job dissatisfaction and stress, which is a significant risk factor for coronary artery disease, hypertension, and ulcers.

Women who work full time inputting information into computers may be at risk for exposure to radiation, electromagnetic fields, and eye strain. Although the electromagnetic fields and radiation near computer terminals fall below government-established limits, it is not known whether these low-level fields are biologic hazards. Glare filters can reduce eye strain but do not affect electromagnetic fields.

Nurses face significant work-related stress because of work characteristics and chemical and physical hazards. Most nurses are women (94%) and have a dual role as wage earner and homemaker. They perceive their pay as inequitable (male nurses earn 10% more than female nurses), have limited opportunities for advancement within the hospital structure, and often find their work task oriented and repetitive. Hospitals are based on authoritarian power models, and many nurses experience a lack of independent decision-making opportunities due to subtle discrimination within this male value dominated environment. Nurses, however, do not seem to have greater stress than other working women. When nurses and other female hospital employees were compared on a stress scale with other employed women, their mean scores were in the average or below-average ranges (Posner et al., 1984).

Substance Abuse

Substance abuse among women in the workplace is a growing problem. Currently about 50% of all alcoholics are women, but less than this percentage are in workplace alcoholism programs. Women use more prescription and over-the-counter drugs than men. Multiple drug use and abuse are increasing, including combining drugs and alcohol. Women are not being reached effectively by traditional identification and referral processes. Most abuse research has focused on male behavioral models rather than female models.

Increased stress levels have been associated with substance abuse. Being a woman and a parent increases stress symptoms, and working exacerbates these problems. The origins, context, and control of employed women's substance abuse differ from those of men and seem related to issues of familial responsibilities, low self-esteem, job and pay discrimination, sex-role conflicts, and stress and conflict management (Vicary et al., 1985).

Women's drinking behavior often changes with time, related to shifting roles, contexts, and circumstances. Younger women show more onset and remission of problem drinking, whereas middle-aged women have more chronic problem drinking. The strongest predictors of alcohol dependence are sexual dysfunction and depression. Other predictors of chronic drinking problems include never being married, part-time employment or unemployment, and cohabitating. Divorce, separation, or children's departure from home are more likely to follow than to precede problem drinking. The onset of problem drinking may be facilitated by long-term use of psychoactive drugs (see Chap. 34; Wilsnack et al., 1991).

Cigarette Smoking

Tobacco use by women carries great health risks. Although smoking rates have dropped substantially for men, the decline among women has been much smaller. Smoking prevalence rates among adolescent and young adult women are beginning to exceed those of men. Smoking by women poses hazards to their own long-term health and has important impacts on reproductive function and the health of children.

The health consequences of smoking can be severe, including such diseases as emphysema, hypertension, coronary artery disease, and lung cancer. The incidence of lung cancer among women is increasing. Female smokers using oral contraceptives are at greatly increased risk for heart attack, especially those older than 35 to 40 years. Smoking during pregnancy retards fetal growth and increases the rates of spontaneous abortion and perinatal mortality. Women who smoke have 50% to 150% higher risk for invasive cervical neoplasia, CIN, and other severe cervical abnormalities (Baron et al., 1990; Mayberry, 1985). As stated previously in the chapter, women who smoke are relatively estrogen deficient; menopause occurs about 1.5 years earlier in smokers, and smokers have two to three times greater risk for osteoporotic fractures of the spine and hip (Baron et al., 1990).

Nonsmokers also are harmed by second-hand smoke, because it contains higher concentrations of toxic chemicals than smoke inhaled into the lungs through a filter. Cigarette smoke is a mixture of particles and gases that contain 3,800 to 4,000 chemicals, of which more than 50 are known carcinogens. Nonsmoking women with normal Pap smears were tested for the presence of nicotine in cervical secretions. Those exposed to tobacco smoke in the home had the highest nicotine levels, with intermediate levels in women exposed only outside the home. Women with no reported exposure had very low nicotine levels (Jones et al., 1991). Even low levels of exposure to tobacco smoke can have systemic effects and may be a risk factor for cervical disease (see Research Highlight).

Nurses continue to smoke at higher rates than other professional women and physicians. About 25% of all nurses smoke, and about 50% of psychiatric and mental health nurses smoke (Charbonneau, 1985). Smoking among women has been related to work characteristics, stress, and concerns about weight. Young adult women are twice as likely as young adult men to report weight gain with smoking cessation and were much more worried about gaining weight when considering quitting. Women feel more social pressure to quit, 70% having been urged by people close to them and 30% by health providers (Pirie et al., 1991).

Nursing Assessment

Stress in women may be assessed by observation and by history taking. A person under severe stress usually manifests it by appearance and behavior: looking drawn, haggard, or poorly groomed and exhibiting a number of behavioral symptoms, such as irritation, fatigue, anxiety, nervousness, confusion, distraction, or depression. Many people express stress through physical symptoms, such as headaches, back pain, constipation or diarrhea, gastric distress, anorexia or overeating, palpitations, hyperventilation, insomnia, and increased susceptibility to infections. Stress assessment and coping strategies tools are helpful (see Assessment Tool: Stress Assessment); involving the client in self-assessment is built into most tools.

RESEARCH HIGHLIGHT

Passive Smoke Increases Nicotine Levels in Cervical Secretions

Women exposed to environmental cigarette smoke have biochemical evidence of nicotine in saliva, serum, and urine. Reports have suggested that the cervical mucus of passive smokers might contain nicotine and its metabolites. This study was designed to measure concentrations of nicotine in cervical lavages taken from cytologically normal, nonsmoking women and compare concentrations in women with passive exposure to smoke and those not exposed.

Subjects were part of a larger study of cervical neoplasia. A sample of 145 nonsmokers with normal cervical cytology on routine Pap smears were interviewed about environmental exposure to tobacco smoke inside and outside the home in the prior 24 hours, time since last exposure, number of smokers in the home and relationships, usual intensity of smoking, and products smoked. A 3 mL saline lavage of the cervix was collected, and laboratory analyses were performed without knowledge of the smoke exposure history. Nicotine was extracted from lavage samples and measured by gas chromatography-mass spectroscopy.

Women were divided into three groups: those exposed to smoke only inside their homes, those exposed only outside their homes, and those not exposed. The study population was 6.3% African American with a median age of 30 years; neither race nor age was associated with environmental tobacco smoke exposure. Nicotine levels were highest among women exposed in the home (0.8 ng/mL), intermediate in those exposed outside the home (0.4 ng/mL), and lowest in those not exposed (0.2 ng/mL). Nicotine values ranged from below the limit of detection (<0.2) to 8.2 ng/mL. No associations were found between nicotine levels and the woman's exposure to number of smokers, smoking intensity, or time of last exposure.

The cervical level of nicotine in these nonsmoking women exposed to passive smoke was lower than in cervical lavages taken from active smokers (median values 11.8 ng/mL). The elevation of nicotine levels in cervical fluid of passive smokers suggests that even low-level exposure to environmental tobacco smoke might result in systemic effects. Passive smoking should be further evaluated as a risk factor for cervical disease.

Critique: This is a well-designed study with a relatively large sample.

Nursing Implications: Nurses need to inform clients of the potential risks associated with passive exposure to environmental cigarette smoke. Women with relatively high levels of passive smoking are encouraged to have at least annual Pap smears.

Jones, C. J., Schiffman, M. H., Kurman, R. et al. (1991). Elevated nicotine levels in cervical lavages from passive smokers. *American Journal of Public Health, 81*(3), 378–379.

Substance abuse may assessed by indicators that are often subtle (Caulker-Burnett, 1994). Early indicators may include depression, dependency, low self-esteem, and learning problems. These are often followed by insomnia, anxiety, worry, inadequacy felt or expressed through poor role performance, few leisure activities, missing appointments, and evasiveness. Late indicators include disrupted social relations, severe depression, inability to work, gastritis, fractures and injuries from falls, suicidal tendencies, and isolation (Box 8-5).

The nurse might observe changes in appearance, heavy perfume or mouthwash, emphasis on somatic complaints (especially menstrually related), and concealing parts of the body (arms, legs). On physical examination, alcoholics may have spider angiomas, a tender or enlarged liver, tachycardia, hypertension, and gastric tenderness. Depending on route of administration, drug users may have tracks on arms or legs.

Smokers usually do not attempt to conceal their cigarette use. Signs that indicate heavy smoking include the smell of smoke on clothing or hair, brown discoloration of index and middle finger, discolored teeth, and thickened or ridged fingernails. Most smokers have changes in lung sounds, such as wheezing or scattered rhonchi that clear with coughing.

Nursing Diagnoses

Possible nursing diagnoses related to stress include the following:

- Ineffective Individual Coping related to
    Inadequate resources (physical, psychological, behavioral)
    Maturational factors (marriage, childbearing, aging)
    Situational factors (work environment, urban living)
    Inadequate psychological resources (poor self-esteem, helplessness, lack of motivation)
- Sleep Pattern Disturbance
- Altered Thought Processes
- Anxiety; Fear; Powerlessness
- Self Esteem Disturbance
- Impaired Communication
- Altered Parenting

Planning and Intervention

Nursing care for the woman under severe stress focuses on assisting her to identify and interpret her stressors and responses to them. The goal is to reduce or reinterpret stress so it becomes possible for the woman to cope effectively. Using counseling and

ASSESSMENT TOOL
Stress Assessment

I. Personal Information
   Age
   Children
   Living arrangements
   Health state
   Financial state

II. Stressors
   Life events
      Relationship change
      Career change
      Illness/death
      Personal illness
      Work problems
      Financial problems
      Family problems
      Legal problems
      Health/body changes
      Psychological stress
   Life conditions
      Living space
      Family relations
      Employment/career
      Financial state
      Health state
      Recreation/activities
      Spiritual values
   Coping strategies
      Eat/drink more/less
      Use alcohol or other drugs
      Sleep more/less
      Exercise more/less
      Use relaxation technique
      Smoke more
      Avoid problem/pretend not there
      Clarify/set goals
      Time management/efficiency
      Make changes in job, relations
      Pray, meditate, seek spiritual help
      Analyze/understand conflicts
      Talk with spouse, friends
      More recreation/activities
      Block out feelings
      Desensitize fears, aversions
      Seek new relations
      Enter therapy/support group
      Other

Marital status
Relatives/friends
Work
Limitations/disabilities

Events that have been experienced in the last 12 months. How important (rank: little to great)

Check if happened	How important
_____	_____
_____	_____
_____	_____
_____	_____
_____	_____
_____	_____
_____	_____
_____	_____
_____	_____
_____	_____

Reasonably consistent patterns in life: Describe usual situation related to each of these that is important.

Usual ways used to cope with stress. Describe how well these work.

BOX 8–5
Red Flags for Substance Abuse

- Frequent missed appointments
- Frequent requests for written excuses from work
- Repeated lost prescriptions (tranquilizers, pain medicine)
- Doctor hopping; having prescriptions from several doctors
- Depressed, agitated appearance
- Recurrent insomnia, nervousness, pain
- Frequent emergency room visits for injuries

CLIENT TEACHING GUIDELINES
Approaches to Stress Reduction

Progressive relaxation uses tensing and relaxing of muscle groups progressively throughout the body to attain a state of deep relaxation. Beginning in a sitting or lying position, the woman takes a few deep breaths, then progressively tenses and relaxes toes, feet, calves, knees, thighs, buttocks, stomach, lower back, chest, upper back, shoulders, arms and hands, neck, face, eyes, and forehead. Next, the entire body is tensed and relaxed, followed by a few deep breaths and a period of stillness.

Guided imagery has the client focus on images that create a relaxed state. Sitting or lying in a comfortable position, the woman closes her eyes and takes several deep breaths. Then she creates a mental image of a scene that she finds satisfying and peaceful, such as a beach, stream, meadow, mountain, or forest. She imagines smells, sounds, textures, colors, and any other aspects of the situation that produce a good feeling. This image may be written, polished, or put on audiotape. It is then played back for relaxation.

Meditation is an approach to quiet the mind and focus on the deep inner silence or peace. A quiet place is needed, and the woman sits comfortably. She may select a word or sound to chant, a symbol or object to gaze at, or music to focus the mind. Meditation is continued for 15 to 20 minutes, with a passive attitude that accepts thoughts and distractions, then gently refocuses attention on the meditation object.

Affirmation uses repeated phrases that affirm a desired attitude, goal, or quality. Many are available in inspirational books, including short prayers. The woman may want to write her own affirmation and keep it where she will see it frequently. A routine is developed in which the affirmation is repeated mentally at set times, such as when awakening, at stop lights, during breaks at work, and at bedtime. An example might be: "I am calm and peaceful within. All good things come to me."

---

teaching skills, the nurse may assist the client in any of these areas: problem solving, decision making, exploring alternative behaviors and strategies, drawing on other internal and external resources, analyzing usual ways of coping, assessing what works and what does not, and learning specific stress reduction techniques.

In the work setting, nurses can identify and evaluate stressors affecting women and develop recommendations or programs for stress management. Some approaches could be flexible work time, child care programs, educational campaigns, stress-reduction workshops, health screening and promotion, time management, conflict management, family problem solving, personal growth groups, fitness programs, stop-smoking programs, assertiveness training, and support groups. When serious problems are identified, such as alcohol or drug abuse, referrals to substance abuse programs are indicated. Psychotherapy or other emotional counseling can be recommended for severe emotional problems.

Many approaches to stress reduction can be used. To obtain maximum benefit, these techniques should be used regularly (see Client Teaching Guidelines: Approaches to Stress Reduction).

Evaluation

The first indication of positive action occurs when the woman identifies stressors and her responses to them. She then chooses an approach and follows the techniques to reduce her stress. Behavior and attitude changes are observed; the woman may report better sleep, thinking more clearly, increased parenting abilities, feelings of empowerment, and decreased anxieties and fears.

Women and Depression

Depression is a disturbance of mood accompanied by changes in activity levels. Nearly 10% of primary care patients experience a major depression, with another 20% to 30% having milder anxiety or depression disorders (Blumenreich, 1993). Most patients with depression are women. Many depressed patients seek care for fatigue, lack of energy, or pain. Depression is a common reaction to stress, illness, and disability. The following are symptoms of depression:

- Insomnia or hypersomnia
- Loss of interest or pleasure in activities
- Feeling sad, blue, down (persistent)
- Feeling worthless, guilty, hopeless, helpless
- Fatigue and loss of energy
- Difficulty concentrating, remembering or making decisions
- Frequent or unexplainable crying spells
- Chronic pain with no obvious cause

- Significant weight loss or gain (>5%)
- Irritability, agitation, or decreased activity
- Thoughts about dying or suicide

Clinical depression, even when milder, is associated with poor physical health and disturbed social and role functioning (Johnson et al., 1992). Risk factors are summarized in Box 8-6. The ability to perform daily tasks is reduced, with more days of disability, which disrupts family and job responsibilities. The person with depression suffers mental, emotional, and physical anguish. Clinical depression often does not resolve spontaneously but requires medical treatment. The greatest consequence of untreated depression is suicide.

Seasonal affective disorder (SAD) is a condition in which mood is affected by changes in season. Symptoms occur during the winter and include mood swings, weight change, low energy, longer time sleeping, and decreased social life. Exposure to ambient light is the critical factor; the farther north from the equator, the greater the prevalence of SAD symptoms. Fluorescent light therapy is the basic treatment, which increases ambient light during the winter season and reduces symptoms (Rosenthal, 1993).

Anxiety or depressive disorders are defined by the American Psychiatric Association and are described briefly in Box 8-7 (American Psychiatric Association, 1994). The role of neurotransmitters, especially serotonin, in affective disorders is well established (Aguglia et al., 1993). Depressed patients have decreased plasma tryptophan, serotonergic function abnormalities, and lower levels of brain serotonin (Risch et al., 1992). Because of these alterations in brain chemistry, antidepressant medications are effective in relieving symptoms and improving mood. Commonly used medications include tricyclics (amitriptyline [Elavil], trazodone [Desyrel], bupropion [Wellbutrin]), selective serotonin reuptake inhibitors (fluoxetine [Prozac], sertraline [Zoloft]), and monoamine oxidase inhibitors (phenlyzine [Nardil], tranylcypromine [Parnate]; American Psychiatric Association, 1993).

Menopause

Approximately 90% of women have regular menstrual cycles until they are 40 years old, but only 10% have regular cycles continuing to 50 years (Nesse, 1989). **Menopause**, defined as the age of the last menstrual period, occurs at the average age of 50 years, with a range usually between 48 and 52 years. Decline in function of the hypothalamic-pituitary-ovarian system occurs for approximately 10 years but is most marked during the 1 to 2 years before cessation of menses. The physiology of menopause is discussed in Chapter 6.

Symptoms

The most common symptoms during the perimenopausal period follow:

- Hot flashes
- Insomnia
- Increased premenstrual tension
- Irritability and mood lability
- Vaginal mucosal thinning with decreased lubrication

Approximately 30% to 40% of women find their lives significantly disrupted by these symptoms (Vliet et al., 1991). Decreased estrogen and vasomotor instability produce rapid dilation or constriction of vasculature, resulting in sudden sensations of heat, often accompanied by sweating and flushed skin. Some women have brief experiences of being cold all over. Decreased estrogen produces atrophic changes of the labia and vaginal mucosa, often resulting in dryness and irritation, making intercourse uncomfortable.

Hormonal Influence

Brain receptors respond to circulating hormones, which influence release of neurotransmitters. Estrogen and progesterone have direct effects on the neurotransmitters (norepinephrine, serotonin, dopamine, acetylcholine) that regulate mood, appetite, sleep, cognition, behavior, and pain perception. Estrogens increase levels of tryptophan, the precursor for serotonin synthesis. Decreased serotonin synthesis and increased metabolic breakdown are seen in the aging process. Reduced serotonin levels are associated with depression, irritability, anxiety, sleep disturbance, and greater pain sensitivity. Endorphin levels also are affected by estrogen and progesterone; declining endorphins caused by decreases in these hormones may precipi-

---

BOX 8-6
Risk Factors for Depression

Prior episodes of depression
Family history of major depressive or bipolar disorder
Personal or family history of suicide attempt
Stressful life events
Lack of social supports
Postpartum period
Current substance abuse
Personal history of sexual abuse
Younger than 40 years when symptoms began
Symptoms of fatigue, chronic pain, sadness, irritability

BOX 8-7
Criteria for Anxiety or Depression Disorders

Major Depressive Disorder

One or more major depressive episodes can be distinguished from the person's usual functioning. Depressed mood exists most of the day, nearly every day, and markedly diminished interest or pleasure in almost all activities. At least four other symptoms of depression must be present. Symptoms must persist for at least two weeks.

Bipolar Illness (Manic-Depression)

Mood cycles occur with discrete episodes of depression and mania. In between episodes, the person may feel perfectly normal. Mania is a persistently elevated mood with less need for sleep, pressured talking, distractibility, flight of ideas, grandiosity, insistent goal-directed activity, agitation, or excesses of pleasurable activities.

Dysthymia

Chronic mild depressive syndrome is present for at least 2 years, with several symptoms of depression. The person may have superimposed major depression (double depression). Dysthymia makes recovery from major depression less likely.

Seasonal Affective Disorder

Seasonal pattern of major depressive episodes occurs with regular temporal relationship between onset and remission of symptoms and particular periods of the year (usually winter in the northern hemisphere).

Generalized Anxiety Disorder

Excessive or unrealistic worry and anxiety about a number of life circumstances occurs for 6 months or more, during which the person is bothered more days than not by these concerns. Three or more of the following six symptoms must be present (with at least some symptoms present more days than not): muscle tension, restlessness, fatigue, difficulty concentrating, irritability, or sleep disturbance.

Panic disorder

Recurrent, unexpected panic attacks occur. In addition, the attacks are followed by at least 1 month of extreme fearfulness of having another attack, worry about implications or consequences of the attack, or significant change in behavior related to the attacks. The panic attack is characterized by a period of intense fear or discomfort, in which four of the following symptoms are present:

- Palpitations, pounding heart, accelerated heart rate
- Sweating
- Trembling or shaking
- Sensations of shortness of breath or smothering
- Feeling of choking
- Chest pain or discomfort
- Nausea or abdominal distress
- Feeling dizzy, unsteady, lightheaded, or faint
- Feelings of unreality or being detached from oneself
- Feelings of losing control or going crazy
- Fear of dying
- Numbness or tingling sensations
- Chills or hot flashes

Source: American Psychiatric Association. (1994). *Diagnostic and Statistical Manual of Mental Disorders, fourth edition (DSM-IV)*. Washington, DC: APA.

---

tate onset of perimenopausal depression and mood changes (Golden et al., 1990; Vliet et al., 1991). Sleep difficulties, mood symptoms, and memory problems may lead to difficulty in coping with psychological stressors in women who previously coped effectively (Vliet et al., 1991; Sarrel, 1989).

Cultural Influence

Cultural perspectives influence women's responses to menopause. As the childbearing years end, women face developmental transitions and enter a new phase of life. In cultures that value youth and reproductive capacity, menopause signifies loss of a socially valued status, which may contribute to depressive symptoms. In cultures where older women have heightened social status (eg, Native American), menopause is not associated with negative reactions. When menopause is viewed as a natural process and not a disease or deficiency state, most women pass through this transition with little difficulty (McCrea, 1983; Kaufert, 1982). Diet and lifestyle affect perimenopausal physiologic changes and symptoms. Japanese women, eating vegetarian diets with soy-based products, rarely have hot flashes. Soy converts to usable estrogens. Women with plant-based diets also have less risk of osteoporosis, while those with high protein diets have greater risk (Heaney, 1993; Recker et al., 1992).

Treatment

Hormone replacement therapy (HRT), discussed later in this chapter, has become the treatment of choice for many menopausal women. However, HRT is contraindicated in some women, and other women may not want to take hormones. Box 8-8 describes alternative therapies for menopause symptoms. In addition, women should be encouraged to eat a healthy diet, get regular exercise, and get plenty of sleep to ease the symptoms of menopause.

Vitamin E: Relieves hot flashes, leg cramps, fatigue
   Dose: 400–800 IU daily
   Food sources: spinach, wheat germ, vegetable oils, peanuts, soy products
Bellergal-S: Relieves hot flashes, sweats, irritability, insomnia, restlessness
   Dose: 1 tablet twice daily
   Contains phenobarbital, ergotamine tartrate, belladonna
   Side effects: sedation, dry mouth, palpitations, tachycardia, urinary retention, blurred vision
   Caution: May be addicting
   Contraindications: hypertension, peripheral vascular disease, coronary artery disease, impaired renal or hepatic function, glaucoma, sepsis
Herbal therapies: Relieves hot flashes, sweats, insomnia, irritability, fatigue
   Oriental herbs: Dong quai, Ginseng
   American herbs: Black cohosh, licorice, dandelion, gentian
   Shephard's purse, elder flower, yarrow
   Other plants: sarsaparilla, wild cherry, yucca, pussywillow, mistletoe, hawthorne, passion flower

Osteopenia and Osteoporosis

With aging, there is a generalized and progressive loss of both trabecular (osseous tissue) and cortical (outer layer) bone:

- **Osteopenia** refers to a condition in which bone mass is substantially lower than the mean level of peak bone mass.
- **Osteoporosis** is an absolute decrease in the amount of bone to a level below that required for mechanical support.

The first sign of osteoporosis often is a fracture with little or no trauma. About 1.5 million fractures are caused by osteoporosis each year in the United States. The lifetime risk for hip fractures in white women is 15%, and about one-third of women older than 65 years will have a vertebral fracture. Hip fractures carry a poor prognosis, leading to death in 12% to 20% of cases and permanent disability in about 75% (Fig. 8-3; Riggs, 1991; Watts, 1991).

Physiology of Bone Growth/Loss

To understand how osteoporosis occurs, it may be helpful to review briefly the three stages of bone mass change over the life span:

1. The first stage is building of bone, which leads to attainment of peak bone mass. After closure of the growth plate at about 20 years, radial growth continues for another 10 to 15 years. Most of the bone mass is acquired by 20 to 30 years.
2. The second stage consists of a slow, age-dependent loss of bone. It begins around 40 years for cortical bone and 45 to 50 years for trabecular bone. This process continues into extreme old age and is probably similar in women and men.
3. In women, a third stage of transient accelerated postmenopausal bone loss is due to decreased estrogen. This is superimposed on the slow stage of bone loss and results in disproportionately more trabecular bone than cortical bone loss.

During the last two stages, it is estimated that the slow phase produces a loss of 25% each from trabecular and cortical bone, and the accelerated phase causes women to lose an additional 10% from trabecular and 25% from cortical components. Women can lose 35% of their cortical bone and 50% of their trabecular bone during a lifetime; men lose about two-thirds these amounts (Watts, 1991; Riggs et al., 1986).

Bone remodeling is a continuous process, in which osteoblasts build bone and osteoclasts resorb it under the control of calcitriol (vitamin D), calcitonin, parathyroid hormone, and bone-produced proteins. The entire cycle takes 90 days, with about 5% of bone surface being remodeled at any given time. During age-related bone loss, there is a remodeling imbalance with an increase in resorption over formation. This results in increased bone turnover, leading to bone loss. In the slow, age-dependent stage, the trabeculae and bone cortex gradually thin. In the accelerated, postmenopausal stage, structural trabeculae and greater trabecular perforation are lost (Riggs, 1991; Lufkin et al., 1989).

Risk Factors for Osteoporosis

The two types of osteoporosis and risk factors for osteopenia and osteoporosis are summarized in Boxes 8-9 and 8-10. Some risk factors are not changeable (eg, sex, race, age, small frame, low body weight). Several changeable risk factors, such as cigarette smoking, heavy alcohol use, high-protein diet, and sedentary lifestyle, also are risk factors for other diseases. Two specific risk factors are menopause and low-calcium diet. Women at particularly high risk for bone fragility are thin, small-framed white women who are sedentary, smoke, and have low calcium intake. About 20% to 25% of white women, and fewer African American women, will develop osteoporosis in the postmenopausal stage of life (Dunnihoo, 1992).

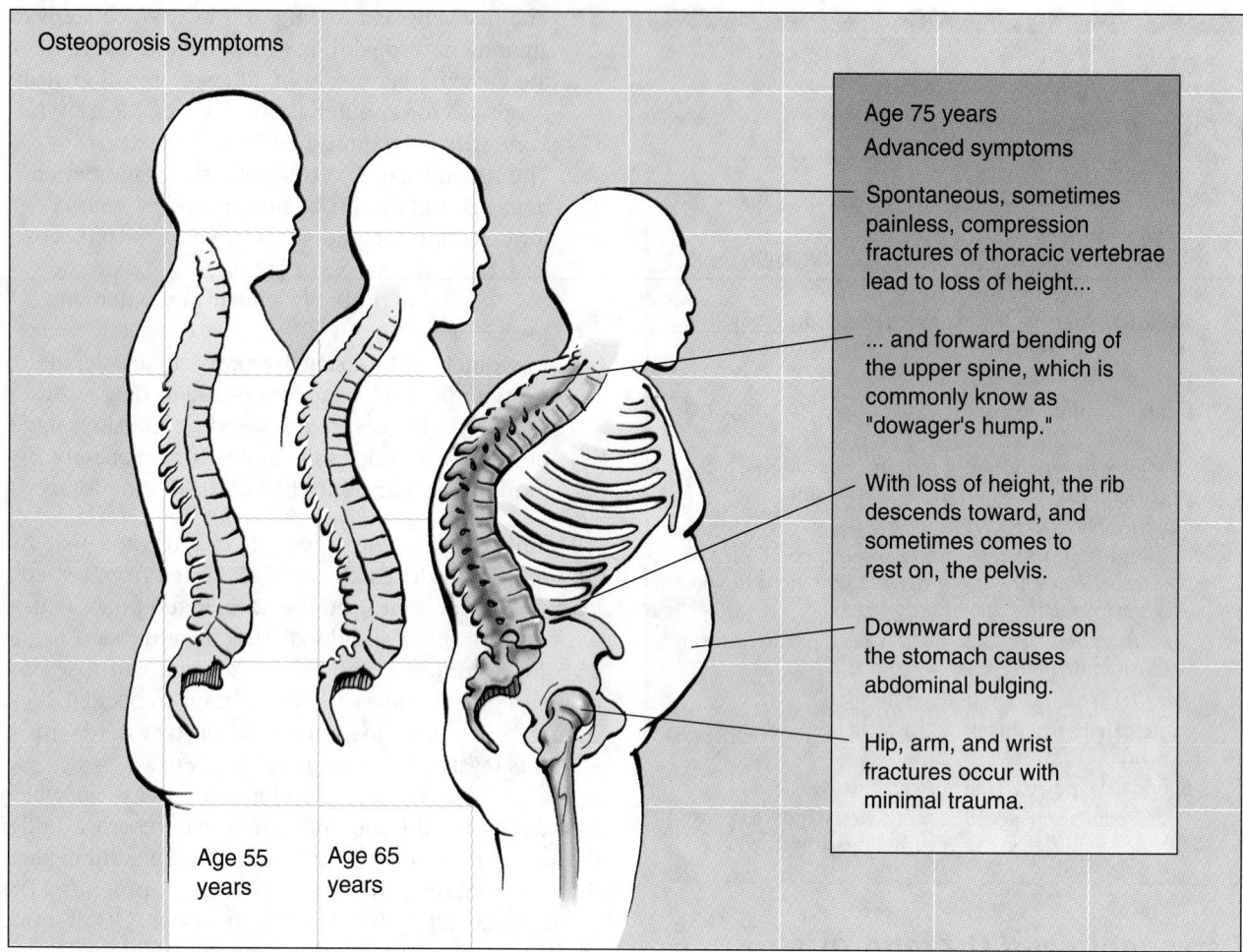

Osteoporosis Symptoms

Age 75 years
Advanced symptoms

Spontaneous, sometimes painless, compression fractures of thoracic vertebrae lead to loss of height...

... and forward bending of the upper spine, which is commonly know as "dowager's hump."

With loss of height, the rib descends toward, and sometimes comes to rest on, the pelvis.

Downward pressure on the stomach causes abdominal bulging.

Hip, arm, and wrist fractures occur with minimal trauma.

Age 55 years

Age 65 years

FIGURE 8–3 Osteoporosis symptoms and progression.

Nursing Assessment

The nurse has an important role in identifying risk factors for osteoporosis (see Box 8-8). Assessment of dietary habits should begin in preadolescence, with attention to adequate calcium and avoidance of excessive protein, caffeine, and alcohol. Use of caffeine, cigarettes, and alcohol is assessed frequently through the woman's life because of their adverse effects on health. Because these habits are lifestyle choices, they can be changed through intervention. Appropriate exercise starting in childhood is important to maximize bone density and prevent bone loss.

Diagnosis and Treatment

Physical examination focuses on the woman's age, race, stature, bone structure, and weight. Obese women have increased supplies of estrogen, even after menopause. The risk of osteoporosis is low among African American women, who have heavier bone structure and greater mass than white or Asian women.

Signs of endocrine or systemic disorders are noted, and further diagnostic testing is undertaken.

Tests for bone mass (bone densitometry) are frequently used to identify women with osteopenia and to assess the extent of osteoporosis. Single or dual photon absorptiometry are most commonly used for spinal and proximal femur measurements. Dual energy x-ray absorptiometry is a more precise refinement of the latter. Quantitative computed tomography is best suited to measure trabecular bone in the spine but is expensive and has high radiation exposure. Bone density is considered abnormal when it falls to 80% or less of young normal values. Ultrasound examination of the patella holds promise of being a low-risk and inexpensive tool for identifying osteoporosis risk (Bourguet et al., 1991).

Treatment for osteoporosis is mostly preventive and consists of balanced diet, good calcium intake, exercise, no smoking, and estrogen replacement therapy in women experiencing menopause. Parenteral salmon calcitonin, sodium fluoride, and intranasal calcitonin have been used for osteoporosis, but they are limited

---

BOX 8-9
Risk Factors for Osteoporosis

Not Changeable	*Changeable or Controllable*
Aging	Low bone mass
Gender (female)	Thin, underweight
Small stature	Cigarette smoking
Asian, white, fair skin	Sedentary (little exercise)
Family history	Low calcium intake
Menopause	Estrogen deficiency
	Excessive alcohol use
	Excessive protein intake
	Excessive caffeine intake
	Drugs (corticosteroids, psychotropics, thyroid, sedatives)
	Previous fractures
	Diseases (thyroid, diabetes, arthritis)
	Oopherectomy

---

by route of administration, safety, and lack of proven efficacy. Intermittent cyclical therapy with etidronate, an organic bisphosphonate compound, has been found to increase spinal bone mass significantly and reduce the incidence of new vertebral fractures in women with postmenopausal osteoporosis (Watts et al., 1990).

Hormone Replacement Therapy in Menopausal Women

Hormone replacement therapy with estrogen alone (ERT) or combined with progestogen (HRT) is widely used to treat changes associated with menopause, including hot flashes, vaginal and urinary tract atrophy, skin changes, and mood changes. Estrogen protects against osteoporosis, as demonstrated in several well-controlled clinical studies (Lichtman, 1991). Receptors for estrogen have been found in human bone cells, supporting the theory that estrogen has a direct effect on osteoblast activity and on reducing osteoclastic resorption. ERT prevents bone resorption by increasing serum levels of calcitonin and maintains bone density, reducing the risk of fractures (Barrett-Conner, 1987).

Women need to begin taking estrogen within 3 years of menopause for maximal effect on preventing bone loss. As soon as women develop symptoms of estrogen deficiency, they are candidates for replacement therapy, even before cessation of menses. Estrogen deficiency can be confirmed by an follicle-stimulating hormone level exceeding 30 mIU/mL (Hulka et al., 1992).

Estrogen protects against fractures to some extent, even if started several years after menopause.

Women may continue taking estrogen indefinitely if there are no complications and the woman finds this acceptable (Bush et al., 1993). At least 5 years of ERT in early menopause appears to reduce hip and arm fractures by 50% and vertebral fractures by 90% (Consensus Development Conference, 1991). Discontinuing therapy may result in resumed bone loss. Continuing ERT for 10 to 15 years stops bone loss; these benefits probably continue beyond age 75 (Hulka et al., 1992).

Common side effects of ERT include resumption of menstrual bleeding, breast tenderness and enlargement, and weight gain. Usually bleeding stops within 6 months to 1 year, but for some women any bleeding is unacceptable. Women with an intact uterus should have combined therapy, either cyclic or continuous, to prevent the risk of endometrial cancer. With a hysterectomy, estrogen alone is used. Client information about HRT is provided in the Client Teaching Guidelines: Hormone Replacement Therapy (HRT).

Cancer Risks

Multiple studies have clearly shown that unopposed estrogen replacement therapy (without progestogen) increases the risk of endometrial cancer five to seven times after 3 years of use. Addition of progestogen reverses this risk by preventing estrogen-produced endometrial hyperplasia (Barrett-Connor, 1987). The relationship between ERT and breast cancer is not as clear. The risk of breast cancer in women who have used ERT is not consistently increased. More than 10 years use may be associated with a small increase in the diagnosis, but not deaths from, breast cancer (Consensus Development Conference, 1991). In American studies, breast cancer relative risk was 1.3 to 2.5, increasing with age and longer use (Bush et al., 1994). A Swedish

---

BOX 8-10
Classification of Osteoporosis

Type I (postmenopausal osteoporosis) affects women within 15 to 20 years after menopause and mainly affects trabecular bone. It may result in fractures of the vertebrae, distal forearm (Colles' fracture), and distal ankle. Vertebral fractures are the crush type and cause pain and deformation.

Type II (age-related osteoporosis) occurs in men and women 70 years or older but is twice as common in women. It usually results in hip and vertebral fractures but may affect the humerus, tibia, and pelvis. Vertebral fractures are the multiple wedge type, leading to dorsal kyphosis (dowager's hump; see Fig. 8-2).

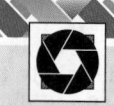

CLIENT TEACHING GUIDELINES
Hormone Replacement Therapy (HRT)

Estrogen (ERT) or combined estrogen-progestogen (HRT) therapy is often recommended for women in the peri-menopausal years. When the ovaries age and produce less estrogen, women often have unpleasant symptoms, such as hot flashes, mood changes, irritability, insomnia, and vaginal dryness. Years of reduced estrogen can cause osteoporosis (thin, fragile bones), which leads to risk of fractures. After menopause, women have greater risk of heart disease, which is partly related to decreased estrogen.

Benefits of HRT/ERT: ERT (for women who have had hysterectomies) and HRT (for those with a uterus) can reduce these symptoms and prevent osteoporosis and heart disease. Estrogen also may protect against Alzheimer's disease.

How to take hormone medications: Dosage regimens may be as follows:

- Conjugated estrogen (Premarin) 0.625 mg minimum to 1.25 mg maximum
  Estrone (Ogen) 1.25–2.5 mg
  Estrace (micronized estradiol) 1.0–2.0 mg
  Ethinyl estradiol 20–40 μg
  Transdermal (estradiol) 50–100 μg
- Medroxyprogesterone acetate (Provera) 2.5–10 mg
- Cyclic combined regimen:
  Estrogen, days 1–25 each month; progestogen, days 13–25 each month

  Estrogen daily: progestogen, days 1–13 each month
- Continuous combined regimen:
  Estrogen daily: progestogen daily (usually 2.5–5 mg)
- Cyclic single regimen:
  Estrogen, days 1–25 each month
- Continuous single regimen:
  Estrogen daily

Contraindications to ERT/HRT: Women with the following conditions should not take estrogen therapy:

- Known or suspected breast cancer
- Undiagnosed vaginal bleeding
- History of thromboembolic disease
- Known or suspected pregnancy
- Thrombophlebitis or thromboembolic disorders
- Known or suspected estrogen-dependent neoplasms

Adverse reactions: These reactions may result from estrogen use:

- Worsening of migraines and other headaches
- Embolic disorders (cardiac, pulmonary)
- Breast tenderness and enlargement
- Nausea, vomiting, cramps, and bloating
- Changes in patterns or recurrence of bleeding
- Enlargement of uterine fibroids (leiomyomata)
- Weight gain, reduced carbohydrate tolerance

---

study found no overall increased risk with several different ERT regimens (Bergkvist et al., 1989). A prospective study of a large cohort of American nurses found a significant increase in breast cancer with current or recent use of ERT; this reversed within 2 years of stopping hormonal therapy (Colditz et al., 1990).

Estrogen Therapy and Coronary Heart Disease

Estrogen therapy has a protective effect against coronary artery disease. Heart disease is a leading cause of death in older women and increases sharply after menopause. A 50% reduction in heart disease has been shown in multiple studies of estrogen effects. Estrogens decrease atherosclerosis by creating a favorable lipid profile, increasing cardiac output and promoting vascular flow. Estrogens increase high-density lipoproteins, which protect vascular walls, and decrease low-density lipoproteins, which promote vascular plaque formation. Direct effects on vascular walls decrease risk of clot formation (Barrett-Connor et al., 1991; Stampfer et al., 1991; Walsh, 1992; Villablanca, 1993). Women with cardiovascular risk factors or disease can derive significant benefit from estrogen therapy.

Estrogen Therapy and Brain Function

Preliminary evidence suggests that estrogen therapy may prevent age-related dementias, such as Alzheimer's disease (Scheck, 1993). Women taking estrogen replacement therapy were 40% less likely to have Alzheimer's disease and related dementias than those not using estrogen. Women with Alzheimer's disease who had been on estrogen therapy performed better on cognitive tests. Animal studies support estrogen's effects on the brain; it improves cognitive function and learning. Estrogen probably protects brain neurons indirectly by maintaining levels of nerve growth factor (NGF). NGF levels of estrogen-deficient animals fell by 45% when estrogen supplements were removed. Estrogen supports formation of connections among neurons within the hippocampus. There are fewer connections in estrogen-deficient animals; these return to normal when estrogen is replaced (Johnson, 1993).

Clinical trials will be needed to demonstrate the effectiveness of estrogen therapy in preventing dementias from developing after menopause and improving cognitive functioning in postmenopausal women with Alzheimer's disease.

Nursing Process for Women Going Through Menopause

The menopause transition has physiologic and psychological effects on women. Mood changes and depression are common and may be related to declining hormone levels and the emotional reaction to the loss of fertility. The nurse can play an important role in helping women cope with the symptoms of menopause. Teaching and counselling about menopause, its symptoms, and medical and alternative therapies are foremost in the arsenal of interventions available to nurses in this area. The Nursing Care Plan: The Woman Experiencing Menopause at the end of this chapter provides specific goals, diagnoses, interventions, and evaluation criteria for helping the woman through this phase of life.

Assessment

The nurse should interview the woman to find out if she is experiencing any physical signs and symptoms of menopause. These might include, but are not limited to, hot flashes, night sweats, headaches, numbness, tingling, insomnia, vaginal dryness, irritability, and mood swings. She also should determine the woman's baseline pattern of menstruation and any changes to that pattern that have occurred. The nurse should ask about risk factors for osteoporosis (see Box 8-9), heart disease, and depression. Finally, assessment of the woman's attitude toward menopause and identification of the key elements of her support system will help the nurse plan appropriate interventions.

Nursing Diagnoses

Nursing diagnoses related to symptoms of menopause include the following:

- Anticipatory Grieving related to loss of childbearing ability
- Self Esteem Disturbance related to physical and emotional changes associated with menopause
- Knowledge Deficit related to normal changes and symptoms of menopause and treatment for symptoms
- Altered Sexuality Patterns related to hormonal changes and decreased vaginal lubrication

Nursing diagnoses related to osteoporosis may include the following:

- Risk for Injury (fractures, complications) related to lack of knowledge about causes, prevention, and treatment for osteoporosis
- Impaired Physical Mobility related to fractures or fear of fractures with bone loss
- Altered Nutrition: Less than body requirements for calcium related to age and inadequate intake of calcium
- Knowledge Deficit related to causes, prevention, and treatment of osteoporosis

Nursing Planning and Intervention

Nursing interventions are aimed at relieving the physical and emotional symptoms of menopause and preventing osteopenia and reducing bone loss with aging and menopause (see the Nursing Care Plan). Primary prevention includes encouraging the woman to discuss her feelings and concerns about the menopause transition. The nurse should emphasize that menopause is a normal part of life. Women should be encouraged not to fear this change. The symptoms of menopause are usually more annoying than serious and can usually be manageable.

Women experiencing menopause should be encouraged to eat a healthy diet, participate in new activities, and get plenty of exercise. Normal sleep patterns are encouraged because fatique often exacerbates the symptoms. These practices of healthy living will lessen the symptoms of menopause and help women feel good about themselves.

Menopause does not mean the termination of a sex life. Women should be encouraged to use water-soluble lubricants to ease vaginal dryness and to practice Kegel exercises to improve muscle tone in the perineal area.

The nurse should provide information about the types of available therapy for treating symptoms of menopause. Women also should be encouraged to discuss the issue of therapy with their doctors.

Nursing actions to assist women in achieving maximal peak bone mass during the years of skeletal maturation may help prevent osteoporosis. Education and counseling focus on diet and exercise from preadolescence through old age, with the goal of ensuring good calcium intake and limiting protein and substances known to affect bone metabolism (caffeine, cigarettes, alcohol). Regular weight-bearing exercise habits are encouraged and modified according to life cycle needs. Dangers of sedentary lifestyles and substance use are emphasized (see Client Education: Preventing Osteoporosis).

Teaching women the major risk factors for osteoporosis and identifying the factors important in family and personal histories will help women take responsibility for their own bone health. Women at higher risk are encouraged to undertake preventive actions as *(text continues on page 186)*

NURSING CARE PLAN
The Woman Experiencing Menopause

Nursing Goals
1. The woman will identify the physical and emotional changes of menopause.
2. The woman will achieve effective relief of symptoms.
3. The woman will understand her risk for osteoporosis, heart disease, and depression and make informed decisions about preventative therapy.
4. The woman and her family will adapt effectively to the menopause transition.

Assessment	*Potential Nursing Diagnosis*	*Intervention/ Rationale*	*Evaluation*
Signs and symptoms of menopause: hot flashes, night sweats, irritability, insomnia, mood swings, depression, headaches, numbness, tingling.	Altered Comfort related to physical and emotional symptoms of menopause. Knowledge Deficit related to menopausal changes. Anxiety related to life change.	Teach range of symptoms *to provide basis for normalization.* Teach physical and emotional processes of menopause and transition *to promote understanding and acceptance.* Listen actively and counsel *to alleviate anxiety and confusion.* Advise possible therapies for symptom relief (estrogen replacement therapy, herbal or vitamin supplements).	Woman states understanding and acceptance of menopausal changes.
Status of menses and hormonal function.	Risk for pain/discomfort related to declining ovarian function.	Assist woman to obtain pain relief *to promote comfort.* Teach physiology of menstrual cessation *to alleviate anxiety and misunderstanding.*	Woman obtains relief of symptoms.
Risk factors for osteoporosis, heart disease, and depression.	Risk for Injury related to osteoporosis, heart disease, and depression. Knowledge Deficit related to risk and prevention.	Assist woman to understand her own risk levels *so informed choices about therapy can be made.* Identify women at risk and make appropriate referrals for treatment *to minimize or prevent development of disease.*	Woman takes action to reduce her risk for osteoporosis, heart disease, and depression; these conditions do not develop or progress.
Attitude toward and conception of menopause.	Self Esteem Disturbance related to role/status change. Situational Low Self Esteem related to menopausal changes. Ineffective Individual Coping related to negative attitudes regarding menopause.	Assist woman to express and clarify her attitudes and conceptions *to bring these to conscious examination.* Counsel regarding positive attitude formation and self-acceptance *to encourage effective coping.*	Woman expresses comfort with postmenopausal self-concept and role. Woman seeks therapy for problematic attitudes or serious depression.

(continued)

NURSING CARE PLAN *(Continued)*
The Woman Experiencing Menopause

Assessment	Potential Nursing Diagnosis	Intervention/ Rationale	Evaluation
Family/Partner reaction and support system.	Family Coping: Potential for Growth Risk for Sexual Dysfunction related to menopausal changes.	Encourage partner/family to express feelings and concerns *to remove misconceptions and bring these to conscious examination.* Encourage emotional support and acceptance *to aid family growth and development.* Identify sexual problems, provide brief counseling, and refer for therapy as indicated *to promote satisfying sexual relationship.*	Family/partner states understanding and acceptance of menopausal changes. Satisfying sexual relationship maintained. Woman states she feels supported and valued by family/partner.

CLIENT EDUCATION
Preventing Osteoporosis

Diet: Bone density can be built in youth by eating calcium-rich foods, such as dairy products; dark green, leafy vegetables; whole grains; tofu; and seafood. Vitamin D is essential for calcium absorption and building bone. Protein intake should be moderate, because high protein intake causes urinary calcium excretion. Vegetable-based diets, even without dairy, are associated with less osteoporosis. Avoid excessive caffeine and alcohol, and do not smoke cigarettes, because these substances rob calcium from the body.

Calcium supplements: Calcium supplements can reduce or stop postmenopausal bone loss, if taken in proper amounts. The following is recommended for women not taking estrogen replacement therapy:

Perimenopause	*Postmenopause*
Calcium 1,000 mg daily	Calcium 1,500 mg daily
Vitamin D 200 IU daily	Vitamin D 200–400 IU daily

Form of Calcium	Elemental Calcium	Side Effects	Considerations
Calcium carbonate	40%	Constipation, gas, bloating, acid rebound	Avoid with hypochlorhydria
Calcium lactate	13%	Less constipating	Avoid if lactose intolerant
Calcium gluconate	9%	Less constipating	Need to take more often
Calcium chloride	27%	Irritates stomach	Used to pickle foods
Bone meal	31%	Irritates stomach	May contain lead; not well absorbed
Dolomite	22%		May contain lead

Exercise: Weight-bearing exercise builds healthy bones in youth and can increase bone mass after menopause. Even in women with osteoporosis, exercise programs have increased bone mass. Exercises that cause muscles to pull against their bony attachments, such as gentle weight training, isometrics, stretching, and range of motion, are effective. Walking, jogging, bicycling, and rowing also will increase calcium levels and help retain bone mass. Women with fragile bones must avoid twisting the spine and stopping active sports suddenly.

early as possible and to have regular medical monitoring, including bone densitometry. The risks and benefits of estrogen or hormone therapy are discussed. Therapy is individualized according to client needs, desires, and individual symptom and risk profile. Calcium supplementation is recommended for perimenopausal women, because it is difficult to consume enough dietary calcium. The risk of kidney stones is minimal unless the woman has a history of renal disease.

Some women may want to avoid ERT, and use natural approaches to prevent osteoporosis and manage the symptoms of menopause. High-dose calcium alone (1,700 mg) can retard bone loss; calcium plus exercise reduces bone loss to only 0.5% per year. Neither is as effective as HRT with exercise, however, which increases bone mass by 2.7% (Prince et al., 1991; Aloia et al., 1994).

Evaluation

Outcomes of effective nursing care include increased knowledge about the symptoms of menopause, prevention and treatment of osteoporosis, and behavior changes to reduce risk of osteoporisis by maximizing bone mass deposition and minimizing bone loss. Women with increased risk factors will seek medical care and assistance to modify their risks whenever possible. The result of effective interventions will be fewer fractures due to osteoporosis, which reduces suffering and disability in older women and promotes healthier aging. Older women's overall health will be improved by exercise, healthy habits, and improved nutrition. Other outcomes to be achieved include acceptance and understanding of menopausal changes by the woman and her partner or family and a positive self-concept on the part of the woman as reported by feelings of satisfaction with herself and her life after menopause.

Summary Points

✔ Wellness care of women occurs primarily in the community. Schedules for periodic screening help detect disease early and prevent development of illness. Screening for breast and cervical cancer is critically important and often done by nurses.

✔ There is considerable variation in normal menstrual patterns. Understanding the normal range is important, especially for young women. Information about menstrual comfort and self-care management must be provided clearly and misconceptions corrected. Healthy attitudes are encouraged.

✔ Cigarette smoking increases women's risk of cancer, cardiovascular, and pulmonary disease. It affects hormone metabolism and increases the risk of osteoporosis. Women should be supported in non-smoking.

✔ Women encounter significant stress in home and work roles. They face particular workplace hazards. Substance abuse can be a result or a cause of stress. Nurses need to identify potential substance abuse and assist women to cope effectively with stress.

✔ Depression is a common problem among women. Risk factors must be identified and women referred for treatment to promote maximal health and well-being.

✔ Menopause is a period of physiologic and psychological transition for women. It is often characterized by physical and emotional symptoms. ERT can relieve symptoms and prevent development of osteoporosis and coronary artery disease. Alternatives to ERT include calcium supplementation and weight-bearing exercise.

REFERENCES

Aguglia, E., Casacchia, M., Cassano, G. B., et al. (1993). Double-blind study of the efficacy and safety of sertraline versus fluoxetine in major depression. *International Clinical Pharmacology, 8,* 197–202.

Aloia, J. F., et al. (1994). Calcium supplementation with and without hormone replacement therapy to prevent postmenopausal bone loss. *Annals of Internal Medicine, 120,* 97–103.

American Cancer Society (1994). Cancer facts and figures, 1994. *American Cancer Society Bulletin,* No 5008.92LE.

American College of Obstetricians and Gynecologists (1989). *Report of task force on routine cancer screening.* Washington, DC: Author.

American Psychiatric Association (1994). *Diagnostic and statistical manual of mutual disorders* (4th ed.). Washington, DC: COG.

Baron, J. A., & Greenberg, R. E. (1989). Cigarette smoking and neoplasms of the female reproductive tract and breast. *Seminar on Reproductive Endocrinology, 7*(4), 335–343.

Baron, J. A., LaVecchia, C., & Levi, F. (1990). The antiestrogenic effect of cigarette smoking in women. *American Journal of Obetetrics and Gynecology, 162*(2), 502–514.

Barrett-Conner, E. et al. (1991). Estrogen and coronary heart disease in women. *Journal of the American Medical Association, 265*(4), 1861–1867.

Barrett-Conner, E. (1987). Postmenopausal estrogen, cancer and other considerations. In S. D. Stellman (Ed.), *Women and cancer* (pp. 179–195). New York: Harworth Press.

Bergkvist, L., Hans-Olov, A., Persson, I. et al. (1989). The risk of breast cancer after estrogen and estrogen-progestin replacement. *New England Journal of Medicine, 321,* 293–297.

Berman, R. L. (1985). Current perspectives in gynecology. *Ciba Clinical Symposium, 37*(1), 2–29.

Blumenreich, P. (1993). Office counseling guidelines for primary care physicians. *Clinical Advances in the Treatment of Psychiatric Disorders, 7*(3), 4–5.

Bourquet, C. C., Hamrick, G. A., Gilchrist, V. J. (1991). The prevalence of osteoporosis risk factors and physician intervention. *Journal of Family Practice, 32*(3), 265–272.

Boyce, J. G., Fruchter, R. G., Romanzi, L. et al. (1990). The fallacy of the screening interval for cervical smears. *Obstetrics and Gynecology, 76*(4), 632–637.

Brown, L. W., & Williams, R. D. (1994). Culturally sensitive breast cancer screening programs for older Black women. *Nurse Practitioner, 19*(3), 21–35.

Burns, C. M. (1994). Toward healthy people 2000: The role of the nurse practitioner and health promotion. *Journal of the American Academy of Nurse Practitioners, 6*(1), 29–35.

Bush, T. L., Dawood, M. Y., Gallagher, C., Hulka, B. S., Lindsey, R., Utian, W. H. (1994). Update: the benefits and risks of HRT. *Patient Care, Supplement, Dec 15,* 23–29.

Bush, T. L., Gambrell, R. D., Miller, V. (1993). More reasons than ever for HRT. *Patient Care, 15,* 103–132.

Capan, P. (1993). Nurse-managed clinics provide access and improved health care. *The Nurse Practitioner, 18*(5), 50–55.

Caulker-Burnett, I. (1994). Primary care screening for substance abuse. *Nurse Practitioner, 19*(6), 42–48.

Champion, V. L. (1991). The relationship of selected variables to breast cancer detection behaviors in women 35 and older. *Oncological Nursing Forum, 19*(4), 733–739.

Charbonneau, L. (1985). Smoking or health: How long can nurses ignore the facts? *Canadian Nurse, 81*(7), 27–32.

Clay, L. S. (1990). Midwifery assessment of the well woman: The Pap smear. *Journal of Nurse Midwifery, 35*(6), 341.

Colditz, G. A. et al. (1990). Prospective study of estrogen replacement therapy and risk of breast cancer in postmenopausal women. *Journal of the American Medical Association, 264*(20), 2648.

Consensus Development Conference (1991). Prophylaxis and treatment of osteoporosis. *American Journal of Medicine, 90,* 107–110.

Cooper, R. A. (1989). Mammography. *Clinical Obetstrics and Gynecology, 32*(4), 768–785.

Dunnihoo, D. R. (1992). *Fundamentals of gynecology & obstetrics* (2nd ed.) Philadelphia: JB Lippincott.

Executive Summary (1992). Nursing's agenda for health care reform. *The American Nurse, 3*(24), 7.

Gitlin, M. J., & Pasnau, R. O. (1989). Psychiatric syndromes linked to reproductive function in women: A review of current knowledge. *American Journal of Psychiatry, 146,* 7–15.

Golden, R. N., & Gilmore, J. H. (1990). Serotonin and mood disorders. *Psychiatric Annals, 20,* 580–586.

Hafner, B. Q., Frandsen, K. J., Karren, K. J., Hooker, K. R. (1992). *The health effects of attitudes, emotions relationships.* Provo, UT: EMS Associates.

Heaney, R. P. (1993). Protein intake and the calcium economy. *Journal of the American Diabetic Association, 93*(11), 1259–1261.

Hein, K. (1984). The first pelvic examination and common gynecological problems in adolescent girls. *Women's Health, 9*(2/3), 47–63.

Hulka, B., Lindsay, M. B., Miller, V. et al. (1992). Health after 50: Hormone replacement. *Patient Care, Supplement,* 5–15.

Johnson, J., Weissman, M., & Klerman, G. (1992). Service utilization and social morbidity associated with depressive symptoms in the community. *Journal of the American Medical Association, 267,* 1478–1483.

Johnson, R. (1993). Estrogen/Alzheimer's link found. *Medical Tribune for Family Physicians, 43*(23), 1–2.

Jones, C. J., Schiffman, M. H., Kurman, R. et al. (1991). Elevated nicotine levels in cervical lavages from passive smokers. *American Journal of Public Health, 81*(3), 378–379.

Kaufert, P. A. (1982). Anthropology and menopause: The development of a theoretical framework. *Maturitas, 4,* 181–193.

Kirschstein, R. L. (1991). Research on women's health. *American Journal of Public Health, 81*(3), 291–293.

Lappe, J. M. (1993). Bone fragility: Assessment of risk and strategies for Prevention. *Journal of Obstetric, Gynecologic, and Neonatal Nursing, 23*(3), 260–268.

Lichtman, R. (1991). Perimenopausal hormone replacement therapy: review of the literature. *Journal of Nurse Midwifery, 36*(1), 30–48.

Lierman, L. M. et al. (1990). Predicting breast self-examination using the theory of reasoned action. *Nursing Research, 39*(2), 97.

Lundeen, S. P. (1985). Nurse-managed centers offer more to patients, nurses. *The American Nurse, 17*(4), 22.

Lufkin, E. G., & Ory, S. J. (1989). Estrogen replacement therapy for the prevention of osteoporosis. *American Family Physician, 40*(3), 205–212.

Mayberry, R. M. (1985). Cigarette smoking, herpes simplex virus type 2 infection, and cervical abnormalities. *American Journal of Public Health, 75*(6), 676–678.

McCrea, F. B. (1983). The politics of menopause: The "discovery" of a deficiency disease. *Social Problems, 31*(3), 111–123.

McGrath, S. (1990). The cost-effectiveness of nurse practitioners. *The Nurse Practitioner, 15*(7), 40–41.

Nesse, R. E. (1989). Abnormal vaginal bleeding in perimenopausal women. *American Family Physician, 40*(1), 185–192.

Pirie, P. L., Murray, D. M., & Luepker, R. V. (1991). Gender differences in cigarette smoking and quitting in a cohort of young adults. *American Journal of Public Health, 81*(3), 324–327.

Posner, I., Lester, D., & Leitner, L. (1984). Stress in nurses and other working females. *Psychological Reports, 54*(1), 210.

American Psychiatric Association (1993). *Practice guidelines for major depressive disorder in adults* (pp. 10–12). Washington, DC: Author.

Prince, R. L. et al. (1991). Prevention of postmenopausal osteoporosis: A comparative study of exercise, calcium supplementation, and hormone-replacement therapy. *New England Journal of Medicine, 325,* 1189–1195.

Recker, R., Davies, M., Hinders, S. et al. (1992). Bone gain in young adult women. *Journal of the American Medical Association, 268,* 2403–2408.

Riggs, B. L. (1991). Overview of osteoporosis. *Western Journal of Medicine, 154,* 63–77.

Riggs, B. L., & Melton, L. J. (1986). Medical progress series: Involutional osteoporosis. *New England Journal of Medicine, 314,* 1676.

Risch, S. C., & Nemeroff, C. B. (1992). Neurochemical alterations of serotonergic neuronal systems in depression. *Journal of Clinical Psychiatry, 53*(Suppl. 10), 3–7.

Rosenthal, N. E. (1993). *Winter blues: Seasonal affective disorder: What it is and how to overcome it.* New York: Guilford Press.

Sarrel, P. (1989). Ovarian steroids and the capacity to function at home and in the work place. Presented at North American Menopause Society Meeting, New York, September 21–23.

Scheck, A. (1993). Estrogen may prevent age-related dementia. *Family Practice News, p. 15.*

Scott, J. R., Disaia, P. J., Hammond, C. B., Spellacy, W. N. (Eds.). (1994). *Danforth's obstetrics and gynecology,* (7th ed.). Philadelphia: JB Lippincott.

Shy, K., Chu, J., Mandelson, M. et al. (1989). Papanicolaou smear screening interval and risk of cervical cancer. *Obstetrics and Gynecology, 74*(6), 838–843.

Stampfer, M. J. et al. (1991). Postmenopausal estrogen therapy and cardiovascular disease. *New England Journal of Medicine, 325*(11), 756–762.

(1990). Women: The road ahead [Special issue]. *Time Magazine, 136*(19), 10–14, 50–52.

U.C. Berkeley Wellness Letter (1994). *Mammograms' let's talk.* School of Public Health, University of California, Berkeley, *10,* 4.

U.S. Department of Health and Human Services (1992). *Healthy people 2000: National health promotion and disease prevention objectives.* Washington, DC: DHHS.

U.S. Department of Health and Human Services (1992). *Healthy people 2000: National health promotion and disease prevention objectives.* Washington, DC: Author.

Vicary, J. R., Mansfield, P. K., Cohn, M. D. et al. (1985). Substance use among women in the workplace. *Occupational Health Nursing, 33*(10), 491–495, 527–530.

Villablanca, A. C. (1993). Coronary artery disease in women. Paper presented at Ambulatory Obstetrics & Gynecology, Lake Tahoe, CA, 32–38.

Vliet, E. L., & Davis, V. L. (1991). New perspectives on the relationship of hormone changes to affective disorders in the perimenopause. *NAACOG's Clinical Issues, 2*(4), 453–471.

Walsh, B. W. et al. (1992). Effects of postmenopausal estrogen replacement on the concentrations and metabolism of plasma lipoproteins. *New England Journal of Medicine, 325*(17), 1196–1204.

Watts, N. B. (1991). Prevention of osteoporosis: The role of primary physicians. *Journal of Family Practice, 32*(3), 261–263.

Watts, N. B., Harris, S. T., Genant, H. K. et al. (1990). Intermittent cyclical etidronate treatment of postmenopausal osteoporosis. *New England Journal of Medicine, 323*(2), 73–125.

Wilsnack, S. C., Klassen, A. D., Schur, B. E. et al. (1991). Predicting onset and chronicity of women's problem drinking: A five-year longitudinal analysis. *American Journal of Public Health, 81*(3), 305–317.

Wysocki, L. M., & Ossler, C. (1983). Women, work and health: Issues of importance to the occupational health nurse. *Occupational Health Nursing, 31*(11), 18–23, 56–61.

Yeh, J., & Barbieri, R. L. (1989). Effects of smoking on steroid production, metabolism, and estrogen-related disease. *Seminars in Reproductive Endocrinology, 7*(4), 326–334.

SUGGESTED READING

Barrett-Conner, E. (1991). Postmenopausal estrogen and prevention bias. *Annals of Internal Medicine, 115,* 455–456.

Burgess, S. (1985). DES daughters: Fighting fear with facts. *American Journal of Nursing, 85*(6), 639–640.

Coleman, E. (Ed.) (1987). *Chemical dependency and intimacy dysfunction.* New York: Haworth Press.

Devor, M. et al (1992). Estrogen replacement therapy and the risk of venous thrombosis. *American Journal of Medicine, 92,* 275–282.

Egan, R. L. (1988). *Breast imaging: Diagnosis and morphology of breast disease.* Philadelphia: W.B. Saunders.

Fillmore, K. M. (1987). Women's drinking across the adult life course as compared to men's. *British Journal of Addiction, 82,* 801–811.

Fiore, M. C., Novotny, T. E., Pierce, J. P. et al (1989). Trends in cigarette smoking in the United States: The changing influence of gender and race. *Journal of the American Medical Association, 261,* 49–55.

Hellberg, D., Nilsson, S., Haley, N. J. et al (1988). Smoking and cervical intraepithelial neoplasia: Nicotine and cotinine in serum and cervical mucus in smokers and non-smokers. *American Journal of Obstetrics and Gynecology, 158,* 910–913.

Kirkpatrick, M. K., Edwards, M. K., & Finch, N. (1991). Assessment and prevention of osteoporosis through use of a client self-reporting tool. *Nurse Practitioner, 16*(7); 16–26.

Klassen, A. D., & Wilsnack, S. C. (1986). Sexual experience and drinking among women in a US national survey. *Archives of Sexual Behaviors, 15,* 363–392.

Lynch, H. T., Watson, P., Conway, T. et al (1988). Breast cancer family history as a risk factor for early onset breast cancer. *Breast Cancer Research and Treatment, 11,* 263.

Makue, D. M., Fried, V. M., & Kleinman, J. C. (1989). National trends in the use of preventive health care for women. *American Journal of Public Health, 79,* 21–26.

Mamon, J. A., & Zapka, J. G. (1985). Improving frequency and proficiency of breast self-examination: Effectiveness of an education program. *American Journal of Public Health, 75*(6), 618–624.

Manolio, T. A., Furberg, C. D., Shemanski, L. et al. (1993). Associations of postmenopausal estrogen use with cardiovascular disease and its risk factors in older women. *Circulation, 88*(part I), 2163–2171.

Orlandi, M. A. (1987). Gender differences in smoking cessation. *Women's Health, 11,* 237–251.

Schnoll, S. H., & Karan, L. D. (1990). Substance abuse. *Journal of the American Medical Association, 263*(19), 2682–2683.

Slattery, M. L., Robison, L. M., Schuman, K. L. et al (1989). Cigarette smoking and exposure to passive smoke are risk factors for cervical cancer. *Journal of the American Medical Association, 261,* 1593–1598.

Stern, P. N., & Harris, C. C. (1985). Women's health and the self-care paradox: A model to guide self-care readiness. *Health Care of Women International 6*(1–3), 151–163.

Verbrugge, I. M. (1986). Role burdens and physical health of women and men. *Women's Health, 11,* 47–77.

Wabrek, A. J., & Gunn, J. L. (1984). Sexual and psychological implications of gynecologic malignancy. *Journal of Obstetric, Gynecologic, and Neonatal Nursing, 13*(6), 371–376.

Woods, N. F., Mitchell, E. S., Lentz, M. J. (1995). Social pathways to premenstrual symptoms. *Research in Nursing Health, 18,* 225–237.

9

Sexual Health and Family Planning

Objectives

- Summarize the development of sexuality from birth to adulthood.
- Discuss components of a sexual history for an adult.
- Identify the possible effects of childbearing on pregnancy as it relates to the couple's sexual history.
- Describe common concerns and problems with sexuality during pregnancy and postpartum.
- Compare and contrast various contraceptive methods according to suitability for use, risks and benefits, and advantages and disadvantages.
- Discuss nursing responsibilities for informed consent and contraceptive counseling.
- Describe the nursing interventions necessary for the client who undergoes sterilization.

Key Terms

Abstinence	Norplant
Basal body	Oral contraceptives
temperature	Sexual desire
Calendar method	Sexual health
Cervical cap	Sexuality
Coitus interruptus	Sterilization
Condom	Symptothermal
Diaphragm	method
Dyspareunia	Tubal ligation
Intimacy	Typical effectiveness
Intrauterine device	Vaginal spermicide
Maximal effectiveness	Vasectomy
Monoclonal antibody	Withdrawal

Sexual Health

Sexuality is an important component of a person's identity. It includes feelings, attitudes, and behaviors that are influenced biologically and culturally. Beginning at birth and continuing through the lifespan, sexuality helps to shape a person's physical, social, emotional, and intellectual responses. An integral component of sexuality is sexual health, which also involves making responsible choices about family planning. The nurse plays a key role in this area, especially with the childbearing couple, through discussion and client education.

This chapter presents a discussion of adult sexual health. Specific aspects and areas of concern, including family planning for the childbearing couple, are addressed. The various methods of contraception are described in detail. Using a nursing process approach, the nurse's responsibilities related to sexual health and family planning are presented and integrated throughout the chapter.

Sexual health can be broadly defined as having the following components:

- Accurate information about the physical, emotional, and social aspects of sexuality
- A well-developed identity, which includes the sexual self, and awareness of attitudes and values surrounding sexuality
- The capacity for intimacy in relationships with others
- The self-esteem to make choices about sexual activities congruent with value system and beliefs
- The use of effective contraception when pregnancy is not sought

- Use of precautions against sexually transmitted diseases (STDs), including safe sex practices and selection of sexual partners
- Awareness of factors that may enhance or detract from the state of sexual well-being (Covington, 1987)

Sexual health is important to a person's well-being. Acceptance of sexuality begins in infancy and early childhood, with positive parental responses to genital exploration and the naming of body parts. Attitudes toward the sexual self and beliefs about sexual expression develop gradually through childhood and adolescence. Responses of parents and other family members to childhood sexual expression, such as sexual play, questions about sex and reproduction, nudity, explicit sexual language, masturbation, and dress, continue to shape developing sexual attitudes and expression. Preparation for puberty and sex education further aid the development of the sexual self. In adolescence, identity formation occurs with incorporation of sexual identity, preferred forms of sexual expression and partner choice, and acceptance of reproductive capacity. (Sexuality in adolescence is discussed further in Chap. 35.)

In early adulthood, the major developmental task is **intimacy.** Intimacy occurs only after identity is established and enough comfort has developed to risk revealing and sharing this identity with another person. Intimacy is freely chosen by consenting, equal people who have worked out their adolescent identity processes. Intimate relationships are characterized by mutuality, mature sharing of sexual pleasures, responsible sex, trust, and respect. Deep emotional sharing occurs with concern for a person's own and the partner's well-being and sexual experience (Masters et al., 1994). Responsible sex involves using effective contraception unless pregnancy is sought and taking precautions against infectious diseases. Healthy adult sexuality and the capacity for intimacy provide the foundation for pregnancy and parenthood.

American culture has seen a rapid increase in knowledge and technology. However, many people still misunderstand sexuality. Some common myths include the following (Stuart et al., 1991):

- Sex during menstruation is harmful.
- Excessive masturbation is harmful.
- The child's sex is determined by the woman.
- Pregnancy can occur only by penile penetration or artificial insemination.
- Simultaneous orgasms are necessary for conception.
- By urinating after intercourse, a woman can prevent pregnancy.
- Older people cannot have sex.

Nursing Assessment

Nurses have an important responsibility in promoting sexual health. When assessing, it is always important for the nurse to be aware of his or her own feelings and attitudes toward a particular area of practice. However, dealing with issues surrounding human sexuality requires a level of self-understanding beyond that of most other areas. Nurses bring their personal experiences, values, and attitudes to the professional relationship, which may either promote or block the process of caring for clients with sexual concerns and problems. A nurse who plans to provide sexual teaching and counseling must become comfortable with sexuality generally and personally. Approaches to developing comfort with sexuality are summarized in Box 9-1.

Taking a sexual history and providing counseling are expected parts of the nursing role. Clients need accurate sex information whether they are seeking contraception, undergoing pregnancy, coping with an illness, or striving to attain a higher level of health. The sexual history identifies actual or potential sexual problems. The process of gathering information about sexual experiences and attitudes demonstrates that the nurse is comfortable talking about sex and gives clients permission to discuss sexual concerns. This supports sexuality as an important expectation of healthcare providers. It is best to have a flexible format so the discussion can follow the client's needs. Forms should be short and simple to keep writing at a minimum and allow the nurse to focus attention on the interaction. A sexual history proceeds from general to specific areas, from common to unusual, and from simple to complex. Conditional statements that assume a range of behaviors are used.

To set the scene for the discussion, the nurse may begin with a general opening statement, such as, "Sexual health is an important part of people's lives. Physical health sometimes affects sexual experiences, and sexual health can affect physical well-being. As part of your health history, I'd like to ask some questions about your sexual health that will help me better understand your health status." It is important to have a quiet, private place to talk and allow enough time for discussion and client education. Confidentiality is essential. The client is assured that all questions are optional. The nurse continually assesses the client's comfort as the history taking progresses.

The sexual history includes the following:

1. Current concerns, questions, or problems
2. Onset and course of problem
   a. Age problem began, gradual or sudden onset, any precipitating events
   b. Changes over time in frequency or intensity
   c. Things with which the problem is associated
2. Ideas, beliefs about cause of problem and why it continues
3. Past treatment and outcome (if any)
   a. Professional treatment (type and results)
   b. Self-treatment (type and results)
4. Expectations for improvement and goals of treatment

See Assessment Tool: Taking an Adult Sexual History for a list of helpful questions to use.

Nursing Diagnoses

Following a thorough assessment, the nurse will be able to identify problems related to sexuality. For a list of possible nursing diagnoses, see Box 9-2.

Nursing Planning and Intervention

Nurses can provide sexual teaching and counseling in many settings, especially in health-promotion classes. Concerns related to sexuality are likely to surface if the atmosphere is comfortable and accepting. The nurse who is prepared to deal with information and feelings about sex will find much opportunity to assist clients.

Although intensive therapy for clients with sexual dysfunctions is usually not within the nurse's role, all nurses caring for the reproductive family can promote sexual health by including sexual teaching and counseling in their nursing care. Sexual health can be promoted by creating a climate conducive to discussing sexuality and sexual concerns, validating the normalcy

---

BOX 9–1
Developing Comfort with Sexuality

The nurse must be personally comfortable with the topic of sexuality to counsel effectively. Some approaches to developing this comfort include the following:

Information and Knowledge	Attitudes and Values
Read books and articles.	Values clarification groups or workshops.
View educational films.	
Attend workshops.	Self-directed values discovery.
Enroll in classes.	
Join discussion groups.	Individual or group counseling.
Read popular books (source of public's information).	

ASSESSMENT TOOL
Taking an Adult Sexual History

As part of the general health history, use these questions about sexual experiences and concerns to help focus your assessment.

1. From where did your information about sex come during childhood and adolescence?
2. How did you find out about sexual intercourse? How did you feel about this?
3. Could you ask parents or another adult questions about sex?
4. Were your early sexual experiences satisfying?
5. How would you describe your current sexual activity?
6. Would you change anything about your current sexual activity? If yes, what would you change?
7. What were things like when they were the best ever sexually?
8. Do you have any health problems you believe are affecting your sexual expression?
9. Do you take any medications that you believe affect your sexuality? If yes, what do you take?
10. Do you have any worries or concerns about sex now?

BOX 9–2
Nursing Diagnoses

- Altered Sexuality Patterns related to
    Acute or chronic illness
    Psychological factors
    Stress
    Fear of pregnancy or sexually transmitted diseases
    Relationship problems
- Sexual dysfunction related to
    Abuse
    Problematic relationships
    Acute or chronic illness
    Lack of knowledge
- Knowledge Deficit related to normal physiologic sexual responses
- Body Image Disturbance related to
    Fear of rejection
    Negative feelings about the body
- Self Esteem Disturbance related to shame and guilt

---

of sexual practices, providing anticipatory guidance for times of altered sexuality patterns, education about various aspects of sexuality, counseling about adapting to changes in usual sexual function, and consultation and referral for more intensive sex therapy (Bancroft, 1989).

Framework for Providing Sexual Care

Sexual care occurs at various levels, determined by the nurse's background and expertise and the origin and severity of the sexual problem of the client. Sexual problems range from those involving gender identity, such as hermaphroditism and transsexualism, to those resulting from misinformation, confusion about the normal sexual response cycle, and minor sexual dysfunctions. The PLISSIT model (Annon, 1976) is a helpful tool to use when providing nursing care for sexuality problems (see Nursing Guidelines: Using the PLISSIT Model).

Knowledge Problems. Lack of knowledge and misinformation are the most common and simple types of sexual problems that occur. Couples may be unaware of altered sexual functions, have the idea that sex might cause injury, or think that oral sex causes an infection.

Fears created by minor unpleasant symptoms may lead to avoidance of sex. The common symptom of painful intercourse can be due to vaginitis causing perineal or vulval irritation or insufficient vaginal lubrication. These usually can be alleviated with medical treatment, explanation of physiologic causes of the pain, and teaching techniques to increase comfort.

Couples need specific information about sex. The couple's own comfort and desires are their best guide when there is no physical problem or contraindication.

Relationship Problems. Communication problems between the partners are the most common types of relationship problems. Sending and receiving messages between people are highly complex symbolic processes. Consequently, people often experience garbled messages and lack of communication.

Good communication regarding sexual needs and preferences is even more difficult than in most interpersonal situations. Some people find it hard to talk about their own sexual feelings or to accept criticism or suggestions regarding sexual performance.

Open and candid discussion of sexual preferences between partners can often dramatically improve satisfaction, but fears about propriety, hurting the other's feelings, not knowing how to say it, or being embarrassed can prevent this communication.

The first step in dealing with common sexual problems is to encourage the couple to talk with each other

> **NURSING GUIDELINES**
> *Using the PLISSIT Model*
>
> **P** *Permission*—Give the client or couple permission to bring up sexual concerns by communicating willingness to discuss these. An opening might be "people often have questions about sexuality practices and dysfunction. Do you have any concerns about this?"
>
> **LI** *Limited information*—Provide well-focused, brief information about changes that can affect sexual functioning and feelings.
>
> **SS** *Specific suggestions*—Provide specific information, instructions or ideas that can help alleviate problems or enhance sexual functioning, such as changes in coital position or techniques.
>
> **IT** *Intensive therapy*—Refer clients or couples who need additional help to an appropriate professional, such as a psychologist, sex counselor, marriage and family counselor, or other specialist.

about what they like and do not like in sex. If they can settle on practices that are comfortable and enjoyable to both of them, often the problem is resolved.

Many other factors can complicate communication about sexual experiences, however. Sex often has a hidden agenda that might involve struggling for power, using sex for manipulation, expressing anger through sexual behaviors, or validating or invalidating male and female sexual roles. Such feelings, whether or conscious or subconscious, can interfere with giving freely to the sexual experience and can lead to sexual dysfunctions.

Problems in the couple's relationship must be worked out before the sexual problem can be resolved. If the nurse is skilled in family or marital counseling, she or he is able to deal with these relationship problems. Because sexual difficulties are part of the symptomatology, it is frequently necessary for the nurse-counselor to have an understanding of sexual physiology and be familiar with basic sex therapy techniques to provide effective care.

Attitude Problems. Attitudes toward sexuality and the sexual self are established through internalized beliefs and values, originating from earliest childhood. They often are rooted in the unconscious levels of the psyche.

The underlying mechanism in the majority of sexual dysfunctions is fear. Whether this fear has its origins in sociocultural values, religious inhibitions and guilt, negative early experiences, familial patterns of dominance and discipline, or temporary functional failures of performance, it is the catalyst that sets into motion the psychodynamics that produce the sexual problem. Fear of inadequacy in sexual performance is the most

significant deterrent to effective sexual functioning because it completely distracts the person from natural responsiveness by blocking reception of sexual stimuli. Both partners may become self-conscious, worrying about their own and each other's sexual performance (Masters et al., 1994).

Specific therapeutic approaches have been developed to help people with sexual problems. These range from intensive residential sexual therapy to short-term behavior modification. Frequently, a process of reeducation is used to modify negative attitudes and counteract inhibitive beliefs. These approaches, combined with effective teaching techniques for sexual stimulation, have a reasonably good success rate.

When deep anxieties, unresolved guilt or conflict, or other psychopathology are present, the person usually receives psychotherapy aimed at the specific problem. Many sex therapists prefer not to explore old conflicts but focus on changing the problematic behavior with a variety of sexual and behavioral techniques. Removal of the symptom often brings immediate relief and may result in satisfactory long-term functioning without the need for extensive insight therapy.

Nurses have become involved in this type of sex therapy after receiving additional education in human sexuality and training in specific techniques for treating sexual problems. This level of sexual counseling is specialty practice often provided by a team, using the cotherapist approach (one therapist of each sex) in an extensive program involving education, attitude change, setting a permissive environment for sexual experiencing, marital counseling or psychotherapy, and appropriate techniques of sex therapy. The scope of nursing practice usually does not include this kind of sexual therapy, unless the nurse has been specially trained and works in a setting that provides these services.

Evaluation

Progress is assessed frequently. It is often necessary to alter approaches, try new approaches, or examine what factors are interfering with satisfactory resolution of the problem. Simple sexual problems may resolve surprisingly rapidly by providing accurate information and altering the context in which sexual activity occurs. However, there may be more deep-seated difficulties, and dealing with an apparently simple problem may reveal conflicts that require specialty referral.

Possible anticipated outcomes for the client with sexuality problems may include the following:

■ The client or couple verbalizes knowledge of the normal physiologic sexual responses.
■ The client or couple seeks therapy or counseling for persistent sexual problems.

- The client or couple identifies positive changes in sexual practices and behavior.
- The client or couple demonstrates ability to communicate openly and honestly about sexuality.

Sexual Health During Childbearing

Sexual expression during childbearing is influenced by physical and emotional changes and beliefs about sex during pregnancy. Difficulties can arise as a result of myths, misconceptions, and a lack of understanding of the physiology and emotional dynamics of couples during pregnancy. Most couples have many questions about sexual activities and their sexual responses during pregnancy. They appreciate the opportunity to discuss these questions. This can prepare them for possible reactions and prevent conflicts in their relationship due to misunderstandings of the physiologic changes and psychodynamics.

The first few months postpartum involve significant change and adaptation for both partners. Partners often experience self-doubt and decreasing self-esteem during the postpartum period, feeling tired, overwhelmed, ignorant, and depressed. Marital difficulties often begin concerning sexuality during the early months after the birth of the first child. The nurse can assist couples to prevent or deal with potential conflicts in their sexual relationship. Understanding and accepting the physiologic and neurohormonal bases for many of the changes in the woman's sexuality may enable the couple to adapt successfully and find satisfying sexual expressions during the postpartum phase.

Nursing Assessment

Assessment of the childbearing client or couple usually begins with the first prenatal visit. During this time, it is important for the nurse to obtain a history of the client's and couple's sexual health. Although the sexual history includes the areas addressed for any client, the nurse must keep in mind the effect of childbearing on sexual expression (see Assessment Tool: Sexual History During Pregnancy).

Nursing Diagnoses

Possible examples of nursing diagnoses related to sexuality during childbearing may involve dysfunction, fear, knowledge, and hormonal changes affecting desire. For a list of possible nursing diagnoses, see Box 9-3.

ASSESSMENT TOOL
Sexual History During Pregnancy

These questions about sexual experiences and concerns can be included as part of the prenatal health history. Most questions are appropriate for both partners, and a joint history-taking session is recommended.

1. How does the pregnancy make you feel?
2. How do you feel about changes in appearance and emotions?
3. How do you feel about each other's experience of the pregnancy?
4. What are your feelings about sex during pregnancy?
5. Has the pregnancy made many changes in your life or in your sexual relationship?
6. How do you think having a baby will change your life? How do you plan to manage these changes?
7. What have you heard about what you should or should not do sexually during pregnancy?
8. Do you feel any different physically now than before you were pregnant? In what ways? What medications do you take? Have you had any recent changes in your health?
9. Are there any concerns or worries about your sexual relationship during pregnancy or afterward?

Nursing Planning and Intervention

Throughout the childbearing process, the nurse performs client education and counseling. Physiologic and psychological aspects of pregnancy are discussed. In addition, any concerns can be addressed.

Common Sexual Concerns During Pregnancy and Postpartum

A wide range of sexual issues may confront couples during pregnancy. Sexual problems of a dysfunctional nature include dyspareunia (painful intercourse), changing and conflicting sexual drives, and male erectile dysfunction. Other issues may relate to lack of sexual desire, breast-feeding and erotic response, and lack of arousal or dyspareunia during the postpartum period. As many as 50% of American couples are estimated to have a sexual dysfunction (Dunnihoo, 1992).

> **BOX 9–3**
> *Nursing Diagnoses*
> _____
>
> - Altered Sexuality Patterns related to
>   Fatigue or discomfort
>   Anxiety and fear about harming the fetus
>   Body changes associated with pregnancy or postpartum
> - Sexual Dysfunction related to
>   Altered body structure
>   Lack of knowledge about pregnancy and sex
>   Diminished vaginal secretions
>   Conflicting sexual drives
> - Knowledge Deficit related to effects of pregnancy on sexual functioning
> - Body Image Disturbance related to pregnancy or postpartum changes

Lack of Sexual Desire and Avoidance of Sex. **Sexual desire**, or the interest in and frequency of sex, varies greatly among people. When sexual desire is persistently low or inhibited, such that it interferes with the sexual relationship, it becomes a sexual dysfunction (Hyde, 1990; Byer et al., 1988). People with low sexual desire usually avoid situations that evoke sexual feelings. When in a sexually arousing situation, they often feel little sexual response or may have negative, unpleasant feelings. Low sexual desire is an increasingly frequent disorder and may be the most common sexual dysfunction.

Fears about harming the fetus or mother may cause some couples to avoid intercourse during pregnancy. Previous birth of an abnormal baby may underlie these fears. Sexual desire may be diminished in either partner by physical and emotional changes of pregnancy and the postpartum period. For couples accustomed to regular intercourse, prolonged abstinence can cause conflicts or emotional distress.

Treatments focus on identifying the cause of low sexual desire and alleviating it when possible. This may involve short-term sex therapy, counseling, or psychotherapy. When discrepancy of sexual desire occurs, treatment includes recognition and acceptance of differences, adapting sexual practices to meet each partner's needs, and counseling for relationship problems.

Nursing intervention includes correcting misinformation about dangers to the fetus or mother and education about changes of pregnancy and the postpartum period. The nurse should encourage discussion of sexual needs and assist the couple with finding sexual practices that are satisfying to both. Intercourse poses no problems even in late pregnancy if there are no complications. Once membranes have ruptured or labor has begun or if vaginal bleeding occurs, intercourse should be avoided to prevent the possibility of orgasm initiating uterine contractions. These couples also should be counseled to avoid oral or manual stimulation that can produce orgasm and initiate premature contractions.

Changes in Sex Drive. Alterations in the woman's sexual responsiveness are common during pregnancy and are vastly different from woman to woman. In early pregnancy, some women experience a heightened sensuality, enjoying sex more and seeking it frequently. Their general level of sensuousness may increase with heightened awareness and responsiveness to stimuli. Other women have decreased sex drive during the first 2 to 3 months of gestation, often because of nausea, bloating, breast soreness, fatigue, and the many other physical changes that occur during pregnancy.

As pregnancy reaches its midpoint, heightened sexuality becomes more common. Many women report an increase in erotic feelings and more interest in sex. Some even report experiencing their first orgasm. Some of this could be explained by the physiologic changes of pregnancy, including increased pelvic vascularity and vasocongestion, which promote building an effective orgasmic platform.

Expectant fathers also experience psychologic processes in pregnancy resembling those of the mother. Fathers may have physical symptoms, alternating periods of emotional stability and well-being and times of anxiety, unexplained fears, and compulsions.

As pregnancy progresses, couples experience changes in body image and self-concept. Most couples find pleasure in these changes and enjoy an expanded sense of self. Sometimes these physical changes of pregnancy can contribute to a negative self-concept or negative body image, which can lead to altered sexual responses or dysfunctions. The woman's emotional lability and fluctuating sexual responses during this time may be confusing to her and her partner.

During the first trimester, several physiologic changes in the woman also affect the sex drive, generating fears and anxieties regarding intercourse: feelings of pelvic fullness and twinges of round ligaments that sometimes cause discomfort during intercourse; occasional spotting, which is common; and different sensations experienced in response to deep penile penetration due to the enlarging soft uterus. Preoccupation with these discomforts, fear, and feelings of different sensations may lead to unpredictable changes in sexual desire and decreased orgasmic response. If there are too many changes from what is usual, both partners may become concerned.

Interventions include educating couples about the following:

- Normal physiologic changes
- Anticipated alterations in sexual response
- Intercourse posing no threat to pregnancy under normal circumstances
- Continuation of their usual sexual activity if there are no pathophysiologic problems

Different techniques of sexual stimulation and orgasmic release for either partner can be used during pregnancy. Sexual techniques may need to be modified because of the increased sensitivity of the woman's breasts and genitals. As the woman's secretions increase and change in character, she should be instructed that maintaining daily hygiene can avoid unpleasant accompanying odors. Vaginal infections, which are common during pregnancy, also can cause irritation and odor. The nurse can provide information about the prevention and treatment of vaginal infections as prescribed by the physician or midwife.

In the second trimester, early in the fourth month, the uterus enlarges rather rapidly and becomes an abdominal organ rather than a pelvic organ. As the abdomen rapidly enlarges, concerns often arise about crushing the fetus during intercourse. There is no danger that this will happen because the fetus is well protected by the uterus and abdominal wall. The enlarging uterus can get in the way about the fifth month if the partners assume face-to-face, prone, and supine positions for intercourse. Modifications in positioning may be needed. As the uterus grows larger, the expectant mother is usually much more comfortable lying on her side, with her uterus supported by a pillow. If she is on her back for any length of time, with the enlarged uterus pressing on the abdominal aorta and the vena cava, she may experience hypotension and lightheadedness. Using a pillow under the hips during intercourse can be helpful to avoid hypotension.

Stress incontinence of urine (losing urine with coughing, sneezing, or orgasm) may occur because the uterus is pressing on the bladder. Some women might confuse this with loss of amniotic fluid and become frightened during intercourse.

Vaginal spotting after intercourse may be related to cervicitis or cervical friability. Although some spotting during pregnancy is normal, spotting and bleeding *can* signal spontaneous abortion and should be evaluated.

During the third trimester, the uterus is distended, and there is increasing pelvic and perineal pressure. Backaches, leg cramps, and shortness of breath may increase the woman's discomfort. Vaginal secretions are increased, and some discharge of colostrum from the nipples may occur. Many couples find intercourse difficult and uncomfortable toward the end of the pregnancy. They may substitute other forms of sexual expression, such as oral or manual sex, caressing, and holding.

Dyspareunia During Pregnancy. **Dyspareunia** (painful intercourse) during pregnancy can be caused by a number of factors. Pressure on the pregnant abdomen may cause a generalized discomfort. Deep penile thrusting may be painful in the presence of pelvic congestion, when the presenting part is deep in the pelvis, or when positions are assumed that exaggerate pressure. Although vaginal secretions are increased during pregnancy, in some instances, there may be a relative lack of lubrication because of inadequate stimulation, which leads to discomfort during intercourse. Irritation of the perineum or introitus, secondary to vaginitis, causes burning or pain on penetration and during intercourse. Cramps and backache may occur after coitus as the result of increased vasocogestion of sexual arousal combined with that of pregnancy. Orgasm may initiate Braxton Hicks contractions, which may continue and cause considerable pain. Aching postcoital pain may result from lack of orgasm to assist removal of the pelvic congestion associated with plateau levels of sexual arousal. If the woman experiences conflicts about having intercourse while pregnant, there may be a psychological overlay with the dyspareunia.

Male Erectile Dysfunction During Pregnancy. Almost all men, at one time or another, fail to have an erection during a sexual encounter. However, this does not indicate significant dysfunction. It is usually connected with being upset, tired, or preoccupied or having too much alcohol. Occasionally, men are unable to attain or maintain an erection during their partner's pregnancy. This is a type of secondary erectile dysfunction. It may be a situational phenomenon with no long-term repercussions, or it may indicate a more significant psychological problem with sexual dysfunction. As men experience emotional upheavals during pregnancy, they may at certain times, because of psychological processes, be disinterested in sex. For some men, a reawakening of maternal relationships and the projection of this relationship onto their pregnant wife create conflicts interfering with erotic response. If the woman's body is perceived as unattractive, sexual arousal may be blocked. This also may occur when the man fears injuring the mother or fetus or if he is feeling a close identification with his partner in vicariously experiencing the pregnancy.

Inability to attain erection on occasion during pregnancy does not indicate a significant sexual problem. Expectations of male performance create enormous pressures on men and often exaggerate fears of inadequacy. This further interferes with sexual arousal, perpetuating the difficulty in having or maintaining erections. A man is considered to have significant erectile dysfunction when he cannot achieve penile erection in 25% of his sexual attempts (Masters et al., 1994).

Breast-Feeding and Erotic Response. The sexual response involving the breasts may cause problems for some couples. The contractile tissues that surround the milk ducts are stimulated during orgasm. Sexual stimulation leading to tissue contraction may produce a "let down" reflex, causing milk to leak or spurt. If this is a concern to the couple, the woman can wear a bra with absorbent pads and avoid pressure on the breast. Breast tenderness also can be a problem during the postpartum period. This is a temporary condition, and the couple can avoid breast stimulation until the soreness subsides.

Another relatively common occurrence is sexual arousal in response to the baby's sucking. This may range from pleasant, mild excitation to orgasm. If women are aware that this is a normal response, they may become comfortable with this experience. However, some women discontinue breast-feeding because they do not feel comfortable with these responses. Women who breast-feed also tend to resume intercourse sooner postpartum than those who do not, presumably because of the increased eroticism associated with breast-feeding.

Postpartum Dyspareunia or Lack of Arousal. During the first 6 months after delivery, the vagina does not lubricate well because of relatively low levels of steroid hormones, which inhibit the vasocongestive response to sexual stimulation. Also, 3 to 6 weeks are needed for healing after childbirth, including the episiotomy; cervical, vaginal, or perineal lacerations; and the site of placental attachment. Couples are usually advised to resume intercourse by the third or fourth postpartum week if the bleeding has stopped and the episiotomy is not painful. Their own comfort and sexual desires are used as the guide for resuming intercourse if there are no contraindications.

Women may be concerned about their lack of sexual response in the months after childbirth. Considering their mothering responsibilities, with the lack of sleep, fatigue, and juggling of activities usually involved, it is not surprising that sexual interest might be low even without the additional factor of the physiologic changes after delivery. Understanding this may alleviate fears and enable women to wait until their hormonal and physical status is fully restored. Residual tenderness of the perineum or vagina also can contribute to painful intercourse and to a lack of interest in sex. Vaginitis resulting from low estrogen levels can create further problems with dyspareunia. Some women believe that pregnancy, labor, and delivery cause damage to the woman's genitalia, which will

permanently affect intercourse. Painful intercourse and lack of arousal during the postpartum period can be taken as evidence that these fears have been realized. The couple needs instruction to assist them with understanding the physiologic processes of childbirth and postpartum and their temporary effects on sexual functioning.

Evaluation

Anticipated outcomes for the client or couple experiencing problems with sexual health during childbearing include the following:

- The couple identifies constructive ways of coping with the effects of pregnancy on sexual health.
- The couple verbalizes concerns and experiences about pregnancy and sexuality.
- The couple identifies acceptable variations and modifications in sexual practices.
- The couple verbalizes satisfaction with sexual activity.

Family Planning

Assisting the couple to select and use an effective contraceptive method is an important nursing function. The nurse must understand his or her own philosophy and beliefs about contraception to avoid presenting biased information. Highly effective contraceptives are available. However, all involve some risk, and their effectiveness may be lowered by inappropriate use.

The ideal contraceptive is 100% safe and 100% effective, inexpensive, simple to use and understand, not directly connected to intercourse, totally reversible at any time, and readily available. No contraceptive method meets all these criteria. Despite the risks involved, people desire the benefits of reproductive choice and must therefore make decisions about methods based on personal values and a full understanding of the risks and benefits involved.

American women, regardless of religious affiliation, approve of and use contraception (Harlap et al., 1991). Having fewer children puts less strain on the family's resources and enhances the family's opportunities for economic and personal advancement.

A well-informed public, supported by changing social values that encourage individual choice and smaller family sizes, expects access to professional advice and contraceptive methods as an integral part of healthcare services.

Motives for contraceptive use are unique. The choice of method and its meaning are individual. Therefore, differences must be respected by the nurse, and the full range of contraceptive possibilities needs to be discussed with each client so that a fully informed and satisfactory choice can be made.

Nursing Assessment

Because family planning deals with sexuality, a private setting is best. Feelings about contraception are explored in a nonjudgmental way. Choices should be summarized to allow the client a method that fits his or her unique circumstances. There is no "best method" of contraception, but there is always a method that can work best in the circumstances at hand.

The choice of a suitable contraceptive depends on factors that can change frequently. These factors include expense, bathroom facilities, frequency of intercourse, sexual practices, number of children, the risk of pregnancy the couple is willing to accept, illness, and physical problems.

Nursing assessment covers the client's knowledge, understanding, and experience using various birth control methods. Information is gathered about general health, menstrual and reproductive histories, sexual patterns, family structures and relationships, and other significant demographic or socioeconomic information. Laboratory work is indicated when the method of choice is sterilization, **intrauterine device** (IUD), or hormonal contraceptives.

Pregnancy prevention ideally involves the participation of male and female partners. This provides an opportunity for the man to share responsibility for fertility control. The discussion includes methods that require the man to assume responsibility, such as a vasectomy, condoms, or symptothermal method.

History

The contraceptive database includes family history, personal health history, menstrual and pregnancy history, and previous contraceptive use.

Family History. Information about diabetes, bleeding or clotting problems, heart problems or high blood pressure, migraine headaches or seizure disorders, kidney or liver disease, anemia, tuberculosis, stroke, cancer, or mental problems should be obtained. This information provides a baseline about diseases for which the client may be at risk. It also helps to identify contraindications to specific methods, especially when hormonal contraceptives are being considered.

Personal Health History. Information about whether the woman has had the problems previously listed, previous hospitalizations, operations, major illness, and current medication use is necessary. Endocrine, cardiovascular clotting problems, migraines, and seizures may contraindicate hormonal contraceptives. Nutritional status and allergies also may affect contraceptive choice.

Menstrual History. Information about menarche, current menstrual pattern problems or concerns, and medication use is collected. Dysmenorrhea and heavy menses may be aggravated by the IUD; oligomenorrhea or hypomenorrhea may contraindicate hormonal methods.

Pregnancy History. Any complications or abnormalities are noted, because these may affect contraceptive use. Women with few pregnancies usually want readily reversible methods. Those with several pregnancies may consider long-term methods or sterilization.

Previous Contraceptive Use. Previous use of and experience with contraceptives are important. Methods that were unsuccessful or created problems or side effects would probably be poor choices unless these were incorrectly used.

To help gather this important information, the nurse can use specific questions to guide the client history (see Assessment Tool: Client History and Contraceptive Selection).

Physical Examination

A focused physical examination is guided by contraceptive choices and positive responses from the history. Breast examination, pelvic examination, a Papanicolaou (Pap) smear, and blood pressure check are usually included. A more thorough physical examination is necessary when hormonal contraceptives, IUD, cervical cap or diaphragm, or sterilization are considered as methods of contraception. The areas covered in physical examination include the following:

- Vital signs: blood pressure, pulse
- Appearance: weight, age
- Head and neck: eyes, thyroid gland
- Chest: lung fields, heart, breasts
- Abdomen: organs, masses, large vessels
- Pelvic: vulva, vagina, cervix, uterus, tubes, ovaries
- Rectal: sphincter tone, masses
- Extremities: varicosities, pulses, circulation
- Skin: lesions, color, pigmentation

Findings and abnormalities in the physical examination that contraindicate or affect use of particular types of contraceptives are described in Table 9-1.

Laboratory Tests

Laboratory tests generally include the following:

- Pap smear (screens for cervical cancer)
- *Chlamydia* and gonorrhea cultures when indicated
- Urinalysis (screens for diabetes, urinary tract infections [UTIs], kidney function)

ASSESSMENT TOOL
Client History and Contraceptive Selection

Question	Rationale
■ When did menarche occur, and have menses been irregular or skipped?	■ Late menarche and irregular menses indicate a possible endocrine abnormality. Therefore, hormonal contraceptives are not used until endocrine status has been investigated.
■ Are menstrual periods heavy with clotting and cramping?	■ The intrauterine device worsens these problems; oral contraceptives improve them. However, extremely heavy flow, particularly in women older than 30 years, needs investigation before the oral contraceptives are prescribed. The diaphragm may be a better choice.
■ Is there a history of severe migraine, cerebral arterial insufficiency, cardiovascular disease, liver disease, severe diabetes, genital or breast cancer, thrombotic problems, high blood pressure, or a family history of stroke?	■ These diseases and disorders are all contraindications for hormonal contraceptives.
■ What type of contraceptive was used before? Was it effective, or did a pregnancy occur?	■ Information is gained here about the probability of the successful use of certain contraceptive methods, and some idea is provided about the client's level of knowledge and understanding of these methods.
■ What are the most important reasons for contraceptive use?	■ This question helps the nurse assess the presence of realistic or unrealistic expectations that can be cleared in discussion. The client is helped to understand the practical benefits of contraception. Goals and priorities can be identified. If the woman feels strongly that pregnancy must be prevented, a highly effective method is indicated. If delay or spacing of pregnancy is actually the goal and the woman is concerned about any alterations in her body physiology and functions, a method with somewhat greater pregnancy risk but no systemic or local alterations would be more appropriate.

■ Complete blood count (rules out anemia and systemic infection gives indication of the condition of the platelets)

■ Liver enzymes (when indicated, impaired liver function, absolute contraindication to oral contraceptives [OCs])

■ Venereal Disease Research Laboratories or other serologic test for syphilis

Other laboratory tests might include a lipid profile if there is cardiovascular risk, hemoglobin electrophoresis if there is risk of hemoglobinopathies, glucose screening to test for diabetes, rubella screening, and herpes smear if indicated.

Nursing Diagnoses

After a thorough assessment, appropriate nursing diagnoses can be identified. See Box 9-4 for a list of possible nursing diagnoses.

Nursing Planning and Intervention

The nursing plan is based on the diagnoses. Intervention focuses on assisting the client or couple through the decision-making process in selecting an appropriate contraceptive method. Knowledge deficits are remedied through teaching about various contraceptives and correcting misinformation as needed. Deci-

TABLE 9-1
Physical Examination Abnormalities Affecting Contraceptive Use

Area Examined	Findings	Disease or Problem
Eyes	Narrow anterior chamber	Glaucoma
	Cupped disks, cup-disk radio abnormalities	Glaucoma
	Arteriolar narrowing, venous nicking	Hypertension, arteriosclerotic vascular disease
	Retinal exudates, hemorrhages	Diabetes, retinal disease
Thyroid	Nodules	Neoplasm
	Diffuse enlargement	Hypothyroidism or hyperthyroidism
Lungs	Crackles, wheezes	Asthma, chronic obstructive pulmonary disease, infection
Heart	Murmurs, arrhythmias	Cardiac disease
Breasts	Masses, lumps, nodules	Neoplasm, fibrocystic breast disease
	Nipple discharge	Neoplasm, hormonal problem
Abdomen	Masses	Neoplasm
	Liver tenderness, enlargement	Hepatic adenoma, hepatitis
Skin	Mottled, brown discoloration	Chloasma
	Pimples, comedomes, cysts	Acne
Legs	Enlarged, tortuous veins	Varicosities
	Weak, absent pulses	Vascular disease
Pelvis	Pelvic relaxation	Cystocele, rectocele
	Small or large cervix	Anatomic variation, trauma
	Posterior cervix	Retroflexed uterus
	Cervical lesions	Neoplasm, infection
	Small or large uterus	Anatomic variation, many pregnancies (large)
	Cervical or uterine tenderness	Infection
	Uterine, ovarian, tubal mass	Neoplasm, infection
	Vaginal discharge, inflammation	Infection
Weight	Greater than 20% above ideal	Obesity
Age	Older than 35	Risk with hormonal methods

sional conflict is reduced by thorough discussion of the risks and benefits of each potential contraceptive choice. Fears need to be expressed, uncertainties clarified, and personal preferences identified. The effec-

BOX 9-4
Nursing Diagnoses

- Health Seeking Behaviors related to family planning
- Knowledge Deficit related to
  Mechanism of action, side effects, and possible complications
  Proper methods of insertion and care
  Reproductive anatomy and physiology
- Risk for Injury related to improper use of method
- Risk for Infection related to inadequate personal hygiene and care of device
- Decisional Conflict related to undesired consequences of contraceptive method
- Altered Sexuality Patterns related to
  Anxiety with using contraceptive method
  Interference with usual sexual practices
  Discomfort from contraceptive method

tiveness of a contraceptive method is of primary concern to clients and professionals. When counseling clients on effectiveness, nurses must be familiar with different effectiveness rates.

Maximal effectiveness is the method's effectiveness in preventing pregnancy under ideal conditions (ie, when it is completely understood and used perfectly). This is the method's lowest failure rate. If a pregnancy occurs, it is due to a failure of the method, not how it is being used. **Typical effectiveness** takes into consideration the method's effectiveness under actual use, in which some people use the method correctly and others use it carelessly or incorrectly. Typical effectiveness rates are lower, because the human error factor is included.

The nurse must avoid using maximal effectiveness figures for preferred contraceptive methods and typical effectiveness figures for methods not favored. This kind of action provides misleading data to the client and may be an attempt to influence choice. Ethical counseling requires consistency in presenting effectiveness data. Some nurses present both sets of figures, so the potential for error in use can be clearly assessed. Figures for maximal and typical effectiveness of common contraceptive methods are shown in Table 9-2.

In assisting clients to select a contraceptive method, the "best method" of contraception is one that a couple will use most consistently and correctly. This is often the one that feels most natural and comfortable. The Assessment Tool: Questions Regarding Contraceptive Effectiveness provides a guide to factors that might lower effectiveness. Any "yes" response indicates potential problems. The method with the fewest "yes" responses would be best for that couple.

Contraceptive Risk

There is a certain amount of risk in every contraceptive method, from the method or the risk of pregnancy due to contraceptive failure or misuse. The mortality associated with pregnancy is greater than that of any commonly used contraceptive method. Often the risk cannot be completely determined in advance. Although in many instances, contraindications can be identified for known health problems or personal characteristics. Still, an apparently healthy woman with no

TABLE 9-2
Effectiveness and Risks of Contraceptives and Pregnancies per 100 Women per Year

Method	Maximal Effectiveness	Typical Effectiveness	Continuing Pregnancies	Deaths due to Pregnancy	Deaths due to Contraception
No contraception			89–90	0.016	0
HORMONAL CONTRACEPTIVES					
Oral contraceptives (combined)	0.1–0.5	2–4	0.5	0	0.003
Low-dose oral progestin	1–1.5	5–10			
Injected progestogen (DMPA)	0.3	0.3			
Hormone implants (Norplant)	0.4	0.4			
INTRAUTERINE DEVICE					
IUD	0.8–2	5	3	0.001	0.001
BARRIER METHODS					
Diaphragm	2–3	13–19	12	0.002	0
Cervical cap*†	5–8	16–18			
Condom*	2–3	10–15			
Spermicides*	3	13–22			
Condom + spermicide	<1	5			
Vaginal sponge*†	5–8	16–28			
FERTILITY AWARENESS METHODS					
Rhythm (calendar)	10–14	21	25	0.005	0
Basal body temperature only	7	21			
Cervical mucus only	2	25			
STERILIZATION					
Laparoscopic tubal ligation	0–0.2	0.4	0.4	0	0.03
Vasectomy	0–0.1	0.15	0.15	0	0
OTHER					
Withdrawal*	3–16	15–25			
Early abortion‡	0	0	0	0	0.003

*Data on continuing pregnancies and deaths due to pregnancy are not available, but typical effectiveness figures indicate these would be in the range found for the diaphragm.

†Data are inadequate for accurate comparisons.

‡Abortion is not a method of contraception but is included here for comparison.

(After Hatcher, R. A., Stewart, F., Trussell, J., et al. [1990]. *Contraceptive technology 1990–1992* [15th ed.]. New York: Irvington Publishers; and Trussell, J. et al. [1990]. Contraceptive failure in the United States: An update. *Studies in Family Planning, 21,* 207.)

ASSESSMENT TOOL
Questions Regarding Contraceptive Effectiveness

Answer "yes" or "no."

1. Am I afraid of using this method of birth control? _____
2. Would I really rather not use this method? _____
3. Will I have trouble remembering to use this method? _____
4. Have I ever become pregnant while using this method? _____
5. Are there reasons why I will be unable to use this method as prescribed? _____
6. Do I still have unanswered questions about this method? _____
7. Has my mother, father, sister, brother, or a close friend strongly discouraged me from using this method? _____
8. Will this method make my periods longer or more painful? _____
9. Will prolonged use of this method cost me more than I can afford? _____
10. Is this method known to have serious complications? _____
11. Am I opposed to this method because of my religious beliefs? _____
12. Have I already experienced complications from this method? _____
13. Has a nurse or doctor already told me not to use this method? _____
14. Is my partner opposed to using this method? _____
15. Am I using this method without my partner's knowledge? _____
16. Will the use of this method embarrass me? _____
17. Will the use of this method embarrass my partner? _____
18. Will my partner or I enjoy sexual activity less because of this method? _____
19. Will this method interrupt love making? _____

Every "yes" response indicates a potential problem with this method of contraception. You will probably be most comfortable with the method getting the fewest "yes" responses.

---

major contraindications to a method can develop serious complications, some of which are life-threatening. Although the incidence of such complications is low, it is the client's right to be well informed about the risks, benefits, and effectiveness of all contraceptive methods.

When the client has experienced prior difficulties with certain methods, intervention focuses on the meanings attached and perceived reasons for problems. The client's health beliefs, values, fears related to physical or psychoemotional harm, and personal reactions to contraceptive experiences are explored. This process assists the client in clarifying values, understanding behaviors, and making personal choices that work better to achieve goals.

Informed Consent

The nurse often is responsible for obtaining informed consent for contraceptive methods or procedures. The important components in providing sufficient information for contraceptive choices include the following:

- Discussing the benefits and risks of each method
- Discussing alternatives, including abstinence and no method
- Supporting the client's rights and responsibility to ask questions about methods
- Explaining the use and results of each method
- Assuring the client that she (or the couple) may choose any method without jeopardizing their right to care

The nurse obtains the client's signature on a consent form, which contains an outline of these components and the information provided. This form must be witnessed by the person obtaining consent and another person of the client's choice.

Legally, the nurse must enter a record of the information covered in the client's chart and make some notation to document client understanding. Often, clients are asked to sign a statement such as, "I have read and discussed the above information about contraception (or the specific method), and I fully understand these points." The importance of a voluntary decision by the clients without coercion or professional bias is evident.

Informed choice is a safeguard for the client and a way of increasing proper contraceptive use. When the woman or couple fully understands the technique; has weighed the possible adverse effects against cost, convenience, and acceptability; and has made a choice based on the method that best meets their needs, the likelihood of discontinuation and misuse is reduced.

Further nursing interventions related to choice and use of specific contraceptive methods are discussed in the section entitled "Contraceptive Methods" later in this chapter.

Evaluation

Evaluation of the contraceptive plan involves observing for desired changes in knowledge, understanding, or behavior in the client. Often evaluation leads to another round of assessment, diagnosis, and planning as problems are refined and better understood.

The most basic level of evaluation is whether or not the client uses the selected method of contraception effectively. Prevention of pregnancy is the basic outcome criterion. Other levels of evaluation consider the client's satisfaction with the method, ease of use, compatibility with lifestyle, acceptability in relation to values and cost, response of sexual partner, and concern with side effects. If difficulties are experienced in any of these areas, the nurse reassesses the situation with the client or couple. A new diagnosis is made, and appropriate intervention is planned and evaluated.

Contraceptive Methods

Numerous types of contraceptive methods are available today. They include hormonal agents, IUDs, barrier methods, fertility awareness methods, sterilazation techniques, and other methods, such as withdrawal and postcoital contraception.

Hormonal Contraceptives

Contraceptives involving preparations of the hormones estrogen and progesterone are available in several delivery systems: OCs ("pills"), long-acting injections, and intradermal implants.

Oral contraceptives are hormonal agents consisting of a combination of estrogen and progestin or progestin alone. Primarily they act at the central nervous system level to inhibit ovulation by suppressing the *follicle-stimulating* hormone (FSH) and luteinizing hormone (LH). Secondarily, endometrial development, tubal motility, and cervical mucus are affected. Under the influence of progestin, the cervical mucus becomes thick, viscous, and unreceptive to spermatozoa.

About 10 million women in the United States and 56 million women worldwide use OCs. The lowest failure rate with consistent and accurate usage of pills is 0.1%. More typical failure rates of average users range from an overall 0.34% to 4.7% for younger users. There is a high attrition rate among pill users. Only 50% to 75% of women starting on OCs are still using them after 1 year. Most women discontinue OCs for nonmedical reasons. Many pregnancies occur after discontinuation because women fail to start other contraception. Because of high discontinuation rates, women starting OCs should be provided with a second method of contraception and encouraged to become familiar with it (Hatcher et al., 1990).

The OCs do not protect against human immunodeficiency virus (HIV) or other STDs. They may contribute to higher STD rates because barrier methods commonly are not used, and women may have increased sexual activity when protected from unwanted pregnancy. Although less gonococcal pelvic inflammatory disease (PID) is found among OC users, lower genital tract infections are more common, especially due to *Chlamydia trachomatis.*

Large number of OCs are available, with differing combinations of estrogen or progestin doses. There are three types:

■ Triphasics, which contain two to three different combinations of estrogen and progestin
■ Combination pills, which contain estrogen and progestin, available at the standard or low (micro) dosage
■ Progestin-only (minipills)

Triphasic Oral Contraceptives

Pills containing two to three different combinations of estrogen and progestins have been available in the United States since 1984. These pills usually increase progestin in three phases during the cycle, and some alter estrogen dosage as well. Triphasic OCs are available in 21- and 28-day regimens. Failure rates have been reported as somewhat higher than for low-dose combination pills (Hatcher et al., 1990). Triphasics have 12% to 20% lower progestin dose than combination pills. This causes fewer metabolic effects on lipids and fewer progestin side effects. They are promoted as more "physiologic" than combination pills, because they more closely approximate the natural hormonal pattern of women. Bleeding patterns may be improved, although spotting and breakthrough bleeding are common with triphasics.

Combination Oral Contraceptives

Combination OCs, containing continuous doses of estrogen and progestin, are available in 21- and 28-day packages. In the 21-day packs, a pill is taken each day for 3 weeks, followed by a week without any pills. In the 28-day pack, a pill is taken every day for 4 weeks, but only those taken during the first 3 weeks have active hormonal ingredients. The pills taken during the last week consist of lactose or ferrous sulfate but no hormones. The purpose of 1 week of nonhormonal pills is to keep the woman in the habit of taking a pill every day and in some instances, to provide an iron supplement for prevention from anemia. Approximately 2 or 3 days after the last pill containing hormone is taken, there is usually a "withdrawal" menstrual flow.

Side Effects and Contraindications. Because most serious side effects are due to estrogen, the trend has been toward reducing this hormonal agent from the original dosage of 80 to 100 mg to doses ranging from 20 to 50 mg. Pills containing 20 to 35 mg of estrogen are used most often. The many types of pills available allow the provider to individualize selection, considering relative estrogen potency and estrogenic and androgenic effects of progestin. Adjustments can be made for side effects that clients experience, such as fluid retention, spotting, and headaches.

Common estrogen-related side effects include breast tenderness, nausea, headaches, spotting, cyclic weight gain, missed periods, and changes in vaginal discharge. More serious estrogen effects include thrombotic and vascular diseases, liver disease, and changes in carbohydrate metabolism. The incidence of these problems is reduced with lower dose OCs and use of newer progestins with less androgenic and estrogenic effects.

Progestin-related side effects include progressive weight gain, depression, acne, oily skin, increased breast size, hair loss or growth, and changes in lipoprotein metabolism. Newer low-dose progestins are associated with improved lipid profiles (increased high-density lipoprotein [HDL] cholesterol), and OCs actually seem to protect against atherosclerosis (Darney, 1993; Godsland et al., 1990). Hypertension, myocardial infarction, and cervical dysplasia are more serious effects attributable to estrogenic and progestogenic components.

The most important risks for thromhotic and vascular diseases are smoking and age. Other risk factors include hypertension, hyperlipidemias, and diabetes. By restricting OC use in women older than 35 years who smoke, most OC-related deaths could be avoided (Darney, 1993; see Box 9-5) Contraindications to OCs include the following:

- Thrombophlebitis, thromboembolic disorders
- Cerebrovascular or coronary artery disease
- Malignancy of the breast or reproductive tract (estrogen-related neoplasia)
- Undiagnosed abnormal genital bleeding
- Marked impairment of liver function
- Pregnancy (known or suspected)

Caution and close follow-up are required when using OCs in women with migraines, hypertension, dia-

---

BOX 9-5
Cigarette Smoking and Hormonal Contraceptives

Oral contraceptives (OCs) in combination with cigarette smoking significantly increase a woman's risk of heart attack, stroke, and clotting problems. These are especially dangerous for women older than 35 years. Women who want to use OCs should discontinue smoking and avoid exposure to secondary smoke. If women continue to smoke, a hormonal method without estrogen is recommended, such as progestin-only pills, implants, or Depo-Provera.

Smoking among OC users has declined during the last decade from 31% to 24%, a rate slightly lower than smoking among women in general (28%). Weight, age, race, and education did not affect the decline in rates of smoking. Women most likely to smoke and use OCs are white, have less than 12 years education, and binge drink.

Smoking among contraceptive users, though declining, remains too high. Given the well-established, serious risk of cardiovascular events, health professionals must do everything in their power to get women using OCs to stop smoking.

Barrett, D. H., et al. (1994). Trends in oral contraceptive use and cigarette smoking. Archives of Family Medicine, 3, 438–443.

---

betes, gallbladder disease, sickle cell disease, and smoking, age (older than 35 years), and cardiovascular risk factors.

Progestin-Only Pills (Minipills)

Oral contraceptives containing only progestins have been available in the United States since 1973. Minipills use the same progestins as those in combination pills but in smaller doses. Their advantage is the avoidance of estrogen-related side effects and complications. Disadvantages include less predictable menstrual patterns and increased irregular bleeding.

Minipills prevent ovulation in only 15% to 40% of cycles. Thus, their contraceptive effect depends on other factors, such as unfavorable cervical mucus, inhibited sperm migration, disturbed endometrial development, and an inadequate luteal phase. Minipills are especially suited for women who are older than 35 years with a history of headaches or mild hypertension or for those who are lactating and experiencing estrogen-related side effects.

Because the progestin dose is low, excellent compliance in taking pills is necessary. Missing one or two tablets of progestin-only pills leads to a much higher risk of accidental pregnancy than with combination pills. Even with perfect compliance, failure rates are higher than those of combination pills. Pregnancies per

100 woman-years are reported at 0.5 to 3.7 in the United States, with higher rates in the first 6 months of use (Hatcher et al., 1990).

Side Effects and Contraindications. Undiagnosed vaginal bleeding is an important contraindication to minipill use. Other contraindications include acute mononucleosis or liver disease. The risk of an ectopic pregnancy also is greater when conception occurs. Because minipills contain no estrogen, theoretically they should not cause serious estrogen-related complications, such as thromboembolic disease and hypertension. However, data are not available to document this advantage (Hatcher et al., 1990).

Side effects include variations in cycle length (both shorter and longer), headaches, weight gain, breast discomfort, and nausea. Less hypertension, dysmenorrhea, and premenstrual syndrome are reported. The side effects of OCs according to excess or deficiency of hormones are shown in Table 9-3.

Different progestins affect lipid fractions in different ways. HDL levels may decrease, low-density lipoproteins (LDL) may increase, and very low density lipoproteins (VLDL) and triglycerides may increase or decrease. It is not clear whether these changes have clinical significance. Minipills have not been associated with an increase in cardiovascular risk (Youngkin, 1993).

Nursing Interventions

When OCs have been selected and a specific type of pill prescribed, nursing care focuses on providing information and education about effective use (Fig. 9-1). Education includes how to start taking the pills, how to develop a reliable routine for taking pills, what to do if pills are forgotten, how to assess spotting and determine when this becomes a problem that needs evaluation, common side effects, and more serious dangers that require immediate medical attention, including systemic effects (see Box 9-6). Women are advised to select and keep handy a backup method of birth control, such as condoms or foam. Women should be reminded that pills provide no protection against HIV and other STDs, and safe sex practices should be discussed. Written information, package inserts, and visual aids enhance the teaching–learning process.

Teaching clients the "ACHES" system of remembering early danger signs is an effective method. Some

---

TABLE 9–3
Hormonal Basis of Side Effects of Oral Contraceptives

Estrogen		Progestin		Androgen
EXCESS	**DEFICIENCY**	**EXCESS**	**DEFICIENCY**	**EXCESS**
Nausea, vomiting	Amenorrhea	Acne, oily scalp	Hypermenorrhea with clotting	Acne
Fluid retention (premenstrual tension, irritability, breast tenderness, corneal swelling, cramping, edema)	Oligomenorrhea	Increased appetite	Late-cycle spotting	Oily skin
	Early-cycle or mid-cycle spotting	Weight gain	Delayed onset of menses	Rashes
	Loss of pelvic tone	Fatigue	Dysmenorrhea	Increased hair growth in male pattern
Increased vaginal discharge	Hot flashes	Depression	Weight loss	Increased interest in sex
Chloasma	Nervousness, irritability	Hair loss		Cholestatic jaundice
Headaches	Decreased interest in sex	Headaches when not taking pills		Increased appetite
Increased breast size		Increased breast size		Pruritus
Weight gain		Increased muscle mass		
Increased cervical ectropion		Increased monilial vaginitis (*Candida*)		
Increased size of fibroids		Breast tenderness not related to fluid retention		
Telangiectasia		Short menses		
Thromboembolic disorders		Relative endometrial atrophy		
Reduction of lactation		Decreased interest in sex		
Possible hypertension		Cholestatic jaundice		
Hepatic adenoma		Decreased carbohydrate tolerance		
		Dilated leg veins		

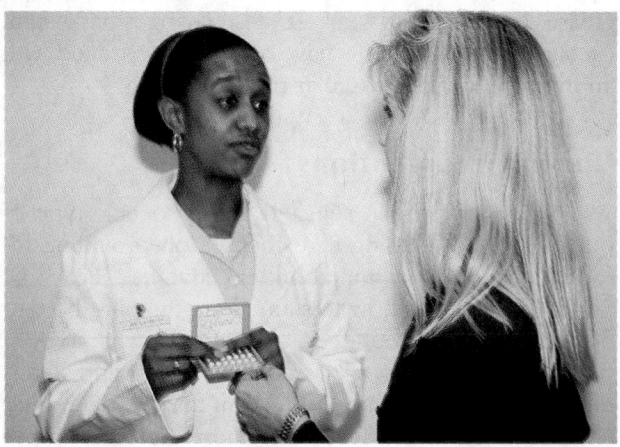

FIGURE 9-1 When the healthcare provider has prescribed a specific type of pill, the nurse should provide information and education about the oral contraceptive and how to effectively use it. During this time the nurse can answer any questions the client might have.

women may experience these symptoms for weeks or months before seeking help. Women should call the clinic or physician right away if any of these danger signals develop (see the Client Education: "ACHES" System: Oral Contraceptive Danger Signs).

A follow-up visit is usually scheduled for 3 to 4 months. Side effects are reviewed with special atten-

tion to headaches, blurred vision, chest pain, and leg pain. The client's experiences and practices using the pills are discussed, and questions are answered. Physical examination includes blood pressure and weight checks. If no difficulties are encountered, another 6-month visit is scheduled, then visits become annual with repeat of the pelvic examination, Pap smear, and breast examination.

Women using OCs who want to stop taking them to become pregnant are instructed on how to do this safely, using another reliable birth control method after stopping OCs until they have two or three normal menstrual cycles. There may be a 1- to 2-month delay in the resumption of menses and ovulation after discontinuing OCs. If pregnancy occurs before normal cycles have been established, it is difficult to assess fetal development accurately.

Norplant Implants

Norplant is a long-acting subdermal hormonal contraceptive approved by the Food and Drug Administration for use in the United States in 1991. The Norplant system consists of six Silastic membrane capsules, each containing 35 mg of levonorgestrel, a type of progestin. All six capsules are inserted subdermally in the woman's upper arm, providing effective contraception

---

BOX 9-6
Systemic Effects of Hormonal Contraceptives

Thrombotic and vascular disease: These are about four times as common in oral contraceptive (OC) users as nonusers, but risk depends largely on age and smoking. Most deaths are from myocardial infarction; fewer are from strokes.

Atherosclerotic cardiovascular disease: Higher doses of OCs have atherogenic effects (decreased HDL, increased LDL, increased blood pressure, decreased glucose tolerance). These do not persist when OCs are discontinued. OC users actually have less atherosclerosis than nonusers, despite lipid elevations during OC use.

Venous thrombotic disease: Although relatively common, venous thrombosis does not cause significant morbidity or mortality among OC users. The risk of venous thrombosis is three times greater in OC users but only 1 in 1,000 women seeks care for symptoms. Although higher dose OCs caused increased production of clotting factors, these effects do not persist after OC discontinuation, and the newer OCs do not have measurable effects on clotting parameters.

Liver disease: Liver enzymes may be increased with OC use, especially at higher doses. Women with impaired liver function or a tendency to form gall stones should avoid OCs. Benign liver adenomas were caused by earlier high-dose OCs but do not occur with low-dose preparations.

Lipoprotein metabolism: Estrogens increase and progestins decrease HDL. Low-dose OCs cause small increases in triglycerides and inconsistent minimal changes in HDL and LDL, which are not clinically significant. The newer progestins appear to have positive effects on lipids (increased HDL, decreased LDL).

Glucose metabolism: There is an initial (first 6 months) increase in insulin secretion with OCs, without an increase in glucose concentration. These changes normalize but do not reverse completely with long-term OC use. OCs do not cause diabetes nor exacerbate clinical disease in diabetic patients.

Cancer: OCs are not implicated in the great majority of cases of breast and cervical cancer. There does not appear to be an increased overall risk of breast cancer, although OCs may promote earlier development of breast cancer in some groups (young women, early menarche, long OC use before first pregnancy). OC users have a small decreased risk and lower death rate from postmenopausal breast cancer. OCs do not seem to increase risk or progression of cervical neoplasia but may combine with cofactors, such as multiple partners and papilloma virus exposure, to increase risk of dysplasia and subsequent cancer. OCs have a strong protective effect against endometrial cancer and decrease the risk of ovarian cancer significantly.

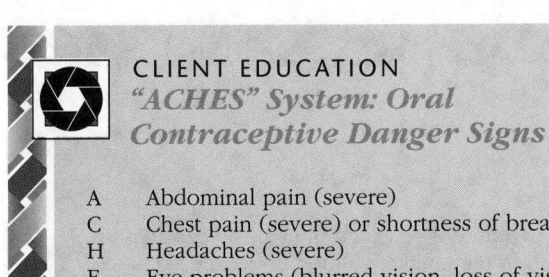

for up to 5 years. Levonorgestrel slowly diffuses through the slender, flexible capsules, providing a constant low dose of hormone. About 50 to 80 µg of the hormone is released daily for the first few weeks, decreasing to 30 to 35 µg daily over the next 2 to 6 months, and gradually reducing to 25 mg/d after 5 years (Franklin, 1990). The capsules are removed after 5 years or at any time the woman desires to reverse the contraceptive effect. Fertility returns to preinsertion levels shortly after the capsules are removed. The Client Teaching Guidelines: Insertion and Removal of Norplant Capsules provides information that the client may want to know about the procedure.

The Norplant system is highly effective in preventing pregnancy. The pregnancy rate for the first year is about 0.2%, with an annual rate of 0.8 per 100 users during 5 years of use. This rate is better than that for the low-dose OCs and approaches that of tubal sterilization, but Norplant is reversible. Pregnancy rates with Norplant gradually increase over 5 years to 2.5 to 3 pregnancies per 100 users. Women who weigh more than 154 lb are more likely to experience pregnancy; their annual pregnancy rate is 1.7 per 100 users over 5 years (Pollack, 1991).

This method is particularly suitable for women who desire long-term but reversible contraception. Good candidates include the following women:

- Have had children but do not want tubal sterilization
- Have had side effects with combined OCs
- Want to delay childbearing for several years but want a rapid return of fertility
- Have experienced contraceptive failure with other methods
- Have difficulty remembering to take daily pills
- Are lactating and at least 6 weeks postdelivery
- Are older than 35 years and smoke
- Are late in their reproductive years and prefer not to use an estrogen-containing method

Norplant's advantages include long-lasting effect, ease of reversibility, lack of interference with intercourse and estrogen side effects, high effectiveness, and no need for user's control. Its disadvantages include the necessity of insertion and removal, visibility under the skin, and menstrual irregularity.

As a progestin-only contraceptive, Norplant's modes of action include suppression of ovulation; thickening of cervical mucus; changes in the endometrium, making it unreceptive to implantation; and more rapid tubal transport of the ovum. With time, about 50% of women using Norplant will have some ovulatory cycles, but this does not increase their risk of pregnancy because of the additional modes of action.

About 80% of women with Norplant insertions continue this method after 1 year (Wehrle, 1994). One-third of women using Norplant complete 5 years; of these, 75% want a second Norplant system. Within 2 years after insertion, 60% of women are having regular cycles of bleeding (Cohall et al., 1993).

The most common side effect is menstrual cycle irregularities, which may include prolonged menstrual flow during the first months of use, bleeding or spotting between periods, or amenorrhea. These usually subside in 3 to 6 months, and a pattern of light and infrequent periods develops. About half of the women using Norplant have changes in their menstrual pattern during the first year, and 10% stop using the method because of this. On average, women continuing to use Norplant have 5 days of bleeding per month with less blood loss, but the bleeding pattern is more irregular.

Some women experience pain or discomfort with insertion and removal. Infection may occur at the insertion site, with expulsion of capsules. This is uncommon and usually associated with improper asepsis. Local reactions, including itching and pain, usually resolve within 1 month but may persist longer. Pregnancy is infrequent, but the capsules must be removed immediately if it does occur. There is no increase in the rate of ectopic pregnancies. No excess cardiovascular complications have been identified with Norplant.

Side Effects and Contraindications. Contraindications to Norplant include the following:

- Undiagnosed vaginal bleeding
- Active thrombophlebitis or thromboembolic disorders
- Pregnancy
- Liver disease
- Coronary artery or cerebrovascular disease
- Breast cancer

Medroxyprogesterone Acetate

Medroxyprogesterone acetate (Depo-Provera) was approved for contraceptive use in 1992. A long-acting injectable form of progesterone, Depo-Provera has been used worldwide for decades by more than 9 million women. Its effectiveness is comparable to that of steri-

CLIENT TEACHING GUIDELINES
Insertion and Removal of Norplant Capsules

Insertion

- Norplant capsules are 34 mm long and 2.4 mm wide, about the size of lead in a pencil.
- The inner surface of the woman's upper arm is used as the insertion site.
- Local anesthetic is injected into the skin at the insertion site in six lines at fanlike positions.
- A small (2-mm) incision is made in the skin with a scalpel, and a trochar is inserted just under the skin.
- The first capsule is inserted through the trochar; the trochar is withdrawn, leaving the capsule in place.

- This procedure is repeated until all six capsules are inserted in the fanlike position under the skin (see Figure).
- The incision is closed using a butterfly skin closure technique; suturing is not necessary.
- The insertion area is covered with a dry compress and gauze to aid in hemostasis.
- The bandage is removed in 3 days.
- The entire procedure takes about 10 minutes.

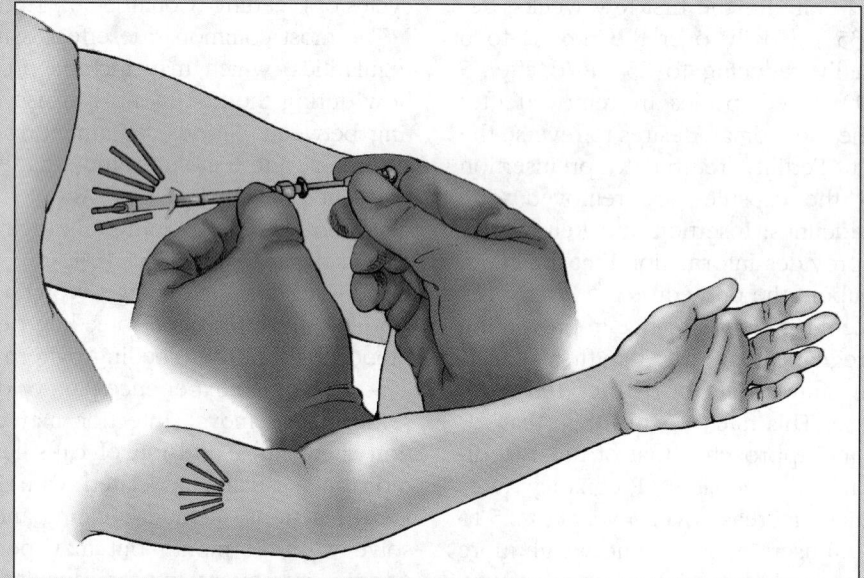

The insertion and placement of Norplant under the skin.

Removal

- A 4-mm incision is made near the end of the implants.
- The implants are pushed downward toward the incision until the ends can be grasped with mosquito forceps.
- The tissue capsule that has formed around the implant is opened with the scalpel, and the tip of

the implant is grasped with another forceps and gently pulled out.
- If the woman wants to continue using Norplant, new implants can be inserted through the same incision, but fanning in the other direction.

---

lization. Depo-Provera has almost immediate contraceptive effect after injection, preventing ovulation and thickening cervical mucus to produce a barrier to sperm penetration.

The contraceptive dose is 150 mg, regardless of weight. The injection is given within 5 days of the beginning of menses. After childbirth, it is given within 5 days of delivery. If the client is breast-feeding, it is given 6 weeks after childbirth. Depo-Provera does not interfere with milk production, and no harmful effects have been seen in children. If given during these times, contraceptive protection begins immediately. If given at any other time, a pregnancy test must be done before administering the injection.

Contraceptive effects last for 3 months. Another injection should be given within 14 weeks of the previous one. If more than 14 weeks since the prior injection, a pregnancy test is necessary. This method is particularly well-suited for the following women:

- Have difficulty remembering daily pills or with other methods
- Have completed childbearing but do not want sterilization
- Have contraindications to estrogen or OCs
- Have chronic health problems (sickle-cell disease, diabetes, renal disease, hypertension, seizure disorder)

- Take teratogenic medications (such as isotretinoin [Accutane]) and antiseizure drugs

Other benefits occur with Depo-Provera use. It reduces the risk of endometrial and ovarian cancer and may improve endometriosis. It decreases seizure activity and sickle cell crises.

Side Effects and Contraindications. The main side effects of Depo-Provera involve changes in menstrual cycles. Most women will have some amenorrhea, spotting, and irregular bleeding. It is impossible to predict which changes will happen in the first few months after injection. With continued use, bleeding usually decreases, with 55% of women having no menstrual bleeding after 1 year of use and 68% after 2 years of use (Depo-Provera Contraceptive Injection, 1993). Other minor side effects include weight gain (average 4 lb/y), hair loss or growth, nausea, dizziness, headaches, mood changes, and possible depression. Decreased libido is possible. An adverse effect on lipid profile, with decreased HDL and increased LDL, has been reported but usually is not clinically important for normal women. This method may not be a good choice for women with dyslipidemias. Cancer risk does not appear to be increased. Bone density may be reduced, but no clinical evidence of osteoporosis or fractures have been reported (National Institute of Child Health and Human Development, 1993).

The following are contraindications to Depo-Provera:

- Active thrombotic problems
- Active liver disease
- Undiagnosed vaginal bleeding
- Known or suspected pregnancy
- History of stroke, myocardial infarction, breast cancer

Caution is necessary when using Depo-Provera in women who have had severe depression. It is not a good choice for women who are distressed with irregular menses or amenorrhea. Because return to fertility is often delayed, women planning to conceive within 6 to 12 months should use another method. Most women will ovulate 9 to 10 months after the last injection. About 70% of women become pregnant within 1 year of stopping Depo-Provera; 85% become pregnant within 2 years. There are no permanent effects on the woman's ability to get pregnant (Cohall et al., 1993).

Systemic Effects of Hormonal Contraceptives

- Thrombotic and vascular disease: These are about four times as common in OC users as nonusers, but risk depends largely on age and smoking status.

Most deaths are from myocardial infarction; fewer are from strokes.
- Atherosclerotic cardiovascular disease: Higher doses of OCs have atherogenic effects (decreased HDL, increased LDL, increased blood ressure, decreased glucose tolerance). These do not persist when OCs are discontinued. OC users actually have less atherosclerosis than nonusers, despite lipid elevations during OC use.
- Venous thrombotic disease: Although relatively common, venous thrombosis does not cause significant morbidity or mortality among OC users. The risk of venous thrombosis is three times greater in OC users, but only 1 in 1,000 women seeks care for symptoms. While higher dose OCs caused increased production of clotting factors, these effects do not persist after OC discontinuation, and the newer OCs do not have measurable effects on clotting parameters.
- Liver disease: Liver enzymes may be increased with OC use, especially higher doses. Women with imparied liver function or tendency to form gall stones should avoid OCs. Benign liver adenomas were caused by high-dose OCs used in the past but do not occur with low-dose preparations.
- Lipoprotein metabolism: Estrogens increase and progestins decrease HDL. Low-dose OCs cause small increases in triglycerides and inconsistent minimal changes in HDL and LDL, which are not clinically significant. The newer progestins appear to have positive effects on lipids (increased HDL, decreased LDL).
- Glucose metabolism: There is an initial (first 6 months) increase in insulin secretion with OCs, without an increase in glucose concentration. These changes normalize but do not reverse completely with long-term OC use. OCs do not cause diabetes nor exacerbate clinical disease in diabetic clients.
- Cancer: OCs are not implicated in the majority of cases of breast and cervical cancer. The overall risk of breast cancer does not appear to be increased, although OCs may promote earlier development of breast cancer in some groups (young women, early menarch, long OC use before first pregnancy). OC users have a small decreased risk and lower death rate from postmenopausal breast cancer. OCs do not seem to increase risk or progression of cervical neoplasia, but may combine with cofactors, such as multiple partners and papillomavirus exposure, to increase risk of dysplasia and subsequent cancer. OCs have a strong protective effect against endometrial cancer and decrease the risk of ovarian cancer significantly.

Intrauterine Device

The IUD is a small, usually flexible appliance that is inserted by a healthcare professional into the uterine cavity. The use of foreign objects placed inside the uterus to prevent pregnancy is an ancient practice.

In the 1950s to 1960s, many IUDs were widely used in the United States; worldwide, about 85 million women use IUDs, 70% of whom are in China. In the early 1980s, 2.2 million women in the United States were using IUDS; about 10% of the reversible contraceptives in use. Since then, IUD use has dropped markedly. Less than 1% of women in the United States choose IUDs, although 98% of those using IUDs are satisfied with this method (Cohall et al., 1993).

Public and professional concern about the serious consequences of pelvic infections associated with IUD use led to withdrawal of many IUDs from the market. The IUD linked with the largest proportion of pelvic infections, subsequent infertility, and lawsuits was the Dalcon Shield. All women with Dalcon Shields have been advised by their producer, AH Robbins, to have these devices removed. In 1985, Robbins declared bankruptcy as a result of Dalcon Shield lawsuits. Pharmaceutical companies gradually discontinued production and sales of IUDs because of numerous lawsuits, declining market shares, liability insurance costs, and loss of profits.

Only two IUDs are now produced and distributed in the United States, the Progestasert and the Copper-T380A (Fig. 9-2). Some women still have older IUDs in place, such as the Lippes Loop.

IUDs prevent pregnancy mainly by preventing fertilization. They inhibit sperm motility and speed ovum tubal transport. Local inflammatory responses and production of prostaglandins disrupt endometrial enzymatic and hormonal activity. With progestin-containing IUDs, there also is endometrial suppression and production of thick cervical mucus that discourages sperm transport.

IUDs are slightly less effective than OCs. The lowest reported pregnancy rate with medicated IUDs (copper, progestin) is about 1%; it is 2% to 3% with unmedicated devices. The first-year failure rate of IUDs in typical users is 6%. Effectiveness depends on type of device, clinician experience with insertion, likelihood of expulsion, ability of the client to detect expulsion, frequency of intercourse, and the client's access to medical services.

The IUD offers continuous protection against pregnancy, does not require daily medication, and does not interfere with intercourse. IUDs can be inserted by the

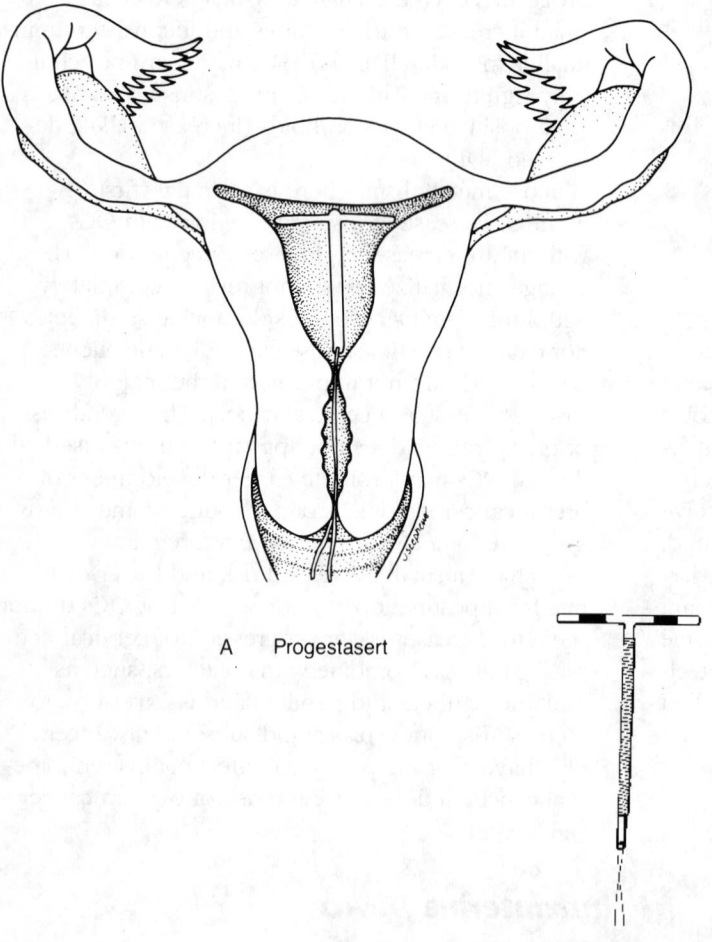

A   Progestasert

B   Copper T-380

FIGURE 9–2 (A) Progestasert-T IUD in place in the uterine cavity. (Childbirth Graphics, Rochester, NY.) **(B)** Copper T-380.

healthcare provider at any time during the menstrual cycle, once pregnancy has been excluded. They may be inserted immediately after an abortion. Contraceptive effects of the IUD are readily reversible once the device is removed. Because IUDs have no systemic hormonal effects, such as those created by OCs, women who are heavy smokers, are older than 35 years, or have histories of cardiovascular disease or diabetes may more safely use them for contraception.

Side Effects and Contraindications

Commonly reported side effects of the IUD include increased menstrual flow, dysmenorrhea, and intermenstrual spotting. Because flow is sometimes excessive, clients should be checked routinely for anemia. Iron supplementation is advisable for IUD users. About 10% to 15% of women have IUDs removed because of increased bleeding.

Pelvic infections can be a serious problem when an IUD is present. PID accounts for the majority of IUD-related deaths and hospitalizations. The IUD itself does not cause PID. Infection is caused by STDs. The IUD should be removed when infection occurs to reduce the risk of serious complications (Hatcher et al., 1990).

If pregnancy occurs when the IUD is in place, removal is recommended because of the increased danger of intrapartum infection and death from sepsis. The risk of spontaneous abortion is somewhat higher when the IUD remains in place (about 50%) than when it is removed when the pregnancy is discovered (25%). When the IUD is left in place during pregnancy, women have a 50-fold greater risk of dying from septic abortion. Flulike symptoms in a woman who becomes pregnant with an IUD in place usually indicate sepsis. Ectopic pregnancy is more common in women with Progestasert-T IUDs (16%–25% incidence compared with 3%–4% with other IUDs).

Another major complication is uterine perforation, which usually occurs when the IUD is inserted. When perforation occurs through the uterine wall into the abdomen, it is generally recommended that the IUD be removed. This can be done with a laparoscope.

Occasionally on insertion, the IUD may produce enough pain and vasovagal stimulation to result in syncope. The nurse should be aware of this complication and should be ready to place the client in a recumbent position if there are any signs of lightheadedness, sweating, or nausea.

About 5% to 20% of women spontaneously expel the IUD within the first year. Signs of expulsion include unusual vaginal discharge, cramping or pain, intermenstrual or postcoital spotting, or painful intercourse for either partner. The IUD string may become longer or the hard tip of the IUD may be felt at the cervical os. Most expulsions occur during menses and may not be noticed. If symptoms of pregnancy occur or the woman cannot find the IUD strings, she should be examined for expulsion. Partially expelled IUDs should be removed. Another IUD can be inserted; the Progestasert-T is a good choice because its progesterone diminishes uterine contractions.

The following are contraindications to IUDs:

- Risk for STD (multiple sexual partners)
- Active, recent, or chronic pelvic infection
- Postpartum endometritis or septic abortion
- Pregnancy
- Endometrial or cervical malignancy
- Valvular heart disease
- Impaired response to infection

Abnormalities of the uterus, such as myomas, polyps, or bicornuate uterus, make insertion difficult. In women with a small uterus (sounding to less than 6 cm) or with marked anteflexion or retroflexion, insertion, although more difficulty, may be accomplished with the smaller devices. Other considerations include severe dysmenorrhea, anemia, Rh-negative blood type, and concern for future fertility.

Nursing Interventions

Once an IUD has been inserted, nursing care focuses on education about signs of complications, side effects, and safety measures to lower risk of infection and pregnancy. The nurse teaches the women how to feel for IUD strings in the upper vagina or at the cervical os. Women are instructed to check the string frequently during the first several months after IUD insertion, right before intercourse, and after each period. Pads and tampons should be examined when removed for an expelled IUD. Backup contraception is advisable for the first month after IUD insertion. The nurse instructs the client in common side effects, which include increased menstrual flow and cramping and intermenstrual spotting. Progesterone IUDs may decrease menstrual flow and cramping.

Nurses should teach clients the "PAINS" system of recognizing early danger signs of the IUD (see Client Education: "PAINS" System: IUD Danger Signs). The physician or clinic should be contacted if any of these danger signs develop. Infection is most likely to occur in the first few weeks after IUD insertion. Nurses must emphasize the importance of immediately reporting symptoms of pain, bleeding, and discharge during this time. Uterine, tubal, or pelvic infections can pose a serious danger to the woman's future health.

The Copper-T IUD must be replaced every 4 years. The Progestasert-T must be replaced every 12 to 18 months. The Lippes Loop, which some women still have, can remain in place until menopause as long as there are no problems.

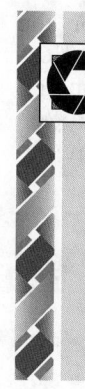

Women using an IUD are advised to wait 3 months after removal before becoming pregnant. This reduces the risk of ectopic pregnancy. Follow-up appointments are scheduled annually to evaluate the client's experience with the IUD and for health maintenance.

Diaphragm

The **diaphragm,** a dome-shaped rubber cap ranging in diameter from 7 to 10 cm, is inserted into the vagina, covering the anterior vaginal wall and cervix before intercourse and providing a vaginal barrier. It must be used with a spermicidal jelly or cream placed inside the diaphragm. The diaphragm holds the spermicidal jelly over the cervix.

When the diaphragm is properly used—each time intercourse occurs, without exception—it has a failure rate of about two pregnancies during the first year per 100 women. Typical use rates vary from 14 to 19 pregnancies per 100 women during the first year. This may be a result of inconsistent use, higher frequency of intercourse, inherent fertility of the couple, or motivation to avoid pregnancy. A diaphragm requires motivation and premeditation, but despite these drawbacks it has gained favor when the risks of hormonal methods and IUDs are compared.

Advantages of the diaphragm include safety, few side effects, and flexibility according to frequency of intercourse. Because it can be inserted up to 2 hours before sex, it is relatively separated from coitus. Once in place, it is unobtrusive because its presence cannot be felt by either partner if it is properly fitted, and less cream or jelly is left in the vagina than with a spermicide alone. Well-motivated women have used the diaphragm effectively to limit pregnancies since the end of the 19th century.

The diaphragm can be an excellent contraceptive for younger, nulliparous women who have intercourse infrequently. With conscientious use, very low pregnancy rates (2 per 100 users per year) can be attained.

Diaphragms are available in a range of sizes and in four styles, including the flat spring, coil spring, arcing spring, and wide seal rim. Each has particular uses de-pending on vaginal tone and pelvic anatomy. The newest version, the wide-seal rim, has a flange on the inner rim that creates a better seal between the diaphragm and vaginal wall. The flat spring is useful with firm vaginal tone, and the coil spring is useful with average vaginal tone. Both can be used with an inserter. The arcing spring is easier to insert manually and is useful with lax vaginal tone, cystocele, or rectocele.

The goal in fitting a diaphragm is to select the largest rim size that is comfortable for the client, taking the above factors into consideration. Sizes that are too small may fail to maintain position covering the cervix, whereas those that are too large may cause vaginal pressure, abdominal pain or cramping, vaginal ulceration, or recurrent UTI.

Diaphragms with spermicide protect against STDs. Spermicides are lethal to organisms causing gonorrhea, herpes, PID, and trichomoniasis. Some protection against *Chlamydia,* hepatitis, toxic shock, and HIV may be provided, but data are incomplete. There is lower risk of cervical dysplasia and cancer among women using diaphragms for more than 5 years (Hatcher et al., 1990).

Complications and Side Effects

There are few serious complications with diaphragm use. Infrequent cases of toxic shock syndrome (TSS) have been reported, and the risk of death is low (0.3 deaths per 100,000 women using barrier contraceptives). Women using the diaphragm should know the danger signs of TSS and should be instructed in TSS precautions (see the display Client Education: Reducing the Risk of Toxic Shock Syndrome). The following are contraindications to diaphragm use:

- History of TSS
- Allergy to latex or spermicide
- Recurrent UTI
- Inability to learn insertion technique
- Abnormalities of vaginal anatomy that prevent satisfactory fit or stable placement (such as uterine prolapse, extreme retroversion, vaginal septum)

Severe pelvic pain (due to herpes, recent episiotomy, PID, tight introitus) precludes using a diaphragm until the condition is resolved. Women must be refitted after each pregnancy but should wait about 12 weeks postpartum before using the diaphragm.

UTIs are twice as common in women who use a diaphragm as in women using OCs. Intravaginal contraceptive methods alter normal vaginal flora and increase enteric organisms, which may explain the risk of UTI. Postcoital voiding may reduce this risk; women with frequent UTIs may be given prophylactic postcoital antibiotic therapy (Cohall et al., 1993). Vaginitis

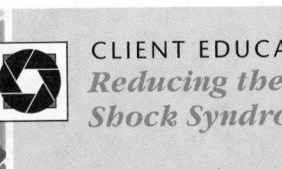

CLIENT EDUCATION
Reducing the Risk of Toxic Shock Syndrome

Toxic shock syndrome (TSS) can occur with the use of the diaphragm and cervical cap. To reduce the risk of TSS with these contraceptives, you should do the following:

- Wash your hands thoroughly with soap and water before insertion or removal.
- Never leave contraceptive in place for more than 24 hours.
- Never use a contraceptive during your menstrual period or if you have any vaginal bleeding or spotting.
- Wait about 12 weeks before using a contraceptive after a full-term pregnancy.
- Watch for TSS danger signs:
    Fever (temperature 101°F or more)
    Diarrhea
    Vomiting
    Muscle aches
    Rash (similar to sunburn)
- Remove the contraceptive right away if you develop these signs, and see your healthcare provider.
- Choose a different type of contraceptive if you have ever had TSS.

(For a more thorough discussion of TSS, see Chap. 11.)

or foul-smelling vaginal discharge may be caused by the spermicide or leaving the diaphragm in the vagina too long. Vaginal trauma or ulceration can result from excessive rim pressure or prolonged wear.

Nursing Interventions

Nursing care focuses on education about effective diaphragm use, safety, and prevention of side effects. After the client has been fitted with an appropriate size and type of diaphragm, the nurse teaches insertion and removal. It is important for the women to feel comfortable with these techniques. Proper placement is critical to effective pregnancy prevention, and correct removal prevents damage to the vaginal mucosa and the diaphragm. Storage techniques to prevent diaphragm deterioration and reduce risk of infection are taught (see the display Client Education: Inserting and Removing a Diaphragm).

Signs and symptoms of TSS and vaginitis are reviewed. The woman is urged to seek care without delay if she has any TSS symptoms. (For a more thorough discussion of TSS, see Chap. 11.) Annual visits are planned for health maintenance and rechecking the diaphragm fit. The need for refitting after significant weight gain (greater than 10 lb), pelvic surgery, and full-term delivery is reviewed. The nurse identifies

clients at high risk for improper diaphragm use and emphasizes consistent and proper use. Higher failure rates have been found in women who have frequent intercourse (four or more times per week).

Cervical Cap

The **cervical cap**, a barrier method of contraception, has a 1¼ to 1½ inch, soft rubber dome with a flexible rim (Fig. 9-3). It fits snugly over the cervix and is held in place by suction between its rim and the base of the cervix. Approximately one-third of the inside of the cap is filled with spermicide. No more spermicide is needed for additional intercourse. When properly positioned, the cap is a barrier to sperm entering the cervix, with spermicidal protection inside, as with the diaphragm. The cap can be inserted several hours before intercourse and should be left in place at least 8 hours after the last act of intercourse. It may be worn 48 hours. If left longer, it causes a strong vaginal odor. The position of the cap must be checked before and after intercourse.

Cervical caps have been widely used in Europe since 1930. The Prentif Cavity-Rim cervical cap was approved for use in the United States in the late 1980s. The cervical cap is similar to the diaphragm in effectiveness, with first-year failure rates from 8 to 27 (average about 16) pregnancies per 100 women who begin using the method. The continuation rate after 12 months for the cap is 59% (Hatcher et al., 1990).

The cervical cap must fit well. If it is too tight, it can cause cervical trauma; if it is too loose, it can be easily dislodged. The position of the uterus and angle of the cervix, shape and size of the cervix, and vaginal muscle tone may affect fitting and use. About 6% of women cannot be satisfactorily fitted with cervical caps.

Complications and Side Effects

Problems may arise due to prolonged cervical exposure to secretions, spermicide, and bacteria trapped within the cap. Trauma to the cervix or vagina from insertion and removal or prolonged retention of the cap could result. There may be an interference with the normal flow of cervical mucus or menstrual blood.

Cervical cap use for more than 3 months causes a higher rate of suspicious abnormal cells on Pap smears compared with diaphragm use. This may be a result of human papillomavirus infection (Mishell, 1989). Women are advised to have a Pap smear before beginning use and repeat Pap smears after 3 months of use and annually thereafter. Vaginal irritation and foul-smelling discharge are associated with prolonged cap use. Cervical abrasions and lacerations can occur with prolonged use and difficult removal.

CLIENT EDUCATION
Inserting and Removing a Diaphragm

Insertion

- The diaphragm is inserted up to 2 hours before intercourse.
- Apply spermicidal jelly or cream to rim and inside of dome.
- Holding dome down, squeeze rim until sides touch (A).
- Stand with one foot propped, squat, or lie down.
- Spread labia, insert folded diaphragm deep into vagina (B).
- Push diaphragm back as far as possible, then tuck front rim up behind the pubic bone inside the vagina (C).
- Check for placement; feel for cervix covered with rubber dome (D).
- For repeated intercourse, add more spermicide without removing diaphragm.
- Leave diaphragm in place for 6 to 8 hours after last intercourse.

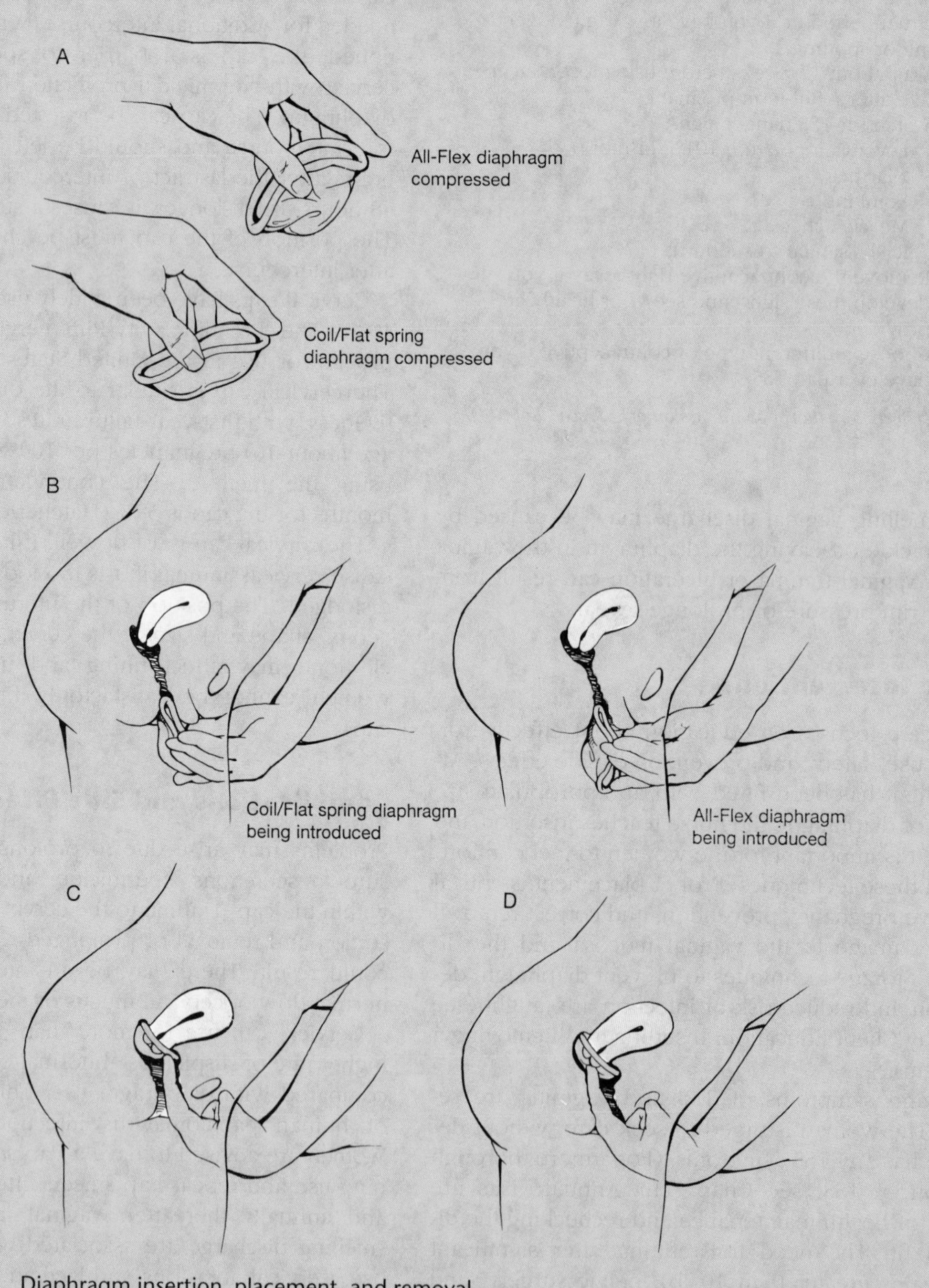

A

All-Flex diaphragm
compressed

Coil/Flat spring
diaphragm compressed

B

Coil/Flat spring diaphragm
being introduced

All-Flex diaphragm
being introduced

C

D

Diaphragm insertion, placement, and removal.

(continued)

CLIENT EDUCATION *(Continued)*
Inserting and Removing a Diaphragm

Removal

- To remove diaphragm, place index finger behind front rim (E); pull down (F).
- If suction is tight, insert finger between pubic bone and rim to break suction, then pull down.
- Clean diaphragm with soap and water, rinse, and dry. Dust with cornstarch or unscented powder; perfumed powders can damage rubber or irritate tissue.
- Store diaphragm in plastic container in cool, dry place.
- Check diaphragm before and after every use for tears and holes.
- Do not use petroleum jelly because it causes deterioration of rubber.

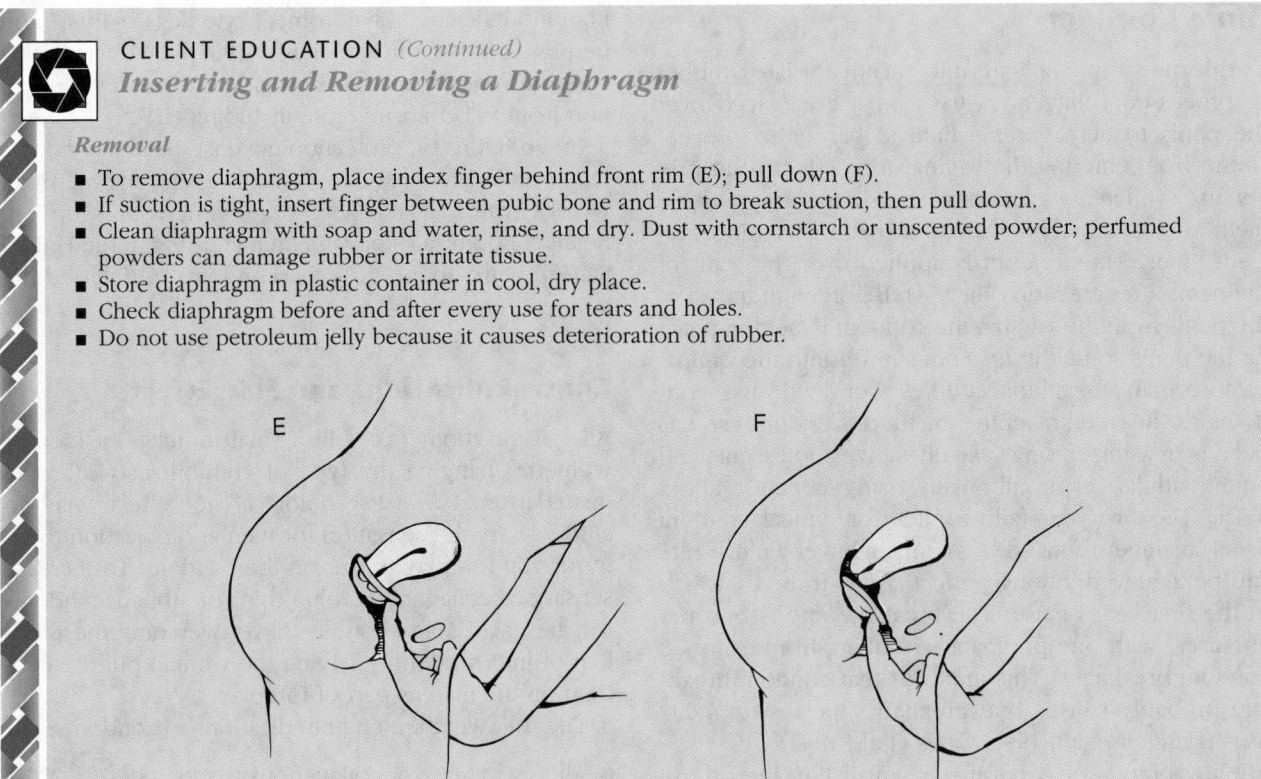

The following are contraindications to cervical cap use:

- History of TSS
- Cervical papillomavirus infection
- Full-term delivery in the past 12 weeks
- Acute PID or cervicitis
- Undiagnosed vaginal bleeding
- Abnormal Pap smear
- Recent cervical surgery
- Cervical neoplasia

- Allergy to rubber or spermicide
- Anatomic abnormalities or variations (extremely shallow or long cervix, severe lacerations)
- Inability to learn insertion and removal

Nursing Intervention

As with the diaphragm, women must practice inserting and removing the cap after they have been fitted. The nurse instructs the client in this, using techniques similar to manual diaphragm insertion and removal. It is critical that the client can identify her cervix and check that the cap is properly attached over the cervix. The cap must not be worn during the menstrual period.

Precautions to reduce risk of TSS are taught by the nurse. The cap should be cleaned with plain, mild soap and water after removal; dried; and placed in its case. Cornstarch, not talcum powder, can be used to dust the cap. The client should check the cap for tears with each use and avoid using petroleum products.

A return visit is scheduled in 3 months for a repeat Pap smear. If the smear is abnormal, use of the cap must be discontinued. An annual gynecologic examination is scheduled, with a Pap smear, recheck of the cervical cap's fit, and review of the woman's experience using the cap. The cap should be refitted after delivery, gynecologic surgery, and any significant weight loss or gain.

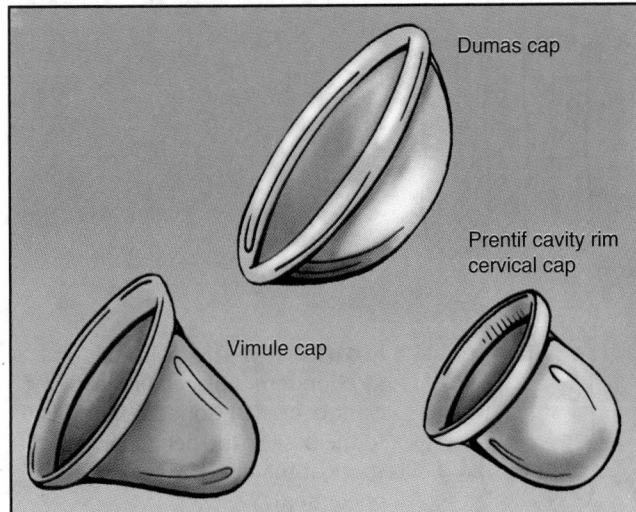

FIGURE 9–3 The cervical cap fits snugly over the cervix and is held in place by suction.

Male Condom

Condoms ("rubbers") are thin sheaths of latex rubber or processed collagenous tissue that are placed over the penis to act as a mechanical barrier to prevent sperm from entering the vagina. Also effective in preventing venereal infections, condoms are a male method of contraception that has been used since ancient times. The condom is applied over the shaft of the penis after erection (Fig. 9-4). Before withdrawal of the penis from the vagina, the condom is held in place on the penis so that it does not slip off into the vagina.

More than 46 million couples worldwide use condoms as their contraceptive method. Condom use has been increasing among sexually active adolescents and young adults, especially with rising concern about STDs. The first-year failure rates for typical condom users average about 12%. A much lower failure rate can be achieved among perfect users, from 1% to 2% in the first year of use. The breakage rate is one per 161 uses, with one pregnancy resulting from every 26 condom breakages. This indicates that condom breakage probably causes one pregnancy per every 4,000 uses (Hatcher et al., 1990; Cates et al., 1992).

Many brands of condoms are available, but all are approximately the same length and width in the United States. Condoms can be straight-sided or tapered, ribbed or smooth, lubricated or nonlubricated, and with or without spermicide. Some have pouches at the tip to collect semen after ejaculation. Lubricated condoms are more popular, and those with spermicides are growing in use. Spermicidal condoms are highly effective at killing sperm within·the condom. About 1% of condoms are made from lamb cecum (collagenous or "skin" condoms). These condoms do not prevent passage of the hepatitis B virus but apparently do trap larger viruses, such as the retrovirus causing acquired immunodeficiency syndrome, cytomegalovirus, and herpes simplex virus (Minuk, 1987). Latex (rubber) condoms with spermicide provide the greatest protection from STD transmission, including HIV.

In addition to protection against STDs, condoms may prevent cervical neoplasia. They are inexpensive, widely available, and accessible without prescription. Retail condom sales have been increasing in the United States, with about 40% of condoms purchased by women.

Contraindications and Side Effects

Allergic reactions occur in a small number of men or women. Changing the type of condom may alleviate this (Barton, 1993). Psychological side effects may include decreased sensation for men and objection to interrupting foreplay to put on the condom. To increase sensation, collagenous, ultra-thin, or ribbed condoms can be used. Many couples have overcome the problem of interruption by having the woman put the condom on the man as part of foreplay.

The following are contraindications to condoms:

- Allergy to latex or collagenous tissue
- Inability to maintain erections
- Inability to use properly

Nursing Intervention

Nursing care includes education about the advantages of condoms and instruction on effective use. The most important rule is to teach clients to use condoms with every sexual activity involving exchange of body fluids or risk of pregnancy. Instructions include choices of types of condoms and procedures for putting the condom on and removing it from the penis. Maximum

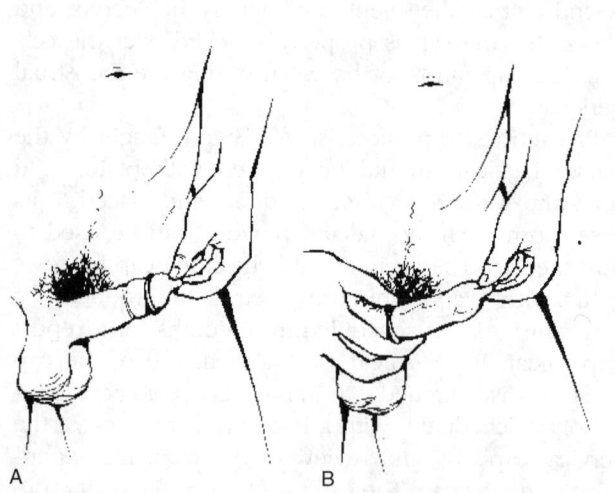

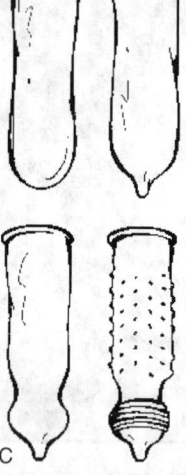

FIGURE 9–4 The male condom. **(A)** Condom is placed on head of erect penis. **(B)** Condom is unrolled to the base of the penis, leaving space at the tip. **(C)** Several types of condoms.

RESEARCH HIGHLIGHT

Condom Use Difficult for Low-Income Minority Youths

Results from a household survey suggest that low income, urban, African American and Hispanic youths may have difficulty using condoms effectively. Rates of human immunodeficiency virus infection are increasing among this population, and negative experiences with condoms leading to decreased use will make this problem worse.

Data came from a household probability sample of African American and Hispanic adolescents and young adults in low-income areas (*n*=1,435), with a response rate of 85% for both groups. Condoms were used by 68%. This subsample was interviewed face to face in neutral settings about experiences with condom use. Interviewers were from these ethnic groups and used a 12-item closed-ended survey developed and pretested for cultural appropriateness. Spanish language was used when indicated.

Negative experiences with condoms were common among the youths studied; 53% reported four or more negative experiences (eg, breakage or slippage, 73%; interrupting lovemaking, 33%; decreased sensation, 45%; condom too tight, 29%). More boys than girls reported problems. More African American boys reported the condom not staying on. Youths who said condoms interrupted sex, made vaginal movement difficult, or reduced sensation were significantly less likely to use a condom at their last intercourse.

Critique: This study suggests that nurses need to focus on education to reduce negative experiences with condoms, teaching specific condom-use skills, and encouraging practice of these skills. Geographic concentration (Detroit area) may limit applicability to other regions.

Norris, A. E., & Ford, F. (1993). Urban, low-income African-American and Hispanic youths' negative experiences with condoms. *Nurse Practitioner*, *18*(5), 40–48.

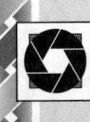

CLIENT EDUCATION
Maximize Protection Against Sexually Transmitted Disease Using Condoms

To attain the best protection against STD, follow these guidelines:

- Use condoms with every intercourse.
- Use only latex condoms.
- Never use petroleum-based lubricants with condoms.
- Apply condoms before any genital-to-genital contact.
- Remove carefully to avoid leakage and post-coital exposure.

protection is offered when the condom is put on before any vaginal penetration occurs. Petroleum products should not be used because they weaken the rubber. Intercourse should not begin until the vagina is well lubricated to avoid tearing the condom from friction. Condoms should be stored in a cool, dry place. Even body heat can cause the rubber to weaken.

Women who rely on condoms are encouraged to insist on their use. Women are at greater risk of reproductive tract damage from STDs than men (see Client Education: Maximize Protection Against Sexually Transmitted Disease Using Condoms). There is a high rate of STD transmission from infected men to their female sex partners. It is the woman's right to insist on condom use and her right to say no to intercourse if her partner refuses to wear a condom. The nurse can discuss alternatives to intercourse that the woman can suggest to her partner if condoms will not be used. Abstinence also is a perfectly acceptable solution.

Female Condom

A polyurethane condom for vaginal use was approved in May 1993. The female condom has flexible rims at each end connecting the prelubricated condom sheath. The closed end is inserted high in the vagina with the rim surrounding the cervix; the open end fits in the introitus (Fig. 9-5). The WPC-33 female condom, made in the United States, may provide better protection against STD and pregnancy than the male condom because it covers a larger surface area, and there is less risk of exposure to seminal fluid (Leeper et al., 1989). Some users find the female condom less convenient and comfortable than the male condom, have difficulty with insertion, or their male partner objects (Sakondhavat, 1990). The pregnancy rate is 208 per year, and the female condom is considered expensive (Cohall et al., 1993).

Vaginal Spermicides

Vaginal spermicide is a physical barrier to sperm penetration that also exerts a chemical action on the sperm. Spermicides are widely used because of their safety and simplicity. These preparations include jellies, creams, foam, suppositories, tablets, and a thin square of film. They are inserted deep into the vagina, covering the cervix, about 5 to 10 minutes before intercourse. Most remain effective for 2 hours. Tablets and suppositories take longer to dissolve, about 10 to 30 minutes. The spermicide used is usually nonoxynol 9, although some preparations use octoxynol 9.

Effectiveness rates vary for vaginal spermicides. First-year failure rates among typical users are about 15% to 30%. Failure rates as low as 2% to 4% in the initial year of use have been found. The most common

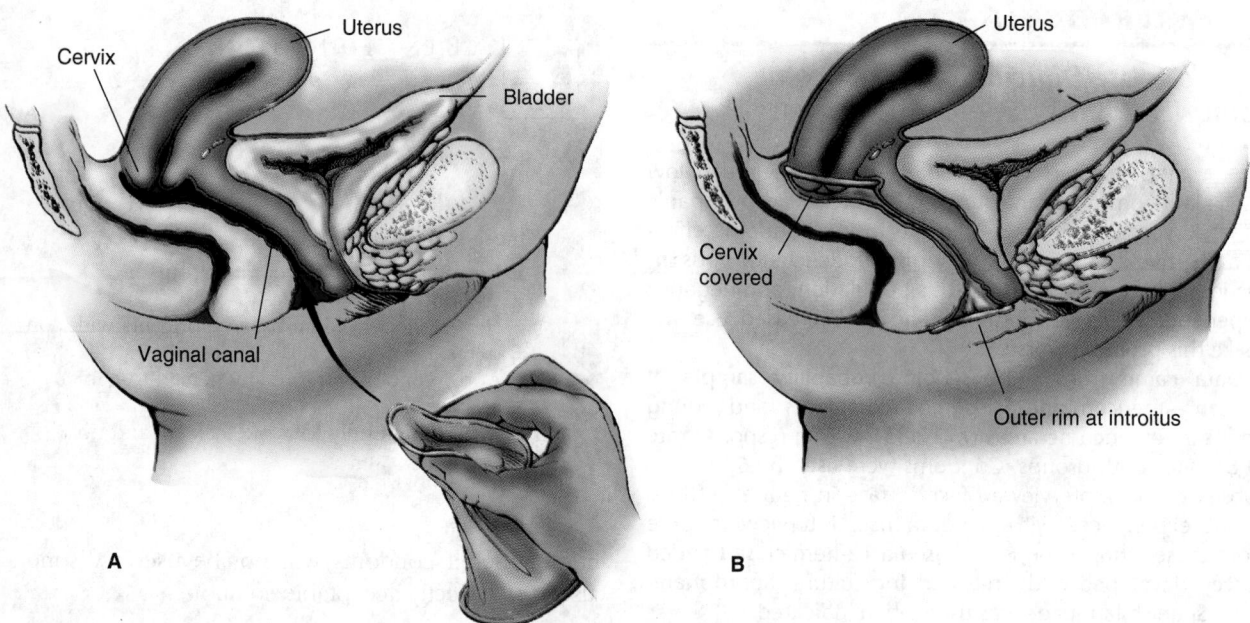

FIGURE 9-5 The female condom. (**A**) The flexible rim on the closed end of the condom (WPC-333) is grasped, and the condom is inserted high in the vagina with the rim around the cervix. (**B**) When in place, the flexible rim at the open end of the condom is at the vaginal introitus.

error leading to pregnancy is not using the method at all. Placing the preparation deep in the vagina and consistent use improve effectiveness (Fig. 9-6).

Vaginal spermicides are readily available in drug stores and markets without a prescription. Spermicides help protect against STD and have been found in vitro to kill organisms responsible for gonorrhea, trichomoniasis, herpes, and chlamydial diseases. Women using spermicides are less likely to develop PID. HIV is killed by spermicides in laboratory tests, but although they may prevent HIV transmission, spermicides should not be relied on as the sole means of prevention.

Contraindications and Side Effects

Rarely, allergies occur in either the man or woman, causing local irritation or inflammation. The tablets or suppositories may fail to melt or foam in the vagina, causing mechanical irritation and discomfort and reducing effectiveness. Spermicides may have an unpleasant taste for couples using oral-genital sex. Some couples object to messiness from the spermicide and the need for additional applications with repeated intercourse.

The following are contraindications to vaginal spermicides:

- Allergy to spermicidal preparation
- Inability to use consistently at the time of intercourse
- Any physical or mental disability causing problems with proper insertion and placement

Nursing Interventions

Spermicide users are educated about proper and consistent use with every episode of intercourse. Time limits between insertion and intercourse are emphasized, as are the need for additional insertions for repeated intercourse. The woman is instructed to wait 6 to 8 hours after intercourse before douching, if she chooses to douche. Spermicides also can be combined with

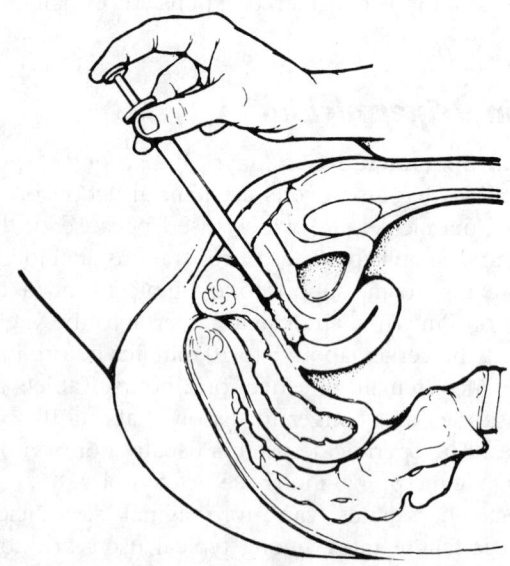

FIGURE 9-6 The user inserts foam or cream near the cervix.

other contraceptives to increase protection, such as condoms, or during midcycle with the IUD and fertility awareness methods.

Spermicides are useful as short-term contraceptives. During the postpartum period, they can be used the first 4 to 6 weeks, until a more effective method can be instituted. They may be recommended as precautionary measures for 2 to 4 weeks after IUD insertion or when starting an OC before these methods can be used alone. When the OC or IUD is discontinued, spermicides can be used until another method is begun or pregnancy is attempted.

Fertility Awareness Methods

Fertility awareness methods involve knowledge of the fertile phase of the menstrual cycle to avoid pregnancy (Roth, 1993). With menstrual cycles that occur regularly, ovulation occurs at about the same time in each cycle (14 days before the beginning of the next menses). The ovum can be fertilized only during the 24 hours after ovulation. Because sperm are capable of fertilizing an ovum for about 48 hours, **abstinence,** refraining from sexual intercourse, at ovulation and for the 2 days before and after (a total of 5 days) would theoretically forestall conception.

In actual experience, regular cycles can vary by 2 days in either direction (28 ± 2 days). With a 4-day range ± 2 days for ovulation, the period of abstinence must be at least 8 days. Due to variability of menstrual cycles, the risk of fertility often is 15 or more days, or about half of the cycle.

Fertility awareness methods determine ovulation by menstrual cycle calendar calculations, changes in the basal body temperature (BBT), symptoms associated with ovulation, and changes in the condition of cervical mucus. These methods are avantageous because they are relatively risk free (no medication or device involved), relatively inexpensive, and acceptable to religious groups. Disadvantages include the need for keeping careful records of menstrual cycles, learning specific details of use, restricting sexual spontaneity, and abstaining (or using another contraceptive method) for about half the menstrual cycle. Some women are unable to recognize ovulation symptoms or cervical mucus changes. Irregular cycles make calendar and BBT methods less reliable.

The first-year failure rates of fertility awareness methods among typical users is 20 to 23 pregnancies per 100 women. Sexual risk taking during fertile days accounts for most pregnancies. First-year failure rates among users who maintain perfect and consistent use can be 2% to 10% (Hatcher et al., 1990).

Calendar Method

The **calendar method** involves using a menstrual calendar to determine periods of fertility. The woman records the length of each menstrual cycle for 8 months. With the first day of bleeding counted as day 1, the earliest fertile day is computed by subtracting 18 days from the length of the shortest cycle. Eleven days are subtracted from the length of the longest cycle to determine the last day of fertility. These two numbers represent the beginning and end of the fertile period. During these days, abstinence, refraining from sexual intercourse, or another method of birth control must be used (Table 9-4).

This method is more effective when the woman has regular menstrual cycles and when used with absti-

TABLE 9-4
Calculating the Interval of Fertility

Number of Days Shortest Cycle	First Fertile Day	Number of Days Longest Cycle	Last Fertile Day
21	3rd day	21	10th day
22	4th day	22	11th day
23	5th day	23	12th day
24	6th day	24	13th day
25	7th day	25	14th day
26	8th day	26	15th day
27	9th day	27	16th day
28	10th day	28	17th day
29	11th day	29	18th day
30	12th day	30	19th day
31	13th day	31	20th day
32	14th day	32	21st day
33	15th day	33	22nd day
34	16th day	34	23rd day
35	17th day	35	24th day

nence or backup contraception through the entire first part of the menstrual cycle to the last fertile day. It may be contraindicated for younger, postpartum, postabortion, and premenopausal women who often have irregular menstrual cycles. Use of the BBT or cervical mucus method can increase effectiveness.

Basal Body Temperature Method

The **basal body temperature**, or resting temperature, of a fertile woman normally rises each cycle just after ovulation. It remains higher until the next menstrual period begins. Most women can observe this temperature change if they take and record their temperature every day with a special thermometer before getting out of bed or beginning any activity, including smoking. The thermometer can be used orally or rectally and should be left in place for 5 full minutes. Temperature is recorded on a special BBT chart (see Chap. 13).

Temperature drops slightly just at ovulation and then rises about 0.4°F to 0.8°F once ovulation has occurred. This rise is sustained until the next menstrual period. Some women have no preliminary drop before the BBT rises. Because ovulation cannot be identified until after it has happened, it is safer to abstain or use another method of contraception until the sustained rise in BBT is seen. The fertile period ends after the BBT has remained elevated for 3 full days.

Many factors, such as illness, nightmares, and changes in daily schedule, can influence BBT. When the pattern of temperature rise is not clear or sustained, it is not safe to have intercourse. This method is more effective when combined with the calendar or mucus methods, which provide earlier signs that ovulation is near.

Cervical Mucus Method

In some women, changes in the character and appearance of cervical mucus occur just before ovulation. One-sided lower quadrant ovulatory pain may be experienced. Typically, there is a rapid increase in the quantity of cervical mucus just before ovulation. Women need to observe their mucus changes for several cycles before relying on this method. The peak of fertility occurs when the vagina feels wet and mucus is abundant, clear, slippery, and stretchable (can be stretched 3–4 inches between the thumb and forefinger). After ovulation, the mucus becomes thick, cloudy, and sticky, or there may be no mucus. When this change is observed, the woman is no longer fertile.

The woman must be careful not to confuse cervical mucus at midcycle with other substances in the vagina, such as semen, lubricants, spermicides, and discharge due to infections. Women who douche cannot observe changes because they wash the mucus away. This

method is more effective when intercourse is restricted to the postovulatory phase of the cycle.

Symptothermal Method

The **symptothermal method** combines the methods for changes in cervical mucus and ovulation symptoms with the BBT method to determine fertility. When using this combination, couples must wait until the fourth day after the peak of slippery mucus and the third day after the sustained rise in BBT before resuming intercourse. If one occurs without the other, safety cannot be assumed, and the couple must await the second event. Other symptoms that help predict ovulation include ovulation pain, midcycle spotting, pelvic or vulvar fullness, and increased libido.

Menstrual calendar calculations and changes in cervical mucus predict onset of the fertile period; ovulation symptoms help identify the peak of fertility, and rise in BBT with thickening of cervical mucus indicates the end of fertility.

Ovulation Predictor Tests

Ovulation predictor tests use **monoclonal antibody** (specific antibody for antigen of the substance to be tested) technology to detect urinary LH. With the sharp rise of LH 12 to 24 hours before ovulation, urinary excretion also rises. The tests detect LH in the urine by a color change; ovulation is expected within 24 hours after the color changes. Other tests use vaginal mucus and chemical indicators to predict fertile days. These tests are not affected by physical activity, illness, or emotional upset. They are available without a prescription for home use and usually include materials for several days of testing.

Nursing Intervention

The nurse educates couples in the effective use of fertility awareness methods. Nursing care includes teaching the use of techniques to measure and record menstrual cycles and changes in cervical mucus and BBT. Individual differences are explored, and precautions are given for situations, such as infections, stress, and travel that may make measurements unreliable. The importance of abstinence during the fertile period or use of another contraceptive is emphasized.

Because fertility awareness methods require close cooperation between sexual partners, the nurse provides counseling about communication and feelings. The couple may need to clarify expectations about sex and work out mutually acceptable solutions. Couples who are reluctant to forego sexual spontaneity or are unable to keep careful records should be advised against using fertility awareness and counseled in another contraceptive method.

Withdrawal

Withdrawal, or **coitus interruptus,** is used by about 6% of American women (Mishell, 1989). Couples using withdrawal have intercourse until ejaculation is impending. The male then withdraws the penis from the vagina and ejaculates completely away from the female's genitals. Withdrawal has certain advantages; it is always available at no cost and requires no devices or chemicals. It does require male awareness of and control over sexual response and careful timing. The woman's sexual experience may be diminished unless she has orgasm before withdrawal or other techniques are used.

The first-year failure rate among typical users is about 18% to 20%. The estimate of the failure rate among perfect users is about 4% in the initial year (Hatcher et al., 1990). Sperm are contained in the pre-ejaculatory fluid that seeps from Cowper's glands during intercourse. After a recent ejaculation, this fluid contains even more sperm, and risk increases with multiple sex acts. Although there are no major physiologic side effects, withdrawal can diminish both partners' sexual pleasure.

Sterilization

Sterilization refers to a surgical procedure that renders the client infertile. For married couples older than 30 years, sterilization is the most common means of birth control. It is now the most prevalent contraceptive method throughout the world (Hatcher et al., 1990). Sterilization techniques used include vasectomy and tubal ligation.

Vasectomy

Vasectomy involves surgical interruption and ligation of the vas deferens. It is a relatively minor operation. Usually performed under local anesthesia, the procedure takes about 15 minutes and can be done on an outpatient basis. It is associated with minimal risk and only slight morbidity (Fig. 9-7).

Short-term complications can include inflammation and pain, hematomas, infections, sperm granulomas, and epididymitis. No changes have been found in levels of testosterone, FSH, or LH in men with vasectomies. However, prostate gland and epididymal secretions may decrease, slightly reducing semen volume. About 50% to 65% of men develop sperm antibodies, but there are apparently no pathologic complications from this.

Most men who have vasectomies are satisfied with their decision and report that sexual performance is unchanged. Less than 2% report decreased sexual performance or other dissatisfaction with vasectomy. Vasectomy failure is the result of recanalization of the ends of the ligated vas deferens. This occurs in 0.4 per 100 cases (Dunnihoo, 1992). Unprotected intercourse before the male reproductive tract is cleared of spermatozoa may result in pregnancy.

Men who remarry and desire more children may request vasectomy reversal. Microsurgical procedures for reanastomosis result in sperm in the ejaculate in almost all cases, but only about 50% of men have successful impregnations (Jarow, 1987). The success of reanastomosis depends on the type of surgical procedure, how long it has been since the vasectomy, and whether sperm antibodies have developed.

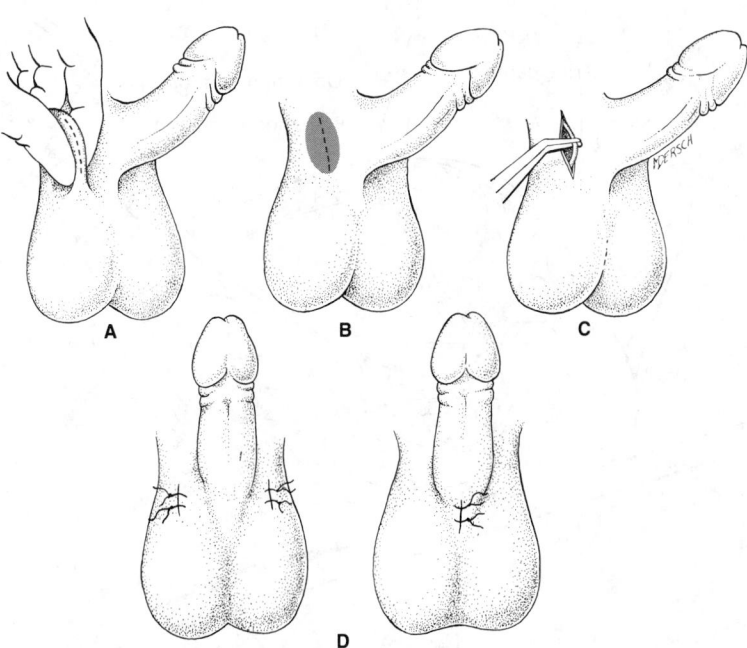

FIGURE 9–7 Vasectomy procedure. **(A)** The vas deferens is identified. **(B)** A small area of the skin and subcutaneous tissue is anesthetized. **(C)** The vas deferens is isolated from surrounding tissue and lifted through the incision then severed and occluded by ligation, coagulation, clip, or burial of cut ends. **(D)** Skin sutures showing one- and two-incision approaches.

Tubal Ligation

Tubal ligation is a surgical procedure designed to block the tubal conduit through which spermatozoa and ova pass. The surgery may be done immediately after delivery with cesarean delivery or as an interval procedure.

Coagulation and interruption of the fallopian tubes can be carried out using a *laparoscopic approach* (Fig. 9-8). This procedure can be done under regional or local anesthesia, hut often a general anesthetic is used. After the abdomen is distended with carbon dioxide, the laparoscopic trocar is introduced through a small incision in the umbilicus. The laparoscope is passed into the peritoneal cavity. Visualization of the adnexa is usually complete. Forceps are used to grasp the fallopian tubes, and a variety of techniques are used to occlude the tubes with a clip, ring, or band; coagulate the tubes; or cut and tie the tubes (resection).

Because the procedure is relatively simple, it can be carried out on an outpatient basis. Although it is associated with a relatively low morbidity, this is considerably higher than for vasectomy.

For a *minilaparotomy* done shortly after delivery, the woman undergoes inpatient or outpatient surgery with usual preoperative procedures (NPO, sedation). A local, regional or general anesthetic may be used. A small, vertical incision is made below the umbilicus, through the abdominal wall. Grasping instruments isolate the fallopian tubes, which may be crushed, ligated, embedded, clipped, or plugged. Discharge usually occurs several hours after recovery from anesthesia.

The *interval minilaparotomy* is done at any time in the menstrual cycle. It uses a small, suprapubic incision below the pubic hair line to enter the abdominal cavity. After preoperative preparation, the fallopian tubes are isolated with grasping instruments and are interrupted as in other tubal ligation methods. It is a 1-day inpatient or outpatient surgical procedure. Tubal ligations also may be done vaginally, but rates of complication, such as infections and hemorrhage, are higher.

Rates of complications associated with tubal ligation range from 0.4% to 1%. Complications include wound infection, hematoma, uterine perforation, bladder or bowel injury, and sterilization failure. Most deaths associated with these procedures are a result of anesthesia; other risks results from sepsis, hemorrhage, and cardiovascular events. The overall case fatality rate is 3 per 100,000; less than that posed by use of OCs or a term pregnancy in a 40- to 45-year-old woman (Hatcher et al., 1990).

After tubal ligation, levels of LH, FSH, testosterone, and estrogen remain within the normal range. No consistent changes occur in the amount of bleeding or in bleeding patterns, and there is no increase in hospital admissions for gynecologic procedures or hysterectomy after sterilization (DeStefano et al., 1983).

Failure rates for tubal ligation range from 0 to 4 per 1,000 procedures. Many failures occur because sterilization is done in the second half of the menstrual cycle, and an already fertilized oocyte implants. Most women are satisfied with sterilization, which is considered a permanent procedure, but a small number (0.4%–3%) request reversal. The client's candidacy for

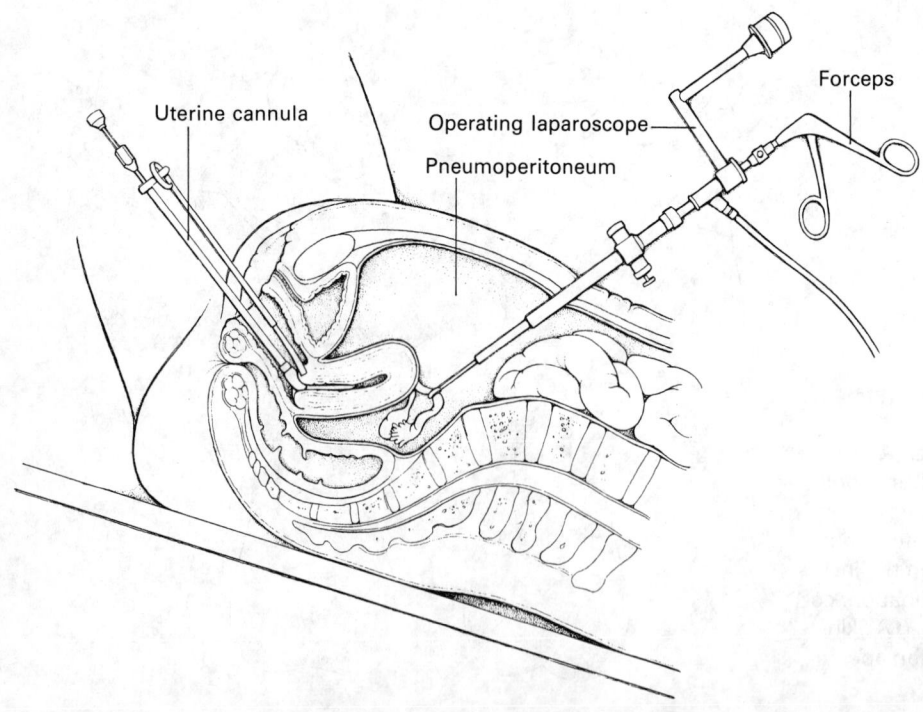

Uterine cannula

Operating laparoscope

Pneumoperitoneum

Forceps

FIGURE 9–8 The one-incision technique for tubal ligation using the laparoscopic approach may be performed on an outpatient basis.

a reversal must be determined according to the amount of tubal damage caused by the sterilization procedure. A laparoscopy to evaluate tubal status is recommended. Surgery for reanastomosis can be done on about 70% of women with tubal ligations, with successful reversals resulting in pregnancy reported at about 15% (Cunningham et al., 1993) to 50% (Dunnihoo, 1992).

Nursing Intervention

Nurses assist the couple or client to make a sound, well-informed decision to have a vasectomy or tubal ligation. Because these usually are considered permanent procedures, the decision to have surgery must be carefully made. The nurse makes certain both partners understand that these methods are considered irreversible. If any doubt about sterilization exists, another contraceptive method should be advised. Family and personal circumstances that could influence the decision are reviewed, including number and ages of children, stability of the marriage, likelihood of future marriage if single, and ability to use reversible contraceptive methods. Information is provided about the procedure, care needed, discomfort, cost, and recovery. See Client Teaching Guidelines: Counseling About Sterilization for a description about a specific counseling technique.

When counseling clients about sterilization, the nurse must keep in mind the following legal regulations:

- Strict adherence to informed consent procedures and voluntary choice are essential, both legally and practically.
- There is no legal requirement for partner or spouse consent.
- When federal and, in some instances, state funds are used, the client must be 21 years or older, mentally competent, and must wait 30 days after signing the consent before the procedure can be performed.

Nursing Intervention for Vasectomy. The nurse teaches self-care measures to the man, including applying ice packs intermittently to the scrotum to reduce swelling and discomfort for several hours after the procedure. A scrotal support is used for several days to reduce traction and discomfort. Men should minimize activity for 2 to 3 days because of scrotal tenderness. Sutures are removed in about 7 days.

The male client may resume intercourse when it is comfortable. Sperm remain present in the sperm ducts proximal to the severed portion after vasectomy. Men are advised that it requires about 15 ejaculations to clear the ducts of sperm. Contraception is needed until the sperm count in the ejaculate is zero on two consecutive tests (Cunningham et al., 1993).

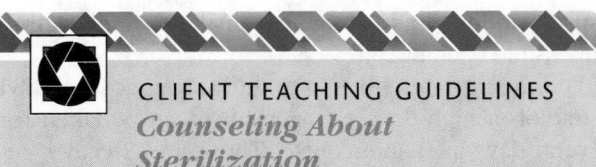

CLIENT TEACHING GUIDELINES
Counseling About Sterilization

The nurse can use the BRAIDED technique in counseling clients who are requesting sterilization procedures for contraception:

B *Benefits:* The procedure is permanent, very effective, relatively inexpensive when years of use are considered, further contraception decisions not needed, comfortable, no chemicals or devices.

R *Risks:* Surgical procedures can have complications or rarely, death. It is expensive in short run; slight chance of future pregnancy (not 100% effective). It is considered permanent, and reversal procedures are expensive and not always successful.

A *Alternatives:* Other forms of reversible contraceptives are discussed; abstinence, chance, pregnancy, and sterilization of the partner are discussed also.

I *Inquiries:* Client is encouraged to ask questions; information is provided to clear myths and misconceptions.

D *Decision to say no:* Client can freely decide not to have sterilization procedure, without experiencing hostility or punishment, such as withdrawal of care or welfare benefits.

E *Explanation:* Sterilization procedure and possible side effects are explained in detail (permanence, cost, where surgery can be done, potential psychological and physiological effects).

D *Documentation:* Written instructions, written risks, and written, signed and witnessed consent for the specific sterilization procedure must be done as part of the informed consent.

(Adapted from Hatcher, R. A., Stewart, F., Trussell, J. et al. [1990]. Contraceptive technology 1990–1992 [15th ed.]. New York: Irvington Publishers.)

Nursing Intervention for Tubal Ligation. Preoperative preparations are carried out and postoperative recovery monitored. Pain relief is administered, orally or by injection. Self-care is taught, including ensuring abdominal support when changing position, minimizing activity for 3 to 4 days, and maintaining hydration and rest. Analgesic medication for use at home usually is prescribed. Sutures are removed in 7 in 10 days. Signs of complications are reviewed, including infection, hemorrhage, and signs of intra-abdominal trauma.

Postcoital Contraception

After unprotected intercourse at midcycle, women may take postcoital OCs to prevent fertilization or implantation. Norgestrel 0.5 mg/ethinyl estradiol 50 μg (Ovral) is most commonly used. Two tablets are taken within 12 to 72 hours of coitus, and two more tablets are taken 12 hours later. This high-dose hormonal therapy causes endometrial sloughing, making implantation impossible (Cohall et al., 1993).

The failure rate is 0.16% to 1.6%. Low-dose ethinyl estradiol or high-dose estrogens also can be taken for several days after intercourse. These are effective, resulting in pregnancy rates of 0.4% and 0.9%, respectively (Hatcher et al., 1990). Side effects include nausea and vomiting. Frequently an antiemetic is given to control these symptoms.

Diethylstilbestrol (DES) 25 mg twice daily for 5 days may be used for postcoital contraception. It must be started within 72 hours after unprotected intercourse. Side effects include nausea and vomiting. Because DES causes teratogenic effects on the fetus, an abortion is recommended if the method fails and pregnancy occurs.

Postpartum Contraception

In the absence of complications, intercourse is commonly resumed 2 to 3 weeks after delivery. The condom is a practical contraceptive method to use during this period. Spermicidal foams and creams are frequently advised, either in combination with the condom or alone. Foams and creams used at this time generally do not contribute to infection.

Insertion of an IUD within the first 6 weeks postpartum is generally not recommended, because the expulsion and infection rates are higher during this time. Estrogen-containing OCs are contraindicated because of the increased incidence of thromboembolic complications associated with their use in the postpartum period. Nursing mothers are usually advised to use progestin-only OCs because lactation may be suppressed with estrogen, particularly higher dose pills. Synthetic hormones are excreted in breast milk, but the amount that actually passes through the milk is small (approximately one-fifth to one-tenth of the mother's dose). Minipills may be given immediately postpartum or at a return visit. These pills have little effect on lactation and do not pose thromboembolic risks.

An effective postpartum contraceptive, DMPA usually given within 5 days of delivery for nonlactating women, and at 6 weeks for lactating women. There does not appear to be any adverse effect on the quality and quantity of breast milk. DMPA may slow uterine involution and increase lochia; therefore, women with anemia should delay beginning this method (Cohall et al., 1993).

Summary Points

✔ Sexual health is an important part of general well-being and contributes to normal developmental processes.

✔ Nurses have a responsibility to promote sexual health and provide education and counseling for sexual concerns and problems. Nurses must be aware of their own values and beliefs about sexuality and present information in a nonjudgmental manner.

✔ Many couples have questions, concerns, and problems related to sexuality during childbearing. Nursing care can alleviate many of these and support normal developmental processes for couples during these phases. Sexual dysfunctions can be identified and referred for therapy.

✔ Contraception to space and prevent pregnancy is widely used among women of every age, socioeconomic, and cultural group.

✔ Before beginning contraception, women should be assessed for contraindications and risk factors and methods examined for individual suitability.

✔ Nurses (and other providers) must examine their own biases regarding contraceptive methods so that these do not interfere with helping the client select the best suited method. Informed consent is obtained before beginning contraception, ensuring that the client is fully aware of conditions of use, risks and benefits, side effects, and complications and voluntarily elects the method without coercion.

✔ Numerous contraceptive methods are available: nonprescription methods include condoms, spermicides, fertility awareness, and withdrawal; prescription methods include hormonal contraceptives (oral, injectable, implants), IUDs, diaphragms, and cervical caps; surgical methods include vasectomy and tubal ligation.

✔ Nurses teach clients the specific steps in using the selected contraceptive, clarify misconceptions, identify concerns, answer questions, and support consistent and effective use.

✔ Sterilization methods are usually permanent; nurses must ensure that clients fully understand this and have made the choice freely and without pressure.

✔ Postcoital contraception involves use of hormonal agents, such as norgestrel/ethinyl estradiol or DES.

REFERENCES

Annon, J. D. (1976). The PLISS+ model: A proposed conceptual scheme for the behavioral treatment of sexual problems. *Journal of Sex Education Therapy, 2,* 211–215.

Bancroft, J. (1989). *Human sexuality and its problems.* New York: Churchill Livingston.

Barrett, D. H. et al. (1994). Trends in oral contraceptive use and cigarette smoking. *Archives of Family Medicine, 3,* 438–443.

Barton, E. C. (1993). Latex allergy: Recognition and management of a modern problem. *Nurse Practitioner, 18*(11), 54–58.

Byer, C. O., Shainberg, L. W., & Jones, K. L. (1988). *Dimensions of human sexuality* (2nd ed.). Dubuque, IA: WC Brown.

Cates, W., & Stone, K. M. (1992). Family planning, sexually transmitted diseases and contraceptive choice: A literature update—Parts I & II. *Family Planning Perspective, 24*, 75–84, 122–128.

Cohall, A. T., Cullins, V. E., Darney, P. D., & Nelson, A. L. (1993). Contraception in the 1990s: New methods and approaches. *Patient Care, July* (Special Suppl.) pp. 1–13.

Covington, T. P. (1987). *Sex care*. New York: Pocket Books.

Cunningham, F. G., MacDonald, P. C., & Gant, N. F. (1993). *Williams obstetrics* (19th ed.). Norwalk, CT: Appleton & Lange.

Darney, P. D. (1993). *New progestins: Will they make a difference? Ambulatory obstetrics and gynecology* (pp. 68–80). UCD-CME conference, School of Medicine, University of California, Davis.

Derman, R. (1994). Selecting an oral contraceptive. *The Female Patient, 19*(8), 25–31.

DeStefano, F., Huezo, C. M., Peterson, H. B. et al. (1983). Menstrual changes after sterilization. *Obstetrics and Gynecology, 62*, 676–681.

Depo-Provera Contraceptive Injection (1993). *Patient information pamphlet*. Kalamazoo, MI: The Upjohn Company.

Dunnihoo, D. R. (1992). *Fundamentals of obstetrics and gynecology*. Philadelphia: J.B. Lippincott.

Franklin, M. (1990). Recently approved and experimental methods of contraception. *Journal of Nurse Midwifery, 35*(6), 365–376.

Godsland, I. F., Crook, D., Simpson, R. et al. (1990). The effects of different formulations of oral contraceptive agents on lipid and carbohydrate metabolism. *New England Journal of Medicine, 323*, 1375–1381.

Harlap, S., Kost, K., & Forrest, J. D. (1991). *Preventing pregnancy, protecting health: A new look at birth control choices in the United States*. New York: Alan Guttmacher Institute.

Hatcher, R. A., Steward, F., Trussell, J. et al. (1990). *Contraceptive technology 1990–1992* (15th ed.). New York: Irvington.

Hyde, J. S. (1990). *Understanding human sexuality* (4th ed.). New York: McGraw-Hill.

Jarow, J. P. (1987). Vasectomy: autoimmunity and reversal. *Journal of the American Medical Association, 257*(15), 2087.

Leeper, M. A., Conrady, M., & Henderson, J. (1989). *Evaluation of the WPC-33 female condom*. Abstract No 6305. Montreal, Canada: 5th International Congress on AIDS.

Masters, W. H., & Johnson, V. E. (1970). *Human sexual inadequacy*. Boston: Little, Brown.

Masters, W. H., Johnson, V. E., & Kolodny, R. C. (1994). *Heterosexuality*. New York: Harper Collier.

Minuk, G. (1987). *Passage of viral particles through natural membrane condoms*. Atlanta, GA: Proceedings of conference: Condoms in prevention of sexually transmitted diseases.

Mishell, D. R. (1989). Contraception. *New England Journal of Medicine, 320*(12), 777.

National Institute of Child Health and Human Development (1993). Preventing unintended pregnancy: The role of hormonal contraceptives. *Clinical Courier, 11*(10), 1–11.

Pollack, A. (1991). Norplant: What you should know about the new contraceptive. *Medical Aspects of Human Sexuality*, 43–38.

Roth, B. (1993). Fertility awareness as a component of sexuality education. *Nurse Practitioner, 18*(3), 40–54.

Sakondhavat, C. (1990). The female condom (letter). *American Journal of Public Health, 80*, 498.

Stuart, G. W., & Sundeen, S. J. (1991). *Principles and practice of psychiatric nursing* (4th ed.). St Louis: Mosby-Year Book.

Wehrle, K. E. (1994). The Norplant system: Easy to insert, easy to remove. *Nurse Practitioner, 19*(4), 47–54.

Youngkin, E. Q. (1993). Progestogens: A look at the "other" hormone. *Nurse Practitioner, 18*(11), 28–40.

10

Common Problems in Women's Health

Objectives

- Discuss the pathophysiology, assessment, and treatment of dysfunctional uterine bleeding, amenorrhea, dysmenorrhea, and premenstrual syndrome.
- Develop a nursing care plan for women with these conditions, focusing on self-care and prevention.
- Differentiate between benign and malignant neoplastic processes of the reproductive system.
- Discuss pathophysiology, assessment, and treatment of neoplasia.
- Develop nursing care plans for women with neoplasia, focusing on self-care, prevention, and consideration of treatment options.
- Explain the emotional impact of cancer and stages of adaptation.
- Describe pathophysiology, assessment, and treatment of pelvic support disorders.
- Develop nursing care plans for women with pelvic support disorders, focusing on self-care and prevention.
- Identify concerns and issues related to reproductive surgery.
- Describe the types of common reproductive surgical procedures.
- Discuss the nursing care involved with the care of a client undergoing reproductive surgery.
- Develop nursing care plans for women undergoing reproductive surgery.

Key Terms

Adjuvant therapy
Amenorrhea
Anovulation
Carcinogenesis
Cystocele
Dysfunctional uterine
    bleeding
Dysmenorrhea
Dysplasia
Endometriosis
Enterocele
Hypomenorrhea
Hysterectomy
Intermenstrual
    bleeding

Low severity pattern
Menorrhagia
Metaplastic process
Metastasis
Neoplasia
Pelvic exenteration
Perimenopause
Premenstrual
    magnification
    pattern
Premenstrual
    syndrome
Rectocele
Sound
Stroma

At various times during a woman's life, problems associated with reproduction functioning can occur. Women may experience problems related to menstrual dysfunctions, disorders or abnormalities of pelvic support structures, breast and genital neoplasms, or surgery on the reproductive tract. When faced with a reproductive health problem, the woman not only experiences the physiologic effects of the disorder, but also the psychosocial effects related to the woman's self-concept. Therefore, nurses providing care to women must be familiar with these common problems and provide appropriate assessment and nursing care.

This chapter focuses on the most common reproductive health problems of women. Menstrual abnormalities, including dysfunctional uterine bleeding (DUB), amenorrhea, and dysmenorrhea; neoplasms of the cervix, ovary, uterus, and breast; disorders of pelvic support, including cystocele, rectocele, uterine prolapse, and urinary incontinence; and reproductive surgery are discussed. The nurse's role in helping the woman deal with the physiologic and psychosocial effects through assessment and intervention is emphasized.

Dysfunctional Uterine Bleeding

Dysfunctional uterine bleeding is abnormally heavy, light, or irregular bleeding. Most problems with DUB are related to endocrine disruptions that alter normal cyclic changes in the endometrium. Abnormal uterine bleeding also may be due to organic disease, such as neoplasms and infections. DUB can be a chronic problem contributing to iron deficiency anemia, or it can be an acute hemorrhagic episode with enough blood loss to cause hypovolemic shock. Table 10-1 lists some examples of age-specific causes of bleeding.

Menorrhagia

Menorrhagia is excessive menstrual flow, usually lasting longer than 7 to 8 days with blood loss of more than 80 to 100 mL. This common gynecologic problem occurs in 15% to 20% of otherwise healthy women (Long et al., 1990). The most common cause is inadequate hormone support for the endometrium. Constant estrogen stimulation produces endometrial overgrowth. There is sporadic and abnormal loss of endometrial tissue, resulting in either prolonged bleeding or irregular sloughing. Administration of medroxyprogesterone acetate (Provera) or combined estrogen-progestin therapy (oral contraceptives) regulates the hormone balance, controls heavy bleeding, and reestablishes the menstrual cycle, usually in 3 to 6 months.

Anovulation, failure of the ovaries to release or produce mature eggs, causes about 90% of DUB, especially in women at the beginning and end of their reproductive years. With anovulation, menstrual patterns are variable, and bleeding may be heavier or lighter than usual. Continued unopposed estrogen secretion occurs with failure to ovulate; thus, the corpus luteum is not formed, which produces progesterone necessary for conversion to a secretory endometrium. Unopposed estrogen stimulation of the endometrium can lead to cystic hyperplasia initially, followed by adenomatous hyperplasia, atypical hyperplasia, and eventually adenocarcinoma (Dunnihoo, 1992).

Anovulation also may result from pituitary adenoma, which produces excess prolactin, disrupting the hypothalamic-pituitary axis. Polycystic ovarian syndrome also causes anovulation related to abnormal gonadotropic secretion and excess androgen activity.

Heavy bleeding may occur with the use of contraceptives. Women occasionally have an episode of heavy bleeding while taking oral contraceptives. After discontinuing oral contraceptives, women may experience increased flow. The use of an intrauterine device (IUD) is associated with a 10% incidence of significant increase in menstrual flow. With persistent menorrhagia, IUD removal or changing oral contraceptives is usually necessary.

Endometrial infections can cause heavy menstrual bleeding because of disturbed clotting mechanisms. Cigarette smoking (Marchbanks et al., 1990) and cervicitis have been associated with an increased risk for pelvic infections. Menses are usually painful and foul smelling. There may be fever, uterine tenderness with

TABLE 10-1
Common Causes of Gynecologic Bleeding

Age 5–13	Age 14–25	Age 25–35	Age 35–45	Age 45+ (Postmenopausal)
Foreign bodies	Pregnancy	Pregnancy	Pregnancy	Estrogen therapy
Self-inflicted lacerations	Oral contraceptives or intrauterine device (IUD)	Oral contraceptives or IUD	Anovulation	Endometrial hyperplasia or polyps
Vaginitis (nonspecific)	Cervical eversion or cervicitis	Cervical eversion or cervicitis	Endometrial hyperplasia	Endometrial carcinoma
Rule out urinary tract infection and rectal bleeding	Anovulation	Cervical polyps	Uterine myoma	Uterine myoma
	Vaginal lacerations or infections	Anovulation	Adenomyosis	Coital injuries related to atrophy
	Foreign bodies	Vaginal lacerations or infections	Endometriosis	
	Cervical polyps	Foreign bodies	Endometrial carcinoma	
		Uterine myoma	Oral contraceptives or IUD	
		Endometrial hyperplasia	Cervical polyps	
		Endometriosis		

enlargement, and mucopurulent cervical discharge. When the tubes or ovaries are involved in pelvic infections, there may be adnexal fullness, masses, or tenderness. When pelvic inflammatory disease (PID) is suspected, cultures are taken for *Neisseria gonorrhoeae* and *Chlamydia* organisms, and a white blood cell count with differential is ordered. PID is treated with antibiotics and if severe, may require hospitalization.

Organic causes of heavy menstrual bleeding include various cervical and uterine lesions, including leiomyomas (fibroids), polyps, endometrial hyperplasia, and malignancies. Leiomyomas usually are detected by palpating an enlarged or irregularly shaped uterus. Polyps and hyperplasias occur more frequently in **perimenopause**, the period from when fertility and menses become irregular through at least 1 year after menopause. There usually is intermenstrual bleeding also. Because of the possibility of a malignancy and similarity of symptoms, these lesions must undergo tissue diagnosis.

Although the incidence is small, systemic disease may cause excessive menstrual bleeding. Blood dyscrasias and liver and renal disease occasionally cause menorrhagia. Obesity may lead to anovulation, eventually resulting in menorrhagia. Various drugs, such as chemotherapy, anticoagulants, steroid hormones, neuroleptics, and major tranquilizers, also may disrupt normal menstrual patterns, causing menorrhagia.

Hypomenorrhea

Hypomenorrhea, short, scant menstrual flow, may result from endocrine dysfunctions. Menstrual flow may be light or consist only of spotting for 1 to 2 days.

Short cycles (17–20 days) may indicate anovulation. Women younger than 30 years with consistent anovulatory cycles are more prone to infertility and are at increased risk for endometrial carcinoma. With normal physical examination and documentation of ovulation (by menstrual calendar, basal body temperature chart, and cervical mucus observation), this menstrual pattern is probably a normal variation. If cycles are anovulatory, further workup is needed to identify potential infertility (see Chap. 13).

Oral contraceptives often cause light menses because they create a relative estrogen deficiency or have an androgenic influence on the endometrium. If other symptoms of estrogen deficiency are not present, this is considered a benign side effect. Unless the woman is troubled by hypomenorrhea, there is no cause for concern.

Cervical stenosis may cause a light menses with dark brown spotting and cramping. The cervical os may appear occluded on pelvic examination, or it may not allow passage of **sound,** an instrument introduced for dilation or detection of foreign bodies. Medical treatment often includes progressive cervical dilatation.

Decreased menstrual flow also may be due to *severe weight loss* and inadequate protein. Eating disorders, such as anorexia or bulimia, may underlie this problem. Some medications and recreational drugs can decrease menstrual flow by inhibiting normal estrogen function.

Endometriosis

About 1% to 7% of women in the United States experience **endometriosis,** a condition in which endometrial tissue is present on the pelvic peritoneum. Endometriosis results from retrograde menstruation, which causes tiny fragments of normal endometrium to implant in the lower peritoneal cavity. The most common sites are the posterior cul-de-sac, ovaries, bladder serosa, fallopian tubes, and large bowel. Women with a longer menstrual flow (more than 8 days) and shorter cycles (less than 27 days) are at greater risk for endometriosis. The condition is estrogen dependent, occurs in women 15 to 44 years old, and is rarely seen before puberty or after menopause. Frequent aerobic exercise has been found to protect against endometriosis, because it decreases the rate of estrogen production (Barbieri, 1990).

The symptoms of endometriosis include painful menses, pelvic pain, cul-de-sac nodularity, adnexal mass, or infertility. Many women have pain with bowel movements and pain with deep penetration during intercourse. Often there is painful, heavy menstrual bleeding that increases with time. On physical examination, the uterus frequently is retroverted and fixed in position. Nodules are found on the rectovaginal septum and cul-de-sac. There also is uterosacral ligament tenderness. The diagnosis is confirmed by direct laparoscopic visualization of lesions, which typically appear as bluish-red blebs or dark power burns (Adamson, 1990).

Medical treatment includes medications for pain relief, such as nonsteroidal anti-inflammatory drugs (NSAIDs), and to suppress estrogen production, such as oral contraceptives, danazol, and nafarelin. Surgical therapy may be done to remove adhesions. Laser surgery may be used to ablate lesions. Occasionally, hysterectomy with oophorectomy is performed. Endometriosis is the second most common reason for hysterectomy, accounting for about 19% of operations (Bachman, 1990).

Intermenstrual Bleeding

Intermenstrual bleeding refers to any bleeding or spotting between menses. It may be due to organic or functional problems. *Midcycle spotting* (mittelstaining), associated with ovulation, is light pink spotting that lasts a few hours to 1 day. This functional condition is caused by a relative estrogen dip at midcycle just before ovulation. It may occur with regularity or only occasionally. When the history and physical examination are normal, other signs of ovulation help confirm the diagnosis. Usually no medical treatment is needed, although small doses of estrogen around the time of ovulation can prevent the spotting.

Vaginitis or cervicitis may cause intermenstrual spotting or light bleeding. These conditions often are associated with increased discharge, itching, spotting after intercourse, or discomfort with intercourse. Pelvic examination may reveal increased vaginal discharge, ery-

thema, cervical discharge, polyp, or inflammation. When vaginitis is diagnosed, medical treatment is specific for the organism (see Chap. 11).

Irregular intermenstrual bleeding may be an early sign of cytologic changes caused by diethylstilbestrol, especially when this occurs in adolescents and young adults. Papanicolaou (Pap) smears and colposcopy are needed for thorough evaluation.

Foreign bodies are another cause of noncyclic intermenstrual spotting. This is more frequent in young girls and adolescents, although it is not uncommon for women to forget a tampon or diaphragm in the vagina for several days. Associated symptoms include lower abdominal cramping, increased foul-smelling vaginal discharge, and pressure. The foreign body usually can be seen on speculum examination and then removed.

When the cause of intermenstrual bleeding is not evident from the history or examination, trauma must be considered. Sexual abuse is a common problem in female children and adult women and is one of the most frequent causes of genital trauma. Sensitive questioning in a supportive, accepting atmosphere may be necessary to obtain a history of abuse. Other causes of trauma may be scratching, falls, and lacerations from using tampons, vaginal sponges, or a diaphragm.

Oral contraceptives may cause breakthrough bleeding at any time in the menstrual cycle. This usually is not cyclic and regular but can be recurrent. The amount of bleeding ranges from light spotting to frank, heavy bleeding and may last from a few hours to several days. Ordinarily, there is little or no pain or cramping. Breakthrough bleeding occurs when endometrial sloughing is incomplete during withdrawal menses, and patches build up with varying thickness until the estrogen levels provided by the oral contraceptive are not enough to maintain the endometrium.

Pregnancy must always be considered as a possible cause of intermenstrual bleeding in women of childbearing age. Even those using contraceptives must be evaluated for pregnancy because of the potential for contraceptive misuse. Some pregnant women continue to have light bleeding at the time their menses would be due.

Endometrial hyperplasia related to hormone imbalances is a frequent cause of sudden, heavy bleeding without a cyclic pattern, particularly in women approaching the cessation of ovarian function. The aging ovary fails to produce estrogen and progesterone with smooth cyclic release in sufficient quantities, and ovulation becomes erratic. Adequate progesterone is necessary to regulate endometrial breakdown during the menstrual phase. When estrogen influences the endometrium in the absence of sufficient progesterone, the endometrium continues to proliferate and grow in thickness. During menses, the endometrium is incompletely sloughed, leading to irregular patches of thick buildup. When the hormone levels no longer support this hyperplastic endometrium, sudden bleeding occurs that can be extremely heavy, have large clots, and last several weeks.

When diagnostic tests show endometrial hyperplasia, treatment may be surgery (dilation and curettage) or hormone therapy. Frequently, a progestational drug, such as medroxyprogesterone acetate, is used during the last part of the menstrual cycle to regulate endometrial breakdown and control bleeding. Acute bleeding episodes can be stopped by administering progesterone or estrogen in high doses, followed by an oral contraceptive or estrogen-progesterone combination to control subsequent menstrual bleeding. Careful monitoring of the client's response to treatment is necessary for premenopausal women with irregular bleeding because of the risk of cancer.

Perimenopausal bleeding is significant because of the increased risk of endometrial cancer. Women in their middle to late 40s and 50s need prompt assessment of any unusual bleeding. Any bleeding or spotting after menopause is potentially serious. Women on hormone replacement therapy (HRT) must be watched carefully for 1 to 2 months; if bleeding does not resolve, an endometrial biopsy is indicated. Women not taking HRT require immediate diagnostic evaluation.

Nursing Assessment

Women with problems related to vaginal bleeding are assessed by taking a menstrual and reproductive history, a history of the bleeding problem, and a personal and family health history. The physical examination includes speculum and bimanual pelvic examination, with specimens and diagnostic tests as indicated.

Menstrual History. The menstrual history establishes the woman's usual pattern and provides a baseline from which to evaluate her current symptoms. To assess the amount of bleeding accurately, the nurse asks if a pad or tampon is needed, how often it is changed, and how saturated it is when changed. Pad or tampon use over a set time, such as 4 hours, can give some idea of the extent of bleeding (see Chap. 27 for estimation of pad saturation).

The history identifies the character of the bleeding:

- Date of onset of bleeding
- How many days of bleeding
- How this relates to the woman's menstrual cycle
- Amount of bleeding (based on tampon or pad use)
- Presence of clots or tissue and odor of discharge
- Pattern of discomfort, pain, cramping, or any associated symptoms

The patterns of pain in relation to bleeding are important: Does pain occur before or after onset of bleeding? Does it continue or cease when bleeding begins and ends? Severity of pain is assessed by how much it affects lifestyle and daily activities. With severe pain, the woman may need to lie down or go to bed or may be unable to continue activities. Less severe pain affects activities to varying degrees. The character of the pain may be described as aching, cramping, sharp, shooting, burning, or piercing.

The presence of foul-smelling vaginal discharge or blood may indicate infection, especially when fever is present. Urinary discomfort or burning may indicate bleeding from the urinary system. The woman is asked about sudden changes in weight, recent major stress or life changes, severe dieting, drug use, signs of pregnancy, other illness, and contraceptive use. History of these symptoms, treatment, and factors that relieve or increase the symptoms can help in assessment. (See Assessment Tool: Menstrual History.)

Physical Examination. The pelvic examination provides data on the condition of the perineum, vagina, cervix, uterus and adnexa, urethra, and rectum. The client may confuse bleeding from hemorrhoids or the urinary meatus with vaginal bleeding. Blood present in the vagina may originate from vaginal, cervical, or uterine structures. Careful inspection may reveal vaginal lacerations or inflammation or cervical polyps, infection, or lesions.

Bimanual examination may reveal uterine enlargement, tenderness, or masses; nodules on the rectovaginal septum, ligaments, or cul-de-sac; or adnexal masses, fullness, or tenderness. Combined with data from the history, pelvic findings can confirm the diagnosis. The nurse may perform or assist in the pelvic examination, depending on skills and expertise (see Chap. 17 for pelvic examination technique).

Diagnostic tests may include the following:

- Pap smear
- Vaginal or cervical smears for culture or microscopic examination
- Hematocrit and hemoglobin
- Complete blood count and differential
- Stool guaiac
- Urinalysis, urine culture
- Pregnancy test
- Gonorrhea or *Chlamydia* culture
- Pelvic ultrasonography or computed tomography (if pelvic mass is identified)

Nursing Diagnosis

After a thorough nursing assessment, the nurse can formulate appropriate nursing diagnoses. Common nursing diagnoses for DUB are listed in Box 10-1.

ASSESSMENT TOOL
Menstrual History

Menarche
  Age menses began _____
  Menstrual pattern first few years:
    Regularity of cycles _____
    Cramping or pain _____
    Length and character of flow _____
  Preparation for menses (extent, who informed her, circumstances)
  _____
  _____
  _____

    Reaction to menarche (feelings, attitudes)
  _____
  _____
  _____

Menstrual cycle characteristics
  Length of cycles (regular, irregular)
  _____
  _____

  Length and character of flow (how many days, amount of blood, clots)
  _____
  _____

  Discomfort or pain with menses:
    When pain begins (days, hours before flow; with onset of flow)
  _____
  _____

    How long pain lasts (hours, days) _____
    Severity of pain (extent of interference with activities, debility)
  _____
  _____

    Medications or remedies used, effectiveness
  _____
  _____

  Use of tampons, pads, sponges, etc.
  _____
  _____

Premenstrual symptoms
  Onset of symptoms (days, hours before flow) _____
  Progression of symptoms (worse, better, when they end) _____
  Types of symptoms and relative severity
  _____
  _____

  Factors associated with symptoms (food, rest, activity)
  _____
  _____

  Medical treatment or self-treatment, results
  _____
  _____

(continued)

ASSESSMENT TOOL *(Continued)*
Menstrual History

Interference with work or daily activities

_____

_____

Effects on spouse, family

_____

_____

Attitudes toward menstruation
   Feelings about menstruation (positive, negative) _____

   Feelings about menstrual symptoms _____

   Perception of relation between menstrual symptoms and woman's status

_____

Feelings about important others' responses to menstrual behaviors

_____

_____

Beliefs about effects of menstrual symptoms on women's cognitive or functional abilities

_____

_____

Knowledge about menstruation
   Physiology of menstrual cycle _____

   Psychology of menstruation _____

   Social constructs related to menstruation _____

   Dysmenorrhea (cause, symptoms, treatment) _____

   PMS (cause, symptoms, treatment) _____

Nursing Planning and Intervention

Nursing care focuses on alleviating knowledge deficits and assisting the woman to understand the problem's cause, clinical course, treatment, and anticipated outcomes. Self-care is encouraged when diet, hot or cold therapy, rest, stress reduction, and exercise can affect the condition or improve symptoms. Anxiety and fear are reduced by providing emotional support, a caring relationship in which feelings can be expressed, empathic listening, and realistic reassurance. Problems involving self-esteem, body image, or sexual dysfunction may be improved by providing reliable information and clarifying misconceptions. The client is encouraged to express her feelings and views of herself. Teaching focuses on the client's resources that will aid in coping.

Education, counseling, and support are provided to assist the woman and family through the medical diagnostic process. The nurse encourages expression of feelings and communication and assists in developing effective coping strategies. When DUB is related to eating disorders, nutritional disruptions, coping difficulties, body image disturbance, and altered thought processes often can occur. Interventions may be complex and long term.

Evaluation

Nursing intervention is evaluated by observing for changes in the woman's behavior, level of knowledge and self-care skills, and perspectives and attitudes. Possible anticipated outcomes include the following:

- The client expresses a clear understanding of the causes, treatment, and outcomes of the bleeding problem. The client demonstrates actions that maximize recovery and prevent recurrences or complications.
- The woman expresses her fears and concerns openly.
- The client develops a plan for integrating changes into her lifestyle.
- The client seeks assistance appropriately from family, health providers, and other community resources.

BOX 10–1

Nursing Diagnoses: Dysfunctional Uterine Bleeding

- Pain related to menstrual dysfunction
- Knowledge Deficit related to the cause of menstrual dysfunction, treatment, and care activities
- Anxiety related to uncertainty of outcome
- Risk for Injury related to possible treatment, surgery, or complications
- Self Care Deficit related to effect of menstrual dysfunction on activity level
- Body Image Disturbance related to psychosocial effects of the menstrual dysfunction or its treatment
- Situational Low Self Esteem related to effects of menstrual disorder
- Altered Sexuality Patterns related to
  - Effects of treatment
  - Menstrual dysfunction's interference with sexual expression
  - Disruption in relationship with significant other
- Sexual Dysfunction related effects of menstrual disorder or its treatment.

Amenorrhea

Amenorrhea refers to the absence of menses, or skipping periods. It is a common problem among women during the reproductive years. *Primary amenorrhea* occurs when a girl reaches 16 years and has never menstruated. The most frequent causes are structural abnormalities, such as gonadal dysgenesis and imperforate hymen; congenital abnormalities, such as absent vagina or uterus; and endocrine abnormalities, such as androgen insensitivity syndrome, prepubertal ovarian failure, congenital adrenal hyperplasia, and hypopituitarism.

Although most girls in the United States menstruate by 12½ to 13 years, menarche may occur much later. The early signs of sexual maturation, breast buds and pubic hair, usually occur about 2 years before onset of menses. If these appear by 14 years, investigation of amenorrhea can be delayed until after 16 years. Body weight is a significant factor influencing onset of puberty. The critical weight for initiation and maintenance of menstruation is 17% to 20% body fat. However, regular menstrual cycles occur in female athletes with as little as 13.7% body fat (Doody et al., 1990).

Secondary amenorrhea occurs when a previously menstruating woman ceases to menstruate. The causes may be organic or functional. *Pregnancy* is probably the most common cause of secondary amenorrhea in women 16 to 45 years old. Oral contraceptives, particularly low-dose estrogen and progestin-only pills, frequently cause women to skip one or more menses.

Amenorrhea related to low levels of gonadotropin and estrogen secretion may be caused by stress, weight loss, anorexia nervosa, exercise, and hypothalamic and pituitary lesions.

Stress, weight loss, anorexia, and exercise are the most common causes of *functional* (hypogonadotropic) *anovulation.* Low gonadotropin levels result from alterations in gonadotropin-releasing hormone (Gn-RH) secretion by the hypothalamus. A hypoestrogenic state results, in which the endometrium does not build up adequately to produce menses. The primary treatment includes counseling directed toward correcting the causes of amenorrhea. Oral contraceptives or estrogen may be given to initiate hormonal cycling, or Gn-RH therapy may be given to encourage adequate endometrial buildup. Estrogen deprivation in young women may contribute to decreased bone density or greater perimenopausal bone loss. Treatment with calcium supplements, calcitonin, bisphosphonates, and vitamin D may be necessary (Chang, 1993).

Ovarian cysts, most commonly follicular and corpus luteum cysts, may cause amenorrhea. When the graafian follicle fails to rupture, it may continue to increase in size and secrete estrogen. The ovary may be enlarged to 4 to 6 cm. Because ovulation does not occur, the luteal phase is not entered and the endometrium continues to proliferate under estrogen influence. Usually these cysts resolve spontaneously in several weeks, and menstruation is restored. Oral contraceptives may be used for one to two cycles to cause involution of the cyst. With corpus luteum cysts, continued progesterone secretion maintains the secretory endometrium, similar to that of early pregnancy. These cysts also tend to regress spontaneously, with regular cycles restored in a few weeks.

Organic causes of secondary amenorrhea include tumors, infections, or cysts that compress or destroy the hypothalamus; pituitary necrosis (Sheehan's syndrome); hyperthyroidism; galactorrhea; hyperprolactinemia; adrenal virilization; intrauterine synechiae (Asherman's syndrome); polycystic ovarian syndrome (Stein-Leventhal); Cushing's syndrome; Kallman's syndrome (idiopathic Gn-RH deficiency) and premature ovarian failure (menopause before 40 years). Various drugs also may induce amenorrhea, including estrogen therapy, general anesthesia, phenothiazines, reserpine, monoamine oxidase inhibitors, opioids, and histamine receptor antagonists.

After anatomic abnormalities and pregnancy are ruled out, serum prolactin levels are evaluated. A progesterone challenge test with medroxyprogesterone acetate (Provera) is administered for 5 days to evaluate estrogen status. Women with normal prolactin levels who have withdrawal bleeding after receiving the progesterone challenge are diagnosed with chronic anovulation with estrogen present. Women who do not have withdrawal bleeding usually have elevated pro-lactin levels and are diagnosed with estrogen absent disorder. Further testing is done to evaluate thyroid (thyroid-stimulating hormone levels) and pituitary (computed tomography, magnetic resonance imaging) function and serum follicle-stimulating hormone (FSH) levels. A client with a low FSH level and normal thyroid and pituitary examinations is classified as having chronic anovulation with estrogen absent, usually due to functional disorders (Doody et al., 1990; Chang, 1993).

Nursing Assessment

Assessment in primary amenorrhea focuses on degree of secondary sexual development and presence of a normal reproductive tract. For secondary amenorrhea, assessment focuses on menstrual patterns after menarche. For example, was a regular cyclic menstrual pattern ever established? How long has this pattern lasted? Onset of amenorrhea and any associated events are important. History of any gynecologic procedures or problems provides cues. Emotional stress, weight loss or gain, altered nutritional patterns, level of exercise, and major life events or changes may be important. The woman's reactions to amenorrhea and its meanings for her and her partner are explored and coping strategies assessed.

During the physical examination, signs of genetic or hormonal disorders are noted, such as exophthalmos and thyroid enlargement (hyperthyroidism), moon faces and hirsutism (Cushing's syndrome), thinning hair and delayed reflexes (hypothyroidism), and deepening voice, breast atrophy, and temporal baldness (virilizing syndromes).

Nursing Diagnosis

Nursing diagnoses are similar to those for the client with DUB. See Box 10-1 for possible examples. They often involve a body image disturbance or problem with self-esteem because many women view their bodies as functioning abnormally when they experience amenorrhea. There may be anxiety or fear about the meanings of the problem and implications about future fertility or femininity. Knowledge deficits are common and are related to the cause, progression, or treatment of the problem. There may be sexual dysfunction, especially in chronic hypoestrogenic or virilizing conditions.

Nursing Planning and Intervention

Nursing care includes education, counseling, reassurance, and increasing or developing options to assist the client to cope with the problem. With serious or permanent disorders, the woman and family may need assistance accepting the problem and integrating it into their lives. The clients should be allowed to grieve about the possible loss of function, such as fertility or menstrual cycles. Threats to well-being, such as cancer or destructive tumors, need to be discussed openly, allowing the client and family to express and work through their feelings.

Evaluation

The possible anticipated outcomes are similar to those for the client with DUB. For more information, see page 233.

Dysmenorrhea

Dysmenorrhea, painful menstruation, is characterized by pain that occurs shortly before the onset of or during menstrual flow, persisting for one to several days during menses. It is one of the most common gynecologic problems, affecting more than 50% of women at some time in their lives and causing incapacitation for 1 to 3 days each month in about 10% of these women. Absenteeism of adolescents from school because of dysmenorrhea is about 25% (Dunnihoo, 1992).

Primary Dysmenorrhea

Primary dysmenorrhea occurs without pelvic pathology, affecting about 50% of women; 10% of women have pain severe enough to incapacitate them for 1 to 3 days each month. The onset is 6 months to 2 years after menarche, with improvement by 25 years and declining incidence after 30 to 35 years. It occurs more frequently in unmarried women. Pregnancy and vaginal delivery may improve discomfort. Exercise does not have a significant effect on incidence (Dawood, 1990). When ovulation is suppressed, dysmenorrhea normally does not occur.

The pain begins a few hours prior to or with the onset of menses, lasting 48 to 72 hours. The pain, located in the suprapubic region, can be sharp, gripping, cramping, or dull and aching. Often there is pelvic fullness or bearing-down sensations that radiate to the inner thighs and lumbosacral area. Some women experience nausea and vomiting, headache, fatigue, dizziness, faintness, diarrhea, or emotional lability during this time.

Increased prostaglandin production and release by the endometrium (mainly PGF_{2a}) during menstruation produce uncoordinated, spasmodic uterine contractions that cause pain. Women with dysmenorrhea have higher intrauterine pressure during the menstrual period and twice as much prostaglandin in their menstrual flow as women without pain. Uterine contractions are more frequent and become uncoordinated or dysrhythmic. With this increased abnormal uterine activity, blood flow is reduced, resulting in uterine ischemia or hypoxia and contributing to pain. Another mechanism of pain is caused by prostaglandin (PGE_2) and other hormones, which hypersensitize sensory pain fibers in the uterus to the action of bradykinin and other chemical and physical pain stimuli (Dawood, 1990).

In women with primary dysmenorrhea, circulating vasopressin levels are higher during menses. Coupled with a concomitant increase in oxytocin levels, higher vasopressin levels cause dysrhythmic uterine contractions that produce uterine hypoxia and ischemia. In some women with primary dysmenorrhea but no increase in prostaglandins, activity of the 5-lipoxygenase pathway is increased. This results in increased biosynthesis of leukotrienes, potent vasoconstrictors that induce uterine muscle contractions (Demers et al., 1985).

Social and psychological factors also may influence symptoms. Women with less acceptance of the female role or higher masculinity traits have reported more menstrual pain. However, women with high femininity traits and homemakers with no outside career ambitions also have reported more menstrual symptoms. Another study supported lack of association between perimenstrual discomfort and traditional or feminist orientations. As income, education, and age increase, there is a tendency for less dysmenorrhea. Negative and positive attitudes toward menses have been associated with dysmenorrhea (Brown et al., 1984).

Medical treatment of primary dysmenorrhea includes oral contraceptives and NSAIDs, which are prostaglandin synthetase inhibitors. Oral contraceptives reduce menstrual fluid volume by suppressing the endometrium and ovulation, thus creating an environment with low prostaglandin levels. A combination estrogen-progestin pill provides relief to 90% of women with dysmenorrhea. NSAIDs, such as ibuprofen, naproxen, and mefenamic acid, inhibit prostaglandin synthesis. Medications are taken as soon as pain begins and continued throughout the first 2 to 3 days of menses.

Secondary Dysmenorrhea

Secondary dysmenorrhea results from organic pelvic disease, such as endometriosis, PID, cervical stenosis, ovarian cysts, uterine myomas, congenital malformations, IUDs, or trauma. Pain usually is present for more than 2 to 3 days during or throughout the entire menses. Women with secondary dysmenorrhea usually have had normal menses previously and are older than

TABLE 10-2
Causes of Secondary Dysmenorrhea

Location	Organic Causes
Vagina	Imperforate hymen
	Transverse vaginal septum
Cervix	Cervical stenosis
Uterus	Congenital malformations
	Uterine myomas or polyps
	Endometriosis (adenomyosis)
	Intrauterine adhesions (Asherman's syndrome)
	Intrauterine device
Fallopian tubes	Pelvic inflammatory disease
Ovaries	Ovarian cysts or tumors
	Endometriosis
Peritoneum	Pelvic congestion syndrome

those with primary dysmenorrhea. Pelvic examination or laparoscopy usually reveals the causes of secondary dysmenorrhea (Table 10-2).

Specific therapy for secondary dysmenorrhea depends on the cause. Women with an IUD can be treated with NSAIDs, because pain is related to increased prostaglandins. NSAIDs can be temporarily helpful with uterine myomas, but surgery is the definitive treatment. Antibiotics are given when infections are present; surgery is used for anatomic and structural abnormalities. Treatment of endometriosis is discussed in a previous section of this chapter.

Nursing Assessment

When a client reports pelvic pain, a thorough assessment is important to determine the cause of the pain because many conditions may cause it. See Box 10-2 for a list of possible causes of pelvic pain. Assessment of dysmenorrhea includes history of menstrual cycle, complaints of pain, and presence of any associated symptoms. The history identifies the following:

- Amount of disruption in daily activities caused by dysmenorrhea
- Role of stress and anxiety as contributing factors to dysmenorrhea
- Lifestyle and habits, such as diet, exercise, and stress reduction, and their effect on dysmenorrhea

The physical examination helps to identify if pelvic disease is the cause of menstrual pain. Diagnostic tests might include cultures, complete blood count, urinalysis, sedimentation rate, pelvic ultrasonography, laparoscopy, hysteroscopy, and hysterosalpingography.

BOX 10–2
Causes of Pelvic Pain

Cyclic, Recurrent Menstrual Pain

Dysmenorrhea (primary, secondary)
Endometriosis
Adenomyosis
Intrauterine device
Endometritis or pelvic inflammatory disease (PID)

Recurrent Pain not During Menses

Midcycle ovulation pain (mittelschmerz)
Ovarian cysts (follicular, corpus luteum)
Ovarian or uterine malignancies
Psychogenic pain

Acute, Severe Nonmenstrual Pain

Ectopic pregnancy, actual or pending rupture
Twisted fallopian tube, ovary, or ovarian cyst
Ruptured ovarian cyst
Appendicitis
Acute PID
Acute lower bowel lesions

Nursing Diagnosis

After collecting assessment information, the nurse identifies appropriate nursing diagnoses. For a list of possible nursing diagnoses, see Box 10-3.

Nursing Planning and Intervention

Nursing care for dysmenorrhea can include a number of nonpharmacologic self-care measures and over-the-counter and prescription medications (see Client Teaching Guidelines: Relief of Menstrual Pain). The client is instructed about any medication, including dosage, frequency, and possible side effects. Information about the condition and its treatment can be provided by education and counseling. B vitamins (particularly B_6) will help to increase protein use and relieve fatigue, tension, and depression. Mild hypoglycemia, which may occur premenstrually, can be helped by small, frequent intakes of protein and complex carbohydrates.

Women with one or more days of significant debility may experience lower self-esteem and less effective role performance. These women may benefit from developing more positive attitudes toward menstruation and toward themselves as normal, healthy women. Explanations of menstrual physiology and psychology can help correct any misconceptions that they might have. Helping them to anticipate and prepare for days when functioning is affected can increase their feelings

BOX 10–3
Nursing Diagnoses: Dysmenorrhea

- Pain related to uncoordinated, spasmodic uterine contractions
- Knowledge Deficit related to condition, treatment, and self-care measures
- Ineffective Individual Coping related to
  - Emotional lability
  - Interference with activities
- Altered Nutrition: Less than body requirements related to nausea, vomiting, or diarrhea and fatigue
- Self Care Deficit related to fatigue and severity of pain
- Body Image Disturbance related to effects on self-care activities and feelings of lack of control
- Situational Low Self Esteem related interference with role performance

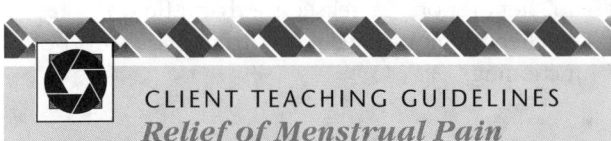

CLIENT TEACHING GUIDELINES
Relief of Menstrual Pain

Self-Care Measures

Heat applied to abdomen (heating pad, hot bath)—causes vasodilation and decreases hypertonic muscle contractions
Massage or effleurage to abdomen—increases pain threshold through secondary stimulus
Exercise—increases blood flow, tones muscles (preventive if done regularly)
Sleep and rest—promotes relaxation, decreases tension
Relaxation techniques (biofeedback, autogenic training, yoga, meditation)—promotes relaxation, decreases tension
Natural diuresis (salt reduction, herbs, vitamins)—reduces congestion

Over-the-Counter Medications

Aspirin or acetaminophen (Tylenol) 650 mg every 4 hours
Ibuprofen (Motrin, Advil, Nuprin) 200 to 400 mg every 4 to 6 hours
Midol or Cope (aspirin for pain, caffeine for diuresis, cinnamedrine to relax uterine muscle)
Other combinations: aspirin or acetaminophen with pamabrom for diuresis, pyrilamine maleate (antihistamine) for sedation or analgesia

Prescription Medications

Mefenamic acid (Ponstel) 250 to 500 mg every 6 hours
Naproxen (Naprosyn) 250 to 500 mg every 6 to 8 hours
Naproxen sodium (Anaprox) 275 to 550 mg every 4 to 6 hours
Ketoprofen (Orudis) 25 to 50 mg every 6 to 8 hours
Meclofenamate (Meclomen) 100 mg three times daily

of control. Assisting the client to find effective methods of pain relief also can help improve self-esteem disturbances.

Dysmenorrhea is one of many stressors. Ineffective coping may be related to other factors in the woman's life. The nurse assists the woman to find ways to remove, reduce, or alleviate causes of stress. Any measures to reduce menstrual pain are helpful. Referrals may be needed for individual or family therapy, social agencies, and increasing social and family networks.

Evaluation

Anticipated outcomes for the client with dysmenorrhea may include the following:

- The client verbalizes relief of pain.
- The client verbalizes knowledge of the condition, treatment, and care.
- The client demonstrates positive coping skills.
- The client reports increased food and fluid intake.
- The client demonstrates return to previous level of functioning.

Premenstrual Syndrome

Premenstrual syndrome (PMS) is a complex set of recurrent, cyclic physical, behavioral, and emotional symptoms. PMS affects 30% to 40% of American women (Smith et al., 1989). Although PMS has been studied since 1930 and the term was coined by Dalton in 1953, much is still unknown about etiology. Several perimenstrual patterns have been identified (see the section, "Variations in Perimenstrual Patterns"; Woods et al., 1994; Mitchell et al., 1991). The PMS pattern has previously been blended with the **premenstrual magnification** (PMM) **pattern**. Women with PMM usually have a medical or psychiatric disorder, such as migraine headaches, seizure disorder, and depression or other affective disorder (Plouffe et al., 1993). Combining PMS and PMM has led to confusion about how these syndromes present and which treatments can be effective. Women with the low severity pattern experience mild symptoms without differences in severity across menstrual cycle phases and frequently do not seek medical treatment.

The commonly used clinical definition for PMS includes the following:

1. Symptoms occur during the luteal phase of the menstrual cycle and resolve within 1 to 2 days after onset of menses; they are recurrent to some degree each month.
2. There is a symptom-free period of at least 1 week during the follicular phase of the cycle.

3. Symptoms are severe enough to interfere with some aspects of lifestyle (Smith et al., 1989; Chihal, 1990; Hsia et al., 1990).

Symptoms in PMS usually appear about 4 to 10 days before menses and improve after the onset of menstrual flow. As many as 200 different recurrent symptoms have been associated with PMS (Dan et al., 1992). The most common PMS symptoms include the following:

- Emotional lability
- Anger, irritability, agitation
- Anxiety, depression, lowered self-esteem
- Decreased interest in work or activities
- Fatigue, lethargy, difficulty concentrating
- Changes in appetite, such as cravings and binge eating, and sleep patterns
- Fluid retention, cramps, pelvic fullness, abdominal bloating, headache, and breast tenderness
- Feelings of panic or loss of control

The American Psychiatric Association includes premenstrual dysphoric disorder in the *Diagnostic and Statistical Manual of Mental Disorders* (1994). In this syndrome, women experience depressed mood, anxiety, affective lability, and decreased interest in activities during most menstrual cycles for at least 1 year. These symptoms regularly occur during the last week of the luteal phase and stop within a few days after onset of menses; there is at least 1 week in which they are entirely absent. Symptoms must be severe enough to markedly interfere with work, school, or usual activities to meet diagnostic criteria.

At least one psychological or physical symptom occurs premenstrually in about 75% of women. Symptoms severe enough to require treatment are much rarer. Premenstrual dysphoric disorder (previously called late luteal phase dysphoric disorder) is estimated to occur in 3% to 5% of women of reproductive age (Jensvold, 1993). Panic, loss of control or violent acts, increased accidents or injuries, and suicidal ideation are infrequent symptoms.

The relationship between the menstrual cycle and psychoemotional symptoms is not clear. Edema, hypoglycemia, declining beta endorphins, or serotonin deficiency may be involved (Menkes et al., 1992). PMS has been described as a "state change" with symptoms of dysphoric mood, fluid retention, and increased autonomic arousal and stress reactivity. These lead to changed perceptions of and responses to the environment and perceived changes in behavior and cognitions. Cyclic changes in ovarian steroids may initiate a cascade of neuroendocrine events that alter stress perceptions and produce symptoms (Woods et al., 1995). Women with PMS do not show decreased cognitive processing or depressive cognitive changes (less recall, slower performance, greater distractibility, decreased problem solving; Rapkin et al., 1989; Haas, 1993).

Variations in Perimenstrual Patterns

Three patterns of menstrual cycle symptoms have been identified:

1. **Low severity patterns**: Symptoms do not vary in severity across different phases of the menstrual cycle.
2. PMS pattern: No or low severity symptoms occur during premenstrual phase.
3. PMM: High severity symptoms occur during postmenses phase that become worse during premenses (Woods et al., 1994).

Causes of Perimenstrual Symptoms

A variety of etiologies are proposed for perimenstrual symptoms. The cause probably involves complex interactions between ovarian steroid hormones, endogenous opioid peptides, central neurotransmitters, prostaglandins, and peripheral autonomic and endocrine systems. Imbalances between estrogen excess and progesterone deficiency have been implicated, but studies have found no difference in a number of gonadotropic hormones in women with and without PMS. Reduced prostaglandin levels occur in the follicular and luteal phases in PMS sufferers. Treatment to increase prostaglandin production, such as evening primrose oil, and to inhibit its action, such as mefenamic acid, have been effective (Chihal, 1990; Smith et al., 1989).

Endogenous opioid peptides, such as endorphins, enkephalins, and dynorphins, which normally increase in peripheral and central concentrations during the luteal phase (Fujimoto et al., 1993), are lower in women with PMS (Tulenheimo et al., 1987; Facchinetti et al., 1987). Because endorphins affect mood, PMS symptoms could be related to an opiate withdrawal syndrome. Estrogens increase endorphin levels, and women with PMS appear to be functionally hypoestrogenic, experiencing vasomotor symptoms that are physiologically identical with menopausal hot flashes (Casper et al., 1987). Altered synchrony in the pulsatile patterns of luteinizing hormone (LH) and progesterone release with endorphin interactions appears to cause progesterone release at a greater rate in women with PMS (Lewis, 1992). Although serotonin deficiency has not been demonstrated as a cause of PMS, treatment with serotonin agonists, such as buspirone, and serotonin uptake inhibitors, such as fluoxitine, has been helpful for some women (Haas, 1993; Menkes et al., 1992).

Nutritional factors may be related to PMS. Many women with PMS report cravings for specific types of food. Fluctuating glucose and insulin levels seem to affect food cravings and may lead to hypoglycemic symptoms. No differences have been found in plasma concentrations of magnesium, zinc, vitamin A, vitamin E, thiamine, or pyridoxine in PMS clients compared with controls (Mira et al., 1988; Haas, 1993).

Women often attribute their perimenstrual symptoms to stress, but only modest relationships have been found with major life events, daily hassles, and chronic stress exposure (Woods et al., 1994; Beck et al., 1990). Autonomic arousal indicated by increased skin conductance and muscle tension and decreased skin temperature occurs premenstrually only for women with a PMS pattern (Woods et al., 1994). Women experiencing a stressful life context who are socialized to expect menstrual symptoms report more perimenstrual symptoms. Depressed mood occurs more often with PMM patterns than with PMS and low severity patterns (Woods et al., 1995).

Medical Therapy

Although many approaches to medical treatment have been used, none has been uniformly successful. Commonly progesterone is prescribed, although clinical trials have failed to demonstrate its superiority over placebos (Peck, 1990). Progesterone may act on cell metabolism in the hypothalamus to decrease catecholamines, resulting in sedative effects. This may underlie reports by women that natural progesterone alleviates their PMS symptoms (Lewis, 1992). Natural progesterone, in oral micronized form or topical cream, appears to balance an estrogen dominance secondary to relative progesterone deficiency in the luteal phase. Endogenous progesterone is a major precursor of cortisone synthesis by the adrenal cortex. Deficiencies lead to heightened limbic system activity through a complex cascade of neuroendocrine and steroid hormone synthesis. This relative imbalance between estrogen and progesterone leads to symptoms of estrogen dominance, such as mood swings, fatigue, feeling cold, and reactivity to stressors (Lee, 1993). Diuretics, such as thiazide, and spironolactone have been used when there is documented evidence of cyclic fluid retention. Oral contraceptives containing progestins have not been effective and may worsen symptoms. Progestin-dominant oral contraceptives, such as Ovral, reduced symptoms in uncontrolled studies.

The Gn-RH agonists, such as leuprolide and naferalin, are effective in improving physical and mental symptoms of PMS. These drugs create a hypoestrogenic state. They usually are intended for short-term use due to risk of osteoporosis with prolonged use. Once gonadotropin suppression is attained, supplemental estrogen or progestin at menopausal replacement doses ("add-back" regimen) is effective in reducing PMS symptoms by 60%. Calcium supplementation also is recommended to maintain bone mineral content (Haas, 1993; Chihal, 1990).

The prostaglandin inhibitor mefenamic acid taken in large doses throughout the luteal phase relieves many PMS symptoms. It is most effective in women who have dysmenorrhea associated with PMS. Evening primrose oil (Efamol), a prostaglandin precursor that increases prostaglandin synthesis, also reduces PMS symptoms in 50% of women. It contains linoleic acid and vitamin E and seems most effective for headache, sweet cravings, increased appetite, fatigue, and insomnia (Peck, 1990).

ASSESSMENT TOOL
Menstrual Symptom Diary

NAME _____   MENSES _____

Date																																				
Day of cycle	1	2	3	4	5	6	7	8	9	10	11	12	13	14	15	16	17	18	19	20	21	22	23	24	25	26	27	28	29	30	31	32	33	34	35	36
Menstruation																																				
Nervous tension																																				
Mood swings																																				
Irritability																																				
Anxiety																																				
Depression																																				
Crying																																				
Forgetfulness																																				
Confusion																																				
Insomnia																																				
Increased naps																																				
Avoid activities																																				
Feel clumsy																																				
Fatigue																																				
Breast tenderness																																				
Abdominal bloating																																				
Swelling—legs, hands																																				
Headaches																																				
Migraine headaches																																				
Hot flushes																																				
Abdominal cramps																																				
General aches																																				
Food cravings—salt																																				
sweets																																				
Skin problems																																				
Weight																																				
BBT																																				

GRADING OF MENSES
1 Light
2 Moderate
3 Heavy
4 Heavy with clots

GRADING OF SYMPTOMS
0 None
1 Mild—does not interfere with activities
2 Moderate—interferes with activities
3 Severe—disabling; unable to function

Other medical approaches to treating PMS include the use of danazol for relief of breast pain, diuretics to reduce fluid retention, clonidine and verapamil for anxiety and irritability, alprazolam to decrease anxiety and improve depression, and buspirone and fluoxitine for mood changes, anxiety, and depression. Some degree of PMS symptom improvement has occurred with most of these treatments (Plouffe et al., 1993).

Nursing Assessment

Assessment identifies the onset and progression of menstrual symptoms and the woman's attitudes and responses with time:

- Age at onset of PMS
- Circumstances surrounding the onset
- Duration
- Precipitating factors
- Type and severity of symptoms
- Timing and interval of symptoms
- Effects on self-esteem, body image, self-concept
- Effects on relationships
- Type and effectiveness of self-help measures
- Type and effectiveness of medical treatment

A helpful assessment tool is a symptom diary, which grades the menses and symptoms for each day of the month. The woman completes a symptom diary for 2 to 3 months, noting carefully the timing, type, and severity of each premenstrual symptom. A review of the symptom diary helps to identify which symptoms are most frequent and troublesome and when so that appropriate therapies can be instituted. (See Assessment Tool: Menstrual Symptom Diary.)

The physical examination identifies any uterine or ovarian enlargement, signs of endometriosis, and structural abnormalities of the reproductive tract. Together with the client's history, an appropriate diagnosis can be made.

Nursing Diagnoses

Nursing diagnoses related to PMS involve the problems that occur as a result of the client's signs and symptom. For a list of possible nursing diagnoses, see Box 10-4.

Nursing Planning and Intervention

The goals of nursing intervention for PMS are to promote a healthy lifestyle, alleviate symptoms, and enhance coping (see Nursing Care Plan: The Woman with PMS). Treatment for PMS varies according to which symptoms are most disturbing to the client. The most effective nursing therapies include dietary, lifestyle, and behavioral adjustments. Between 36% and 75% of women with PMS obtain significant symptomatic relief

---

BOX 10-4
Nursing Diagnoses:
Premenstrual Syndrome

- Pain related to uterine cramping and spasms
- Anxiety related to
  - Misconception about Premenstrual Syndrome (PMS)
  - Stress of disorder
  - Interference with activities
- Ineffective Individual Coping related to effects of PMS
- Fluid Volume Excess related to fluid retention
- Knowledge Deficit related to causes, contributing factors, treatment, and self-care measures
- Altered Nutrition: Less than body requirements related to decreased appetite and abdominal bloating
- Altered Nutrition: More than body requirements related to cravings or binge eating
- Body Image Disturbance related to emotional effects of PMS and interference with activity level
- Altered Sexuality Patterns related to
  - Interference with normal activities and sexual expression
  - Effects of PMS
  - Disruption in relationship with significant other

---

with these interventions (Goodale et al., 1990; Haas, 1993). Relaxation techniques may be helpful in managing discomfort. They also are helpful in managing the PMS symptoms of irritability, depression, and anxiety. Information is provided about the physiology and psychology of PMS. Any misconceptions about sociopsychological factors and PMS are corrected.

Nutritional counseling focuses on avoiding caffeine, chocolate, and other xanthine derivatives because of their tedency to increase mood and emotional symptoms. Less red meat and fat and more complex carbohydrates, vegetables, whole grains, legumes, and fiber promote health and reduce symptoms. Sodium should be reduced, especially premenstrually when fluid retention occurs. Use of alcohol and tobacco should be curtailed. Adequate fluids and natural diuretics, such as cranberry or grapefruit juice, are helpful.

Hypoglycemia symptoms, such as fatigue, headache, dizziness, and food cravings, can be relieved by avoiding sweets and refined carbohydrates and by eating a diet high in protein and complex carbohydrates. Frequent, small meals help to keep blood glucose levels more stable.

Vitamin B_6 (pyridoxine), a coenzyme in the synthesis of certain neurotransmitters, is often recommended to reduce irritability and depression. In large doses (>1 g/d), vitamin B_6 can cause peripheral neuropathy. Data on effectiveness of vitamin B_6 are contradictory. Other vitamins, such as vitamins A and E, and minerals, such as calcium, magnesium, chromium, tryptophan, have

NURSING CARE PLAN
The Woman with Premenstrual Syndrome (PMS)

Nursing Goals
1. Woman identifies symptoms of PMS and assesses symptom patterns and associated factors.
2. Woman initiates actions to reduce symptoms and debility from PMS.
3. Woman learns and implements self-care to prevent and minimize effects of PMS.
4. Woman seeks appropriate care for family or sexual problems associated with PMS.

Assessment	Potential Nursing Diagnosis	Intervention/ Rationale	Evaluation

Menstrual history
  Menarche, menstrual patterns, reactions, preparation
  Menstrual cycle character and symptoms
  Attitudes toward menstruation
  Knowledge about menstruation
	Knowledge Deficit related to menstrual physiology and psychology	Teach menstrual physiology and psychology *to promote understanding.*
		Clarify myths, misconceptions *to reduce confusion and anxiety.*
		Provide information and data on social and psychological factors *to provide normalization.*
			Client describes correct understanding of menstrual physiology and psychology; myths and misunderstandings are cleared.

Physical and pelvic examination negative for pathology	Self Esteem Disturbance related to negative attitudes and perceptions toward menstruation	Provide education and counseling about menstruation as normal female functioning *to encourage acceptance.* Reduce PMS symptoms *to promote comfort.* Suggest group therapy *to build positive attitudes and correct social stereotypes.*	Client accepts normality of menstruation and symptoms. Client states positive attitudes and corrects former stereotypes.
Specific PMS symptoms Pain, cramping	Pain	Prescribe mild analgesics (acetylsalicylic acid, acetaminophen) *for pain relief.* Apply dry or moist heat *for pain relief.* Teach relaxation techniques *to reduce pain perception.* Encourage regular exercise *to increase tone.*	Client says pain and cramping are decreased.

Fluid retention:
  Breast tenderness
  Abdominal bloating
  Peripheral edema
  Weight gain
	Fluid Volume Excess
	Altered Nutrition: More than body requirements (sodium)
		Reduce or avoid sodium in foods *to reduce fluid retention.*
		Drink 1 quart of water daily *for good hydration.*
		Use natural diuretics (teas, cranberry and grapefruit juice) *to reduce fluid retention.*
			Client states she has less bloating, and her symptoms are improved.

Depression, irritability, mood swings, frustration, impaired concentration, nervousness, anxiety, emotional instability	Altered Nutrition: More than body requirements (xanthines)	Eliminate or reduce caffeine, chocolate, other xanthines; increase vitamin B_6, calcium, magnesium *to reduce symptom aggravation.*	Client adopts nutritional patterns and feels better.

(continued)

NURSING CARE PLAN *(Continued)*
The Woman with Premenstrual Syndrome (PMS)

Assessment	Potential Nursing Diagnosis	Intervention/ Rationale	Evaluation
		Stress regular exercise *to increase tone.*	Client develops coping strategies and performs daily activities more effectively.
		Teach relaxation techniques *to reduce pain perception.*	
	Ineffective Individual Coping related to PMS symptoms and stress	Counsel on lifestyle adjustments, limit setting, self-management practices *to enhance coping.*	
Headaches Hypoglycemia-like symptoms: fatigue, dizziness, food cravings, hunger	Altered Nutrition: Less than body requirements for protein and complex carbohydrates; more for simple carbohydrates	Avoid sweets and simple or refined carbohydrates; eat diet high in protein and complex carbohydrates *to control energy metabolism.*	Client adopts new nutritional patterns and feels better.
		Eat several small meals each day *to increase energy availability.*	
		Do not skip meals, *to avoid hypoglycemic dips.*	
		Snack on fresh fruit or vegetables *to control weight.*	
Family conflicts or sexual problems	Ineffective Family Coping related to effects of PMS symptoms on communications and functions	Provide relief of PMS symptoms *to promote comfort.*	Family communicates well, copes more effectively, and redistributes functions.
		Provide education and counseling of family about menstrual physiology and psychology and PMS causes and symptoms *to promote understanding.*	
		Teach effective communication techniques to family *to reduce stress.*	
		Involve family in care (diet, exercise, relaxation, rest) *to encourage support.*	
		Refer for family therapy *to enhance dynamics.*	
	Sexual Dysfunction	Provide relief of PMS symptoms *to promote comfort.*	Couple establishes a satisfying sexual relationship.
		Provide education and counseling on sexual response and patterns *to promote understanding.*	Couple makes accommodations to premenstrual problems.
		Refer for sexual counseling for more complex sexual problems.	

been used, but data on their effectiveness are scant (Chihal, 1990).

Regular exercise can reduce stress and cramping and improve depression and moodiness by increasing endorphins. Relaxation techniques can reduce physical and emotional symptoms, helping to improve self-concept and functioning (see Research Highlight).

Education and counseling can help alleviate negative attitudes. Group therapy has been effective in correcting stereotypes and providing positive feminine

RESEARCH HIGHLIGHT

Relaxation Response Helps Premenstrual Syndrome

Stress appears to exacerbate the symptoms of premenstrual syndrome (PMS), including negative life events and daily stressors, which have been related to increased severity of premenstrual negative affect, pain, and water retention. Increased physiologic responsivity to stress during the luteal phase contributes to PMS symptomatology. The relaxation response is a physiologic process elicited by sitting quietly with eyes closed, focusing attention on a repetitive mental activity, and ignoring distracting thoughts. It produces lower heart and respiratory rate, blood pressure, and oxygen consumption and more alpha and theta activity on EEG. These changes are compatible with decreased sympathetic nervous system arousal and decreased end-organ responsivity to norepinephrine.

The purpose of this study was to determine whether daily practice of the relaxation response would reduce the severity of physical and emotional premenstrual symptoms. Subjects were menstruating women with regular cycles, not breast-feeding or using oral contraceptives, who had not experienced a major traumatic life event or psychiatric illness in the past 6 months and were not taking prescription medications. Those who exhibited an appropriately high level of premenstrual-only symptoms after a 2-month screening phase were eligible for the study. A sample of 46 women was randomly assigned to one of three groups: daily symptom charting only, symptom charting plus reading leisure material, and symptom charting plus relaxation response practiced for 15 to 20 minutes twice daily. Subjects were followed for 5 months and administered the Holmes and Rahe Life Stress Inventory at the end of the study.

The relaxation response group showed significantly greater improvement (58%) than the charting only (17%) and reading groups (27%) for physical symptoms measured daily and emotional symptoms and symptoms of social withdrawal measured retrospectively. The reading group had more improvement than the charting-only group. Women with more severe symptoms showed greatest improvement.

Critique: The study is limited by small sample size and nonrepresentative sampling techniques. Although results may not be widely generalizable, regular practice of the relaxation response seems to be an effective treatment for physical and emotional premenstrual symptoms. Nurses can include teaching this simple method of relaxation to their clients as an approach to decreasing PMS symptoms and promoting comfort and well-being.

Goodale, I. L., Domar, A. D., & Benson, H. (1990). Alleviation of premenstrual syndrome symptoms with the relaxation response. *Obstetrics and Gynecology, 75*(4), 649–655.

---

models. Counseling to set limits, respect needs, and accept realistic limitations can help improve exaggerated self-expectations ("superwoman syndrome"). Self-management practices can be used to postpone decisions or prepare for important events that will fall in the premenstrual phase (Woods et al., 1995, Peck, 1990).

When PMS causes significant debility, providing relief of symptoms aids recovery. As the woman is better able to carry out daily activities, emotional reactions often improve. Family therapy is indicated for dysfunctional family patterns. Sexual problems related to PMS often improve when PMS symptoms are reduced. More complex sexual dysfunctions need referral for sexual therapy. For a list of helpful instructions, see Client Education: Self Care for PMS.

Evaluation

Nursing care for PMS is effective when symptoms improve, attitudes become more positive, and ability to perform work and family roles increases. Less stress premenstrually indicates a successful therapeutic program. Possible anticipated outcomes include the following:

■ The client reports a decrease in pain and associated symptoms of PMS.

■ The client verbalizes correct information about the causes, contributing factors, treatment, and self-care measures.

■ The client demonstrates positive coping mechanisms.

■ The client demonstrates skill with self-care measures, incorporating them into her lifestyle.

■ The client reports improved self-esteem, body image, and sexuality patterns.

■ The client demonstrates ability to remain at current level of functioning during an episode of PMS.

Neoplasia

Neoplasia refers to new tissue growth, also called tumors. Most body tissues are capable of neoplastic changes. *Benign neoplasias* are well-organized, slowly growing cells that do not invade other tissues. They usually are not life-threatening. *Malignant neoplasias*, also called cancer, are disorganized, rapidly growing cells, often invading surrounding tissues. Cancers can spread far from the original tumor site, a process called **metastasis.** Most malignant neoplasias are potentially life-threatening. Certain tumor types are more dangerous and aggressive than others.

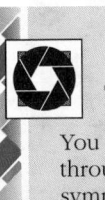

CLIENT EDUCATION
Self-Care for PMS

You often can reduce the symptoms of PMS through self-care measures appropriate to their symptom complex. Use the following as a guide to help you.

Fluid retention (breast tenderness, abdominal bloating, peripheral edema):
   Cook without salt, or avoid salting cooked foods.
   Use fresh or frozen vegetables instead of canned.
   Eliminate foods high in sodium (pickles, potato chips, pork, catsup, sauces, prepared soups and other foods, soy sauce).
   Drink 1 quart of water daily.
   Use natural diuretics (teas, cranberry and grapefruit juice).

Depression, irritability, mood swings:
   Get adequate sleep (at least 7–8 hours per night; more may be needed).
   Get regular exercise (walk about 2 miles/d, swim, bicycle).
   Use multivitamin and multimineral supplements daily.
   Be sure to take at least 100 mg of vitamin B_6 per day or eat foods high in B_6 (corn, whole wheat, yeast, tomatoes, sunflower seeds, peanuts).
   Increase intake of calcium, magnesium, and chromium.
   Develop support systems (friends, spouse, women's group) for expressing feelings.
   Use relaxation techniques (yoga, autogenic training, progressive relaxation, biofeedback, visualization, imagery, meditation).

Headaches and hypoglycemia-type symptoms:
   Avoid sweets and refined carbohydrates.
   Eat diet high in protein and complex carbohydrates.
   Eat several small meals per day.
   Avoid caffeine, chocolate, xanthine derivatives.
   Do not skip meals.
   Snack on fresh fruit or vegetables.

Malignant neoplasia can have profound effects on physiologic functioning, self-concept, coping ability, sexuality, family functioning, and spirituality. Benign neoplasias provide many similar challenges, especially during the diagnostic process but do not have the powerful threat to life and well-being. Nurses can assist women and families through these difficult experiences, providing education, support, and compassion.

Cervical Neoplasia

Changes in cervical cells are common, with a range of histologic characteristics. Cells at the squamocolumnar junction, also called the transformation zone, frequently undergo repair processes, transforming from columnar (endocervical) cells to squamous epithelial (ectocervical) cells throughout the years of gonadotropic hormone activity. Neoplastic changes first occur at the squamocolumnar junction (Fig. 10-1).

Cervical cancer develops primarily in young and middle-aged women. It is the most common cancer in women younger than 35 years (Schaffer et al., 1992; Silverberg, 1990). There is a strong association between cervical intraepithelial neoplasia (CIN) and human papillomavirus (HPV) types 16 and 18, which may progress rapidly (within 3 years) to invasive disease (Dunnihoo, 1992). Herpes simplex virus type 2 and cytomegalovirus infections also may preceed CIN. These viruses alter nuclear deoxyribonucleic acid of immature cervical cells. Exposure to semen from many different sexual partners encourages initiation of the neoplastic process (Beal, 1990). The combination of HPV, herpes, and smoking has an additive effect in producing atypical cells (Schaffer et al., 1992).

Pap smear reports describe the degree of cervical epithelial change (Box 10-5). All grades of **dysplasia,** abnormal cellular growth, through carcinoma are part of the same process, called CIN (DiSaia et al., 1992). Cellular changes of cervical neoplasia follow a gradual course, existing for 10 to 15 years before invasive cancer develops. Preinvasive neoplasia (CIN and carcinoma in situ [CIS]) can usually be treated effectively. HPV is not readily detected by Pap smears, so women

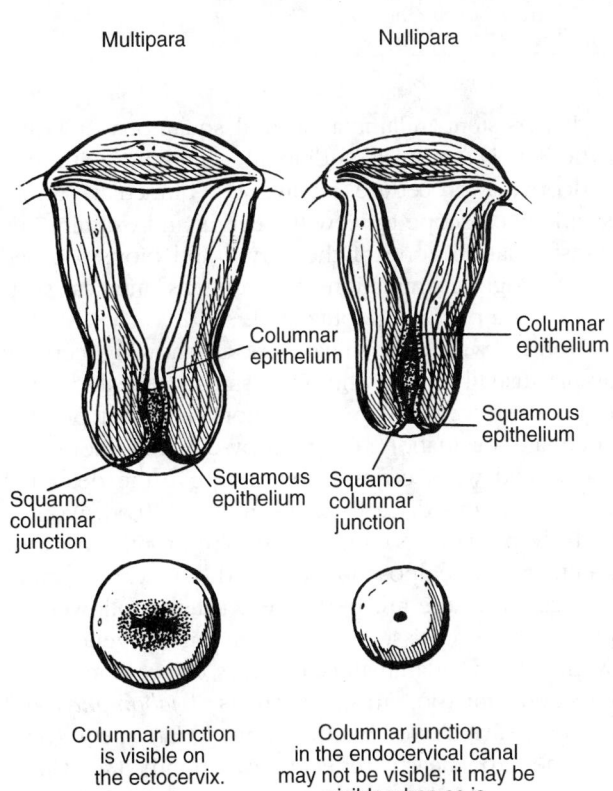

FIGURE 10–1 Squamocolumnar junction.

BOX 10–5
Papanicolaou Smear Cytology Reports

Laboratories may report Pap smears by different classification systems. Descriptive systems are preferrable. The National Cancer Institute and American College of Obstetricians and Gynecologists have replaced Pap classifications with the Bethesda system for vaginal or cervical cytology.

Original Papanicolaou Classification

Class I: Normal cells

Class II: Slightly abnormal, usually inflammatory change; a repeat Pap smear should be done

Class III: More serious cellular abnormality; usually biopsy needed

Class IV: Distinctly abnormal cells, possibly malignant; biopsy required

Class V: Malignant cells

Descriptive Papanicolaou Cytology Reports: Cellular characteristics

- Within normal limits (benign)
- Inflammatory atypia, may be reactive, metaplastic, or infectious with some organisms identifiable (*Candida, Trichomonas*)
- Squamous cell abnormality
  - Atypical squamous metaplasia
- Koilocytosis (atypical cells associated with viral infection)
  - Dysplasia (reactive, low grade, high grade) or cervical
  - intraepithelial neoplasia (cervical intraepithelial neoplasia [CIN] I, mild; CIN II, moderate; CIN III, severe; or carcinoma in situ [CIS])
- Squamous cell carcinoma
  - Invasive carcinoma

- Glandular cell abnormality (endometrial cells)
  - Atypical glandular cells
  - Adenocarcinoma
- Estrogen effect: high, moderate, low

Bethesda System

Statement of specimen adequacy (satisfactory, unsatisfactory, less than optimal)

General categorization of diagnosis (within normal limits, other)

Descriptive diagnosis

- Inflammatory changes (cervical or vaginal diseases suggested by cytology are listed)
- Atypia reserved for cytology of undetermined significance (not for inflammatory, preneoplastic, or neoplastic changes).
- Reactive or reparative changes
- Epithelial cell abnormalities
  - (1) Low-grade squamous intraepithelial lesion (SIL) with
    Changes consistent with human papillomavirus
    Changes consistent with mild dysplasia and CIN I
  - (2) High-grade SIL with
    Changes consistent with CIN II to III or CIS
- Nonepithelial malignant neoplasia
- Hormonal effects

---

with persistent inflammation and squamous or koilocytic atypias require additional screening with colposcopy, a procedure involving a binocular stereoscopic microscope to view the cervix and examine the transformation zone of the cervix and biopsy. Based on cytologic examination of specimens, medical therapy can be planned (Montz et al., 1992).

Women with Pap smear reports showing cervical atypia usually have the Pap smear repeated in 3 months. However, Pap smear alone may not provide adequate evaluation. Colposcopy-directed biopsy or acetic acid wash examinations improve the detection of more serious disease (Slawson et al., 1994). Women with dysplasia (CIN) and CIS require prompt management. Initially colposcopy, directed biopsy, and endocervical curettage are performed, usually followed by procedures for tissue destruction and regeneration. Women with inflammatory changes or presence of an infectious microorganism, such as *Trichomonas* and *Candida,* are treated with the appropriate medication, and the Pap smear is repeated in 3 months (see Chap. 11). If atypia still is present, colposcopy and directed biopsy are done.

Medical Treatment

Medical treatment depends on the extensiveness of the CIN. If endocervical cells are free of disease and the cervical cytology reports mild, moderate, or severe dysplasia or CIS, techniques are used that completely destroy the surface of the transformation zone and penetrate at least 4 to 5 mm to destroy any possible extensions of cellular dysplasia. Cryosurgery, laser therapy, conization, or electrocautery are all effective techniques that can be performed on an outpatient basis or in surgical centers (Box 10-6).

When CIN has progressed to the microinvasive stage (no more than 3 mm penetration into submucosal tissues), surgical conization is the initial treatment. It is used when colposcopy and biopsy fail to reveal the source of abnormal cells and when the upper margin of the transformation zone cannot be visualized. Depending on the extent of invasion, a hysterectomy may follow conization.

Invasive cervical cancer is staged according to extent of involvement of the **stroma,** the tissue forming the framework of the organ, and whether there is vaginal

BOX 10-6
Surgical Treatment of Cervical Dysplasia

Cryosurgery

Nitrous oxide or carbon dioxide is used to freeze ecto-cervical tissue, causing tissue necrosis and sloughing. A double freeze method is preferred, usually done 1 week after menses to allow generation of new tissue before the next menstrual period. Cryosurgery can be done without anesthesia in the physician's office or outpatient clinic. It usually is not painful, although some cramping may be felt. Heavy, watery discharge for several weeks is normal; while present, the woman should avoid tampons and sexual intercourse. Healing may take 2 to 3 months.

Laser Therapy

In laser therapy, the invisible, highly concentrated light beam is absorbed by tissue fluid; this energy is converted to heat, causing rapid fluid evaporation and tissue death. Laser therapy is appropriate when boundaries of the lesion are visible on colposcopy, and the endocervical curettage is negative. It can be done in the physician's office or outpatient clinic without anesthesia; bleeding is minimal. Women may feel minor cramping and slight discharge for 5 to 7 days. Tampons and sexual intercourse should be avoided for 2 weeks. Healing usually is complete by 6 weeks.

Loop Electrosurgical Excision Procedure (LEEP)

An electric current in a thin wire loop electrode is used to excise the transformation zone of the cervix. These loops come in different sizes for shaving off thin slices with fine wire or an entire lesion with thicker wire. The loop is inserted to the desired depth, then swept sideways across the area to be excised. A 5-mm ball electrode can be used to coagulate the crater base and provide hemostasis. The amount of bleeding and thermal damage is regulated by electrosurgical generators, blending current between cutting and coagulating. Tissue removed by LEEP is suitable for histologic examination.

Conization

Surgical conization with a knife blade removes a cone-shaped specimen of tissue, the size and length determined by the extent of the cervical lesion. It is done when the boundaries of the lesion cannot be seen on colposcopy. A significant amount of normal tissue also is removed to ensure excision of the entire lesion. Conization can be done as an outpatient or inpatient procedure, using local or general anesthesia. Long, profuse menstrual periods often occur during the subsequent two to three cycles. Anesthesia risks and postoperative infection and hemorrhage are possible complications.

---

or pelvic wall extension, rectal or bladder extension, kidney involvement, and distant metastases (Box 10-7). Treatment consists of hysterectomy (simple or radical), radiotherapy, or chemotherapy, depending on the extent of the disease, the woman's age and general health, and the presence of other abnormalities.

Stage IA cancer of the cervix is treated with either hysterectomy or radiotherapy, because the cancer is confined to the cervix. Stages IB and IIA are treated with a total hysterectomy and bilateral lymphadenectomy. Stages IIB through IVB involve spread of cancer beyond the cervix to other organs, and the treatment of choice usually is radiotherapy (DiSaia et al., 1992; Baird et al., 1991).

Radiotherapy to the cervix can be done externally or by intracavitary or interstitial-intravacitary implants. External radiation therapy to the pelvis or lymph nodes provides more homogeneous doses to the pelvis, while avoiding skin damage. Treatment with the radiation sensitizer, hydroxyurea, improves survival rates. Complications of radiotherapy include radiation cystitis or proctitis, rectovaginal and vesicovaginal fistulas, and bone marrow suppression.

Metastatic cervical cancer may be treated with chemotherapeutic agents, such as cisplatin, but response rates are low or short lasting. Clients treated with radiation or chemotherapy who have a pelvic re-currence may undergo a partial or complete **pelvic exenteration** (removal of the rectum, vagina, bladder, uterus, and cervix) with construction of ureterostomy and colostomy.

Squamous cell carcinoma antigen (*SCC antigen*) a cancer marker, can detect recurrence or identify treatment failure early. Using radioimmunoassay, it monitors serum levels of the antigen. SCC antigen test is very specific (94.3%), making it a useful way to monitor known disease. However, its low sensitivity (53.3%) does not lend the test to screening (Dunnihoo, 1992).

Nursing Management

Nursing care includes providing education and information to resolve any knowledge deficits and reduce anxiety and fear. The nurse supports the client's self-care ability to promote health and prevent complications. The nurse needs to identify how the client and her partner view her reproductive ability and the meaning each associates with it. For some women, severe self-esteem and body image problems can arise when they can no longer have babies. Their spouses often hold similar attitudes that devalue nonprocreative women. Interventions should focus on helping the client and her partner accept the physical and psychological changes associated with the disorder and

---

BOX 10–7
Staging for Cervical Cancer

Stage 0	Carcinoma in situ, intraepithelial carcinoma
Stage I	Carcinoma is strictly confined to the cervix.
IA	Microinvasive carcinoma (early stromal invasion)
IB	All other cases of stage I (occult cancer = occ)
Stage II	Carcinoma extends beyond the cervix but has not extended to the pelvic wall. The carcinoma involves the vagina but not as far as the lower third.
IIA	No obvious parametrial involvement
IIB	Obvious parametrial involvement
Stage III	Carcinoma has extended to the pelvic wall. On rectal examination, there is no cancer-free space between the tumor and the pelvic wall. The tumor involves the lower third of the vagina.
IIIA	No extension to the pelvic wall
IIIB	Extension to the pelvic wall or hydronephrosis or nonfunctioning kidney
Stage IV	Carcinoma has extended beyond the true pelvis or has clinically involved the mucosa of the bladder or rectum.
IVA	Spread of carcinoma to adjacent organs
IVB	Spread to distant organs

Nomenclature of the International Federation of Gynecology and Obstetrics.

---

find other qualities for which the woman can be valued. Even when the loss of the uterus and reproductive capacity does not significantly diminish the client's self-esteem or body image, the woman needs encouragement about her other valued roles as a person. Women experiencing severe pain with menses and disruption in routines may view treatment, such as a hysterectomy, with relief.

If cancer is diagnosed, many women find the threat to life vastly more important than the loss of reproductive capacity. Nursing interventions then focus on helping the client express fear, place realistic parameters on expectations, clarify values and spiritual supports, enhance family and community resources, and find personal strengths for coping.

Prevention. A key aspect of nursing care includes education about reducing the risk factors for cervical cancer (see Chap. 8). Young women need to be informed that early sexual activity and multiple sexual partners place them at increased risk for cervical cancer. Avoiding sexually transmitted disease exposure can reduce risk. The importance of regular, frequent Pap smears should be emphasized, with a screening interval of 1 to 2 years. Women are informed that screening intervals longer than this increase their risk of more advanced cervical cancer.

Diet may be a factor in the development of cervical cancer. Low intake of vitamin A, beta carotene, vitamin C, or folic acid has been associated with an increased prevalence of cervical neoplasia (Lichtman, 1990). Vitamin A and its precursors inhibit the steps in the chain of **carcinogenesis** (development of cancer), controlling cellular differentiation, or blocking the effects of transforming growth factors. Retinoids may stimulate immunologic defense mechanisms, thus interfering with carcinogenesis. Vitamin C helps to maintain normal epithelium and protects against the effects of potential carcinogens. It alters the structure of carcinogens and prevents access of carcinogens to the target tissue by competitive inhibition. Folate may inhibit or stimulate specific enzymes that are important for cells undergoing mitosis (Schneider et al., 1989; Lichtman, 1990).

Vitamin A has been found to revert the **metaplastic process** in which one adult cell is replaced by another adult cell. Cervical cancer begins with the metaplastic process in the transformation zone of the cervix. Studies have shown that there is a marked deficiency or absence of vitamin A binding proteins in cervical neoplastic tissues and that beta carotene has a protective effect against cervical cancer (Schneider et al., 1989). Most studies show a consistent inverse association between vitamin consumption and risk of cervical neoplasia. Nurses can advise women of the importance of adequate vitamin intake, especially vitamins A and C, through diet or nutritional supplements.

Benign Ovarian Neoplasia

Approximately 75% of ovarian masses are benign. Common benign ovarian neoplasia among women 20 to 40 years old include functional ovarian cysts, cystadenomas, cystic teratomas, fibromas, endometriomas (chocolate cysts), and tuboovarian pregnancies (ectopic pregnancies). Half of these masses are functional cysts. Unless quite large, ovarian masses usually cause no symptoms and often are discovered incidentally during an examination. When present, symptoms may include lower abdominal discomfort or aching and feelings of fullness, pressure, dyspareunia, or discomfort with menstruation or defecation. Tuboovarian pregnancies cause acute abdominal pain prior to and during rupture and are discussed in Chapter 31.

Functional cysts, which include follicular and corpus luteum cysts, usually are smaller than 3 cm and frequently resolve on their own in 1 to 2 months. Women with small ovarian cysts are re-examined in 1 to 2 months. Oral contraceptives may be used for one to two cycles to suppress ovarian function, aiding cyst resorption. Ovarian masses that do not resolve, which are larger than 3 cm, cause persistent pain, or have suspicious characteristics require further evaluation. Transvaginal ultrasonography can identify the type of lesion, such as solid, cystic, septated, and mixed; the presence of free pelvic fluid; and uterine characteristics. Suspicious masses are examined by laparoscopy or laparotomy and removed if indicated. If the woman is older than 40 years or the mass is larger than 6 to 7 cm, surgical removal is more likely.

Nursing Management

Nursing care includes client education about the treatment process, including rationale for 1 to 2 months' observation of small ovarian masses. Women are informed that oral contraceptives protect against ovarian masses and reduce the incidence of cancer. If surgery is indicated and an ovary is removed, the nurse should explain about the ability of the other ovary to function. Information about the possibility of future conception is discussed, taking into account the condition of the remaining ovary.

Ovarian Cancer

One out of 70 women will develop ovarian cancer in her lifetime. A lethal neoplasm, ovarian cancer causes more deaths than endometrial and cervical cancers combined. The frequency of malignant ovarian neoplasms increases with each decade of life, from 4% in women younger than than 30 years to about 50% in women older than 60 years. Before menopause, 15% of ovarian masses are malignant; after menopause, 45% are malignant (Plaxe et al., 1993). Risk factors for ovarian cancer include:

- High-fat diet (doubles risk)
- Smoking, drinking alcohol
- Environmental pollutants

- history of two first-degree relatives with breast or ovarian cancer (50% risk)
- Personal history of colon, breast, or endometrial cancer

Certain factors protect a woman from ovarian cancer. These include multiparity and prolonged use of oral contraceptives (more than 1 year). Pregnancy and oral contraceptives temporarily remove the stimulation of FSH and LH, probably preventing formation of epithelial inclusion cysts and their subsequent malignant transformation.

Screening and Detection

Ovarian cancer is generally silent, making early diagnosis difficult. More than two-thirds of women have metastatic disease (stage III to IV) at initial diagnosis. Women with stage I disease (limited to the ovaries) have a 73% 5-year survival rate, while those with stage IV (distant metastasis) have a 5% 5-year survival rate (Box 10-8.)

In women younger than 30 years, there is a higher incidence of low-grade tumors, supporting a preclinical phase of ovarian cancer that might be detected by screening. However, no accurate and feasible screening tests are available. Abdominal ultrasonography is a sensitive test for detecting morphologic changes that suggest cancer, but the false-positive rate is high. Vaginal ultrasonography provides improved ovarian imaging but often misses large masses extending above the true pelvis.

CA 125, a tumor marker using monoclonal antibodies, is found in serum of more than 80% of women with nonmucinous epithelial ovarian cancer. Only 23% of women with stage I ovarian cancer have elevated CA 125, and values can be elevated with menstruation, endometriosis, leiomyoma, PID, hepatitis, and other inflammatory processes. CA 125 is not sensitive or specific enough to use for screening, but at levels above 65 U/mL in combination with a pelvic mass, it is highly predictive of malignant disease. Because ovarian cancers are heterogeneous, it is difficult to find a common tumor marker. Complementary markers to CA 125, such as *CA 54/61, NB/70K,* and *urinary gonadotropin fragment* can increase detection rates (Coates, 1993; Plaxe et al., 1993).

The most common ovarian cancers are cystadenocarcinomas and adenocarcinomas, which may be solid or cystic. Ovarian metastasis from other primary cancers may occur. In early stages, ovarian cancer may feel no different on examination than benign cystic or solid ovarian masses. Later, cancers may become fixed, heavy, and hard and have ill-defined margins. Malignant tumors frequently are nontender and cause few symptoms except vague pelvic fullness or aching.

BOX 10–8
Staging for Ovarian Cancer

Stage I	Growth is limited to the ovaries.
Ia	Growth limited to one ovary, no ascites, no tumor on external surface, capsule intact
Ib	Growth limited to both ovaries, no ascites, no tumor on external surfaces, capsule intact
Ic	Tumor either stage Ia or Ib, but with tumor on the surface of one or both ovaries, capsule ruptured, ascites present containing malignant cells, or positive peritoneal washings
Stage II	Growth involves one or both ovaries with pelvic extension.
IIa	Extension or metastasis to uterus or tubes
IIb	Extension to other pelvic tissues
IIc	Tumor either stage IIa or IIb, but with tumor on the surface of one or both ovaries, capsule ruptured, ascites present containing malignant cells, or positive peritoneal washings
Stage III	Tumor involves one or both ovaries, with peritoneal implants outside the pelvis or positive retroperitoneal or inguinal nodes. Superficial liver metastasis equals stage III. Tumor is limited to true pelvis but with histologically proven malignant extension to small bowel or omentum.
IIIa	Tumor grossly limited to true pelvis, with negative nodes but with histologically confirmed microscopic seeding of abdominal peritoneal surfaces
IIIb	Tumor of one or both ovaries with histologically confirmed implants on abdominal peritoneal surfaces, not exceeding 2 cm diameter; Nodes negative
IIIc	Abdominal implants greater than 2 cm diameter or positive retroperitoneal or inguinal nodes
Stage IV	Growth involves one or both ovaries with distant metastases. If pleural effusion is present, there must be positive cytology for stage IV. Parenchymal liver metastases equals stage IV.
Special Category	Unexplored cases thought to be ovarian carcinoma are in a special category.

Large tumors or ascites can increase abdominal size, but this often is attributed to midlife weight gain. Gastrointestinal symptoms may include heartburn, bloating, anorexia, and food intolerance. Abnormal vaginal bleeding may occur. Late signs of cancer are pelvic pain, cachexia, and anemia.

Medical Diagnosis and Treatment

Medical diagnosis is based on tumor characteristics and results of diagnostic tests. Surgical removal of the tumor with pathologic examination establishes the diagnosis and stage based on the international system for staging ovarian cancer. Tests of vaginal, pleural, or peritoneal fluids; lung and bone scans; blood tests; and radiographic studies of chest, kidneys, and gastrointestinal system complete the diagnostic workup and guide selection of therapy.

Ovarian cancer is treated according to stage of the disease. Surgical removal of as much of the tumor as possible is done. This can range from simple removal of one ovary to a radical hysterectomy and bilateral salpingo-oophorectomy. Node biopsy or removal and dissection of malignant tissue implants from abdominal organs and omentem are part of this "debulking procedure." Radiation is used less often because it is not as effective as chemotherapy. Chemotherapy is used for most ovarian cancers, because many are diagnosed with stage II to IV disease. Agents used, often in combination, include the following:

- Cisplatin (Platinol)
- Carboplatin (Paraplatin)
- Cyclophosphamide (Cytotoxan)
- Cisplatin and doxorubicin (Adriamycin)

Intraperitoneal chromium phosphate may be used in stage I and II disease. Following chemotherapy, a second-look surgery often is performed, which evaluates the response to therapy and permits restaging. Benefit of this procedure in terms of survival is unclear.

Nursing Management

Nursing care includes client teaching, physical and emotional support during procedures, and emotional support to cope with fear and anxiety. During hospitalization, physiologic monitoring and technical procedures are done, and comfort measures are provided. The nurse offers support for family coping and adjustment, allowing them to express and deal with their fears and helping to coordinate resources for family support and recovery. Throughout, the nurse assists the client and family to clarify values and spiritual supports and find personal strengths for coping. The woman and family can be expected to go through the phases of grief and loss when facing life-threatening illness. If the client is terminally ill, care alternatives, such as hospice, home care, and multilevel care facilities that can support quality of life and peaceful death, are explored. These alternatives promote function as long as possible, provide pain relief, encourage interaction with loved ones, and offer emotional and spiritual support.

Uterine Neoplasia

Uterine masses often present as an enlarged or irregularly shaped uterus. Among women of childbearing age, pregnancy must always be considered with uterine enlargement. Infections, adenomyosis, polyps, fibroids, hyperplasia, and malignancy are among the common causes of uterine enlargement.

Endometrial carcinoma is the third most frequent malignancy in women. Ninety percent of endometrial carcinomas are adenocarcinomas. The peak incidence is between 50 and 70 years, and it is more common in postmenopausal women. The etiology of endometrial cancer is unclear. It may be triggered by metabolic abnormalities involving pituitary hyperactivity and impaired glucose metabolism. There is a 2- to 10-fold increase in endometrial cancer with prolonged exogenous estrogen use, especially in postmenopausal women. This risk of cancer is neutralized by addition of progestins in hormone replacement therapy (Lacey, 1991).

Risk factors for endometrial cancer include the following:

- Hormonal imbalance (unopposed estrogen)
- Obesity
- Nulliparity or infertility
- Late onset of menopause
- Diabetes mellitus
- Hypertension

Medical Treatment

Benign conditions, such as uterine fibroids that are not enlarging significantly, are managed conservatively by regular evaluation with pelvic examination and diagnostic tests. If the fibroids enlarge or other symptoms cause concern, surgery may be done with tumor resection or hysterectomy. The management of conditions causing DUB is discussed earlier.

Endometrial cancer is treated according stage and the woman's age and health status (Box 10-9).

For early stages of adenocarcinoma (stage I), total abdominal hysterectomy with bilateral salpingo-oophorectomy (TAH-BSO) is the usual treatment. Stage II cancers, which extend beyond the corpus to the cervix, are treated with TAH-BSO accompanied by lymph node dissection, which is followed by radiation therapy. Stages III and IV are usually treated with intrauterine radiation or external radiotherapy. Chemotherapy and hormone therapy in various combinations also may be used.

Nursing Management

Assessment of uterine neoplasia focuses on the identification of risk factors and evaluating the client's signs and symptoms.

- Fever, abdominal pain, nausea, and anorexia indicate an infection.
- Urinary frequency, nausea and vomiting, breast tenderness, and amenorrhea suggest possible pregnancy.
- Irregular menses and abnormal bleeding are the most common symptoms of endometrial cancer.

Postmenopausal bleeding, a hallmark symptom, requires immediate investigation because cancer more frequently occurs in this age group. Pelvic examination is done to determine size, shape, and consistency of the uterus and to evaluate the ovaries and adnexa. Depending on symptoms and risk factors, endometrial biopsy or fractional curettage of the endocervix and endometrium often is done. More than 80% of endometrial cancers will be diagnosed with these methods. The Gravlee Jet Washer is another diagnostic aid used in women older than 35 years. This method obtains endometrial cells by washing the uterine cavity with normal saline in a collecting system.

Clinical findings often diagnose benign uterine masses, such as fibroids or adenomyosis. Diagnostic tests may include a pregnancy test, biopsy, or curettage. White blood cell count with differential and erythrocyte sedimentation rate aid in the diagnosis of infections.

Nursing care for women with uterine masses follows the approaches described for cervical, ovarian, and breast neoplasia and for women having reproductive surgery.

Nursing intervention is effective when the woman can express a clear understanding of the health problem and its cause, treatment, and outcomes. The client undertakes measures to prevent illness or complications, such as behavioral changes, including weight loss, medication compliance, and control of diabetes and hypertension. Expressing fears and concerns, positive attitude, and family support and following through on referrals for counseling or social support indicate effective emotional responses.

Benign Breast Neoplasia

Women with breast neoplasia may experience a wide variety of signs and symptoms. They may have pain, lumps, nipple discharge, skin rashes or discolorations, or changes in breast size or shape. Distinguishing be-

---

BOX 10-9
Staging for Endometrial and Breast Cancer

Endometrial Cancer

Stage I	The carcinoma is confined to the uterine corpus.
IA	Length of the uterine cavity, 8 cm or less
IB	Length of the uterine cavity, more than 8 cm
Stage II	The carcinoma involves the corpus and the cervix.
Stage III	The carcinoma has extended outside the uterus but not outside the true pelvis.
Stage IV	The carcinoma has extended outside the true pelvis or has involved the mucosa of the bladder or rectum.

The stage I cases are subgrouped by histologic type of adenocarcinoma as follows:

G1	Highly differentiated adenomatous carcinomas
G2	Differentiated adenomatous carcinomas with partly solid areas
G3	Predominantly solid or undifferentiated carcinomas

Classification system developed by the International Federation of Gynecology and Obstetrics.

The TNM* System of the American Joint Committee for Cancer Staging

Breast Cancer

Stage I
(T) Tumor less than 2 cm diameter
(N) Nodes in axilla, if present, not felt to contain metastasis
(M) No distant metastases

Stage II
(T) Tumor less than 5 cm diameter
(N) Nodes in axilla, if present, not fixed
(M) No distant metastases

Stage III
(T) Tumor greater than 5 cm or tumor of any size with skin invasion or attachment
(N) Nodes in supraclavicular area
(M) No distant metastases

Stage IV
(T) Tumor of any size with extension to chest wall and skin
(N) Any amount of nodal involvement
(M) Distant metastases present

*T, tumor; N, nodes; M, metastases.

---

tween benign and malignant breast conditions is often complex and difficult. Any sign or symptom that cannot be identified readily as a benign problem should receive diagnostic evaluation (Table 10-3).

Women often feel lumps during breast self-examination (BSE), or masses are detected by providers during routine health screening. Unless masses are quite large with suspicious characteristics, evaluation by mammography or ultrasonography is often the initial diagnostic evaluation. Mammography results showing no malignant characteristics or ultrasonography results indicating cystic lesions usually support a benign tumor. However, distinct breast masses that do not resolve must receive biopsy or surgical excision.

Fibrocystic disease is the most common benign breast problem among women 25 to 45 years old. It usually subsides with menopause. This condition, also called *chronic cystic mastitis* or *mammary dysplasia,* is probably estrogen related because its symptoms follow menstrual cycles and decrease after menopause. Fibrocystic change is characterized by multiple, usually bilateral breast lumps that become more tender prior to menses. The lumps are usually firm, mobile, well defined, and tender to palpation. They increase in size premenstrually, can fluctuate rapidly in size, and regress after menses. The most common location is the upper outer breast quadrants, although the lumps may occur in any area of breast tissue. Nipple discharge is rare.

Lumps that are unusual in size, shape, consistency, or behavior should have aspiration or biopsy. Mammography usually is done, because it is difficult to distinguish cystic lumps from early breast cancer. Ultrasonography and needle aspiration can identify cysts typical of fibrocystic disease.

TABLE 10-3
Characteristics of Breast Neoplasia

	Fibrocystic Disease	Fibroadenoma	Cancer
Usual age	30–55, regresses after menopause	15–20+, occurs up to 55	30–80, peak incidence 42–48
Number	Usually multiple; may be single	Usually single; may be multiple	Usually single, but may coexist with other lesions
Shape	Round	Round, discoid, or lobular	Irregular or stellate
Consistency	Soft to firm, bumpy nodular breasts	Usually firm; may be soft	Firm or hard
Delimitation	Usually well delineated	Well-delineated, clear margins	Not clearly delineated from surrounding tissue
Mobility	Mobile	Very mobile, slippery	May be fixed to skin or underlying tissue
Tenderness	Often tender	Usually nontender	Usually nontender but not always
Retraction signs	Absent	Absent	Often present

Fibroadenoma is the third most common type of breast tumor (following fibrocystic changes and carcinoma). It occurs primarily in women in their teens and early 20s. In adolescents, the cause is associated with breast hypertrophy during the pubertal growth spurt. The lump is typically well defined, firm and rubbery, freely movable, rounded, and nontender. A solitary nodule ranging from 1 to 5 cm is common, but multiple tumors occur in about 15% of cases. These tumors respond to hormones and can increase rapidly. Risk of breast cancer is increased in a small subset of women with fibroadenoma. When fibroadenomas have complex histology or there is adjacent tissue with proliferative disease, risk of breast cancer is doubled. Family history of breast cancer augments this risk (Dupont et al., 1994).

Diagnosis of fibroadenoma is based on tumor characteristics identified during examination. If there are unusual characteristics, a biopsy or mammogram may be necessary. Watchful observation with eventual surgical excision is the usual course of treatment. Although cancer is unlikely, it cannot be completely ruled out in any discrete lump.

Intraductal papillomas are small tumors, 2 to 3 mm in size, most commonly located in a major subareolar collection duct. They have a central fibrovascular stalk with delicate papillae and are often too small to palpate. Tumors are usually single but may be multiple and can occur in any age group. The most common presenting symptom is serosanguineous nipple discharge. During examination, the location of the affected duct may be found by gently pressing with the fingertip at successive points around the circumference of the areola. A point may be found where pressure produces the discharge. Samples of discharge are collected on a slide and sent for cytologic examination. A small lump or thickening may be felt. If no lump is palpable and the lesion cannot be localized, mammography is used to locate the papilloma.

Although papillomas are usually benign, low-grade malignancy may exist. The lesion must be excised and examined histologically. Excision is the definitive treatment for papillomas, and follow-up is necessary because they may recur. Multiple lesions are more difficult to manage, requiring several excisions.

Nursing Management

Pain is common for many women who have quite severe cyclic breast discomfort. In addition, the client may have a knowledge deficit related to the medical condition, diagnostic procedures, and treatments. Many women have little knowledge of breast physiology and cyclic changes. The client may be upset regarding the pain or potential loss of body part or function. Women often fear cancer when they experience breast lumps, with the specter of surgery, life-threatening disease, and loss of body part or function.

Nursing care focuses on pain relief, education, and emotional support. The woman is advised to wear a good supportive brassiere both day and night and to avoid trauma to the breasts. Dietary factors may aggravate breast pain. The client is instructed to avoid chocolate, coffee, and black tea and reduce sodium intake. When pain is acute, ice packs to the tender areas may help, and mild analgesics, such as salicylates or anti-inflammatory medications may be used. The hormone inhibitor danazol (Danocrine) provides relief of pain and nodularity for 70% to 80% of women. Danazol's side effects include menstrual pattern changes and weight gain (Guiliano, 1991).

Women are taught BSE so that they can identify unusual lumps or changes in their breasts. By explaining the relationship of fibrocystic disease to the monthly cycle, the nurse can help alleviate fears of cancer while reinforcing the need for further evaluation of suspected abnormalities. Providing support for emotional responses to the threat of cancer can dissipate fears and develop effective coping strategies. Women with fibrocystic changes are encouraged to have regular breast examinations by a physician or nurse practitioner and periodic mammography.

Breast Cancer

Breast cancer is the leading cause of cancer deaths in women. One woman in eight will develop breast cancer during her lifetime. Each year, more than 180,000 new cases are diagnosed, and more than 46,000 deaths from breast cancer are reported (American Cancer Society, 1993). The incidence of breast cancer is increasing more than 1.5% per year (Rippon, 1993; Boring et al., 1991). Women are most likely to develop breast cancer after 35 years, with the peak incidence between 40 and 60 years. Individual risk increases steadily with age. Theories of causality include hormonal mechanisms involving endogenous steroids, viral agents, genetic transmission, and immunologic deficiencies.

Risk factors for breast cancer include the following:

- Age (75% of breast cancers occur after 40 years)
- Race (white women have higher risk than nonwhite)
- Breast cancer in first-degree female relatives
- Nulliparity
- Early menarche (before 12 years)
- Late menopause (more than 30 years after menarche)
- First pregnancy after 30 years
- Oophorectomy before 40 years
- Obesity, diet high in fat and protein, low in selenium
- Personal history of cancer, especially in other breast
- Radiation exposure

Genetic risk factors occur in families with a strong history of breast cancer. When two or more first-degree relatives have breast cancer, a woman's risk is increased threefold. Familial breast cancer accounts for about 25% of all breast cancers. A more specific genetic linkage occurs in hereditary breast cancer, which results from an autosomal dominant gene. It is characterized by early age of onset (average 44 years), high degree of bilateral breast cancer, multiple sites of primary cancer with integral tumor patterns, and improved survival rates. About 9% of all breast cancer is hereditary. The risk of transmission by an affected woman is 50%. Biomolecular studies of cancer support the concept of suppressor genes (antioncogenes) that protect against the development of cancer. Inactivation or loss (deletion from a chromosome) is one of several steps leading to malignant transformation. Chromosome 17 is a genetic locus for hereditary breast cancer (Friedman et al., 1995). The *BRCA1* gene is commonly found in clients with family histories of breast and ovarian cancer (Shattuck-Eidens et al., 1995). Women with the *BRCA1* gene have more than an 85% lifetime chance of getting breast cancer (King et al., 1994; Breo, 1993).

Hormone therapy increases the risk of breast cancer among postmenopausal women. This increased risk of invasive breast cancer is greatest among women older than 55 years who have used hormone therapy for 5 or more years. Estrogen alone, estrogen plus progestin, and progestins alone all appear to increase the risk of breast cancer. Estrogen stimulates the proliferation of epithelial cells in the breast, and progestins may enhance this process. Risk increases steadily with age; after 5 years of hormones, breast cancer risk increases almost 40% in women 55 to 59 years and more than 70% in women older than 60 years (Colditz et al., 1995). Women older than 55 years must carefully consider risks and benefits of hormone therapy, especially if they have few risk factors for heart disease.

The two most common types of breast cancer are adenocarcinomas and ductal carcinomas, arising from ductal or lobular epithelial cells. They are frequently multicentric; about half have multiple sites of the primary lesion, often are microscopic in size, and are only identifiable by pathologic examination. Invasion and metastasis occur early, and by the time a breast cancer is palpable (about 1 cm), micrometastases are almost certainly present. It takes between 3 months and 2½ years for breast cancer to grow 1 cm size. It may take as long as 30 years for malignancies to progress from a single cell to a palpable mass. Invasion first occurs in surrounding tissue, then through the ductal system, lymph channels, and circulatory system to distant metastatic sites, such as bones, liver, and lungs (Fig. 10-2).

Medical Diagnosis

A breast mass is the most common sign of breast cancer. It is usually discovered by the woman or her sexual partner. In early stages, the lump is usually single, firm, and dense; movable or fixed to skin or underlying tissue; and poorly delineated or irregular. The most frequent location is the upper outer quadrant of the breast. Other signs that usually appear later may include nipple discharge or retraction, skin edema or dimpling, breast asymmetry, and enlarged axillary lymph nodes. Breast cancer is usually nontender, but pain or tingling can occur.

Mammography can detect about 90% of breast cancers. Malignant masses classically appear as star shaped with radiating fibrils, or they may be irregular and poorly defined. Malignant calcifications may appear as tiny rods (0.25–1.5 mm), or they may be pointed. Isolated, clustered microcalcifications are the most common mammographic sign of occult malignancy (Kopans et al., 1993). Mammography often detects

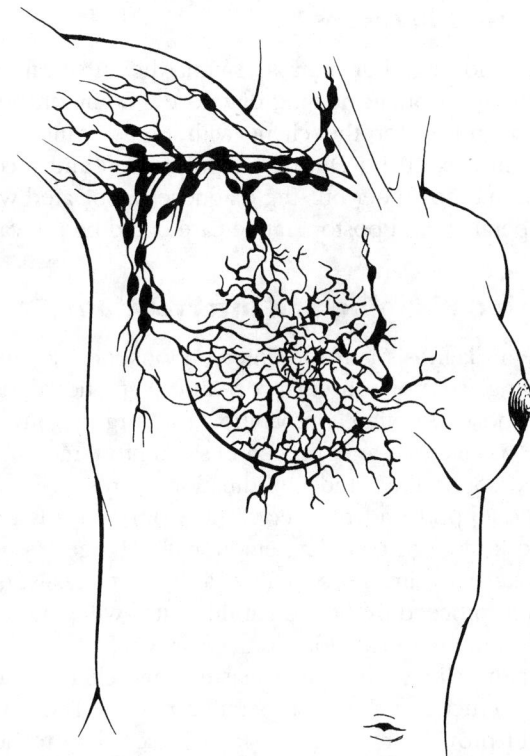

FIGURE 10–2 Lymphatics of breast and axilla by which breast cancer spreads.

small breast cancers as much as 2 years before they can be palpated on breast examination.

With a suspicious breast mass, biopsy must be performed despite mammographic results. Mammography may not reveal cancer in a very dense breast, and it often misses medullary type cancers. Needle or aspiration biopsy withdraws a core of tumor cells or cystic fluid for microscopic examination. Incisional biopsy, which can be done under local anesthesia, removes a portion of tumor for cytologic examination.

If biopsy confirms malignancy, staging is done to determine if the disease is local (confined to the breast) or if metastasis has occurred. Chest x-ray, lung scan, blood tests (primarily for alkaline phosphatase or hypercalcemia), and computed tomography scan of liver and bones are done. Node biopsies may be indicated. This information on metastasis permits staging of the tumor and directs therapy (see Box 10-9). Carcinoembryonic antigen may be used as a marker for recurrent breast cancer.

Medical Treatment

Surgical treatment for breast cancer ranges from local excision of the tumor to total resection of the breast, chest wall muscles, and axilla. The extent of surgery depends on the clinical staging of the disease, the histologic characteristics of the tumor, and other considerations, such as age and health status. Conservative

breast surgery combined with radiotherapy or chemotherapy yields survival rates similar to those with more extensive mastectomy. Partial mastectomy or modified radical mastectomy, both with axillary dissection and radiation therapy, are most common for earlier stage breast cancer. Radiation therapy also is used as an adjunct to local excision, to shrink large tumors to operable dimensions, and as primary treatment for inflammatory breast cancer or inoperable tumors. For small breast cancers treated with breast-conserving surgery, radiotherapy used as **adjuvant therapy** (additional treatment given to eliminate microscopic disease and promote cure or improve client response) appears to protect against recurrences (Fisher et al., 1993; Veronesi et al., 1993; Box 10-10).

BOX 10–10
Types of Surgery for Breast Neoplasia

Radical mastectomy (Classical, Halsted). Through a vertical incision, the entire breast is removed with a significant margin of skin around nipple, areola, and tumor. The pectoralis major and minor muscles are removed, the axillary vein is dissected, and the axillary lymph nodes are dissected. A skin-thin surgical flap is left, but depending on the amount of skin removed, skin grafting may be necessary.

Extended radical mastectomy. Includes the above procedure plus excision of the internal mammary lymph nodes. Some sections of the ribs must be removed to reach the internal mammary nodes. The supraclavicular nodes also may be removed. This operation is rarely done today.

Modified radical mastectomy. The entire breast and most of the axillary lymph nodes are removed, but the pectoralis muscles are preserved. Some surgeons dissect the entire axillary chain, whereas others leave the upper third intact. The axillary vein is stripped.

Simple (or total) mastectomy. The entire breast is removed, but the axillary nodes and pectoralis muscles are not. Some surgeons biopsy the last lymph node in the tail of the breast. If it has been invaded, either the axilla is irradiated or a radical mastectomy is done.

Partial mastectomy (segmental resection, wedge resection). The tumor and a wide segment of surrounding breast tissue, underlying fascia, and overlying skin are removed, usually about one-third of the breast. Some surgeons also dissect the axillary nodes.

Lumpectomy, tylectomy, or local excision. The tumor and 3 to 5 cm of tissue on either side are removed, retaining other breast tissue and skin.

Subcutaneous mastectomy. Breast tissue, including the axillary tail, is removed through an incision beneath the breast. All breast skin, including the nipple and areola and a small button of tissue under the nipple, remains. A silicone implant is inserted, either during the initial surgery or several months later.

Medical oncology uses antineoplastic drugs and endocrine therapy to affect tumor growth. Chemotherapy often is preferred as adjuvant therapy to surgery when there is axillary node involvement. The systemic effects of drugs halt microscopic metastatic disease and can lengthen the period before relapse. For advanced breast cancer, chemotherapy is primarily palliative. When breast tumors are hormone sensitive, their growth can be retarded by using estrogen, androgen, or progestin, depending on tumor receptors.

With cancer localized to the breast, the 5-year survival is 90%. With axillary node involvement, this drops to 40% to 50%. Women with hormone-receptor positive tumors and those who are young at onset have poorer prognosis. With comparable disease, women in their early 30s have only a 44% disease-free 5-year survival, compared with 72% when older than 40 years (delaRochefordiere et al., 1993).

Breast Reconstruction

Breast reconstruction following mastectomy is frequently done, and many surgeons give special attention to skin preservation at the time of surgery. Reconstruction may be performed at the time of mastectomy, or it may be done later. Silicone implants were used previously, but problems with leakage and its complications have curtailed this method. Saline implants are most common, but interest is growing in autologous tissue reconstruction. Autologous methods use tissue from the abdomen or latissimus dorsi muscle, taking a flap of underlying tissue and placing it beneath the preserved breast skin. Nipple reconstruction also can be done (Kopans et al., 1993). Women with breast implants and reconstruction need annual examinations and mammograms, including the affected breast.

Nursing Assessment

Nursing assessment focuses on the following:

How long the lump, thickening, or other symptom has been present and whether it has changed

Character of breast pain, if present

Presence and characteristics of nipple discharge

Presence of rash or eczema on the nipple

History of breast trauma and family history of cancer risk

The woman's and family's emotional responses and resources for coping are identified. Physical examination involves assessing any skin changes (dimpling, erythema, rash), nipple discharge, and thickening or lumps. The woman should be examined in sitting and supine positions.

Nursing Diagnoses

After a thorough nursing assessment, the nurse can formulate appropriate nursing diagnoses. Common nursing diagnoses for the client with breast cancer are listed in Box 10-11. During hospitalization and recovery, numerous other nursing diagnoses associated with preoperative and postoperative care could be relevant.

Nursing Planning and Intervention

Once a diagnosis is made, interventions include client teaching, support during procedures, emotional support and counseling, preparation for surgery, physiologic monitoring and procedures, comfort measures, family counseling, and coordination of resources for family support and recovery. The woman needs time to work through complex, emotionally charged issues, such as body image, sexuality, and mortality. Nurses need to proceed as the woman indicates willingness to address these issues (Johnson, 1994).

For the client who has a mastectomy, client education is crucial in the postoperative period. The nurse should provide information slowly, according to how the client is progressing and adapting to her surgery. Often written instructions are helpful because of the

---

BOX 10–11
Nursing Diagnoses: Breast Cancer

- Knowledge Deficit related to condition, diagnostic tests, and treatment options
- Ineffective Individual Coping related to effects of diagnosis of cancer
- Body Image Disturbance related to potential loss of body part or function
- Self Esteem Disturbance related to loss of body part and associated femininity
- Fear related to
  - Anticipated pain
  - Surgery
  - Life-threatening disease and prognosis
  - Loss of body part or function
- Anxiety related to
  - Life-threatening illness
  - Side effects of treatment
  - Effects on relationship with partner
- Pain related to postoperative surgical incision
- Powerlessness related to outcome of disease and its effect on activities
- Altered Family Processes related to
  - Surgery
  - Impact of disease on family
  - Life-threatening effects of disease
- Altered Sexuality Patterns related to
  - Mastectomy
  - Fear of rejection from partner

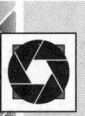

CLIENT EDUCATION
Care After Mastectomy

Use the following to help you after your mastectomy:

- *Incision Care.* Change dressings after washing hands, using clean technique. Inspect the incision for redness, swelling, drainage, or separating edges. Avoid constricting circulation, shaving axilla, and using depilatory creams and strong deodorants. Be aware that sensation around the wound may be absent or decreased, perhaps permanently. (Tingling or discomfort often precedes return of normal sensation.) After the wound heals, gentle massage with cocoa butter or other balm soothes the tissue and increases familiarity with new chest contours.
- *Care of drains.* Drains often remain in place for a period after discharge. In the hospital, practice emptying, measuring, and recording drain output. Usually, the reservoir is emptied every 8 hours. Drink plenty of fluids because keeping fluid intake up promotes healing. When drainage has decreased adequately, the physician will remove the drain.
- *Arm exercises.* (1) Climbing wall: Facing wall with feet close, place palms against the wall, with bent elbows, at shoulder level. Move both hands up wall together, until incision pain occurs. Then move hands down, and repeat. Your goal is to be able to completely extend your elbow up wall. (2) Arm swinging: Dangle both arms down while bending from waist. Swing arms together left-to-right, then in circles parallel to floor in both directions. (3) Pulling rope: Hang rope over hook or shower rod, grasp each end and alternately pull, raising affected arm until incision pain occurs. Keep shortening rope until your affected arm is raised almost directly overhead. (4) Elbow spread: Clasp hands behind neck, raise elbows to chin level slowly, then spread apart until pain occurs.
- *Care of affected arm.* Avoid constricting clothing. Keep your affected arm supported, not dependent,

and protect it during activities such as cooking, gardening, and sewing. If your sensation is decreased, position your arm carefully to avoid burns and bumps.
- *Activity and rest.* Normal energy takes at least 6 weeks to return. Extra rest is needed with naps for the first 2 weeks. Restful sleep at night is important to restore strength. You can resume activities, such as cooking, driving, and cleaning, slowly. Walk every day because walking will build strength. Increase the distance slightly to improve your endurance.
- *Emotional adjustment.* Over the weeks and months following mastectomy, you may experience different emotional phases. Each woman adjusts individually. Be aware that periods of discouragement and sadness are normal. As your physical strength returns, your emotions and mood usually will improve. It is helpful to devote the year after surgery to developing a healthy lifestyle and full recovery.
- *Sexuality.* Sexual relations can be resumed when both partners are ready and both feel desired, loved, and trusted. Changes in your self-image may pose challenges to how you express yourself sexually. You and your partner should try looking at the incision, touching it, and learning to accept the shape of your chest. Learning from other women's experiences, by reading or through groups, can help you accept the changes in your body.
- *Health promotion.* Good health practices will promote recovery and increase chances of staying well. Eat a nutritious diet, rest, exercise, and stress management promote health. Be sure to follow your physician's advice. Regular follow-up visits, medication, and adhering to treatment; monthly breast self-examination; and regular mammography of the other breast contribute to maintaining health.

physiologic and psychological stresses following surgery (see Client Education: Care After Mastectomy).

The nurse plays a key role in client education for prevention of cancer recurrence. Regular follow-up examinations, mammography of the other breast, and monthly BSE are important. Following good health practices, such as maintaining a low-fat diet, taking antioxidants, and exercising regularly, will increase the likelihood of staying well (Brinton, 1994). A periodic screening and surveillance protocol are recommended for women from families with a history of breast cancer, including BSE, provider examinations, baseline mammography by 25 years and annual mammography after, and tests for other forms of cancer.

Evaluation

Possible anticipated outcomes for the client with breast cancer may include the following:

- The client verbalizes information about the disease and its treatment.
- The client demonstrates positive coping mechanisms.
- The client demonstrates acceptance of diagnosis and treatment.
- The client or family verbalizes feelings and concerns openly.
- The client returns to previous level of functioning following treatment.
- The client is assisted to a peaceful and dignified death.

Disorders of Pelvic Support

Alterations in pelvic support result primarily from childbearing. During vaginal delivery, the muscles of the pelvic diaphragm (levator ani, pubococcygeus) separate, with stretching of the fascia and damage to deep support structures. Lacerations of perineal and rectal muscles reduce the integrity of the perineal body. Pelvic trauma and age-related musculoskeletal changes also contribute to problems with pelvic support. Pelvic relaxation is a late effect, appearing during perimenopause. Pelvic relaxation can affect the urethra, bladder, vagina, uterus, and rectum.

Cystocele, Rectocele, and Enterocele

Cystocele refers to the descent of a portion of the posterior bladder wall and trigone into the vagina. Relaxation of the anterior vaginal wall results from stretching or laceration of vesicovaginal fascia by birth of a large baby or multiple births. Cystoceles develop gradually, protruding into the vagina with stretching and increased bladder capacity. Urinary incontinence is the most common symptom. However, this only occurs when musculofascial support of the urethra also is damaged. Typically, women may feel vaginal pressure

and have difficulty emptying the bladder. On pelvic examination, bulging of the anterior vaginal wall is observed (Fig. 10-3*A*).

Rectocele is herniation of the anterior rectal wall into the vagina, caused by disruption of the rectovaginal fascia during childbirth. Small rectoceles are asymptomatic. Large ones cause difficult bowel movements, rectal fullness, bearing down sensations, and perianal pressure. Constipation and irregular bowel habits aggravate this problem. Some women may need to apply digital pressure vaginally to support the rectovaginal bulging to defecate. On pelvic examination, bulging of the posterior vaginal wall is observed (see Fig. 10-3*B*).

Enterocele is herniation of the rectouterine pouch into the rectovaginal septum. It appears as a bulging mass as the bowel descends into the posterior fornix or upper posterior vaginal wall. Usually enteroceles are associated with other pelvic support disorders, appearing in multiparous women during perimenopause. Factors that increase intra-abdominal pressure contribute to the etiology. Symtoms include aching, vagi-

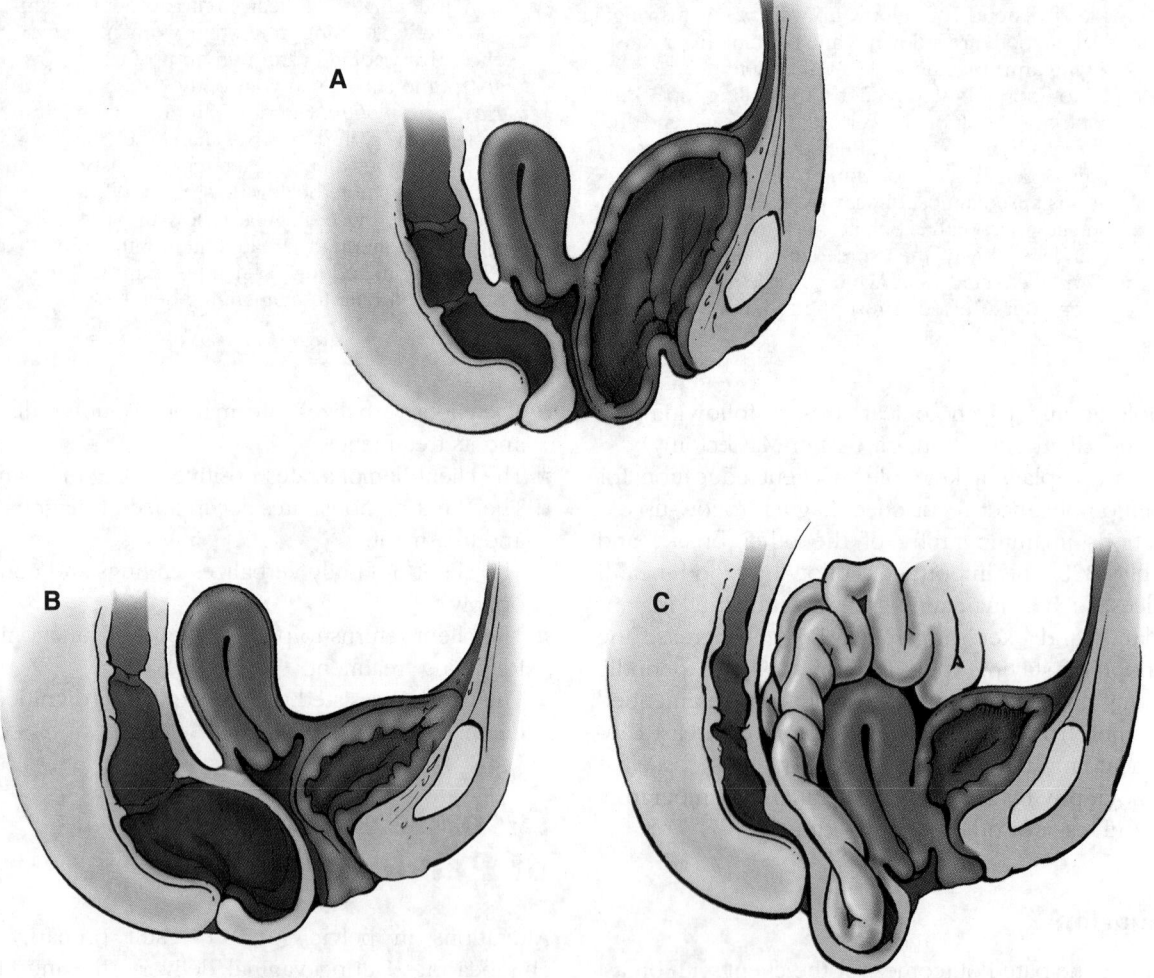

FIGURE 10-3 Disorders of pelvic support. (**A**) Cystocele. (**B**) Rectocele. (**C**) Enterocele and prolapsed uterus.

nal pressure, and fullness. Gastrointestinal symptoms are rare (see Fig. 10-3*C*).

Treatment

Small to moderate cystoceles are treated with a vaginal pessary to support the bladder and urethra (Fig. 10-4). The client is instructed how to perform Kegel isometric exercises to tighten the pubococcygeus muscles. If the woman is postmenopausal, estrogen replacement therapy may be ordered.

Surgery is needed for large cystoceles or if there is significant urinary incontinence, urinary retention, or recurrent bladder infections. Anterior vaginal colporrhaphy is the most effective surgical procedure (see the section, "Reproductive Surgery").

Until the woman has completed childbearing, rectoceles are treated by supporting bowel function. Increased fluid intake, stool bulking, regular elimination habits, diet high in roughage, and occasional stool softeners or laxatives usually are effective in correcting constipation. A large round ball or doughnut type pessary may be needed to improve symptoms. When the rectocele is large enough to make fecal evacuation difficult, or it protrudes enough to cause discomfort or tissue breakdown, surgical repair is indicated. Posterior colpoperineorrhaphy is usually able to correct the condition (see the section, "Reproductive Surgery").

Uterine Prolapse

In uterine prolapse, the uterus sags downward into the vagina. It results from childbirth injuries to the endopelvic fascia, with stretching of the uterosacral and cardinal ligaments that help support the uterus. Lacerations or damage to the levator ani and perineal body contribute to general pelvic relaxation. Uterine prolapse,

cystocele, and rectocele often occur together. Obesity; chronic cough, such as with asthma or chronic bronchitis; and large uterine or ovarian tumors may promote uterine prolapse.

The degree of uterine prolapse parallels the extent of weakening of supporting structures. In slight prolapse, the uterus descends partially into the vagina; in moderate prolapse, it descends to the introitus; and in marked prolapse (procidentia), the cervix and uterus protrude beyond the introitus, inverting the vagina (Fig. 10-5).

Symptoms of prolapse include pelvic heaviness, low backache, lower abdominal discomfort, dyspareunia, and a feeling of something falling out. With more pronounced prolapse, women may feel a lump just inside the vagina or at the introitus. On examination, the cervix is observed descending in the vagina or at the introitus. Compression and distortion of the bladder may lead to residual urine with incontinence or urinary tract infection.

Treatment

Treatment may be with vaginal pessary, postmenopausal estrogen replacement, or surgery. Selection of the surgical procedure depends on the degree of prolapse, presence of cystorectocele, desire for pregnancy and preservation of vaginal function, and age. Usually a composite operation is necessary. Uterine syspension, even with ventrofixation of the corpus to the abdominal wall, is not usually effective in treating prolapse (see the section, "Reproductive Surgery").

Urinary Incontinence

Urinary incontinence is involuntary leakage of urine that occurs when intravesical pressure exceeds the

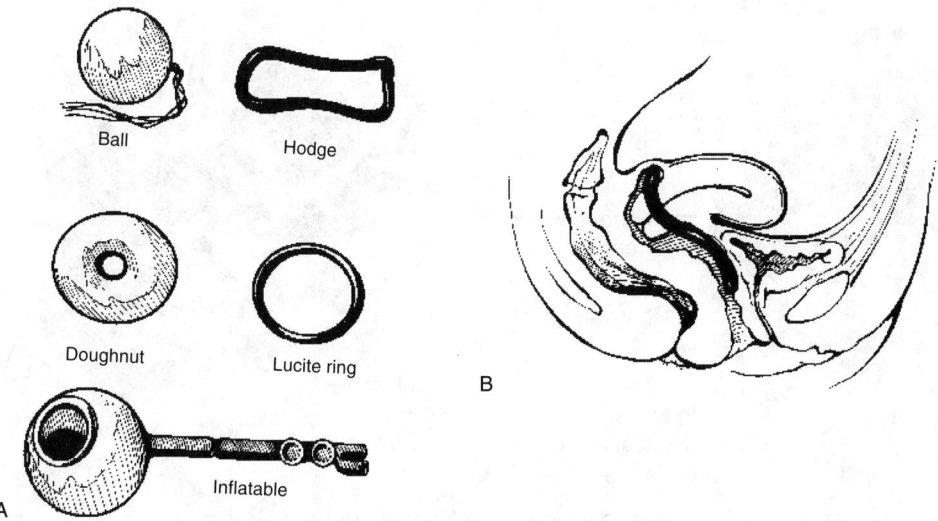

FIGURE 10-4 (A) Several types of pessaries. **(B)** Hodge pessary in place, holding cervix backward and upward in the pelvis.

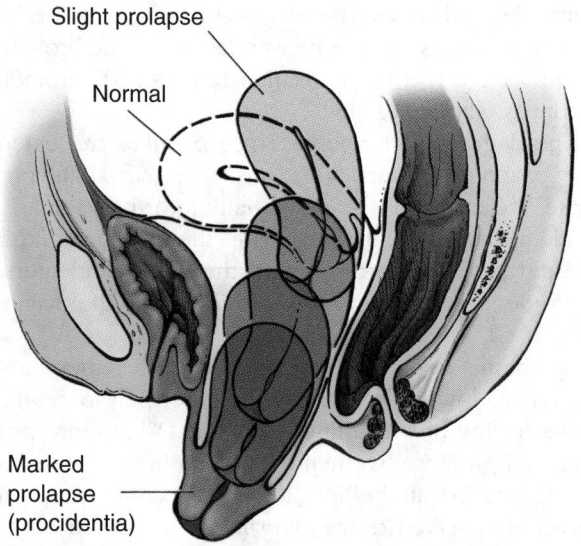

FIGURE 10-5 Stages of uterine prolapse, from slight to marked.

maximum urethral pressure in the absence of detrusor muscle contraction. About 50% of all women experience incontinence occasionally, and 10% experience it regularly. Incontinence prevents many women from fully enjoying social and sexual relationships, activities, and careers. More than 30% of women in nursing homes are incontinent; it is often a major reason for placement (Robertson et al., 1991). Recurrent urinary tract infections, perineal irritation, unpleasant odor, vaginal discharge, and dyspareunia are common effects.

Urinary stress incontinence results from injury to vesicourethral structures during childbirth. Increased intra-abdominal pressure, such as during coughing, sneezing, or lifting, exerts pressure on the bladder and proximal urethra. Normally, the sphincter at the upper urethra is able to withhold urine. Changes in the urethrovesicular angle, anatomic descent of the proximal urethra, and failure of neuromuscular support following birth injury lead to inability of the sphincter to withstand increased pressure (Fig. 10-6). Other factors associated with weakening the urethral sphincter closure mechanism include estrogen deficiency, scarring, infection, neuropathies (diabetes, multiple sclerosis), and some medications (prazosin, alpha-adrenergic blockers).

Cystocele or urethrocele occurs in 75% of women with stress incontinence. Poor urethral support can be demonstrated by cystography, ultrasonography, and tests of urinary leakage with straining (observing urine flow, saturation of pad). Cystometrogram is used to rule out detrusor instability. Nonsurgical treatment consists of Kegel exercises; pessaries; postmenopausal estrogen replacement; elimination of ganglionic or alpha-adrenergic blocking agents, such as methyldopa, prazosin, and guanethidine; and use of alpha-adrenergic agonists, such as phenylpropanolamine, pseudoephedrine, and imipramine. Regular, scheduled voiding; weight loss; and cough or straining management are advised. Periurethral injection of polytetrafluorethylene or glutaraldehyde provide support of the urethral sphincter; repeat injections may be needed (Harris, 1993). Surgical correction is often necessary, with a 75% to 85% success rate in carefully selected clients. Abdominal and vaginal procedures are used, depending on concommitant problems, such as cystorectocele, age, history, and severity of incontinence.

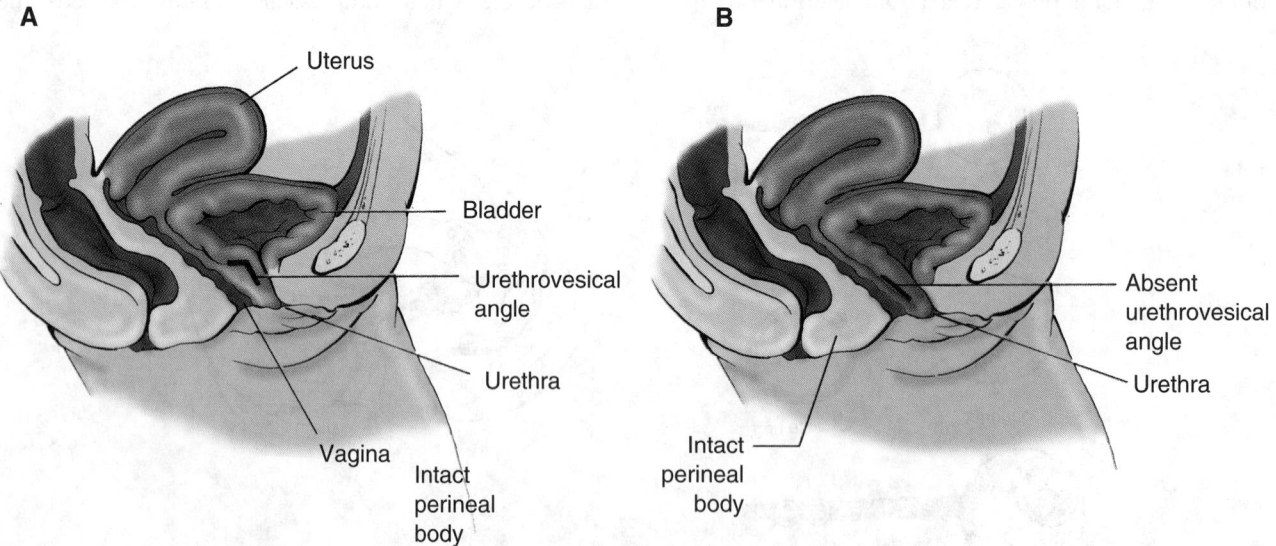

FIGURE 10-6 Urethrovesical angle in stress incontinence. **(A)** Normal urethrovesical angle. **(B)** Absent or flat urethrovesical angle.

Nursing Management

Prevention of pelvic support disorders may be encouraged by teaching intrapartum and postpartum exercises. Kegel isometric exercises are designed to strengthen the levator and perineal muscle groups (see Appendix C). Helping the client maintain normal weight is important because obesity predisposes a client to decreased pelvic muscle tone. Nutrition and exercise counseling can help women develop a program for weight management. Control of chronic cough, and avoidance of repeated straining during bowel movements or by improper lifting can be helpful. Good bladder habits are reinforced, including adequate fluid intake, regular voiding, and complete bladder emptying. Measures to prevent urinary tract infections are taught, such as front-to-back wiping after bowel movements, voiding before and after intercourse, using cotton-crotch underpants, and avoiding tight-fitting pants.

If a client is suspected of having a pelvic support disorder, pelvic muscle strength needs to be evaluated. Pelvic muscle strength can be assessed by the following:

- Digital examination: The women squeezes vaginal muscles against examiner's fingers during pelvic examination.
- Urine stream interruption test: The woman is instructed to void normally; 5 seconds into the void, she interrupts urine flow by contracting pelvic muscles. The examiner uses a stopwatch to time how long it takes to stop the stream of urine. Women who can stop their urine stream in 2 seconds or less have significantly lower urinary incontinence (Sampselle, 1993).

If a problem is noted, appropriate treatment can be started.

Reproductive Surgery

Numerous women will undergo minor or major surgical procedures related to the reproductive system. Many of these procedures are discussed elsewhere in this text (dilation and curettage, tubal ligation, elective abortion, cervical cryosurgery, laser surgery, endometrial or endocervical curettage). Common major surgical procedures for pelvic structures are included here.

Hysterectomy

Hysterectomy is the removal of all or a portion of the uterus by abdominal or vaginal procedures. Often ovaries (oopherectomy) and tubes (salpingectomy) are removed during these procedures. Hysterectomy is used to treat various problems, including DUB, endometriosis, adenomyosis, chronic PID, leiomyomata, and cancers of the cervix, endometrium, and ovary.

Commonly, TAH-BSO is done. About 650,000 women undergo this procedure annually in the United States (Stovall et al., 1990). Abdominal procedures are preferred for women with previous pelvic surgery (because of adhesions and scarring), endometriosis, malignancy (to permit staging and tumor debulking), adnexal disease, gastrointestinal symptoms, and uterus larger than 12 to 16 cm. A midline abdominal or suprapubic incision may be used, depending on the suspected pathology and extent of abdominal exploration indicated. Abdominal procedures have disadvantages, however, including scarring, slower postoperative recovery with more pain, greater alteration in bowel function, and higher rate of complications than with vaginal procedures.

Partial hysterectomy is removal of the uterine corpus and usually the cervix and fallopian tubes. In the past, procedures left the cervix in place, but this is rarely done today. The ovaries are left in place to preserve hormone function.

Vaginal hysterectomy is removal of the uterus by transvaginal approach. This is the preferred route for women with cystocele or rectocele, uterine prolapse, a uterus with less than 12 cm benign lesion, and prolapse of urethrovesical angle. Women who are elderly, obese, debilitated, or have heart or lung disease tolerate vaginal procedures better. Advantages include less anesthesia, earlier ambulation, shorter recovery time, less blood loss, and no visible scarring. However, there is increased risk of deep vein thrombosis with vaginal hysterectomy (DiSaia et al., 1990).

Oopherectomy is removal of one or both ovaries. It is done for severe PID, ectopic pregnancy, ovarian tumors or cysts, and malignancies. When a hysterectomy is done for reasons other than malignancy, most surgeons recommend leaving ovaries in place in premenopausal women. This allows continued endogenous estrogen secretion, reducing the need for estrogen replacement to prevent development of surgical menopause and osteoporosis. In women 40 years or older, an oopherectomy may be done because of increasing risk of ovarian cancer.

Surgical Repair of Pelvic Support Disorders

Anterior vaginal colporrhaphy is the most effective surgical procedure for correcting cystocele. The anterior vaginal wall herniation is resected, and the vesicovaginal fascia is drawn together (plicated) to support the bladder. This procedure is often combined with vaginal hysterectomy and posterior colpoperineorrhaphy.

Posterior colpoperineorrhaphy is often combined with procedures to correct uterine prolapse. The posterior midline incision includes the perineum and posterior vaginal wall, high enough to rule out enterocele (bowel herniation into cul-de-sac). The rectovaginal fascia is plicated and extra vaginal tissue removed. It is usually curative for large rectoceles.

Composite procedures involve a combination of vaginal hysterectomy, colporrhaphy, and colpoperineorrhaphy. Enterocele also must be corrected if present. Vaginal length must be preserved when continued vaginal function is important. In the extreme elderly, if vaginal preservation is not important, narrowing and shortening the upper vaginal walls during the composite procedure is highly effective in correcting urinary incontinence. Abdominal hysterectomy may be combined with the other two procedures, but this is cumbersome and lengthy.

Abdominal incontinence procedures place sutures in periurethral or paravaginal tissue to elevate the urethrovesical junction by attaching to strong structures, such as the periosteum of the symphysis pubis (called a *Marshall-Marchetti-Krantz procedure*) or Cooper's ligaments (called a *Burch procedure*).

Vaginal incontinence procedures are adaptations of the anterior colporrhaphy, which alone has a poor outcome. Variations use more defined and permanent anatomic structures, such as the pubourethral ligaments, periosteum of the pubic ramus, or pubococcygeus muscle, rather than the vesicovaginal fascia to provide support for the bladder.

Sling procedures may correct incontinence when standard surgical procedures do not succeed. Rectal fascia, fascia lata, or round ligaments are passed under the urethra to provide support at the urethrovesical junction and partially obstruct the upper urethra. While some clients can then void normally, others need intermittent self-catheterization or external abdominal pressure over the bladder to void.

Nursing Assessment

Nursing assessment for the client facing reproductive surgery involves a thorough history and physical examination. Included with the nursing history is the client's menstrual history, which helps to identify specific areas of reproductive concern. As with any client facing surgery, possible risks also can be identified.

Nursing Diagnosis

Once a thorough history and physical examination are obtained, nursing diagnoses can be formulated. Possible nursing diagnoses for women having reproductive surgery are listed in Box 10-12.

BOX 10–12
Nursing Diagnoses: Women Having Reproductive Surgery

- Knowledge Deficit related to reasons for procedure, hospitalization, recovery, and outcomes
- Knowledge Deficit related to preoperative or postoperative experiences
- Fear or Anxiety related to uncertainty of outcomes, anesthesia, life-threatening disease
- Pain related to surgery
- Risk for Infection related to surgery
- Body Image Disturbance related to loss of function or body part
- Sexual Dysfunction related to change in body image or loss of body part

---

Nursing Planning and Intervention

Women facing reproductive surgery need to understand the reasons for the surgical procedure, expected benefits, risks of surgery, and effects on childbearing and sexuality. Obtaining a second opinion often is beneficial, especially for elective surgery and when there may be a controversy about treatment, for example, in cases of early cervical and breast cancers. Thorough informed consent is necessary, with signed and witnessed written consent documents.

The woman's concerns about fear of anesthesia, fear of death or disability, postoperative pain, length of recovery, financial impact of hospitalization, and family arrangements are addressed. Knowledge deficits about the procedure, hospital course, and recovery are resolved by preoperative teaching. She is encouraged to express her fears and is helped to set realistic parameters and find effective support resources. Body image, sexuality, and self-esteem concerns are alleviated through supportive listening and enhancing postsurgical recovery and functioning.

Preoperative Care

Information is provided about the surgical procedure and consequences, particularly on sexuality and reproductive function. Anesthesia risks, postoperative and recovery processes, and return to normal function are discussed. Arrangements for care of children and home are encouraged. Immediate preoperative care includes nothing by mouth for 8 hours before surgery; enema and douche as indicated; abominal, pubic, or perineal shave; emptying bladder by voiding or catheter insertion; and administering medications or intravenous fluids.

Postoperative Care

Following surgery, vital signs are monitored frequently, at least every 4 hours. Bleeding and pain are assessed, fluid intake and output are measured, and medications or fluids are administered. Comfort is promoted by positioning and frequent turning, leg exercises, deep breathing, and pain relief with analgesics. Early ambulation is promoted, and diet is progressed as tolerated. Bowel and bladder function are monitored. When the urinary catheter is removal, the client is assisted to void. Stool softeners to prevent straining or laxatives to prevent constipation may be given. Perineal discomfort from vaginal procedures may relieved by sitz baths, heat lamps, or ice packs.

The nurse observes the client for postoperative complications. Hemorrhage, urinary problems, wound infections, and deep vein thrombosis occur more often with vaginal procedures. Paralytic ileus, pulmonary embolism, atelectasis, pneumonia, wound infections, and dehiscence may occur with abdominal procedures.

The nurse observes the client closely for psychological responses to surgery. The client is encouraged to express any anxiety, depression, disturbed self-esteem, and worry about sexual and reproductive function. Processes of grieving for loss of body parts or cancer are supported. Women are helped to develop realistic expectations of their recovery and return to full functioning. Anticipating physical and emotional responses can reduce anxiety and promote adjustment.

Following hysterectomy, women can expect the following postoperative effects:

- Fatigue and weakness
- Painful intercourse until vaginal walls are stretched (after vaginal hysterectomy)
- Decreased appetite and bowel irregularity
- Temporary decreased vaginal sensation (after vaginal hysterectomy)
- Phantom uterine pain and cramping

Discharge Preparation

Women need 3 to 4 months for full recovery from hysterectomy and most other major pelvic surgery. They must avoid heavy housework and lifting and active sports for 1 month. Tub baths, douching, and sexual intercourse can be resumed in 3 to 6 weeks. Lengthy sitting may lead to increased pelvic congestion and should be discouraged. Emotional lability may be common for several weeks. Depression may occur with more serious conditions, such as cancer. Referrals for counseling may be indicated. Women are taught signs of complications, urged to seek medical care early, and encouraged to keep follow-up appointments. Sexual adjustment may be enhanced by using vaginal lubricants and gentle positions for intercourse, focusing on clitoral orgasm, and emphasizing more generalized sensuality.

Evaluation

Nursing care is effective when the woman understands and accepts the surgical procedure and prepares optimistically for hospitalization. Pain control, comfort, resumption of body functions, and prevention of complications signify successful postoperative care. Eventual return to full physical and social functioning, positive self-concept, enjoyable sexual expression, and integration of the surgical experience are long-range signs of effective care.

Summary Points

- ✔ DUB is common during reproductive years. It may be related to hormone dysfunction, structural abnormalities, neoplastic processes, infections, medication use (eg, hormonal contraceptives), behaviors, or endocrine abnormalities.

- ✔ Self-care is important for most nonpathologic bleeding and may involve nutrition, exercise, stress management, attitude management, weight control, and emotional support.

- ✔ Benign neoplasias account for most cellular changes and tumors of reproductive organs. Many resolve spontaneously or can be watched closely. Women with risk factors for cancer or persistent suspicious neoplasia must have further diagnostic evaluation.

- ✔ Malignant neoplasias increase with age and are associated with specific risk factors. Early diagnosis and treatment are associated with better outcomes in terms of recurrence and survival. Controversy exists about treatment options for early stage breast and ovarian neoplasia.

- ✔ Potential for significant self-esteem and functional disruption and threat to life are major issues related to malignant neoplasia.

- ✔ Disorders of pelvic support result from childbirth injuries. Decreased pelvic support usually appears perimenopausally, as muscle tone decreases with aging and diminished estrogen secretion. Surgery often is necessary for adequate relief of symptoms and restoration of function.

- ✔ Major reproductive surgery poses challenges for many women, with implications for self-worth and sexuality. Women need to understand physiologic and emotional consequences of such procedures as hysterectomy and repairs for pelvic support disorders.

REFERENCES

Adamson, G. D. (1990). Diagnosis and clinical presentation of endometriosis. *American Journal of Obstetrics and Gynecology, 162*(2), 568–569.

American Cancer Society (1993). *Cancer facts and figures—1993.* Atlanta, GA: Author.

American Psychiatric Association (1994). *Diagnostic and statistical manual of mental disorders* (4th ed.). Washington, DC: Author.

Bachman, G. A. (1990). Hysterectomy: A critical review. *Journal of Reproductive Medicine, 35*(9), 839–862.

Baird, S. B., McCorkle, R., & Grant, M. (1991). Cancer nursing: A comprehensive textbook. Philadelphia: W.B. Saunders.

Barbieri, R. L. (1990). Etiology and epidemiology of endometriosis. *American Journal of Obstetrics and Gynecology, 162*(2), 565–567.

Beal, M. W. (1990). Cervical cytology. *Clinical Issues in Perinatology and Women's Health Nursing, 1*(4), 470.

Beck, L., Gervitz, R., & Mortola, J. (1990). The predictive role of psychosocial stress on symptom severity in premenstrual syndrome. *Psychosomatic Medicine, 52*, 536–543.

Boring, C. C., Squires, T. S., & Tong, T. (1991). Cancer statistics, 1991. *CA Cancer Journal for Clinicians, 41*(1), 19.

Breo, D. L. (1993). Altered fates—counseling families with inherited breast cancer. *Journal of the American Medical Association, 269*, 2017–2022.

Brinton, L. A. (1994). Ways that women may possibly reduce their risk of breast cancer. *Journal of the National Cancer Institute, 86*(18), 11–12.

Brown, M. A., & Woods, N. F. (1984). Correlates of dysmenorrhea: A challenge to past stereotypes. *Journal of Obstetric, Gynecologic, and Neonatal Nursing, 13*(4), 256–265.

Casper, R. F., Graves, G. R., & Reid, R. L. (1987). Objective measurement of hot flushes associated with the premenstrual syndrome. *Fertility and Sterility, 47*, 341.

Chang, R. J. (1993). *Hormone replacement therapy: Therapeutic considerations of various estrogen deficiency states* (pp. 91–98). In Ambulatory obstetrics and gynecology update, School of Medicine, University of California, Davis.

Chihal, H. J. (1990). Premenstrual syndrome: An update for the clinician. *Obstetrics and Gynecology Clinics of North America, 17*(2), 457–479.

Coates, T. (1993). *Ovarian cancer screening: The role of ultrasound.* Ambulatory obstetrics and gynecology conference, UCD School of Medicine, University of California, Davis, Jan 17–19, 13–27.

Colditz, G. A., Hankinson, S. E., Hunter, D. J. et al. (1995). The use of estrogens and progestins and the risk of breast cancer in postmenopausal women. *New England Journal of Medicine, 332*(24), 1589–1593.

Colditz, G. A. et al. (1990). Prospective study of estrogen replacement therapy and risk of breast cancer in postmenopausal women. *Journal of the American Medical Association, 264*(20), 2648.

Dan, A. J., & Lewis, L. L. (Eds.) (1992). *Menstrual health in women's lives.* Univ of Illinois Press, Urbana & Chicago.

Dawood, M. Y. (1990). Dysmenorrhea. *Clinical Obstetrics and Gynecology, 33*(1), 168–178.

delaRochefordiere, A. et al. (1993). Age as prognostic factor in premenopausal breast carcinoma. *Lancet, 342*, 1039–1043.

Demers, L. M., Hahn, D. W., & McGuire, J. L. (1985). Newer concepts in dysmenorrhea research: Leukotrienes and calcium channel blockers. In M. Y. Dawood, J. L. McGuire, & L. M. Demers (Eds.), *Premenstrual syndrome and dysmenorrhea.* Baltimore: Urban and Schwartzenberg.

Disaia, P. F., Creasman, W. T. (1992). *Clinical gynecologic oncology,* 4th ed. St. Louis: Mosby Yearbook.

Doody, K. M., & Carr, B. R. (1990). Amenorrhea. *Obstetric and Gynecologic Clinics of North America, 17*(2), 361–367.

Dunnihoo, D. R. (1992). Menstrual problems. In *Fundamentals of gynecology and obstetrics* (pp. 622–627). Philadelphia: J.B. Lippincott.

Dupont, W. D. et al. (1994). Long-term risk of breast cancer in women with fibroadenoma. *New England Journal of Medicine, 331*, 10–15.

Facchinetti, F., Martignoni, E., Petraglia, F. et al. (1987). Premenstrual fall of plasma β-endorphin in patients with premenstrual syndrome. *Fertility and Sterility, 47*, 570.

Fisher, B. et al. (1993). Lumpectomy compared with lumpectomy and radiation therapy for the treatment of intraductal breast cancer. *New England Journal of Medicine, 328*, 1581–1586.

Friedman, L. S., Ostermeyer, E. A., Lynch, E. D. et al. (1995). 22 genes from chromosome 17q21: Cloning, sequencing, and characterization of mutations in breast cancer families and tumors. *Genomics, 25*(1), 256–263.

Fujimoto, V. Y., Spencer, S. V., Rabinouici, J. et al. (1993). Endogenous catecholamines augment the inhibitory effect of opioids on luteinizing hormone secretion during the midluteal phase. *American Journal of Obstetrics and Gynecology, 169*(6), 1524–1530.

Giuliano, A. E. (1991). The breast. In M. L. Pernoll (Ed.), *Current obstetric and gynecologic diagnosis and treatment* (pp. 1148–1168) (7th ed.). Norwalk, CT: Appleton & Lange.

Goodale, I. L., Domar, A. D., & Benson, H. (1990). Alleviation of premenstrual syndrome symptoms with the relaxation response. *Obstetrics and Gynecology, 75*(4), 649–655.

Guiliano, A. E. (1991). The breast. In *Current obstetric & gynecologic diagnosis & treatment,* 7th ed. Norwalk, CT: Appleton & Lange.

Haas, G. G. (1993). *Premenstrual syndrome, new treatment strategies* (pp. 60–67). In Ambulatory obstetrics and gynecology update. School of Medicine, University of California Davis.

Harris, T. (1993). *Genuine stress incontinence: Office evaluation and new treatments.* Ambulatory obstetrics and gynecology conference, UCD School of Medicine, University of California, Davis, Jan 17–19, 99–115.

Hsia, L. S. Y., & Log, M. H. (1990). Premenstrual syndrome: Current concepts in diagnosis and management. *Journal of Nurse Midwifery, 35*(6), 351–357.

Jensvold, M. F. (1993). Psychiatric aspects of the menstrual cycle. In D. E. Stewart & N. L. Stotland (Eds.), *Psychological aspects of women's health care: The interface between psychiatry and obstetrics and gynecology* (pp. 165–191). Washington, DC: American Psychiatric Press.

Johnson, J. R. (1994). Caring for the woman who's had a mastectomy. *American Journal of Nursing, 94*(5), 25–31.

King, M. C. et al. (1994). Inherited breast and ovarian cancer—what are the risks? What are the choices? *Journal of the American Medical Association, 269*, 1975–1980.

Kopans, D. B., Marchant, D. J., & Osborne, M. P. (1993). Breast cancer: Vigilance, not panic. *Patient Care, 27*(18), 135–164.

Lacey, C. G. (1991). Premalignant and malignant disorders of the uterine corpus. In M. L. Pernoll (Ed.), *Current obstetric and gynecologic diagnosis and treatment* (pp. 955–973) (7th ed.). Norwalk, CT: Appleton & Lange.

Lee, J. R. (1993). *Natural progesterone: The multiple roles of a remarkable hormone.* Sebastopol, CA: BLL Publishing.

Lewis, L. L. (1992). PMS and the progesterone controversy. In A. Dan, & L. Lewis (Eds.), *Menstrual health in women's lives* (pp. 61–72). University of Illinois Press, Urbana & Chicago.

Lichtman, R. (1990). The cervix. In R. Lichtman & S. Papera (Eds.), *Gynecology: Well-woman care* (pp. 249–260). Norwalk, CT: Appleton & Lange.

Long, C. A., & Gast, M. J. (1990). Menorrhagia. *Obstetrics and Gynecology Clinics of North America, 17*(2), 343–359.

Marchbanks, P. A., Lee, N. C., & Peterson, H. B. (1990). Cigarette smoking as a risk factor for pelvic inflammatory disease. *American Journal of Obstetrics and Gynecology, 162*(3), 639–644.

McKeon, V. A. (1989). Estrogen replacement therapy: Current guidelines for education and counseling. *Journal of Gerontology Nursing, 16*(10), 6.

Menkes, D. B. et al. (1992). Fluoxetine treatment of severe premenstrual syndrome. *British Medical Journal, 305,* 346–347.

Mira, M., Stewart, P. M., & Abraham, S. F. (1988). Vitamin and trace element status in premenstrual syndrome. *American Journal of Clinical Nutrition, 47,* 636.

Mitchell, E., Woods, N., & Lentz, M. (1991). Recognizing PMS when you see it. Criteria for PMS sample selection. In D. Taylor & N. Woods (Eds.), *Menstruation, health, and illness* (pp. 89–102). New York: Hemisphere.

Montz, F. J., Monk, B. J., Fowler, J. M., & Nguyen, L. (1992). Natural history of the minimally abnormal papanicolaou smear. *Obstetrics and Gynecology, 80,* 385.

Peck, L. (1990). Premenstrual syndrome. In R. Lichtman & S. Papera (Eds.), *Gynecology: Well-woman care* (pp. 333–343). Norwalk, CT: Appleton & Lange.

Plaxe, S. C. et al. (1993). Profiles of women age 30–39 and age less than 30 with epithelial ovarian cancer. *Obstetrics and Gynecology, 81,* 651–654.

Plouffe, L., Stewart, K., Craft, K. et al. (1993). Diagnostic and treatment results from a southeastern academic center-based premenstrual syndrome clinic: The first year. *American Journal of Obstetrics and Gynecology, 169*(2), 295–307.

Rapkin, A. J., Chang, L. C., & Reading, A. E. (1989). Mood and cognitive style in premenstrual syndrome. *Obstetrics and Gynecology, 74*(4), 644–649.

Rippon, M. B. (1993). Breast cancer prevention trial: Preliminary results. In *Ambulatory obstetrics and gynecology update* (pp. 28–31). School of Medicine, University of California, Davis.

Robertson, J. R., & Hebert, D. B. (1991). Gynecologic urology. In M. L. Pernoll (Ed.), *Current obstetric and gynecologic diagnosis and treatment* (pp. 851–865) (7th ed.). Norwalk, CT: Appleton & Lange.

Sampselle, C. M. (1993). Using a stopwatch to assess pelvic muscle strength in the urine stream interruption test. *Nurse Practitioner, 18*(1), 14–20.

Schaffer, S. D., & Philput, C. B. (1992). Predictors of abnormal cervical cytology: Statistical analysis of human papillomavirus and cofactors. *Nurse Practitioner, 17*(3), 46–50.

Schneider, A., & Shah, K. (1989). The role of vitamins in the etiology of cervical neoplasia: An epidemiological review. *Archives of Obstetrics and Gynecology, 246,* 1–13.

Shattuck-Eidens, D. et al. (1995). A collaborative survey of 80 mutations in the BRCA1 breast and ovarian cancer susceptibility gene: Implications for presymptomatic testing and screening. *Journal of the American Medical Association, 273,* 535–541.

Silverberg, E. (1990). Cancer statistics. *Cancer, 40*(9).

Slawson, D. C. et al. (1994). Should all women with cervical atypia be referred for colposcopy: a HARNET study. *Journal of Family Practice, 38,* 387–392.

Smith, S., & Schiff, I. (1989). The premenstrual syndrome—diagnosis and management. *Fertility and Sterility, 52*(4), 527–543.

Stovall, T. G. et al. (1990). Hysterectomy for chronic pelvic pain of presumed uterine etiology. *Obstetrics and Gynecology, 75*(4), 676.

Tulenheimo, A., Laafikainen, T., & Salminen, K. (1987). Plasma β-endorphin immunoreactivity in premenstrual tension. *British Journal of Obstetrics and Gynaecology, 94,* 26.

Veronesi, U. et al. (1993). Radiotherapy after breast-preserving surgery in women with localized cancer of the breast. *New England Journal of Medicine, 328,* 1587–1591.

Woods, N. F., Lentz, M. J., Mitchell, E. S., & Kogan, H. (1994). Arousal and stress response across the menstrual cycle in women with three perimenstrual symptom patterns. *Research in Nursing and Health, 17,* 99–110.

Woods, N. F., Mitchell, E. S., & Lentz, M. J. (1995). Social pathways to premenstrual symptoms. *Research in Nursing and Health, 18*(3), 225–237.

11

Infectious Diseases

Objectives

- Describe the process of nursing care for women with sexually transmitted diseases.
- Identify risk factors, risk reduction, and prevention for various types of sexually transmitted diseases.
- Contrast types of viral hepatitis, nursing care, and implications for childbearing.
- Discuss care of human immunodeficiency virus-infected women and implications for childbearing.
- Describe types of urinary tract infections and the process of nursing care.
- Identify signs, symptoms, and prevention of common contagious diseases, and discuss implications for childbearing.
- Describe signs, symptoms, risk factors, prevention, and nursing care of women with toxic shock syndrome.
- Summarize standard precautions used by healthcare workers to reduce the risk of contracting and transmitting infectious diseases.

Key Terms

AIDS	HIV
Bacterial vaginosis	Human papillomavirus
Candida (Monilla)	Mycobacterium
albicans	tuberculosis
Chlamydia trachomatis	Pneumocystis carinii
Cystitis	PID
Cytomegalovirus	Rubella
Escherichia coli	Syphilis
Genital herpes	Toxic Shock
Gonorrhea	syndrome
Hepatitis	Toxoplasmosis
Histoplasma	Trichomonas vaginalis

BOX 11-1
High-Risk Groups—Infectious Diseases

High-Risk Groups for Sexually Transmitted Diseases (STDs)

Younger than 20 years

Sexually active

Multiple sexual partners

Sexual partner who has multiple sexual contacts

History of STD

Sexual partner diagnosed with STD

Prostitutes

High-Risk Factors for Hepatitis B

IV drug users

Recipients of blood products

Prostitutes

Women with multiple sex partners

Women with a history of liver disease

Women who have occupational exposure to blood and blood products (healthcare workers, laboratory technicians, and so forth)

Indochinese refugees

Women of Asian descent or women born in Haiti or South Africa

High-Risk Groups for Human Immunodeficiency Virus Infection and Acquired Immunodeficiency Syndrome

History of IV drug use or current use

Long-term residence or birth in area with high prevalence of HIV infection or AIDS

Received blood transfusion between 1978 and 1985 (before HIV screening was standard practice)

Diagnosed with another sexually transmitted disease

History of frequent sexual partners or prostitutes

Past or present sexual partner who is IV drug user, bisexual, or HIV infected; has signs or symptoms of AIDS; has frequent sexual partners; or who has received a blood transfusion between 1978 and 1985

Infectious diseases cause a wide range of illnesses in women and are especially dangerous during pregnancy. Some infectious diseases cause serious complications in the fetus, such as congenital anomalies, blindness, or intrauterine death. The woman's life may be threatened by some types of infections, such as hepatitis or human immunodeficiency virus (HIV). Many infectious diseases can be prevented, either by immunizations or by safe sex practices. Education is often the key to prevention. The nurse plays a crucial role by increasing clients' awareness of high-risk behaviors.

Sexually Transmitted Diseases

Sexually transmitted diseases (STDs) are spread through sexual contact. Many STDs can be successfully treated if detected early. However, some are chronic or incurable. The presence of an STD during pregnancy makes the pregnancy high-risk, requiring continuous monitoring and treatment. The incidence of many STDs is increasing, especially among adolescents (Box 11-1). In addition, resistant strains of infectious microorganisms are developing that are difficult to treat.

Nursing Assessment

Women with STDs may be asymptomatic in early stages of the infection. However, physical examination may reveal signs of infection, such as elevated temperature and heart rate. The skin is observed for rashes, lesions, and evidence of intravenous (IV) drug use (check for needle tracks on forearms, legs, and feet). Abdominal and pelvic examination may reveal tenderness to palpation, erythema, edema, discharge (vagina, cervix), and uterine, tubal, or ovarian enlargement (Box 11-2 and Assessment Tool: Physical Examination for Sexually Transmitted Diseases).

The risk of contracting an STD is increased when women have multiple sexual partners, partners who are IV drug users, or bisexual partners and when the woman is an IV drug user. History of an STD also increases risk. Type and duration of treatment are important in assessing for recurrence or inadequate therapy.

During pregnancy, standard laboratory tests are performed to screen for the more common sexually transmitted and infectious diseases (syphilis, gonorrhea, and *Chlamydia*; Table 11-1). Specimens of discharge or lesions are obtained, and blood tests are taken as indicated by the history and physical examination.

BOX 11–2
Symptoms of Sexually Transmitted Diseases

- Increased or foul-smelling vaginal discharge
- Itching or burning (vaginal, vulval)
- Lesions of vulva, labia
- Enlarged lymph nodes in the groin, axilla, or neck
- Pain or burning on urination
- Skin rash or oral lesions
- Fever, malaise, fatigue, anorexia
- Abdominal discomfort
- Changes in menstrual patterns

Nursing Diagnoses

Nursing diagnoses for STDs may include the following:

- Risk for Infection related to specific STD risk factors
- Risk for Infection Transmission (to sexual partners, fetus)

- Knowledge Deficit related to risk of STD transmission
- Knowledge Deficit related to progress and effects of infection, treatment, and prevention
- Anxiety or Fear related to effects of infectious process and treatment
- Pain related to effects of illness, diagnostic tests, and treatments
- Altered Family Processes related to effects of STD on sexual and emotional relations
- Body Image Disturbance related to changes caused by infection
- Self Esteem Disturbance with diminished role performance and negative effects on personal identity

Planning and Intervention

The primary goal of nursing care is to prevent the occurrence and transmission of STDs. Education is the major strategy in prevention. The nurse helps women identify factors that increase the risk of STDs and methods of prevention and transmission (see Client Educa-

ASSESSMENT TOOL
Physical Examination for Sexually Transmitted Diseases

Pelvic examination
  Inspection of vulva and perineum for lesions, erythema, discharge, edema
  Speculum examination of vagina and cervix; note:
    Vaginal discharge (color, amount, odor, other characteristics)
    Vaginal mucosa (erythema, edema, ulcerations, lesions)
    Cervical discharge (color, amount, odor, other characteristics)
    Cervical mucosa (erythema, edema, lesions, ulcerations, ectropion, erosion, petechiae)
  Bimanual examination; note:
    Cervical tenderness, irregularity
    Uterine tenderness, enlargement, irregularity
    Adenexal tenderness, enlargement, fullness; masses of ovaries, tubes, or in cul-de-sac
    Rectovaginal examination for condition of posterior uterine wall, rectovaginal septum, cul-de-sac, uterosacral ligaments
Specimens
  Pap smear (cervix, herpetic lesions)
  Saline mount (*Candida, Trichomonas, Gardnerella, Chlamydia,* PID)
  Potassium hydroxide mount (*Candida, Gardnerella*)

Gonorrhea culture (Thayer-Martin)
Herpes simplex type 2 culture (if media and procedures available)
Chlamydia culture (if media and procedures available)
Abdominal examination
  Superficial and deep palpation for condition of organs, tenderness, masses
  Palpation of groin lymph nodes
  Auscultation of bowel sounds
Vital signs
  Temperature
  Pulse
  Respiration
  Blood pressure
Skin
  Rashes (characteristics and distribution)
  Lesions (ulcers, nodules, warts, scars, tracks)
  Color (jaundice, pallor, erythema)
  Texture (hydration, scaling, wasting)
Lymph nodes
  Size, number, location
  Tenderness
  Heat
  Erythema

TABLE 11–1
Laboratory Tests for Infectious Diseases

Laboratory Test	Source/Site	Infectious Disease
Wet mount/potassium hydroxide	Vaginal discharge	*Candida, Trichomonas,* bacterial vaginosis
Venereal Disease Research Laboratory (VDRL)/rapid plasma reagent (RPR)	Blood	Syphilis
Gonorrhea culture	Cervix, rectum	Gonorrhea
Chlamydia culture	Cervix	*Chlamydia trachomatis*
Hemagglutination-inhibition antibodies	Blood	Rubella
Urinalysis, urine culture	Urine	Urinary tract infection
Tuberculin skin test	Skin	Tuberculosis
Hepatitis antigens and antibodies	Blood	Hepatitis
Toxoplasmosis antibody	Blood	Toxoplasmosis
Cervical or vaginal culture	Cervix, vagina	Group B *Streptococcus*
Viral culture	Cervix, genital lesions	Herpes simplex I and II
Enzyme-linked immunosorbent assay	Blood	*Chlamydia,* gonorrhea HIV infection or AIDS
Western blot test	Blood	Confirm HIV infection
Immunofluorescent test, rapid immunofluorescent protein assay (RIPA)	Blood	Confirm HIV infection Detect HIV infection from small amounts of viral genetic material (DNA/RNA)
Polymerase chain reaction	Blood (serum)	

tion: Preventing Transmission of Sexually Transmitted Diseases). Because many STDs are treated more effectively if detected early, education emphasizes early signs and symptoms and the importance of seeking medical attention as soon as these occur.

As part of prevention, nurses teach general health measures that promote overall good health and enhance immune system function (see Client Teaching Guidelines: General Health Measures for Preventing Sexually Transmitted Diseases). When teaching the client, the nurse should explain that lifestyle modifications may be necessary to implement some of these practices.

If the woman has contracted an infection, nursing care focuses on facilitating effective treatment, reducing complications and progression of the disease, and preventing further spread of the infection. Many STDs can be treated with antibiotics or other medications. If treatment includes medications, the nurse stresses the importance of taking medications as directed, completing the course of treatment, and following other directions, such as refraining from alcohol or dairy products when taking certain medications. The nurse can facilitate compliance with medication regimens by reviewing expected minor side effects, such as diarrhea and gastric upset, and advising remedies to ease these. Women must be clearly informed of potential allergic reactions, such as hives and respiratory distress.

Many STDs cause local vulvar inflammation and pain, with discomfort during intercourse (dyspareunia) or urination (dysuria). The nurse teaches measures that provide relief, such as sitz baths or topical steroid creams. Women should avoid intercourse or use a condom for 2 to 3 days to relieve pain and inflammation

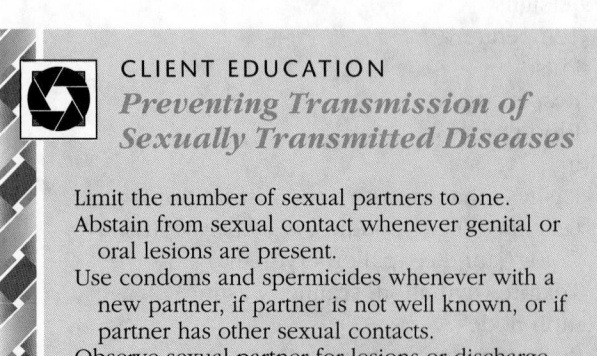

CLIENT EDUCATION
Preventing Transmission of Sexually Transmitted Diseases

Limit the number of sexual partners to one.
Abstain from sexual contact whenever genital or oral lesions are present.
Use condoms and spermicides whenever with a new partner, if partner is not well known, or if partner has other sexual contacts.
Observe sexual partner for lesions or discharge, or ask about symptoms, and be prepared to say no if these are present.
Be responsible with sexual partner(s): advise about history of STD, and avoid contact if symptoms and signs are present.

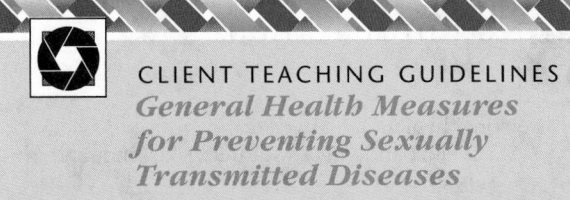

CLIENT TEACHING GUIDELINES
General Health Measures for Preventing Sexually Transmitted Diseases

- Eat a balanced whole food diet.
- Limit fat and simple sugar intake.
- Get adequate rest.
- Get plenty of exercise.
- Engage in satisfying life work.
- Participate in enjoyable "healthy" activities.
- Develop a support network.
- Avoid harmful substances (ie, alcohol and cigarettes).

and prevent transmission of the disease. In addition, sexual partner(s) should receive simultaneous treatment to prevent recurrence of the disease. It would be best for women to avoid intercourse or use condoms with all STDs (though there is controversy about bacterial vaginosis). Sexual partners may not be treated with bacterial vaginosis or *Candida (Monilla)* vaginitis (some controversy exists about whether these should be called STDs).

The nurse explains diagnostic tests and procedures, answers questions, and provides reassurance. Nurses often help in collecting and processing specimens.

The Nurse as Counselor

The woman who contracts an STD often feels anxious or fearful about the outcome for herself and if pregnant, her fetus. The nurse provides support for women to discuss and express feelings, fears, and expectations. A nonjudgmental, accepting attitude and an empathic manner are important. Pregnant women are usually concerned about the danger that an infectious disease may cause the fetus. An assessment of fetal risk is discussed with the woman, and opportunity is provided for her to express fear, guilt, and other emotions. Options, including abortion, are discussed when infections occur early in pregnancy and there is a high probability of fetal damage.

Educating expectant parents about STDs is an important part of nursing care, but information alone is not enough. Strategies that empower women to act on the information are critical. The nurse encourages women to understand that they have control over their bodies and can make choices about participating sexually. Supporting women to be active participants in their physical examinations, assisting them to learn about reproductive and sexual processes, and encouraging comfort with genital anatomy are ways to help women become empowered (Killion, 1994).

Counseling regarding modification of sexual practices is often indicated. If the couple practices high-risk sexual behaviors, the nurse teaches ways to practice safer sex, such as limiting the number of partners and using condoms (see Chap. 9). The nurse emphasizes that there is risk of reinfection after successful medical treatment if the woman's sexual partner(s) is infected and remains untreated.

There are special considerations when counseling clients with HIV because of severe complications, the eventual fatal outcome, and the risk of transmission. Nurses teach how HIV is transmitted and how to prevent transmission. Nurses also dispel common myths regarding transmission. Education also includes the expected progression of the disease, how it affects the immune system, and methods of treatment. Referral to HIV or acquired immunodeficiency syndrome (AIDS) support groups helps women cope with this serious disease and offers strategies for living as fully as possible.

Evaluation

The ideal outcome of nursing intervention in STD is prevention, Nursing care is effective when women demonstrate an understanding of how STDs are transmitted, what specific measures are necessary to avoid unsafe sex practices and reduce exposure to STDs, and how to maintain a health-promoting lifestyle. Nursing interventions for early detection are effective when women recognize symptoms of an STD early and seek prompt medical care. With successful treatment, the disease resolves within the expected time, and there are no complications or sequelae for the woman or fetus during pregnancy.

Teaching is effective when women take steps to prevent transmission of STDs, comply with treatment regimens, take the full course of medications, and use measures for symptom relief. Intervention for emotional needs is successful when women express their feelings, receive support, and take necessary actions with confidence and hope. If the woman decides to terminate a pregnancy, she is able to accept her choice without guilt or remorse.

Types of Sexually Transmitted Diseases and Therapy

Vaginal Infections

Candida (Monilia) Vaginitis

This common vaginal infection is caused by the fungus ***Candida albicans,*** which is widely distributed in nature and often found on the skin and mucous membranes. It occurs more frequently in women who are pregnant, have diabetes, and take higher dose estrogen oral contraceptives because of its ability to thrive in well-estrogenized, high-glycogenic vaginal tissue. Women taking systemic antibiotics are more susceptible to *Candida* due to suppression of normal vaginal flora and changes in pH and enzymes. Stress decreases resistance to *Candida* vaginitis, as do some hygiene practices, such as douching, using perfumed or medicated sprays and soaps, or wearing nylon underwear. Many women use natural remedies to relieve the uncomfortable symptoms of vaginitis (see Client Education: Preventing Vaginitis, Client Education: Natural Remedies for Vaginitis, and Table 11-2).

Symptoms. Discharge is typically white, thick, curdy, and adherent to the cervix and vaginal walls. Thin, milky, and more confluent whitish discharge is not uncommon. Itching, especially of the vulva and perineum, ranges from moderate to severe. The labia and vulva may be bright red, swollen, sensitive to touch, and painful during intercourse.

Diagnosis. Usually saline and potassium hydroxide (KOH) mounts are prepared from vaginal or labial secretions (Fig. 11-1). Microscopic examination shows the hyphae and spores of *C. albicans*. On saline mount, the vaginal epithelial cells appear normal; there are numerous lactobacilli (normal flora) and few white blood cells (WBCs).

Treatment. Vaginal tablets or creams, such as mycostatin (Nystatin), miconazole (Monistat), clotrimazole (Gyne-Lotrimin, Mycelex), terconazole (Terazol), and ticonozole (Vagistat), are prescribed for insertion once daily for 7 to 14 days. Shorter regimens are available: Terazol-3 and butoconazole (Femstat) in a 3-day regimen and Mycelex G-500 and Vagistat 6.5% in a single treatment. Some vaginal creams are available without prescription (eg, Monistat, Gyne-Lotrimin).

Persistent or chronic *Candida* vaginitis may be treated with oral antifungal medications, such as mycostatin (Nystatin), ketoconazole (Nizoral), or fluconazole (Diflucan). A single oral dose of fluconazole is as effective as 3 days of intravaginal clotrimazole. Prophylactic oral fluconazole once monthly can control recurrent infections (The Medical Letter, 1994). This treatment may cause liver toxicity; therefore, liver function tests should be done after 30 days of therapy.

The nurse teaches the client to insert creams or tablets at bedtime to maximize the effectiveness of the medication. A minipad can be advised during the day to absorb drainage. Women should not use tampons during treatment because they absorb the medication. Douching should be avoided, and intercourse

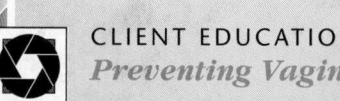

CLIENT EDUCATION
Preventing Vaginitis

Personal hygiene
Wash labia and vulva with mild soap (not antiseptic) daily.
Dry external genitals and perineum thoroughly.
Wipe front-to-back after voiding and bowel movements.
Wash hands before inserting tampons, diaphragm, and contraceptive creams.
Avoid or minimize douching (once per week, use water or mild solutions).
Avoid deodorants, perfumed sprays or lotions, powders, antiseptic soaps, perfumed toilet paper.
Change tampons and pads every 1 to 4 hours, depending on flow.
Avoid using superabsorbent tampons, or use only during heaviest flow.
Wear cotton underclothing; avoid tight-fitting clothing in genital area.
Sexual practices
Limit the number of sexual partners, or have one partner.
Ask or check sexual partner for symptoms (penile disharge, lesions, dysuria); avoid sex or use condom with spermicide if present.
Know the sexual partner (history of genital infections or STD, other sexual contacts).
Avoid intercourse when you have symptoms (increased discharge, itching or burning, lesions, pain).
Avoid oral–genital contact if vulvar or mouth lesions are present in either partner.
Avoid anal–vaginal penetration or use different condoms for each.
General health status
Eat well-balanced, nutritious meals, and avoid less-healthful foods (sweets, red meats, salty foods, saturated fats).
Get regular exercise.
Get enough sleep (6–8 hours per night).
Find time each week for personal interests and hobbies.
Recognize sources of stress at home and work, and find methods to reduce stress (progressive relaxation, autogenic training, yoga, biofeedback, meditation, imagery, quiet time).
Maintain satisfying relationships and friendship networks.

is preferably stopped or a condom used during the course of treatment. If vulvar inflammation and itching are severe, antifungal or steroidal creams can be applied for several days. If *Candida* vaginitis is recurrent, the male partner should be examined and skin scrapings taken if inflammation is found at the base of the penis or perineum. Antifungal treatment is prescribed if indicated.

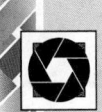

CLIENT EDUCATION
Natural Remedies for Vaginitis

Women are increasingly interested in self-care that includes preventing or minimizing vaginitis, and they are using natural remedies for therapy. The following natural remedies have been suggested or used by women. Little research supports these approaches, and effectiveness is variably reported. However, such approaches are compatible with the lifestyle and philosophy of growing numbers of women.

Candida (Monilia) Vaginitis

Douche with white vinegar, 1 tablespoon/pint water, one to two times each day for 1 week.

Douche with acidophilus culture, 2 tablespoons/pint water, one to two times each day for 1 week.

Apply acidophilus yogurt or buttermilk to labia, vulva, or intravaginally every 2 to 3 hours, as needed, for relief of itching and burning (may assist growth of normal flora).

Take sitz baths every 2 to 4 hours as needed for relief of itching, burning, and swelling of labia and vulva.

Make tea of equal parts of uva ursi, parsley root, dandelion root, and burdock root; use 1 oz of herbs per pint of water in decoction. Drink ½ to 1 cup tea every 2 hours.

Douche with solution of equal parts goldenseal, chaparral, comfrey root, and kava kava; use 1 oz herbs per pint water, simmer gently for 30 minutes, strain, cool, and add 1 tablespoon vinegar per pint. Douche once daily for 1 to 3 days.

*For use in bacterial vaginitis also.

Use boric acid capsules once daily in vagina or every other day until symptoms resolve.

Trichomonas Vaginitis

Douche with solution of equal parts of chaparral and chamomile; use 1 oz of herbs per pint water, steep for 20 minutes, strain, and cool. Douche two to three times each day for 1 or 2 weeks.

*Combine powders of *Echinacea*, goldenseal, chaparral, and squawvine in equal parts; fill gelatin capsules. Take 2 capsules three times each day before meals; also take 1 teaspoon garlic oil with meals.

Bacterial Vaginitis

Douche with white vinegar, 1 tablespoon/pint water, once each day for 1 week.

Douche with solution of 1 teaspoon goldenseal and 1 clove minced garlic steeped in 1 quart boiling water, strained and cooled. Use daily for 1 week.

Insert Betadine gel or solution intravaginally two times each day for 1 week.

Trichomonas Vaginalis

A unicellular protozoan flagellate, **Trichomonas vaginalis** is nearly always transmitted through sexual intercourse. In women, it usually infects the vagina and Skene's ducts; in men, it can be present in the lower genitourinary tract and may cause prostatitis.

Symptoms. Vaginal discharge is typically yellow green, frothy or bubbly, and copious with a strong, foul odor. The cervix and upper vagina often have tiny petechiae due to inflammation. With severe inflammation, the vaginal wall, cervix, and vulva may be edematous and erythematous. Moderate to severe itching is common, and some women have dysuria or dyspareunia secondary to inflammation. *Trichomonas* infections can be mild, with great variation in symptoms. For example, discharge can be thin, slight, whitish yellow, and without the typical foul odor.

Diagnosis. During pelvic examination, discharge samples are placed on a saline mount and examined microscopically as soon as possible. Motile trichomonads are usually seen. Under high power, these oval organisms are about two to three times the size of WBCs, and their flagella may be seen moving. Lactobacilli are usually

absent, many WBC are present, and a range of vaginal intermediate and parabasal epithelial cells are usually present. Routine Pap smears often indicate presence of trichomonads. Even in asymptomatic women, these vaginal pathogens should be treated.

Treatment. Medical treatment for *Trichomonas* vaginitis consists of metronidazole (Flagyl), 2 g orally in a single dose or 250 mg tid for 5 to 7 days. The single dose may not be as effective as longer treatment, but it facilitates compliance. The woman's sexual partner should be treated simultaneously, usually with the 2-g single dose. Trichomonal infections frequently cause symptoms of urethritis in men (Krieger et al., 1993). When taking metronidazole, alcohol must be avoided because it may cause abdominal cramps, nausea, vomiting, headaches, and flushing. Lactating women can be treated with 2 g metronidazole but should not breast-feed for 24 hours after therapy. Metronidazole is contraindicated during the first trimester of pregnancy and should be avoided throughout. Clotrimazole vaginal cream or tablets at bedtime for 7 days can provide symptomatic relief for pregnant women (Deutchman et al., 1994).

Local vulvar inflammation can be treated with sitz baths or steroid creams. Dysuria related to urethral in-

TABLE 11-2
Common Types of Vaginitis: Characteristics and Treatment

Type of Vaginitis	Erythema and Itching	Discharge	Saline Mount	Potassium Hydroxide Mount	Culture or Other	Medication or Other Treatment
Candida albicans (Monilia)	Vulva, labia, perineum, thighs Mild to severe	Mild to moderate Curdy white pH <5.0	Hyphae or spores Many lactobacilli	Hyphae or spores	Dextrose agar I colonies	Antifungal vaginal tablets or cream (eg mycostatin, miconazole, clotrimazole)
Trichomonas vaginalis	Severe vulval itching, ±erythema Petechiae of cervix and vagina	Copious Yellow-green frothy pH >5.0	Trichomonads Few lactobacilli Many white blood cells (WBC)	Negative	None	Metronidazole (Flagyl) orally* (treat sexual partner)
Bacterial vaginosis	Mild to moderate	Mild to moderate Homogeneous Gray, foul pH >5.0	Clue cells Small rods Many WBCs Few lactobacilli	Positive whiff test	Blood agar ± colonies	Metronidazole orally* (treat sexual partner) or vaginal gel Clindamycin vaginal cream
Chlamydia trachomatis (cervicitis)	None to mild	Slight to moderate, varies	Many WBCs Few lactobacilli	Negative	Pap smear with inclusion bodies *Chlamydia* culture ELISA, DFA, PCR tests	Erythromycin, doxycycline, azithromycin, ofloxacin (treat sexual partner)

*Metronidazole is contraindicated during the first trimester of pregnancy; use in later pregnancy is controversial and should preferably be avoided.

flammation responds to these treatments also. If intercourse is painful owing to inflammation, it should be avoided for 2 to 3 days to allow healing.

Bacterial Vaginosis

Bacterial vaginosis is caused by *Gardnerella vaginalis,* a short, gram-negative rod (coccobacillus) often seen in combination with *Mobiluncus* species, *Mycoplasma hominis,* and anaerobic bacteria, such as nonfragilis *Bacteroides* species. These are common in vaginal flora but cause symptoms when they crowd out the *Lactobacillus* species.

Symptoms. Symptoms include increased vaginal discharge that is typically thin, gray white, and homogeneous. The discharge has a fishy odor, particularly after sexual intercourse and during menstruation. Vulvar and vaginal inflammation are uncommon. Symptoms often are minimal, but infection may have serious consequences, including cervicitis, pelvic inflammatory disease (PID), intra-amniotic infection, postpartum en-

dometritis, posthysterectomy vaginal cuff cellulitis, preterm labor, and recurrent urinary tract infections (UTIs; Deutchman et al., 1994; Secor, 1994).

Diagnosis. During pelvic examination, the discharge is easily wiped from the vaginal wall. Adding 10% KOH to the discharge produces an unpleasant fishy odor owing to production of two malodorous amines, putrescine and cadaverine. A saline mount is taken and examined microscopically. Diagnosis is made when clue cells are present; these are vaginal epithelial cells that appear stippled due to growth of *Gardnerella* and other organisms. Lactobacilli usually are absent, and vaginal epithelial cells are mature. Vaginal pH is >5.0. Cultures are not useful.

Treatment. Medical treatment is with metronidazole, 500 mg orally twice a day for 7 days or 2 g orally in a single dose (slightly less effective). Clindamycin 300 mg orally tid for 7 days is an alternative. Clindamycin phosphate vaginal cream 2% (Cleocin) at bedtime for 7 days or metronidazole vaginal gel (MetroGel) at

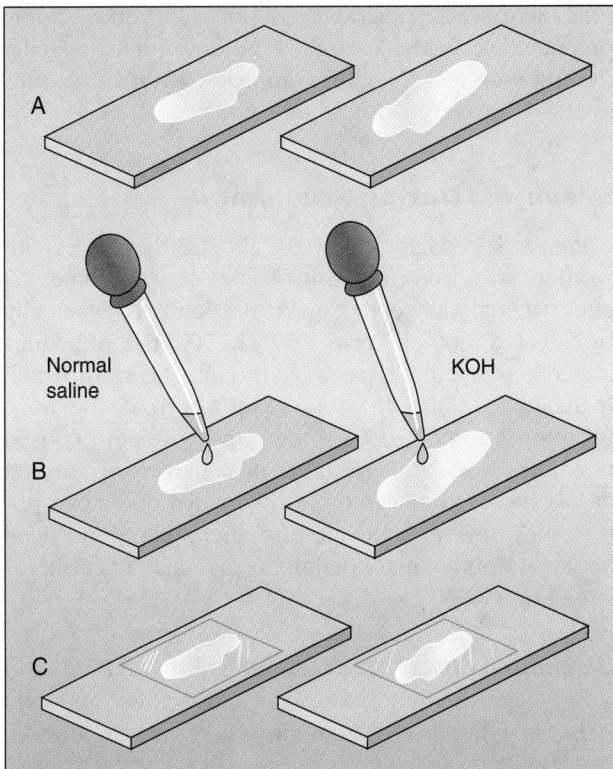

FIGURE 11–1 Preparation of wet mount of vaginal discharge for microscopic examination. (**A**) Using a cotton-tipped applicator or Pap stick, drops of the vaginal discharge are placed on two separate glass slides and spread thinly. (**B**) One drop of normal saline is added to one specimen for microscopic examination for *Trichomonas vaginalis*. One drop of 10% to 20% potassium hydroxide (KOH) is added to the other specimen for microscopic examination for *Candida albicans*. (**C**) Separate coverslips are placed over each specimen. Slides are examined under high- and low-power lenses of microscope.

bedtime for 5 days may be used (Bowie et al., 1994). These vaginal treatments have 90% cure rates and few adverse reactions. When metronidazole is used, advice is given about avoiding alcohol. The woman's sexual partner(s) may be treated simultaneously with the above dosage of metronidazole, especially in recurrent infections, though little benefit has been found (Bowie et al., 1994). Male sexual partners with symptoms of urethritis should be tested for other STDs; there is controversy about whether *Gardnerella* causes infection in men (Hatcher et al., 1990).

Human Papillomavirus

Condyloma (genital warts) are sexually transmitted skin lesions caused by **human papillomavirus** (HPV). There has been a dramatic rise in HPV infections in the last 20 years, with estimated overall incidence at about 17% (Schaffer et al., 1992). Young women (younger than 35 years) have the highest rate of infection by HPV. Cervical HPV rates of 33% and combined cervix

and vulva rates of 46% have been reported in this age group. In women older than 35 years, the rate decreases to 5% to 10% (McCance, 1994).

Risk factors for HPV are younger age, multiple sexual partners, and failure to use condoms. HPV is difficult to eradicate and is easily transmitted. About 67% of exposed sexual partners develop condyloma. Therefore, condoms should be used to reduce transmission of HPV to sexual partners. There are about 70 types of papillomavirus. The skin is commonly infected by HPVs 1, 2, 3, and 4; while mucosa is usually infected by HPVs 6, 11, 16, and 18 (McCance, 1994).

Symptoms. Lesions may be large, cauliflower-like clusters or tiny, single, closely grouped or widely dispersed bumps. Condyloma are usually multiple, although single lesions can occur and are usually found on the vulva, vagina, cervix, and rectum.

Association With Cervical Cancer

Certain strains of HPV are causative factors in cervical cancer (oncogenic strains). HPV 16 and 18 account for about 80% of cervical cancers; other types also may pose a high risk (Box 11-3). Women older than 35 years infected with an oncogenic strain are more likely to have cancer or significant dysplasia (McCance, 1994). In addition, a link has been found between HPV, smoking, and cervical cancer. Women with HPV should be counseled not to smoke, because this may greatly increase their risk of cervical cancer (Corwin, 1996).

Benign lesions, such as genital warts, are largely due to HPV 6 and 11. Low-grade dysplasias, such as cervical intraepithelial neoplasia I (low-grade squamous intraepithelial lesions [SIL]; SIL in the Bethesda system) caused by other strains, rarely ever progress to malignant disease.

Human Papillomavirus During Pregnancy

Pregnant women may be infected with HPV. Cervical, vaginal, and vulval lesions may increase in size during pregnancy and occasionally become so large that they interfere with vaginal delivery. Condyloma frequently

---

BOX 11–3
Genital Human Papillomavirus (HPV) and Associated Cancer Risk

Low risk: HPV 6, 11, 34, 40, 42–44, 53–55, 57–59
High risk: HPV 16, 18, 30, 31, 33, 35, 39, 45, 51, 52, 56

HPV 6 and 11 account for 80% of genital condylomas; HPV 16 and 18 account for 80% of cervical cancers.

regress after pregnancy and may become subclinical. Newborns exposed perinatally to condyloma may develop laryngeal papillomatosis, with most cases occurring between the ages of 2 and 4 years. About one-fourth of cases occur during infancy. The presenting symptoms are hoarseness and a croupy cough. Laryngeal papillomas are treated by excision.

Diagnosis and Treatment. Condyloma can be diagnosed by visualization of anal, vulvar, or vaginal lesions; colposcopy; biopsy; and occasionally Pap smears. Approved treatments include the following:

- Podophyllin 10% to 25% in tincture of benzoin
- Trichloroacetic acid 80% to 90%
- Cryotherapy with liquid nitrogen or cryoprobe
- Electrodessication or electrocautery

Self-treatment of external condyloma can be done with Podofilox (Condylox) 0.5% topical solution. Laser therapy and surgery may be needed for extensive lesions. Alpha-interferon has been used but is not recommended by the Centers for Disease Control and Prevention (CDC) because of its low success rate, high toxicity, and high cost. Fluorouracil cream also is not recommended by the CDC because it has not been adequately evaluated (Bowie et al., 1994). Podophyllin application is contraindicated in pregnancy because of teratogenic effects and reported maternal and fetal deaths. Cryotherapy is most commonly used during pregnancy.

Chlamydia

Infections caused by ***Chlamydia trachomatis*** have high prevalence among adolescents and young adults. More than 4 million cases occur annually, making *Chlamydia* the most common STD in the United States (Clinical Update, 1994). *Chlamydia* is an intracellular organism that infects the lower genital tract of women and men, causing urethritis, cervicitis, PID, and proctitis. Risk factors include the following (Guide to Clinical Preventive Services, 1989):

- Age 24 or younger
- Multiple sexual partners
- New sexual partner (in previous 2 months)
- Friable cervix
- Nonbarrier method of contraception or no contraception

Symptoms. As many as two-thirds of cervical infections due to *Chlamydia* are asymptomatic. In about 25% of infections, a symptom complex of pelvic pain, fever, tenderness, and mucopurulent cervical discharge indicates salpingitis or PID. About half of these clients also are infected with gonorrhea. Resultant salpingitis and PID increase the incidence of infertility and ectopic pregnancies. In the urethral syndrome, there is acute dysuria with less than 10^5 colonies; *Chlamydia* causes about 30% to 40% of these infections.

Chlamydia During Pregnancy

Chlamydia cervicitis occurs in about 30% of pregnant women, increasing the risk of late-onset endometritis after vaginal delivery. Newborns delivered vaginally by infected mothers have a 60% to 70% risk of acquiring infection during passage through the birth canal. Inclusion conjunctivitis of the newborn is the most common infection, occurring in up to 50% of exposed newborns and often resulting in conjunctival scarring and corneal vascularization. Chlamydial neonatal ophthalmia is several times more frequent than gonorrheal neonatal ophthalmia. Pneumonia also may occur in infected neonates.

Diagnosis. *Chlamydia* cultures are expensive and slow. Direct immunofluorescent monoclonal antibody stain, enzyme-linked immunosorbent assay (ELISA), and polymerase chain reaction (PCR) tests provide more rapid diagnosis. These tests have a high degree of accuracy in populations in which chlamydial infection is higher (8%–10% incidence). ELISA and PCR tests have been developed that can be used on urine and genital swab specimens.

Treatment. Many chlamydial infections cause no symptoms but can have serious consequences. Therefore, the CDC recommends treating women and their partners whenever *Chlamydia* is detected. Treatment regimens include the following:

- Doxycycline hyclate 100 mg orally bid for 7 days
- Azithromycin 1 g orally in single dose
- Erythromycin 500 mg orally qid for 7 days
- Ofloxacin 300 mg orally bid for 7 days
- Sulfisoxazole 500 mg orally qid for 10 days

During pregnancy, doxycycline, erythromycin estolate, and ofloxacin are contraindicated. Another erythromycin or sulfisoxazole (except near term) may be used, but sulfisoxazole is less effective. Amoxicillin or clindamycin also may be effective treatments (Bowie et al., 1994; The Medical Letter, 1994). Newborns are routinely treated prophylactically against ocular chlamydial infections. Topical erythromycin or tetracycline ointments are used. Applying a 1% silver nitrate solution is not an effective prophylactic against ocular chlamydial infections (Traboulsi et al., 1994). Chlamydial pneumonia and conjunctivitis in the neonate are treated with systemic erythromycin (The Medical Letter, 1994).

Genital Herpes

Two types of herpes simplex viruses (HSV) that are immunologically and clinically distinct may infect the genital tract. HSV-1 is mainly seen as "cold sores" of the lips but can cause genital eruptions. HSV-2 causes 85% of genital herpes lesions and usually is sexually transmitted. HSV-2 is one of the most rapidly spreading STDs, with up to 20 million American adults infected. Most people infected with HSV-2 have no history of genital herpes lesions. Seroprevalence rates vary widely and are higher with increasing age, lower income and education levels, multiple sexual partners, African American or Hispanic race, and female gender. In adults older than 30 years, HSV-2 antibodies occur in 25% of white women and 60% of African American women (Mertz, 1993).

Symptoms. The incubation period for primary infections is 3 to 14 days. After this incubation period, the woman with HSV-2 will develop painful vesicles in the vulva and perineal areas. These lesions will rupture, ulcerate, and then scab over and heal without scarring (Fig. 11-2). The cervix and vagina can be infected with asymptomatic lesions that may shed for several months. The infected woman usually has flulike symptoms with achiness, fever, headache, and inguinal adenopathy. Cytologic smears reveal large multinucleate cells with eosinophilic inclusion bodies. Unsuspected herpes is occasionally diagnosed as an incidental finding by Pap smear. The initial herpes symptoms usually disappear within 3 weeks; however, recur-

rences are frequent during the next 6 months. Between recurrences, the virus resides in the sensory sacral ganglia, where it remains indefinitely. Subsequent eruptions tend to be smaller and more localized than the initial infection. Physical, emotional, and psychological stress or illness often trigger recurrences.

Diagnosis. Diagnosis may be confirmed by viral cultures or antibody titers using ELISA techniques. Multinucleated giant cells on a Pap smear also support the diagnosis of HSV infection.

Herpes Infection During Pregnancy

Approximately 1% to 2% of pregnancies are complicated by HSV infection. Most genital infections in pregnancy are caused by HSV-2. Maternal infection is rarely transmitted transplacentally to the fetus, but when this occurs in the first trimester, spontaneous abortion or severe fetal abnormalities may result. After the 20th week of gestation, infection increases the risk for premature birth but not for fetal abnormalities. The fetus is most likely to be infected after rupture of the membranes or during the course of delivery, because the virus can be transmitted through lesions in the genital tract. Detection of active herpes infections before delivery is most important, because disseminated neonatal herpes has a 50% mortality rate, and ocular and central nervous system (CNS) damage occurs in about two-thirds of the survivors (Dunnihoo, 1992).

If genital herpes lesions are present, delivery is usually by cesarean to protect the fetus from exposure to

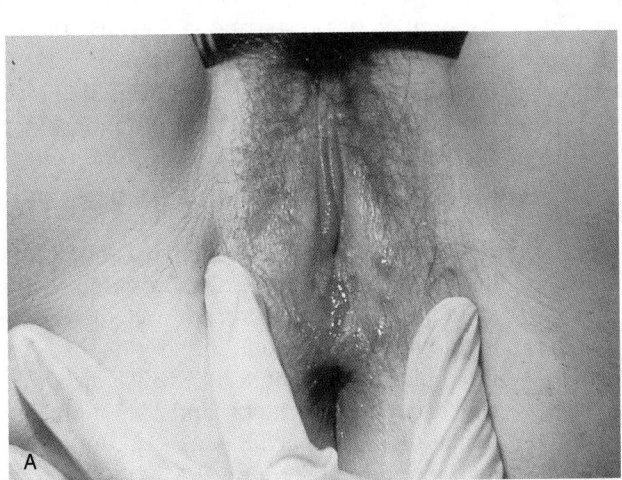
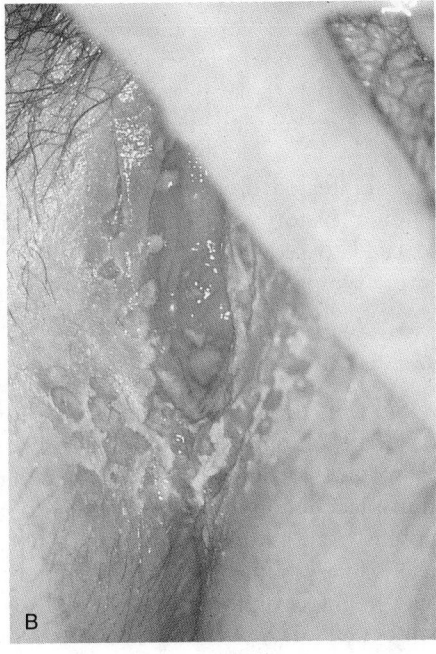

FIGURE 11–2 (A) Initial vesicular appearance of vaginal herpetic lesions. **(B)** Coalescence typical of vulvovaginal herpes simplex infection. (Source: CDC Still Pictures Archive)

the virus during passage through the birth canal. With ruptured membranes and active genital herpes lesions, risk of fetal infection is greater.

Treatment. In nonpregnant women, acyclovir (Zovirax) 200 mg orally five times daily or 400 mg three times daily for 10 days often facilitates healing of lesions and decreases duration and severity of symptoms in primary infections. For recurrent infections, acyclovir 200 mg five times daily for 5 days or 800 mg twice daily for 5 days seems to reduce symptoms when started within 2 days after appearance of lesions. Chronic suppressive therapy with 400 mg acyclovir twice daily can be effective in reducing recurrences. Suppressive therapy is continued for 1 year; it is then stopped, and the recurrence rate is monitored.

The use of acyclovir during pregnancy has not been defined as safe for the fetus. The Food and Drug Administration (FDA) recommends against its use "unless the potential benefit justifies the potential risk." Studies of pregnant women inadvertantly exposed to acyclovir reported no increased risk of fetal abnormalities and no unusual pattern in type of defects found (The Medical Letter, 1994). The main goal of care is to prevent neonatally acquired herpes infection. Pregnant women with a history of herpes or with infected partners are monitored carefully in the third trimester to detect active infection. Serial viral cultures of the cervix and external genital area may be taken. Transplacental infections may account for many of these. Risk of transmitting genital herpes is high (33%–50%) in neonates during vaginal delivery in women with first episode infections. It is low (3%) when the mother has developed antibodies through previous HSV infections, whether neonates are exposed through asymptomatic shedding or actual lesions (Mertz, 1993).

Broad-spectrum antibiotic therapy is often prescribed to treat secondary infection. Perineal comfort may be promoted by taking sitz baths two to three times per day and keeping the infected region clean and dry.

When an uninfected pregnant woman has a sexual partner with a history of genital herpes, condoms should be used to reduce the possibility of transmission, even in asymptomatic phases of the disease.

Syphilis

Syphilis can be transmitted through exposure to infected exudate during sexual contact, by contact with open wounds or infected blood, or congenitally through transplacental inoculation. The rate of acquisition of syphilis from an infected partner is about 30%. The disease is rarely transmitted sexually after the person has had the infection for 2 years. Syphilis is caused by the spirochete *Treponema pallidum*. More than

30,000 new cases of primary and secondary syphilis occur annually. The incidence of all stages of syphilis increased dramatically from 1985 to 1990 (from 28 to 54 cases per 100,000 population), then decreased slightly. Congenital syphilis also increased during this time (from 7 to 92 cases per 100,000 live births), then remained near 100 cases in the early 1990s. The prevalence of HIV infection among people with syphilis is increasing (Clinical Guidelines, 1995a).

Symptoms. Syphilis can occur at any stage during pregnancy. The primary stage, which lasts 1 to 6 weeks, is characterized by classic lesions (chancres), which are deep and painless ulcers often found on the genitalia, lips, or rectal area. In the secondary stage of syphilis, which lasts 2 to 10 weeks, a macular rash appears on the entire body. In the latent, or third, stage, diagnosis is based on a positive serology, and the infection is usually subclinical. Early latent stage is 1 year from onset of the infection, and late latent stage occurs after 1 year and may last indefinitely. About one-third of cases progress to late latency. Cardiovascular, neurologic, cutaneous, and visceral tissue damage may occur during late syphilis.

Syphilis During Pregnancy

Syphilis can be acquired by the fetus of an infected woman when transmitted through the placenta as early as the sixth week of pregnancy. However, clinical manifestations of the disease in the fetus usually do not occur unless infection is present in the woman after 16 weeks' gestation. The risk of prematurity, perinatal death, and congenital syphilis is greater during primary or secondary syphilis, when recurrent episodes of spirochetemia occur (Dunnihoo, 1992).

Congenital syphilis is a systemic infection with a wide range of presentations. At birth, there may be no sign of disease, or the newborn may be severely affected with hepatosplenomegaly, hemolytic anemia, osteochondritis, bullous skin eruptions containing spirochetes, and "snuffles" (rhinitis due to nasal mucosal involvement).

Diagnosis. Diagnosis of primary and secondary syphilis is made by darkfield microscope identification of spirochetes in samples from a chancre or skin lesion. Serologic tests include nontreponemal tests (VDRL, rapid plasma reagent [RPR]), which are quantifiable but less accurate in primary and late syphilis, and treponemal tests for specific antibody (fluorescent treponemal antibody absorption [FTA-ABS], microhemagglutination assay for antibodies to *T. pallidum* [MHA-TP]), which are highly sensitive. A small number of pregnant women have a biologic false-positive test, requiring serology titers.

Treatment. Parenteral penicillin G remains the drug of choice for treating all stages of syphilis. Dosage may differ by stage of disease:

- Less than 1 year duration, single dose of 2.4 million U benzathine penicillin G intramuscularly (IM)
- More than 1 year's duration, three doses of 2.4 million U benzathine penicillin G IM weekly for 3 weeks
- Neurosyphilis, 10 to 14 days of IV penicillin G or procaine penicillin IM plus oral probenecid
- Penicillin allergy in nonpregnant clients, erythromycin

The previous treatment regimens are followed during pregnancy. However, erythromycin is not used because it does not effectively cross the placental barrier and cure the fetal infection. For pregnant women with penicillin allergy, hospitalization and desensitization are necessary so they can receive penicillin (Bowie et al., 1994).

Gonorrhea

Gonorrhea is caused by the gram-negative coccus *Neisseria gonorrhoeae,* which most commonly infects the mucosa of the lower genital tract. The endocervical glands, urethra, anus, and oropharynx may be sites of infection. Gonorrhea is spread by sexual contact. The prevalence of gonorrhea has declined steadily in the United States since 1986. However, 1 million new infections occur yearly, with rates higher for minority adolescents and young adults, especially in the inner cities (Bowie et al., 1994).

Symptoms. Symptoms of dysuria, frequency, and purulent vaginal discharge appear 3 to 5 days after exposure. When infection spreads to the fallopian tubes and ovaries (salpingo-oophoritis), symptoms include lower abdominal pain, fever, and leukocytosis. About 6% of clients are asymptomatic. Tubal infection may result in scarring and subsequent infertility. Reinfections occur in 11% to 30% of women with a history of gonorrhea.

Diagnosis. Diagnosis is by culture on a Thayer-Martin medium or Gram-stained cervical smear with intracellular gram-negative diplococci. An immunoassay test for antibodies can be done. In some populations, about 45% of women with gonorrhea also have chlamydial infections.

Gonorrhea During Pregnancy

Although gonorrhea usually causes few symptoms during pregnancy, it can result in serious postpartum and neonatal infections. Routine gonorrhea testing is rec-

ommended in early pregnancy and should be repeated at 28 weeks' gestation in high-risk populations.

Gonorrhea infection during pregnancy increases the risk of septic abortion, chorioamnionitis, premature delivery, premature rupture of membranes, and intrauterine growth retardation. When the woman is infected at delivery, 30% to 35% of newborns contract gonorrhea during passage through the birth canal. Risk is increased with prolonged rupture of membranes. Gonorrhea in the newborn most often causes ophthalmic infections. Infections of nasopharyngeal passages, vagina, anus, ear canals, and scalp abscesses (from fetal monitoring electrodes) also may result.

Treatment. Increasing numbers of gonorrhea strains are penicillinase producing and tetracycline resistant. Some strains resistant to fluoroquinolones (ciprofloxacin, ofloxacin) have recently been found (CDC, 1994). CDC recommendations for uncomplicated urethral, endocervical, or rectal infections are dual therapy with one of the following:

- Ceftriaxone sodium (Rocephin) 125 mg IM single dose
- Cefixime (Suprax) 400 mg orally single dose
- Ciprofloxacin HCL (Cipro) 500 mg orally single dose
- Ofloxacin (Floxin) 400 mg orally single dose
- Spectinomycin HCL (Trobicin) 2 g IM single dose combined with doxycycline 100 mg orally bid for 7 days

The fluoroquinolones should not be used in pregnant women and those younger than 18 years. No single-dose regimen for gonorrhea is effective against coexisting *Chlamydia* infection; therefore, 7 days of doxycycline (not used during pregnancy) or a single dose of azithromycin is added. Gonorrhea infections during pregnancy are treated with ceftriaxone 125 mg IM or other cephalosporin (spectinomycin 2 g IM if allergic), plus erythromycin base 500 mg orally qid for 7 days. In the neonate, prophylaxis against gonococcal ophthalmia has historically been accomplished by topical application of 1% silver nitrate. However, erythromycin and tetracycline ointment are used most frequently because they are effective prophylaxics against gonococcal and chlamydial ophthalmia infections (Traboulsi et al., 1994). Newborns who are infected perinatally need treatment with parenteral antibiotics.

Pelvic Inflammatory Disease

A more complicated infection, **PID** involves the uterus, fallopian tubes, and ovaries. Causative organisms may include *N. gonorrhea, C. trachomatis, M. hominis,* gram-negative facultative bacteria, anaerobes, and streptococci. More than 10% of women of reproductive age have been treated for PID. This is probably an underestimate because of poor reliability of the diagnosis; many women have atypical or no symptoms (Soper, 1994). Ascending infection from the vagina, cervix, or uterus leads to widespread pelvic infection.

Symptoms. Symptoms of PID include lower abdominal pain; fever; increased menstrual cramping; heavy, foul-smelling menstrual flow; and malaise. Women often report dyspareunia and painful defecation. Examination findings include cervical or uterine tenderness and adnexal fullness and tenderness.

Complications of PID may include tubo-ovarian abscess, pelvic abscess, tubal occlusion, and infertility. In 15% to 30% of clients with PID, infectious perihepatitis (Fitz-Hugh–Curtis syndrome) may occur. Symptoms include pleuritic right upper quadrant pain that limits chest expansion and usual PID symptoms and findings. Pathophysiologic changes are inflammation of Glisson's capsule of the liver and of the undersurface of the diaphragm, with development of adhesive bands.

Diagnosis. Diagnostic tests may include the following:

- Gram-stained cervical smear with intracellular gram-negative diplococci (gonorrhea)
- Cervical specimen for gonorrhea and *Chlamydia* enzyme immunoassay (EIA)
- WBC showing leukocytosis (WBC >10,000/mm²)
- C-reactive protein and erythrocyte sedimentation rate elevation
- Laparoscopy

Treatment. Medications effective against all possible causative organisms are recommended; no single agent is usually sufficient. The CDC recommends multiple drug therapy as follows: Outpatient antibiotic therapy includes cefoxitin 2 g IM plus probenecid 1 g orally or ceftriaxone 250 mg IM. This is combined with doxycycline 100 mg orally bid for 14 days. Alternatives include ofloxacin 400 mg PO bid for 14 days plus either clindamycin hydrochloride 450 mg orally qid for 14 days or metronidazole 500 mg orally bid for 14 days (Bowie et al., 1994).

Acutely ill clients, particularly those with pelvic or tubo-ovarian abscess and Fitz-Hugh–Curtis syndrome, often need hospitalization. Hot sitz baths relieve pain and promote comfort and healing. The client should be placed in a semi-Fowler position to allow drainage of mucopurulent discharge. The following broad-spectrum intravenous antibiotics are used while the client is hospitalized:

- Regimen A: cefoxitin 2 g IV q6h or cefotetan 2 g IV q12h. Continue for at least 48 hours after the client is afebrile. This is combined with doxycycline 100 mg q12h orally or IV for 10 to 14 days.
- Regimen B: clindamycin 900 mg IV q8h for at least 48 hours after the client is afebrile. This is combined

with gentamycin, loading dose 2 mg/kg IV or IM, then 1.5 mg/kg q8h until discharge. After discharge, administer doxycycline 100 mg orally q12h for 10 to 14 days or clindamycin 450 mg orally qid for 10 to 14 days.

Studies have found other drug regimens to be effective. Single-agent therapy with ciprofloxacin seems equally effective as combinations of cefotetan and doxycycline, cefoxitin and doxycycline, or clindamycin with an aminoglycoside (Walker et al., 1993). Ampicillin-sulbactam (no longer recommended for PID by the CDC) has been found equally effective and well tolerated as cefoxitin plus doxycycline (McGregor et al., 1994).

Hepatitis

Several viruses make up the hepatitis family, and each one has the potential to cause acute liver disease. The types of hepatitis include the following:

- Hepatitis A virus (HAV)
- Hepatitis B virus (HBV)
- Hepatitis C virus (HCV)
- Delta hepatitis (HDV)
- Hepatitis E (HEV)
- HSV, cytomegalovirus (CMV), and Epstein-Barr virus

Acute clinical hepatitis without a demonstrable virus is called non-A, non-B, non-C hepatitis. Some hepatitis infections can become chronic.

Most types of hepatitis are spread by blood, blood products, or body fluids. Because hepatitis is a viral infection, it is difficult to treat with simple medications. Therefore, the best protection against hepatitis is prevention (see Client Education: Preventing Hepatitis).

Hepatitis B

The most common cause of acute and chronic hepatitis is HBV. It is transmitted through sexual contact and body fluids (blood, saliva, breast milk, vaginal fluid, and semen). The risk of contracting HBV increases with the number of sexual partners, use of IV drugs, and frequent exposure to body fluids. Groups at increased risk for contracting HBV include homosexuals; IV drug users; clients who frequently require use of blood products, such as during hemodialysis; and healthcare workers. Prison inmates and homeless shelter occupants have high prevalence rates of HBV. Certain population groups have higher prevalence rates, because HBV is endemic among Alaskan natives, Pacific islanders, Haitians, and sub-Saharan Africans (CDC, 1995d; see Box 11-1).

Symptoms. Infection with HBV results in liver infection with a wide range of clinical manifestations. Many

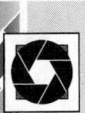
clients are asymptomatic or have vague flulike symptoms. Classic symptoms include fatigue, nausea, anorexia, abdominal pain, low-grade fever, and in 25% of cases, jaundice. HBV infection can become chronic, ranging from an asymptomatic carrier state to persistent hepatitis, cirrhosis, or hepatocellular carcinoma (Tsukuma et al., 1993). About 5% to 10% of infected adults develop persistent hepatitis (CDC, 1990a). There is no effective treatment for HBV infection; immunization is the only protection against the disease.

Diagnosis. The diagnosis of HBV is made by serologic testing to identify antigen and antibody systems. Hepatitis B surface antigen (HBsAg) may be identified in the serum 7 to 14 days following exposure and persists for an indefinite period. Hepatitis B surface antibody present with HBsAg indicates noninfectious state. Several other antigen (HBcAg, HBeAg) and antibody (anti-HBc) tests are used to evaluate the stage and progression of the infection. In the United States, about 0.1% to 0.5% of the population are HBV carriers (Dunnihoo, 1992).

Hepatitis B Virus in Pregnancy. All high-risk pregnant women are screened for HBsAg, but some authorities recommend routine prenatal screening for all women.

About 18,000 newborns are born to HBsAg-positive women annually in this country. Transmission of HBV to the fetus may occur transplacentally or during passage through the birth canal. In women with acute and chronic carrier state disease, vertical transmission to the fetus occurs in about 65% of pregnancies, especially during the third trimester. Premature births are increased, and the newborn may become a chronic carrier or may develop fulminant hepatic disease, often resulting in death.

Information about pregnant clients with positive HBsAg should be communicated to obstetric and pediatric staffs so that the newborn can receive prompt treatment and health workers can take appropriate precautions. HBV infection can be prevented in 85% to 95% of newborns by administering hepatitis B immune globulin (HBIG; 0.5 mL IM) as soon as possible after birth, preferably within the first 12 to 48 hours, along with the first dose of HBV vaccine (0.5 mL IM). This is followed by doses of HBV vaccine at 1 and 6 months of age.

Treatment. Active immunization with HBV vaccine is recommended for all high-risk groups, healthcare workers, and as a routine immunization in newborns. HBV vaccine is administered in three doses; the first two are given 1 month apart, and the third is given in 6 months.

After exposure of nonimmunized people to HBV infection, prophylactic treatment with HBIG is recommended as soon as possible, no longer than 14 days after exposure. This is followed by three doses of hepatitis B vaccine to provide active immunity.

Hepatitis A Virus

About 38% of acute hepatitis cases in the United States are caused by HAV. It is called "infectious hepatitis" because it is readily transmitted by close physical contact, through contaminated food and water, and by sexual contact.

Symptoms. Symptoms include abrupt onset of flulike syndrome with abdominal pain, fever, malaise, anorexia, nausea, vomiting, jaundice, and pruritus. The period of greatest infectivity is the 2 weeks preceding onset of jaundice. Incubation usually takes 15 to 20 days. HAV is more severe in adults than in children. Transplacental (vertical) transmission of HAV infection to the fetus occurs rarely.

Diagnosis. Diagnosis is by detection of anti-HAV antibodies in serum. Liver function tests often are elevated (aspartate transaminase [AST], alanine aminotransferase [ALT]), as are alkaline phosphatase, cholesterol, and bilirubin. Life-long immunity is conferred by HAV infection with presence of immunoglobulin G (IgG)-type anti-HAV antibodies. About 30% to 50% of adults will show serologic evidence (antibodies) of previous HAV infection (Dunnihoo, 1992).

Treatment. In February 1995, the FDA approved the world's first vaccine against HAV. The vaccine, called Havrix, is made from inactivated hepatitis virus. According to the manufacturer of the vaccine, one dose is 96% effective. Nonimmunized people who come in close contact with a person infected with HAV should be given serum immunoglobulin (0.02 mL/kg IM) within 14 days of exposure. This provides successful prophylaxis in most instances. The only treatment for people who have contracted HAV is rest and good nutrition.

Hepatitis C Virus

About 90% of hepatitis cases not caused by HAV or HBV are due to HCV. HCV infection usually results from a blood transfusion or exposure to blood or blood products. The virus also can be transmitted by the fecal–oral route but rarely by sexual intercourse (Sodeyama et al., 1993). The incubation period is 6 to 7 weeks, with symptoms similar to HAV and HBV infections. HCV is usually milder than HAV or HBV, although it leads to chronic infection (70%) and cirrhosis (20%) more often (Brown et al., 1994). Fulminant HCV has 70% to 80% mortality. Long-term probability of liver failure is 18% (Koretz et al., 1993). Transplacental (vertical) transmission of HCV to the fetus is rare. Although most newborns of HCV-positive mothers have antibodies at birth, these are passively transferred from the mother. By 2 to 5 years, less than 10% of children have anti-HCV antibodies (Wejstal et al., 1992).

Hepatitis E Virus

All cases of HEV in the United States can be attributed to immigrants or visitors from endemic areas (Mexico, developing countries). HEV is primarily transmitted by contaminated food and water. It usually causes an acute, self-limiting icteric illness without chronic infection or liver disease. Most disturbing is its high mortality rate among pregnant women (20%), usually in the third trimester. No explanation has been found for this increased mortality risk (Brown et al., 1994). The only treatment for HEV is rest and good nutrition.

Delta Hepatitis

In conjunction with HBV infection, HDV occurs as a coinfection or superinfection. It is usually found in people with multiple parenteral exposures, such as IV drug users, hemophiliacs, and those having repeated blood transfusions. Homosexuals also are at increased risk. Chronic infection results in about half of the cases (Mandell et al., 1990). There is no treatment for HDV. A person with this virus should be encouraged to get plenty of sleep and to eat nutritious food.

Human Immunodeficiency Virus and Acquired Immunodeficiency Syndrome

Overview

While most of the infectious diseases previously discussed are serious and possibly life-threatening if not properly treated, HIV infection usually leads to death within several years. **HIV** causes a gradual decline of immune system function, resulting in **AIDS** when specific opportunistic infections develop (Table 11-3). AIDS was first identified among homosexual men in 1981, and within the decade, it spread to epidemic proportions among this group. During the 1980s, the disease seriously began to affect the heterosexual population as well. In fact, although heterosexuals represented only 1.4% of AIDS cases in 1985, they represented 10% by 1991. At first, the disease spread so quickly because no one knew what it was or how it was transmitted. Therefore, no specific precautions were taken. The rapid spread of the infection during this decade and the continued high rate of infection transmission are attributed to the length of time a per-

TABLE 11-3
Centers for Disease Control Classification System for Human Immunodeficiency Virus (HIV) Infection

Group	Description
I	Acute HIV infection (mononucleosis-like syndrome) with documented seroconversion for HIV antibody
II	Asymptomatic infection, seropositive but no signs or symptoms of infection
III	Persistent generalized lymphadenopathy, defined as ≥1-cm nodes at two or more extrainguinal sites, persisting for >3 mo
IV	Other AIDS-related diseases
A	Constitutional disease: unexplained fever, diarrhea, weight loss
B	Neurologic disease: unexplained dementia, neuropathy, or myelopathy
C	Opportunistic infections: viral, fungal, parasitic, bacterial, other
D	Opportunistic neoplasms: Kaposi's sarcoma, lymphoma
E	Other conditions (including chronic lymphocytic interstitial pneumonitis)

son can be HIV infected without knowing it. Some people do not develop opportunistic infections of AIDS for up to 7 years and unknowingly pass the virus to many others during this time.

As the knowledge of the disease increased, so did the massive prevention campaign. Starting in the mid-1980s, the CDC and the Surgeon General released a document that outlined universal precautions to prevent the transmission of HIV (see Nursing Guidelines: Preventing Transmission of HIV Infection [Standard Precautions]). In addition, public campaigns encouraged condom use as a way to prevent the spread of the virus (see Research Highlight). Today millions of dollars are allocated to HIV and AIDS research, prevention, and the search for a cure.

Recently, a second type of HIV was found, and HIV has been separated into HIV-1 and HIV-2. HIV-1 causes most infections in Europe and the Western hemisphere. HIV-2 is a retrovirus endemic in West Africa, more closely related to the simian immunodeficiency virus than HIV-1. Only a few cases have been found in other areas. There is a high degree of immunologic cross-reactivity between HIV-1 and HIV-2. Current HIV-1 screening tests (ELISA) detect between 42% and 92% of HIV-2 infections. HIV-2 infection can be confirmed by HIV-2 specific Western blot test, the radioimmunoprecipitation assay, or the PCR tests.

Transmission

Prevention of HIV transmission is critical to reduce the incidence and spread of AIDS. HIV is transmitted through blood and body fluids, transplacentally, and through breast milk. The primary mode of transmission is sexual. Condom use is a major means of preventing sexual transmission of HIV. Compared with the risk associated with vaginal intercourse, the risk of transmission increases with anal intercourse and probably decreases with oral–genital contact. HIV also is transmitted through transfusions of HIV-contaminated blood and sharing of needles used for IV drugs. Healthcare workers may contract the virus by needle prick or accidental mucous membrane contact with HIV-containing blood or body fluids (see Box 11-1).

Clinical Course

A retrovirus, HIV substitutes its own RNA and DNA for a portion of the T4 cell's DNA. T4 cell replication produces new infected cells, and eventually these cells release additional virus that in turn infects more T4 cells. After exposure to HIV, some people experience a flu-like or mononucleosis-like syndrome, but others have no symptoms. From 6 weeks to 1 year after exposure, HIV antibodies appear in the serum and can be detected by ELISA, which is usually confirmed by a Western blot test. The appearance of HIV antibodies is called seroconversion. People who test positive for HIV are able to transmit the infection to others.

Although producing no symptoms, the virus continues to destroy T4 cells and slowly alters immune system functioning. Within 6 months to 1 year, chronically swollen lymph nodes usually develop as the body attempts to combat HIV through overproduction of B cells (abundant in the lymph nodes). In about 3 to 5 years, there is a persistent drop of T4 cells to less than $400/mm^3$. The person begins to lose the ability to mount an effective cellular immune response to patho-

---

NURSING GUIDELINES
Preventing Transmission of Human Immunodeficiency Virus Infection (Standard Precautions)

Infectious diseases spread by blood, blood products, and body fluids pose special risks for healthcare providers. To minimize the risk of disease transmission, the Centers for Disease Control and Prevention recommend that healthcare workers take these precautions with all clients, not only those known to be HIV infected.

1. Wear disposable latex gloves for any contact with blood, body fluids, mucous membranes, and non-intact skin. This includes blood contact during procedures or surgery, drawing blood, handling IVs, and changing peripads, chux pads, diapers, or dressings. If a glove tears, remove it, wash hands, and put on a new glove. Double gloves offer better protection than single gloves, particularly during surgical procedures.
2. Wash hands after removing gloves and before contact with another client.
3. Wear protective coverings during procedures in which splashing of blood or body fluids is possible. A plastic apron, gown, mask, and eye or face shield should be worn in addition to gloves for such procedures as surgery, vaginal or cesearean birth, amniotomy, vaginal examination, and newborn care. Full-size glasses or goggles are acceptable eye shields.
4. Newborn suctioning should be done with mechanical suction devices or bulb syringes and mucus extractors attached to wall suction at low settings. Mouth-operated devices, such as DeLee mucus traps should not be used. Direct mouth-to-mouth resuscitation should be avoided.
5. Syringes and needles should be handled carefully to avoid accidental needle punctures. Needles should not be bent, returned to protective caps, or broken. Special hazardous waste containers are used for disposal of needles and syringes.
6. Resuscitation procedures should use disposable masks, mouthpieces, and ventilation equipment that do not permit exchange of secretions.
7. During cleaning procedures for blood and body fluids, gloves and appropriate protective coverings should be worn.

Condom Use After AIDS Education and Publicity

An extensive public health campaign in the mid-1980's promoted condom use, particularly latex condoms containing spermicide, unless in a mutually monogamous relationship. Condom sales were counted at about 550 drug stores across the United States from 1984 to 1988, using a national probability sample stratified by size, geographic region, and relative urbanization. Condom sales at the drug stores were audited every 2 months and compared to the same period 1 year earlier to control for seasonal variation. Publicity over this time period was monitored by counting the number of articles regarding condom use in three different newspapers' indexes across the country.

Drug store condom sales grew slowly from 1984 to 1988, except for a 20% increase in 1987. Between 1986 and 1987, sales of all latex condoms increased 25% and those with spermicide increased 116%. Natural membrane condom sales increased 7.8%. Sales of condoms in areas with a high incidence of AIDS were growing virtually throughout the study period. Sales increases in other areas did not begin until early 1987 and stopped increasing in summer of 1988. In both high-risk and other areas of the United States, condom sales grew rapidly throughout 1987 and early 1988 after the release of the Surgeon General's report in November 1986. Newspaper publicity about condoms (which were rarely mentioned before the report) increased to a peak in February 1987, with 182 items appearing in 19 newspapers. Newspaper items continued through 1988, but slowly diminished.

The 20% increase in drug store condom sales during the year after the Surgeon General's report indicates that Americans responded to his message about AIDS prevention. The greatest increase was in latex condoms with spermicide, which cost more but provide additional protection against HIV transmission.

Critique: This well-designed national study demonstrates that public education can be effective in reducing risk-taking behavior. Nurses can continue individual client and community education to prevent STDs with some assurance of effectiveness.

(Moran, J. S., Janes, H. R., Peterman, T. A. et al: (1990). Increase in condom sales following AIDS education and publicity, United States. *American Journal of Public Health, 80,* 607–608.)

gens and neoplasia. Usually within another 2 to 5 years, the breakdown of cell-mediated immunity is evident by opportunistic infections caused by *C. albicans,* herpes simplex, CMV, papovavirus, **Histoplasma,** *Toxoplasma,* **Pneumocystis carinii,** and others. Oral hairy leukoplakia and neoplasms suh as Kaposi's sarcoma and lymphoma often occur. People with later stages of HIV infection are susceptible to tuberculosis

(TB) and other bacterial infections, including *Legionella* and *Salmonella.* When the T4 cell count drops to 100/mm³ or less, death usually ensues within 2 years (Fig. 11-3; Redford et al., 1989).

There is no cure, although some drugs, such as zidovudine (Retrovir; formerly called azidothymidine), appear to delay progression. Research is focused on finding a vaccine to provide immunity against HIV infection.

Incidence

About 1 million people were estimated by the CDC to be HIV infected in 1991, with 60,000 to 90,000 new cases expected annually (CDC, 1990b). In 1993, the criteria for reporting AIDS cases expanded to include conditions that occur earlier in the course of HIV infection. With the expanded definition, cumulatively 441,528 cases of AIDS and 270,870 deaths from AIDS have been reported (CDC, 1995a). The World Health Organization estimates about 15 million people worldwide have been infected with HIV since the epidemic began. More than 10 million cases have arisen from heterosexual spread. Of these, 95% have occurred in developing countries, especially in Africa and Asia (Ronald, 1995).

In the United States, AIDS is the fourth leading cause of death in young women (25–44 years old; CDC, 1995b) and the third most common cause of death in this age range among both sexes (Clinical Guidelines, 1995b).

According to sociodemographic data, infection is more prevalent in urban areas, accounting for 29% of deaths among young men in New York, 28% in New Jersey, and 61% in San Francisco (Selik et al., 1993). However, the AIDS epidemic also is spreading to rural America. AIDS cases increased 37% annually in rural areas, compared with 5% increases in large urban areas. In many rural areas, there is little information about HIV infection and an overwhelming fear of people infected with HIV or AIDS. Ignorance and fear seriously hamper efforts to treat people with HIV and AIDS and work against prevention (AIDS Commission, 1990). In 1994, African Americans and Hispanics accounted for 57.7% of all AIDS case, while non-Hispanic white people accounted for 41.1%. This was the first year that the African American and Hispanic populations surpassed the non-Hispanic white population in the number of AIDS cases (CDC, 1995a).

Human Immunodeficiency Virus Infection in Women.

In the United States, more than 13% of all AIDS cases occur in women, with new infections occurring at a greater rate among women compared with men. More than 100,000 women in the United States are estimated to be HIV infected. Nearly 38% of AIDS cases in

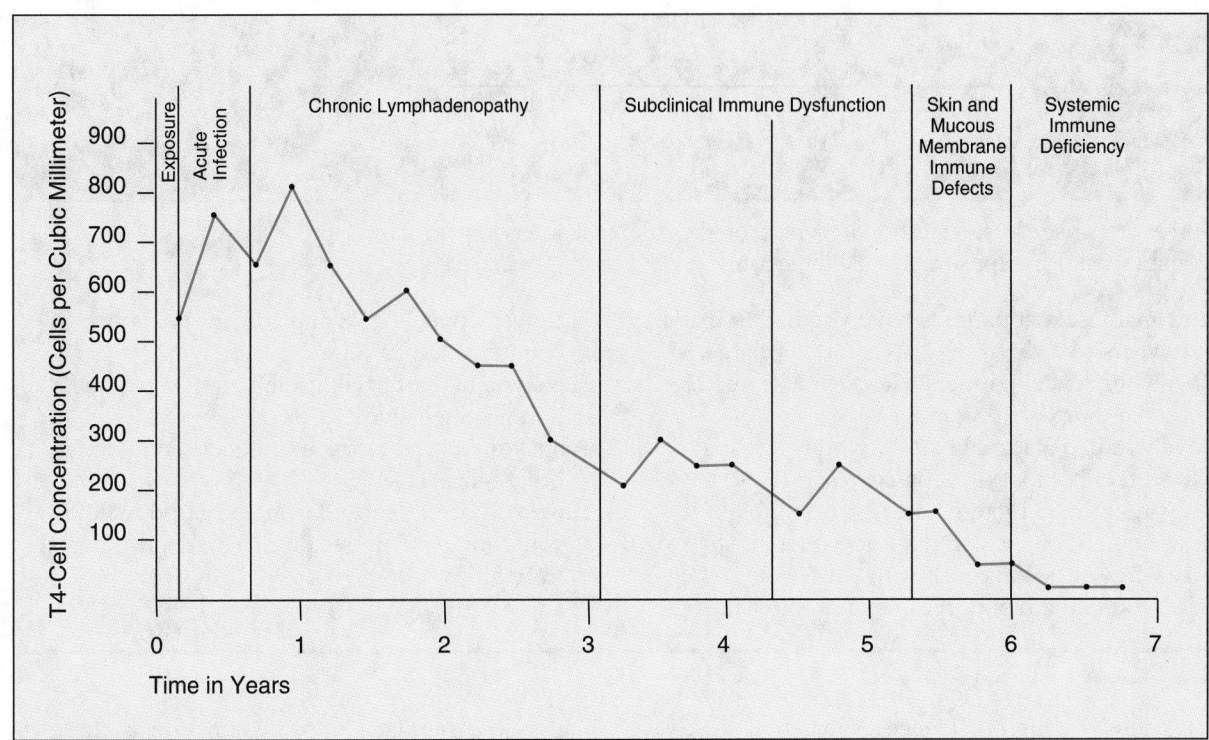

FIGURE 11-3 Decline in T4 cells in HIV/AIDS disease progression. Seroconversion occurs about 3 months after exposure to HIV, with a drop in T4 cells, then a rebound. Chronic lymphadenopathy develops around 9 months, and a long, slow decline of T4 cells occurs. As the T4 cell count falls below 400/mm³ at about 3 years, delayed hypersensitivity occurs. Gradually, the ability to mount a cellular immune response fails, with early signs, such as thrush and oral hairy leukoplakia. When the T4 count falls below 100/mm³ (shortly before 6 years), opportunistic infections and neoplasms occur, leading to death usually within a few years

women are a result of heterosexual transmission. This risk is especially severe among minority groups; more than 77% of AIDS cases occur in African American and Hispanic women. Infection rates for African American women are 16 times greater and for Hispanic women, 7 times greater than for white women. AIDS among women is primarily associated with injecting drug use and heterosexual contact with an at-risk partner. Heterosexual contact is the most rapidly increasing mode of transmission (CDC, 1995b).

Adolescents are particularly susceptible to HIV infection, because they often undertake high-risk behavior out of a false sense of invulnerability. The adolescent population (ages 13–21) accounts for 1% of all AIDS cases, with another 1 million to 1.5 million individuals estimated to be HIV infected. Epidemiologic data suggest that the epidemic of HIV infection in the adolescent population will continue to grow at an alarming rate if effective measures are not found to check it. The number of adolescents with AIDS doubles every 14 months. Adolescents' HIV seroprevalence rates have increased 500% in some areas of the country during a 5-year period ending in 1992 (Nelson, 1995).

Human Immunodeficiency Virus Infection and Pregnancy

During prenatal assessment, women should be screened for potential exposure to HIV (see Assessment Tool: Assessing Women's Risk for Human Immunodeficiency Virus Exposure). Most women infected with HIV are in their reproductive years, and the incidence of HIV in pregnancy is increasing. Women often are unaware of HIV risk and become infected as teenagers. They may remain undiagnosed until a perinatally infected child becomes ill (CDC, 1990c).

Pregnancy may cause clinical symptoms of HIV to accelerate. While pregnant women develop symptoms of HIV infection sooner than nonpregnant women, there is no difference in how soon they develop or die from AIDS (Deschamps et al., 1993). Early indications of possible HIV infection include persistent *Candida* infections, anogenital condyloma, and herpes simplex. These often occur when there is T-cell dysfunction (Dunnihoo, 1992). HIV infection may cause premature rupture of membranes, fetal death, preterm birth, and low birth weight (Lindberg, 1995; Wiesenfeld et al.,

ASSESSMENT TOOL
Assessing Women's Risk for Human Immunodeficiency Virus (HIV) Exposure

Nurses can use these questions as part of the prenatal interview to assess the woman's risk for exposure to HIV infection:

How many sexual partners have you had in the last 10 years?

Have your sexual partners had several sexual partners in the past 10 years?

Have you had a sexual partner who is bisexual or who had homosexual contact since 1978?

Do you have anal intercourse?

Have any of your sexual partners had a positive HIV test or become sick with AIDS?

Have you had a blood transfusion in the United States between 1978 and 1985 or in another country since 1978?

Have you had artificial insemination using untested donor semen since 1978?

Have you or your sexual partners used IV street drugs since 1978?

Have you been exposed to blood or body fluids in your work (eg, nurse, physician, dentist, dental hygienist)?

1994). There is a high incidence of infectious diseases during pregnancy in seropositive women, including bacterial pneumonia, UTIs, *Pneumocystis carinii* pneumonia, toxoplasmosis, STDs, postoperative abscess, and postpartum endometritis (Lindberg, 1995).

Perinatal Transmission. Nearly 85% to 90% of all AIDS cases and virtually all new HIV infections among children can be attributed to perinatal transmission. The estimated prevalence nationally of HIV infection in childbearing women is 1.7 HIV-infected women per 1,000 childbearing women. About 7,000 HIV-infected women give birth annually, with perinatal transmission rates (vertical transmission) ranging from 13% to 40%. The average transmission rate is 25% (CDC, 1995c; Lindberg, 1995; Clinical Practice Guidelines, 1994). This means that a newborn of a woman with HIV has a 60% to 86% chance of being born without HIV infection. The rate of perinatal transmission is expected to continue to rise (Lindberg, 1995).

Several factors affect perinatal transmission. Premature newborns are more likely to be born infected with HIV than full-term newborns. Identical twins are more likely to be infected or uninfected concordantly; while fraternal twins have the same rate as singletons. Vitamin A deficiency is associated with higher rates of perinatal transmission. Newborns of symptomatic mothers are twice as likely to be born infected than those of asymptomatic mothers. Mothers with lower CD4 cell counts have higher perinatal infection rates. Those with CD4-CD8 ratios greater than 0.90 have less than half the rate of transmitting HIV to their newborns as women whose ratios were less than 0.60. When *p24 antigen* is present in maternal blood during preg-

nancy, the perinatal transmission rate is three times higher than when it is not detectable (Lindberg, 1995; European Collaborative Study, 1992).

Newborns delivered by cesearean section are slightly less likely to be infected with HIV than those born vaginally (14% versus 20%). Invasive procedures, such as episiotomy, internal fetal monitoring, fetal scalp sampling, use of forceps, and vacuum extraction, during labor and delivery increase the risk of perinatal transmission in some settings (Lindberg, 1995; European Collaborative Study, 1992).

Zidovudine administered to asymptomatic seropositive women during pregnancy and labor and to the newborn reduced perinatal transmission rates by about two-thirds (Lindberg, 1995). The United States Public Health Service has issued recommendations regarding use of zidovudine to decrease the risk of perinatal transmission (CDC, 1994a):

- Asymptomatic women with CD4 lymphocyte counts above 200 who have not yet taken zidovudine can decrease the risk of perinatal transmission to about 8%.
- Pregnant women with HIV who have low CD4 counts, are more than 34 weeks' gestation, have already received zidovudine treatment, or have symptoms can be treated again, but the benefits of therapy are not known.

Diagnosis in the Newborn. Maternal antibodies (anti-HIV IgG) cross the placenta and are present in the newborn's serum for up to 18 months. Most newborns of seropositive mothers are themselves seropositive, although only 10% to 30% are actually infected with HIV.

Uninfected newborns gradually lose their passively acquired maternal antibodies (Proffitt et al., 1993). It is difficult to diagnose HIV infection in seropositive newborns using antibody tests because of transfer of maternal antibodies. Early diagnosis and immediate treatment of HIV-infected newborns is critical because of their poor prognosis.

In seropositive newborns, PCR tests may be used to detect actual HIV infection. This DNA technique permits analysis of tiny amounts of genetic material by amplification of the infecting organism's DNA or RNA. The amplification is rapid and dramatic; up to 100 million copies of a target nucleic acid sequence can be made in 3 hours (Baer et al., 1995). Precise gene amplification permits detection of HIV in its DNA proviral form from as few as one to two genomic copies per milliliter serum. The HIV PCR test is very sensitive and specific, about 20 times more sensitive than tissue culture isolation of HIV (Proffitt et al., 1993).

Newborns who acquire HIV infection in utero may characteristically exhibit microcephaly, growth failure, patulous lips, prominent boxlike forehead, flattened nasal bridge, wide inner canthus, blue sclerae, and mild obliquity of eyes. These newborns have a high mortality rate. The median age for onset of AIDS symptoms in children is 9 months, and 82% develop symptoms by 3 years. These symptoms include failure to thrive, rcurrent infections, Epstein-Barr infections, interstitial lymphocytic pneumonia, hepatosplenomegaly, and neurologic abnormalities. Encephalopathy with delayed development or loss of cognitive and other skills occurs in 50% to 90% of children with AIDS (Pizzo, 1990).

Clinical Management

Screening. The Institute of Medicine has recommended that HIV screening should be offered to but not required of all pregnant women. Women must have the right to consent to or refuse HIV testing, because the diagnosis has powerful psychological and social consequences (Institute of Medicine, 1991). The United States Public Health Service recommends that all pregnant women be counseled and encouraged to be tested for HIV infection as early in pregnancy as possible. They should be provided access to other HIV prevention and treatment services (eg, drug treatment and partner notification services). HIV testing of pregnant women and their fetuses should be voluntary, using legal consent procedures (CDC, 1995c).

The HIV-1 testing algorithm recommended by the Public Health Service is as follows:

- Initial screening with FDA-licensed EIA
- For repeatedly reactive EIA tests, confirmatory testing with FDA-licensed Western blot or immunofluorescence assay (IFA)

- Indeterminate Western blot results resolved with an IFA test
- Definitive diagnosis of HIV infection in newborns, use of PCR tests or virus culture

Home HIV testing may be available in kits that require a finger prick; a drop of blood is then placed on filter paper and sent to a laboratory for EIA testing. Results would be obtained by telephone. The home testing would be anonymous, with identification by preassigned number only. Negative results would be reported by a recording, and positive results would be reported by a trained counselor who would discuss the test and its implications and provide referrals to medical and community services. Several home-sampling kits have been considered by the FDA. Use of home sampling for HIV is supported by the CDC and public health officials in several states. Opposition to home testing is primarily based on concern for psychological risk if sufficient counseling is not available (Bayer, 1995).

Pregnant women at risk for HIV infection should be screened in early pregnancy and again in the third trimester. Risk factors may include the following:

- IV drug use (woman, sexual partner)
- Multiple sexual partners
- Sexual partner with high-risk characteristics
- STD during current pregnancy (gonorrhea, syphilis, *Chlamydia,* HBV, prolonged herpes)
- Oropharyngeal or chronic vaginal candidiasis
- TB
- CMV
- Toxoplasmosis

Treatment. Many antiviral medications are used to treat HIV, although none is effective at eradicating the infection. These drugs act on reverse transcriptase or interfere with synthesis of proviral DNA (Box 11-4).

In HIV-infected pregnant women, CD4 counts should be determined on presentation for prenatal care, with repeat testing as follows:

- >600 cells/μL, repeat count not needed
- 200 to 600 cells/μL, repeat each trimester
- <200 cells/μL, repeat every 3 months to monitor antiretroviral therapy or initiate new preventive therapies against infections as indicated by clinical symptoms

When CD4 counts are less than 500 cells/μL, pregnant women should be offered antiretroviral therapy with zidovudine. Risks and benefits of early zidovudine therapy are discussed. Increased morbidity has been found during pregnancy with CD4 counts less than 200 cells/μL. Anemia has occurred in newborns of treated mothers, but no fetal malformations were reported (Clinical Practice Guideline, 1994). Opportunistic infections can occur during pregnancy and are generally treated with the recommended drugs, although

BOX 11–4
Drugs Used to Treat AIDS

Zidovudine (Retrovir, ZVD, AZT)

- p24 antigen titers decrease.
- CD4 T cells increase.
- Opportunistic infections decrease.
- Progression of AIDS slows, and survival length increases.
- Use in asymptomatic HIV-infected clients controversial.
- Resistance to the drug often develops.
- Side effects include anemia, neutropenia, nausea, vomiting, headache, fatigue, confusion, malaise, myopathy, and hepatitis.
- Teratogenicity in pregnancy is not well studied, but some data found the drug well-tolerated and not associated with fetal malformations or other untoward effects (*The Medical Letter,* 1993).

Didanosine (DDI, Videx)

- Used in clients who cannot use zidovudine
- Decreases p24 antigens
- Increases CD4 T-cells
- Leads to weight gain in clients with AIDS and ARC
- Clinical deterioration delayed when used after zidovudine
- Side effects: peripheral neuropathy, acute pancreatitis, gastrointestinal disturbances, and hepatic failure.

Zalcitabine (DDC, Hivid)

- Used in clients with advanced disease
- Often used in combination with zidovudine
- Side effects: peripheral neuropathy, rash, stomatitis, esophageal ulceration, fever, and pancreatitis.

little is known about the adverse effects of these drugs on the mother or fetus.

Nursing Diagnoses

Nursing diagnoses for pregnant women who are HIV positive or have AIDS may include the following:

- Risk for Infection transmission (to fetus, sexual partners)
- Knowledge Deficit related to HIV and AIDS (disease progression, transmission, long-term effects on woman and fetus)
- Anxiety or Fear related to effects of HIV or AIDS and eventual death
- Risk for Infection due to impaired immune system function
- Pain related to opportunistic infections, side effects of medications
- Self Esteem Disturbance related to stigma of the disease
- Altered Nutrition: Less than body requirements

- Ineffective Family Coping related to HIV risk for family members, sexual transmission implications

Nursing Intervention and Evaluation

When a pregnant woman is HIV positive, counseling includes instruction in safe sex practices and information on sexual and perinatal transmission. Latex condoms, used correctly and consistently, provide protection against HIV transmission. Breakage and slippage rates for condoms are 1% to 2% with proper use (CDC, 1993b). Abortion and sterilization services are offered when appropriate. Because HIV infection is frequently associated with other STDs, the woman who is HIV positive is tested for syphilis, gonorrhea, *Chlamydia,* and HBV. Baseline antibody titers are drawn for rubella, chickenpox, CMV, and toxoplasmosis, because these infections are common in HIV clients and can cause serious illness. Tuberculin skin testing (purified protein derivative [PPD]) is done, and vaccination status is determined.

Because many women infected with HIV are IV drug users, assessment for substance abuse must be performed, and treatment should be provided. The nurse carefully evaluates symptoms and discomforts of pregnancy (ie, anorexia, fatigue, weight loss, vaginitis), because these may be evidence of HIV disease progression. Nutritional counseling is important to promote health. The woman is counseled about getting adequate sleep, rest, and exercise and and reducing stress to support immune system functioning. The use of alcohol and cigarettes is discouraged because these may interfere with medical treatments and further stress the immune system. Although the risk of HIV transmission through breast milk is not well known, the woman is advised not to breast-feed because the virus has been isolated from breast milk.

Emotional support by a nonjudgmental nurse assists the childbearing family in coping with the devastating impact HIV or AIDS can have. Knowing the mother and infant face decreased life expectancy and that other family members are at risk often creates feelings of helplessness, anger, fear, or despair. Social isolation may occur due to the rejection and condemnation often associated with a diagnosis of HIV. Family and sexual counseling are often necessary, and the woman and family may be referred to mental health or HIV and AIDS support groups.

Nursing care is effective when the woman can express her fears and uncertainties and examine the implications of HIV and AIDS for herself, the fetus, and her family. She uses information to obtain counseling and other assistance. Self-care is undertaken to promote health and reduce risk of disease transmission (see Nursing Care Plan: The Woman With HIV Infection/AIDS).

NURSING CARE PLAN
The Woman With HIV Infection/AIDS

Nursing Goals
1. The woman will understand the disease process and approaches to treatment.
2. The woman will have opportunities to discuss her fears, concerns, and feelings with supportive people.
3. The woman will remain well and delay disease progression as much as possible.
4. Nutrition and weight will be maintained.
5. Precautions will be taken to prevent transmission of HIV infection to others.
6. Opportunistic infections in the woman will be avoided or minimized.
7. Family members will understand the disease, avoid risk of transmission, and cope appropriately.

Assessment	Nursing Diagnoses	Intervention/Rationale	Evaluation
Determine woman/family's knowledge of HIV/AIDS disease process and treatment.	Knowledge Deficit related to HIV/AIDS disease process, treatment program	Provide information about disease effects, progression, monitoring CD4 count, medical treatment and results *to alleviate knowledge deficit*	Woman can describe what to expect from medical treatment, and course of the disease.
Physical/emotional signs of fear and anxiety (ie, crying, shakiness, tachycardia, verbalizing worry or confusion)	Anxiety/Fear related to HIV/AIDS	Provide opportunities for woman to discuss her fears, concerns, feelings, offer support, counseling, caring. Refer for therapy or community group support *to reduce anxiety/fear and enhance coping.*	Woman expresses her fears and feelings and expresses being supported. Woman uses community resources and receives assistance. Woman carries out daily activities effectively.
Determine knowledge of HIV infection transmission, sexual practices, possible exchange of blood or body fluids (toothbrush, razors, etc). Now pregnant or planning to become pregnant.	Risk for Infection transmission (sexual partners, close family members, fetus)	Provide information about transmission of HIV infection and ways to prevent transmission, *to encourage safe sex and avoid household exposures.*	Woman identifies ways to prevent transmission and implements these. Pregnancy is avoided.
Determine feelings about herself related to AIDS infection	Self-Concept Disturbance related to stigma of the disease	Provide opportunities for woman to express her self-perceptions and reinforce positive self-valuation *to enhance self-concept.*	Woman expresses self-acceptance.
Measure weight, compare with usual weight, note trends. Take diet history and observe her nutritional practices	Altered nutrition: Less than body requirements.	Counsel about diet and nutrition, with high-protein and -calorie foods *to maintain weight and health*.	Woman follows recommended diet and maintains normal weight or gains if underweight
Observe for signs of opportunistic infections (vaginal, skin, lungs) such as fever, discharge, rash, cough	Risk for Infection due to impaired immune system	Report signs of infection, to physician promptly; encourage woman to seek early treatment.	Infections diagnosed early and treated effectively
Determine if discomfort, pain, and decreased function occur during infections or from medications.	Altered Comfort due to infection or side effects of medication.	Suggest comfort measures to reduce swelling, itching, nausea, and pain	Discomforts are minimized and resolved rapidly.

(continued)

NURSING CARE PLAN *(Continued)*
The Woman With HIV Infection/AIDS

Assessment	Nursing Diagnoses	Intervention/Rationale	Evaluation
Observe family dynamics, expressions of fears, feelings, coping patterns	Ineffective Family Coping	Provide opportunities for family members to express fears, feelings and problems *to reduce tensions*. Refer for family therapy *to help resolve dysfunctions*.	Family communicates clearly, provides support and love to all members, copes and functions adequately

Urinary Tract Infections

Acute lower UTI (**cystitis**) is one of the most common bacterial infections in women. Most initial and infrequent UTIs are caused by ***Escherichia coli*** (80%–90%). *Staphylococcus saprophyticus* and *C. trachomatis* cause most of the remaining cases. Upper UTI (pyelonephritis) occurs less frequently and is difficult to distinguish from a lower UTI. The most common bacteria causing upper tract infection include the Enterobacteriaceae species, most commonly *E. coli* but also *Klebsiella, Proteus, Enterococci, Pseudomonas,* and *Staphylococcus* species.

During pregnancy, anatomic changes and hormonal effects cause narrowing of the lower ureter and renal pelvis and dilation of the upper ureter. These changes result in stasis of urine, delayed emptying, and an increased risk of infection. This risk increases as pregnancy progresses and continues into the puerperium.

Assessment

Symptoms of lower UTI include the following:

- Pain or burning on urination (dysuria)
- Urgency
- Frequency
- Discolored urine (dark, cloudy, bloody)
- Suprapubic cramping

Symptoms of upper UTI can include those listed above and the following systemic symptoms:

- Lower to midback (flank) pain
- Fever, chills
- Anorexia
- Nausea, vomiting
- Malaise

Nursing assessment includes information about voiding practices, changes in sexual partners or activities, genital hygiene practices, and use of topical soaps, sprays, or lotions.

Physical examination includes vital signs, particularly temperature, as indicators of infection. Suprapubic tenderness on palpation or flank pain on percussion may be present. The nurse obtains a clean catch, midstream urine specimen for chemical and microscopic analysis and culture if indicated.

Urinalysis shows presence of leukocytes, red blood cells, and bacteria. Urine culture with >100,000 colonies/mL indicates significant infection.

Nursing Diagnoses

Common nursing diagnoses include the following:

- Pain related to UTI
- Altered Urinary Elimination
- Knowledge Deficit related to treatment and prevention of UTIs
- Anxiety or Fear about the effects of UTI

Planning and Intervention

Nursing care focuses on promoting effective treatment of UTI and preventing recurrences. Careful instructions are provided about taking medications correctly and completing the course of treatment. Women are counseled to increase fluid intake to 8 to 10 glasses of liquids daily and to void promptly and thoroughly. Good bladder hygiene is emphasized with proper front-to-back wiping techniques. Factors that may predispose women to urinary infections are identified and eliminated, such as perfumed soaps and sprays. The woman is counseled to avoid sexual practices that traumatize the urethra or spread intestinal bacteria toward the vagina and urinary meatus.

Evaluation

Nursing care is effective when the UTI is successfully treated and symptoms resolve, the woman understands and eliminates contributing factors, and good bladder hygiene is followed. The client reports her anxieties or fears are relieved, and she is able to implement appropriate self-care.

Asymptomatic Bacteruria

Approximately 2% to 12% of pregnant women have asymptomatic bacteruria (ASB). Risk factors for ASB include sickle cell trait, toxemia, and diabetes mellitus. Poor hygiene and incorrect wiping after bowel movements also contribute to risk. Women with decreased uromucoid, a hydrophilic polysaccharide that interposes water between bacteria and cell surface membranes, have more frequent UTIs. Uromucoid is less in the absence of estrogen, such as during menopause. Postmenopausal women who use estrogen therapy have fewer UTIs (Dunnihoo, 1992).

The ASB is identified by urine culture with >100,000 colonies/mL of a single organism in a clean catch urine specimen. With elevated counts less than 100,000/mL, repeated cultures demonstrating the same organism are necessary to diagnose ASB. The most common causative organisms are *E. coli, Enterobacter* species, and *Klebsiella.*

Detecting ASB during pregnancy is important because if left untreated, 25% to 30% of cases will progress to pyelonephritis (acute upper UTI). Bacteruria is usually present during the first trimester and persists until after delivery in about 80% of untreated women, often leading to postpartum endometritis. Routine screening for ASB in all pregnant women is recommended. Urine cultures early in the second trimester detect nearly all women with bacteruria. ASB in pregnancy is treated with antibiotics, including trimethoprim-sulfamethoxazole (Bactrim DS) bid, sulfisoxazole (Gantrisin) 1 g qid, amoxicillin 250 mg tid, nitrofurantoin 50 to 100 mg qid, or cephalexin 250 to 500 mg qid, all for 10 days. Persistent infections should be treated with continued antibiotic suppression. At least one negative repeat urine culture should be obtained during pregnancy and after delivery (Box 11-5).

Cystitis and Urethritis

Acute lower UTI (cystitis, urethritis) affects 10% to 20% of women each year and occurs in 1% to 2% of women during pregnancy. Detection and treatment of ASB in pregnant women would prevent about one-third of acute lower UTIs from developing. Occasionally, pregnant women have severe hemorrhagic cystitis with hematuria. UTI during pregnancy increases the risk of low birth weight, prematurity, premature labor, hypertension and preeclampsia, maternal anemia, and amnionitis (Schieve et al., 1994). Urinalysis shows WBC, red blood cells, and bacteria; urine culture is positive for bacteria.

BOX 11-5
Management of Asymptomatic Bacteruria (ASB) in Pregnancy

Screening
Urine culture and sensitivity on initial prenatal visit or early in second trimester

Antibiotic Treatment
Sulfisoxazole
Nitrofurantoin
Ampicillin
Cephalexin

Follow-Up
Monthly urine culture and sensitivity tests
Monitoring for symptoms of infection affecting lower or upper urinary tracts
Antibiotic suppression for persistent or recurrent infection
Teaching bladder hygiene and prevention of infection

Treatment is with antibiotics, including sulfisoxazole, nitrofurantoin, amoxicillin, or cephalexin or other cephalosporins as described previously. Single-dose therapy for nonpregnant clients may be used as follows:

- Trimethoprim-sulfamethoxazole two to three tablets
- Amoxicillin 3 g
- Cefalexin 3 g
- Sulfisoxazole 1 to 2 g
- Nitrofurantoin 400 mg

The nurse should teach the woman good bladder hygiene. This includes voiding every 2 hours, drinking 8 to 10 glasses of water daily, and wiping properly. Allowing the bladder to become overdistended by holding urine predisposes women to infections. Repeat cultures are performed to determine the effectiveness of treatment and to detect recurrent infections.

Pyelonephritis

This acute upper UTI occurs in 1% to 3% of women during pregnancy, usually in the late second or early third trimesters or in the postpartum period. Usually pregnant women with acute pyelonephritis had ASB early in pregnancy (Pernoll, 1991). Urine culture and sensitivities are performed to identify appropriate antibiotic treatment. Pregnant women with pyelonephritis are best treated in the hospital with hydration and parenteral antibiotics (broad-spectrum penicillins, third-generation cephalosporins, ticarcillin-clavulanate, aminoglycosides). With effective antibiotics, temperature usually returns to normal in 3 to 5 days. Medication is continued for 14 days, with repeat urine cultures to fol-

---

BOX 11–6
Management of Acute Pyelonephritis in Pregnancy

Hospitalization
IV hydration
IV antibiotic therapy
Monitoring vital signs and urinary output
Urine and blood cultures
Monitoring for multisystem dysfunction
Follow-up urine cultures, continuing after discharge
Continuous suppressive antibiotic therapy for persistent or recurrent infections

---

low progress. Hydration includes at least 3,000 mL of fluids daily; this may need to be supplied intravenously if the client is vomiting. Urinary output is monitored because renal function is significantly reduced during the acute phase of infection.

Women with pyelonephritis are at increased risk for premature labor, anemia, and septic shock. Control of the infection reduces the likelihood of these complications. Follow-up urine cultures are done because recurrences of infection may indicate renal abnormalities or systemic disease. Persistent or recurrent infection requires long-term antibiotic treatment until after delivery, usually with an agent such as nitrofurantoin (Dunnihoo, 1992; Box 11-6).

Chronic Renal Disease

Chronic glomerulonephritis and nephrosis occur infrequently in pregnancy. The condition is serious, and the outcome for the woman and fetus depends on the severity of renal disease and the presence of hypertension. With hypertension, fetal survival is 55% compared with 93% without hypertension. This is because hypertension causes decreased placental perfusion and increased risk of infarcts and abruptio placentae. Proteinuria, edema, anemia, and pregnancy-induced hypertension are often present with chronic renal disease. Impaired kidney function can lead to renal insufficiency or failure. Preexisting hypertension is a risk factor for renal disease. Treatment focuses on controlling hypertension, maintaining fluid and electrolyte balance, maintaining adequate protein levels, and restricting sodium (Dunnihoo, 1992).

Other Infectious Diseases

Other infectious diseases, primarily viral and bacterial, may affect the woman or fetus during pregnancy. Their effects range from inconsequential to life-threatening.

In addition, many diseases, particularly viral infections, can cause significant congenital abnormalities in the newborn. Immunizations are available for many common contagious diseases. This mode of primary prevention is often the only approach to avoiding the consequences of infection.

Assessment

An immunization history is obtained as part of the woman's health or prenatal evaluation. Although most women have either had childhood communicable diseases (rubella, rubeola, mumps, chickenpox) or have been immunized for them, a small percentage remain susceptible to these infections as adults. If symptoms of communicable disease develop, the nurse assesses possible sources of exposure, such as contact with ill children or known epidemics in the community. Common symptoms of communicable diseases include the following:

- Fever
- Nasal discharge
- Sore throat
- Cough
- Malaise
- Anorexia
- Occasionally nausea and vomiting
- Skin rash or enlarged lymph nodes

A physical examination is performed. Vital signs are taken, and any temperature elevation is noted. The nasal mucosa, pharynx, and tympanic membranes are examined for signs of infection (redness, swelling, discharge). When the client has a cough and expectoration, the lungs are auscultated for abnormal sounds. The skin is inspected for rash; if present, its color, characteristics, and distribution are noted. Examination also includes the degree and location of lymphadenopathy.

Nursing Diagnoses

Diagnoses for communicable diseases may include the following:

- Risk for Infection related to nonimmunity
- Risk for Infection transmission
- Knowledge Deficit related to causes, consequences, and treatment of the infection
- Anxiety or Fear related to the effects of the infection on the fetus
- Risk for Altered Health Maintenance related to lack of knowledge about prevention of infectious diseases

Planning and Intervention

Communicable diseases are usually spread by droplet or airborne transmission, although some are spread by water, vector, or direct contact. The nurse identifies women at risk for communicable diseases and other infections during pregnancy and provides education and counseling about risk reduction. Many vaccines cannot be administered during pregnancy because of the risk to the fetus. Therefore, the woman is alerted to her nonimmune status and advised to avoid exposure to communicable diseases. The importance of immunization after delivery is emphasized.

When the pregnant woman has contracted a communicable disease, the nurse and other members of the healthcare team explain the expected course and effects of the disease. The length of communicability is carefully described, and the woman is taught how to avoid exposing others. If the potential effects on the fetus are serious, the nurse provides the opportunity for the woman to express her fears and concerns in a caring, supportive environment. Options for terminating the pregnancy are discussed when fetal anomalies are probable or have been identified. The woman is supported in making and feeling satisfied with her decision.

Symptomatic relief during the course of the illness includes adequate rest and fluids. Natural remedies for relieving a stuffy nose, sore throat, and nausea may be suggested (see Chap. 17). Medications are avoided or minimized during pregnancy. However, if the physician prescribes antibiotics or medications for symptom relief, the nurse reviews how to take the medications and stresses the importance of completing the course of treatment.

Evaluation

Nursing care is most effective when communicable diseases are prevented or their spread is minimized. Teaching and counseling are effective when the woman can describe her risks for communicable diseases and knows ways to reduce risk and avoid exposure. She expresses her anxieties or fears and reports an understanding of the disease process and its potential effects. She obtains symptomatic relief or completes the course of prescribed medications.

Influenza

The occurrence of influenza infection during pregnancy poses serious maternal and fetal morbidity risks and has been correlated with higher premature labor and abortion rates. Symptoms of influenza include high fever, muscle aches and back pain, sore throat, and prostration.

The pregnant woman is no more likely than the nonpregnant woman to contract influenza. However, she is more susceptible to pneumonia developing secondary to influenza. This is especially true if she is in the third trimester because the diaphragm is elevated, and respi-

ration is compromised. Maternal mortality increases significantly when this complication occurs. In an epidemic involving a specific strain of influenza virus, immunization with a killed or attenuated virus vaccine is indicated. Nonspecific polyvalent vaccines are probably ineffective.

Measles (Rubeola)

Pregnant women who contract measles may be more likely to have spontaneous abortions and premature labor. No congenital defects have been reported, although the typical skin rash has been noted on newborns. However, premature newborns are particularly prone to adverse sequelae from measles infection, such as pneumonia and encephalitis.

Measles epidemics that occurred in the United States between 1989 and 1991 were largely due to underimmunization. Improved vaccination efforts in preschool children produced marked declines in measles cases by mid-1993 (CDC, 1993c). Guidelines issued by the CDC to reduce measles include a second vaccination for older children and college entrants, because children receiving the vaccine before 15 months are probably not adequately immunized. It also is recommended that pregnant women with no firm history of the disease or of immunization should receive immune globulin within 6 days of exposure to measles (CDC, 1989b).

Rubella

Approximately 10% of women of childbearing age are susceptible to **rubella** (German measles). There is a high incidence (74%) of congenital abnormalities in newborns whose mothers contracted rubella during the first 4 months of pregnancy. There is also evidence that infection occurring late in the second trimester causes congenital abnormalities. The most common defects include heart disease, hearing loss, cataracts, and psychomotor retardation (see Chap. 42). Other effects of infection in early pregnancy include abortion, premature delivery, and intrauterine fetal death. Abortion is usually recommended when rubella is contracted in early pregnancy.

It is extremely important to verify rubella infection. This is done on the basis of hemagglutination-inhibition antibodies, complement-fixing antibodies, and rubella-specific IgM antibodies. Each of these follows a typical pattern, which in combination allows an accurate diagnosis. If rubella infection during pregnancy is verified, gamma globulin is not recommended because this does not appear to prevent viremia and fetal involvement.

Rubella antibody titer is done routinely as part of the prenatal panel. A titer of 1:8 or more indicates that the woman is immune. When the titer is less, the woman is susceptible and is advised to avoid contact with ill people and to seek immediate medical care if she develops a viral syndrome with a rash. Rubella vaccination is not recommended during pregnancy because the virus has been recovered from fetal tissues after vaccination. Although the vaccine virus is less teratogenic than the wild virus, abnormalities have occurred with vaccination during pregnancy. A nonpregnant woman who is vaccinated for rubella should not become pregnant for at least 3 months.

Chickenpox (Varicella)

Varicella during pregnancy is rare. However, if it does occur, it is likely to be severe. If varicella pneumonia or necrotizing angitis (bacterial gangrene of blood vessels) develop as complications, the infection is often fatal for the pregnant woman. Other complications include myocarditis, hepatitis, nephritis, and encephalitis. Treatment of varicella infection includes maintaining adequate oxygenation, controlling bacterial superinfection, and administering acyclovir. Herpes zoster (shingles) is another manifestation of varicella in pregnant women. It is quite rare and does not increase risk for the woman or fetus (Dunnihoo, 1992).

Maternal chickenpox during the first trimester is associated with congenital malformations, such as limb defects, skin scars, Horner's syndrome, and low birth weight. If the fetus is exposed to the virus just before delivery, there is a serious risk of disseminated visceral and CNS disease. Specific varicella-zoster globulin administered to the woman may be life-saving for the fetus.

Mumps

Infection with the mumps virus (parotitis) during pregnancy can cause spontaneous abortion or premature labor. Fetal death and abnormalities, such as endocardial fibroelastosis, have been reported. Evidence of diffuse necrotic villitis and viral inclusions in chorionic and fetal tissues verifies that the mumps virus crosses the placenta. If a mumps epidemic occurs, an administration of hyperimmune mumps gamma globulin may be a protective measure for nonimmune pregnant women.

Tuberculosis

In North America and other industralized countries, TB has been dramatically increasing since 1985. This is largely due to the spread of HIV (Nunn et al., 1993). There is a strong link between AIDS and TB; 11% of all TB cases are HIV positive, and 4.3% of all AIDS clients have TB. In the United States, homelessness, drug abuse, deterioration of living conditions among the poor, lack of accessible healthcare, and immigration have contributed to this situation. Most new TB cases occur in the 25- to 44-year age group. Two-thirds of this group are racial and ethnic minorities, many of whom are immigrants (Rieder at al., 1993).

Pathophysiology. Mycobacterium tuberculosis is carried on droplets in the air and is spread by coughing or sneezing. It enters the body through the airways. If the immune system fails to stop the infection, bacteria spread and multiply primarily in the lungs. However, the skin, lymph nodes, bones, and kidneys can be infected. The risk of contracting TB is greater when a person is exposed to or has prolonged close contact with clients with active lung cavitations. The risk for infection also is increased in a person with a condition that weakens immune system functioning (ie, diabetes, cancer, malnutrition, AIDS). In about 10% of those exposed, infection progresses to disease. TB may remain dormant for many years and become active when resistance is lowered. This risk remains present for the remainder of an infected person's life.

Treatment. Treatment with the antituberculosis drugs streptomycin, isoniazid (INH), rifampicin, ethambutol, or pyrazinamide usually provides good control of the disease. Streptomycin may cause congenital nerve deafness in an infant. Multidrug-resistant TB has become a serious problem in some U.S. cities, especially among HIV-positive clients. Failure to take TB drugs for the required 6 months has allowed bacterial mutation, leading to resistant strains (Tripathy, 1993). Multidrug-resistant TB associated with AIDS raises the specter of a potentially untreatable, lethal infection that can easily be transmitted (Edlin et al., 1992).

Tuberculosis and Pregnancy. During pregnancy, TB is not associated with abortion, premature labor, or stillbirth. The disease is seldom acquired congenitally. Pregnancy should be undertaken only when TB has been inactive for 2 years. There is increased risk that latent lesions will become active if pregnancy overtaxes the woman's resistance. Maintenance of proper nutrition and rest help to prevent activation of latent lesions.

Screening of all pregnant women for TB using PPD is recommended. In high-risk groups or if there is clinical indication of disease, testing should be repeated later in pregnancy. Newborns of mothers with active TB infection are isolated from the mother and others who may be contagious until the disease is controlled. Breast-feeding is acceptable if the mother has been effectively treated. Most infants who develop TB in their first year of life are infected by an adult family member or household contact (Vallejo et al., 1994).

Poliomyelitis

Poliomyelitis is a virus that causes paralytic illness. It can be prevented by vaccination. In the United States, nearly 90% of the population has been immunized and the last confirmed case of polio occurred in 1991. However, any unimmunized people in western countries are at risk for infection due to people immigrating from areas where paralytic polio is still endemic, such as India, Asia, and sub-Saharan Africa (CDC, 1994b).

Maternal infection with polio during the first trimester may result in abortion, intrauterine growth retardation, and congenital abnormalities. Infection of the fetus during passage through the birth canal is possible. Nonimmunized pregnant women should be immunized with Salk vaccine (killed virus), which confers immunity for about 2 years. Immunization with Sabin's vaccine (attenuated live virus) is contraindicated during pregnancy.

Cytomegalovirus

Approximately 60% of the general population have antibodies to CMV by age 35 to 40. Transmission occurs by close contact, sexual intercourse, breast-feeding, and transplacentally. CMV has been isolated in cervical secretions, breast milk, urine, tears, and saliva. Most infections in adults are mild and go unnoticed. Women younger than 25 years with small children at home have the greatest risk of acquiring CMV infection. About 4 to 8 weeks after infection, fever, fatigue, and malaise with splenomegaly and atypical lymphocytes may occur. There is no effective treatment for the disease.

Congenital CMV infection is common; it annually affects about 40,000 newborns in the United States. Congenital infections occur in 0.5% to 2.0% of all neonates, but only 5% to 10% manifest evidence of disease. In women who are seropositive prior to pregnancy, less than 1% transmit the virus transplacentally, and most of these newborns do not have clinically serious disease.

The rate of seroconversion during pregnancy (acquiring a primary infection) is about 1% to 2%. Primary infection in pregnancy increases the risk of congenital CMV. In fact, 30% to 50% of fetuses become infected with CMV during the first trimester if the woman acquired the virus after becoming pregnant. Of these fetuses, 10% to 15% exhibit clinical manifestations. CNS abnormalities, microcephaly, hydrocephaly, cerebral calcification, deafness, chorioretinitis, hepatosplenomegaly, jaundice, hemolytic anemia, and convulsions may result. Fetuses infected during passage through the birth canal may not manifest symptoms at the time of birth. However, blindness, epilepsy, mental retardation, spastic diplegia, hearing loss, and optic atrophy may develop later. As many as 4,000 infants may be severely damaged by CMV infection each year (Dunnihoo, 1992).

Diagnosis of CMV infection may be confirmed by urine culture, urinalysis showing cells with intranuclear inclusion bodies (fluorescent antibody [FA] or complement fixation [CF] tests), and indirect hemagglutination and ELISA tests specific for CMV antibodies.

Toxoplasmosis

Toxoplasmosis is caused by the protozoan *Toxoplasma gondii,* which is transmitted to humans in raw meat, unpasturized goat milk, or cat feces. There are no symptoms of infection in 90% of adults who are exposed to toxoplasmosis. When symptoms do occur during the acute infection stage, they resemble influenza accompanied by lymphadenopathy.

Fetal infection usually occurs as a result of maternal parasitemia during the initial acute attack, but it also may occur in chronic carrier states. About 25% of women in the United States show evidence of having been infected with *T. gondii.* When toxoplasmosis is acquired in early pregnancy, abortion occurs frequently. If it is acquired later in pregnancy, about 50% of the fetuses have a higher perinatal mortality rate and increased risk of having the following disorders:

- CNS calcifications
- Microcephaly
- Hydrocephaly
- Chorioretinitis
- Hepatosplenomegaly
- Jaundice
- Mental retardation

Indirect immunofluorescent, Sabin-Feldman dye, and ELISA tests are used to diagnose toxoplasmosis. Treatment consists of pyrimethamine (Daraprim) and folinic acid. Sulfonamides also are given. Pyrimethamine is teratogenic and should not be used in the first trimester. Pregnant women should avoid exposure to substances capable of transmitting *T. gondii.*

Group B Streptococcal Disease

Caused by *Streptococcus agalactiae,* GBS often leads to significant infection during the perinatal period. This infection causes serious effects in the mother and infant. There are five serotypes of GBS: Ia, Ib, Ic, II, and III. Approximately 33% of pregnant women are colonized by GBS, and up to 70% of newborns of colonized mothers also will be colonized. The heavier the maternal colonization, the more likely the newborn will be affected by GBS.

Colonization by GBS can be chronic or intermittent. No differences in colonization have been found related to age, race, or parity. Sites of colonization include the cervix, vagina, and rectum. Vaginal colonization usually occurs from rectal transfer and may be spread sexually. During pregnancy, GBS can cause bacteruria, bacteremia, intra-amniotic infection, and chorioamnionitis. This may lead to premature rupture of membranes and premature labor, possibly resulting in fetal demise or a seriously infected premature newborn (Dinsmoor, 1990). Postpartum, GBS can cause endometritis with high fever developing in the first 24 hours. Bacteremia and wound infection also may occur.

Diagnosis. Prenatal screening for GBS is done by vaginal or cervical cultures at 26 to 32 weeks' gestation. GBS cultures are recommended for pregnant women admitted for premature or prolonged rupture of membranes, premature labor, fever during labor, and multiple births (Committee on Infectious Diseases, 1992). An EIA test for GBS antigen provides rapid detection (30 minutes), but sensitivity may be low, leading to false-negatives, particularly in lightly colonized women (Gallagher et al., 1994).

Group B Streptococcal Disease in the Neonate. Early-onset (before 7 days after birth) neonatal disease is caused equally by all serotypes of group B streptococci. It occurs in 2 to 4 per 1,000 births and has a 50% or greater mortality rate. Late-onset neonatal disease is usually caused by serotype III. Rates of infection are 1 to 2 per 1,000 births, and the mortality rate is up to 30%. Factors associated with early onset include prolonged labor, premature delivery, premature rupture of membranes, and overt maternal infection with fever. Sepsis may be apparent at birth or may not appear until after 1 week. Infections may lead to pneumonia, bacteremia, meningitis with residual neurologic or developmental deficits, or death. Late-onset disease occurs after 7 days and may cause meningitis, bacteremia, and bone and joint infections. Infants surviving late-onset GBS have increased risk for permanent neurologic or developmental problems (Fletcher et al., 1990).

Treatment. Treatment regimens for GBS include the following:

- Prenatal: Ampicillin 500 mg orally qid for 7 days given in the third trimester (reduces colonization prior to delivery). Erythromycin is used for penicillin-sensitive clients. Sexual partners may be treated with ampicillin to prevent recolonization. Use of condoms is recommended.
- Intrapartum: Ampicillin 2 g IV initially, followed by 1 to 2 g IV q6h during labor (reduces mother–newborn transmission and postpartum endometritis). Erythromycin or clindamycin is used with penicillin allergy.
- Neonatal with evidence of infection: Parenteral ampicillin 75 mg/kg q12h plus gentamicin 2.5 mg/kg q12h starting within 2 hours after birth and continuing for 10 days (see Chap. 42).

Toxic Shock Syndrome

Toxic shock syndrome (TSS) is a multisystem infectious disease caused by toxin-producing strains of *Staphylococcus aureus*. The toxin enters the bloodstream through microulcerations in the vaginal or cervical mucosa usually caused by tampons or reflux of menstrual blood from the uterus and out through the fallopian tubes onto the peritoneum, due to obstruction of menstrual flow by tampons. The incidence of TSS is 6.2 per 100,000 menstruating women per year. Most (95%) of cases occur in menstruating women using tampons, though the disease can occur in men and nonmenstruating women (Dunnihoo, 1992; Box 11-7).

Pathophysiology and Disease Process

Although most women have antibodies to *S. aureus,* only a small number ever develop TSS. The organism is found in normal vaginal flora in 9% of women and in urethral cultures in about 5% of men without the disease. When TSS occurs, the organism invades tissue and produces an endotoxin and an exotoxin TSST-1 with pyogenic effects. The exotoxin and endotoxin stimulate the release of tumor necrosis factor-a (TNF-a) from monocytes and peritoneal macrophages. TNF-a is probably the primary mediator of TSS symptoms and gram-negative sepsis. Synthesis of IgM antibodies is suppressed, and altered capillary permeability leads to extravasation of fluid. Venous blood volume is reduced, cardiac blood return is diminished, and tissue perfusion is impaired. These factors lead to hypoxia and renal and CNS abnormalities. Release of thromboplastin from damaged organs leads to thrombocytopenia and coagulopathy.

Toxic shock syndrome can be a serious, life-threatening systemic disease with acute onset, which rapidly progresses to hypotensive shock and a moribund state. Severe TSS is characterized by abrupt onset of high fever, vomiting, and diarrhea. This may be accompanied by a sore throat, myalgia, headache, and confu-

---

BOX 11-7
Risk Factors for Toxic Shock Syndrome

- Women 15 to 24 years who use tampons
- Chronic vaginal infections
- Poor perineal hygiene
- Use of high-absorbancy tampons
- Skin or incisional infections
- Postpartum endometritis
- Low estradiol levels (postpartum, menstruation)

sion. Within 24 to 48 hours, the condition may progress to hypotension and shock. A fine, erythematous maculopapular rash develops that resembles sunburn on the skin begins to desquamate about 10 days later. The acute phase of TSS lasts 4 to 5 days, and convalescence takes place over 1 to 2 weeks. Disseminated intravascular coagulation (DIC), thrombocytopenia, and adult respiratory distress syndrome (ARDS) may occur.

Laboratory tests show elevated SGOT, SGPT, blood urea nitrogen, creatinine, WBC, and bilirubin, with decreased platelets. Blood, throat, and cerebrospinal fluid cultures are negative for other diseases, as is serology. TSS must be distinguished from diseases with similar rashes, such as Rocky Mountain spotted fever, leptospirosis, measles, and scarlet fever (Box 11-8).

Medical Treatment

Hospitalization is required for most cases of TSS, especially those with severe symptoms. Medical treatment includes intravenous fluid replacement, cardiorespiratory support, maintenance of blood pressure, and antibiotic therapy for penicillinase-producing *S. aureus.* Electrolytes may be supplemented, and renal dialysis

may be needed. Pulmonary and peripheral edema and ascites may result from extravasation of fluids and needs intensive management.

Prognosis and recovery are related to severity and complications of the disease. The leading causes of mortality are ARDS, uncontrollable hypotension, and DIC. Most women fully recover, but some have residual damage, including impaired intellectual, neuromuscular, renal, or cardiac function. The recurrence rate of menstrual-related TSS is about 30%, usually at the next menstrual cycle. Treatment with antistaphylococcal antibiotics reduces recurrences.

Nursing Assessment

To prevent TSS, nurses should assess tampon and barrier contraceptive use. Early signs of TSS, which may resemble upper respiratory infections, must be identified. When TSS has occurred, the nurse assesses the client's response to medical therapy and her abilities to cope emotionally with the impact of this illness. Family responses and adaptations to the illness experience also are assessed.

Nursing Diagnosis and Intervention

During the acute phase of TSS, nursing diagnoses may include the following:

- Altered Tissue Perfusion
- Ineffective Breathing Patterns
- Decreased Cardiac Output
- Impaired Gas Exchange
- Fluid Volume Deficit or Excess
- Self-Care Deficit
- Pain related to dehydration, equipment
- Knowledge Deficit related to illness, treatment, prevention
- Fear, Anxiety, Powerlessness

Nursing care implements life-supportive and monitoring measures of the medical treatment regimen. Potential complications must be identified early to initiate effective treatment. Measures to prevent complications include adequate ventilation, repositioning, and ambulation to decrease risk of pneumonia and clotting disorders. To promote comfort and pain control, nursing care includes administering pain medications and providing comfort measures, such as positioning, moisturizing lip creams, mouth care, and ice chips to relieve dry oral mucosa. Supportive care is provided for alterations in bowel and urinary elimination. The nurse encourages the woman to express feelings and reactions to the illness. As recovery progresses, she is assisted in performing appropriate self-care to regain some mastery over the body.

BOX 11-8
Centers for Disease Control and Prevention Case Definition for Toxic Shock Syndrome

Fever (temperature > 38.8°C)

Rash (diffuse erythematous macular)

Desquamation (10 days after onset, mainly of palms and soles)

Hypotension (including orthostatic syncope or dizziness)

Involvement of three or more systems:

Gastrointestinal (vomiting, diarrhea)

Muscular (severe myalgias, creatinine phosphokinase > three times normal)

Renal (blood urea nitrogen or creatinine > two times normal, >5 WBCs per high-power field without urinary tract infection)

Hepatic (SGOT, SGPT, total bilirubin > two times normal)

Hematologic (platelets < 100,000)

Central nervous system (disorientation, altered sensorium, headache)

Respiratory (adult respiratory distress syndrome)

Differentiation from similar-appearing infectious diseases (Rocky Mountain spotted fever, leptospirosis, measles, streptococcal scarlet fever)

Negative blood, throat, and cerebrospinal fluid cultures for other pathogens

Nurses should educate women about TSS prevention. The most important preventive measure for women to practice is avoiding high absorbency tampons and prolonged tampon use (see Client Education: Preventing Toxic Shock Syndrome). Women who have had TSS should never use tampons and need to be taught how to recognize early symptoms because they are at risk for a recurrence of TSS (Eschenbach, 1990).

Evaluation

An outcome of effective nursing care is that women will understand the cause of TSS and alter tampon and contraceptive practices that increase their risk. Women who develop TSS will recognize the illness early, seek medical care promptly, and avoid complications.

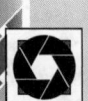

CLIENT EDUCATION
Preventing Toxic Shock Syndrome

Toxic shock syndrome may be a life-threatening infection associated with use of tampons and barrier contraceptives. Women can minimize their risk of this disease by following these guidelines.

Tampon Use

- Avoid using superabsorbent tampons.
- Change tampons every 2 to 4 hours.
- Wash hands before inserting tampons.
- Be sure tampons are clean.
- Use napkins or pads at night and during light flow instead of tampons.
- Do not use during first 6 weeks postpartum.

Barrier Contraceptive Use

- Wash hands before inserting diaphragm or cervical cap.
- Be sure contraceptive device is clean.
- Do not use contraceptive devices during menstrual period.
- Remove contraceptive device at recommended time.
- Do not use during first 6 weeks postpartum.

Identify TSS Symptoms Early

- Call your healthcare provider if you are menstruating or have been using a barrier contraceptive method and develop these symptoms:
  - High fever (102°F [38.8°C])
  - Vomiting and diarrhea
  - Skin rash
  - Sore throat, headache, muscle aches
  - Dizziness, disorientation (hypotension)

Women Who Have Had TSS

- Never use tampons or barrier contraception.
- Watch for recurrence of symptoms during menstruation.

Summary Points

✔ Sexually transmitted diseases occur frequently. They affect many women, their sexual partners, and often the fetus during pregnancy. Risk factors for STDs include age (young adult), multiple sex partners, infrequent or no condom use, and alcohol or drug use.

✔ Standard precautions are used to minimize the risk of disease transmission in healthcare workers. These precautions include wearing barriers to protect against exposure (eg, gloves, aprons, masks, eye shields), washing hands after client contact, using mechanical suctioning (no mouth activated systems), and handling needles and knife blades properly.

✔ Common vaginal infections include moniliasis (*Candida*), trichomonas, and bacterial vaginosis. These are diagnosed by microscopic examination of vaginal discharge and treated with vaginal or oral medication. Except for bacterial vaginosis, upper genital tract disease is infrequent.

✔ Chlamydial infection is often difficult to detect; infection may ascend from the cervix and involve the tubes and ovaries. This may lead to PID and danger of sterility. Diagnosis is by culture or immunoassay; treatment is with doxycycline.

✔ Genital herpesvirus infection usually causes recurrent eruptions affecting the vulva and cervix. Diagnosis is by culture; treatment is with acyclovir to control or reduce symptoms. There is no cure.

✔ Gonorrhea often causes minimal symptoms. The infection often ascends to the tubes and ovaries, causing PID. Diagnosis is by culture or immunoassay; treatment is with ceftriaxone and doxycycline.

✔ Condyloma (genital warts) is caused by a skin virus transmitted by sexual contact. It may affect the vulva, vagina, and cervix. There is increased risk of cervical cancer with condyloma. Treatment is by cryotherapy, chemocautery, electrocautery, or excision.

✔ Syphilis may have a long latency period, cause serious multisystem disease in later stages, and cause fetal abnormalities. Diagnosis is by serologic tests; treatment is with penicillin.

✔ Hepatitis is caused by several types of viruses with various routes of transmission. Disease ranges from mild to life-threatening. There is no treatment, but immunization is available for HAV and HBV. Health workers are at risk for contracting HBV and possible other types. Universal precautions should be used when providing care.

✔ Acquired immunodeficiency syndrome is a life-threatening disease with no cure. The virus causes severe immunosuppression, leading to opportunistic infections that are difficult to control. Diagnosis is by antibody or antigen tests; treatment with zidovudine and other antiretroviral agents can delay progression. The fetus can be infected. Because HIV is spread by blood and body fluids, health workers are at risk, and universal precautions should be used when providing care.

✔ Urinary tract infections include urethritis, cystitis, pyelonephritis, and chronic renal disease. These infections are common in women; ASB should be treated because it can lead to pyelonephritis, especially during pregnancy. Sulfonamides are first-line treatment; many antibiotics may be used.

✔ Contagious diseases (eg, measles, mumps, varicella, influenza, CMV) may be mild in women but cause congenital abnormalities in the fetus. Immunizations are available for many contagious diseases. There often is no effective treatment because most are viral infections.

✔ Group B streptococcal infections occur by vaginal colonization and may be transmitted vertically (transplacentally) or through the birth canal to the fetus. GBS can cause early postpartum (puerperal) endometritis in the mother and septicemia in the infant.

✔ Tuberculosis is an increasing problem, particularly among immigrants. The incidence of TB and HIV infections occurring simultaneously is an important link in the increasing number of cases of multidrug-resistant TB. Pregnancy should be avoided until TB has been arrested for 2 years, because it may reactivate the disease.

✔ Toxic shock syndrome is a streptococcal infection that can cause severe systemic disease. Risk is increased by using tampons (especially superabsorbant types) and barrier contraceptives. Treatment includes hospitalization for control of fluid-electrolyte balance and administration of IV antibiotics.

REFERENCES

AIDS Commission raises alarm on epidemic in rural areas. (1990) *The Nation's Health, 22*(9), 1, 12.

Baer, D., Schuman, A. J., & Soloway, H. B. (1995). Lab diagnosis: On the cusp of change. *Patient Care, 29*(16), 61–66.

Bayer, R. (1995). Home testing for HIV: Has its time come? *Patient Care, 29*(16), 66–69.

Bowie, W. R., Hammerschlag, M. R., & Martin, D. H. (1994). STDs in '94: The new CDC guidelines. *Patient care, 28*(7), 29–53.

Brown, E. A., Hidenori, K., & Schiff, E. R. (1994). Hepatitis C & E: how much of a threat? *Patient Care, May 15*, 105–117.

Centers for Disease Control (1989) Recommendations of the Immunization Practices Advisory Committee. Measles prevention: Supplementary statement. *MMWR, Morbidity and Mortality Weekly Report, 38*(1), 11–14.

Centers for Disease Control (1990a). Protection against viral hepatitis—Recommendations of the Immunization Practices Advisory Committee (ACIP). *MMWR, Morbidity and Mortality Weekly Report, 39*(2), 16–19.

Centers for Disease Control (1990b). HIV prevalence estimates and AIDS case projections for the United States: Report based upon a workshop. *MMWR, Morbidity and Mortality Weekly Report, 39*(16), 1–15.

Centers for Disease Control (1990c). AIDS in women—United States. *MMWR, Morbidity and Mortality Weekly Report, 39*(47), 845–846.

Centers for Disease Control (1991). Mortality attributable to HIV infection/AIDS—United States, 1981–1990. *MMWR, Morbidity and Mortality Weekly Report, 40*(3), 41–55.

Centers for Disease Control (1994). Recommendations of the U.S. Public Health Service Taks Force on the use of zidovudine to reduce perinatal transmission of human immunodeficiency virus. *MMWR, Morbidity and Mortality Weekly Report, 43*(RR-11), 1–20.

Centers for Disease Control (1995a). Update: Acquired immunodeficiency syndrome—United States, 1994. *MMWR, Morbidity and Mortality Weekly Report, 44*(4), 64–67.

Centers for Disease Control (1995b). Update: AIDS among women—United States, 1994. *MMWR, Morbidity and Mortality Weekly Report, 44*(5), 81–84.

Centers for Disease Control (1995c). U.S. Public Health Service recommendations for human immunodeficiency virus counseling and voluntary testing for pregnant women. *MMWR, Morbidity and Mortality Weekly Report, 44*(RR-7), 1–15.

Centers for Disease Control (1995d). Update: Recommendations to prevent hepatitis B virus transmission—United States. *MMWR, Morbidity and Mortality Weekly Report, 44*(3), 574–575.

Clinical update (1994). Chlamydial infection: Formulating a plan of attack. *Clinician Reviews, 4*(7), 94–101.

Clinical Practice Guideline, No. 7. (1994). Evaluation and management of early HIV infection. USDHHS, PHS, Agency for Health Care Policy and Research, AHCPR Pub. No. 94-0572, Rockville, MD.

Clinical Guidelines (1995a). Sexually transmitted diseases and HIV infection. *The Nurse practitioner, 20*(2), 66–71.

Clinical Guidelines (1995b). Adult counseling for sexually transmitted diseases and HIV infection. *The Nurse Practitioner, 20*(10), 76–79.

Committee on Infectious Diseases and Committee on Fetus and Newborn, American Academy of Pediatrics (1992). Guidelines for prevention of group B streptococcal (GBS) infection by chemoprophylaxis. *Pediatrics, 90*(5), 775–778.

Corwin, E. (1996). *Handbook of pathophysiology* (p. 669). Philadelphia: Lippincott-Raven.

Deschamps, M. M. et al. (1993). A prospective study of HIV-seropositive asymptomatic women of childbearing age in a developing country. *Journal of Acquired Immune Deficiency Syndrome, 6*, 446–451.

Deutchman, M. E., Leaman, D. J., & Thomason, J. L. (1994). Vaginitis: Diagnosis is the key. *Patient Care, 28*(14), 39–61.

Dinsmoor, M. J. (1990). Group B streptococcus still poses a challenge. *Contemporary OB/GYN, 35*, 93–105.

Dunnihoo, D. R. (1992). *Fundamentals of gynecology and obstetrics* (p. 150). Philadelphia: J.B. Lippincott.

Edlin, B. R. et al. (1992). An outbreak of multidrug-resistant tuberculosis among hospitalized patients with the acquired immunodeficiency syndrome. *New England Journal of Medicine, 326*, 1514–1521.

Eschenbach, D. A. (1990). Pelvic infections and sexually transmitted diseases. In J. R. Scott et al. (Eds.), *Danforth's obstetrics and gynecology* (6th ed.). Philadelphia: J.B. Lippincott.

European Collaborative Study (1992). Risk factors for mother-to-child transmission of HIV-1. *Lancet, 39*, 1007–1012.

Fletcher, J., & Gordon, R. (1990). Perinatal transmission of bacterial sexually transmitted diseases. Part II: Group B streptococcus and chlamydia trachomatis. *Journal of Family Practice, 30*, 689–696.

Gallagher, R. J., & Fuller, C. A. (1994). Group B streptococcal disease: A life-threatening infection in the newborn. *Journal of the American Academy of Nurse Practitioners, 6*(8), 357–361.

Gilstrap, L. C., & Wendel, G. D. (1988). Urinary tract infections in pregnancy: Presentations and approaches. *PA—Physicians Assist,* 107–112.

Guide to Clinical Preventive Services (1989). *Report of the US Preventive Services Task Force.* Baltimore: Williams & Wilkins.

Hatcher, R. A., Stewart, F., Trussell, J. et al. (1990). *Contraceptive technology 1990–1992* (15th ed.). New York: Irvington Publishers.

HIV Guidelines Panel (1994). Quick reference guide for clinicians: Managing early HIV infection. *Journal of the American Academy of Nurse Practitioners, 6*(2), 65–81.

Institute of Medicine (1991). Offer pregnant women test for HIV antibodies. *The Nation's Health, XXI*(3), 2, March.

Killion, C. (1994). Pregnancy: A critical time to target STDs. *MCN: American Journal of Maternal Child Nursing, 19*(3), 156–161.

Krieger, J. N. et al. (1993). Clinical manifestations of trichomoniasis in men. *Annals of Internal Medicine, 118*, 844–849.

Koretz, R. L. et al. (1993). Non-A, non-B post-transfusion hepatitis: Looking back in the second decade. *Annals of Internal Medicine, 119*, 110–115.

Lindberg, C. E. (1995). Perinatal transmission of HIV: How to counsel women. *MCN: American Journal of Maternal Child Nursing, 40*(4), 207–212.

Mandell, G. L., Douglas, R. G., & Bennett, J. E. (Eds.) (1990). *Principles and practice of infectious diseases* (pp. 1006–1016) (3rd ed.). New York: Churchill Livingstone.

McCance, D. J. (1994). Human papilloma viruses. *Infectious Disease Clinics of North America, 8*(4), 751–764.

McGregor, J. A., Crombleholme, W. R., Newton, E. et al. (1994). Randomized comparison of ampicillin-sulbactam to cefoxitin and doxycycline or clindamycin and gentamicin in the treatment of pelvic inflammatory disease or endometritis. *Obstetrics and Gynecology, 83*, 998–1004.

Medical Letter (1994). Drugs for sexually transmitted diseases. *The Medical Letter,* 36/913, 1–6.

Mertz, G. J. (1993). Epidemiology of genital herpes infections. *Infectious Disease Clinics of North America, 7*(4), 825–839.

MMRW (1993a). Pregnancy outcomes following systemic prenatal acyclovir exposure—June 1, 1984–June 30, 1993. Oct. 22, 42, 806–809.

MMRW (1993b). Update: barrier protection against HIV infection and other sexually transmitted diseases. Aug 6, 42, 589–591.

MMRW (1993c). Measles—United States, first 26 weeks, 1993. Oct. 29, 42, 813–816.

MMRW (1994a). Decreased susceptibility of *Neisseria gonorrhoeae* to fluoroquinolones—Ohio and Hawaii. May 13, 43, 325–327.

MMRW (1994b). Progress toward global eradication of poliomyelitis, 1988–1993. July 15, 43, 499–503.

Nelson, J. A. (1995). HIV in adolescents. *MCN: American Journal of Maternal Child Nursing, 20*(1), 34–37.

Nunn, P., & Kochi, A. (1993). A deadly duo—TB and AIDS. *World Health, 4*, 7–9.

Pernoll, M. L. (Ed.) (1991). *Current obstetric and gynecologic diagnosis and treatment.* Norwalk, CT: Appelton & Lange.

Pizzo, P. A. (1990). Pediatric AIDS: problems within problems. *Journal of Infectious Diseases, 161*, 316.

Proffitt, M. R., & Yen-Lieberman, B. (1993). Laboratory diagnosis of human immunodeficiency virus infection. *Infectious Disease Clinics of North America, 7*(2), 203–216.

Redford, R. R., & Burke, D. S. (1989). HIV infection: The clinical picture. In *The science of AIDS: Readings from Scientific American Magazine* (pp. 63–74). New York: W.H. Freeman.

Rieder, H., & Raviglione, M. (1993). TB revisits the industrialized world. *World Health, 4*, 20–21.

Ronald, A. R. (1995). Slowing heterosexual HIV transmission. *Infectious Disease Clinics of North America, 9*(2), 287–296.

St. Louis, M. E. et al. (1993). Risk for perinatal HIV-1 transmission according to maternal immunologic, virologic, and placental factors. *Journal of the American Medical Association, 269*, 2853–2859.

Schaffer, S. D., & Philput, D. B. (1992). Predictors of abnormal cervical cytology: Statistical analysis of human papillomavirus and cofactors. *Nurse practitioner, 17*(3), 46–50.

Schieve, L. A., Handler, A., Hershow, R. et al. (1994). Urinary tract infection during pregnancy: Its association with maternal morbidity and perinatal outcome. *American Journal of Public Health, 84*, 405–410.

Secor, R. M. (1994). Bacterial vaginosis: A common infection with serious sequelae. *Advance for Nurse Practitioners, 2*(4), 11–15.

Selik, R. M. et al. (1993). HIV infection as leading cause of death among young adults in US cities and states. *Journal of the American Medical Association, 269*, 2991–2994.

Sodeyama, T. et al. (1993). Detection of hepatitis C virus markers and hepatitis C virus genomic-RNA after needlestick accidents. *Archives of Internal Medicine, 153*, 1565–1573.

Soper, D. E. (1994). Pelvic inflammatory disease. *Infectious Disease Clinics of North America, 8*(4), 821–840.

(1993). Drugs for AIDS and associated infections. *The Medical Letter, 35*(904), 79–86.

(1994). Drugs for sexually transmitted diseases. *The Medical Letter, 38*(913), 1–6.

Trabousli, E. I., & Maumenee, I. H. (1994). Eye problems. In F. A. Oski et al. (Eds.), *Principles and practice of pediatrics* (pp. 878–897). Philadelphia: J.B. Lippincott.

Tripathy, S. P. (1993). Multidrug-resistant tuberculosis. *World Health, 4*, 19.

Tsukuma, H. et al. (1993). Risk factors for hepatocellular carcinoma among patients with chronic liver disease. *New England Journal of Medicine, 328*, 1797–1801.

Vallejo, J. G. et al. (1994). Clinical features, diagnosis, and treatment of tuberculosis in infants. *Pediatrics, 94*, 1–7.

Walker, C. K. et al. (1993). Pelvic inflammatory disease: Meta-analysis of antimicrobial regimen efficacy. *Journal of Infectious Diseases, 168*, 969–916.

Wejstal, R. et al. (1992). Mother-to-infant transmission of hepatitis C virus. *Annals of Internal Medicine, 117*, 887–890.

Wiesenfeld, H. C., & Sweet, R. L. (1994). Perinatal infections. In J. R. Scott et al. (Eds.), *Danforth's obstetrics and gynecology* (7th ed.). Philadelphia: J.B. Lippincott.

12

Clinical Interruption of Pregnancy

Objectives

- Describe the factors affecting abortion services and availability.
- Discuss reasons women seek termination of pregnancy.
- Describe the impact of clients' rights and professional responsibility as they relate to abortion.
- Identify the key areas of nursing intervention necessary for the client undergoing an abortion.
- Discuss possible long-term physiologic and psychological sequelae of abortion.
- Compare and contrast the methods of pregnancy termination.
- Identify potential complications of abortion procedures and methods of prevention.
- Develop a plan of nursing care for women seeking and undergoing abortion.

Key Terms

Abortifacient
Amnioinfusion
Curettage
Dilation and
evacuation (D&E)

Dilation and curettage
(D&C)
Elective abortion
Laminaria
Mifepristone

Women have long sought **elective abortion** procedures to deliberately end a pregnancy, regardless of whether their culture approved or disapproved of this practice. Abortion is sought by women for a variety of reasons, including health, economics, marital status, family stability, the circumstances of conception, personal goals, age, and many other social and psychological factors. Although accurate abortion statistics are difficult to obtain, especially in countries where the procedure is illegal, it is estimated that 30 to 60 million pregnancies are intentionally ended each year throughout the world (Henshaw, 1990).

This chapter describes the current controversy surrounding elective abortion, including legislation and the issues of clients' rights, professional responsibility, and financing of abortion services. Nursing care of the client receiving an abortion, including the long-term sequelae, is discussed using a nursing process framework. The various types of abortion procedures used during the first and second trimester are presented.

Controversy About Abortion

Attitudes toward elective abortion and the availability of abortion procedures are strongly influenced by prevailing societal values. Whether the society's approach is permissive or restrictive depends on several factors: culture, economy, and ecology. For example, the existence of a predominant religion in a country can affect abortion laws and practices, as can the country's economic or sociopolitical system, population trends, level of technology, and standard of living. There also are critical ethical and legal implications associated with abortion (see Chap. 5 for a complete discussion).

The abortion rate in the United States is about 26 per 1,000 women of reproductive age, with slightly more than 1.5 million legal abortions performed annually (Henshaw et al., 1994). The rate of abortion is higher for nonwhite women (57%) than for white women (21%), although the number of abortions is smaller for nonwhite women because they constitute a smaller proportion of the population. Younger women have abortions more frequently, with peak incidence in the early to mid-20s. Abortion rates have increased markedly among minority women 15 to 30 years years (Henshaw, 1992). About 28% of all pregnancies are terminated by legal abortion (Costa, 1991).

In the United States, about half of all abortions are done within 8 weeks of the woman's last menstrual period (LMP). Ninety percent of abortions occur within 12 weeks of the LMP, with less than 1% done after 20 weeks of the LMP. The performance of legal abortions in early pregnancy has reduced morbidity and mortality. The mortality rate from abortions is 0.6 per 100,000 legal abortions (Henshaw, 1990). Nearly 90% of abortions are performed in nonhospital settings.

Legislation

The U.S. Supreme Court decision in 1973 (Roe versus Wade) legalized abortion, allowing elective abortions during the first trimester in all states. The decision was left up to the judgment of the woman and her physician during this time. Individual states were responsible for regulating second-trimester abortions and mandating additional regulations about the procedure.

Although abortion continues to be legal, gradual changes since Roe versus Wade have occurred through several Supreme Court decisions and state laws. In 1980, the Hyde Amendment (U.S. Congress, 1976) was upheld as constitutional by the U.S. Supreme Court. It prohibited the expenditure of federal funds for abortion services except when continuing the pregnancy would threaten the woman's life. With the Webster decision (U.S. Supreme Court, 1989), states were able to restrict use of public employees and facilities for abortion services or counseling (Chavkin et al., 1990). Rust versus Sullivan (U.S. Supreme Court, 1991) upheld federal regulations prohibiting Title X clinics (federally funded) from engaging in abortion counseling, referral, or advocacy (Harrison et al., 1991; Rhodes, 1990). This "gag rule" was lifted by presidential action in 1992, allowing family planning clinics to counsel women about abortion (Frankel, 1992). In July 1992, the Supreme Court ruled in Casey versus Planned Parenthood of Pennsylvania that states could allow a 24-hour waiting period from counseling to the performance of the procedure. It also provided for a mandatory notification of at least one parent if the client was younger than 18 years old.

Abortion is viewed with misgivings by many because of religious and personal attitudes. Abortion is not a substitute for pregnancy prevention. The procedures necessary for pregnancy termination, although generally safe, are associated with a higher morbidity than most contraceptive methods.

RESEARCH HIGHLIGHT

General Public Not as Polarized on Abortion as Surveys Imply

Most surveys of the public's attitudes toward abortion use a single, general item that offers three or four policy options. Surveys using only a few items overstate the strength of respondents' positions at either end of the scale (no restrictions on abortion versus abortion not permitted at all). This study used data from a CBS News/New York Times national survey, which included a wide variety of abortion-related questions. There were 1,347 respondents in six states. Responses were compared with the General Social Survey (GSS), which includes six specific items asking if abortion should be legal under various concrete circumstances (physical or social problems) and a more general item asking if abortion should always be legal.

The general questions elicited more all-or-none responses than did the specific questions. A series of items asking respondents to consider specific circumstances resulted in more respondents favoring abortion under some circumstances. Respondents appeared to take a position on general questions closest to where they place themselves when give a scale of seven specific circumstances. General questions with only one middle category induced respondents favoring strong restrictions to take the most conservative position and those favoring few restrictions to take the most

liberal option. With no middle category, there was a larger contingent who would place no restrictions on abortion. However, GSS-type items reveal that a large majority of respondents support some limitations on abortion.

The study concluded that general abortion questions with only one middle category produce higher estimates of respondents holding liberal and conservative views on abortion than do GSS-type specific questions. Descriptions of public opinion drawn from single items are misleading. Although the majority of people support legal abortion, most favor some restrictions. Of the minority who oppose legal abortion, many hedge on this position, depending on circumstances. This indicates that the general public is not as polarized as survey data suggest and that there is a substantial middle ground for a political compromise on abortion.

Critique: This sophisticated content-analysis study used a large national sample based in six states. Well established instruments (GSS, National Election Study) were used. Data were reported in percentages and inter-relationships between scale items evaluated by correlation analysis. Results are more believable than single-item, general question data. Nurses can use this information in their community and organizational work when seeking compromise in groups dealing with abortion issues.

Cook, E. A., Jelen, T. G., & Wilcox, C. (1993). Measuring public attitudes on abortion: Methodological and substantive considerations. *Family Planning Perspectives, 25*(3), 118–145.

Abortion remains a highly controversial issue in the United States. Since 1973, opponents have tried many strategies to restrict or prevent legal abortions. State legislatures have attempted to give the spouse veto power over the woman's abortion decision. Some have enacted laws requiring parental notification of abortion request by teenagers (Rogers et al., 1991). Restricting access to abortion counseling or services by preventing use of federal or state funds has impacted poor and minority women. Harassment of abortion providers has been an attempt to discourage professionals and clients. Between 80% and 90% of abortion facilities have experienced some form of the following types of harassment:

■ Picketing outside clinics
■ Vandalizing or bombing facilities
■ Tracing the identity of clients
■ Jamming telephone lines
■ Scheduling massive no-show appointments
■ Blocking clients' entrance to clinics
■ Picketing homes of staff members
■ Using death threats and murdering providers

These activities interfere with abortion services, making them more difficult and costly to provide because of the increased expenditures for security, legal ser-

vices, and insurance. The number of abortion providers has decreased, especially hospitals and physicians offices. Specialized abortion clinics perform about 70% of all abortions (Henshaw et al., 1994). Threats of violence against abortion providers make them less likely to work at abortion facilities, and these clinics are targeted by antiabortion protesters (Jerry, 1995).

Clients' Rights and Professional Responsibility

As professionals, nurses are committed to responding in a caring, competent manner to the needs of their clients. Women seeking abortion services have the right to expect and receive empathic, supportive, and nonjudgmental care from nurses. Nurses, as people and as professionals, have the right to their values, beliefs, and ethical perspectives. For many nurses, moral convictions and personal ethics dictate that abortion is unacceptable and that any participation in the care of clients seeking abortion violates these convictions. In this instance, the rights of clients and the rights of nurses are in conflict. The nurse has the right to refuse to participate in the care of clients seeking abortion to keep with personal moral and ethical beliefs. Most nurses with such beliefs avoid working in facilities that provide abortions. Only when a client's life is in immediate danger would it be necessary for nurses to assist women undergoing abortion, even if this violates the nurse's beliefs. Other nurses may choose to present alternatives to the client through counseling and referral services. Although nurses are entitled to their own perspectives on abortion, in general, the professional's responsibility is to advise the client of all options and expected outcomes and to assist her in making a personally satisfactory decision. The woman's perspective should be respected, although it may differ from the nurse's perspective.

The Association of Women's Health, Obstetrics, and Neonatal Nurses (formerly the Nurses' Association of the American College of Obstetricians and Gynecologists), in their position paper, described the rights of nurses and women undergoing abortion, giving guidelines for conflict resolution between professional responsibilities and personal ethics:

- Women have the right to expect and receive supportive, nonjudgmental care when undergoing elective abortion.
- Nurses have the right to refuse to assist with abortions or sterilizations in keeping with their own moral or religious beliefs, unless the woman's life is in danger.

Nurses need to examine their values and beliefs carefully and decide whether to participate in the care of clients seeking abortion. Conflicts, doubts, and confusion on the nurse's part frequently can be communicated to the client, possibly causing additional distress. Self-honesty and values clarification are important for the nurse; honoring the self must be done before effective, caring services can be provided to the patient (see Chap. 5).

Financing Abortion Services

As a result of the Hyde Amendment and Webster decision, federal funds (Medicaid) for support of abortion services have been withdrawn. As a result, many poor women have experienced restricted access to abortions except in some of the more populous states, such as California and New York, which have maintained more liberal standards for abortions and have paid for services with state funds.

Although the restrictions on publicly funded abortions did not completely eliminate use of federal funds, they have had a major impact. The number of federally subsidized abortions has decreased significantly (Daley et al., 1993). In states with restrictive policies, public financial support for abortions for poor women has been virtually eliminated. Poor women may raise the money to pay for their own abortions by diverting funds from something else, such as rent, utility bills, food, or clothing. They may borrow from friends or relatives, rely on charity, or travel out of state, risking delay and complications. Although the health of these women and their families has suffered, they have not been deterred from obtaining abortions. Even in states where federal funds were cut off, 65% to 80% of Medicaid-eligible women obtained legal abortions; an undetermined number received them illegally (Petchesky, 1990).

The accessibility of facilities that perform abortions also is an important factor. Nearly all abortions in the United States are done in metropolitan areas (about 98%). Most nonmetropolitan counties do not have any services. The number of hospitals that offer abortion services also has declined. This partially has been offset by an increase in free-standing clinics that perform about two-thirds of all abortions (Henshaw et al., 1990). Abortion rates vary dramatically by state, due to availability of abortion services, proportion of Hispanic population (which has above average abortion rates), degree of urbanization, and state policies related to public payment for abortion services for low-income women. States with the highest abortion rates include California, New York, Hawaii, Nevada, New Jersey, Delaware, and District of Columbia. Those with the lowest abortion rates include Wyoming, South Dakota, West Virginia, Idaho, Mississippi, Arkansas, and Indiana (Henshaw et al., 1990).

Many women travel to bordering states to obtain an abortion when there are no services in their home state. The distance women must travel is important in determining whether they can obtain services when needed. Information is more difficult to obtain when facilities are distant. Travel expenses may be prohibitive for poor women, including the costs of overnight lodging and loss of pay due to absence from work. Health risks are greater, because diagnosis and treatment of postabortion complications can be delayed. Privacy is jeopardized because of the need to be away from home and work for a longer time. Nationally, about 6% of abortions are performed on nonresidents of the state providing the service. Liberal states provide abortion services for a large proportion of nonresidents. More than half of the abortions done in the District of Columbia and 40% of those performed in Kansas, Kentucky, and North Dakota were for nonresidents (Henshaw et al., 1990).

The inequity in access to abortion services continues to worsen with the shift from hospital to clinic providers. The overall effect has been to reduce abortion services in states and counties where they were already limited. Women in many parts of the country must travel long distances to obtain abortions, resulting in considerable personal hardship and often delaying the procedure until later in pregnancy, when the risks are greater.

Care of the Client Undergoing an Abortion

The nurse is often a key professional, providing counseling to women considering abortion. Assisting the woman to consider alternatives and make responsible decisions about an unwanted pregnancy is part of client education and support. The nurse may offer initial discussion and assistance in problem solving to women or couples facing the problem of an undesired conception.

Nursing Assessment

Nursing assessment includes data about the client's physiologic, psychological, and social status. The nurse often encounters clients at an early stage in decision making and can provide valuable assistance in considering alternatives and arriving at an acceptable choice. The history follows the format used with women seeking contraception (see Chap. 9). Special attention is focused on the menstrual and obstetric history, medical and family history for conditions that increase surgical risk, contraceptive use, and abortion history.

The nurse assesses the woman's or couple's decision-making processes, with particular attention to expressions of ambivalence, confusion, or conflict. This process usually begins as soon as the woman suspects she may be pregnant, although some women may have thought through their desires and choices before becoming pregnant. Timing is critical in the abortion decision. An abortion should occur within the first 8 weeks of gestation to minimize the risk of complications, so the nurse must focus carefully on any decisional conflicts. Interventions to assist the client in resolving any conflicts or confusion need to be planned and instituted at the earliest possible time. The woman may want her partner or other significant person to be involved in the decision-making process. It is important to honor her wishes about involvement of important people, because this contributes to overall satisfaction with the decision.

An exploration of psychological factors is particularly important, especially signs of ambivalence or conflict. See Box 12-1. In most societies, the highest value placed on women is their role as mothers. Powerful systems of reinforcement operate to make motherhood central to women's lives. Because of the complex meanings and values associated with reproduction and motherhood, a decision to interrupt a pregnancy is rarely taken without some conflict.

Even if the outcome of pregnancy (a child) is consciously unwanted, the woman may on some level desire to be pregnant as a symbol of potency, vitality, or reconnection with primal inner forces. Although preg-

---

BOX 12-1
Psychological Factors in Pregnancy and Abortion

Purpose for Becoming Pregnant (complex meanings and values associated with reproduction and motherhood)
- Symbol of potency, vitality, or reconnection with primary inner forces
- Symbol of man's virility, potency
- Manipulation of relationships with particular people
- Maturity, sexuality, self-concept
- Elimination of feelings of inadequacy or doubts about femininity
- Avoidance of facing loss of reproduction capacity in the older woman

Purpose for Interrupting Pregnancy
- Marital status
- Quality of man–woman relationship
- Realization that motives for pregnancy were not appropriate
- Poor physical health (risk to life)
- Poor mental health (drain on energies, unable to cope)
- Educational or professional goals
- Conception too early in marriage
- Conception too soon after birth of previous child
- Emotionally unable to handle parenthood
- Financially unable to handle parenthood
- Rape or incest resulting in pregnancy
- Hereditary genetic defects
- Possible fetal anomalies
- Possible reactions of peers, family, community

---

nancy can be completely accidental, it can be used to affect relationships with important people in the woman's life, such as parents, husband, or lover. Examples of motives for pregnancy include the following:

- A teenage girl may become pregnant to demonstrate her maturity, prove her sexuality, or bolster her self-concept as a woman. Pregnancy may result because her romantic ideals of motherhood and man–woman relations preclude the use of contraceptives, which implies premeditated sexual activity.
- Pregnancy may result from youthful sexual experimentation, clouded mental functioning (substance use), or sexual risk taking when neither partner assumes responsibility for contraception.
- A woman at any age may use pregnancy as a means of alleviating feelings of inadequacy or doubts about her femininity. A woman entering menopause may conceive to reinforce her sexual self-image or avoid facing the loss of reproductive capacity.
- Pregnancy may be used to force a man into marriage. This is a poor basis on which to build a lifetime relationship.

- In marriages that are in trouble and facing dissolution, pregnancy may be used as an attempt to prevent a breakup or improve the relationship.
- A woman may become pregnant, even though she does not truly desire a child, to meet her partner's expectation, for example, if the man's sense of masculinity or potency requires that she become pregnant.

Reasons Women Seek Abortions

Although pregnancy may have been sought, the woman may find she cannot face the responsibilities of caring for and raising a child. Pregnancy in many cases does not produce the desired result, and the woman realizes motives for the pregnancy were misguided. She may elect abortion as the most feasible solution under the circumstances.

Poor physical or mental health can lead a woman to interrupt her pregnancy if it poses a risk to her life or a stress on her already depleted energies. A life crisis or emotional upheaval may lead a woman to feel incapable of coping with pregnancy and motherhood until her life becomes less chaotic.

Abortion also may be chosen when a pregnancy is untimely. Education or professional goals may have a higher priority at the time, or pregnancy may occur too early in a marriage or too soon after the birth of a child. The couple may feel emotionally or economically unable to manage parenthood. They choose to strive for a higher standard of living and greater social opportunity for themselves and their present children and are unwilling to be subjected to the increased material hardship of providing for another child.

Abortion may be sought for genetic reasons, even if pregnancy and the child are desired. Patients are becoming better informed about their genetic risks. Screening techniques are used to detect such conditions as Tay-Sachs disease, hemophilia, Down syndrome, sickle cell disease, and other genetic abnormalities. Awareness of fetal anomalies caused by rubella, exposure to radiation, and teratogenic drugs may cause some women to elect abortion if they were exposed during the first trimester.

Availability of fetal diagnostic techniques may lead to pressures to detect and abort abnormal fetuses. With limited social support for disabilities, parents may feel burdened with emotional and economic care of disabled children. Many women feel little choice but to abort defective fetuses whose disabilities would drain personal and societal resources (Rothman, 1990). Some women decide to continue pregnancy even with fetal abnormalities, using this time for practical and emotional preparation. For many, fetal diagnosis of abnor-

malities offers an opportunity to relieve suffering and the burden of chronic diseases and genetic disorders (Jackson, 1990).

Physical Examination and Diagnostic Tests

A focused physical examination is performed, with particular attention to signs of current illness, risk factors that might increase the potential for complications, the condition of the pelvic organs, and stage of gestation. An accurate estimation of uterine size is made, and the gestational age is estimated and compared with that obtained using the LMP. The position of the uterus (eg, anteversion, retroversion) is important for safe execution of the uterine evacuation procedure. The presence of physical structures that might interfere with the abortion procedure, such as uterine fibroids or adnexal masses, is carefully assessed.

Diagnostic tests usually include the following:

- Pregnancy test (urine or serum) to confirm pregnancy
- Hemoglobin or hematocrit to rule out anemia
- Blood type and Rh factor (Rh-negative women receive Rh immune globulin if not already sensitized)
- Screening for sexually transmitted diseases:
    Gonorrhea and *Chlamydia* cultures or immunoassay
    Syphilis (VDRL, STS)
    Wet mounts for *Monilia* and *Trichomonas*
    Human immunodeficiency virus
    Hepatitis B virus

Abdominal or transvaginal ultrasonography can detect ectopic pregnancies, molar pregnancies, women who are not pregnant, and pregnancies at a later gestational stage than clinical examination indicates (Kaali et al., 1990).

Nursing Diagnosis

Following the nursing assessment, the nurse is able to identify problems and formulate appropriate nursing diagnoses. A list of possible nursing diagnoses is shown in Box 12-2.

Nursing Planning and Intervention

Nursing intervention assists the patient to consider her alternatives, understand requirements for various abortion procedures, examine supports and resources, understand her reactions, express emotional needs, and locate or take advantage of facilities or financing methods. The nurse provides education about abortion procedures, preparation, recovery, complications, and

BOX 12-2
Potential Nursing Diagnoses

- Knowledge Deficit related to the following:
  - Options available and abortion procedures indicated
  - Self-care
  - Abortion experience
  - Complications
  - Sexual activity
  - Contraception
  - Community resources
- Ineffective Coping related to the following:
  - Depression
  - Feelings of failure
  - Feelings of sadness, worry, and fear
  - Moral or ethical conflict
  - Negative self-concept
  - Disapproval by others
  - Inadequate problem solving
  - Inadequate support systems
- Anticipatory Grieving related to loss of the pregnancy
- Altered Sleep Patterns related to anxiety or depression
- Altered Family Processes related to stress, communication difficulties
- Anxiety related to abortion procedures and consequences
- Decisional Conflict related to mixed motives regarding pregnancy
- Self Esteem Disturbance with negative feelings, shame or guilt, feeling unable to deal with events and make decisions
- Spiritual Distress related to religious or personal ethical conflicts
- Pain related to the abortion procedure
- Risk for Injury related to the following:
  - Post-abortion infection
  - Hemorrhage
- Risk for infection related to retained products of conception

contraception (see Nursing Care Plan: The Woman/Couple Interrupting a Pregnancy).

Exploring Alternatives

Many women need help to think beyond their first reaction to the unwanted pregnancy. They need to be encouraged to consider other options available to them. Many women often feel ambivalent and confused because of pressure from family or their own social values. The nurse must encourage the woman to make the decision for herself. There is less regret and emotional sequelae when the choice is the woman's and is not perceived as having been forced on her by other people. Exploring alternatives realistically helps

clarify the situation, placing manageable boundaries within which the decision can be made. Women often need help thinking through what each choice means, not only for present feelings and relations, but also for future circumstances, goals, and needs. The choices should be considered from a practical and an emotional and values standpoint. The nurse encourages a carefully weighed choice.

While the counseling is in progress, tests are carried out to confirm the pregnancy and determine the length of gestation. Based on the results, the type of abortion procedure indicated is discussed. These factors alone may influence the decision. Simply knowing that the pregnancy has progressed beyond the time when simple evacuation can be used and that the abortion may actually involve labor and expulsion of the fetus may cause a woman to decline abortion. Understanding the nature of the procedure required is essential to informed decision making (Fig. 12-1).

Educating About Procedures and Experiences

Information about the abortion procedure and what women usually experience is an important nursing intervention. The type of procedure is determined by the length of gestation, the experience of the physician, and the medical evaluation of patient suitability for the procedure. While teaching the client about the procedure and what to expect, the nurse needs to take into account any factors that increase physiologic and psychological risk. The procedures, pain experience, and possible complications are discussed.

Surgical Methods. In the United States, surgical methods are most commonly used, including vacuum curettage, **dilation and evacuation** (D&E), **dilation and curettage** (D&C), and hysterotomy or hysterectomy.

- Vacuum (suction) curettage is the most widely used procedure, generally done before 9 weeks' gestation. This method can be done in an office setting through 16 weeks' gestation when there is appropriate backup available for handling complications.
- D&E extends the vacuum curettage into the second trimester, using cervical dilation to accommodate removal of fetuses ranging from 13 through 20 weeks' gestation.
- The traditional D&C uses a sharp, metal curette to remove the uterine contents. It is used infrequently because it is more painful and causes more blood loss with greater cervical dilation.
- Hysterotomy and hysterectomy are used when concomitant sterilization or other gynecologic surgery is necessary.

NURSING CARE PLAN
The Woman/Couple Interrupting a Pregnancy

Nursing Goals
1. Woman/couple reaches acceptable decision regarding continuing or interrupting a pregnancy.
2. Woman seeks early confirmation of pregnancy and first-trimester abortion to minimize risk and trauma, or seeks early prenatal care if pregnancy is to be continued.
3. Woman/couple understands procedures as indicated by gestational age and clarifies misunderstandings or fears.
4. Woman/couple obtains psychological counseling if indicated.
5. Woman/couple obtains information about effective contraception to avoid future unwanted pregnancy.

Assessment	Potential Nursing Diagnoses	Intervention/ Rationale	Evaluation
Menstrual history and last menstrual period, use of contraceptives Assist in physical examination, collection of specimens, pregnancy tests to determine length of gestation Understanding of physiology of conception and contraceptive methods Consideration of alternatives to abortion Pregnancy and health history to identify special needs and risks	Knowledge Deficit related to options available, procedures, normalcy of emotions, self-care, post-procedure care, expected bleeding or cramping, signs and symptoms of complications, resumption of sexual activity, contraception, sexuality, community resources, follow-up care Altered Comfort: Pain related to abortion procedure Risk for Infection related to tissue trauma	Advise of length of gestation and what type of procedure this indicates; discuss various types of abortion procedures, time in hospital or if outpatient, techniques and what the experience entails, risks and complications *to provide information on which to base decision.* Explore alternate choices (ie, have abortion or continue pregnancy and either keep the baby or give baby for adoption) and meanings these have for woman, partner, and family *to support decision making.* Assist during procedures; minimize tissue trauma and risk of infection; provide pain relief, support, and clarification; and keep client informed of process *to encourage cooperation and successful procedure.* Advise of postabortion complications, when to seek medical care, preventive measures, and when to resume activities and sex *to promote recovery and prevent complications.* Discuss contraception follow-up visits, and emotional reactions *to avoid future unwanted pregnancy.*	Able to reach decision about pregnancy termination with which woman/couple feels comfortable Accepts requirements of various procedures as indicated by gestational age Affirms understanding of process of conception and effective use of contraceptive method Returns for follow-up visit and institutes contraceptive method Feels accepting of abortion if undertaken; no serious emotional problems Seeks prenatal care if abortion decided against Avoids future unwanted pregnancies

(continued)

NURSING CARE PLAN *(Continued)*
The Woman/Couple Interrupting a Pregnancy

Assessment	Potential Nursing Diagnoses	Intervention/ Rationale	Evaluation
		For midtrimester abortion, monitor during labor, provide pain relief and supportive care, and facilitate presence of companion if desired *to encourage successful procedure.*	
Circumstances surrounding unwanted conception Level of ambivalence or certainty about abortion decision Involvement of partner, family, parents, and sources of support Presence of crisis, need for further psychological counseling	Ineffective Individual Coping leading to depression related to unresolved emotional responses (guilt, regret) Self-Concept Disturbance related to pregnancy Altered Family Processes related to the effects of abortion on relationships (disagreements, marital and personal conflicts, adolescent identity problems) Altered Sexuality Patterns related to stress or conflict, pain, fear	Initiate referral to psychological counseling if indicated *to deal with psychological problems.* Provide opportunity to express emotional responses, conflicts, problems *to relieve stress and tension.* Initiate referral to psychological or sexual counseling if indicated *to deal with problems.* Provide opportunity to express emotional responses, conflicts, problems *to relieve stress and promote resolution.*	Initiates psychological counseling if emotionally distressed Expresses emotional responses openly, seeks resolution to conflicts and problems Initiates psychological/sexual counseling if emotionally distressed Expresses emotional responses openly, seeks resolution to conflicts and problems

Most women who undergo suction or vacuum curettage experience pain during and after the uterine evacuation. Women's pain experience varies widely. Abortion pain is ranked as moderately intense. Preabortion depression is the principal predictor of pain intensity during abortion and is significantly correlated with other measures of emotional distress, such as anxiety, ambivalence, fear, greater pain expectancy, and tendency toward emotionality. Women who are younger and less educated report higher levels of pain, as do those with moral conflicts and concerns about others' judgment. Other factors associated with higher levels of pain include dysmenorrhea, a retroverted uterus, and early (5–7 weeks) or later gestations (more than 16 weeks) that require additional dilation and aspiration (Belanger et al., 1989).

In many clinics, **laminaria,** dried seawead substance, is inserted shortly before the abortion procedure. This material readily absorbs moisture and expands to dilate the cervix over a 6-hour period. It is relatively painless and effective, slowly dilating the cervix to facilitate the curettage procedure and decreasing the chance of cervical laceration (Fig. 12-2).

Local anesthesia, such as a paracervical block, is administered in most settings, often accompanied by a mild analgesic or sedative.

Early abortion under local anesthesia is well tolerated by most women, especially those who are clear about their desire to terminate pregnancy, are more mature and well educated, and do not have anatomic or physiologic variations contributing to more intense pain experiences. Women who are ambivalent or depressed before the procedure, are younger, have moral and social concerns, have low pain threshold, and have other anatomic or physiologic factors may require additional pain management to ensure a comfortable and safe abortion. This might include additional narcotic analgesia or a general anesthetic (Belanger et al., 1989).

Complications. Complications from early abortions are extremely infrequent, and compared with childbirth, legal abortion is remarkably safe. The most frequent complications include hemorrhage, infection, and retained products of conception. Deaths due to abortion range from 0.5 per 100,000 abortions in the first trimes-

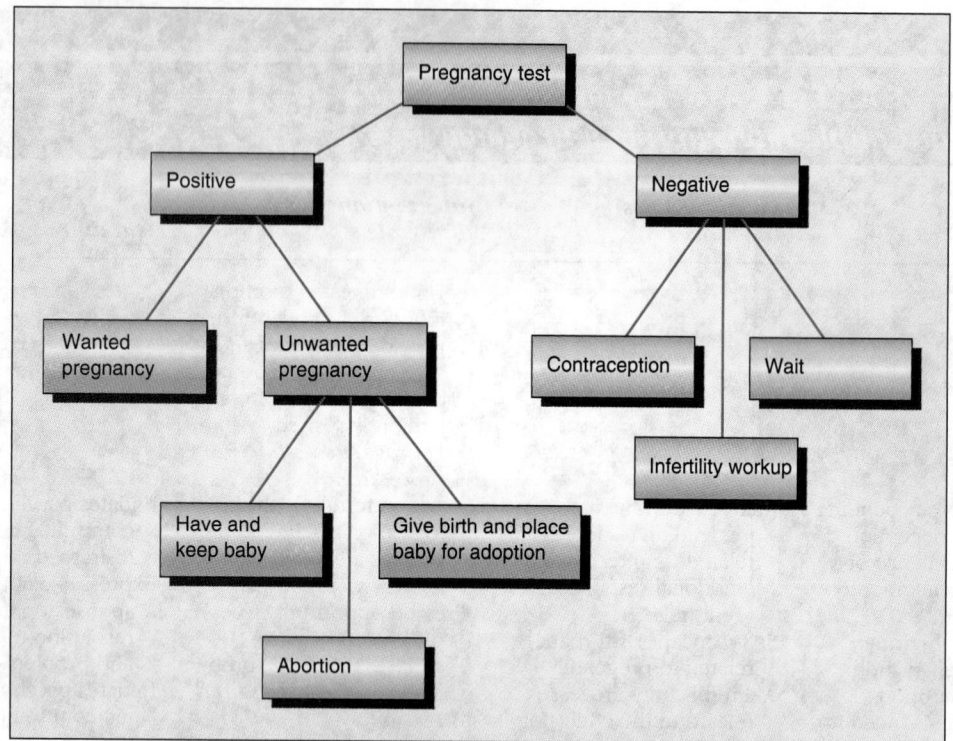

FIGURE 12-1 Decision tree for pregnancy alternatives.

ter to 10 per 100,000 abortions during the late second trimester. Younger women have fewer complications than older women. Complications are fewer in early pregnancy (less than 12 weeks) and in healthy patients who are not ambivalent about having the abortion performed. Providers with specific training and more experience have fewer complications. The number of resident physicians receiving abortion training has declined.

Treatment for Complications. Oxytocic drugs, usually methergine, are administered for heavy postabortion bleeding. If hemorrhage occurs, the physician searches for the cause (ie, retained products, uterine perforation, cervical laceration) and corrects it, often surgically. Infections are treated with broad-spectrum antibiotics. Retained tissue may cause severe cramping, fever, or abnormal discharge. The uterus must be evacuated completely and antibiotics given as indicated (Turk, 1990).

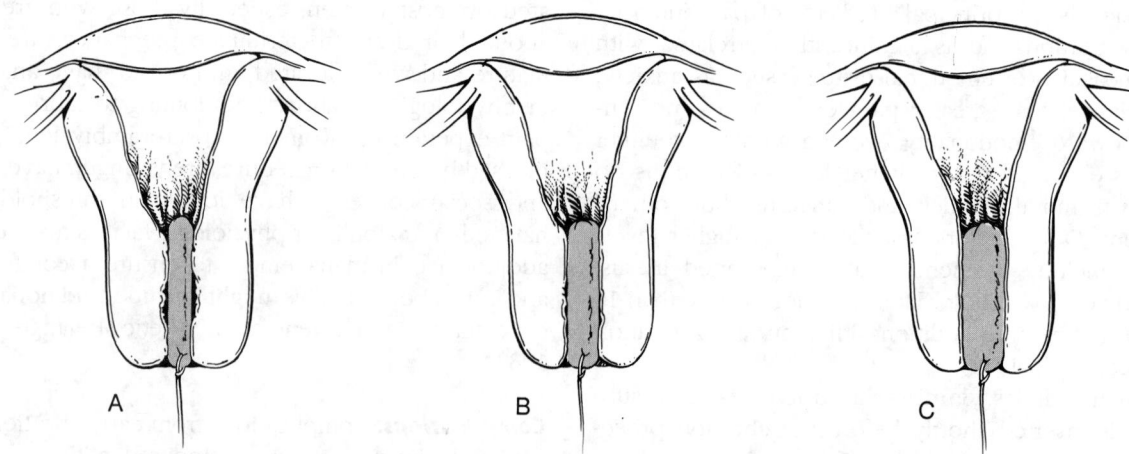

FIGURE 12-2 Laminaria used for cervical dilation. (**A**) Inserted in cervical canal beyond internal os. (**B**) Hygroscopic material absorbs fluid and distends. (**C**) Maximum distention and cervical dilation in 6 to 12 hours.

Providing Supportive Care

Nursing intervention focuses on emotional support and creating a caring environment. Most nursing diagnoses for pregnancy termination involve psychological factors and emotional distress. The nurse assists the client to identify and express feelings, supports positive self-evaluations and coping behaviors, mobilizes support systems, helps the client learn new coping skills, and assists in exploring value conflicts and value clarification techniques. The nurse teaches constructive problem-solving techniques and assists the client to use her personal strengths and previous experiences. Discussing alternatives and encouraging a fully informed decision are the core of nursing interventions.

When family processes are altered, the nurse assists the family to acknowledge feelings about the situation, communicate openly about perceptions and feelings, expand understanding of the other family members' experiences, and identify and use family strengths. The family is helped to appraise the situation, identify choices and consequences, and find sources of additional professional or social assistance.

Preventing Complications

The nurse teaches the patient to recognize and prevent postabortion problems. The most common complications include infection, retained products of conception, intrauterine blood clots, continuing pregnancy, cervical or uterine trauma, and bleeding.

Infection is the most common problem, and the nurse teaches the woman to identify the signs of infection and report these promptly to the provider or clinic. The woman also is taught how to prevent infection after the abortion (see Client Education: Minimizing the Risk of Postabortion Infections).

The woman is instructed about what to expect physiologically and emotionally after abortion. This assists her to recognize normal postabortion reactions and to know when to seek help for possible complications. Emotional responses are discussed, and parameters for normal postabortion feelings are identified (see Client Education: What to Expect After Abortion).

Follow-up Care

A follow-up office visit is scheduled for 2 weeks after the abortion, at which time contraceptives are prescribed if not already begun. The client's adjustment to termination of pregnancy and her partner's or family's reactions can be discussed; referrals are made if needed for psychological, social, or economic reasons.

Two weeks after an abortion, uterine size should be normal, and bleeding usually should have ceased. The

---

CLIENT EDUCATION
Minimizing the Risk of Postabortion Infections

Taking good care of yourself after your abortion can make a big difference in the way you feel. These things can bolster your general health and help to prevent infection.

- Listen to your body, and keep alert to signs of infection. Take your temperature twice each day. Call the clinic if it is over 100.4°F, which could indicate infection.
- Avoid inserting anything into the vagina.
- Do not use tampons until your first normal period. Use only pads.
- Do not take tub baths, use hot tubs or douches, or go swimming for at least 2 weeks.
- Do not have vaginal intercourse or oral-vaginal sex for at least 2 weeks. Other forms of love making are fine.
- Eat foods that are good for you. Vegetables, protein, and whole grains help you recover more quickly.
- Get enough sleep and rest. This allows your body to use its energy to heal. Avoid putting pressure on yourself for a few weeks.
- Exercise sensibly. If your usual exercises cause increased bleeding, stop them for 1 week.
- Call the clinic if you experience any of the following:
    - Fever over 100.4°F
    - Prolonged heavy bleeding
    - Severe cramping or one-sided abdominal or pelvic pain
    - Change in odor (foul) of vaginal discharge
    - Passing large clots or white-gray tissue
- When you call the clinic, have the following information available:
    - Your temperature taken within the last hour
    - Number of pads used during the last 2 hours
    - Any medicine taken (such as aspirin, acetaminophen) and how long ago
    - The telephone number of your pharmacy

---

client is evaluated for any signs of complications or for continuing pregnancy (ongoing symptoms of pregnancy, enlarged uterus). Concerns about long-term sequelae of abortion are discussed.

Long-Term Sequelae of Abortion. Data on physiologic complications of legal elective abortions show that risks are minimal. The overall complication rate for first-trimester abortions is about 1% (Hakim-Elahi et al., 1990). In second-trimester abortions, a 10% to 15% rate of complications occurs. Early first-trimester abortions have 0% to 1% longer term sequelae, such as subsequent infertility, ectopic pregnancy, spontaneous abor-

CLIENT EDUCATION
What to Expect After Abortion

Bleeding

Bleeding similar to that of your menstrual period, lasting about 1 week, is the most usual pattern after abortion. Every woman is an individual, and the amount of bleeding varies. Some women have almost no bleeding; others have heavier than usual bleeding. Excessive bleeding would be soaking through several pads in 2 to 3 hours, having a very heavy flow for more than 2 days, and bleeding that lasts more than 2 weeks.

Cramping

It is not unusual to have cramping for a few days after the abortion. Aspirin, acetaminophen, or heat to the abdomen usually relieves the cramps.

Clots

Blood clots may or may not be expelled after an abortion. These are usually dark red or brown. Cramping may get worse as the uterus is trying to expel clots. Cramps usually stop once the clots are expelled. Severe persistent cramps and clots that are gray-white may indicate complications.

Menstruation

The next normal menstrual period usually begins in 4 to 6 weeks, although a few women have a period in 2 weeks. If birth control pills are started right after an abortion, the next period should occur 2 to 3 days after the last active pill in the pack. If menstruation has not occurred by 8 weeks, medical evaluation is indicated.

Breast Soreness

Some women may have breast tenderness for the first few days after an abortion. Occasionally there may be a little milk the second through fourth day, which stops in a few days.

Contraception

Pregnancy can occur before your next period. You should decide on a contraceptive method and be prepared to use it as soon as you resume intercourse. If you have not selected another method, you should insist that your partner use a condom or use foam. Using both together is most effective.

Medications

If your provider has given you medications (antibiotics are most common), be sure to take all the pills as directed. If you notice a rash or hives, call the clinic right away.

Feelings

Many women experience strong feelings after an abortion. You may feel great relief and elation that you have made a difficult decision and come to terms with yourself, or you may feel sadness and a sense of loss. This is a normal feeling, and you may want to talk to someone close about how you feel. Sometimes women experience feelings that seem beyond their control, such as depression or anger. Discussing your feelings with friends or seeing a counselor can provide important support.

---

tions, premature delivery, and low–birth-weight babies. Risk of problems with subsequent pregnancy appears related to use of traumatic procedures (eg, sharp curettage), but social and geographic factors confound the data (Costa, 1991).

Studies show that psychological problems after induced abortion are rare. Distress and depression are more commonly reported before the abortion than after it. Relief and happiness are much more common in the weeks after abortion of an unwanted pregnancy. When women do have negative reactions after abortion, these are mainly related to uncertainty about having the abortion, delay in decision making, lack of support from others, and need to terminate a wanted pregnancy (ie, for fetal defects). Most psychological sequelae are short-lived (Adler et al., 1990; Rogers, et al, 1989).

Urban African American adolescent women undergoing abortion were found to experience less negative change than a control group that continued their pregnancies. After 2 years, the young women who terminated their pregnancies were far more likely to have graduated from high school or still be in school at the appropriate grade level. They also were better off economically and had not experienced greater levels of stress or anxiety. The teenagers who obtained abortions were less likely than those continuing pregnancy to have a subsequent pregnancy and were more likely to practice contraception. They did well on several measures of psychological well-being (Zabin et al., 1989).

When abortion is legal and socially accepted, deciding to have an abortion usually does not cause major psychological trauma. Psychological sequelae generally are of short duration and reflect the circumstances surrounding abortion and attitudes conveyed by peer groups, family, and health providers. Americans' attitudes toward abortion have become more accepting during the last decade (Gallop et al., 1990).

Evaluation

Nursing care is successful when the woman makes an informed decision (whether to interrupt or to continue the pregnancy), feels comfortable with her decision, and follows through with appropriate care (whether for abortion or prenatal care). She has adjusted well if she expresses emotional responses openly and seeks resolution to her conflicts and problems. Effective care results in her returning for a follow-up visit and using a suitable contraceptive method to prevent further unwanted pregnancies.

If the woman continues to experience emotional distress, problems with self-esteem, ineffective coping, or altered family processes, care is effective when she initiates psychological counseling (individually or for the family), as appropriate. Additional nursing intervention may be necessary for unresolved problems or if counseling assistance has not been sought.

Abortion Procedures

The approach to pregnancy termination varies according to gestational age. Before the 12th week, abortion is a relatively uncomplicated vaginal procedure, using vacuum curettage, D&E, or D&C. Prior dilation of the cervix is achieved with laminaria, prostaglandin gels, or magnesium sulfate sponges. Prostaglandins may be used in the form of vaginal suppositories, intramuscular injections, or transcervical instillation to induce abortion.

Beyond the 12th week, interruption requires more complex procedures. D&E, the most frequently used method, is safest between 13 and 16 weeks, but has an increased rate of morbidity and mortality than if it was done in the first trimester.

Amnioinfusion in used for pregnancies 16 weeks and beyond. It is most effective at 16 to 18 weeks' gestation. The amnioinfusion solution may be prostaglandin, hypertonic saline (20%), or urea. Providers are performing an increasing percentage of second-trimester abortions using a combination of techniques for their dilating, fetocidal, and uterine contracting effects. For example, laminaria may be used for dilation, intrauterine instillation of urea may be used for fetocidal effects, and prostaglandin may be used for uterine-contracting effects (Turk, 1990).

Vacuum (Suction) Curettage

The procedure of choice for the termination of early pregnancy is vacuum **curettage,** which is cleansing of a surface using a spoon-shaped instrument (Fig. 12-3). The cervix is gently dilated over 6 to 24 hours before the procedure with laminaria or prostaglandin gel. The laminaria, when placed in the cervical canal, expands gradually by absorbing fluid. A local anesthetic (paracervical block) or a spinal anesthetic may be used for the curettage procedure. The cervix is dilated with graduated dilators, and a suction curette is placed into the endometrial cavity to the fundus. Suction is ap-

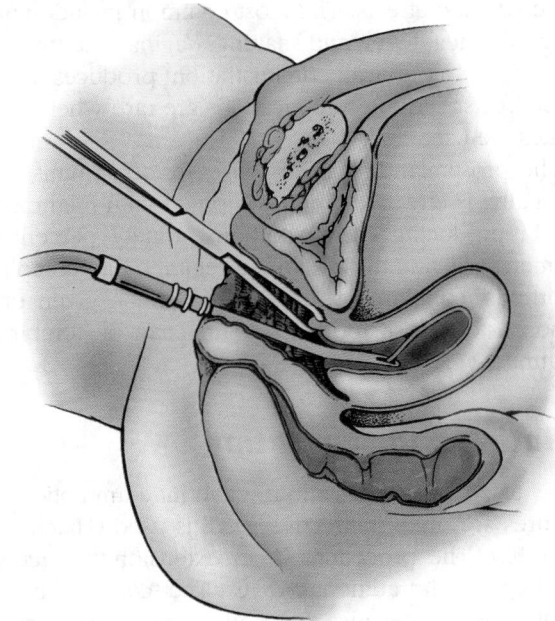

FIGURE 12–3 Vacuum curettage.

plied, usually by an electric pump, and the products of conception are evacuated into a container. These are usually sent to the pathology laboratory for confirmation of the pregnancy and to rule out unusual conditions, such as hydatidiform mole. Generally, recovery takes from 2 to 3 hours, during which time the client is observed for excessive bleeding.

Insertion of a laminaria several hours before the procedure can reduce the need for mechanical cervical dilation and may decrease the incidence of cervical lacerations. The most common complications following a vacuum curettage are infection, hemorrhage, retained products of conception or blood clots in the uterus, and cervical or uterine trauma.

Dilation and Curettage

Occasionally, D&C, which requires a surgical (sharp) curette, is used for first-trimester abortions. However, it requires greater amounts of anesthesia and preoperative precautions. The cervix must be dilated more than for vacuum curettage, and there is a greater risk of cervical laceration and blood loss. This technique is widely used and known by family physicians, general practitioners, and obstetrician-gynecologists.

Prostaglandins

Prostaglandins, a group of fatty acid compounds, are effective **abortifacients** (agents that induce abortion) at any stage of pregnancy. The exact mechanisms by which they work are not clearly understood. Oral administration is impractical because of the high incidence of side effects. The most common include vomiting, diarrhea, fever, and shaking. Vaginal, intramuscular, and transcervical administration produces fewer side effects. Serious complications are rare when these routes are used.

The prostaglandin analog *misoprostol,* administered vaginally, is effective when combined with methotrexate in producing early abortions. Ninety percent of women receiving the combined regimen had complete abortions, compared with 47% of women given only misoprostol. Most aborted the first day of combined treatment (Creinin et al., 1994).

Dilation and Evacuation

At 13 to 20 weeks' gestation, when intra-amniotic procedures are often ineffective, D&E is used (Hatcher et al, 1990). The procedure is an extension of vacuum curettage and traditional D&C. The cervix requires greater dilation because the products of conception are larger. Usually laminaria is inserted for gradual cervical dilation before the procedure. After administration of a paracervical block or general anesthesia, graduated metal dilators are introduced until the cervix is adequately dilated. A large suction cannula (14–16 mm) is used to remove pregnancy tissue. Forceps or crushing instruments may be needed to remove fetal tissue completely.

After the uterus has been emptied, a sharp curette is often used to explore the cavity for any remaining tissue. All fetal parts must be removed before oxytocic agents are administration. Some providers administer prophylactic antibiotics to reduce the risk of infection. The most common complications include infections, retained products, hemorrhage, and cervical injury.

These abortions are less stressful for women than amnioinfusion abortions using a substance to induce labor and fetal expulsion. Because D&E often requires a destructive procedure, the psychological impact of second-trimester abortion may be transferred from the woman to the physician.

Hypertonic Saline

When pregnancy has progressed beyond the 16th week, termination may be done by instilling *hypertonic saline* into the amniotic cavity. This procedure is most easily carried out when there is sufficient fluid in the amniotic cavity to be identified and aspirated. The bladder is emptied, and the client is placed in the supine position. The skin is prepped and draped with sterile towels and infiltrated with a local anesthetic over the injection site. An 18-gauge spinal needle is inserted through the uterus into the amniotic cavity. About 200 mL of amniotic fluid is withdrawn, and the same volume of hypertonic saline (20%–25% solu-

tion) is injected into the amniotic cavity over about 15 minutes.

After a latent period of several hours, labor usually ensues, and the fetus and part or all of the placenta are delivered within 24 to 72 hours. If the placenta cannot be extracted completely after delivery, a curettage is carried out to complete the abortion. During the course of labor, the contractions can cause considerable discomfort. As the cervix dilates, the patient should be medicated at intervals. Generally, a substantial amount of emotional support is needed during this process. The previable fetus is usually dead at the time of delivery, but at this later stage of gestation, it has human form.

Oxytocin infusion is often used as an adjunct to saline abortion to decrease the time needed for completing the process. Oxytocin is used in a manner similar to that used for induction of labor (see Chap. 37), except that a more concentrated solution is used. The oxytocin infusion is started 6 to 12 hours after amnioinfusion of saline and continued for up to 24 hours. Use of oxytocin longer than this period may result in water intoxication. If hypertonic saline fails to induce contractions, a repeat dose must be administered.

Use of hypertonic saline is contraindicated in severe hypertension. Complications most often include hemorrhage, infection, and retained placenta. Occasionally, more serious complications occur as a result of the intravenous injection of saline, including hypernatremia, amniotic fluid embolism, disseminated intravascular coagulation, and necrosis of the myometrium from saline entering the uterine musculature.

Hypertonic Urea

A 30% solution of urea can be used to terminate second-trimester pregnancies using the same technique as described for the hypertonic saline infusion. This agent is advantageous because it is relatively safe, low cost, and highly fetocidal. When used alone, however, urea has a high failure rate for inducing successful abortions. It is usually combined with prostaglandins, which stimulate uterine contractions and induce labor, with delivery occurring within 12 hours. Oxytocin also may be used to stimulate and continue effective labor.

Intra-amniotic Prostaglandin F2-Alpha

Instillation of prostaglandin F2-alpha ($F_{2\alpha}$) into the amniotic cavity by a similar amniocentesis technique is another method of inducing midtrimester abortions. It has a lower complication rate than saline instillation between 16 and 20 weeks and a more rapid onset of labor with subsequent expulsion. Medication can be used to control the gastrointestinal side effects (nausea and vomiting). Women with asthma or pulmonary disease are at increased risk for problems because the drug can cause marked bronchospasm.

When used as the only agent, 40 to 45 mg of prostaglandin $F_{2\alpha}$ is instilled by intra-amniotic infusion. Labor is usually shorter than with saline solution, and related complications are avoided. Its disadvantages include the potential for delivering a live fetus, the cost of the medication, and risk of complications, such as cervical lacerations and retained products of conception.

Vaginal Prostaglandin E_2

Prostaglandin E_2 prepared as a vaginal suppository is used in patients to induce abortions and to assist evacuation in patients with missed abortions. The 20-mg vaginal suppositories have a high incidence of gastrointestinal side effects and often affect the thermoregulatory mechanism, causing some patients to have a temperature elevation. Other complications are similar to those with prostaglandin $F_{2\alpha}$.

Hysterotomy

When other methods of midtrimester abortion fail or if D&E, saline, or prostaglandins are contraindicated for various reasons, a hysterotomy or minicesarean section may be performed. The operation is major surgery and may be done abdominally or vaginally. This procedure requires the standard preoperative preparations and general or spinal anesthesia. The morbidity and mortality from this procedure are greater than for other techniques, and a live fetus may be delivered. Advantages of this method include the opportunity for concomitant sterilization by tubal ligation or hysterectomy and treatment of pelvic disease. Mortality rates for several methods of pregnancy interruption are summarized in Table 12-1.

RU 486 (Mifepristone)

Mifepristone is a progesterone antagonist that has been investigated as an early abortifacient and a mid-cycle contraceptive. The action of RU 486 prevents implantation of a fertilized ovum by blocking the effects of progesterone. Taken within 10 days of the expected onset of the missed period, up to 8 weeks after conception, it is highly effective in producing an abortion. Mifepristone decreases cervical resistance to dilation in pregnant and nonpregnant women, facilitating abortions and gynecologic procedures (Gupta et al., 1990).

The effectiveness of mifepristone is related to length of gestation, human chorionic gonadotropin (hCG) levels, and the patient's weight. Obese women with higher hCG levels (or longer gestations) have increased failure rates. Complete abortion after adminis-

TABLE 12-1
Mortality Rates for Abortion Procedures*

Type of Procedure	Mortality Rate
Vacuum aspiration or curettage	
< 8 weeks	0.2
9–10 weeks	0.3
11–12 weeks	0.6
16–20 weeks	3.7
> 20 weeks	12.7
Intra-amniotic infusions	4.9
Hysterotomy or hysterectomy	58.9

*Deaths per 100,000 abortions, with relative risk based on index rate for vacuum curettage abortions.

(Henshaw, S. K. [1990]. Induced abortion: A world review, 1990. *Family Planning Perspectives, 22* [3], 102–108.)

tration of RU 486 occurs in 85% to 94% of women up to the 10th week of gestation (U.K. Multicentre Trial, 1990). Administration of 600 mg of RU 486 causes complete expulsion in 60% of patients overall. The addition of prostaglandins accomplishes abortions in 95% to 100% of patients (Dunnihoo, 1992). Failure to induce abortion is <4%; incomplete abortions, 2%; and mortality, 1 per 100,000 users (Lader, 1991).

The medication is well tolerated with fewer gastrointestinal side effects than prostaglandins and less severe cramping. Women beyond 50 days' gestation have more painful contractions using RU 486 than those in earlier pregnancy. Severe or prolonged bleeding are the main complications. About 9% of women experience severe bleeding in the 2 days after the medication. A small number of women experience hemorrhage that requires curettage and blood transfusion (U.K. Multicentre Trial, 1990).

Mifepristone is widely used in Europe. It offers a reasonable alternative to surgical abortions by vacuum or sharp curettage, which require some form of anesthetic and often analgesia. Women who express fear of surgery or anesthesia often prefer this method (Henshaw et al., 1993).

RU 486 is not yet approved for use in the United States. There has been some public controversy about its safety and efficacy (The Debate, 1987). The Population Council conducted clinical trials of RU 486 in this country in spring 1995 to obtain Food and Drug Administration approval (Newsline, 1994). In reaction to the trials, a coalition of antiabortion groups boycotted products made by affiliates of Roussel Uclaf (the French manufacturer of RU 486; Drug Update, 1994). This political and economic battle regarding the rights of the unborn has been described as limiting options for meeting women's healthcare needs (Regelson et al., 1990).

Other Uses of Mifepristone

This medication softens and dilates the cervix, suppresses breast tumors, blocks ovulation, and opposes endometrial proliferation. RU 486 has shown benefit in treating patients with breast and endometrial cancer, endometriosis, Cushing's disease, and inoperable meningioma. It may be useful in uterine evacuation after fetal death and has been considered for contraception in women 35 to 50 years old (Donaldson et al., 1994; Costa, 1991). Other gynecologic uses may include intrauterine device insertion and removal, endometrial sampling, laser treatment of cervical lesions, and diagnostic curettage (Gupta et al., 1990).

Summary Points

✔ Women seek to terminate pregnancy for various personal, psychological, social, and economic reasons. Fetal diagnosis that identifies congenital or genetic abnormalities often leads to the decision to abort.

✔ Since abortion was legalized in 1973, many state laws and Supreme Court decisions have created restrictions on abortion availability. This especially impacts poor women who rely on federal and state programs for their healthcare. In some states, abortion is virtually unavailable, forcing women to travel to other states to obtain services.

✔ For most women and their partners, making the decision to terminate pregnancy is stressful and difficult. Emotional support and full exploration of options is important in assisting couples to make the decision that is best for them.

✔ The immediate complication rates and long-term sequelae of abortion, both physiologic and psychological, are low when abortion is legal and women receive supportive, accepting care.

✔ Procedures for terminating pregnancy during the first trimester can be done in clinics and outpatient facilities. Complication rates are low, and recovery usually is rapid.

✔ In the second trimester, abortions are more regulated, and the complication rates are higher. Most second-trimester procedures involve labor and expulsion or surgery, requiring short-term hospitalization and careful monitoring.

✔ Mifepristone (RU 486) is a highly effective oral abortifacient widely used in Europe. Now in clinical trials in the United States, it provides a nonsurgical abortion option that is simple to administer.

REFERENCES

Adler, L. E. et al. (1990). Psychological responses after abortion. *Science, 248*, 41–44.

Belanger, E., Melzack, R., & Lauzon, P. (1989). Pain of first-trimester abortion: A study of psychosocial and medical predictors. *Pain, 36*, 339–350.

Chavkin, W., & Rosenfield, A. (1990). A chill wind blows: Webster, obstetrics, and the health of women. *American Journal of Obstetrics and Gynecology, 163*(2), 450.

Costa, M. (1991). *Abortion: A reference handbook* (pp. 81–87). Santa Barbara, CA: ABC-CLIO.

Creinin, M. D., & Vittinghoff, E. (1994). Methotrexate and misoprostol vs misoprostol alone for early abortion: A randomized controlled trial. *Journal of the American Medical Association, 272*, 1190–1195.

Darney, P. D., Landy, V., MacPherson, E. (1987). Abortion training in U.S. obstetric and gynecology residency programs. *Family Planning Perspectives, 19*(4), 158–162.

Donaldson, K., Briggs, J., & McMaster, D. (1994). RU 486: An alternative to surgical abortion. *Journal of Obstetric, Gynecologic, and Neonatal Nursing, 23*(7), 555–559.

Drug update (1994). US RU-486 trials likely in fall. *The Female Patient, 19*(9), 78.

Dunnihoo, D. R. (1992). *Fundamentals of gynecology and obstetrics* (2nd ed.). Philadelphia: J.B. Lippincott.

Forrest, J. D., & Henshaw, S. K. (1987). The harassment of U.S. abortion providers. *Family Planning Perspectives, 19*(1), 9–13.

Frankel, D. H. (1992). USA: Victory over the gag rule for family planning groups. *Lancet, 340*(8829), 1215.

Gallop, G., & Newport, F. (1990). Americans shift toward pro-choice position. *The Gallop Poll Monthly, April,* 2.

Gupta, J. K., & Johnson, N. (1990). Effect of mifepristone on dilatation of the pregnant and nonpregnant cervix. *Lancet, 1*, 1238.

Hakim-Elahi et al. (1990). Complications of first-trimester abortion: A report of 170,000 cases. *Obstetrics and Gynecology, 76*(1), 129.

Hatcher, R. A. et al. (1990). *Contraceptive technology: 1990–1992* (15th ed.). New York: Irvington.

Harrison, L. K., & Naylor, K. L. (1991). The laws that affect abortion in the United States and their impact on women's health. *Nurse Pract, 16*(1), 53–59.

Henshaw, R. C. et al. (1993). Comparison of medical abortion with surgical vacuum aspiration: Women's preferences and acceptability of treatment. *British Medical Journal, 307*, 714–717.

Henshaw, S. K. (1990). Induced abortion: A world review, 1990. *Family Planning Perspectives, 22*(2), 76–89.

Henshaw, S. K., & Van Vort, J. (1990). Abortion services in the United States, 1987 and 1988. *Family Planning Perspectives, 22*(3), 102–108.

Jackson, L. G. (1990). Commentary: Prenatal diagnosis: The magnitude of dysgenic effects is small, the human benefits, great. *Birth, 17*(2), 80.

Kaali, S. G., Csakany, G. M., Szigetavari, I. et al. (1990). Updated screening protocol for abortion services. *Obstetrics and Gynecology, 76*(1), 136–138.

Newsline (1994). California clinic takes part in first U.S. trials to test RU-486. *Nurseweek, 7*(23), 4–5.

Regelson, W. et al. (1990). Beyond "abortion": RU 486 and the needs of the crisis constituency. *Journal of the American Medical Association, 264*(8), 1026.

Rhodes, A. M. (1990). Issue update: Abortion. *MCN, 15*, 289.

Rogers, J. L. et al. (1989). Psychological impact of abortion: Methodological and outcomes summary of empirical research between 1968 and 1988. *Health Care Women International, 10*(4), 347.

Rogers, J. L. et al. (1991). Impact of the Minnesota parental notification law on abortion and birth. *American Journal of Public Health, 81*(3), 294.

Rothman, B. K. (1990). Commentary: Women feel social and economic pressures to abort abnormal fetuses. *Birth, 17* (2), 81.

The debate (1987). Abortion pill (RU 486). We should test this drug in the USA. Opposing view: Abortion pill. Keep this chemical killer out of the USA. *USA Today, January 15*, 10A.

Turk, P. (1990). Abortion. In R. Lichtman & S. Papera (Eds.), *Gynecology: Will-woman cure* (pp. 451–463). Norwalk, CT: Appleton & Lange.

U.K. Multicentre Trial (1990). The efficacy and tolerance of mifepristone and prostaglandin in first trimester termination of pregnancy. *British Journal of Obstetrics and Gynaecology, 97*, 480.

Zabin, L. S., Hirsch, M. B., & Emerson, M. R. (1989). When urban adolescents choose abortion: Effects on education, psychological status and subsequent pregnancy. *Family Planning Perspectives, 21*(6), 248–255.

SUGGESTED READING

Costa, M. (1991). *Abortion: A reference handbook* (pp. 81–87). Santa Barbara, CA: ABC-CLIO.

Donaldson, K., Briggs, J., & McMaster, D. (1994). RU 486: An alternative to surgical abortion. *Journal of Obstetric, Gynecologic, and Neonatal Nursing, 23*(7), 555–559.

Henshaw, S. K. (1992). Abortion trends in 1987 and 1988: Age and race. *Family Planning Perspectives, 24*(2), 85–86, 96.

Henshaw, S. K., & Van Vort, J. (1994). Abortion services in the United States, 1991 and 1992. *Family Planning Perspectives, 24*(3), 100–106, 112.

Daley, D., & Dold, R. B. (1993). Public funding for contraception, sterilization and abortion services, fiscal year 1992. *Family Planning Perspectives, 25*(6), 244–251.

Jerry, R. A. (1995). Protesters should target abortion clinics. In Cozic, C., & Petrikin, J. (Eds.), *The abortion controversy* (pp 183–188). San Diego: Greenhaven Press.

Lader, L. (1991). *RU 486* (pp. 37–39). Menlo Park, CA: Addison-Wesley.

Petchesky, R. P. (1990). *Abortion and woman's choice* (pp. 155–161). Boston: Northeastern University Press.

Turk, P. (1990). Abortion. In R. Lichtman & S. Papera (Eds.), *Gynecology: Will-woman cure* (pp. 451–463). Norwalk, CT: Appleton & Lange.

13

Management of Infertility

Objectives

- Discuss male and female factors involved in infertility.
- Explain the nursing process as it relates to infertility evaluation.
- Describe current medical testing and treatments for infertile couples.
- Examine ethical and psychological factors involved with assisted reproductive technologies.

Key Terms

Amenorrhea
Assisted reproductive
  technology
Azoospermia
Coitus
Cryptorchidism
Diagnostic
  laparoscopy
Galactorrhea
GIFT
Hysterosalpingogram
Infertility
In vitro fertilization

Menstrual cycle
Motility
Nulliparous
Oligomenorrhea
Ovulation
Spermatogenesis
Sterility
Therapeutic artificial
  insemination
Varicocele
ZIFT

BOX 13-1
Definitions

Primary infertility: A pregnancy has never occurred.
Secondary infertility: At least one prior pregnancy has occurred, but a successful pregnancy at the current time has not been realized.
Relative infertility or impaired fertility: A set of conditions that may impede or postpone pregnancy but often can be corrected.
Sterility: Conception cannot occur, and the causative factor cannot be reversed.

Childbearing is often considered a matter of choice. Many couples, reaching a certain point in their relationship, decide to discontinue using contraception and attempt a pregnancy. After 5 to 6 months of unprotected intercourse and without any other variables, 70% to 80% of women will conceive. However, pregnancy does not occur for about 15% of women (Hatcher et al., 1994). Some sources speculate that 30% of women in this country will at some point experience the inability to become pregnant when they desire to do so (Gray et al., 1994). Demographic studies indicate that most women who seek infertility advice, testing, or treatment are white, educated, older than 30 years, **nulliparous** (no biologic children), married, and of a higher socioeconomic position (Wilcox et al., 1993).

The number of infertile couples has risen in recent years. This can be linked to several factors. Women of the "baby boomer" generation (individuals born in the 1950s and 1960s) are now in the latter part of their own childbearing cycles. Characteristically, this group postponed pregnancy in favor of career. This postponement may compound infertility problems because some disorders, such as endometriosis, tend to worsen with time. An increased acceptance of multiple sexual partners and the correlating increase in incidence of sexually transmitted diseases (STDs) place more women at risk of tubal damage and pelvic scarring. Likewise, men may be rendered sterile after infections, such as gonorrhea. Exposure to environmental toxins also may contribute to the rise in impaired fertility (Gray et al., 1994; Maroulis, 1993; Speroff et al., 1989). The different types of infertility are defined in Box 13-1.

Nursing Assessment

Inability to initiate a pregnancy is usually due to an abnormality of the anatomy or physiology of the reproductive system. Conception requires the completion of a specific set of events within a specific time frame. Therefore, infertility investigation requires the examination of both partners and their ability to function as a unit.

When the infertile couple is treated as a whole, neither partner feels singled out. Both people must be evaluated in a systematic, cohesive, and compassionate manner. There is no substitute for a carefully planned clinical assessment. Unless the underlying cause is discovered, treatment may be ineffectual, time consuming, and unsuccessful.

Initiating Investigation

One year of unprotected **coitus** without conception is the general criterion for an **infertility** evaluation. However, because fertility declines with age, couples in their 30s who have not conceived after 6 months are being aggressively evaluated. Younger couples who demonstrate an increased risk of infertility, such as a history of STD or endometriosis, also benefit from earlier testing (Cefalo, 1990).

A comprehensive infertility workup includes examination of all factors involved in conception and assessment of the reproductive anatomy and physiology of both partners, including the following:

- The hypothalamic-pituitary-ovarian axis
- Fallopian tube function
- Cervical and endometrial environments
- The hypothalamic-pituitary-testicular axis
- Sperm production and motility

The evaluation also must consider the frequency and methods of coitus and each partner's emotional state.

TABLE 13-1
Summary of Physiologic Factors of Infertility and Methods of Testing

Factor	Test	Timing in Cycle
Male factors 　Sperm	Semen analysis	Anytime; suggested as initial study
Male–female factor 　Mucus–sperm compatibility	Postcoital test	At time of ovulation, done 2–12 h after intercourse
Female factors 　Ovulation	Serum progesterone	Luteal phase, day 21–24 of 28-day cycle
Uterine environment	Endometrial biopsy	Luteal phase, day 21–24 of 28-day cycle
Tubal function	Hysterosalpingogram	Within 2–3 days of end of menstruation
	Diagnostic laparoscopy with tubal dye study	Before ovulation

These factors and their related diagnostic tests are summarized in Table 13-1.

The Initial Interview

Couples in the beginning stages of an infertility evaluation are often fearful, embarrassed, and anxious. These feelings may be due to beliefs that they are abnormal because they cannot conceive or due to a realization that the evaluation will include discussion of their intimate relationship and close examination of their reproductive anatomy. The initial interview can set the stage for cooperation and motivation. By creating a nonjudgmental and empathic atmosphere, the nurse assists the couple in adjusting to the evaluation process. The nurse's acknowledgment of their frustration, fear, and anxiety helps the couple accept their situation and the offered assistance.

The initial infertility interview typically includes the following:

- A comprehensive health history of both partners. Many agencies find that self-assessment tools are helpful in eliciting information pertinent to childbearing (see Assessment Tools: Medical History Form for Men and Medical History Form for Women).
- Details of menstrual history, past pregnancies, past gynecologic or medical illnesses, surgical procedures, and contraceptive use
- Data relating to personal habits (diet, sleep patterns, tobacco, alcohol, or drug use)
- Data about the couple's sexual habits, including timing, frequency, and positioning for coitus (Hawkins et al., 1993)

Some nurses are uncomfortable discussing sexual issues with clients. Nurses who are comfortable with their own sexuality and have experience dealing with these issues generally have less difficulty discussing details of a couple's sexual life. By first collecting sexually unrelated data, an atmosphere of trust can be established. Once that occurs, the interview can proceed to more sensitive areas, such as frequency and methods of coitus and sexual satisfaction.

Assessing Male Fertility Factors

Problems relating to sperm production and motility account for 35% to 40% of all infertility cases. Evaluation of the male is simple and straightforward and should be one of the first steps in the process.

Physical Examination

Physical abnormalities of the male genitals may immediately reveal a possible cause of decreased sperm count or motility as a cause of infertility. Physical abnormalities may include the following:

- **Cryptorchidism** (undescended testes)
- Hypoplastic testes (as a result of a genetic XXY disorder)
- Testicular atrophy (a sequelae of postpubescent mumps)
- **Varicocele** (varicose veins of the scrotum)
- Previous herniorrhaphy (and resulting scar tissue)
- Other structural anomalies

Semen Analysis

Laboratory evaluation of semen is essential to the infertility evaluation. Careful instructions to the client will avoid erroneous results of this test. Although clinical laboratories may differ in their specific instructions, there is a general set of guidelines to ensure obtaining (*text continues on page 326*)

Name: Date:
Address: Tel.:
Occupation: Age: Religion:
Employer: Ins.:
Bus. Tel.:   Cert. No.:
Referred by: Gr. No.:
Birth Place: Name Rel./Friend:
Birth Date: Address:

All previous occupations: List all states or countries in which you have lived:

Education: Please encircle the last   Grade   5   High School   1 2 3 4   Post Grad. _____ yrs.
              grade you completed   6   7   8   College   1 2 3 4   Degrees

CHIEF COMPLAINTS
Please list all symptoms you have NOW.   P. I. Please do not write in this space.
1. _____
2. _____
3. _____
Routine checkup—no symptoms [ ]

FAMILY HISTORY		Age	If Living Health	Age at death	If Deceased Cause	Please Encircle — Has any blood relative had			Who
Father						Cancer	no	yes	
Mother						Tuberculosis	no	yes	
Brother or sister	1.					Diabetes	no	yes	
	2.					Heart trouble	no	yes	
	3.					High blood pressure	no	yes	
	4.					Stroke	no	yes	
	5.					Epilepsy	no	yes	
Husband or wife						Mental illness	no	yes	
Son or daughter	1.					Suicide	no	yes	
	2.					Congenital deformities	no	yes	
	3.					NOTE:			
	4.								
	5.								
	6.								
	7.								

NOTE:

This is a confidential record of your medical history and will be kept in this office. Information contained here will not be released to any person except when you have authorized us to do so.

PERSONAL HISTORY
ILLNESS: Have you had
(Please Encircle all Answers no or yes)

Measles or German measles	no	yes
Chickenpox or mumps	no	yes
Whooping cough	no	yes
Scarlet fever or scarlatina	no	yes
Pneumonia or pleurisy	no	yes
Diphtheria or smallpox	no	yes
Influenza	no	yes
Rheumatic fever or heart disease	no	yes
Arthritis or rheumatism	no	yes
Any bone or joint disease	no	yes
Neuritis or neuralgia	no	yes
Bursitis, sciatica or lumbago	no	yes
Polio or meningitis	no	yes
Bright's disease or kidney infection	no	yes

Gonorrhea or syphilis	no	yes
Anemia or jaundice	no	yes
Epilepsy	no	yes
Migraine headaches	no	yes
Tuberculosis	no	yes
Diabetes or cancer	no	yes
High or low blood pressure	no	yes
Nervous breakdown	no	yes
Food, chemical or drug poisoning	no	yes
Hay fever or asthma	no	yes
Hives or eczema	no	yes
Frequent colds or sore throat	no	yes
Frequent infections or boils	no	yes
Any other disease	no	yes
ALLERGIES: Are you allergic to		
Penicillin or sulfa	no	yes
Aspirin, codeine or morphine	no	yes

Mycins or other antibiotics	no	yes
Merthiolate or mercurochrome	no	yes
Any other drug	no	yes
Any foods	no	yes
Adhesive tape	no	yes
Nail polish or other cosmetics	no	yes
Tetanus antitoxin or serums	no	yes
INJURIES: Have you had any		
Broken bones	no	yes
Sprains or dislocations	no	yes
Lacerations (extensive)	no	yes
Concussion or head injury	no	yes
Ever been knocked out	no	yes
TRANSFUSIONS: Have you ever had		
Blood or plasma transfusion	no	yes

Weight: now _____ one year ago _____
Max _____ when _____ Height _____

Please review the section you have just completed and wherever you answered "yes" fill in the year (guess if necessary) and also where there is more than one illness to a line encircle the ones you have had. Example: Chickenpox or mumps .... 1961 .... no yes

(continued)

SURGERY: Have you had

Tonsillectomy .... no yes
Appendectomy .... no yes
Any other operation (give details) no yes

Give DETAILS below of all hospitalizations for surgery or illness including name and address of Doctor and Hospital . . . .

Have you ever been advised to have any surgical operation which has not been done? [1] no [2] yes what ....

Systems: Please check those you have had.

Eye disease [ ], Eye injury [ ], Impaired sight [ ], Ear disease [ ], Ear injury [ ], Impaired hearing [ ],
Trouble with: Nose [ ], Sinuses [ ], Mouth [ ], Throat [ ], Have you checked any in this group? .... no yes
Fainting spells [ ], Loss of consciousness [ ], Convulsions [ ], Paralysis [ ], Frequent or severe headaches [ ], Dizziness [ ], Depression
or anxiety [ ], Hallucinations [ ], Have you checked any in this group? .... no yes
Enlarged glands [ ], Goiter or enlarged thyroid [ ], Skin disease [ ], Have you checked any in this group? .... no yes
Chronic or frequent cough [ ], Chest pain or angina pectoris [ ], Spitting up of blood [ ], Night sweats [ ], Shortness of breath [ ],
Palpitation or fluttering heart [ ], Swelling of hands, feet, or ankles [ ], Varicose veins [ ], Extreme tiredness or weakness [ ], Have you
checked any in this group? .... no yes

Kidney disease or stones [ ], Bladder disease [ ], Albumin, sugar, pus, etc. in urine [ ], Difficulty in urinating [ ], Awake to urinate
nightly [ ], Have you checked any in this group? .... no yes

Stomach trouble or ulcers [ ], Indigestion [ ], Liver or gallbladder disease [ ], Colitis or other bowel disease [ ] Appendicitis [ ],
Hemorrhoids or rectal bleeding [ ], Constipation or diarrhea [ ], Recent change in bowel action or stools [ ], Recent change in appetite
or eating habits [ ], Have you checked any in this group? .... no yes

HABITS: Do you

Sleep well? .... no yes
Use alcoholic beverages .... no yes
   Every day? .... no yes
Smoke? .... no yes
   How much? ....
Exercise enough .... no yes
Is your diet well balanced? .... no yes

List any drugs or medications you take regularly or frequently:

_____
_____
_____
_____
_____
_____
_____

MARITAL HISTORY

Prior marriage? ....
Was pregnancy achieved? ....

When? (Dates) ....
Any other proof of fertility? ....
....
....
....

Is sex entirely satisfactory? ....
Reaction of wife: ....

Estimated frequency of coitus (intercourse) per month: ....
Remarks: ....
....
....
....
....
....
....

INFERTILITY STUDIES

	Result	Date	Where Done
Semen analysis			
Thyroid tests:			
Hormone tests:			
Medicines given:			
Other tests:			

Name: Date: Unit No.:
(Nee):   Tel.:   Husb.:
Address: Age: Ins.:   Occupation: Age:
Occupation: Cert. No.:   Employer
Employer: Gr. No.:   Bus. Address:
Bus. Tel.:   Name Rel./Friend: Bus. Tel.:
Referred by: Address: Religion: Husb.   Wife:
Birth Place: [ ] Single   [ ] Divorced
Birth Date: [ ] Married   [ ] Widow (er)

All previous occupations: List all states or countries in which you have lived:

Education: Please encircle the last   Grade   5   High School   1 2 3 4   Post Grad. _____ yrs.
grade you completed   6   7   8   College   1 2 3 4   Degrees

Date of last physical exam.   P. I. Please do not write in this space.

Chief Complaints: Please list all symptoms you have NOW.
1. _____
2. _____
3. _____
Routine checkup—no symptoms [ ]

FAMILY HISTORY	Age	If Living Health	Age at death	If Deceased Cause	Please Encircle Has any blood relative had		Who
Father					Cancer	no yes	
Mother					Tuberculosis	no yes	
Brother or sister 1.					Diabetes	no yes	
2.					Heart trouble	no yes	
3.					High blood pressure	no yes	
4.					Stroke	no yes	
5.					Epilepsy	no yes	
Husband or wife					Mental illness	no yes	
Son or daughter 1.					Suicide	no yes	
2.					Congenital deformities	no yes	
3.							
4.							
5.							
6.							

NOTE: This is a confidential record of your medical history and will be kept in this office. Information contained here will not be released to any person except when you have authorized us to do so.

PERSONAL HISTORY
ILLNESS: Have you had
(Please Encircle all Answers no or yes)

Measles or German measles	no yes	Gonorrhea or syphilis	no yes	Mycins or other antibiotics	no yes
Chickenpox or mumps	no yes	Anemia or jaundice	no yes	Merthiolate or mercurochrome	no yes
Whooping cough	no yes	Epilepsy	no yes	Any other drug	no yes
Scarlet fever or scarlatina	no yes	Migraine headaches	no yes	Any foods	no yes
Pneumonia or pleurisy	no yes	Tuberculosis	no yes	Adhesive tape	no yes
Diphtheria or smallpox	no yes	Diabetes or cancer	no yes	Nail polish or other cosmetics	no yes
Influenza	no yes	High or low blood pressure	no yes	Tetanus antitoxin or serums	no yes
Rheumatic fever or heart disease	no yes	Nervous breakdown	no yes	INJURIES: Have you had any	
Arthritis or rheumatism	no yes	Food, chemical or drug poisoning	no yes	Broken bones	no yes
Any bone or joint disease	no yes	Hay fever or asthma	no yes	Sprains or dislocations	no yes
Neuritis or neuralgia	no yes	Hives or eczema	no yes	Lacerations (extensive)	no yes
Bursitis, sciatica or lumbago	no yes	Frequent colds or sore throat	no yes	Concussion or head injury	no yes
Polio or meningitis	no yes	Frequent infections or boils	no yes	Ever been knocked out	no yes
Bright's disease or kidney infection	no yes	Any other disease	no yes	TRANSFUSIONS: Have you ever had	
		ALLERGIES: Are you allergic to		Blood or plasma transfusion	no yes
		Penicillin or sulfa	no yes	Weight: now _____ one year ago _____	
		Aspirin, codeine or morphine	no yes	Max _____ when _____ Height _____	

Please review the section you have just completed and wherever you answered "yes" fill in the year (guess if necessary) and also where there is more than one illness to a line encircle the ones you have had. Example: Chickenpox or mumps ....1961 .... no (yes)

(continued)

SURGERY: Have you had   no   yes   Give DETAILS below of all hospitalizations for surgery or illness including name and address of
Tonsillectomy .... no   yes   Doctor and Hospital . . . .
Appendectomy .... no   yes
Any other operation (give details)   no   yes

Have you ever been advised to have any surgical operation which has not been done? [1] no   [2] yes   what ....

Systems: Please check those you have had.
Eye disease [ ], Eye injury [ ], Impaired sight [ ], Ear disease [ ], Ear injury [ ], Impaired hearing [ ],
Trouble with: Nose [ ], Sinuses [ ], Mouth [ ], Throat [ ], Have you checked any in this group? .... no   yes
Fainting spells [ ], Loss of consciousness [ ], Convulsions [ ], Paralysis [ ], Frequent or severe headaches [ ], Dizziness [ ], Depression
or anxiety [ ], Hallucinations [ ], Have you checked any in this group? .... no   yes
Enlarged glands [ ], Goiter or enlarged thyroid [ ], Skin disease [ ], Have you checked any in this group? .... no   yes
Chronic or frequent cough [ ], Chest pain or angina pectoris [ ], Spitting up of blood [ ], Night sweats [ ], Shortness of breath [ ],
Palpitation or fluttering heart [ ], Swelling of hands, feet, or ankles [ ], Varicose veins [ ], Extreme tiredness or weakness [ ], Have you
checked any in this group? .... no   yes
Kidney disease or stones [ ], Bladder disease [ ], Albumin, sugar, pus, etc. in urine [ ], Difficulty in urinating [ ], Awake to urinate
nightly [ ], Have you checked any in this group? .... no   yes
Stomach trouble or ulcers [ ], Indigestion [ ], Liver or gallbladder disease [ ], Colitis or other bowel disease [ ], Appendicitis [ ],
Hemorrhoids or rectal bleeding [ ], Constipation or diarrhea [ ], Recent change in bowel action or stools [ ], Recent change in appetite
or eating habits [ ], Have you checked any in this group? .... no   yes

---

HABITS: Do you

Sleep well? .... no   yes
Use alcoholic beverages ...... no   yes
    Every day? .... no   yes
Smoke? .... no   yes
    How much? ....
Exercise enough .... no   yes
Is your diet well balanced?   no   yes

List any drugs or medications you
take regularly or frequently:
_____
_____
_____
_____
_____
_____

OBSTETRICAL-GYNECOLOGICAL REVIEW

Age at first menstruation _____ Age at first coital
experience _____ Number of living children (at present) _____
Number of pregnancies _____
Number of live births _____ Number of multiple
pregnancies _____
Number of stillbirths (more than 20 weeks) _____
Number of abortions, miscarriages (20 weeks or less) _____
Number of children dead _____ Age of oldest child _____
Number of births with deformities _____

GYNECOLOGICAL HISTORY

Are menstrual cycles regular? .... Are your periods similar? ....
Interval between periods ....
Length of flow .... Date of last menstrual cycle ....
Amount of flow .... [1] Light   [2] Moderate   [3] Heavy
Was the quality, quantity, and duration of flow for this last cycle similar in
comparison with previous cycles? ....
    [1] No (specify how it differed) ....
    .... [2] Yes
Has there been any bleeding in between periods? ....
    [1] No   [2] Yes (specify) ....

Were any medications taken during cycle? ....
    [1] No   [2] Yes (specify)
Dysmenorrhea (menstrual discomfort)
    [1] None   [2] Intermittent   [3] Constant
Type of menstrual discomfort experienced
    [1] None   [3] Dull   [5] Cramp
    [2] Sharp   [4] Ache   [6] Backache

PREMENSTRUAL SYMPTOMS

Bloating .... no   yes
Breast tenderness .... no   yes
Pelvic pain .... no   yes
Backache .... no   yes
Headache .... no   yes
Irritability .... no   yes
Edema .... no   yes
Acne .... no   yes

INTERMENSTRUAL DISCHARGE

Type [1] None   [3] Yellow [5] White
     [2] Tan   [4] Bloody [6] Other (specify)
Amount .... Scant Heavy
Itching .... no   yes
Odorless .... no   yes
Frequent .... no   yes
Regular pattern .... no   yes

MARITAL HISTORY

Prior marriage? .... when? (Dates) ....   Was pregnancy achieved? ....
Is sex entirely satisfactory? ....   Dyspareunia (discomfort during coitus): no .... yes ....
Estimate frequency of coitus (sexual   Does coitus occur during menses?   Yes .... No ....
intercourse) per month: ....
Reaction of husband: ....   On which days of flow? ....
Remarks: ....   Is this consistent? ....
....
....

(continued)

INDICATE THE INFORMATION FOR ANY OF THE FOLLOWING STUDIES WHICH YOU HAVE HAD.

	Date	Result	Doctor
Basal body temperature record:	....	....	....
Biopsy test:	....	....	....
Thyroid test:	....	....	....
Gas (Rubin) test:	....	....	....
X-ray of uterus and tubes:	....	....	....
Postcoital test: (survival of seed in your secretions)	....	....	....
Cautery of cervix:	....	....	....
Hormone test:	....	....	....
Inseminations:	....	....	....
Medicines given:	....	....	....
Other:	....	....	....

(Courtesy of Division of Human Reproduction, Hospital of the University of Pennsylvania, Philadelphia, PA)

---

the maximum information from the specimen (see the Client Education: Semen Analysis).

The semen analysis is performed on a fresh ejaculate that is collected by masturbation after the couple abstains from intercourse for several days. The entire specimen is collected in a clean, dry container and immediately transported to the testing facility. During transport, the specimen should be kept warm by placing the container under the arm or next to the skin in some manner. Laboratory personnel need to know the time of collection because seminal fluid coagulates immediately after ejaculation and reliquefies within 20 to 30 minutes. For an accurate analysis, the ejaculate must be in the liquefied state to ensure an even distribution of spermatozoa in the counting chamber.

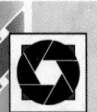

CLIENT EDUCATION
Semen Analysis

To evaluate the quality of the semen accurately, a specimen must be collected in a specific manner. Please follow these instructions carefully.

1. Collect the specimen at approximately the same time as your usual sexual schedule.
2. Do not use any lubricants while collecting the specimen.
3. Masturbate and ejaculate into a clean and dry plastic or glass container with a tight-fitting lid. Cap tightly. Note the time of collection.
4. Keep the specimen at body temperature by placing it under your arm or next to your chest while you are transporting it to the laboratory. Do not use artificial heating or cooling sources.
5. Transport immediately to the laboratory. The specimen must be analyzed within 1 hour of collection.

Factors Affecting Semen Analysis. The specimen is analyzed for volume, density, number of mature sperm, percentage of motile sperm, quality of motility, and percentage of abnormal forms. White blood cells and bacteria should not be present in the specimen (Table 13-2). An alteration in the normal values of any one or more of these factors can contribute to an abnormal semen analysis.

Spermatogenesis is an ongoing process of sperm maturation that requires approximately 60 to 90 days. Therefore, a single abnormal semen analysis should not be interpreted as a threat to the couple's fertility. Normal results or information requiring further investigation may be obtained by performing repeat analyses, collected at 60- to 90-day intervals (Speroff et al., 1989).

An increase in volume of sperm may indicate a lower sperm concentration; a volume less than 1 mL may indicate inability of the semen to reach the cervix during coitus. A minimum count of 20 million sperm/mL (with normal motility) is considered adequate for achieving a pregnancy. However, pregnancies have been documented with lower counts.

Along with the number of sperm, the following must be analyzed:

- **Motility.** Greater than 60% of the living spermatozoa should move for up to 2 hours after ejaculation. Living sperm that do not move cannot penetrate the waiting egg.
- Abnormal forms (double-headed sperm, immature forms). If more than 40% of the total count is abnormal, there may be a spermatogenesis defect. This requires further investigation.
- **Azoospermia** (absence of sperm in the ejaculate)

If testicular biopsy indicates sperm production, a blockage of the vas deferens should be considered.

TABLE 13–2	
Normal Values for Semen Analysis	
Volume	2–5 mL
Liquefaction	Complete in 20–30 min
Count	>20 million per mL
Motility	>60% mobile after 1 h
	>50% mobile after 2 h
Morphology	<40% of total
White blood cells	None
Bacteria	None to few

Blockage may be the result of a previous infection, such as tuberculosis or gonorrhea (Box 13-2) or a prior vasectomy performed for sterilization purposes. Patency of the vas deferens may be restored by microsurgery. Genetic abnormalities must be ruled out if testicular biopsy indicates no sperm production. Total aspermia, although rare, does indicate that the man is incapable of fathering a child. **Therapeutic artificial insemination** with donor sperm may be considered.

Excess heat to the testes, without physical abnormality or prior viral infections, can affect semen quality. Men who habitually wear tight-fitting underwear and pants often have decreased sperm counts. Constant use of hot tubs and spas also has been found to lower sperm counts. Elimination of these habits can bring increased sperm count and motility. Exposure to pesticides, herbicides, and other toxic chemicals adversely affects the quality and quantity of sperm. Some medications, recreational drugs (especially marijuana), and cigarette smoking also can decrease the number and motility of the sperm (Speroff et al., 1989).

Another factor is the ability of sperm to penetrate the cervical mucus and maintain motility. This is evaluated

---

BOX 13–2
Sexually Transmitted Diseases (STDs)
and Infertility (Male)

Male STDs can impair infertility. Bacterial infections (especially *Chlamydia* and gonorrhea) can produce scarring of the epididymis and other structures, causing obstruction. Gram-negative bacteria (such as *Escherichia coli*) can impair sperm motility.

Because the semen analysis is an early component of the infertility workup, these sequelae are often identified quickly. Culturing of seminal fluid is indicated if there are any signs or symptoms of infection. Prompt treatment of any STD will prevent long-term consequences.

(Shaban, S. [1995]. Male infertility. Monograph URL. Atlanta, GA: Atlanta Reproductive Health Center.)

---

by means of the *postcoital examination,* or Sims-Huhner test, which analyzes the interaction between the cervical mucus and the semen. If fewer than 15 to 20 sperm are found in the postcoital specimen, techniques of intercourse should be investigated. The ejaculate may not be placed deep enough in the vagina for sperm movement toward the cervix. Couples should be encouraged to use positions that allow deep penetration during intercourse. Other causes may include impotence or hypospadias, a condition in which the urethra is improperly positioned on the shaft of the penis instead of at the glans (see the Client Teaching Guidelines: Postcoital Examination).

If a couple has a normal semen analysis and an abnormal postcoital test, further investigation is indicated. The man may have had an isolated retrograde ejaculation, in which sperm are released into the urinary bladder instead of the ejaculate. This is often due to emotional anxiety about having to perform coitus

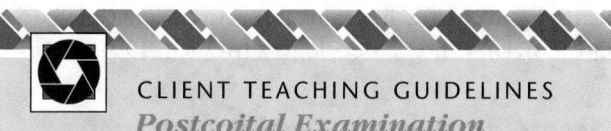

CLIENT TEACHING GUIDELINES
Postcoital Examination

This examination is scheduled to coincide with the time of ovulation when the cervical mucus is clear, abundant, and receptive to spermatozoa. The couple should be instructed to have unprotected intercourse 2 to 12 hours before the test; the woman should remain in bed 10 to 15 minutes after coitus. Couples also should be instructed to refrain from using lubricants or douches after coitus because some of the chemicals contained in these agents can reduce sperm count or motility.
The procedure can be performed in the office and requires less than 10 minutes.

Client preparation: The client is prepared in a similar manner as for a regular gynecologic examination.

Explanation of procedure: The cervix is exposed using a speculum, and a sample of cervical mucus is collected by aspirating it from the endocervical canal by way of a thin polyethylene tube. The cervical mucus is examined grossly for quality, quantity, and spinnbarkeit (ability to form a continuous, stretchy thread). Spinnbarkeit is evaluated by stretching the mucus between the tips of a forceps or gloved fingers until the mucus thread breaks. Spinnbarkeit is considered normal if the mucus stretches 8 to 10 cm. Mucus also is immediately examined under a microscope by placing a drop or two on a glass slide and covering it with a cover slip. In a normal test, 15 to 20 living motile sperm are seen in each high-powered field.

Adverse effects: None known.
The most common cause for abnormal test results is performing this examination at the wrong time of the menstrual cycle by using basal body temperature charting or urine testing for the luteinizing hormone (LH) surge.

From Hawkins, J. et al. (1993) and Star, W. et al. (1995).

on command and on schedule. A second postcoital test should be performed.

Cross-penetration testing is available to define the causes of abnormal postcoital tests. In this test, the man's semen and the woman's mucus are tested against donor semen and mucus, previously established as normal. Sperm motility and ability to penetrate cervical mucus are examined. This test evaluates whether the semen or the mucus is the causative factor. Inability of the sperm to penetrate the cervical mucus can be rectified with medications or by direct insemination of semen into the uterus. These are discussed later in this chapter.

If sperm are found, but they are not moving or are dead, the seminal fluid and the cervical mucus may be incompatible. Antisperm antibodies, produced either by the man or woman, may be found. Sophisticated immunologic testing is required to document this condition. Temporary condom use or short-term oral steroid therapy for the man can reduce the antibody count and lead to successful insemination (American College of Obstetricians and Gynecologists [ACOG], 1994).

Assessing Female Fertility Factors

The woman's role in fertility is far more complex than the man's. In addition to **ovulation,** specific events must occur on schedule for a pregnancy to implant and continue. These factors must be evaluated in a systematic and timely fashion to determine the cause of infertility.

Physical Examination

A complete physical examination should be the starting point for any infertility evaluation. Factors influencing fertility include the following:

- Disease processes (thyroid disorders, diabetes, hypertension, cardiovascular disease, kidney disorders, infection)
- Nutritional status and body-fat ratio. A body-fat ratio of less than 10% can indicate malnutrition or overtraining and may result in anovulation (Green et al., 1988).

Pelvic examination may add evidence of reproductive problems:

- Ovarian masses, such as cysts, may interfere with ovulation.
- Thickening of the adnexa may indicate past pelvic infections and resultant scarring. Pelvic tenderness may be a sign of a chronic subacute infection. Screening for *Chlamydia* and gonorrhea should occur during the physical examination (Box 13-3).
- Nodularity along the uterosacral ligament or a fixed, retroflexed uterus is often linked to endometriosis.

BOX 13-3
Sexually Transmitted Diseases (STDs) and Infertility (Female)

Although STDs often cause acute illness, long-term sequelae also must be considered. Many organisms cause infection and inflammation in the female pelvis. This fosters formation of scar tissue on the ovaries, fallopian tubes, uterus, and surrounding tissues. These filmy, weblike adhesions can impair fertility by blocking the fallopian tubes, destroying the tubal fimbria, or decreasing pelvic organ mobility.

Unfortunately, even with asymptomatic or subclinical STDs and pelvic inflammatory disease (PID), adhesions may form. The woman may never know that she has or had a subacute episode, yet her fertility may be impaired or even destroyed. Approximately 12% of women with just one episode of PID will be infertile, while more than 50% of women with three or more episodes will be infertile. The risk of ectopic pregnancy increases sevenfold after one PID event.

The human papillomavirus (HPV; causative agent of genital warts) can indirectly impair fertility. HPV also is a contributing factor to cervical intraepithelial neoplasia (CIN, formerly called dysplasia) and cervical cancer. Treatment for CIN may involve surgical removal of the affected area. However, this procedure also can remove vital mucous-forming glands in the cervix. Surgical treatment also may compromise the muscular integrity of the cervix, making it incapable of supporting the weight of a growing pregnancy.

Prevention of STDs is the best defense against impaired fertility. However, prompt and appropriate treatment can minimize long-term effects.

(Star, W., Lommel, L., & Shannon, M. [Eds.] [1995]. Women's primary health care, protocols for practice. *Washington, DC: American Nurses' Publishing.)*

- Cervical anomalies may have resulted from exposure in utero to diethylstilbestrol, a synthetic nonsteroidal estrogen that was widely used to prevent miscarriage and premature labor.
- Chronic cervical inflammation (cervicitis) or cervical dysplasia can decrease the amount and quality of cervical mucus.

A Pap smear is performed, and any abnormal results are investigated. Correction of minor cervical problems may result in successful conception.

Assessing Ovulation

Ovulatory failure is one of the most common causes of infertility, accounting for about 20% of all reproductive problems (Hatcher et al., 1994). Women display an amazing range of ovulatory patterns, from the expected ovulation once per cycle to ovulation only two or three times per year. Obviously, infrequent ovulation hinders fertility. For women older than 35 years, the pattern and quality of ovulation decrease with time, predisposing them to impaired ovulation and reduced fertility (Maroulis, 1993).

Clues to the measure and effectiveness of ovulation can be gathered by taking a careful menstrual history, recording basal body temperature, and examining cervical mucus. The menstrual history may reveal irregular cycles or episodes of amenorrhea, which indicate infrequent ovulation or dysfunction within the hypothalamic-pituitary-ovarian axis. Shifts of basal body temperature without ovulatory peak point to ovulatory problems. Cervical mucus that does not change to a clear, stringing consistency (spinnbarkeit) during ovulation also can indicate ovulatory disorders (Cunningham et al., 1993).

Diagnostic Tests of Ovulation. The following tests are used to assess ovulation:

■ Serum progesterone levels are determined from blood tests conducted during the luteal phase. This phase occurs approximately 7 days before the expected onset of menses or between day 21 and 24 of a 28-day cycle. Serum progesterone levels greater than 4 ng/mL indirectly indicate ovulation.

■ Endometrial biopsy documents the normal predictable and progressive hormonal and structural changes in the endometrium after ovulation (Fig. 13-1). If phasing of the endometrial stroma is not in sinc with the day of the **menstrual cycle** (ie, the number of days elapsed since the prior menses) or if it reflects a lagging maturation of 2 or more days behind the predicted day, the fertilized egg may not properly implant in the uterine lining. This increases the possibility of spontaneous abortion. This disor-

der, termed *luteal phase defect*, is discussed later in the chapter (see the Client Teaching Guidelines: Endometrial Biopsy).

■ Urinary luteinizing hormone (LH) levels are another indication of ovulation. Recent advances in monoclonal antibody technology have resulted in the development of simple home testing kits for LH levels. LH is known to peak shortly before ovulation. Therefore, testing levels of LH can assist in the prediction of the day of ovulation for appropriately timed coitus or insemination (Vermes et al., 1987). Urine is tested daily beginning shortly before the expected day of ovulation. A color change of the kit's reagents indicates the concentration of urinary LH. This test has greatly simplified the timing of inseminations or planned coitus.

Assessing Uterine Factors

The uterine environment is closely allied with ovulatory function. The endometrium must be in harmony with hormonal patterns, and uterine structure must allow

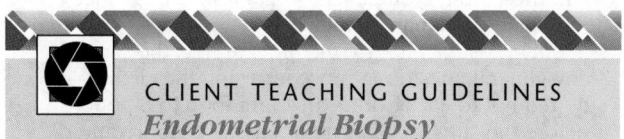

CLIENT TEACHING GUIDELINES
Endometrial Biopsy

The endometrial biopsy can easily be performed in less than 5 minutes in the doctor's office. It is scheduled during the woman's luteal phase, approximately 7 days before expected onset of menses or between days 21 and 24 of a 28-day menstrual cycle.

Client preparation for the procedure is the same as for a regular pelvic examination. Some physicians premedicate women with a nonsteroidal anti-inflammatory medication (ibuprofen, naprosyn sodium) about 1 hour before the procedure to help reduce cramping.

Explanation of procedure: After the position of the uterus is determined, a slender pipette is introduced through the cervix to the uterine cavity (see Fig. 13-1). This indicates the depth or size of the uterus. The pipette is pulled along the walls of the uterus in several places, and samples of the uterus are obtained by gentle suction. These collected samples are evaluated by a pathologist to determine the depth of the secretory glandular structure and linked to the exact day of the cycle. The biopsy also helps rule out chronic inflammation and the presence of fibroid tumors.

Adverse effects: Mild to moderate uterine cramping may occur during the procedure but usually subsides within 5 to 10 minutes. The client is able to drive home and can return to work or normal activities immediately.

Clients should be instructed to avoid strenuous activities or lifting for 24 hours and not to douche or have intercourse for 72 hours after the test.

If the client experiences excessive bleeding (more than one pad saturated per hour), fever, or significant pain, she should notify her physician.

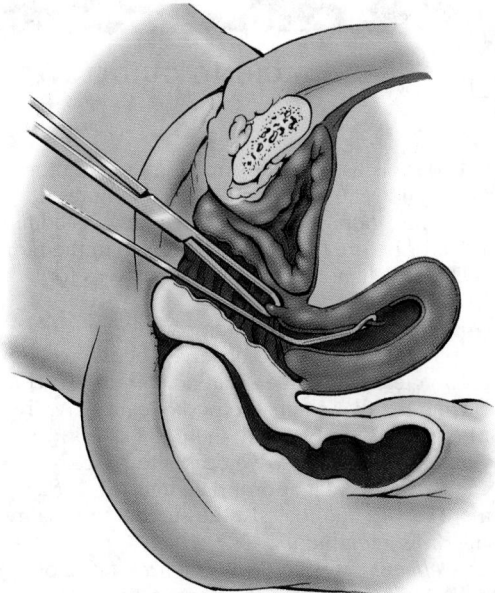

FIGURE 13-1 Endometrial biopsy samples the lining of the uterus to determine hormonal levels of the endometrial tissue.

successful implantation and embryonic growth. Potential uterine-related problems include the following:

- Asherman's syndrome, chronic inflammation of the uterus, can result in adhesions that restrict muscular growth associated with pregnancy. It is associated with chronic and habitual abortion. Clients with this disorder often have a history of repeated dilation and curettage for therapeutic abortion or diagnostic evaluation, with or without a postoperative infection (Cefalo, 1990).
- Benign fibroid tumors distort the uterine cavity and restrict implantation and growth of a pregnancy. They also can contribute to repeated spontaneous abortion. Myomectomy, or surgical removal, is best accomplished when the fibroids are within the en-

dometrial cavity or no deeper than the myometrium. Hormonal treatment is possible in selected clients.
- Congenital malformations can affect the size and shape of the uterus, tubes, and vagina. Some of these are surgically correctable.

Assessing Tubal Factors

The fallopian tubes are more than just a passageway between the ovary and uterus. They are involved in the retrieval of the ovum from the ovarian follicle, provide an environment in which fertilization can occur, and are the means by which the fertilized egg is transferred to the uterine environment. Any insult to tubal structures can diminish fertility by impeding transport of the ovum (Cunningham et al., 1993). The most common problems include the following:

- Adhesions or scar tissue resulting from infections, including acute gonorrheal salpingitis, *Chlamydia,* nonspecific pelvic inflammatory disease, infections related to intrauterine device use, rupture of physiologic ovarian cysts, or peritonitis from a ruptured appendix
- Endometriosis, a condition in which the endometrial tissue displaces into the peritoneal cavity and bleeds each month in synchrony with the endometrium

Diagnostic Tests for Tubal Defects. Evaluation of tubal function requires visualization of the structures. This can be accomplished by hysterosalpingogram and diagnostic laparoscopy (see Client Teaching Guidelines: Diagnostic Laparoscopy and Hysterosalpingogram).

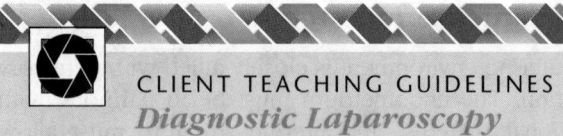

CLIENT TEACHING GUIDELINES
Diagnostic Laparoscopy

This surgical procedure is performed under general anesthesia in the outpatient surgery unit. The procedure takes less than 30 minutes.

Client preparation for the procedure is the same as any general anesthesia procedure, and the client is required not to eat or drink anything for 6 to 8 hours before the surgery. Shaving or enema is not required for most clients.

Explanation of procedure: The surgeon is able to inspect the reproductive organs and surrounding tissue by inserting a laparoscope (fiberoptic telescope) through a small incision made near the umbilicus. Carbon dioxide is introduced into the abdominal cavity, which causes the abdomen to balloon, enhancing the field of vision. A second small incision is made above the pubic hairline through which a calibrated wand is passed. This wand can be fitted with microsurgical instruments that allow the surgeon to manipulate the organs, cut adhesions, or take selected biopsies as needed. Tubal patency can be evaluated by injecting dye through the cervix while the surgeon observes the dye passing through the fimbriated ends of the tubes. No spillage of dye into the tubes indicates the tubes are blocked. The client is generally kept in the hospital for 4 to 6 hours after the surgery and is discharged when she is awake and able to tolerate oral fluids, demonstrates no significant bleeding from the incisions, and is able to urinate. The client should not drive for 24 hours after receiving the general anesthesia and should arrange for someone to drive her home after discharge. The client should be able to return to work within 2 to 3 days.

Adverse effects: The client may experience tenderness at the incision sites and bloating of the abdomen, often manifesting as pain to one or both shoulders. The gas insufflation often allows residual gas to become trapped beneath the diaphragm, causing shoulder pain. Discomfort may last for 1 to 2 days after surgery. Codeine and codeine analogues are effective in controlling pain.

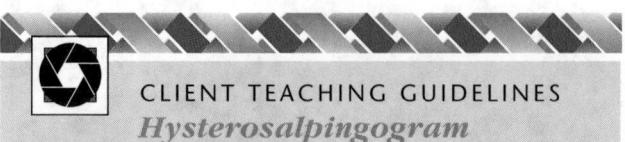

CLIENT TEACHING GUIDELINES
Hysterosalpingogram

This procedure is usually performed in the radiology department and requires about 20 to 30 minutes.

Client preparation: Ibuprofen or naprosyn is administered 1 hour before the procedure. Once in the radiology suite, the client is prepared the same as for a pelvic examination.

Explanation of procedure: Radiopaque dye is infused through the cervix and observed by fluoroscopy to enter the uterus and tubes. Patency of tubes is confirmed when the dye enters the peritoneal cavity. If one or both tubes are blocked, the point of occlusion can be observed when the dye ceases to progress further. X-rays are taken at appropriate intervals for a permanent record and to assist the surgeon if tubal reconstruction is attempted.

Adverse effects: Cramping may last for 1 to 2 hours after the procedure. Most women can return to work the same day or the next day without any significant pain or discomfort.

- **Hysterosalpingogram** (Fig. 13-2) is an x-ray procedure performed to assess for tubal blockage. During this procedure, dye is passed through the fallopian tubes to determine the exact location of blockage. This procedure can have a curative effect by removing minor adhesions and stimulating ciliary action within the tubes.
- **Diagnostic laparoscopy** (Fig. 13-3) is a minor outpatient surgery. Advances in fiberoptic technology allow the physician to see inside the uterus with a hysteroscope or laparoscope. Using these instruments, the physican has direct visualization into the pelvic area, which assists with the diagnosis of intrauterine adhesions, fibroid tumors, and other uterine anomalies. Hysteroscopes and laparoscopes have video capabilities, which allow better visualization and magnification of the surgical field for close examination (ACOG, 1994).

Nonmedical Factors Inhibiting Fertility

Not all cases of infertility are related to medical problems (see Client Education: Increasing Fertility). Sometimes a couple may engage in sexual habits and preferences that are inadvertently detrimental to conception. It is extremely important for the nurse to gather as much information as possible regarding these practices so that the couple can alter them. Some nonmedical factors may include the following:

- **Lubricants** (petroleum or water-soluble lubricant jelly) may inhibit sperm motility or may actually be a spermicide (Hatcher et al., 1994).
- **Postcoital douches** or the woman rising immediately after intercourse can remove the semen pool from the vagina.

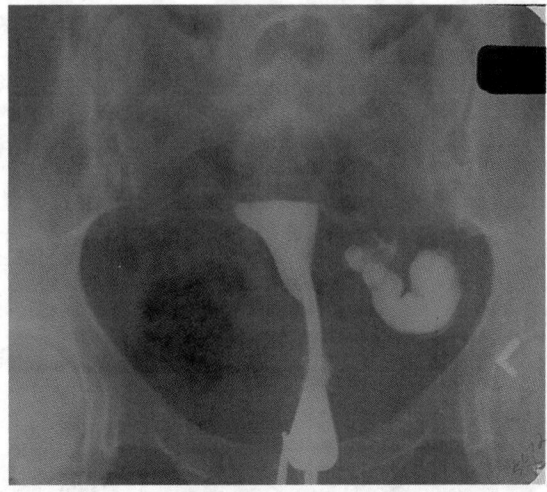

FIGURE 13–2 Hysterosalpingogram of the abdomen of a woman suffering from blocked fallopian tubes. In this client, the right tube (left on image) is blocked near the uterus—the central, pale triangular feature. No contrast medium appears to have penetrated through the obstruction. The left tube is obstructed at a point further from the womb, and dilatation (enlargement) has occurred.

- **Premature ejaculation** can prevent semen from being able to reach the cervix. While this can be embarrassing and frustrating for the man, it can be overcome with specific exercises and alternative positions for coitus.
- **Psychological factors,** such as job or financial stress, family illness, depression, and fatigue, may decrease fertility. The stress and frustration of being unable to conceive may further inhibit the couple's chances to conceive. The stress and anxiety surrounding intercourse and the rigorous time schedules imposed by some infertility treatments may create tension and emotional distress between couples.

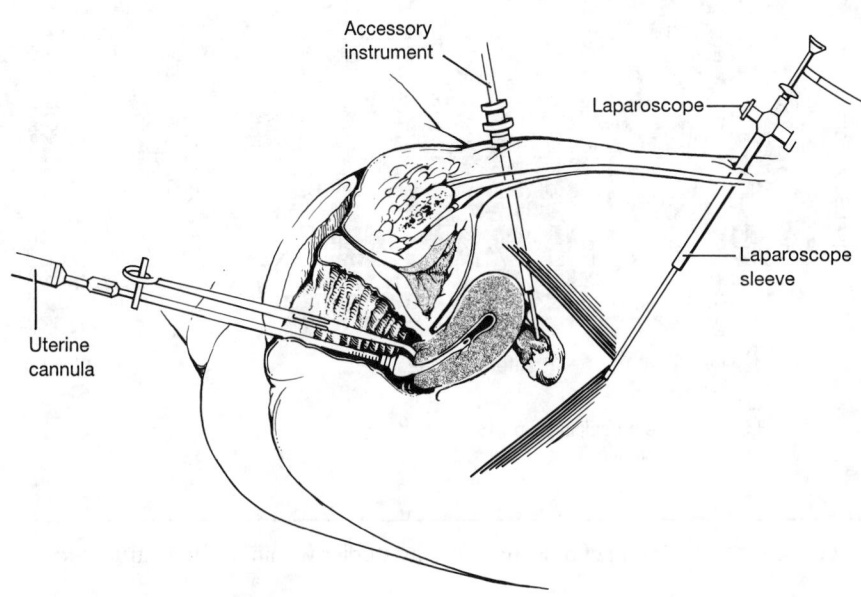

FIGURE 13–3 Diagnostic laparoscopy permits the direct visualization of pelvic organs. Tubal patency also can be evaluated during this procedure.

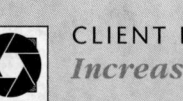

CLIENT EDUCATION
Increasing Fertility

There are several simple things you can do to increase your chances of becoming pregnant.

1. Stay healthy. Maintain good nutrition, reduce stress, and get regular exercise. Avoid alcohol, tobacco, and recreational drugs.
2. Encourage communication with your partner. "Trying" to get pregnant can become a chore and increases stress. Relax. Talk about your expectations and desires.
3. Do not stress conception as the product of sexual relations. Enjoy being with your partner.
4. Do not use lubricants or douches before, during, or after intercourse. They can have an adverse affect on the sperm and the cervical mucus.
5. Do not rise to urinate immediately after intercourse. Remain flat in bed or elevate your hips slightly to allow the sperm to reach the cervix. You may rise after 20 to 30 minutes.
6. Maximize your chances of pregnancy by timing intercourse around the time of ovulation. Have coitus at intervals of 36 to 48 hours during the midpoint of your cycle. There are several methods to help you identify your fertile time. Your healthcare provider can assist you in learning about these methods.

Although research does not confirm this correlation, the act of seeking medical assistance may relieve emotional stress for some couples. There have been cases of previously infertile couples conceiving after just one or two visits to the doctor. This also has been observed in couples who decide to adopt a child. It is presumed that once the stress of scheduled intercourse is relieved, sexual activity can proceed in a more relaxed atmosphere on the couple's own schedule, therefore enhancing the chances for conception (Hatcher et al., 1994; ACOG, 1994).

- **Lack of knowledge about sexuality or reproductive anatomy and physiology** also can hinder fertility. It is important for the nurse or health provider to educate the couple about how to enhance the possibilities of natural conception (eg, basal body temperature, mucus quality assessment, positions for optimum semen pool).
- **Physical problems** may prevent intercourse (tight hymenal ring, a rigid perineal body, or vaginismus). They are often correctable.

Timing of Testing Procedures

When testing procedures are outlined, couples usually want to proceed in the safest, fastest, and least expensive manner to find out what may be causing their infertility.

Many baseline testing procedures are done at a specific point in the menstrual cycle. With proper planning, these studies can be accomplished in one cycle, allowing diagnostic conclusions to be reached as soon as possible. Using a basal body temperature chart, Figure 13-4 shows the schedule of baseline testing within one cycle. At the end of this cycle, all diagnostic data can be evaluated to plan for further testing or treatment.

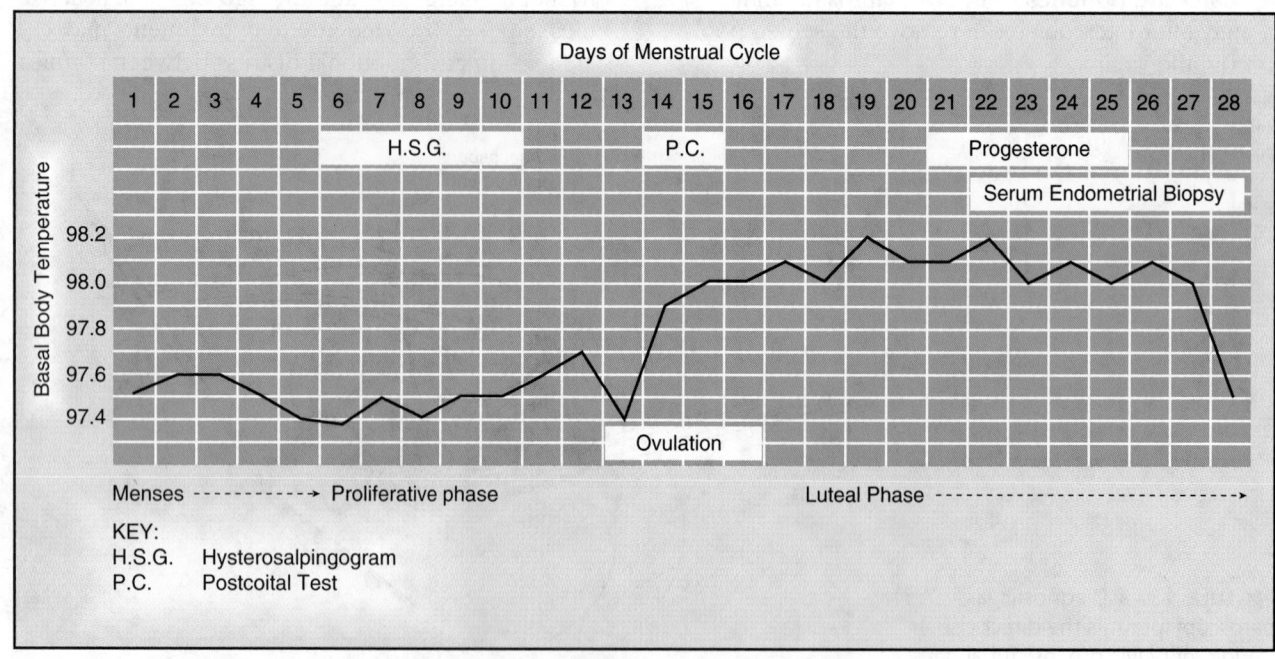

FIGURE 13–4 Timing of baseline infertility studies within one menstrual cycle.

Nursing Diagnosis and Intervention

Childbearing often is seen as one of the most basic of life's achievements. For those who cannot achieve a pregnancy, feelings of failure, depression, isolation, guilt, and anger accompany their desire for a child. Acknowledgement of these intense feelings aids the couple in their quest for solutions and acceptance of the testing procedures (see Nursing Care Plan: The Infertile Couple).

The nurse can easily set a stage for a healthy provider–client relationship through an attitude of acceptance. In many healthcare facilities, the nurse gathers the initial history and may even order baseline tests. By providing clear explanations, the nurse can help the couple maintain realistic expectations and accept the gathered information. Nursing diagnoses are related to investigation of fertility disorders and may be seen at any point in this process (Box 13-4).

The goal of an infertility evaluation is not solely a completed pregnancy. Establishing an acceptable treatment plan and a realistic prognosis are equally important. If a couple is unable to conceive and carry their own biologic child, options are presented to aid them for fulfilling their desire for a family. These options may include **assisted reproductive technology** (ART), such as **in vitro fertilization** (IVF), gamete or zygote intrafallopian transfer (GIFT or ZIFT) procedures, artificial insemination, surrogate parenting, and adoption.

Infertility evaluation and treatment can be a time- and resource-consuming process. It should proceed on a schedule that meets the needs of the couple. If at any point they elect to stop, they must be allowed to do so. They should be advised of the consequences of their decision, but the decision must be theirs. At some point, many couples elect to remain a family of two. This is their option (Cefalo, 1990; Hatcher et al., 1994).

Couples may decide to continue evaluation and treatment. Whereas most baseline testing can be accomplished in a short time, treatment may be a long process. Financial, emotional, and physical drain may influence couples to proceed slowly or to stop completely for a period of time. Reproductive technology is changing rapidly, and new doors are constantly opening for those who may have been considered irreversibly sterile.

Client education is often the nurse's responsibility. The nurse must understand the process as a whole to inform clients of needed testing procedures and their purposes and possible outcomes. From this framework, the nurse can provide factual information that allows the couple to make informed decisions that reflect their desires, resources, and acceptance of the situation (Box 13-5).

It is not unusual for infertile couples to suggest and request treatment that may be inappropriate for them. They bring stories of what worked for friends, neighbors, or families. The nurse's knowledge and empathic understanding can assist the couple in letting go of hopes that may not be appropriate for their situation.

The nurse can aid the couple in their ongoing acceptance of their fertility dilemma. Many couples experience a grief reaction to news that childbearing may be difficult or impossible for them. Common themes of denial, anger, guilt, bargaining, and finally, resolution are often displayed by the infertile couple. Nonjudgmental acceptance of their emotional state can provide the best atmosphere in which the couple can grow and move toward final acceptance.

Isolation is a common feeling of infertile couples. They may find it difficult to share their feelings and emotions with their peers, who seem to conceive and carry pregnancies without problem. Isolation is a result of the couple's sense of personal failure, inadequacy, and decreased self-image. Again, the nurse can be of greatest value by encouraging open communication between partners and with the healthcare team.

Support groups have made important inroads in the area of psychological care for infertile couples. Resolve, Inc., a national support group for infertile couples, has chapters around the country in which couples can find support and guidance as they seek answers to their reproductive predicaments. Resolve also is a national resource center, gathering and disseminating information about the latest developments in infertility treatment. Information about Resolve and various infertility treatments also is available for home computer users through the internet.

Medical Interventions

Reduced Sperm Count or Motility

There are several treatments for reduced sperm count or decreased sperm motility, including surgical treatment of varicoceles, reduction of heat to the scrotum, hormonal treatments with clomiphene citrate to increase sperm count, and artificial insemination.

In cases of nonreversible decreased count or motility, direct insemination with the man's sperm is performed. Therapeutic artificial insemination with husband's sperm (TAI-H) is indicated when count and motility are below normal ranges. In cases of aspermia, therapeutic artificial insemination with donor sperm can be used. In both situations, semen is directly delivered to the cervix by means of a cup device, similar to

NURSING CARE PLAN
The Infertile Couple

Nursing Goals
1. Obtain a complete assessment through history taking, records, and behavioral observation.
2. Provide thorough explanation as necessary of infertility conditions and options for remedial help.
3. Allay anxiety through information and emotional support.

Assessment	*Potential Nursing Diagnoses*	*Intervention/ Rationale*	*Evaluation*
Couple's knowledge about the reproductive process	Knowledge Deficit related to sexual anatomy or physiology	Take complete history regarding this area *to form database* Provide accurate information as needed *to enhance client understanding* Allow time for feedback and questions *to enhance client knowledge*	Couple demonstrates that they have accurate information
Couple's knowledge and technique regarding sexual behavior	Knowledge Deficit related to foreplay or coital techniques	Same as above	Same as above
Couple's family coping styles (eg, cohesiveness, blaming, sharing responsibility)	Ineffective Coping styles	Take complete history in this area *to supplement database* Observe family interaction *to assess mutual support* Clarify observations *to enhance client understanding* Provide feedback on coping behaviors *to enhance insight*	Couple demonstrates realistic appraisal of the situation
Couple's general lifestyle including substance use, nutrition	Knowledge Deficit related to impact of lifestyle on fertility	Take complete history (use self-assessment form as necessary) *to supplement database* Clarify misinformation *to increase client understanding* Provide feedback on lifestyle and habits *to enhance insight*	Couple can verbalize accurate information and make positive changes as indicated
Feelings of self-esteem	Lowered Self Esteem related to inability to conceive	Clarify misinformation *to enhance client understanding* Provide reinforcement of positive feelings and attitudes *to strengthen self-esteem*	Couple demonstrates more positive attitude
Degree of anxiety or fear regarding conditions and treatment options	Anxiety or fear related to the unknown and treatment procedures and outcomes	Provide adequate time for questions *to enhance client understanding* Provide accurate information and clarification of treatment procedures as indicated *to enhance client knowledge* Provide opportunity to verbalize concerns *to provide support* Provide referrals as necessary *to provide comprehensive care* Schedule tests and procedures carefully with the clients' interests in mind *to enhance client's comfort*	Couple indicates that their fear and anxiety have lessened Couple follows through with regimen

---

BOX 13-4
Potential Nursing Diagnoses

Knowledge Deficit related to sexual anatomy or physiology

Knowledge Deficit related to foreplay or coital techniques

Ineffective Coping

Knowledge Deficit related to impact of lifestyle on infertility

Situational Low Self-esteem related to inability to conceive

Anxiety or Fear related to tests, treatment, procedures, and outcome.

Additional nursing diagnoses may include the following:

Spiritual Distress

Impaired Communication

Altered Family Process

Social Isolation

Grieving related to actual or perceived loss

Powerlessness

Altered Sexual Patterns

BOX 13-5
Nursing Interventions for the Couple Undergoing Fertility Evaluation

---

- Provide the couple with factual information to assist in their decision-making process.
- Empower the couple in the establishment of realistic expectations at each point in the process.
- Provide the couple with emotional support critical to the successful completion of evaluation and treatment, regardless of the final outcome.

---

a diaphragm or cervical cap (Fig. 13-5*A*). This is left in place for several hours, which allows the cervix to rest in the seminal pool. If cervical mucus is suspect, semen can be injected directly into the uterine cavity by means of a slender flexible plastic catheter (see Fig. 13-5*B*). This procedure is called intrauterine insemination. With both procedures, the semen is processed with an albumin solution to concentrate the sperm, remove bacteria, and enhance motility (Speroff et al., 1989).

Timing of insemination greatly depends on ovulation. With the use of basal body temperature charts or home ovulation predictor kits, inseminations can occur immediately before ovulation.

Donor insemination has changed due to the possibility of transmitting the human immunodeficiency virus (HIV). Donors are carefully screened for HIV and other STDs, and each specimen is tested extensively. Specimens are frozen and held for 6 months' quarantine. This has raised the price of donor sperm significantly, and success rates are somewhat lower with frozen sperm (Speroff et al., 1989).

Cervical Problems

Although TAI-H is used to bypass cervical mucus, some cervical problems can be treated.

- Chronic inflammation, cervicitis, and cellular abnormalities can be treated with cryosurgery (freezing). When the cervix heals, the epithelium should return to its normal mucus-producing patterns. Medications are available to restore vaginal and cervical pH to normal levels.

- Medications may be tried to improve the characteristics of cervical mucus. These include guaifenesin (increases mucus flow), doxycycline (reduces bacterial contamination), and sodium bicarbonate douches (decreases the acidity).

- In women who produce scanty amounts of cervical mucus, oral hormonal supplementation may increase mucus volume and make it more hospitable to sperm. These treatments have limited success (ACOG, 1994).

Ovulation Problems

Ovulation failure is not always the result of ovarian pathology. The cause may be at any point in the hypothalamic-pituitary-ovarian axis or may be a disorder of the thyroid or adrenal glands. Clients with suspected ovarian-related infertility must be screened for deficiencies of these endocrine glands.

A *serum prolactin* is ordered if a client exhibits **galactorrhea,** spontaneous breast milk discharge; **oligomenorrhea**, irregular menses with long cycles; or **amenorrhea**, the absence of menstruation. The cause may be a pituitary adenoma, a space-occupying tumor of the anterior pituitary. An elevated serum prolactin, without evidence of pituitary enlargement, may indicate hyperprolactinemia. This is often successfully treated with bromocriptine, a dopamine receptor agonist. This drug lowers prolactin levels, allowing the resumption of ovulation.

Clomiphene citrate (Clomid, Serophene), an estrogen antagonist, is the drug of choice for women with decreased serum progesterone levels and evidence of continuing estrogen production. This medication enhances follicular development and induces ovulation. To titrate clomiphene to the individual's needs, clients should have serum progesterone levels measured after the first cycle. If no increase is shown, the dosage is increased for the next cycle, and the serum progesterone measurement is repeated. This procedure is followed until ovulatory progesterone levels are reached. Clients also should be examined each cycle for the presence of ovarian cysts. If a cyst develops, the drug should be discontinued for one cycle. Cysts that do not sponta-

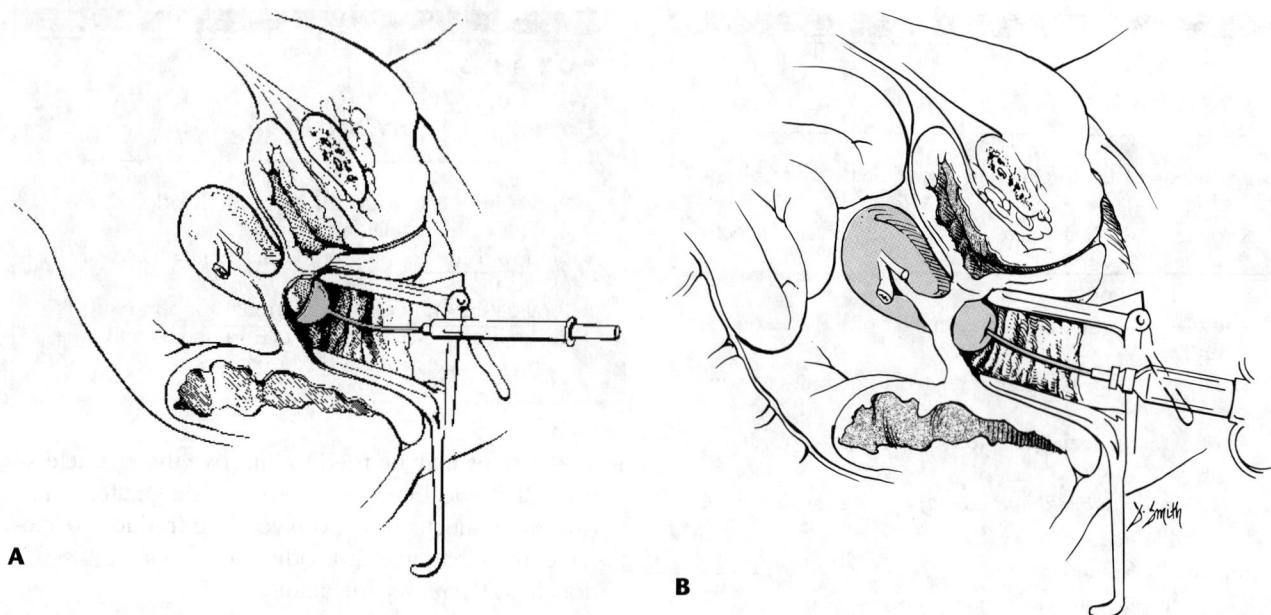

FIGURE 13-5 Artificial insemination. (**A**) Semen is placed in direct contact with the cervix by means of a cervical capping device. (**B**) Prepared semen is injected directly into the uterine cavity.

neously resolve may require surgical drainage. Twins result from clomiphene therapy in about 10% of cases.

Human menopausal gonadotrophin or menotrophin (hMG, Pergonal, Humegon, Metrodin) is used for ovulatory failure at the hypothalamic-pituitary level. These drugs stimulate follicular development, often resulting in the maturation of several follicles simultaneously. With daily hormonal and sonographic monitoring, follicular age can be determined. Ovulation is induced with an injection of human chorionic gonadotrophin, and intercourse or insemination is planned accordingly. Mature follicles also can be harvested for IVF with embryo transfer (IVF-ET), GIFT, ZIFT, or other ART procedures (detailed at the end of this chapter).

Because the use of menotrophins can induce multiple follicles, women receiving this treatment have a higher incidence of multiple gestations. Because of the high infant mortality associated with gestations of three or more fetuses, careful monitoring and consistent care are essential. Hyperstimulation of the ovaries also is possible with ovulation induction. This potentially dangerous condition can be prevented with careful monitoring and dose titration.

Uterine Problems and Habitual Abortion

Congenital anomalies of the uterus, fibroid tumors, and intrauterine scarring may contribute to habitual abortion more than to infertility. These problems often are surgically correctable. Use of the hysteroscope has en-

hanced the ability to correct uterine anatomy without incising the body of the organ.

Habitual abortion also may be caused by asynchronous hormone levels. Asynchronous hormone levels cause inadequate amounts of progesterone to be secreted during the luteal phase; without adequate levels of progesterone, the endometrium cannot support a gestation. This problem, luteal phase defect, can be treated by administering progesterone by injection or vaginal suppository as soon as pregnancy is confirmed. Therapy is continued at least until the 16th week, when the placenta is mature enough to support the pregnancy with its own hormone production. Early detection of pregnancy is essential to preserve the gestation.

The presence of antiphospholipid antibodies, especially anticardiolipins, also may contribute to habitual abortion. These antibodies may interfere with prothrombin activity, predisposing the client to thrombosis, placental infarction, and increased coagulation that affects the fetus. Immunologic testing and treatment are available (Ament, 1994).

Tubal Problems

Success in correcting tubal occlusion depends greatly on the extent of damage to the adnexa. Severe endometriosis, extensive scarring from repeated infections, or recurrent ectopic pregnancies make correction of defects difficult. However, microsurgery may be successful if the tubal structures are minimally compromised or if minor adhesions impede the fimbria.

Advances in microsurgery, plastic surgery, and laser procedures have increased the success rate of tubal reconstruction. Reanastomosis and reimplantation are possible depending on the location of the occlusion. However, due to the structure and size of the tube, there is a greater than 50% failure rate.

Tubal ligation or fulguration done as sterilization procedures can be reversed, but these procedures have the same dismal failure rate. Postoperative inflammation may decrease the tubal lumen to such an extent that the fertilized egg is too large to pass through to the uterus. Women undergoing any tubal surgery must be advised of the increased risk and signs and symptoms of ectopic pregnancy.

Techniques of Assisted Reproductive Technology

No longer are all children conceived within the body of their biologic mothers. Several techniques have been developed that mix ovum and sperm and transfer the mixture to the woman's body. Significant controversy has arisen about these techniques. However, the American Fertility Society regards these procedures as an acceptable alternative for couples who would otherwise be infertile due to untreatable reproductive disorders. These techniques hold promise for women older than 35 years or who require donor oocytes for pregnancy (Maroulis, 1993).

In Vitro Fertilization. The first technique developed was IVF-ET. In 1978, the birth of Louise Brown in England heralded the beginning of this new era in reproductive medicine (Navot et al., 1989). IVF-ET involves overstimulation of the ovaries with clomiphene or hMG so that multiple follicles are developed. When mature (determined by ultrasonography), the eggs are harvested by way of laparoscopy or needle aspiration and fertilized in vitro with washed sperm. When the oocytes reach the four- to eight-cell stage, they are transferred to the uterus.

Gamete Intrafallopian Tube Transfer. A simpler procedure than IVF-ET, GIFT produced its first success in 1984. With **GIFT,** multiple follicles are produced and harvested by laparoscopy. They are mixed with the treated sperm and immediately introduced into a tubal segment known to be patent. Fertilization occurs in the tube, and the embryo then moves to the uterus. Some tubal function is required for GIFT. The most promising results have occurred with women using donor oocytes (due to ovarian failure or advanced maternal age). Some centers report as high as 56% of transfers resulting in pregnancies.

Zygote Intrafallopian Tube Transfer. A variation on GIFT, **ZIFT** is appropriate when proof of fertilization is essential (severe male factor infertility or immunologic infertility). Pregnancy rates vary but are usually quoted at about 20% to 25% (Balmaceda et al., 1993).

Surrogate Embyro Transfer. Ovum transfer or surrogate embryo transfer is a more complicated procedure. A donor ovum is used in this process. The donor and recipient are matched genetically, medically, and psychologically. Their menstrual cycles are synchronized using oral hormones. After synchronization and at the time of ovulation, the donor is inseminated with the biologic father's sperm. Five days later, the donor's uterus is lavaged, and the fertilized ovum is retrieved. It is then transferred to the recipient's uterus.

Financial and Ethical Considerations Concerning Assisted Reproductive Technology

With all four techniques, success rates and cost of procedures vary from institution to institution. Generally, less than 20% of all attempts result in normal pregnancies. Attempts may range over many cycles and cost several thousand dollars each. Despite enthusiastic claims from proponents of ART, these procedures are costly in terms of resources and human input. When a pregnancy is not achieved, a sense of failure may be shared by the fertility team and the couple, and the level of disappointment can be significant (Maroulis, 1993; ACOG, 1994).

As techniques for assisting infertile couples improve and are refined, healthcare providers must repeatedly examine their own belief systems, ethics, and morals to determine what they deem appropriate and acceptable. Some may believe that no cost should be spared or no technique left untried in the quest for a successful pregnancy. Others may feel that these elaborate techniques are challenging nature and that humans have no right to interfere with a natural process. ART entails expensive treatment protocols, and critics argue that this successfully bars many couples from obtaining it. Insurance companies generally do not pay for infertility treatment or pay at a greatly reduced rate, therefore creating another barrier to care.

While these opinions reflect the ends of the spectrum, there are varying views in between. Some providers may feel that one technique is morally acceptable but another is not. It behooves the infertile couple to seek healthcare providers who share similar beliefs, ethics, and morals. Also, it is beneficial for each healthcare provider to define his or her own limits and boundaries of acceptable treatment. See Chapter 5 for further discussion on ethical and legal considerations prior to conception.

Unexplained Infertility

Occasionally, in spite of normal results in every diagnostic testing procedure and one or many corrective surgical procedures, a couple fails to conceive. This is perhaps more devastating than infertility that can be linked to a physical cause. It is difficult to give up, but at some point many couples voluntarily end testing and attempts to conceive. Providers must accept that decision.

Alternatives to Childbearing

After years of testing and attempting to conceive, many couples look for a solution outside of biologic parenting. Adoption is a viable alternative. Although the number of infants available for adoption has decreased, adoption remains a satisfactory solution for some couples (Cefalo, 1990).

Adoption can be an open agreement between biologic and adoptive families. A birth mother can work with an attorney or physician to select a family for her child. Communication between the two parties can be as limited or as open as desired. Agencies specializing in open adoption can provide psychological counseling for the birth mother to assist her adaptation to the adoption. Should the birth mother wish no contact with the adoptive family, closed adoptions also are available. Most government and church agencies encourage the birth mother to have no contact with her child after its birth.

Foster parenting is another option for couples. As "temporary" parents, couples have a chance to impact the lives of many children, while serving as a vital link between birth parents and adoptive parents. County social service departments can provide information about requirements, reimbursement, and outcome criteria.

Childlessness may be the final alternative. After exploring various treatments and opportunities, couples may decide to remain childless. For some, the stress of testing and treatment becomes unbearable. For others, the economic drain is simply impossible.

A person's worth as an individual does not rest on the ability to conceive and bear children. For the childless couple, self-fulfillment may come from career pursuits, altruistic activities, or other creative projects. Each woman, man, couple, and family must find their own meaning in the creative process of life (Northrup, 1994).

The Future

In 1994, researchers reported the successful implantation of a pregnancy initiated with injection of a single sperm into a human egg. This process, called intracytoplasmic sperm injection or single-sperm injection, is used in cases of severe male infertility. Most techniques are experimental, expensive, and accessible to only a small segment of the population. The overall success rate is limited.

However, research in infertility continues at a rapid pace. Those once believed to be infertile may have another chance as each discovery is made.

The future holds promise and conflict in the area of infertility. Nurses will need to assist clients in making appropriate decisions, while maintaining a sense of economic and philosophic responsibility.

Summary Points

✔ Infertility is a complex problem that affects the biopsychosocial and spiritual health of many couples. Infertility may be due to male or female factors or a combination of hormonal, structural, and developmental problems.

✔ The nursing process can be applied to the evaluation and treatment of the infertile couple, thus providing comprehensive and appropriate care.

✔ Treatment goals include correcting physical problems, assisting ovulation or fertilization, and normalizing response patterns of the client and family.

✔ The advent of ART has given childless couples another chance at parenthood but not without serious ethnical, philosophic, and economic dilemmas.

REFERENCES

Ament, L. (1994). Anticardiolipin antibodies: A review of the literature. *Journal of Nurse-Midwifery, 39*(1), 19–24.

American College of Obstetrics and Gynecologists (1994). *Precis V: An update in obstetrics and gynecology.* Washington, DC: Author.

Balmaceda, J., & Manzur, A. (1993). Current status of GIFT. *Contemporary OB/GYN, 38*(12), 59–72.

Cefalo, R. C. (1990). *Clinical decisions in obstetrics and gynecology.* Rockville, MD, Aspen.

Cohen, J., Alikani, M., Munne, S., & Palmero, G. (1994). Micromanipulation in clinical management of fertility disorders. *Seminars in Reproductive Endocrinology, 3*(12), 151–168.

Cunningham, F. G., MacDonald, P. C., Gant, N. F., Leveno, K. J., & Gilstrap, L. C. (1993). *Williams obstetrics* (19th ed.). Norwalk, CT: Appleton & Lange.

Gray, R. H., & Fuentes, A. (1994). Infertility epidemiology: current scene. *Contemporary OB/GYN, 39*(5), 70–81.

Green, B. B., Weiss, N. S., & Daling, J. R. (1988). Risk of ovulatory infertility in relation to body weight. *Fertility Sterility, 50,* 721.

Hatcher, R. A., Trussell, J., Stewart, F., Steward, G. K., Kowal, D., Guest, F., Cates, W. L., & Policar, M. (1994). *Contraceptive technology* (16th ed.). New York: Irvington Publishers.

Hawkins, J., Roberto, D., & Stanley-Haney, J. (1993). *Protocols for nurse practitioners in gynecologic settings*. New York: Tiresias Press.

Maroulis, G. (1993). Fertility, pregnancy, and the older woman. *Contemporary OB/GYN, 38*(5), 101–123.

Navot, D., & Laufer, N. (1989). Assisted reproductive technology: A clinical appraisal. *Journal of Reproductive Medicine, 34*, 3.

Shaban, S. (1995). *Male infertility. Monograph URL*. Atlanta, GA: Atlanta Reproductive Health Center.

Speroff, L., Glass, R. H., & Kase, N. G. (1989). *Clinical gynecologic endocrinology and infertility* (4th ed.). Baltimore: Williams & Wilkins.

Star, W., Lommel, L., & Shannon, M. (Eds.) (1995). *Women's primary health care, protocols for practice*. Washington, DC: American Nurses' Publishing.

Vermes, M., Kletzky, O. A., Davajan, V. et al. (1987). Monitoring techniques to predict and detect ovulation. *Fertility Sterility, 47*, 259.

Wilcox, L., & Mosher, M. (1993). Use of infertility sevices in the United States. *Obstetrics and Gynecology, 82*(1), 122–127.

Northrup, C. (1994). Women's bodies, women's wisdom. New York: Bantam.

RESOURCES

Association of Women's Health, Obstetric and Neonatal Nurses
700 14th St. NW
Suite 600
Washington, DC 20005-2019
800-376-8499

American College of Obstetricians and Gynecologists
409 12th Street SW
Washington, DC 20024-2188

American Fertility Society
1209 Montgomery Highway
Birmingham, AL 35216-2809
205-978-5000

RESOLVE, Inc.
1310 Broadway
Somerville, MA 02114-1731
617-623-1156

14

Genetic Counseling and Diagnosis During Pregnancy

Objectives

- Discuss the mechanisms for genetic transfer of traits and disorders.
- Define the process and significance of prenatal diagnosis.
- Describe the role of the nurse or counselor in prenatal diagnosis.
- Discuss the ethical considerations of prenatal diagnosis.

Key Terms

Amniocentesis
Aneuploidy
Autosomal recessive
Chorionic villus
  sampling
Gamete
Genotype
Hemoglobinopathy
Karyotype
Meiosis

Mitosis
Monosomy
Mosaicism
Nondisjunction
Phenotype
Teratogenic
Translocation
Trisomy
Ultrasonography
X-linked recessive

With increasing accuracy, prenatal genetic diagnosis provides valuable information about the health of a fetus. Although this process often detects potential problems, it also provides vital information and reassurance for the expectant couple. In the last 5 years, great strides have been made in identifying genetically based disorders.

Genetic diagnostic services are no longer confined to major medical centers or to a select percentage of the pregnant population. The physician or nurse involved in prenatal care can provide basic genetic counseling and testing services and should have the information to make necessary referrals.

As data about genetic counseling have increased, public awareness also has increased, and clients are more likely to request such services.

Genetic Counseling

The science of genetics is concerned with disease processes that can be passed from one generation to the next or that are related to a defect in chromosomal reproduction. The range of genetic problems is considerable. Some are incompatible with life; others may cause little disruption to the life process.

Genetic counseling integrates family history with available information about the fetus to determine the risk of genetic disease in the fetus. This communication process supplies the family with necessary information to make informed decisions and offers options for treatment.

During genetic counseling and diagnosis, many aspects of this process are examined. These include the genetic mechanisms involved, the extent of the risk to the fetus, medical considerations, treatment options, and the impact of the possible diagnosis on future childbearing and the family unit. This can be an emotional time for parents as they question their future and

that of their children. The role of the healthcare provider is to present factual information concerning testing, risks, and outcome expectations, while supporting the family as they reach decisions.

Genetic counseling is a multidisciplinary service. It involves a team of geneticists, obstetricians, nurses, counselors, and laboratory personnel who facilitate the process.

Cellular Reproduction

Before nurses can provide information about genetic problems to clients, they must understand the basic mechanisms involved in reproduction. Human reproduction is a complex process involving the union of the genetic material of both parents. This union produces a fetus similar, but not identical, to the biologic parents.

A normal human cell contains 46 chromosomes (diploid number of 2N). There are 22 pairs of autosomes and one pair of sex chromosomes (XX for the girl and XY for the boy; Fig. 14-1*A* and *B*). Each chromosome is constructed of protein matter supporting deoxyribonucleic acid (DNA) strands containing thousands of genes. Whereas chromosomes were first identified in the 1870s, it was not until the 1950s that the normal human **karyotype** of 23 paired chromosomes was identified. This led to subsequent investigation of the cellular aspects of certain genetic disorders (Miller, 1990).

Mechanisms Involved in Cellular Reproduction

Mitosis (Fig. 14-2*A*) is the process in which cell division yields exact replication of the parent cells. **Meiosis** (Fig. 14-2*B*) is the means by which **gametes** are created. One half of the parents' genetic information is contained in a gamete.

Inherited Traits and Disorders

Chromosomal Abnormalities

Chromosomal abnormalities result when mitosis and meiosis do not occur in a normal fashion. Several types of chromosomal abnormalities are described below:

- **Nondisjunction** (Fig. 14-3) is the unequal distribution of chromosomes to the daughter cells during mitosis or meiosis. This accounts for the majority of numeric chromosome abnormalities.
- **Aneuploidy** is the result of numeric chromosome errors. This usually results in major developmental

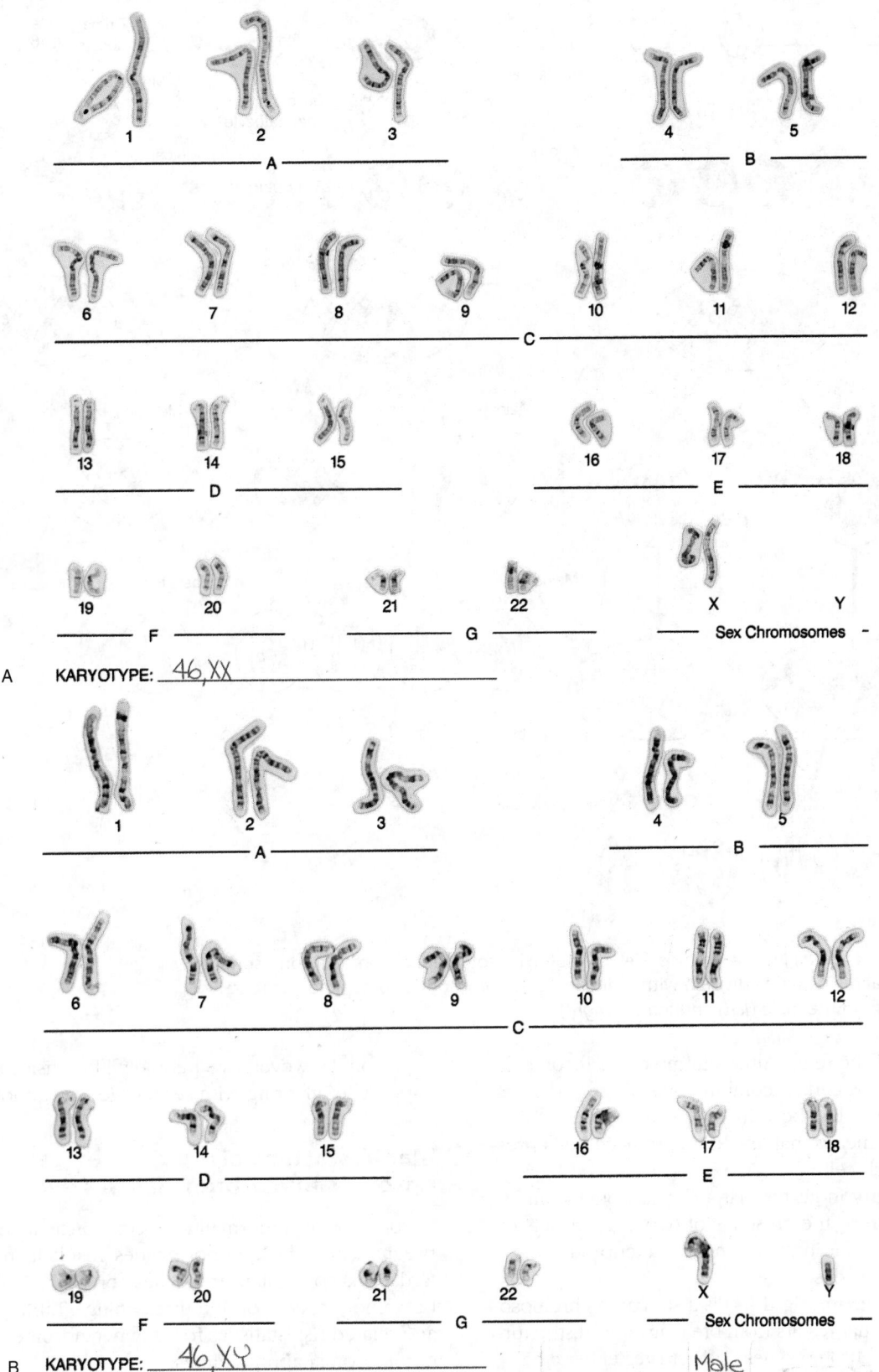

FIGURE 14–1 Karotype of (**A**) normal human girl and (**B**) normal human boy. (Courtesy of the Prenatal Diagnostic and Imaging Center, Sacramento, CA. Frederick W. Hansen, MD, Medical Director.)

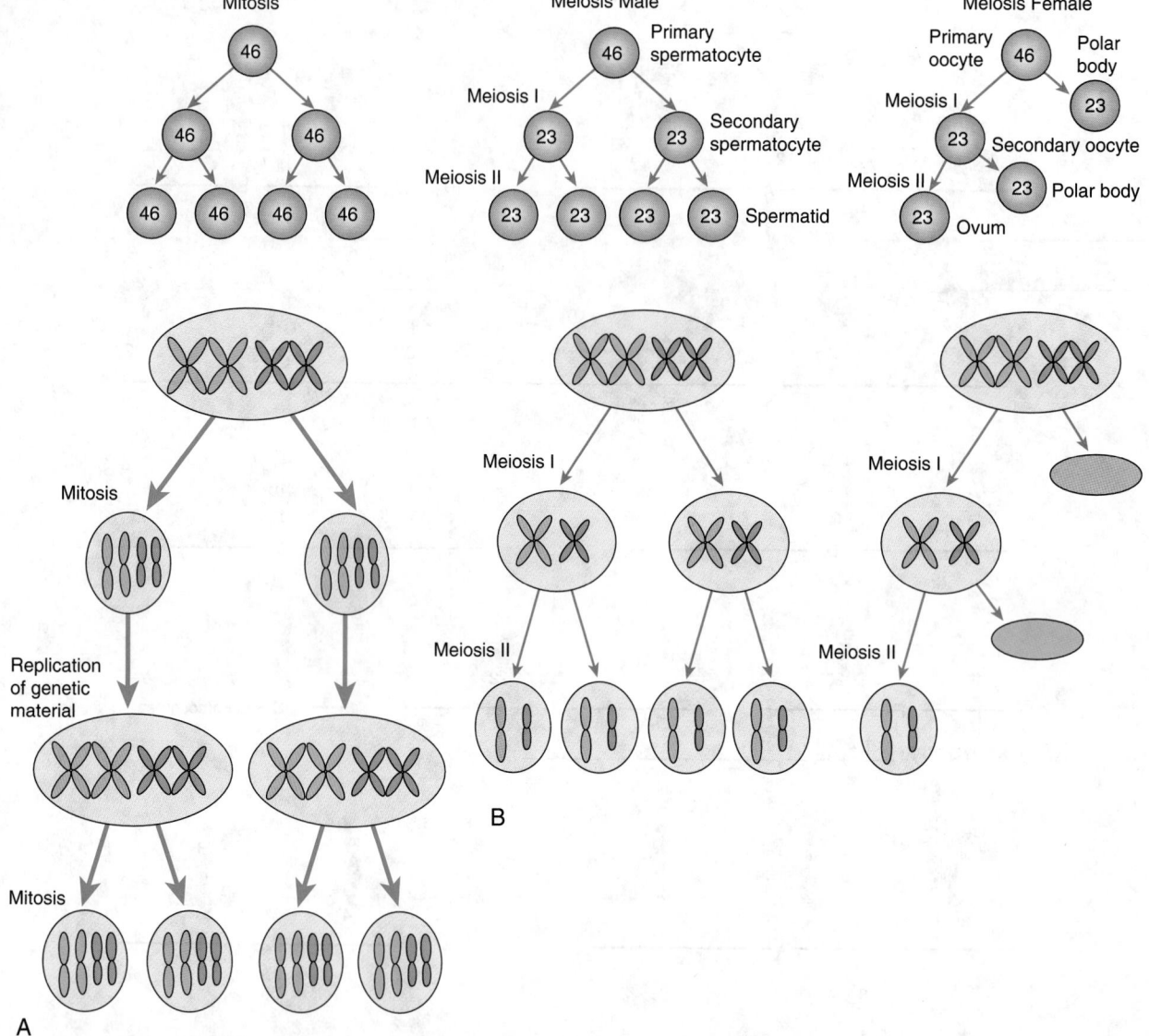

FIGURE 14–2 **(A)** Normal mitosis. Cell division with total replication of chromosomes. **(B)** Normal meiosis. Cell division with reduction of chromosomes to haploid number. Normal meiosis in the male (*left*) and female (*right*).

defects of the fetus. Although many are incompatible with life, certain combinations of these defects can result in live-born infants.

- **Trisomy** means that an extra chromosome is present in each cell.
- **Monosomy** indicates that a chromosome is missing.
- **Mosaicism** is the presence of two or more sets of cells that differ in their genetic makeup but arise from single cells.
- **Translocation** (Fig. 14-4) is a structural chromosomal error that results from breakage and restructuring of the chromosomes. This creates either a balanced carrier of the defect or an unbalanced carrier (Fig. 14-5). If translocation occurs without loss of genetic information, the carrier does not suffer major phenotype consequences if paired with a normal

person. However, two people with translocation can produce offspring with serious genetic abnormalities.

Manifestations of Chromosomal Abnormalities

Chromosomal abnormalities occur once in every 400 pregnancies. These abnormalities result in mental retardation, congenital anomalies, or both. Defects can be minor, major, or life-threatening. Table 14-1 lists age-related risk statistics for Down syndrome and other chromosomal abnormalities.

Trisomy 21. This is the presence of an extra chromosome in the 21st pair, resulting in a fetus affected with Down syndrome (Fig. 14-6). Children affected with

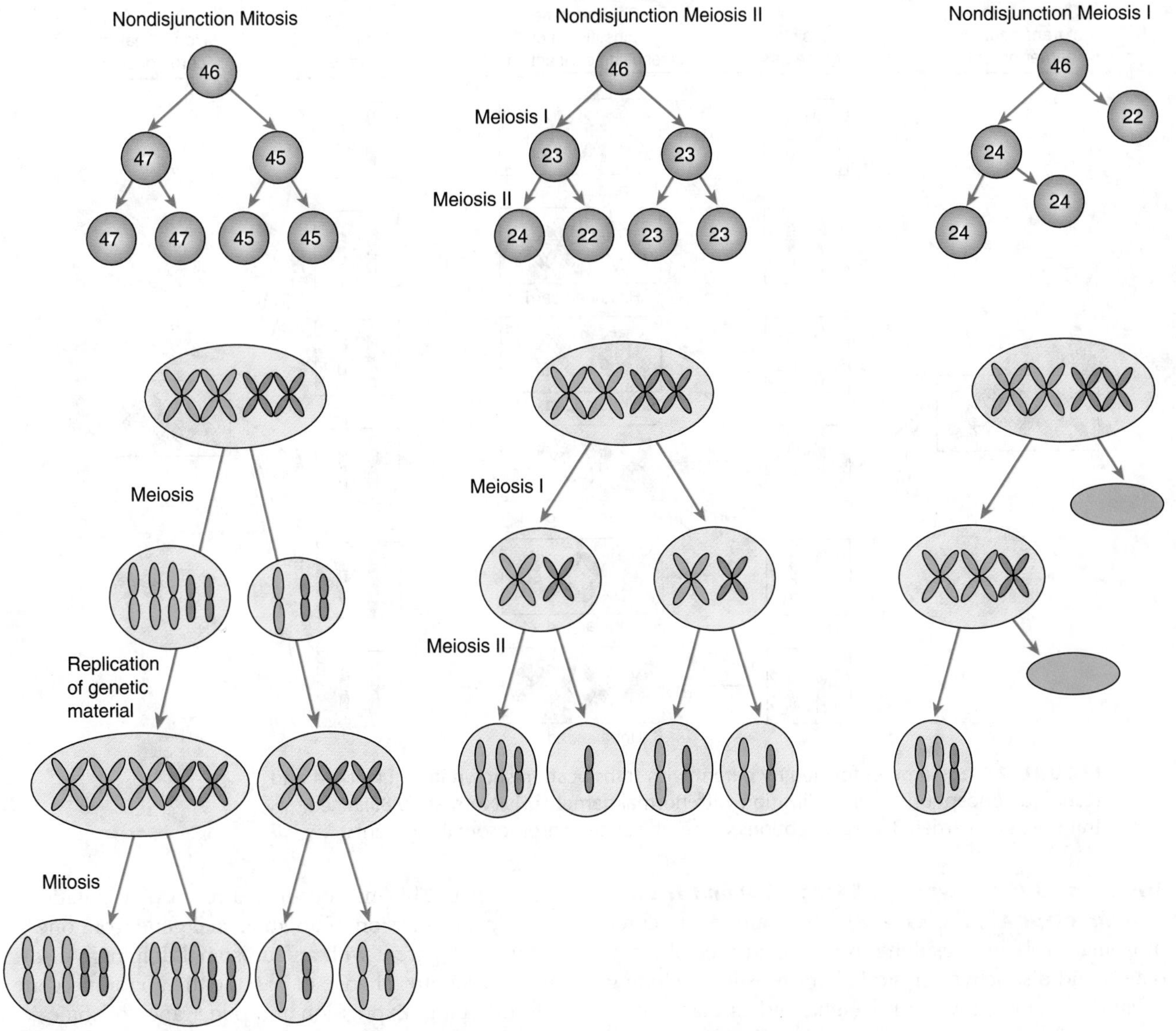

Nondisjunction Mitosis

Nondisjunction Meiosis II

Nondisjunction Meiosis I

FIGURE 14–3 Nondisjunction in mitosis and meiosis. Upper portion demonstrates the segregation of chromosomes numerically, and lower portion depicts the segregation of two of the 23 chromosome pairs. (*Left*) Mitosis, two mitotic divisions with nondisjunction occurring in the first, and the error passed through the subsequent division. (*Center*) Meiosis in the male, with nondisjunction occurring in the second division of meiosis, resulting in normal and abnormal spermatids. (*Right*) Meiosis in the female, with nondisjunction occurring in the first division of meiosis resulting in an abnormal ovum.

Down syndrome have the characteristic physical features of low-set, small ears; increased epicanthal folds; cardiac defects; and poor muscle tone. Mental impairment can range from moderate to severe. Mosaic Down syndrome results when two cell lines are af-fected, one normal and one with trisomy 21. Children with this disorder may have physical characteristics of trisomy 21 with a wide range of IQ impairment (Miller, 1990; Cunningham et al., 1993; Hoekelman, 1987; Robinson et al., 1993).

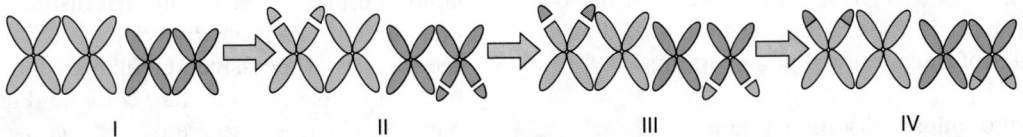

FIGURE 14–4 Mechanism of reciprocal translocation. (**I**) Two normal chromosome pairs. (**II**) Breakage of one member of each pair. (**III**) Exchange of broken segments. (**IV**) Reunion to form balanced rearrangement (translocation).

Chromosomes of translocation carrier parent	Possible gametes	Chromosome constitution of resulting conception	Normal gametes	Normal parental chromosomes

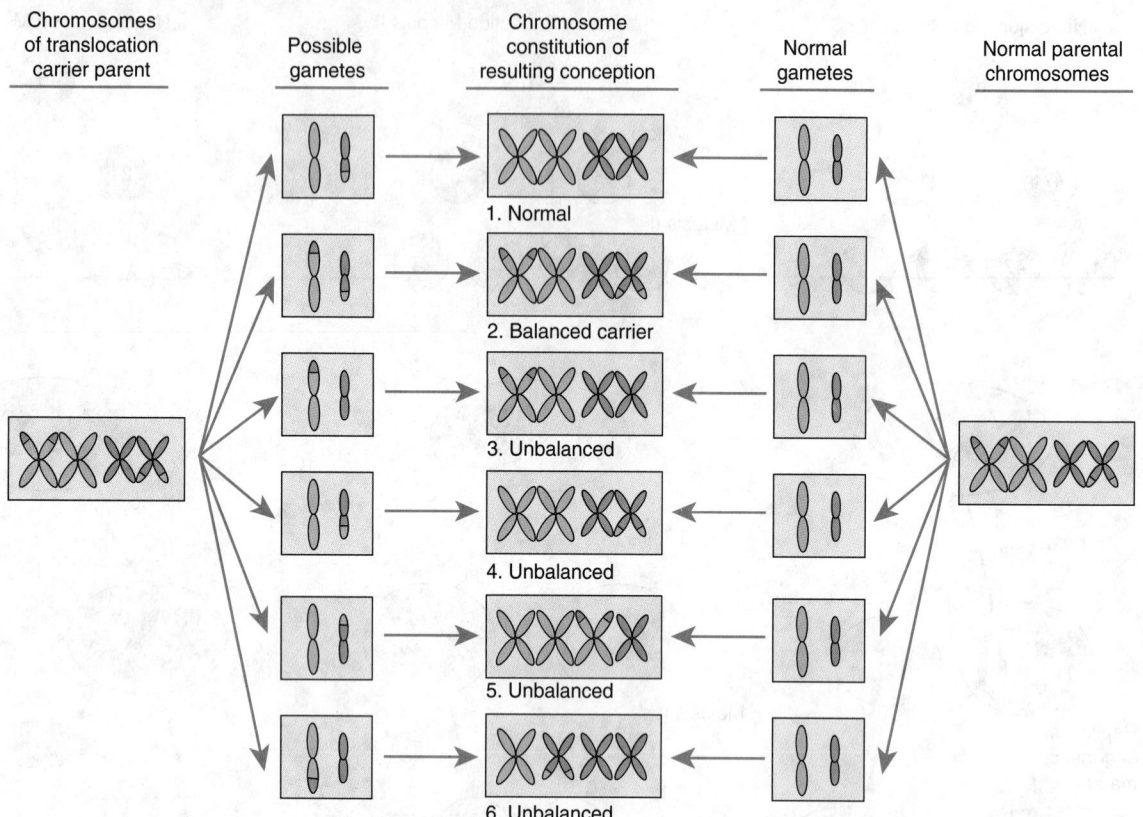

1. Normal

2. Balanced carrier

3. Unbalanced

4. Unbalanced

5. Unbalanced

6. Unbalanced

FIGURE 14–5 Gametes formed by parent with translocation shown in Figure 14–4 and resulting conceptions after fertilization with normal gametes. 1. Normal. 2. Balanced translocation carrier. 3–6. Conceptions with unbalanced chromosomal segments.

Trisomies 13 (karyotype 47, XX/XY +13) and Trisomy 18 (karyotype 47, XX/XY +18). These are severe chromosomal problems resulting in profound mental retardation and distinctive physical characteristics, including facial deformities, low birth weight, and cardiac abnormalities. These newborns often fail to thrive, and 10% will not survive their first year of life.

Turner's syndrome (karyotype 45, X) and Klinefelter's syndrome (karyotype 47, XXY). These are nondisjunctive disorders that result in delayed or absent sexual maturity, short stature, mild retardation, or behavioral abnormalities. This defect is suspected clinically and confirmed with karyotyping (Hoekelman, 1987; Robinson et al., 1993).

Mendelian Disorders

Many genetic disorders result from mechanisms described by Mendel. These are classified according to characteristics of the abnormal gene pattern:

■ Autosomal dominant disorders (Table 14-2) are those in which the presence of a single abnormal gene results in phenotypical changes or disease, despite the normalacy of the other member of the

gene pair. This may occur as a result of a mutation or by transmission of an abnormal gene from one parent. A parent with an autosomal dominant disorder has a 50% chance of passing the abnormal gene to offspring. Expression and penetrance of some dominant genes vary greatly. Diagnosis of autosomal dominant disorders is sometimes possible only after birth.

■ **Autosomal recessive** disorders (Table 14-3) are those in which both members of the gene pair are abnormal (homozygous). During meiosis, this abnormal gene is passed to the gamete. However, if the other parent has normal genetic structure, the abnormal gene contributed by the affected parent usually is not expressed. The offspring, however, are carriers of the defect and are termed heterozygous for the abnormal gene. If both parents carry recessive genes for a specific disorder, one child in four is affected with that disorder, and one child in two is a carrier. Figure 14-7 depicts the process of recessive inheritance. Other genetic traits, such as eye color, hair color, and left or right hand dominance, also are passed to offspring in this manner.

■ **X-linked recessive** disorders (Table 14-4) are present only on the X chromosome. In normal women,

TABLE 14-1
Age-Related Risk of Down Syndrome and Chromosome Abnormalities

Maternal Age	Risk of Down Syndrome	Total Risk for Chromosomal Abnormalities*
20	1/1667	1/526*
25	1/1250	1/476*
30	1/952	1/384*
35	1/385	1/192
36	1/294	1/156
37	1/227	1/127
38	1/175	1/102
39	1/137	1/83
40	1/106	1/66
41	1/82	1/53
42	1/64	1/42
43	1/50	1/33
44	1/38	1/26
45	1/30	1/21
46	1/23	1/16
47	1/18	1/13
48	1/14	1/10
49	1/11	1/8

*47,XXX excluded for ages 20–30 (data not available).
(Reprinted with permission from Cefalo, R. C. [Ed.] [1990]. *Clinical decisions in obstetrics and gynecology* [p. 158]. Rockville, MD: Aspen Publishers. © 1990.)

one X chromosome in each pair is inactive and may be visualized as a *Barr body*, a chromatin mass found in the periphery of the cell nucleus. The inactivation of the X chromosome is random (ie, some of the maternally inherited X chromosomes are active in some cells, and paternally inherited X chromosomes are active in others). A woman with an X-linked disorder has some active abnormal genes, but unless the majority of normal genes are inactivated, the disease will not be manifest. During reproduction, if the abnormal gene is active and passed to the gamete, the male offspring will manifest the disorder because the X chromosome in each male cell is active. Female offspring may be carriers of the disorder. Half of the offspring will either be carriers or will manifest the disorder.

Manifestations of Mendelian Disorders

Single-gene defects account for a considerable number of genetic problems associated with mendelian disorders. Careful history taking and appropriate genetic testing can identify fetuses affected with these disorders.

Osteogenesis imperfecta (OI). This manifests with dental defects, increased susceptibility to long bone fractures, and otosclerosis. It is often detected in infancy. Intelligence is usually normal and with comprehensive care, prognosis for those with the milder forms is usually good. OI is classified as one of four types based on osseous fragility and other markers.

Marfan syndrome. This is an autosomal dominant defect, affecting the skeletal, ocular, and cardiac systems. Those affected are usually tall with long extremities and are prone to aortic aneurysms and detachment of the retina and myopia. Life expectancy is normal with medical or surgical intervention.

Cystic fibrosis (CF). This is a severe multisystem autosomal recessive disease. It is marked by pancreatic enzyme deficiency, chronic obstructive and infective pulmonary disease, and increased concentrations of sodium in the sweat. CF clients have a decreased life expectancy in spite of increasing treatment modalities. The marker gene for CF was identified in 1985, and carrier testing is available for families at risk (Robinson et al., 1993; Harrington et al., 1992).

Phenylketonuria (PKU). This is an autosomal recessive disease that affects metabolism of the enzyme phenylalanine. Maintaining a diet of foods low in phenylalanine has been found to prevent the mental retardation associated with this disorder. All newborns are tested for PKU.

Sickle cell anemia. This is a **hemoglobinopathy** that primarily affects African Americans. It is an autosomal recessive condition that manifests a wide range of clinical symptoms from mild to life-threatening. Sickle cell trait is a carrier state found in less than 10% of African Americans. All African American women should be screened for this trait during prenatal care.

Hemophilia A and B. These are bleeding disorders that prevent adequate clotting because of a missing blood factor. They are X-linked recessive diseases mostly affecting men. Hemophiliac children are monitored and treated with prophylactic administration of the missing blood factor. Life expectancy is increasing.

Duchenne's muscular dystrophy. This is a severe, debilitating, fatal, X-linked disease. Male children who are affected suffer muscle hypertrophy as a result of a defect in creatinine phosphokinase metabolism. Carrier testing and prenatal diagnosis are now available (Robinson et al., 1993).

Fragile X syndrome. This is an X-linked disorder that frequently causes mental retardation. Affected children

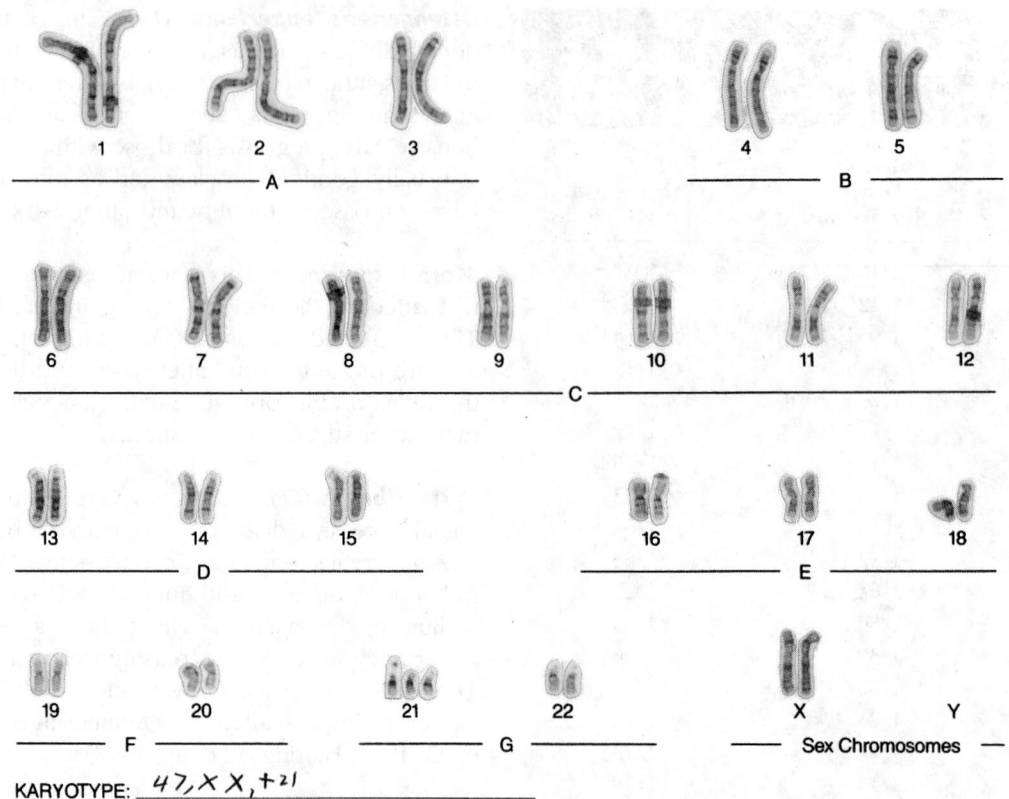

KARYOTYPE: 47, X X, +21

FIGURE 14-6 Karotype of trisomy 21 or Down syndrome. (Courtesy of the Prenatal Diagnostic and Imaging Center, Sacramento, CA. Frederick W. Hansen, MD, Medical Director.)

TABLE 14-2
Autosomal Dominant Traits

PRINCIPAL CHARACTERISTICS
- Every affected child has at least one affected parent (except mutations).
- An affected person need only be heterozygous for the given allele.
- Male and female offspring are equally affected.
- There are affected people in several generations.
- There is a 50% risk of involvement of each sibling of an affected person if the parent is affected.

EXAMPLES OF AUTOSOMAL DOMINANT DISORDERS

Achondroplasia

Acute intermittent porphyria

Adult polycystic kidney disease

Apert's syndrome

Crouzon's syndrome

Familial hypercholesterolemia

Hereditary hemorrhagic telangiectasia

Hereditary spherocytosis

Huntington's disease

Idiopathic hypertrophic subaortic stenosis

Marfan syndrome

Myotonic dystrophy

Neurofibromatosis

Noonan's syndrome

Osteogenesis imperfecta

Polydactyly

Treacher Collins syndrome

Tuberous sclerosis

von Willebrand's disease

(Adapted from Cunningham, F. C., MacDonald, P. C., & Gant, P. C. [1993]. *Williams Obstetrics* [19th ed.]. Norwalk, CT: Appleton & Lange.)

TABLE 14–3
Autosomal Recessive Traits

PRINCIPAL CHARACTERISTICS

- Each parent of an affected person must carry at least one mutant allele (normal parents are carriers).
- Every affected person is homozygous for the given allele.
- People possessing a single mutant allele do not show the trait.
- Either sex may be affected.
- There is a 25% risk of involvement of the siblings of an affected person.
- The disease tends to be rarer and more severe than dominantly inherited conditions.

EXAMPLES OF AUTOSOMAL RECESSIVE DISORDERS

Albinism	Galactosemia
α-Thalassemia	Hemochromatosis
β-Thalassemia	Hereditary emphysema
Congenital adrenal hyperplasia	Homocystinuria
Cystic fibrosis	Phenylketonuria
Familial Mediterranean fever	Sickle cell anemia
Friedreich's ataxia	Tay-Sachs disease
	Wilson's disease

(Adapted from Cunningham, F. C., MacDonald, P. C., & Gant, P. C. [1993]. *Williams Obstetrics* [19th ed.]. Norwalk, CT: Appleton & Lange.)

---

display a variety of physical manifestions, including, low intelligence, behavioral problems, vision disorders, and even autism. Carrier testing is available.

Multifactoral Defects

Many common birth defects are multifactoral. This implies a genetic predisposition to a lower threshold for development abnormalities. Several genes in combination may account for this disposition. Also, genetic interplay may have a cumulative effect by adding factors, such as family history, chance of mutations, and adverse affects of certain environmental factors (eg, exposure to toxic chemicals or radiation, use of recreational drugs). In affected families, the risk of occurrence increases with each child.

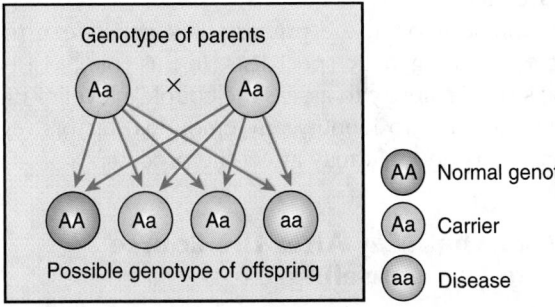

FIGURE 14–7 Recessive inheritance (A, normal gene; a, abnormal gene; AA, normal genotype; Aa, carrier; aa, disease). Note that the frequency of aa children when both parents are Aa carriers is 1:4, or 25%.

Manifestations of Multifactoral Defects

It is difficult to describe the full range of defects due to the high number of possible genetic combinations. Some of the more common multifactoral defects are described below.

Neural Tube Defects. Neural tube defects (NTDs), such as anencephaly, spina bifida, and encephalocele, are thought to occur between days 26 and 28 of gestation when the neural tube normally closes. Although the exact cause is unknown, it is hypothesized that folic acid metabolism, genetic mutations, and environmental factors are involved. NTDs are classified by the affected skeletal location:

- Anencephaly is the failure of the development of the skull and brain. *The cerebral hemispheres are either completely missing or severely reduced in size.* It is the most severe NTD and is incompatible with extrauterine life.
- Myelomeningocele (spina bifida) indicates a defect in the spinal vertebra with the protrusion of meninges or spinal cord. The degree of disability depends on the size of the defect, its location, and its contents. The introduction of maternal serum α-fetoprotein (MS-AFP) testing has increased the chances of perinatal diagnosis of affected pregnancies. With prompt neurosurgical intervention and aggressive management, the prognosis for af-

TABLE 14–4
X-linked Recessive Traits

PRINCIPAL CHARACTERISTICS

- Affected people are nearly always men.
- The mother is usually a carrier, and she transmits the disease to 50% of her sons.
- One half of carrier mothers' daughters will be carriers.
- Affected men transmit their mutant allele to each of their daughters and none of their sons.
- The uninvolved sons do not transmit the disease.

EXAMPLES OF X-LINKED DISORDERS

Chronic granulomatous disease	Glucose 6-phosphate dehydrogenase deficiency
Color blindness	Hemophilia A and B
Fabry's disease	Hypophosphatemic rickets
Fragile X syndrome	Kinky-hair syndrome

(Adapted from Waechter, E. W., Phillips, J., & Holaday, B. [1985]. *Nursing care of children* [10th ed.]. Philadelphia: J.B. Lippincott and Cunningham, F. C., MacDonald, P. C., & Gant, P. C. [1989]. *Williams*

fected children is improving, but the likelihood of serious and permanent handicaps continues.

- Encephalocele *is the protrusion of brain substance and meninges through an opening in the skull.*

Facial deformities. These include cleft lip or palate and may be genetic in origin or the result of exposure to certain chemicals during gestation. Several medications have been identified in connection with these problems. Extremely high-resolution ultrasound may prenatally detect a cleft lip. The presence of this defect should be viewed as a marker for the possibility of other syndromes and associated defects, and a complete examination should be conducted. When occurring as an isolated event, cleft lip and palate are surgically correctable with a high degree of cosmetic and functional success.

The Nursing Process in Genetic Services

The nurse involved in maternity services is vital to the process of genetic screening, testing, and diagnosis. Most genetic services occur in an outpatient setting. Therefore, the nurse often has brief, sporadic contact with the expectant couple. However, the value of these visits can be maximized by application of the nursing process at each appropriate point in the genetic testing schedule.

As the nursing role expands, some nurses further their education and become specialists in the field of genetics. Multidisciplinary centers offering full-spectrum genetics services use physicians, geneticists, and counselors. Genetic counselors are now master's prepared and board certified. Nurses in this role can

effectively use the nursing process to enhance the care provided. The nurse-counselor often integrates aspects of the medical and nursing disciplines and can use the nursing process to design information-gathering techniques, teaching plans, and appropriate emotional support. The nursing process also enables the counselor to evaluate the client's outcome accurately.

Nursing Assessment

The nurse providing prenatal care is often involved in initial client contact and assessment. Within early phases of prenatal care, factors that can potentially impact on the pregnancy are identified. The nurse must be aware and knowledgeable about predisposing conditions and procedures and resources available for prenatal diagnosis. Ideally, factors affecting the genetics of a fetus should be identified before conception. However, it cannot be assumed that potential parents are aware of specific risks. Therefore, care is often sought after pregnancy occurs. Timely diagnosis and intervention are vital.

The nurse is often the primary liaison between the couple and the genetic specialists. In this role, it is the nurse's responsibility to assess the couple's level of understanding and to identify any emotional factors (eg, fear and anxiety) that may affect the process.

Factors That May Alter the Course of Genetic Counseling

- Identify the knowledge base. Public awareness of genetic problems has increased, and self-referral for testing is common. Increased awareness affects the client's perception of and response to testing. The nurse ascertains what information the family has gathered and what sources were used. This allows for clarification and correction of misinformation.

- Explore feelings about the pregnancy. The nurse must determine if the pregnancy was planned or if there is some ambivalence surrounding the event. If these feelings are not addressed, the focus of the client during counseling may be diverted and clouded by denial and anxiety.
- Investigate how the information gathered in the testing process will be used. The nurse must stress that genetic testing is designed to provide information, explore possibilities, and create a plan of treatment that is acceptable to the client, while remaining medically and ethically sound. It is important to clarify that prenatal diagnosis is as more than a means to justify abortion. It is the means by which clients can make informed choices through use of appropriate resources.

Identifying the Couple at Risk

Most pregnancies consist of a normal gestation followed by the birth of a healthy and intact newborn. However, genetic predispositions, familial health problems, environmental factors, and maternal influences can alter the chances of a positive outcome.

The initial prenatal interview can identify clients at risk for genetic disorders. A brief screening questionnaire (Box 14-1) can be used to discover some risk factors. Using this information as a baseline, the nurse asks for specific information related to the couple's history. The following information should be reviewed in detail with the couple:

- Maternal age. The risk of having a child with chromosomal abnormalities (especially Down syndrome) increases with maternal age. Women 30 years and older at the time of birth are particularly at risk (see Table 14-1). At 35 years, the risk of fetal loss from invasive genetic testing (ie, amniocentesis) equals that of the risk of having a child with abnormalities (0.5%).
- Ethnic background. Certain genetic diseases are found within the population of people with specific ethnic backgrounds. For example, Tay-Sachs disease is found in offspring of Eastern European Jews, Mediterranean people have an increased risk of being afflicted with thalassemia, and African Americans have an increased chance of carrying the sickle cell trait. If a history of these disorders exists, a pedigree (or genogram) is helpful to analyze the familial pattern (Fig. 14-8).
- Family history. If there is a family history of certain diseases (eg, hemophilia, Huntington's disease, cystic fibrosis), birth defects (eg, neural tube defects, abdominal wall defects, congenital heart disease), or

mental retardation, the chance that future children will have these problems may increase. A careful family history also may alert the client to other potential health risks, such as breast or ovarian cancer, diabetes, and heart disease.
- Reproductive history. A history of previous stillbirths, several (two or three) spontaneous abortions, and children with birth defects or genetic diseases may indicate an increased risk for the fetus. Available medical records should be reviewed, and appropriate referrals for testing (ie, parental chromosome studies) should be recommended.
- Maternal disease. Women with diabetes, thyroid disease (especially untreated hyperthyroidism), metabolic disease (PKU), heart disease, or seizure disorders may have an increased chance of bearing children with similar defects and may expose their children to **teratogenic** effects of necessary medications.
- Environmental hazards. Exposure to harmful chemicals or radiation, use of certain medications, use of recreational drugs, frequent use of hot tubs and spas, and a history of poor nutrition before pregnancy increase the chance of genetic problems.

Counseling After Specific Indications Are Identified

When specific indications are identified, the family should be advised of the availability of genetic testing and diagnosis. Although most people are aware of the reasons for genetic testing, many do not know what to expect in the process. The counselor must maintain a reassuring, nonjudgmental attitude, while providing factual information. Although the family makes the final decision to test, the nurse must be able to support them throughout the decision-making and testing processes.

Once baseline information obtained by the assessment process is analyzed, the family is referred for appropriate testing. Timely contact with the family minimizes anxiety and maximizes options dependent on gestational age. The assessment process includes information regarding normal genetic reproduction and the mechanisms involved in genetic disease. Testing procedures are outlined, and rationales are explained. Risks, benefits, limitations, and accuracy of each of the tests are explained. Explanations should be tailored to the needs and educational level of the client. Information about post-testing evaluation and counseling also is included in the process.

Nursing Diagnosis

The stress of pregnancy is often increased when there is a need for genetic testing. Although the final deci-

BOX 14–1
Sample Prenatal Genetic Screen*

Name _____ Patient # _____ Date _____

1. Will you be 35 years or older when the baby is due?   Yes _____ No _____
2. Have you, the baby's father, or anyone in either of your families ever had any of the following disorders?
   - Down syndrome (mongolism)   Yes _____ No _____
   - Other chromosomal abnormality   Yes _____ No _____
   - Neural tube defect (ie, spina bifida [meningomyelocele or open spine], anencephaly)   Yes _____ No _____
   - Hemophilia   Yes _____ No _____
   - Muscular dystrophy   Yes _____ No _____
   - Cystic fibrosis   Yes _____ No _____

   If yes, indicate the relationship of the affected person to you or to the baby's father: _____
3. Do you or the baby's father have a birth defect?   Yes _____ No _____
   If yes, who has the defect and what is it? _____
4. In any previous marriages, have you or the baby's father had a child, born dead or alive, with a birth defect not listed in question 2 above?   Yes _____ No _____
   If yes, what was the defect and who had it? _____
5. Do you or the baby's father have any close relatives with mental retardation?   Yes _____ No _____
   If yes, indicate the relationship of the affected person to you or to the baby's father: _____
   Indicate the cause, if known: _____
6. Do you, the baby's father, or a close relative in either of your families have a birth defect, any familial disorder, or a chromosomal abnormality not listed above?   Yes _____ No _____
   If yes, indicate the condition and the relationship of the affected person to you or to the baby's father: _____
7. In any previous marriages, have you or the baby's father had a stillborn child or three or more first-trimester spontaneous pregnancy losses?   Yes _____ No _____
   Have either of you had a chromosomal study?   Yes _____ No _____
   If yes, indicate who and the results: _____
8. If you or the baby's father are of Jewish ancestry, have either of you been screened for Tay-Sachs disease?   Yes _____ No _____
   If yes, indicate who and the results: _____
9. If you or the baby's father are African American, have either of you been screened for sickle cell trait?   Yes _____ No _____
   If yes, indicate who and the results: _____
10. If you or the baby's father are of Italian, Greek, or Mediterranean background, have either of you been tested for β-thalassemia?   Yes _____ No _____
    If yes, indicate who and the results: _____
11. If you or the baby's father are of Philippine or Southeast Asian ancestry, have either of you been tested for α-thalassemia?   Yes _____ No _____
    If yes, indicate who and the results: _____
12. Excluding iron and vitamins, have you taken any medications or recreational drugs since being pregnant or since your last menstrual period (including nonprescription drugs)?   Yes _____ No _____
    If yes, give name of medication and time taken during pregnancy: _____

*Any patient replying "yes" to questions should be offered appropriate counseling. If the client declines further counseling or testing, this should be noted in the chart. Given that genetics is a field in a state of flux, alterations or updates to this form will be required periodically.

(Reprinted with permission from the American College of Obstetricians and Gynecologists [1987]. Antenatal diagnosis of genetic disorders. ACOG Technical Bulletin, 108, 3.)

sion to proceed with testing is the couple's choice, the decision-making process is a time of increased anxiety and concern. Appropriate nursing diagnoses allow the nurse to plan suitable intervention to support the couple at this critical time (Box 14-2).

Nursing Planning and Intervention

Nursing care planning should emphasize interventions that gather needed information (eg, completing the intake history), increase the couple's knowledge and

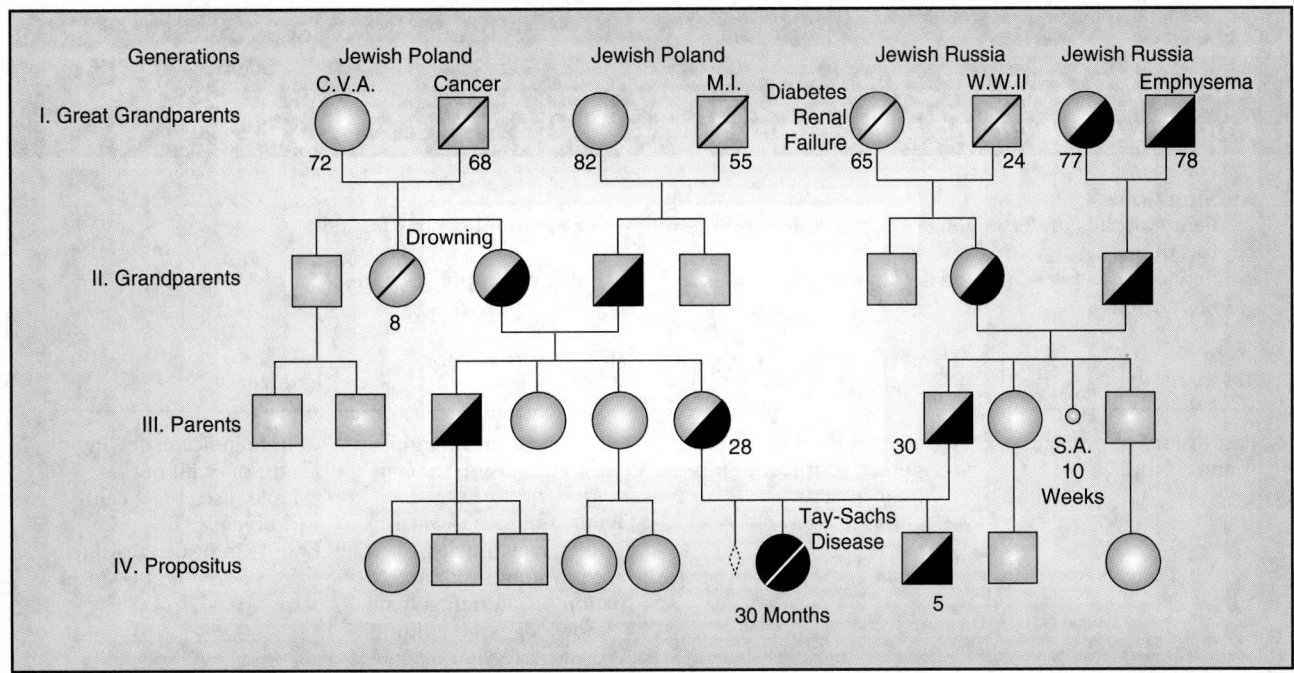

Generations

I. Great Grandparents

II. Grandparents

III. Parents

IV. Propositus

○ Female

□ Male

◇ Pregnancy/Sex unknown

○ Abortus

FIGURE 14–8 Sample pedigree demonstrating recessive inheritance of Tay-Sachs disease and the carrier state. Slanted line (/) through symbol represents deceased individual. Carriers are depicted by partially blackened symbol. Affected individual is depicted by totally blackened symbol.

BOX 14–2
Potential Nursing Diagnoses

- Knowledge Deficit related to pregnancy and genetic disorders
- Fear and Anxiety related to the testing process and outcome
- Powerlessness
- Self Esteem Disturbance
- Altered Family Processes
- Anticipatory Grieving related to possible outcome or perceived loss
- Decisional Conflict

Associated diagnoses may include the following:

- Ineffective Individual or Family Coping
- Spiritual Distress related to conflicting beliefs or crises
- Situational Low Self Esteem

---

understanding of the testing process (eg, providing information and answering questions), and minimize the effects of fear and anxiety while supporting the couple.

The nurse also should have the necessary information to make referrals to other agencies. In every situation, the nurse must allow the couple to make their own decisions and must support whatever decision they make (see Nursing Care Plan: Families Involved in Genetic Counseling).

Nursing Evaluation

Nursing care can be evaluated by assessing the couple's willingness to participate in, and ability to make necessary decisions during, the testing process. The couple's openness, rapport, and participation are measures of their adaptation to the genetic testing process.

NURSING CARE PLAN
Families Involved in Genetic Counseling

Nursing Goals
1. Client indicates understanding of the need for and the process of indicated genetic testing procedures.
2. Client demonstrates appropriate physical, emotional, and psychological responses to testing outcome.

Assessment	Potential Nursing Diagnoses	Intervention/ Rationale	Evaluation
Past history of pregnancy and so forth	Anxiety related to actual or perceived threat to biologic integrity	Take general health and obstetric history *to form database.* Obtain attitudes toward pregnancy, nuclear-family composition, initiation of referral, general knowledge and attitude toward prenatal diagnosis *to assess client understanding*	Couple indicates feeling of rapport with nurse Couple discusses health problems Couple indicates readiness for referral and counseling
Genetic history of extended family Psychological status of pregnancy	Altered Family Processes related to birth history of previous pregnancy or of other family members	Obtain multigeneration family pedigree (when necessary, request medical records, arrange appropriate consultations, and perform laboratory studies) *to supplement database.*	Couple understands implications of high-risk factors Couple understands vocabulary used by nurse-counselor Couple freely discusses genetic history of family Couple weighs advantages and risks for their situation
Need for counseling related to prenatal diagnosis and amniocentesis Knowledge related to ultrasound and amniocentesis	Knowledge Deficit related to purpose of tests and procedures of examinations	Provide precise, detailed information (eg, ultrasonography and its purposes, length of time for procedures and results) in objective, nonjudgmental manner *to enhance client understanding* Brief overview of initial counseling (by nurse-counselor and physician) *to enhance client understanding* Assist client to examination table; position and drape client; direct father to best position to observe ultrasound *to enhance client's comfort*	Couple asks additional questions to clarify details Mother is comcortable and at ease. Father feels included in procedure Parents continue to develop rapport with nurse-counselor
Understanding of outcome of tests	Knowledge Deficit related to outcome of tests	Review possible after-effects and complications; provide couple with phone number for answering service (24-hour availability) *to provide support*	Couple expresses reduced anxiety Couple exercises control in receiving information

(continued)

NURSING CARE PLAN *(Continued)*
Families Involved in Genetic Counseling

Assessment	Potential Nursing Diagnoses	Intervention/ Rationale	Evaluation
		Arrange per couple's preference (call directly, referring physician call with results, or arrange return visit to review results with nurse-counselor or physician) *to decrease anxiety related to results*	Couple indicates that they feel diagnosis is accurate
		Arrange appointment with couple to return for detailed objective discussion of findings; be prepared to answer any questions regarding diagnosis, prognosis, and pregnancy termination *to assess client's understanding and acceptance*	Couple evaluates options and makes decisions
		Suggest referral to appropriate parent support groups *to provide ongoing support*	

Prenatal Genetic Diagnostic Testing

Tremendous advances have been made in the field of genetic testing in the last 5 years. Progress in molecular genetics, DNA testing, and fetal medicine has allowed diagnosis of many more conditions. Testing procedures have become increasingly available, are safely conducted earlier in the gestation, and are demonstrating increased accuracy. Basic screening procedures are often performed in the obstetrician's office and are part of primary care (Cunningham et al., 1993).

Certain tests are performed by analyzing the maternal blood for fetal information. Other testing procedures fall into two categories. Those that describe the **phenotype** (observable characteristics) or the **genotype** (genetic composition) of the fetus. Although the latter is preferable in many cases, the former is usually more accessible and more widely used.

Maternal Serum α-Fetoprotein Testing

The MS-AFP test screens maternal blood for the presence and volume of circulating AFP. This substance is a normal by-product of pregnancy, produced first by the yolk sac and then by the fetal liver. It is excreted by the fetal kidneys as urine and circulates with the amniotic fluid. Some crosses the placenta into the maternal bloodstream and is detectable in the second trimester (Cunningham et al., 1993).

The blood sample for the MS-AFP test must be drawn between the 15th and 20th weeks of gestation (optimally between the 16th and 18th weeks). Coupled with a precise gestational age, the client's level of AFP can be compared with the predicted level for that week of pregnancy. An elevated AFP level in maternal serum can be attributed to many factors: underestimated gestational age, twins, correctable defects (omphalocele, gastroschisis), or open neural tube defects (spina bifida, meningocele). It also may signal an increased chance of preterm labor, intrauterine growth retardation, impending intrauterine fetal demise, or premature rupture of membranes. A decreased level of AFP is predictive of trisomies in approximately 20% of cases (Robinson et al., 1989; Drugan et al., 1989).

A newer version of this test, the MS-AFP[3] or "triple marker," is now available in limited areas. This test measures levels of serum AFP, hCG, and unconjugated estradiol (UE3) to assess for neural tube defects and certain chromosome abnormalities. Data suggest that the MS-AFP[3] test is more accurate than the standard AFP test in detecting Down syndrome and trisomy 18. Therefore, this test may be more appropriate for clients older than 35 years (Wald et al., 1988; Palomaki et al. 1992).

The American College of Obstetricians and Gynecologists recommends that screening programs for MS-AFP should be established with an integrated system of referral, quality control, genetic counseling, appropriate follow-up, and sonographic facilities with specific capabilities (Cunningham et al., 1993).

Because MS-AFP is only a screening test, it does not diagnose neural tube defects or chromosomal abnormalities. An abnormal level indicates a need for further testing (ultrasonography and amniocentesis with measurement of amniotic fluid, AFP, and chromosomal analysis). False-positives and -negatives of MS-AFP testing do occur. However, with appropriate follow-up testing, defects can be detected with a high degree of accuracy (Callen, 1994).

Ultrasonography

Ultrasonography (or sonogram) uses high-frequency sound waves to detect differences in tissue density (Fig. 14-9). Structure and form of the fetus are visible as a two-dimensional image. Ultrasound can be used to determine fetal viability in early pregnancy because the fetal heart beat is visible at approximately 6 weeks' gestation. It also can be used to guide amniocentesis or other procedures. One of its greatest merits is in assessing the fetus for visible anomalies (Box 14-3).

Most physicians' offices offer on-site ultrasonography screening for their pregnant clients. Many genetic problems can be detected with routine ultrasound. However, anomalies can be missed with routine scanning, and referral to perinatal centers with higher level scanning capabilities must be available to confirm suspicious findings (Callen, 1994; Horger et al., 1989; Rosendahl et al., 1989).

No concrete evidence of ultrasonography causing harm to mother or fetus has ever been validated, and

> ### BOX 14-3
> *Comprehensive Ultrasound Examination of the Fetus*
>
> - **Measurement** of the head, abdomen, and long bones (for estimation of gestational age and fetal weight)
> - **Inspection** of the thorax, heart, and abdomen (to evaluate stomach, bladder, kidneys, liver, and circulation)
> - **Survey** of the bony skeleton, including the head (to determine structural integrity)
> - **Evaluation** of the placenta (for size and location)
> - **Estimation** of the amniotic fluid volume (to determine the presence of oligohydramnios or hydramnios)
>
> *(Callen, P. W. [Ed.] [1994]. Ultrasonography in obstetrics and gynecology. Philadelphia: W. B. Saunders.)*

benefits continue to be defined. Obvious deformities (eg, hydrocephalus, spina bifida, and omphalocele) and subtle defects (eg, Turner's syndrome, heart defects) can be detected and evaluated using sonography. When used with amniocentesis, most genetic defects can be discerned (Horger et al., 1989; Rosendahl et al., 1989; Hogge et al., 1989; Callen, 1994).

Amniocentesis

Amniocentesis, the aspiration of fluid from the amniotic sac, is a relatively safe and simple outpatient procedure. It is traditionally performed between 14 and 18 weeks of gestation, although it can be performed before the 14th week. Box 14-4 lists indications for performing an amniocentesis.

Amniotic fluid contains desquamated cells from the fetus that can be cultured and analyzed for karyotype, metabolic disorders, DNA patterns, and a variety of other components. Cells found in the amniotic fluid are fetal in origin and contain genetic information identical to the fetus (Cunningham et al., 1993; Callen, 1994; Robinson et al., 1993).

The list of diagnoses possible with amniocentesis includes chromosomal abnormalities (including translocation, aneuploidy), autosomal disorders, X-linked disorders, metabolic diseases, enzyme defects, hematopoietic diseases, and immunodeficiencies. Specialized tests have been developed to diagnose many of these conditions.

Amniocentesis Procedure

Questions and concerns about amniocentesis should be addressed before the procedure. The client is asked to sign an informed consent outlining the procedure, including risks, benefits, and limitations. Fetal loss is

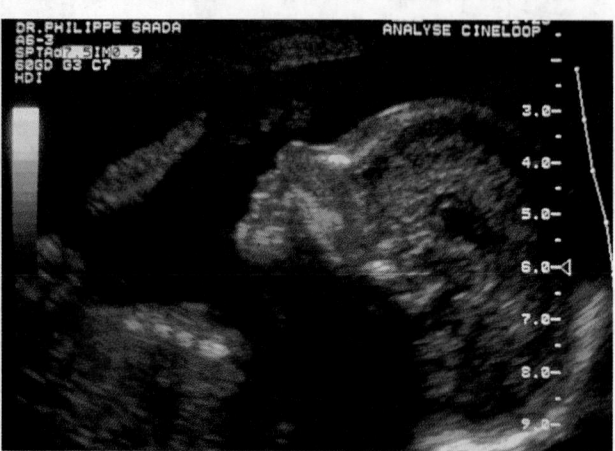

FIGURE 14-9 Color ultrasound scan of a profile of the head of a human fetus, age 5 months.

BOX 14–4
Indications for Amniocentesis

- Maternal age of 35 years or older at the time of the birth
- Previous child diagnosed with a chromosomal abnormality or certain birth defects (including spina bifida)
- Parent with a diagnosed chromosomal abnormality, especially translocation errors or autosomal recessive disease
- Woman diagnosed with an X-linked disorder
- Familial history of neural tube defects
- Abnormal MS-AFP level in the current pregnancy
- Fetal abnormalities identified by ultrasonography

(Cephalo, R. C. [1990]. Clinical decisions in obstetrics and gynecology. Rockville, MD: Aspen. Simpson, L. & Goldbus, M. [1992]. Genetics in obstetrics and gynecology. [2nd ed.]. Philadelphia: W. B. Saunders.)

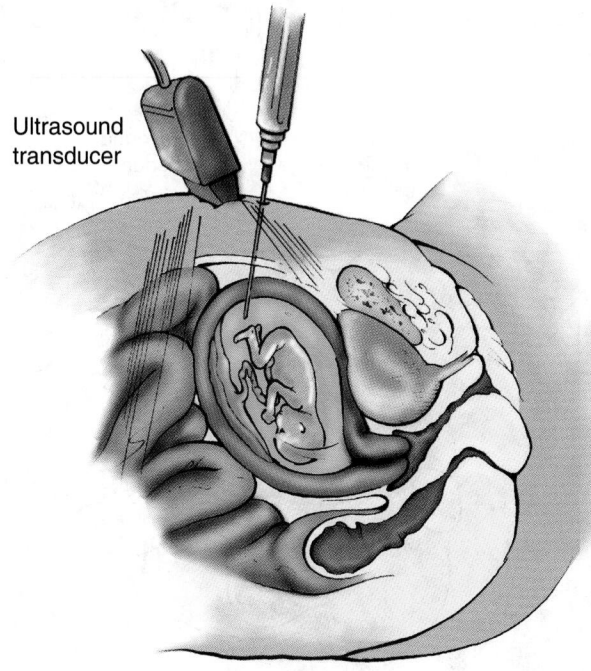

Ultrasound
transducer

FIGURE 14–10 Amniocentesis. Amniotic fluid is withdrawn for analysis by transabdominal needle aspiration. Continuous ultrasound monitors fluid sac and fetus.

possible after amniocentesis, and the client must be aware of the chance of this event (approximately 0.5% or 1 in 200). The procedure is explained in detail to reduce anxiety.

Before the procedure, the client fills her bladder (to enhance the ultrasound image) and is instructed to rest on an examining table in the supine position with legs extended. An ultrasound is performed to locate the fetus, placenta, and an adequate pocket of amniotic fluid. The skin over the selected site is prepared with an antiseptic solution, and the abdomen is prepped as a sterile field. Local anesthesia is often used to decrease pain during the procedure. After the anesthesia takes effect, a 20- to 22-gauge spinal needle with trochar is inserted through the skin and into the amniotic sac using ultrasound surveillance as guidance. The client may experience some pressure or mild cramping during the procedure (Fig. 14-10).

Once the amniotic sac is entered, the trochar is removed and fluid is aspirated. The first 1 or 2 mL is discarded to prevent contamination from maternal skin and tissues. Generally 10 to 30 mL of amniotic fluid is aspirated in one or two sterile syringes. These fluid specimens are labeled and taken to the laboratory.

The needle is withdrawn, and direct pressure is applied to the site. The puncture site is dressed, and the client is allowed to rest. Ultrasound or fetal monitoring is continued for a short time to ensure fetal well-being and reassure the mother.

The client is advised to observe for complications of the procedure, including vaginal bleeding, leakage of amniotic fluid, severe cramping, or fever. Intercourse and heavy lifting should be avoided for 24 hours after the procedure. The client should be advised that cell cultures take 7 to 10 days for incubation, processing, and evaluation. She should be advised concerning test result availability and how she will be contacted. If a repeat amniocentesis is required, she should be assured of prompt notification.

Chorionic Villus Sampling

Although amniocentesis has been proven a safe and precise method of collecting fetal cells for analysis, in some circumstances, earlier diagnosis is desired. Amniocentesis is not advised before the 12th week due to the small size of the gestational sac. **Chorionic villus sampling** (CVS) is an alternative method of collecting fetal genetic information.

Today, most major medical centers with genetic specialty units offer this technique as an alternative to amniocentesis. CVS is performed in the first trimester before the pregnancy becomes physically visible. Earlier diagnosis of genetic problems provides more decision-making time for the client and allows for first-trimester therapeutic abortion if necessary.

Chorionic Villus Sampling Procedure

In CVS, chorionic tissue is aspirated from the placenta site. It is done vaginally or abdominally. A polyethylene catheter (for the vaginal approach) or a spinal needle (for the abdominal approach) is inserted, using ultrasound as a guide, and a small amount of placental and chorionic tissue is collected (Fig. 14-11). The tissue is processed and evaluated in a manner similar to that of amniocentesis.

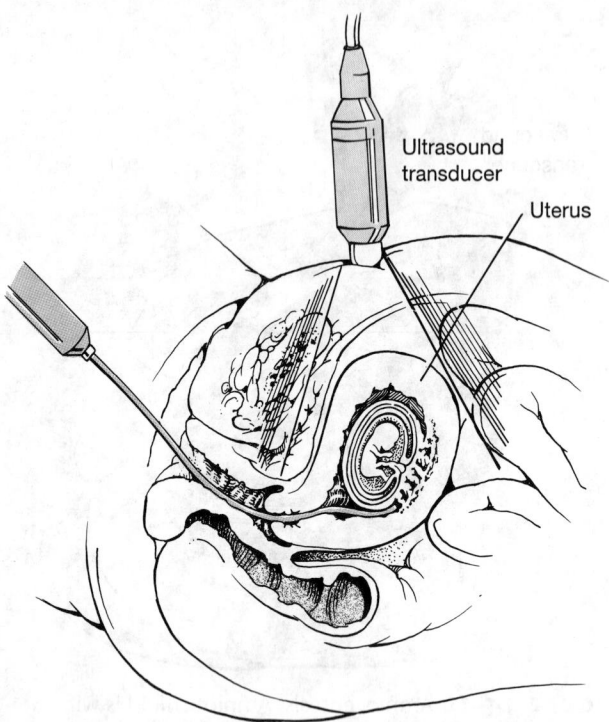

Ultrasound transducer

Uterus

FIGURE 14–11 Chorionic villus sampling of placental and chorionic material with transvaginal catheter and with direct ultrasound guidance.

Risk Factors for Chorionic Villus Sampling

Recent literature suggests that CVS may carry some risks not associated with amniocentesis. However, more research is needed to confirm these factors:

- Multiple attempts to retrieve sufficient tissue are associated with increased fetal loss (Wade et al., 1989).
- A retroverted uterus adds an additional risk factor for loss (Silver et al., 1994).
- Multiple cases of fetal limb reduction have been reported following CVS (Martins et al., 1993; National Institute of Child Health and Human Development, 1993).
- The chance of contamination with maternal cells is increased.
- AFP cannot be measured.

Nursing Considerations for Counseling and Intervention After Diagnosis

When a genetic diagnosis has been made, the couple must plan appropriate interventions, with the assistance of the genetic team. These interventions are based on the diagnosis, its potential for life-changing consequences, and its overall prognosis.

Genetic counseling fosters an intimate relationship between the client and the genetic team. The counselor is often the primary contact throughout the process. By creating an open, honest atmosphere and relationship between client and provider, the counselor can provide the maximum amount of information and emotional support for the expectant couple.

After genetic testing has been sucessfully completed, the client's anxiety shifts from the procedures to the the results. Fears of an abnormal result may intensify during this time. Therefore, emotional support from the counselor and genetics team is crucial. The couple should be advised that telephone communication to the couselor is available whenever they need to discuss their fears or apprehensions.

Some prenatal diagnosis centers relay results by phone (especially when the results indicate a normal pregnancy). Other centers advise a consultation with the client's obstetrician for the results. News of a normal baby brings relief and joy to most couples. They feel reassured about the pregnancy and the immediate future. This is an appropriate time to plan continued prenatal care and inform the family of the need for follow-up, because genetic diagnosis is confirmed with birth.

When amniocentesis yields a positive result (presence of an abnormality), the couple must decide the fate of the pregnancy. If the couple decides to terminate the pregnancy, they often request that it be performed immediately. The method of termination must be selected with the mother's safety in mind. Parents who decide to terminate an abnormal pregnancy undergo a grieving process. The counselor assists these families by advising them of possible physical and emotional sequelae (eg, depression and marital discord). Close continuing contact with the couple can minimize these problems and facilitate their resolution. Appropriate referrals for support groups or psychological counseling should be available if necessary.

However, couples may elect to continue the pregnancy and learn to deal with a newborn with special needs. The counselor can provide referral to support groups and specialized medical care. For example, a family expecting a newborn with spina bifida may be referred to a tertiary care center for prenatal care and planned cesarean delivery, followed by immediate neurosurgery for the newborn. Referral to neural tube defect support groups also is appropirate because they provide practical information on caring for an affected child. The parent-to-parent approach is especially beneficial.

Prenatal diagnosis is not confirmed until the newborn arrives or the pregnancy is terminated. Careful physical examination of the newborn (or products of conception) aids in the identification of defects and their cause. Laboratory analysis of karyotype, enzyme, hematologic, and metabolic factors may be necessary. The parents should be advised of the results of testing and the implications for future childbearing.

Summary Points

✔ Healthcare providers must understand the basic mechanisms involved in cellular reproduction and the role that these play in the realm of genetics.

✔ As technology advances, more genetically transmitted disorders are being investigated and identified. These advances enable healthcare providers to identify more accurately parents at risk for certain diseases and afflictions.

✔ The nurse is in a position to provide unbiased and factual information to the family at risk. The nurse-genetic counselor is often the primary contact with the family throughout the process of prenatal diagnosis.

✔ Genetic information may produce an ethical dilemma regarding the fate of an affected pregnancy. Within legal limits, parents now can choose to continue or terminate a high-risk pregnancy. All options must be explored within the context of prenatal diagnosis.

The author wishes to acknowledge the generous contributions to this chapter provided by Frederick W. Hansen, MD, Medical Director; Marcia Ehinger, MD, Clinical Geneticist; and Michelle De-Haven, MS, Genetic Counselor, of the Prenatal Diagnostic and Imaging Center, Sacramento, CA.

REFERENCES

Callen, P. W. (Ed.) (1994). *Ultrasonography in obstetrics and gynecology*. Philadelphia: W.B. Saunders.

Cefalo, R. C. (1990). *Clinical decisions in obstetrics and gynecology*. Rockville, MD: Aspen.

Clark, S. L., & DeVore, G. R. (1989). Prenatal diagnosis for couples who would not consider abortion. *Obstetrics and Gynecology*, *73*, 1035–1036.

Cunningham, F. G., MacDonald, P. C., Gant, N. F., Leveno, K. J., & Gilstrap, L. C. (1993). *Williams obstetrics* (19th ed.). Norwalk, CT: Appleton & Lange.

Drugan, A., Dvorin, E., Koppitch, R. D. et al. (1989). Counseling for low maternal serum alpha-fetoprotein should emphasize all chromosome anomalies, not just Down syndrome. *Obstetrics and Gynecology*, *73*, 271–274.

Harrington, D., Fujimura, F., & Venne, V. (1992). A Guide to Genetic Testing for Cystic Fibrosis. *The Female Patient*, *17*(12), 22c–22i.

Hoekelman, R. A. (1987). *Primary pediatric care*. St Louis: C.V. Mosby.

Hogge, W. A., Thiagarajah, S., Ferguson, J. E. et al. (1989). The role of ultrasonography and amniocentesis in the evaluation of pregnancies at risk for neural tube defects. *American Journal of Obstetrics and Gynecology*, *161*, 520–524.

Horger, E. O., & Tsai, C. C. (1989). Ultrasound and the prenatal diagnosis of congenital anomalies: A medicolegal perspective. *Obstetrics and Gynecology*, *74*, 617–619.

Jennings, J. C. (1990). Prenatal tests: Helping the patient decide. *OBG Management*, 61–71.

Martins, M., & Johnson, A. (1993). Does chorionic villus sampling cause limb defects? *Genetics and Teratology*, *2*(1)1–3.

Miller, W. A. (1990). Medical genetics. In K. J. Ryan, R. Berkowitz, & R. L. Barbieri (Eds.), *Kistner's gynecology* (5th ed.). Chicago: Year Book Medical Publishers.

National Institute of Child Health and Human Development (1993). Report on workshop on chorionic villus sampling and limb and other defects (October 20, 1992). *American Journal of Obstetrics and Gynecology*, *169*(1), 1–6.

Palomaki, G. E. et al. (1992). Prospective intervention trial of a screening protocol to identify fetal trisomy 18 using maternal serum AFP, UE3, and hCG. *Prenatal Diagnosis*, *12*, 925–930.

Robinson, L., Grau, P., & Crandall, B. F. (1989). Pregnancy outcomes after increasing maternal serum alpha-fetoprotein levels. *Obstetrics and Gynecology*, *74*, 17–19.

Robinson, A., & Linden, M. G. (1993). *Clinical genetics handbook* (2nd ed.). Boston: Blackwell Scientific Publications.

Rosendahl, H., & Kivinen, S. (1989). Prenatal detection of congenital malformations by routine ultrasonography. *Obstetrics and Gynecology*, *73*, 947–951.

Silver, R., MacGregor, S., Muhlback, L., Kambick, M., & Ragin, A. (1994). A comparison of pregnancy loss between transcervical and transabdominal chorionic villus sampling. *Obstetrics and Gynecology*, *83*(5), 657–660.

Simpson, L., & Goldbus, M. (1992). *Genetics in obstetrics and gynecology* (2nd ed.). Philadelphia: W.B. Saunders.

Thompson M., McInnes, R., & Huntington, F. W. (1991). *Genetics in medicine* (5th ed.). Philadelphia: W.B. Saunders.

Wade, R. V., & Young, S. R. (1989). Analysis of fetal loss after transcervical chorionic villus sampling—A review of 719 patients. *American Journal of Obstetrics and Gynecology*, *161*, 513–519.

Wald, N. J. et al. (1988). Maternal serum screening for Down syndrome in early pregnancy. *British Medical Journal*, *297*(6653), 833–87.

Wright, D. J., Brindley, B. A., Foppitch, F. C. et al. (1989). Interpretation of chorionic villus sampling laboratory results is just as reliable as amniocentesis. *Obstetrics and Gynecology*, *74*, 739–743.

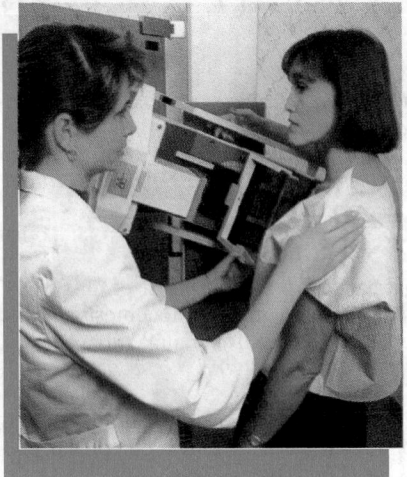

Assessment and Management of Women's Health

Critical Thinking Exercises

1. Latisha Hammond is a 34-year-old mother of three who arrives for her biannual check up. She has used oral contraceptives successfully for a total of 7 years. Her physical examination is normal. She smokes a half pack of cigarettes per day and has smoked for 15 years. After being at home for the last 5 years, she has just started a new job as an account executive for a major sales firm. She states, "I'm so overwhelmed with my new job, taking care of the children, housework, and being a wife."

   What health promotion issues would you identify as problematic and how would you counsel Latisha?

2. Carol Dane is a 32-year-old single mother of two children, ages 6 and 4. Three months ago, she had a Pap smear showing atypical cells. She comes to the women's health clinic for the results of a repeat Pap smear. Based on the results of the repeat Pap smear, cancer of the cervix is suspected. The client is visibly upset and crying. She states, "What am I going to do? If I have to have a hysterectomy, I won't be a woman anymore. Am I going to die? What will happen to my kids?"

   Determine the priority nursing diagnoses for Carol and propose appropriate intervention strategies specific for this client.

3. You are a nurse working in an inner city community health clinic. You notice an increase in the number of clients being treated for STDs. You know that the spread can be prevented by safe sex practices that avoid exchange of body fluids. You also know that condoms, a major factor in preventing STD transmission, are used erratically, especially by high-risk groups. You decide to start an education program for teaching clients about STDs.

   Formulate a teaching plan based on an analysis of the factors that increase a woman's risk for STDs and the behaviors and attitudes common to those at increased risk. Include any cultural and socioeconomic considerations that may be appropriate.

4. Ms. Tower, is a 29-year-old nulligravida. She and her partner have been trying to get pregnant and have not been using any contraception for about a year. They are now interested in pursuing an infertility program. Outline the intake interview and develop appropriate client teaching strategies for addressing the procedures to be performed for this evaluation.

5. A client, age 39, comes for her first prenatal visit. During the initial assessment, the client states that she has two healthy daughters and a son with Down syndrome. Outline the genetic counseling for this client, including possible testing procedures and client teaching strategies.

Multiple Choice Questions

1. When preparing a teaching plan for a client, the nurse includes information that intercourse should be avoided during pregnancy:

   A. After the 3rd month
   B. When the uterus is large enough to press on the vena cava
   C. If vaginal bleeding or loss of amniotic fluid occurs
   D. If slight cramping occurs

2. A client has used a diaphragm for the past couple of years. Which of the following assessment findings would alert the nurse to the need for possible refitting?

   A. Surgery with general anesthesia
   B. Surgery on the pelvic organs
   C. No pregnancies since first fitting
   D. Weight gain of 5 lbs

3. A client asks the nurse about using a douche. The nurse is correct in replying:

   A. "Douche regularly especially during menses."
   B. "Douching is essential to prevent infection."

C. "Douching is an effective method of contraception; use it often."

D. "Douching is unnecessary; daily showering or bathing is adequate."

4. A client is diagnosed with SAD. During assessment, the nurse identifies which of the following as a characteristic?

A. Increased active time
B. Symptoms appearing during the summer
C. Increased exposure to ambient light
D. Mood swings

5. A client comes to the clinic after finding a lump in her breast. If breast cancer is suspected, which of the following findings might the nurse also note:

A. Breast dimpling
B. Edges of lump well delineated
C. Normal sized axillary nodes
D. Breast symmetry

6. When caring for the client with HIV, it is essential for the nurse to:

A. Wear a mask to bathe the client
B. Use gloves when changing perineal pads
C. Recap nondisposable needles
D. Wear a gown and gloves to obtain a client history

7. Prior to discharge following an elective abortion, the nurse instructs the client to report which of the following?

A. Periodic cramping
B. Vaginal discharge without odor
C. Temperature above 100.4 degrees F
D. Passage of small dark brown clots

8. A pregnant client undergoes diagnostic testing for possible neural tube defects. The nurse prepares the client specifically for:

A. VDRL
B. CVS
C. MSAFP
D. Ultrasound

9. A couple is found to be carriers of a gene for cystic fibrosis. They ask what is the chance that their children will affected. The nurse's correct response is:

A. 25%
B. 50%
C. 75%
D. 100%

Study Questions

1. When should a woman perform BSE?

2. Identify six nonmodifiable risk factors for osteoporosis.

3. List four common sexual concerns during pregnancy and postpartum.

4. Define the "ACHES" system of danger signs for oral contraceptives.

5. Define endometriosis.

6. Describe the difference between primary and secondary amenorrhea.

7. Name the most common cancer found in women under age 35.

8. State the breast condition that usually subsides with menopause.

9. List four risk factors for breast cancer.

10. Identify the characteristics of the vaginal discharge seen with monilial vaginitis.

11. What possible complications may arise if gonorrhea is present during pregnancy?

12. State the primary mode of HIV transmission.

13. List the commonly used surgical methods for abortion.

14. Define trisomy.

15. When should an MS-AFP blood sample to obtained?

16. Identify when CVS sampling is done.

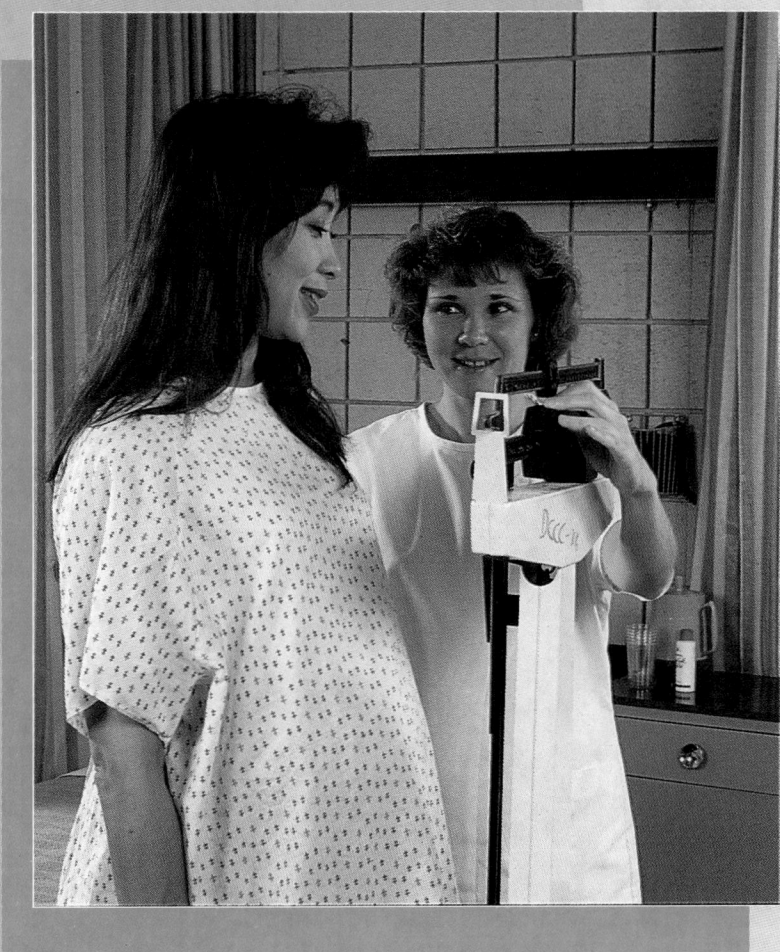

Assessment and Management in the Antepartum Period

IV

15

Biophysical Aspects of Normal Pregnancy

Objectives

- Define early physiologic signs and symptoms of pregnancy.
- Explain the use of and rationale for various pregnancy testing methods.
- Discuss biophysiologic changes that occur with pregnancy.

Key Terms

Ballottement	Presumptive signs
Chadwick's sign	Primigravida
Colostrum	Probable signs
Hegar's sign	Quickening
Morning sickness	Striae gravidarum
Positive signs	

The average length of human pregnancy is 267 days, or 38 weeks from the time of conception. During this time, the woman's body undergoes many changes to accommodate the growing fetus. Largely orchestrated by the endocrine system through the hormones, these changes arise in response to fetal needs for additional space, nourishment, waste removal, and protection from injury. Profound emotional adjustments in the woman also occur. The psychosocial and emotional components of pregnancy adaptation are discussed in Chapter 16. This chapter focuses first on the biophysical changes that are signs and symptoms of pregnancy and are helpful for pregnancy diagnosis. It then explores many of the other biophysical adaptations that occur as the pregnancy continues.

Pregnancy Testing

There are many signs and symptoms of pregnancy, and biochemical advances have made early pregnancy testing accessible, affordable, quick, and reliable (Table 15-1). Today, many women do not wait for the physical signs of pregnancy. Gone are the days of animal colonies maintained for testing purposes (the "rabbit test") and delays of up to 3 days for results. Current pregnancy tests can provide accurate results in as little as 3 to 5 minutes.

Detection of Human Chorionic Gonadotropin

Fertilization of the ovum initiates profound biochemical changes in the human system. The early formation of chorionic villi from the implanted embryo causes secretion of human chorionic gonadotropin (hCG), which can be detected and measured in maternal serum and urine.

After implantation, the level of hCG rises rapidly and predictably. It can be detected in as few as 8 to 9 days after fertilization by ultrasensitive assays. More commonly, the presence of hCG is detected in maternal urine at about the time of the first missed menses, or 2 weeks after ovulation and conception.

The hCG contains alpha (α) and beta (β) subunits. α-hCG is similar to the pituitary hormones; β-hCG has a unique molecular structure specific to pregnancy. Tests that identify β subunits do not cross-react with other gonadotropins.

In the first trimester of normal pregnancy, the levels of β-hCG will double every 48 to 72 hours. In an abnormal gestation, the levels will rise to a certain point then level off or decline (Hatcher et al., 1994). Use of ultrasound plus serial measurements of β-hCG can identify nonviable and ectopic gestations before they develop into a medical emergency (see Chaps. 31 and 37).

Accuracy of pregnancy testing relies on the following:

- The sensitivity and specificity of the testing procedure
- The amount of circulating hCG based on the time elapsed since conception
- The accuracy of the performance of the testing method used (user reliability)

Home Pregnancy Testing

In the last 10 years, monoclonal antibody testing has brought pregnancy testing out of the laboratory and into the home. Home testing provides the added elements of privacy and accessibility. In theory, home testing should enable a woman to identify her pregnancy in its earliest stages and therefore make appropriate decisions or lifestyle changes in a timely manner.

Home tests often carry the disclaimer that the results should be confirmed by a health professional (ie, have another test performed). This is prudent advice, because home testing does not have the same specificity as professional testing. The user's ability to read and follow the instructions, especially regarding the timing of the test, can lead to errors in as many as 20% to 30% of the tests performed. The most common error occurs as a result of performing the test too early for an accurate result (Hatcher et al., 1994).

Signs and Symptoms of Pregnancy

Although it is now possible to diagnose pregnancy before physical signs are present, some signs and symptoms that indicate pregnancy can be observed or reported within a few weeks of conception. The signs of pregnancy are traditionally divided into three groups:

TABLE 15-1
Comparison of Pregnancy Testing Methods

Type of Test	Specificity	Uses	Example/Brands
Immunometric test (urine)	Specific for beta hCG Detects hCG levels as low as 5–50 mLU/mL Positive for 98% of women within 7 days of implantation	Screening test Qualitative test; gives yes/no result	ICON II Testpack
Agglutination inhibition test (urine)	Specific to whole hCG Possible crossreaction with other pituitary hormones Accurate 18–21 days after conception	Screening test Qualitative test only	Pregnosis Pregnosticon
Beta subunit hCG radioimmunoassay (RIA) (serum)	Specific for beta hCG Detects hCG levels as low as 5 mLU/mL Accurate 7 days after fertilization (before missed menses)	Quantitative Can identify pregnancy loss, ectopic pregnancy when serial measurements are performed	Tandem ICON Commercial laboratories have individual names for this test
Home test kits (urine)	Brands differ High incidence of test performance error May have error rate as high as 38%	Qualitative Positive results should be confirmed with more specific and controlled test	First response Clear Blue easy Daisy II

(Additional information adapted from Hatcher, et al, 1994)

presumptive, probable, and positive. These are listed in Box 15-1 and discussed below.

Presumptive Signs

Presumptive signs of pregnancy include signs and symptoms that suggest but do not prove that a woman is pregnant. Presumptive signs are not enough to diagnose pregnancy, but they often are the first clues that a pregnancy may exist. Presumptive signs include the following:

- Abrupt menstrual cessation in a woman who in the past has had predictable menstrual cycles. A woman may miss an occasional menstrual cycle for a variety of reasons, including hormonal imbalances, some chronic and systemic illnesses, psychological and emotional stress, low body fat ratio (as seen with eating disorders or in highly trained athletes), and as a side effect of some medications. In the absence of these conditions, however, and if two consecutive cycles are missed, pregnancy must be considered. Amenorrhea, or the cessation of menstruation for a prolonged period, is fully discussed in Chapter 10.
- Continued bleeding during pregnancy is abnormal, usually associated with pregnancy complications or

BOX 15-1
Signs and Symptoms in Pregnancy

Presumptive signs:

1. Menstrual suppression
2. Nausea, vomiting, and "morning sickness"
3. Frequent urination
4. Breast tenderness
5. Perception of fetal movement, or "quickening"
6. Dark blue discoloration of the vaginal mucous membrane (Chadwick's sign)
7. Fatigue

Probable signs:

1. Enlargement of the abdomen
2. Changes in the size, shape, and consistency of the uterus (Hegar's sign)
3. Fetal outline, distinguished by abdominal palpation and detection of a fetal part vaginally by ballottement
4. Softening of the cervix
5. Braxton Hicks contractions

Positive signs:

1. Fetal heart sounds
2. Fetal movements felt by examiner
3. Visualization of the fetus by ultrasound or, rarely, roentgenogram

an undiagnosed disorder of the reproductive system (Cunningham et al., 1993).

- Nausea and vomiting. Approximately 50% of women will experience varying degrees of gastrointestinal distress in early pregnancy. **Morning sickness** refers to nausea typically occurring early in the day and subsiding after a few hours. It also may occur episodically during the day or in response to hunger. It is most common from 6 to 16 weeks of pregnancy.
- Frequent urination. Early hormonal changes of pregnancy can cause bladder irritability and increased sensitivity of the lower bladder and trigone. As the uterus grows, it pushes on the bladder, creating the sensation of a bladder full of urine. As the pregnancy progresses, the uterus rises out of the pelvis, and this sensation decreases. The hormonal effects also decrease with time.
- Breast tenderness. Many women can predict the onset of menstruation with the degree of breast tenderness they experience. The breast changes of early pregnancy may feel like an exaggeration of these changes and may be accompanied by a tingling feeling.
- Perception of fetal movement, or "quickening." **Quickening** is an ancient term derived from the idea that life was infused into a fetus at approximately 20 weeks' gestation. It refers to the first perceptions of fetal movement as discerned by the mother. It was said that at that moment, the unborn "became alive" and was often the first tangible evidence of pregnancy.
- Quickening is still used in obstetric terminology and is often described as a fluttering low in the abdomen. While it can be detected as early as 16 weeks, most women first perceive fetal movement between 18 and 22 weeks. Quickening can be easily confused with intestinal gas. Women with thick abdominal walls may feel movement to a lesser degree than thinner women.
- Vaginal changes. After about 8 to 10 weeks' gestation, discoloration of the vaginal mucous membrane can be observed. Elevated hormone levels thicken the vaginal mucosa, and increased vascularity, especially in the cervix, lends a blue-purple cast to the tissues. This finding, termed **Chadwick's sign**, is most noticeable in **primigravidas** (woman who are pregnant for the first time) and is easily contrasted to the normal pink vagina and cervix. It is only a presumptive sign of pregnancy, however, because other conditions that create pelvic congestion also can cause coloration changes.
- Vaginal secretions also increase in response to the pregnancy. Other organs in the pelvis reflect changes due to pregnancy and prepare the structures for labor and birth.

- Fatigue. Extreme fatigue or lack of energy is a common symptom of early pregnancy although its cause is not entirely clear.

Probable Signs

Probable signs of pregnancy are objective findings that are usually detected at 12 to 16 weeks' gestation. These findings, when combined with presumptive symptoms, strongly suggest pregnancy:

- Abdominal changes. The increasing size of the uterus causes a gradual increase in abdominal girth. At 12 weeks, the pregnant uterus can be palpated just above the pubic symphysis. At 15 weeks, it can be found midway between the symphysis and umbilicus, and at 20 weeks, the fundus can be palpated at the level of the umbilicus. At term, the fundus can be found at the ensiform cartilage. Abdominal enlargement can be due to a variety of causes, including tumor formation, edema, and body fat accumulation. These conditions usually do not cause the progressive and predictable changes in uterine size.
- Uterine changes. In the first 12 weeks of pregnancy, the uterus becomes more globular, enlarged, soft, and spongy. **Hegar's sign** describes the extreme softening of the lower uterine segment to the point where it can be compressed almost to the thinness of paper (Table 15-2). An experienced examiner can identify this sign and support the diagnosis of pregnancy (Fig. 15-1).
- Fetal outline. At about 24 weeks' gestation, the outline of the fetus is evident to the experienced examiner. Fetal back, extremities, and head become more defined as the gestation proceeds. Uterine or other pelvic tumors usually do not have the same distinct outlines but need to be considered in diagnosis.
- **Ballottement.** From 16 to 24 weeks' gestation, the fetus is small compared with the amount of amni-

TABLE 15–2
Uterine Changes in Pregnancy

	Nonpregnant	Pregnant
LENGTH	6.5 cm	32 cm
WIDTH	4 cm	24 cm
DEPTH	2.5 cm	22 cm
VOLUME	2 mL	More than 1,000 mL
WEIGHT	50 g	1,000 g
WALL THICKNESS	1 cm	2 cm (thins to 5 mm at term)

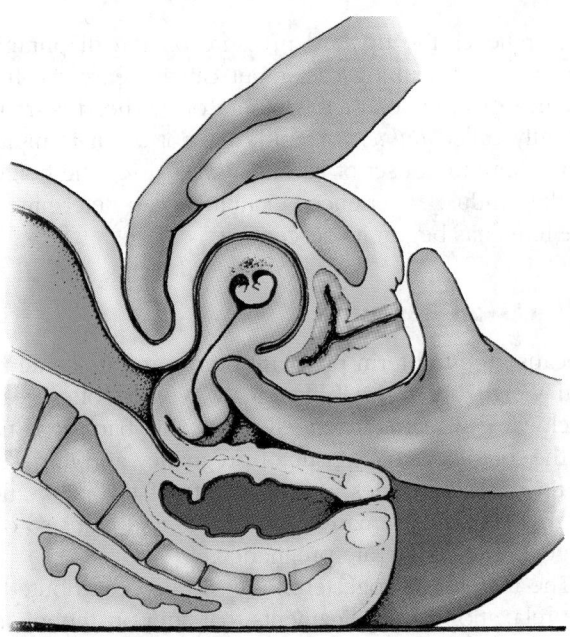

FIGURE 15-1 Hegar's sign.

otic fluid. During a vaginal examination, a sudden tap on the presenting part makes the fetus rise in the amniotic fluid, rebound to its original position, and tap the examining finger (ballottement). When elicited by an experienced examiner, ballottement (from the French *balloter*, to toss up like a ball) is the most certain of the probable signs.

- Cervical changes. At about 8 weeks' gestation, the cervix begins to soften, and the external os exhibits the consistency of an ear lobe or lips (*Goodell's sign*). In comparison, the nonpregnant cervix feels similar to the tip of the nose.
- Braxton Hicks contractions. From the early weeks of pregnancy, the uterus contacts every 5 to 10 minutes. These contractions, called Braxton Hicks after a famous British obstetrician of the 1800s, are not always perceived by the woman; they are usually painless and can be palpated in the later months of pregnancy. By first contracting and then relaxing, the uterine muscles elongate, thus enlarging the uterus to accommodate the growing fetus.

Positive Signs

While most pregnancies are diagnosed on the basis of hCG testing or one or more of the signs defined previously, there remain only three **positive signs** of pregnancy. These findings are the only means of detecting the presence of a fetus:

- The detection of fetal heart sounds
- Fetal movements felt by the examiner
- Visualization of the fetus

The appearance of one or more of these positive signs removes any doubt of the diagnosis. Many factors can cause false readings of a laboratory test, and on rare occasions, the other signs may be simulated by nonpregnant pathologic states.

Fetal Heart Sounds

Electronic Doppler monitoring allows the patient and practitioner to hear heart sounds as early as the 8th to 10th week. The first experience of hearing the unborn's heartbeat can be an exciting and emotional time for the woman and her partner.

The use of Doppler ultrasound, which detects the contractions and valve closures of the fetal heart, has replaced the fetoscope (head stethoscope) for auscultation purposes.

Fetal heart sounds usually range from 120 to 160 beats/min, with an average of 130 to 140 beats/min. They are best heard over the fetus' back.

Two other sounds are often detected:

- Funic (from the Latin *funis* for umbilical cord) souffle (a blowing murmur or whizzing sound): This soft, blowing murmur of blood rushing through the umbilical cord is synchronous with the fetal heart (120–160 beats/min).
- Uterine souffle: This rushing sound of blood moving through the large vessels of the uterus is synchronous with the mother's pulse (approximately 70–80 beats/min).

Fetal Movements Felt by Examiner

Fetal movements reported by the patient may be misleading in the diagnosis of pregnancy. However, when an experienced examiner feels the characteristic thrust or kick of the fetus against the hand, this is positive evidence of pregnancy. Often this can be felt after the end of the fifth month.

Visualization of the Fetus

Visualizing a pregnancy through ultrasonography is increasingly the method of choice for confirming early pregnancies (see Chap. 39). An intrauterine sac is often detectable as early as 30 days after conception, and a beating fetal heart can be seen at 7 to 8 weeks. Sonography is invaluable for the diagnosis of spontaneous abortion and ectopic pregnancy and can often detect extrauterine gestation before the condition becomes life-threatening (Callen, 1994; Catlin et al., 1991; Schurz et al., 1990).

Both transabdominal and transvaginal sonography are used to diagnose pregnancy, evaluate fetal structure, and date the gestation. It has become a standard within prenatal care and provides clients with a clear visual image of their fetus. This may enhance the bonding process that continues throughout pregnancy and into the neonatal period. There is widespread support for use of ultrasound for antepartum diagnostic procedures and for general improvement of maternal and fetal health (Callen, 1994; Ringa et al., 1989).

On rare occasions, an x-ray of the maternal abdomen, ordered for other diagnostic purposes, reveals an advanced and unsuspected pregnancy. However, because of the potential hazards of ionizing radiation and because the fetus can be outlined sonographically, x-rays are rarely used to diagnose pregnancy today.

Physiologic Changes of Pregnancy

From the moment of conception, many changes begin to take place in the pregnant woman's body. While the reproductive system undergoes the most extreme change to accommodate fetal growth, all other body systems must adapt as well. Most of the changes resolve during the postpartum period.

Bodily Changes Associated With Uterine Growth

Between the 12th and 14th weeks of pregnancy, the growing uterus rises out of the pelvis and can be palpated above the symphysis pubis. It rises progressively to reach the umbilicus at approximately 20 weeks and almost impinges on the xiphoid process at term (Fig. 15-2).

Effects on the Abdominal Wall

In most pregnancies, the uterus is rotated to the right as it rises out of the pelvis. This dextrorotation is probably caused by the presence of the rectosigmoid colon on the left. As the uterus becomes larger, it comes in contact with the anterior abdominal wall and displaces the intestines to the sides of the abdomen.

The umbilicus is pushed outward until the third trimester, when its depression is completely obliterated, and it forms merely a darkened area in the smooth and tense abdominal wall. Later, it rises above the surrounding integument and may project slightly outward.

When the abdominal wall is unable to withstand the tension created by the enlarging uterus, the abdominal recti muscles may become separated in the median line. This separation, termed *diastasis recti*, can be so slight that it goes unnoticed, or it can be quite wide.

In primigravidas, the fetal head descends into the pelvic cavity 2 to 4 weeks before labor begins. As a result, the uterus sinks to a lower level and falls forward.

This relieves the upward pressure on the diaphragm and makes breathing easier but can increase the frequency of urination. This descent of the head is traditionally called *lightening*, and may not occur in multiparas until the onset of labor. By measuring the height of the fundus, experienced examiners can determine if the fetus has begun its descent.

Effects on Posture

Because the full-term pregnant uterus and its contents can weigh up to 12 lb, pregnant women often lean backward to maintain equilibrium. This backward tilt of the torso is characteristic of pregnancy and imposes strain on the muscles and ligaments of the back and thighs. This causes many of the aches and pains so often experienced in late pregnancy.

The increased progesterone levels also contribute to the relaxation of the ligaments that support the joints. As pregnancy progresses, relaxation of the sacroiliac joints and the pubic symphysis creates a certain amount of pelvic instability, producing additional strain on the back muscles and thighs. These changes account for the swayback waddling gait often observed in late pregnancy and in the early postpartum period.

Changes in Metabolism

Metabolic changes of pregnancy reflect the increased demands of the growing fetus on the body. Weight gain, associated with the presence of the fetus, placenta, fetal membranes, and amniotic fluid, is minimally affected by metabolic changes.

Pregnancy has a marked influence on carbohydrate metabolism. In general, levels of fasting blood sugar are lower, and insulin requirements are elevated in many women. This mechanism may actually induce *gestational diabetes mellitus*, which is responsible for babies of high birth weight (macrosomia) and other complications (see Chap. 31).

The products of conception contain more protein than fat or carbohydrates, and plasma protein levels are altered. During pregnancy, albumin concentration decreases and fibrinogen levels increase, whereas immunoglobulin levels fall somewhat. In the latter half of pregnancy, there is an increase in plasma lipid, including total lipids, cholesterol, phospholipids, free fatty acids, and lipoproteins. Table 15-3 lists the common laboratory values and the expected changes in pregnancy.

Breast Changes

In the second month, the breasts become larger, fuller, and more tender (Fig. 15-3), and the client may report feelings of stretching, tingling, and heaviness. The nipple becomes elevated, and the *areola*, the pig-

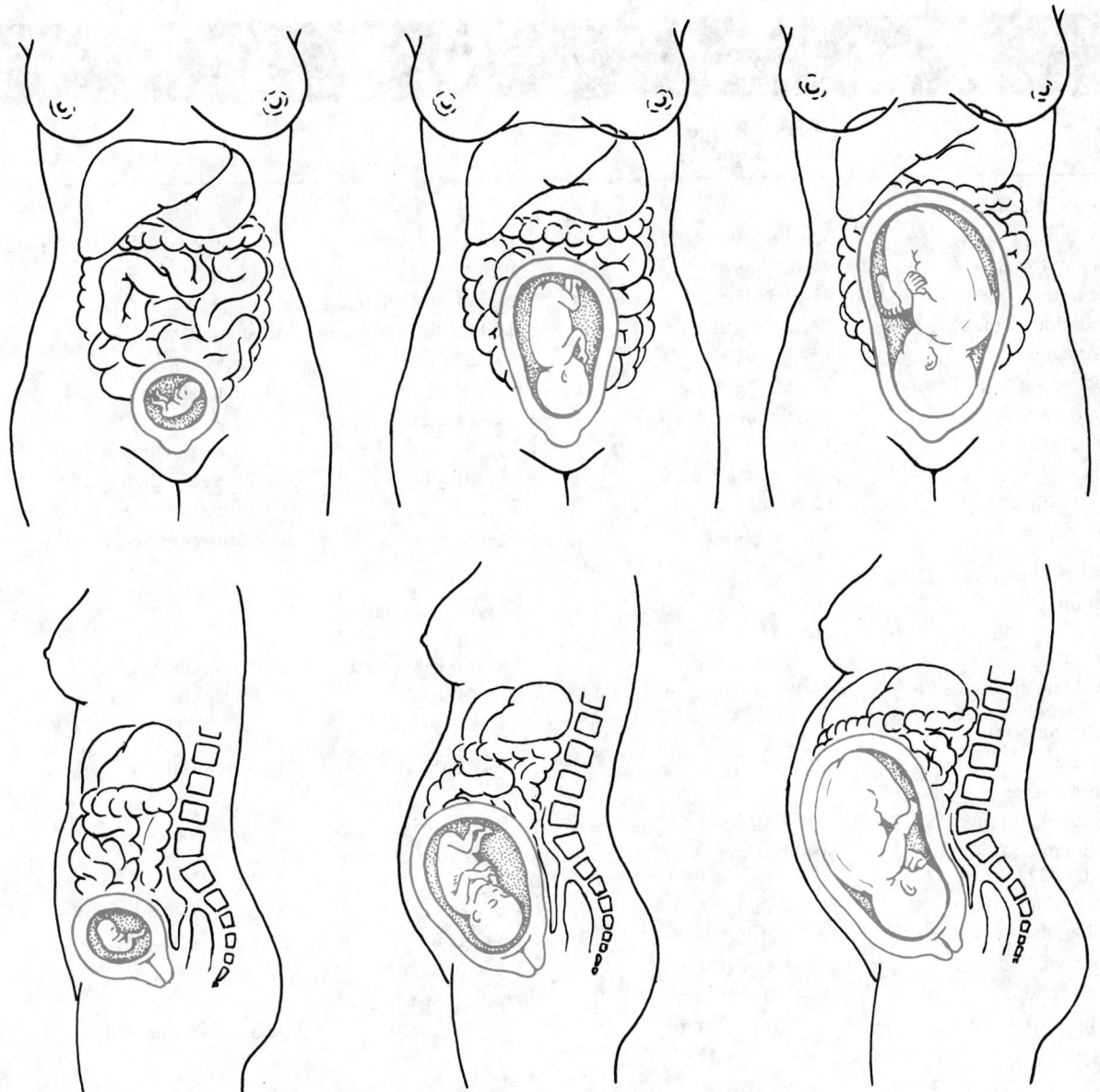

FIGURE 15–2 Front (top) and lateral (bottom) views of the relative size of the growing uterus, showing the fetus at 4, 5, and 9 months of gestation. The fundus reaches a height between the symphysis pubis and the umbilicus by the fourth month (15–16 weeks), is about the level of the umbilicus at the fifth month (20 weeks), and almost impinges on the xiphoid process at about the ninth month of gestation.

mented area around the nipple, darkens and enlarges from 3 cm (1½ in) to 5 to 6 cm (2–3 in). A secondary areola may be present if the woman has never before nursed a child. Tiny glands around the areola enlarge and may protrude. The blood supply to the breast tissue increases, and surface vessels become more pronounced.

These changes prepare the tissue for lactation; **colostrum**, the watery precursor to breast milk, may appear. Colostrum will be produced throughout the pregnancy and play a critical role in the newborn's immunologic defense mechanism. Composed of protein, fat, and minerals, it also contains immunoglobulin A

(IgA), which protects the infant's gastrointestinal system by preventing attachment of bacteria to the mucosal surface.

Breast changes are most pronounced in primigravidas and do not fully revert to the prepregnant state until after the birth of the child. In women who have been pregnant and who have nursed an infant, the breast changes are less profound.

Reproductive System Changes

All the internal organs of the reproductive system undergo significant adaptation during pregnancy.

TABLE 15–3
Common Laboratory Values in Pregnancy

Test	Normal Range (Nonpregnant)	Change in Pregnancy	Timing
SERUM CHEMISTRIES			
Albumin	3.5–4.8 g/dL	↓ 1 g/dL	Most by 20 weeks, then gradual
Calcium (total)	9–10.3 mg/dL	↓ 10%	Gradual fall
Chloride	95–105 mEq/L	No significant change	Gradual rise
Creatinine (female)	0.6–1.1 mg/dL	↓ 0.3 mg/dL	Most by 20 weeks
Fibrinogen	1.5–3.6 g/L	↑ 1–2 g/L	Progressive
Glucose, fasting (plasma)	65–105 mg/dL	↓ 10%	Gradual fall
Potassium (plasma)	3.5–4.5 mEq/L	↓ 0.2–0.3 mEq/L	By 20 weeks
Protein (total)	6.5–8.5 g/dL	↓ 1 g/dL	By 20 weeks then stable
Sodium	135–145 mEq/L	↓ 2–4 mEq/L	By 20 weeks then stable
Urea nitrogen	12–30 mg/dL	↓ 50%	First trimester
Uric acid	3.5–8 mg/dL	↓ 33%	First trimester, rise at term
URINARY CHEMISTRIES			
Creatinine	15–25 mg/kg per day (1–1.4 g/d)	No significant change	
Protein	Up to 150 mg/d	Up to 250–300 mg/d	By 20 weeks
Creatinine clearance	90–130 mL/min per 1.73 m^2	↑ 40%–50%	By 16 weeks
SERUM ENZYMATIC ACTIVITIES			
Amylase	23–84 IU/L	↑ 50%–100%	Controversial
Transaminase			
Glutamic pyruvic (SGPT)	5–35 mU/mL	No significant change	
Glutamic oxaloacetic (SGOT)	5–40 mU/mL	No significant change	
Hematocrit (female)	36%–46%	↓ 4%–7%	Bottoms at 30–34 weeks
Hemoglobin (female)	12–16 g/dL	↓ 1.5–2 g/dL	Bottoms at 30–34 weeks
Leukocyte count	4.8–10.8 × 10^3/mm^3	↑ 3.5 × 10^3/mm^3	Gradual
Platelet count	150–400 × 10^3/mm^3	Slight decrease	
Erythrocyte count	4.0–5.0 × 10^6/mm^3	↑ 25%–30%	Begins 6–8 weeks
SERUM HORMONE VALUES			
Coritsol (plasma)	8–21 µg/dL	↑ 20 µg/dL	Peaks 28–32 weeks then constant to term
Prolactin (female)	25 ng/mL	↑ 50–400 ng/mL	Gradual, peaks at term
Thyroxine, total (T$_4$)	5–11 g/dL	↑ 5 mg/dL	Early sustained
Triiodothyronine, total (T$_3$)	125–245 ng/dL	↑ 50%	Early sustained

The Uterus

As already stated, the uterus softens, becomes more globular, and increasing in size and volume to accommodate the fetus, placenta, and amniotic fluid.

The uterus forms new muscle fibers during the early months of pregnancy, and the existing muscle fibers enlarge and elongate considerably. This hypertrophy of the uterus is probably due to the estrogen stimulation on the muscle fibers. Fibroelastic tissue develops between preexisting muscle fibers and forms a network around various muscle bundles. This strengthens the uterine walls and enables the uterus to contract during labor.

The muscle fibers are arranged in three layers:

- External hoodlike layer, arching over the fundus
- Middle layer of interlacing network supporting the blood vessels
- Internal layer of circular fibers around the ostia and internal os

The Cervix

The cervix begins to soften at about 8 weeks due to increased vascularity, edema, and hyperplasia of the cervical glands. The mucous glands of the cervix prolifer-

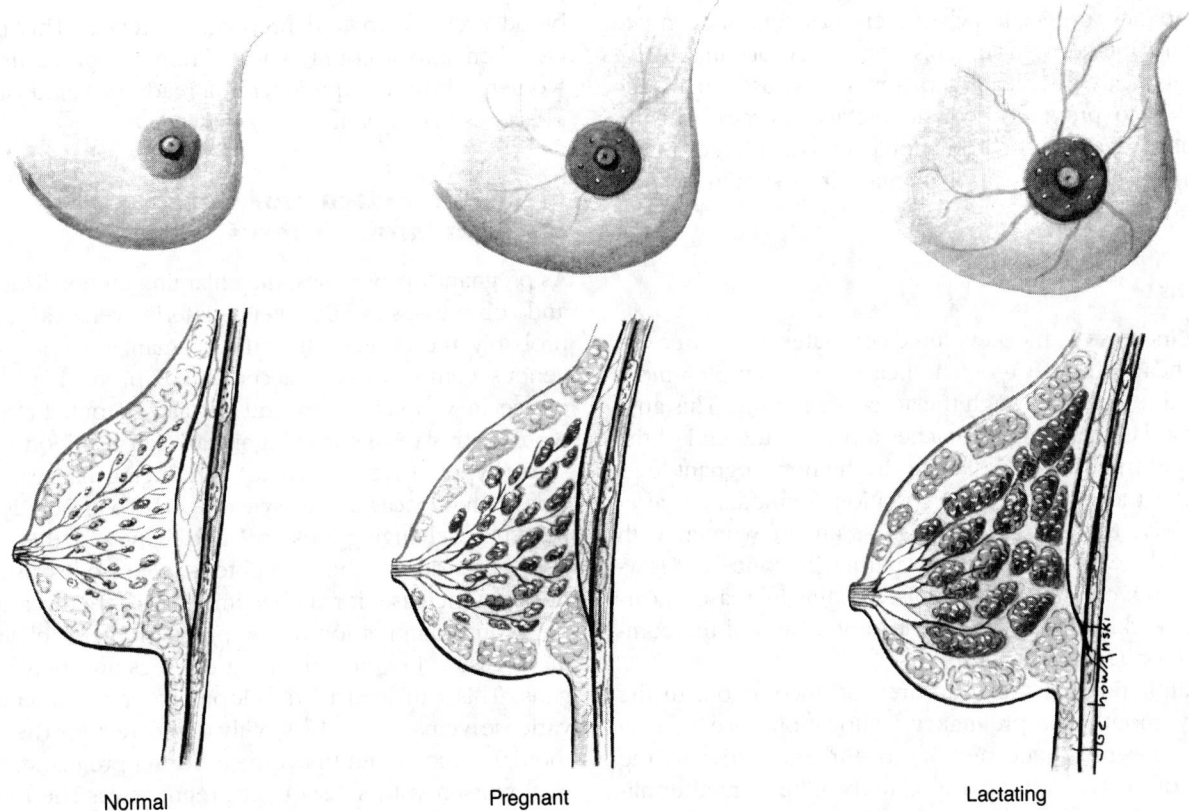

FIGURE 15–3 Breast changes during pregnancy. (Whitley, N. [1985]. *Manual of clinical obstetrics.* Philadelphia: J.B. Lippincott.)

ate and become distended with mucus. They form a structure resembling a honeycomb, making up about half of the entire structure of the cervix. This creates a mucous plug (Fig. 15-4) that seals the uterus from contamination by vaginal bacteria. At the end of pregnancy, this mucous plug is expelled, along with a small amount of blood, called the *bloody show*. This event often precedes labor but does not predict impending birth.

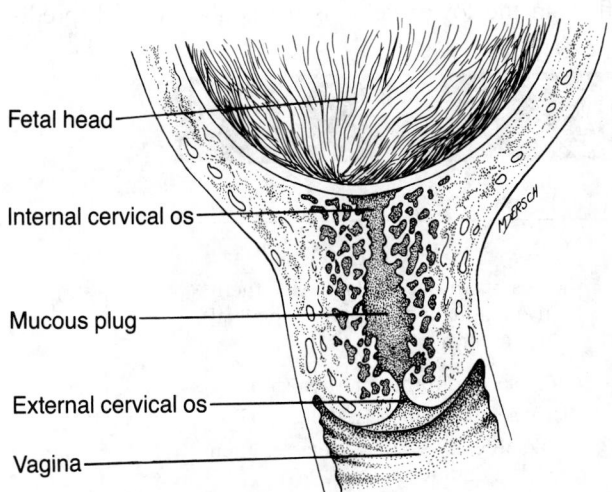

Fetal head

Internal cervical os

Mucous plug

External cervical os

Vagina

FIGURE 15–4 Cervix with mucous plug.

Circulatory System Changes

Blood

The average minimal hematologic values for nonpregnant women and pregnant women are 12 g of hemoglobin, 3.75 million erythrocytes, and 35% hematocrit. If there are adequate iron reserves in the body or if sufficient iron is supplied from the diet, these values will remain relatively stable throughout pregnancy.

Blood volume is increased about 50% during pregnancy, and the bone marrow increases production of red blood cells. Thus, the actual concentration of red blood cells should be more or less the same as under nonpregnant conditions. However, the plasma component may increase more rapidly than the red cell mass, leading to a fall in hematocrit beginning early in pregnancy.

Iron Needs

Many women experience a borderline iron-deficiency anemia as a result of menstruation. Poor dietary intake can compound this problem. When a woman becomes pregnant, anemia can worsen as the blood volume increases and red cell production accelerates. These changes place an increased demand on bodily iron stores. Iron-deficiency anemia is often present before pregnancy, especially when there has been inadequate dietary intake of iron. This commonly occurs among clients with poor eating patterns or those financially unable to provide adequate dietary sources. The increased demand for iron should be considered during prenatal care, and supplementary iron should be provided as indicated.

Heart

The increase in blood volume correlates to its effect on the heart (Table 15-4). The heart has about 50% more blood to pump through the aorta per minute. This augmented cardiac output reaches a peak at the end of the second trimester and declines to the nonpregnant level during the last weeks of gestation. Immediately after delivery, there is a sharp rise again. In women with normal hearts, this is of no particular concern. However, in women with heart disease, this increase in cardiac workload may add to the seriousness of the complication (see Chap. 32).

Palpitations of the heart are not uncommon. In the early months of pregnancy, palpitations are usually due to sympathetic nervous disturbance; toward the end of gestation, they are related to the intra-abdominal pressure of the enlarged uterus.

Blood Pressure

The arterial blood pressure of the pregnant woman is affected by her position. Pressure in the brachial artery is highest when she is sitting and is lowest when she is in the lateral recumbent position. Ordinarily, arterial blood pressure falls during the second or early third trimester of pregnancy and rises slowly thereafter.

Systolic pressure falls slightly during pregnancy, whereas diastolic pressure decreases more markedly. These changes are due to the increased cardiac output and reduced peripheral resistance typical of pregnancy. Toward the end of pregnancy, vasoconstrictor tone usually increases, resulting in a normal rise of blood pressure toward prepregnant levels. This must be taken into account when caring for preeclamptic women who are experiencing already elevated blood pressures (Villar et al., 1989).

Mechanical Circulatory Effects of the Enlarging Uterus

As pregnancy progresses, the enlarging uterus displaces and compresses the iliac veins, inferior vena cava, and probably the aorta. When the woman is supine, this venous compression is accentuated, producing a decrease in venous return and cardiac output. In some women, this results in a significant fall in blood pressure (hypotensive syndrome), producing nausea, dizziness, and occasionally syncope. Hypotension is relieved by changing position and lying on the side. Heart rate during these hypotensive episodes usually does not increase; it may become slower (bradycardia).

Venous compression by the pregnant uterus elevates the pressure in veins, draining the legs and pelvic organs. This can lead to development or worsening of varicose veins in the legs, vulva, and rectum (hemorrhoids), which often first appear during pregnancy and may worsen with subsequent pregnancies. The rise in venous pressure is a major cause of edema in the lower extremities that often occurs in later pregnancy. Decreases in plasma oncotic pressure also contribute to edema. The hypoalbuminemia associated with pregnancy shifts the balance of the colloid osmotic pressure in favor of fluid transfer from the intravascular to the extravascular space. This mechanism of edema may be more important than venous compression (Valenzuela, 1989). Extracellular volume, consisting of intravascular and interstitial components, increases throughout pregnancy, creating a physiologic extracellular hypervolemia. Maternal interstitial volume has its greatest increase during the last trimester, contributing to edema.

Because of venous compression, the rate of blood flow in the lower veins is markedly reduced, predis-

TABLE 15-4
Cardiovascular Changes in Pregnancy

Parameter	Amount of Change	Timing
Arterial blood pressures		
Systolic	↓ 4–6 mm Hg	Lowest values at 20–24 weeks, then rise gradually to prepregnancy values at term
Diastolic	↓ 8–15 mm Hg	
Mean	↓ 6–10 mm Hg	
Heart rate	↑ 12–18 beats/min	Early second trimester, then stable
Stroke volume	↑ 10%–30%	Early second trimester, then stable
Cardiac output	↑ 33%–45%	Peaks in early second trimester, then stable until term

posing pregnant women to thrombosis. The effects of compression of the vena cava are partially offset by development of paravertebral collateral circulation that permits blood from the lower extremities to bypass the partly occluded vena cava.

During late pregnancy, the uterus partially compresses the aorta and its branches, which may account for lower pressure in the femoral artery compared with the brachial artery. Aortic compression is accentuated during labor contractions and may cause fetal distress when the woman is in the supine position.

Regional Blood Flow

Blood flow to most regions of the body increases during pregnancy. In the uterus, kidneys, and skin, the blood flow increases with gestational age. This enhances the ability of the kidneys to eliminate waste materials better and the skin to regulate heat production. Both of these processes require large amounts of plasma, which is one reason for the disproportionate increase of plasma over red blood cells in the expansion of blood volume during pregnancy.

Respiratory System Changes

The major respiratory changes in pregnancy are caused by the mechanical effects of the enlarging uterus, the increased total body oxygen consumption, and the respiratory stimulant effects of progesterone (Table 15-5). As pregnancy progresses, the enlarging uterus places pressure upward toward the lungs and elevates the position of the diaphragm. This results in lower intrathoracic pressure and decreased resting lung volume, creating a decreased functional residual capacity (FRC) in the lungs. Reductions in the expiratory reserve volume and the residual volume of the lungs contribute to the reduced FRC. The movement of the diaphragm

and the thoracic muscles is not impaired by the enlarging uterus; thus, the vital capacity of the lungs is unchanged.

Oxygen Consumption and Ventilation

With pregnancy, total body oxygen consumption increases about 15% to 20%, primarily due to increased needs of the uterus and its contents. More oxygen is required for increased renal and cardiac work, with small increments needed for work of the respiratory muscles and the breasts. During pregnancy, the increases in cardiac output and alveolar ventilation are greater than those needed to meet increased oxygen consumption. Therefore, despite the rise in total oxygen consumption, the arteriovenous oxygen difference and arterial PCO_2 fall, indicating hyperventilation. Progesterone increases ventilation, making the respiratory center more sensitive to CO_2.

In hyperventilation of pregnancy, the PCO_2 falls to a level of 27 to 32 mm Hg, producing respiratory alkalosis. There is a corresponding rise in arterial PO_2 to about 106 to 108 mm Hg in the first trimester, with a slight downward trend as pregnancy progresses. To compensate for the alkalosis, there is increased renal bicarbonate excretion, leading to a final pH between 7.40 and 7.45.

Dyspnea in Pregnancy

Dyspnea is common during pregnancy. While the respiratory rate does not change during pregnancy, there is a rise in minute ventilation, reflecting about a 40% increase in tidal volume at term. The increased size of the uterus and corresponding displacement of abdominal contents also may affect respiration, while airway resistance is generally unchanged. This also may be related to greater differences between nonpregnant and

TABLE 15–5
Changes in Lung Volume and Capacity During Pregnancy

Test	Description	Change in Pregnancy
Respiratory rate	Breaths per minute	Unchanged
Inspiratory capacity	Maximum volume air inspired from resting level	Increased about 5%
Tidal volume	Volume air inspired and expired each breath	Rises through pregnancy 40% increase (0.1–0.2 L)
Functional residual capacity	Volume air in lungs at resting expiratory level	Decreased about 18%
Vital capacity	Maximum volume air forcibly inspired	Unchanged, may be small decrease at term
Minute ventilation	Volume air inspired or expired in 1 min	Increased about 40%
Expiratory reserve volume	Maximum volume air expired after normal expiration	Decreased about 15%
Residual volume	Volume air remaining after maximum expiration	Decreases considerably

pregnant PCO_2 levels in susceptible women. There are no substantial differences in pulmonary function tests between pregnant women with dyspnea and those who do not experience this symptom.

Gastrointestinal System Changes

Besides morning sickness, several gastrointestinal system changes occur during pregnancy.

Mouth and Gums

Vascular swelling of the gums is called epulis of pregnancy. The gums become hyperemic and softened, with an increased tendency toward bleeding after brushing the teeth. These changes do not lead to an increased incidence of tooth decay and usually regress spontaneously after delivery. Additional vitamin C in the diet may decrease the tendency. Consultation with a dentist should be encouraged if the bleeding gums becomes a persistent problem.

Stomach and Intestines

The intestines and stomach are displaced upward by the enlarging uterus. These positional changes may alter the physical findings in certain diseases, such as appendicitis. The appendix is usually displaced somewhat laterally and upward and at times may be located as high as the right flank. This also accounts for the increase in gastric reflux and the resulting sensation of "heartburn."

Motility and Muscle Tone. The motility in the gastrointestinal tract is decreased, resulting in a prolonged gastric emptying time and a longer intestinal transit time. A generalized relaxation of the smooth musculature of the gastrointestinal tract occurs under the influence of progesterone. Constipation and heartburn often result.

Muscular tone around the stomach and esophagus is altered, resulting in lower intraesophageal pressures, higher intragastric pressures, and slower esophageal peristalsis. All of these changes contribute to gastroesophageal reflux.

Digestion

Appetite may be decreased in early pregnancy in association with nausea. As the digestive system becomes accustomed to its new conditions, the appetite is increased. Because of organ displacement and diminished tone, stomach emptying time is decreased, and feelings of "fullness" are increased. Women may need small, frequent meals, rather than three large meals. Diet teaching should focus on food quality rather than quantity to provide optimal nutrition.

Adequate dietary intake of fiber and fluids can help to decrease constipation.

Liver and Gallbladder

No characteristic changes in liver morphology occur during normal pregnancy, but some of the laboratory tests for hepatic function are altered:

- Total alkaline phosphatase activity in serum doubles, reaching levels that would be abnormal in the nonpregnant state. This is caused by the effect of alkaline phosphatase isoenzymes produced by the placenta.
- Serum cholinesterase activity normally falls during pregnancy.
- Leucine aminopeptidase activity (serum) is markedly elevated.
- Gallbladder function is affected by decreased tone and distention, leading to prolonged emptying time and incomplete evacuation. This may account for the increased predisposition to gallstones during pregnancy.

Urinary and Renal System Changes

Along with the customary increase in frequency of urination, the renal system undergoes several physiologic changes:

- The urine in pregnancy usually is increased in amount and has a lower specific gravity.
- There is a decrease in the renal threshold for glucose, and urine may test positive for sugar, even without other symptoms of diabetes. While "spilling sugar" or lactosuria is common, it should be investigated within the course of prenatal care.
- Renal function tests may be altered, including the following:
  Decreased plasma creatinine
  Decreased urea concentrations
  Decreased urine concentration
- The ureters become markedly dilated in pregnancy, particularly the right ureter. (This change apparently is due in part to the pressure of the gravid uterus on the ureters as they cross the pelvic brim and in part to a softening that the ureteral walls undergo as the result of endocrine influences. This does not appear to be accompanied by decreased ureteral peristalsis. Ureteral dilatation begins in the first trimester and is present in 90% of women at term. It usually resolves within 4 to 6 weeks after delivery, although it may persist until the 12th to 16th postpartum week.)
- Renal plasma flow and the glomerular filtration rate begin to increase in early pregnancy, reaching a plateau by midpregnancy at about 40% above nonpregnant levels. This persists unchanged until term.

The exact mechanism of these changes is unclear; although partially related to the increased plasma volume in pregnancy, the renal changes reach a peak relatively early in pregnancy, before the maximum increase in plasma volume occurs.

- Plasma concentrations of renin, renin substrate, and angiotensin I and II are increased during pregnancy. Renin levels remain elevated throughout pregnancy; some of this elevated renin may represent a different, high molecular weight form or inactive form of the enzyme. The uterus and kidneys can produce renin, and high concentrations of renin are found in the amniotic fluid. The role of renin in amniotic fluid is not fully understood.

- The bladder usually functions efficiently during pregnancy. The urinary frequency experienced in the first few months of pregnancy is caused by hormonal effects and pressure exerted on the bladder by the enlarging uterus. Mechanical frequency is observed again when lightening occurs before the onset of labor. Urinary tract infections, especially cystitis, are not uncommon during pregnancy and may be related to urinary stasis and inadequate emptying of the bladder.

Endocrine System Changes

Placenta

The placenta functions as the major endocrine gland during pregnancy, secreting four hormones that are vital to maintaing the pregnancy. The early chorionic villi of the implanted ovum secrete hCG, which prolongs the life of the corpus luteum. The result is the continued production of estrogen and progesterone, which are necessary to maintain the endometrium. During pregnancy, hCG appears in maternal blood and is excreted in the mother's urine, allowing diagnosis of pregnancy by tests previously discussed.

The chorionic cells of the placenta produce another unique hormone, human chorionic somatomammotropin, which also is known as human placental lactogen (hPL). This hormone is detectable in placental cells as early as the third week after ovulation and is found in maternal serum by the sixth week. It influences somatic cell growth of the fetus and facilitates preparation of the breasts for lactation.

In addition, the placenta takes over the production of estrogen and progesterone from the ovaries and after the first 2 months of gestation, becomes the major source of these two hormones. The increase in these hormones in the maternal organism is thought to be responsible for many important changes that take place during pregnancy, such as the growth of the uterus and the development of the breasts. In the breasts, the development of the duct system is promoted by estrogen, and the development of the lobule-alveolar system is promoted by progesterone.

Pituitary Body

The pituitary gland enlarges somewhat during pregnancy but is not essential for the maintenance of pregnancy.

The *anterior lobe* of this small gland, located at the base of the brain, is called the "master clock," which, under the influence of the hypothalamus, controls the menstrual cycle. In addition to gonadotropins, the anterior lobe secretes hormones that act on the thyroid and adrenal glands and another hormone that influences the growth process. Production of these hormones continues during the pregnancy. Gonadotropins, on the other hand, are no longer cyclically released. The estrogen and progesterone produced by the placenta inhibit their release from the pituitary gland.

The *posterior lobe* of the pituitary secretes an oxytocic hormone, *oxytocin*, which has a strong stimulating effect on the uterine muscle. Extracts of the pituitary gland that contains oxytocin are widely used in obstetrics for the following:

- To stimulate or augment contractions during labor (see Chap. 36)
- To stimulate the uterus to contract after delivery, thereby diminishing postpartum hemorrhage (see Chap. 22)
- To stimulate lactation

Thyroid Gland

During pregnancy, there is slight to moderate enlargement of the thyroid. This hypertrophy of thyroid tissue is not associated with increased thyroid activity, although an elevation in the basal metabolic rate increases throughout the course of pregnancy. This is a reflection of the increased oxygen consumption as a result of the metabolic activity of the products of conception.

Other parameters for the measurement of thyroid function display changes. The serum protein-bound iodine, butyl extractable iodine, and thyroxine (T_4) levels increase, and the elevated levels are maintained until shortly after delivery. The increase is not due to increased thyroid activity, but to an elevation in the level of thyroid-binding protein normally present in the blood. Thus, although the amount of circulating thyroid hormones and therefore the total concentration of hormone are elevated, the actual amount of unbound or available hormone remains within normal limits.

The triiodothyronine (T_3) uptake test displays decreased values in pregnancy, which indicates an increase in the binding of circulating triiodothyronine. A similar increase in the level of thyroid-binding proteins is seen in the nonpregnant client after the administration of estrogen, and it is likely that in pregnancy, the increase is a reflection of the high level of circulating estrogen.

Adrenals

The *adrenal cortex* hypertrophies during pregnancy, and its activity increases. The actual secretion of cortisol by the adrenals is unchanged, although the metabolism of cortisol is altered as a result of the influence of estrogen. There is an increase in the production by the adrenal glands of aldosterone, the hormone responsible for the retention of sodium by the kidneys. This increase begins early in pregnancy and continues throughout. The result of the increase is a decreased ability of the kidneys to handle salt during pregnancy, leading to some fluid retention and either occult or overt edema.

Ovaries

The *ovaries*, except for the activity of the corpus luteum of pregnancy, remain relatively quiescent. Gonadotropin levels are low, because their release is inhibited by the estrogen and progesterone produced by the placenta. Thus, follicular activity in the ovary is suppressed, and there is no further ovulation until after delivery.

Integumentary System Changes

The vast hormonal changes in pregnancy often result in some skin and other integumentary system changes.

Striae Gravidarum

"Stretch marks," termed **striae gravidarum**, are elongated streaks of pink to red, often found on the abdomen and breasts of a pregnant woman. Any time the skin is subject to rapid stretching (growth spurts, sudden weight gain, development of rapidly growing tumors), the underlying connective tissue can stretch, rupture, and atrophy, leaving characteristic scars. Striae usually fade to a silvery blue after delivery. They cannot be prevented, and they tend to run in families.

Pigment Changes

Many women will develop a darkened line from the mons pubis to umbilicus during pregnancy. This area of increased pigmentation is termed *linea nigra* and fades after pregnancy. *Chloasma,* or the "mask of pregnancy," is increased facial pigmentation, especially noticeable over the nose and cheeks. It also is seen with women who use oral contraceptives or experi-ence some collagen-vascular disorders (systemic lupus). While these areas tend to fade after pregnancy, some women will retain the added pigmentation. Women with darker skin will experience more pronounced skin changes than those with fair skin.

Spider Hemangiomas

Fair-skinned women tend to develop fiery-red blemishes with branching legs coming from a central body. These are probably due to the increase in circulating estrogens. They have no clinical significance and tend to fade after delivery.

Sweat Glands

Sebaceous glands, sweat glands, and hair follicles are more highly active during pregnancy due to the hormonal increases. Pregnant women can be reassured that increased perspiration is normal and will revert to normal after birth.

Immunologic Response in Pregnancy

From the immunologic standpoint, pregnancy is an example of a tissue graft that does not cause a rejection response. The presence of the fetus in the uterus can be compared with an organ transplant, in which organs of two different people are grafted together. Problems with immunologic rejection of grafted tissue from another person often occur, but in pregnancy, several mechanisms permit tolerance of the fetal "graft" and successful continuation of the gestation (Table 15-6).

During pregnancy, the woman's immune system remains intact and protects the woman and fetus from infection. Pregnancy is a time of enhanced and specialized immune function as the immune system undergoes significant changes to prevent host (woman) versus graft (fetus) rejection. Cellular immunity is mediated by T cells and B cells, each serving a specific purpose in the protection of the body. In response to an assault on the host, T and B cells eliminate the foreign antigen (American College of Obstetrics and Gynecologists [ACOG], 1994).

The primary sites where maternal immunologic defenses are modulated in response to the fetus are the uterus, regional lymphatics, and placental surface.

The Uterus

The uterus has decreased or altered afferent lymphatic systems that allow it to modify the host response to tissue grafts. The T cells' role is to mediate the cellular response to foreign tissue by acting to help or suppress

TABLE 15–6
Mechanisms of Maternal Immunologic Tolerance of Fetal "Graft"

Maternal		Fetal	
SYSTEMIC	**UTERUS AND LOCAL LYMPHATIC SYSTEMS**	**PLACENTA**	**SYSTEMIC**
None (normal cell mediated immunity)	Privileged immunologic site	Separation of the maternal-fetal circulations, including tight local barriers	Unidentified humoral and cellular immunosuppressive elements
	Localized, nonspecific suppression induces tolerance and generates suppressor T cells	Lack of expression of the major histocompatibility antigen (HLA) at the maternal-fetal interface	
		Nonspecific local immunosuppression through placental proteins and hormones	
		Immunoabsorbent effect of placental proteins and hormones	
		Production of masking and blocking antibodies	
		Generation of immune cell blockage	

the immune response; they are altered locally in the uterus during pregnancy. Pregnancy-related suppressor T cells, which decrease the maternal lymphocyte response, have been found. These T cells, in conjunction with actions by the placenta, can create an altered local immunologic environment.

Regional Lymphatics

The woman and fetus each have independent lymphatic systems. Because there is no communication between them, antibodies formed in the mother's immune system do not reach the fetus unless there is a defect in the placental barrier.

Placental Surface

The placenta is an interface between the maternal and fetal systems. The separate vascular compartments of the placenta effectively protect the fetus from direct contact with the maternal immunologic defense system. Tight trophoblastic intercellular junctions and a fibrinous covering of the trophoblast allow control of cellular and molecular exchange between mother and fetus. Also, the placenta does not have the major histocompatibility (human leukocyte) antigens that are needed for maternal lymphocytes to initiate an effective immunologic response (Cunningham et al., 1993). Several placental proteins and steroids, including pregnancy-specific β_1 glycoprotein, hPL, and hCG,

have been shown to suppress the local (uterine) immune response in pregnancy. The placenta is immunoabsorbent, decreasing the response against the fetus by trapping maternal immune components.

While tolerating the existence of the fetal "graft," the maternal immune system provides the usual protective responses to infection, including phagocytosis and the inflammatory response. T-cell immunity is slightly decreased, while the B cells are more active during pregnancy. Immunoglobulin levels do not reflect measurable change in pregnancy.

- Maternal IgG is the only immunoglobulin able to cross the placenta. It becomes the major component of the fetal immunoglobulin in utero and provides significant passive immunity to the fetus and neonate.
- IgM, IgA, IgD, and IgE do not cross the placenta and do not provide any direct harm or benefit to the fetus.
- IgA is secreted in maternal colostrum and provides additional gastrointestinal immunity (especially against *Escherichia coli*) to the breast-fed newborn (ACOG, 1994; Adelsberg, 1985; Medearis, 1986).

Summary Points

✔ Even though there are many signs and symptoms of pregnancy, advanced testing techniques now make it possible and feasible to diagnose pregnancy before physical symptoms occur. Testing is available in the home or healthcare agencies but with a wide range of accuracy.

✔ Pregnancy stimulates great anatomic and physiologic changes in the human system. All body systems are affected to some degree, and normal physiology is altered to support the growing fetus.

✔ The adaptations of pregnancy occur on every level of the mother's physiology, from intracellular to multisystemic.

REFERENCES

Adelsberg, B. R. (1985). Immunology of pregnancy. *Mount Sinai Journal of Medicine, 52,* 5.

American College of Obstetrics and Gynecologists (1994). *Precis V, an update in obstetrics and gynecology.* Washington, DC: Author.

Callen, P. W. (Ed) (1994). *Ultrasonography in obstetrics and gynecology.* Philadelphia: W.B. Saunders.

Catlin, A., & Wetzel, W. (1991). Ectopic pregnancy: Implications for nurse practitioners. *Nurse Practitioner, 16*(1), 38–46.

Cunningham, F. G., MacDonald, P. C., Gant, N. F., Leveno, K. J., & Gilstrap, L. C. (1993). *Williams obstetrics* (19th ed.). Norwalk, CT: Appleton & Lange.

Hatcher, R. A., Trussell, J., Stewart, F., Steward, G. K., Kowal, D., Guest, F., Cates, W. L., & Policar, M. (1994). *Contraceptive technology* (16th ed.). New York: Irvington Publishers.

Medearis, A. L. (1986). Immunology of pregnancy. In N. F. Hacker & J. G. Moore (Eds.), *Essentials of obstetrics and gynecology* (pp 47–83). Philadelphia: W.B. Saunders.

Ringa, V., Blondel, B., & Breart, G. (1989). Ultrasound in obstetrics: Do the published evaluative studies justify its routine use? *International Journal of Epidemiology, 18,* 489.

Schurz, B., Wenzl, R., Eppel, W. et al. (1990). Early detection of ectopic pregnancy by transvaginal ultrasound. *Archives of Gynecology and Obstetrics, 248,* 25–29.

Villar, J., Rapke, J., Markush, L. et al. (1989). The measuring of blood pressure during pregnancy. *American Journal of Obstetrics and Gynecology, 161*(4), 1019–1024.

Valenzuela, G. J. (1989). Is a decrease in plasma oncotic pressure enough to explain the edema of pregnancy? *American Journal of Obstetrics and Gynecology, 161*(6), 1624–1627.

16

Psychosocial Aspects of Pregnancy

Objectives

- Develop an understanding of the influence that culture has on perceptions of pregnancy and its management.
- Develop the ability to differentiate between crisis, stress, and role transition when assessing the meaning and impact of pregnancy on the client and her partner.
- Identify the cognitive and emotional tasks that the mother and father must accomplish as a result of taking on the role of "pregnancy."
- Describe the cognitive and emotional reactions that occur in the mother and father during a pregnancy.
- Using the nursing process, develop expertise in making accurate family assessments for the pregnant woman or couple.

The family is society's most basic unit that has survived through the centuries because it serves vital human needs. There are many different styles of family living and many different ways in which the family relates to society. Whatever the form, the family will no doubt continue to exist as long as humans continue to populate this planet. Naturally, childbearing plays an important role in the family, and the family, likewise, has a major influence on each new generation's perceptions of pregnancy, childbearing, and childrearing.

Cultural Influences on Perceptions of Pregnancy

Each member of a family assumes roles that are in part dictated by cultural expectations. Each member's perceptions of these roles vary according to the manner of socialization and the kind of interaction he or she has had with others. As society evolves and changes, so do the various role expectations. Each successive generation may hold different expectations as they adapt to changing times and needs, although there are always socially imposed limitations.

So it has been with childbearing. Pregnancy and birth are important events in most cultures. However, attitudes toward these processes vary considerably among different cultures and even within one society. In some cultures, birth is a social event, with open attendance by all friends and family. In other cultures, it is conducted in secrecy. Similarly, pregnancy may be seen as a normal uneventful preparatory phase to a desired change in status signifying achievement; conversely, it may be viewed as mysterious, the harbinger of possible disaster, or an atonement for simply being a lowly woman (Berk, 1993; Gilliss et al., 1989).

Pregnancy in the American Culture

Two competing views of pregnancy exist in American culture. One views pregnancy and childbirth as "crisis"

situations; the other regards it as a normal role transition experience. Each of these attitudes rests on different assumptions that, if carried to their logical conclusions, have different implications for the delivery of healthcare. Unfortunately, assumptions and terminology have not always been clearly articulated, and when the rhetoric has been uncritically accepted and applied to the healthcare environment, some peculiar innovations and traditions have been incorporated into the delivery of care. This chapter examines the "crisis" and the "normal" orientations to pregnancy and their impact on the delivery of maternity and perinatal care in American culture.

Pregnancy as Crisis

Pregnancy, particularly a couple's first pregnancy, represents a critical period in the evolution of a family. Until the 1970s, this period was often described by researchers in many fields as a period of crisis (Bibring, 1955; Caplan, 1960; Coleman et al., 1971; Shainess, 1963). Chertok (1960), for instance, wrote of pregnancy as a progressively developing crisis, with labor and delivery as the peak of the crisis, because parturition results in separation of the mother and child and isolation from significant others. This view was based largely on experiential or clinical impressions; there were many flaws in research design and analysis, including small samples skewed to the pathologic end of the normal–abnormal continuum and a lack of control groups (McCubbin et al., 1983; Gilliss et al., 1989).

Other research led to the formulation of the concept of "normal crisis of parenthood," a contradiction in terms. Although the original focus of this crisis research was parenthood, often pregnancy became intermingled with the general research in this area with little empirical basis. The early work of Le Masters (1957), Dyer (1963), and Hobbs (1963) laid the foundation for this unfortunate extrapolation. Unfortunately, these early writings have remained in the literature, and their concepts of parenthood and pregnancy as "crisis situations" for parents continue to influence thinking and often the delivery of care.

Pregnancy as a Stressor

In many of the early conceptual formulations, both psychological and sociologic, a "crisis" was considered to be a critical event but one that was not necessarily totally psychologically or interpersonally disruptive. However, the authors' true meaning was often subverted because they did not precisely define their terms.

In the original stress research on the family as exemplified by Hill (1958) and Hill et al. (1960), the term **crisis** signified a sharp, decisive change in experience for which old patterns of behavior become inadequate.

Thus, there was an interruption in the family's routine, and new patterns of interaction had to be developed. There also was the implication that resolution and reintegration were not only possible (ie, "normal"), but expected and well within the family's capabilities without outside intervention. This view did not include the idea of collapse or immobilization, which with time, have been attributed to crises.

In the 1980s and 1990s, researchers have done much to clarify and refine concepts, definitions, and measurements of family stress, particularly regarding the conceptualization of stressors, crisis, and role transition; and where pregnancy fits into the total process (Belsky et al., 1984; Steffenmeier, 1982; Gay et al., 1988; Gilliss et al., 1989). In the newer, more refined conceptualizations, pregnancy is considered a potential **stressor** (something that can produce stress) that provides input into the entire equation of the role transition from nonparent to parent, and its impact depends on a variety of factors.

Clearly, there has been some confusion in the last 50 years in the way the term *crisis* has been applied to the events of pregnancy, childbirth, and parenthood. This has sometimes led to pregnancy being viewed as disruptive and potentially damaging emotionally or psychologically. Recent research indicates that pregnancy is a time of transition but is not necessarily disruptive.

Pregnancy as a Role Transition

In a classic paper, Rossi (1968) suggested that the term *normal crisis* was a misnomer as applied to parenthood because the concepts of "normal" and "crisis" are basically incompatible—one implies a natural successful resolution and the other indicates the possibility of nonresolution. She suggested that parenthood be viewed as a role transition and be based on a stage-task conceptual framework, such as found in the work of Erickson (1959), Benedek (1959), and Hill (1958). This type of orientation puts parenthood and other phases of the reproductive cycle, including pregnancy, into a development task formulation and allows these phenomena to be seen as essentially normal or usual. It also respects the fact that deviation, stress, or disruption can occur, depending on a variety of circumstances. This orientation is most commonly accepted and used by current researchers (Whall et al., 1991; Feetham et al., 1993; Friedman, 1992; Pruett, 1987; Fuller et al., 1993; Mercer et al., 1994). Chapter 26 discusses this concept as applied to the postpartum period, when parenthood becomes tangible.

Life-Span Cycles and Role Transition in Pregnancy

By viewing the total life span in terms of a developmental task interaction, people's life spans can be viewed as having cycles composed of stages or phases, each with its unique tasks. As the various cycles occur, social roles develop out of interaction with others in the social network. By analogy, social roles may be said to have cycles, and each stage in the cycle has its set of tasks and adjustments. Family researchers have outlined four broad stages in a role cycle that have implications for pregnancy and parenthood (Rossi, 1968; Reeder, 1994).

- *Anticipatory stage*. Almost all social roles have some kind of formal or informal training, either through formal schooling, role modeling, or watching others. This stage socializes or trains the potential actor for the role that he or she is to assume. As its name implies, this stage precedes the assumption of the role and may take place years ahead of the actual role assumption.
- *Honeymoon stage*. This is the time immediately after the full assumption of the role. Intimacy and exploration occur as the person tries to adjust the "fit" of his or her personality to the role demands. Reality testing takes place rather than the fantasizing that often accompanies the anticipatory phase.
- *Plateau stage*. This is the protracted middle period of a role cycle during which the role is fully exercised. In this phase, people validate themselves as adequate or inadequate depending on how well they and others see themselves performing in the role.
- *Disengagement or termination stage*. This period immediately precedes and includes the actual termination of the role. For some roles, this stage is tangible. The marital role, for instance, can end abruptly with death or divorce. Similarly, pregnancy ends with labor or the termination of the pregnancy. For other roles, such as parenthood, the distinction is much less clear because there is little cultural prescription about when authority and obligations end. Box 16-1 summarizes these life cycle stages.

BOX 16–1
Stages in the Role Cycle

Anticipatory stage—Formal or informal training for the role; socializes the incumbent-to-be; may take place years before; no role modeling for the "pregnant" role

Honeymoon stage—Immediately follows the assumption of the role; exploration and adjustment to the "fit" of the role to the incumbent; reality testing

Plateau stage—Role is fully exercised; validation of role adequacy

Disengagement or termination stage—Immediately precedes and includes role termination; sometimes tangible (pregnancy); sometimes less distinct (parenthood)

Pregnancy as a Social Role

Although there have been many attempts to describe the various stages of pregnancy, the emotional reactions, and the developmental tasks that need to be accomplished, there are no definite boundaries, expectations, and prescriptions for the pregnant role. How are pregnant women supposed to act? What kinds of behaviors are really expected? Does the woman act ill, or is pregnancy essentially a well state? Is it "business as usual," or are there special restrictions or exemptions that may be claimed? Healthcare providers often have their own expectations of what pregnancy ought to be and what behavior is to be expected; however, in the American culture, there is no distinct or identifiable pregnant role. In the absence of any such role, there are certain alternatives. One alternative is to treat pregnancy as nothing different—like having a new hair cut or acquiring a new house. People remark and compliment and then go on about their business without change in the relationship. This attitude is difficult, however, because pregnancy has enormous positive and negative emotional significance and requires expression and acknowledgment from others. Moreover, as pregnancy advances, it interferes to some degree with normal activity in many cases. Hence the pregnant woman and those with whom she interacts require a distinctive pattern of pregnancy "rights" and "duties" (Reeder, 1993).

In the absence of a defined role, the woman and relevant others attempt to allocate or assign some other role that will fit. One possibility is to anticipate the mother role. Classes for expectant parents that involve physical and emotional preparation for labor, hands on feeding, diapering, bathing, burping, and so forth probably serve more to anticipate the mother role and solve the problems of the pregnant nonrole than they do to improve mothering behaviors. Another alternative is to emphasize the disabling aspects of pregnancy and allocate the sick role. This may be easier for the health providers who care for the woman, because the ways of dealing with the sick person are well routinized and in these days of defensive medicine, impart a feeling of safety for those concerned. There are costs to this approach, however, because often the client's orientation to pregnancy differs from the provider's, and difficulties in the delivery of care can develop (Reeder, 1993).

One way to analyze the pregnant role is to examine its structure and function according to the stages in the role cycle outlined previously:

- *Anticipatory stage.* Being pregnant is an anticipatory stage in a role transition to parenthood. This can cause confusion at the outset. As she enters the anticipatory stage of the pregnant role, the woman attempts to learn the role by observing family and friends and recalling how other significant people in her life acted when they were pregnant. She also takes cues from her physician, who may overtly or covertly influence her thinking, even to the extent of regarding pregnancy as a "sick" or "well" state (Reeder, 1993). As indicated previously, there is little socialization or role modeling for the pregnant role in our American culture; little girls play at being mothers but not usually at being pregnant. Thus, although certain behaviors directly relate to women and their fetuses during pregnancy and are essential for the collective well-being of the entire family, the prescriptions for these activities are hard to categorize and vary considerably in different social classes. They include, for example, assuming positive personal health habits, cutting down on certain activities (or increasing certain activities, such as exercise, to maintain fitness), prompt and consistent attendance to prenatal care, and adequate nutrition practices.

- *Honeymoon and plateau stages.* The honeymoon and plateau stages of the role cycle come quickly after the anticipatory stage. The showers, coffee klatches, and conversations with the woman's mother, pregnant friends, and new mothers help the woman adjust the "fit" of the pregnant state to her personality. Some women find that they adore being pregnant. They feel at one with the earth and see themselves at the center of the universe. They find that they seem to bloom physically and emotionally. Others find the condition almost unbearable. They feel unwell and ugly and cannot wait to be "unpregnant." By far, the more usual are those women who come to accept the condition, enjoy the positive aspects, and tolerate the discomforts and inconveniences. They see it as a necessary stepping stone to another larger role change.

- *Disengagement stage.* With the newborn's birth comes a relatively sudden disengagement stage. There are few cultural norms concerning when the duties and privileges of pregnancy end and parenting begins, although in the space of a few hours the mother is obviously "unpregnant." This role ambiguity can make the transition from pregnancy to actual parenthood difficult for some. (See the list of suggested readings for articles that examine this issue in depth.)

The Meaning and Effect of Pregnancy on the Couple

Pregnancy is a unique experience in which a sexual union between a man and a woman leads to the creation of a new life. This new life results in the creation of many new and unprecedented relationships.

The Mother

Although the normal woman may love her partner greatly and desire a child, she still must make major developmental changes to become a mother. In the process of childbearing, she is creating from the union of herself and her mate another individual inside herself who must ultimately grow to become a separate person. Hence, the coming newborn represents the synthesis of three distinct entities: the mother's relationship to her partner, the mother's relationship to the newborn as a representative of herself, and the mother's relationship to the unique individual that is the newborn (Fig. 16-1). As with puberty, when the person can never again be a child, or menopause when the person can never again reproduce, with pregnancy, the person can never become a completely single unit again. As long as the child lives, it never ceases to exist as a representative of the woman, her mate, and itself.

Psychodynamics of Pregnancy

The pregnant woman must accomplish several psychological and cognitive tasks in pregnancy in addition to the physiologic restructuring that takes place. As her body adapts to the physiologic demands of the fetus, she must adapt to the idea of being a mother of one or more children and to the incorporation of another person into her family and social sphere (Tulman et al., 1990; Coffman et al., 1994). The psychological tasks of pregnancy are summarized in Box 16-2 and described in the following section.

Psychological and Cognitive Tasks of Pregnancy. One of the first tasks the woman must accomplish is to believe she is pregnant and incorporate the fetus into her

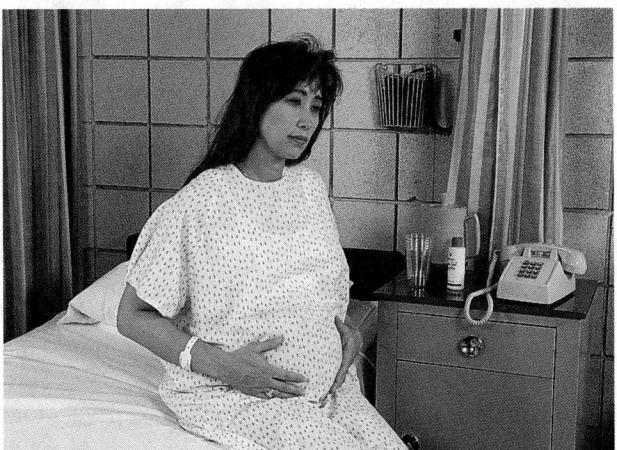

FIGURE 16-1 The mother can never again be a single unit. Her baby represents her relationship to her partner, her relationship to her baby as a representative of herself, and her relationship to the unique individual who will soon become a separate person outside herself.

BOX 16-2
*The Woman's Psychological
Tasks of Pregnancy*

1. Incorporation of the fetus into her own body image
2. Perception of the fetus as a separate object
3. Readiness to assume the caretaking relationship with the newborn

---

body image. Although she may be ambivalent initially about whether this is the "right time" for the pregnancy, she usually gradually resolves this cognitive dissonance and becomes enthused about the coming child. The experience of fetal movement generally dispels doubts about the readiness or desire for a child at this time in her life. It is also a reality marker that the woman is carrying a child. She may have had a sonogram, which also is a reality marker. As the woman feels the fetus move and her body change in subtle and apparent ways, she begins to realize that the fetus inside her is a real and separate being, complete with its own boundaries and identity. There is still turmoil and a great range of behavioral displays: mood swings, introspection, and physical and psychological weariness. These are among the many descriptions of the emotional instability of pregnancy. However, there is evidence that the physiologic and hormonal changes of pregnancy contribute to the woman's mood swings (Mercer, 1986; Berk, 1993). (The Research Highlight describes some research on maternal-fetal attachment.)

The woman's second task is to prepare for the physical separation, the birth. As with all aspects of pregnancy, there are many different responses. Many women are eager to give birth; they are tired of being pregnant. Some even state they are frightened to have this intrusive "invader" within them. However, others do not want to let the fetus go; they anticipate delivery as a loss of a loved object, and this anticipation may actually cause depression. Nevertheless, the task must ultimately be resolved, because every fetus "lost" to a healthy delivery is a newborn gained (McKay et al., 1991; Hofmeyr et al., 1990).

A third task is to resolve the identity confusions that accompany role transition and prepare for the smooth functioning of the family after birth. Researchers studying the period of pregnancy suggest that as the woman progresses in pregnancy, she becomes one with "mother," the primitive memory of the omnipotent being who nurtured her. Moreover, she becomes increasingly likely to evaluate her partner with respect to his appropriateness as a father. She may criticize his current behavior patterns to bring them more into line with her idea of what constitutes an ideal father (Mercer et al., 1994; Hofmeyr et al., 1990). Fishbein (1984)

RESEARCH HIGHLIGHT

Maternal-Fetal Attachment

Although the development of a relationship between a woman and her fetus most likely begins during pregnancy, the correlates of maternal-fetal attachment are poorly understood. In this study, the authors examined the influence of family functioning on maternal-fetal attachment in a convenience sample of White, Hispanic, African American, and Asian women of varied socioeconomic status who attended a clinic in a large metropolitan city. The authors surveyed 339 pregnant women in their last trimesters with the Family Adaptability and Cohesion Scales III. (FACES III), Maternal-Fetal Attachment Scale (MFA), and a demographic interview. On the basis of correlational and regression analyses, the demographic variables of parity, ethnicity, age, education, and occupation of primary wage earner correlated significantly with maternal-fetal attachment. Multiple regression analysis revealed that parity, ethnicity, and occupation explained 12% of the variance in the MFA scores. The FACES III total score and the subscale scores of adaptability and cohesion also correlated significantly with the scores on the MFA and explained an additional 3% of the variance in the MFA beyond that explained by the demographics.

Critique: The study is well written and fairly easy to read. It would have been strengthened by a randomization of the sample, although the sample size was adequate. Hence, generalizations to an entire population cannot be made. The scales and their subscales are not easy to understand to the neophyte consumer of research. The authors have done an adequate job of explaining their findings in understandable terms, although they made no reference to the reliability and validity of their instruments.

The article is useful in introducing these scales, which are reliable and valid to the practicing nurse, and in demonstrating the use of these scales in family assessment. The findings further verify the importance of family interaction on the cognitive-emotional functioning of the woman during pregnancy.

Fuller, S. G., Moore, L. R., & Lester, J. W., (1993). Influence of family functioning on maternal-fetal attachment. *Journal of Perinatology, 13*(6), 453–463

the other hand, the merger may be experienced as a trap (Mercer, 1986; May 1994). This resolution of identity confusion requires energy, commitment, and work.

Cognitive and Emotional Reactions in Pregnancy. In addition to the psychological tasks of pregnancy, the woman has certain cognitive and emotional reactions during the different trimesters of her pregnancy. Although not every woman has every reaction, research has shown that a certain pattern occurs with fair regularity. Box 16-3 summarizes these reactions according to the work of Gay (1988), Mercer (1986), Mercer et al. (1994), Berk (1993), and Fishbein (1984). (See the list of suggested readings for in-depth reading on this topic.)

The Father

Men undergo far less social preparation for parenthood than women do, and there is little to prepare them for pregnancy except for the childbirth education classes that they may attend with their mates. Experience with fathers who have actively involved themselves in pregnancy indicates that men, like women, go through various phases during the pregnancy, although these may not be as definitive and pronounced (Richman, 1982; Pruett, 1987). As more attention is given to the father and more research efforts directed toward his experiences, researchers are beginning to find out and redefine what the pregnancy experience means for him. For instance, some of the earlier research relating to body image change in fathers and the *couvade syndrome* (described in a subsequent section) has been modified (Lamb et al., 1982; Taubenheim et al., 1988; Fawcett et al., 1986; Drake et al., 1988).

The First Trimester

The introduction to pregnancy comes with the confirmation of the diagnosis of pregnancy. This places fathers almost immediately into a honeymoon stage. The reactions are as many and varied as with women. There may be unclear feelings because the intellectual focus is on the impending fatherhood, rather than the immediate state of pregnancy (Jordan, 1990; Grossman, 1987). Like his partner, he must assimilate the fact that the fetus is his. He does not have the gross physiologic changes to help him in this as the woman does, although some men experience some of the same physical symptoms of early pregnancy (known as couvade syndrome). How men accomplish this psychological task is still unclear and has been the topic of some fascinating research (Pruett, 1987; Richman, 1982; Lamb et al., 1982; Pruett, 1993; Jordan, 1990).

We do know that there may be guilt reactions about getting the partner pregnant or causing her to be sick

and Coffman et al. (1994) found that agreement between the partners about the expectations of the father role was important in reducing the father's anxiety during pregnancy. Similarly, the father watches his partner become transformed into "mother" as her body changes and her behavior tends toward "nesting" (McKay et al., 1991). He is simultaneously confronting his own feelings and aspirations as he metamorphoses into the father role. Pregnancy may be the first occasion in the relationship when the partners realize the extent to which they are interdependent psychologically, socially, and economically. On one hand, this represents a physiologic union that can be mystical; on

---

BOX 16–3
Maternal Cognitive and Emotional Reactions to Pregnancy

First Trimester

Ambivalence

- Initial uncertainty about the timing of the pregnancy
- Physical discomforts: urinary frequency, nausea, fatigue, restlessness and sleeplessness at night
- Uncertainty about herself and partner's role adequacy as parents
- Uncertainty about material considerations

Fears and Fantasies

- Speculation and anticipation about new role assisted by fantasies: imagines and role plays what her newborn will be like, how she and her partner will cope, what her new life will be like
- Concerns about the future enhanced by fear and anxiety; if severe and unremitting, can be physically debilitating (rise in catecholamine levels)

Second Trimester

Feeling of Well-Being

- Decrease in physical symptoms and unwellness
- Fear and anxiety forgotten as fetus moves (if pregnancy progresses normally)

Introversion, Self-Engrossment, Introspection

- Concentration of woman on her own needs and those of her fetus
- Fascination with pregnancy and birth process; conscious of children's behavior
- Examination of her relationship with her own mother as she develops her own sense of maternal identity

- Appears egocentric, daydreams frequently
- Begins to exhibit "nesting" behavior: getting things ready for the newborn and herself in anticipation of the birth

Mood Swings and Emotional Lability

- Preoccupation and mood swings troublesome to those around her; needs extra love, attention, and understanding

Third Trimester

Physical Discomfort Returns

- Fatigue, heaviness, urinary frequency, sleeplessness, clumsiness

Psychosocial Dimensions Expand

- Self-image changes; feelings of awkwardness and clumsiness

Heightened Introversion

Heightened Concerns

- Fears for her own well-being and "performance" during labor
- Fears for the well-being of the fetus

Contemplation of her Assumption of the Maternal Role

- Fantasizing of hypothetical situations involving parenthood
- Obsession with labor and delivery, desire for pregnancy to be over
- Increased nesting behavior: finishing touches on efforts

(Adapted from the work of Gay [1988]; Mercer [1986, 1994]; Berk [1993]; Fishbein [1984].)

---

and uncomfortable. On a more positive note, there may be feelings of pride at his virility or mutual pride that "We did it!" There also may be feelings of distance between the man and his partner as the woman continues through her introverted first trimester. Jealousy, worry about the change in sexual relationships, and concern about his own competence as a man and provider may occur (Strickland, 1987; Drake et al., 1988; Richman, 1982; Pruett, 1993).

The Second Trimester

The first perceptible movement of the fetus generally creates a profound feeling that the fetus is real; most men can recall the time they "first felt the baby move" or viewed the fetus through ultrasound. In the second trimester, more thought is given to what it means to be a father, and the plateau stage is entered. Men observe children and pregnant women more intently and become more acutely aware of their partner's growing uterus. A myriad of thoughts and concerns may sweep over the father just as with the mother. Often these

center on his ability to provide for the expanding family. However, there also is concern and thought about how well he will be able to "father" the new progeny and meet the newly evolving expectations of the mother (Richman, 1982; Grossman, 1987; Pruett, 1987).

The Third Trimester

As with pregnancy for the woman, a good deal of literature describes this period as a "crisis" time for fathers. However, evidence indicates that psychologically healthy men cope without major problems. What is clear, however, is that pregnancy requires as much adjustment for the man as it does for the woman (Jordan, 1990; Richman, 1982; Pruett, 1993).

As is true for the woman, labor and delivery mark the disengagement or termination stage of the role transition of pregnancy for the father. How these proceed can have a profound effect on the father. Most health providers who have had experience with pregnant couples believe that men who take an active part in the pregnancy by attending childbirth and parent education classes, participating in preparations for the newborn, and so on are more likely to participate in the birthing with positive psychological outcomes, and this strengthens the parental bond (Fig. 16-2).

Laboring for Relevance

In a recent study using grounded theory, Jordan (1990) used the term *laboring for relevance* to describe the essence of the experience of expectant and new fatherhood. This concept encompasses intrapersonal and interpersonal aspects. The man labors to perceive the paternal role as relevant to his sense of self and his repertoire of roles. He labors to incorporate the paternal role into his self-identity as a salient and integrated component of his personhood and to be seen as relevant to childbearing and childrearing by others. Jordan suggests that laboring for relevance is a three-part process that consists of the following:

- Grappling with the reality of the pregnancy and newborn
- Struggling for recognition as a parent from mate, coworkers, friends, family, newborn, and society
- "Plugging away" at the role of involved fatherhood

Each subprocess is developmental, and the focal trajectory is the man's movement toward becoming an involved father. The driving force is the unfolding reality of the newborn. As with any process, the laboring for relevance processes occur within the larger contextual environment of interpersonal interactions and the larger society. People within the father's environment, the *recognition providers,* promote or impede his development (Fig. 16-3).

Jordan also found that in general, men tend not to be recognized as parents but as helpmates or breadwinners, which interfered with validation of the reality of the pregnancy and later the newborn. They felt somewhat excluded from the childbearing experience by their mates, healthcare providers, and society. Moreover, they found themselves without models to assist them in taking on the role of active and involved parent. This type of study is helpful for gaining insight into the male experience of pregnancy and fatherhood and into designing interventions and supports to promote involved paternal behavior. Subsequent, replicative research must confirm these initial findings.

Body Image and the Couvade Syndrome

Body image refers to the way a person pictures his or her body. It is a composite of attitudes, feelings, and perceptions that each person has regarding how his or her body appears. In the 1960s and 1970s, researchers examined this topic to provide explanations for the appearance of pregnancy symptoms in spouses and partners of pregnant women. Early studies examined changes in body image in the man and the woman and found similarities. Fawcett's (1978) early work suggested that not only the woman experienced a change in body image perception as she grew during pregnancy, but her mate as well. These early data also showed that the couple's ability to identify with one another played a mediating role in the process (Drake et al., 1988). Subsequently, more tightly designed, longitudinal studies by the same researcher and others found that although the woman definitely experienced

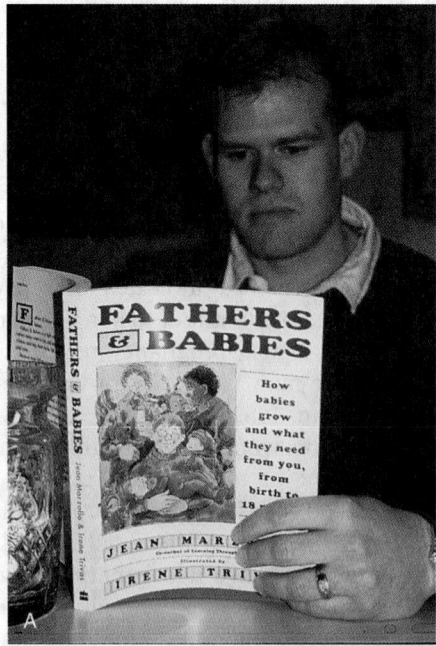

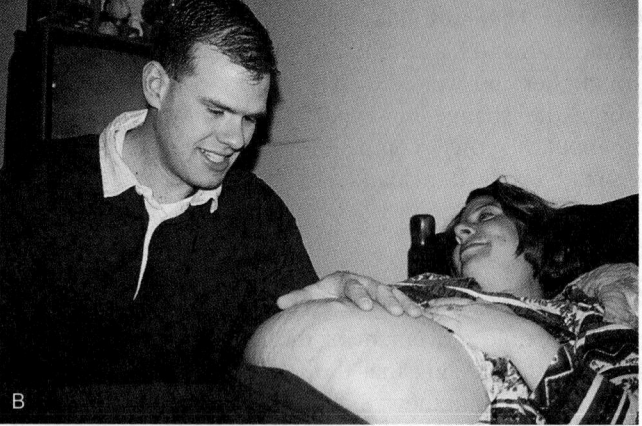

FIGURE 16–2 Fathers who take an active role in the pregnancy are more likely to participate in the birthing with positive psychological outcomes. **(A)** Books, videos, and parent education classes help fathers prepare for their child's birth. **(B)** Bonding with the unborn child is an important aspect of preparing for fatherhood.

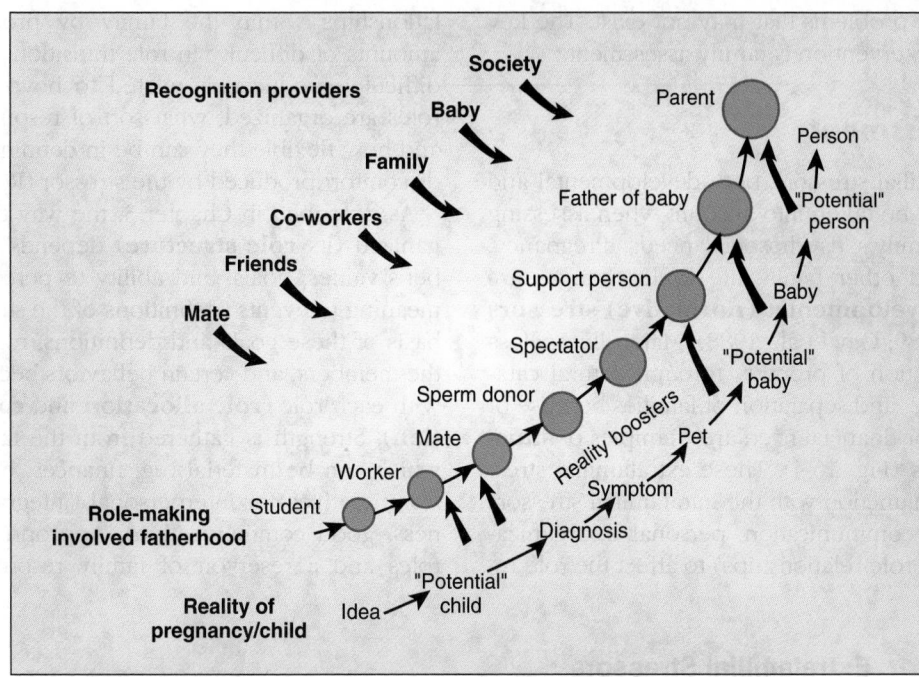

FIGURE 16–3 Model of male experience of expectant and new parenthood.

changes in perceived body space and global body attitude, her partner lacked significant identification with her on these dimensions and did not experience these changes (Fawcett et al., 1986; Drake et al., 1988; Berk, 1993). Thus, although there is some identification on other dimensions of the pregnant state, no significant evidence proves that the man's perception of body image changes.

In the 1960s and 1970s, research was directed to the study of men who were afflicted with pregnancy-related symptoms. This phenomenon was dubbed the **couvade syndrome** because of its resemblance to some aspects of the primitive ritual couvade. In primitive cultures, couvade consists of the man's lying-in and simulation of his mate's labor and delivery and the observation of certain proscribed dietary rituals after the birth (Treathowan, 1972).

The most frequently exhibited couvade symptoms are alimentary and mimic symptoms common in pregnancy, such as nausea, vomiting, alterations in appetite, weight gain, abdominal pain, backache, leg cramps, elusive toothaches, and other aches and pains in different parts of the body (Strickland, 1987). Many studies beginning in the 1960s have consistently documented that husbands have a variety of these signs and symptoms (Treathowan et al., 1965; Lamb et al., 1982; Drake et al., 1988; Garbarino, 1993). In a longitudinal study of 91 expectant fathers, Strickland (1987) found that men who were working class, African American, or reported that pregnancy was not planned experienced more pregnancy-related symptoms during pregnancy. White expectant fathers reported an increase in

somatic symptoms as pregnancy progressed; African American men, on the other hand, indicated a decrease. However, African American men consistently reported more symptoms than white men. Moreover, symptom manifestation in expectant fathers was positively associated with anxiety.

The observation has been made and documented that the man's close proximity to the woman influences his response to the pregnancy. Some researchers have found that the more closely the man identifies with his mate, the more intensely he experiences changes in his own body during pregnancy (Lamb et al., 1982; Grossman, 1987; Pruett, 1993). These findings have withstood the test of multiple studies and replication over several decades—unlike the findings about changes in body image. Thus, we can see what a momentous physiologic, psychological, and emotional milestone pregnancy can be for the woman and her mate.

Applying the Nursing Process to the Psychosocial Aspects of Normal Pregnancy

The nurse collaborates with other members of the health team by providing emotional support, counseling, and teaching to the pregnant couple. Treating pregnancy as a role transition rather than a crisis helps emphasize the normality of the condition. Care is structured to support the resources of the couple rather than looking for problems that may not exist. The key to appropriate intervention is family assessment.

Family Assessment

Certain extrafamilial stressors, both developmental and situational, must be taken into account when assessing the pregnant family's psychosocial needs. Pregnancy, parenthood, and other family life cycle changes are examples of **developmental (normative) stressors** (Gilliss et al., 1989; Gay et al., 1988). Major illness, loss of a job, destruction of property through natural catastrophes, divorce, and separation of families because of job obligations or financial need are examples of **situational stressors** (Fig. 16-4). These extrafamilial stressors work in conjunction with the intrafamilial stressors (eg, inadequate communication, personal disorganization, inadequate role relationships) to affect the role re-

lationships within the family by producing varying amounts of difficulty in role transition. The amount of difficulty produced is related to how well the family roles are organized, what sort of resources they have, and how flexible they can be in defining positively the discomfort produced by the stressor (Reeder, 1994).

As described in Chapter 3, the way the family is organized (its **role structure**) depends on each member's values, goals, and ability to perceive and attach meaning to events (definitions of the situation). On the basis of these goals and definitions, roles are given to the members, and certain behaviors become associated with each role (**role allocation** and **role differentiation**). Strength is gathered from the family resources, which can be material (eg, finances, material support from relatives) or interpersonal (integration, cohesiveness, good communication). Appropriately structured roles and a reservoir of family resources buffer the

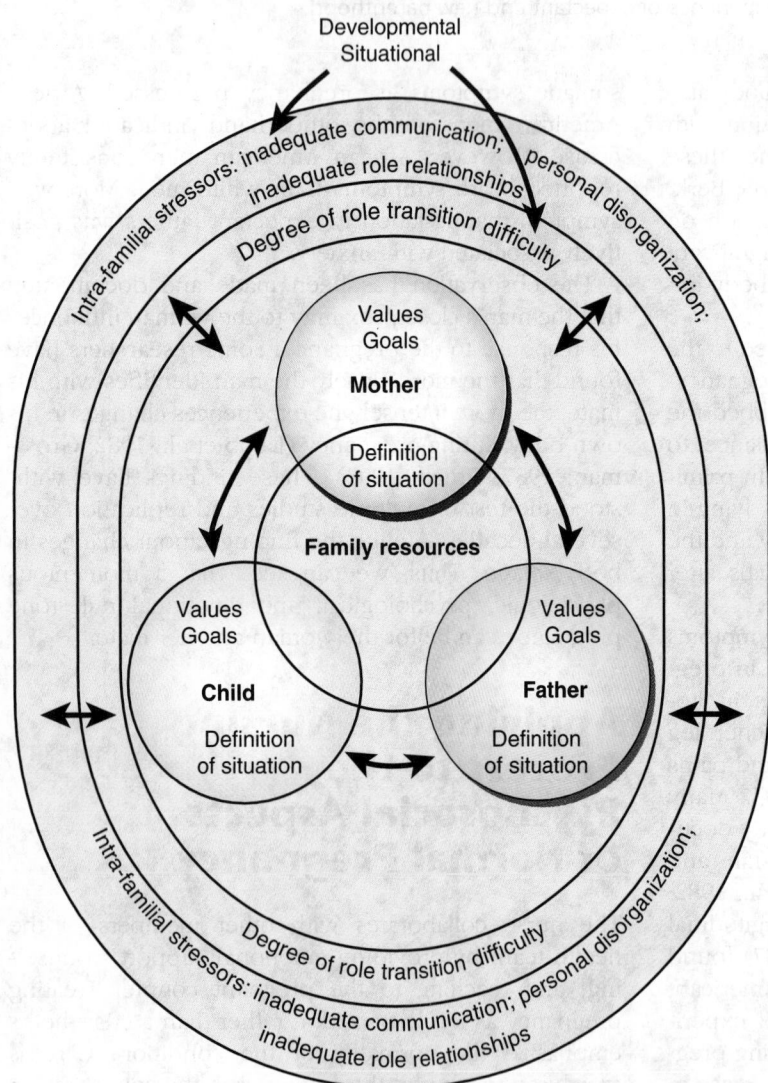

Extrafamilial Stressors

FIGURE 16–4 Model of family interaction during role transition and components of assessment.

family from the impact of the various stressors and make role transition easier.

McCubbin (1983) has pointed out that a family infrequently copes with only one stressor at a time. Preexisting or new stressors can accrue, often because of the immediate stressor, causing what McCubbin calls a "pile up" of stressors. This calls for the garnering of new resources to consolidate with the old and the redefinition of the current emerging situation. According to McCubbin's formulation, this results in the adaptation of the family along a continuum of good adaptation (**bonadaptation**) through poor adaptation (**maladaptation**). A schematic rendering of McCubbin's

model can be seen in Fig. 16-5. The Assessment Guidelines: Assessment of Psychosocial Aspects of Pregnancy includes the types of questions the nurse would ask during an assessment aimed at developing a family care plan.

Nursing Diagnoses

Assessment helps the nurse determine if members of the family are fulfilling their expected role behaviors appropriately. If they are fulfilling expected roles, the nurse can anticipate the potential problems for the remainder of the pregnancy or postpartum period. If they

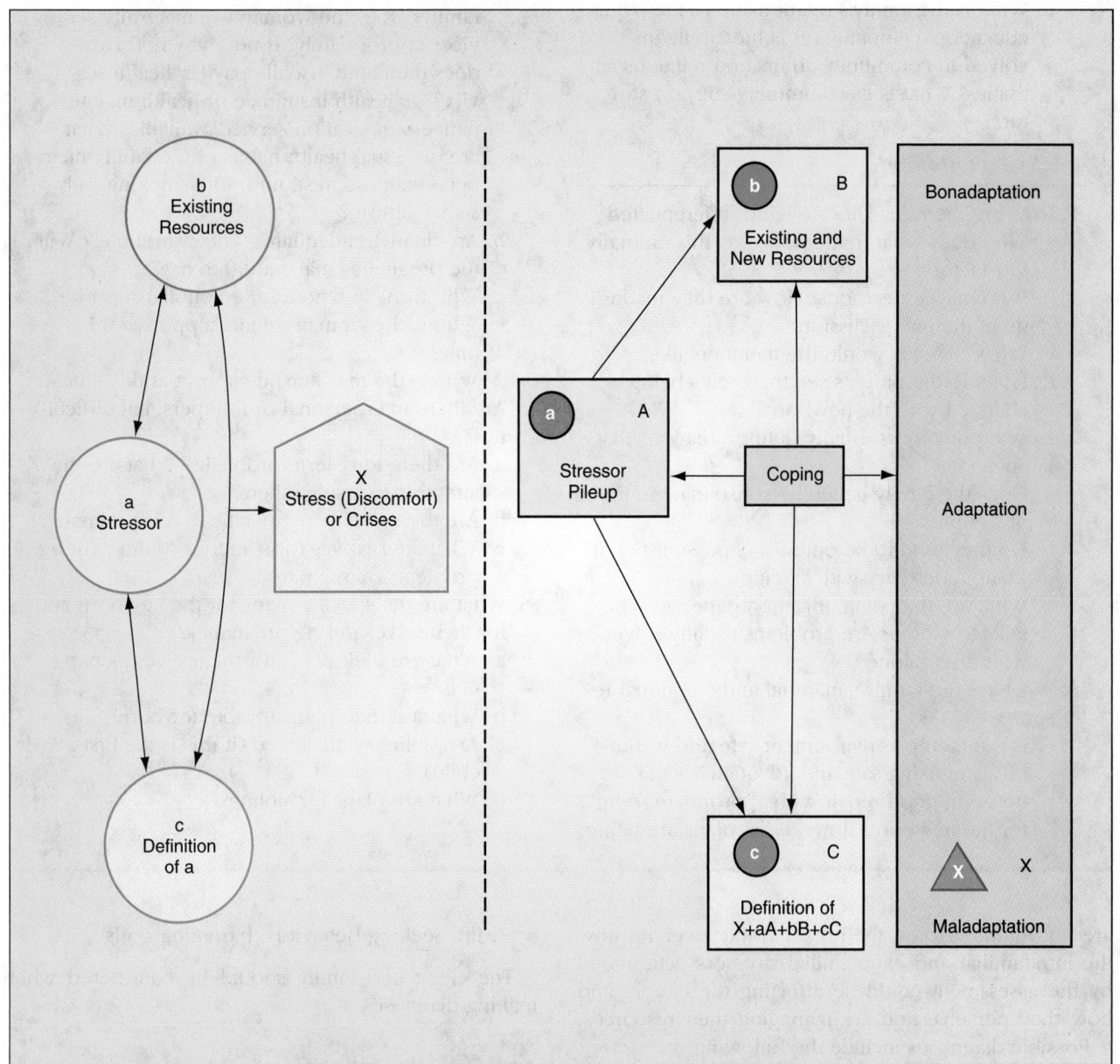

FIGURE 16–5 Modification of the McCubbin model for the family stress process (double ABCX). (McCubbin HI, Sussman JM, Patterson M [eds]: *Social Stress and the Family,* p 12. New York, Haworth Press, 1983.)

ASSESSMENT GUIDELINES
Assessment of Psychosocial Aspects of Pregnancy

Family Composition

1. Who are the family members? (Include the extended family.)
   a. What are their ages? What are their relationships to one another?
   b. Where do they live? Do they interact frequently?
   c. Are they "close" emotionally if not physically?
   d. What is the family's relationship to the larger educational community? Is the family involved in community affairs and religious activities? What is its community support structure?

Family Functioning

1. How are the roles allocated and differentiated?
   a. Who does what in the house? Is this mutually satisfactory?
   b. Who makes decisions? How are they made? Is there mutual discussion?
   c. What changes would the members like?
   d. How do the parents see their roles being changed with the newborn?
2. How do members usually define situations that happen?
   a. Does the family generally consolidate in time of trouble?
   b. Do they tend to be optimistic, pessimistic, or do attitudes vary with situations?
   c. What are the communication patterns? Who talks to whom? Are problems usually solved with discussion?
3. What are the family's material and emotional resources?
   a. Is the family's environment safe and healthful? Is housing safe and adequate? Is the house in good repair with appropriate room for the newborn? If not, what plans are being

made to remedy the situation? Is the housing environment structured to prevent accidents? If not, what plans are being made to remedy this?
   What is the general health status of the family? Have there been or are there now illnesses? If so, has appropriate medical (or dental) care been sought? Is there a regular source of medical and dental care for the family? Does the woman use maternity services appropriately? If not, why not? How does the family usually pay for health services? Is health insurance or health maintenance organization service available? What are the usual health habits of the family members (exercise, rest, nutrition, smoking, substance abuse)?
   b. Are finances adequate? Who contributes? Will the pregnancy make a difference?
   c. Who turns to whom for emotional support? Who is the woman's main support at this time?
   Who is the man's main support at this time?
4. Are there interpersonal or intrapersonal difficulties?
   a. Are there long-term problems? What are the attempts to resolve them?
   b. Are there problems specific to this pregnancy?
   c. What alternatives for solutions to the existing problems do the parents see?
5. What are the specific plans for the newborn and for themselves during pregnancy?
   a. What are their plans for themselves as parents?
   b. What are their plans for the newborn?
   c. Are siblings anticipated (if this is the first child)?
   d. What are plans for siblings?

---

are not fulfilling roles, the nurse would ascertain how the intrafamilial and extrafamilial stressors determined by the assessment could be affecting the couple and how they perceive and are managing their resources. Possible diagnoses include the following:

■ Altered Family Processes related to the family's difficulty in integrating new roles
■ Ineffective Individual Coping related to financial worries associated with the growing family

■ Health Seeking Behaviors, parenting skills

The client and family should be considered when making diagnoses.

Planning and Intervention

The nurse who is planning interventions should keep in mind that the rationale behind each intervention is aimed at helping the parents define possible stressors and resources within their family unit and developing strategies for coping with existing or possible disruptive elements. By helping parents become aware of their resources and supporting them in their decision making, the nurse can minimize a great deal of stress associated with this role transition. Parents need to validate their impressions of what is happening to them, physically and emotionally, with an outside person. Family, friends, and healthcare professionals can be useful in this way. The nurse should encourage the parents to use their network of family and friends if this network can supply material and emotional support.

Evaluation

Intervention can be evaluated as effective if the family unit is perceived by the nurse and the family as drawing together, there is open discussion of problems and experiences, concrete plans are made for the newborn's arrival, and the parents have a realistic perception that the newborn will change their lives and that adjustment is possible for this momentous new role.

Summary Points

✔ Orientations and attitudes toward pregnancy and childbearing vary between and within cultures. In some cultures, birth is seen as a social event to be enjoyed by the mother, family, and friends and is viewed as an essentially normal phenomenon. In other cultures, birth is viewed as mysterious, a harbinger of possible disaster, or atonement for being a lowly woman.

✔ The notion of parenthood and pregnancy as crisis situations has never been empirically documented; however this orientation is embedded in the thinking about these events. Pregnancy has been documented as stressful for some people under some circumstances, but the stress is usually able to be resolved and does not routinely result in incapacitation or immobility. The idea of pregnancy as a role transition is the most current and reliable orientation and is examined in this chapter. The four stages in a role cycle (anticipatory, honeymoon, plateau, and disengagement) that have implications for pregnancy are discussed in detail.

✔ During pregnancy, the mother must accomplish a variety of psychological and cognitive tasks preparatory to taking on the role of mother. As these tasks are accomplished, they result in various cognitive and emotional reactions in the woman that are perceived by the man in particular.

✔ The man also "experiences" pregnancy although not in the same way as his mate. He has a variety of cognitive and emotional reactions as the trimesters progress. It has been documented that he often experiences physical symptoms and maladies as the pregnancy progresses; this phenomenon has been called the couvade syndrome.

✔ When assessing the psychosocial aspects of pregnancy, it is necessary to consider the whole family, not just the woman. A care plan provides an illustration.

REFERENCES

Belsky, J., & Rovine, M. (1984). Social network contact, family support, and the transition to parenthood. *Journal of Marriage and the Family, 46*(6), 455–462.

Benedek, T. (1959). Parenthood as a developmental phase. *Journal of the American Psychoanalytical Association, 7*(8), 389–417.

Berk, B. (1993). Body image and pregnancy: Bridging the mind-body connection. *Journal of Perinatology, 13*(4), 300–304.

Bibring, G. L. (1955). A study of the psychological processes in pregnancy and of the earliest mother–child relationship. *Psychoanalytic Study of the Child, 16*(4), 9–72.

Caplan, G. (1960). Patterns of parental response to the crisis of premature birth: A preliminary approach to modifying the mental health outcome. *Psychiatry, 23*(7), 365–374.

Chertok, L. (1960). *Motherhood and personality.* London: Tavistock.

Coffman, S., Levitt, M. J., & Brown, L. (1994). Effects of clarification of support expectations in prenatal couples. *Nursing Research, 43*(2), 111–117.

Coleman, A. P., & Coleman, L. (1971). *Pregnancy: The psychological experience.* New York: Herder and Herder.

Drake, M. L., Verhulst, D., & Fawcett, J. (1988). Spouse's body image changes during and after pregnancy. A replication in Canada. *IMAGE, 20*(2), 88–95.

Dyer, E. D. (1963). Parenthood as crisis: A restudy. *Marriage and Family Living, 25*(5), 196–201.

Erickson, E. (1959). Identity and the life cycle: Selected papers. *Psychological Issues, 1*(2), 1–171.

Fawcett, J. (1978). Body image and the pregnant couple. *MCN: American Journal of Maternal Child Nursing, 3*(4), 227–233.

Fawcett, J., Bliss Holtz, V., & Hass, J. (1986). Spouses' body image changes during and after pregnancy. *Nursing Research, 35*(3), 220–223.

Feetham, S. L., Meister, S. B., Bell, J. M., & Gilliss, C. L. (1993). *The nursing of families: Theory/research/education/practice.* Newbury Park, CA: Sage Publications.

Fishbein, E. G. (1984). Expectant fathers' stress—due to the mothers' expectations. *Journal of Obstetric, Gynecologic, and Neonatal Nursing, 13*(5), 325–328.

Friedman, M. M. (1992). *Family nursing: Theory and practice* (3rd ed.). Norwalk, CT: Appleton & Lange.

Fuller, S. G., Moore, L. R., & Lester, J. W. (1993). Influence of family functioning on maternal-fetal attachment. *Journal of Perinatology, 13*(6), 453–463.

Garbarino, J. (1993). Reinventing fatherhood. *Families in Society: The Journal of Contemporary Human Services, 74*(1), 51–54.

Gay, J. T., & Douglas, A. B. (1988). Reva Rubin revisited. *Journal of Obstetric, Gynecologic, and Neonatal Nursing, 17*(6), 394–399.

Gilliss, C. L., Highly, B. L., Roberts, B. M., & Martinson, I. M. (1989). *Toward a science of family nursing*. New York: Addison Wesley.

Grossman, F. (1987). Separate and together: Men's autonomy and affiliation in the transition to parenthood. In P. Berman & F. Pedersen (Eds.), *Men's transitions to parenthood*. Hillsdale, NJ: Erlbaum.

Hill, R., & Hansen, D. A. (1960). The identification of a conceptual framework utilized in family study. *Marriage and Family Living, 22*(4), 299–311.

Hill, R. (1958). Generic features of families under stress. *Social Casework, 39*(2), 32–54.

Hobbs, D. J., Jr. (1963). Parenthood as crisis, a third study. *Journal of Marriage and the Family, 27*(5), 367–372.

Hofmeyr, G. J., Marcos, E. F., & Butchart, A. M. (1990). Pregnant women's perceptions of themselves: A Survey. *BIRTH, 17*(4), 205–209.

Jordan, P. L. (1990). Laboring for relevance: Expectant and new fatherhood. *Nursing Research, 39*(1), 11–16.

Lamb, G. S., & Lipkin, M., Jr. (1982). Somatic symptoms of expectant fathers. *MCN: American Journal of Maternal Child Nursing, 7*(2), 110–115.

Le Masters, E. E. (1957). Parenthood as crisis. *Marriage and Family Living, 19*(4), 352–355.

May, K. A. (1994). Impact of maternal activity restriction for preterm labor on the expectant father. *Journal of Obstetric, Gynecologic, and Neonatal Nursing, 23*(3), 246–251.

McCubbin, H. I., Sussman, M. B., & Patterson, J. M. (Eds.) (1983). *Social stress and the family: Advances and developments in family stress theory*. New York: Haworth Press.

McKay, S., & Barrows, T. (1991). Holding back: Maternal readiness to give birth. *MCN: American Journal of Maternal Child Nursing, 16*(5), 251–254.

Menninger, W. C. (1943). The emotional factors in pregnancy. *Bulletin of the Menniger Clinic, 7*(4), 15–24.

Mercer, R. T. (1986). *First-time motherhood: Experience from teens to forties*. New York: Springer.

Mercer, R. T., & Ferketich, S. L. (1994). Predictors of maternal role competence by risk status. *Nursing Research, 43*(1), 38–43.

Pruett, K. D. (1987). *The nurturing father*. New York: Warner Books.

Pruett, K. D. (1993). The paternal presence. *Families in Society: The Journal of Contemporary Human Services, 74*(1), 46–50.

Reeder, S. J. (1993). *Childbearing in the American culture: Paper/seminar presentation*. Los Angeles: UCLA School of Nursing.

Reeder, S. J. (1994). *Theoretical orientations to crisis and stress in the family: Seminar presentation*. Los Angeles: UCLA School of Nursing.

Richman, J. (1982). Men's experiences of pregnancy and childbirth. In L. McKee & M. O'Brien (Eds.), *The father figure*. London: Tavistock Publications.

Rossi, A. S. (1968). Transition to parenthood. *Journal of Marriage and the Family, 30*(2), 26–39.

Shainess, N. (1963). The structure of the mothering encounter. *Journal of Mental Disease, 136*(5), 146–161.

Steffenmeier, R. H. (1982). A role model of the transition to parenthood. *Journal of Marriage and the Family, 44*(6), 319–347.

Strickland, O. (1987). The occurrence of symptoms in expectant fathers. *Nursing Research, 36*(3), 184–189.

Taubenheim, A. M., & Silbernagel, T. (1988). Meeting the needs of expectant parents. *MCN: American Journal of Maternal Child Nursing, 13*(2), 110–113.

Treathowen, W. H., & Conlon, M. F. (1965). The couvade syndrome. *British Journal of Psychiatry, 11*(1), 57–66.

Treathowan, W. H. (1972). The couvade syndrome. In J. G. Howell (Ed.), *Modern perspectives in psycho-obstetrics* (pp. 66–93). New York: Brunner/Mazel.

Tulman, L., & Fawcett, J. (1990). Functional status during pregnancy and the postpartum: A framework for research. *IMAGE, 22*(3), 191–194.

Whall, A. L., & Fawcett, J. (1991). *Family theory development in nursing: State of the science and art*. Philadelphia: F.A. Davis.

SUGGESTED READINGS

DeJoseph, J. F. (1993). Redefining women's work during pregnancy: Toward a more comprehensive approach. *BIRTH, 20*(2), 86–93.

Garbarino, J. (1993). Reinventing fatherhood. *Families in Society: The Journal of Contemporary Family Services, 74*(1), 51–54.

Lerum, C. W., & LoBiondo-Wood, G. (1989). The relationship of maternal age, quickening, and physical symptoms of pregnancy to the development of maternal–fetal attachment. *BIRTH, 16*(3), 13–17.

Maloni, J. A., McIndoe, J. E., & Rubenstein, G. (1987). Expectant grandparents class. *Journal of Obstetric, Gynecologic, and Neonatal Nursing, 16*(4), 26–29.

Muller, M. E., & Ferketich, S. (1993). Factor analysis of the maternal fetal attachment scale. *Nursing Research, 42*(3), 144–147.

Stainton, M. C. (1990). Parents' awareness of their unborn infant in the third trimester. *BIRTH, 17*, 92–96.

Stainton, M. C. (1994). Supporting family functioning during a high-risk pregnancy. *MCN: American Journal of Maternal Child Nursing, 19*(1), 24–28.

17

Nursing Care in the Prenatal Period

Objectives

- Identify and describe components of prenatal assessment.
- Formulate nursing diagnoses for early and later pregnancy.
- Outline the recommended schedule for healthcare visits during pregnancy.
- List warning and danger signs in pregnancy.
- Develop nursing care plans for a client in each trimester of pregnancy.
- Describe nursing approaches to maintaining the pregnant woman's health and promoting comfort.
- Discuss nursing management of minor pregnancy discomforts, emphasizing the nurse's role in client teaching.
- Summarize components of prebirth preparation.
- Summarize components of preparation for the baby.

Key Terms

Colostrum	Leopold's maneuvers
Dependent edema	Live, killed, or
Estimated date of	inactivated vaccines
delivery (EDD)	McDonald's technique
Fetal activity	Morning sickness
assessment	Nägele's rule
Fetal drug vulnerability	Para
Fetal heart rate (FHR)	Pregnancy health
Fundal height	maintenance
Gravida	Toxoids and
Kegel exercises	immunoglobulins
Last menstrual period	Trimesters of
(LMP)	pregnancy
Layette	

Pregnancy is a normal physiologic process. Most pregnancies do not require significant intervention by health professionals, because the natural reproductive process unfolds according to biologic patterns. Normal pregnancy does significantly alter psychophysiologic systems, which can affect the woman's and fetus' health status. The most frequent stressors reported by women during pregnancy are related to physical symptoms, body image, welfare of the fetus, changes in living patterns, emotional disturbances, and worries about problems in pregnancy, labor, and delivery (Affonso et al., 1990).

Prenatal Care: Trends and Goals

Age and Pregnancy

The current trend is toward pregnancy at both ends of the age spectrum. Teenage pregnancy has increased in the last 20 years; more than 60% of teenage girls are sexually active, accounting for nearly one-fifth of pregnancies and more than one-third of unmarried births in the United States (Dunnihoo, 1992). Pregnancy in teenagers carries greater risk of physiologic and psychosocial complications and requires many medical and social resources (see Chap. 35). During the last decade, increasing numbers of women have been postponing childbearing until their late 30s and 40s. If this trend continues, 1 in 12 babies will be born to women older than 35 years by 2000 (University of California Berkeley Wellness Letter, 1994). Women who are older than 35 years have a higher risk for sponta-

neous abortion, birth defects, and other complications of pregnancy (Dunnihoo, 1992). The incidence of low birth weight or premature delivery in older women does not appear to be increased. Fertility declines quickly after 40 years, and genetic abnormalities in the fetus increase. Genetic counseling is advised for older couples planning pregnancy (see Chap. 14).

Goals of Prenatal Care

Prenatal care is concerned with the physical, emotional, and social needs of the woman, the fetus, her partner, and any other children in the family. Goals include protecting the life and health of the woman and fetus and ensuring a satisfying and growth-promoting experience for the woman and family. Prenatal care takes into consideration the sociocultural conditions in which the family lives (ie, its economic status, educational level, community setting, nutrition, support systems, and cultural perspectives).

Most prenatal care takes place in the expectant woman's community, which may include her home, a clinic, or a private physician's office. Goals are accomplished through the combined efforts of the expectant parents, the physician, the nurse, and other members of the health team. Emphasis is on increasing the knowledge and expanding the abilities of the expectant parents and family; in this way, all members may experience pregnancy in a positive way, the health of the woman and infant is promoted, and the family transition to include its new member proceeds smoothly.

Nurses provide essential prenatal care to women and their families. An ongoing relationship is established with regular contact and opportunity to assess client and family needs. Nursing responsibilities for prenatal care include physiologic and psychosocial assessment, education, and counseling for pregnant women and their families and identification of needs for other types of services with appropriate community and specialty referrals. Care Path: Clinical Obstetric Prenatal provides an example of a client's ongoing antepartal care schedule.

Initial Prenatal Evaluation

The prenatal workup consists of a thorough health history, a physical examination, and laboratory tests. Prenatal forms summarize data and serve as a flow sheet for continuing visits throughout pregnancy. Advanced practice nurses (nurse practitioners or clinical specialists) often obtain the history, order diagnostic tests, conduct the physical examination, and provide com-

Name _____

This care path is a guideline and is not intended to create a standard of care. This guideline may be modified based on individual client's needs.

	Consults Date	Proced/Tests Date	Pt/Family Ed Date	Routine visits	Meds Date	Other Date	Initials
Pre-concep-tion	MD RD, prn RN, prn MSW, prn	PAP, breast exam Hx/family hx screen for Sickle cell, TaySach prn	Wellness ed. Nutrition Self br. exam Abstain from Tob, ETOH, etc	Yearly and prn	PNV FeSO-4 Folic acid		
Week 1–8	MD RD RN MSW	Preg test, prn Initial labs HIV, prn Sickle cell, prn	Given prenatal hand-book Additional info:	1/Mo. First 32 Weeks, and prn	PNV, FeSO-4 ⌐		
Week 8–12	MD RD, prn RN, prn MSW	PAP, breast exam DNA probe Urine tox.					
Week 12–16	MD RD, prn RN, prn MSW, prn	Order MSAFP to be done in weeks 15–17					
Week 16–20	MD RD, prn RN, prn MSW, prn	Order U/S to be done in weeks 18–22	Refer to childbirth/VBAC class				
Week 20–24	MD RD, prn RN, prn MSW, prn	Order 1 hr GTT, H&H ~ 24 weeks	Epidural class Breastfeed or bottle				
Week 24–28	MD RD, prn RN, prn MSW, prn	GBS 28 weeks, prn	Additional info.		(Rhogam 28 wks prn)		
Weeks 28–32	MD RD, prn RN, prn MSW, prn		S/Sx PTL				
Weeks 32–36	MD RD, prn RN, prn MSW, prn	Vag exam at 36 wks if ctx	S/Sx labor	Bi-monthly		NST, prn Fetal/pelvic index, prn	
Weeks 36–40	MD RD, prn RN, prn MSW, prn			Weekly til del.			
Week 40–del.	MD RD, prn RN, prn MSW, prn						
Post-partum	MD RD, prn RN, prn MSW, prn	PAP, breast exam	Care of self PP (care of infant) Family planning Wellness	(2 wks for C/S) 6 weeks	(Rhogam prn) (Rubella prn)		

Client Problems Identified:

_____

_____

_____

CLIENT IDENTIFICATION

plete prenatal management. Nurses usually conduct client education and orientation to prenatal services. The nurse's initial contact with the client is particularly important. By greeting the woman in a pleasant, interested, and professional manner, the nurse communicates a personalized approach to care. When the client experiences positive regard, she is more likely to keep return visits and discuss her concerns.

Diagnosis of Pregnancy and Estimating Date of Delivery

Early, accurate diagnosis of pregnancy is done by radioassay and immunologic pregnancy tests, which often confirm pregnancy before or shortly after the first missed menstrual period. Although highly sensitive and specific, these tests occasionally are inaccurate. The absence of menses and the other presumptive, probable, and positive signs and symptoms support the diagnosis of pregnancy (see Chap. 15).

An accurate **estimated date of delivery (EDD)** is important, because this allows the nurse and physician to assess the progress of gestation and evaluate term pregnancy more readily. A correct and definite date for the last menstrual period facilitates determining EDD, but many women do not keep careful menstrual records or have regular periods. Delivery date may be calculated by **Nägele's rule** based on **last menstrual period (LMP)**, progressive measurements of the height of the fundus (**McDonald's rule**), and ultrasonography to measure fetal growth (Box 17-1).

Assessment

Nursing assessment begins with the initial visit to confirm pregnancy and continues throughout the prenatal period at each contact with the pregnant woman and her family. The nurse often is responsible for prenatal assessment. In the initial interview, a relationship of confidence, trust, and respect can be established, which facilitates care throughout pregnancy. When the woman's partner or other family members are present, the nurse establishes a therapeutic relationship with them as well. During visits, the interaction among family members and methods of family coping style and support are assessed. Social support has been found to be exceedingly important in positive experiences and outcomes of pregnancy. Emotional disequilibrium and anxiety during pregnancy decrease with good social support systems. Psychosocial measurements demonstrate increased health among women who receive social support during pregnancy (Albrecht et al., 1989; Oakley et al., 1990).

History

The prenatal history covers many areas, including the following:

- Personal characteristics (age, marital status, occupation, ethnicity, religion, family members in the home)
- Family history of problems that could affect pregnancy

BOX 17-1
Estimated Date of Delivery (EDD)

Nägele's Rule

Count back 3 months from the first day of the last menstrual period (LMP) and add 7 days. Correct for year if necessary.

EDD = LMP − (3 months) + 7 days

Considerations for using Nägele's rule: Assumes a 28-day menstrual cycle with conception occurring on the 14th day. Adjustments must be made for shorter or longer cycles.

McDonald's Rule for Fundal Height

Height of fundus (cm) × 2/7

= gestation in lunar months

Height of fundus (cm) × 8/7

= gestation of pregnancy in weeks

Considerations in using fundal height measurements: Such factors as hydramnios, multiple gestation, very large fetus, and obesity affect the accuracy of measurement. For

women weighing more than 200 lb, subtract 1 cm from the measurement obtained. Technique can vary measurements; providers need to standardize approaches when more than one person takes serial measurements.

Ultrasonography

Four methods for estimating fetal age are the following:

- Determination of gestational sac dimensions (used as early as 6–10 weeks; fetus appears in sac about 7–8 weeks after the LMP, fetal heart activity appears by 9–10 weeks, and fetal movement is seen by 11 weeks)
- Measurement of crown-rump length (between 7 and 14 weeks)
- Measurement of femur length (after 12 weeks)
- Measurement of biparietal diameter (BPD) of fetal head (after 12 weeks, BPD is frequently used for diagnosis of term pregnancy. Fetal weight and BPD are well correlated, and at 36 weeks BPD should be about 8.7 cm. At term, the BPD is usually greater than 9.8 cm.)

- Personal health history, including menstrual history
- History of prior pregnancies, including prenatal, labor, and neonatal and postpartum complications (Terms related to the pregnancy history are summarized in Box 17-2.)
- History of the present pregnancy
- Data about the fetus' father
- Habits including use of tobacco, alcohol, drugs, and caffeine
- Attitudes about the pregnancy, whether positive or problematic
- Prenatal classes attended and birth plans

The prenatal health history also should elicit information about the client's previous experience with pregnancy or childbearing; her expectations and concerns about this pregnancy, birth, and care of the newborn; and her apparent willingness or disinclination to prepare herself in the areas that need attention. The nurse should elicit information about the woman's financial and social resources (eg, family, extended network of family and friends).

It is important for the nurse to assess any *cultural beliefs* about pregnancy that might have an impact on the woman's activity level, nutritional intake, or relationship with healthcare providers during her pregnancy. Many cultural customs revolve around pregnancy; although few *prescriptive beliefs* (which describe positive

activities), *restrictive beliefs* (which limit choices), or *taboos* (restrictions with serious supernatural consequences) are likely to cause any real danger to the woman or fetus, some may cause a woman to unnecessarily limit her activity and her exposure to some aspects of life (Andrews et al., 1995). Many of these beliefs also may affect the kind of support from family and close friends that the woman is likely to receive. Knowing this information in advance will help the nurse plan care in a way that is most suited to the woman's individual needs. The Assessment Tool: Prenatal History provides a sample of a prenatal history form.

Physical Examination

A thorough physical examination is performed to establish a baseline for the woman's general state of health and to evaluate the pregnancy. This examination may be conducted by advanced practice nurses. Vital signs are taken. The Assessment Tool: Components of Prenatal Physical Examination summarizes the techniques for examination along with normal and abnormal findings.

During the physical examination, the nurse is alert to clues that indicate a need for information, support, or follow-up. Often a client hesitates to discuss concerns with a physician because she considers them too trivial, but she may feel comfortable discussing them with the nurse. To promote comfort, the nurse ensures that the woman has adequate cover during the examination and has emptied her bladder because a full bladder is uncomfortable and may interfere with the pelvic examination.

Attention is paid to the teeth and throat, thyroid gland and lymph nodes, lungs, heart, breasts, skin, extremities, and abdomen. Characteristic changes of pregnancy are noted, and signs of infection or systemic disease are identified if present. Indications of high-risk pregnancy are identified, such as obesity, underweight for height, hypertension, severe varicosities, preeclampsia, or inappropriate uterine size for dates.

Pelvic Examination. Pelvic examination includes speculum and bimanual examination and provides data to confirm the pregnancy and determine the length of gestation, pelvic characteristics, and any abnormalities that might lead to complications. Specimens are obtained to screen for cervical cancer, infections, and sexually transmitted diseases.

- During speculum examination, the characteristics of the vaginal and cervical mucosa are examined, and vaginal discharge is evaluated. Unusual lesions are identified and biopsies taken; smears for vaginitis and tests or cultures for gonorrhea and *Chlamydia*

BOX 17–2
Terms Related to Pregnancy History

Gravida: A woman who has been or is pregnant

Primigravida: A woman who is pregnant for the first time

Primipara: A woman who has given birth once to a fetus that has reached the stage of viability

Multigravida or multipara: A woman who has given birth to two or more fetuses that have reached the stage of viability

In a health history, a woman's pregnancies are recorded in terms of gravida and para. *Gravida* refers to the number of pregnancies the client has experienced, regardless of outcome. *Para* refers to the number of pregnancies carried to viability (more than 20 weeks' gestation) regardless of the number of fetuses delivered. Most facilities also designate the number of term pregnancies, premature births, abortions, and living children as follows:

G Gravida

T Term births

P Premature births

A Abortions

L Living children

ASSESSMENT TOOL
Prenatal History

Name _____ Date _____
Address _____ Phone number _____
_____ Date of birth _____
Physician _____

I. Health History

Family History

Health status of parents, siblings (if deceased, note cause of death):
_____
_____
_____
_____

Occurrence or history of the following diseases in parents, siblings, and close relatives:

diabetes mellitus ____   hypertension ____   renal disease ____   vascular disease ____
tuberculosis ____   cardiopulmonary ____   neuromuscular disease ____
complications of pregnancy or congenital anomalies (specify) _____
psychiatric disorders (specify) _____
cancer (specify) _____

Personal and Health History

Personal characteristics:
age _____   habits:
racial/ethnic background _____   smoke _____
relationships (husband, partner, children,   alcohol ____   drugs ____
support networks) _____   exercise _____
_____   relaxation _____
_____   misc. _____

Medical history:
childhood diseases: _____
_____

immunizations (including rubella): _____
_____

hospitalizations (reasons, years): _____
_____

surgery (type, year): _____
_____

blood transfusions: _____
drug sensitivities: _____
allergies (foods, allergens): _____
_____

diseases: vascular disease ____   endocrinopathy ____
diabetes mellitus ____   sexually transmitted disease ____ severe anemia ____
rheumatic fever ____   asthma ____   blood dyscrasias ____
cardiopulmonary ____   psychiatric disorders ____   malnutrition ____
hypertension ____   cancer ____   malignancy ____
tuberculosis ____
renal/urinary tract disease ____
injuries (especially to pelvic organs or structures): _____
_____

(continued)

ASSESSMENT TOOL *(Continued)*
Prenatal History

Menstrual history:
   age at menarche ____
   describe present cycle (interval between menses ____, amount of flow ____, pain ____, clots ____,
      intermenstrual bleeding) ____:
   problems and procedures (eg, D&C ____, conization, ____, irregular bleeding ____, amenorrhea ____):
Sexual history:
   sexual learning and understanding of sexual functions: _____
   _____
   _____
   sexual self-concept and identity: _____
   _____
   _____
   attitudes toward sexuality, particularly as affected by pregnancy: _____
   _____
   _____
   current sexual practices and satisfaction with these: _____
   _____
   _____
   contraceptive history and practice: _____
   method _____ effective/satisfied with use _____ problems _____
   method _____ effective/satisfied with use _____ problems _____
   method _____ effective/satisfied with use _____ problems _____
   sexually transmitted diseases and treatment: _____
   type of STD _____ date _____ Rx _____
   type of STD _____ date _____ Rx _____
   type of STD _____ date _____ Rx _____

II. Pregnancy History

Past Obstetric History

Year	Length Gest	Probs During Preg	Onset Labor	Length Labor	Complications Labor

Current Pregnancy

Last menstrual period (LMP): _____ Prior menstrual period (PMP): _____
Date fetal movement first felt: _____
Symptoms: nausea ____ urinary frequency ____ headache ____ leukorrhea ____
edema ____ constipation ____ bleeding ____ abdominal pain ____
others _____

Drugs or medications taken since pregnancy began: _____
_____

Exposure to communicable disease (especially rubella if not immune): _____
_____
_____

(continued)

ASSESSMENT TOOL *(Continued)*
Prenatal History

Illnesses since beginning of pregnancy (eg, colds, flu): _____
_____
Occupation: _____ Possible workplace exposure to toxins: _____
Reactions and adaptation to pregnancy (Was pregnancy planned? Is woman pleased or concerned?): _____
_____
_____
Reactions of partner and family: _____
_____
_____

Data about father:
   age _____   height _____   weight _____
   racial/ethnic origins: _____
   health status: _____
   medical history: _____
_____
_____
   response to pregnancy: _____
_____
_____
   relationship with client and family: _____
_____
_____
   occupation: _____ potential health hazards: _____
Interviewed by: _____ Date: _____
Comments:

---

are taken. Pap smears to screen for cervical cancer are done routinely.

- The bimanual examination provides information about the following:
  - Consistency of the cervix
  - Size, shape, and consistency of the uterus
  - Condition of the fallopian tubes and ovaries
  - Configuration of the bony pelvis

Uterine size is useful in determining length of gestation, and pelvic measurements enable a clinical appraisal of potential pelvic contractions that might lead to cephalopelvic disproportion in labor. Other abnormalities of the birth canal, such as soft-tissue masses, also can be identified (Procedure 17-1).

Laboratory Tests

Laboratory tests are done early in pregnancy to provide data about the physiologic changes in pregnancy and to identify risks or problems (Table 17-1). The approximate timing of tests is as follows:

- Initial visit or as early as possible:
  - Clean-catch urinalysis, urine culture
  - Cultures or tests for gonorrhea, *Chlamydia*
  - Complete blood count
  - Blood type, Rh factor, and antibody screen
  - Serologic test for syphilis
  - Rubella antibody screen
  - Hepatitis B antigen
  - Human immunodeficiency virus antibody screen (optional, done only with client's permission and counseling)
  - Pap smear
  - Tuberculosis skin test
- 6 to 12 weeks' gestation:
  - Chorionic villus sampling for fetal chromosomal abnormalities (optional)
- 10 to 12 weeks' gestation:

ASSESSMENT TOOL
Components of Prenatal Physical Examination

Part Examined, Examination Technique	Normal Findings	Abnormal Findings
Head and Neck		
Inspection with otoophthalmoscope, and visual inspection of mouth Palpation of nodes, thyroid	Hyperemia of nasal and buccal mucous membranes, slight diffuse enlargement of thyroid	Enlarged lymph nodes; thyroid tenderness, nodules or irregular enlargement; lesions of eyes or mouth; caries and abscesses of teeth; ear infections
Chest and Heart		
Auscultation with stethoscope, percussion and inspection	Lungs clear; heart in regular rhythm (occasionally a soft, short functional murmur due to hemodynamic changes of pregnancy)	Adventitious lung sounds (crackles, wheezes, rhonchi), irregular cardiac rhythm, nonphysiologic murmurs
Breasts		
Palpation and inspection of nipples, breasts, and axilla	Enlargement of breasts with increased vascular patterns; darkened areola with prominent tubercles; thin, yellow fluid secreted from nipples in later pregnancy	Masses or nodules; bloody or serosanguineous nipple discharge; nipple lesions; erythema
Skin		
Inspection and palpation	Pigmentation changes (linea nigra, mask of pregnancy); enlargement of nevi; appearance of spider angiomas; mottled erythema of hands	Pallor, jaundice, rash, skin lesions
Extremities		
Visual inspection and palpation, percussion with reflex hammer	Mild pretibial and ankle edema in third trimester, slight edema of hands in hot weather	Limitations of motion; varicosities; more than slight pretibial, hand, or ankle edema; hyperreflexia and clonus
Abdomen		
Palpation, inspection, auscultation, percussion	Enlarged uterus; palpation of fetal outline in later pregnancy; fetal heart sounds; contractions in last trimester	Uterus too large or too small for dates; absence of fetal heart sounds beyond 10 wk (using Doppler); transverse lie of fetus; fetal head in fundus; tonic uterine contractions; enlarged liver or spleen

(continued)

ASSESSMENT TOOL *(Continued)*
Components of Prenatal Physical Examination

Part Examined, Examination Technique	Normal Findings	Abnormal Findings
Pelvis		
Speculum examination, bimanual examination with inspection and palpation; collection of specimens	**Speculum examination:** Bluish discoloration of mucosa of vagina and cervix, congested cervix, ectropion in multigravidas, increased leukorrhea	**Speculum examination:** Yellow, purulent, frothy, cheesy white or homogeneous gray, foul-smelling discharge; friable, bleeding lesions of cervix; vaginal lesions; bleeding from cervical os, amniotic fluid
	Bimanual examination: Cervix soft, admits a finger or two (depending on gravida and length of pregnancy); uterus soft and enlarged; fetal head or parts may be felt in lower uterine segment; gynecoid pelvic configuration	**Bimanual examination:** Cervix dilated and effaced (unless labor has begun); cervical or vaginal masses; excessive amniotic fluid (uterus unusually enlarged); adnexal masses or fullness; rectal masses; hemorrhoids; contractions of the pelvic inlet, midpelvis, or outlet
	Pap smear: Squamous metaplasia, negative or normal; adequate or increased estrogen; endocervical cells present; hyperplasia considered borderline	**Pap smear:** Inflammation; presence of *Trichomonas* or fungi; diminished or absent estrogen; atypical or suspicious cells; atypical hyperplasia; dysplasia, neoplasia, or carcinoma

Ultrasonography for gestational age (crown–rump length; optional, commonly done)

■ 15 to 19 weeks' gestation:
Amniocentesis to detect certain genetic abnormalities (optional)
α-fetoprotein to screen for neural tube defects (optional)

■ 16 to 26 weeks' gestation:
Ultrasonography for gestational age (biparietal diameter; optional)

■ 24 to 28 weeks' gestation:
Screening for diabetes with 50 mg oral glucose (optional)
3-hour glucose tolerance test if elevated blood sugar on screening test (optional)

■ First trimester:
Hemoglobin electrophoresis for hemoglobinopa-

thy (ie, sickle cell anemia or trait, thalassemias; optional, done when indicated)

Ultrasonography is used frequently to provide information about gestational age, fetal position, multiple pregnancy, placental location, and growth retardation and to detect several fetal abnormalities. Ultrasound also may identify the sex of the fetus; parents are usually asked if they want to know this information. Studies have not found harmful fetal effects of pulsed or continuous ultrasound in over 25 years of use (Jack et al., 1987; Cunningham et al., 1993).

Women older than 35 years have increased risk for fetal abnormalities. Diagnostic procedures in early pregnancy to detect such abnormalities as Down syndrome, neural tube defect, and other chromosomal dis-

(text continues on page 411)

PROCEDURE 17-1
Pelvic Examination and Pap Smear

Overall Objective: Evaluate condition of pelvic structures, progress of pregnancy, and obtain specimens for diagnostic testing

Preparation

Nursing Actions	*Rationale*
1. Explain procedure to woman and rationale for what will be done.	Explanations reduce anxiety and promote cooperation.
2. Instruct woman to empty bladder before beginning examination.	This promotes comfort and accuracy of evaluation.
3. Assist woman into supine position on exam table with lower extremities flexed and rotated outward. Her heels should be supported in stirrups, which are level with the table about 1–2 ft in front of her buttocks.	This position promotes accuracy of evaluation.
4. Assist woman to relax by encouraging her to breathe naturally. Have her press the small of her back down on the table to avoid arching. Direct guidance to relax can be given for clenching fists (eg, "let your hands go limp—very limp—like a rag doll's. That's it—very limp.") or for holding the breath (eg, "Keep breathing naturally.")	If the woman is anxious, she may tense her abdominal, pelvic, and thigh muscles, closing her thighs. If she arches her back, the pelvis is tilted downward, making the pelvic exam difficult. Direct guidance from the nurse promotes relaxation.

Speculum Examination

Objective: To inspect the vagina and cervix and obtain specimens

Nursing Actions	*Rationale*
1. Assemble equipment, including stool, light source, vaginal speculum, gloves, swabs, cotton balls, slides, lubricating jelly, and specimen collection material. Label slides with the client's name. Provide data about the woman's age, LMP, pregnancy or postpartum status, gynecologic surgery, and use of hormones.	This promotes efficiency and facilitates interpretation.
2. With gloved hands, inspect and palpate the external genitalia, including the urethra and Skene's and Bartholin's glands.	This helps to detect abnormalities.
If any unusual discharge is present, a specimen may be obtained for culture or microscopic examination.	The specimen can be checked for infection.
3. Insert warmed speculum into the vagina.	This distends the folds and provides a clear view of the cervix (see accompanying figure). Lubricating jelly distorts the cells.
If a Pap smear is to be taken, do not use lubricating jelly. Instead, the speculum may be rinsed with tepid water to facilitate insertion. Occasionally, the dilation of the vagina by the speculum may cause an unpleasant stretching sensation.	

(continued)

PROCEDURE 17–1 *(continued)*
Pelvic Examination and Pap Smear

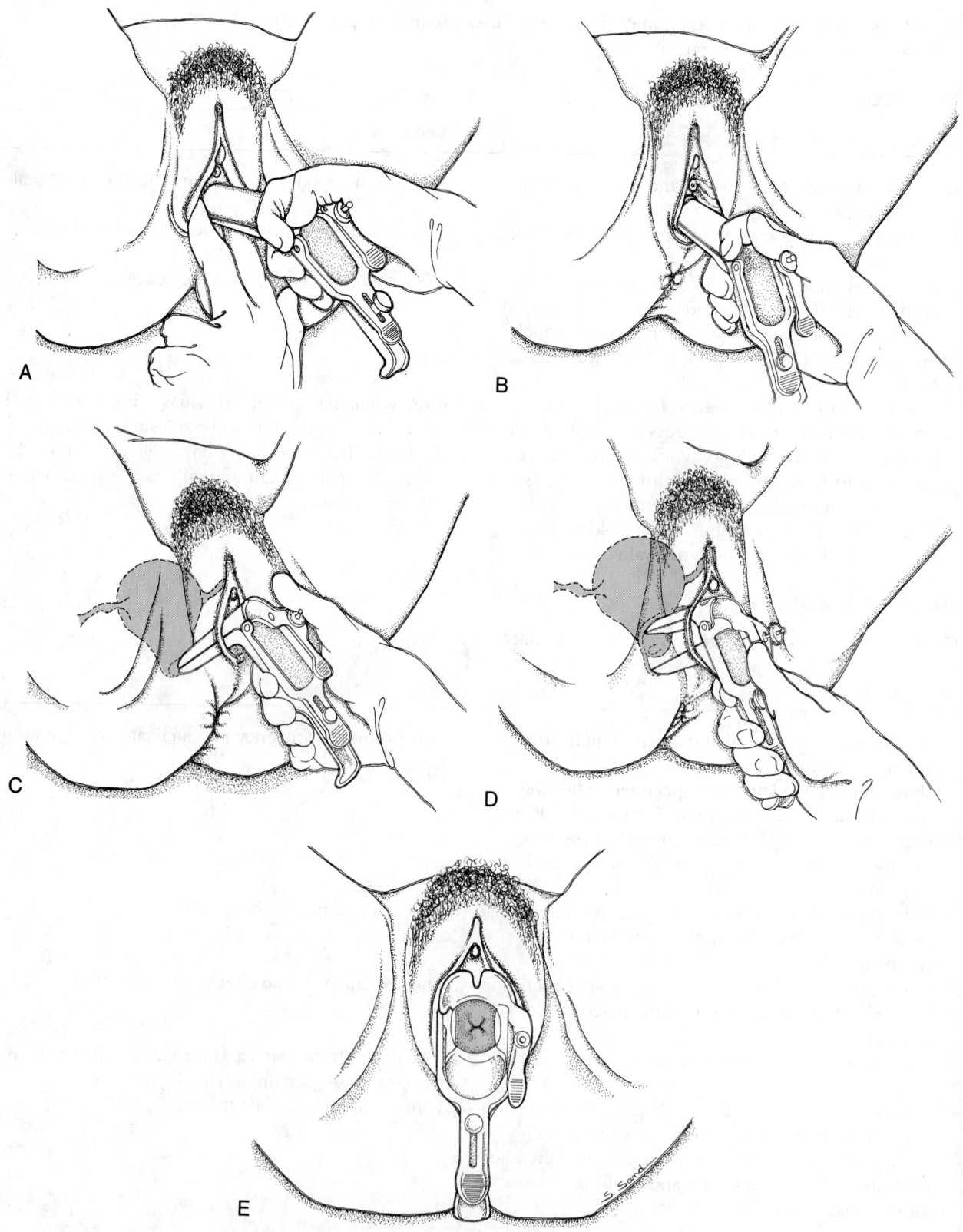

Insertion of the speculum. (**A**) Opening the introitus. (**B**) Oblique insertion Period of the speculum. (**C**) Final insertion of the speculum. (**D**) Opening the blades of the speculum. (**E**) View of the cervix through the speculum.

PROCEDURE 17–1 *(continued)*
Pelvic Examination and Pap Smear

Preparation

Nursing Actions	*Rationale*
4. Visualize the cervix. Normally the cervix of the primigravida is pink or bluish and smooth, with a dimple for the os. The cervix of a multigravida may have an irregular os owing to lacerations from previous deliveries (see accompanying figure). Ectropion is often present around the os in multigravidas; this is a darker pinkish-red, bumpy tissue composed of columnar epithelium, which lines the endocervical canal. Unless infection is present, this tissue is considered a normal variant during the years of active estrogen secretion.	Note color and character.

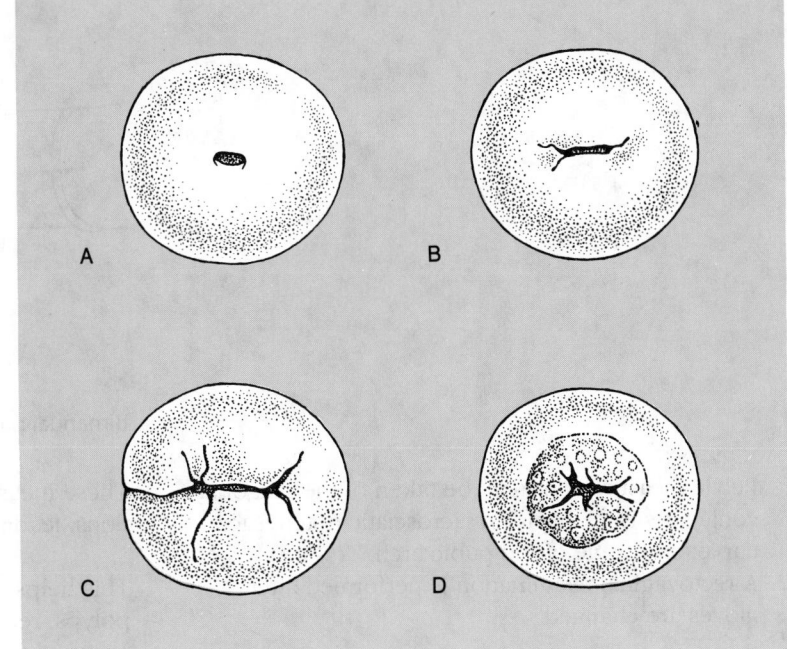

Common appearance of the cervix. (**A**) The nulliparous cervical os is small and either round or oval. (**B**) After childbirth, the os presents a slitlike appearance. (**C**) Difficult deliveries may tear the cervix, producing permanent lacerations. (**D**) Ectropion, often present in multigravidas, is a pinkish-red, bumpy tissue composed of columnar epithelium. (Redrawn from Bates, B. [1979]. *A guide to physical examination* [2nd ed.]. Philadelphia: J.B. Lippincott.)

A specimen may be taken. Any discharge that is purulent, greenish, frothy, or foul in odor is abnormal and may indicate infection.	Microscopic examination or culture is done.
5. Withdraw the speculum after specimens have been obtained, keeping blades collapsed.	Keeping the blades collapsed avoids distending the vulva and causing discomfort.

(continued)

PROCEDURE 17–1 *(continued)*
Pelvic Examination and Pap Smear

Bimanual Examination

Objective: To assess size, shape, and consistency of the uterus, fallopian tubes, and ovaries, and to determine pelvic architecture

Nursing Actions	Rationale
1. Lubricate the index and middle fingers of one gloved hand, and from a standing position, gently insert fingers into the vagina. Place the other hand on the adomen, midway between the umbilicus and pubis to palpate cervix, uterus, and adnexa between the adominal and vaginal hand (see accompanying figure).	This procedure determines the size, consistency, and contour of these organs and the relationship of the uterus to the pelvis.

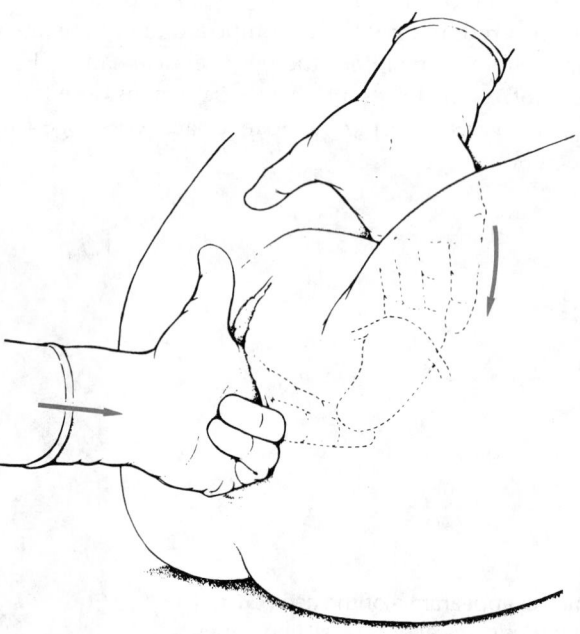

Bimanual palpation of the uterus.

Nursing Actions	Rationale
Pelvic measurements can be taken of the diagonal conjugate, ischial spines, sacrosciatic notch, sacral curve, and angle of the pubic arch.	These measurements identify potential pelvic contractions, leading to delivery complications.
2. A rectovaginal examination is performed after gloves are changed.	This helps to determine the presence of hemorrhoids, polyps, rectocele, or other abnormalities. Gloves are changed to prevent spreading any vaginal infection to the rectum.
3. When the exam is completed, the client should be assisted to a sitting position and disposable tissues should be offered to the client.	These actions promote comfort and allow the client to wipe her perineum.

Papanicolaou (Pap) Smear

Objective: To obtain a specimen of cervical cells for cancer screening

Nursing Actions	Rationale
1. The Pap smear is obtained during speculum examination. Excess mucus is removed from the cervix with a dry cotton swab.	The removal of excess mucus allows for a more accurate specimen sample.

PROCEDURE 17–1 *(continued)*
Pelvic Examination and Pap Smear

Nursing Actions	*Rationale*

2. A saline-moistened Dacron applicator or cytobrush is introduced into the endocervical canal (see accompanying figure).

A specimen of cells is obtained.

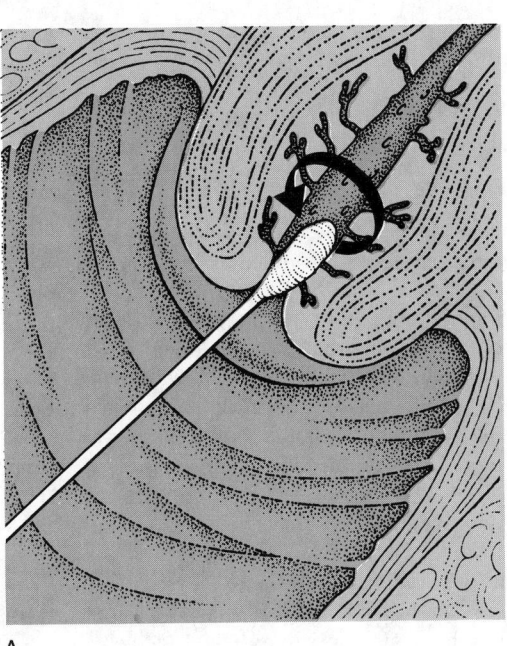 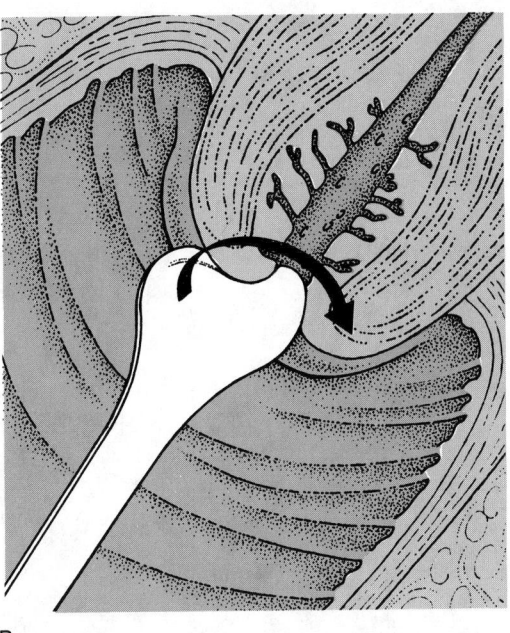

A   B

The Pap smear. (**A**) Obtaining the endocervical sample. (**B**) Obtaining the ectocervical sample.

The applicator or cytobrush is rotated clockwise 360 degrees, withdrawn, and rolled on a glass slide. The smear is fixed immediately with commercial fixatives or immersed in 95% ethyl alcohol.

This distributes the cells.

This prevents the specimen from drying, which distorts the cells.

3. A wooden or plastic spatula is used to obtain the ectocervical sample. The longer end is introduced slightly into the cervical os, pressed, and turned in a full circle firmly several times.

This action scrapes the tissue of the squamocolumnar junction (where the endocervical epithelium meets that of the ectocervix). This is the area where most malignancies arise and can be seen as a color change of cervical epithelium.

The specimen is smeared on a glass slide as above. Some providers place both endocervical and ectocervical specimens on one slide.

4. A vaginal pool sample also may be taken by introducing the rounded end of the spatula into posterior vaginal fornix or by aspirating fluid with a vaginal pipette.

This allows any endometrial cells present in the vagina to be included in the evaluation for malignancy.

TABLE 17–1
Laboratory Tests During Pregnancy

Test	Source of Specimen	Purpose
URINE		
Urinalysis	Clean voided urine	Sugar (glycosuria)—screen for diabetes
Sugar		Albumin (proteinuria)—screen for preeclampsia, kidney stress, or renal problems
Albumin		
Microscopic		RBCs, WBCs, epithelial cells, casts, microorganisms—screen for renal disease, urinary tract infection
Urine culture	Clean voided urine	Diagnose urinary tract infections; often done routinely on all pregnant women; done when urinary symptoms are present to identify organism
BLOOD		
CBC	Venous blood	
Hematocrit (HCT) and hemoglobin (HGB)		HCT and HGB—screen for anemia
White blood cell count and differential (WBC w/Diff.)		WBC w/diff.—identify infectious processes; screen for blood dyscrasias, folic acid deficiency
Platelets		Platelets—assess blood-clotting mechanisms
Serologic test for syphilis (RPR, VDRL)	Serum	Screen for syphilis (if positive must confirm with FTA-ABS)
Rh factor and blood type	Venous blood	Determine the blood type and Rh factor (positive or negative): blood type is important in case of hemorrhage; Rh factor alerts providers to possible incompatibility disease in fetus
Rh titers	Venous blood	Done when mother is Rh negative and father is Rh positive to assay danger to fetus (signified by rising titer)
Rubella antibodies	Venous blood	Determine if mother has been exposed previously to rubella and has built up antibodies (ie, is immune or not)
α-fetoprotein (AFP)	Serum	Screen for neural tube defects between 15th and 20th weeks of gestation
Glucose (blood sugar)	Venous blood	Screen for gestational diabetes (if elevated, 3-h glucose tolerance test is done)
Hemoglobin electrophoresis	Blood	Diagnose hemoglobinopathies (eg, sickle cell anemia, thalassemias)
BUN, creatinine, total protein, electrolytes	Serum	Evaluate renal function and diagnose renal disease
Hepatitis B antigen (HBsAg)	Serum	Infection by hepatitis B virus
HIV antibody assay (ELISA—enzyme-linked immunosorbent assay)	Serum	Infection by human immunodeficiency virus
CERVICAL/VAGINAL		
Beta streptococcus	Cervical discharge	Diagnose beta streptococcus infection; often done routinely as many women are asymptomatic
Gonorrhea culture	Cervical discharge	Diagnose gonorrhea; often done routinely because gonorrhea is frequently asymptomatic in women
Pap smear	Cervix, vagina	Screen for cervical intraepithelial neoplasia; herpes simplex type 2
Chlamydia culture	Cervical discharge	Diagnose *Chlamydia trachomatis*, often done routinely because infections may be asymptomatic and often occur with gonorrhea infections
Herpes simplex culture	Skin lesions	Diagnose herpes simplex if lesions are present on vulva, labia, buttocks
OTHER		
Tuberculin skin test	Applied to skin	Screen high-risk women for tuberculosis
ECG, chest x-ray	Heart, lungs	Evaluate cardiac and pulmonary function
Ultrasonography	Uterine contents	Evaluate gestational age, fetal position, multiple pregnancy, placental location, growth retardation, fetal abnormalities
Chorionic villi sampling (CVS)	Placental villi	Detect fetal chromosomal disorders, some metabolic disorders
Amniocentesis	Amniotic fluid	Detect fetal chromosomal disorders, some metabolic disorders

orders are recommended. Procedures include chorionic villus sampling, which involves transcervical or transabdominal aspiration of placental samples, and amniocentesis, which involves intra-abdominal aspiration of amniotic fluid samples (see Chap. 39).

Identification of Increased Risk During Pregnancy

Any condition that might adversely affect the health of the woman or fetus during pregnancy, labor, or delivery places the pregnancy in a high-risk category (Box 17-3). Various psychosocial and developmental factors can place the mother and father at high risk for parenting difficulties (Box 17-4). The nurse assesses the family structure, communication, supports, and coping behaviors to identify strengths and stressors.

BOX 17-3
Indicators of High-Risk Pregnancy

Social-Behavioral Factors

Age (less than 16 or greater than 35)
Poverty, low income
Nutritional (underweight, overweight, poor diet)
Substance use (tobacco, alcohol, drugs)
High-risk sexual behavior
High risk for family or environmental violence
Work exposure to toxins

Health Conditions—Deviations in Health

Chronic illness (diabetes, cardiovascular disease, renal disease, respiratory disorders, blood dyscrasias, others)
Sexually transmitted disease (current, history of)
Other infectious diseases (urinary tract, communicable diseases)

Pregnancy-Related Conditions

Previous pregnancy complications (preterm birth, recurrent abortions, ectopic pregnancy, operative delivery, breech delivery, prolonged labor, infection, hemorrhage, stillbirth, gestational diabetes, hydatidiform mole)
Previous newborns with birth defects
Previous low–birth-weight newborns, macrosomia
Multiple pregnancy
Gestational diabetes
Rh or ABO sensitization
Recent previous delivery (less than 1 year)
Uterine or ovarian tumors
Bleeding problems
Reproductive tract abnormalities (contracted pelvis, vaginal septum, septate uterus)

BOX 17-4
Indicators of High-Risk Parenting

Unplanned pregnancy
Single parent, limited support systems
Adolescent pregnancy
Substance abuse by parents (alcohol, drugs)
Psychiatric history or mental retardation in parents
Ambivalence or negativity about pregnancy or parenthood
History of abuse as a child
Previous stillbirth, neonatal death
Extreme desire for child of particular sex
Severe marital discord, spousal abuse
Previous child relinquished for adoption
Previous child with anomalies, chronic illness
History of abusing and neglecting previous child
Multiple recent moves, no permanent living plan, homeless
Several small children close together in age

Pregnancy

Nursing Diagnoses in Early Pregnancy

Nursing diagnoses during early pregnancy may include the following:

- Health Seeking Behaviors related to lack of knowledge about emotional and physiologic changes of pregnancy, what to expect during the course of prenatal care, self-care during pregnancy, and family adjustments
- Altered Nutrition: Less than body requirements related to nausea and vomiting during the first trimester
- Anxiety related to physical changes of pregnancy, fear of pregnancy loss, emotional reactions to being pregnant, and concerns for safety
- Altered Comfort related to breast tenderness, lower abdominal achiness, and the need for frequent urination in early pregnancy
- Altered Health Maintenance related to insufficient knowledge of effects of tobacco use (alcohol use, drug use) on self and fetus
- Altered Sexuality Patterns related to early pregnancy discomforts, nausea and vomiting, or emotional reactions
- Altered Family Processes related to the family's response to the pregnancy
- Ineffective Individual Coping related to addictions, emotional disturbances, adolescent parents, physical illness, inadequate financial resources, or abusive family patterns

NURSING GUIDELINES
Prenatal Teaching Checklist

Pregnancy and Health Status

Date   *Initials*

_____   _____   Prenatal history and physical examination results discussed
_____   _____   Prenatal laboratory panel results discussed
_____   _____   Medications and teratology discussed
_____   _____   Nutritional counseling
_____   _____   Preferred weight gain _____
_____   _____   Emotions of pregnancy
                      The following minor problems discussed:
_____   _____   Constipation or hemorrhoids
_____   _____   Backache
_____   _____   Stretch marks
_____   _____   Difficulty sleeping
_____   _____   Ankle edema
_____   _____   Nausea and vomiting
_____   _____   Heartburn
_____   _____   Varicosities
_____   _____   Headache
_____   _____   Stuffy nose and allergies
                      The following danger signs discussed:
_____   _____   Vaginal bleeding
_____   _____   Swelling of face and fingers
_____   _____   Severe continuous headaches
_____   _____   Dimness or blurring of vision
_____   _____   Flashes of light before eyes
_____   _____   Severe abdominal pain
_____   _____   Persistent vomiting
_____   _____   Chills and fever
_____   _____   Sudden escape of fluid from vagina

Preventive Health Care

_____   _____   Smoking discussed
_____   _____   Activity, exercise, travel, working discussed
_____   _____   Sexual activity discussed
_____   _____   Accident prevention
_____   _____   Dental care
_____   _____   Alcohol discussed
_____   _____   Community health resources
_____   _____   Contraception discussed. Plans: _____ birth control pills, _____ IUD, _____
                      diaphragm, _____ foam and condom, _____ tubal ligation, _____ vasectomy, _____
                      rhythm or ovulation, _____ vaginal sponge, _____ none

Preparation for Labor, Delivery, and Parenthood

_____   _____   Prenatal classes discussed
_____   _____   Enrolled in class: date _____ type _____
_____   _____   Hospital arrangements discussed (visit and register)
_____   _____   Breast-feeding versus bottle feeding discussed
_____   _____   Type selected _____ Breast care taught _____
_____   _____   Management of labor and delivery discussed
                          Anesthesia/analgesia _____
                          Prepared childbirth _____
_____   _____   Partner in delivery room discussed. Yes _____ No _____
_____   _____   Signs of labor discussed (when to go to hospital)
                      Instructed on what to do about the following:
_____   _____   Ruptured membranes
_____   _____   Bleeding
_____   _____   Fever
_____   _____   Fetal monitoring equipment discussed
_____   _____   Circumcision discussed
_____   _____   Special requests related to birth _____
_____   _____   Infant care
_____   _____   Rooming-in
_____   _____   Pediatrician
_____   _____   Layette

Planning and Intervention

At the initial prenatal visit, counseling and education in response to knowledge deficits should be brief and focused on immediate and short-term needs. The mother's questions are answered, and an overview is given of the process of prenatal care. Explanations are provided about testing and diagnostic procedures, when these are to be done, why, and what to expect. Current problems, such as alterations in comfort (nausea and vomiting, frequent urination, breast and abdominal pain) are addressed. The nurse interprets any treatments ordered by the physician and ascertains the client's understanding and ability to follow the prescribed regimen. Problems with immediate effects on maternal or fetal well-being are handled during the first visit.

Smoking

If the woman is currently smoking, nursing intervention focuses on supporting her to stop smoking or reduce cigarette consumption as much as possible. Adverse effects of smoking increase with daily cigarette consumption; even some decrease is beneficial. The nurse educates the client about risks of tobacco use for the fetus, other children at home, herself, and others. Regardless of race, adequacy of prenatal care, or mother's educational level, fetuses of smoking mothers have increased risk for low birth weight (Centers for Disease Control [CDC] Reports, 1993; Raine et al., 1994).

The nurse describes the benefits of quitting and outlines strategies to stop smoking (see Chap. 34). Many approaches are available, ranging from stopping "cold turkey" to ongoing smoking cessation groups and residential programs. Some success has been reported using self-help smoking cessation programs with pregnant women (Ershoff et al., 1989; Mayer et al., 1990).

Alcohol and Drug Use

Alcohol use during pregnancy presents significant risk for fetal alcohol syndrome and other more subtle developmental disorders. Evidence of maternal alcohol use during the initial assessment requires immediate nursing intervention. The objective is to assist the pregnant women to stop drinking, because no safe level of alcohol use during pregnancy has been established (Dunnihoo, 1992). The use of street drugs and abuse of over-the-counter and prescription medications also call for early nursing intervention to stop or control use during pregnancy. Alcohol and drug use during pregnancy are covered in detail in Chapter 34.

Depending on the duration of pregnancy, the nurse reviews important danger signs with the client and discusses when to contact the health provider. In early pregnancy, indicators of complications include vaginal bleeding, abdominal cramping, persistent and frequent nausea and vomiting, and elevated temperature. It is better to postpone further routine health teaching and counseling about weight gain, diet, exercise, sexuality, and other areas until a subsequent visit, when the mother is not so overloaded with new stimuli.

Evaluation

Nursing care is effective when the client expresses increased understanding of pregnancy and prenatal care, states that her questions have been adequately answered, and follows through with prenatal care, such as diagnostic tests and return visits. The client is able to describe symptoms of pregnancy complications and what to do if these occur. Interventions to improve family processes and coping strategies are considered effective when family members communicate well and provide or receive needed support. When alterations in health maintenance are diagnosed (smoking, alcohol, or drug use), nursing intervention is effective when the client acknowledges the risks to herself and the fetus and participates in developing a plan for stopping the substance use. Subsequent evaluation of the level of substance use is necessary with each visit.

The focus of nursing care for the pregnant woman evolves and changes as the woman's pregnancy progresses. One way to make sure all the crucial health teaching topics have been covered is to use a teaching checklist, such as the one provided in the Nursing Guidelines: Prenatal Teaching Checklist.

Continuing Care During Pregnancy

Regular return visits are scheduled throughout pregnancy to monitor maternal and fetal status, institute treatment and further diagnostic tests as necessary, and offer ongoing support and education. The usual schedule of visits is once a month until the 28th week, every 2 weeks until the 36th week, and weekly from the 37th week until delivery. Low-risk women may have visits scheduled less often without adversely affecting pregnancy outcome (Walker, 1993). Visits are scheduled more frequently if problems arise.

Assessment

A schedule of assessment priorities throughout pregnancy is provided in the Assessment Guidelines: Continuing Assessment During Pregnancy. Physiologic and psychological adaptations to pregnancy, measures of fetal well-being, signs or symptoms of complications,

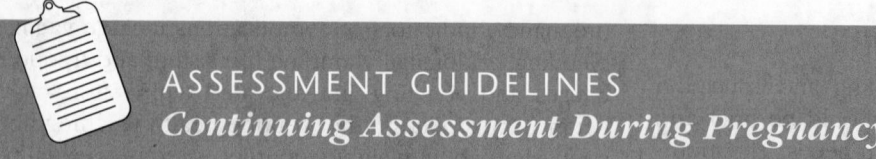

ASSESSMENT GUIDELINES
Continuing Assessment During Pregnancy

Schedule of Return Visits

Once per month, 1–28 weeks' gestation
Every 2 wk, 27–36 weeks' gestation
Every week, 37–40 weeks' gestation

Weeks' Gestation	Assessment	Rationale
Every visit	*Weight*	*Evaluate fetal growth, screen for maternal edema, pregnancy-induced hypertension (PIH), undernourishment*
	Blood pressure (BP)	*Screen for PIH*
	Fundal height (McDonald's Rule)	*Evaluate fetal growth*
	Leopold's maneuver	*Determine fetal position*
	Fetal heart rate (FHR)	*Evaluate fetal well-being*
	Edema	*Screen for PIH, fluid retention*
	Symptoms	*Identify problems, discomforts*
	Adjustment	*Identify problems, provide support*
	Nutrition	*Determine adequacy of diet*
	Urinalysis	*Glucose screen for gestational diabetes, protein screen for PIH*
6–12 wk	**Chorionic villus sampling*	*Detect fetal chromosomal abnormalities*
10–12 wk	*Ultrasound*	*Determine fetal age, development (crown–rump)*
	*Hemoglobin (Hgb) electrophoresis	*Detect sickle cell, thalassemias, other hemoglobinopathies*
15–20 wk	*α-Fetoprotein*	*Detect fetal neural tube defects*
	*Amniocentesis	*Detect fetal genetic abnormalities*
	Ultrasound	*Determine fetal age, development (biparietal diameter)*
24–28 wk	*Glucose 50 mg*	*Detect gestational diabetes*
32–34 wk	*Hematocrit/Hgb*	*Detect anemia*
37–40 wk	*Pelvic examination*	*Identify cervical changes preceding labor onset*

*For clients at risk.

compliance with medical regimens, and preparations for parenthood are assessed at each visit. The nurse assesses the following:

- How the client and family are adjusting to the pregnancy

- Any concerns, questions, or reported problems (Fig. 17-1)
- Physical symptoms, such as weight gain, edema, bleeding, constipation, headaches, dysuria
- Weight, blood pressure, temperature
- **Fundal height** and **fetal heart rate (FHR)**

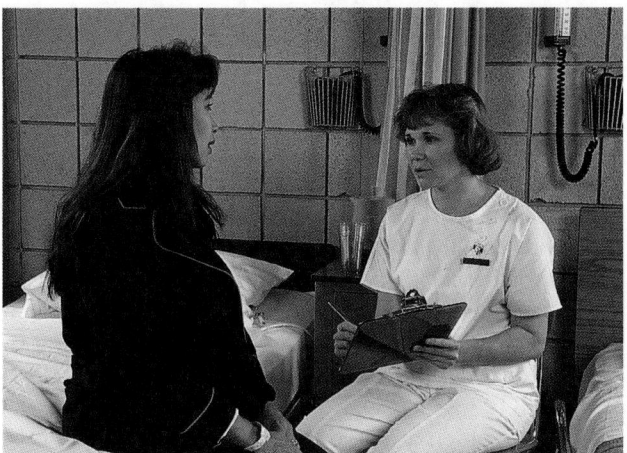

FIGURE 17–1 During follow-up visits throughout the pregnancy, the nurse asks what physical symptoms the client has been experiencing, how the client and her family are adjusting to the pregnancy, and if the client has any concerns, questions, or problems.

- Face, hands, legs, and feet for edema or varicosities
- Urine for glucose and protein

Weight is plotted on a graph or flow sheet, and deviations from expected progression are noted and explored. Vaginal examinations are usually not done on return visits until the client is about 2 or 3 weeks from EDD to assess the status of the cervix, fetal presentation, and the degree of engagement.

Abdominal Examination

Abdominal examination is useful for providing information about the position of the fetus after the 13th week of gestation. **Leopold's maneuvers** (see Chap. 20) help determine position and presentation of the fetus, and auscultation of the fetal heart rate provides an indication of fetal condition. **Fetal activity** is assessed by asking the mother about the frequency of fetal movements.

Fundal Height

The height of the fundus is measured to determine fetal growth in relation to uterize size and weeks of gestation (McDonald's technique). A pliable but not stretchable paper tape measure is used to measure the distance from the upper border of the symphysis pubis to the top of the uterine fundus. Frequently the tape measure is curved over the mother's abdomen, although some providers hold it straight between the fingers with the hand at a right angle to the top of the fundus (Fig. 17-2; see Box 17-1).

Nursing Diagnoses in Later Pregnancy

Nursing diagnoses in the second and third trimesters may include the following:

- Health Seeking Behaviors related to self-care methods to reduce common discomforts and preparation for labor, delivery, and parenthood
- Health Seeking Behaviors related to proper use of seat belts and body mechanics for pregnancy
- Anxiety related to the increasing discomforts of later pregnancy and approaching labor
- Sleep Pattern Disturbance related to physiologic changes and physical discomforts of pregnancy

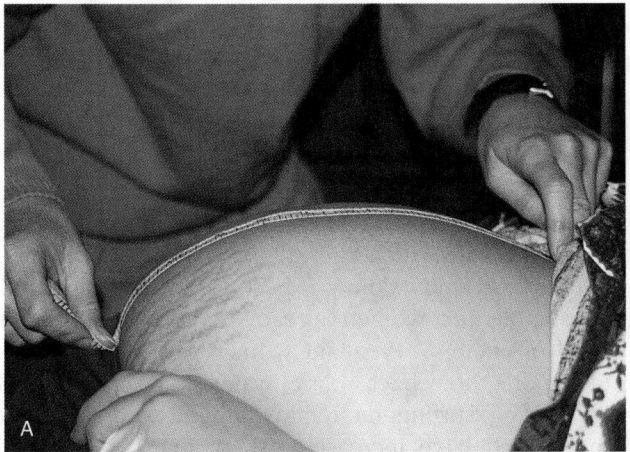
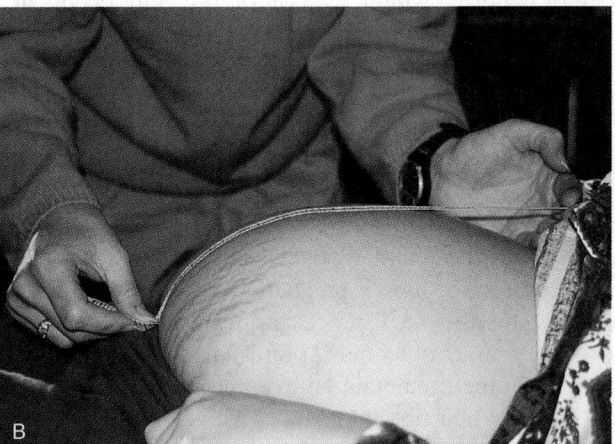

FIGURE 17–2 Measurement of fundal height (McDonald's technique) during a home visit. (**A**) The tape measure is curved over the mother's abdomen. (**B**) The tape measure is held straight between the fingers with the hand at a right angle to the top of the fundus.

■ Activity Intolerance related to changes in center of gravity and increased weight

Planning and Intervention

Nursing interventions include techniques of teaching, support, advice, self-care preparation, direct physical care, and referral or coordination of services. The nurse helps the woman and family understand and adapt to physiologic and emotional changes of pregnancy, deal with minor discomforts effectively, recognize and avoid potentially serious complications, plan for parenthood and integration of the newborn into the family, understand and comply with the medical regimen, and attain optimal health status (see Nursing Care Plan).

Weight Gain

During early pregnancy, the fetus gains 1 g daily; 90% of its weight is gained after the fifth month, with half of this weight acquired during the last 8 weeks. The nurse explains pregnancy weight patterns to help the woman understand why increased weight is necessary for normal fetal development (see Chap. 18). Recommended weight gain during pregnancy is summarized in Box 17-5 (National Institute of Medicine, 1990).

Maternal weight gain is positively and significantly associated with birth weight and exerts a direct influence on pregnancy outcome. During the second and third trimesters, the client should gain about 1 lb per week. Underweight mothers frequently have lower birth-weight newborns. About 17% of white and 27% of African American women with full-term pregnancies gain less than 20 lb (CDC Reports, 1993). Obese women may have more difficult labors, but pregnancy outcomes are good (Abrams et al., 1990). The influence of maternal weight gain on birth weight occurs at all levels of prepregnancy body mass, age, parity, and education (Seidman et al., 1989; Frentzen et al., 1988; Haiek et al., 1989).

Weight gain of 20 to 40 lb has been associated with good pregnancy outcome (full term, appropriate size for gestational age) in women with underweight, normal, and overweight prepregnant body mass. Fewer women with pregnancy weight gain at the lower end (20–22 lb) have good pregnancy outcomes. Higher weight gain (40–45 lb) does appear consistent with good pregnancy outcome (Abrams et al., 1990).

Many women maintain an average weight gain of 4 to 7 lb after their first pregnancy, with redistribution of adipose tissue and increased waist-to-hip ratio. These changes persist and are greater than those occurring because of age alone. Increased waist-to-hip ratio is associated with higher risk for cardiovascular disease

(Smith et al., 1994; Manson et al., 1994). The Research Highlight describes some of these findings in more detail.

Rest, Recreation, and Sleep

Rest and sleep are essential to health. Pregnant women tire more readily and may show symptoms of fatigue, such as irritability, apprehension, worry, and restlessness. Pregnant women are advised to get as much sleep as needed; this varies by individual. Napping or resting for a half hour every morning and afternoon is beneficial.

Not all women are able to have regular rest periods. The woman who works throughout her pregnancy and the mother of preschool children may have difficulty getting adequate rest. The nurse searches with the woman for minutes in her busy day that can be used for rest. Counseling the family may be necessary to provide rest times. Resting might include lying down or sitting comfortably to relax the body, mind, abdominal muscles, legs, and back. Stretching out whenever possible makes it easier for the heart to pump blood to the extremities. During the last months of pregnancy, a small pillow supporting the abdomen while the pregnant woman lies on her side helps relieve discomfort.

Conscious relaxation can be used by the pregnant woman. Various techniques are available, including progressive relaxation, breathing exercises, attention focusing, imagery, and forms of meditation. Practiced regularly, relaxation is refreshing, energizing, and effective in counteracting stress. If the woman does not already practice relaxation, the nurse can teach her a simple technique. Relaxation techniques are discussed in Chapter 19; exercises are given in Appendix C.

Exercise

Exercise during pregnancy is usually beneficial, depending on the woman's state of health, conditioning, and stage of pregnancy. Exercise provides a diversion, reduces anxiety and tension, quiets the mind, promotes sleep, helps decrease constipation, and stimulates the appetite, all of which are valuable aids to the pregnant woman. Moderate exercise involving large muscle groups, such as walking, cycling, swimming, and cross-country skiing, is best. Jogging or running is acceptable for women already conditioned for this level of exercise. Pregnant women should avoid contact sports, horseback riding, water skiing, racquetball, ice skating, surfing, mountain climbing, and scuba diving, which have increased risk of injury or hypoxia (Sady et al., 1989; Freyder, 1989). Client Education: Exercise During Pregnancy lists guidelines for advising pregnant women about exercise.

NURSING CARE PLAN
The Pregnant Woman

Nursing Goals
1. Women have early and regular prenatal care.
2. Women and families understand the progress of pregnancy and adapt to changes.
3. Women learn self-care and health maintenance during pregnancy.
4. Women are able to alleviate minor discomforts of pregnancy.
5. Women can identify potential or actual complications and seek appropriate care.

Assessment	*Potential Nursing Diagnoses*	*Intervention/ Rationale*	*Evaluation*
Physiologic status of pregnancy (vital signs, weight, urine, fundal height, fetal heart rate and activity, symptoms, test results)	Knowledge Deficit of effects of pregnancy on body systems Knowledge Deficit of fetal growth and development Concomitant medical conditions	Take general health history and obstetric history, physical examination, and laboratory tests as part of prenatal workup with regular return visits *to monitor maternal and fetal development.*	Client repeats EDD. Client understands implications of minor health problems and complications.
Psychosocial status of pregnancy (responses to pregnancy, family adaptations, knowledge of psychosocial effects)	Knowledge Deficit related to effects of pregnancy on psychosocial domain Knowledge Deficit of effects of pregnancy on sexuality Self Esteem Disturbance related to effects of pregnancy on biopsychosocial patterns	Discuss attitudes toward pregnancy, knowledge, expectations, family and personal resources, coping mechanisms, and economic situation; teach and provide support *to facilitate adaptation to pregnancy.*	Client discusses expectations of pregnancy. Client realizes who support people are. Client clarifies her understanding of (or lack of) information.
Health maintenance needs (self-care, diet, rest and exercise, substance use, medications, sexuality)	Health Seeking Behaviors achieve successful pregnancy outcome Knowledge Deficit of nutritional requirements Knowledge Deficit of hazards of smoking, alcohol, drugs Altered Health Maintenance related to increased psychophysical needs	Teach ways to promote health and well-being during pregnancy, avoid/ reduce toxic exposure, use self-care measures *to enhance health and reduce risk of complications.* Refer to community resources *to obtain necessary care* when problems are identified.	Client acknowledges areas needing improvement. Client seeks information on changing behavior. Client follows through on referrals, recommendations, and treatment plans.
Minor discomforts (symptoms in specific systems: genitourinary, gastrointestinal, urinary, musculoskeletal, neurologic)	Alteration in Comfort: nausea or vomiting, heartburn, constipation, headaches, hemorrhoids, flatulence, backache, dyspnea, leg cramps, vaginal discharge, carpal tunnel syndrome Activity Intolerance related to fatigue and dyspnea Risk for Infection, vaginal, due to hormonal changes	Teach about occurrence and alleviation of minor discomforts, self-care and natural approaches *to reduce discomfort and promote health.* Refer to physician or community resources if difficulties persist or if significant interference with daily activities occurs *to obtain further care.*	Client identifies discomforts. Client understands remedies for symptoms. Client receives comfort from remedies. Client follows through on referral.

(continued)

NURSING CARE PLAN *(Continued)*
The Pregnant Woman

Assessment	Potential Nursing Diagnoses	Intervention/ Rationale	Evaluation
Preparation for parenthood (knowledge of effects of pregnancy, fetal development, prenatal routines, preparing for delivery and child care)	Knowledge Deficit of fetal growth and development Knowledge Deficit of effects of pregnancy on body systems Knowledge Deficit related to effects of pregnancy on psychosocial domain Knowledge Deficit of childbirth preparation resources	Teach growth and development of the fetus, progression of pregnancy, physical and emotional changes, prenatal management routines, and preparation for childbirth; refer to community sources providing these educational services (ie, childbirth classes, nutritionist).	Couple attends childbirth classes. Couple indicates understanding of fetal development, effects of pregnancy, and prenatal routines. Couple makes plans for labor and delivery. Couple makes plans for infant care at home.
Indicators of complications of pregnancy (ie, rising blood pressure, facial edema, bleeding, excessive weight, inappropriate fundal measurements for dates)	High risk for pregnancy complication (related to specific symptoms) Anxiety and Fear related to potential complication	Notify physician *to obtain additional physical data and laboratory tests to evaluate problems,* explain to client the meaning of signs and symptoms and the plan *to reduce anxiety and facilitate care.*	Client affirms understanding of complications. Client cooperates with treatment. Client controls signs and symptoms of complications.
Indicators of stress and psychosocial problems (ie, missed appointments, noncompliance, affect, direct expression of concerns, acting out behavior of children, complaints)	Risk for Self Esteem Disturbance related to pregnancy or other life situations Risk for Altered Parenting or Family Processes related to psychosocial problems High risk for pregnancy complication (related to specific behaviors)	Identify sources of problems (economic, psychosocial, cultural, or conflicts within healthcare systems) *to determine focus of intervention.* Counsel and refer as needed for more intensive therapy; use community resources for socioeconomic, cultural problems; work with agency and health team *to improve client relations.*	Client keeps appointments. Client follows through on referrals. Client implements suggestions and recommendations. Client reports recommendations have been helpful. Client affirms improvement of problems.

Exercise is limited with such high-risk conditions as maternal heart disease, preterm delivery, multiple gestation, previous SGA infants, placenta previa, bleeding, incompetent cervix, ruptured membranes, or history of repeated spontaneous abortions (Scott et al., 1994). Maternal hyperthermia from exercise may contribute to fetal anomalies in the first trimester. During exercise, uterine blood flow is reduced as blood is shunted to the muscles. Fetal hypoxia does not occur from this, but decreased ability to dissipate heat through the placenta may be problematic for the fetus (Fishbein et al., 1990).

The fetus can tolerate strenuous maternal exercise when women are accustomed to this level of activity and continue exercise programs into their pregnancies. New strenuous exercise should not begin during pregnancy. In physically fit women, the ventilatory reserve and cardiovascular changes of pregnancy contribute to increased fetal tolerance of the circulatory and respiratory challenges of strenuous maternal exercise (Paisley et al., 1988; Woodward, 1981).

Prenatal exercises are standard components of childbirth education, with the intention to strengthen abdominal muscles, relax muscles of the pelvic floor, teach the pelvic tilt, stretch and adduct the thighs, and limber specific body parts (see Chap. 19 and Appendix C).

BOX 17–5
Recommended Weight Gain During Pregnancy

- Total 25 to 35 lb for normal weight women (90%–120% weight for height)
- 28 to 40 lb for underweight women (<90% weight for height)
- 15 to 25 lb for overweight women (120%–135% weight for height)

Bathing and Skin Care

The glands of the skin are more active during pregnancy with increased perspiration, which can result in irritation or odor. Elimination through the skin is an important method of removing body waste products. The woman should take a bath or a shower daily for cleansing; these also are refreshing and relaxing. A possible danger from tub baths during the last trimester of pregnancy is that the heavy weight of the large abdomen may affect the pregnant woman's balance, making climbing in and out of the bathtub awkward. Therefore, the likelihood of slipping or falling in the bathtub is increased. Rubber mats or hand grips can prevent falls. Baths should not be taken when there is vaginal bleeding or after rupture of the membranes to avoid infection.

Breast Care

Care of the breasts during pregnancy is an important preparation for breast-feeding.

Early in pregnancy, the breasts begin to secrete **colostrum** and should be bathed daily with a clean washcloth and warm water. Soap, alcohol, and other drying cleansers reduce integrity of the nipple tissue, because they remove the protective skin oils and leave the nipple more prone to damage. Rubbing the nipples with a bath towel or rolling them between thumb and forefinger during the last trimester of pregnancy can help toughen them in preparation for breast-feeding. The position of the thumb and finger should be gradually shifted around the circumference of the nipple until a complete circuit has been made. Because nipple stimulation can produce uterine activity by releasing oxytocin from the posterior pituitary, women with a history of preterm labor should consult their healthcare provider before engaging in any nipple preparation activities.

Clothing

During pregnancy, clothes should be comfortable and nonconstricting. Most women can dress in their usual

RESEARCH HIGHLIGHT

First Pregnancy Adds and Redistributes Weight

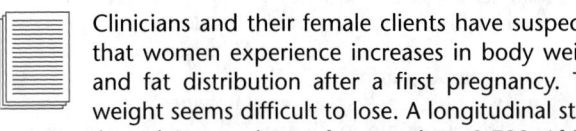

Clinicians and their female clients have suspected that women experience increases in body weight and fat distribution after a first pregnancy. This weight seems difficult to lose. A longitudinal study was conducted in a cohort of more than 2,700 African American and white women who were part of the ongoing Coronary Artery Risk Development in Young Adults (CARDIA) study. During a 5-year period, weight changes were compared in 925 nulliparous women and women who had a single pregnancy during the study period and were at least one year postpartum on follow-up (89 primiparas, 114 multiparas).

Statistical adjustments were made for baseline weight, age, education, smoking status, physical fitness, baseline physical activity, and changes in activity. During the 5-year period, primiparas of both races gained 4 to 7 lb more than nulliparas. African American women had greater weight increases than white women. Primiparas had greater increases in waist to hip ratio (WHR) that were independent of weight gain. WHR in African American primiparas was twice that of African American nulliparas; this difference was eightfold between white subjects. Weight gain and fat distribution in multiparas were similar to those in nulliparas.

Researchers concluded that first pregnancy is associated with adverse adiposity changes that persist and are greater than those occurring because of age alone, independent of demographic and behavioral factors. Though the weight gain is modest, it persists and may predispose to additional weight gain. Increased WHR is linked with higher risk for cardiovascular disease.

Critique: This well-designed, longitudinal study had a large sample and adjusted for confounding variables. The associations found between first pregnancy and changes in body weight and fat distribution appear reliable. Nurses can use this information to support moderate weight gain control measures, such as diet and exercise, after childbirth.

Smith, D. E., Lewis, C. E., Stampfer, M. J. (1994). Longitudinal changes in adiposity associated with pregnancy: The CARDIA study. *Journal of the American Medical Association, 271,* 1747-1751.

manner until their clothes become uncomfortable. Maternity specialty shops and department stores carry a wide variety of maternity clothes. Maternity clothes are designed to be comfortable and hang from the shoulders to avoid constriction. Fashion designers have created maternity clothing that is attractive and that helps women feel confident about their appearance. The expectant woman can dress according to climate and temperature for her comfort.

Pregnant women should avoid clothing or accessories that constrict movement or circulation. Tight

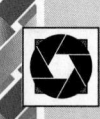

CLIENT EDUCATION
Exercise During Pregnancy

- Exercise of any kind should not be fatiguing and should be combined with periods of rest.
- Consult with provider about current or new exercise program.
- Avoid high-risk sports and activities.
- Decrease intensity of exercise as pregnancy progresses.
- Exercise at least three times per week for 15- to 30-minute intervals, with maximum pulse rate 140 to 150 beats/min.
- Wear supportive bra and shoes.
- Drink liquids before and after exercise to avoid dehydration.
- Avoid vigorous exercise in hot weather to prevent hyperthermia.
- Stretch and warm up before exercise (prepare joints and muscles for activity); cool down with mild activity (avoid pooling of blood).
- Stop activity and consult provider if symptoms occur (palpitations, shortness of breath, dizziness, abdominal pain, bleeding, numbness and tingling, no fetal movement).
- Avoid sitting or standing for long periods.

belts, garters, knee socks, knee-high stockings, panty girdles, garter belts, and tight stretch pants can be constricting. Particularly dangerous are round garters, rolled stockings, and tight knee-high stockings that might restrict circulation in the lower extremities. These can aggravate varicose veins, cause edema of the lower legs and feet, and produce venous stasis.

Clothing that fits snugly in the perineal area, such as tight pantyhose and stretch pants, can contribute to vaginal infections and heat rash (miliaria). Pantyhose are preferable to hose held up by garters or tight waist garter belts but should not be constricting and should have cotton crotches.

Breast Support

Pregnant woman benefit from wearing a well-fitted bra to support the breasts in a normal uplifted position. Proper support of the breasts is conducive to good posture and helps to prevent backache. The cup must be large enough with the underarm built high enough to cover all the breast tissue. Wide cotton shoulder straps afford more comfort for the woman who has large and pendulous breasts. The size of the bra is determined by breast size, but in most instances, it is approximately two sizes larger than that usually worn. The mother who is planning to breast-feed can buy nursing bras with drop flaps over the nipples, which can be worn during the latter months of pregnancy and during the postpartum period for as long as she is nursing her baby.

Shoes

Comfortable, well-fitted shoes are essential for the expectant woman. The postural changes that occur as the woman's abdomen enlarges may be aggravated by wearing high-heeled shoes, leading to backache and fatigue. Low-heeled shoes should be worn during working hours and for daytime activities. For more fashionable attire, a 2-inch heel is acceptable if the woman does not develop backache from the increased lordosis induced by the heels and if she can maintain adequate balance. Shoes should provide adequate support to the arch and sides of the foot to promote comfort.

Abdominal Support

If the woman's abdomen is large or if previous pregnancies have caused abdominal muscle relaxation, a well-fitted maternity girdle gives support and comfort. The purpose of the girdle is support, not constriction of the abdomen. When putting the girdle on, the woman should lie on the bed rather than stand and should fasten it from the bottom upward so support is provided to the uterus from below. Abdominal support provided by a maternity girdle can help relieve backache, prevent fatigue, and assist in maintaining good posture.

Bowel Habits

Pregnant women with regular bowel habits often experience little change in elimination. Those who have a tendency toward constipation become noticeably more irregular during pregnancy because of decreased physical exertion, relaxation of the bowel and smooth muscle systems, and pressure of the enlarging uterus. The presenting part of the fetus exerts pressure on the lower bowel, especially during the latter part of pregnancy. Iron supplementation during pregnancy is an additional contributing factor to constipation.

Constipation may be prevented or alleviated by maintaining regular bowel elimination, drinking a large amount of fluids daily, and maintaining a diet that contains several daily servings of fresh fruit, raw vegetables, and whole-grain breads and cereals, particularly products with whole bran. Vegetable fiber and psyllium seed preparations (eg, Citracel or Metamucil) add bulk to stool to promote elimination. If these measures are not effective, a stool softener, such as dioctyl sodium sulfosuccinate, or a mild laxative, such as milk of magnesia, may be recommended. Harsh laxatives and purgatives are contraindicated. Mineral oil should not be used because it prevents absorption of fat-soluble vitamins (A, D, E, and K) from the gastrointestinal tract. Lack of vitamin K can lead to hemorrhagic disease of the newborn.

Hemorrhoids

Pregnancy often causes hemorrhoids (anal varicosities), partially as a result of constipation. Maintaining regular bowel habits, keeping the stool soft, and avoiding straining with bowel movements can help prevent or minimize hemorrhoids. Passage of hard fecal material can injure the rectal mucosa and cause bleeding from fissures or hemorrhoids. Hemorrhoids may become thrombosed or protrude through the anus. The little bumps and nodules seen in a mass of hemorrhoids are the distended portions of the affected vessels. As with varicosities in other areas, they are caused by pressure that interferes with return venous circulation and are aggravated by constipation. Standing for long periods and wearing constricting clothing are aggravating factors. Hemorrhoids often cause discomfort during pregnancy and due to pressure at the time of delivery, may cause great distress during the postpartum period.

Prevention and treatment of constipation can minimize the severity of hemorrhoids. When internal hemorrhoids protrude through the rectum, the mother can be instructed to replace them carefully by pushing them gently back into the rectum with her finger. Use of petrolatum or mineral oil aids insertion; a finger cot can be used to cover her finger. Assuming the knee–chest position or elevating the buttocks on a pillow facilitates replacement through gravity.

Application of an icebag or cold compresses wet with witch hazel or Epsom salt solution provides relief for inflamed hemorrhoids. The physician may order analgesic or astringent suppositories, stool-bulking agents, or stool softeners. Sitz baths several times daily promote comfort and healing. Surgery is seldom performed during pregnancy. Doing **Kegel exercises** regularly helps prevent and control hemorrhoids (see Client Education: Kegel Exercises).

Sexuality During Pregnancy

Expectant couples often have questions about sexual practices during pregnancy. The nurse responds to their needs for information, creating an accepting climate in which to discuss sexual concerns. Many different views about discussing sexuality are found among people of different cultural backgrounds. The nurse respects cultural perspectives, while offering the opportunity to discuss sexual concerns. Being willing to explore and respond to sexual concerns and having knowledge of appropriate sources of referral for sexual counseling are part of the maternity nurse's role (see Chaps. 6 and 9).

Maternal Assessment of Fetal Activity

Fetal well-being may be monitored by the woman at home by counting fetal movements. Presence of fetal movement is reassuring; the average number of weekly movements, calculated from 12-hour daily recording periods, increases from 200 at 20 weeks' gestation to a more than 500 at 32 weeks. Fetal movements gradually decrease to about 280 per week at term. Large daily variation occurs, with as few as four to 10 movements per 12-hour day in normal pregnancies (Cunningham, et al., 1993). During the last 10 weeks of gestation, the fetus has alternating rest and activity cycles lasting 90 minutes each (Connors et al., 1988). There is considerable variation in fetal movement patterns. Fetal activity is affected by sound, cigarette smoking, blood glucose levels, time of day, drugs, and fetal sleep states. Significant decrease or absence of fetal movements has been noted by most women who experienced stillbirth (Calhoun, 1990).

Beginning at 27 weeks' gestation, pregnant women are taught to count the number of fetal movements occurring in a 30-minute period, twice daily. This is best

---

CLIENT EDUCATION
Kegel Exercises

Tightening and relaxing the pubococcygeal muscle keeps the vagina toned, increases the strength of the perineum, and helps prevent or control hemorrhoids. This contributes to the strength of the pelvic sling in supporting the fetus, increases sexual pleasure, and enhances urinary control.

The muscle that is used to stop the flow of urine is the pubococcygeal muscle. Practice stopping urine by squeezing this muscle several times to become familiar with it. When lying down, insert one finger into the vagina and contract the pubococcygeal muscle; note the feeling of contraction around your finger.

1. Squeeze the pubococcygeal muscle for 3 seconds, relax for 3 seconds, and squeeze again. Begin with 10 three-second squeezes per day, and increase gradually until you are doing 100 twice daily.
2. Squeeze and release, then squeeze and release alternately as rapidly as you can. This is called the "flutter" exercise.
3. Bear down as during a bowel movement, but concentrate on the vagina instead of the rectum. Hold for 3 seconds.

Kegel exercises can be done anywhere and anytime. The increased control gained over the pubococcygeal muscle is useful throughout pregnancy, during labor, during intercourse, and to prevent loss of vaginal tone with aging. This exercise, done regularly, is useful for the rest of your life.

done at least 1 hour after eating, while lying on the side to provide optimal placental–fetal circulation. Five or six movements should occur in 30 minutes. If there are less than three movements, the woman should continue counting for 1 hour. If there are questions or as routine monitoring, the woman can count and record movements for 8 to 12 hours. Further evaluation is indicated when the woman counts the following:

■ Fewer than three fetal movements in 1 hour
■ Fewer than 10 fetal movements in 12 hours
■ No fetal movements in the morning

If fetal activity is decreased, further evaluation includes nonstress or contraction stress testing, ultrasound, and tests for pulmonary maturity. Very low activity counts or a trend toward decreased motion usually is significant. The mother may report that the fetus' movements are slowing, and it takes longer each day to note 10 movements. This is expected in the last 4 weeks of gestation but may be abnormal earlier in pregnancy. If fetal movements cease entirely for 12 hours, the "fetal alarm signal" occurs and immediate evaluation is needed. Maternal awareness of fetal movements appears to be 90% accurate when compared with simultaneous real-time ultrasound demonstration of fetal activity (Gabbe, 1986).

General Health Maintenance in Pregnancy

During pregnancy, women are encouraged to continue their usual activities, unless these are not conducive to health and well-being. Although pregnancy creates numerous psychophysiologic changes, women with positive attitudes and good health adapt without undue stress. Many find these changes interesting and enjoyable. During the months of prenatal care, the nurse has many opportunities to reinforce health-promoting behaviors. (Specific nursing interventions related to psychosocial needs are discussed in Chapter 16.)

Employment

Women frequently continue work during pregnancy. The type of work, level of physical activity, environmental risks or occupational hazards, and obstetric or medical problems of the woman affect whether and how long she should continue working during pregnancy. When there are no risk factors, work does not increase late pregnancy complications, preterm delivery, or low birth weight (Henriksen et al., 1994). Avoidance of work environments that expose the pregnant woman to fetotoxic substances is a major consideration.

Research has shown that women working in strenuous manual jobs have a higher incidence of preterm or small-for-gestational age fetuses than office workers or homemakers. This may be due to decreased uteroplacental blood flow as blood is shunted to muscles, or it may result from socioeconomic factors; poor women are rarely office workers (Launer et al., 1990). Women whose jobs require prolonged standing, repeated stooping and bending, climbing ladders or stairs, and heavy lifting have more placental infarcts, spontaneous abortions, and lower birth-weight newborns (McDonald et al., 1988).

Jobs requiring manual labor increase risk when physical activity continues for hours, good balance is necessary, or prolonged standing is required. Positions that require constant sitting can be tiring. Adequate rest periods and opportunities to stand and walk should be provided for pregnant women employed in such positions.

The nurse discusses the woman's work environment and identifies sources of possible risk. Education and counseling by the nurse help the woman make an informed decision about the risks and benefits of continuing to work in a potentially hazardous environment. Steps to minimize or avoid risky activities or fetotoxic substances can be identified. Guidelines for employment of pregnant women have been developed by the U.S. Children's Bureau (Standards for Maternity Care and Employment).

Travel

Travel does not increase risk of abortion or preterm labor if there are no medical or pregnancy complications. Pregnant women are advised to avoid trips that will cause undue fatigue or stress. The obstetrician or nurse-midwife should be consulted about extensive travel at any time during pregnancy. The availability of medical care must be considered when traveling to remote areas. Many insurance plans do not cover delivery or hospitalization for premature labor in foreign countries (Barry et al., 1989). Travel should be avoided with history of bleeding, pregnancy-induced hypertension, multiple gestations, or in the last weeks of pregnancy.

Air Travel

For traveling long distances, flying is recommended. Metal detectors used for airport security are not harmful to the fetus. Sitting in airline seats for long periods is tiring, uncomfortable, and may increase risk of venous thrombosis. Pregnant women need to walk around in the airplane for 15 minutes every hour. Low humidity in airplane cabins (about 8% humidity) promotes water loss; pregnant women should drink water liberally during flights to prevent dehydration. Nonsmoking flights are recommended to avoid elevated carboxyhemoglobin levels. In the United States, women in the last month of pregnancy are not permitted on airlines without a statement from their obstetrician. Most foreign airlines do not allow women beyond the 35th week of gestation to fly. In late pregnancy, flying is contraindicated in women with severe anemia, sickle cell anemia, or history of thrombophlebitis (Dunnihoo, 1992).

Automobile Travel

Automobile travel can be tiring and may aggravate minor discomforts of pregnancy. Rest periods of 15 minutes should be taken at least every 2 hours to avoid fatigue and increase circulation by providing the chance to stretch and walk. The pregnant woman should wear seat belts, both lap and shoulder, during all automobile travel. Risks of injury and death to the woman and fetus are increased when seat belts are not used. Placental separation can occur with an automobile accident, because the force of the collision alters the contours of the uterine muscle and displaces placental attachment (Crosby, 1983). The shoulder belt reduces the extent of traumatic flexion of the pregnant woman's body, decreasing the risk of placental separation (Krozy et al., 1985).

Proper placement of seat belts during pregnancy is important. The lap belt is worn low and under the abdomen. The shoulder belt is worn above the uterus and below the neck, with the woman sitting upright and using a headrest to minimize flexion-extension injuries (Fig. 17-3). Most pregnant women do use seat belts, but some do not. One survey found 88% to 90% of pregnant women used seat belts 100% of the time when driving or as passengers, but 22% of them used seat belts incorrectly. Some women believed wearing seat belts increased the risk of injuring the fetus. Less than half had been advised by a health professional on seat belt use and technique during pregnancy (Hammond et al., 1990).

Immunizations During Pregnancy

As a rule, immunizations are best avoided during pregnancy. Several factors enter into the decision about immunizing a pregnant woman against an infectious disease, including the possibility of disease exposure, the effect on woman and fetus if the disease is contracted, susceptibility to the disease, and risk to the fetus from the immunization. **Immunoglobulins, toxoids,** and

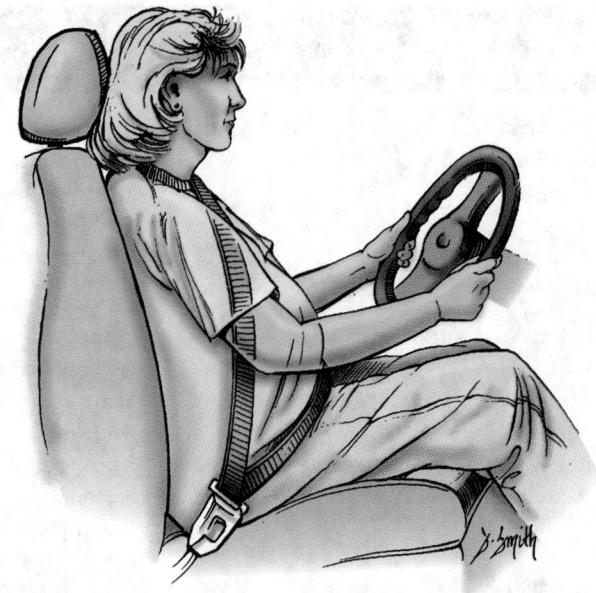

FIGURE 17–3 Pregnant women should wear seat belt with shoulder strap above the uterus and below the neck and lap belt low and under the abdomen.

killed or inactivated vaccines are safe during pregnancy. Vaccines made from live organisms must not be given during pregnancy unless the risk of exposure and illness clearly outweighs the risks of the vaccine itself.

The live virus MMR vaccine (measles, mumps, and rubella) is contraindicated during pregnancy. There is a well-established risk for serious fetal abnormalities from these diseases. About 10% of reproductive age women are susceptible to rubella, either because they were never vaccinated or their immunity has waned. The Centers for Disease Control have monitored fetal effects of rubella vaccination since 1971. In over 300 susceptible women who were immunized within 3 months of conception and whose pregnancies went to term, there were no fetal abnormalities (Cunningham et al., 1993). Pregnancy should be avoided for 3 months after rubella vaccination, even though there is no documentation of congenital rubella syndrome (CRS; Scott et al., 1993).

Pregnant women with chronic cardiac, pulmonary, or metabolic diseases should be evaluated carefully for immunization against influenza and pneumonia. Recommendations for travel immunizations during pregnancy by the American College of Obstetricians and Gynecologists with updates are summarized in Table 17-2.

The nurse advises the pregnant woman to minimize exposure to infectious diseases when traveling. Any febrile illness or rash should be reported to the physician without delay. Clients are educated about updating

TABLE 17–2
Immunizations During Pregnancy

LIVE VIRUS VACCINES (USUALLY CONTRAINDICATED DURING PREGNANCY)

Measles (rubeola)	Teratogenic; not given during pregnancy
Mumps	Measles immunoglobulin given for postexposure prophylaxis
Rubella	Teratogenic; not given during pregnancy
Poliomyelitis	Usually not given during pregnancy unless increased risk of exposure
Yellow fever	(endemic areas)

INACTIVATED/KILLED VIRUS VACCINES (MAY BE GIVEN DURING PREGNANCY IF INDICATED)

Influenza	Given when risk increased (severe pulmonary, cardiac disease or diabetes)
Haemophilus influenzae	Same indications as for nonpregnant clients
Pertussis	Same indications as for nonpregnant clients
Rocky Mountain spotted fever	Same indications as for nonpregnant clients
Rabies	Same indications as for nonpregnant clients
Hepatitis B	Not approved for use in pregnancy; benefits of vaccination may outweigh risks; must be negative for B antigen
Hepatitis A	Given postexposure or for travel to endemic areas

LIVE BACTERIAL VACCINES (USUALLY CONTRAINDICATED DURING PREGNANCY)

Bacillus of Calmette-Guerin	Not given during pregnancy
Tularemia	Not given during pregnancy

INACTIVATED OR KILLED BACTERIAL VACCINES (GIVEN DURING PREGNANCY WHEN INCREASED RISK OF EXPOSURE OR TO CONFER IMMUNITY IF INDICATED)

Pneumococcus	Given when risk increased (chronic cardiac, pulmonary, or metabolic disease)
Meningococcus	Same indications as for nonpregnant clients
Cholera	Given for travel to endemic areas
Typhoid	Given for travel to endemic areas
Typhus	Given for travel to endemic areas
Plague	Given for travel to endemic areas
Tetanus	Toxoid given if no primary series or booster within 10 years (same as non-pregnant client)
Diphtheria	

IMMUNOGLOBULINS (GIVEN DURING PREGNANCY FOR POSTEXPOSURE PROPHYLAXIS)

Hepatitis B	After exposure, hyperimmune globulin given with vaccine, then vaccine alone at 1 and 6 mo, infants of infected mothers also treated
Hepatitis A	After exposure, pooled immune globulins given
Measles	After exposure, pooled immune globulins given
Tetanus	After exposure, hyperimmune globulin given with vaccine (toxoid) in unvaccinated women
Varicella	After exposure, hyperimmune globulin given; infants of infected mothers also treated
Rabies	After exposure, hyperimmune globulin given

immunizations after delivery to reduce future risk. After receiving live organism vaccinations, clients are advised to avoid conception for the recommended time.

Care of Teeth

Good dental care is important during pregnancy. The teeth should be brushed at least twice daily, and flossed four to five times per week. An alkaline mouthwash may be used if desired. Gum hypertrophy, tenderness, ptyalism, heartburn, nausea, and vomiting may cause pregnant women to neglect dental practices; the nurse needs to encourage regular dental care despite discomforts.

A dental checkup in early pregnancy is recommended, with dental repair as indicated. The best time for routine, minor procedures is from the fourth to the seventh month, when the woman usually is less nauseated and feeling well. Any extensive dental work is better postponed until after delivery. If extensive care is necessary, the dentist and obstetrician or nurse-midwife should consult about management. Diagnostic dental x-rays should be avoided during pregnancy or delayed until late pregnancy. A lead apron over the abdomen provides protection.

The old saying, "For every child a tooth," based on a belief that the fetus takes calcium from the woman's teeth, has no real scientific basis. An adequate diet during pregnancy supplies the fetus with calcium and phosphorus in sufficient amounts to build bones and teeth.

Nursing Management of Minor Discomforts

Most women experience the minor discomforts of pregnancy to some degree in the course of a normal pregnancy. Not all women have these discomforts, and some go through the entire prenatal period without any. Although the discomforts are not serious, their presence detracts from the woman's feeling of comfort and well-being. In many instances, they can be avoided by preventive measures or reduced by healthful practices once they do occur (Table 17-3).

Gastrointestinal Discomforts

Nausea

Nausea and vomiting (**morning sickness**) are the most common discomforts of the first trimester of pregnancy. Nausea occurs in about half of all pregnant women; of these, about one-third experience some vomiting. Symptoms usually appear during the fourth to the sixth week and last until about the 12th week. Usually, symptoms occur in the morning only, but a small percentage of women may have nausea and vomiting throughout the entire day.

Altered hormonal status with high levels of human chorionic gonadotropin and progesterone is involved in producing these symptoms through effects on gastrointestinal smooth musculature. Changes in carbohydrate metabolism and other metabolic processes also may contribute to these symptoms.

Typically, morning sickness starts with a feeling of nausea when the woman arises. Vomiting often occurs when food is taken. By noon, the woman feels better and may have no further episodes until the next morning. The nausea may happen in the afternoon or in the evening. In a few women, nausea and vomiting may persist throughout the day and become worse in the afternoon. In the majority of women, this problem lasts from 1 to 3 months and then suddenly ceases. There may be slight loss of body weight but no other signs or symptoms.

Nursing Care. The nurse assesses patterns of nausea and vomiting and then suggests methods of relief. Nau-

sea in the early morning may be relieved by dry toast, plain popcorn, or crackers eaten slowly before getting up. Moving slowly and avoiding sudden position changes and rapid head turning help prevent nausea related to postural hypotension. The smell of certain foods may cause nausea and should be avoided. Eating frequent, small meals throughout the day, even every 2 hours, is helpful. Liquids (including soups) and dry foods should be separated by 1 to 2 hours. Meals should be high in protein or complex carbohydrates to stabilize blood sugar levels, avoiding hypoglycemia.

Greasy and spicy foods should be avoided, because these contribute to heartburn and excessive acid, both of which aggravate nausea. Sweet lemonade, ginger ale, cola, or spearmint, raspberry, or peppermint tea are often helpful after vomiting. An acupressure wrist band with a small button pressing on the inner wrist meridian may provide relief. Vitamin B_6 (pyridoxine, 10 to 30 mg daily) may be helpful in controlling nausea (Varner, 1990).

Pregnancies differ, and what may help one person may not benefit another. The trial-and-error method often is necessary to obtain results. If persistent vomiting develops or vomiting continues beyond the fourth month, this may signal a serious complication called hyperemesis gravidarum (see Chap. 31).

Heartburn

Heartburn results from diminished gastric motility, relaxation of the cardiac sphincter, and reverse peristaltic waves that cause regurgitation of the stomach contents into the esophagus. Irritation of the esophageal mucosa produces symptoms of burning discomfort behind the lower sternum, often radiating upward along the course of the esophagus. Heartburn is a gastrointestinal, not cardiac, condition with symptoms that include pain, belching, nausea, and epigastric pressure. Stress, tension, emotional disturbances, worry, fatigue, and improper diet may contribute to heartburn. Dietary fat, coffee, and cigarettes tend to make heartburn worse because they stimulate acid secretion in the stomach and irritate the mucosa. Eating several small meals daily instead of three large ones may help prevent heartburn. Wearing clothes that are loose around the waist is helpful. When heartburn occurs, it may be relieved with small sips of water, milk, or a carbonated drink. Lying down makes regurgitation worse, so it is best to sit upright. Relaxing and breathing deeply for several minutes may help. The "flying exercise" also is suggested: Sitting tailor fashion, the arms are raised and lowered quickly, bringing the hands together over the head; this is repeated several times.

When antacids are used, those with an aluminum hydroxide (Amphojel) or magnesium hydroxide (Maalox) base should be taken. Many over-the-counter

TABLE 17–3
Natural Remedies for Minor Discomforts of Pregnancy

Prevention	Natural Remedies	Medicines Not to Be Used[a]
NAUSEA AND VOMITING		
Eat high-protein meals and fruit and drink fruit juices to avoid hypoglycemia. Eat several small meals daily. Avoid fried foods. Drink liquids between meals rather than with meals. Get out of bed slowly, avoid sudden movements. Eat dry bread or crackers before rising (keep by bed). Eat yogurt or drink milk at night or before rising.	Eat dry bread or crackers. Sip soda water. Take a walk in fresh air. Drink spearmint, raspberry leaf, or peppermint tea.	Antihistamines (contained in most antinausea medicines)
HEADACHE		
Get enough sleep at night and enough rest during the day. Do not go for long periods without eating. Drink plenty of fluids. Avoid things that contribute to headaches (eg, eye strain, stuffy rooms, cigarette smoke, rushing around).	Apply a cool, wet washcloth to forehead and back of neck (some prefer warm cloth). Massage neck, shoulders, face, scalp, forehead. Take a walk in fresh air. Take a warm bath. Find a quiet place and relax. Meditate or do yoga.	Narcotic analgesics Aspirin, Excedrin, Percogesic, Cope Advil
DIFFICULTY SLEEPING		
Exercise daily. Take a warm bath at bedtime. Drink hot water with lemon or warm milk at bedtime. Do not eat a large meal within 2–3 h of bedtime. Decrease noise and lights. Do relaxation exercises. Use pillows under knees, back, or abdomen. Avoid caffeine.	Relax and do not worry about not sleeping; even lying in bed is restful to the body. Read for a while. Follow suggestions under prevention.	Sleeping aids (Sleep-Eze, Nytol, Sominex, Compoz, and so forth) Sedatives Tranquilizers
STUFFY NOSE AND ALLERGIES		
Avoid allergens. Do not smoke cigarettes; avoid smoke-filled rooms.	Breathe steam from hot shower, pot of boiling water, or vaporizer or humidifier. Drink plenty of liquids. Use salt-water nose drops (¼ tsp salt in 1 cup warm water). Use warm, moist towel on sinuses; massage sinuses.	Antihistamines (in most cold remedies—Contac, Coricidin, Allerest, Dristan, and so forth)
HEARTBURN		
Avoid foods known to cause gastric upset. Avoid greasy, fried foods. Avoid highly seasoned foods.	Take small sips of water. Sip carbonated beverage. Sit upright.	Sodium base antacids (eg, Maalox, Alka-Seltzer, Fizrin, Soda Mint, baking soda)

(continued)

TABLE 17–3 *(Continued)*
Natural Remedies for Minor Discomforts of Pregnancy

Prevention	Natural Remedies	Medicines Not to Be Used*
HEARTBURN		
Eat several small meals daily. Avoid coffee and cigarettes. Wear loose clothes at waist. Drink 6–8 glasses water daily.	Relax and breathe deeply for several minutes. Do the "flying exercise." Use aluminum-base antacids.	
FATIGUE		
Get enough sleep and rest. Take naps during the day. Pace daily life to provide for extra rest. Eat well-balanced meals. Exercise regularly.	Take the time to rest when the body demands it. Sit with feet up whenever possible. Follows suggestions under Prevention.	Caffeine (eg, coffee, tea, cola drinks, stay-awake pills) Amphetamines
LEG CRAMPS		
Get enough calcium (milk, dark green leafy vegetables, supplements). Exercise regularly. Keep the legs warm. Take a warm bath at bedtime. Do not point the toes when stretching.	Sit down, straighten the leg; point or pull toes upward toward the knees. Massage the cramped muscle. Walk around when able. Soak cramped muscle in warm water or use heating pad.	Quinine Muscle relaxants
CONSTIPATION		
Drink plenty of fluids (6–8 glasses of water daily). Exercise regularly. Eat raw vegetables, cooked fruit (eg, prune juice), 3 Tbsp bran daily, whole grain bread and cereal, oatmeal, brown rice. *Caution*—raw apples and coffee increase constipation. Chew food thoroughly. Have good bowel habits (do not force bowel movements; go when having the urge; take time for bowel movements; raise feet on stool to reduce strain).	Drink either hot or very cold liquid on an empty stomach. Follow suggestions under Prevention. Use bulk-producing laxatives (eg, Metamucil, Effersyllium).	Laxatives that are other than bulk producing (best to avoid all laxatives; at least use only twice per week; taking too many laxatives causes more constipation)
VARICOSE VEINS		
Exercise regularly. Avoid tight or binding clothes (especially garters, knee-length stockings). Wear full-length support hose when standing or walking for a long time. Avoid sitting or standing for a long time. Wear shoes with well-padded soles to absorb shock.	Lie with feet raised several times daily. Lie with feet against wall. Wear elastic support hose (put on before rising).	No medications
HEMORRHOIDS		
Prevent constipation and straining during bowel movements. Follow good bowel habits.	Sit in warm tub for 15–20 min three to four times daily.	Local anesthetic creams (Preparation H, Americaine, Anusol)

(continued)

TABLE 17–3 *(Continued)*
Natural Remedies for Minor Discomforts of Pregnancy

Prevention	Natural Remedies	Medicines Not to Be Used*
HEMORRHOIDS		
Do not sit for a long time on the toilet.	Apply dilute lemon juice or vinegar compresses; use Tucks or witch hazel compresses.	
Do Kegel exercises regularly.	Use bulk-producing laxatives to keep stool soft.	
BACKACHE		
Maintain good posture.	Do prenatal exercises (especially the pelvic tilt and knee–chest twist).	Analgesics
Bend from knees when lifting.	Apply heat to the lower back.	Aspirin, ibuprofen
Wear supportive shoes with low heels.	Have a back rub or back massage.	
Exercise regularly.	Rest the back.	
Do prenatal exercises or yoga.		
Maintain normal weight gain.		
EDEMA		
Eat high-protein foods.	Sit in warm bathtub or hot tub for 20–30 min.	Diuretics (prescriptions and over-the-counter water pills)
Avoid highly salted foods.	Lie or sit with legs raised as much as possible.	
Avoid standing for long periods.	Follow suggestions under prevention.	
Avoid tight clothing and constrictions of legs.		
Rest and elevate legs two to three times daily for 20 min.		

*In severe cases, the physician may prescribe a medication after weighing the benefits to the woman and risks to the fetus.

---

remedies contain sodium, which promotes water retention and could lead to edema. Women are advised to avoid Alka-Seltzer and baking soda (sodium bicarbonate), which are high in sodium ions.

Flatulence

Flatulence results from decreased gastrointestinal motility with delayed emptying, and pressure on the large bowel from the enlarging uterus. Bacterial action on foods in the intestines produces gas. Eating small amounts of food and masticating well may prevent this feeling of distress after eating. Regular daily elimination is important, and foods that form gas should be avoided (eg, beans, parsnips, corn, sweet desserts, fried foods, cake, and candy).

Backache

Most pregnant women experience some degree of backache. As pregnancy advances, the woman's posture changes to compensate for the weight of the growing uterus. The shoulders are thrown back as the enlarging abdomen protrudes, and to maintain body balance, the inward curve of the spine is exaggerated.

Relaxation of the sacroiliac joints, along with postural changes, causes varying degrees of backache after excessive strain, fatigue, bending, or lifting.

Pregnant women can prevent back strain through good posture and body mechanics and avoidance of fatigue. Appropriate shoes worn during periods of activity and a supporting girdle may be helpful. The key to good posture is to sit, stand, walk, and lie in a way that minimizes the hollow or curvature of the lower back. To do this, the abdominal and gluteal muscles are contracted and those of the lower back are relaxed, while the pelvis is tilted slightly upward and forward. The pelvic tilt exercise brings the pelvis into this alignment (see Chap. 19).

Sitting posture can be improved by using arm rests, foot supports, and a pillow for the back. The tailor position or semilotus position used for yoga helps relieve back pain. The woman should always bend from the knees rather than the back when lifting, keeping the spine straight. Avoiding forward leaning while doing chores and adjusting the height of the work surface to maintain proper posture when standing or sitting reduce back strain.

Daily exercises, such as walking, swimming, and stretching, are effective ways of preventing backache.

The knee–chest twist is a particularly beneficial exercise (see Chap. 19). When backache occurs, it may be relieved by applying a heating pad or hot water bottle to the lower back, having a back rub, or taking a warm bath.

Dyspnea

Difficult breathing or shortness of breath occasionally results from pressure on the diaphragm by the enlarged uterus. Dyspnea may interfere with sleep and comfort during the last weeks of pregnancy. It is relieved by lightening (settling of fetus into pelvis in late pregnancy) in primigravidas. Lying down makes dyspnea worse, and pillows used for propping in a semisitting posture may promote breathing and sleep. During the day, breathing is promoted by sitting straight and assuming good posture when standing.

Nasal Stuffiness

Congestion of nasal mucosa often results from elevated estrogen levels, which occur once pregnancy is well established. Mucosal edema causes nasal stuffiness, discharge, and obstruction. Epistaxis (nosebleed) may occur from hyperemic capillaries, aggravated by frequent blowing of the nose. Use of saline nose drops and steam or cool air vaporizors may relieve nasal stuffiness. When stuffiness interferes with sleep, women may self-medicate with nasal decongestant sprays. These provide temporary relief, but if used too frequently (more than 3 days), rebound edema results, exaggerating the nasal congestion. Their use is discouraged.

Varicose Veins

Varicose veins may occur in the lower extremities and extend to the vulva or into the pelvis. Varicosities are enlargements or pouches in veins due to thinning and stretching of the walls from abdominal pressure. Higher levels of abdominal pressure increase the incidence of varicosities of the lower extremities and the vulva. These distended areas often occur at short intervals along the course of the blood vessel, giving it a knotted, lumpy appearance. There is a hereditary tendency for varicosities, which is enhanced by weight gain, advancing age, multiple pregnancy, and activities that require prolonged standing or sitting.

During pregnancy, pressure from the enlarged uterus on the large pelvic and abdominal veins interferes with return of blood from the lower extremities. Symptoms include dull, aching pain in the legs due to distention of the deep vessels. A fine purple network of superficial veins may be seen. Varicosities appear as a tortuous mass of bluish or purplish veins, which may extend along the course of the veins of the legs, labia majora, vulva, vagina, and uterus.

Nursing Care. Varicose veins may be minimized by eliminating constricting garters, stockings, or other clothing that causes pressure on the legs or thighs. Maintaining normal weight and regular exercise helps prevent varicosities. The right-angle position relieves and decompresses varicosities; the woman lies on the floor with her buttocks and heels resting against a wall, legs extended upward (see Chap. 19). This position is assumed for 2 to 5 minutes several times a day. This position may be too difficult in late pregnancy because of pressure against the diaphragm. Support pantyhose can be used to support weak-walled leg veins. Pregnant women should avoid prolonged periods of standing or sitting and should avoid crossing legs at the knees and cross instead at the ankles. Pregnant women should sit with legs elevated whenever possible, being careful to avoid pressure points against the legs, which interfere with circulation, particularly in the popliteal space. Many women who must walk or stand for long periods wear support hose prophylactically. *Varicosities of the vulva* may be relieved by placing a pillow under the buttocks and elevating the hips or assuming the elevated Sims' position several times a day (Fig. 17-4). Pressure should be reduced by sitting and lying down as often as possible and minimizing standing.

Leg Cramps

Leg cramps are painful spasmodic muscular contractions that may occur at any time during the pregnancy but more often in late pregnancy. They are more frequent at night after going to bed but also occur during the day. Possible causes are calcium deficiency, pressure from the enlarged uterus on pelvic nerves and vasculature supplying the lower extremities, fatigue, chilling, tension, and calcium or phosphorus imbalance. Extension of the foot (pointing the toes) can provoke gastrocnemius muscle spasm, causing leg cramps.

Immediate relief may be obtained by forcing the toes upward and by putting pressure on the knee to straighten the leg. This stretches the gastrocnemius muscle, encouraging release of the spasm. Hot packs, massage, flexing the foot, and walking help relieve discomfort.

To prevent leg cramps, pregnant women can elevate the feet, keep the extremities warm, and avoid pointing the toes. Regular exercise promotes good circulation in the legs, and taking a warm bath before bedtime can improve circulation at night.

With frequent, severe leg cramps, the health provider may recommend reducing phosphorus intake. Milk contains calcium and phosphorus, and 1 quart

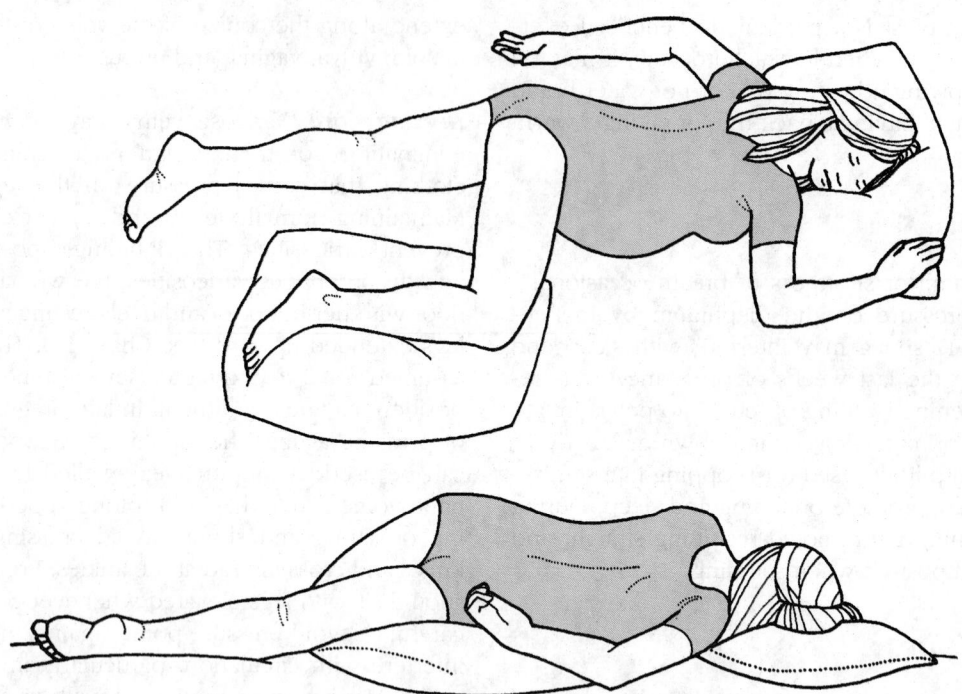

FIGURE 17-4 Sims' position for varicosities of the vulva and rectum.

daily (usual recommendation during pregnancy) may cause excess phosphorus in some women. Limiting milk to 1 pint daily with calcium lactate supplements or taking 1 quart of milk daily with aluminum hydroxide gel can reduce phosphorus intake. Aluminum hydroxide gel absorbs phosphorus and eliminates it through the intestinal tract, preventing its action on calcium and subsequent leg cramps.

Edema

Swelling of the lower legs and ankles is common during pregnancy, due to reduced venous return from lower extremities. Edema is aggravated by prolonged standing or sitting (**dependent edema**) and by hot weather. Providing abdominal support, resting frequently, elevating the feet, or taking the right-angle position often gives relief. Edema may be reduced by avoiding highly salted foods, eating high-protein foods, and avoiding tight clothing. Women who must remain standing or sitting for long periods need to elevate the legs for about 20 minutes every 2 to 3 hours and change position frequently. Dorsiflexion of the feet frequently while sitting helps contract leg muscles and stimulate circulation.

Resting with legs elevated has been the standard treatment for edema during pregnancy. Immersion in warm water is a safe and more rapid method than rest to mobilize extravascular fluid in pregnant women. A tub bath appears as effective as 1 hour of rest in reducing edema during pregnancy (Katz et al., 1990).

Edema of the ankles, feet, and even hands is common, particularly in late pregnancy. It can signal complications, however. *Edema is one of the signs of preeclampsia or pregnancy-induced hypertension.* Sudden weight gain of more than 2 lb/wk, edema of the face and sacrum, and proteinuria could indicate complications and must be brought to the physician's attention.

Vaginal Discharge

Increased vaginal discharge (leukorrhea) usually is physiologic, due to increased mucus production by endocervical glands and vaginal mucosal hyperplasia. Leukorrhea is white, consisting of mucus and exfoliated vaginal epithelial cells. Usually there is no odor, irritation, itching, or discomfort unless hygiene is poor. Increased acidity of vaginal secretions predisposes pregnant women to candidal infections. Thick, white, cottage cheese-like discharge with profuse vaginal and perineal pruritus may indicate yeast infection (condidiasis, *Monilia*). Clients should not self-medicate for possible vaginal infection but should seek medical care. Yellow or greenish, foul-smelling, irritating discharge may indicate bacterial vaginal infections (see Chap. 11).

Daily bathing or showering is advised for cleanliness and to prevent irritation or vaginal infections. Cotton underpants and cotton-crotch pantyhose promote air circulation and absorb moisture, reducing irritation and risk of infection. Douching is discouraged during pregnancy.

Carpal Tunnel Syndrome

Edema or adipose tissue deposition during pregnancy can produce carpal tunnel syndrome (CTS). This syndrome results from compression of the median nerve as it passes under the transverse carpal ligament of the wrist. Symptoms include numbness, tingling, or burning of the volar aspect of the thumb pad and several fingers. The affected hand(s) may be slightly weaker. Usually CTS is bilateral in pregnancy but may be unilateral. Repetitive hand motion can provoke or worsen CTS. When due to edema during pregnancy, CTS disappears after delivery.

Treatment is with a flexion splint worn during sleep and avoidance of aggravating motion. When symptoms are intense, clients may need cortisone injections into the carpal tunnel area. Rarely, surgery is performed to release the median nerve in retractive cases (Dunnihoo, 1992).

Drug Use During Pregnancy

All medication should be avoided or minimized during pregnancy. No medication (prescribed or over-the-counter) should be taken without the provider's knowledge and approval. Because of the rapid formation of fetal organ systems and development of cellular functions, the first trimester is a particularly susceptible time. However, ingestion of drugs at any time during pregnancy can potentially damage the fetus. The impact of a drug on the developing fetus may range from no measurable effect to such marked toxicity that the embryo is killed (aborted). Sublethal doses of drugs may result in gross anatomic defects or permanent metabolic or functional deficit.

Periods of Vulnerability

The first critical period is during the initial 13 days of gestation, when the conceptus is either killed or not affected by the chemical agent—an "all or nothing" effect. From days 13 to 56 of gestation (days 31–71 after the LMP) organogenesis is taking place, with formation of the various organ systems (Dunnihoo, 1992; Niebyl, 1990). During this time, chemical insult may produce congenital abnormalities (teratogenic effects). For the remainder of pregnancy, chemical agents, toxins, or infections can affect the fetus in subtle ways, damaging intellectual, behavioral, or organ system functioning.

Drugs and other chemical agents undergo various interactions in the body before combining with specific tissue receptors, through which they manifest their pharmacologic effect. The effects of drugs are influenced by route of administration, extent and rate of absorption, volume of distribution, rate and methods of metabolic degradation, and interactions with other compounds. Dosage and timing of ingestion in relation to organogenesis are critical. The Food and Drug Administration has categorized drugs according to possible teratogenic effects (Box 17-6).

The incidence of detectable congenital abnormalities increases from about 3% at birth to more than 7% at 1 year. This indicates that many minor anomalies are not detected until later in life (Dunnihoo, 1992). Health providers should document all medication or chemical exposures just prior to and during pregnancy. Some prescription drugs are well known for teratogenicity; others are suspect, but evidence is not definitive (see Appendix E). Many antibiotics, including penicillin de-

---

BOX 17–6
Drugs in Pregnancy: Food and Drug Administration Risk Categories

- *Category A* Controlled studies in women fail to demonstrate a risk to the fetus in the first trimester (and there is no evidence of risk in later trimesters), and the possibility of fetal harm appears to be remote.
- *Category B* Either animal reproduction studies have not demonstrated a fetal risk and there are no controlled studies in pregnant women, or animal reproduction studies have shown an adverse effect (other than a decrease in fertility) that was not confirmed in controlled studies in women in the first trimester (and there is no evidence of a risk in later trimesters).
- *Category C* Either studies in animals have revealed adverse effects on the fetus (teratogenic, embryocidal, or other effect) and there are no controlled studies in women, or studies in women and animals are not available. Drugs in this category should be given only if the potential benefit justifies the potential risk to the fetus.
- *Category D* There is positive evidence of human fetal risk, but the benefits from use in pregnant women may be acceptable despite the risk. The drug may be needed in a life-threatening situation or for a serious disease when safer drugs cannot be used or are ineffective.
- *Category X* Studies in animals or human beings have demonstrated fetal abnormalities, there is evidence of fetal risk based on human experience, or both, and the risk of the use of the drug in pregnant women clearly outweighs any possible benefit. The drug is contraindicated in women who are or may become pregnant.

(Based on information from Yaffe, S. J. [1990]. Introduction. In G. G. Briggs, R. K. Freeman, & Yaffe, S. J. [Eds.], Drugs in pregnancy and lactation [p. xiii]. Baltimore: Williams and Wilkins; and Food and Drug Administration labeling and prescription drug advertising. [1979]. Content and format for labeling for human prescription drugs. Federal Register 44 (June 26), 37434–37467.)

rivatives, erythromycins, and cephalosporins, may be used in pregnancy. Sulfa drugs should not be used during late pregnancy, because these can lead to hyperbilirubinemia if present in the newborn at delivery. Aminoglycosides, tetracyclines, chloramphenicol, metronidazole, trimethoprim, and nitrofurantoin should not be used. Whenever drugs are considered for pregnant women, the benefits must be carefully weighed against potential risks for the fetus.

About half of all drugs taken during pregnancy are over-the-counter products used to relieve symptoms. Most commonly used are preparations for nasal congestion, backache, headache, constipation, hemorrhoids, and heartburn. Some of these products can be dangerous. Aspirin inhibits prostaglandin synthesis and decreases uterine contractility and may delay onset of labor or prolong pregnancy or labor. It decreases platelet aggregation, which increases risk of bleeding. Nonsteroidal anti-inflammatory agents, such as ibuprofen and naproxen, may cause premature closure of the fetal ductus arteriosus and decreased amniotic fluid with prolonged use. One or two doses for short-term pain relief will not cause these problems (Gazaway et al., 1993). While no fetal effects have been found for antihistamines, decongestants, or cough suppressants, their use generally is not recommended during pregnancy. Acetaminophen (Tylenol) causes prostaglandin inhibition, which is rapidly reversed and cleared; often it is used for pain relief with no apparent harmful effects in pregnancy (Dunnihoo, 1992).

Prebirth Preparation

During the last few months of pregnancy, expectant women and families usually make preparations for labor, delivery, and newborn care. The nurse presents and reviews with them the following:

■ Recognizing signs of true versus false labor (see Chap. 21)

■ When to go to the hospital
■ Approaches to pain control
■ Supplies to bring for labor and postpartum
■ Planning for care of children at home
■ Signs of complications (see Client Teaching Guidelines: Danger Signs During Pregnancy)
■ Care of the newborn

Hospital Arrangements

Most hospitals offer tours of the maternity suite to expectant parents. Preregistration may be required, and orientation materials provide information about where to come when labor begins, visiting policies, what to bring, and planning for discharge. Becoming familiar ahead of time with the surroundings where the client will deliver the newborn reduces anxiety. Carrying out the details of the hospital admission during late pregnancy, rather than when the woman is in labor, can be reassuring and eliminates one possible cause of stress.

Community Resources

Prenatal classes offering extensive preparation for childbirth and parenting are widely available in most communities. Expectant parents are encouraged to attend classes (see Chap. 19). For those unable to attend formal classes, the nurse teaches as much basic prebirth preparation as possible in the healthcare setting.

When emotional and social problems are identified during pregnancy, the nurse makes referrals to community resources (eg, community health nurse, community services, counseling, social agencies). A home visit by the community health nurse may be helpful, because the family's home and surroundings can be assessed. The social worker works closely with the nurse, helping the pregnant woman and family cope with problems and transitions. These may include single parenthood, care of children during the mother's hospital stay, housekeeping arrangements, or financial assistance.

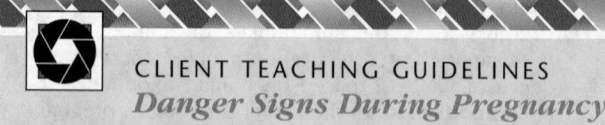

CLIENT TEACHING GUIDELINES
Danger Signs During Pregnancy

The pregnant woman should immediately report any of the following signs or symptoms to her healthcare provider:

Signs or Symptom	Potential Cause
Severe, persistent vomiting	Hyperemesis gravidarum
Fever, chills, dysuria	Infection
Abdominal pain, vaginal bleeding	Spontaneous abortion or miscarriage
Fluid drainage from vagina	Premature rupture of membranes
Decrease in fetal movements	Fetal compromise, anoxia
Swelling around face, fingers, over sacrum	Pregnancy-induced hypertension (PIH) or preeclampsia
Headache, blurred vision	PIH/preeclampsia

Preparation for the Newborn

The newborn's **layette** and equipment are assembled during later pregnancy, according to the family's interests and economic circumstances.

Layette

Newborn clothing should be comfortable, lightweight, and easy to put on and launder. The materials used must be fire resistant and nonirritating. Clothes that open down the full length and fasten with grippers are easier to put on. Clothing should not inhibit normal movements. The layette should include the following:

- Five to six shirts
- Three to four dozen diapers (or arrangements with diaper service)
- Four to six receiving blankets
- Three to six nightgowns
- Four to six waterproof diaper pads
- Two to three heavier blankets
- Two to four soft towels
- Two to four soft washcloths
- Two to three sweaters
- Several bibs
- Several socks, booties

Diapers

The selection of diapers is based on comfort (soft and lightweight), absorbency, cost, and washing and drying qualities. Commercial diaper services offer the company's diapers or will clean the mother's own. Disposable diapers are frequently used for convenience, but they may be more expensive than cloth diapers or a diaper service.

Nursery Equipment

Expense, space, and future plans all influence the selection of nursery equipment. Furniture should be suitable for and appealing to the child as he or she grows and develops. Equipment usually includes the following:

- Basket, bassinet, or crib
- After about 2 months, a crib, which should have bars close enough together to prevent the baby's head from being caught between them and should be painted with nonleaded paint
- Mattress that is firm (not hard), flat, and smooth; waterproof-covered or protected by a waterproof sheeting
- Sheets for mattress
- Chest or separate drawers for clothes
- Cotton crib blankets

- Bathtub (plastic tub is safe and easy to clean); some mothers adapt the kitchen or bathroom sink for the baby's bath
- Diaper pail that is large enough for at least 1 day's supply of soiled diapers
- Table or tray for holding supplies (eg, cotton balls, unscented soap, moisturizers, wipes)
- Chair (many mothers prefer rocking chairs)
- Nursery night light

Bottle-Feeding Equipment

- Five to six bottles (4 and 8 oz)
- Five to six nipples (various shapes can be helpful to determine newborn's sucking preferences)
- Brushes for cleaning bottles and nipples

Breast-Feeding Equipment

- Breast pump and cleaning equipment
- Four or five bottles and nipples for storing breast milk and supplemental feedings

Traveling Equipment

- Diaper bag with pockets for bottles, wipes, extra clothes, and so forth
- Stroller
- Car seat (Federally approved)
- Collapsible playpen

Summary Points

✔ Pregnancy is a normal process with extensive psychophysiologic changes. Most healthy families adapt well and experience positive growth during pregnancy and birth.

✔ Prenatal assessment is comprehensive, including physical, psychological, social, and emotional components. Screening for selected maternal and fetal problems is conducted at specific times during gestation.

✔ Care during pregnancy follows a regular schedule, with periodic screening and ongoing monitoring of physiologic changes, psychological adaptations, and social needs.

✔ Nurses have primary responsibility to provide teaching and anticipatory guidance through the stages of pregnancy and in preparation for birth and parenting.

✔ Exposure to teratogenic substances must be minimized. Pregnant women need information about dangers of substance use, workplace and household hazards, self-medication, and prescription drugs.

✔ Physiologic and anatomic changes during pregnancy may cause various minor discomforts. The nurse provides teaching about prevention and self-care measures to prevent or relieve these discomforts.

REFERENCES

Abrams, B., & Parker, J. D. (1990). Maternal weight gain in women with good pregnancy outcome. *Obstetrics and Gynecology, 76*(1), 1–7.

Affonso, D. D., & Mayberry, L. J. (1990). Common stressors reported by a group of childbearing American women. *Health Care for Women International, 11,* 331–345.

Albrecht, S. A., & Rankin, M. (1989). Anxiety levels, health behaviors, and support systems of pregnant women. *Maternal-Child Nursing Journal, 18*(1), 49–59.

Andrews, M. M., & Boyle, J. S. (1995). *Transcultural concepts in nursing care* (2nd ed.). Philadelphia: J.B. Lippincott.

Bates, B. (1995). *A guide to physical examination* (6th ed.). Philadelphia: J.B. Lippincott.

Calhoun, S. (1990). Ask the experts: Daily fetal movement counts. *NAACOG Newsletter, 17*(8), 6.

Centers for Disease Control Reports (1993). Pregnancy risks determined from birth certificate data—United States, 1989. *The Female Patient, 18*(3), 75–76.

Connors, G., et al. (1988). Maternally perceived fetal activity from twenty-four weeks' gestation to term in normal and at-risk pregnancies. *American Journal of Obstetrics and Gynecology, 158,* 294.

Crosby, W. M. (1983). Traumatic injuries during pregnancy. *Clinical Obstetrics and Gynecology, 26*(4), 902.

Cunningham, F. G., MacDonald, P. C., Gant, N. F., et al. (1993). *William's obstetrics,* (19th ed.). Norwalk, CT: Appleton & Lange.

Dunnihoo, D. R. (1992). *Fundamentals of gynecology and obstetrics* (2nd ed.). Philadelphia: J.B. Lippincott.

Ershoff, D. H., Mullen, P. D., & Quinn, V. P. (1989). A randomized trial of a serialized self-help smoking cessation program for pregnant women in an HMO. *American Journal of Public Health, 79,* 182–187.

Fishbein, E. G., & Phillips, M. (1990). How safe is exercise during pregnancy? *Journal of Obstetric, Gynecologic, and Neonatal Nursing, 19*(1), 45.

Frentzen, B., Dimperio, D. L. et al. (1988). Maternal weight gain: Effect on infant birth weight among overweight and average-weight low income women. *American Journal of Obstetrics and Gynecology, 159,* 1114–1117.

Freyder, S. C. (1989). Exercising while pregnant. *Journal of Orthopedic Sports Physical Therapy, 10,* 358.

Haiek, L., & Lederman, S. A. (1989). The relationship between maternal weight for height and term birth weight in teens and adult women. *Journal of Adolescent Health Care, 10,* 16–22.

Gabbe, S. (1986). Antepartum fetal evaluation. In S. Gabbe, J. Neiby, & J. Simpson (Eds.), *Obstetrics: Normal and problem pregnancies.* New York: Churchill Livingstone.

Gazaway, P. M., Niebyl, J. R., Repke, J. T. et al. (1993). Antibiotics, analgesics, arthritis drugs in pregnancy. *Patient Care, November 30,* 71–82.

Hammond, T. L. et al. (1990). The use of automobile safety restraint systems during pregnancy. *Journal of Obstetric, Gynecologic, and Neonatal Nursing, 19,* 339.

Henriksen, T. B., Savitz, D. A., Hedegaard, M., & Secher, N. J. (1994). Employment during pregnancy in relation to risk factors and pregnancy outcome. *British Journal of Obstetrics and Gynaecology, 101*(10), 858–865.

Jack, B. W., & Empkie, T. M. (1987). Routine obstetric ultrasound. *American Family Physician, 35*(5), 173–182.

Katz, V. L., Ryder, R. M., Cefalo, R. C. et al. (1990). A comparison of bed rest and immersion for treating the edema of pregnancy. *Obstetrics and Gynecology, 75*(2), 147–151.

Krozy, R. E., & McColgan, J. J. (1985). Automobile safety, pregnancy and the newborn. *Journal of Obstetric, Gynecologic, and Neonatal Nursing, 14,* 11.

Launer, L. J. et al. (1990). The effect of maternal work on fetal growth and duration of pregnancy: A prospective study. *British Journal of Obstetrics and Gynaecology, 97,* 62.

Leaf, D. A. (1989). Exercise during pregnancy. *Postgraduate Medicine, 85*(1), 233.

Manson, J. E., Colditz, G. A., & Stampfer, N. J. (1994). Parity, ponderosity, and the paradox of a weight-preoccupied society. *Journal of the American Medical Association, 271,* 1788–1790.

Mayer, J. P., Hawkins, B., & Todd, R. (1990). A randomized evaluation of smoking cessation interventions for pregnant women at a WIC clinic. *American Journal of Public Health, 80,* 76–78.

McDonald, A. et al. (1988). Fetal death and work in pregnancy. *British Journal of Industrial Medicine, 45,* 148.

National Institute of Medicine, Subcommittee on Nutritional Status and Weight Gain During Pregnancy (1990). *Nutrition during pregnancy. Part I-Weight gain. Part II-Nutritional supplements.* Washington, DC: National Academy of Sciences.

Niebyl, J. R. (1994). Teratology and drugs in pregnancy and lactation. In J. R. Scott et al. (Eds.), *Danforth's obstetrics and gynecology* (7th ed.). Philadelphia: J.B. Lippincott.

Oakley, A., Rajan, L., & Grant, A. (1990). Social support and pregnancy outcome. *British Journal of Obstetrics and Gynaecology, 97,* 155.

Paisley, J. P., & Mellion, M. B. (1988). Exercise during pregnancy. *American Family Physician, 38*(5), 143.

Raine, T., et al. (1994). The risk of repeating low birth weight and the role of prenatal care. *Obstetrics and Gynecology, 84,* 485–489.

Sady, S. P. et al. (1989). Aerobic exercise during pregnancy: Special considerations. *Sports Medicine, 7*(6), 357.

Scott, J. R., DiSaia, P. J., Hammond, C. B., Spellacy, W. N. (Eds.). (1994). *Danforth's obstetrics and gynecology,* 7th Edition. Philadelphia: J. B. Lippincott.

Seidman, D. S., Ever-Hadani, P., & Gale, R. (1989). The effect of maternal weight gain in pregnancy on birth weight. *Obstetrics and Gynecology, 74*(2), 240–246.

Smith, D. E., Lewis, C. E., Caveny, J. L. et al. (1994). Longitudinal changes in adiposity associated with pregnancy: The CARDIA study. *Journal of the American Medical Association, 271,* 1747–1751.

University of California Berkeley Wellness Letter (1994). Having babies at any age. *School of Public Health, 11*(1), 6.

Varner, M. (1994). General medical and surgical diseases in pregnancy. In J. R. Scott et al. (Eds.), *Danforth's obstetrics and gynecology* (7th ed.). Philadelphia: J.B. Lippincott.

Walker, D. S. (1994). *Evaluation of an alternative prenatal care visit schedule for low risk pregnant women.* Ann Arbor, MI: UMI Dissertation Services.

Woodward, S. L. (1981). How does strenuous maternal exercise affect the fetus? A review. *Birth and Family Journal, 8*(1), 17–24.

18

Nutritional Care in Pregnancy

Objectives

- Discuss the importance of maternal nutrition during pregnancy to the well-being of the woman, fetus, and newborn.
- Describe methods for assessing nutritional status and dietary patterns of the pregnant woman.
- Identify the possible risk factors associated with nutritional problems.
- Discuss the nutrient needs for the pregnant client.
- Relate weight gain during pregnancy to maternal well-being and pregnancy outcomes.
- Summarize the nutritional knowledge needed by the nurse to provide appropriate dietary counseling to pregnant clients.
- Compare nutritional needs and concerns of the pregnant adolescent with those of pregnant adults and nonpregnant adolescents.

Key Terms

Aflatoxins	Ketonemia
Anthropometric	Minerals
measurements	Pica
Body mass index	Protein
Carbohydrates	Recommended dietary
Complete protein	allowances
Dietary faddism	vegan
Essential amino acids	Vegetarianism
Fat	Vitamins
Food additives	
Gynecologic age	

Nutrition plays a key role in the outcome of pregnancy. A woman's nutritional status at conception and the quality of the diet she consumes during the subsequent months help to determine her health and well-being and that of her fetus. Although ensuring optimum nutrition for all childbearing women may not eliminate all the problems of pregnancy, it is an important step.

If counseling is to be effective and the results lasting, the nurse needs to elicit the client's cooperation. This cooperation may be facilitated by involving her in the planning; considering her needs, background, preferences, and attitudes and those of her family; providing information; encouraging and reinforcing appropriate choices and preparation; providing gentle but firm limit setting when indicated; and giving careful, thorough explanation regarding the rationale behind the advice.

If the pregnant woman is helped to understand the importance of good nutrition for herself and her fetus, she may be more motivated now than at any other time in her life to improve her dietary habits. She should be encouraged to continue her new interest in nutrition after the newborn arrives. These improvements can have long-lasting effects on her family. Not only does improved nutrition promote better health for the family, it also can have a positive effect on future pregnancies of the mother and her children.

This chapter uses a nursing process framework to discuss the nutritional care of the pregnant client. Necessary components of assessment, including information about dietary intake, nutritional status, dietary factors, food choices and possible nutritional risk factors are presented. Examples of nursing diagnoses related to pregnancy and nutrition are identified. Specific information related to dietary counseling, including adequate weight gain, nutrient needs, dietary planning,

available resources, and supplementary programs, is described to inform the reader of key areas of nursing planning and intervention. Special nutritional concerns for the pregnant adolescent client also are presented. The chapter concludes with a discussion of how to evaluate the effectiveness of nutritional care interventions, including a listing of possible client outcomes.

Importance of Nutrition During Pregnancy

The importance of maternal nutrition during pregnancy has long been recognized. A report in 1970 from the National Academy of Sciences, which reviewed studies of reproductive experiences, concluded that adequate prenatal nutrition is one of the most important environmental factors affecting the health of pregnant women and their newborns (Committee on Maternal Nutrition, 1970).

Nutritional advice for pregnant women has been a consistent component of prenatal care, but the advice given has varied widely. At times, diets have been severely restricted, while at other times, women have been encouraged to eat large quantities. Specific nutrients, such as protein or salt, have sometimes been restricted and at other times increased. Guidelines continue to change according to the nutritional wisdom of the time, but current emphasis is on a varied diet consisting of adequate amounts of known nutrients.

Animal studies often show a direct relationship between maternal diet and pregnancy outcome. However, studies to determine direct cause-and-effect relationships between specific nutrients and specific problems are not possible in humans. Some general correlations have been found in naturally occurring situations. For example, chronic malnutrition in developing countries and in low-income populations of developed countries has been shown to be related to reproductive problems, including difficulties during pregnancy, labor, and delivery; increased perinatal mortality; and low birth weight and other problems of the newborn (Worthington-Roberts, 1993b).

Some historic events also have demonstrated the effects of nutritional deprivation under conditions that would not have been set up purposely. During World War II, a 7-month food embargo of western Holland decreased the population's average daily food ration to fewer than 750 calories. In a retrospective study, women who were pregnant or who conceived during this time were shown to have a higher incidence of stillbirth and neonatal mortality and decreased newborn birth weight (Rosso et al., 1979). Similar effects on pregnancy were found during the siege of Leningrad in 1941 and 1942.

ASSESSMENT TOOL
Nutritional Questionnaire for Pregnant Women

Name: _____ I.D.#: _____ Date: _____

Please answer the following questions by checking the appropriate box "yes" or "no" or by filling in the blank. Answer only the questions that apply to you. All information is confidential.

1. a. How many times have you been pregnant?
   b. If you have children, list their birth dates and birthweights below.

   Birth date and birthweight   Birth date and birthweight

   _____   _____

   _____   _____

   _____   _____

2. Do you now have or have you ever had any of the following?

Yes No		Yes No		Yes No	
☐ ☐	Abnormal Pap smear	☐ ☐	Liver disease/hepatitis	☐ ☐	Premature infant
☐ ☐	Allergy/asthma	☐ ☐	Tuberculosis	☐ ☐	Infant weighing less than 5½ lb (2500 g)
☐ ☐	Anemia	☐ ☐	Venereal disease	☐ ☐	Infant weighing more than 8 lb 13 oz. (4000 g)
☐ ☐	Cancer	☐ ☐	Miscarriage		
☐ ☐	Diabetes	☐ ☐	Twins/triplets	☐ ☐	Infant with medical problems
☐ ☐	Heart disease	☐ ☐	Cesarean delivery		
☐ ☐	High blood pressure	☐ ☐	Excessive bleeding during/after delivery	☐ ☐	Infant death
☐ ☐	Intestinal problems				
☐ ☐	Kidney disease				
☐ ☐	Other _____				

3. Have you had any of the following during this pregnancy?

Yes No		Yes No		Yes No	
☐ ☐	Nausea	☐ ☐	Diarrhea	☐ ☐	Stress
☐ ☐	Vomiting	☐ ☐	Heartburn	☐ ☐	Cold or flu
☐ ☐	Constipation or hemorrhoids	☐ ☐	Leg cramps	☐ ☐	Other illness _____

4. a. Before this pregnancy, what was your usual weight? _____ Pounds/kilos ☐ Don't know

   b. If you have been pregnant before, how much weight did you gain during your last pregnancy?

   _____ Pounds/kilos   _____ Don't know

   c. How much weight do you expect to gain during this pregnancy?

   _____ Pounds/kilos   _____ Don't know

5. a. How often do you exercise (besides housework, child care)? _____

   b. What types of exercise do you do? _____

   (continued)

ASSESSMENT TOOL *(Continued)*
Nutritional Questionnaire for Pregnant Women

6. During your pregnancy, have you wanted to eat any of the following?

Yes No   Yes No   Yes No
☐ ☐ Ice or freezer frost   ☐ ☐ Laundry starch   ☐ ☐ Plaster
☐ ☐ Cornstarch   ☐ ☐ Dirt or clay   ☐ ☐ Other: _____

7. Are there any foods that you avoid eating?   ☐ Yes   ☐ No   If yes, what: _____
_____ Why? _____

8. Are you now on any of these special diets?

Yes No   Yes No   Yes No
☐ ☐ Diabetic   ☐ ☐ Low salt   ☐ ☐ High protein
☐ ☐ Low fat   ☐ ☐ Weight loss   ☐ ☐ Other: _____

If yes, who suggested the diet? _____

9. a. Are you a vegetarian?   ☐ Yes   ☐ No

    b. If yes, do you consume milk products (milk, cheese, yogurt) and/or eggs?   ☐ Yes   ☐ No

10. During this pregnancy, are you taking the following?

Yes No   Yes No   Yes No

☐ ☐ Prenatal vitamin-mineral formula   ☐ ☐ Antihistamines or cold remedies   ☐ ☐ Birth control pills
                     ☐ ☐ Other prescription drugs
☐ ☐ Iron   ☐ ☐ Laxatives or antacids   ☐ ☐ Marijuana/cocaine
☐ ☐ Other vitamins   ☐ ☐ Other nonprescription drugs   ☐ ☐ Other drugs
☐ ☐ Other minerals
☐ ☐ Aspirin

11. How many cups of the following liquids do you usually drink per day?

_____ Water   _____ Sodas with sugar   _____ Coffee
_____ Juice   _____ Diet soda, diet punch   _____ Tea
_____ Milk   _____ Punch, Kool-Aid, Tang   _____ Other: _____

12. a. How often do you drink beer, wine, hard liquor, or mixed drinks? ☐ Daily ☐ Weekly ☐ Monthly

    b. When you drink, how many drinks do you have? ☐ One ☐ Two ☐ Three ☐ More

    c. During this pregnancy, how many times have you had more than four drinks on any single occasion?

_____

13. How many cigarettes do you smoke each day?

☐ Do not smoke   ☐ Fewer than 10 cigarettes   ☐ 11–20 cigarettes   ☐ More than 20 cigarettes

14. What is the highest grade or year of regular school you have completed?

☐ Less than 6 years   ☐ Two-year college (14 years)
☐ Elementary school (6 years)   ☐ Four-year college (16 years)
☐ Junior high school (9 years)   ☐ Graduate school (17+ years)
☐ High school (12 years)

(continued)

ASSESSMENT TOOL *(Continued)*
Nutritional Questionnaire for Pregnant Women

15. Do you live: ☐ Alone ☐ With own family ☐ With other people

16. Check if you have the following: ☐ Stove ☐ Oven ☐ Refrigerator

17. a. Do you plan your own meals? ☐ Yes ☐ No
    b. Do you buy your own food? ☐ Yes ☐ No
    c. Do you prepare your own food? ☐ Yes ☐ No

18. How would you describe the type and amount of food in your household?
    ☐ Enough of the kind you want   ☐ Sometimes not enough
    ☐ Enough, but not always the kind you want   ☐ Often not enough

19. Are you receiving any of the following?
    ☐ Food stamps   ☐ Medi-Cal   ☐ Donated food/meals
    ☐ WIC   ☐ AFDC/welfare   ☐ Other: _____

20. a. How do you plan to feed your baby?
    ☐ Breast-feed   ☐ Both breast and formula
    ☐ Formula-feed   ☐ Other: _____

    b. Have you ever breast-fed or tried to breast-feed before? ☐ Yes ☐ No

    c. If yes, how long did you breast-feed? _____

    d. Why did you stop breast-feeding? _____

(Nutrition During Pregnancy and the Postpartum Period: A Manual for Health Care Professionals. Sacramento, Maternal and Child Health Branch, WIC Supplemental Food Branch, California Department of Health Services, 1989)

Programs such as the Special Supplemental Food Program for Women, Infants, and Children (WIC) in the United States and the Higgins Nutrition Intervention Program in Canada were developed to improve the nutritional status of pregnant women. These programs have been studied in an attempt to demonstrate the effects of improved nutrition on the pregnancies of women whose nutritional status was deficient. Although results have varied, most studies have generally substantiated the belief that improving maternal nutrition during pregnancy is important for optimal maternal and fetal outcome (Trouba et al., 1991). Studies that have attempted to determine the effects of nutrition on mental development have experienced difficulty differentiating between prenatal and postnatal nutritional effects. The critical period for brain cell development begins during pregnancy and continues during the first year of life. The development of brain cells in a nutritionally deprived fetus may be decreased, but if opti-

mum nutrition is provided after birth, the effects may be reversible (Winick, 1979).

Records show that children whose conception, gestation, or birth occurred during the 1944 to 1945 Dutch famine but who had mothers who were well-nourished before and after the famine had significantly lower birth weights than was expected for that population in nonfamine times. Intelligence tests later in life, however, failed to show significant differences between famine and nonfamine subjects (Stein, 1975). In other study populations in which malnutrition during and after pregnancy was associated with other forms of environmental deprivation, mental retardation and severe, long-lasting behavioral effects, such as learning disabilities, were more frequent. The Montreal Diet Dispensary study indicates that improved nutrition during pregnancy and lactation improved the mental development of the children in the study, compared with siblings who were born before the mother received supplements (Higgins, 1973).

ASSESSMENT TOOL
Dietary Intake (24-hour recall)

Do Not Write In This Space
Intake Summary

Name		Age	Height	Weight	Animal protein	Veg. protein	Milk products	Breads/cereals/grains	Vit C frt/veg	Vit A frt/veg	Other fruits/veg	Fats/sweets/other foods
Time	Place	Amount	Foods Eaten									
Influences on Diet, Comments and Follow-up			Servings Eaten									
			Servings Needed									
			Difference									
Condition/ Diagnosis	Visit No.	Weeks Gestation	Date	Interviewer								

Sample Instructions for Completing A 24-Hour Diet Recall

1. Please write down everything, all foods and liquids, that you consumed during the last 24 hours—from the time you awakened yesterday morning until you awakened this morning.
2. Indicate the amount actually eaten, not how much was put in the dish.
3. Use measuring cups or spoons to describe the amount. For example:
   1 cup cornflakes
   ½ cup milk (whole)
   1 tsp sugar
4. For pieces of food that do not fit into a cup or spoon, write down the size. For example:
   1 tortilla (6 in across)
   1 piece cheese (3 × 3 × ¼ in)
5. Tell what is in a mixed food. For example:
   1 cup stew (¼ cup meat, ¼ cup potato, ¼ cup carrot, ¼ cup gravy)
6. Describe preparation method. For example:
   1 chicken drumstick (fried in shortening, no flour or batter)
7. Remember to write down the little things like butter, jelly, sugar, gravy, or salad dressing.
8. Remember to write down the snacks and drinks between meals.

(Nutrition During Pregnancy and the Postpartum Period: A Manual for Health Care Professionals. Sacramento, Maternal and Child Health Branch, WIC Supplemental Food Branch, California Department of Health Services, 1989)

Assessment

Each pregnant woman brings with her a unique nutritional background. Many factors influence her daily food intake and her nutritional status. To help these women choose the best possible diets during their pregnancy, the nurse needs to be aware of the factors, their effect on each person, and ways of obtaining information about them.

Assessing Dietary Intake

Gathering information about the client's food habits and actual food intake requires a comfortable atmosphere that allows the woman to discuss her concerns about food and diet and to provide information about her current dietary patterns. Nutritional assessment requires information about what is eaten, the quantities consumed, and the method of preparation. Information regarding purchasing practices also is needed; for

ASSESSMENT TOOL
Nutritional Assessment for Pregnant Women

Source   Date

Identification

Nutritional Risk Factors

Very overweight ☐	Hypovolemia ☐	Medical/obstet. complications ☐
Underweight ☐	Prev. obstet. complications ☐	Low income ☐
Inadequate gain ☐	Adolescence ☐	Substance abuse ☐
Excessive gain ☐	High parity ☐	Pica ☐
Anemia ☐	Short inter-preg. interval ☐	Psychological problems ☐

Visit 1

Date _____

Week gest. _____

Weight _____

BP _____

Comment _____

Alb _____

Glu _____

Ket _____

Edema _____

Dietary Assessment

Daily avg. from _____ days:

Food Group	Min. Amt./ Serv.	Amt./ Serv. Eaten	Sugg. Change
Animal protein	6 oz.	_____	_____
Vegetable protein	1	_____	_____
Milk products	3	_____	_____
Breads/cereals/grains	7	_____	_____
Vit. C-rich frt./veg.	1	_____	_____
Vit. A-rich frt./veg.	1	_____	_____
Other fruit/veg.	3	_____	_____

Excessive: ☐ Fat   ☐ Sugar   ☐ Salt
            ☐ Caffeine   ☐ Alcohol

Comments:

Prenatal Weight Gain Grid

Age (at conception) _____

Prepregnant weight: _____

Height (w/o shoes) _____

Desirable weight: _____

% Desirable weight: _____

Body mass index: _____

Term weight goal: _____

(Weight Gain (lb) vs. Weeks Gestation grid)

Laboratory Observations

TEST	Values			
	Date	Date	Date	Date
Hemoglobin (g/dl)				
Hematocrit (%)				
MCV (μ^3 or fL)				
Cervical cytology				
1-hour oral glucose load				

(continued)

Visit 2

Date _____
Week gest. _____
Weight _____
BP _____
Comment _____
Alb _____
Glu _____
Ket _____
Edema _____

Dietary Assessment

Daily avg. from ____ days:

Food Group	Min. Amt./Serv.	Amt./Serv. Eaten	Sugg. Change
Animal protein	6 oz.		
Vegetable protein	1		
Milk products	3		
Breads/cereals/grains	7		
Vit. C-rich frt./veg.	1		
Vit. A-rich frt./veg.	1		
Other fruit/veg.	3		

Excessive: ☐ Fat ☐ Sugar ☐ Salt ☐ Caffeine ☐ Alcohol

Comments:

Visit 3

Date _____
Week gest. _____
Weight _____
BP _____
Comment _____
Alb _____
Glu _____
Ket _____
Edema _____

Dietary Assessment

Daily avg. from ____ days:

Food Group	Min. Amt./Serv.	Amt./Serv. Eaten	Sugg. Change
Animal protein	6 oz.		
Vegetable protein	1		
Milk products	3		
Breads/cereals/grains	7		
Vit. C-rich frt./veg.	1		
Vit. A-rich frt./veg.	1		
Other fruit/veg.	3		

Excessive: ☐ Fat ☐ Sugar ☐ Salt ☐ Caffeine ☐ Alcohol

Comments:

Visit 4

Date _____
Week gest. _____
Weight _____
BP _____
Comment _____
Alb _____
Glu _____
Ket _____
Edema _____

Dietary Assessment

Daily avg. from ____ days:

Food Group	Min. Amt./Serv.	Amt./Serv. Eaten	Sugg. Change
Animal protein	6 oz.		
Vegetable protein	1		
Milk products	3		
Breads/cereals/grains	7		
Vit. C-rich frt./veg.	1		
Vit. A-rich frt./veg.	1		
Other fruit/veg.	3		

Excessive: ☐ Fat ☐ Sugar ☐ Salt ☐ Caffeine ☐ Alcohol

Comments:

(Nutrition During Pregnancy and the Postpartum Period: A Manual for Health Care Professionals. Sacramento, Maternal and Child Health Branch, WIC Supplemental Food Branch, California Department of Health Services, 1990)

example, who does the shopping, and what factors determine choices? Many useful tools have been developed to assist in data collection to make an accurate assessment of the client's usual dietary intake.

Many useful tools have been developed to assist in data collection to make an accurate assessment of the client's usual dietary intake. Three are included in this text (see Assessment Tools). The *Nutritional Questionnaire for Pregnant Women* is designed to be completed by the client at her first prenatal visit. The *Dietary Intake (24 hour recall)* form can be used by the client or caregiver to record what the client recalls having eaten during the past 24 hours; as a food diary for the client to record her intake for 2 to 3 days; or as a dietary history for the caregiver to record answers to questions about the client's food intake for a usual day. The *Nutritional Assessment for Pregnant Women* provides space to record ongoing assessment and progress from visit to visit.

Regardless of which assessment tool is used, some questions may not be applicable to all client populations, and some may require further clarification during the interview. The client should be instructed that when she is recording information, whether for a 24-hour recall or a food record or diary, she should include the time, place, type, and amount of food eaten. She also should be instructed to avoid recording intake on holidays or days with atypical diet patterns. Instructions should be given for writing down amounts of each food as accurately as possible. When using a food diary, the importance of recording everything as soon after eating as possible should be stressed. Some women have difficulty remembering to write things down, but even if the diary is incomplete, it can still provide useful information.

Assessing Nutritional Status

A number of methods can be used to assess a woman's nutritional status. The following are examples.

Anthropometric measurements include various objective, noninvasive measurements of body size and composition. Height and weight are the most common measurements taken. Comparing height with pregravid weight gives an estimate of body build, which is useful in determining standard weight and identifying the underweight person. Recording weight at intervals throughout the pregnancy also allows comparison of the person's weight gain pattern with the recommended pattern (see prenatal weight gain grid on the Assessment Tool: Nutritional Assessment for Pregnant Women) (Fig. 18-1). Measurement also can include the use of tape measures and calipers for arm muscle circumference and skin fold thickness, but these are not necessary for most women and are not done routinely.

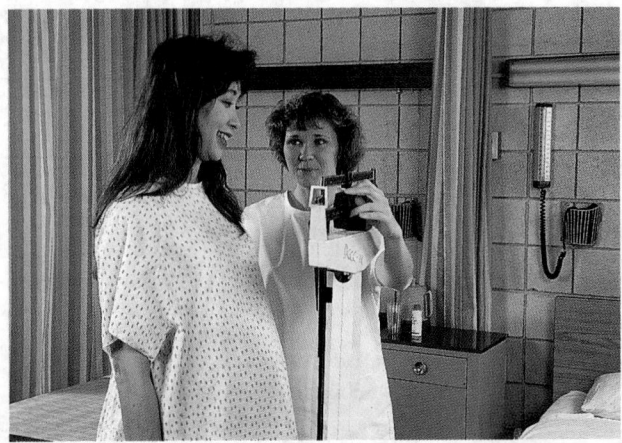

FIGURE 18–1 Recording weight at intervals throughout pregnancy allows the nurse to determine if the client's weight gain pattern compares with the recommended pattern.

Laboratory tests are used to determine the presence of adequate amounts of certain nutrients. Hemoglobin and hematocrit are measured routinely to evaluate the woman's iron status and need for supplements. The serum folacin level may be used as an indicator of the adequacy of nutritional intake. Determination also might be made of serum albumin, total serum protein, and serum vitamin B_{12}. Additional hematologic values may be obtained when assessing specific nutrient-related problems (California Department of Health Services, 1990).

General physical assessment of the pregnant woman can provide useful information in assessing nutritional status. Alone, the signs may not be reliable indicators, but together and with laboratory tests and dietary history, they can provide useful clues for further investigation (Table 18-1).

Assessing Individual Dietary Factors Involved in Food Choices

Assessment of factors involved in how an individual chooses what, when, where, and how much to eat provides important information for nutritional counseling. The factors on which food choices are based include psychological aspects of nutrition; stage of growth and development; religious, racial, or ethnic background; specific dietary patterns; and food allergies (Table 18-2).

The *psychological aspects* of nutrition are important determinants of food choice but are not easily analyzed. Food preferences result from a combination of heritage, superstition, custom, knowledge, and opportunity. Pregnant women may crave or reject certain foods, due more to symbolic meanings of the food

TABLE 18-1
Selected Clinical Signs for Nutritional Evaluation

Body Area	Clinical Signs	Possible Nutritional Implications
Hair	Dull, dry, sparse, shedding, or lightening of normal color	Protein-calorie malnutrition (Also may be due to hypothyroidism)
Face	General lightening of skin color	Protein-calorie malnutrition
	Scaling with dry, greasy, gray, or yellowish threadlike material around nostrils; also on bridge of nose, eyebrows, and back of ears; sebaceous gland ducts plugged	Riboflavin, niacin, or pyridoxine deficiency (Also may be due to poor hygiene)
Eyes	Pale conjunctivae	Iron, folate, or B_{12} deficiency
	Redness of membranes; redness and fissuring of eyelid corners	Riboflavin and niacin deficiency
	Dryness of membranes; dullness of cornea	Vitamin A deficiency
Lips	Cracks, redness, and flaking at corners of the mouth; scars at corners of the mouth; important only if bilateral	Riboflavin, niacin, iron, and pyridoxine deficiency (also results from poor dentures, herpes, and syphilis)
	Vertical cracks on lips, usually in center of the lower lip; red, swollen, and inner mucosa appearing to extend out onto the lip; may be ulcerated.	Riboflavin and niacin deficiency (Also may occur from environmental exposure)
Tongue	Pale	Iron deficiency
	Purplish red (magenta)	Riboflavin deficiency
	Taste buds atrophied; tongue smooth, pale, and slick (even when slightly scraped)	Folate, niacin, riboflavin, iron, or B_{12} deficiency (Also may occur in non-nutritional anemia)
	Tongue beefy, red, painful, and taste buds atrophied; usually hypersensitivity, burning, and even taste changes, especially when eating; oral mucosa possibly red and swollen.	Niacin, folate, riboflavin, iron, B_{12}, pyridoxine, and tryptophan deficiency
Teeth	Carious or missing	Excessive intake of carbohydrate (sucrose) or alcohol, poor hygiene, or multiple nutrient inadequacies (eg, calcium)
	Mottled enamel	Fluorine excess
Gums	Swollen, bleeding	Vitamin C deficiency (Also may be caused by chronic overdoses of hydantoinates [eg, Dilantin], poor hygiene, and lymphoma)
Glands	Thyroid enlargement (goiter)	Iodine inadequacy or toxicity (Also may be caused by cysts, tumors, and hyperthyroidism)
Skin	Dry, flaking, or scaly; skin like sandpaper	Vitamin A or essential fatty acid deficiency (also occurs with fungus infection, syphilis, and so forth)
	Petechiae (small purple spots or hemorrhages under the skin)	Vitamin C and vitamin K deficiency (also occurs in hematologic disorders, trauma, liver disease, and anticoagulant overdose)
	Poor turgor or tone; pressure sores	Multiple nutrient inadequacies, especially of protein and vitamin C
	Xanthomas (fat deposits under the skin, around joints, and under the eyes)	Increased serum levels of low-density lipoproteins or very low-density lipoproteins with resultant hyperlipoproteinemia
Nails	Brittle, ridged, or spoon-shaped	Iron deficiency (Also may occur in thalassemia)
Abdomen	Edematous	Protein-calorie malnutrition
Extremities	Muscle wasting	Protein-calorie malnutrition
	Edematous	Protein-calorie malnutrition

(continued)

TABLE 18–1 *(Continued)*
Selected Clinical Signs for Nutritional Evaluation

Body Area	Clinical Signs	Possible Nutritional Implications
Nervous system	Listless and apathetic	Protein deficiency
	Mental irritability and confusion	Protein deficiency
	Sensory loss	Thiamin deficiency
	Motor weakness (inability to squat and then stand three to four times in a row)	Thiamin deficiency
	Loss of vibratory sense (significant only if bilateral)	Thiamin and B_{12} deficiency (or other cause of peripheral neuropathy)
	Loss of ankle and knee jerks (significant only if absolute and bilateral)	Thiamin and B_{12} deficiency (or other cause of peripheral neuropathy)
	Calf tenderness (significant only if bilateral)	Thiamin deficiency (or deep vein thrombosis and other causes of peripheral neuropathy)

Source: Maternal and Child Health Branch, WIC Supplemental Food Branch, California Department of Health Services (1990). *Nutrition during pregnancy and the postpartum period: a manual for health care professionals.* Sacramento: Author.

than to any physiologic factors. It is crucial that the meaning that food has for the client be explored and that her feelings and attitudes be respected.

The *stage of growth and development* of the client also may influence her food choices. For instance, foods enjoyed by adolescents are often different from those enjoyed by adults, and older gravidas may have developed distinct dietary patterns that are resistant to change.

The *religious, racial, and ethnic background* of the client and her family also is an important consideration in nutritional assessment and counseling. Regional or national food preferences may be different from the standard American diet usually portrayed in diet plans. Knowing the client's ethnic background can be helpful in understanding her dietary habits. However, there is much variation within ethnic groups related to such factors as climate, growing conditions, geographic relocation, intermarriage, and individual differences. Therefore, assumptions should not be made about a client's food habits based only on surname or language spoken.

An *individual dietary pattern,* **vegetarianism,** has become the dietary choice of an increasing number of people. Some abstain from eating meat for religious or health reasons, whereas others choose the vegetarian way to make more efficient use of the world's resources or to economize on their food bills. Vegetarian diets vary in the extent to which they exclude animal sources of protein; therefore, information about whether the individual follows a lacto-ovovegetarian, lactovegetarian, or "pure" vegetarian (**vegan**) diet, excluding all animal sources of protein, is important.

Food allergies or intolerances can develop to a number of different foods. Adjustments in the diet may be required to avoid these foods while obtaining adequate amounts of essential nutrients. Intolerance to the milk sugar lactose is a particular problem during pregnancy because it is difficult to meet the pregnant woman's need for calcium, protein, and certain vitamins and minerals without using milk.

Assessing Nutritional Risk Factors

Certain factors place women at risk for nutritional problems related to pregnancy and require special attention to nutritional needs. These factors can be grouped into categories that help focus the assessment. These categories, which are further defined in Table 18-3, include the following:

- Age
- Obstetric history
  High parity or frequent conceptions
  Previous obstetric complications
- Current pregnancy complications
- Medical history
- Maternal weight
- Socioeconomic status
- Ethnic or language differences
- Psychological conditions
- Dysfunctional dietary patterns
  Dietary faddism
  Pica
  Excessive use of alcohol, drugs, or tobacco

TABLE 18–2
Assessing Individual Dietary Factors Involved in Food Choices

Category	Factor	Significance
Psychological aspects	Hunger	Individuals have a basic instinct to seek food for survival.
	Appetite	A learned response to hunger is determined, in part, by the person's previous experiences with eating. Worry, fear, and preoccupation with troublesome or difficult problems may result in either an increase or a decrease in appetite. Appetite may be stimulated by situations that encourage feelings of calm, contentedness, mild elation, or ego stimulation.
	Heritage, superstition custom, knowledge, opportunity	Food preferences are passed along from one generation to the next by the process of training and imitation. Unique methods of food preparation, food selection, combinations, and prejudices are embodied in this training. The serving of good food also enhances congeniality and hospitality.
	Symbolic meanings of food	Women may crave or reject certain foods. This may be related to the pregnant woman's close identification of food with mother, fears that certain foods can "mark" the fetus, or beliefs that specific foods give the fetus strength or other desirable characteristics.
Stage of growth and development	Adolescence	Food choices influenced by adolescent eating patterns. Client may exert independence by rejecting "healthy foods" associated with "home" and "dependency." Client may have strong desire to be free and to select "forbidden," often non-nutritious foods.
	Older gravidas	Women may have set dietary patterns related to lifestyle. Use of medications or dietary restrictions may increase at upper end of age range interfering with food choices.
Religious, racial, and ethnic background		Certain foods may be highly valued, and others may be excluded from the diet, according to laws or customs of the religious or cultural group. Methods of food preparation also may be different. Some differences are beneficial and others detrimental. During counseling, the nurse can encourage beneficial practices and assist in finding acceptable substitutes for those that are detrimental to the health of the mother, fetus, or newborn. Those new to the United States may need assistance to find sources of their accustomed foods or alternatives.
Individual dietary pattern: vegetarianism	Lacto-ovo	Meat is excluded, but eggs, dairy products and sometimes fish, poultry, and liver are included.
	Lacto	All animal protein sources except dairy products are excluded.
	Vegans	All animal sources of protein are excluded. Women need to obtain enough high-quality protein. Also, diets may be lacking in other nutrients. Caloric intake may be low, leading to low prepregnancy weight and low pregnancy weight gain. Women may not get enough calcium in their diets and run the risk of developing a vitamin B_{12} deficiency, because this vitamin is found only in foods of animal origin.
Food allergies and intolerances		This may lead to avoidance of foods containing essential nutrients. Women may need assistance with adjustments in diet to avoid these foods and still obtain adequate nutrition for pregnancy.

Nursing Diagnosis

Nutritional assessment of the pregnant woman can lead the nurse to a variety of nursing diagnoses that can be used in planning and implementing care. Most of these nursing diagnoses would involve the diagnostic category Altered Nutrition and would be related to different factors that might put the woman or fetus at increased risk for problems. For a list of possible nursing diagnoses, see Box 18-1.

Planning and Intervention: Dietary Counseling

During the reproductive cycle, the nurse has many opportunities to assist the client with the improvement of her nutritional status. Drawing from the information obtained during assessment, the nurse can work with

TABLE 18–3
Nutritional Risk Factors

Category	Factor	Significance
Age	Adolescence	Increased nutritional needs; possible poor food habits
	Older gravidas	Possible increased incidence of other risk factors
Obstetric history	High parity or frequent conceptions	Depletion of maternal nutrient stores
	Previous obstetric complications	Possible nutritional relationship may recur
Medical history	Preexisting medical problems such as anemia, cardiac disease, diabetes, hypertension, and infections	May affect ingestion, use, or absorption of nutrients
Complications of current pregnancy	Development of complications, such as anemia, preeclampsia, or gestational diabetes	Development of nutritional deficiencies due to increased nutritional needs
Maternal weight	Low prepregnancy weight—defined as 10% or more under the standard weight for height or a BMI of less than 19.8.	Increased pregnancy problems; increased rate of prematurity; newborns with low birth weight, lower Apgar scores, and increased neonatal morbidity
		Improved outcome with improved nutrition and adequate weight gain during the pregnancy
	Insufficient weight gain during pregnancy—weight that falls below prepregnant weight in first trimester, a gain of 2 lb/mo or less, or less than 0.5 lb/wk in the second and third trimesters.	Correlated with low–birth-weight newborns and may indicate poor maternal or fetal nutrition
	Obesity prior to pregnancy—divided into two categories: *Overweight:* a weight 20% above the standard weight for height (BMI 26.0–29.0) *Very overweight:* greater than 35% over the standard weight for height (BMI 29.0).	Increased risk for developing problems, such as hypertension, gestational diabetes, and thrombophlebitis May indicate poor nutritional habits
	Excessive weight gain during pregnancy—not well defined; lack of agreement on whether it is a risk factor May be defined as weight gain 35% above prepregnancy weight	Increased risk of hypertension, preeclampsia, difficult labor, and cesarean section. Weight loss more difficult during postpartum, with increased risk of continuing obesity.
Dysfunctional dietary patterns	**Dietary faddism** (very restrictive diets or diets that concentrate on certain foods or food groups to the exclusion of others), for example, macrobiotic diet, Atkins diet, Stillman diet	Diets often inadequate to meet fetal or maternal nutritional needs
	Pica (the craving for and ingestion of non-nutritive substances, such as clay, laundry starch, raw flour, or rice)	Displacement of nutritious foods, often related to iron deficiency anemia; possible toxic reactions to substance ingested
	Excessive use of alcohol, drugs, or tobacco	Interference with appetite and with use of some nutrients; possible low–birth-weight newborns and withdrawal symptoms (alcohol and drugs)
Socioeconomic status	Low income	Limited ability to buy sufficient food; possible chronic malnutrition; increased likelihood of low–birth-weight newborns
Cultural or ethnic group	Ethnic or language differences	Interference with ability to find usual foods; misinterpretation of dietary instructions
Psychological conditions	Depression, anorexia nervosa	Possible reduced caloric and nutrient intake, leading to poor maternal weight gain, possible low–birth-weight newborns, and increased perinatal mortality

---

BOX 18–1
Nursing Diagnoses

- Altered Nutrition: Less than body requirements related to
  - Inadequate understanding of nutritional needs during pregnancy
  - Nausea and vomiting of early pregnancy
  - Cultural or ethnic influences on dietary patterns
  - Inadequate monetary resources for proper food purchase
  - Substance abuse
  - Self-imposed dietary restrictions
  - Inadequate calorie intake
  - Food allergies or intolerance
  - Fear of retained weight after birth of newborn
- Altered Nutrition: More than body requirements related to:
  - Overeating
  - Unnecessary use of supplements in megadoses
  - Decline in physical activity as pregnancy progresses
  - Poor understanding of nutrient needs during pregnancy
- Constipation related to
  - Inadequate intake of fiber foods
  - Decline in physical activity as pregnancy progresses
- Risk for Fluid Volume Deficit related to inadequate fluid intake
- Risk for Infection related to malnutrition
- Knowledge Deficit related to
  - Nutritional needs of pregnancy
  - Changes in body systems with pregnancy and need for increased nutrients
  - Effect of nutrition on fetal growth and development

---

individuals or groups of clients to plan and implement nutritious food choices (see the Nursing Care Plan).

The responsibility for initial and ongoing dietary evaluation and counseling varies from one prenatal setting to another. Dietitians or nutritionists, if available, may see all clients at least one time or may limit their services to seeing high-risk clients. They also may consult with staff concerning other clients. In the absence of a nutritionist or dietitian, the primary responsibility for nutrition counseling may rest with the nurse. Whether it is the nurse's primary responsibility or a shared responsibility with other members of the healthcare team, the nurse plays an important role because he or she usually sees the client at each visit and is available to answer questions. If more than one person is involved in the counseling, it is important to be consistent with the nutritional information taught and the advice given. Nutrition counseling ideally begins at the first prenatal visit, during the assessment of dietary intake.

As the nurse and the woman plan together, the client's likes and dislikes are recognized. Preferred foods that provide essential nutrients are encouraged. Suggestions may be given for adding certain foods or modifying existing methods of selecting or preparing them. Encouraging the woman to participate in the planning and allowing her choices whenever possible, helping her to increase her knowledge of nutrients, encouraging and reinforcing correct choices or willing adaptations, and giving firm guidance when indicated all help the client and nurse achieve their respective goals.

Many women already eat an adequate diet. They may only need reinforcement of their dietary habits and encouragement to continue what they are doing. For women whose dietary intake is not adequate or whose history indicates one or more risk factors, consistent counseling toward optimum nutritional intake is vitally important.

The nurse needs to be tolerant and nonjudgmental, respecting the client's right to reject dietary information if she chooses. This may be difficult for the nurse because healthcare providers traditionally expect their advice to be followed. However, more may be gained in the long run by accepting the "client's right to choose." A client is more likely to seek care from people she feels respect her views, even when these views differ from those of the provider.

Dietary counseling should be an ongoing aspect of prenatal care. It is not enough to talk about it at the first visit and hand out a suggested diet plan or food guide. There should be some discussion of nutrition at each follow-up visit, with reinforcement or additional suggestions as needed. Periodic use of diet recall or a food diary can be helpful in assessing the extent to which the suggestions are being followed. Information on specific areas that may be helpful in counseling includes weight gain and pregnancy, nutrient needs, dietary planning, available resources, and supplemental food programs.

Nutrient Needs

A brief review of basic nutrition may be helpful to the nurse when teaching her clients about good nutrition during pregnancy. All foods are made up of a combination of classes of nutrients: carbohydrates, protein, fat, vitamins, minerals, and water. Carbohydrates, protein, and fat constitute the group called "energy nutrients" because they contribute energy or calories to the diet. Vitamins, minerals, and water do not contribute to the caloric content of food.

Recommended Dietary Allowances

The Food and Nutrition Board of the National Research Council sets standards for the daily intake of calories and nutrients by people in the United States. These **recommended dietary allowances** (RDAs) are defined

NURSING CARE PLAN
The Pregnant Woman and Her Nutritional Needs

Nursing Goals
1. Client is free of nutritionally related problems, such as preeclampsia or anemia.
2. Client demonstrates implementation of suggested dietary changes through use of dietary recall or food diary.
3. Client's weight gain is adequate and follows recommended pattern.
4. Client's fetus or newborn demonstrates adequate growth and well-being.

Assessment	Potential Nursing Diagnosis	Planning and Intervention	Evaluation
Nutritional status	Altered Nutrition: Less than body requirements related to inadequate caloric intake or inadequate financial resources or dysfunctional dietary patterns	Use assessment tools *to determine individual client needs.*	Nutritionally related problems, such as preeclampsia and anemia are absent.
Physical indicators			
Prepregnant weight			
Pregnancy weight gain		Provide dietary counseling in the following areas as needed *to assist client in attaining optimal nutritional status during pregnancy:*	Repeat dietary recall or food diary indicates use of daily food guide and implementation of suggested changes.
Laboratory values (hemoglobin, hematocrit)			
Current dietary habits			
Daily food intake	Altered Nutrition: Less calcium than pregnancy requirements related to lactose intolerance	Involve client in planning.	
Individual factors in food selection		Consider individual needs, preferences, attitudes, family needs, and cultural or ethnic background.	Weight gain is adequate and follows recommended pattern.
Nutritional risk factors	Knowledge Deficit regarding nutritional needs during pregnancy related to lack of information		Fetal growth and well-being follow optimal pattern.
Client understanding of nutrition		Provide information about nutrient needs.	
Importance of good nutrition during pregnancy	Altered Nutrition: Inadequate weight gain related to self-imposed limitation of calories	Encourage and reinforce appropriate food choices and preparation.	
Important nutrients		Plan menus with client, including foods she likes and can afford and is able to prepare.	
Importance of weight gain		Give careful, thorough explanation of rationale for any suggested changes *to increase client understanding.*	
		Teach importance of weight gain *to help client accept changing eating patterns and body image.*	
		Use and discuss weight gain grid at each visit *to keep client aware of progress.*	
		Refer to dietitian when appropriate *to provide additional nutritional counseling in particular situations.*	

as "the levels of intake of essential nutrients that, on the basis of scientific knowledge, are judged by the Food and Nutrition Board to be adequate to meet the known nutrient needs of practically all healthy persons" (National Research Council, 1989). The 10th edition of the RDAs, published in 1989, provides the most recent recommendations (Table 18-4). RDAs are based on reference individuals, using actual height and weight medians for the American population of the designated age. Allowances vary according to age and during pregnancy and lactation. They are meant to be used as a basic reference and adjusted according to individual need.

Carbohydrates

The main function of **carbohydrates** is to produce energy. They are necessary in adequate amounts to spare protein for growth needs. Glucose, one form of carbohydrate, is the major fuel of the body. All other forms of carbohydrates are converted to glucose in the body. The main sources of carbohydrates in the diet are fruits, vegetables, and grain products. The unrefined sources contribute valuable fiber. Sugars and sweets also are sources of carbohydrates but are often called empty calories because they do not contribute many nutrients to the diet.

Fat

Fat is a concentrated source of energy, yielding more than twice as many calories per gram as carbohydrates. As pregnancy progresses, there is an increased breakdown of fat to use as a maternal fuel source so that more glucose will be available for fetal needs. Besides supplying energy, fat in the diet provides essential fatty acids and supplies and carries the fat-soluble vitamins A, D, E, and K. Also, fats, such as butter, margarine, and salad oil, add to the palatability of food.

Protein

The main function of **protein** is to build and repair all body cells. An increased amount is needed during pregnancy for growth and maintenance of maternal and fetal tissues. Proteins are made up of different combinations of the more than 20 amino acids. Eight of these cannot be synthesized by the body and are called **essential amino acids,** which must be supplied by the diet. All eight must be present in the correct proportion at the same meal to be used by the body.

Proteins that contain adequate amounts of all eight essential amino acids are called **complete proteins.** Most animal sources fall into this category. Most vegetable protein sources are deficient in one or more of the essential amino acids. However, when a vegetarian diet is well balanced and a wide variety of foods is in-

cluded, protein quality (the percent of protein the body is able to use) is usually adequate (California Department of Health Services, 1990).

Vitamins

Vitamins are organic substances that are essential to life and must be supplied by the diet in minute amounts daily. They are directly involved in regulating the metabolism of carbohydrates, protein, and fat, and they assist in regulating reactions by which body tissues are maintained. Many reactions in the body require more than one vitamin, and the lack of any one can interfere with the function of another. Most vitamins cannot be synthesized by the body. Vitamins are usually grouped according to whether they are soluble in fat or in water. Their solubility affects the way they are handled by the body (Table 18-5).

Fat-Soluble Vitamins. Fat-soluble vitamins A, D, E, and K are closely related to lipids in the body, and their functions are generally related to body structure (see Table 18-5). They are stored by the body, therefore large doses, especially of vitamins A and D, can be toxic. Excesses usually come from excessive supplementation, not from food sources.

Water-Soluble Vitamins. Water-soluble vitamins, including vitamin C and the B complex vitamins, are not stored in any significant amount. Therefore, deficiencies can develop more easily than with the fat-soluble vitamins (see Table 18-5). Vitamin C (ascorbic acid) is an important structural agent involved with bone, tooth, and collagen formation and acts as an antioxidant to protect other nutrients from destruction. The B complex actually consists of a number of different vitamins that are essential to good nutrition and are coenzyme factors in cell metabolism. The Food and Nutrition Board lists allowances for four of the B complex vitamins: thiamine (vitamin B_1), riboflavin (vitamin B_2), niacin (vitamin B_6), folacin (folic acid), and vitamin B_{12}.

Folic acid is one of the B vitamins that has received increasing attention in recent years. Maternal serum folate levels are often low during pregnancy, but megaloblastic anemia, a sign of folic acid deficiency, is seldom seen. In a number of recent studies, periconceptual supplementation with multiple vitamins containing folic acid substantially reduced the risk of having a newborn with a neural tube defect (see Research Highlight). This was true whether the women had previous newborns with neural tube defects or whether first-time occurrences were being studied (Romanczuk et al., 1994). To be effective, the folic acid supplement needs to be taken before conception, or prior to the time the neural tube usually closes at about 6 weeks'

(text continues on page 454)

TABLE 18–4
Recommended Dietary Allowances* During Pregnancy and Lactation

Recommended Energy Intake for Women:

Age or Condition	Weight† KG	Weight† LB	Height† CM	Height† IN	Average Energy Allowance (kcal) PER KG	Average Energy Allowance (kcal) PER DAY
11–14	46	101	157	62	47	2,200
15–18	55	120	163	64	40	2,200
19–24	58	128	164	65	38	2,200
25–50	63	138	163	64	36	2,200
Pregnant (first trimester)						+0
Pregnant (second and third trimester)						+300
Lactating (first 6 mo)						+500
(second 6 mo)						+500

Recommended Protein, Vitamin, and Mineral Allowances

	Women 19–24 y	Women 25–50 y	Pregnant	Lactating FIRST 6 MO	Lactating SECOND 6 MO
PROTEIN (g)	46	50	60	65	62
FAT-SOLUBLE VITAMINS					
Vitamin A (μg RE)‡	800	800	800	1,300	1,200
Vitamin D (μg)§	10	5	10	10	10
Vitamin E (mg α TE)‖	8	8	10	12	11
Vitamin K (μg)	60	65	65	65	65
WATER-SOLUBLE VITAMINS					
Vitamin C (mg)	60	60	70	95	90
Thiamine (mg)	1.1	1.1	1.5	1.6	1.6
Riboflavin (mg)	1.3	1.2	1.6	1.8	1.7
Niacin (mg NE)#	15	15	17	20	20
Vitamin B_6 (mg)	1.6	1.6	2.2	2.1	2.1
Folate (μg)	180	180	400	280	260
Vitamin B_{12} (μg)	2.0	2.0	2.2	2.6	2.6
MINERALS					
Calcium (mg)	1,200	800	1,200	1,200	1,200
Phosphorus (mg)	1,200	800	1,200	1,200	1,200
Magnesium (mg)	280	280	320	355	340
Iron (mg)	15	15	30	15	15
Zinc (mg)	12	12	15	19	16
Iodine (μg)	150	150	175	200	200
Selenium (μg)	55	55	65	75	75

*The allowances expressed as average daily intakes over time, are intended to provide for individual variations among most normal people as they live in the United States under usual environmental stresses. Diets should be based on a variety of common foods to provide other nutrients for which human requirements have been less well defined.

† Weights and heights of reference individuals are actual medians for the U.S. population of the designated age. The use of these figures does not imply that the height-to-weight ratios are ideal.

‡ Retinol equivalents. 1 retinol equivalent = 1 µg retinol or 6 µg β-carotene.

§ As cholecalciferol. 10 μg cholecalciferol = 400 IU of vitamin D.

‖ α-Tocopherol equivalents. 1 mg d-α tocopherol = 1 α-TE.

#1 NE (niacin equivalent) is equal to 1 mg of niacin or 60 mg of dietary tryptophan.

(Adapted from National Research Council (US) Subcommittee on the Tenth Edition of the RDAs. [1989]. *Recommended dietary allowances*. Washington, DC: National Academy Press.)

TABLE 18–5
Vitamins and Minerals

	Function	Sources	Comments
FAT-SOLUBLE VITAMINS			
A	■ Assists in maintaining the integrity of the mucous membrane, which increases the body's resistance to infection ■ Is essential for normal skeletal and tooth development ■ Plays a role in night vision	Dark green and deep yellow vegetables and fruits are the best sources of vitamin A. Foods such as milk are fortified with vitamin A. (It is found in foods in the form of the precursor, Carotene.)	This is teratogenic in large doses when used as nutritional supplement or in topical form used to treat acne.
D	■ Plays important role in the absorption and use of calcium and phosphorus in skeletal and tooth bud formation	Egg yolk, liver, and some fish contain small amounts of vitamin D. Most milk is fortified with 400 IU per quart. It can be produced by the body from sunlight on the skin, but this is not a reliable source.	Reliability of sunlight as a source is decreased due to variability of exposure and interferences, such as smog or dust. Excessive amounts may be harmful during pregnancy.
E	■ Is primarily an antioxidant ■ Reduces oxidation of the polyunsaturated fatty acids, helping to maintain the integrity of cell membranes ■ Is involved in certain enzymatic and metabolic reactions	Vegetable fats and oils; leafy, green vegetables; grains, nuts, and egg yolks contain vitamin E.	Needs are believed to increase during pregnancy, but deficiency in humans is rarely seen.
K	■ Acts as an essential factor in the formation of prothrombin, therefore necessary for normal blood clotting	Leafy, green vegetables and pork liver are excellent dietary sources. Also it is synthesized by bacteria of the lower intestinal tract.	Dietary deficiency usually is not a problem.
WATER-SOLUBLE VITAMINS			
B Complex	■ Serve as components of enzymes and coenzymes in many reactions in the body, such as cell respiration, glucose oxidation, and energy metabolism	These are not all found together in the same foods; however, if the diet includes milk, organ and other meats, eggs, whole grain or enriched cereals and breads, legumes, and dark green vegetables, most are probably present. Vitamin B_{12} is only found in foods of animal origin.	Requirements are increased to meet the increased metabolic and growth needs of pregnancy.
Folic acid	■ Is involved in deoxyribonucleic acid (DNA) and ribonucleic acid (RNA) synthesis: when lacking, cell division unable to proceed normally	Leafy, green vegetables; other green vegetables; liver, yeast; legumes; nuts; and whole grains are good sources.	As much as 80% of the vitamin may be destroyed in cooking or storage, so supplementation is often advised. Needs are increased during pregnancy for growth of the fetus and expansion of maternal blood volume.
C	■ Is essential for the formation of collagen (sometimes called the "cement" that holds the body's cells and tissues together) ■ Plays an important role in building strong bones and teeth, healing wounds, and aiding the ability of the body to withstand the stresses of injury and infection ■ Is easily destroyed by exposure to air, overcooking, or cooking in too much water	This is found in fresh vegetables and fruits, especially citrus fruits. Good sources include fresh strawberries, cantaloupe, pineapple, guavas, tomatoes, and the green vegetables. Also it is found in other fruits and vegetables in sufficient quantity.	Exact amount needed in diet to promote optimum health is not known. It probably varies from person to person. Infections and stress may increase requirements.

(continued)

TABLE 18–5 *(Continued)*
Vitamins and Minerals

	Function	Sources	Comments
MINERALS			
Calcium	• Is an important constituent of bone and teeth • Can be used by the body for functions such as normal blood clotting, promoting muscle tone, and regulating the heart beat	Sources include cheese, eggs, oatmeal, vegetables, and milk. A quart of milk supplies 1.2 g of calcium.	Two-thirds of calcium in fetus is deposited during last month of pregnancy, but mother's daily requirement is increased during entire course of pregnancy to prepare adequate storage for this demand.
Phosphorus	• Is an essential constituent of all cells and tissues of the body	Milk provides an abundant source of phosphorus. Other protein-rich food, eggs, meat, cheese, oatmeal, and green vegetables, also provide adequate amounts.	Diet providing adequate amounts of protein will also provide sufficient phosphorus.
Iron	• Is one of the chief components of hemoglobin (the substance in the blood responsible for carrying oxygen to the cells) • During pregnancy, is needed to manufacture hemoglobin for fetal red blood cells and maternal red blood cells	Meats; wheat germ; egg yolks; seafood; green, leafy vegetables; nuts; and legumes contain iron. Foods rich in ascorbic acid appear to enhance absorption of dietary, but not supplemental, iron.	This is transferred to fetus in moderate amounts during the first two trimesters and accelerated during last trimester, when the fetus builds its reserve. Dietary sources and limited maternal stores often are not adequate for pregnancy. Daily supplementation is usually recommended, after 12th week of gestation.
Iodine	• Is needed in small amounts for health of woman and fetus	This is obtained readily from seafood and cod liver oil in most localities. Iodized salt is recommended when iodine is lacking in water supply.	Water supply and the vegetables grown are poor in iodine in certain localities around the Great Lakes and in parts of the Northwest.
Zinc	• Plays an active role in metabolism as a component of insulin and other key cell enzymes • Is active in the synthesis of DNA and RNA	Meats, fish, egg yolks, and most other protein foods have a relatively high zinc content. A diet meeting the RDA for protein also should furnish sufficient amounts of zinc.	This essential trace element is widely distributed in tissue. Deficiency is linked to congenital malformations and labor and delivery complications, including prolonged labor. Also a deficiency is thought to predispose to bacterial infections of the amniotic fluid, which may lead to preterm labor and birth.
Sodium	• Maintains fluid balance, acid–base balance, and muscular irritability • Also regulates cell permeability and nerve impulse transmission	This is present in foods of animal origin and in some vegetables. Major dietary source is table salt and processed foods.	There is increasing recognition of importance of adequate sodium intake during pregnancy. Clinical and laboratory data indicate that the sodium requirement is increased during pregnancy. Restriction can be harmful by reducing circulating blood volume. Expanded blood volume increases needs during pregnancy to maintain normal blood levels. Usual diet of most women in the United States easily meets daily 2 to 3 g requirement. Increased salt intake usually is not needed during pregnancy, but restriction can cause problems.

The Relationship Between Folic Acid and Prevention of Neural Tube Defects

Early studies demonstrating the relationship between folic acid and the prevention of neural tube defects were done by supplementing women who had a previous child with a neural tube defect. The current study looked instead at the possibility of decreasing the incidence of neural tube defects in newborns of women who had not had a previous child with the problem by providing vitamin supplementation prior to conception and during the first 6 weeks of gestation.

This study was a randomized controlled trial of women planning a pregnancy. For most of them, it was their first pregnancy. The women were randomly assigned to receive either a vitamin supplement containing 0.8 mg of folic acid in addition to 11 other vitamins, four minerals, and three trace elements, or a supplement containing three trace elements and a low dose of vitamin C. These supplements were taken daily for at least 1 month before conception and continued at least until the date of the second missed menstrual period.

Of the women who agreed to participate in the study, the outcome of pregnancy related to the presence or absence of neural tube defects was known for 2,104 women who received the vitamin supplement and 2,052 who received the trace element supplement. In the vitamin supplement group, there was an incidence of 13.3 congenital malformations per thousand births, with no neural tube defects. In the trace mineral group, the incidence of congenital malformations was 22.9 per thousand births, with six neural tube defects. These results lead the authors of this study to recommend that all women take a vitamin supplement containing folic acid when planning a pregnancy.

Critique: This study is important because it extends the possibility of the prevention of neural tube defects to all pregnancies, rather than a specific group of pregnant women. It has significance for nurses, because they often have the opportunity to assist clients in planning their diets to included important nutrients and to reinforce the client's use of recommended supplements.

Czeizel, A. E. et al (1992). Prevention of the first occurrence of neural-tube defects by periconceptional vitamin supplementation. *New England Journal of Medicine, 327*, 1832–1835.

gestation (Willett, 1992). The RDA of 0.4 mg of folic acid was found to be sufficient. Although the relationship between folic acid and neural tube defects is a significant finding, a cause and effect relationship has not been established. The actual cause of neural tube defects is not known (Romanczuk et al., 1994).

Minerals

At least 14 mineral elements are essential for good nutrition. Some, calcium and phosphorus, for example, are present in the body in relatively large amounts (greater than 5 g). Others, called trace elements, such as iron and zinc, are present in minute amounts (less than 5 g). The **minerals** are constituents of vital body materials, and some are regulators and activators of body functions. Minerals of special importance during pregnancy include calcium, phosphorus, iron, iodine, zinc, and sodium (see Table 18-5).

Sodium intake during pregnancy has long been a subject of controversy. In the past, like calorie restriction, sodium restriction was thought to be an important factor in the prevention of pregnancy-induced hypertension. Clinical and laboratory data since that time have indicated that the sodium requirement is increased during pregnancy. Restriction, therefore, can be harmful when imposed indiscriminately. An adequate renal and placental blood flow demands an adequate circulating blood volume. When there is a stringent reduction in sodium intake, there is a reduction in circulating blood volume, which is not tolerated well during pregnancy and is dangerous for the woman and fetus. Thus, the routine restriction of salt is no longer practiced. The use of diuretics for reducing edema, previously thought to be associated with sodium retention caused by excessive salt in the diet, also has been discontinued.

Vitamin and Mineral Supplements

There is no universal agreement about the use of vitamin and mineral supplements during pregnancy. Ideally, the diet should supply all the nutrients needed so supplements are not necessary. Some physicians prescribe a multivitamin and mineral supplement as a precaution against deficiencies. The Subcommittee on Dietary Intake and Nutrient Supplements During Pregnancy of the Food and Nutrition Board (Institute of Medicine, 1990) considers supplementation during pregnancy an intervention, to be used only when specifically indicated. They point out that supplementation can create imbalances, because increasing one nutrient often changes the requirement for other nutrients. There also may be unidentified essential nutrients that supplementation could affect adversely.

Iron and folacin are the most frequently recommended supplements, because they are difficult to obtain by diet alone. The Subcommittee for an Implementation Guide (Institute of Medicine, 1992) recommends a low-dose supplement of 30 mg/d of elemental iron for the woman who is not anemic. For the anemic woman, a supplement of 60 to 120 mg/d is recommended. Iron tablets taken between meals are absorbed more completely than those taken with food. Because large doses of iron appear to depress plasma zinc in pregnant women, zinc supplementation may be needed when a supplement of more than 30 mg/d of elemental iron is taken. If zinc is given, the Subcommittee recommends the addition of a 2-mg copper supplement to offset zinc's depressive effect on copper absorption (Institute of Medicine, 1992).

Folic acid is recommended for 4 weeks prior to conception and during the first 3 months of pregnancy (Institute of Medicine, 1992). Supplementation prior to and in early pregnancy has been found to protect against neural tube defects in women who had a previously affected pregnancy (MRC Vitamin Study Research Group, 1991) and first occurrences (Czeizel et al., 1992; see the Research Highlight). If there is any evidence of an inadequate dietary intake, folic acid may be given throughout the pregnancy.

Certain conditions or habits of the pregnant woman may increase requirements for certain nutrients. For example, women who are carrying more than one fetus or who smoke cigarettes, drink alcohol, or use illicit drugs may require additional supplementation. Special attention also needs to be given to the adequacy of calcium and vitamin D intake for pregnant women younger than 25 years, because their bone mineral density is still increasing (Institute of Medicine, 1990). Calcium supplements might be advised for women who drink little or no milk, and vitamin B_{12} might be needed by the vegan who eats no animal protein (Williams, 1993). If any vitamin or mineral supplements are used, it is important for the woman to understand that these are in addition to, not instead of, her recommended dietary intake.

Megadoses of Vitamins and Minerals. A megadose is an amount of a nutrient that is at least 10 times greater than the RDA. Some people think that if a little vitamin supplementation is good, a lot is even better. As more is learned about vitamins and their uses in the body, it is becoming more apparent that doses in excess of body requirements may cause chemical imbalances that can lead to adverse effects. Toxic effects have been seen in people consuming large amounts of certain vitamins. Evidence of detrimental effects during pregnancy is limited, but the embryo or fetus is thought to be particularly vulnerable to toxic effects of vitamin and mineral megadoses (Worthington-Roberts, 1993b). One reason for this is that the placental transport system concentrates some nutrients in fetal blood in an effort to make sure that the fetus has a sufficient amount. Thus, excessive maternal intake exposes the fetus to unusually high levels. Another reason is that the excretory capacity of the fetus is limited. Susceptibility to damage is greatest during early pregnancy when organ systems are developing (Worthington-Roberts, 1993b).

The fat-soluble vitamins, especially vitamins A and D, have been linked to birth defects by human case reports and animal studies. Some newborns whose mothers took doses of vitamin A greater than 25,000 IU/d for a prolonged period during pregnancy have been born with urinary tract malformations and other congenital anomalies (Worthington-Roberts, 1993b). Retinol or preformed vitamin A also has been shown to be teratogenic. Carotene, the vitamin A precursor found in foods, does not appear to be harmful, even in large amounts, primarily because it is not efficiently absorbed and converted to vitamin A (Institute of Medicine, 1990).

Vitamin D has the smallest margin of safety of any of the vitamins. Among the adverse conditions associated with an excess intake during pregnancy are neonatal hypercalcemia, premature closure of fontanels, craniofacial abnormalities, and calcification of soft tissues (Worthington-Roberts, 1993b).

Although water-soluble vitamins are not stored in the body in the same way as fat-soluble vitamins and are therefore not toxic, some have been shown to have adverse effects when taken in excessive amounts. There is some evidence that the fetus may become accustomed to the high levels during pregnancy and show withdrawal symptoms after birth. Some newborns of women who took large amounts of vitamin C during pregnancy have shown scurvy-like symptoms when their high prenatal intake was cut off at birth (Worthington-Roberts, 1993b).

To help avoid potential dangers of vitamin overdosage, questions about vitamin supplementation should be included in the initial dietary assessment of the pregnant woman. As with other aspects of dietary counseling, the nurse can assist the expectant woman in planning a diet that includes appropriate amounts of nutrients and avoids excesses.

Water and Other Fluids

Water, often omitted when nutrients are listed, is an essential nutrient. It is an important solvent that is necessary for digestion, nutrient transport to the cells, and removal of body wastes. It also is a lubricant and helps to regulate body temperature.

Fluids should be taken freely. The woman should drink an average of six to eight glasses daily. Water and juices are good choices. Some beverages contain ingredients that should be used sparingly in the prenatal diet. For example, regular soft drinks contain many empty calories, dietetic soft drinks contain artificial sweeteners, and cola, tea, and coffee contain caffeine (see section entitled "Food Additives"). Women who drink large quantities of any of these beverages should be counseled to decrease their intake.

Although there is no definite evidence that tea and coffee should be eliminated from the prenatal diet, women are usually advised to at least cut down. Using decaffeinated coffee or tea and removing the teabag promptly when brewing regular tea help to decrease the amount of caffeine per cup.

Planning the Diet

The nurse can use many tools when helping the pregnant woman plan a nutritious diet and follow basic guidelines for good nutrition during pregnancy. Planning a menu to include all the essential nutrients would seem impossible if each nutrient had to be considered individually. Fortunately, nutrients are found in foods in certain combinations, allowing foods to be divided into groups according to the major nutrients they supply to simplify the planning. The specific groups and the actual number of servings suggested are less important than finding a guide to which the woman can relate (Institute of Medicine, 1992). Two currently used guides for grouping foods and planning food intake are the daily food guide for women (Table 18-6) and the food guide pyramid.

Both guides use essentially the same basic food groups:

- Protein food group, including meat, poultry, beans, and nuts
- Milk product group, including milk, yogurt, and cheese
- Fruits and vegetables group
- Breads, cereals, and grains group, which also includes pasta and rice
- Fats, oils, and sweets, which should be included in the diet, but used sparingly

The food guide pyramid, developed by the U.S. Department of Agriculture for use by the general popula-

tion, may be more familiar to pregnant women, because it has been widely publicized and is found on the packages of many foods. However, examples of materials to use for the pregnant woman are limited. A WIC pamphlet (U.S. Department of Agriculture Food and Nutrition Service, 1994) provides recommendations for the number of daily servings from each food group during pregnancy and lactation (Fig. 18-2).

The daily food guide has been extensively adapted for use in teaching pregnant women about prenatal nutrition and menu planning and is used in many prenatal clinics. The Client Education displays in this chapter are based on the daily food guide but can be used with the food guide pyramid with only minor modifications in the fruits and vegetables and breads, cereal, and grains groups. A comparison of the number of daily servings recommended from each group is shown in Table 18-7.

The nutritional teaching guides are helpful in selecting foods from each food group. The woman is encouraged to eat the number of servings recommended from each food group every day (see Client Education: Nutritional Teaching Guides). The sample meal plan illustrates how the guide can be used. Note that the food guide is a framework for the menu but does not limit the foods that can be included (see Client Education: Sample Meal Plan for Pregnant or Lactating Women-Moderate-Calorie Diet).

Assisting the client whose ethnicity affects her dietary habits can be challenging. Table 18-8 lists some of the preferred choices in each food group for various ethnic groups. Using the Client Education: Sample Menus to Meet the Daily Food Requirements During Pregnancy for Ethnic Groups, the nurse can assist the

TABLE 18-6
Daily Food Guide for Women

Food Group	Minimum Number of Servings		
	NONPREGNANT ADOLESCENT GIRL	NONPREGNANT ADULT WOMAN	PREGNANT/LACTATING ADOLESCENT/ADULT WOMAN
Protein foods	5*	5*	7*
Milk products	3	2	3
Breads, cereal grains	7†	6†	7†
Fruits and vegetables:			
Vitamin C-rich	1	1	1
Vitamin A-rich	1	1	1
Other	3	3	3

*Each serving is equivalent to 1 oz of animal protein; at least one serving should be from the vegetable protein list (two servings during pregnancy or lactation).
†At least four servings should be from whole grains
(California Department of Health Services, MCH/WIC [1990]. *Nutrition during pregnancy and the postpartum period: Manual for health care professionals.* Sacramento, CA: Author.)

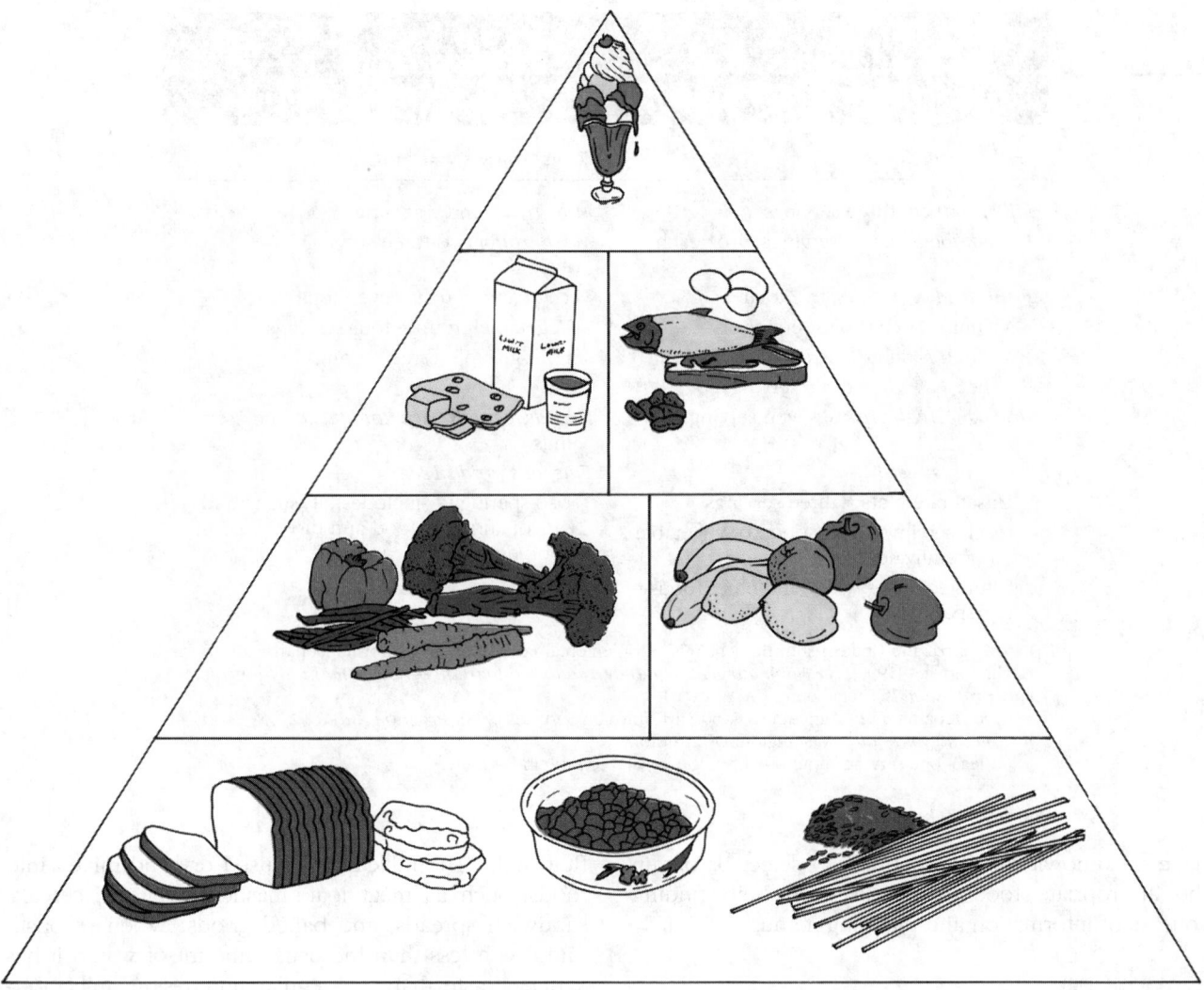

FIGURE 18-2 The food guide pyramid. A guide to daily food choices modified for pregnancy. (Courtesy of U.S. Department of Agriculture Food & Nutrition Service from *Eating for You & Your Baby*, 1994.)

woman in deciding where ethnic foods fit into the plan. Intake of specific nutrients varies depending on the foods selected, but using the daily food guide leads to an average intake of adequate amounts of most of the essential nutrients. The woman should be counseled to include additional nutritious food to meet her caloric needs (California Department of Health Services, 1990).

Protein Foods

Six or seven ounces of protein-rich foods, such as beef, pork, lamb, veal, organ meats, or vegetable protein sources are recommended daily. At least one serving should come from vegetable sources, such as legumes (eg, dried beans, peas, and lentils) or nuts. In addition to providing amino acids, the protein foods are good sources of many vitamins and minerals. In keeping with

current concerns about limiting the intake of fat to 30% of calories consumed, protein-rich foods can be distinguished as those that are low in fat (<5 g per serving) and those that are high in fat (>5 g per serving).

Often the family's budget restricts the quantity and variety of protein foods, especially meat. Choosing a leaner and possibly tougher grade of meat may require changes in cooking methods, but it may be less expensive. The substitution of cheese, peanut butter, poultry, fish, or legumes as protein sources also may be suggested to decrease cost.

Women who follow a vegetarian diet, especially vegans, may need assistance in meeting their protein needs. Vegetarian diets can be adequate in protein if they are well balanced. Knowledge about the complementarity of protein foods (Table 18-9), while not essential, helps to ensure the presence of complete proteins. Some people who adopt vegetarian diets do not

TABLE 18-7
Comparison of Daily Food Guide and Food Guide Pyramid Recommended Minimum Amounts During Pregnancy and Lactation

Daily Food Guide*	Food Guide Pyramid†
Milk products: three servings	*Milk group:* three servings
Protein foods: seven servings (1 oz each)‡	*Meat group:* two-three servings (2-3 oz each)
Fruits and vegetables: five total	*Vegetable and fruit:* seven total
Vitamin C rich = one serving	Vegetable group = four servings
Vitamin A rich = one serving	Fruit group = three servings
Other = three servings	
Breads, cereal, grains: seven servings	*Breads, cereals, rice, and pasta:* nine servings
Fats, oils, sweets:	*Fats, oils, and sweets:*
Unsaturated fats = three servings (each serving = 1 teaspoon of vegetable oil or equivalent)	Use sparingly—includes fat, sugar, and oil contained in food and those used in cooking and at the table
Saturated fats, sweets, and other foods—use sparingly	

*(Maternal and Child Health Branch, WIC Supplemental Food Branch, California Department of Health Services [1990]. *Nutrition during pregnancy and the postpartum period: A manual for health care professionals.* Sacramento, CA: Author.)

†U.S. Department of Agriculture Food and Nutrition Service [1994]. *Program Aid No. 1198: Eating for you and your baby.* Washington, DC: Author.

‡At least one serving should be from the vegetable protein list daily.

have the knowledge or resources to select or obtain the appropriate foods and will need help finding sources of information and planning menus.

Milk and Milk Products

Three 1-cup servings of fluid milk daily, or the equivalent, is recommended for the expectant woman. Milk has been called nature's most nearly perfect food, and it is an invaluable source of nutrients during pregnancy. It contains vitamins, such as vitamin A and riboflavin, and minerals, such as calcium and phosphorus, that are needed for fetal development. Milk's high content of calcium and phosphorus is in the correct proportions and in a digestible form that permits optimum use by the woman and fetus. It also is an excellent source of protein that is readily digested and easily absorbed.

When a woman indicates that she does not drink milk or drinks very little, it is important to explore the subject with her and find out the basis for the avoidance. She may not like milk or may not tolerate it well. After the cause is established, a plan can be developed with her to make milk more palatable or to include adequate substitutes.

Instant nonfat or whole dry milk may be used in a variety of ways to provide an adequate intake. Approximately 5 tablespoons of dried skim milk equals 1 pt of fluid milk. The milk may be used dry and mixed into foods, such as meat loaf, mashed potatoes, cereals, sandwich spreads, and baked goods. When reconstituted with less than the usual amount of water, it has a richer taste than the regular liquid skim milk. Certain condiments and flavorings, such as vanilla, nutmeg, or cinnamon, can enhance the flavor of milk. Some clients may prefer evaporated milk, buttermilk, or nonfat or low-fat milk instead of whole milk. Milk also can be taken in some other form, such as in soups or custards.

Other dairy products, such as cottage cheese, ricotta cheese, farmer's cheese, hoop cheese, yogurt, and the hard cheeses, also are adequate substitutes. One ounce of cheese contains approximately the same amount of minerals and vitamins as a large glass of whole milk. However, the total protein and fat content varies and must be considered when making substitutions. Cream cheese has a high percentage of fat and a low calcium content, so it is not a good substitute for the other cheeses. Also, products such as "cheese foods" and "cheese spreads" are diluted and contain fewer nutrients per serving.

Lactose Intolerance. Many adults, especially Hispanics, African Americans, Asians, and Native Americans, have difficulty digesting milk because of an insufficient amount of the enzyme lactase in the small intestine. Lac-

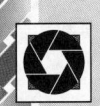

CLIENT EDUCATION
Nutritional Teaching Guides

Food Group	One Serving Equals		Male/non pregnant female	Pregnant*/ breast- feeding
			Recommended Minimum Servings	
Protein Foods Excellent sources of protein, vitamin B$_6$, iron, and zinc. Animal protein supplies vitamin B$_{12}$. Vegetable protein is a good source of folic acid, magnesium, and fiber.	**Animal Protein:** 1 oz cooked lean meat, fish, poultry, or seafood 1 egg 2 hot dogs 2 slices luncheon meat 2 oz or 3 links sausage 2 fish sticks	**Vegetable Protein:** ½ cup cooked dry beans 3 oz tofu 1 oz or ¼ cup peanuts, pumpkin, or sun- flower seeds 1½ oz or ⅓ cup other nuts 2 tbsp peanut butter	5 Have at least 1 serving from vegetable protein	7
Milk Products† Excellent sources of protein and calcium. In addition, milk products are good sources of vit- amins A, B$_{12}$, riboflavin, and zinc. Fortified fluid milk contains 100 IU of vitamin D per cup.	1 cup milk or yogurt 1 cup milkshake 1½ cups cream soups (made with milk) 1½ oz or ⅓ cup grated brick-type cheese (like cheddar or jack)	1½ slices presliced American cheese 4 tbsp parmesan 2 cups cottage cheese 1 cup pudding or custard 1½ cups ice cream or frozen yogurt	2 (3 for teens)	3
Breads, Cereals, Grains All provide carbohy- drates and some pro- tein, as well as thi- amine, riboflavin, niacin, and iron. Whole grains provide addi- tional vitamin B$_6$, folic acid, vitamin E, magne- sium, zinc, and fiber.	1 slice bread 1 dinner roll ½ bun, bagel, English muffin or pita 1 small tortilla ¾ cup dry cereal ½ cup granola	½ cup cooked cereal, noodles, or rice 4 tbsp wheat germ 1 4-in pancake or waffle 1 muffin 8 medium crackers 4 graham cracker squares	6 Have at least 4 servings from whole-grain products	7
Vitamin C-Rich Fruits and Vegetables Excellent sources of vit- amin C and fiber. They also supply vitamins A, B$_6$, and folic acid.	6 oz orange, grapefruit, tomato, vegetable juice cocktail, or fruit juice enriched with vitamin C 1 orange, kiwi, mango ½ grapefruit, cantaloupe ¼ papaya 2 tangerines, tomatoes	½ cup strawberries, broccoli, brussels sprouts, cabbage, cau- liflower, snow peas, sweet peppers, or tomato puree 2 tbsp fresh or ½ cup cooked hot peppers	1	1

†See Nondairy Calcium-Rich Foods below.

(continued)

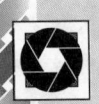

CLIENT EDUCATION *(continued)*
Nutritional Teaching Guides

Food Group	One Serving Equals		Recommended Minimum Servings	
			Male/non pregnant female	*Pregnant*/ breast-feeding*
Vitamin A-Rich Fruits and Vegetables Excellent sources of beta-carotene and vitamin A. Most are good sources of fiber. The dark green vegetables also supply good amounts of vitamin B_6, folic acid, and magnesium	6 oz apricot nectar or vegetable juice cocktail 3 raw or ¼ cup dried apricots ¼ cantaloupe or mango ½ papaya 1 small or ½ cup sliced carrots	½ cup greens (beet, chard, collards, dandelion, kale, mustard, spinach) ½ cup pumpkin, sweet potato or winter squash 2 tbsp raw or cooked hot peppers 2 tomatoes	1	1
Other Fruits and Vegetables Provide carbohydrates and fiber as well as smaller amounts of other essential vitamins and minerals	6 oz fruit juice 1 medium or ½ cup sliced fruit (apple, banana, berries, cherries, grapes, peach, pear) ½ cup pineapple or watermelon ½ cup dried fruit	½ cup sliced vegetable (asparagus, beets, green beans, celery, corn, eggplant, mushrooms, onion, peas, potato, summer squash) ½ artichoke 1 cup lettuce	3	3

Folic Acid-Rich Foods

These foods are rich in folic acid, a B-vitamin especially important during pregnancy because of its role in growth and repair. Pregnant women should have at least four servings daily of these foods.

Protein Foods

Beans: baked, garbanzo, kidney, navy, pinto, pork'n'beans	Peanuts
Lentils	Split peas
Liver	Sunflower seeds
	Yeast, nutritional

Fruits and Vegetables

Asparagus	Lettuce: bibb, Boston, endive, romaine

Nondairy Calcium-Rich Foods

Each of the following is approximately equivalent in calcium to one serving from the milk products group (250–300 mg calcium):

Almonds	4 oz
Beans: baked, pork'n'beans	2 cups
Broccoli, fresh cooked	1½ cups
Greens: turnip, cooked	1½ cups
Greens: bok choy, collard, dandelion, cooked	2 cups
Greens: kale, mustard, cooked	3 cups
Molasses, blackstrap	2 tbsp
Oranges	5 medium
Salmon (with bones)	½ cup canned

(continued)

Folic Acid-Rich Foods		*Nondairy Calcium-Rich Foods*	
Avocado	Orange	Sardines	5 medium or 2½ oz
Beets, fresh	Orange juice	Tofu (must be processed with calcium salt)	9 oz
Broccoli	Peas	Tortillas, corn	7 medium
Brussels sprouts	Pineapple juice		
Cabbage	Spinach		
Corn	Tomato juice		
Greens: collards, mustard	Vegetable juice		

**All pregnant women should have at least four servings of the foods rich in folic acid.
(California Department of Health Services, MCH/WIC: Nutrition During Pregnancy and the Postpartum Period: A Manual for Health Care Professionals, 1990).*

tase is responsible for breaking down lactose (milk sugar) into glucose and galactose. If the available lactase is not sufficient to hydrolyze the amount of lactose ingested, fermentation occurs in the large intestine and causes abdominal cramps, diarrhea, bloating, and flatulence.

Not every woman who says "I don't like milk" or "Milk doesn't agree with me" is lactose intolerant. On the other hand, it is counterproductive to encourage the truly lactose-intolerant person to drink more milk if it causes symptoms. Besides causing discomfort, increased loss of nutrients, including calcium, in the feces can lead to a negative calcium balance and other deficiencies. When counseling these women, special attention should be directed to meeting calcium, protein, vitamin, and mineral requirements. Certain dairy products, such as aged and soft cheeses, are lower in lactose and can be used in place of fluid milk. Some women may find that due to improved efficiency of lactose absorption during pregnancy, they are able to tolerate small amounts of fluid milk at a time (California Department of Health Services, 1990). Also, ingesting milk and milk products in combination with other foods may help lactase-deficient women tolerate them better. Women who consume less than the recommended number of servings of milk products can be advised to substitute foods from the nondairy calcium-rich list included in the Client Education: Nutritional Teaching Guides.

Bread, Cereal, and Grains

A minimum of seven to nine servings should be included from this group daily. At least four of these should be whole-grain products, which contain vitamins and minerals not found in refined flour and not replaced by the enriching process. The germ of the grain, removed in the refining process, also contains protein of value comparable to that from animal sources. Wheat germ can be purchased separately and eaten as a cereal or added to foods, such as baked goods or meat loaf, to increase the nutritional value.

Cereal products are a primary source of energy in the diet, and they make an important contribution to every nutrient need except calcium, ascorbic acid, and vitamin A. Whole-grain cereal and breads also add fiber to the diet to help promote gastrointestinal elimination.

Vegetables and Fruits

Five or more servings of fruits and vegetables, some raw, should be included in the diet daily. Fruits and vegetables contain variable amounts of vitamins and minerals, and most are excellent sources of fiber. Breaking the vegetable and fruit group into the subgroups of vitamin C rich, vitamin A rich, and other helps to ensure that vitamins A and C are adequately included in the diet.

Vegetables. Vegetables are rich sources of iron, calcium, and several vitamins. The dark green vegetables are good sources of vitamin A, folacin, and iron. The deep yellow fruits and vegetables also are good sources of vitamin A. Fresh or frozen vegetables can be used interchangeably. Canned vegetables may be used if necessary, but some nutrients are lost in the cooking and canning process.

CLIENT EDUCATION

Sample Meal Plan for Pregnant or Lactating Women—
*Moderate-Calorie Diet**

Meal	Menu	Protein	Milk	Grains	Vit. C	Vit. A	Other
Breakfast	2 cups puffed wheat			1			
	8 oz low-fat milk		1				
	1 banana						1
	1 bran muffin			1			
	1 tsp. butter**						
Snack	¼ cup frozen strawberries, sweetened				½		
Lunch	2 slices whole-wheat bread			2			
	2 oz tuna, canned in oil, drained	2					
	2 tsp. mayonnaise**						
	1 carrot, raw					1	
	4 oz low-fat milk		½				
Snack	4 graham cracker squares			1			
	4 oz lowfat milk		½				
Dinner	4 oz ground beef	4					
	½ cup refried beans	1					
	¾ oz American cheese		½				
	2 flour tortillas			2			
	½ cup corn, frozen						1
	1 medium tomato, sliced				½		
Snack	½ cup peaches, canned light syrup						1
	6 oz low-fat yogurt, fruited		1				
	TOTALS	7	3	7	1	1	3

*2218 Kcal in basic diet
**This food is optional and represents extra calories added to the basic diet.
(Adapted from Nutrition during Pregnancy and the Postpartum Period: A Manual for Health
Care Professionals. Sacramento, Maternal and Child Health Branch WIC Supplemental Food
Branch, California Department of Health Services, 1990)*

Careful preparation and cooking of vegetables helps to retain the maximum vitamin and mineral content. Presoaking should be avoided. Steaming and stir-frying are preferred methods of cooking. Steamer baskets to fit standard size pans are widely available. Some vegetables contain incomplete proteins that can add to the total protein intake.

In addition to their value as nutrient agents, vegetables play an important role in the diet as laxative agents because their fibrous framework increases the bulk of the intestinal content and thereby stimulates elimination.

Fruits. Citrus fruits, such as oranges, lemons, and grapefruit, are the best sources of vitamin C. Most of these fruits also supply vitamins A and B. Tomatoes also are an excellent source of vitamin C; the amount eaten, however, must be twice that of the citrus fruits to supply the same amount of the vitamin. Other fruits, raw and cooked, such as prunes, raisins, and apricots, contain vitamins and important minerals, such as iron and copper. Fruits contain some incomplete proteins but only supplement the other proteins. Fruits may stimulate a lagging appetite and counteract constipation. They may be eaten plain or combined in salads,

TABLE 18–8
Ethnic Dietary Characteristics

Ethnic Group	Protein Foods	Milk and Milk Products	Grain Products	Vegetables and Fruits	Counseling Suggestions
Mexican American	Variety of meats; poultry, legumes, eggs	Not usual part of adult diet as beverage; small quantities of cheese in cooking	Tortillas and rice, staples	Tomatoes, chili peppers, fried potatoes, other raw or boiled vegetables, oranges, apples, bananas	Increase consumption of cheese and milk in cooking and milk as beverage. Encourage variety of vegetables eaten raw or cooked for short time in small amount of water. Decrease consumption of carbonated beverages and other empty calorie foods. Encourage use of enriched flour for tortillas.
Puerto Rican	Beans, chicken, pork, beef, eggs; ham butts and sausage used for flavoring, not as a protein source	Limited use—"cafe con leche" may contain 2–5 oz of milk	Rice; French bread, rolls, crackers, increasing use of cereals	Pumpkins, carrots, green peppers, tomatoes, sweet potatoes, special boiled root vegetables, canned fruits and nectars	Encourage milk and cheese. Suggest meat source with bean meal. Urge more leafy, green vegetables. Increase use of citrus and other fresh fruits and use of whole grain or enriched breads, cereals, and rice.
African American and Southern	Beef, pork, chicken; legumes as accompaniment	Some milk, buttermilk, cheese, ice cream	Rice, biscuits, white and corn bread	Greens, sweet potatoes, okra, cabbage, corn, green beans, usually boiled; seasonal fruits, limited citrus	Increase milk and decrease carbonated beverages. Encourage whole-grain cereals and bread. Decrease water and time for cooking greens and other vegetables. Eat some raw vegetables. Increase vitamin C sources.
Chinese	Fish, chicken, pork, legumes, eggs, nuts	Ice cream, flavored milk, some milk in cooking	Rice, millet, noodles	Variety of vegetables, often stir-fried with minimal nutrient loss; many fruits, usually fresh	Increase serving size of protein foods, or use as snacks. Increase calories. Encourage dairy products in cooking and use of tofu (soybean curd). Discourage washing rice because of nutrient loss.

(continued)

TABLE 18–8 *(Continued)*					
Ethnic Dietary Characteristics					
Ethnic Group	**Protein Foods**	**Milk and Milk Products**	**Grain Products**	**Vegetables and Fruits**	**Counseling Suggestions**
Southeast Asian	Legumes, fish, fish sauce, eggs, poultry, beef, organ meats, pork	Ice cream, milk (infrequently)	Rice, French bread, noodles	Variety of fresh, uncooked vegetables and fresh fruit	Describe combinations of foods in terms of meals with rice at the center. Reinforce use of vegetable protein, such as mung beans, and calcium-rich foods, such as fermented fish sauce, soft shelled crabs, and small whole fish. Increase calories.
Japanese	Variety of meat and fish, eggs, nuts, legumes, tofu (soybean curd)	Milk and milk products limited	Polished rice, some wheat products	Variety of fruits and vegetables	Encourage use of dairy products to overcome major dietary problem. Use calcium and vitamin D supplements if necessary. Avoid par-cooking of vegetables and washing of rice to avoid nutrient loss.

added to cereals or plain yogurt, and served as between-meal snacks or in desserts, such as gelatins and puddings.

Food Quality

Women need to be reminded to select foods that are fresh and of good quality, because they are safer and more appealing. Foods that have been on the shelf a long time are more likely to begin to deteriorate or become rancid, interfering with their nutritive value. **Aflatoxins**, produced by fungal growths on a wide variety of foodstuffs, have been implicated in mental retardation when consumed during pregnancy (Worthington-Roberts, 1993a). Warning pregnant women against eating any foods that are fermented, moldy, rotten, discolored, or malodorous can help them avoid potentially contaminated foods.

Food Additives

Food additives are substances added directly or indirectly to a food that become a component of the food or affect its functional characteristics. Some additives are necessary in our food supply to prevent spoilage and ensure that certain products are safe to eat. Other additives improve the flavor, odor, texture, color, or the nutritional quality of foods.

The FDA monitors additives and bans those that cause cancer or other problems in animals. The safety of additives is controversial. Nitrates and nitrites, for example, can be converted by the body to nitrosamines, which have been shown to be teratogenic and carcinogenic in rats, but they are still used to preserve processed meats and other foods until adequate substitutes can be found.

The safety of artificial sweeteners has been questioned in recent years. The use of saccharin as an additive in commercial products has decreased markedly since it was linked with the development of bladder cancer in animal studies. There is no real evidence that other artificial sweeteners, such as aspartame (Nutra-Sweet), are harmful, but most dietitians recommend that they be used with caution during pregnancy. The safety of BHA and BHT, which are used in many foods, including cereals, oils, and snack foods, has been questioned.

Caffeine is not really an additive; however, it is a substance of potential concern to the pregnant woman. Although studies show conflicting results, caffeine has been teratogenic and mutagenic in some experiments on rats and mice. There is insufficient evidence to label

CLIENT EDUCATION

Sample Menus to Meet the Daily Food Requirements During Pregnancy for Ethnic Groups

			Food Groups					
Mexican	African-American	Lacto-Ovovegetarian	Protein	Milk	Grains	Vit. C	Vit. A	Other
Breakfast ½ cup oatmeal	1 slice whole grain toast	½ cup Wheatena			1			
1 sweet roll (pan dulce)	½ cup grits	½ cup granola cereal			1			
1 cup low-fat milk Sugar*	1 cup whole milk Margarine, bacon*	1 cup nonfat milk Margarine*		1				
Lunch Tostadas: 2 oz chicken breast	Chiliburger: 2 oz hamburger	Soup and Salad: 1½ cups lentil soup	} 3					
½ cup refried beans	½ cup chili beans	1 egg hard boiled (in salad)						
2 corn tortillas	1 hamburger bun, white	2 whole-grain rolls			2			
Fresh chili salsa: ½ tomato + ½ tbsp. chili pepper	Cole slaw: ½ cup cabbage + dressing*	Salad: 1 fresh tomato				½		
1 cup romaine lettuce	½ cup french fries	1 cup romaine lettuce						1
¾ oz jack cheese	½ cup vanilla milkshake	½ cup nonfat milk		½				
Dinner Bistec ranchero: 3 oz chuck steak	Pork chops: 3 oz pork chop	Stuffed pita: ½ cup kidney beans	} 4					
½ cup kidney beans	½ cup baked beans	6 oz tofu						
¼ cup red potatoes	½ cup mashed potatoes	½ cup hummus ½ cup mushrooms						1
Fresh chili salsa: ½ tomato + ½ tbsp. chili pepper	½ medium orange	¼ cup tomato purée				½		
2 corn tortillas	2 whole-grain rolls	1 pita, whole-wheat			2			
½ fresh mango	½ cup mustard greens	½ cup carrots, raw					1	
Snacks Licuado: 1 cup low-fat milk	1 cup fruit yogurt	Smoothee: 4 oz nonfat milk + ½ cup yogurt		1				
1 cup banana + sugar, vanilla*	15 small grapes	1 banana + honey*						1
¾ cup corn flakes	8 whole-wheat crackers	8 whole-wheat crackers			1			
½ cup low-fat milk	¾ oz American cheese	¾ cups frozen yogurt		½				
		TOTALS	7	3	7	1	1	3

Each menu meets the minimum number of servings for all groups in the Daily Food Guide for Women. One extra serving from the breads/cereals/grains group is included in each menu to follow customary eating habits.

*Indicates foods that provide extra calories only.

(continued)

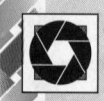

CLIENT EDUCATION
Sample Menus to Meet the Daily Food Requirements During Pregnancy for Ethnic Groups (Continued)

Chinese	Japanese	Southeast Asian	Protein	Milk	Grains	Vit. C	Vit. A	Other
Breakfast								
1 egg, soft-boiled	1 egg, hard-boiled	1 oz pork stir-fried	1					
1 cup oatmeal, cooked	1 cup steamed rice	1 cup rice noodles			2			
1 cup low-fat milk	1 cup low-fat milk	½ cup evaporated milk (in decaf coffee)		1				
Lunch Chicked and soup noodles:	Soup and Salad:	BBQ beef:						
2 oz chicken, boiled	2 oz beef, boiled	2 oz beef strips, grilled	2					
Soy sauce, ginger*	Miso soup broth*	Lemon grass, garlic, oil*						
1 cup noodles, boiled	1 cup buckwheat noodles (soba)	1 cup rice noodles			2			
½ cup snow peas	½ cup broccoli	6 oz orange juice				1		
½ cup bean sprouts, onions	1 cup head lettuce, white radish	1 cup green leaf lettuce						1
Jasmine tea*	Seasoned rice vinegar*	Fish sauce, hot red pepper*						
Dinner Mongolian beef:	Teriyaki salmon:	Stir-fry chicken and cabbage:						
3 oz beef strips	3 oz fresh salmon fillet, broiled	3 oz chicken	3					
Garlic, soy sauce, green onions*	Shoyu marinade*	Fish sauce, chili*						
1 cup white rice, steamed	1 cup white rice, steamed	1 cup white rice, steamed			2			
2 medium plums	½ cup cucumber salad	½ cup bean sprouts						1
½ cup bok choy, stir-fried	½ cup carrots	Soup: ½ cup mustard greens					1	
Soup: 3 oz tofu	3 oz tofu (in soup)	1 oz pork	1					
Parsley, chicken broth*	1 cup miso soup with onion*	Broth*						
Snacks								
1 cup low-fat milk	1 cup low-fat milk	½ cup evaporated milk (in decaf coffee)		1				
1 medium apple	15 small grapes	1 medium banana						1
8 whole-wheat crackers	8 whole-wheat crackers	8 whole-wheat crackers			1			
		TOTALS	7	2	7	1	1	3

Each menu contains at least the minimum number of servings for each food group in the Daily Food Guide for Pregnant Women, except the milk products group. Women who are able to drink milk or who will take lactose-reduced milk can include more milk products to meet the need for calcium. Additional calcium is supplied by broccoli, greens, and tofu.

None of these menus supplies the recommended four servings from whole grains, and the Southeast Asian menu does not include the recommended two servings of vegetable protein, because the menus reflect usual cultural practices. Women should be encouraged to eat more whole-grain breads or crackers and vegetable protein to meet the recommended number of two servings each.

*Indicates foods that provide extra calories only or are used for seasonings.

(California Department of Health Services, MCH/WIC: Nutrition During Pregnancy and the Postpartum Period: A Manual for Health Care Professionals. 1990)

TABLE 18-9
Complementary Plant Protein Sources

Food	Amino Acids Deficient	Complementary Protein
Grains	Isoleucine Lysine	Rice + legumes Corn + legumes Wheat + legumes Wheat + peanuts + milk Wheat + sesame + soybean Rice + sesame Rice + brewer's yeast
Legumes	Tryptophan Methionine	Legumes + rice Beans + wheat Beans + corn Soybeans + rice + wheat Soybeans + corn + milk Soybeans + wheat + sesame Soybeans + peanuts + sesame Soybeans + peanuts + wheat + rice Soybeans + sesame + wheat
Nuts and seeds	Isoleucine Lysine	Peanuts + sesame + soybeans Sesame + beans Sesame + soybeans + wheat Peanuts + sunflower seeds
Vegetables	Isoleucine Methionine	Lima beans Green peas Brussels sprouts } + sesame seeds or Brazil nuts or mushrooms Cauliflower Broccoli Greens + millet or converted rice

(After Lappé, F. M. [1983]. Diet for a small planet [2nd ed.] New York: Ballantine, 1983.)

it as a teratogen in humans; however, a recent study did indicate that the risk of intrauterine growth retardation is increased with heavy caffeine consumption (Fenster et al., 1991). Avoidance or cautious use of caffeine during pregnancy is advised.

Teratogenicity of substances in the diet is usually considered to be dose related. Therefore, although it may be impossible to eliminate additives from the diet, reducing the amount during pregnancy would lower the risks. Until more is known, it is wise to encourage the pregnant woman to read labels carefully and choose products with as few additives as possible.

Weight Gain and Pregnancy

Recommendations for weight gain during pregnancy have varied through the years from unlimited weight gain to severe limitations for all pregnant women. Current trends are to encourage weight gain based on individual characteristics and needs.

The pregnant woman's weight, as measured by prepregnancy weight for height and serial weight measurements during the pregnancy, has been found to have clinical value in assessing gestational weight gain (Institute of Medicine, 1990). This can be expressed as a percentage of a standard or by comparing weight with height as **body mass index (BMI),** defined as weight (kg) divided by height (meters)^2.

Components of Weight Gain

For some time, it was taught that maternal weight gain was adequate if it consisted only of the amount necessary for the products of conception. Anything over that amount was thought to be stored by the mother as "unwanted fat." The exact components of weight gain and the proportions of each are not known and probably vary from one pregnancy to another. A possible distribution of average weight gain is shown in Table 18-10. These figures are rough estimates only, and if

TABLE 18–10
Components of Weight Gain During Pregnancy

Components	Average Weight Gain	
	LB	KG
FETAL		
Fetus	7.5	3.4
Placenta	1.0	0.45
Amniotic fluid	2.0	0.9
MATERNAL		
Uterus (weight increase)	2.5	1.1
Breast tissue (weight increase)	3.0	1.4
Blood volume (weight increase)	4.0 (1,500 mL)	1.8
Maternal stores (fat)	4.0–8.0	1.8–3.6
Total	24–28	10.85–12.65

(Sources: Williams, S. R. [1990]. *Essentials of nutrition and diet therapy* [6th ed.]. St. Louis: C.V. Mosby; Worthington-Roberts, B., & Williams, S. R. [1993]. *Nutrition in pregnancy and lactation* [5th ed.]. St. Louis: C.V. Mosby.)

actual weights of the various components could be measured, they would undoubtedly differ for each pregnant woman. The largest variation occurs in the "maternal stores" component, which consists mainly of extra adipose tissue. This is no longer thought of as unwanted but is considered necessary to provide maternal energy reserves during pregnancy, labor, and delivery and lactation (Williams, 1993). In some analyses, part of the maternal gain is credited to increased lean muscle mass (California Department of Health Services, 1990).

Most of the gain during the second trimester is related to maternal tissues, whereas the fetus gains the most during the third trimester. The pattern of total weight gain is believed to be much more important than the actual amount of weight gained. The usual pattern consists of a 1- to 2-kg (2–4 lb) weight gain during the first trimester, followed by an average, fairly steady, gain of about 0.4 kg (0.9 lb) per week during the last two trimesters (Institute of Medicine, 1990).

The prenatal weight gain grid, included as part of the Assessment Tool: Nutritional Questionnaire for Pregnant Women, indicates recommended patterns of weight gain. It can be used to plot the pregnant woman's weight gain and to detect deviations from expected patterns. For example, a sudden, sharp increase in weight after the 20th week may indicate excessive water retention and the onset of pregnancy-induced hypertension. Inadequate weight gain or weight loss also can be noted.

Calorie Intake and Weight Gain

Calories provide the energy requirements for the body and are needed to maintain bodily processes, thermal balance, and physical activity. Caloric allowances are established to provide adequate energy and to support growth and body weight levels appropriate for the health and well-being of the fetus and woman.

In the past, attempts were made to limit maternal weight gain during pregnancy by restricting caloric intake to prevent and control preeclampsia. However, controlled studies have not supported the belief that caloric intake as reflected by weight gain causes preeclampsia. To the contrary, evidence shows that limiting weight gain decreases essential nutrient intake, which is thought to be one of the contributing factors in the development of preeclampsia. During pregnancy, there is an increased need for calories to meet the energy requirements for building fetal and placental tissue and for maintaining the woman's tissue requirements. The RDA during the second and third trimesters of pregnancy is 300 kcal/d above the woman's usual RDA. For the individual woman, actual needs could vary according to many factors, including her size and activity. Average energy intake needs are met by a daily intake of 45 kcal/kg of pregnant body weight and for optimal protein use should not fall below 36 kcal/kg (Williams, 1993). In a study group at the Montreal Diet Dispensary, additional calories are recommended for specific conditions, such as protein deficiency, underweight, and special conditions of stress (Worthington-Roberts, 1993b).

One of the main risks to the newborn is low birth weight and the problems that accompany it. The outcome for the newborn has been shown to improve as the birth weight increases. Many studies have shown the relationship between maternal weight gain and birth weight. These findings, coupled with concern about relatively high U.S. perinatal mortality, have led to the recommendation of more liberal weight gain for the woman during pregnancy.

The 1990 recommendations for weight gain during pregnancy from the Food and Nutrition Board of the National Academy of Sciences suggest a total gain of 25 to 35 lb for women whose prepregnancy weight falls within the normal weight range (Institute of Medicine, 1990). These recommendations also emphasize individualization of weight gain goals based on the woman's prepregnant weight for height and other individual factors. For women who are underweight, the recommendation is 28 to 40 lb, and for those who are moderately overweight, 15 to 25 lb (Table 18-11). Higher weight gains also may be appropriate for those who tend to have smaller babies, such as young adolescents, African American women, women who smoke, and those with multiple pregnancies. Very short women and those who

TABLE 18-11
*Recommended Total Weight Gain Ranges for Pregnant Women**

Prepregnancy Status	Prepregnancy Weight for Height Category	BMI	Recommended Total Gain	
			LB	KG
Underweight	<90% of desirable weight	<19.8	28–40	12.5–18
Desirable weight	90%–120% of desirable weight	19.8–26	25–35	11.5–16
Moderately overweight	121%–135% of desirable weight	26–29	15–25	7–11.5
Very overweight	>135% of desirable weight	>29	≥15	≥7.0
Overall Range			15–40	7–18

*For women 18 years and older with a singleton pregnancy.
Women 17 years or younger, women carrying twins or triplets, African American women, or women who smoke should strive for gains above these ranges, irrespective of their prepregnancy weight. Short women (<5 ft, 2 in or <157 cm) should strive for gains at the lower end of the range.
(Sources: Maternal and Child Health Branch, WIC Supplemental Food Branch, California Department of Health Services [1990]. *Nutrition during pregnancy and the postpartum period: A manual for health care professionals.* Sacramento: Author.
National Academy Press [1992]. *Nutrition during pregnancy and lactation: An implementation guide.* Washington, DC: Subcommittee for a Clinical Application Guide, Committee on Nutritional Status During Pregnancy and Lactation, Food and Nutrition Board.)

are very overweight may do well with lower weight gains. Studies have found that the very overweight have the lowest perinatal mortality when they gain 15 to 16 lb (Worthington-Roberts, 1993b).

It is sometimes tempting for the obese client to try to lose weight during pregnancy, but this should be discouraged. When caloric intake is low enough to cause weight loss, maternal fat stores are catabolized for energy, resulting in **ketonemia,** ketone bodies in the blood, which may adversely affect the fetus. Also, environmental contaminants stored in the fat may be released during the process and affect the fetus. Emphasizing nutritious foods, rather than weight reduction, may help improve dietary habits and lead to easier weight reduction after pregnancy.

Promoting Adequate Weight Gain

The need for counseling about weight gain varies from one client to another. Some women have been counseled to restrict weight with previous pregnancies or have heard about this practice from friends and believe it is the best way. They may need reassurance that gaining more than 20 lb can be beneficial for themselves and the baby. Other women may think that they can limit the size of the fetus and have an easier delivery if they eat less. They can be helped to understand that limiting intake does not guarantee a smaller newborn, and if the woman's nutritional status is poor, the labor and delivery might be difficult regardless of the size of the newborn.

Some women are weight conscious and may resist gaining adequate weight because of fears that they will

not be able to lose it after the newborn arrives. Careful explanation of the distribution of the additional weight and the importance of good nutrition to the outcome of pregnancy may help them accept the weight gain. They also may benefit from information about recent studies that show that for women who gain weight within the recommended guidelines, the average difference between prepregnancy and postpartum weight was 2.3 lb for white women and slightly higher for African American women (Keppel et al., 1993).

Women who gain weight rapidly during the first two trimesters may reach what they consider to be maximum gain by the seventh month. If they attempt to cut down on what they eat to try to avoid gaining any more weight, they may be deprived of adequate nutrients at the time when fetal brain cells are growing the fastest and when the fetus is depositing a protective layer of fat. These women need encouragement to continue eating adequately.

Making Calories Count

Making calories count emphasizes the importance of eating only foods that contribute necessary nutrients to the diet. "Empty calories" are to be avoided, especially if the woman's appetite is poor, or her food dollar is limited. The obese woman also benefits from this kind of instruction, not only during pregnancy, but also in planning a weight reduction program after pregnancy. "Eat to appetite" may be a good slogan to promote adequate weight gain during pregnancy, but it is valid only when the woman is taught which foods to eat to obtain the most nutrients.

The woman whose diet consists mainly of food such as doughnuts, candy bars, and soda pop may satisfy her appetite; however, her nutritional status suffers, and she gets a poor return for her food dollar. This does not mean that desserts must be eliminated from the diet. Custard, made from eggs and milk, is an example of a nutritious dessert. The nutritive value of other desserts, such as baked goods, can be improved by using whole grain flour, adding wheat germ, and reducing the amount of refined sugar.

Resources

The nurse should be aware of available resources for nutritional counseling, education, and support. This helps to keep nutritional education up to date and enables the nurse to make appropriate referrals.

When consultation with a nutritionist is advisable and one is not available on the clinic or hospital staff, it may be possible to locate one in the area through the local community health department or a home economist's office. Publications, visual aids, charts, and other materials may be secured from city, county, and state health departments. The March of Dimes Birth Defects Foundation also provides many teaching aids and reminders about nutrition during pregnancy.

The U.S. Government Printing Office is another invaluable source of publications. The Food and Nutrition Board, National Research Council, Council on Foods and Nutrition, American Medical Association, American Home Economics Association, and American Public Health Association are all professional organizations that offer additional resources. The above associations are only a few of the resources that the nurse and physician have to assist their clients in planning for adequate nutrition.

Supplemental Food Programs

A source of nutritional help for some pregnant women is WIC. This program was initiated in 1973 to provide food for low-income families at critical times of growth and development. Funds for the program come from the U.S. Department of Agriculture and are administered at the state and local levels by state health departments (Rush, 1989).

At the local level, specific foods are provided for pregnant women, lactating women, infants, and children up to 5 years of age who are determined to be at risk nutritionally and who otherwise would be unable to afford an adequate diet. Food vouchers or supplemental foods are distributed at designated health clinics. The WIC program also provides education, which is mandated to be an integral part of the program. The educational component of the program uses a variety of teaching methods, including lectures, films, group or individual discussions, and written material. It is planned to take into account socioeconomic, educational, and cultural factors and the level of understanding of the recipients.

Special Nutritional Concerns for the Pregnant Adolescent

If the pregnant client is an adolescent, nutritional concerns arise that need to be highlighted in her care. Adolescents have repeatedly been shown to have poorer pregnancy outcomes than older pregnant women. This has sometimes been attributed to a competition for nutrients between the growth requirements of the adolescent and those of the fetus. Current information, however, indicates that except for those of low **gynecologic age** (number of years past onset of menarche), the adolescent's nutrient needs are not very different from those of other pregnant women (Food and Nutrition Board, 1990; Nutritional Research Council, 1989; Winick, 1989). However, the pregnant adolescent is at higher nutritional risk. She is more likely to begin pregnancy in poor nutritional status as evidenced by being underweight, iron deficient, and consuming inadequate amounts of calcium and other important nutrients.

Factors leading to inadequate nutrition for the pregnant adolescent include the desire to be slim, peer food practices, and resistance to adult advice. Eating nutritionally may be of low priority to the pregnant adolescent, who may be much more concerned about meeting her social and emotional needs. Because adolescent pregnancy is most common among the poor and socially disadvantaged, and therefore among those least likely to receive needed medical and social support, the risk for poor nutritional status is further increased. Appropriate referrals to WIC and other resources, such as classes and programs for pregnant adolescents, are important (Winick, 1989).

Food Selection

The teenager's food choices often include many "fast foods" and non-nutritious snacks. This leads to a low intake of fresh fruits and vegetables, which in turn limits the intake of vitamins and minerals, especially vitamins A and C. If milk and milk products are avoided, there may be a lack of certain B-complex vitamins and vitamin D, in addition to inadequate intake of calcium and protein.

Weight Gain

The levels of protein and energy intake and the pregnancy weight gain needed to promote optimal intrauterine growth for the fetuses of adolescent mothers are matters of ongoing study. Theoretically, the ideal weight gain would include the usual pregnancy recommendation, plus, for the girl who is still growing, the amount she would have gained in the process of maturation during the 9-month period if she had not become pregnant. Younger adolescents (12–15 years) would therefore be expected to gain more than older adolescents (16 and older), whose growth rate would have slowed down or stopped (Rees et al., 1993). Chronologic age, however, is less important in this regard than gynecologic age, the girl's individual growth pattern, her prepregnancy weight for height, and her level of activity. Weight-conscious teenagers may resist continuous weight gain, especially if they have gained a lot in early pregnancy. They need extra help in understanding the importance of weight gain throughout the pregnancy and dieting's potential dangers to the fetus during this time when extra nutrients are needed.

Eating Disorders

Weight consciousness and equating thinness with attractiveness have led to an increased incidence of eating disorders. Anorexia nervosa and bulimia are found most frequently in the adolescent and young-adult age groups. Fertility is usually reduced in an anorectic female, who is rarely able to conceive or carry a pregnancy. Bulimia, which is becoming more common among teenagers, is less likely than anorexia to affect fertility. However, the nutritional state of the bulimic, through her binging and purging and use of diuretics, is far from optimum in spite of near-normal body weight. Because recognition of bulimia is relatively recent, little research is available on how best to manage the pregnant bulimic female (Williams et al., 1993).

Some possible effects of bulimia, besides the nutritional deficits, are tooth decay and possible esophageal damage caused by repeated vomiting, hemorrhoids, occult bleeding, metabolic acidosis caused by the continual use of laxatives, and fluid and electrolyte imbalances resulting from diuretic abuse (Davis et al., 1994). Theoretically, the primary additional problem during pregnancy is the effect on the fetus from the potentially detrimental changes in its biochemical environment that results from maternal binging, vomiting, and purging (Williams et al., 1993).

To provide sufficient nourishment to support the pregnancy and attempt to avoid detrimental effects on the fetus, the bulimic woman needs psychological intervention and nutritional support. The nurse's primary role is detection of the problem and referral to an appropriate source for psychological help.

Counseling

The pregnant adolescent benefits most from counseling designed to meet her individual needs. Many teenagers do eat nutritionally sound diets and only need reinforcement of their good eating habits and information about additional pregnancy needs. Others need more specific assistance. Although some may respond to the appeal to eat well for a healthy baby, to many pregnant teenagers, the fetus does not seem real until late in the pregnancy or after the birth. Stressing the girl's own growth and development needs may be a more effective way of gaining their interest. When pregnant teenagers are well nourished throughout their pregnancy, they are much less likely to develop complications and much more likely to produce a healthy newborn.

Evaluation

The nurse can use the evaluation phase of the nursing process to improve the effectiveness of nutritional care for the pregnant client. Evaluation is ongoing, and revisions in the nursing care plan are made throughout the pregnancy in response to the evaluation. Possible anticipated outcomes may include the following:

- The client gains weight appropriately throughout the pregnancy.
- The client demonstrates knowledge of nutritional needs.
- The client verbalizes appropriate food choices.
- The fetus demonstrates adequate growth and development for age.
- The client delivers a full-term, healthy newborn of adequate size without complications.

Summary Points

✔ Maternal nutrition during pregnancy impacts on the well-being of the woman, the developing fetus, and later, the development of the infant. Adequate weight gain during pregnancy helps to provide better pregnancy outcomes.

✔ The nurse can play a key role in nutritional assessment of pregnant women. Areas to be assessed include dietary intake, nutritional status, factors involved in food choices, and nutritional risk factors.

✔ Nutritional counseling is an important nursing role before, during, and after pregnancy.

✔ Knowledge of nutrient needs of pregnant women and how adequate nutrients can be incorporated into the diet is essential for nurses who counsel women.

✔ The best source of nutrients is from the woman's diet. Supplementation is recommended when dietary intake is inadequate. The most frequently recommended supplements are iron and folic acid.

✔ Adequate weight gain during pregnancy helps to provide better pregnancy outcomes. The recommended amount of weight gain during pregnancy is influenced by the woman's prepregnant weight for height and other individual characteristics and needs.

✔ Ethnic and cultural dietary characteristics are important factors to include when planning the diet.

✔ Government agencies provide a number of resources, services, and publications to help pregnant women obtain optimal nutritional status.

✔ Pregnant adolescents may have increased nutrient needs, but they also may have decreased intake due to their food habits or peer pressure.

REFERENCES

California Department of Health Services (1990). *Nutrition during pregnancy and the postpartum period: A manual for health care professinals.* Sacramento: Author.

Committee on Maternal Nutrition, Food and Nutrition Board, National Research Council (1970). *Maternal nutrition and the course of pregnancy.* Washington, DC: National Academy of Sciences.

Czeizel, A. E., & Dudas, I. (1992). Prevention of the first occurrence of neural-tube defects by periconceptional vitamin supplementation. *The New England Journal of Medicine, 327,* 1832–1835.

Davis, J., & Sherer, K. (1994). *Applied nutrition and diet therapy for nurses* (2nd ed). Philadelphia: W.B. Saunders.

Fenster et al. (1991). Caffeine consumption during pregnancy and fetal growth. *American Journal of Public Health, 81,* 458–461.

Higgins, A. (1973). Montreal diet dispensary study. In *Nutritional supplementation and the outcome of pregnancy* (pp. 93–110). Washington, DC: National Academy of Sciences.

Institute of Medicine (1990). *Nutrition during pregnancy: Part I, weight gain; Part II, nutrient supplements.* Committee on Nutritional Status During Pregnancy and Lactation, Food and Nutrition Board. Washington, DC: National Academy Press.

Institute of Medicine (1992). *Nutrition during pregnancy and lactation; An implementation guide.* Subcommittee for a clinical application guide, Committee on Nutritional Status During Pregnancy and Lactation, food and Nutrition Board. Washington, DC: National Academy Press.

Keppel, K. G., & Taffel, S. M. (1993). Pregnancy-related weight gain and retention: Implications of the 1990 Institute of Medicine guidelines. *American Journal of Public Health, 83,* 1100–1103.

MRC Vitamin Study Research (1991). Prevention of neural tube defects: Results of the Medical Research council vitamin study. *Lancet, 338,* 131–137.

National Research Council (US) Subcommittee on the Tenth Edition of the RDAs (1989). *Recommended dietary allowances.* Washington, DC: National Academy Press.

Primrose, T., & Higgins, A. (1971). A study in human antepartum nutrition. *Journal of Reproductive Medicine, 7,* 257–264.

Rees, J. M., & Worthington-Roberts, B. S. (1993). Nutritional needs of the pregnant adolescent. In B. Worthington-Roberts & S. R. Williams (Eds.), *Nutrition in pregnancy and lactation* (5th ed.) (pp. 280–315). St. Louis: C.V. Mosby.

Romanczuk, A. N., & Borwn, J. P. (1994). Folic acid will reduce risk of neural tube defects. *MCN: American Journal of Maternal Child Nursing, 19,* 331–334.

Rosso, P., & Cramoy, C. (1979). Nutrition and pregnancy. In M. Winick (Ed.), *Nutrition—Pre and postnatal development* (p. 176). New York: Plenum Press.

Rush, D. (1989). Effects of changes in protein and calorie intake during pregnancy on the growth of the human fetus. In I. Chalmers, M. Enkin, & M. J. N. C. Keirse (Eds.), *Effective care in pregnancy and childbirth* (pp. 255–280). New York: Oxford University Press.

Stein, Z. (Ed.) (1975). Famine and human development: The Dutch hunger winter of 1944-1945. New York: Oxford University Press.

Trouba, P. H., Okereke, N., & Splett, P. L. (1991). Summary document of nutrition intervention in prenatal care. *Journal of the American Dietetic Association,* (Suppl.), 521–526.

U.S. Department of Agriculture, Food and Nutrition Service (1994). *Eating for you and your baby* (Program Aid No. 1198). Hyattsville, MD: Author.

Willett, W. C. (1992). Folic acid and neural tube defect: Can't we come to closure? *American Journal of Public Health, 82,* 666–668.

Williams, S. R. (1993). Nutrition assessment and guidance in prenatal care. In B. Worthington-Roberts & S. R. William (Eds.), *Nutrition in pregnancy and lactation* (5th ed.) (pp. 206–238). St. Louis: C.V. Mosby.

Williams, S. R., & Trahms, C. M. (1993). Management of pregnancy complications and special disease conditions of the mother. In B. Worthington-Roberts, & S. R. Williams (Eds.), *Nutrition in pregnancy and lactation* (5th ed.) (pp. 239–279). St. Louis: C.V. Mosby.

Winick, M. (1979). Malnutrition and mental development. In M. Winick (Ed.), *Nutrition—Pre and postnatal development* (p. 52). New York: Plenum Press.

Winick, M. (1989). *Nutrition, pregnancy, and early infancy.* Baltimore: Williams & Wilkins.

Worthington-Roberts, B. (1993a). Prenatal nutrtion: Additional dietary and lifestyle concerns. In B. Worthington-Roberts & S. R. Williams (Eds.), *Nutrition in pregnancy and lactation* (5th ed.) (pp. 173–205). St. Louis: C.V. Mosby.

Worthington-Roberts, B. (1993b). Prenatal nutrition: General issues. In B. Worthington-Roberts & S. R. Williams (Eds.), *Nutrition in pregnancy and lactation* (5th ed.) (pp. 87–172). St. Louis: C.V. Mosby.

19

Education for Pregnancy and Parenthood

Objectives

- Describe the characteristics of adult learners.
- Describe the concepts in the cone of learning.
- List the conditions that are considered contraindications to exercise during pregnancy.
- List the four principles related to Lamaze breathing strategies.
- Describe and demonstrate the following Lamaze breathing patterns: cleansing breath, slow paced breathing, modified paced breathing, and breathing for birth.
- Define habituation, and describe how it influences which breathing patterns to use.
- Identify postpartum factors that influence teaching and learning.

The increased involvement of childbearing couples in all phases of the reproductive cycle benefits not only the parents as receivers of care, but also nurses as givers of care. A concerned and knowledgeable woman follows a more healthful regimen during pregnancy. A prepared woman and an involved partner can cope positively with the stresses of labor, enriching their relationship and promoting psychological maturation. Parents who are informed and who actively seek understanding of their child's numerous needs for comfort, security, and stimulation during the early formative years can attain a happier, more satisfying parent–child relationship and foster optimal growth and development of the child. Thus, nurses working with childbearing families have a unique opportunity to make a positive impact on the family's health and well-being that could last for many years.

The cornerstone of client education is recognition and respect for the learning needs of clients. The nurse may design a program with the right content, but if it does not meet the family's learning needs, it is pointless and ineffective. The nurse must develop skills to assess these learning needs accurately.

Factors in Parent Education

Many factors need to be taken into consideration when planning childbirth and parenting education programs. Understanding the woman's needs and interests and recognizing the changes that occur in the prenatal period and during labor and postpartum are essential. Before any teaching can begin, the nurse also must have some understanding of the client's background and cultural practices. Finally, the nurse should be aware of the characteristics of adult learners (unless his or her client is an adolescent) and plan teaching with these characteristics in mind.

Psychological Tasks of Pregnancy and Women's Interests

Nurses have long observed that pregnant women ask different kinds of questions and express different con-

cerns in early pregnancy than in later periods of gestation. Professional interest in the many behavior changes characteristic of pregnant women has led to identification of the specific and unique psychological tasks that appear to be a universal phenomenon of pregnancy (see Box 16-2). These tasks are necessary to cope with the numerous changes. In addition, research has confirmed that most pregnant women experience certain cognitive and emotional reactions during the different pregnancy trimesters, as described in Chapter 16 (see Box 16-3).

During early pregnancy, when the woman is working through the idea of being pregnant, informational needs center on validating the pregnancy, understanding physical changes, and recognizing normal emotions and feelings. In midpregnancy, a woman begins to identify the fetus as a unique person and is receptive to information about fetal growth and development and about maintaining her own health and the health of the fetus. As pregnancy draws to an end, the woman becomes concerned about preparing for the newborn's arrival and becomes interested in preparation for childbirth, infant behavior, and caretaking activities, including feeding, handling, and bathing. By tailoring the information to the different interests of each group and providing women with the opportunity to express their own learning needs, nurses can conduct meaningful prenatal educational programs. Box 19-1 lists learning needs by trimester.

Importance of Labor and Postpartum Processes

Although the experience of labor is undoubtedly significant for the woman's self-concept, maternal–newborn bonding, and possibly the couple's relationship, little data are available to substantiate what impact nursing intervention during labor might have on these perceptions. Advocates of prepared childbirth believe that women move more rapidly into the caretaking role when they are actively participating in their labor. There is some empirical evidence that fathers who act as labor partners during some of their children's births but not for others develop stronger and more recognizable paternal feelings toward the infants whose labors and births where they participated.

Effective client teaching must take into account what is known about the processes that occur during labor and the puerperium and individual variation and specific need. Because the labor experience is so important, health professionals have an obligation to assist parents in preparing for it and supporting them during this stressful time. When labor has started, a certain amount of teaching is possible, and sensitive care can be helpful, but this is not as effective as prenatal preparation. Other physiologic and psychological changes that occur during the puerperium are part of

BOX 19-1
Learning Needs of Expectant Parents

First Trimester
Physical changes of pregnancy
Emotional changes of pregnancy
Sexuality
   Changing relationships
   Sexual concerns
Minor discomforts of pregnancy
   Frequent urination
   Nausea
   Leg cramps
   Vaginal discharge
   Fatigue
Danger signs
   Vaginal bleeding
   Persistent vomiting
Nutrition
General hygiene
   Rest and sleep
   Exercise
Use of drugs
   Smoking
   Alcohol
   Over-the-counter (OTC) drugs
   Prescription drugs
Fetal development
Financial considerations
How to use the healthcare system
Resources for pregnancy and child-
   birth
Myths about pregnancy and childbirth

Second Trimester
Physical changes of second trimester
Emotional changes of second tri-
   mester
Sexuality
   Changing needs
   Sexual concerns
Minor discomforts of pregnancy
   Backache
   Varicose veins
   Braxton Hicks contractions
   Leg cramps
   Vaginal discharge
   Constipation
   Round ligament pain
Danger signs
   Vaginal bleeding
   Abdominal pain
   Edema of face, hands, feet
   Severe headache
   Visual disturbances
   Rupture of membranes
Nutrition
General hygiene
   Rest and sleep
   Exercise
Use of drugs
   Smoking
   Alcohol
   OTC drugs
   Prescription drugs
Fetal growth
Preparation for newborn
   Feeding methods
   Physical arrangements
   Selection of pediatrician
   Infant care

Third Trimester
Physical and emotional changes of
   third trimester and postpartum
Sexuality
   Changing needs
   Sexual expression (different
      methods)
   Sexual concerns
   Problem solving
Minor discomforts of pregnancy (also
   see second trimester)
   Frequent urination
   Dyspnea
   Fatigue
Danger signs (also see second tri-
   mester)
   Rupture of membranes (before 38
      weeks)
Nutrition
   Rest and sleep
   Exercise
Use of drugs (see second trimester)
Fetal growth
Breastfeeding
Support systems
Preparation for childbirth
   Fears and anxieties
   Father involvement
   Issue of choice
   Anatomy and physiology of child-
      birth
   Comfort measures
   Pain management
   Variation in labors
   Hospital routines
   Obstetric interventions
   Special needs of multiparas
Parenting
   Lifestyle changes
   Role changes
   Role conflict
   Balancing family demands
   Maternal role acquisition
   Maternal development tasks
Preparation for newborn
Family planning

*While there is strong research support for some of these learning needs, others are based on healthcare
professionals' beliefs of what expectant parents need to know. The most appropriate time for the introduction of these topic areas in childbirth education classes is undetermined from a scientific perspective.
There is a need for the systematic documentation of the learning needs of expectant parents and the best
time during pregnancy to discuss them from the parents' perspective and from that of health professionals.*

(This Table is adapted from Nichols, F. [1988]. The content. In F. Nichols, & S. Humenick (Eds.). Childbirth education: Practice research, and theory. *Philadelphia: W.B. Saunders.)*

the process undergone by the mother and must be taken into consideration when planning postpartum education. For further details of these physiologic and psychological changes and their relation to teaching, refer to Chapters 25 and 26.

Socioeconomic and Cultural Factors

The learning process varies according to culture and the socioeconomic situation. Mothering practices in lower income groups are influenced by economic circumstances that limit equipment, supplies, and mobility; by the organization of the family group and the authority structure; and by the accumulated folk knowledge that establishes specific practices for many common activities and problems of childrearing. Standard educational programs about breast-feeding or formula preparation, clothing and supplies for the infant, integration of the newborn into the family, and the mother's nutritional and rest needs may be meaningless to low-income mothers because of a lack of resources and a different value system. Family and friends are generally viewed as more reliable consultants for health concerns than professionals, whose assistance is sought only when community knowledge cannot solve the problem. Sometimes the use of language precludes useful exchange of information. In some cultures the grandmother's word about infant care is often law, and she may be the major caretaker of the infant. Teaching given solely to the mother may be of little consequence to the actual care given to the infant. Different cultural groups also have unique approaches to childrearing and patterns of assistance to new mothers. The nurse must understand different cultural and income lifestyles if effective prenatal and postpartum teaching is to occur. The approach to teaching used with these groups probably needs to shift from the giving of information to assessing present practices and supplementing these practices when necessary with information presented in a form that can be understood and accepted.

Characteristics of Adult Learners

According to Knowles (1980), adult learners differ from other learners. Because the majority of expectant and new parents with whom the nurse comes into contact are adults, it is important to take these differences into consideration. According to Aukamp et al. (1988), the adult learner has the following characteristics:

1. Independent and self-directed in learning. The nurse serves, therefore, as a facilitator, resource person, and encourager in the learning situation as opposed to being the total director of learning.
2. Previous experiences that are rich resources for learning. Students learn faster and better when the teacher relates new class material to past experiences and builds on previous knowledge. Learners can also be resources for others in the classroom situation. The teacher is not, therefore, the source of all knowledge in the classroom.
3. Readiness to learn that is based on current social roles and tasks. Life situations influence the adult's readiness to learn. For example, a stressful life situation because of inadequate money can hinder readiness to learn, whereas other life situations, such as pregnancy, can increase the adult's eagerness to learn. The nurse needs to be sensitive to the life situations of learners and work with the adult to overcome any barriers to learning.
4. Desire to learn things that have immediate application. Adults often are motivated to attend classes because of a particular need. If the class can be structured so that the learner can immediately use some of the information in life situations, this enhances the learning process. Information presented on the first night of class on coping with the discomforts of pregnancy and how to develop basic relaxation skills are examples of information that the adult learner can use immediately.
5. Preference for a problem-oriented learning approach as opposed to a subject-oriented learning approach. Adults want to learn how to solve real-life problems; thus, they are often less interested in information presented in a subject-oriented format. When a nurse teaches fetal development by describing the anatomy and physiology of conception and subsequent development, the nurse is using a subject-centered approach. When the nurse teaches about pregnancy from the perspective of expectant parents' tasks and sensations of pregnancy while weaving in a description of the developing fetus, he or she is using a problem-centered approach to teaching fetal development. In this approach, learners can more readily apply the information to their own situation.

Time also is important to adults. Classes should start and end on time. Adults need to feel they are getting something of value out of their learning experience. Classes should be organized so that early in the first class, each learner feels his or her presence in class is important because of the material that was discussed. Ideally, each learner should come away from each class thinking it is a good thing he or she did not miss this class because important things were learned, and each minute of class time was well spent.

The Cone of Learning

In addition to all the other factors just discussed, the nurse educator must take into consideration the learning cone before planning content (Fig. 19-1). The cone of learning describes the amount of learning that occurs with increasing amounts of involvement. Taking this into account, it is clear that if learning is to occur,

the nurse must do more than merely present the content and hope the client remembers.

Types of Education for Pregnancy, Labor, and Postpartum

Knowledge about pregnancy and parenthood is influenced by an accumulation of experiences through infancy, childhood, adolescence, and maturity. Schools

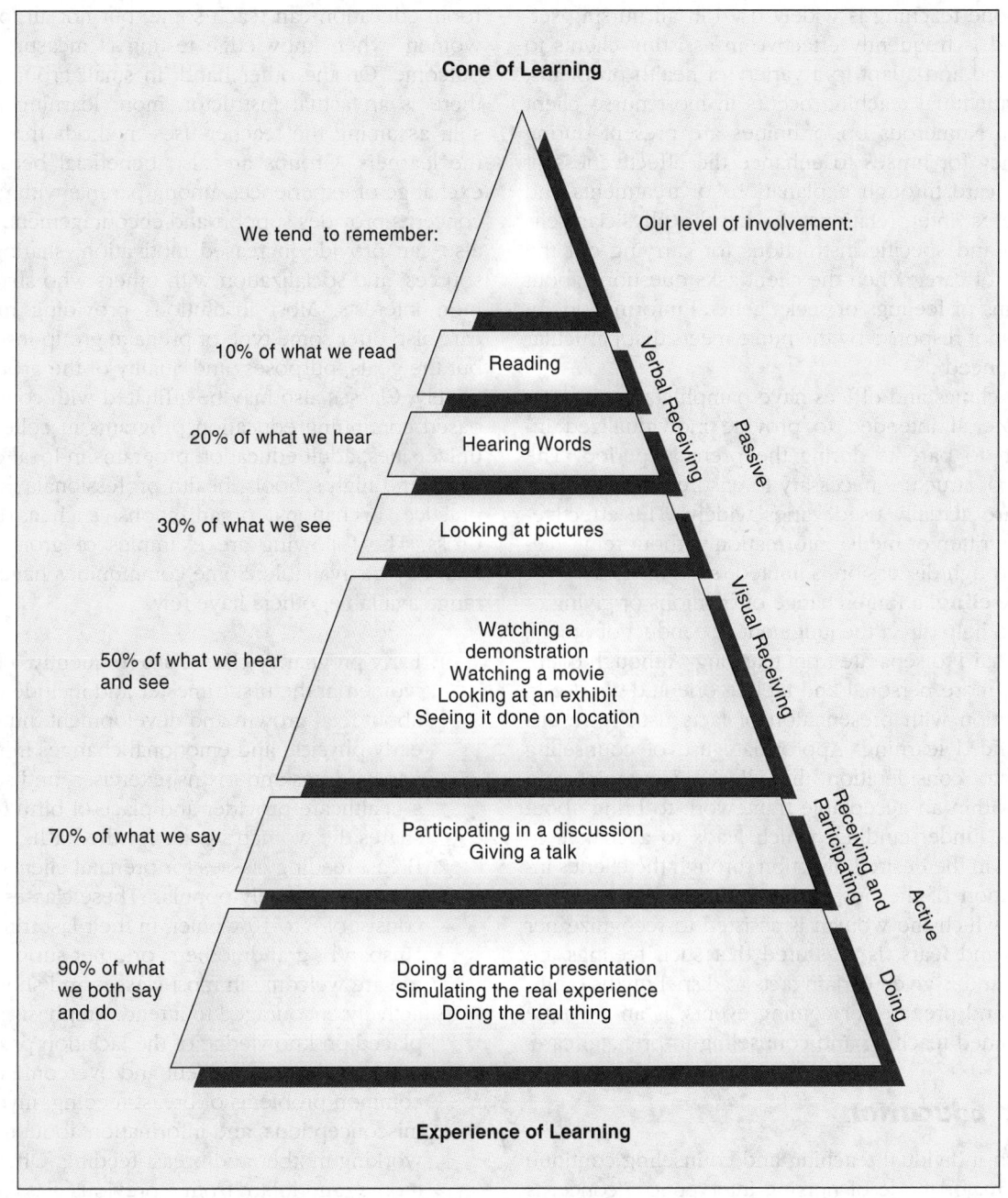

Cone of Learning

We tend to remember:

Our level of involvement:

10% of what we read	Reading
20% of what we hear	Hearing Words
30% of what we see	Looking at pictures
50% of what we hear and see	Watching a demonstration / Watching a movie / Looking at an exhibit / Seeing it done on location
70% of what we say	Participating in a discussion / Giving a talk
90% of what we both say and do	Doing a dramatic presentation / Simulating the real experience / Doing the real thing

Verbal Receiving — Passive

Visual Receiving

Receiving and Participating — Active

Doing

Experience of Learning

FIGURE 19–1 Cone of learning.

are increasingly incorporating information about child-bearing and parenthood into health education and family life courses. Classes about pregnancy, sexuality, and parenthood are becoming more common in high school and university curricula, and they are more widely available in continuing education and private adult educational programs. Couples bring a wealth of previous learning to their experience of childbearing; some of it is useful and positive and some frightening and inaccurate. With the advent of pregnancy, preparation for parenthood begins in earnest.

Individual Teaching and Counseling

One-to-one teaching is widely used in all nursing settings and is frequently effective in assisting clients to understand and adapt to a variety of health problems. Some individual teaching occurs in most nurse–client contacts. Numerous opportunities are present during pregnancy for nurses to enhance the effectiveness of medical care through explanations of treatments and procedures, interpretations of what the physician tells parents, and specific instructions for carrying out the regimen of care. When the client asks questions about symptoms or feelings or seeks general information, an on-the-spot response by the nurse meets that particular learning need.

Some clinics and offices have pamphlets or audiovisual material intended to provide individualized instruction to parents during the prenatal period. The amount of structure necessary to ensure that these materials are actually used varies widely. The effectiveness of written or media information without reinforcement through discussion is limited (see Fig. 19-1).

Counseling, an interchange of opinions or giving of advice to help direct the judgment or conduct of others, is often hard to separate from teaching. Although counseling is more personal and feeling oriented, its use in combination with presentation of facts usually results in enhanced learning. Appropriate use of counseling takes into consideration the client's viewpoint and works within an acceptable framework to bring about increased understanding, which leads to a change in behavior in the desired direction through the client's internalization of the new goals. Individualized nursing care, in which the woman is assisted to recognize her feelings and fears, is reassured that such feelings are normal, and is given certain facts to dispel myths or anticipate and prepare for coming events, is an example of combined teaching and counseling in prenatal care.

Group Education

Although individual teaching and counseling continue to be a major mode of nursing intervention, concerns for more efficient use of the health professional's time have led to different ways to teach greater numbers of pregnant women and their partners. It is common in waiting rooms where pregnant women are waiting for their prenatal appointments to have educational video-tapes playing continuously or available in another room. However, teaching and learning are not synonymous, and as Figure 19-1 makes clear, learning requires active participation. In a study conducted in a clinic waiting room, nulliparas and women younger than 20 years had the same score on a knowledge test whether or not the videotapes were shown (Freda et al., 1994). Other groups did demonstrate learning, leading the authors to conclude that passive waiting room education can teach some, but not all, pregnant women, when knowledge testing is measured as an outcome. On the other hand, in small groups, where there is an actual instructor, more learning may result, assuming the teacher uses methods that involve the learners. Groups are also beneficial because the exchange of experiences among parents with common concerns provides support and encouragement. Groups also can provide increased motivation, sharing of resources, and socialization with others who share common interests. Most institutions providing maternity care also offer some type of prenatal group instruction, but the goals, purposes, and quality of the groups vary widely. Classes also may be affiliated with community-based continuing education programs in colleges and universities, adult education programs in local communities and high schools, health professionals in private practice, or national organizations, such as the Red Cross. The following are examples of group classes that may be available. Some communities have a wide range available; others have few.

1. Early pregnancy classes are frequently offered to women in the first trimester and include content about fetal growth and development, nutrition, early physical and emotional changes in pregnancy, drugs and toxins, exercises, and selecting a healthcare provider and place of birth that shares the woman's goals for the birth.
2. Breast-feeding classes for prenatal clients are becoming extremely popular. These classes usually consist of 8 to 10 women in their last trimester. Husbands, grandmothers, or other support people are welcome in most classes and should be actively encouraged to attend. Emphasis is placed on knowledge of the lactation process, nutrition, how to prevent and overcome the common problems of breast-feeding, myths and misconceptions, and information about the working mother and breast-feeding. Often, a mother and infant from a previous class return

to demonstrate proper positioning, manual expression, and how to use breast pumps. These classes are often taught by certified lactation educators or certified lactation consultants who are either hired by a hospital to teach or are in private practice in the community.

3. Baby care classes usually include the father and interested family members and cover safety, crying, parenting tips, car seats, buying clothes, circumcision, handling the infant, and feeding. Some classes have each of the participants bathe, diaper, and dress a life-size and weight doll. This hands-on experience is valuable.

4. Sibling preparation classes help prepare the sibling for the newborn by discussing pregnancy, birth and newborns, and the sibling's role as a big brother or sister.

5. Prenatal and postpartum exercise classes are beneficial for the woman.

6. Yoga classes provide breathing and relaxation skills useful for pregnancy and labor.

7. Lamaze and other birth preparation classes.

8. Vaginal birth after cesarean classes are specialized classes for women who have had a previous cesarean who are attempting a vaginal birth with the current pregnancy. In many areas, however, the special needs of this group are met with standard childbirth education classes, supplemental reading, and individual discussion with the teacher.

9. Mothers and infants groups provide support and information to new mothers.

10. Parenting groups can offer advice on common parenting issues.

11. Breast-feeding and returning to work classes are designed for the special concerns and needs of these groups of women.

12. Infant and child cardiopulmonary resuscitation (CPR) classes are offered because most parents do not know how to perform CPR on infants or children. These classes can be valuable for parents of young children.

13. Emergency situations classes for your child care provider are relatively new in some areas. These innovative classes cover infant and child CPR, the Heimlich maneuver, when to call 911, basic first aid, poison control, common childhood illnesses, home safety, what to do in case of fire or earthquake, and kidnapping awareness.

14. Grandparent classes discuss the grandparenting role and how infant care has changed.

These educational programs can enhance, strengthen, and broaden the care and services provided by the physician and maternity nurse.

Education for Achieving Comfort During Pregnancy

The Nursing Process

During the many weeks of prenatal care, the nurse has many opportunities to help the woman be more comfortable throughout her pregnancy. Aches and pains are so common during pregnancy that many women are unaware that remedies are available (see Chap. 17).

Assessment

Prenatal assessment should include observation of posture (see Client Education: Posture Checklist), a thorough history of the client's discomforts, and what, if anything, she has found to relieve them.

Nursing Diagnoses

Possible nursing diagnoses associated with the woman's comfort during pregnancy follow:

- Pain in lower back related to weak abdominal muscles, poor posture, improper body mechanics in conjunction with physical changes of pregnancy
- Sleep Pattern Disturbance related to knowledge deficit about pillow placement for increased relaxation and comfort during pregnancy
- Pain in upper back related to poor posture in pregnancy
- Discomfort related to swelling of feet and ankles with pregnancy
- Pain related to leg cramps from pressure of uterus on nerves in lower extremities
- Constipation related to diminished peristalsis and pressure of the growing uterus during pregnancy
- Shortness of breath related to pressure on diaphragm by enlarged uterus
- Health Seeking Behaviors related to relief of common discomforts of pregnancy

Interventions and Rationale

Having identified the woman's discomforts, the next step is to plan client teaching strategies to help alleviate them. The nurse must first be sure that specific problems are not related to pathophysiology (eg, swelling of feet and ankles may be related to preeclampsia or shortness of breath may be related to cardiac difficulties). Any reported problem that indicates pathophysiology should be reported to the woman's

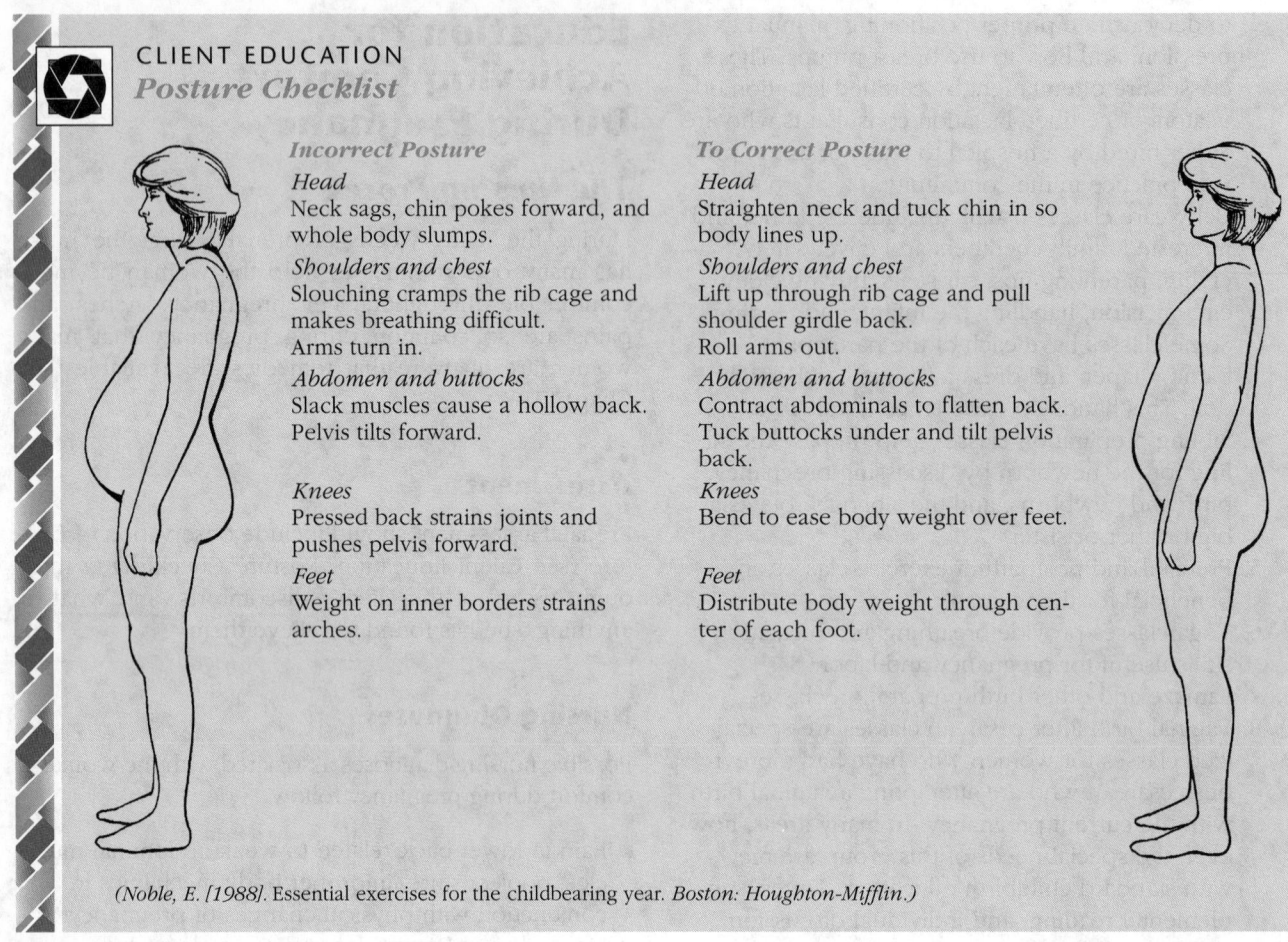

CLIENT EDUCATION
Posture Checklist

Incorrect Posture

Head
Neck sags, chin pokes forward, and whole body slumps.

Shoulders and chest
Slouching cramps the rib cage and makes breathing difficult.
Arms turn in.

Abdomen and buttocks
Slack muscles cause a hollow back.
Pelvis tilts forward.

Knees
Pressed back strains joints and pushes pelvis forward.

Feet
Weight on inner borders strains arches.

To Correct Posture

Head
Straighten neck and tuck chin in so body lines up.

Shoulders and chest
Lift up through rib cage and pull shoulder girdle back.
Roll arms out.

Abdomen and buttocks
Contract abdominals to flatten back. Tuck buttocks under and tilt pelvis back.

Knees
Bend to ease body weight over feet.

Feet
Distribute body weight through center of each foot.

(Noble, E. [1988]. Essential exercises for the childbearing year. Boston: Houghton-Mifflin.)

physician. Using the information found in the Client Education: Posture Checklist and Client Education: Principles for Activities of Daily Living During Pregnancy, the nurse can plan appropriate interventions for the client.

Evaluation

The nurse must be realistic in the evaluation of the outcome of the nursing interventions. It is unlikely that all the woman's discomforts can be relieved, but some improvement, even temporary, should be expected. On the other hand, a reassessment may point to a misdiagnosis and lead to a more effective nursing intervention.

Posture and Body Mechanics

Maintaining correct posture and practicing good body mechanics are important to avoid some of the common discomforts of pregnancy. As pregnancy progresses, body proportion and weight distribution are altered. As the body's center of gravity is gradually shifted forward, the abdominal muscles often relax, and the natural curvature of the spine becomes exaggerated,

shortening the muscles of the lower back. The woman often compensates for this by leaning backward slightly at the waist, which shifts her weight to her heels when walking. This results in an awkward, waddling gait and frequently contributes to backaches, particularly of the lower back. The woman should be encouraged to be mindful of her posture, and she should be given information on correcting her body alignment (see Client Education: Posture Checklist). Some exercises, such as the pelvic tilt, which strengthens the muscles of the abdomen and lower back, are also helpful for correcting poor posture and relieving backaches (see Appendix C). When sitting, the woman should choose a solid-backed chair with arms and use lumbar support, such as a rolled towel to support the lower back. Also, many commercially available abdominal supports may increase comfort. She should discuss this with her physician before purchase.

The importance of practicing good body mechanics should also be taught. **Body mechanics** involve the efficient use of the body to distribute weight and stress evenly among several muscle groups rather than overtaxing a particular muscle group with undue strain. For example, pregnant women should be instructed to

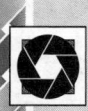

CLIENT EDUCATION
Principles for Activities of Daily Living During Pregnancy

- Activities need to be varied (walking, standing, sitting).
- Walking back and forth is preferable to standing still.
- Standing posture should be with one leg forward so that weight can be shifted easily and efficiently from foot to foot and the body can be turned comfortably.
- Walking posture should be head erect, back upright, and abdomen tucked.
- Use a footstool when sitting.
- When climbing stairs, the entire foot should be placed on stair and leg muscles should be used to lift self up each step without leaning forward.
- Stooping and lifting should be avoided; if stooping is necessary, it is best to squat down and reach and lift, with feet wide apart and back straight.
- When carrying bulky packages (eg, groceries), the load should be balanced, not excessive in size, and held in front if possible. A cart that rolls easily should be used for heavy loads.

avoid stooping when lifting or reaching for low objects. Bending forward or stooping may put the woman off balance and requires the muscles of the back to assume the burden of returning the trunk (and any weight that is lifted) to an erect posture. A squatting posture, hands and knees, or on all fours is much preferred when reaching for low objects. The woman should be instructed to squat with the back straight and the body properly aligned. Any weight to be lifted should be pulled close to the body, and the muscles of the thighs and legs should be used to raise the body to an erect posture.

Good body mechanics relate directly to good posture. Throughout daily activities, such as household chores, walking, and climbing stairs, the woman should be encouraged to keep the back straight (but not rigid) and the body in proper alignment. Learning to maintain correct posture and practicing good body mechanics often require a considerable amount of conscious thought

and practice at first. It is not unusual for a person who has previously had poor posture to feel strange or even uncomfortable when her body is in proper alignment. However, it should be emphasized that good posture and body mechanics are beneficial throughout life, and the lessons learned during pregnancy may carry over to a more healthful future (see Client Education: Principles for Activities of Daily Living During Pregnancy).

Comfort Positions

Pregnant women often find it difficult to relax because they are unable to find a comfortable position or because heartburn, backaches, or other common discomforts interfere with their ability to relax. Many positions are effective in providing comfort and relieving some of the discomforts of pregnancy. A comfort method for sleeping is illustrated in Figure 19-2.

A position that is effective for one woman may not necessarily work for another. For example, some women find the squatting position relaxing and effective in relieving backaches; others find a pushing posture or some other position or exercise more effective. Women should be encouraged to try a variety of positions until they find what works best for them (Table 19-1).

Education Related to Exercise During Pregnancy

Exercises performed during pregnancy increase circulation, improve muscle tone, aid in prevention of fatigue, promote physical comfort, and encourage good posture.

The Nursing Process
Assessment

Before encouraging a pregnant women to begin an exercise program, the nurse should consider several factors in the assessment. Has the woman's lifestyle been active or sedentary? Does she have any of the contraindications to exercise during pregnancy (Box 19-2)?

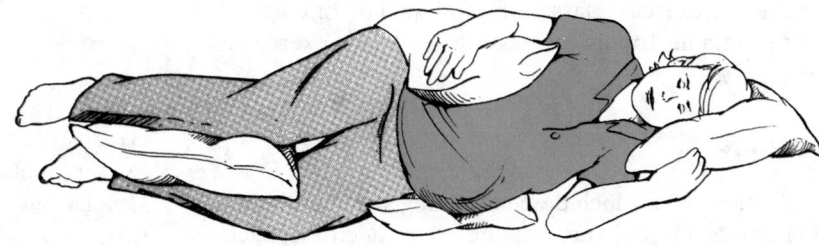

FIGURE 19–2 Comfort positions are positions in which the body is in alignment, with no body part resting on any other body part.

TABLE 19-1
Exercises and Positions to Relieve Common Discomforts of Pregnancy

Discomfort	Exercise or Position
Swelling of feet, ankles	Leg elevating
Leaking urine when coughing, laughing	Pelvic floor contraction
Heaviness in pelvis	Pelvic floor contraction
Hemorrhoids and swelling around vagina	First trimester—hips elevated Later in pregnancy—all fours
Cramps in legs	Leg elevating; calf stretching
Tired legs	Leg elevating, calf stretching
Varicose veins in legs	Leg elevating, calf stretching
Shortness of breath	Good posture, good body mechanics, rib cage lifting, shoulder circling
Low backache	Pelvic rocking, good posture, pushing position, squatting
Middle backache	Pushing position
Upper backache	Shoulder circling, good posture
Numbness in arms and fingers	Shoulder circling, lying on side; checking neck and upper back posture
Abdominal muscle spasm (stitch)	Pelvic rocking, deep abdominal breathing

Is she already involved in an exercise program? How many times a week and for how long does she exercise? How strenuous is the exercise? What kinds of exercises does she perform?

Each woman needs to be individually evaluated before beginning an exercise program. She should be instructed about the general warning signs and symptoms that should always signal her to stop exercising and contact the physician (Box 19-3).

Interventions and Rationale

The nurse can plan teaching activities or refer the woman to some of the many books and videotapes available that deal specifically with exercise and pregnancy. Some hospitals have physical therapists who specialize in pregnancy. The community may offer pregnancy exercise classes of good quality, or community swimming pools may be available for exercising (Fig. 19-3).

Evaluation

Evaluation would include determining whether the exercises are helpful (eg, whether they decrease back-

BOX 19-2
Contraindications to Exercise

Pregnancy-induced hypertension
Preterm rupture of membranes
Preterm labor during the prior or current pregnancy or both
Incompetent cervix or cerclage
Persistent second- or third-trimester bleeding
Intrauterine growth retardation

ACOG (1994)

ache due to weak abdominal muscles and increase physical stamina). The nurse also should evaluate any signs or symptoms that should be reported to the obstetric care provider (see Box 19-3). Frequency and duration of exercise periods should be evaluated.

General Guidelines for Exercise

According to the American College of Obstetricians and Gynecologists (ACOG), "an exercise prescription in pregnancy should be individualized and should be based on a health assessment. There are no data in humans to indicate that pregnant women should limit exercise intensity and lower target heart rates because of potential adverse effects" (ACOG, 1994). For women with no risk factors for adverse maternal or perinatal outcome, the following recommendations apply:

1. During pregnancy, women can continue to exercise and derive health benefits even from mild to moderate exercise routines. Regular exercise (at least three times per week) is preferable to intermittent activity.

BOX 19-3
Warning Signs and Symptoms During or After Exercising

The following signs and symptoms should always signal the woman to stop exercising and contact the physician

Pain	Faintness
Bleeding	Tachycardia
Dizziness	Back pain
Shortness of breath	Pubic pain
Palpitations	Difficulty walking

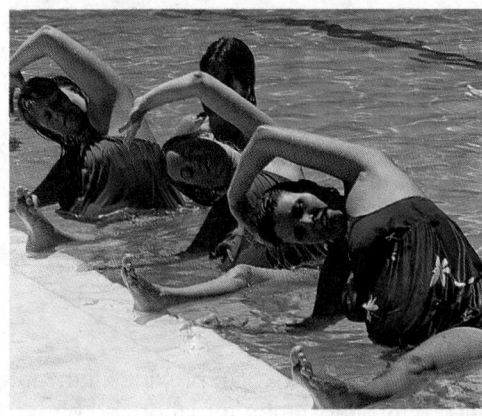

FIGURE 19–3 Swimming is an excellent form of exercise for the pregnant woman.

2. Women should avoid exercise in the supine position after the first trimester. The supine position is associated with decreased cardiac output in most pregnant women, and the remaining cardiac output will be preferentially distributed away from splanchnic beds (including the uterus) during vigorous exercise. Prolonged periods of motionless standing should also be avoided.

3. Women should be aware of the decreased oxygen available for aerobic exercise during pregnancy. They should be encouraged to modify the intensity of their exercise according to maternal symptoms. Pregnant women should stop exercising when fatigued, and they should not exercise to exhaustion. Non–weight-bearing exercises, such as cycling or swimming, will minimize the risk of injury and facilitate the continuation of exercise during pregnancy.

4. Pregnant women should avoid types of exercise in which loss of balance could be detrimental to maternal or fetal well-being, especially in the third trimester. Further, any type of exercise involving the potential for even mild abdominal trauma should be avoided.

5. Pregnancy requires an additional 300 kcal/d to maintain metabolic homeostasis. Thus, women who exercise during pregnancy should be particularly careful to ensure an adequate diet.

6. Pregnant women who exercise in the first trimester should augment heat dissipation by ensuring adequate hydration, wearing appropriate clothing, and maintaining optimal environmental surroundings during exercise.

7. Many of the physiologic and morphologic (structural) changes of pregnancy persist 4 to 6 weeks postpartum. Thus, prepregnancy exercise routines should be resumed gradually based on a woman's physical capability (ACOG, 1994).

The recommendations listed previously are intended for women who do not have any additional risk factors for adverse maternal or perinatal outcome. Medical or obstetric conditions may lead the physician to recommend modifications to those general recommendations. The conditions listed in Box 19-2 should be considered contraindications to exercise during pregnancy. In addition, women with certain other medical or obstetric conditions, including chronic hypertension or active thyroid, cardiac, vascular, or pulmonary disease, should be evaluated carefully to determine whether or what sort of exercise program is appropriate (ACOG, 1994).

In the absence of obstetric or medical complications, women who have achieved cardiovascular fitness prior to pregnancy should be able to maintain safely that level of fitness throughout pregnancy and the postpartum period. Many women may have to modify their specific exercise regimens, however. Some research has found lower birth weights among offspring of women who continue to exercise vigorously throughout pregnancy; however, no data confirm that with the specific exceptions mentioned, moderate exercise during pregnancy within the limits described has any ill effect on the fetus. In addition, while maternal fitness and sense of well-being may be enhanced by exercise, no level of exercise during pregnancy has been conclusively shown to be beneficial in improving perinatal outcome (ACOG, 1994).

Some prenatal exercises are presented in Appendix C. Note that ACOG recommends avoiding exercises done on the back after the fourth month of pregnancy. All the exercises included in the appendix except straight curl-ups can be done easily in positions other than on the back. (The straight curl-up, as noted in Appendix C, is not for "late starters.")

Women who wish to continue exercise during pregnancy should be taught to watch for symptoms of dyspnea and dizziness, in which case exercise on the back is contraindicated. Women who have no symptoms may want to alternate back exercises with those that can be done in other positions. Strenuous exercises on the back are not advisable in any case.

Preparation for Labor and Birth

Whether or not the maternity nurse is involved in offering classes for parents, education for childbirth must be part of the professional repertoire. This information can be used for individual teaching or for reinforcing what has been learned from other sources. Including the father or partner in this instruction helps to promote understanding of the woman's needs during the childbearing process.

The Nursing Process

Women become increasingly concerned about the impending labor and birth during the last trimester and are especially receptive to learning about that process. The nurse has the responsibility of helping the woman and her labor partner prepare for that momentous event.

Assessment

Assessment concerning preparation for labor and birth covers several areas. Is there someone the woman would like to have with her to help her during labor? If the father is unwilling or unavailable, can she count on a friend or relative to be with her? What previous labor experience do the woman and the labor support person have? What have they read about the labor process? Are they planning to attend childbirth education classes? If they are not, why not? Has the woman (and her partner) given any thought to any of the items discussed in the Client Education: Choices in Childbirth? Many women do not know that they have any choices or are not willing to do the research necessary to delve into this area. Others have great difficulty establishing a dialogue with their care provider that may involve assertiveness skills to obtain compromises. The nurse can be helpful as a consumer advocate by encouraging the client to think about options and suggest reading materials.

Nursing Diagnoses

Most nursing diagnoses in this area relate to a lack of information or knowledge about the labor and childbirth process. Some possible nursing diagnoses include the following:

- Health Seeking Behaviors related to labor process
- Fear related to myths about childbirth or "horror stories" heard from others
- Anxiety related to lack of knowledge about hospital routines and personnel
- Ineffective Individual Coping related to lack of support and labor information

Interventions and Rationale

Having determined the woman's needs and knowledge deficits, the nurse can plan ways to assist the woman to take responsibility for her own learning. Books and audio and video materials are available about labor and how to prepare for coping with labor

and birth (Box 19-4). The nurse can assist the woman to choose a quality childbirth class and in the event that the woman cannot attend such a class, assist her in learning relaxation, imagery, breathing, and pushing techniques. If the woman comes to labor not knowing how to relax and not knowing any breathing techniques, the nurse can teach her some on-the-spot techniques.

Evaluation

It is unlikely that the nurse can provide all the information concerning preparation for labor and birth for any one client, let alone for the many clients seen. This is why organized classes were developed and so many books have been written. However, the nurse can do a great deal for most clients, including dispelling misinformation and confirming accurate information.

Choices in Childbirth

In most areas of the United States today, women and their partners have many choices surrounding their birth experience. Some parents-to-be decide to choose their birth attendant and allow the birth attendant to make all the other choices, either because they do not want to decide or do not know about their options. Other expectant parents decide what they want in a birth experience and find a birth attendant and facility who can help them achieve the experience they want. The Client Education: Choices in Childbirth gives some specific labor and birth options expectant parents may want to consider. (To obtain a detailed pamphlet entitled "Planning Your Baby's Birth," see Box 19-4.)

The Dick-Read Method: The Beginning of Childbirth Preparation

The late Grantly Dick-Read, a British obstetrician, emphasized certain psychological aspects of labor—that "fear is in some way the chief pain-producing agent in otherwise normal labor." Dick-Read suggested that the woman builds up a state of tensions because she is frightened, and these tensions create an antagonistic effect on the muscular activity of normal labor, resulting in pain. The pain causes more fear, which further increases the tensions, and so on, creating a vicious circle.

Dick-Read's approach included an educational component to help women comprehend the physiologic processes of labor, exercises to improve muscle tone, and techniques to assist in relaxation and prevent the fear-tension-pain mechanism. These three components are included in most childbirth preparation pro-

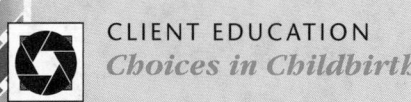

CLIENT EDUCATION
Choices in Childbirth

The two lists below do not represent an "either–or" situation. Most parents choose their options from both pathways. Very few doctors or midwives practice completely in accordance with either pathway. Consider and discuss each option and then decide which you prefer. Flexibility is necessary to ensure that the birth plan will apply in difficult or complicated labors and normal and typical labors.

Medical Pathway

(Which of these are routines, and which are options in your hospital or birth center?)

Labor
- Mother in wheelchair on arrival at hospital
- Shave, minishave, or clipping of perineal hairs
- Enema

- Partner asked to leave during preparation and examinations
- Limit to one support person during labor and birth
- Confinement to bed or one position
- Induction of labor
  Methods: stripping membranes, amniotomy, oxytocin
- Intravenous fluids for hydration and energy
- Frequent vaginal examinations

- Electronic fetal heart monitor
- Pain relief through medication

Birth
- Lithotomy position or semisitting in labor bed for pushing
- Prolonged breath holding and bearing down for expulsion
- Limit of 2 hours on second stage, then forceps, vacuum, or cesarean birth
- Delivery table for birth
- Lithotomy position with stirrups for birth

- Mother not allowed to touch sterile field
- Catheterization in second stage
- Episiotomy

- Forceps or vacuum extraction

After Birth
- Intubation or suctioning
- Immediate care of newborn done out of sight of mother (eg, identification, Apgar, heat lamp, replace hemostat with cord clamp)
- Limit of 15–20 minutes on third stage followed by manual extraction of the placenta
- Pitocin drip or injection for contraction of uterus after placenta is delivered

Newborn
- Newborn to isolette or nursery for 4–24 hours; mother to recovery room for observation
- Eye drops—silver nitrate applied shortly after birth

- Newborn's first feeding—glucose water by nurse

- Newborn in nursery except for scheduled 4-hour feedings
- Circumcision

Physiologic Pathway

- Mother walks to labor and delivery
- No shaving or clipping of hair
- Bowels emptied spontaneously or enema self-administered at home
- Partner present throughout labor and delivery

- Presence of other friends, relatives, and siblings
- Freedom to walk and change position as desired
- Spontaneous labor
  Alternatives: making love, breast stimulation
- Drinking fluid or eating as desired
- Vaginal examinations when requested by woman or for medical reasons
- Listening to fetal heart with fetal stethoscope
- Relaxation, emotional support, massage, breathing

- Choice of position and freedom to move

- Mother follows her urge to push

- Allow for longer second stage and position variations to help progress
- Birth in labor bed, birth chair, or bean bag
- Sidelying, all fours, squatting, standing with leg up, semireclining with back support, no stirrups
- Mother allowed to touch newborn's head as it crowns
- No catheterization and frequent voiding in first stage
- No episiotomy: massage, warm compresses, slower delivery, coaching to pant out newborn, support to perineum
- Late episiotomy with no anesthetic
- Spontaneous delivery

- Waiting to see if newborn can handle own mucus
- Care done on mother's abdomen. Newborn skin to skin with mother with heat lamp or blanket over them
- Delay in nonessential routines
- Allow for longer time for placenta; allow mother to move around, nurse; let cord drain
- Evaluation of uterus before using uterine stimulant
- Breast-feeding

- Newborn held by mother or partner on delivery table or in recovery
- Omit eye drops or delay administration up to 2 hours, or use of other agent as alternative
- Colostrum by mother who plans to breast-feed or plain water given by mother
- Demand feeding, newborn to mother when crying
- Twenty-four hour rooming in
- No circumcision

(continued)

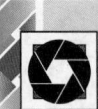

CLIENT EDUCATION *(Continued)*
Choices in Childbirth

The Unexpected

Cesarean Birth

- Scheduled surgery
- Mother without her support person in surgery
- General anesthesia
- Spinal or epidural
- Screen to prevent viewing surgery

- Mother not allowed to wear contacts or glasses
- Newborn sent to intensive care nursery

Premature or Sick Newborn

- Newborn cared for by professionals

- Newborn rushed to intensive care

- Newborn sent to another hospital or another part of hospital
- Newborn transported to hospital with intensive care unit
- Limited visits to newborn from mother only
- IV, gavage, and bottle feeding

Possible Options

- Surgery after labor begins
- Partner present to support mother

- Screen lowered at time of birth or newborn held up for parents to see
- Mother allowed to wear contacts or glasses
- Partner allowed to hold newborn and mother to see newborn, if newborn is not in distress
- Mother allowed to breast-feed in recovery if her and her newborn's condition permits

- Parents involved in care of newborn, diapering, touching, talking to newborn in incubator, feeding newborn
- Mother allowed to hold and see newborn, if not distressed
- Newborn close to mother in same part of hospital

- Partner goes with the transport team; mother goes if able
- Partner or extended family allowed to see newborn
- Mother allowed to express her colostrum for the newborn and encouraged and helped to get started at breast-feeding

(Adapted from Simpkin, P., & Reinke, C. [1980]. Planning your baby's birth. *Seattle: The Pennypress.)*

grams developed after Dick-Read's work became well known.

Early Resistance

At first, the prepared childbirth movement in the United States earned a bad name due to publicity about its more overzealous advocates. "Painless childbirth" was held up as a goal by some extremist groups, and the woman who did experience pain and resorted to pain medication during labor was made to feel like a failure. This can be extremely destructive to the woman's self-concept at a time when she needs positive reinforcement in her abilities to achieve and perform competently. Fortunately, current thinking recognizes the variability in individual responses to stress and the differing character of individual labors; it teaches that pain medication may be desired and does not signify failure.

In addition, in the early years, many obstetricians and labor room nurses resisted prepared childbirth. Couples who had been trained in a particular method often had to oppose staff pressures in their attempt to use the relaxation and breathing techniques they had

learned. Practices that are standard now, such as laboring in a semiupright position instead of lying flat, having ice chips or sips of water, eliminating the perineal shave, holding and putting the newborn to breast immediately after birth, and constant presence of the father or partner throughout labor and birth at one time caused much staff consternation and were often vetoed. Although prepared childbirth advocates had long been reporting the increased satisfaction the couple experienced when these methods were used, it took economic consumer pressure to bring about widespread acceptance of prepared childbirth. Research on the effectiveness of coping strategies taught in childbirth education programs has provided support for their continued use (see Research Highlight).

Father or Partner Involvement

The Dick-Read method, and its successor prepared childbirth programs, include the father or a significant other as an active participant in helping the woman cope with labor. The father or support person is made to feel involved and useful and through learning the physiologic and emotional processes of pregnancy, of-

BOX 19–4
Resources for Pregnancy and Childbirth

Relaxation Tapes for Childbirth Preparation (Audio cassettes)

"Letting Go of Stress" by Emmet Miller and Steve Halpern, Halpern Sounds, 1980

Four different 15-minute relaxation techniques; excellent for general use or pregnancy

"The Relaxation Rhythm: Pregnancy," "The Relaxation Rhythm: Labor," Vered Productions, 1994

Two different 15-minute, guided relaxation tapes; each with 15 minutes of music on side two.

Music for Relaxation and Labor (Audio cassettes)

"Celtic Harp" by Patrick Ball, Fortuna Records

"Fairy Ring" by Mike Rowland, Sona Gaia Productions

"Pachabel Canon in D," "With Ocean" by Invincible Recordings

"Seascapes" by Michael Jones, Narada Productions

"Silverwings" by Mike Rowland, Antiquity Records

"Solace" by Mike Rowland, Antiquity Records

Videotapes

"Postnatal Exercise Program," American College of Obstetricians and Gynecologists (ACOG), Feeling Fine Programs, Inc., 1985 (55 minutes, color, VHS)

"Pregnancy Exercise Program," ACOG, Feeling Fine Programs, Inc., 1985 (51 minutes, color, VHS)

"Modern Moves for Pregnancy Fitness," by Elize St. Charles and Associates (60 minutes, VHS)

Follows ACOG guidelines; an innovative conditioning and stress-reduction program that combines traditional yoga stretching with contemporary nonimpact exercise for use before and after childbirth.

"Special Delivery," by Injoy Productions (42 minutes, VHS)

Couples discussing birthing options; three labors and births.

"A Birth Class: Focus on Labor and Delivery," 1991, (120 minutes, VHS)

Perfect as a supplement to regular childbirth preparation classes or for those who are unable or unwilling to attend classes; stages of labor, preparation for pain, and comfort measures by well-known childbirth educators Beth Shearer and Cathy Romeo.

Comprehensive Mail-Order Catalogue of Books, Pamphlets, Audiotapes and Videotapes

ASPO/Lamaze, (800) 368-4404

Birth and Life Bookstore, (800) 443-9942

International Childbirth Education Association, (800) 624-4934

RESEARCH HIGHLIGHT

Most Effective Coping Strategies Taught During Childbirth Education Classes

Previous research indicates that much progress has been made in establishing a scientific knowledge base for coping strategies taught in childbirth education classes. Minimal research, however, has been done to document the effectiveness of the coping strategies used by prepared women during labor and birth.

This descriptive study was designed to determine which coping strategies women perceived as most effective during childbirth. Fifty seven primiparas were interviewed within 24 hours of birth. Using a specifically designed instrument, women rated the effectiveness of a list of coping strategies. The coping strategies learned in Lamaze classes with the highest mean score were labor companion support, pushing techniques, information, breathing techniques, relaxation, and birth choices. When the women were asked to choose *the* most helpful strategy during childbirth, the following received the highest number of responses: breathing techniques, labor companion support, and information.

Critique: Considering the lack of control for possible influencing variables, such as class content or emphasis by different instructors, labor and delivery staff influence, and the high use of epidurals on the use or effectiveness of Lamaze coping strategies, further research is needed in this area. Nurses should continue to assess the effectiveness of an individual woman's coping strategies during childbirth and support her in using those she perceives as most helpful at a given time.

Koehn, M. (1992). Effectiveness of prepared childbirth and childbirth education. *The Journal of Perinatal Education, 1*(2), 35–43.

---

ten gains an appreciation of the woman's experience. If the labor support person is the father, this also provides a chance to explore feelings about the parental role and to prepare psychologically for parenthood (Fig. 19-4).

Labor companions also may play another important role in labor. An important study by Klaus et al. (1986) found that women who received constant companionship and support in labor, even from strangers, had shorter labors with fewer cesareans, less oxytocin augmentation, and fewer overall perinatal problems. In another study, the women rated medication during labor as less important than the presence of a labor companion (Koehn, 1992).

Selecting a Class

Although most prepared childbirth classes are based on the same principles, they can differ in emphasis. Couples must know how to shop around for a teacher and class that suit their particular needs (Box 19-5).

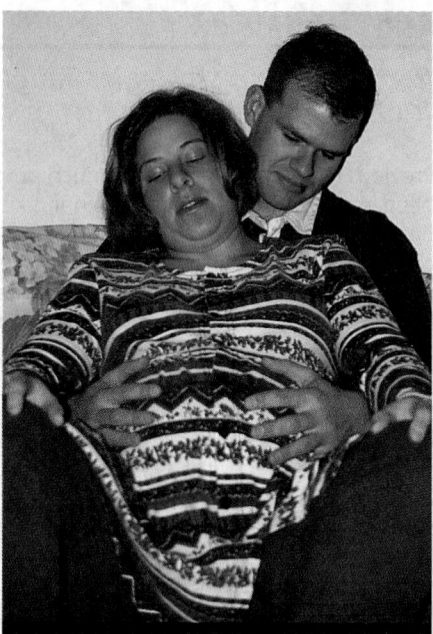

FIGURE 19-4 The labor support person can learn about pregnancy and prepare for labor along with their partner. This couple is practicing some of the breathing and relaxation techniques they learned in childbirth preparation class.

Lamaze or Psychoprophylactic Method

The psychoprophylactic method, or Lamaze method, is the most widely used prepared childbirth method in the United States today. It was first promoted by two Russian doctors, Nicolaiev and Velvovsky.

The rationale of the program was based on Pavlov's concept of pain perception and his theory of conditioned reflexes (ie, the substitution of favorable conditioned reflexes for unfavorable ones).

The theory intrigued a Paris obstetrician, Ferdinand Lamaze, who studied Russian-trained mothers-to-be in a Leningrad clinic. Lamaze returned to France and began to prepare his clients in *psychoprophylaxis*, or mental prevention of pain in childbirth. He gradually introduced certain adaptations, the most important of which was the rapid, shallow breathing that came to characterize the Lamaze method. (This breathing has since been changed.)

As the technique spread throughout Europe and Latin America, the *Lamaze method* and psychoprophylaxis became synonymous. The late Marjorie Karmel was perhaps the most responsible for introducing this technique to America. There are programs in psychoprophylaxis throughout the country. Many are under the auspices of the American Society for Psychoprophylaxis in Obstetrics, Inc. (ASPO), which was founded through joint efforts of Karmel, Elisabeth Bing, and others.

BOX 19–5
Variables to Consider When Selecting a Childbirth Class

1. Professional credentials of instructor and type of training as a childbirth educator
2. Class size
   a. Eight couples or less—ideal for group interaction and supervised practice
   b. More than 12 couples—limited group interaction, limited supervised practice, and decreased relaxation skills mastered by couple
3. Location of class
   a. Home—usually limits class size and provides informal, relaxed atmosphere
   b. Office, school, church, or hospital—class size may escalate, and atmosphere may be less than ideal
4. Total hours of class time for the fee
5. Amount of supervised practice time per session
6. Fee payment by couple
   a. Directly to instructor—instructor accountable to consumer
   b. To group or sponsoring health facility—instructor accountable to agency for content (ie, content may not be consumer oriented but is what health facility wants couple to know)

Several changes have occurred in the original Lamaze method as a result of research. Class content, slower and more flexible breathing techniques, and theories of learning and motivation constitute the major changes. Class content originally dealt mostly with exercises, relaxation, breathing techniques, and the normal labor and birth experience. Childbirth educators have added information on such subjects as nutrition, infant feeding, cesarean birth, benefits and risks of medical interventions, variations from usual labor, sexuality, early parenting, and coping skills for the postpartum period.

Relaxation

The use of relaxation as a coping skill during labor is the foundation of all the childbirth education techniques. Many authorities regard the ability to release tension under stress as the most important skill taught or learned in childbirth education classes. It is the core of all other skills, including breathing and expulsion techniques (Shrock, 1988). Humenick (1980) found that prenatal relaxation skill achievement was significantly related to medication used in childbirth. She also found that larger childbirth class size correlated negatively with achievement of relaxation skill for expectant mothers (Humenick et al., 1981).

Tensing during labor is a natural response to the contracting uterus. Tension, however, causes exhaustion and oxygen depletion, lowers the pain threshold, and prolongs labor. Adrenaline, the hormone that accompanies the fear-tension-pain syndrome, inhibits the effects of oxytocin, which causes the uterus to contract. This interference with oxytocin actually makes the contractions of the uterus less effective and prolongs labor.

Learning to relax involves an active building of awareness of the state of the muscles, either tensed or relaxed, and a conscious control by the mind of that state. It is a learned activity, a process of isolating muscle groups, differentiating between tenseness and relaxation, and letting go of or totally releasing muscle groups. Relaxation is an active involvement of mind over body, which requires awareness, concentration, and practice.

Constant practice or repetition of a relaxation technique is necessary to maintain a conditioned response of this nature. Continued practice establishes patterns that can be used when thought processes become cloudy in active labor.

The skill of relaxation is not only helpful for birth, but is a lifelong skill that can be used during the daily stresses of life. The many ways of teaching relaxation, include progressive relaxation, focusing, meditation, and touching. Some of the methods are listed in Table 19-2.

To begin teaching relaxation, it is important to start with the simple techniques and after they are mastered, to move to the more complex. A simple, general body relaxation technique is presented to begin (see Conditioned Relaxation in Appendix C), followed by tense-release relaxation, and finally a neuromuscular dissociation technique. All of these techniques are described in detail in Appendix C.

Many people find an audio cassette recording of a relaxation technique helpful to supplement their practice with their partner (see Box 19-4). It is also possible for a person to record her own relaxation tape by reading the exercise slowly into a tape recorder. A quick way to teach relaxation to untrained women in labor is presented in the section entitled "Jaw Relaxation" in Chapter 23 (see Nursing Care Plan: Couples Participating in Training for Relaxation for Pregnancy, Labor, and Birth or Life Stress).

Imagery

Coupled with relaxation, imagery can be a powerful coping mechanism for labor. Also called **visualization, imagery** is a form of daydreaming with direction and purpose. It is a conscious experience in which a person maintains a focus on an object of concentra-

tion. The physiologic basis of how imagery decreases pain is not understood, though several theories have been proposed. It is known that when a person is in a highly relaxed state, electroencephalographic (EEG) recordings show brain waves in the alpha state and sometimes in the theta state. The alpha state is most easily created in a relaxed person. This state allows a person to use the functions of the right brain more efficiently (Bressler, 1979).

The brain is divided into two hemispheres with separate functions. It is thought that the different hemispheres allow the brain to access the central nervous system with two different and separate methods of communication. Access to the somatic nervous system is thought to be verbal, and access to the autonomic nervous system is thought to be the language of imagery, dreams, and intuition. The autonomic nervous system prepares the body for action through the sympathetic nervous system (SNS) and prepares the body for rest through the parasympathetic nervous system (PNS). When the PNS is activated, a feeling of tranquility occurs as the breathing and heart rates slow. The person who can learn to influence the activities of the body that previously were thought to be out of one's control can benefit by stress reduction and pain control techniques (Bressler, 1979).

To start a learning session on imagery, the nurse must first create an atmosphere in which relaxation can occur (Steffes, 1988). The room should be quiet, with the lights lowered. Participants are encouraged to find a comfortable position. Music may help to set the right mood (see Box 19-4 for some music suggestions). The next task is to orient those present to the activity. This includes explaining what sensations to expect and emphasizing the need to just "let things happen." Occasionally, as people relax, they experience new or unusual feelings, which may include a feeling of losing control. The group, however, needs to be reassured that they will always remain in control and that to gain control, they first must learn to let go. It is important to set a low achievement level and allow anyone who does not want to participate to refrain from doing so. Once the group is oriented, the relaxation process begins. Generally, any relaxation technique or breathing exercise can be used in part or whole (see the breathing techniques described below and Conditioned Relaxation in Appendix C). When the group is relaxed, the next step is to begin the exercise in imagery (see Imagery Exercises in Appendix C).

When the nurse is working with women in labor, it is helpful to be able to assist with imagery, whether or not the laboring woman is trained in imagery techniques. To do this effectively, the nurse must be comfortable with imagery and have a spontaneous dia-

TABLE 19–2
Approaches to Teaching Relaxation

Name and Type	Description	Feedback
Progressive relaxation (modifies muscular responses)	Systematically tensing and releasing muscles;, developed by Edmond Jacobson; modified by J. Wolpe into a 6-week approach with home practice	Primary feedback is initially described as the awareness of participant who focuses on the sensation of tensing and relaxing each muscle. Either a coach or electromyograph can provide feedback.
Neuromuscular dissociation (modifies muscular responses)	Follows progressive relaxation by asking the participant to tense some muscles and relax others simultaneously; introduced in this country by Elisabeth Bing	The coach checks relaxation (see Appendix C) and tension was introduced by Karmel and Bing—not mentioned in books by either Fernand Lamaze or Irwin Chabon.
Autogenic training (mental control modifying muscular and autonomic systems responses)	Training through suggestions, including "my right arm is heavy" or "my left arm is warm"; includes slowing of the heart and respiration and cooling of forehead; developed by J. Schultz and W. Luther	Feedback is initially described as the awareness of the participant with no outside feedback; has been used with biofeedback equipment, thermometers, and so forth.
Meditation (modifies vascular and neurotransmitter responses)	Defined by Herbert Benson as dwelling on an object (repeating a sound or gazing at an object) while emptying all thoughts and distractions in a quiet atmosphere in a comfortable position; used in transcendental meditation and yoga	Concentration on a focal point and on breathing patterns would be forms of meditation by Benson's definition. Participant can monitor self but also receives coach's feedback on both activities.
Visual imagery	Includes techniques such as visualizing oneself on a warm beach or as a bag of cement or going down a staircase; often precedes introduction of other kinds of relaxation; may also be used to visualize and potentially affect specific body parts as in cancer therapy; may be used in desensitization in which one relaxes while visualizing a potentially threatening situation; used in labor rehearsals	
Touching and massaging	A way for one person to calm another; evidence of actual transfer of energy taking place in some forms of touching; In childbirth preparation, associated with muscular relaxation (Sheila Kitzinger)	Feedback from coach includes informing when muscle tension is felt, necessitating advanced coaching. Coaches may need first to discern relaxation by moving a limb.
Biofeedback	Electromyograph used to measure neuromuscular tension Thermometer used to measure skin temperature at extremities Galvanic skin reflex used to record conductivity changes because of the action of sweat glands at the surface of the skin Electroencephalograph used to distinguish alpha, beta, and theta waves in the brain	Feedback from all these machines is in one or more of these forms: visualization of a meter, listening to a sound, or watching a set of flashing lights.

(Humenick, S. [1984]. Teaching relaxation. *Childbirth Educator, 3*(4), 47.)

logue, perhaps a loose memorization of one from a book, ready to use.

Breathing Techniques

Lamaze breathing techniques are presented here, because Lamaze is the most widely used in the United States right now. Modifications in these techniques over the years may result in regional differences, but the principles are the same. Box 19-6 summarizes the ASPO-Lamaze standard of practice for breathing strategies as of 1993 (ASPO, 1993). Two paced breathing strategies are taught to promote optimal psychophysiologic responses. Each is preceded and ended with a cleansing breath, a relaxed, effortless breath that is a signal for focus of attention.

NURSING CARE PLAN
Couples Participating in Training for Relaxation for Pregnancy, Labor, and Birth or Life Stress

Nursing Goals
1. Woman verbalizes understanding of importance of relaxation techniques.
2. Partner is willing to assist woman to learn and practice relaxation techniques.
3. Woman practices on regular basis.
4. During practice sessions observed by the nurse, woman shows evidence of relaxation.
5. Couple appears to work together as a team.

Assessment	Potential Nursing Diagnoses	Intervention/ Rationale	Evaluation
1. Knowledge of benefits of relaxation in pregnancy, labor, and birth and life stress management a. ↑ O_2 to fetus and uterus b. ↓ Fatigue c. ↓ Pain perception d. ↑ Feeling of competency and mastery e. Aids breathing for labor and expulsion of fetus f. Facilitates labor process g. ↓ Blood pressure and stress disease h. Enhances feeling of well-being	Knowledge Deficit related to relaxation skills	After assessing information level, explain benefits of relaxation *to raise knowledge level*. Include benefits for right now, labor, birth, and later life. Give other examples in everyday life that may be familiar, for example, "tension headache" (tension causes ↑ pain).	Woman verbalizes understanding. Woman may add some benefits she thinks of during the discussion. Woman has no further questions.
2. Past use of relaxation techniques, meditation, or yoga in any life situation and its effectiveness		Build on what she already knows *to develop a knowledge base*. You may be able to omit more basic techniques if she is currently skilled in a technique. Encourage her to use what she knows best or what has worked in the past.	
3. Partner's or friends' willingness to help her learn and practice new skill 4. Motivation to practice consistently, 15–20 min/d, three to five times per week	Noncompliance related to a. Partner's knowledge deficit about importance of relaxation skills b. Powerlessness c. Learning deficit: ineffective teaching	Include partner in teaching when possible. Discuss health benefit for partner. Have partner participate by doing relaxation with woman as you teach. Teach partner how to assess woman's level of relaxation and how to give positive nonjudgmental feedback to her. Explain that it will take time and daily practice (15–20 min) to be effective in labor or stress.	Woman practices three times a week.

(continued)

NURSING CARE PLAN (*Continued*)
Couples Participating in Training for Relaxation for Pregnancy, Labor, and Birth or Life Stress

Assessment	Potential Nursing Diagnoses	Intervention/ Rationale	Evaluation
		Motivate by making sure couple understands benefits and physiologic consequences resulting from unnecessary tension. Help couple plan specific home practice schedule with self-reward system *to help motivate.*	
		Tailor teaching to individual, or with class, provide multimodal approach (see Table 19-4).	
5. Client's ability to relax during technique		1. Week 1: Start with basic whole body relaxation. (see Conditioned Relaxation—Appendix C).	Couple practices, evidenced by verbal reports and by woman's increasing ability to relax as observed by nurse during practice sessions:
6. Client's ability to tense and release during technique		2. Week 2: Progress to tense-release exercise. (see Tense-Release Relaxation—Appendix C).	a. Relaxed jaw
7. Couple's ability to work together			b. Slow, regular breathing
8. Woman's ability to learn imagery		3. Week 3: Progress to neuromuscular disassociation exercise. (see Appendix C).	c. Smoothed out facial muscles
9. Woman's ability to integrate relaxation, imagery, and previously learned paced breathing techniques		4. Week 4: Add imagery exercises (see Appendix C).	d. Legs rolled out and flexed; arms flexed
		5. Week 5: Have client integrate relaxation, breathing, and imagery during practice contractions.	Couple acts as team during observed practice session.
			Partner assists with woman's learning, practice, and evaluation; gives appropriate feedback during practice.

Slow Paced Breathing. In assisting women to learn slow paced breathing, the nurse needs to help the couple determine the woman's normal breathing rate. Clinically, in most women, one half the normal rate is six to nine breaths per minute. Whether the woman breathes in or out through her nose or mouth or in any combination is her choice. Because of the enhanced relaxation and improved oxygenation that occurs with slow paced breathing, women should be encouraged to use this breathing for as long as it works well during labor. Throughout labor and before changing breathing patterns, women should be assessed for the need to change positions, relax more completely, urinate, and so forth to decrease pain. With time, habituation

may make slow paced breathing less effective. **Habituation** is the decreased response to a repeated stimulus. Changing positions, walking, imagery, and changing music tapes help decrease habituation to this breathing technique, but most women eventually need to change to a breathing pattern that causes an alerting response (Rose et al., 1988).

Modified Paced Breathing. The second breathing technique, modified paced breathing, mediates the stress response of advancing labor by pacing the respirations at a controlled rate. Modified paced breathing is performed as an upper chest breath. It is not confined to the throat, and the chest does not move vigorously.

The ASPO/Lamaze faculty has reviewed and updated the standard of breathing. This standard restates the changes made in ASPO/Lamaze techniques by the faculty. We continue to teach two rates of breathing, with patterned breathing a variation of the modified paced breathing, which incorporates rhythm and cognition.

Subject: Breathing Strategies

Purpose: Paced breathing strategies promote optimal psychophysiologic responses to stressors. Respiration modulates and is modulated by the central nervous system and the autonomic nervous system.

Principles

General principles related to all breathing strategies include the following:

- Maintenance of adequate oxygenation of woman and fetus
- Enhancement of the opening of airways and elimination of the inefficient use of muscles to decrease the cost of breathing
- Provision of a means of attention focusing
- Definition of the rate and pattern based on an individual's own respiratory physiology

Types of Breathing Patterns

"Cleansing" breaths: The "cleansing" breaths are effortless, relaxed breaths to a comfortable depth, similar to a sigh, taken at the beginning and end of contractions. They are signals for a focus of attention.

Slow paced breathing: This is a slow, rhythmic breathing pattern at a repetitive rate that is comfortable for each woman. The slowest rate for this breathing pattern should be no less than one-half the woman's normal breathing rate.

Modified paced breathing: Modified paced breathing is done at a slightly faster rate than slow paced breathing. The rate should be no greater than twice the woman's normal respiratory rate. A variation is the use of the modified pace interspersed with soft blows to create a pattern. This is called patterned paced breathing.

Breathing for birth: A variety of choices in breathing patterns may be used during birth:

- Open glottis with vocalization at will
- Open glottis with slow exhalation
- Short breath holding (5–6 seconds)

ASPO/Lamaze Educational Council (1993), Genesis, ASPO/Lamaze

Telling the woman to breathe at a level at which she feels comfortable may help her determine how deeply she needs to breathe to meet her own physiologic needs. A delicate balance should be sought—breathing deep enough to obtain adequate ventilation but not so shallow as to move only "dead air." Breathing should not be rapid enough to cause hyperventilation. The respiratory rate should not exceed twice the woman's normal rate. This rate has been observed empirically to be a safe upper limit. The choice of mouth or nose breathing is the woman's; if mouth breathing is her choice, however, the nurse needs to help her protect the mucous membranes by offering fluids, ice, or mouth rinses at regular intervals. Sounds ("hee" or "haw") should be avoided because these are made by tightening the vocal cords and contracting the intercostal muscles. Relaxation is always the core on which paced breathing patterns are built (Rose et al., 1988). A variation of modified paced breathing is the use of the modified pace interspersed with soft blows to create a pattern. A common pattern taught in Lamaze classes is the 3 to 1, that is, three breaths in and out plus a soft blow. This pattern is repeated through the contraction. Clients may be taught other patterns (eg, 2 to 1, 4 to 1) or make up their own.

Modified paced breathing provides an altering mechanism to the brain that decreases habituation. Once this has been achieved, a return to slow paced breathing may be appropriate. Both of the two breathing techniques may be used at any time in labor without regard for any phase of dilation. The decision as to how best to use them is left up to the laboring woman (Rose et al., 1988).

Breathing Techniques for Birth. In the second stage of labor, the woman may assume any physiologic position (see Chap. 22). As the second stage proceeds, the nurse often monitors the progress of the descent of the fetus. If 20 minutes pass without progress, the woman should be assisted to change positions.

Often there is a lull at the end of the first stage when women do not feel the urge to push. This pause is physiologic and allows the woman to rest. The urge to push is felt only when the head is low enough to stimulate the stretch receptors in the pelvic floor.

Pushing with a closed glottis (Valsalva's maneuver) results in severe cardiovascular effects. This causes a high intrathoracic pressure, preventing venous return and causes a falling blood pressure, a decrease in cardiac output, and a disrupted blood flow to the uterus. Visible signs of straining include red face and tight neck muscles. When women are not directed to hold their breath, spontaneous pushing with a partially open glottis results. In spontaneous pushing, the air is audibly exhaled. Moans, grunts, and groans are the normal sounds of birth. If no sound is heard, it means the breath is being held, and the body is tense (Noble, 1988). Noble suggests the following for expectant women in the second stage:

- Do not strain. Let go and flow with the contraction.
- Relax the pelvic floor throughout second stage. Do not tense the muscles when you feel rectal pressure,

the vagina stretching, or the gaze of many eyes! Relax *all* sphincters and the mouth, too—with your lips and jaws parted.

- Direct the push low down and in front—increase the pressure in your abdomen, not in your face. Do not strain so that you screw up your eyes; you might miss the moment of birth.
- Always take one or two deep breaths to refuel at the start and the end of a contraction. Exhale slowly as you bear down.
- Push only as long and hard as you feel the urge to do so. Avoid prolonged pushes, which affect your breathing, circulation, and the baby's heart rate.
- When asked to refrain from pushing at any time, immediately relax the head back and pant. Keep it light and brisk. Do not blow out hard and pull in the abdominals at this time.

Breathing and Relaxation Techniques for Untrained Women

Not all women arriving in the labor and delivery suite have attended childbirth education classes, and labor nurses must be able to impart as much of this information as possible before contractions become too uncomfortable.

If possible, teach the woman slow paced breathing. When contractions become uncomfortable, help her do the breathing. You can do the breathing with her (she focuses on your face) or verbally coach her through it.

As labor progresses, if she needs it, teach her the following simple version of modified paced breathing:

1. As the contraction begins, have the woman focus her attention on your face.
2. The woman takes a big relaxing sigh.
3. She breathes in and out through her nose or mouth at a rate of about 20 to 30 breaths per minute. You might "conduct" her breathing with rhythmic hand signals to help her pace herself.
4. The contraction ends. The woman takes another big sigh. Relaxation techniques for untrained women are described in more detail in Chapter 23.

Other Childbirth Methods

Several approaches to prepared childbirth other than the Lamaze method are popular in specific geographic regions or even in pockets of a particular city. Although these programs may vary in specific techniques, they have many more points in common than differences. During the last 20 years, there has been a blending of methods, all of which share the following basic beliefs:

- Fear enhances the perception of pain but may diminish or disappear when the parturient knows about the physiology of labor.
- Psychic tension enhances the perception of pain, but the parturient may relax more easily if childbirth takes place in a calm and agreeable atmosphere and if good human contacts have been established between her and the personnel attending to her.
- Muscular relaxation and a specific type of breathing diminish the pain of labor.

Postpartum Teaching

Parenthood often constitutes a stress in the developmental processes of mothers and fathers. The postpartum period is particularly stressful because of the numerous physical changes the mother undergoes, the incomplete integration of her pregnancy and labor experiences, the changing roles that must occur within the family complex, and the uncertainty of the nature of the early mother–infant relationship. Fatigue, confusion, feelings of helplessness and inadequacy, and depression often complicate this period. Isolation from the extended family, lack of community resources, economic strains, and pressures on the woman to resume her full previous role within the family as rapidly as possible create additional stresses. Factors that may influence teaching and learning in the postpartum period are outlined in Table 19-3.

The nurse working on the postpartum unit has a unique opportunity to intervene early in the developing mother–infant relationship and to assist the parents to anticipate and plan for the first few critical weeks at home. If the mother can attain a level of confidence in her ability to perform caretaking tasks and begin to recognize her newborn's behavioral messages, a good foundation can be laid, and later difficulties can be minimized.

The needs of the hospitalized postpartum woman may conflict with the nursing staff's needs to maintain the routine or provide the teaching they believe necessary. Shorter postpartum stays also complicate planning. Mothers progress at different speeds in assuming the caretaking role and have individualized concerns. Finding a way to respond to individual needs yet conduct an efficient postpartum educational program is a major challenge to postpartum nurses.

As always, the nurse needs to prioritize client teaching, especially because most women leave the hospital less than 24 hours after birth. The nurse must know about community-based resources for the newly post-

TABLE 19–3
Factors Influencing Teaching and Learning

Factor	Implications
Infant's condition	Preparation of the parents of a preterm newborn or newborn with significant neonatal problems differs considerably from that of parents of the healthy, full-term newborn.
Parental age	Parental age reflects development status. For example, the adolescent may need more concrete examples and may be less able to assimilate written material.
Marital status	Marital status may influence the paternal role. Whether married or not, there is need to determine desired paternal involvement. Father should be included in caretaking activities when interested. Marital instability usually increases the anxiety level and makes teaching more difficult.
Parity	When there are siblings, the family usually needs more of a review of child care than actual teaching. Some teaching should be directed at interaction with the other children and meeting their needs and the newborn's.
Socioeconomic status	Socioeconomic status influences the parents' ability to provide material things for the newborn, and it usually influences childrearing practices.
Educational levels of the parents	Appropriate vocabulary should be used for verbal instruction and written material.
Experimental readiness	Previous learning transfers to the new situation. Insight enables the learner to apply older learning to a new situation.
Health beliefs and behaviors of the family	When health beliefs deviate from the usual, teaching may be difficult, and more time may be required to convince the family of the need to change.
Emotional state of the learner	Some anxiety may enhance the learning process, but high anxiety militates against learning. Efforts should be made to lower high anxiety levels before proceeding with instruction. Attempts should be made to help parents work through feelings about their child's illness before attempting to teach.
Physical state of the learner	Physical discomfort may preclude or reduce learning.
Parental questions	The type of questions asked indicates learning needs.
Parental motivation	Motivated parents are usually easier to teach. The nurse needs to find ways of stimulating the apparently unmotivated.
Interest in the infant	Lack of interest in the newborn makes teaching very difficult. When interest appears slight, there should be exploration of apparent disinterest.

partum woman and her family. For specific postpartum teaching content, see Chapters 25 and 27.

Individual Teaching

Part of the postpartum nurse's daily responsibility is to provide individual instruction and support to mothers. This can range from information about infant sleep and activity patterns, growth and development, and how to dress the newborn for different types of weather to sibling rivalry, contraception, and organizing the household to get the necessary tasks done. Mothers' concerns may be small and particular, such as getting the newborn to stay awake and suck well, or they may be larger and more general, such as the changes in her own and the father's lifestyle after the birth. The nurse needs to be informed about a wide variety of topics, including contraception, sexuality, family dynamics, infant care, and involutional physiology.

Individual teaching allows the nurse to respond to the personal questions and concerns of mothers and to relate information to the particular situation. Reinforcement of mothering skills is particularly effective on an individual basis, as is counseling regarding family problems or emotions. However, the nurse may not have the time to give each mother the amount of individual teaching and counseling needed. Because of this, hospitals often rely on videos played on every room television, although their effectiveness may be questionable (Freda et al. 1994). Even though stays are short, many hospitals continue to offer postpartum group education of a limited variety.

Group Education
Postpartum Classes

The organization of classes for postpartum mothers and fathers differs considerably from one institution to another. Each unit must work out the most convenient time for staff and parents and a method of communication to ensure maximum attendance. Sometimes a conference room on the unit is used, or a large room can be adapted and extra chairs brought in. The teachers may be postpartum nurses only, or they may be nursery nurses, physicians, social workers, dietitians, or physical therapists. Many media aids can be used, ranging from videos to flip charts, books, or other printed material. Closed-channel television, which can be viewed by each mother in her room, is also used as a method of postpartum group instruction.

The content of postpartum teaching generally includes content about the mother and her needs and information about the care of a newborn. Content about the mother should include getting enough rest, postpartum blues, family adjustment to a newborn, involutional physiology, pericare, breast care, sexuality, contraception, nutrition, and postpartum exercises. Mothers should be instructed in bathing and dressing the newborn, breast-feeding or bottle feeding, holding and handling, cord care and care of the circumcision, routine tests (eg, the phenylketonuria [PKU] test), and the normal range of newborn behaviors, including sleeping and crying. Some classes may include time for the mother to practice what she has just been taught while the nurse is available for assistance.

Some postpartum units organize special classes for mothers with particular needs (eg, breast-feeding classes). The mothers are instructed in techniques of breast-feeding, and possible problems and their prevention are discussed. Experienced mothers can be encouraged to attend, because they are most helpful to new mothers who have never breast-fed before. Common situations that breast-feeding mothers might encounter are discussed, and group solutions are developed. Having the telephone number of the nurse or La Leche League (1-800-La Leche) for consultation if problems arise after discharge is helpful to mothers and promotes continued success with breast-feeding. Many hospitals are hiring certified lactation educators and consultants to provide specialized service and expertise to this growing population of clients.

Outpatient Classes

With 6- to 24-hour discharge common in most areas, the postpartum nurse has little time for postpartum teaching. In addition, the new mother can only absorb so much. For these reasons, nurses and other health professionals are increasingly aware of the need to extend services to parents after discharge from the hospital. These services may be provided through the public health department, hospital-affiliated clinics, private physicians' offices, a community liaison nurse from the

postpartum unit, or community-based health professionals in private practice.

Postpartum nurses should be able to inform new parents about how they can contact these community resources for postpartum education. Some hospitals provide clients with lists of these classes, or the client can contact a childbirth educator who frequently knows about these resources (Box 19-7).

Postpartum Exercise

During the puerperium, the 6 weeks after childbirth, the body undergoes major changes. Postpartum exercises are important in restoring muscle tone and the woman's figure. Often the exercises recommended during the prenatal period are also useful in the postpartum exercise program (see Appendix C). Many communities offer special exercise classes for pregnant and postpartum women. A group setting is often beneficial because motivation and learning are enhanced. In an uncomplicated birth, simple exercises should begin during the first postpartum day. If the woman had an abdominal delivery or extensive perineal repair, the beginning exercises may differ. The physician should be consulted before resuming fitness activities, such as jogging.

The nurse's role in parent education is a challenging one and requires much thought and preparation. The rewards for the nurse are equally great—hearing the

---

BOX 19–7
Outpatient Hospital or Community-Based Postpartum Services

Parenting groups: Usually both parents attend. Some innovative corporations are now offering these classes.

Mother–infant support groups: These are often divided by age of infant or child and can extend for several years.

Exercise classes: Usually these include pregnant and postpartum women and their infants.

La Leche League: This breast-feeding support group is for pregnant and postpartum mothers and their infants.

Warm line for parenting concerns: nonmedical parenting issues are discussed. Usually this is hospital based under the auspices of pediatric or psychiatric departments.

Breast-feeding warm line: This may be hospital or community based. La Leche League has a phone support system and groups (1-800-LALECHE).

Breast-feeding and working classes: These may be hospital, community, or even corporate sponsored.

grateful comments of parents and having participated in a special, memorable event in their lives.

Summary Points

✔ Adult learners differ from other learners in several critical ways. Nurses must take these important differences into consideration when planning educational content for expectant and new parents.

✔ Learning is increased by actively involving the learner in the experience by participating and doing. Verbal and visual receiving is passive involvement and produces lower levels of retention.

✔ In the absence of either obstetric or medical complications, pregnant women who have achieved cardiovascular fitness prior to pregnancy should be able to maintain that level of fitness safely throughout the pregnancy, although depending on the individual's needs and the physiologic changes associated with pregnancy, she may have to modify her specific exercise regimen.

✔ Breathing techniques are rated by women as one of the most effective coping strategies for labor. Nurses need to be able to teach and assist all (not just pregnant and female) clients in using these techniques, whether they are coping with labor or any difficult treatment or procedure.

✔ During the postpartum period, several factors influence the client's ability to take in and learn what the nurse wants to teach. Failure to consider these factors can make educational content irrelevant to parents.

REFERENCES

American College of Obstetricians and Gynecologists (1994). *Technical Bulletin 189: Exercise during pregnancy and the postpartum period.*

American Society for Psychoprophylaxis in Obstetrics (1993). Washington, DC: ASPO/Lamaze Education Council.

AuKamp, V., Humenick, S., & Freerick, A. (1988). The Learner. In F. Nichols & S. Humenick (Eds.), *Childbirth education: Practice, research and theory.* Philadelphia: W.B. Saunders.

Barnett, M. & Humenick, S. (1982). Infant outcomes in relation to second stage labor pushing method. *Birth, 9,* 221.

Bressler, D. (1979). *Free yourself from pain.* New York: Simon and Schuster.

Caldeyro-Barcia, R. (1979). The influence of maternal bearing down efforts during second stage on fetal well-being. *Birth Fam J, 6,* 17.

Freda, M., Fogarassy, M., Davini, D., Devore, N., Damus, K., & Merkatz, I. (1994). Are they watching? Are they learning? Prenatal video education in the waiting room. *The Journal of Perinatal Education, 3*(1), 20–28.

Humenick, S. (1980). Assessing the quality of childbirth education: Can teachers change? *Birth Fam J, 7,* 82–90.

Humenick, S., & Marchbanks, P. (1981). Validation of a scale to measure relaxation in childbirth education classes. *Birth Fam J, 8,* 141.

Klaus, M., Kennell, J. H., Robertson, S. S., & Sosa, R. (1986). Effects of social support during parturition on maternal and infant morbidity. *British Medical Journal, 293*(6547), 585–587.

Knowles, M. (1980). *The modern practice of adult education.* Chicago: Association Press.

Koehn, M. (1992). Effectiveness of prepared childbirth and childbirth satisfaction. *The Journal of Perinatal Education, 1*(2), 35–43.

Krauth, D., & Haloburo, E. (1986). Effect of pushing techniques in birthing chair on length of second stage labor. *Nursing Research, 35,* 49.

Noble, D. (1988). *Essential exercises for the childbearing year.* Boston: Houghton-Mifflin.

Rose, A., & Hilbers, S. (1988). Relaxation: Paced breathing techniques. In F. Nichols & S. Humenick (Eds.), *Childbirth education: Practice, research and theory.* Philadelphia: W.B. Saunders.

Shrock, P. (1988). The basis of relaxation. In F. Nichols & S. Humenick (Eds.), *Childbirth education: Practice, research and Theory.* Philadelphia: W.B. Saunders.

Steffes, S. (1988). Relaxation: Imagery. In F. Nichols & S. Humenick (Eds.), *Childbirth education: Practice, research and theory.* Philadelphia: W.B. Saunders.

SUGGESTED READINGS

Bing, E. (1994). *Six practical lessons for an easier childbirth.* New York: Bantam Books.

Enkin, M., Keirse, M., & Chalmers, I. (1995). *A guide to effective care in pregnancy and childbirth,* 2nd Edition. New York: Oxford University Press.

Nichols, F., & Humenick, S. (Eds.) (1988). *Childbirth education: Practice, research and theory.* Philadelphia: W.B. Saunders.

Noble, E. (1995). *Essential exercises for the childbearing year.* Boston: Houghton-Mifflin.

Simkin, P. (1989). *The birth partner: Everything you need to know to help a woman through childbirth.* Boston: Harvard Common Press.

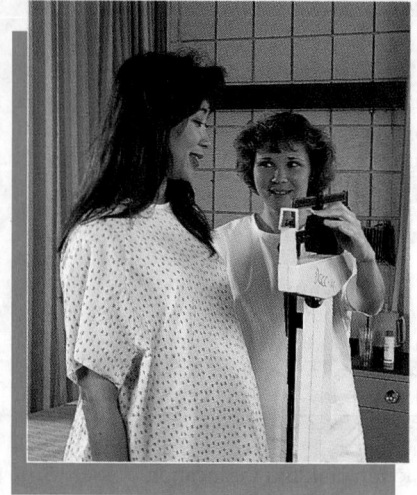

IV

Assessment and Management in the Antepartum Period

Critical Thinking Exercises

1. You are running a pregnancy support group for first time mothers. Many of the participants are talking about different complaints they are experiencing. You are hearing statements such as "I have to constantly run to the bathroom"; "My rings are getting tight"; and "My back hurts and I get leg cramps at night." You plan to focus the next class on the common discomforts of pregnancy.

    How would you meet the needs of this group, include specific suggestions for dealing with these discomforts in your teaching plan?

2. Sue Hart has come to the clinic for her first antepartal visit. She is 17 years old, unmarried, and 17 weeks pregnant. She is presently unemployed and is receiving governmental financial assistance. She lives at home with her mother and two sisters. Sue is overweight and smokes one and one half packs of cigarettes per day. She wants to keep the baby and relates that her mother will help her care for it.

    Following your antepartal assessment, formulate appropriate nursing diagnoses for this client and outline a specific plan to address these nursing diagnoses.

3. You are teaching a group of pregnant women in the WIC program about nutrition. There are several Mexican-American women in the group. After reviewing the nutritional needs of pregnancy, one of the women expresses concern that she doesn't drink milk.

    What information do you need to assess this client, and how would you intervene? Include a meal plan for this client based on her ethnic dietary preferences that would meet her nutritional requirements of pregnancy.

4. Shelly and Jeff Crane come to the healthcare facility for a first trimester checkup. During the visit, the couple voice concerns about planning for labor and delivery. Jeff states, " We want to do it naturally, but

what if Shelly has too much pain?" Shelly says, "I don't want any medication at all, no matter what. It will hurt the baby."

    When preparing to address this couple's concerns, what areas need to be addressed and how would you address them?

Multiple Choice Questions

1. When assessing a client with morning sickness, the nurse understands that it is most common during:

    A. First month
    B. First 6 weeks
    C. Fourth to 12th weeks
    D. Eighth to 20 weeks

2. During her first visit to the clinic, a client confides that she is afraid to have a baby. The most appropriate response by the nurse would be:

    A. "Modern obstetrics make having a baby so safe that you have absolutely nothing to fear."
    B. "Perhaps if you discussed this with a psychiatrist, he would help you."
    C. "Many women feel this way, so I wouldn't be concerned about it if I were you."
    D. "I can understand that you might be afraid. What is it that you are worried about?"

3. The nurse instructs the client complaining of low backache about which exercise to relieve this complaint:

    A. Shoulder circling
    B. Pelvic floor contraction
    C. Calf stretching
    D. Pelvic rocking

4. As part of an initial evaluation to confirm pregnancy, the nurse would identify which of the following as a presumptive sign?

    A. Breast enlargement
    B. Reports of backache

C. Abdominal striae

D. Braxton Hicks contractions

5. Which of the following suggestions would the nurse give for food choices that are high in protein?

A. Broccoli

B. Beans

C. Cottage cheese

D. Pasta

6. During the second trimester, the nurse would expect a client to:

A. Anticipate labor and delivery

B. Realistically prepare for childbirth

C. View the fetus as a separate being

D. Feel ambivalent about the pregnancy

7. A client is approximately 12 weeks pregnant and mentions to the nurse that she hasn't felt the baby move yet. The nurse correctly responds by saying:

A. "Make sure you tell your doctor when she examines you."

B. "You may not feel movement for another 3 months."

C. "It's too early; you should begin to feel something in about 6 to 8 weeks."

D. "You probably aren't aware of what the movement feels like since this is your first baby."

8. When developing a meal plan for the pregnant client, the nurse keeps in mind that total daily caloric intake should be increased by:

A. 100 to 200 calories

B. 200 to 300 calories

C. 300 to 400 calories

D. 400 to 500 calories

9. A client reports drinking three to four cups of coffee and two to three cans of cola per day. The nurse understands that excessive caffeine intake has been associated with:

A. Intrauterine growth retardation

B. Abruptio placentae

C. Pregnancy-induced hypertension

D. Premature labor

10. A client attending a childbirth education class is learning to relax by picturing herself lying on a warm sunny beach. This is an example of:

A. Progressive relaxation

B. Biofeedback

C. Imagery

D. Neuromuscular dissociation

11. A client at her ideal body weight when becoming pregnant is expected to gain:

A. 10 lb

B. 20 lb

C. 30 lb

D. 40 lb

12. A client reports intermittent painless contractions of her uterus at about 5 1/2 months. The nurse interprets this as:

A. Braxton Hicks contractions

B. Signs of true labor

C. Danger sign

D. Premature labor

13. A client's last menstrual period (LMP) was March 15. What is her estimated date of delivery (EDD)?

A. January 8

B. December 22

C. November 8

D. October 22

14. A client complains of heartburn. The nurse instructs the client to:

A. Lie down immediately after eating

B. Take small sips of a carbonated drink

C. Take some baking soda

D. Eat three large meals a day

Study Questions

1. List the positive signs of pregnancy.

2. During pregnancy, what change occurs in cardiac output?

3. List three cognitive and emotional responses to pregnancy during the second trimester.

4. Define couvade syndrome.

5. When does the nurse screen for diabetes?

6. When is the best time for the client to monitor fetal movement?

7. Identify the physiologic basis for the discomfort of nasal stuffiness.

8. What happens to fat as pregnancy progresses?

9. Which vitamin has the smallest range of safety?

10. During the first trimester, how much weight does a pregnant woman usually gain?

11. List the two types of paced breathing techniques.

12. Define leukorrhea.

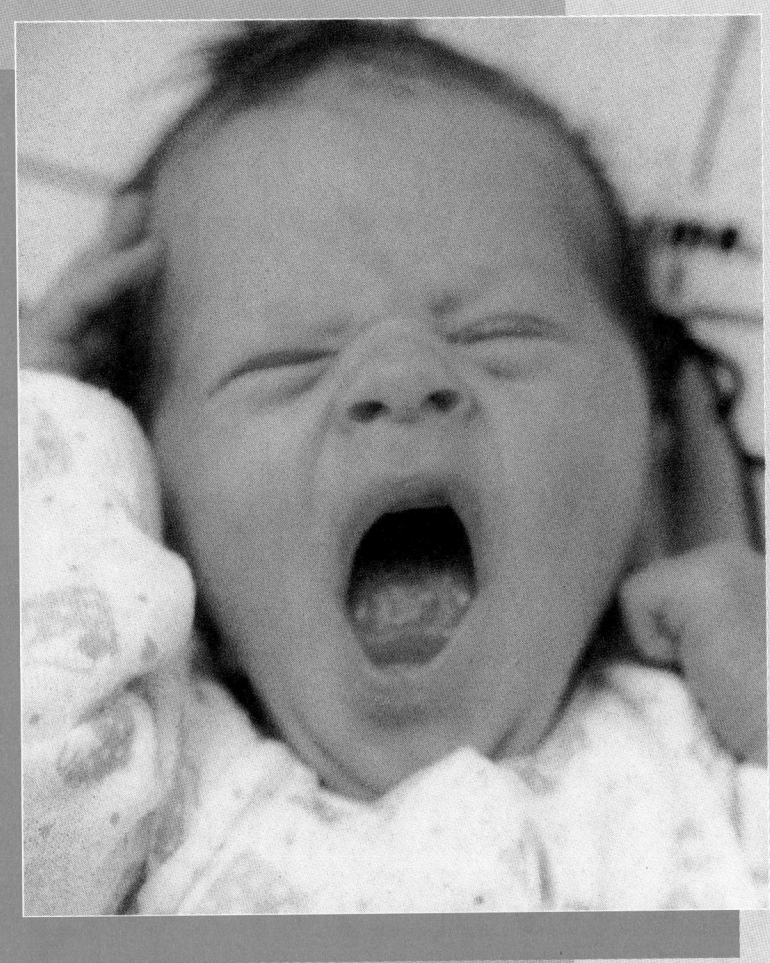

Assessment and Management in the Intrapartum Period

V

20

Assessment of the Passageway and Passenger

Objectives

- Describe the anatomic structure of the female pelvis.
- Compare the four types of pelves.
- Describe the internal pelvic measurements.
- Define fetal lie, attitude, presentation, and position.
- Identify the major bones, fontanels, sutures, and diameters of the fetal skull.
- Describe the procedure for performing Leopold maneuvers.

Labor, or **parturition,** is the physiologic process by which regularly occurring uterine contractions result in progressive effacement and dilation of the cervix. These cervical changes permit passage of the fetus and other products of conception from the uterus through the birth canal, resulting in delivery. The process of labor involves four components that must be well coordinated for normal labor to progress and birth to occur. Commonly known as the "four Ps," they include the powers (forces) of labor, passenger, passageway, and psyche. The **powers,** involuntary uterine contractions assisted by maternal pushing efforts during the second stage, must be of adequate strength with coordination of muscle activity. These forces propel the fetus or **passenger** through the birth canal or **passageway**. The passenger must be a size and shape to undergo the necessary maneuvers to pass through the varying dimensions of the birth canal. The passageway must be of adequate size and configuration, not presenting any undue obstacles to the descent, rotations, and expulsion of the newborn. The **psyche** or maternal psychological response may affect the woman's progress during labor and possibly weaken the forces. For example, maternal catecholamines are secreted when the laboring woman is anxious. Release of these stress hormones inhibits uterine contractions and impairs placental blood flow. The passageway and passenger are discussed in this chapter and the powers and psyche in Chapter 21. When nature tries to propel the fetus through the birth canal and fails to do so, some problem in the powers, passenger, passageway, or coordination of these components exists. Such disruptions in the labor process are discussed in Chapter 36.

The Passageway

The entire childbirth process centers on the safe passage of the fully developed fetus through the pelvis. Slight irregularities in the structure of the pelvis may delay the progress of labor, and any marked deformity may render delivery through natural passages impossible.

True Pelvis

True and false pelves were discussed briefly in Chapter 6. The difference between the two is illustrated in Figure 20-1. The true pelvis, or lower part, is the focus of this chapter. It forms the bony canal through which the fetus must pass during labor and birth and is di-

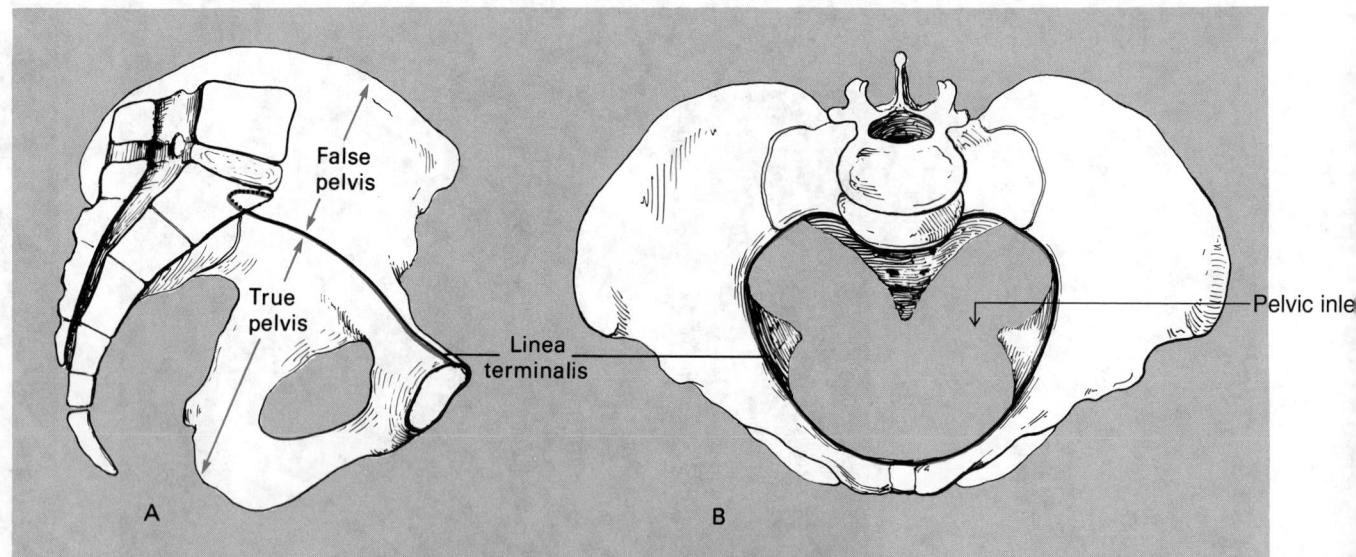

FIGURE 20-1 (**A**) Side view of true and false pelvis. (**B**) Front view showing linea terminalis (pelvic brim).

vided into three parts: an *inlet* or brim, an *outlet*, and a *cavity*.

Pelvic Inlet

Continuous from the sacral promontory and extending along the ilium on each side in circular fashion is a ridge called the *linea terminalis*, or brim (see Fig. 20-1*A*). This forms the boundary for the inlet or entryway through which the fetal head must pass to enter the true pelvis.

The **pelvic inlet**, sometimes called the *pelvic brim* or *superior strait*, divides the false pelvis from the true pelvis. It is heart-shaped, and the promontory of the sacrum forms a slight projection into it from behind (see Fig. 20-1*B*). Generally, it is widest from side to side and narrowest from back to front (ie., from the sacral promontory to the symphysis). The fetal head enters the inlet of the average pelvis with its longest diameter (anteroposterior) in the transverse diameter of the pelvis (Fig. 20-2*A*). In other words, the greatest diameter of the head accommodates itself to the greatest diameter of the inlet (see Fig. 20-2*B*).

Pelvic Outlet

As viewed from below, the *pelvic outlet* is a space bounded in front by the symphysis pubis and the pu-

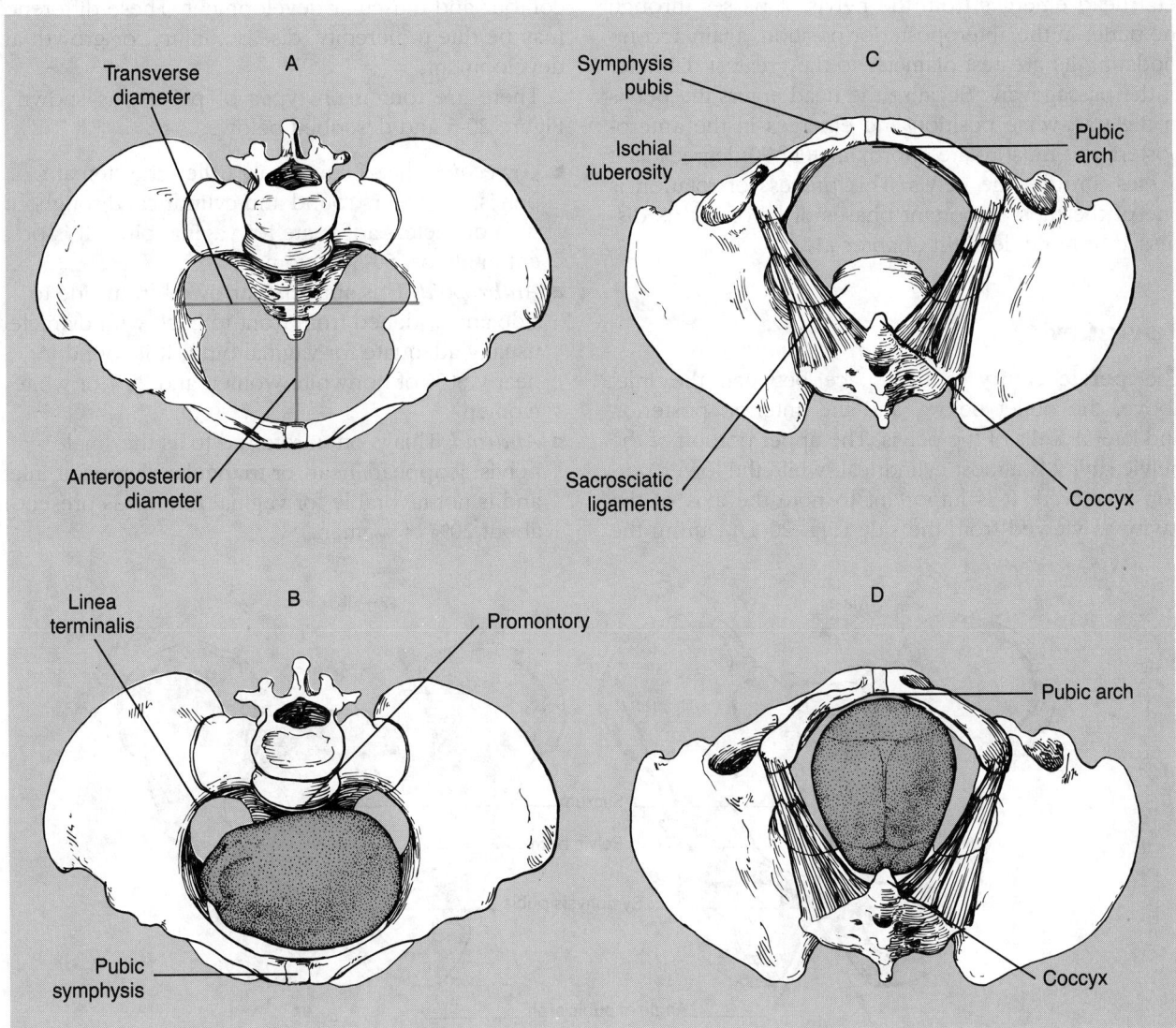

FIGURE 20-2 Views of pelvic inlet and outlet with fetal head in place. (**A**) Inlet of normal female pelvis showing transverse and anteroposterior diameters. (**B**) Largest diameter of the fetal head passes through the largest diameter of the inlet; therefore, it enters transversely. (**C**) Pelvic outlet and sacrosciatic ligaments. (**D**) Largest diameter of the fetal head passes through the largest diameter of the outlet; therefore, it passes through anteroposteriorly.

bic arch, at the sides by the ischial tuberosities, and behind by the coccyx and the greater sacrosciatic ligaments (see Fig. 20-2*C*). The front half of the outlet resembles a triangle. The base of the triangle is the distance between the ischial tuberosities; the other two sides of the triangle are represented by the pubic arch. From an obstetric point of view, this triangle is of great importance because the fetal head must use this space to exit from the pelvis and the mother's body (see Fig. 20-2*D*). Women have a wide pubic arch, whereas men have a narrow arch (Fig. 20-3).

In the typical female pelvis, the greatest diameter of the inlet is the transverse (from side to side), whereas the greatest diameter of the outlet is the anteroposterior (from front to back; see Fig. 20-2*A* and *C*). As the fetal head emerges from the pelvis, it passes through the outlet in the anteroposterior position, again accommodating its greatest diameter to the greatest diameter of the passageway. Because the head enters the pelvis in the transverse position and emerges in the anteroposterior, it must rotate approximately 90 degrees as it passes through the pelvis. This process of rotation is one of the most important phases of labor and is discussed in more detail in Chapter 21.

Pelvic Cavity

The **pelvic cavity** is the space between the inlet above, the outlet below, and the anterior, posterior, and lateral walls of the pelvis. The upper portion of the pelvic cavity is almost cylindrical, while the lower portion is curved. It is important to note the axis of the cavity as viewed from the side (Fig. 20-4). During the birth process, the head must descend along the downward axis until it almost reaches the level of the ischial spines and begins to curve forward. The axis of the cavity determines the direction that the fetus takes through the pelvis in the process of birth. Labor is complicated by this curvature in the pelvic canal because the fetus has to accommodate itself to the curved path and to variations in the size of the cavity at different levels.

Pelvic Variations

The pelvis presents great individual variations: no two pelves are exactly alike. Even women with average pelvic measurements may have pelves that differ in contour and muscular development. These differences may be due to heredity, disease, injury, or growth and development.

There are four main types of pelves, as shown in Figure 20-5 and described below:

- *Gynecoid*: This is commonly called the "female" pelvis; it appears round and cylindrical throughout with diameters adequate for vaginal birth. It is present in almost 50% of women.
- *Anthropoid*: This appears narrowed from side to side and widened from front to back with diameters usually adequate for vaginal birth. It is found in nearly 50% of nonwhite women and 25% of white women.
- *Android*: This is often referred to as the "male" pelvis; it appears heart or triangular shaped at inlet and is not favorable for vaginal birth. It is present in about 20% of women.

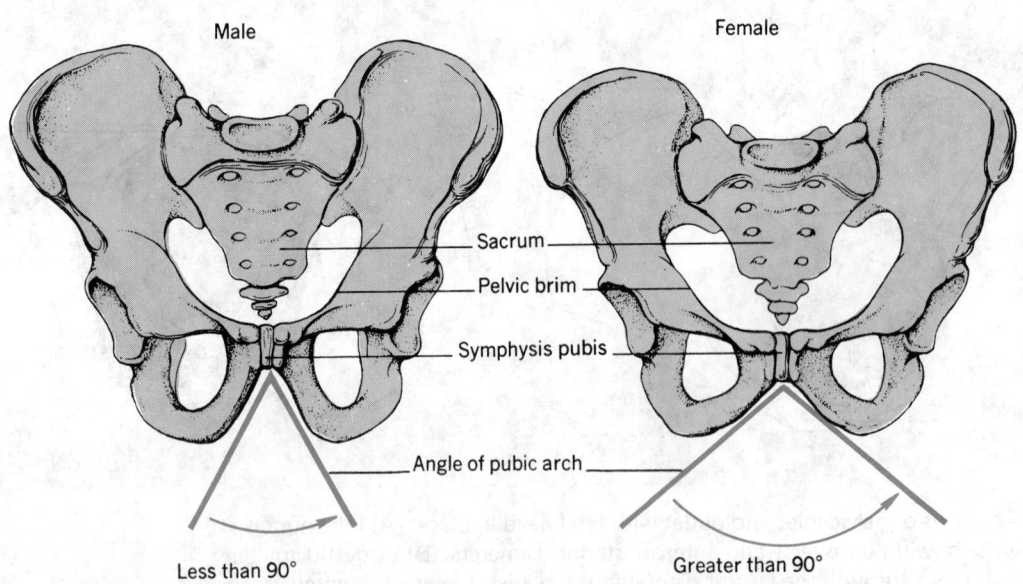

Male   Female

Sacrum

Pelvic brim

Symphysis pubis

Angle of pubic arch

Less than 90°   Greater than 90°

FIGURE 20–3 Comparison of the male and female pelvis. (*Left*) The male pelvis is narrow and compact; the pelvic arch is less than a right angle. (*Right*) The female pelvis is broad and capacious; the pubic arch is greater than a right angle.

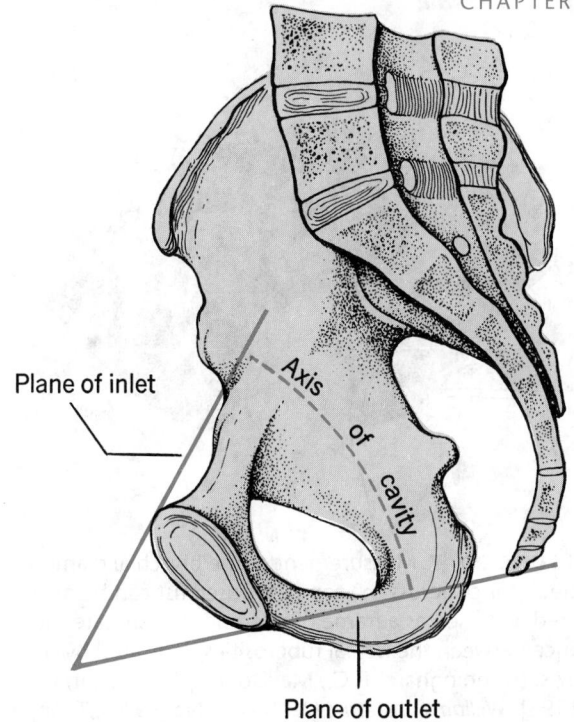

Plane of inlet

Axis of cavity

Plane of outlet

FIGURE 20-4 Pelvic cavity showing plane of inlet and outlet. The direction the fetus takes through the pelvis is determined by the axis of the cavity.

■ *Platypelloid*: This appears flattened from front to back and widened from side to side with diameters usually not favorable for vaginal birth. It is found in less than 3% of women.

The manner in which the fetus passes through the birth canal, and consequently the type of labor, varies considerably in each pelvic type. In addition, many variations result from abnormal narrowing of one or another of the diameters. These contracted pelves are described in Chapter 36.

During pregnancy, relaxation of the pelvic joints results from hormonal influences. Use of a modified squatting position during the second stage of labor shortens the second stage of labor (Golay et al., 1993). In this position, the woman can increase the diameter of her pelvic outlet by as much as 0.5 to 2.0 cm and can improve the efficiency and effectiveness of her pushing efforts.

Assessment: Pelvic Measurements

The pelvis of every pregnant woman should be measured accurately during the prenatal evaluation to determine whether anything may complicate the birth. It is most useful to know in advance whether there are any abnormalities in the size or configuration of the pelvis; this information is most readily and appropriately obtained well in advance of the onset of labor.

Types of Pelvic Measurements

Internal pelvic measurements, taken manually, are an important means of estimating the size of the pelvis and identifying variations from normal (eg, small or flattened) that may cause complications during labor and birth. These are optimally performed during the 34th to 36th week of gestation when increased joint mobility and soft-tissue distensibility make the procedures easier and more comfortable for the client (Scott et al., 1994). In many abnormal pelves, the most

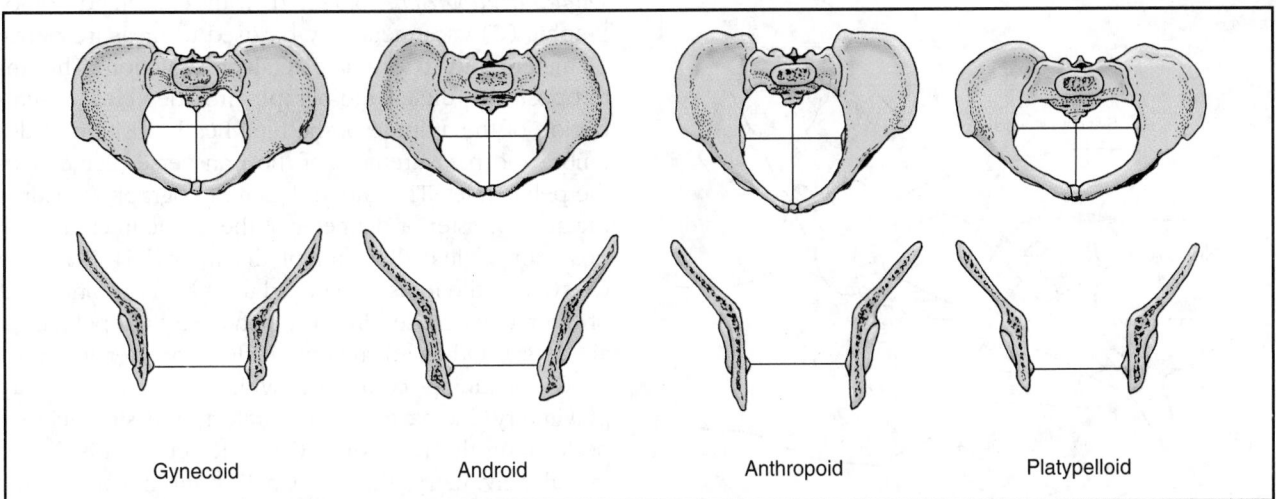

Gynecoid   Android   Anthropoid   Platypelloid

FIGURE 20-5 Caldwell-Maloy classification of pelvic types. (*Top*) The typical shape of the inlet for each type is shown. A line has been drawn through the widest transverse diameter, dividing the inlet into an anterior and posterior segment. The longitudinal line illustrates the anteroposterior diameter of the inlet. (*Bottom*) The typical interspinous diameter of each type is depicted.

marked deformity affects the anteroposterior diameter of the inlet (Scott et al., 1994).

Pelvic measurements may be performed by obstetricians or by advanced practice nurses who have been specially trained in the measurement techniques. Before obtaining specific pelvic measurements, the clinician should carefully explain the procedure to the woman. The contour of the pelvis is then evaluated by palpation. The woman is first placed on her back on the examining table, with her knees drawn up and her feet supported by stirrups. Two fingers are then inserted into the vagina (Fig. 20-6). The evaluation includes assessment of the height of the symphysis pubis, the shape of the pubic arch, the motility of the coccyx, the inclination of the anterior wall of the pelvis, and the prominence of the ischial spines (Fig. 20-7). The types of pelvic measurements obtained and the related assessment procedures are described in the Assessment Guidelines display.

X-Ray Pelvimetry

Although x-ray pelvimetry was used frequently in the past, it is now often performed only if vaginal birth is anticipated for a breech presentation. Pelvimetry also may be indicated for evaluating women with a history of injury or disease that could have affected the bony pelvis. The method subjects the maternal ovaries and fetal gonads to a certain amount of radiation; however, the slight risk from exposure appears justifiable whenever information critical to the welfare of the fetus or woman is likely to be obtained (Cunningham et al., 1993).

Many different pelvimetry techniques have been developed to provide exact measurement of the inlet, the

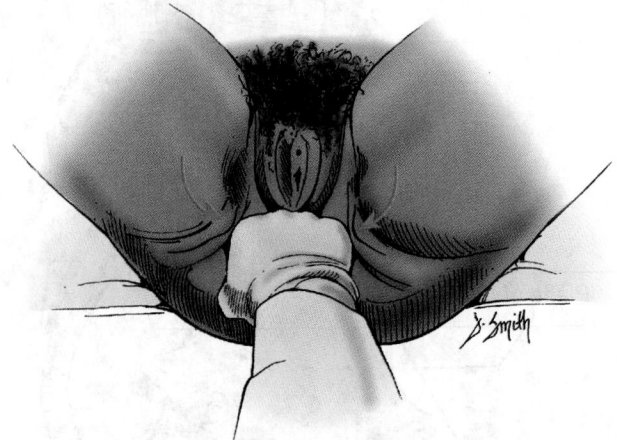

FIGURE 20–7 Measurement of the bi-ischial diameter. The distance across the top of a closed fist can be measured and used as a frame of reference to estimate the distance between the ischial tuberosities, indicated by the arrows. (Cunningham, F. C., MacDonald, P. C., Gant, N. F.: [1993]. *Williams obstetrics* [19th ed.]. Norwalk, CT: Appleton & Lange.)

interischial spinous diameter of the midpelvis, and the anteroposterior dimensions of the pelvis, including the obstetric conjugate. It also is possible to gain an impression of the size of the fetal head through pelvimetry.

Other Techniques: Computed Tomography, Magnetic Resonance Imaging, and Ultrasound

Digital radiographs obtained with computed tomographic (CT) scanners may be used to measure pelvic diameters and to evaluate fetal presentation. The anteroposterior digital radiograph provides clear visualization of the attitude of the fetal head, position of the limbs, and measurement of the transverse diameter of the pelvic inlet. The lateral digital radiograph measures the anteroposterior diameter of the pelvic inlet and the posterior sagittal diameter of the midpelvis. With the CT system, the fetus is exposed to only about one-third of the radiation used in x-ray pelvimetry (Kopelman et al., 1986). Other advantages include greater accuracy of CT scanning compared with conventional x-ray pelvimetry, increased client comfort, and simplicity in performing the procedure (Twickler et al., 1992). For digital pelvimetry, the woman lies supine on the CT table, which is positioned so the geometric center of the pelvis corresponds with the geometric center of the CT gantry circle. The procedure generally takes less than 10 minutes.

Magnetic resonance imaging is another method for obtaining accurate pelvic measurements and complete

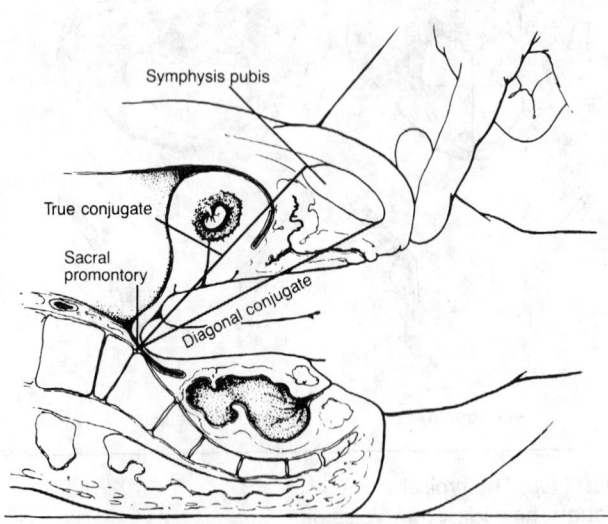

FIGURE 20–6 Method of obtaining diagonal conjugate diameter.

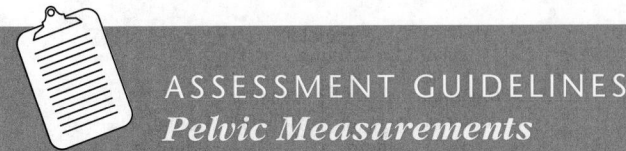

ASSESSMENT GUIDELINES
Pelvic Measurements

Measure	*Definition and Description*	*Assessment Procedure*
Diagonal conjugate (pelvic inlet)	1. The distance between the sacral promontory and the lower margin of the symphysis pubis 2. The most important pelvic measurement 3. In abnormal pelvis, diameter may be shortened	1. Insert two fingers into the vagina. 2. Press fingers inward and upward as far as possible until the middle finger rests on the sacral promontory. 3. Mark the point on the back of the hand just under the symphysis by putting the index finger of the other hand on the exact point (see **Fig. 20-6**). 4. Withdraw fingers and measure distance from the tip of the middle finger to the point marked (*conjugate measurement*). 5. Use a rigid measure scale or pelvimeter to determine distance. Note: If distance $\geq$ 11.5 cm, pelvic inlet is assumed to be adequate for childbirth.
True conjugate or conjugate vera *(pelvic inlet)*	1. The distance between the upper margin of the symphysis pubis and the sacral promontory; direct measurement only by x-ray study 2. The smallest anteroposterior diameter of the inlet through which the fetal head must pass; normally $\geq$ 10 cm	This measurement is derived from the diagonal conjugate measurement by 1. Subtracting 1.5–2.0 cm from the length of the diagonal conjugate 2. Using 1.5 cm in the above formula if the ht and inclination of the symphysis pubis is average *or* 2 cm if the symphysis pubis is high and has a marked inclination
Obstetric conjugate (pelvic inlet)	1. The anteroposterior diameter that begins at the tip of the sacral promontory and ends on the inner surface of the symphysis pubis, a few millimeters below its upper margin 2. The shortest diameter through which the fetal head must pass in descending through the true pelvis	1. This measurement cannot be directly obtained by pelvic examination; it is rarely distinguished from the conjugate vera except in pelvimetry. 2. Normally measures $\geq$ 10 cm.
Bi-ischial diameter or intertuberous diameter *(pelvic outlet)*	1. The diameter between the ischial tuberosities 2. The transverse diameter of the pelvis outlet; normally > 8 cm	1. Place client in lithotomy position with legs widely separated. 2. Place a closed fist against the perineum between the innermost and lowermost aspect of the ischial tuberosities, on a level with the lower border of the anus (**Fig. 20-7**). 3. Note distance between these landmarks on closed fist. 4. Compare size of closed fist with distance obtained to determine measurement.

imaging of the fetus. Although this method eliminates exposure to ionizing radiation, it is expensive, time-consuming, and requires equipment unavailable in many healthcare settings.

Ultrasound provides important information on fetal well-being, but accurate measurement of maternal pelvic diameters has not been achieved with this method.

The Passenger

Even in an adequately sized pelvic outlet, the birth may be difficult if the fetus is too large or in a difficult position. There are various means of assessing the fetal head, lie, attitude, presentation, and position.

Fetal Head

From an obstetric viewpoint, the head is the most important part of the fetus. If it can pass through the pelvic canal safely, there is usually no difficulty in delivering the rest of the body, although occasionally the shoulders may cause trouble.

The cranium, or skull, is made up of eight bones. Four of the bones—the sphenoid, the ethmoid, and the two temporal bones—lie at the base of the cranium, are closely united, and are of little obstetric interest. On the other hand, the four bones forming the upper part of the cranium—the frontal, the occipital, and the two parietal bones—are of great importance. These bones are not knit closely together at the time of birth but are separated by membranous interspaces called **sutures.** The intersections of these sutures are known as **fontanels** (Fig. 20-8).

This formation of the fetal skull allows the bones to overlap each other slightly during labor. This diminishes the size of the head during its passage through the pelvis. This process of overlapping is called "molding," and after a long labor with a large baby and a snug pelvis, the head often is so definitely molded that several days may elapse before it returns to its normal shape.

The most important sutures of the skull are identified below:

- The *sagittal suture* is located between the two parietal bones and runs anterioposteriorly; it connects the two fontanels and separates the skull into the left and right halves.
- The *frontal suture* is located between the two frontal bones.
- The *coronal sutures* are located between the frontal and parietal bones and extend transversely left and right from the anterior fontanel.
- The *lambdoid suture* is located between the posterior margins of the parietal bones and the upper

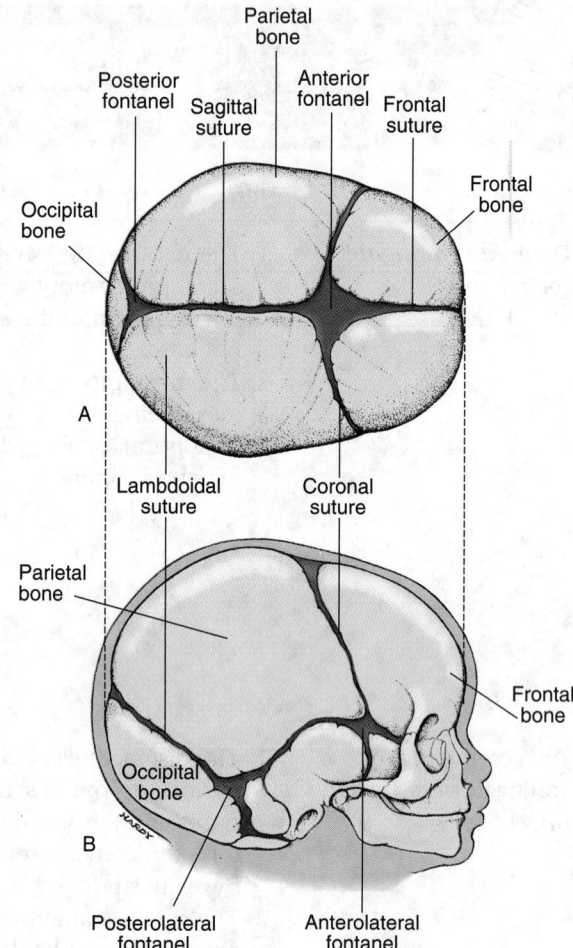

FIGURE 20–8 Fetal skull showing fontanels, bones, and sutures. (**A**) Superior aspect. (**B**) Lateral aspect.

margin of the occipital bone and extends transversely left and right from the posterior fontanel.

The important fontanels are the anterior and posterior. The *anterior fontanel* is large and diamond shaped and is located at the intersection of the sagittal and the coronal sutures; the small triangular *posterior fontanel* lies at the junction of the sagittal and lambdoid sutures. The sutures and the posterior fontanel ossify shortly after birth, but the anterior fontanel remains open until the child is older than 1 year, constituting the familiar "soft spot" just above the forehead of an infant.

By feeling or identifying one or another of the sutures or fontanels and considering its relative position in the pelvis, the nurse is able to determine accurately the position of the head in relation to the pelvis.

Fetal Skull Measurement

The principal measurements of the fetal skull are shown in Figure 20-9. The most important transverse diameter is the biparietal; it is the distance between the biparietal protuberances and represents the greatest width of the head. It measures, on an average, 9.5 to 9.8 cm.

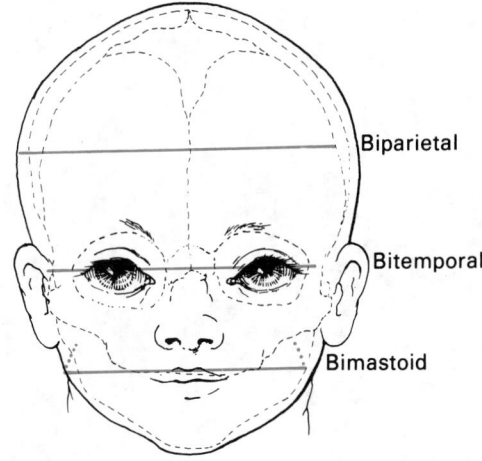

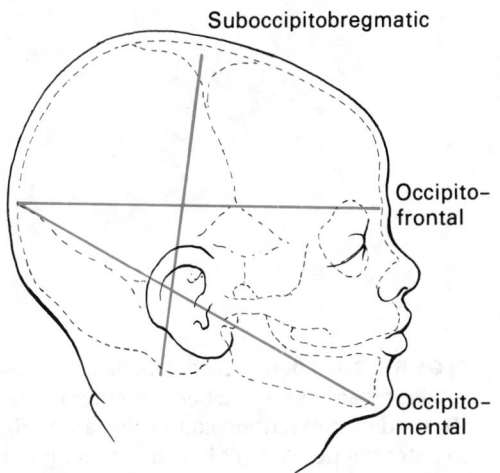

FIGURE 20-9 Fetal skull showing various diameters.

There are three important anteroposterior diameters of the fetal skull:

- *Suboccipitobregmatic*: Extends from the undersurface of the occiput to the center of the anterior fontanel and measures about 9.5 cm
- *Occipitofrontal*: Extends from the root of the nose to the occipital prominence and measures about 12 cm
- *Occipitomental*: Extends from the chin to the posterior fontanel and averages 13.5 cm

When the head is in complete flexion and the chin is resting on the thorax, the smallest diameter, the suboccipitobregmatic, presents itself into the pelvis; if the fetal head is extended or bent back (flexion is absent), the greatest anteroposterior diameter presents itself to the pelvic inlet. The more the head is flexed, the smaller the anteroposterior diameter that enters the pelvis (Fig. 20-10).

Fetal Lie

The term **fetal lie** refers to the relationship of the long axis (spine) of the fetus to the long axis of the mother.

The *longitudinal lie*, in which the fetal and maternal spines are parallel, is present in more than 99% of labors at term. This is the optimal position for vaginal delivery (Cunningham et al., 1993). In a *transverse lie*, the long axis of the fetus is approximately perpendicular to that of the mother. The common causes of the transverse lie are abnormal relaxation of the abdominal wall due to grand multiparity, pelvic contraction, and placenta previa. In an *oblique lie*, the fetus forms an acute angle in relation to the axis of the mother. An oblique lie is usually converted during the course of early labor to a longitudinal or a transverse lie. Transverse and oblique lies ultimately prevent the fetus from entering the bony pelvis, and if left unconverted, they necessitate a cesarean delivery.

Fetal Attitude

The **fetal attitude** refers to the relationship of the fetal parts to one another. The most striking characteristic of the fetal body conformation is flexion. The spinal column is bowed forward, the head is flexed with the chin against the sternum, and the arms are flexed and folded against the chest. The lower extremities also are flexed, the thighs on the abdomen, and the calves against the posterior aspect of the thighs. In this state of flexion, the fetus assumes a roughly ovoid shape, occupies the smallest possible space, and conforms to the shape of the uterus. In this attitude, the fetus appears approximately half as long as if it were completely stretched out.

Fetal Presentation

The term **presentation**, or presenting part, designates the portion of the fetus' body that lies nearest the internal cervical os, which is felt during a vaginal examination. By palpating the presenting part on an abdominal examination, the nurse can determine the fetal lie (see Procedure 20-1). Fetal presentation may be one of the following:

- **Head** or **cephalic presentation** is observed in 96% to 97% of all fetuses. Cephalic presentations are divided into groups according to the relation of the fetus' head to its body. The most common is the vertex presentation, in which the head is sharply flexed so that the chin contacts the thorax and the vertex is the presenting part. Face presentation, in which the neck is sharply extended so that the occiput and back come in contact, is less often observed (approximately 1 in 550 births).
- **Breech presentation** occurs in 3% to 4% of cases at term. The incidence increases in preterm fetuses and multiple gestation and in women with a history of breech birth. In breech presentations, the thighs

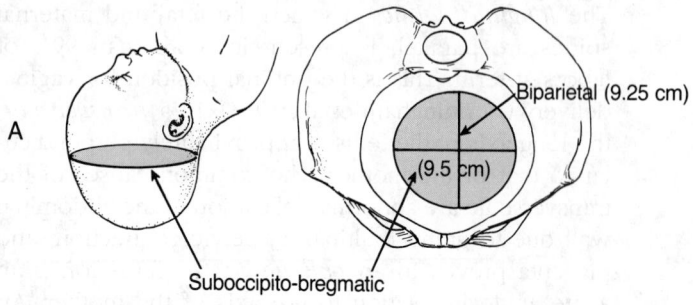

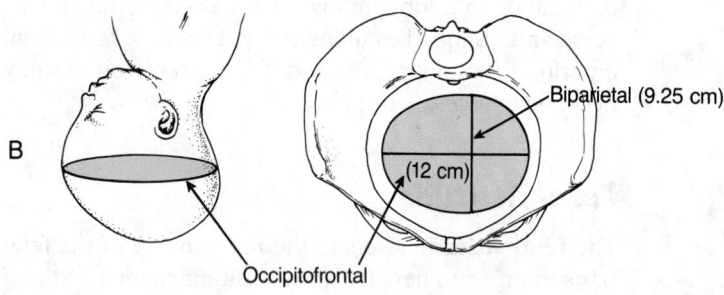

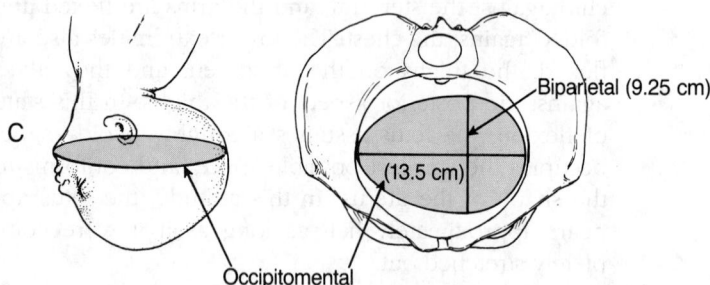

FIGURE 20–10 (A) Complete flexion allows the smallest diameter of the head to enter the pelvis. **(B)** Moderate extension causes the larger diameter to enter the pelvis. **(C)** Marked extension forces the largest diameter against the pelvic brim, but the head is too large to enter the pelvis.

may be flexed and the legs extended over the anterior surface of the body (frank breech), the thighs may be flexed on the abdomen and the legs on the thighs (full breech), or one or both feet may be the lowest part (foot or footling breech).

- **Shoulder presentation** occurs when the fetus lies crosswise in the uterus so that the shoulder is the presenting part. This is relatively uncommon, and with rare exceptions, the spontaneous birth of a fully developed child is impossible in a "persistent transverse lie." The condition is associated with multiparity, abdominal laxity, uterine and fetal anomalies, and low-lying placenta.

The term **asynclitism** refers to an oblique presentation of the fetal head in labor. The fetal head is laterally flexed and therefore the sagittal suture is not oriented in the midplane of descent. *Anterior asynclitism* exists when the anterior parietal bone is designated the point of presentation, and *posterior asynclitism* exists when the posterior parietal bone presents. This malposition increases the diameter of the fetal head entering the pelvis and causes fetal dystocia. There may be several causes of asynclitism, including overzealous attempts at induction of labor through amniotomy before the fetal head enters the pelvic inlet and pelvic structural abnormalities (Perkins, 1987). The condition may sometimes be corrected by vacuum extraction, or a cesarean birth may be necessary. The prognosis for a vaginal birth is more favorable for anterior asynclitism than for posterior asynclitism.

Fetal Position

In addition to knowing the presenting part of the baby, it is important to know the exact position of the presenting part in relation to the pelvis. This relationship is determined by finding the position of certain points on the presenting surface and relating these to the four imaginary divisions or quadrants of the pelvis—the left anterior, left posterior, right anterior, and right posterior. These divisions aid in indicating whether the presenting part is directed toward the right or left side and toward the front or back of the pelvis.

Certain points on the presenting surface of the fetus have been arbitrarily chosen as points of direction

PROCEDURE 20-1
Leopold Maneuvers

Overall Objective: To determine fetal position by systematic abdominal palpation

Nursing Action	*Rationale*
Preparation:	
■ Explain procedure to woman and rationale for what is being done.	Explanation of procedure relieves anxiety and promotes cooperation.
■ Instruct woman to empty bladder before beginning procedure, if she has not recently voided.	Emptying the bladder increases client comfort, prevents uterine distension and ability to palpate fetal parts in suprapubic area.
■ Instruct woman to lie flat on her back, with her knees flexed slightly. Place a small pillow or rolled towel under one side.	Flexing knees relaxes the abdominal muscles. Tilting the uterus with a pillow or towel prevents supine hypotension.
■ Wash hands with warm water.	Handwashing helps to prevent transmission of microorganisms.

First Maneuver

Objective: To determine if fetal head or breech is in fundus

1. Observe woman's abdomen before beginning palpation.	Inspection allows for identification of asymmetry, bulging prominences, and indentations.
2. Stand at the foot of the examining table, facing the woman, and gently place both hands flat on the abdomen.	Overstimulation by the fingers may cause the abdominal muscles to contract.
3. Palpate upper abdomen with both hands as shown in Figure A.	Palpation of upper abdomen enables determination of what is lying at the fundus.
4. Determine if the mass palpated is the head or buttocks by observing the relative consistency, shape and mobility.	The head is round and hard, the transverse groove of the neck may be felt. The breech has no groove and feels softer and more angular.
5. Assess ballottement (the ability of the head to be moved back and forth against the examining fingers).	The head moves independently of the body, but the breech moves only with the trunk.

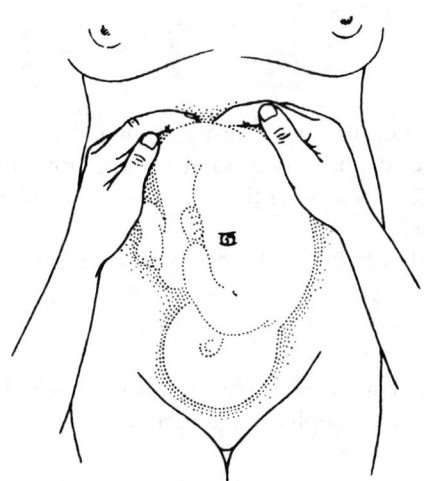

A. First Maneuver

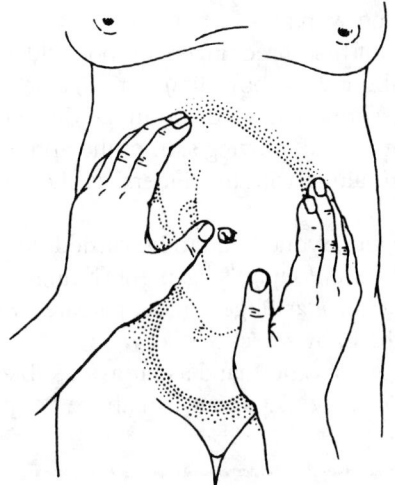

B. Second Maneuver

(continued)

PROCEDURE 20-1 *(continued)*
Leopold Maneuvers

Nursing Action	*Rationale*

Second Maneuver

Objective: To locate the back of the fetus in relation to the right and left sides of the woman.

1. Facing the woman, place the palmar surfaces of both hands on either side of the abdomen and apply gentle but deep pressure.
2. Hold one hand still while using the flat surface of the fingers on the other hand to gradually palpate the opposite side from the top to the lower segment of the uterus as shown in Figure B.
3. Palpate the fetal outline.
4. Reverse actions of the hands to palpate the other side (ie, the hand that was used to palpate remains steady, and the other hand palpates).

This action allows the uterus to be held steady while palpation is performed to determine the fetal outline.

The back feels like a smooth, hard, convex surface.
The knees and elbows feel like numerous angular nodulations.

Third Maneuver

Objective: To determine if the fetal head is at the pelvic inlet and to determine its mobility

1. Gently grasp the lower portion of the abdomen, just above the symphysis pubis, between the thumb and the fingers of one hand.
2. Press thumb and fingers together in an attempt to grasp the presenting part, as shown in Figure C.

A movable body is felt, usually the head, when the presenting part is not engaged in the pelvis.

Fourth Maneuver
(Omit if fetus is in breech presentation)

Objectives: To determine if the fetal head is well flexed and how far it is distended in the pelvis; to confirm location of fetal back

1. Stand facing woman's feet.
2. Place tips of first three fingers on both sides of the midline about 2 in above Poupart's ligament.
3. Exert pressure downward and in the direction of the birth canal, moving skin of the abdomen downward along with the fingers, as shown in Fig. D.
4. Allow fingers of one hand to be carried downward well under the Poupart's ligament (if fingers meet no obstruction); as fingers glide, palpate over the nape of the baby's neck.
5. Slide fingers of other hand as far as possible (obstruction usually met about 1 in above Poupart's ligament).

The obstruction met is the brow of the baby, often called the "cephalic prominence." Location of this landmark tells how far the head has descended in the pelvis.
The brow should be on the opposite side from the fetal back.

A posterior position of the occiput is suggested by an easily palpated cephalic prominence

PROCEDURE 20-1 *(continued)*
Leopold Maneuvers

Nursing Action	*Rationale*
Note: If the head is floating or poorly flexed, this maneuver may yield little information.	In the uncommon face presentation, the cephalic prominence and back are on the same side.

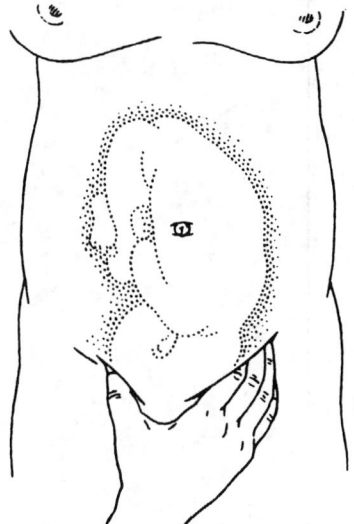

C. Third Maneuver

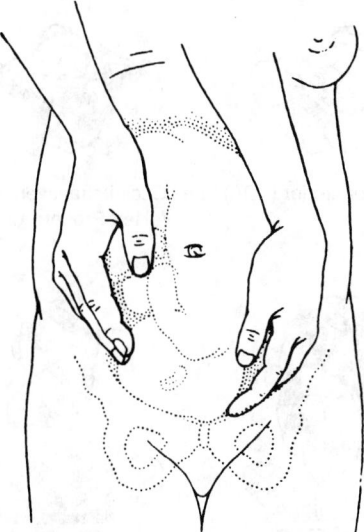

D. Fourth Maneuver

when determining the exact relationship of the presenting part to the quadrants of the pelvis. The guiding point is the occiput in vertex presentations, the sacrum in breech presentations, the chin (mentum) in face presentations, and the scapula (acromion process) in shoulder presentations.

Position has to do with the relationship of some arbitrarily chosen portion of the fetus to the right or the left side of the mother's pelvis. Thus, in a vertex presentation, the back of the head (occiput) may point to the front or back of the pelvis. The occiput rarely points directly forward or backward in the median line until the second stage of labor but is usually directed to one side or the other.

The various positions are usually expressed by a series of abbreviations (summarized in Box 20-1), which represent the left to right orientation of the fetal presenting part to the mother, indicated by R for right, L for left; the actual fetal presenting part, indicated by O for occiput, M for mentum (chin), and S for sacrum; and the front to back orientation of the fetal presenting part to the maternal pelvis, indicated by A for anterior (front) and P for posterior (back). Thus, LOA (left occipitoanterior) indicates that the occiput is directed toward the left side of the mother and toward the front

part of the pelvis; LOT (left occipitotransverse) indicates that the occiput is directed straight to the left side of the mother with no deviation toward the front or back of the maternal pelvis. ROP (right occipitoposterior) indicates that the occiput is directed toward the

BOX 20-1
*Standard Abbreviations Used
to Describe Fetal Position*

Orientation to Side of Maternal Pelvis
L   (left)
R   (right)
T   (transverse)

Fetal Presenting Part
O   (occiput)
M   (mentum or chin)
S   (sacrum)

Orientation of the presenting part to the pelvis
A   (anterior or front)
P   (posterior or back)

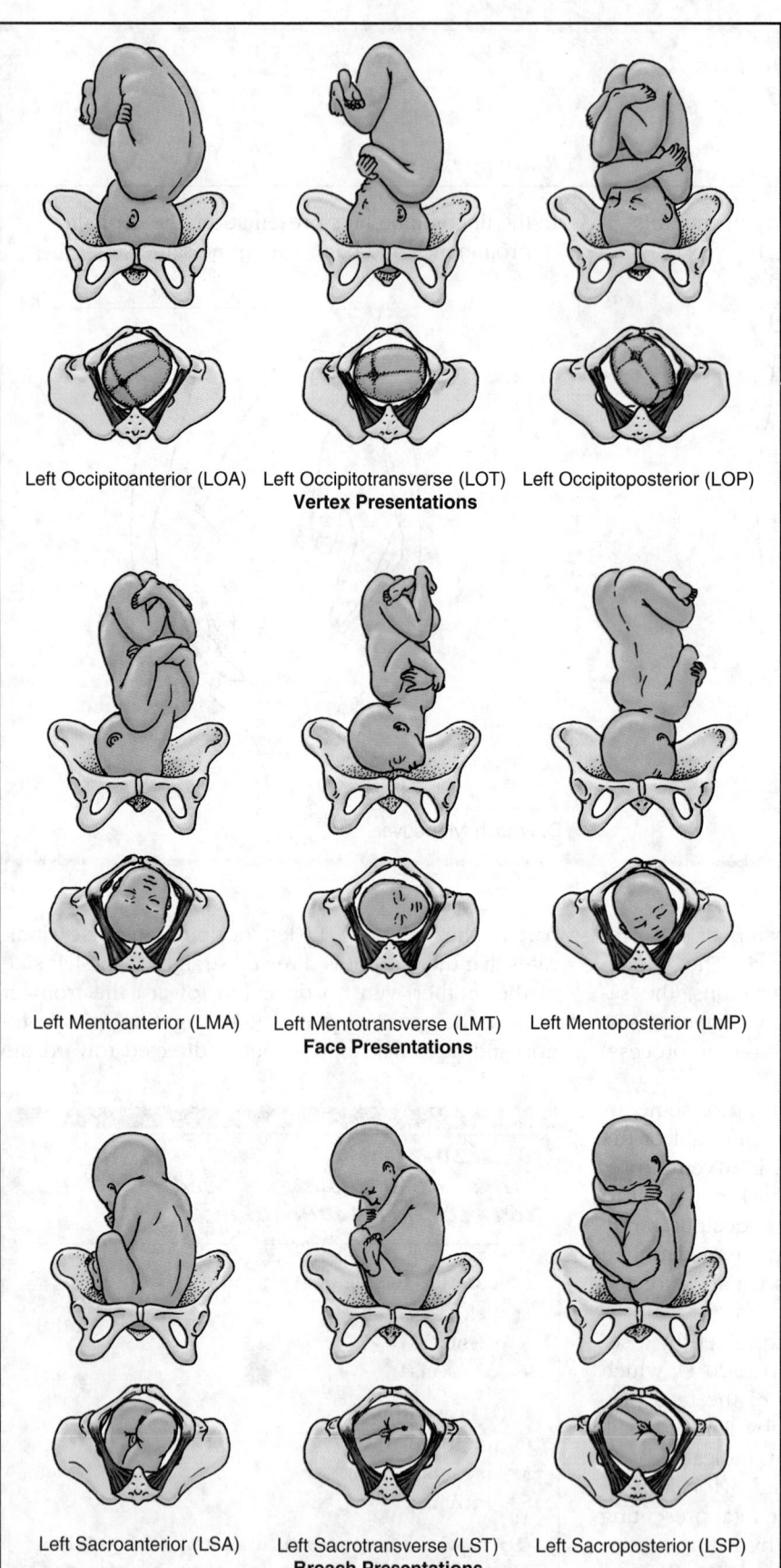

Left Occipitoanterior (LOA)   Left Occipitotransverse (LOT)   Left Occipitoposterior (LOP)
Vertex Presentations

Left Mentoanterior (LMA)   Left Mentotransverse (LMT)   Left Mentoposterior (LMP)
Face Presentations

Left Sacroanterior (LSA)   Left Sacrotransverse (LST)   Left Sacroposterior (LSP)
Breach Presentations

FIGURE 20–11 Fetal presentations. (Redrawn from Benson, R. C. [1980]. *Handbook of obstetrics and gynecology,* [7th ed]. Los Altos, CA: Lange Medical Publications.)

back or posterior right quadrant of the maternal pelvis. The occipital anterior positions are considered the most favorable for mother and baby, and of these, the LOA position is most common.

This system of terminology is used for vertex, face, and breech presentations, as illustrated in Figure 20-11. Although it is customary to speak of all "transverse lies" of the fetus simply as shoulder presentations, the following terms are sometimes used to express position in the shoulder presentation: left acromiodorso-anterior (LADA; the fetal acromion is to the mother's left and the back is anterior); left acromiodorso-posterior (LADP); right acromiodorso-anterior (RADA); and right acromiodorso-posterior (RADP).

Assessment

Assessment of fetal position is made in five ways: abdominal palpation, vaginal examination, combined auscultation and examination, ultrasound, and in certain cases, roentgenogram. The first three are discussed in this chapter; ultrasound is discussed in Chapter 39.

Palpation. It is extremely helpful to palpate the abdomen before listening to the fetal heart tones. The region of the abdomen in which the fetal heart is heard varies according to the presentation and the extent to which the presenting part has descended. The location of the fetal heart sounds does not give important information as to the presentation and the position of the fetus, but it sometimes reinforces the results obtained by palpation. To determine fetal position by abdominal palpation, a systematic examination using the four **Leopold maneuvers** is performed (see Procedure 20-1). If the fetus is in a cephalic presentation, the breech will be felt in the fundus. If the presentation is breech, the head will be felt in the fundus (see Research Highlight).

Vaginal Examination. During the vaginal examination, the nurse identifies the fontanels and the suture lines of the fetal skull. Before the onset of labor, the vaginal examination gives only limited information about the position of the fetus because the cervix is closed and the landmarks on the fetal head are not palpable. However, during labor, after dilatation of the cervix, important information about the position of the fetus and the degree of flexion of its head can be obtained by palpating and identifying the fontanels through the dilated os. When the head is well flexed, the nurse can easily identify the posterior fontanel by palpating the junction point of the sagittal suture and the two lambdoid sutures. The anterior fontanel, located well within the birth canal, is diamond shaped and has four sutures that lead to it: the sagittal posteriorly, two coronal laterally, and the frontal. The nurse

RESEARCH HIGHLIGHT

How Accurate Are Leopold Maneuvers for Screening?

 This prospective study conducted at the University of New Mexico Women's Ultrasound Clinic was designed to measure the accuracy of Leopold maneuvers to screen for fetal malpresentation.

A comparative, descriptive design was used in which each subject was her own control. The sample included 150 women; nearly one-half were nulliparous. Inclusion criteria required an estimated gestational age of at least 27 weeks and single gestation. Leopold maneuvers were performed by experienced and specially trained nurse midwives (blinded to the medical indication for ultrasound) who categorized fetal presentation as cephalic or noncephalic (breech or shoulder). This was followed by an ultrasound examination to determine fetal presentation. Results revealed that the Leopold maneuvers were performed with high sensitivity (88%), specificity (94%), positive predictive value (74%), and negative predictive value (97%) in a population with a 17% frequency of fetal malpresentation. Based on these results, it was concluded that the maneuvers used by experienced clinicians can be effective as a screening tool for fetal malpresentation, particularly when ultrasound is not readily available.

Critique: This study would have been strengthened by analyzing the relationship between accuracy of findings and weeks of gestation. A larger sample size would have increased generalizabiltiy of findings. Data were not provided on the types of presentations associated with performance error.

(Lydon-Rochelle, M., Albers, L., Gorwoda, J., Craig, E., & Qualls, C. [1993]. Accuracy of Leopold maneuvers in screening for malpresentation: A prospective study. *Birth, 20,* 132–134.)

can develop the skill of identifying these landmarks on the fetal skull by palpating the skull of the newborn after birth. The steps of a vaginal examination are described and illustrated in Chapter 22.

Auscultation. The location of the fetal heart sounds, as heard through the fetoscope, Doppler transducer, or external fetal heart monitor, yields helpful but not wholly dependable information about fetal position. Certainly, it never should be the sole means of diagnosing fetal position. Ordinarily, the heart sounds are transmitted through the convex portion of the fetus, which lies in intimate contact with the uterine wall; therefore, the nurse will hear them best through the fetus' back in vertex and breech presentations and through the thorax in face presentation.

In cephalic presentations, the nurse will hear the fetal heart sounds loudest midway between the umbilicus and the anterior superior spine of the ilium (Fig. 20-12). In general, in LOA and LOP positions, the fetal

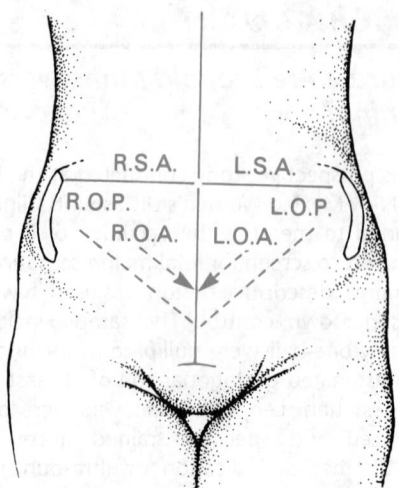

FIGURE 20–12 Fetal heart tone locations on the abdominal wall indicate possible corresponding fetal positions and the effects of the internal rotation of the fetus.

heart sounds are loudest in the left lower quadrant. A similar situation applies to the ROA and ROP positions. In posterior positions of the occiput (LOP and ROP), the sounds are often loudest well down in the side of the maternal abdomen toward the anterior superior spine. In breech presentation, the fetal heart sounds usually are loudest at the level of the umbilicus or above. The procedure for assessing fetal heart tones is discussed in Chapter 40.

Summary Points

✔ Four inter-related components influence the process of labor. These include the powers or forces (uterine contraction and maternal pushing), the passenger (the fetus), the passageway (birth canal) and the psyche (emotional responses).

✔ Fetal size and shape must be small enough and positioned favorably to pass through the birth canal, which likewise must be of adequate size and configuration.

✔ The four main pelvic types include the gynecoid, anthropoid, android, and the platypelloid. The round, cylindrical gynecoid pelvis, which is present in nearly 50% of women, is optimal for vaginal births.

✔ Several pelvic measurements are assessed during pregnancy. Examples include the diagonal conjugate, the true conjugate (conjugate vera), the ob-

stetric conjugate, and the bi-ischial diameter (inter-tuberous diameter). The most important pelvic measurement is the diagonal conjugate, which is the distance between the sacral promontory and the lower margin of the symphysis pubis.

✔ The fetal head has several important landmarks, such as the satigittal, frontal coronal, and lamb-doid sutures. The anterior and posterior fontanels form at the intersection of different sutures and are palpated by vaginal examination to determine the position of the fetal head in relation to the pelvis.

✔ The most common fetal presentation is the head or cephalic presentation (96%–97% or all births). The breech and shoulder presentations complicate the intrapartum process.

✔ Leopold maneuvers provide a systematic method for assessing fetal position using external abdominal palpation. If the fetus is in the cephalic presentation, the breech will be felt in the fundus.

✔ The fetal heart rate may be assessed using a fetoscope, Doppler transducer, or external electronic monitor. In cephalic presentations, fetal heart sounds are heard loudest midway between the umbilicus and the anterior superior spine of the ilium.

REFERENCES

Cunningham, F. G., MacDonald, P. C., & Gant, N. F. (1993). *Williams obstetrics* (19th ed.). Norwalk, CT: Appleton & Lange.

Golay, J. G., Vedam, S., & Sorger, L. (1993). The squatting position for the second stage of labor: Effects on labor and on maternal and fetal well-being. *Birth, 20*(2), 73–78.

Kopelman, I. N., Duff, P., Karl, R. T., Schpiel, A. H., Reed, J. A. (1986). Computerized tomographic pelvimetry in the evaluation of breech presentation. *Obstetrics & Gynecology, 68*, 455–458.

Perkins, R. (1987). Fetal dystocia. *Clinical obstetrics and gynecology, 30*, 56–88.

Scott, J. R., DiSaia, P. J., Hammond, C. B., & Spellacy, W. N. (1994). *Danforth's obstetrics and gynecology* (7th ed.). Philadelphia: J.B. Lippincott.

Thubisi, M., & Moodley, J. (1993). Vaginal delivery after previous caesarea section: Is X-ray pelvimetry necessary? *British Journal of Obstetrics and Gynaecology, 100*, 421–424.

Twickler D. M., Clarke, G., & Cunningham, F. G. (1992). *Diagnostic imaging in pregnancy. Williams obstetrics* (18th ed.). Norwalk, CT: Appleton & Lange.

21

The Process of Labor and Birth

Objectives

- Summarize four theories proposed to explain the onset of labor.
- Identify the premonitory signs of labor.
- Differentiate the signs of true versus false labor.
- Describe the four stages of labor and the related uterine activity and maternal behavioral changes.
- Discuss fetal position changes (cardinal movements) that are involved in the process of labor and birth.
- Identify the signs of placental separation.
- Differentiate between primary and secondary powers of labor.
- Identify and describe the three phases of a uterine contraction.
- Describe maternal and fetal physiologic responses to labor.

Key Terms

Acme	Frequency
Active phase	Fundus
Cardinal movements	Increment
Cervical dilatation	Intensity
Cervical effacement	Internal rotation
Contractions	Latent phase
Crowning	Lightening
Decrement	Physiologic retraction
Descent	ring
Duration	Placental expulsion
Engagement	Premonitory signs
Extension	Primary powers
External rotation	Second stage of labor
First stage of labor	Secondary powers
Flexion	Third stage of labor
Fourth stage of labor	Transition phase

Labor refers to the series of processes by which the products of conception are expelled out of the uterus and through the birth canal. Related terms include childbirth, parturition, accouchement, and confinement. The actual birth is called *delivery* in medical terminology; however, the word "birth" reflects a more humanistic approach to childbearing and is used in this text.

Chapter 20 identified the four necessary elements in labor and birth as the 4 Ps: the passageway, passenger, powers (or force), and psyche. The passageway and passenger also were described in Chapter 20 in terms of assessment and preparation for labor and birth. This chapter discusses the powers and psyche as part of the labor and birth process.

As described in Chapter 15, the pregnant uterus grows due to *hypertrophy* (enlargement) of existing muscle cells and to a lesser degree, *hyperplasia* (production of new muscle fibers and fibroelastic tissue). During labor, each of these cells is activated by a series of chemical reactions to begin rhythmic, highly coordinated, and forceful (involuntary) uterine **contractions**; these result in effacement and dilatation of the cervix and voluntary bearing down efforts that ultimately cause expulsion of the infant. It is still not known what simulates these uterine cells to begin labor contractions. Various theories have been proposed, but current research findings suggest that a combination of several maternal and fetal mechanisms are involved in initiating the onset of labor and supporting the labor process (Goff, 1993).

Theories of Labor Onset

The onset of labor usually occurs when the fetus is mature enough to cope with extrauterine conditions but not large enough to cause mechanical problems in labor. Most research on why labor begins, however, has focused on the balance between the levels of hormones that seem to stimulate labor contractions and the levels of hormones that tend to relax the uterine muscles. The following theories are among the most widely accepted as possible explanations for labor onset.

Estrogen-Progesterone Theory

This theory proposes that the estrogen-progesterone ratio is important in maintaining pregnancy and initiating parturition. The levels of both hormones regulate changes in concentrations of oxytocin receptors in the uterus. In animal research, decreased circulating progesterone has been shown to facilitate uterine contractility by increasing gap junction formation and increasing prostaglandin E_2 (PGE_2) formation; estrogen promotes the development of gap junctions and increases local synthesis of PGE_2 (Zlatnik, 1994). For many years, it was believed that the onset of labor results from progesterone withdrawal at a time of relative estrogen dominance; however, substantial evidence does not show that a demonstrable withdrawal of progesterone exists when labor commences (Cunningham et al., 1993).

Oxytocin Theory

The oxytocin theory suggests that oxytocin stimulates contractions of the uterus by acting directly on the myometrium and indirectly to increase the production of prostaglandins in the decidua. The uterus becomes increasingly sensitive to oxytocin as pregnancy advances. Research findings provide inconsistent support for this theory. Although some studies link increasing levels of oxytocin to onset of labor, others do not indicate that levels of this hormone increase before labor or through the first stage (Soloff, 1988; Padayachi et al., 1988). The highest concentration of oxytocin-like activity in the blood has been found during the second stage of labor. Because humans and other mammals go into labor normally after removal or destruction of the hypophysis, which secretes oxytocin, it is unlikely that this hormone alone initiates the labor process.

Fetal Endocrine Control Theory

The fetal endocrine control theory proposes that at the appropriate time of fetal maturity, the fetal adrenal glands secrete corticosteroids that trigger the mechanisms leading to labor. Fetal steroids stimulate the release of precursors to prostaglandins, which in turn produce uterine labor contractions (Casey et al., 1985). Shortly before labor, the sensitivity of the fetal adrenal glands to adrenocorticotropic hormone, produced by the pituitary, increases, causing a rise in the production of cortisol. The release of corticosteroids during periods of stress has been suggested as one cause of premature labor. This may occur when the fetus is compromised, such as preeclampsia or uterine overdistention due to multiple pregnancies or hydramnios.

Prostaglandin Theory

The prostaglandin theory hypothesizes that human labor is initiated by a sequence of events, including the release of lipid precursors, possibly triggered by steroid action; release of arachidonic acid from these precursors, perhaps at the site of the fetal membranes; increased prostaglandin synthesis from the arachidonic acid; and increased uterine contractions as a consequence of prostaglandin action on the uterine muscle (Bennett et al., 1990; Sahmay et al., 1988). Study of the mechanisms of prostaglandin synthesis has shown that arachidonic acid, the obligatory precursor to prostaglandin, increases markedly in comparison with the other fatty acids in the amniotic fluid of women in labor (Reddi et al., 1987). Prostaglandins have been effective in inducing uterine contractions at any stage of gestation (Cunningham et al., 1993; Granstrom et al., 1990; Shaala et al., 1989). They are produced by the uterine decidua, umbilical cord, and amnion. Research findings vary concerning whether the concentration of prostaglandins increases in the amniotic fluid and maternal blood just before labor onset (Ilancheran et al., 1990; Liggins et al., 1980). However, prostaglandin levels are known to be high during and after labor.

Premonitory Signs of Labor

During the last few weeks of pregnancy, a number of changes indicate that labor is approaching (Box 21-1). **Premonitory signs** refer to symptoms experienced before the onset of true labor. Lightening occurs about 10 to 14 days before birth, particularly in primigravidas. This alteration is brought about by a settling of the fetal head into the pelvis. Lightening may take place suddenly so that the woman arises one morning entirely relieved of the abdominal tightness and diaphragmatic pressure that she had experienced previously. In multigravid women, lightening is more likely to occur after labor begins. Unfortunately, the relief in

---

BOX 21-1
Premonitory Signs of Labor

"Lightening" or descent of fetal head into pelvis
Braxton Hicks contractions
Cervical softening, effacement, and sometimes dilatation
Increased vaginal discharge
Show
Sciatic nerve pressure
Greater frequency of urination
Spurt of energy
Occasional rupture of the membranes

---

the upper abdomen is often followed by signs of greater pressure in the lower abdomen, such as shooting pains down the legs from pressure on the sciatic nerves, an increase in the amount of vaginal discharge, and greater frequency of urination due to pressure on the bladder.

Cervical changes, called "ripening," also occur before the onset of labor. The changes may include softening, effacement (shortening and thinning), and occasional dilation of the cervix to 1 to 2 cm. Weight loss, caused by hormone-induced electrolyte shifts, is common in the last days of pregnancy and may range from 0.5 to 1.5 kg (1–3 lb).

True Versus False Labor

False labor contractions may begin as early as 3 or 4 weeks before the actual delivery of the fetus. They are merely an exaggeration of the intermittent uterine contractions (Braxton Hicks) that have occurred throughout the entire gestation, but now they may be accompanied by discomfort. The differences between false and true labor are described in Table 21-1.

Restlessness and sleepless nights may result from the more intense uterine contractions, leading to increasing tension and fatigue. In some women, this is counterbalanced by the spurt of energy that occurs 1 to 2 days before labor begins.

Show

Another sign of impending labor is the pink vaginal discharge commonly termed "show." The mucous plug that has filled the cervical canal during pregnancy (and that contains accumulated cervical secretions) may be expelled when the cervix softens in the last days of pregnancy. The pressure of the descending presenting part of the fetus causes the minute capillaries in the cervix to rupture. This blood is mixed with the mucus,

TABLE 21–1
Differentiating Between True and False Labor

False Labor	True Labor
No or little change in cervix	Progressive cervical dilatation and effacement
Discomfort, usually in low abdomen and groin	Discomfort starting in back and sweeping around abdomen
Contractions occur at irregular intervals	Contractions occur at regular intervals
No increase in frequency and intensity of contractions	Progressive increase in frequency, intensity, and duration of contractions
Intervals between contractions remain long	Intervals between contractions gradually shorten
Walking has no intensifying effect on contractions, often gives relief	Contractions intensify by walking

creating a pink tinge. The "show" must be differentiated from a substantial discharge of blood, which may indicate an obstetric complication.

Rupture of the Membranes

Occasionally, rupture of the membranes is the first indication of approaching labor. After the membranes rupture, there is always the possibility of a prolapsed cord if the presenting part does not adequately fill the pelvic inlet. This is more likely if the fetus presents as a footling breech, by the shoulder, or in the vertex presentation but with the fetus not descended far enough into the true pelvis before the rupture of the membranes. Pregnant women should be advised to notify their prenatal healthcare provider when the membranes rupture to determine whether immediate hospitalization is necessary.

Four Stages of Labor

The process of labor is divided into four stages (Table 21-2).

- The **first stage of labor**, the dilating stage, begins with the onset of regular labor contractions and ends with the complete dilatation of the cervix. This stage may be subdivided into three phases: latent, active, and transition.
- The **second stage of labor**, the pelvic stage, begins with the complete dilatation of the cervix and ends with the delivery or birth of the newborn.

- The **third stage of labor**, the placental stage, begins with the birth of the newborn and terminates with the delivery of the placenta.
- The **fourth stage of labor**, the recovery stage, begins with the delivery of the placenta and extends to the first 1 to 4 hours postpartum.

Duration of Labor

Although there is some degree of variation, the average length of labor can be estimated based on studies of records of several thousand primigravidas and multiparas. In the classic study of labor duration, Friedman (1978) reviewed the time spent in the first and second stages of labor for a group of 500 women under normal conditions with good outcomes. The results of this study and others like it are summarized in Figure 21-1. The average duration of a primigravida's first labor is about 14 hours: approximately 13 hours in the first stage, 5 minutes to 1 hour in the second stage, and 10 minutes in the third stage. The average duration of multiparous labors is approximately 6 hours shorter than for first labors (7 hours and 20 minutes in the first stage, 15 to 30 minutes in the second stage, and 10 minutes in the third stage).

First Stage of Labor

During the first stage of labor, full dilatation of the cervix (10 cm) is slowly accomplished. The progress of cervical dilatation is more rapid in multiparas than primiparas (see Fig. 21-1). The first stage of labor is divided into the latent phase (prodromal labor), the active phase, and the transition phase. The **latent phase**, from the onset of uterine contractions, takes many hours and accomplishes cervical softening, effacement, and slight (3–4 cm) dilatation. With the beginning of the **active phase**, uterine contractions increase in intensity and duration and occur more frequently (every 3–5 minutes). This phase ends when cervical dilatation has reached approximately 7 cm. The **transition phase** is when the cervix is undergoing complete dilatation (8–10 cm) and is characterized by intense uterine contractions that occur every 2 to 3 minutes.

When cervical dilatation is 5 cm, the woman has progressed well beyond the halfway time point in labor, even though 10 cm represents full dilatation. At that point, the average labor is more than two-thirds over.

The active period begins with the *acceleration phase*, proceeds to the *phase of maximum slope*, and ends with the *deceleration phase* (see Fig. 21-1). In the active phase of labor, the nulliparous woman's cervix should dilate at least 1.2 cm/h, and the multiparous woman's cervix should dilate at least 1.5 cm/h.

TABLE 21-2
Summary of Stages of Labor

Stage	Definition	Duration	Uterine Activity	Maternal Behavior and Manifestations
First stage (dilating stage)	Period from first true labor contractions to complete cervical dilatation	Varies with phase and parity		
Latent phase	Begins at true labor onset and ends with onset of active labor; 0→3–4 cm	Approximately 8.6 h for the nullipara and 5.3 h for the multipara	Mild, often irregular contractions 5–30 min apart, 10–30 s duration; cervix becomes softer and thinner, 0 to 3–4 cm dilatation	Laboring woman is generally excited, alert, talkative or quiet, calm, or anxious; may experience abdominal cramps, backache, rupture of membranes, pain controlled fairly well, may ambulate
Active phase	Begins with onset of active labor and progresses into transition; 4–7 cm	Approximately 4.6 h for the nullipara and 2.4 h for the multipara	Moderate to strong uterine contractions every 2–5 min; 30–90 s duration; cervical dilatation for nulliparas of 1.2 cm/h and for the multipara, 1.5 cm/h true for transition also	Laboring woman generally feels increasing discomfort, perspiring, nausea and vomiting, flushed; experiences trembling of thighs and legs, pressure on bladder and rectum, backache, circumoral pallor, amnesia between contractions; transition may be more apprehensive, fear losing control, self-focused; may become irritable, urge to push, rectal pressure
Transition phase	8–10 cm dilatation	*		
Second stage (pelvic stage)	Period from complete cervical dilatation to delivery of newborn	Approximately 1 h for the nullipara and ¼–½ h for the multipara	Strong uterine contractions every 2–3 min, 45–90 sec duration; intra-abdominal pressure is exerted	May experience decreased pain, pressure on rectum, bulging perineum, urge to bear down, often excited and eager, grunting sounds or expiratory vocalization
Third stage (placental stage)	Period from delivery of newborn to delivery of placenta and membranes	5–30 min	Strong uterine contractions; uterus changing to globular shape; intra-abdominal pressure exerted	Focus on newborn, excited about birth, feeling of relief
Fourth stage	Period from delivery of placenta and membranes to first 4 hours postpartum	4 h	Uterus firm at level of two fingerbreadths above umbilicus	Exploration of newborn; family integration begins; newborn alert and responsive

*Transition is not seen as a separate phase of labor in the medical model.

Two important changes occur in the cervix during the first stage of labor: effacement and dilatation.

Cervical Effacement

Cervical effacement is the thinning and shortening of the cervical canal from a structure 2 to 3 cm in length and about 1 cm thick to one in which no canal at all exists, except a circular orifice with almost paper-thin edges. The edges of the internal os are drawn several centimeters upward, so that the former endocervical canal becomes part of the lower uterine segment (Fig. 21-2). In primigravidas, effacement is often complete before dilatation begins, but in multiparas it is rarely complete; dilatation proceeds with rather thick cervical edges.

The terms *obliteration* and *taking up* of the cervix are synonymous with effacement. Effacement is mea-

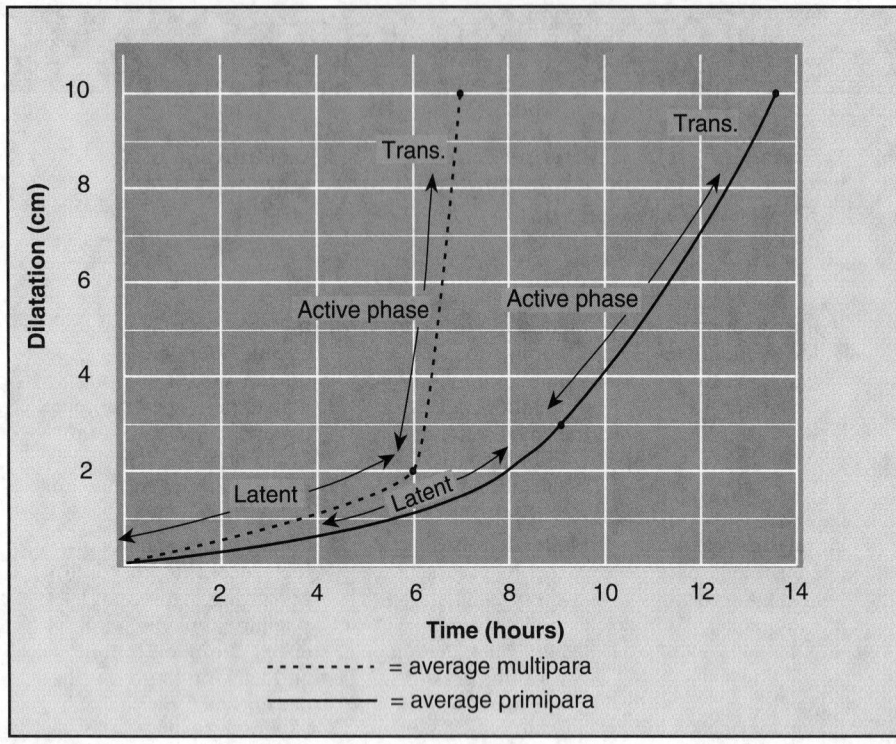

FIGURE 21–1 Composite of the average dilatation curve for nulliparous and multiparous labor. The first stage is divided into a relatively flat latent phase and a rapidly progressive active phase. The active phase has three identifiable component parts: an acceleration phase, a linear phase of maximum slope, and a deceleration phase.

sured during pelvic examination by estimating the percentage by which the cervical canal has shortened. For example, in a cervix 2 cm long before labor, 50% effacement has occurred when the cervix measures 1 cm in length.

Dilatation of the Cervix

Cervical dilatation is enlargement of the cervical os from an orifice a few millimeters in size to an aperture large enough to permit the passage of the fetus (ie, a diameter of about 10 cm). When the cervix can no longer be felt, dilatation is said to be complete.

Although the forces concerned in dilatation are not well understood, several factors appear to be involved. The muscle fibers around the cervix are so arranged that they pull on its edges and draw it open. Mechanical stretching of the cervix intensifies uterine activity (*Ferguson's reflex*). Release of endogenous oxytocin may mediate this process. The uterine contractions cause pressure on the amniotic sac, and this burrows into the cervix in a pouchlike fashion, exerting a dilating action (see Fig. 21-2). In the absence of the membranes, the pressure of the presenting part against the cervix and the lower uterine segment has a similar effect.

Measurement of cervical dilatation in centimeters is done during pelvic examination through digital estimation of the diameter of the cervical opening. Because dilatation of the cervix in the first stage of labor is solely the result of involuntary uterine contractions, the

process cannot be expedited through maternal efforts, such as bearing down. The woman should be discouraged from bearing down until the cervix is dilated 10 cm because the process may exhaust her and cause the cervix to become edematous.

Influence of Catecholamines

During labor, stress hormones known as catecholamines (ie, epinephrine [adrenaline] and norepinephrine [noradrenaline]) are produced in the brain, nerve endings, adrenal medulla, and other body organs. In several classic studies, researchers demonstrated that women in early labor produce catecholamines at their usual prelabor level if they are relatively free of anxiety (Lederman et al., 1978; Sosa et al., 1980; Simkin, 1986a). As labor advances, catecholamine levels are likely to rise in response to increasing stress, pain, or intrapartum complications (Simkin, 1986a). Normal catecholamine production in the laboring woman is beneficial because it prepares the body for action and expenditure of energy; however, excessive amounts may have deleterious effects on labor and the fetus. These include decreased efficiency of uterine contractions, longer labor, and shunting of blood away from the uterus and placenta (Simkin, 1986a; Lederman et al., 1979).

The fetus also produces increasing amounts of catecholamines (predominantly norepinephrine) in response to the stress of normal labor and the temporary hypoxia caused by normal contractions. Production of

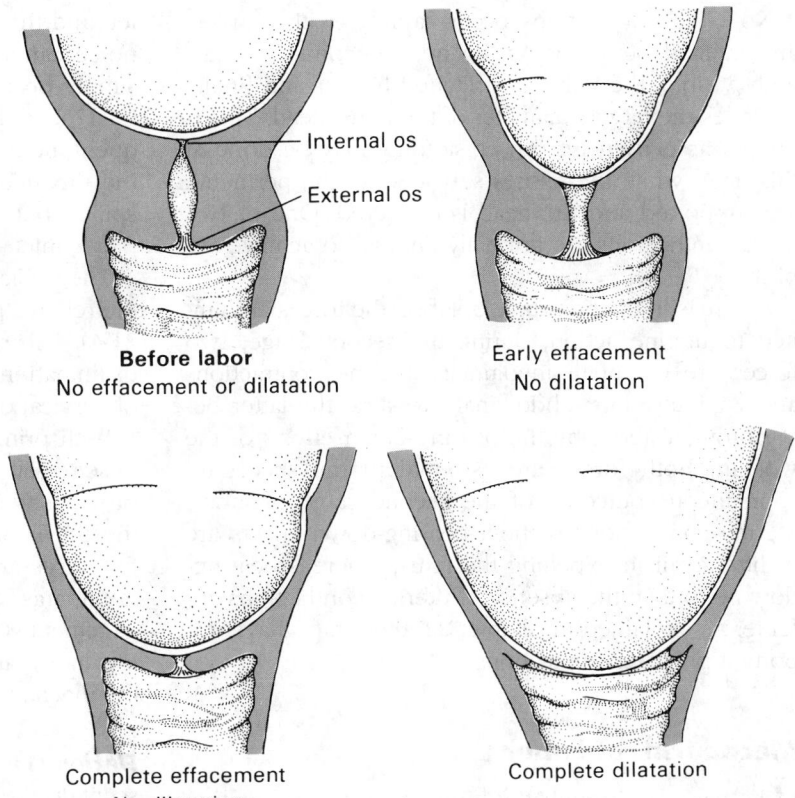

Internal os

External os

Before labor
No effacement or dilatation

Early effacement
No dilatation

FIGURE 21–2 Stages in cervical effacement and dilatation.

Complete effacement
No dilatation

Complete dilatation

fetal catecholamines causes more blood to shunt to vital organs, increases oxygen uptake, and helps to prevent fetal hypoglycemia (Lagercrantz et al., 1985; Phillippe, 1983; Fox, 1979). A drop in fetal heart rate (FHR) assists in oxygen conservation. The result of these processes is that the fetus is able to obtain as much oxygen as before labor even though there is less oxygenated blood available during contractions (Simkin, 1986a).

Maternal disorders of the prenatal or intrapartum period (see Chaps. 31, 32, and 36) may cause catecholamine production by the fetus to exceed physiologic bounds. This can lead to problems in the newborn, such as respiratory distress, cold stress, metabolic acidosis, and hyperbilirubinemia (Simkin, 1986).

Second Stage of Labor

During the second stage of labor, the contractions increase in intensity, last 50 to 70 seconds, and occur at intervals of 2 or 3 minutes. If they have not already ruptured, the membranes often do so during the early part of this stage, with a gush of amniotic fluid from the vagina. In rare cases, the newborn is born in a *caul*, which is a piece of the amniotic membrane that envelops the newborn's head.

As the fetal head or presenting part descends and reaches the perineal floor, pressure of the presenting part on the sacral and obturator nerves causes the woman to feel the urge to push, and the muscles of the abdomen are brought into play. With contractions in progress, the woman strains or "bears down" with all her strength so that her face becomes flushed and the large vessels in her neck become distended. As a result of this exertion, she may perspire profusely. During this stage, the woman directs all her energy toward giving birth. There is a marked pressure in the area of the perineum and rectum, and the urge to bear down is usually beyond her control. When the fetal presenting part distends the pelvic floor, stretch receptors trigger the release of endogenous oxytocin. Thus, the urge to push is more influenced by the fetal station than by cervical dilatation (Cosner et al., 1993).

Toward the end of the second stage, the pressure of the fetal head well down in the vagina causes the anus to become patulous and everted, and often small particles of fecal material may be expelled from the rectum with each contraction. As the head descends further, the perineal region begins to bulge, and the perineal skin becomes tense and glistening. At this time, the scalp of the fetus may be detected through a slitlike vulvar opening. With each subsequent contraction, the perineum bulges more, and the vulva becomes more dilated and distended by the head; the opening is gradually converted into an ovoid and at last into a circle. With the cessation of each contraction, the opening becomes smaller, and the head recedes from it until it advances again with the next contraction.

Now the contractions occur rapidly, with scarcely any interval between. As the head becomes increasingly visible, the vulva is stretched further and finally encircles the largest diameter of the fetus' head. This is known as **crowning**. An episiotomy may be done at this time, while the tissues surrounding the perineum are supported and the head is delivered. One or two more contractions are normally enough to achieve the birth.

Whereas in the first stage of labor, the forces are limited to uterine action, during the second stage, two forces are essential: involuntary uterine contractions and voluntary intra-abdominal pressure, the latter being brought about by the bearing-down efforts of the woman. Both forces are essential to the successful spontaneous outcome of the second stage of labor; uterine contractions without bearing-down efforts are of little avail in expelling the fetus, whereas bearing-down efforts in the absence of uterine contractions are futile. As explained in Chapter 22, these facts have important practical implications.

Mechanism of Labor

In its passage through the birth canal, the presenting part of the fetus undergoes certain positional changes, called **cardinal movements**, that constitute the mechanism of labor. These movements are designed to adapt the smallest possible diameters of the presenting part to the contours and varying diameters of the pelvic canal so that it encounters as little resistance as possible.

The mechanism of labor consists of a combination of movements, several of which may occur at the same time. As they occur, the uterine contractions bring about important modifications in the attitude of the fetus, especially after the head has descended into the pelvis. This adaptation of the fetus to the birth canal involves the following movements: descent, flexion, internal rotation, extension, external rotation (restitution), and expulsion (Fig. 21-3).

For purposes of instruction, the various movements are described as if they occurred independently.

Descent. The first requisite for the birth is **descent**. When the fetal head has descended so that its greatest biparietal diameter is at or has passed the pelvic inlet, the head is said to be **engaged**. This provides a clear indication that the pelvic inlet is large enough to accommodate the widest portion of the fetal head and is of adequate size. For the average fetal head, the linear distance between the occiput and the plane of the biparietal diameter is less than the distance between the pelvic inlet and the ischial spines. Thus, when the occiput is at the level of the ischial spines, its biparietal diameter has usually passed the pelvic in-

let, and the vertex is therefore engaged. However, the nurse cannot assume that **engagement** has occurred simply because the vertex is at the spines. When the fetal head has been molded markedly, with consequent increase in the distance between the occiput and the biparietal diameter, the vertex may be felt at the spines, but its greatest diameter may still be above the pelvic inlet.

The ischial spines are used as a landmark to describe the relative position of the fetal head in the pelvis (Fig. 21-4). This relationship is evaluated during each pelvic examination and recorded, along with the assessment of cervical dilatation and effacement.

With primigravidas, engagement often precedes the onset of labor. This is called **lightening**, as described previously. Because the vertex is frequently deep in the pelvis at the onset of labor, further descent does not necessarily begin until the second stage of labor. In multiparas, however, descent often begins with engagement. Once having been inaugurated, descent is inevitably associated with the various movements of the mechanism of labor.

Flexion. **Flexion** occurs early in the process of descent, as the head meets resistance from the soft tissues of the pelvis, the pelvic floor, and the cervix. The head may become so flexed that the chin is in contact with the sternum; as a consequence, the smallest anteroposterior diameter (the suboccipitobregmatic plane) is presented to the pelvis.

Internal Rotation. The head enters the pelvis in the transverse or diagonal position. When it reaches the pelvic floor, the occiput is rotated and lies beneath the symphysis pubis. In other words, with **internal rotation**, the sagittal suture is in the anteroposterior diameter of the outlet. Although the occiput usually rotates to the front, occasionally it may turn toward the hollow of the sacrum. If anterior rotation does not take place, the occiput usually rotates to the direct occipitoposterior position, a condition known as persistent occipitoposterior. Because this represents a deviation from the normal mechanism of labor, it is discussed in Chapter 36.

Extension. After the occiput emerges from the pelvis, the nape of the neck becomes arrested beneath the pubic arch and is a pivotal point for the rest of the head. **Extension** of the head ensues, and the frontal portion of the head, the face, and the chin are born.

External Rotation. After the birth of the head, it remains in the anteroposterior position only a short time, then turns to one or another side of its own accord in a process called *restitution*. When the occiput originally was directed toward the left of the woman's pelvis, it

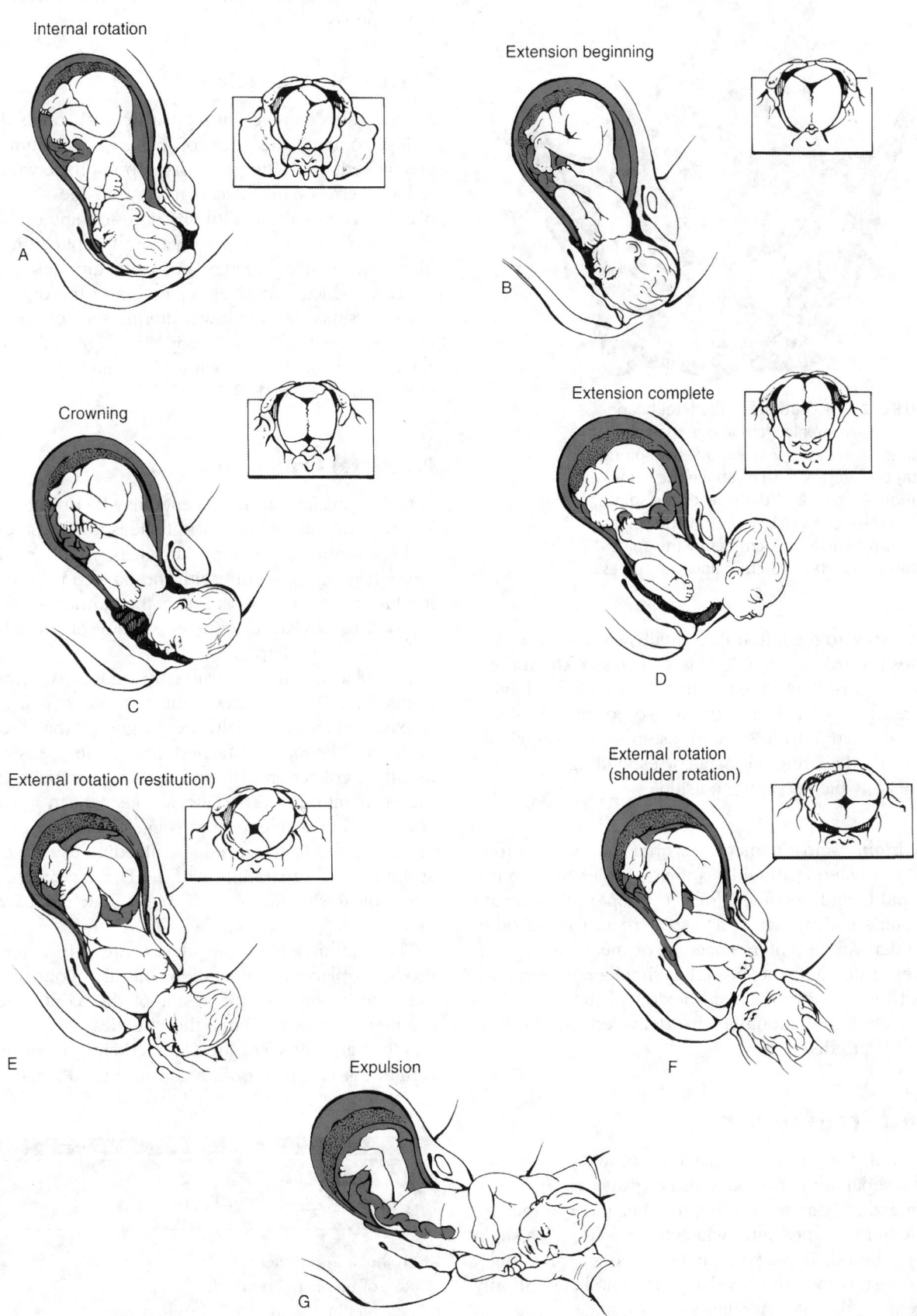

FIGURE 21–3 Mechanism of delivery for a vertex presentation.

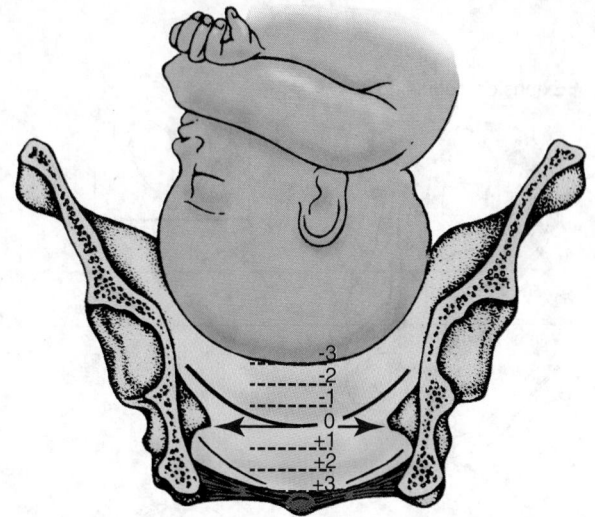

FIGURE 21–4 Stations of the fetal head:
–3 station—vertex is 3 cm above the spines.
–2 station—vertex is 2 cm above the spines.
–1 station—vertex is 1 cm above the spines.
0 station—vertex is at the level of the spines.
+1 station—vertex is 1 cm below the spines.
+2 station—vertex is 2 cm below the spines.
+3 station—vertex is 3 cm below the spines.

rotates toward the left. If it originally was to the right, it rotates toward the right. This is known as **external rotation** and is due to the fact that the shoulders, having entered the pelvis in the transverse position, undergo internal rotation to the anteroposterior position, as did the head. This brings about a corresponding rotation of the head, which is on the outside.

Expulsion. Almost immediately after the external rotation, the anterior shoulder appears under the symphysis pubis and becomes arrested temporarily beneath the pubic arch to act as a pivotal point for the other shoulder. As the anterior margin of the perineum becomes distended, the posterior shoulder is born, assisted by an upward lateral flexion of the newborn's body. Once the shoulders are delivered, the body is quickly extruded.

Third Stage of Labor

The third stage of labor is made up of two phases, placental separation and **placental expulsion**.

Immediately after the birth, the remainder of the amniotic fluid escapes, after which there is usually a slight flow of blood. The uterus can be felt as a firm globular mass just below the level of the umbilicus. Shortly thereafter, the uterus relaxes and assumes a discoid shape. With each subsequent contraction or relaxation, the uterine shape changes from globular to discoid un-

til the placenta has separated, after which the globular shape persists.

Placental Separation

As the uterus contracts at regular intervals on its diminishing content, the area of placental attachment is greatly reduced. The great disproportion between the reduced size of the placental site and the size of the placenta brings about a folding or festooning of the maternal surface of the placenta, and separation takes place. Meanwhile, bleeding occurs within these placental folds, which expedites separation of the organ. The placenta sinks into the lower uterine segment or upper vagina as an unattached body. The signs of placental separation usually occur within 5 minutes after the birth of the infant (Box 21-2).

Placental Expulsion

Actual expulsion of the placenta may be brought about by the woman bearing down if she is not anesthetized. If this cannot be accomplished, it is usually achieved through gentle pressure with the hand on the uterine fundus. Excessive pressure on the fundus should be avoided to obviate the rare possibility of inversion of the uterus (see Chap. 36).

The placenta may extrude by one of two mechanisms (Fig. 21-5). Schultze's mechanism, evident in approximately 80% of deliveries, signifies that the placenta has become detached first at its center, and usually a collection of blood and clots is found in the sac of membranes. The Duncan mechanism is seen in about 20% of deliveries and suggests that the placenta has separated first at its edges. Bleeding usually occurs at the time of separation with the Duncan mechanism. No clinical significance has been attached to either mechanism.

The contraction of the uterus after birth not only produces placental separation, but also controls uterine hemorrhage. As the result of this contraction of the uterine muscle fibers, the countless blood vessels within their interstices are clamped shut. Even then, a certain amount of blood loss in the third stage is un-

BOX 21–2
Signs of Placental Separation

Globular and firmer uterus
Rise of uterus in abdomen
Lengthening of umbilical cord into vagina
Sudden gush of blood

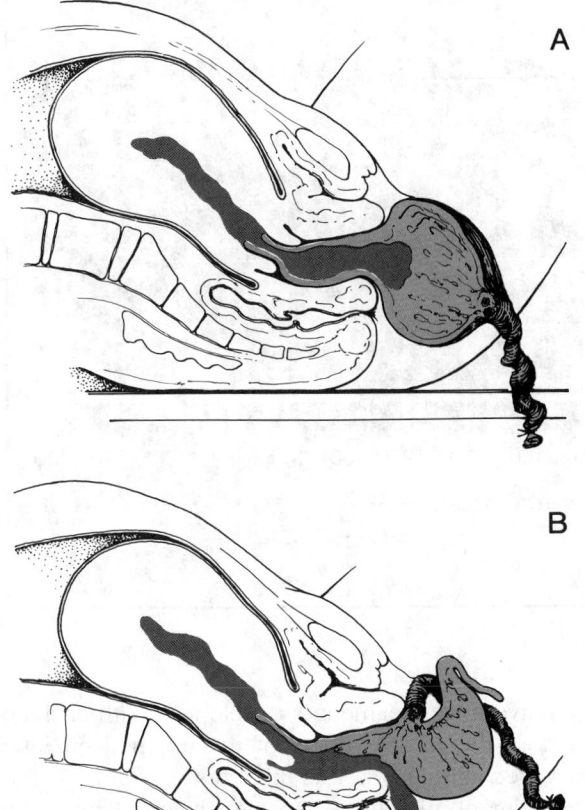

FIGURE 21-5 Expulsion of the placenta by (**A**) Schultze's mechanism, whereby the placenta is turned inside out within the vagina and is delivered with the glistening fetal surfaces to the outside, and by (**B**) the Duncan mechanism, whereby the placenta is rolled up in the vagina and is delivered with the maternal surface to the outside.

avoidable, commonly amounting to about 500 mL or less. One of the goals of labor management is to keep this bleeding to a minimum.

Fourth Stage of Labor

The first 4 hours postpartum, sometimes referred to as the fourth stage of labor, is the time that physiologic stability is restored. During this period, myometrial contraction and retraction, accompanied by vessel thrombosis, operate effectively to control bleeding from the placental site. However, potential risks exist for hemorrhage, urinary retention, hypotension, and side effects of anesthesia.

This period also is important for initial formation of the mother–newborn relationship and consolidation of the family unit. Early parental interactions with the newborn and each other are believed to affect the quality of their subsequent relationships (see Chap. 22).

The Powers of Labor

Recall from Chapter 20 that the powers of labor provide the force for expulsion of the fetus and placenta from the uterus. Primary and secondary powers work together in this effort. The **primary powers** consist of involuntary uterine contractions that provide the force in the first stage of labor. The **secondary powers** are maternal pushing efforts that augment the involuntary contractions in a coordinated effort. These voluntary efforts come in response to the urge to push and are generally effective only in the second stage of labor. In the first stage of labor, pushing efforts can be counterproductive to cervical dilatation.

Uterine Contractions

To expel the fetus, the uterus goes through a series of contractions (the intermittent shortening of a muscle). Each contraction includes three phases: a period when the intensity of the contraction increases (**increment**), a period when the contraction is at its height (**acme**), and a period of diminishing intensity (**decrement**). Figure 21-6 illustrates these phases and the key characteristics of contractions. The **duration** of contractions normally ranges from 30 to 90 seconds, averaging about 1 minute. The strength, or **intensity**, of the contraction is measured in mm Hg. Normal spontaneous contractions often exert pressures of about 60 mm Hg; however, they may vary between 20 and 75 mm Hg. Cervical dilatation most likely will not occur with pressures of less than 25 mm Hg above resting tone (see Fig. 21-6; Berg et al., 1992).

The contractions of the uterus during labor are intermittent, with periods of relaxation between, resembling the systole and the diastole of the heart. **Frequency** refers to the time between the beginning of one contraction to the beginning of the next. The interval between contractions, often called the resting phase, diminishes gradually from about 10 minutes early in labor to about 2 or 3 minutes in the second stage. These periods of relaxation not only provide rest for the uterine muscles and for the mother, but also are essential to the welfare of the fetus. During the myometrial relaxation that follows the contraction in normal labor, there is a rebound phenomenon during which the uteroplacental blood flow increases above the control levels. Thus, the transfer of oxygen and other essential nutrients to the fetus is not significantly compromised. When contractions consistently last longer than 90 seconds (tetanic) or occur more frequently than every 2 minutes, placental function may be disrupted, resulting in a decrease in fetal oxygenation and presenting potential danger to the fetus from intrauterine hypoxia.

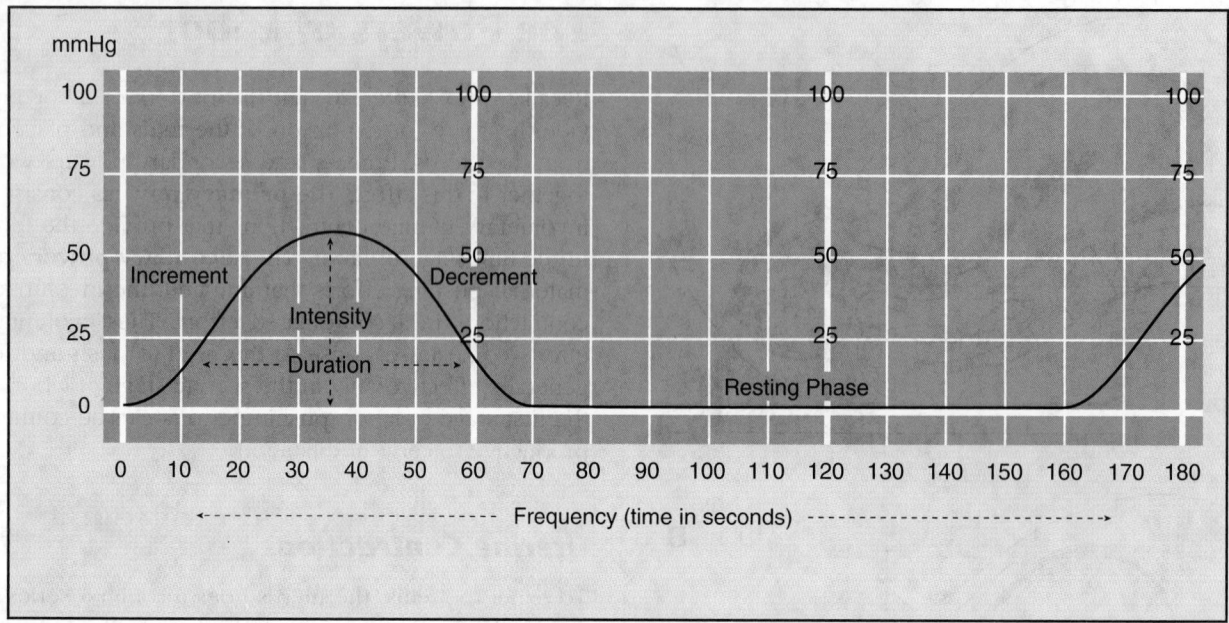

FIGURE 21-6 Phases and characteristics of uterine contractions.

Labor contractions are involuntary; their action is independent of the woman's will and of extrauterine nervous control. The myometrium contracts by the sliding of actin and myosin filaments and requires adenosine triphosphate and calcium (Hacker et al., 1992). Estrogen promotes the growth of actin and myosin until by full term, the myometrial cells have adequate actomyosin to accomplish the work of labor. The smooth muscle contraction of the uterus is triggered primarily by hormonal stimuli and does not require the innervation needed for skeletal muscle contraction. Receptors for oxytocin and prostaglandins are found in the myometrial cell membrane. The efficiency of uterine contractions is facilitated by the existence of cell-to-cell contacts, known as *gap junctions* in myometrial tissue, which promote synchronous contractions of smooth muscle cells. During labor, the gap junctions increase in number and size. Prostaglandins assume a key regulatory role; PGE_2 and PGF_2 are powerful stimuli of myometrial contractions. These hormones cause the rapid appearance of myometrial gap junctions and induce the maturational changes of cervical ripening (Cunningham et al., 1993). Effective uterine contractions also depend on adequate cellular electrolyte exchange of calcium, sodium, and potassium.

During labor, the uterus is differentiated into two identifiable portions, the upper and lower uterine segments. The upper segment, known as the **fundus**, contains the greatest concentration of myometrial cells and is the active, contractile portion of the uterus. Its function is to expel the uterine contents. The uterus displays a decreasing gradient of intensity of contractions from the fundus downward. As labor progresses,

a passive lower segment is developed. With each contraction, the muscle fibers of the upper segment retract, becoming shorter as the fetus descends. The upper segment, therefore, becomes thicker. Fibers of the lower segment stretch, and consequently it becomes thinner. The distinct boundary between the upper and lower uterine segments is called a **physiologic retraction ring**.

The degree of discomfort experienced during labor varies considerably among individuals. The woman who anticipates a painful experience generally has more discomfort than the woman who is prepared for what can be a positive experience. To allay preexisting fear, the nurse should refer to uterine contractions as contractions, not *pains*.

Maternal Pushing

After the cervix is dilated fully, the power most important in expulsion of the fetus is the secondary power produced by increased intra-abdonimal pressure as the woman pushes or bears down. Most women experience an overwhelming urge to push when the fetal head or presenting part reaches the pelvic floor and full cervical dilatation is achieved. Increased abdominal pressure is created by deep inhalation, then purposefully contracting the abdominal muscles with the glottis closed. Bearing down efforts should coincide with uterine contractions, and the woman should be encourage to rest between contractions. Although pushing is a necessary complement to uterine contractions in the second stage of labor, it accomplishes little in the first stage and may cause cervical edema. In the third stage of labor, spontaneous expulsion of the placenta is again aided by the woman's bearing-down efforts.

Maternal Responses to Labor and Birth

The process of labor and birth is associated with a number of physiologic and psychological changes in the childbearing woman. These changes vary considerably according to the duration and intensity of the labor, the amount of panting by the woman, room temperature, and fluid replacement. Preparation for childbirth may positively influence maternal responses by decreasing anxiety and improving maternal work efforts (see Chap. 19).

Physiologic Responses

Cardiovascular

During labor, cardiac output increases by 40% to 50% compared with prelabor levels and by about 80% to 100% compared with prepregnancy levels (Hacker et al., 1992). This increase in cardiac output is due to catecholamine release brought about by pain and to abdominal and uterine muscle contraction. With the contraction of the uterus, approximately 300 to 500 mL of blood is shifted to the central blood volume (Sullivan et al., 1985). In a classic study, Hendrick and Quilligan (1956) demonstrated that pain and anxiety alone can increase cardiac output by 50% to 60%. Because uterine contractions can cause significant compression of the aorta and iliac arteries, much of the increase in cardiac output is distributed to the upper extremities and head (Gabbe et al., 1991). With each uterine contraction, the blood flow in the branches of the uterine artery that supply the intervillous space decreases roughly in proportion to the magnitude of the contraction. This decrease is not related to significant alteration in the systemic perfusing pressure, but rather to a localized increase in the vascular resistance within the uterus (Assali, 1989). Systemic venous pressure increases as blood is returned from the engorged uterine veins. In the first stage, there is an average rise of 10 mm Hg systolic and 5 to 10 mm Hg diastolic during contractions but little change between contractions; in the second stage, there is a rise of 30/25 mm Hg during contractions and 10/5 to 10 mm Hg between contractions (Beischer et al., 1986). If the woman is pushing strongly, there is a compensatory and often dramatic fall in blood pressure as bearing down stops at the end of the contraction. Other changes in labor include a slow but steady rise in pulse rate to about 100 beats/min by the second stage of labor. Pulse rate may be further increased by dehydration, hemorrhage, anxiety, pain, and certain drugs (eg, terbutaline).

Because of the cardiovascular changes that occur during uterine contractions, the most accurate period for assessment of maternal vital signs is between contractions. Positioning has a great effect on cardiac output. Turning the laboring woman from side to back is associated with a 25% to 30% decrease in cardiac output.

Respiratory

In labor, women exhale more CO_2 with each breath. During strong uterine contractions, rate and depth of respirations are increased in response to the greater demand for oxygen arising from the higher metabolic rate. The mean $PaCO_2$ falls from 32 mm Hg at the start of labor to 22 mm Hg at the end of the first stage (Beischer et al., 1986). Maternal breath holding associated with pushing during the second stage of labor may result in less CO_2 being expired. A common problem is maternal *hyperventilation*, causing the $PaCO_2$ levels to fall below 16 to 18 mm Hg (Beischer et al., 1986). This condition may be manifested by tingling of the hands and feet, numbness, and dizziness. If shallow breathing is excessive, the opposite situation may result because the tidal volume is low. Excessive or prolonged maternal pushing during the second stage can similarly cause a drop in oxygen secondary to breath holding.

Gastrointestinal

Gastrointestinal motility and absorption are reduced during active labor, and stomach emptying time is delayed. These effects may be exaggerated after narcotic administration. Many women experience nausea and vomiting as labor progresses, particularly during the transition phase of the first stage of labor. Other discomforts may include dehydration and dry lips and mouth that result from mouth breathing. Because of the risks of vomiting and nausea, many birthing facilities restrict oral intake during labor. Ice chips are commonly provided to laboring women to relieve discomforts from dry lips and mouth. Some facilities allow clear liquids, juices, and ice pops. Many facilities maintain fluid intake per the intravenous route.

Renal

Laboring women may be unaware that their bladder is full due to the intensity of uterine contractions and pressure of the presenting part or the effects of regional anesthesia. However, a full bladder may restrain fetal descent and can lead to trauma of the bladder mucosa during the birth process. Prevention (by reminding the woman to void during a lengthy first stage) is crucial.

Renal system adaptations also include diaphoresis and increased insensible water loss through respirations.

Hematopoietic

Vaginal delivery of a full-term newborn results in a mean blood loss of 500 mL, whereas an uncomplicated cesarean birth results in a mean maternal blood loss of 1,000 mL. The hypervolemia of pregnancy helps to compensate for this blood loss. During labor, blood coagulation time deceases slightly, but plasma fibrinogen levels are elevated. Leukocyte count normally increases as labor progresses.

Fluid and Electrolyte

The plasma levels of sodium and chloride may decrease as a result of reduced gastrointestinal absorption, panting, and diaphoresis (perspiration) during labor and birth. Polyuria (frequent urination) is common. Reduced intake of oral fluids due to nausea and vomiting, discomfort, and the administration of analgesics or anesthesia may further change fluid and electrolyte balance.

Pain

The pain associated with labor and birth is part of the normal physiologic response to several factors. During the first stage of labor, pain is primarily caused by dilatation of the cervix and distension of the lower uterine segment. Pain during the second stage of labor is mainly caused by distension and possible disruption of the lower vagina and perineum. Perception of pain is influenced by a variety of factors. Pain mechanisms and methods for relieving pain are discussed in detail in Chapter 23. Pain and discomfort also vary a great deal from woman to woman. However, a pattern of responses is common to each phase and stage, as described below.

At the beginning of the first stage, during the latest phase, the contractions are short, slight, 5 to 10 minutes or more apart, and lasting 20 to 30 seconds. The woman may not experience any particular discomfort and may be walking around comfortably between contractions. Early in the first stage, the sensation is usually located in the small of the back, but as time goes on, it sweeps around, girdle-like, to the anterior part of the abdomen. The contractions recur at shortening intervals, every 3 to 5 minutes, becoming stronger and lasting longer.

When labor has progressed to the active phase, the woman often prefers to remain in bed; ambulation may no longer be comfortable. She becomes intensely involved in the sensations within her body and tends to withdraw from the surrounding environment. The duration of each contraction ranges from 30 to 90 seconds, averaging about 1 minute.

As cervical dilatation progresses to 8 to 9 cm, the contractions reach peak intensity, and the woman enters the transition phase. Transition is usually short, but it also often is the most difficult and painful time for the woman due to frequent (every 2–3 minutes) and lengthy (often lasting 90 seconds) contractions. The woman may become irritable and lose control. There is usually a marked increase in the amount of show due to rupture of capillary vessels in the cervix and the lower uterine segment.

Psychological State (The Psyche)

Psychological responses to the experience of labor vary widely and are influenced by a number of factors. Of particular importance is the woman's cultural background. People from diverse cultural backgrounds may differ in their beliefs about how the laboring woman should behave, the presence of support people, and the nurse's role. For example, in the orthodox Jewish faith, religious scriptures require modesty, such that even the husband may be prohibited from observing his wife when she is immodestly exposed (Lutwak et al., 1988). Within other cultures, the use of touch may be an issue of concern. The findings from a recent qualitative study (Khazoyan et al., 1994) revealed that adult Latina women desire their partners to be with them throughout labor and delivery, to show "love," and to demonstrate understanding and patience.

Preparation for childbirth often varies and may dramatically influence the coping skills of the laboring woman and her partner (see Chap. 19). In a classic study, Mercer, Hackley, and Bostrom (1983) found that the mate's emotional support during childbirth was a major predictor of positive perceptions of the experience. Maternal confidence in coping with labor has been found to contribute to women's perception of pain during labor (Lowe, 1991). Similarly, expectations may influence psychological responses to labor. Heaman, Beaton, Gupton, and Sloan (1992) observed that high-risk pregnant women expected more medical interventions and more difficulty coping with pain during their labor and birth than low-risk pregnant women. For both groups of women, anxiety was negatively associated with childbirth expectations.

In a well known series of classic studies, Lederman et al. (1978, 1979) investigated the relationship between psychological factors in pregnancy and labor variables, such as plasma epinephrine and progress in labor. Anxiety in labor and plasma epinephrine were related to FHR pattern in active labor (Lederman et al., 1981). Duration of labor was related to plasma epinephrine and norepinephrine levels in multiparas; longer labors were associated with higher catecholamines, which were related to measures of patient anxiety (Lederman et al., 1985). Other researchers have similarly found that women who experienced extreme pain or distress may be more likely to experience an inefficient labor (Wuitchik et al., 1989).

Fetal Responses to Labor and Birth

The experience of labor and birth leads to several changes in fetal position, attitude, and compression of the presenting part; these adaptations are discussed in Chapter 20. Additional physiologic adaptations are described in the following section.

Cardiovascular System

The FHR is regulated by the interplay of the sympathetic and parasympathetic divisions of the autonomic nervous system and chemoreceptors and baroreceptors. The normal range of FHR is between 120 and 160 beats/min during labor. The FHR rhythm is fairly stable, and variability fluctuates 5 to 10 beats/min. Beat-to-beat changes (short-term variability) are mediated through the vagal reflex (parasympathetic nervous system). When the vagal reflex is stimulated, the FHR declines; when the sympathetic nervous system is stimulated, the FHR increases. The autonomic nervous system receives information on oxygen status from the chemoreceptors (sensory nerve cells in the aortic arch, carotid bodies, and brain), which can trigger the sympathetic nervous system to increase FHR to improve perfusion to the affected area. The baroreceptors (pressure-sensitive nerve endings in the walls of the internal and external carotid arteries) provide input on blood pressure. A rise in blood pressure causes the baroreceptors to signal the parasympathetic nervous system to decrease cardiac output and blood pressure rapidly, thereby slowing the FHR.

During uterine contractions, FHR usually does not change significantly if placental function is adequate. Blood flow to the intervillous spaces ceases when uterine tension reaches 50 mm Hg pressure. The healthy fetus is able to rely on oxygen reserves in the intervillous space under normal circumstances. FHR may drop during a contraction if there is cord compression, stretching, or pressure on the fetal head (causing stimulation of the vagus nerve and decreased cerebral blood flow). If uteroplacental function is inadequate, the FHR may drop after the onset of the contraction and not return to baseline until after the contraction is finished (late deceleration). Mild hypoxia causes an increase in FHR; however, with more severe hypoxia, the FHR decreases.

Acid–Base Balance

Normal values for fetal serum pH range between 7.25 and 7.35 during labor. As birth approaches, there is a slow fall in pH, largely because uterine contractions inhibit placental exchange, but partly because the pH of the woman also falls at this time (Beischer et al., 1986). Maternal pushing in the second stage of labor may further decrease pH by causing a mild hypoxia. Fetal pH values between 7.20 and 7.25, obtained by scalp samples, are considered preacidotic, and values below 7.20 are considered frank acidosis. The normal pCO_2 is usually in the 40 to 50 mm Hg range. Research findings suggest that fetuses demonstrating FHR accelerations in response to scalp sampling or to sound stimulation have a pH above 7.20 (Clark et al., 1982; Rice et al., 1986; Smith et al., 1986).

Breathing and Movement

During labor, there is a sharp decrease in the time spent by the fetus in breathing activity (30%–40% to about 1%; Beischer et al., 1986). Movement of the trunk is basically unchanged but may decrease when the membranes rupture. Sleep–wake cycles continue to occur, even as labor progresses. During the quiet sleep state, FHR variability and fetal breathing movements decrease.

Nursing Management During Labor and Birth

The nursing management in relation to labor and birth is briefly introduced. A more detailed presentation of the dimensions of effective nursing care and applications of the nursing process is presented in Chapter 22. Nursing interventions related to labor and birth include the following:

- Anticipatory guidance and education of the pregnant woman and her family about the process of labor and delivery
- Instruction on how to differentiate signs of true versus false labor
- Ongoing assessment during the intrapartum period for changes in cervical effacement, dilatation, and station of the fetus
- Ongoing assessment and appropriate interventions to ensure the safety of mother and newborn
- Explanation about the physiologic changes occurring during labor to alleviate anxiety and help the woman and her support person gain control over the experience
- Administration of appropriate pharmacologic and nonpharmacologic interventions to relieve pain

- Education and support to correct inappropriate breathing patterns that result in hyperventilation or breath holding during pushing
- Provision of information to the laboring woman and her support person about labor progress, procedures, and medications
- Administration of comfort measures and assistance with personal hygiene

Summary Points

✔ Several maternal and fetal mechanisms have been proposed as key factors in initiating the onset of labor (parturition) and to support the labor process. The theories proposed relate to estrogen and progesterone balance, oxytocin stimulation, prostaglandin activity, and fetal endocrine control.

✔ Premonitory signs of labor include lightening or descent of the fetal head into the pelvis; Braxton Hicks contractions; increased vaginal discharge; cervical softening, effacement, and sometimes dilatation; show; greater frequency of urination; and occasional rupture of the membranes.

✔ True labor is distinguished from false labor (exaggerated Braxton Hicks contractions) by the presence of regular uterine contractions leading to progressive cervical dilatation and effacement. The intervals between contractions shorten as labor progresses.

✔ Labor is divided into four stages: The first stage extends from the time of onset of true labor to complete cervical dilation (10 cm) and consists of three phases: latent, active, and transition. The second stage spans from complete dilatation of the cervix to birth. The third stage extends from birth to expulsion of the placenta. The fourth stage includes the first 4 hours postpartum.

✔ The average duration of first labors is about 14 hours; approximately 1 hour of this period constitutes the second stage and 10 minutes, the third stage.

✔ The mechanism (cardinal movements) of labor involves fetal descent, flexion, internal rotation, extension, external rotation, and expulsion.

✔ Signs of placental separation include change in uterine shape and position in the abdomen, lengthening of the umbilical cord, and a sudden gush of blood.

✔ During labor and birth, involuntary contractions of the uterus occur intermittently, with periods of relaxation. The interval between contractions diminishes, and the intensity of contractions increases as labor progresses. Each uterine contraction has an increment, acme, and decrement.

✔ Gap junctions in the myometrial tissue increase the efficiency of uterine contractions. Prostaglandins assume a key regulatory role in the process of labor.

✔ Many physiologic and psychological adaptations involving the cardiovascular, respiratory, gastrointestinal, and other systems occur in the laboring woman. These changes vary based on the duration and strength of the labor, breathing techniques used, room temperature, degree of discomfort, and fluid replacement.

✔ The psyche or maternal psychological response must allow the woman to cope with uterine contractions and the physical demands of labor and birth. Examples of factors that influence the psyche include cultural background, previous experience, anxiety, and presence of a support person. Preparation for childbirth may positively influence maternal responses by decreasing anxiety and improving maternal work efforts.

✔ The healthy fetus is able to adapt positively to the process of labor as long as uteroplacental circulation is adequate.

REFERENCES

Adams, J. Q., & Alexander A. M. (1958). Alterations in cardiovascular physiology during labor. *American Journal of Obstetrics and Gynecology, 12,* 542–549.

Assali, N. S., Dilts, P. V. Jr, Plentl, A. A., Kirschbaum, T. H., & Gross, S. J. (1968). Physiology of the placenta. In N. S. Assali (Ed.), *Biology of gestation* (Vol. 1) (pp. 185–289). New York: Academic Press.

Assali, N. S. (1989). Dynamics of the uteroplacental circulation in health and disease. *American Journal of Perinatology, 6*(2), 105–109.

Beischer, N. A., & Mackay, E. V. (1986). *Obstetrics and the newborn* (2nd ed.). Philadelphia: W.B. Saunders.

Bennett, P. R., Chamberlain, G. V., Patel, L., Elder, M. G., Myatt, L. (1990). Mechanisms of parturition: The transfer of prostaglandin E_2 and 5-hydroxyeicosatetraenoic acid across fetal membranes. *American Journal of Obstetrics & Gynecology, 162*(3), 683–687.

Berg, T. C., & Rayburn, W. F. (1992). Effects of analgesia on labor. *Clinical Obstetrics and Gynecology, 35*(3), 457–463.

Casey, M. L., & MacDonald, P. C. (1985). Initiation of labor in women. In G. Hugzar (Ed.), *The biochemistry and physiology of the uterus and labor.* Cleveland, OH: CRC Press.

Casey, M. L., Winkel, C. A., Porter, J. C., MacDonald, P. C. (1983). Endocrine regulation of the initiation and maintenance of parturition. *Clinics in Perinatology, 10,* 709–721.

Chard, T., & Gibbens, G. L. (1983). Spurt release of oxytocin during surgical induction of labor in women. *American Journal of Obstetrics and Gynecology, 147,* 678–680.

Clark, S., Gimovsky, M., & Miller, F. (1982). Fetal heart rate response to fetal scalp blood sampling. *American Journal of Obstetrics and Gynecology, 33,* 706–708.

Cosner, K. R., & deJong, E. (1993). Physiologic second stage labor. *MCN: American Journal of Maternal Child Nursing, 18*, 38–43.

Cunningham, F. G., MacDonald, P. C., & Gant, N. F. (1993). *Williams obstetrics* (19th ed.). Norwalk, CT: Appleton & Lange.

Fox, H. A. (1979). The effects of catecholamines and drug treatment on the fetus and newborn. *Birth and the Family Journal, 6*, 157–165.

Friedman, E. A. (1978). *Labor and clinical evaluation and management* (2nd ed.). New York: Appleton-Century-Crofts.

Fuchs, A. R., Fuchs, F., Husselein, P., Soloff, M. S., Feinstrom, M. J. (1982). Oxytocin receptors and human parturition: A dual role of oxytocin in the initiation of labor. *Science, 215*, 1396–1398.

Gabbe, S. G., Niebyl, J. R., & Simpson, J. L. (1991). *Obstetrics normal and problem pregnancies.* New York: Churchill Livingstone.

Goff, K. J. (1993). Initiation of parturition. *MCN: American Journal of Maternal Child Nursing, Sept.-Oct* (Spec. Suppl.), 7–13.

Granstrom, L., Akman, G., & Ulmsten, U. (1990). Myometrial activity after local application of prostaglandin E_2 for cervical ripening and term labor induction. *American Journal of Obstetrics and Gynecology, 162*(3), 691–694.

Hacker N. F., & Moore, J. G. (1992). *Essentials of obstetrics and gynecology.* Philadelphia: W.B. Saunders.

Heaman, M., Beaton, J., Gupton, A., & Sloan, J. (1992). A comparison of childbirth expectations in high-risk and low-risk pregnant women. *Clinical Nursing Research, 1*, 252–265.

Hendrick, C. H., & Quilligan, E. J. (1956). Cardiac output during labor. *American Journal of Obstetrics and Gynecology, 71*, 953–972.

Ilancheran, A., & Ratnam, S. S. (1990). Effect of oxytocics on prostaglandin levels in the third stage of labour. *Gynecologic and Obstetric Investigation, 29*, 177–180.

Khazoyan, C. M., & Anderson, N. L. (1994). Latinas' expectations for their partners during childbirth. *MCN: American Journal of Maternal Child Nursing, 19*, 226–229.

Lagercrantz, H., & Slotkin, T. A. (1985). The "stress" of being born. *Scientific American, 12*, 100–107.

Lederman, E., Lederman, R. P., Work, B. A., & McMann, D. S. (1981). Maternal psychological and physiologic correlates of fetal-newborn health status. *American Journal of Obstetrics and Gynecology, 139*, 956–958.

Lederman, R. P., Lederman, E., Work, B. A., & McMann, D. S. (1978). The relationship of maternal anxiety, plasma catecholamines, and plasma cortisol to progress in labor. *American Journal of Obstetrics and Gynecology, 132*, 495–500.

Lederman, R. P., Lederman, E., Work, B. A., & McMann, D. S. (1979). Relationship of physiological factors in pregnancy to progress in labor. *Nursing Research, 28*, 94–97.

Lederman, R. P., Lederman, E., Work, B. A., & McMann, D. S. (1985). Anxiety and epinepherine in multiparous women in labor: Relationship to duration of labor and fetal heart rate pattern. *American Journal of Obstetrics and Gynecology, 153*, 870–877.

Liggins, G., & Novy, M. (1980). Role of prostaglandins, prostacyclin, and thromboxanes in the physiologic control of the uterus and in parturition. *Seminars in Perinatology, 4*, 45–66.

Lowe, N. (1991). Maternal confidence in coping with labor. *Journal of Obstetric, Gynecologic, and Neonatal Nursing, 20*, 457–463.

Lutwak, R., Ney, A. M., & White, J. (1988). Maternity nursing and Jewish law. *MCN: American Journal of Maternal Child Nursing, 13*, 44–46.

Mahan, C. S., & McKay, S. (1984). Are we overmanaging second stage labor? *Comtemporary Obstetrics and Gynecology, 24*, 37–63.

Mercer, R. T., Hackley, K. C., & Bostrom, A. G. (1983). Relationship of psycholsocial and perinatal variables to perception of childbirth. *Nursing Research, 32*, 202–207.

Noble, E. (1981). Controversies in maternal effort during labor and delivery. *Journal of Nurse Midwifery, 26*, 37–63.

Norr, K. L., Block, C. R., Charles, A. G., & Meyering, S. (1980). The second time around: Parity and birth experience. *Journal of Obstetric, Gynecologic, and Neonatal Nursing, 9*, 30–36.

Padayachi, T., Norman, R. J., Dhavaraj, K., Kemp, M., Joubert, S. M. (1988). Serial oxytocin levels in amniotic fluid and maternal plasma during normal and induced labour. *British Journal of Obstetrics and Gynaecology, 96*(9), 888–893.

Phillippe, M. (1983). Fetal catecholamines. *American Journal of Obstetrics and Gynecology, 146*(7), 840–855.

Reddi, K., Norman, R. J., Dappe, W. M., Machathe, C. T., Kemp, M., Joubert, S. M. (1987). Amniotic membrane production of prostaglandin F_2 alpha is reduced in dysfunctional human labor: Results of in vivo and in vitro studies. *Journal of Clinical Endocrinology Metabolism, 65*, 1000–1005.

Rice, P. E., & Benedetti, T. J. (1986). Fetal heart rate acceleration with fetal blood sampling. *Obstetrics and Gynecology, 68*, 469–472.

Sahmay, S., Coke, A., Hekim, N., Atasu, T. (1988). Maternal, umbilical, uterine and amniotic prostaglandin E and F_2 alpha levels in labour. *Journal of Internal Medicine Research, 16*(4), 280–285.

Saling, E., & Schneider, D. (1967). Biochemical supervision of the foetus during labour. *Journal of Obstetrics and Gynaecology of the British Commonwealth, 74*, 799–811.

Seitchik, J., & Castillo, M. (1983). Oxytocin augmentation of dysfunctional labor, II. Uterine activity data. *American Journal of Obstetrics and Gynecology, 145*, 526–529.

Shaala, S., Darwish, E., Anwar, M., Rocca, M., Ismail, A. A. (1989). Cervical prostaglandin injection: A novel method of administration for ripening the cervix and induction of labor. *International Journal of Gynaecology and Obstetrics, 30*(3), 221–223.

Simkin, P. (1986a). Stress, pain, and catecholamines in labor: Part 1. A review. *Birth, 13*, 227–233.

Simkin, P. (1986b). Active and physiologic management of the second stage: A review and hypothesis. In S. Kitzinger & P. Simkin (Eds.), *Episiotomy and the second stage of labor* (pp. 7–21). Seattle: Pennypress.

Smith, C., Nguyen, H., Phelan, J., & Paul, R. (1986). Intrapartum assessment of fetal well-being: A comparison of fetal acoustic stimulation and acid base determinations. *American Journal of Obstetrics and Gynecology, 155*, 726–728.

Soloff, M. S. (1988). The role of oxytocin in the initiation of labor, and oxytocin-prostaglandin interactions. In D. McNellis, J. R. G. Challis, P. C. MacDonald, Robertson, S., Urrutia, J. (Eds.), *Cellular and integrative mechanisms in the onset of labor: An NICHD workshop.* Ithaca, NY: Perinatology Press.

Sosa, R., Kennell, J., Klaus, M. et al. (1980). The effect of a supportive companion on perinatal problems, length of labor, and mother-infant interaction. *New England Journal of Medicine, 303*(11), 597–600.

Sullivan, J. M., & Rammanathan, K. B. (1985). Management of medical problems in pregnancy-severe cardiac disease. *New England Journal of Medicine, 313,* 304.

Thorburn, G. D., & Challis, J. R. G. (1979). Endocrine control of parturition. *Physiology Review, 59,* 863–866.

Tulchinsky, D., & Giannopoules, G. (1983). Estrogen/progesterone receptors and parturition. In P. C. MacDonald & J. C. Porter (Eds.), *Initiation of parturition: Prevention of prematurity* (pp. 153–159). Columbus, OH: Ross Laboratories.

Vorherr H. (1972). Disorder of uterine functions during pregnancy, labor, and puerperium. In N. S. Assali & C. R. Brinkman III (Eds.), *Patho-physiology of gestation: Maternal disorders* (Vol. 1) (pp. 146–268). New York: Academic Press.

Wathes, D. C., & Porter, D. G. (1982). Effect of uterine distension and oestrogen treatment on gap junction formation in the myometrium of the rat. *Journal of Reproductive Fertility, 65,* 497–505.

Wuitchik, M., Bakal, D., & Lipshitz, J. (1989). The clinical significance of pain and cognitive activity in latent labor. *Obstetrics and Gynecology, 73*(1), 35–42.

Zlatnik, F. J. (1994). Normal labor and delivery. In J. R. Scott, P. J. Desaia, C. B. Hammond, & W. N. Spellacy (Eds.), *Danforth's obstetrics and gynecology* (7th ed.). Philadelphia: J.B. Lippincott.

22

Management of Normal Labor

Objectives

- Describe the primary role of the labor and delivery nurse.
- Define labor and identify the conditions that allow it to proceed as a healthy process for both the mother and fetus.
- Describe the main characteristics of the birth process for the fetus.
- Describe what is necessary to facilitate the birth process for the woman and fetus.
- Discuss the normal course of immediate postpartum recovery.
- Identify the main goals of nursing care at each stage of labor.
- Describe primary nursing interventions in each of the four stages of labor.

Key Terms

Episiotomy	Oxytocics
Estimated date	Primipara
of delivery	Semi-Fowler position
Fetal heart rate	Show
Fundal height	Sims' position
Meconium	Valsalva's maneuvers

Parturition is a unique, exciting, wondersome yet sometimes worrisome experience for the woman and her partner and for their healthcare providers. For the woman or couple, labor looms as a critical period in the process of childbearing; they often consider labor as the end of a long drawn-out process rather than the beginning of a new role. Hence, many women attribute enormous significance to events during labor and to the people who are helpful to them at this time. The goal of perinatal nursing is to facilitate maximum physical and emotional well-being in the woman and her fetus. This includes the maternal transitions throughout pregnancy, birth, and recovery and the fetus' transition to becoming a newborn, but it also includes participation of the father and other support people in the birth experience. The nursing interventions used to achieve this goal are purposeful but flexible and are based on thorough assessments and nursing diagnoses to meet the individual needs of the mother, newborn, and family. The nurse must be familiar with the normal physiology of labor and deviations from the norm (discussed in Chapters 20, 21, and 36) to provide safe and supportive care.

This chapter describes the environment and care that accompany a labor and delivery carried out in a conventional labor and delivery unit (including the labor-delivery-recovery [LDR] room option and the labor room-delivery room option) within a hospital setting. Labor and delivery care varies depending on the facility's policies and procedures but tends to be accompanied by increasing amounts of technological intervention and more restriction on the woman's activity. However, other changes in the delivery of maternity care have worked to make childbearing a more "natural" and family-centered experience for everyone involved.

Not long ago, "conventional" meant admission to a labor room, transfer to a delivery room, recovery in a recovery room, and a final transfer to a postpartum or maternity floor. Now, however, many women labor, deliver, and recover in one room. After recovery is complete, the client is transferred to a postpartum unit.

In some hospitals, labor, delivery, recovery, and postpartum care can occur in one room.

Professional organizations, such as the Association of Women's Health, Obstetrics, and Neonatal Nurses (AWHONN) and others, are publishing documents supporting changes in perinatal care to incorporate family-centered care concepts in every aspect of perinatal service (American Academy of Pediatrics and American College of Obstetricians and Gynecologists [AAP/ ACOG], 1992; Nurses Association of American College of Obstetricians and Gynecologists [NAACOG], 1991). Medical center personnel must look at the traditional procedures and determine whether they are based on sound scientific research and are in the best interest of the client and her family. Above all, the family should not lose their rights to determine their own care when they enter the hospital. They have choices and options in care, and the professional is there to support choices that are not injurious.

Labor

Prelude to Labor

The prodromal signs that herald the onset of labor begin several weeks before true labor commences. As discussed in Chapter 21, lightening may occur any time during the last 4 weeks of pregnancy; in **primiparas** (first pregnancy > 20 weeks), it usually occurs about 10 to 14 days before labor. In multiparas, lightening may not occur until labor has begun. This is the time for the woman to tend to last-minute preparation details, such as arrangements for care of the other children or the functioning of the household while she's away. Walks in the fresh air are a good way to release extra tension without creating fatigue. The expectant woman should be encouraged to achieve a happy balance between activity and rest. As the **estimated date of delivery** (EDD) approaches, the nurse should explore with the woman her preparations for coming to the hospital. The woman or couple should determine approximately how long it takes to reach the hospital and what alternate transportation is available in an emergency. The entrance to the hospital they should use and admission procedures also are important topics. Many hospitals offer a monthly maternity tour to acquaint clients with their birthing facilities so that expectant couples can become more familiar with the surroundings and hospital staff.

Onset of Labor

Early in the third trimester, the client should be informed about what to do when labor starts and of certain situations that would necessitate a visit to the hos-

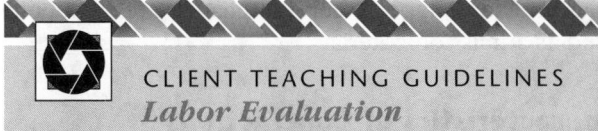

CLIENT TEACHING GUIDELINES
Labor Evaluation

The woman needs to call her physician or midwife and prepare to go to the hospital for evaluation when the following occur:

- There is a regular uterine contraction pattern, increasing in intensity.
- Spontaneous rupture of the membranes occurs.
- There is bright-red vaginal bleeding.
- There is a decrease in fetal movement (less than three movements per hour).
- Anything occurs that her clinician has instructed her to report.

pital for evaluation. The client should be encouraged to report early in labor and not wait at home to see if it is true or false labor. Most physicians instruct their clients to notify them if the labor contractions become regular. A primipara, for instance, may be given instructions to wait at home until contractions are every 5 minutes for 2 hours, whereas the multipara would be instructed to come to the hospital much sooner. Other situations of which the woman needs to be advised include breaking of the "bag of waters" or any vaginal bleeding. Clarify that the breaking of the amniotic sac may result in only a small intermittent leak or a gush of fluid from the woman's vagina. In either situation, the physician or midwife should be notified, and the woman should come to the hospital (see Client Teaching Guidelines: Labor Evaluation).

When the woman first becomes aware of the contractions, they may be irregular or regular in frequency, anywhere from 15 to 30 minutes apart, and last only 20 to 30 seconds. Because these are of mild intensity, however, she usually can continue with whatever she is doing, except that she must be alert to time the subsequent contractions to have specific information when she calls the physician. The client must know when it is appropriate to go to the hospital in relation to her uterine contraction pattern.

Admission to the Hospital

The woman who has received adequate prenatal care also has received instruction on what to anticipate when she comes to the hospital to have her baby. If this is her first hospital experience, it will be much easier for her if she has been told about the necessary preliminary procedures, such as any vulvar and perineal preparation, the methods of examination used to ascertain the progress of labor, pain relief measures, and the usual routines in the course of labor.

If the woman has not had adequate prenatal preparation, her labor may be advanced at the time of admission, and she may not know what to expect. The nurse must reassure this woman and orient her to the process of labor and the physical environment as quickly as possible. The ability of the nurse to make decisive clinical judgments in this situation, especially with regard to establishing priorities of care, cannot be overstated.

Every hospital has its own admission procedure. However, the differences are in details only, because the principles are the same everywhere: asepsis and antisepsis, careful monitoring of the woman for any deviations from normal, and supportive care.

Admission Information

After making the woman comfortable, the nurse needs to proceed with the admission as quickly as possible. When admitting procedures are done early in labor, before contractions have become very intense, the woman is able to respond with relative ease. It may be more difficult for her to answer questions if her labor is further along.

The nurse initiates the admitting process by determining the following:

1. Is the client in true labor, and if so, how far has she progressed?
2. What is the current status of the woman and fetus?
3. Is there a high-risk condition present?
4. Is there a history of high-risk conditions during the prenatal period or prepregnancy chronic diseases?
5. What preparation has she had for childbirth, and what support systems are available to assist her through labor?

As part of the admission procedure determined by hospital policies and physician orders, the nurse may be doing perineal shaves or enemas, setting up electronic fetal monitoring, starting intravenous fluid therapy, and requesting laboratory tests (eg, hematocrit, hemoglobin, type and screens, and urinalysis or a minimum of dipstick test for protein, glucose, and acetone). A detailed look at assessment during the admission of a woman in labor follows.

Assessment

Nursing History

Nursing practice is guided by professional standards, and in the course of admitting the laboring woman, the nurse must document the name of the client, the reason for admission, the date and time of arrival, the time the physician was notified, and the time the client was seen by the physician (AAP/ACOG, 1992; NAACOG, 1991). For the client whose admission was planned, the prenatal record is usually sent from the doctor's office or clinic to the labor and delivery unit at approximately 36 weeks; this record should be checked by the admitting nurse. The following information may be transcribed from the prenatal record to the admission form: EDD or "due date," any prenatal problems, blood group and Rh factor, irregular antibody detection, rubella immunity, vaginal cultures, serology, hepatitis screen, and any diagnostic or therapeutic measures taken.

A good nursing history and physical examination help the admitting nurse evaluate the client's high-risk status. If any factors that place the woman or fetus at risk are found, the physician is notified. Such factors might alter the type of labor and birth experience the client desires. (See Chapter 36 for a discussion of high-risk labor.) Clients who are not in need of acute, immediate care should have a more detailed history, covering the following information: onset, frequency, duration, and intensity of contractions; status of membranes; vaginal bleeding; fetal activity; history of allergies; time and content of last ingestion; current medications; and recent exposure to and/or presence of infections (eg, herpes). The fetus is evaluated by noting the gestational age, fetal position, and heart rate. Nursing personnel with advanced skills may perform the initial pelvic examination (first noting that there is no abnormal bleeding, status of membranes, and fetal position) to determine cervical dilatation, effacement, and fetal position and station (see Chaps. 20 and 21).

The nurse spends a great deal of time with the client after admission and is expected to monitor the general character of the labor contractions and the other manifestations of labor. First, it must be determined whether the client is actually in labor. Friedman (1978) has pointed out that no fixed or uniformly applicable rules can be used to determine true labor at the bedside. Technically, it can be assumed that the client is in true labor if her contractions continue without interruption and result in dilatation of the cervix. In practice, however, many different types of contractions may be apparent; thus, the differential points between true and false labor contained in Table 21-1 are to be used only as *guidelines* for assessing the state of the woman's labor. Many practitioners, especially in busy regional labor and delivery units, use the criterion for active labor (>2–3 cm cervical dilatation) as the labor decision factor to decide the need for immediate hospital admission for term gestation, instructing clients in early labor (<3–4 cm) to return when contractions are stronger. Preterm clients need a different criterion to prevent the advancement of labor without surveillance. Therefore, the presence of contractions every 10 minutes for 1 hour and some type of cervical change are frequently used as admission criteria.

Characteristics of Contractions

The frequency, duration, and intensity of the contractions should be monitored closely and recorded regardless of whether a monitor is used (see Fig. 21-7):

- The *frequency* of contractions is timed from the beginning of one contraction to the beginning of the next and is noted as occurrence per interval in minutes (eg, uterine contraction q3 min).
- The *duration* of a contraction is timed from the moment the uterus first begins to tighten until it relaxes again and is measured in seconds (eg, uterine contraction q3 min × 60 sec).
- The *intensity* of a contraction may be mild, moderate, or strong at its acme. Because this is a relative factor, intensity is difficult to interpret unless the nurse is at the woman's bedside palpating the uterus during contractions. The nurse uses the pads of the fingertips, palpating the woman's abdomen over the uterine fundus during the contraction to judge intensity. With internal uterine monitoring, intensity can be quantified in terms of mm Hg (eg, uterine contraction q3 × 60 sec at 50 mm Hg).

During a *mild* contraction, the uterine muscle becomes somewhat tense but can be indented with gentle pressure. During a *moderate* contraction, the uterus becomes moderately firm, and a firmer pressure is needed to indent. During a *strong* contraction, the uterus becomes so firm that it has the feel of woodlike hardness, and at the height of the contraction, the uterus cannot be indented when pressure is applied by the examiner's finger.

General Physical Condition and Vital Signs

The nurse begins by asking the client why she came to the hospital. Do not assume that the onset of regular contractions is the client's chief complaint; leaking amniotic fluid or a decrease in fetal activity also may have prompted this visit. The nurse should give the woman time to express in her own words her reason for admission. The use of open-ended questions to elicit this information is beneficial, although more direct questions may be necessary later to clarify information. The chief complaint is recorded in the client's own words.

Temperature, Pulse, and Respiration. Temperature and respiration should be normal. If temperature is more than 37.2°C (99.6°F) orally or if the pulse and respiration become rapid, the physician or birth attendant should be notified. The temperature and respiration are taken every 4 hours or more frequently if indicated (AAP/ACOG, 1992). Conditions that warrant closer observation are rupture of the membranes and the presence of a fetal tachycardia. Temperature is taken every 2 hours after rupture of membranes (ACOG, 1992).

The pulse in normal labor is usually in the 70s or 80s and rarely exceeds 100. Sometimes the pulse rate on admission is slightly increased because of the excitement of coming to the hospital, but this returns to normal shortly thereafter. A persistent pulse over 100 suggests exhaustion or dehydration. Pulse rates are recorded every 4 hours (AAP/ACOG, 1992).

Blood Pressure. Significant hemodynamic occurrences are observed during labor and birth that affect the blood pressure value. As mentioned in Chapter 21, with every contraction of the uterus, approximately 300 to 500 mL of blood is shifted to the central blood volume, causing increases in cardiac output. Other conditions leading to significant increase in cardiac output are anxiety and pain, especially in the primipara. Hendricks et al. (1956) have shown in a now-classic study, that pain and anxiety alone can increase cardiac output by 50% to 60%.

For the client without recognized high-risk factors, the blood pressure should be taken and recorded every hour (AAP/ACOG, 1992). To obtain accurate blood pressure, the nurse needs to be aware of the hemodynamic alterations involved with contractions and must work with the client to relieve her pain and anxiety. Blood pressures start to rise approximately 5 to 8 seconds preceding a contraction, returning to resting level when the contraction subsides (Elkayam et al., 1982). Hence, the nurse should take the client's blood pressure and pulse after a contraction, well before the next one starts.

No research-based recommendations can help the nurse with the choice of position when obtaining a blood pressure during labor. Most experts agree that the blood pressure taken with the client on her left side is the one to use for clinical diagnosis and management. If the nurse gets a blood pressure reading initially that needs to be reevaluated because it is either higher or lower than expected, the cuff should be deflated and a waiting period of 2 minutes observed. At this time, the nurse should assess factors that may be contributing to the atypical reading. Is the reading elevated because of pain or anxiety, or is it low as the result of regional anesthesia, supine position, systemic medication, or hemorrhage? The second reading can be taken in the same arm, and if the deviation from the expected norm still exists, this information is reported. The student should be aware that the person being told the information, whether physician or staff nurse, will want other information to evaluate the client. For instance, for an elevation in blood pressure, the expe-

rienced nurse evaluates the client for signs and symptoms of pregnancy-induced hypertension, knowing that a certain number of women are asymptomatic during their pregnancy but develop the disease when in labor.

When epidural anesthesia is given in labor, blood pressures in some facilities are evaluated every minute for the first 10 minutes, then every 5 minutes for 10 minutes, then every 15 minutes or until stable. The application of the "Dynomap" automated blood pressure device can facilitate use of a frequent monitoring protocol. The blood pressure may be taken every 30 minutes or as directed by the department of anesthesia protocols at that particular hospital. The nursing protocol for evaluating a client after epidural anesthesia is usually outlined in the labor and delivery policy book.

Fetal Evaluation

It cannot be stressed enough that when caring for the pregnant woman, the nurse is treating two clients, the woman and the fetus. This is especially important to remember when admitting the laboring woman. The nurse must perform the following assessment measures to establish fetal well-being:

1. Determine the EDD.
2. Measure the fundal height of the uterus, and correlate the height with the gestational age.
3. Determine fetal position by abdominal palpation.
4. Auscultate fetal heart tones to determine the baseline and any periodic changes.
5. Determine presence of fetal movement.

Estimated Date of Delivery. The EDD can be obtained from the prenatal record. A term pregnancy is one that has achieved 38 weeks' gestation and has not exceeded 42 weeks. As explained in Chapter 17, the date of the client's last normal menstrual period allows the nurse to calculate the EDD using Nägele's rule. The EDD is truly an estimate, because the exact day of ovulation and conception is rarely known; no more than 5% of viable pregnancies end on their EDD, but most women who do reach term deliver within 7 days of their due date. Many pregnancies also are dated using ultrasound, which can provide a more accurate gestational age estimate at the time of admission (Halle, 1993).

Fundal Height. Even though determination of **fundal height** using a tape measure is not a common practice on admission, the labor and delivery nurse should be able to perform this measurement and know its significance (see Chap. 17). Another method used by experienced nurses is to palpate the fundal height while keeping in mind the relationship of fundal height to gestational age. Finding an abnormally low or excessively high fundal height does not necessarily indicate an unhealthy fetus but cues the nurse to look for the reason for the deviation from normal.

Abdominal Palpation: Leopold's Maneuvers. The fetal position should be confirmed before the initial vaginal examination (NAACOG, 1991; AAP/ACOG, 1992). Performing Leopold's maneuvers in a systematic manner enables the nurse to assess fetal position and makes locating the fetal heart tone easier. In cephalic and breech presentations, the fetal heart is best heard through the fetal back because it is the fetal part in closest contact with the uterine wall (see Chap. 20 for procedure and illustrations).

Fetal Heart Rate. **Fetal heart rate** (FHR) should be determined early in the admission process. Under normal circumstances, the heart rate of a term fetus, determined by the atrial pacemaker, usually ranges between 120 and 160 beats/min (Freeman et al., 1991). However, many term and post-term well-oxygenated fetuses have a stable baseline rate between 10 and 20 beats/min below this range, because the baseline rate decreases as the fetal neurologic system matures (Murray, 1988).

The evaluation of FHR in labor is of great importance. Although it is not clear that electronic fetal monitoring of the low-risk woman provides any better results than intermittent auscultation, a 15- to 20-minute initial evaluation with an external electronic fetal monitor is recommended and has become accepted practice in many hospitals and birthing centers (Zlatnik, 1994). AWHONN (1992) states that the baseline FHR and response to contractions should be evaluated and documented throughout labor. After the initial evaluation and confirmation of low-risk status, intermittent FHR should be evaluated every 15 to 30 minutes during the active and transition phases of the first stage of labor and every 5 to 15 minutes in the second stage of labor.

Intermittent FHR assessment can be obtained using a number of methods, including a Doppler unit (Doptone), an external electronic fetal monitor, or a fetoscope. The Doptone is a portable electronic instrument that emits ultrasound waves, which when reflected off the fetal heart, produce echoes or "clicks." Used like a stethoscope, the Doppler is effective in finding the FHR when the FHR is difficult to hear with a fetoscope or hard to locate by external monitor. The Doppler unit also is usually able to detect the FHR no matter what the maternal position; thus, it allows for freedom of positioning and ambulation. However, using the Doppler does not allow the nurse to detect FHR variability. In addition, when assessments must be made every 5 or 15 minutes, this method may become more intrusive

than continuous monitoring (or difficult to carry out in a busy unit).

The external electronic fetal monitor allows for either intermittent or continuous monitoring of FHR. It uses an ultrasound transducer much like the portable Doppler, but it also includes a *tocotransducer,* which records the frequency and duration of uterine contractions when strapped on the uterine fundus. Its advantages include reliability, ability to evaluate FHR variability, and avoidance of the need to interrupt the woman for auscultation. It usually displays a readout of the FHR and produces a continuous graphic display of the FHR, which makes it a permanent record of the FHR patterns. Used as a continuous monitoring system, this method does limit the woman's mobility during labor and could increase her discomfort or anxiety level. Continuous electronic FHR monitoring is used if any abnormalities are found on the initial admission monitoring or if the pregnancy is considered high risk because of medical or obstetric complications. Use of the external electronic fetal monitor (and intrauterine monitoring) is discussed in more detail in Chapter 40.

The fetoscope is a modified stethoscope that contains a head attachment to enhance conduction of fetal heart sounds. Although inexpensive and noninvasive, the fetoscope is used much less frequently than in the past because it can detect only gross abnormalities in FHR. It is most effective when used during and immediately following a uterine contraction.

When checking the fetal heart sounds with a fetoscope, the nurse listens and counts the rate for 1 full minute (or for 15 seconds and then multiplies by 4). Checking the rate before, during, and after a contraction is important so that any slowing or irregularities may be detected. It may be difficult to hear the sounds during a contraction because the uterine wall is tense, and it is more difficult for the woman to lie still during this period.

The student in the clinical area should be working with a staff nurse and not be totally responsible for evaluation of the FHR. If the student nurse notices a slowing of the FHR, he or she should notify the staff nurse for further evaluation of the fetus, and the staff nurse determines if the pattern warrants notification of the birth attendant. Interpretation of FHR patterns and appropriate nursing interventions for decelerations are covered in Chapter 40.

Amniotic Fluid Status

The nurse must establish whether the woman's membranes are intact. Ruptured membranes are significant for the following reasons:

■ If the presenting part is not engaged in the pelvis (0 station), there is the possibility of a prolapse of the cord and consequent cord compression and fetal distress.

- Labor is likely to occur soon after rupture if the pregnancy is at or near term.
- If the fetus remains in the uterus 24 hours or more after the membranes rupture, especially when associated with multiple vaginal examinations, protracted labor, or intrauterine monitoring, there is an increased probability of intrauterine infection that is especially harmful to the fetus, even if the woman is given antibiotics (Gabbe, 1986).

Ruptured membranes are often difficult to diagnose unless the fluid is seen escaping from the vagina. Moreover, no tests are completely reliable. Those most widely used involve testing the pH (acidity or alkalinity) of the vaginal fluid. The amniotic fluid pH is generally 7 to 7.5, whereas vaginal secretions are in the range of 4.5 to 5.5; urine's pH is 5.5 to 6.5 (Zuspan et al., 1988). The nitrazine tests use test papers similar to litmus paper. These papers are impregnated with a dye that reacts with the vaginal material and can be compared with a standard color chart (Box 22-1). Bloody show can confound the reading, giving a false reading of ruptured membranes when the membranes are intact, because maternal blood (pH 7.35–7.45) is basic like amniotic fluid (Berne et al., 1993; Cunningham et al., 1993).

Some clients come in wearing a peripad or have wet underclothing that may be tested with the nitrazine. If the client presents to the unit with a term gestation, whether in labor or not, and a history of leaking fluid from the vagina, determination of ruptured membranes is often made with a sterile speculum examination.

The nurse may assist the physician with this procedure, or with advanced preparation on the technique, the nurse may be incorporating it into his or her practice. A sterile speculum is inserted into the vagina to visualize the cervix. At this time, sterile cotton swabs are used to take samples of vaginal secretions from the cervical os to test with nitrazine and make a slide to check for ferning. The practitioner also looks for fluid leaking from the cervix, vaginal pooling, color of the fluid, and any cervical dilatation. The slide prepared for the fern test needs to dry for 5 to 7 minutes before it is examined under the microscope. Because of the sodium chloride content in amniotic fluid, the dried specimen, if truly amniotic fluid, looks like clusters of fern leaves. The client and support person should be informed of the test results; if the membranes are ruptured, the report will be a positive fern test, and if they are not ruptured, the report will be negative.

Once it has been determined that the membranes are ruptured, some physicians may wait up to a certain time for labor to start on its own; others may start an oxytocin infusion. With both options, delaying or minimizing the number of vaginal examinations can lower the chance of introducing bacteria into the uterine cavity.

Meconium Staining. Passage of fetal colonic contents, called **meconium,** may result in a staining of the amniotic fluid to yellow or brownish-green. The reason it has been associated with fetal distress is that hypoxia can relax the fetal bowel, causing meconium passage. The passage of meconium may or may not indicate fetal distress, because it is a natural physiologic process for postmature fetuses. It can range in viscosity from thin to thick and may be particulate. Whether the placental membranes or fetal skin are stained at birth depends on the length of exposure in utero to the meconium in the amniotic fluid. However, its presence, color, and consistency are *always* documented in the nursing notes; arrangements are made for tracheal intubation prior to the first breath at birth, and the physician is notified of its presence.

Initial Vaginal Examination

Abdominally assessing fetal position, assessing for abnormal vaginal bleeding, and assessing amniotic fluid status are all recommended nursing practices before the initial vaginal examination. In many teaching institutions, the physician or resident may assume responsibility for the vaginal examination, but in other facilities, the nurse performs this assessment (Fig. 22-1).

To begin the procedure, the client lies on her back with her knees flexed and heels together; her knees fall outward laterally. The nurse drapes the client so that she is well protected, leaving the perineal region exposed. The examiner puts on sterile gloves. Before the fingers are introduced into the vagina, the labia are opened wide with the nurse's nondominant hand to minimize possible contamination of the examining fingers should they come in contact with the inner surfaces of the labia and the margins of the hymen. The index and middle fingers are lubricated with K-Y Jelly;

BOX 22-1
Nitrazine Test Color Interpretation

Membranes Probably Intact

Yellow:	pH 5.0
Olive yellow:	pH 5.5
Olive green:	pH 6.0

Ruptured Membranes

Blue green:	pH 6.5
Blue gray:	pH 7.0
Deep blue:	pH 7.5

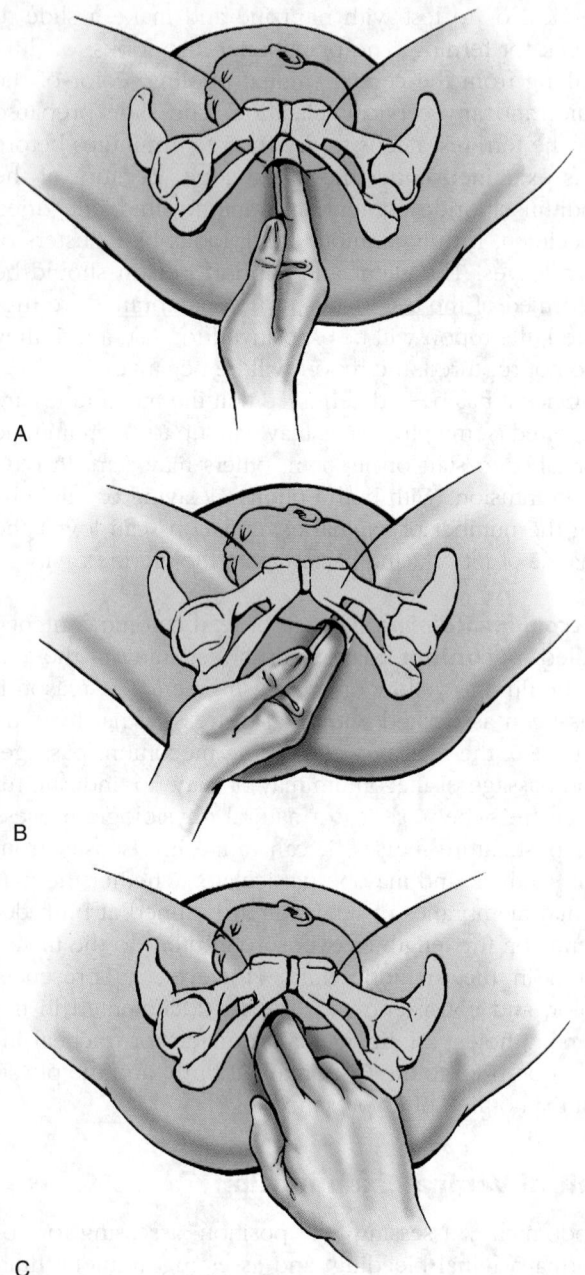

FIGURE 22–1 Vaginal examination. **(A)** Determining the station and palpating the sagittal suture. **(B)** Identifying the posterior fontanel. **(C)** Identifying the anterior fontanel. Note the first and second fingers are the examining fingers. The examiner must be careful not to touch the rectal area with the fourth and fifth fingers. The examiner also must be careful with placement of the thumb by not applying too much pressure to the mons pubis.

it is important not to touch the lubricant tube with the fingers. An assistant can squeeze the lubricant onto the examiner's fingers. The index and middle fingers of the examining hand are gently introduced into the vagina, and the following are assessed:

- Cervical effacement
- Cervical dilatation
- Position of the cervix
- Fetal station
- Presenting part and fetal position

Nursing Diagnoses

During the admission process, the nurse begins to gather data and develop the care plan. Differentiating normal conditions from developing problems requires critical thinking skills and the ability to analyze several findings. Any finding in isolation may have several implications, from benign to deleterious, and only in association with other presenting findings can the correct interpretation of the physiologic or pathophysiologic process be made. Various medical diagnoses of high-risk perinatal problems are discussed in the chapters covering maternal and perinatal complications. As a professional healthcare provider and client advocate, today's registered nurse needs to be able to differentiate normal from abnormal findings and to classify these findings, in collaboration with the physician, into the commonly known high-risk conditions. The following is a list of potential nursing diagnoses that may be used independently by the nurse.

Potential physiologic problems include:

- Risk for Infection related to premature rupture of membranes
- Altered Tissue Perfusion: placental perfusion to fetus decreased due to supine position
- Sleep Pattern Disturbance

Potential psychosocial problems include:

- Pain related to uterine contractions
- Anxiety related to unfamiliar hospital surroundings
- Fear related to impending labor and birth
- Knowledge Deficit: expectations in labor related to lack of specific information regarding labor process
- Knowledge Deficit: appropriate relaxation techniques related to lack of specific teaching on techniques
- Ineffective Individual Coping related to lack of support systems

The birth of a newborn is viewed as a major life event. When developing the care plan, the labor and delivery nurse should keep in mind the needs of other family members who may be accompanying the woman, including the father, grandparents, aunts, uncles, and friends. From the psychosocial nursing diagnoses listed previously, the second, third, fifth, and sixth might apply to other family members.

Intervention and Rationale

The labor and delivery nurse is faced with the problem of providing high-quality care in a short amount of time. It is important to use whatever time is available to develop a therapeutic relationship and provide an atmosphere of receptivity to the family's needs. The ability to determine needs lies in the perceptions that underlie the assessment and diagnosis portions of the nursing process. The nurse's facility with therapeutic communication plus technical understanding and skill are key to implementing effective care.

Psychosocial Considerations

A good deal of time and effort has been spent in nursing research to determine the needs of clients, especially the needs above and beyond those related directly to physiologic and pathologic conditions. These needs have generally been classified as "emotional" or "psychosocial." Whatever their label, they are especially important for consideration with the maternity client and support system.

Establishment of the Nurse–Client Relationship. Admission to the maternity unit may be a woman's first acquaintance with hospitals as a client. Her immediate reaction may be one of strangeness, loneliness, and homesickness, particularly if she arrives alone or if a significant other is not permitted to stay with her in the labor room. Regardless of the amount of preparation for this event, whether she is happy or unhappy and whether she wants the baby or not, every woman enters labor with a certain amount of normal tension and anxiety. Moreover, some women are thoroughly afraid of the whole process. This may be attributed in part to limited preparation for childbearing or to prior exposure to stories that emphasized the dangers or mysteries of childbirth. If she has had children previously, she may have had difficult or fear-producing experiences. All these factors make the woman's fear understandable.

First Impressions. The kind of greeting the client and her partner or support person receive as they enter the labor and delivery unit is extremely important and sets the tone for future interaction with the health team. Many hospitals allow the expectant father and other support people whom the woman may want to have with her during labor and delivery.

Support Person. Women rarely have babies without a support person present. This person can be the father of the baby, a family member (eg, mother or sister), or a close friend (Fig. 22-2). This person may have at-

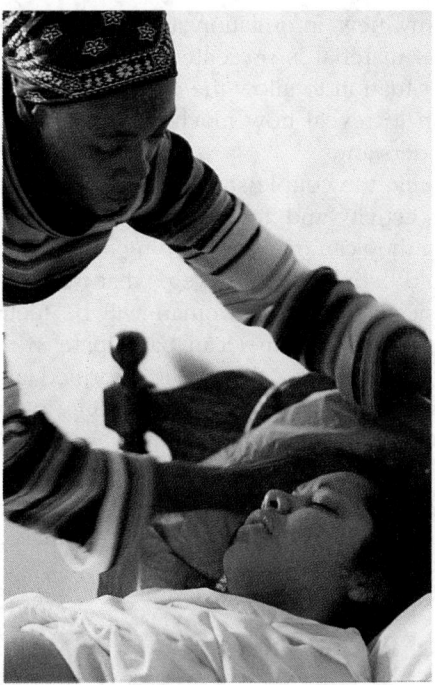

FIGURE 22–2 A support person is very important to the woman in labor. This person can be the father of the baby, a family member (eg, mother or sister), or a close friend.

tended prepared childbirth classes with the client and may be ready to assume the role of coach during the labor and delivery. The opposite also is true; the support person may not have attended classes and needs, as does the client, teaching about ways to relax and cope with labor.

Culture may dictate the amount of involvement the support person is to have in the birth experience. The nurse needs to assess the family and be respectful of their choice and not judgmental if their choice differs from what the nurse and other staff feel is the appropriate way for the family to respond.

Orientation. The woman and her support person need to know what is expected of them and what they can expect. The woman can be helped, if necessary, to change to the hospital gown and can be made comfortable in a chair or if she wishes, in bed.

The nurse can begin an orientation to the process of labor and to equipment and the general environment. There is no set form for this orientation. The nurse must first explore what the parents know about the environment and the labor process to judge what needs to be introduced or reinforced and the most appropriate time to accomplish this. An easy conversational manner may be used rather than a rapid-fire explanation.

The rationale for any procedures or restrictions is always given. The client must not be overloaded with too many stimuli at one time and should be allowed to absorb any new information and explanation before additional material is presented. The nurse can structure the situation to allow the client to "feed back" information to reveal how much the woman or couple really understands.

Generally, the couple should know the limits of the woman's activity and any restrictions of food and fluids. What they can expect regarding the progress of labor should be included also (eg, what will be happening physically, how the woman will be feeling, and how she and her partner can participate in the labor experience). Keeping the client informed about her progress in labor is a priority in nursing intervention.

As implied, this orientation continues throughout the entire course of labor and delivery. The nurse determines when and how each phase is to be instituted, according to the cues given by the woman and her support person.

Physical Preparation

Physical preparation protocols vary greatly among hospitals and birthing centers. At one time, the routine preparation for labor and birth soon after admission included shaving the perineum and administering an enema. It was thought that shaving the perineal area would improve hygiene (and reduce the chance of postpartum infection) and that the enema would help to eliminate the presence of stool in the rectum, which might impede the descent of the presenting part, and ensure that no stool would be expelled during childbirth, which might contaminate the newborn or episiotomy. However, experience and research have called both these routines into question, and many practitioners do not routinely practice them; some practitioners believe that shaving may actually increase the risk of infection and that an enema is likely to cause unnecessary embarrassment and discomfort in early labor and cannot guarantee that no bowel contents will be expelled during delivery. In addition, with childbearing clients participating much more fully in the decision-making process, their interest in a more natural birthing experience and rightful questioning of these uncomfortable procedures has resulted in their being used much less frequently (Zlatnik, 1994).

Perineal Shave. Shaving or clipping the perineal hair continues in some institutions. Some physicians may require only clipping the hair, while others may simply have the area washed well with a bacteriostatic soap. When the perineum is to be shaved, a pad is placed under the buttocks, and the client assumes the same position she was in for the vaginal examination. Lighting must be optimal, and the nurse asks the woman if she has any warts or moles of which the nurse should be aware before shaving. The nurse wears gloves for this procedure, as with other procedures that involve potential contact with blood and other body fluids, for the client's and the nurse's protection.

Enema. In some institutions, the decision to give an enema is left to the nurse's clinical judgment. In other hospitals, an enema is still required. In any case, it is wise for the nurse to ascertain during the history taking if the client has had a recent bowel movement. If the client is constipated, an enema can be helpful. However, if she is having diarrhea, the procedure is certainly not necessary, and the possibility of an infection must be considered.

Enemas, when given, must be given during early labor. They are absolutely contraindicated during rapid or advanced labor and in clients with a history or presence of vaginal bleeding, unengaged vertex, nonvertex lie, history of placenta previa or abruptio, or nonreassuring FHR. Any time the nurse feels the benefits of an enema do not outweigh the risk of administration, the physician should be notified and the enema should not be given.

Small-volume enemas (for example, Fleet) are commonly used. The nurse uses the same principles when administering the enema as for any other client. However, it may be more difficult to insert the tube because of the pressure of the presenting part of the fetus or because of hemorrhoids that may accompany pregnancy.

Hemorrhoids or the strength of the contractions may make the enema uncomfortable for the client, and it is essential that she be informed that the nurse is aware of the possible discomfort. To aid in comfort, the nurse can stop the enema infusion during the contractions by pinching the tubing or ceasing to squeeze the disposable enema container. The client is encouraged to hold the enema as long as possible before expelling. The nurse needs to chart that the procedure has been done and the results of the enema.

First Stage of Labor

The first stage of labor (dilating stage) begins with the first symptoms of true labor and ends with the complete dilatation of the cervix. The physician depends heavily on the accuracy of the nurse's bedside examinations and timely reports of the client's condition from admission onward throughout labor. In most community level I and II hospitals, if no high-risk problems exist, most private physicians delegate normal bedside care to the nurse, according to standing orders initiated following the physician's phone order to admit the client. Depending on the length of labor and the physician's other simultaneous responsibilities (eg, office hours, surgery), the physician may or may not see the client until the time of the actual birth. In university-affiliated level III medical centers and health maintenance organizations, residents and attendings are usually on 24-hour in-house call and frequently perform their own assessments; the nurse needs to coordinate the various evaluations to minimize duplication of any invasive assessments that could increase the woman's risk of infection and level of discomfort.

During labor, assessments of the FHR and vaginal examinations determine whether the fetus is in good condition and that the woman is making steady progress. Furthermore, the rate of progress often gives some indication as to when birth is to be expected. During this stage, the nurse is in constant attendance, safeguarding the welfare of the woman and fetus and notifying the physician of the progress of labor.

Assessment

Assessment during the first stage of labor includes vaginal examination and assessment of contractions, show, vital signs, and FHR.

Vaginal Examination

The frequency with which vaginal examinations are required during labor depends on the individual case; often one or two such examinations are sufficient, whereas in some instances, more are required. In the presence of ruptured membranes, it is especially important to limit the number of vaginal examinations to protect against infection. In the presence of vaginal bleeding, placenta previa must first be ruled out before a vaginal examination can safely be done, or perforation of the placenta could be a catastrophic consequence.

The nurse who stays with the woman constantly becomes increasingly skillful in the ability to follow the progress of labor by careful evaluation of the character of the uterine contractions, the amount of show, the progressive descent of the area on the abdomen where fetal heart sounds are heard, and the woman's overall response to her physical labor. Experienced labor and delivery nurses know to suspect an imminent birth when a woman says that she feels she needs to have a bowel movement. Instead of helping the woman to the bathroom, they lift the bed sheet and see if the fetal head is crowning.

Uterine Contractions

Many young women approach childbirth with fear of pain. It is no easy task to dispel this age-old fear, but throughout the childbirth experience, a conscious effort must be made to instill a wholesome point of view about the laboring experience. The nurse should avoid the use of the word *pain* whenever possible because of the connotation of the word.

Sociocultural factors play an important part in the meaning, interpretation, and expression of pain for clients. Although pain is basically a physiologic phenomenon, the meaning pain has and the kinds of responses to pain that are deemed appropriate are partly culturally determined. Cultural orientations, social conditioning, and sociocultural sanctioning mold patterns of response to painful experiences that are modal (ie, occur most frequently) in a group, and these modal patterns are meaningful in terms of the values and beliefs of a particular group. Therefore, the culture or subculture from which a person comes conditions the formation of her particular reaction patterns to pain.

However, as labor progresses, the contractions become increasingly intense. Therefore, it is the nurse's responsibility to help the woman distinguish between the fear and anticipation of pain and the discomfort or actual pain that she may be experiencing. The nurse needs to help her cope effectively and provide pharmacologic and nonpharmacologic interventions to decrease discomfort.

Timing the Contractions. Frequency, duration, and intensity of the contractions should be monitored closely and recorded, whether or not an electronic fetal monitor is used. As labor progresses, the character of the contractions changes. They become stronger in intensity, last longer (30–60 seconds), and come closer together (every 2–3 minutes). If the monitor is not being used, one effective method the nurse can use when timing contractions is to keep her fingers lightly on the fundus. The fingers are recommended because they are more sensitive than the palm. However, for some people, the whole hand is helpful. Enough of the fingers should be used to ensure adequate contact with the abdomen: Too slight a contact does not enable the nurse to evaluate the contractions accurately.

Assessing contractions in this manner enables the nurse to detect the beginning of the contraction by the gradual tensing and rising forward of the fundus and to feel the contraction through its three phases until the uterus relaxes again. The inexperienced nurse can get some idea of how a contraction feels under her fingertips by contracting her own biceps. First, the forearm should be extended and the fingertips of the hand on the opposite side placed on the biceps. The arm is gradually flexed until the muscle becomes hard, held a few seconds, and gradually extended. This should take about 30 seconds to simulate a uterine contraction.

The nurse should not rely on the woman to indicate when a contraction begins, because often she is unaware of it for perhaps 5 or 10 seconds, sometimes even until the contraction reaches its acme. It is important to observe the frequency and duration of the contractions and to be assured that the uterine muscle relaxes completely after each contraction.

As the labor approaches the transition phase, the contractions become stronger, last about 60 seconds, and occur at 2- to 3-minute intervals. *A pattern of contractions lasting longer than 90 seconds not followed by a rest interval with complete relaxation of the uterine muscle (hyperstimulation, tetanic contractions, or hypertonus) should be reported to the physician immediately.* The implications for the woman and her fetus can be severe (see Chap. 36).

Show

Show is a mucoid discharge from the cervix that is present after the mucous plug has been dislodged. As progressive effacement and dilatation of the cervix occur, the show becomes blood tinged due to the rupture of the superficial capillaries. The presence of an increased amount of bloody show—blood-stained mucus (not actual bleeding)—suggests that rapid progress may be taking place, and the client should be reassessed. Often in conjunction with the increase in bloody show are strong uterine contractions and the urge to push. If by vaginal examination the woman is found to be close to delivery, the physician is notified.

If the increased vaginal bleeding is associated with maternal tachycardia, increased uterine tone and fundal height, decreased hematocrit, or nonreassuring FHR pattern, physician notification and a further workup are warranted to rule out abruptio placentae, uterine rupture, or fetal-maternal hemorrhage. A fetoplacental bleed may not cause a large volume of vaginal bleeding but may be a significant blood loss for the fetus, which at term has an umbilical blood flow of 120 mL/min per kilogram or only 420 mL/min in an average size 3.5-kg (7.7 lbs) term fetus (Arnold-Aldea et al., 1990). Fetoplacental hemorrhage of more than 10 mL has been associated with significant fetal morbidity (Knuppel et al., 1990), with fetal deaths being reported with massive fetomaternal hemorrhages (>30% loss) of more than 150 mL (Laube, 1986). The technique for detecting fetal red blood cells in maternal circulation is known as the Kleihauer-Betke test (Knuppel et al., 1990; Kleihauer et al., 1957).

Vital Signs

Temperature, pulse, and respiration should be evaluated on admission and every 4 hours in normal labor when membranes are intact or more frequently as necessary, depending on the clinical situation and treatments used. The blood pressure also should be evaluated on admission and reassessed regularly as the client's condition warrants (AAP/ACOG, 1992). If membranes have ruptured, it would be wise to evaluate the temperature every 2 hours to screen for the development of amnionitis.

Fetal Heart Rate

Assessment of FHR constitutes one of the most important responsibilities during the intrapartum period. The selection of method and frequency of assessment should reflect the client's condition, department policy, and recommendations of professional organizations. Whether using electronic FHR monitoring or intermittent auscultation with uterine palpation, it is recommended that for low-risk clients, the nurse assesses, interprets, and records FHR every 30 minutes after a contraction in the active phase of the first stage of labor and every 15 minutes in the second stage of labor (AAP/ACOG, 1992).

With high-risk clients, the recommendations are different, but the practitioner still has the choice of electronic fetal monitoring or intermittent auscultation. During the active phase of the first stage of labor, the FHR is evaluated and recorded at least every 15 minutes. During the second stage of labor, the FHR is evaluated and recorded every 5 minutes (AAP/ACOG, 1992).

The electronic fetal monitor is widely used in the hospital setting to assess fetal well-being and evaluate uterine contractions during labor. A thorough discussion of this device can be found in Chapter 40.

As mentioned previously, the fetus must be assessed before and after ambulation, enema administration, artificial rupture of membranes, and the administration of analgesia or anesthesia. It is important to assess FHR immediately after the rupture of membranes because there is a possibility that with the gush of water, the cord may be prolapsed, and any indication of fetal distress from the pressure on the umbilical cord can be detected by a decrease in the FHR. Also, manipulation of the fetal membranes and cervix can stimulate prostaglandin release, mainly $PGF\alpha_2$, causing an increase in myometrial intracellular free calcium by opening calcium channels and by releasing calcium from intracellular stores (Fuchs et al., 1991). Because calcium is the primary trigger for muscle contractility, the result of the artificial rupture of membranes may result in an episode of excessive uterine activity, which could temporarily compromise uteroplacental circulation.

Nursing Diagnoses

Updating the nursing care plan for the client in labor is an ongoing process. Attending to the immediate needs of the client, ensuring comfort, and maintaining maternal and fetal well-being may be the primary areas the nurse is addressing; other identified diagnoses may not be readdressed until the fourth stage of labor or during the postpartum period. Below is a list of possible nursing diagnoses that may be used during the first stage of labor. Related nursing interventions and evaluation criteria are found in the Nursing Care Plan: The Woman/Family During First Stage of Labor.

NURSING CARE PLAN
The Women/Family During First Stage of Labor

Nursing Goals
1. Client is able to verbalize her progress in labor.
2. Client acknowledges increase in comfort by verbal and nonverbal communication when comfort measures are done by the nurse and support person(s).
3. Client, support person, and family continue to demonstrate adequate knowledge of physical surroundings, procedures, and expectations.
4. Support person and family indicate knowledge of client's progress in labor.

Assessment	Potential Nursing Diagnoses	Intervention/ Rationale	Evaluation
Monitor labor, contractions, fetal heart rate (FHR), vital signs.	Altered Tissue Perfusion: placental, secondary to maternal position	Check vital signs regularly per hospital policy and clinical needs *to evaluate labor progress and on-going maternal-fetal health status.* Attach fetal monitor, or time contractions *to evaluate labor progress and on-going maternal-fetal health status.* Check FHR for rate, accelerations, variability, decelerations *to evaluate labor progress and on-going maternal-fetal health status.* Avoid supine position *to prevent compression of aorta and vena cava by gravid uterus.*	Woman has vital signs within normal limits. FHR maintains normal rate. Woman's labor progresses.
Monitor intake and output.	Fluid Volume Deficit related to decreased fluid intake. Altered Oral Mucous Membrane related to mouth breathing. Altered Nutrition: Less than body requirements related to restriction of intake during labor	Give ice chips prn *to prevent dehydration and assure normal kidney function.* Maintain adequate parenteral intake (125 mL/h) *to prevent dehydration and assure normal kidney function.* Encourage voiding q2–3 h; catheterize if needed *to prevent dehydration and assure normal kidney function.* Record intake and output *to prevent dehydration and assure normal kidney function.* Encourage use of lip balm *to prevent dehydration and assure normal kidney function.* Provide mouth care *to prevent dehydration and assure normal kidney function.* Instruct and reinforce proper breathing techniques.	Woman's mouth and lips are moist. Woman's bladder remains normal.

(continued)

NURSING CARE PLAN (Continued)
The Women/Family During First Stage of Labor

Assessment	Potential Nursing Diagnoses	Intervention/ Rationale	Evaluation
Determine which comfort measures are most helpful.	Altered comfort; pain related to labor contractions Self Care Deficit related to immobility during labor (toileting, hygiene)	Rub back and change client's position and linen as necessary *to facilitate pain relief and promote endurance.* Apply cool wash cloth to face *to facilitate pain relief and promote endurance.* Encourage rest *to facilitate pain relief and promote endurance.* Encourage frequent voiding, giving assistance to bathroom or with bedpan *to facilitate pain relief and promote endurance.* Give analgesia if client requests and as ordered by physician *to facilitate pain relief and promote endurance.*	Client breathes appropriately with contractions. Client relaxes between contractions. Client states what comfort measures are most helpful.
Determine client's need for explanations and emotional support as indicated.	Sleep Pattern Disturbance related to labor Ineffective Individual Coping related to inappropriate relaxation and breathing patterns	Keep explanations and instructions short and simple *to promote effective coping of client and family.* Encourage woman to sleep and rest between contractions *to promote effective coping of client and family.* Decrease environmental stimulus *to promote effective coping of client and family.*	Couple changes breathing patterns to coincide with stage of labor. Couple follows instruction with minimum of difficulty. Client rests when able.
Determine support person's ability to coach and support the client. Determine support person's needs.	Knowledge Deficit related to coaching role Ineffective Individual and Family Coping related to hospitalization for the onset of labor Ineffective Family Coping related to client being in pain.	Allow couple time together *to promote effective coping of client and family.* Encourage support person's participation in care *to promote effective coping of client and family.* Explain labor process to client and support person as things progress *to promote effective coping of client and family.* Keep support person(s) in waiting room up to date *to promote effective coping of client and family.*	Support person assists woman in coping with labor. Support person feels a part of the labor process. Client benefits from support person's presence and support.

(continued)

NURSING CARE PLAN *(Continued)*
The Women/Family During First Stage of Labor

Assessment	Potential Nursing Diagnoses	Intervention/ Rationale	Evaluation
		Assist client in changing breathing techniques as labor progresses *to promote effective coping of client and family.* Identify and reinforce adaptive coping behavior *to promote effective coping of client and family.* Provide support to the coach (refreshments, breaks), and reinforce appropriate behavior *to promote effective coping of client and family.*	

Possible psychosocial problems include:

- Health Seeking Behaviors related to
  Hospital procedures
  Process of labor
  Adaptive relaxation techniques
- Fear related to lack of knowledge about or control over impending labor and birth
- Ineffective Individual Coping related to
  Inappropriate relaxation and breathing patterns
  Lack of support systems
  Hospitalization
- Ineffective Family Coping related to
  Client being in pain
  Hospitalization

Possible physiologic problems include:

- Altered Fetal Tissue Perfusion: uteroplacental, or cord blood flow, decreased
- Fluid Volume Deficit related to decreased fluid intake, restricted oral intake in labor
- Sleep Pattern Disturbance related to timing and length of labor
- Pain related to uterine contractions
- Altered Oral Mucous Membrane related to mouth breathing
- Altered Nutrition: Less than body requirements related to labor and decreased oral intake
- Self Care Deficit related to immobility during labor (toileting, hygiene)

Intervention and Rationale

As previously emphasized, the nurse must have an empathic, nonjudgmental, and supportive attitude toward the woman to interpret the progress of labor and perform certain technical procedures skillfully. It should be pointed out that "supportive care" includes not only emotional support, but also aspects of physical care that contribute to the woman's well-being and comfort and hence to her emotional equilibrium. The nursing staff must not just walk into the labor room, review the fetal monitor, and walk out.

The Effective Use of Touch

Many of the physical care activities that nurses perform consist, in part at least, of "laying on of hands." This type of communication can be a way of demonstrating the nurse's concern and empathy, especially when verbal communication is difficult or impossible. This contact can take the form of a back rub, stroking the client's brow, and so forth. Many of the relaxation techniques practiced in the prepared childbirth classes rely on the use of touch. Even the intrusive procedures that are so often painful or distasteful, if done with gentleness and skill, show the client that her dignity and integrity are respected.

However, touch should not be used indiscriminately; excessive or inappropriate touching is offensive to some people. The need varies from person to person, and the woman indicates which type of touch is helpful and who is the most appropriate person to give it. The nurse must use professional judgment regarding its use, and rapport with the client helps to indicate a correct decision. It also is an effective means of incorporating the partner into the care and support of his or her significant other.

In the late active phase, the woman may need someone to hold onto during the severe contractions. The woman responds less well to other physical contact, such as stroking and sponging; she may even say, "Leave me alone." However, if it is helpful for her to have someone's hand to hold, she should be encouraged to do this.

Supportive Milieu

The woman who has attended prenatal classes that have included exercise and relaxation techniques is usually better prepared for labor, but nevertheless she needs to be coached in using the techniques that enable her to cooperate with the natural forces of labor. During early labor, the client usually prefers to move around the room and frequently is more at ease sitting in a comfortable chair. She can be permitted and encouraged to do this and whatever else seems to be most relaxing and pleasant to her if there are no contraindicating conditions.

Once labor is well established, the laboring woman should not be left alone. The morale of women in labor is sometimes hopelessly shattered when they are left by themselves for long periods, regardless of whether or not they have been prepared for labor during pregnancy. During labor, most women are more sensitive to the behavior of those around them, particularly in relation to her perception of how much concern healthcare personnel show for her safety and well-being. As labor progresses, there is a normal narrowing of the phenomenal field, an "inward turning," which results in easy distortion of stimuli and perception. For instance, careless remarks dropped in conversation often are misinterpreted as indicative of negligence or lack of feeling. Comments and laughter overheard in the corridor outside the client's room may contribute to her uneasiness. Therefore, the nurse must be on guard against unfortunate happenings of this kind.

The nurse should be aware that her own anxieties in the situation may be communicated to the client. The process of labor and the forthcoming birth produce normal anxieties that are no more than a healthy anticipation of the events to come (in client and nurse). Thus, most clients tolerate their labor better if they are told the kind of progress that is being made and are assured that they are doing a good job working with their contractions. This is part of the continuing orientation to the labor process that was mentioned previously.

The nurse should not underestimate the usefulness of suggestion for the woman in labor. Because the woman responds readily to suggestions, especially in early labor, the nurse can use suggestibility to great advantage in her supportive care. The groundwork can be laid at this time for the more complicated instructions that may be necessary later in labor concerning relaxation, breathing techniques, and the management of pain.

Assisting With Maternal Birthing Positions

Many hospitals attach an electronic fetal monitor to the client routinely for fetal assessment during labor. The woman must be in bed for this equipment to function appropriately. This, of course, limits her mobility. The reason for the use of the monitor needs to be explained to the client so that she can understand why her activity is restricted and will not become unduly alarmed. If the client asks to ambulate, the nurse must get an order from the physician. Most facilities allow ambulation if the initial FHR tracing is reassuring, the presenting part is engaged or the bag of waters is intact, and ambulation is not contraindicated because of a high-risk condition or treatment. The woman should come back to the labor room for periodic auscultation of the FHR (ie, every 30 minutes). The newer fetal monitors with improved electronics allow for better tracings on the external mode and allow more maternal movement to positions of comfort. Changes in position and transducer adjustments should be noted on the strip chart.

If monitors are not used and no contraindicating high-risk conditions exist, the client can be encouraged to assume any position that is comfortable for her, such as side, semisitting, squatting, all fours, or sitting (Fig. 22-3). Generally, women should avoid laboring on

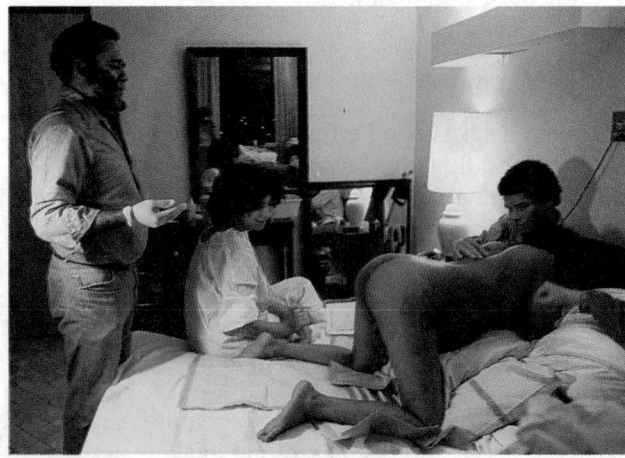

FIGURE 22-3 The woman in labor should be encouraged to assume any position that is comfortable for her.

their back, because the weight of the gravid uterus could theoretically compress the major maternal vessels. With vena caval occlusion, the return of blood to the heart is decreased, and this might result in a fall in maternal cardiac output, maternal hypotension, and decreased uterine blood flow. Compression of the aorta against the spine or iliac vessels as they cross the pelvic brim might result in decreases in uterine blood flow without maternal hypotension (Freeman et al., 1991). Thus for many clients, contractions become stronger and less frequent when the woman changes position from her back to her side, because the uteroplacetal perfusion improves (Fig. 22-4; Caldeyro-Barcia et al., 1960).

Fortunately, many women do not have significant major vessel compression while on their backs; with close fetal surveillance and adequate uterine progress, most clients could assume the supine position if this is their preferred position of comfort, as long as no complications arise. Allowing a woman to assume a comfortable position may help reduce her anxiety, which can have profound beneficial physiologic effects.

Many women and birth attendants prefer the left lateral **Sims' position** for laboring. The woman lies on her left side with her left leg extended and her right knee flexed at her side or pulled up against the abdomen or with both knees flexed. Pillows may be used for support and to prevent pressure. Women who prefer this position report that it increases comfort and is less intrusive. The position promotes placental blood flow and prevents supine hypotension. Contractions may be more intense and less frequent (more efficient). Because the perineum is more relaxed, the need for an episiotomy and the potential for perineal lacera-

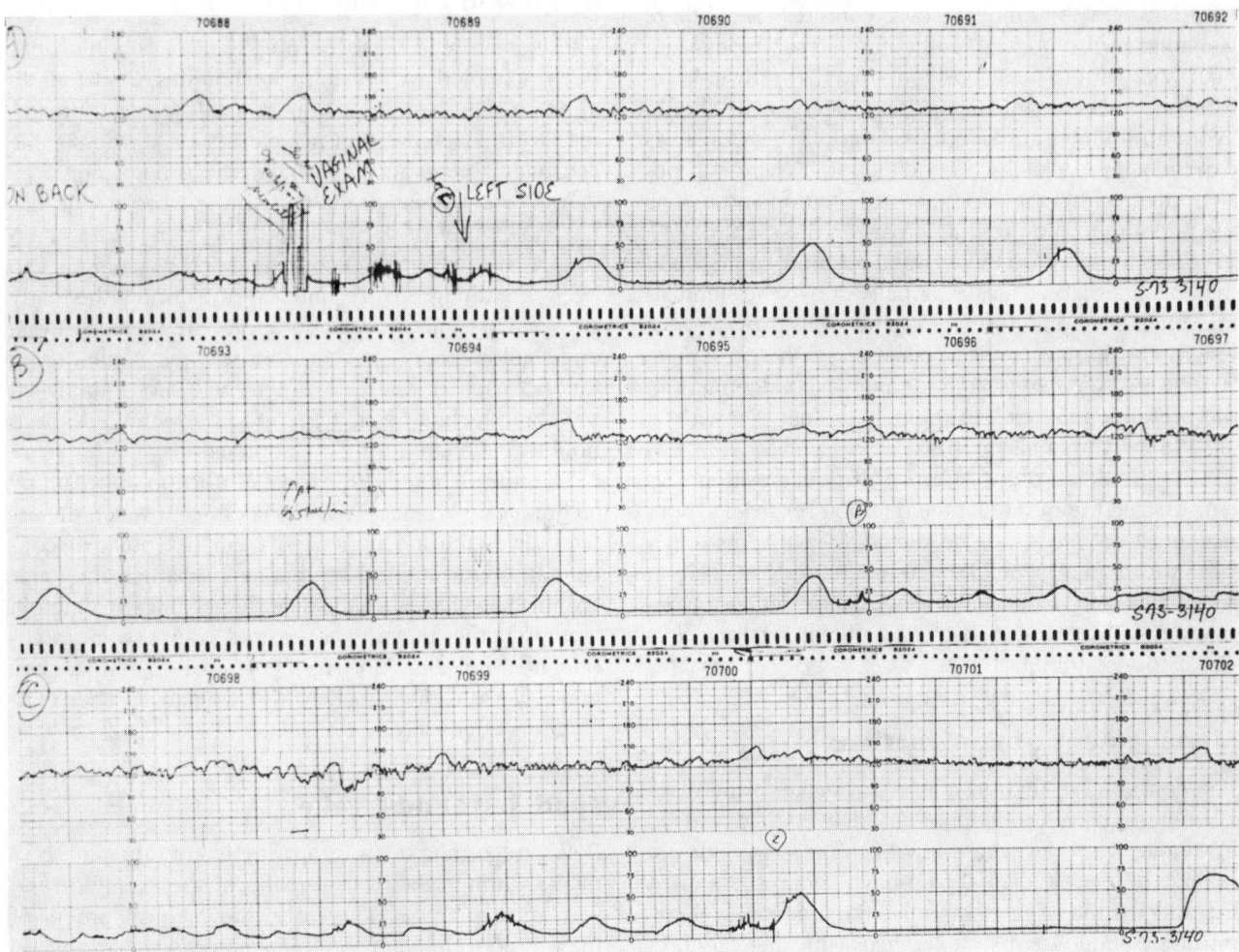

FIGURE 22-4 Uterine contractions. (**A**) Frequent uterine contractions are occurring. When the client is turned to her left side, the contractions become less frequent and increase in strength. (**B**) The woman has turned and is lying on her back; the contractions have become frequent and smaller. (**C**) Again on her left side, the contractions are spaced out as in A. (Freeman, R., & Garite, T. [1981]. *Fetal heart rate monitoring.* Baltimore: Williams & Wilkins.)

tions is reduced. Disadvantages include the fact that access to the birth process for the attendant is reduced and it may be more difficult to obtain a consistent FHR.

The squatting position may be preferred by some women because it makes positive use of gravity, although some birth attendants object to a position that makes the perineum somewhat inaccessible and increases the difficulty of fetal monitoring and use of instruments. Squatting may not be a position the woman wishes to keep for a long time, because knees and hips can grow tired after a while.

Position changes during labor can improve maternal comfort; the woman may find that she prefers various positions at various points in the labor, and the nurse should help her to assume whichever position seems most comfortable and safe for the woman and fetus. Frequent position changes may help with promoting fetal rotation and descent. Sometimes a position change will help to relieve mild fetal distress if the distress is caused by umbilical cord compression. If there is evidence of umbilical cord compression, monitoring FHR with various fetal positions may help provide information about which positions the woman should avoid and which are safe to assume. If the woman is experiencing backache, or back labor, a change in positioning may help to promote fetal rotation and relieve the pressure of the presenting part on the sacrum.

For some women, the upright position while walking enhances labor. This is partially due to the stimulating effect on the intensity of contractions, the effect of gravity on the improved application of the presenting part against the cervix, and the improved alignment of the presenting vertex into the pelvic canal (Fenwick et al., 1987; Flynn et al., 1978).

This discussion of the effects of various positions has emphasized the point that the decision regarding "optimal position" needs to be dictated by the maternal-fetal effects in a given client at a certain time in labor; it often is a dynamic inter-relationship, requiring ongoing modifications to maintain optimal maternal-fetal circulatory conditions.

Management of Contractions

The contribution that the nurse can make in the management of pain during labor and delivery is discussed in Chapter 23. However, a few of the major points are reiterated here. Studies of pain have demonstrated that the anticipation of pain can raise the anxiety level significantly and lower pain tolerance. Thus, the client reacts sooner to even minimal pain stimuli. The pain is subjectively intensified and even a slight amount of pain seems great. Furthermore, other sensations may be misinterpreted as pain (eg, pressure, stretching), which explains why the digital examinations and even the pressure of the nurse's fingers on the abdomen as

she manually times contractions cause women to recoil in pain. Every intervention becomes painful, and the heightening of the anticipation of pain increases the response to pain; soon a vicious cycle is established.

The nurse can help to break this cycle or prevent it from becoming established by intervening at the anticipation–anxiety junction. This is done by reminding the client that a contraction is over (and the pain is gone) and that because another contraction is not expected for several minutes, this is the time for her to rest and relax. The anxiety related to the anticipation of pain is lowered or eliminated (the woman knows that she will be free from pain for several minutes and can rest), and the subjective intensification is diminished. It is obvious that the nurse or some other reliable person should be in continuous attendance to do this.

Breathing Techniques

The woman who has been prepared for childbirth has been schooled in breathing techniques, such as diaphragmatic breathing or rapid, shallow costal breathing. With coaching from her partner or her nurse, she is usually able to accomplish conscious relaxation.

A different situation exists with the woman who has had no childbirth preparation. It is often best to help such a client relax by encouraging and coaching her to keep breathing slowly and evenly during the early contractions and to assume a pattern of more rapid and shallow breathing that is most comfortable during the late active phase. Women with no training in breathing techniques may need to be reminded not to hold their breath during the contractions.

The nurse should not expect perfection in breathing techniques with these (or any) clients; however, the activity gives the inexperienced woman a point of concentration and the feeling that she is participating and "controlling" her labor to some degree. Most women in labor, whether they are "prepared" or not, want to cooperate. The calm, kind, firm guidance of an interested nurse can do much to help the woman use her contractions effectively.

Food and Fluid Intake

Beliefs regarding the appropriateness of fluid and food intake during labor vary greatly in the literature and in clinical practice. Therefore, the medical orders of the physician in charge and in some cases the anesthesiologist need to be ascertained before proceeding. In the hospital setting, it is customary to limit oral intake to ice chips. If the client is admitted in the latent phase of labor, the physician may order a clear liquid diet. The client in active labor is usually not given solid or liquid foods because many women experience nausea and vomiting during labor and delivery. The other concern is the potential risk of aspiration of gastric contents. Gastric emptying is slower in pregnancy than in the nonpregnant state, and labor may contribute to a slowing in gastric contents. Proponents of allowing women in labor to eat might consider limiting this practice to healthy women with no risk factors and to labors that are unmedicated (Douglas, 1988). It is common practice in American hospitals to limit the oral intake to women in labor to ice chips, clear fluids, or even nothing.

Nursing interventions to combat the dry mouth and potential for dehydration are to provide mouth care and offer clear fluids or ice chips. The nurse may increase client comfort by using a washcloth to moisten the mouth and lips; use of lip balm also is encouraged. The woman may be encouraged to brush her teeth or rinse her mouth with mouthwash, normal saline, or water.

Intravenous fluid administration for all labors is common practice in hospitals. Administration of an IV in early labor is probably not necessary, and delayed start of an IV may be an intervention that allows women more freedom for ambulation. Intravenous solutions are started for the following reasons:

- Prevention of dehydration, electrolyte imbalance, and acidosis
- A "life line" for emergencies
- Usually required before the administration of analgesia, anesthesia
- Administration of oxytocin prophylactically after the delivery to prevent uterine atony

Bladder Care

The client should be encouraged to void at least every 3 hours (AAP/ACOG, 1992). The laboring woman often attributes all of her discomfort to the intensity of uterine contractions and therefore is unaware that the pressure of a full bladder has increased her discomfort. With epidural anesthesia, she may be unable to sense bladder fullness. In addition to causing unnecessary discomfort, a full bladder may be a serious impediment to labor or the cause of urinary retention in the puerperium. If the distended bladder can be palpated above the symphysis pubis and the client is unable to void, the physician should be notified. Straight catheterization may be prescribed in such cases.

Progression of Active Phase of Labor

As labor progresses into the active phase, the woman's mood changes and she "gets down to business." She begins to concentrate on her breathing techniques and needs assistance from her support person. She needs help to get in a position of comfort. Regardless of how diligently the woman has practiced the various breathing and relaxing techniques during pregnancy or the level of her understanding about the physiology of labor, the woman's confidence may waiver somewhat during active labor. Encouragement should be given to the woman and her partner or support person. The nurse remains with the client, providing care in an organized, calm manner; instructions need to be short and direct. Nursing care measures include mouth care, keeping ice chips available, placing a cool washcloth on the woman's forehead, keeping the perineum clean and dry, lowering the lights and keeping the environment quiet, providing counterpressure on the sacral area during contractions, and updating the physician and family members on the progress. Also, the nurse may want to suggest that the woman's partner take some nourishment before the actual birth. As labor progresses (ie, 8–10 cm), the nurse should continue to encourage correct breathing techniques and assist the client not to bear down prematurely, which may cause cervical swelling. The client should be reassured that she will soon be completely dilated and will be ready to start to push.

Second Stage of Labor

The second stage of labor begins with complete dilatation of the cervix and ends with the birth. The complete dilatation of the cervix can be definitely confirmed only by a vaginal examination. However, the experienced nurse is often able to suspect complete dilatation by observing changes in the client's behavior, particularly if these findings are correlated with knowledge of the client's parity, the speed of any previous labors and the present labor, and the anticipated size of the newborn.

The median duration of the second stage of labor has been shown to be 50 minutes for the primipara and 20 minutes for the multipara (Cunningham et al., 1993). The length of the second stage can vary considerably, but by clinical risk category, it has traditionally been considered prolonged if more than 2 hours (O'Brien et al., 1991). However, if descent is progressive and electronic fetal monitoring used for close surveillance, a longer second stage can be a safe option and operative intervention may not be necessary (Cohen, 1977). To determine if the duration of second stage is significantly increasing the risk of birth injury, the nurse must always keep in mind "who" is going through this process. Characteristics such as a large fetus (≥ 9 lbs), a post-term pregnancy (≥ 41 weeks), a smaller size woman (≤ 5 feet), or a more difficult presentation (eg, occiput posterior) *in-*

crease the likelihood of cephalopelvic disproportion or fetal distress. If these conditions occur, a cesarean birth may be necessary to prevent second stage birth injuries.

Assessment

Certain behavioral and physical signs and symptoms herald the onset of the second stage of labor. The nurse should watch for these carefully (Box 22-2). Prompt reporting of these manifestations allows enough time to prepare the woman for the birth without rushing and provides an opportunity to cleanse and drape the woman properly. If these signs are overlooked, a precipitous birth may occur without benefit of medical attention. In the traditional setting, in which different rooms are used for labor and the delivery, the primigravida is usually not taken to the delivery room when the cervix is fully dilated and may push in the labor room for some time before transfer. She may not be transferred to the delivery room until perineal bulging or the beginning of crowning is observed. In contrast, the multipara is taken to the delivery room much sooner, often at 7 to 8 cm of dilatation. The use of epidural anesthesia during labor usually delays transfer of the multipara also, and she may even push in the labor room for a while, much like the primigravida.

Nursing Diagnoses

As the client begins the second stage of labor, she begins to realize that the dilatation phase of labor is done. The final part of labor, the pushing stage, is about to begin. Below is a list of potential nursing diagnoses:

- Ineffective Individual Coping related to physical exhaustion with labor
- Pain related to lower fetal position and uterine contractions
- Fear related to new surroundings (if moved to a delivery room)

Intervention and Rationale

Methods for Bearing Down

During the second stage of labor, the client is asked to exert her abdominal forces and bear down. In most cases, bearing-down efforts are involuntary, reflexive, and spontaneous in the second stage of labor, but there is a voluntary component as well. If the woman has had epidural anesthesia, she may not be able to bear down easily on demand, because she will not feel the urge to push. However, she should be encouraged to try.

Positions and Pushing Efforts. The positions used during the second stage of labor must allow the presenting

---

BOX 22–2
Signs and Symptoms of Second Stage

1. The client begins to bear down of her own accord; this is caused by a reflex when the head begins to press on the perineal floor.
2. Her mood of increasing apprehension, which has been building since the contractions began, deepens; she becomes more serious and may appear bewildered by the force of the contractions.
3. There is usually a sudden increase in show, which is more blood tinged.
4. The client may become increasingly irritable and unwilling to be touched; she may cry if disturbed.
5. The client may vomit or report that she feels nauseous.
6. The woman thinks that she needs to defecate. This symptom is due to pressure of the head on the perineal floor and consequently against the rectum.
7. Although she has been "working" successfully with her contractions during most of her labor, the uncertainty that she has been experiencing (since 6–8 cm cervical dilatation) as to her ability to cope with the contractions may become overwhelming; she is frustrated and feels unable to manage if left alone.
8. The membranes may rupture, with discharge of amniotic fluid. This, of course, may take place any time but occurs most frequently at the beginning of the second stage.
9. The woman may be saying at this time that she wants to be "put to sleep" or have a cesarean section owing to the increased pain and the desire for labor to be done. The woman's consciousness is somewhat altered because of the pain, her enforced concentration, and possibly medication; therefore, any coaching needs to be short and explicit and may need to be repeated with each contraction. The nurse also must be firm but gentle in setting limits with the woman, so that she can conserve her energy for the second stage. Thrashing about and continued crying only lead to exhaustion, and the woman needs the firm guidance of a skillful person to help her to maintain control.
10. The perineum begins to bulge and the anal orifice begins to dilate. This is a late sign, but if signs numbered 1, 3, 5, and 7 occur, it should be watched for with every contraction. Only a vaginal examination or the appearance of the head can definitely confirm the suspicion.

Zlatnik, F. (1994). Normal labor and delivery. In Scott, J., DiSaia, P., Hammond, C., Spellocy, W. (Eds). Danforth's obstetrics and gynecology. 7th edn. Philadelphia: J.B. Lippincott.

part to be in alignment with the axis of the pelvis. The student may find that in the hospital setting, the semi-Fowler and lateral positions are frequently used. Other positions, such as squatting, kneeling, standing, and semisitting, are becoming more popular but require the staff to be flexible in their provision of care (Fig. 22-5; Golay et al., 1993; Biancuzzo, 1993). It is valuable when assessing appropriate positioning to take into consideration the radiologic studies that have shown that squatting increases the diameter of the pelvic outlet by as much as 0.5 to 2.0 cm (Borell et al., 1967; Russell, 1969).

Previously, the bearing-down efforts were thought to be best when the client used long and sustained pushes with no audible sounds made. This methodology is being changed in conjunction with research showing the disadvantage on woman and fetus with repetitive **Valsalva's maneuvers.** Caldeyro-Barcia's (1979) recommendations include the following:

■ Short pushes of no longer than 6 to 7 seconds
■ Physiologic pushing: pushing only with the urge to

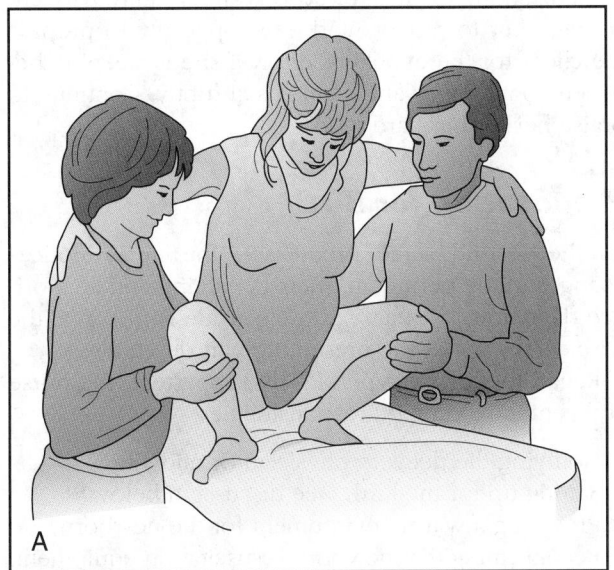

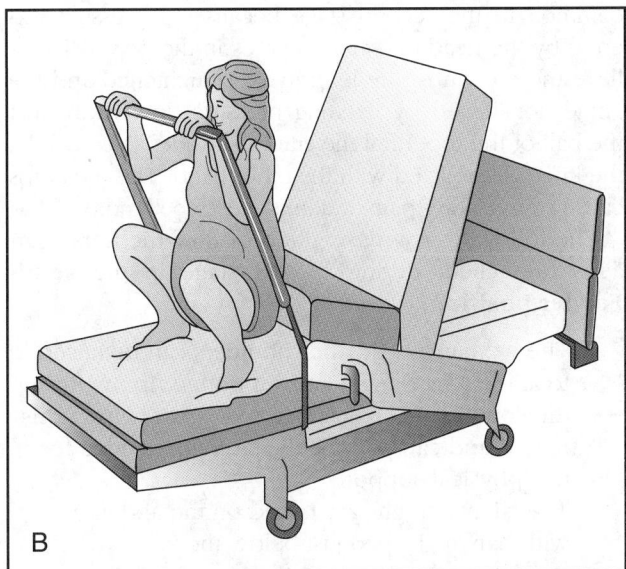

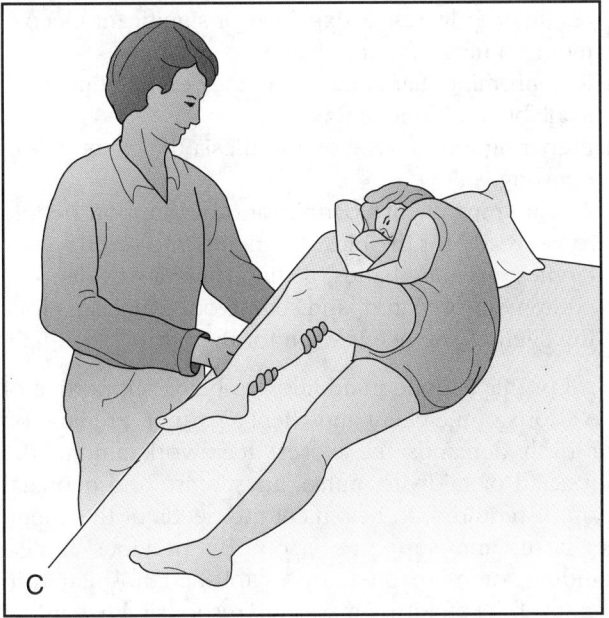

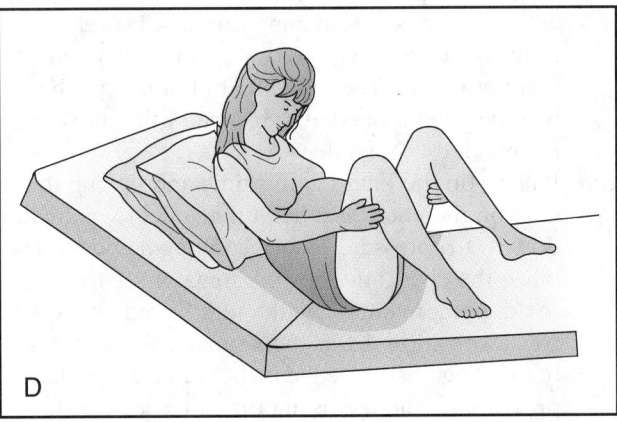

FIGURE 22–5 Positions for pushing during the second stage of labor. (**A**) Squatting with help. (**B**) Squatting with squat bar. (**C**) Pushing in side-lying position. (**D**) Pushing in sitting position.

push or approximately three to five times during each contraction
- Pushing with an open glottis and slight exhale

The woman should be encouraged to listen to her body. Caregivers may treat all clients the same in this stage, but it is incorrect to assume that all labors are the same. The uterus decides the amount of effort and the timing of that effort during the second stage (Carr, 1983). The nurse should review with the couple the type of pushing method they learned in prepared childbirth classes and adapt as necessary. The nurse should facilitate a quiet environment and encourage total relaxation between contractions. Muscular cramps in the legs are common in the second stage because of pressure exerted by the head on certain nerves in the pelvis. To relieve these cramps, the leg can be straightened and the ankle dorsiflexed by exerting pressure upward against the ball of the foot until the cramp subsides. Meanwhile, the knee is stabilized with the other hand. These cramps cause excruciating pain and must never be ignored.

The following is a description of how the nurse can assist the client during second stage in the **semi-Fowler position:**

1. The woman's head and shoulders can be raised to a 45-degree angle and supported firmly during the contraction. The father is of great help in this regard and can provide the strength needed for this physical support.
2. The client's thighs are flexed on the abdomen, with hands grasped just below the knees when a contraction begins.
3. The client can be encouraged to work with the urge to push, using short, 5-second pushes, with the glottis open. She should be instructed that the action is similar to straining during a bowel movement or trying to blow up a balloon that will not inflate. The long breath-holding pushes may be used if needed to hasten birth, but should be avoided if possible.
4. Pulling on the knees at this time and flexing the chin on the chest, is a helpful adjunct to maintain downward pressure of the diaphragm and to stabilize the chest and the abdominal musculature.
5. In addition, maintaining the legs flexed as for the "push" position deters the woman from pushing her feet against the table or bed. Avoiding such pressure on the feet is important because it discourages tensing of the gluteal muscles and contributes to further relaxation of the pelvic floor.

Psychosocial Support

During the second stage, the woman becomes increasingly involved in the whole birth process. The seemingly panicky frustration of the late active phase subsides a bit (with appropriate coaching and reassurance), and the client may experience a sense of relief that the expulsive stage has begun. The desire to push and bear down is strong—uncontrollable, in fact—and the client generally gets enormous satisfaction with each push. Some clients, however, experience acute pain and need all available help and encouragement to continue bearing down. In most instances, there is complete exhaustion after each expulsive effort, and the woman often drops off to sleep, only to be roused by the next contraction. Because consciousness is still altered, it may be difficult for the woman to follow directions readily even though she may want to. Repeated, short, explicit directions are required to encourage her to rest or work but especially to prepare the client for the expulsive effort if she is sleeping between contractions and awakens abruptly. Continue to praise her for her hard work.

Preparation for Birth

As the second stage progresses, the nurse notices changes in the perineum, such as bulging and anal orifice dilatation; if a fetal scalp electrode is in place, the wire comes out as the presenting part descends.

Regardless of the type of delivery system, the nurse at this time has certain responsibilities:

- Notifying the delivery physician or midwife
- Setting up for the birth (see discussion below)
- Providing a warm environment for the newborn
- Reconfirming that newborn resuscitation equipment is present and functioning
- Notifying the neonatal team to attend the birth if respiratory distress is expected or significant meconium staining of amniotic fluid is present
- Reconfirming that adult emergency equipment is available and functioning
- Preparing for the type of anesthesia the client is requesting
- Assisting the client's partner or other support people to get ready for the birth: changing into scrub clothes, washing hands, getting camera or video equipment prepared, and setting out eyeglasses for the client if she needs them for the birth

All of this is done in addition to being supportive of the efforts of the client and client's partner. Preparation for birth demands the closest teamwork among the physician or midwife, nurse, anesthetist, and neonatal team, if required, to best meet the needs of the client, newborn, and support person. By previous understanding, or more often by established hospital routine, each has their own specific responsibilities in the delivery room.

The primary focus for the nurse has been on direct client care. Now she must enlarge her focus to include the physician and other allied professionals (ie, more activities require the assistance of these people than was necessary during the first stage of labor). Thus, the nurse must be sensitive not only to the cues sent by the woman, but also to those relayed by the other personnel.

As stated previously, many women now are able to labor, deliver, and recover in the same room and thus do not have to be transferred to a delivery room when birth is imminent. Set-ups vary considerably from birthing room to delivery suite and from hospital to hospital. There are some general considerations for the preparation of each at the time of delivery, however.

Preparation of the Birthing Room

Most birthing rooms have a bed that can be adapted for birth by removing or lowering a small section at the bottom of the bed. Stirrups are available if needed. The birth attendant and all healthcare personnel wear sterile gloves and use sterile equipment, but scrub attire is usually not required. Good handwashing techniques are essential, however. Although every institution has its own set of protocols, the nurse is generally responsible for making sure that at least the following pieces of equipment are on hand when birth seems imminent

For the birth:

- Sterile gloves
- Prep set for perineal scrub prior to birth
- Cord set (eg, scissors, clamps)
- Sterile towels, drape, gown (often in a disposable pack)
- Warm sterile water

For the newborn:

- Radiant warmer for the newborn
- Sterile, warmed infant blankets
- Bulb syringe
- Suction equipment
- Oxygen
- Laryngoscope
- Resuscitation set with necessary emergency equipment

Preparation of the Delivery Room

In no two hospitals is the delivery room setup or the procedure for birth precisely the same. Therefore, observation and experience in a particular institution are the basis for becoming acquainted with the physical layout and the method of care offered. The following, however, gives a general idea of the equipment and materials used in a typical setting.

The delivery table or bed is designed so that its surface is actually composed of two adjoining sections, each covered with its own mattress. This permits the client to lie on her back in the supine position or with her head and back elevated; if it is not possible to raise the back section, a large wedge-type pillow or regular bed pillows can be used until the woman must put her legs up into stirrups or into the lithotomy position. The woman is still at risk for hypotension due to compression of the gravid uterus on the inferior vena cava. To avoid this, the nurse may want to wedge or tilt the woman using folded towels or a sandbag under her right hip to shift the uterus off the vein and maintain venous return. The table is "broken" by a mechanical device. The retractable or lower end of the table drops and is rolled under the main section of the table, allowing ready access to the perineal region. If the client will deliver in the dorsal recumbent position, the lower portion of the table can remain in place.

The table opposite the foot of the delivery table, the back table, contains the principal sterile supplies and instruments needed for normal childbirth, including sterile gowns, drapes, towels, sponges, basins, and cord set. The cord set is a group of instruments used for clamping and cutting the umbilical cord: two Kelly clamps, a pair of bandage scissors, and a cord clamp. Other instruments often are included because it may be necessary for the birth attendant to perform an episiotomy or to repair lacerations. Other instruments frequently included are two Kelly clamps, two Allis clamps, one mouse-tooth tissue forceps, two sponge sticks, two tenacula, one needle holder, and straight scissors. The nurse adds to this setup sterile gloves of the correct size, bulb syringe, syringe with large-bore needle for cord blood sample, and if needed, local anesthesia tray with anesthetic solution, catheter, and suture.

A single- or double-bowl solution stand or basin rack is used to hold warm sterile water or normal saline. Depending on the birth attendant's preference, the nurse may be asked to put an antimicrobial solution into the basin. If the double-bowl stand is used, the other basin may be used to place the placenta; this depends on the facility's preference. A prep set used to prepare the perineal area needs to be set up. Prep sets range from a small basin with sponges, to which the nurse must add antimicrobial solution and warm sterile water, to a prep set that the manufacturer prepares, requiring only that the nurse open it, put on the sterile gloves, and do the prep. To prepare for the newborn, a radiant warmer and a resuscitator are present with the necessary emergency equipment.

Asepsis and Antisepsis

Any person with a communicable disease or any person who has been in contact with a communicable disease should be excluded from maternity service until examined by a physician. Only after a physician has certified that the employee is free from infections should he or she be allowed to return to duty. Personnel with evidence of upper respiratory tract infections or open skin lesions, diarrhea, or any other infectious disease also should be excluded. Furthermore, all people working in the maternity area should have a pre-employment physical examination and rubella titers and such interim examinations as may be required by the hospital.

Of prime importance in the second stage of labor are strict asepsis and antisepsis throughout the entire birth. To this end, everyone in a formal delivery room wears clean scrubs and cap. Those actually participating in the childbirth are in sterile attire. Masking includes nose and mouth, but most facilities have reevaluated the need for a mask for a normal birth and do not require one. Caps are to be adjusted to keep *all* hair covered. If the nurse scrubs to assist the doctor, the strict aseptic technique is observed. The hands are scrubbed as carefully as for a surgical operation. Scrubbing the hands should be started sufficiently early to allot full time for the scrub and to don gown and gloves. In many hospitals, caps and masks are no longer required. Most physicians still wear caps and masks, however, because of the need to repair the episiotomy.

Transfer of the Woman to the Delivery Room

For women who are to be transferred to a delivery room for the birth, transfer occurs when birth appears imminent. Transfer to the delivery room can be a stressful time for the woman; contributing factors include temperature, environment, bed, and potential staff changes. One of the greatest benefits of maternity centers with the LDR method of care is that this transfer is not necessary.

If the woman's partner has chosen not to accompany the woman to the delivery room, time is allowed for them to bid each other a temporary goodbye. This kind of planning not only is supportive, but also enables both to cooperate more fully. If the support person is going to the delivery room, he or she should be changed into appropriate scrubs, cap, and mask, if needed, and ready with camera equipment, if appropriate.

Care should be taken to have only one person instruct or coach the woman at any one time. When birth is imminent, her attention is limited, as previously illustrated, and the sound of several voices at one time is confusing.

The nurse should know what type of anesthesia will be used before the actual transfer to the delivery room. The immediate positioning of the client in the delivery room depends on the type of anesthesia used, so this information is essential to the functioning of the team.

Positioning for Anesthesia

If regional anesthesia is to be administered, the client is usually turned on her side. If she is given a saddle block, she may be placed on her side or assisted to a sitting position on the side of the delivery table, with her feet supported on a stool and her body leaning forward against the nurse. Her back should be toward the operator and bowed (the position requires flexion of the neck and the lumbar spine). This principle of cervical and lumbar flexion is used also in the side-lying position (see Chap. 23). A caudal or epidural anesthesia may be started in the labor room.

Although the positioning and the administration of the anesthesia take only a few minutes, the woman may be extremely uncomfortable because of the severity of the contractions at this time; she can be assured that this discomfort is only temporary. The FHR and the maternal blood pressure are checked every 5 minutes or so. In addition, the woman's head should be elevated with at least two pillows to help prevent the anesthetic level from rising beyond the desired height. To allow the anesthetic level to stabilize, the nurse waits for instructions from the anesthetist before putting the woman's legs in stirrups or performing any other manipulations. Local or pudendal anesthesia is administered with the woman in the lithotomy position.

Positioning for Birth

An important nursing responsibility is helping the woman obtain a position that is safe and as comfortable as possible. There is no one perfect position for delivery, although many hospitals and birth attendants prefer the lithotomy position with or without stirrups because it allows for the most access to the perineum and control over the birth process. Any position that aids in the bearing-down efforts of the woman, promotes fetal descent and rotation, and avoids supine hypotension should be encouraged. Modern delivery tables allow for a variety of positions that allow for good visualization of the process and good access. The nurse and support person often will stand at either side of the woman and support her back in a semisitting position, at the same time steadying her legs (Zlatnik, 1994). The woman may grasp her legs at the knees as she did during the pushing phase of the second stage. This position allows visualization of the perineum and adequate prepping and draping of the area.

Before the woman's legs are placed in stirrups or leg holders of some type, cotton flannel boots that cover the entire leg are put on. When the legs are placed in the stirrups or holders, care is taken not to separate the legs too widely or to have one leg higher than the other. Both legs are raised or lowered at the same time, with a nurse supporting each leg if the woman is unable to help in the positioning. Failure to observe

RESEARCH HIGHLIGHT

The Effects of Maternal Squatting Position on Second Stage of Labor

This cohort study was designed to evaluate the effects of the maternal squatting position for the second stage of labor on the evolution and progress of labor and on maternal and fetal well-being. Outcomes from 200 squatting births, randomly selected from a sample of 1,000, were compared with 100 semirecumbent births, randomly selected from a sample of 300. Data collection was by chart review. Results revealed that the mean length of the second stage of labor was 23 minutes shorter for primiparas and 13 minutes shorter for multiparas in the squatting group than women in the semirecumbent group. When the rates of oxytocin induction during the second stage were compared, the semirecumbent group required more medication to enhance contractions than the squatting group (p = 0.0016). Significantly fewer and less severe perineal lacerations occurred, and fewer episiotomies were performed in the squatting group (p = 0.0001). No significant differences were found between groups for third-stage complications and newborn complications. Based on these results, it was concluded that upright positions increase the efficiency and effectiveness of maternal expulsive efforts, resulting in significantly shorter second stages for primiparas and multiparas. This has consequential implications for maternal and fetal well-being.

Critique: The findings of this study should be considered in light of several limitations. The research design was historic and involved a nonexperimental approach with retrospective data analysis. This design limits generalizations of findings to larger samples. The samples were recruited from two different settings, level II and III hospitals, that reportedly had similar protocols but may have differed in terms of physical environment and professionals employed. Data collection techniques were not standardized because many clinicians without prior training for this study were recording duration of the stages of labor. The methods for implementing positional interventions may have differed widely among caregivers. The reader is given no information about possible effects of confounding variables (eg, use of medications, childbirth preparation).

Golay, J., Vedam, S., & Sorger, L. (1993). The squatting position for the second stage of labor: Effects on labor and on maternal and fetal well-being. *Birth, 20*, 73–87.

these principles may strain the ligaments of the pelvis, with consequent discomfort in the puerperium. Care should be taken to avoid pressure on the popliteal space and to angle the stirrups so that the feet are not dependent.

If stirrups are used during the birth, the client can be given handles to grip and pull on, which aid her in her bearing-down efforts. The stirrups support the legs and should be covered with a towel for the woman's comfort, before placing her legs in them.

Preparing the Perineum

When the woman is positioned on the birthing or delivery table or bed, the nurse carries out the procedure for cleansing the vulva and the surrounding area (Fig. 22-6). If the birth is to be conducted with the client in the recumbent position, this may be done with the knees drawn up slightly and the legs separated. Once the birth attendant has scrubbed and donned sterile gown and gloves, the client is draped with towels and sheets appropriate for the purpose.

After the client has been prepared for birth, catheterization, if needed, is carried out. Sometimes it is difficult to catheterize a client in the second stage of labor because the fetus' head may compress the urethra. If the catheter does not pass easily, it should not be forced. If available, a mirror may be positioned so the couple can view the birth.

Birth

As the fetus descends the birth canal, pressure against the rectum may cause fecal material to be expelled. Sponges (as a rule with saline solution) may be used to remove any fecal material that may escape from the rectum.

Fundal pressure should not be used to accomplish spontaneous birth or to bring the head deeper into the birth canal. Severe fundal pressure may cause uterine damage or rupture.

As soon as the head distends the vaginal orifice to a diameter of 6 or 8 cm (crowning) a towel may be placed over the rectum while forward pressure is exerted on the newborn's chin with one hand, at the same time that downward pressure is applied to the occiput by the other hand. This technique, called the Ritgen maneuver (Fig. 22-7), provides control of the head as it emerges and directs the extension phase of birth so that the head is born with the smallest diameter presenting. The head is usually delivered between contractions and as slowly as possible. At this time, the woman may complain about a "splitting" sensation caused by the extreme vaginal stretching as the head is born.

Control of the head by the Ritgen maneuver, extension, and slow delivery between contractions help to prevent lacerations. If a tear seems to be inevitable, an incision called an **episiotomy** may be made in the perineum. This prevents lacerations and facilitates the delivery.

Immediately after the birth of the head, the mouth and nose are routinely suctioned with the bulb syringe. If there has been meconium-stained amniotic fluid, the oropharynx also must be suctioned with a DeLee suction catheter attached to a mucus trap while the head is still on the perineum to prevent meconium aspiration at the time of the first breath.

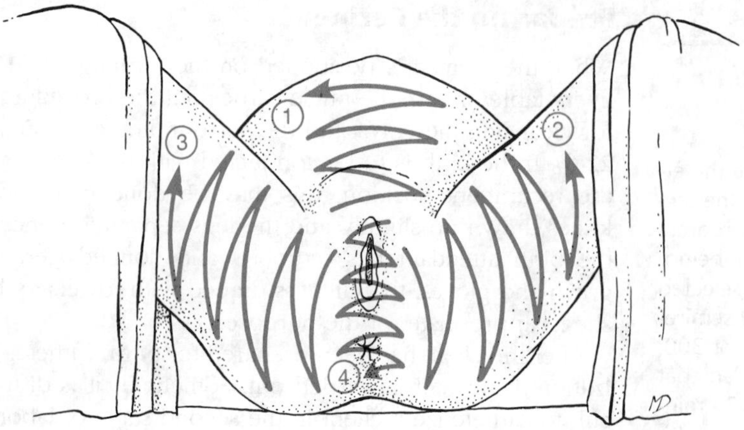

FIGURE 22-6 Perineal preparation. A recommended method when cleansing the perineum. Use a new sponge or gauze square for each numbered area; clean the rectal area last. To finish the procedure, blot the perineum dry with a sterile towel or rinse with warm sterile water.

After suctioning, a finger is passed along the occiput to the newborn's neck to feel whether a loop or more of umbilical cord encircles it. If such a coil is felt, it should be gently drawn down and if loose enough, slipped over the newborn's head. This is done to prevent interference with the oxygen supply, which could result from pressure of the shoulder on the umbilical cord. If the cord is too tightly coiled to permit this procedure, it must be clamped and cut before the shoulders are delivered; the newborn must be extracted immediately before asphyxiation results.

The anterior shoulder is usually brought under the symphysis pubis first and then the posterior shoulder is delivered, after which the remainder of the body follows without particular mechanism. The exact time of the birth should be noted. The newborn usually cries immediately, and the lungs gradually become expanded. The pulsations in the umbilical cord begin to diminish about this time. Birth is illustrated in Figure 22-8.

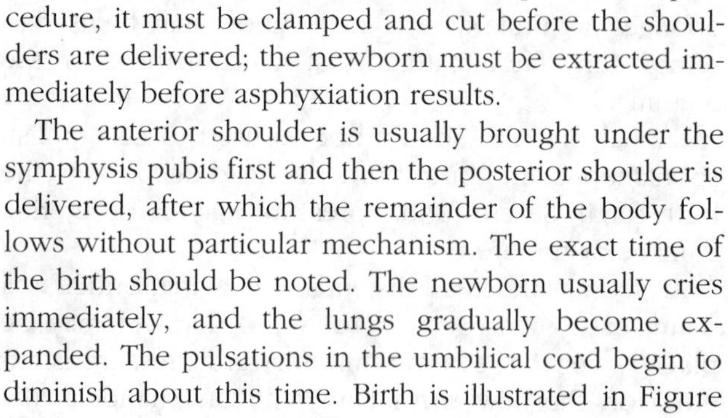

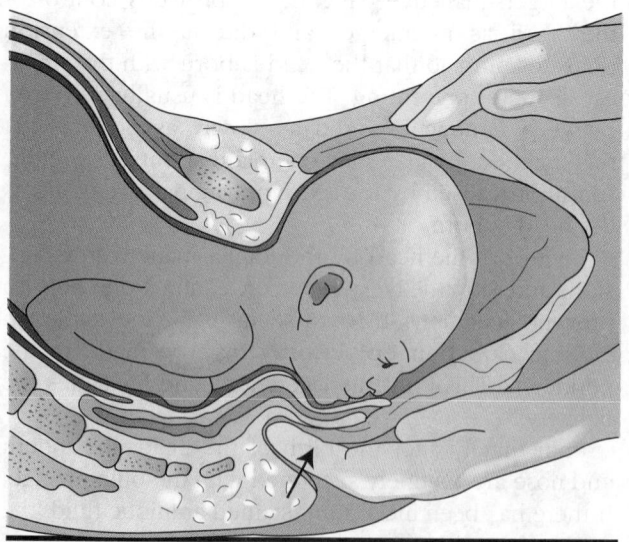

FIGURE 22-7 Ritgen maneuver as it appears in median section. Arrow shows direction of pressure.

Clamping the Cord

The cord usually is clamped before pulsations cease to prevent transfusion from the placenta and hyperviscosity in the newborn (hematocrit >65%; Fig. 22-9). The cord is cut between the two Kelly clamps, which have been placed a few inches from the umbilicus; the umbilical clamp is then applied. Many umbilical clamps are available. The delivery room nurse must assess and document the numbers of vessels present in the cord (two arteries and one vein), because a single artery is associated with congenital anomalies, most often renal (Endo et al., 1993).

Episiotomy

An episiotomy is an incision of the perineum made to facilitate delivery (Fig. 22-10). The incision is made with blunt-pointed straight scissors about the time that the head distends the vulva and is visible to a diameter of several centimeters. The incision may be made in the midline of the perineum, a median episiotomy, or it may be begun in the midline and directed downward and laterally away from the rectum, a mediolateral episiotomy. In the latter instance, the incision may be directed to either the right or the left side of the woman's pelvis.

If a laceration seems to be inevitable as the fetus' head distends the vulva, the physician chooses to incise the perineum rather than allow that structure to sustain a traumatic tear. This operation has traditionally been used to serve the following purposes:

- It substitutes a straight, clean-cut surgical incision for the ragged, contused laceration that otherwise may ensue; such an incision is easier to repair, but the belief that it heals better than a tear and is less painful appears not to be true (Larson et al., 1991).
- The direction of the episiotomy can be controlled, whereas a tear may extend in any direction, sometimes involving the anal sphincter and the rectum. However current research by several investigators

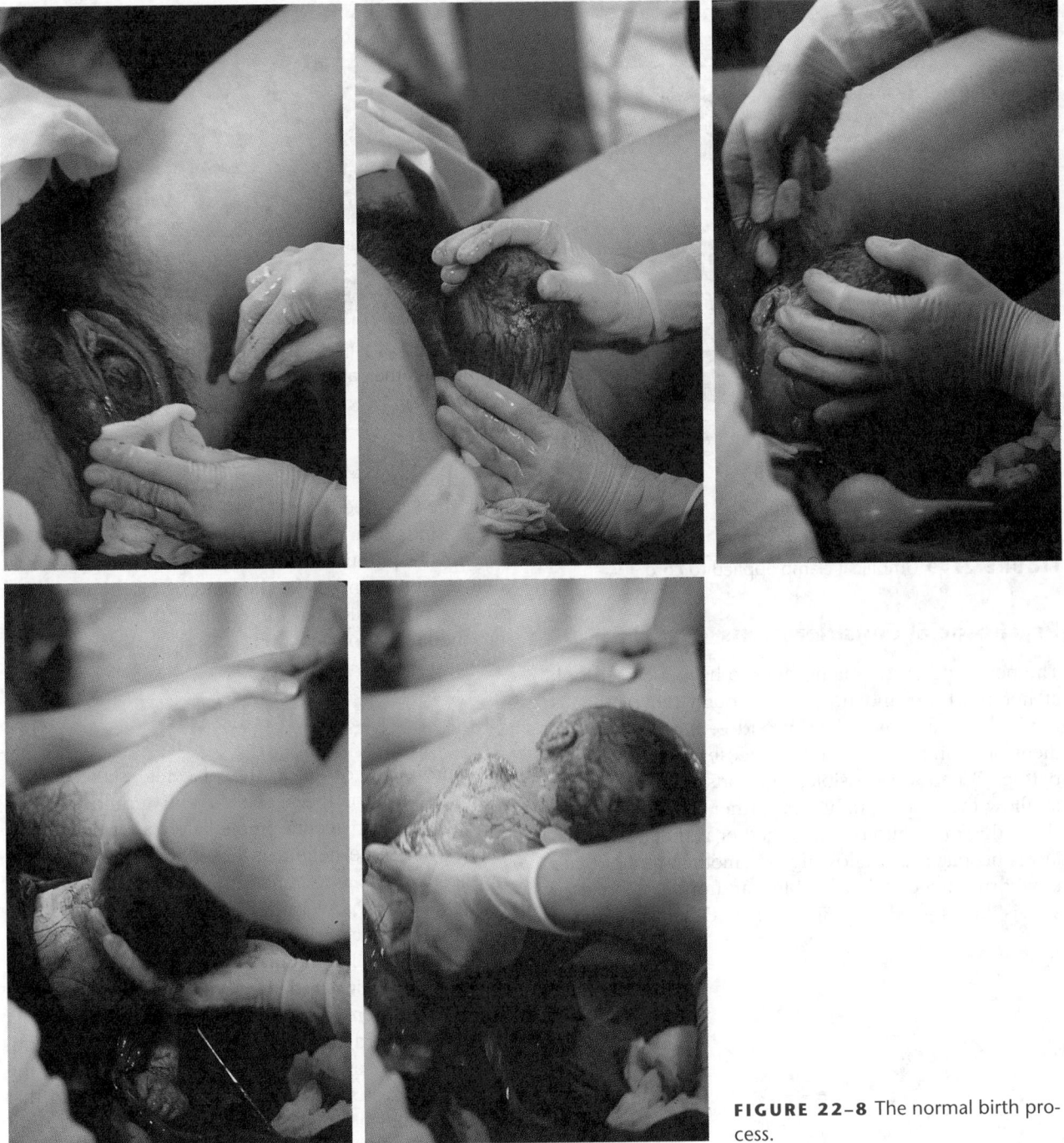

FIGURE 22–8 The normal birth process.

has shown that routine episiotomy is associated with an increased incidence of anal sphincter and rectal tears (Gass et al., 1986; Borgatta et al., 1989; Wilcox et al., 1989).

■ Inordinate stretching and tearing of the perineal musculature is avoided, and the incidence of subsequent perineal relaxation with cystocele or rectocele may be reduced, although this association has never been proven. Because the episiotomy is usually done at the time of maximal perineal distention, this benefit might be limited (Goodlin, 1983).

■ The operation shortens the duration of the second stage of labor.

In view of these previously held beliefs about the multiple advantages, many physicians use episiotomy routinely in the delivery of the primigravida, although based on new findings, routine use is not recommended (Cunningham et al., 1993). It is now believed that the procedures should be applied selectively for appropriate indications, such as occiput posterior or shoulder dystocia.

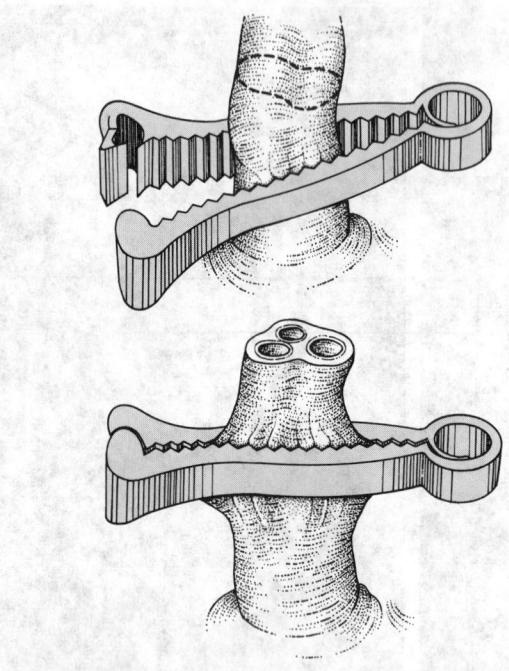

FIGURE 22-9 Umbilical clamp applied to cord.

Psychosocial Considerations

The new mother is usually eager to have a closer look at her newborn and hold it. Although the mother is tired, she is usually elated, proud of her accomplishment of giving birth, and eager to share this with her partner. Whenever possible, all efforts should be made to allow the mother, father or partner, and newborn to share this momentous time together if they so desire. More hospitals are allowing the mother to hold her newborn immediately after birth and put it to breast if she is breast-feeding (Fig. 22-11). Other institutions

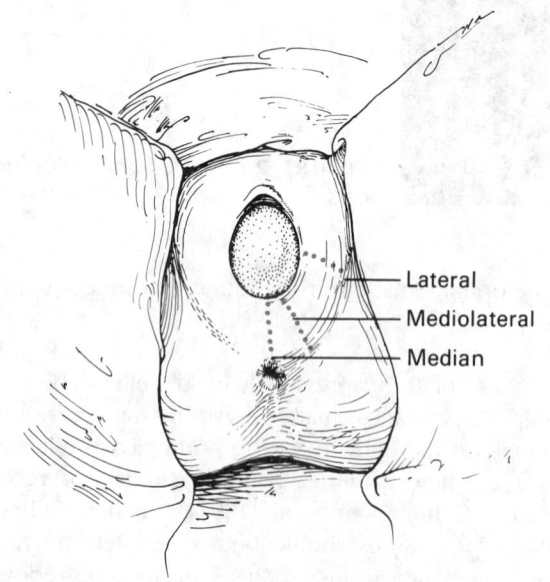

FIGURE 22-10 Types of episiotomies.

Lateral
Mediolateral
Median

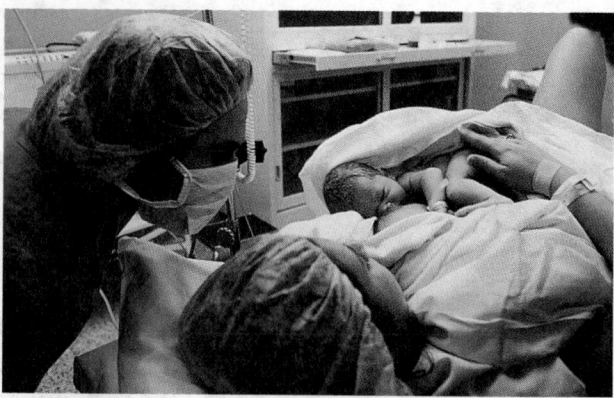

FIGURE 22-11 Immediate bonding between the mother, partner or father, and infant should be encouraged whenever possible.

have the mother wait to hold the newborn or nurse it until she has been transferred to the recovery room. These kinds of arrangements provide more opportunities for the parents to have a close, thorough look at their newborn and to let the triad begin the necessary process of bonding and integrating the new member into the family constellation.

Third Stage of Labor

The third stage of labor, the placental stage, begins after the birth of the newborn and terminates with the birth of the placenta. Immediately after delivery of the newborn, the height of the uterine fundus and its consistency are ascertained by palpating the uterus through a sterile towel placed on the lower abdomen. The physician places his or her hand on top of the sterile drape and holds the uterus gently, with the fingers behind the fundus and the thumb in front. So long as the uterus remains hard and there is no bleeding, the policy is ordinarily one of watchful waiting until the placenta is separated. No massage is practiced; the hand simply rests on the fundus to make certain that the organ does not balloon out with blood.

Placental Separation and Delivery

Because attempts to deliver the placenta before its separation from the uterine wall are not only futile but may be dangerous, it is most important that the signs of placental separation be well understood. The signs that suggest that the placenta has separated are as follows:

- The uterus rises upward in the abdomen because the placenta, having been separated, passes downward into the lower uterine segment and the vagina, where its bulk pushes the uterus upward.

- The umbilical cord protrudes 3 inches or more farther out of the vagina, indicating that the placenta also has descended.
- The uterus changes from a discoid to a globular shape and becomes, as a rule, more firm.
- A sudden trickle or spurt of blood often occurs.

These signs are apparent sometimes within a minute or so after the birth of the newborn and usually within 5 minutes and occur within 15 minutes in 95% of all deliveries (O'Brien et al., 1991). Prolonged placental separation, known as "retained placenta," has been defined by some as a duration of third stage longer than 30 minutes, because incidence of hemorrhage (>500 mL estimated blood loss) increases significantly after that length of time (Combs et al., 1991). This abnormally firm adherence of the placenta to the uterus is termed "placenta accreta," and further discussion and treatment options are presented in Chapter 38.

When the placenta has separated and the uterus is firmly contracted, the client is asked to bear down so that the intra-abdominal pressure helps expel the placenta. If this fails, or if it is not practical because of anesthesia, gentle pressure is exerted downward with the hand on the fundus, and the placenta is gently guided out of the vagina. This procedure, known as placental expression, must be done gently and without squeezing (Figs. 22-12). Placental expression should never be attempted unless the uterus is hard; otherwise, the organ may be turned inside out. This is one of the gravest complications of obstetrics and is known as *inversion of the uterus*. Once the placenta is expelled, it is carefully inspected to make sure that it is intact. If a piece is left in the uterus, it may cause subsequent hemorrhage.

Use of Oxytocics

After the separation and delivery of the placenta in the third stage of labor, hemostasis along the inner uterine surface is achieved at the placental site by contraction of the myometrium, causing vasoconstriction of the uterine spiral arteries. Oxytocin (Pitocin, Syntocinon), ergonovine maleate (Ergotrate), or methylergonovine maleate (Methergine) may be administered at the physician's request to stimulate uterine contractions and control bleeding. All oxytoxic agents exert their action by mobilizing calcium required for the contractile process in myometrial cells and for transmitting the signal of excitation from the cell membrane to the contractile machinery inside the cell (Fuchs et al., 1991).

Oxytoxic agents are used widely in the normal third stage of labor, but the timing of their administration differs greatly in various hospitals. However waiting until after the placenta is delivered is the common practice in the United States, because it might hamper management of undiagnosed second twin or placenta acreta (O'Brien et al., 1991). These **oxytocics** are not necessary in most cases, but their use is considered ideal from the viewpoint of minimizing blood loss and the general safety of the mother.

Oxytocin causes marked uterine contractions for the first 5 to 10 minutes, after which normal rhythmic contractions of amplified degree return with intermittent periods of relaxation. It is the most frequently used drug, because it has been shown in controlled trials that when dilute intravenous oxytocin is administered through the mainline intravenous solution (10–20 U/L), it was superior to intravenous or intramuscular ergometrine (Sorbe, 1978).

Oxytocin's most important side effect is its antidiuretic effect, which can cause water intoxication if administered intravenously in a large volume of electrolyte-free aqueous dextrose solution. Fortunately, the antidiuretic effect disappears within a few minutes after the infusion is discontinued.

Ergonovine is an alkaloid of ergot and is a powerful oxytocic; it stimulates uterine contractions and exerts an effect that may persist for several hours. When it is administered intravenously, the uterine response is almost immediate and within a few minutes for the intramuscular or oral administration. This response is sustained with no tendency toward relaxation. *However, this drug does cause an elevation in blood pressure.* Intravenous route should be considered only with emergencies. More recently, a semisynthetic derivative of ergonovine, methylergonovine maleate, has

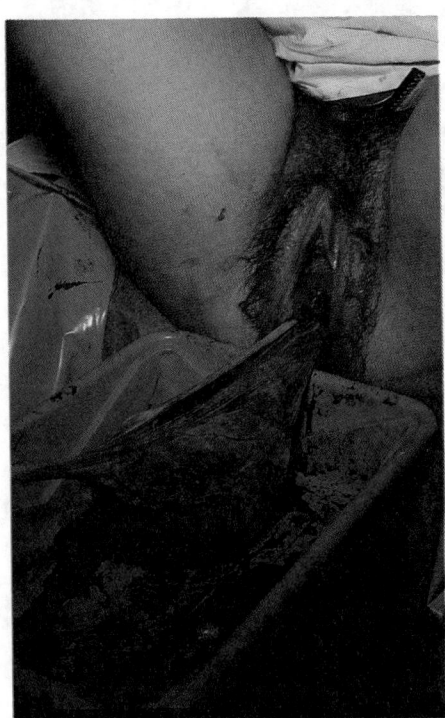

FIGURE 22–12 Delivering the placenta.

been used. It is thought to cause less elevation in blood pressure when given parenterally.

Both forms of ergonovine when given intravenously may cause transient headache and to a lesser extent, temporary chest pain, palpation, and dyspnea. These side effects are less likely to occur with intramuscular administration of the drug, which is the usual route of administration. The usual doses are ergonovine, 0.2 mg intramuscularly or intravenously, and methylergonovine, 0.2 mg intramuscularly or intravenously.

The choice of the oxytocic also depends on the anesthetic agent administered. Oxytocin is contraindicated for use with drugs that have a sympathomimetic action.

Lacerations of the Birth Canal

During the process of a normal delivery, lacerations of the perineum and vagina may be caused by rapid and sudden expulsion of the head, excessive size of the newborn, and friable maternal tissues. In other circumstances, they may be caused by difficult forceps deliveries, breech extractions, or contraction of the pelvic outlet in which the head is forced posteriorly. Some tears are unavoidable, even in the most skilled hands, but control of the head is extremely important to deter perineal lacerations.

Perineal lacerations usually are classified in three degrees according to the extent of the tear:

- First-degree lacerations involve the fourchette, the perineal skin, and the vaginal mucous membrane without involving any of the muscles.
- Second-degree lacerations involve (in addition to skin and mucous membrane) the muscles of the perineal body but not the rectal sphincter. These tears usually extend upward on one or both sides of the vagina, making a triangular injury.
- Third-degree lacerations extend completely through the skin, the mucous membrane, the perineal body, and the rectal sphincter. This type is often called a complete tear. Frequently, these third-degree lacerations extend a certain distance up the anterior wall of the rectum.

Some classifications refer to a laceration that extends into the rectum as a fourth-degree tear.

First- and second-degree lacerations are extremely common in primigravidas; their high incidence is one of the rationales for the use of the episiotomy. Fortunately, third-degree lacerations are far less common. All three types of lacerations are repaired by the physician immediately after the delivery to ensure that the perineal structures are returned approximately to their former condition. The technique used for the repair of

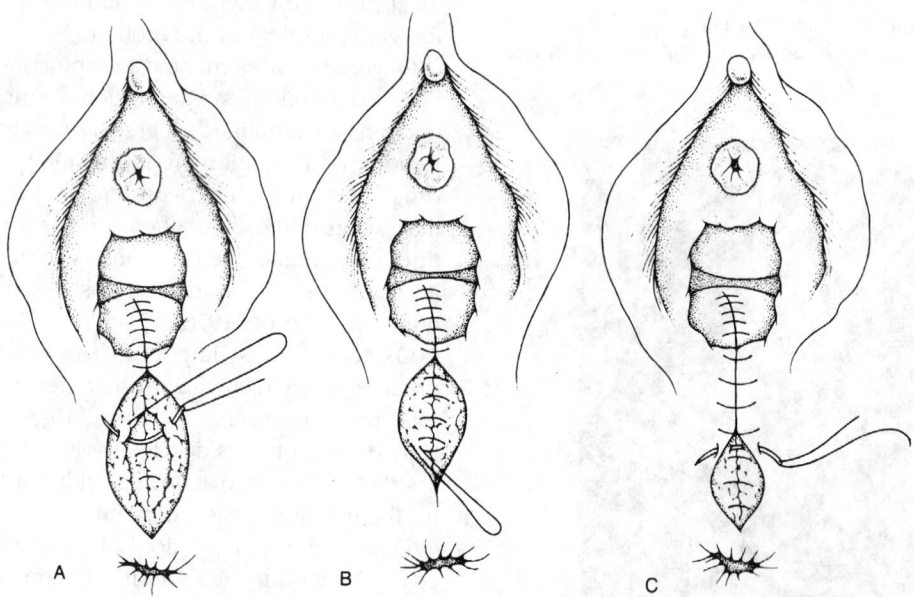

FIGURE 22–13 Repair of median episiotomy. (**A**) Chromic catgut 2-0, or preferably 3-0, is used as a continuous suture to close the vaginal mucosa and submucosa. (**B**) After closing the vaginal incision and reapproximating the cut margins of the hymenal ring, the suture is tied and cut. Next, three or four interrupted sutures of 2-0 or 3-0 catgut are placed in the fascia and muscle of the incised perineum. (**C**) Repair of complete perineal tear. The rectal mucosa has been repaired with interrupted, fine chromic catgut sutures. The torn ends of the sphincter ani are next approximated with two or three interrupted chromic catgut sutures. The wound is then repaired, as in a second-degree laceration or an episiotomy.

a laceration is virtually the same as that used for epis-iotomy incisions, although the former is more difficult to do because of the irregular lines of tissue that must be approximated.

Episiotomy and Laceration Repair

There are many equally satisfactory methods used for episiotomy repair (Fig. 22-13). The suture material ordinarily used is a fine chromic catgut, either 2–0 or 3–0. A round needle and continuous suture are used to close the vaginal mucosa and fourchette; the continuous suture is set aside while several interrupted sutures are placed in the levator ani muscle and the fascia. The continuous suture is again picked up and used to unite the subcutaneous fascia. Finally, the round needle is replaced by a large, straight cutting needle, and the running suture is continued upward as a subcuticular stitch.

Fourth Stage of Labor

The fourth stage can be defined as starting after the delivery of the placenta and ending when the mother's physical status has stabilized. This usually occurs within 1 to 2 hours. The weary work of labor is completed, and the mother and father or partner should be commended by the nurse on the good job they did. Questions can be answered, and any labor occurrences can be clarified. This may not be adequate, and at a later time, the couple may still need their delivery nurse to clarify the labor and birth process. This stage is a transitional period for the new parents, and many important physical and psychological tasks begin at this time.

After the delivery has been completed and the episiotomy or lacerations, if present, have been repaired, the drapes and the soiled linen are removed and the lower end of the delivery table is replaced. If stirrups have been used, the mother's legs are lowered simultaneously to prevent cramping or twisting of the extremities. A sterile perineal pad is applied, and the mother is given a clean gown and covered with a warm blanket to avoid chilling. If the delivery occurred in an LDR, the mother and normal newborn stay for their immediate 1- to 2-hour postpartum recovery in the same LDR; if a traditional delivery room was used, they are transferred to another room known as the postpartum recovery area. Some institutions still require that all newborns be taken to the nursery at this time, and mother and newborn recover separately.

Assessment

Postpartum care begins immediately after the delivery; mother and newborn are making adjustments that need to be assessed. If problems arise, actions need to be taken promptly to ensure well-being. (Immediate Care of the newborn is addressed in Chapter 24.) The first maternal assessment is to be done in the delivery room before transfer. If the delivery has taken place in the LDR, assessment begins as soon as the mother's legs are down and the warm blanket has been placed on her. The immediate postpartum checks, performed every 15 minutes for the first hour, include blood pressure, pulse, respirations, massaging the fundus and observing the vaginal flow, inspecting the perineum, and assessing for bladder distention. A temperature reading is usually taken within the first hour (Box 22-3).

Meticulous assessment is essential, because the mother is at great risk at this time for postpartum hemorrhage and development of a hematoma. If a change in nursing staff occurs (the labor and delivery nurse is not the recovery room nurse), a complete report is given. The report includes name of the physician who delivered, method of delivery, presence of an episiotomy, presence of lacerations, type of anesthesia, intravenous bottle solution and number, amount of oxytocin in the bottle (or if not used, any medications she received to decrease bleeding), method of newborn feeding, time of last voiding, sex of the newborn, summary of the labor, any pertinent items that need to be observed and any pertinent medical history, and any medical orders that need to be carried out immediately.

During the first hour, with every assessment, the fundus is massaged and its condition and position are documented (eg, one fingerbreadth above the umbilicus and firm or boggy and massaged to firm). Vaginal bleeding is assessed and documented in regard to amount, color, and presence of clots or foul odor. The amount of bleeding is noted: scant, light, moderate, or heavy. Problems arise when amounts are not standardized and when measurement differs among nurses. The following is a suggested standardized method to record vaginal flow. It can be implemented to ensure accurate documentation of the flow and reflection of the client's condition (Jacobson, 1985).

■ Scant: blood on tissue only when wiped or less than 1-inch stain

---

BOX 22–3
Fourth-Stage Assessments

■ Vital signs
■ Fundus
■ Amount of lochia, presence of clots
■ Perineum
■ Bladder distention
■ Family interaction

- Light: less than 4-in stain on peripad
- Moderate: less than 6-in stain on peripad
- Heavy: saturated peripad within 1 hour

This subject is discussed further in Chapter 27, with an illustration of peripads.

Nursing Diagnoses

During the third and fourth stages of labor, the nursing goal of maintaining maternal and newborn well-being is ongoing. At this time, the nurse may be able to address and plan for some of the diagnoses identified in the admitting process to which he or she was unable to attend during the actual labor and birth of the newborn. Once the nurse has confirmed that physical systems are stabilized and that the woman is comfortable, he or she can begin to prepare the client for the new (or renewed) role of mothering. Possible nursing diagnoses at this stage include the following:

- Pain related to involution of uterus, episiotomy
- Sleep Pattern Disturbance related to length of labor
- Altered Nutrition: Less than body requirements related to nothing by mouth status during labor and delivery
- Altered Parenting related to inexperience, lack of role models
- Grieving related to labor and delivery not occurring the way client wanted it to be, newborn not desired sex, pregnancy over
- Risk for Infection: vaginal, perineal related to bacterial invasion secondary to trauma during labor and delivery and episiotomy
- Health Seeking Behaviors related to newborn care, newborn behavior, self-care, normal postpartum physiologic occurrences
- Risk for Fluid Volume Deficit related to uterine hemorrhage

Intervention and Rationale

Nursing interventions at this stage focus on anticipation of potential complications and providing supportive and positive care that promotes family interaction.

Management of Potential Complications

Hypothermic Reactions. Chilling accompanied by uncontrollable shaking often occurs in the early period after birth. It is uncomfortable and sometimes embarrassing or frightening for the client, but it is self-limiting (usually not more than 15 minutes) and is not considered an ominous sign. The exact etiology of this shaking has not been determined, although several explanations have been offered: sudden release of intra-abdominal pressure after birth; nervous and exhaustion responses related to the stress of childbirth; disequilibrium in the internal and external body temperature, resulting from the waste products of muscular exertion; break in aseptic technique (which predisposes to infection); minute circulatory amniotic fluid emboli; and previous maternal sensitization to elements of fetal blood.

Clean, dry, warm gowns and blankets and a warm, nondrafty environment help in the prevention and control of this phenomenon. Warm fluids by mouth can be given and are much appreciated for their hydrating and energy-giving effects.

Postpartum Hemorrhage. Constant massage of the uterus during the period immediately after birth is unnecessary and undesirable. However, if the organ shows any tendency to relax, it is to be massaged immediately with firm but gentle circular strokes until it contracts effectively. *Relaxation of the uterus is a prime cause of postpartum hemorrhage, and surveillance of the uterus and the amount of bleeding is of extreme importance at this time.*

Because the prevention of postpartum hemorrhage is such a crucial factor in the health and well-being of the mother, clients at risk to develop this condition should be identified quickly. The most predictive factors associated with postpartum bleeding are conditions that have tired or overstretched the uterine muscle or otherwise interfered with its ability to continue actively contracting:

- Rapid labor
- Prolonged first and second stages of labor
- Operative delivery (ie, forceps extraction)
- Overdistention of the uterus (hydramnios, multiple pregnancy, overly large newborn)
- Previous uterine atony or associated previous postpartum hemorrhage
- Advanced maternal age and high parity
- Other hemorrhagic complications, such as abruptio placentae or placenta previa
- Induced labor
- Heavy medication during labor or general anesthesia
- Preeclampsia and eclampsia

The nurse has an intravenous infusion with an oxytocic for immediate administration ready in the event that the attendants suspect hemorrhage is imminent.

Psychosocial Considerations

Emotional Reactions. Immediately after childbirth, or perhaps later, the parents, particularly the mother, may relieve tension by giving way to some emotional displays, such as laughing, crying, talking incessantly, or expressing anger (if all has not gone well or as expected). These emotions often are unexpected, and a calm, accepting, nonjudgmental attitude on the part of the nurse is effective in allaying any embarrassment.

The nurse must remember that the client is beginning a period that is enormously important; she is a "mother" with all its concomitant responsibilities. This is not the end, but the beginning of a new role. In addition, she is physically and emotionally exhausted from the labor and birth and is at risk for potential sleep and rest disturbance.

Several comfort measures can be used to restore calm and to help the mother relax enough to get some much needed rest and sleep. A soothing back rub, change of gown and linen, a quiet conversation with the nurse or the father or partner in which the client is allowed to ventilate her feelings, and an environment conducive to rest may be helpful. In addition, if she is stable after the first hour, a warm beverage can be offered to help relaxation. Because the mother is apt to be extremely hungry and thirsty, this is welcome nourishment.

Many mothers do not have an emotional outburst, although most do experience some degree of excitement and elation when the birth is accomplished. Any of the above nursing activities also are suitable for them. Some clients experience a great need for sleep and drop off as soon as they know that the newborn is normal and healthy. If the client is sleeping continuously or intermittently, she should be allowed to do so, being disturbed only for nursing observations that are necessary. When she indicates readiness, her newborn can be presented and she can be allowed to examine and explore it to her heart's content.

Mothers who have not been conscious during childbirth may have rather different reactions from those who have participated in the birth process. Often they do not seem to believe that childbirth has taken place or that the newborn shown to them is really theirs. They question again and again, "Is it really all over?" "Tell me again, is it a boy or a girl?" "Did I have the baby?" The apparent alteration in awareness seems to be related to the anesthesia and the unconsciousness. These mothers may need more firm reassurance and contact with their newborns to help them realize that they have had a baby. Even though the repeated questioning may become annoying, the nurse must recognize that this is necessary for the mother to begin the important process of disengagement from the symbiotic relationship that she had with her fetus during pregnancy. She must establish the newborn as a real entity outside her body rather than inside. All mothers have this task to perform, but it may be harder for the mother who delivered under heavy anesthesia, because as far as she is concerned, she was not "there" when it all happened.

Family Interactions. As we know, the couple's attachment to the newborn does not spring unbound at the time of birth. At the birth, there may be excitement about the sex, the color and amount of hair, and other physical characteristics, but attachment develops with time, as in any other relationship. Attachment is defined as a "unique relationship between two people which is specific and endures through time" (Klaus et al., 1982). Parental attachment may have started before conception and continued through the pregnancy; it is enhanced with the actual birth and intensifies during the next weeks (Klaus et al., 1982).

The nurse attending the birth and giving care in recovery can assist the couple with the first interactions. The nurse may help the mother with her first breastfeeding or the father as he holds the newborn the first time. These interactions are important as the beginning foundation for their family relationship continues to develop.

Assessment of Family Integration. Rising (1974) has pointed out that there is a certain openness about the fourth stage of labor that may not occur again during the postpartum period. This openness allows the nurse to make assessments regarding the couple's ability to proceed with integrating the newborn smoothly into the family. If family units are identified for potential alteration in parenting, the nurse should set aside more time to be with the couple to reinforce any positive responses that they might demonstrate and to give encouragement. Listening attentively as the couple relives their recent experience and encouraging verbalization of these feelings can be helpful. Most importantly, the nurse should pass on the client's care plan to ensure continuity in care. The postpartum nursing staff can work closely with community health nurses or arrange for other follow-up care to encourage appropriate adjustment for the family. This is a time when the nurse needs to use all the observational skills, time, and laying on of hands to foster initial integration and begin prescribing future care aimed at consolidating the family unit. The topic of parent–infant attachment is discussed more thoroughly in Chapter 26.

Summary Points

✔ The primary role of the labor and delivery nurse is to ensure maternal-fetal well-being during the childbirth process, provide adequate biopsychosocial support, and respond in a timely and appropriate manner to any complications.

✔ Labor is the process of rhythmic uterine contractions causing cervical dilatation and descent of the fetal presenting part. Most labors progress normally because the placental reserve and umbilical cord vasculature are designed in a healthy term pregnancy to supply adequate perfusion to the fetus during labor, and the usual fetopelvic dimensions allow passage of the fetus down the birth canal.

✔ Birth is the transition of the fetus from the intrauterine environment to extrauterine life as a newborn. Special equipment, drapes, and supportive delivery techniques are used to facilitate this process. The incorporation of significant others and a participating, observant client help to make this birth event a rewarding and significant experience for all involved.

✔ Immediate postpartum recovery is an important maternal physiologic transition time and a critical family bonding time. Close surveillance and supportive measures facilitate optimal outcome for mother and newborn.

REFERENCES

American Academy of Pediatrics and American College of Obstetricians and Gynecologists (Eds.) (1992). *Guidelines for perinatal care* (3rd ed.). Elk Grove Village, IL and Washington, DC: Author.

Adams, J. Q., & Alexander, A. M. (1958). Alterations in cardiovascular physiology during labor. *American Journal of Obstetrics and Gynecology, 12,* 542–549.

Arnold-Aldea, S., & Parer, J. (1990). Fetal cardiovascular physiology. In R. Eden & F. Boehm (Eds.), *Assessment and care of the fetus: Physiological, clinical, and medicolegal principles* (pp. 29–42). Norwalk, CT: Appleton & Lange.

Berne, R., & Levy, M. (1993). *Physiology* (3rd ed.). St. Louis: C.V. Mosby.

Biancuzzo, M. (1993). Six myths of maternal posture during labor. *MCN, American Journal of Maternal Child Nursing, 18,* 265–269.

Borell, U., & Fernstrom, I. (1967). The mechanism of labor. *Radiology Clinics of North America, 5,* 73–85.

Borgatta, L., Piening, S., & Cohen, W. (1989). Association of episiotomy and delivery position with deep perineal laceration during spontaneous delivery in nulliparous women. *American Journal of Obstetrics and Gynecology, 160,* 294.

Caldeyro-Barcia, R. (1979). The influence of maternal bearing-down efforts during second stage on fetal well-being. *Birth and Family Journal, 6,* 117–121.

Caldeyro-Barcia, R., Noriega-Guerra, L., Cibils, L. et al. (1960). Effects of position change on the intensity and frequency of uterine contractions during labor. *American Journal of Obstetrics and Gynecology, 80,* 284.

Carr, K. (1983). *Management of the second stage of labor (NAACOG Update Series No. Lesson 9 [1]).* Washington, DC: Nurses Association of American College of Obstetricians and Gynecologists.

Centers for Disease Control (1988). *Morbidity and mortality weekly report* (No. 37 [24] 377–382). Bethesda, MD: Author.

Cohen, W. (1977). Influence of the duration of the second stage of labor on perinatal outcome and puerperal morbidity. *Obstetrics and Gynecology, 49,* 266.

Combs, D., & Laros, R. (1991). Prolonged third stage of labor: Morbidity and risk factors. *Obstetrics and Gynecology, 77,* 863.

Cunningham, M., MacDonald, P., Gant, N., Leveno, K., & Gilstrap, L. (Eds.) (1993). *Williams obstetrics* (19th ed.). Norwalk, CT: Appleton & Lange.

Douglas, M. (1988). Commentary: The case against a more liberal food and fluid policy. *Birth, 15*(2), 93–94.

Elkayam, V., & Gleicher, N. (Eds.) (1982). *Cardiac problems in pregnancy.* New York: Alan R. Liss.

Endo, A., & Nishioka, E. (1993). Neonatal assessment. In C. Kenner, A. Brueggemeyer, & L. Gunderson (Eds.), *Comprehensive neonatal nursing* (pp. 265–293). Philadelphia: W.B. Saunders.

Fenwick, L., & Simkin, P. (1987). Maternal positioning to prevent or alleviate dystocia in labor. *Clinical Obstetrics and Gynecology, 30,* 83–89.

Flynn, A. et al (1978). Ambulation in labor. *British Medical Journal, 2,* 591–593.

Freeman, R., Garite, T., & Nageotte, M. (1991). *Fetal heart rate monitoring* (2nd ed.). Baltimore: Williams & Wilkins.

Friedman, E. A. (1978). *Labor, clinical evaluation and management.* New York: Appleton-Century-Crofts.

Fuchs, A., & Fuchs, F. (1991). Physiology of parturition. In S. Gabbe, J. Niebyl, & J. Simpson (Eds.), *Obstetrics: Normal and problem pregnancies* (pp. 147–174). New York: Churchill Livingstone.

Gabbe, S. (1986). Antepartum fetal evaluation. In S. Gabbe, J. Niebyl, & J. Simpson (Eds.), *Obstetrics: Normal and problem pregnancies* (pp. 269–322). New York: Churchill Livingstone.

Garite, T. (1985). Achieving good outcomes when membranes rupture prematurely. *Contemporary Obstetrics and Gynecology, 25,* 96–105.

Gass, M., Dinn, C., & Styes, S. (1986). Effect of episiotomy on the frequency of vaginal outlet lacerations. *Journal of Reproductive Medicine, 31,* 240.

Golay, J., Vedam, S., & Sorger, L. (1993). The squatting position for the second stage of labor: Effects on labor and on maternal and fetal well-being. *Birth, 20*(2), 7378.

Goodlin, R. (1983). On protection of the maternal perineum during birth. *Obstetrics and Gynecology, 62,* 393.

Halle, J. (1993). Diagnostic evaluation of high-risk pregnancies. In S. Mattson & J. Smith (Eds.), *Core curriculum for maternal-newborn nursing* (pp. 157–184). Philadelphia: W.B. Saunders.

Hendricks, C. H., & Quilligan, E. J. (1956). Cardiac output during labor. *American Journal of Obstetrics and Gynecology, 71,* 953–972.

Howard, B., Goodson, J., & Mengert, W. (1953). Supine hypotensive syndrome in late pregnancy. *Obstetrics and Gynecology, 1,* 371.

Jacobson, H. (1985). A standard for assessing lochia volume. *Maternal-Child Nursing, 10,* 174–175.

Kantor, H., Rember, R., Tabio, P., & Al, E. (1965). Value of shaving the pudendal-perineal area in delivery preparation. *Obstetrics and Gynecology, 25,* 509–512.

Klaus, M., & Kennell, J. (1982). *Parent-infant bonding.* St. Louis: C.V. Mosby.

Kleihauer, E., Braun, H., & Betke, K. (1957). Demonstration of fetal hemoglobin in erythrocytes by elution. *Klin Wochenschr, 35,* 637.

Knuppel, R., & Angel, J. (1990). Diagnosis of fetal-maternal hemorrhage. In R. Eden & F. Boehm (Eds.), *Assessment and care of the fetus: Physiological, clinical, and medicolegal principles* (pp. 417–424). Norwalk, CT: Appleton & Lange.

Landry, K., & Kilpatrick, D. (1977). Why shave a mother before she gives birth? *Maternal-Child Nursing, 2*(3), 189–190.

Larson, P., Platz-Cristensen, J., Bergman, B., & Wallstersson, G. (1991). Advantage or disadvantage of episiotomy compared with spontaneous perineal laceration. *Gynecological and Obstetrical Investigation, 31,* 213.

Laube, D. (1986). Fetomaternal hemorrhage and fetal outcome. *American Journal of Obstetrics and Gynecology, 155,* 917.

Lederman, R. (1978). The relationship of maternal anxiety, plasma catecholamines, and plasma cortisol to progress in labor. *American Journal of Obstetrics and Gynecology, 132,* 1978.

Long, A. (1967). Unshaved perineum at paturition. *American Journal of Obstetrics and Gynecology, 99,* 1967.

Mahan, C., & Mc Kay, S. (1983). Preps and enemas: Keep or discard? *Contemporary Obstetrics and Gynecology, 22*(5), 241.

Murray, M. (1988). *Essentials of electronic fetal monitoring: Antepartum and intrapartum fetal monitoring.* Washington, DC: Nurses Association of American College of Obstetricians and Gynecologists.

Nurses Association of American College of Obstetricians and Gynecologists (1992). *Nursing responsibilities in implementing intrapartum fetal heart rate position statement.* Washington, DC: Author.

Nurses Association of American College of Obstetricians and Gynecologists (1991). *Standards for Obstetric, Gynecologic and Neonatal Nursing (4th Edition).* Washington, DC: Author.

O'Brien, W., & Cefalo, R. (1991). Labor and delivery. In S. Gabbe, J. Niebyl, & J. Simpson (Eds.), *Obstetrics: Normal and problem pregnancies* (pp. 427–455). New York: Churchill Livingstone.

Rising, S. (1974). The fourth stage of labor: Family integration. *American Journal of Nursing, 74,* 870–874.

Russell, J. (1969). Moulding of the pelvic outlet. *Journal of Obstetrics and Gynaecology of British Commonwealth, 76,* 817–820.

Sorbe, B. (1978). Active pharmacologic management of the third stage of labor. *Obstetrics and Gynecology, 52,* 269.

Sweeney, W. (1963). Perineal shaves and bladder catheterization: Necessary and benign or unnecessary and potentially injurious? *Obstetrics and Gynecology, 21,* 291–294.

Wilcox, L., Strobino, D., Brauffi, G., & Dellinger, W. (1989). Episiotomy and its role in the incidence of perineal lacerations in a maternity center and a tertiary hospital obstetrics service. *American Journal of Obstetrics and Gynecology, 160,* 1047.

23

Pain Management During Childbirth

Objectives

- Discuss the two major theories concerning pain.
- Define pain, pain experience, pain expression, pain intensity, pain tolerance, and suffering.
- Describe the unique nature of pain associated with labor and childbirth.
- Identify the psychological variables affecting pain.
- Discuss the areas to assess for the client in labor who is experiencing pain.
- List specific noninvasive coping strategies for the sensory-discriminative, motivational-affective, and cognitive-evaluative systems.
- Discuss how to avoid habituation when using coping strategies.
- Devise a plan of care using noninvasive strategies for the client in labor.
- Identify appropriate nursing implications for each type of obstetric analgesia and anesthesia.
- Describe the types of regional blockade used in obstetric analgesia and anesthesia.
- Discuss the nurse's role when caring for a client requiring a cesarean delivery and obstetric analgesia and anesthesia.

Key Terms

Acupressure
Analgesia
Anesthesia
Cognitive-evaluative system
Doula
Dysphoria
Effleurage
Endorphins
Epidural anesthesia
Epidural space
Hypnosis
Imagery
Intensity of pain
Intrathecal
Motivation-affective system
Pain tolerance

Pain experience
Paracervical block
Patient-controlled analgesia
Perceived control
Pudendal nerve block
Regional blockade
Self-efficacy
Sensory-discriminative system
Subarachnoid blockade
Suffering
Therapeutic touch
Transcutaneous electric nerve stimulation (TENS)
Transition

Uterine muscle contractions associated with labor are unique in that they usually are painful. The pain of labor, a subjective experience, is caused by ischemia of the uterine muscle; stretching and traction of the uterine ligaments; traction on the ovaries, fallopian tubes, and peritoneum; pressure on the urethra, bladder, and rectum; and distention of the lower uterine segment, pelvic floor muscles, and perineum. Other causes of labor pain are discussed in this chapter.

Nurses who provide care for the family in labor have a special and unique role. Unlike nurses who work in other hospital settings, they are privileged to watch a normal physiologic process culminating in the miracle of birth, an event that transforms the lives of the parents and of those who assist in the process. Nurses, in return, have the responsibility of helping decrease the pain that usually accompanies this process. The chapter focuses on defining the pain of childbirth, the theories behind it, and the various factors that affect a person's pain experience. In addition, nonpharmacologic and pharmacologic methods of pain management are discussed.

Pain Theory

Pain is a mysterious and complex phenomenon with underlying mechanisms that have yet to be fully explained. Although there have been several theories regarding pain, the early work of Melzack et al. (1965) is a classic, accepted theory. This theory and the role that the endorphins play in the theory of pain are discussed below.

Melzack's Contributions

Perhaps the most important contribution of Melzack's work is the possible explanation it offers for the individuality of the pain experience. One conclusion has been clear for many years: When comparable stimuli are applied to several people, one person may perceive intense pain, another moderate pain, and still another no pain at all. This suggests that mechanisms involve numerous factors that may determine the existence of pain and influence the nature of a painful experience. These factors may include not only stimulation of pain fibers, but also cutaneous stimulation, other sensory input, thoughts, and feelings.

As a basis for understanding and devising pain relief measures, Melzack has defined three interacting components of pain that affect a person's repsonse to pain. These components are the **motivational-affective system** (a central interpretation of the message in the brain affected by the person's feelings, memories, experiences, and culture), the **cognitive-evaluative system** (central interpretation of the pain messages affected by a person's knowledge, attention, use of cognitive strategies, and cognitive evaluation of the situation), and the **sensory-discriminative system** (communicates information to the brain regarding physical sensations). Figure 23-1 shows the interactive relationship of these systems.

Endorphins

In 1975, it was discovered that opiate-like substances occur naturally within the body. These substances have been called **endorphins**. To date, several endorphins have been isolated, but many more exist. Their role in the cause and alleviation of pain has not yet been clarified.

Endorphins influence the transmission of impulses interpreted as painful. Endorphins may be neurotransmitters or neuromodulators that inhibit the transmission of pain messages. Thus, the presence of endorphins at the synapse of nerve cells results in a decrease in the sensation of pain. Failure to release endorphins allows pain to occur. Opiates, such as morphine, work in the same manner as endorphins by inhibiting transmission of pain messages by attaching to opiate receptor sites of nerves in the brain and spinal cord (Pittman et al., 1980).

Endorphin levels differ from one person to another, explaining in part why some people feel more pain than others. People with a high endorphin level feel less pain. Also, for example, people with a low endorphin level prior to surgery require more analgesia postoperatively than people with a higher level of endorphin. Differences in endorphin levels may be inherited, which may explain differences in pain sensitivity found between groups of people (Terenius, 1981).

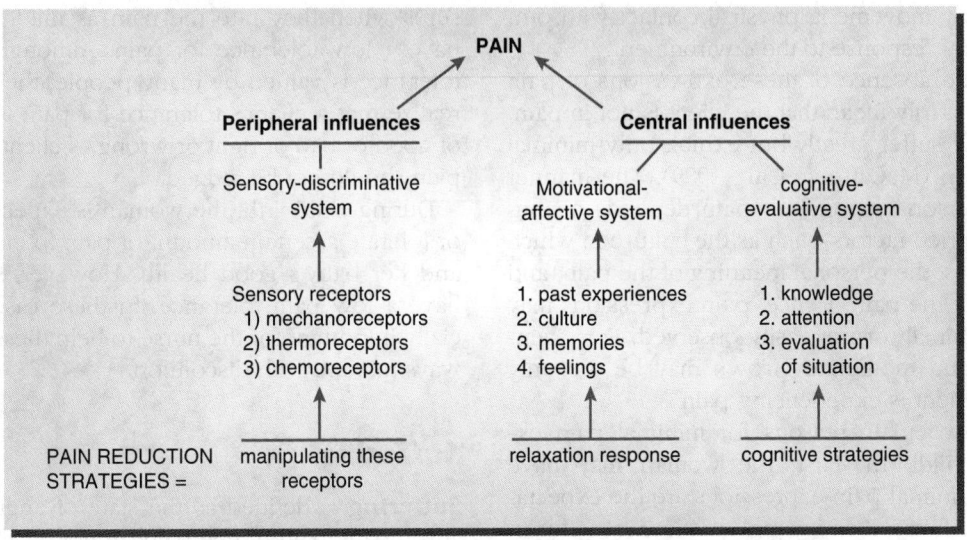

FIGURE 23–1 Interacting components of pain. Cognitive-evaluative-system. (Adapted from Hilbers, S., & Gennaro, S. [1986]. *Nonpharmacologic pain relief. NAACOG Update Series, vol. 5, lesson 15.* Princeton, NJ: Continuing Professional Center.)

Certain situations, such as stress and pregnancy, cause an increase in endorphin levels. Therefore, the endorphin level varies within the individual from one situation to another. During pregnancy and birth, the mother and fetus may have a decreased sensitivity to pain because of increased endorphin levels (Terenius, 1981).

At 36 weeks of pregnancy, women with positive attitudes toward their pregnancies have been found to have higher blood endorphin levels. Women at delivery were found to have an endorphin blood level 30 times that of nonpregnant women (Newnham, 1984) and those levels have been found to be 20 times higher in women with prolonged, difficult labor than those with uncomplicated labor (Kimball, 1979). It also was found that endorphin levels rose progressively with increasing intensities of labor pain. Highest levels were seen in the first few minutes after delivery, dropping rapidly within the first 4 hours postpartum (Bacigalupo et al., 1990).

Various pain relief measures may depend on endorphins. For example, it is possible that certain kinds of client teaching or stimulation of the skin, such as massage, can increase endorphins, which in turn relieves pain (West, 1981). Some people speculate that acupressure decreases pain by releasing endorphins, but there has been no research to support this hypothesis.

Definitions of Pain

Pain is a personal, subjective experience, differing from one person to another and varying within the same person from one time to the next. The client's de-finition of pain can be defined as whatever the person experiencing the pain says it is, existing whenever the person says it does. It is crucial for the nurse to adopt this client definition of pain and believe what the client says. Nurses may tend to believe clients only when they know the physical cause of pain (McCaffery et al., 1989). This hampers the understanding of the subjective pain experience. For example, if a woman in labor complains of severe pain, she must be believed, even if there seems to be no physical cause for such a painful labor. The temptation to judge the woman's discomfort by the results of electronic monitoring must be avoided. Clients also may communicate pain in nonverbal ways. In some clients, a marked increase in rate and depth of respirations may alert the nurse to the intensification of discomfort.

Pain Experience

The phrase **pain experience** encompasses all of the client's sensations, feelings, and behavioral responses, including physiologic activities, such as blood pressure changes. The pain experience also may refer to any or all of the three phases of pain: anticipation, presence, and aftermath. In addition, it may include the client's actions and the impact that others have on the client during the pain experience.

Pain Expressions

Clients who show signs of acute pain, such as perspiration, muscle tension, or moaning, are obviously in pain. The nurse is usually able to observe expressions of client pain in one or more of the following categories of behavioral response: physiologic, verbal, vocal, facial, body movement, physical contact with others, and general response to the environment.

However, the absence of these expressions of pain does not necessarily mean that the client is not in pain. The client may suffer greatly but exhibit only minimal pain expression (McCaffery et al., 1989). The manner in which a person responds to pain depends on numerous and varied factors, such as the culture in which the person lives, the personal meaning of the pain, and the intensity of the pain. Hence, pain expressions may be absent, minimal, or not easily observed. For example, a slight and momentary frown may be the only sign that the client is experiencing pain.

There are two main reasons for minimal pain expression in childbirth. First, the woman may have learned that minimal pain expressions are the expectations of the culture. For example, in some cultures, women pause briefly from work to give birth and resume work shortly after birth. In other cultures, women remain quiet with relaxed facial expressions during childbirth. This lack of expression of pain does not necessarily mean that pain is absent.

Activities learned from methods of preparing for childbirth also may minimize expressions of pain. For example, relaxation techniques and breathing patterns reduce muscle tension and moaning, which are two signs of acute pain.

Pain Intensity

Intensity of pain refers to the severity of the sensation itself. To determine the degree of pain, the client may be asked to rate the intensity on a numeric scale, such as zero to 10, with zero being no pain at all and 10 being the worst possible pain. An alternative to using numbers is to use a series of words for rating pain intensity, such as none, mild, moderate, severe, and very severe. When a client does not exhibit many expressions of pain, it is important to use a rating scale to convey the intensity of pain. If the use of a scale is explained early in labor, the woman may feel comfortable using this method throughout labor and birth.

Pain Tolerance

The presence and intensity of a pain sensation, as indicated by expressions of pain, must be differentiated from the client's tolerance for that pain. **Pain tolerance** may be defined as the duration or intensity of pain that the client is willing to endure without pain relief.

Pain tolerance differs markedly from one person to another. Some clients state that the pain sensation is severe, yet they are willing to tolerate the pain without requesting pain relief. These clients have a high tolerance for pain. Other clients request pain relief mea-

sures when they rate the pain as mild. These clients have a low tolerance for pain. Although a high pain tolerance is valued by many people, the nurse should realize that a client's tolerance for pain is not a matter of good or bad or right or wrong. A client's response to pain should not be judged.

During childbirth, the woman is expected to endure or tolerate a certain amount of pain to ensure her own and her baby's good health. However, some women have a low pain tolerance. In these cases, it is especially important for the nurse to help these women find ways to cope with discomfort.

Suffering

Suffering is defined as the state of anguish that may accompany pain. When pain cannot be eliminated, it is imperative for the client to receive whatever assistance is necessary to prevent or diminish feelings of suffering. Women fear the suffering aspect of pain most and nurses can most affect this aspect.

Uniqueness of Pain During Childbirth

The discomfort and pain of childbirth are unique. Hence, the childbirth experience has a high potential for achieving satisfactory pain relief. Studies suggest that anxiety is reduced if the person knows when pain will occur and how long the discomfort will last. Ordinarily, the woman knows labor will occur, she knows the expected date within a few weeks, and she knows that labor usually lasts many hours but not many days.

Even more helpful is the information the woman has once labor actually has begun. By looking at a watch, she can determine the usual length of her contractions and predict when the next one will occur. In addition, she knows that contractions generally become more intense and more frequent as labor progresses. Furthermore, although her pain may increase in intensity, she is usually not in constant discomfort. Between contractions, there are periods of relative comfort, even during the final phase of labor contractions.

The woman also knows the reason for her discomfort. She knows it is a normal process of muscle contractions and stretching that will result in the birth of her newborn. Most women recognize the onset of labor and do not fear that something harmful or life-threatening is happening.

The discomfort of labor also is unique because there is a tangible end-product—the newborn. The birth of the newborn is accompanied by deep personal involvement, both emotional and physiologic, regardless of whether the baby was planned or not. When the newborn arrives, the pain of labor subsides drastically, and the event is characterized by physical and psychological closure. Few episodes of pain end so dramatically.

The Pain of Labor

Most women have at least some worries about pain in labor. A recent study found that 67% of women were a "bit worried," 12% "very worried," and 23% "not at all worried" about the pain of labor (Green, 1993). When asked if the reality of labor pain was as bad as had been described to them by others, 29% of women said others made it seem less painful than it was, 31% said others made it seem more painful than it was, and 40% said others accurately described the level of pain (Yarrow, 1992). Conflicting information was reported about whether women get more or less pain than they expected. Another researcher reported that 106 primiparas' scores on expected pain and actual pain did not differ significantly. However, 60% of them had epidurals, suggesting that these women did not so much underestimate pain as underestimate their ability to tolerate it (Reynolds, 1990).

Variability is probably the most striking feature of pain during labor. There is variability not only in overall intensity, but also in the progression of pain intensity and the location of pain during labor. In one study, some women showed the expected rising curve of pain intensity, but others experienced increases and decreases in pain intensity throughout labor; some had high pain intensity levels early in labor, and others had low levels up to the time of birth. Location of pain also varied. Some women had widespread pain over a large part of the abdomen, back, and perineum, whereas others had localized areas of pain (Melzack, 1984).

During the first stage of normal labor, pain or discomfort may result from involuntary contraction of the uterine muscle. Contractions tend to be felt in the lower back at the beginning of labor. As labor progresses, the sensation encircles the lower torso, covering the back and abdomen. Contractions are frequently described as waves of pain that come and go rhythmically. Each wave increases to a certain height or intensity and then decreases until it disappears. Contractions usually last about 45 to 90 seconds. As labor progresses, the intensity of each contraction increases, resulting in a greater intensity of pain.

The quality of the pain varies and is difficult to describe. A labor contraction is usually described as a feeling of deep aching. Words commonly chosen by women in labor to describe their pain include sharp, cramping, aching, throbbing, stabbing, hot, shooting, heavy, tiring, exhausting, intense, and tight (Melzack, 1984).

The interval between contractions shortens as labor proceeds. Early labor contractions are about 5 to 20 minutes apart. As labor progresses, contractions occur 3 to 5 minutes apart. Prior to pushing, the intervals between contractions may be only a few seconds long. This period, when the cervix is about 7 to 10 cm dilated, is called **transition.**

Most women perceive the uterine contractions during transition as being at the peak of intensity, pain, and difficulty. Of course, women may certainly experience pain during the actual birth. However, most women say that pushing is a relief.

The predominant sensations during birth occur in the vaginal and perineal area and can be described as pressure, stretching, splitting, and burning. Women usually have an overwhelming desire to push. Pushing may relieve discomfort. Also, the pressure of the baby's head causes a degree of numbness in the perineum.

In addition to uterine contractions, approximately 25% of women in labor have to cope with the discomfort of back labor. This occurs when the fetus is in a posterior position. With each contraction, the occiput presses on the woman's sacrum, causing extreme discomfort as the intensity of contractions increases. Back labor is considerably more painful for the woman compared with labor in which the fetus is in an anterior position. Both pharmacologic and nonpharmacologic methods assist women with labor pain. Often a combination of both is used, and the nurse must understand her role in the use of analgesia and anesthesia with the obstetric client.

Psychological Variables That Affect Pain

A range of psychological variables have been identified that influence a client's perceptions and reports of pain. Fear and anxiety, expectancy, cognitive appraisal, self-efficacy, and perceived control influence the reports and experience of acute pain (Turk et al., 1992; VanDalfsen et al., 1990).

Fear and Anxiety. Anxiety has been demonstrated to be a cause and a correlate of pain reports. Anxiety can initiate a sequence of physiologic changes that provoke muscle spasm, vasoconstriction, visceral disturbances, and release of pain-producing substances. Findings in laboratory and clinical settings during the last 30 years have demonstrated that heightened anxiety levels have been associated with higher pain ratings and increased analgesic requirements.

Expectancy. Anticipation of pain can lead to an increase in perceived pain. Hall et al. (1954) show that when the word "pain" was included in their instructions to laboratory subjects, the subjects demonstrated significantly lower thresholds for and greater sensitivity to a noxious thermal stimulus than when exposure to the stimulus was preceded by a neutral instruction omitting the word "pain." Byron et al. (1975) report that 77% of clients with advanced cancer reported complete pain relief for 4 or more hours from pharmacologic preparations that included no active analgesic medication. This well-known placebo effect has been replicated in many other studies.

Cognitive Appraisal. Diversity of people's responses to threatening events or ambiguous sensations is often attributable to variations in the appraisal process. A person's appraisal influences emotional arousal and behavioral response to a situation. "Waiting for it to get worse" increases the probability that expected changes will be perceived.

Self-Efficacy. **Self-efficacy** is defined as a personal conviction that one has the the power to produce an effect by successfully performing required behaviors in a situation. A person's self-efficacy determines whether the behavior will be initiated, how much effort will be expended, and how long effort will be sustained in the face of obstacles and adverse experiences (Bandura 1977; VanDalfsen et al., 1990). If women feel there is little they can do to control the pain of labor, they will expend minimal effort trying to use pain reduction strategies.

Perceived Controllability. **Perceived control** refers to the belief that one has control (whether actual or not) over a situation. Several clinical studies indicate that perceived control is sufficient to produce significant pain relief (Thompson, 1981; Holyrod et al., 1984; Hill et al., 1986).

The Nursing Process

During labor, the nursing process is likely to be repeated many times as the nurse assesses the pain experience; forms potential nursing diagnoses; plans, implements, and evaluates strategies; reassesses; and continues in the feedback loop of the process.

Assessment

Essential to using any noninvasive intervention is assessment. No one intervention is a panacea. Rather they must be customized to the needs, attitudes, and beliefs of the individual. The Pain Medications Preference Scale (Table 23-1) can be used prenatally to assess what a woman wants to do concerning pain medications. It briefly gives the nurse or support

person(s) information about how active their role will be. If avoiding or minimizing pain medications is the woman's goal, nurses must be ready to answer the challenge and know how to help her with other pain reduction strategies. This enthusiasm, however, must be tempered with the knowledge that goals can change and everyone, including the nurse, must be able to adapt as labor progresses.

Assessment of Contractions

When assessing the woman in labor, the sensations should always be called *contractions*, not pains. The characteristics of uterine contractions include onset, frequency, duration, intensity, description of sensation, and attitude toward contractions. During assessment, it is important to note the time when labor began (*onset*), because prolonged labor intensifies the painful experience. Prolonged labor not only is uncomfortable, but it also fatigues and discourages the parents and makes it more difficult to cope with labor.

Contractions that occur regularly and increase in frequency and intensity indicate a normal labor pattern. Information about the contractions can be used to assure the parents that progress is being made. To obtain detailed information about the *intensity of contractions*, the nurse may ask the woman to rate the contraction on a scale of mild, moderate, strong, or very strong.

It is helpful to encourage the woman to describe other characteristics of the contraction, such as where the sensation begins and where it is felt most intensely. This information suggests the need for specific pain relief. For example, if contractions begin and are felt most intensely in the lower back, rubbing that area and applying pressure or ice may provide considerable comfort.

Assessment of Anxiety or Fear

As the woman is discussing her contractions, she may reveal her *attitude* toward labor. The degree of fear or anxiety she may have is especially important because these feelings profoundly affect pain. High anxiety or fear decreases pain tolerance and increases perceived pain intensity. These feelings also increase muscle tension and painful stimuli during labor by interfering with contractions.

Anxiety or fear during labor may be related to worry about how pain will be managed and how labor is progressing. Throughout the assessment, the nurse should inform the mother of various pain relief measures that may be used to alleviate any anxiety. Concern about labor progression or the effectiveness of the contractions may be partially diminished if the nurse keeps

TABLE 23–1
Pain Medications Preference Scale

You and your partner may use this scale to determine your preferences regarding the woman's use of pain medications in labor. Begin with each of you choosing the number that best matches your feelings, and then compare. If you are not in close agreement, discuss why and come to an agreement. The woman's preferences are more important and must prevail if you cannot agree. The right hand column describes what help she needs.

Number	What It Means	How the Birth Partner Helps
+10	A desire that she feel nothing; a desire for anesthesia before labor begins.	This is an impossible extreme; if she is a +10, she has no interest in helping herself in labor. Help her accept that she will have some pain.
+9	Fear of pain; lack of confidence that mother will be able to cope; dependence on staff for pain relief.	Follow recommendations for +10. Suggest she discuss fears with caregiver or childbirth educator.
+7	Definite desire for anesthesia as soon in labor as the doctor will allow it or before labor becomes painful.	Be sure the doctor is aware of her desire for early anesthesia; learn whether this is possible in your hospital. Inform staff when you arrive.
+5	Desire for epidural anesthesia before transition (7–8 cm. dilation). Willingness to cope until then, perhaps with narcotic medications.	Encourage her in breathing and relaxation. Know comfort measures. Suggest medications to her in labor as she approaches active labor.
+3	Desire to use pain medications but would like as little as possible. Natural childbirth is not a goal.	Plan to be active as a birth partner to help her keep medication use low. Use comfort measures. Help her get medications when she wants them. Suggest reduced doses of narcotics or a "light" epidural block.
0	No opinion or preference. This is a rare attitude among pregnant women; not uncommon among birth partners.	Become informed. Discuss medications. Commit yourself to helping her decide her preferences. If she has no preference, let the staff manage her pain.
-3	Would prefer that pain medications be avoided but only if labor is short or easy. Wants medication otherwise.	Do not suggest that she take pain medications. Emphasize coping techniques. Do not try to talk her out of pain medications.
-5	Strong preference to avoid pain medications, mainly for fetus' benefit. She is actively preparing (practicing labor-coping skills and reading outside childbirth class) and learning comfort measures but will accept medications for difficult labor.	Prepare yourself for a very active role, and if possible, invite or hire an experienced labor support person to accompany and help the two of you. Practice together in advance. Thoroughly learn how to help her relax and breathe in pattern. Know the comfort measures. Do not suggest medications. If she asks, try other alternatives. Have her checked for progress. Ask her to try five more contractions without medication. Be firm, confident, and kind. Maintain eye contact and talk her through each contraction. Get help from others.
-7	Very strong desire for natural childbirth for sense of personal gratification and to benefit fetus. She will be disappointed if she uses medications.	Follow the recommendations for -5, but with even greater commitment; interpret requests for pain medication as an expression that she needs more help. Use the take charge routine. Only if that does not work do you stop trying to help her cope without medications.
-9	Wants medication to be denied by staff, even if she asks for it.	This is difficult for you to be responsible for her satisfaction. Promise to help all you can, but the final decision is not yours. It is hers.
-10	Will not use medication even for cesarean delivery.	An impossible extreme. Encourage her to learn about complications that require painful interventions. Help her get a realistic understanding of risks and benefits of pain medications.

(Adapted from Simkin, P. [1989]. *The birth partner: Everything you need to know to help a woman through childbirth*. Boston: Harvard Common Press.)

the woman informed of signs of progress, such as effacement, increasing cervical dilatation or regularity of contractions, and descent and rotation of the fetus.

Assessment of Pain Relief Methods Used by Parents

Some women have been instructed on the use of pain relief methods, such as relaxation, breathing techniques, and positioning, and are practiced in using them. The nurse should assess their effectiveness, be prepared to assist with their use, or suggest others that may be helpful. Other women have not been formally trained in using pain reduction strategies in labor and require assistance and training from the nurse. Specific methods of nonpharmacologic pain relief methods are discussed in the section, "Nursing Planning and Interventions."

Assessment of Labor Support

The father is usually the support person during labor if the couple has attended childbirth preparation classes. When the father is absent, a friend, relative, childbirth educator, or doula may be in attendance. After identifying the support person, the nurse finds out if that person has been with the woman prior to hospital admission and if the woman wants the person to remain with her throughout labor and birth. From this point on, the woman's support person will be referred to as the father for convenient discussion.

The nurse should assess the father's attitude and desires. It is possible that although the woman might want the father to remain with her, the father may be reluctant and fearful. The nurse also should determine what the father has done for the woman prior to admission, what (if any) preparation the parents have had, what they have planned for the remainder of labor, and whether they have practiced what they plan to do. Sometimes the father simply stays near the woman, touching her gently and offering verbal encouragement. In other instances, the father is expected to take an active role in pain relief measures, such as massaging the back or abdomen, applying counterpressure, or assisting with relaxation and breathing techniques (Fig. 23-2).

Assessment of Medication Use

When the woman is admitted, the nurse should ask whether she has taken any medications or other substances for pain relief, such as aspirin, codeine, or an alcoholic beverage. The nurse writes down any substances that were taken, what time they were taken, and how much was taken. The physician must be informed.

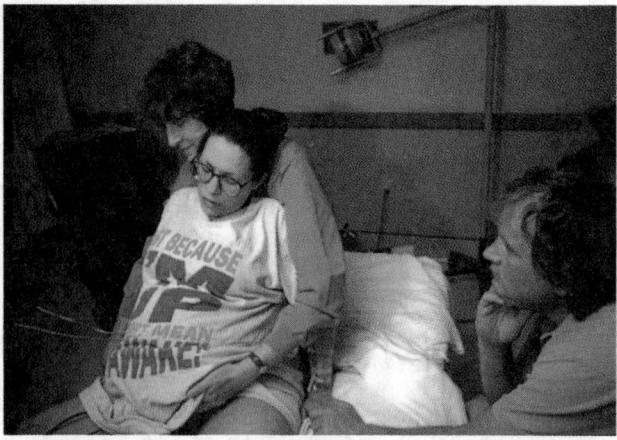

FIGURE 23-2 Fathers can take an active role in pain relief measures by massaging the back or abdomen, applying counterpressure, or assisting with relaxation and breathing techniques.

It is always possible that the woman has taken an illegal drug, such as marijuana, cocaine, heroin, or a drug of unknown composition. The woman who used illegal drugs may fear legal action taken against her or disdain from the healthcare team. To increase the likelihood of obtaining an honest answer from a woman who has used an illegal drug, the nurse should always stress that the questions about medication are important and are used to determine what other medications can be used safely.

It also is important to inquire about what analgesics and anesthetics are being considered for use during labor. The woman may have no knowledge about the medication process, or she and the father may have discussed several possibilities with the physician.

Assessment of Problems in Addition to Labor

Additional Causes of Physical Discomfort. The process of labor may not be the only source of discomfort for the woman. Other discomforts may be associated with the pregnancy itself, a chronic illness, or a recent illness or injury.

Pregnancy may cause or increase heartburn, hemorrhoids, or varicose veins in the legs or vagina, all of which can be extremely uncomfortable when added to the discomforts of labor. Chronic illnesses (ie, arthritis or allergies) and acute illness or injury (ie, influenza, broken bones or sprains, and cuts) cause additional pain and discomfort and may require careful positioning and different pain relief techniques.

The nurse should assess any sources of discomfort not related to labor so that appropriate actions can be taken to provide relief. Any treatment used prior to the onset of labor should be identified. If the woman has found effective means of handling discomfort, she should able to use these same methods during labor whenever possible.

Other Concerns of the Parents. Because the precise time for the onset of labor is rarely predictable, significant activities or plans may be interrupted by labor. For example, the onset of labor may interfere with the father's job requirements, causing him to worry about the possibility of losing his job if he does not report to work. If the parents have other children, they may be anxious about what will happen to them during their absence. Hospitalization and the physician's fees, particularly if complications arise, are major concerns.

Parents may be fearful about the condition of the woman or the fetus whether or not there is a reason for this fear. The onset of labor may precipitate many feelings about this. In addition, there may have been an unexpected change in some aspect of the parents' plans for childbirth. Their physician may be out of town, or labor may have progressed so rapidly that they were unable to reach the hospital of their choice. The development of complications may have changed their wish for a birth without medical interventions.

Assessment of Goals and Expectations Regarding Labor

Parents usually have expectations regarding labor. The nurse may encounter extremes in parents' expectations related to pain and pain relief techniques. Some women expect severe pain and ask to be heavily medicated throughout labor. Other women expect minimal to moderate pain and want to deliver without medication. Parents may believe that the techniques they have been taught to use during labor, such as breathing patterns, are sufficient assistance. Other parents expect to use the methods they were taught in combination with medication.

Parents' expectations of the nurse and physician also need to be determined. Some expectant parents are fearful of certain medical interventions, such as forceps or episiotomies. Some parents, particularly mothers, want to observe the effects of their pushing and the birth of the newborn. Many birth rooms have mirrors for this purpose. The parents may have brought a camera to take pictures in the labor and delivery rooms. They also may want someone to take a picture of them with their newborn immediately after birth. Some parents want to tape record or videotape the birth.

A mother almost always wants to touch and hold the newborn as soon as possible. The mother may plan on holding the newborn before the cord is cut. She also may expect to be allowed to breast-feed the newborn immediately after birth.

Throughout the assessment, the nurse should encourage the parents to express their goals and expecta-

tions. The nurse also should be alert to differences between the desires of the mother and father. For example, the father may not want to witness the birth, although the mother wants him with her. In other instances, the mother may not want the father present. In addition, the father may think the mother is unrealistic in her plans for little or no medication. Another type of problem may arise with a father who forcefully tries to impose his own goals on the mother, who does not share his values. In the situation in which the father does not want the mother to admit pain or to seek assistance with pain relief measures, the nurse may find that she obtains more accurate information when the father is absent from the room. The opposite type of situation also may exist. The woman may feel perfectly capable of handling the pain and discomforts of labor, but the father may become insistent that she be medicated to relieve the pain. When the nurse observes such differences, he or she should help the parents become aware of them and formulate compatible goals.

When assessing the parents' goals, the nurse notes whether these goals have been discussed with the physician. Some goals may be contraindicated for medical reasons. Other goals may require the awareness and cooperation of the physician. In addition, hospital policy sometimes places limitations on the parents. For instance, some labor rooms are so small that the hospital may have a policy of including only the father.

As labor progresses, the nurse continues to assess the client for any changes in goals and expectations. Some aspects of the labor situation may change dramatically, such as the nature of the contractions. There may be a sudden need for modification of pain relief methods. Also, the discomforts and concerns extraneous to labor may be resolved or suddenly may appear when none had existed before. The Assessment Guidelines display provides some guidelines to use when assessing the client's pain experience.

Nursing Diagnoses

Because comfort and pain relief are the focus of this chapter, nursing diagnoses are related to pain and its relief. Box 23-1 lists possible diagnoses.

Nursing Planning and Interventions

The International Childbirth Education Association's motto is "freedom of choice based on knowledge of alternatives." It is the nurse's role to ensure that the client and her support person(s) clearly understand the pain reduction choices they have for labor, including

ASSESSMENT GUIDELINES
Factors in Assessing the Pain Experience During Labor

Use the following as a guide when assessing the client's pain during labor.

I. Contractions:
   Onset
   Frequency
   Duration
   Intensity
   Description of sensation, location
   Attitude toward contractions
II. Assessment of anxiety and fear:
   Attitude toward labor
   Pain management
   Progressing labor
III. Pain relief methods used by parents for labor:
   Relaxation techniques
   Breathing patterns
   Positioning
   Other strategies
IV. Support people:
   People to assist or be present during labor
V. Medication use:
   Over-the-counter medications
   Alcohol
   Illicit drugs
VI. Current problems of woman other than labor

Pregnancy related
Chronic illness
Recent illness or injury
Methods of handling above; effectiveness of methods
VII. Parents' current concerns other than labor:
   Activities or plans interrupted by labor
   Care of children at home
   Financial arrangements
   Condition of woman or fetus
   Unexpected change in childbirth plans
   Plans and needs for assistance regarding above
VIII. Parents' goals and expectations regarding labor:
   Provisions for pain relief
   Father's presence/others
   Concerns about medical interventions
   Watching or photographing birth
   Holding, breast-feeding
   Differences between mother and father regarding goals and expectations
   Which of the above not possible or not discussed with physician

---

BOX 23–1
Nursing Diagnoses

- Pain related to
  - Contractions
  - Progression of labor and impending birth
  - Ineffective coping measures
- Knowledge Deficit related to
  - Absence of participation in childbirth education classes
  - Physiology of labor and birth
  - Coping techniques for pain relief
- Fear and anxiety related to
  - The unknown of labor and birth
  - Anticipation of uncontrollable pain
  - Personal well-being and well-being of fetus
  - Lack of support during labor
  - Perceived loss of control
- Powerlessness related to
  - Inability to manage increasing labor pain
  - Inability to control the process of labor and birth

the benefits and the risks. For some, the risks of even the most popular regional anesthesias may be too great (Chalmers et al., 1995; Thorp et al., 1989; Sepkoski et al., 1992; Thorp et al., 1993; Fehder, 1993; Kennell, 1994). For others, passive pain relief is the goal. The nurse must support the client's informed choices.

In some parts of the country or specific hospitals, regional anesthesia is the first choice for pain management. In other areas and hospitals, nonpharmacologic pain reduction strategies are more common, with or without supplements of pain medications. Even in labor and delivery areas that routinely provide more drugs than support, a significant number of women enter these areas wanting to avoid, or at least significantly minimize, the use of drugs (Green, 1993).

The labor nurse informs the laboring woman and her support person(s) about any new or untried pain reduction strategies to enhance what they already know. Labor is an acute event, so the nurse must be actively involved in assisting the woman and her partner(s) in using pain reduction strategies throughout the labor

process. Good pain relief does not necessarily mean total elimination of painful sensations. In fact, complete abolition of pain is rarely a realistic goal. It is more helpful and reasonable to aim for a decrease in the intensity or perception of pain. The latter is closely related to another possible goal of increasing the woman's tolerance for pain. The Nursing Guidelines display lists possible guidelines for pain relief measures.

Three important principles guiding pain management and relief include decreasing the pain impulses that reach the cortex of the brain, managing anxiety, and decreasing habituation (use of the same techniques repeatedly).

The interaction between anxiety and pain may become a spiraling process. Pain may cause anxiety, which may increase the intensity of pain. Insufficient input or monotonous stimuli may cause pain to worsen. If pain returns or increases, it may be due to advancing labor, or it may be due to habituation. The nurse must know how to avoid habituation. Ways to avoid habituation include changing positions, changing from imagery to focusing on an external point, changing music, changing to a different breathing technique, or alternating massage techniques. The combinations of strategies are practically limitless. If and when new strategies become less effective, the woman can go back to previous methods.

The commonly held belief that pain management is the key to satisfaction in childbirth has been challenged by several authors (Humenick, 1981; Green, 1993). Research studies that compared the amount of pain reported by women found no correlation between reported pain and satisfaction with their childbirth experience (Davenport-Slack et al., 1974; Frank, 1973; Wilmuth, 1975; Morgan et al., 1982; Green, 1993;

Chamberlain et al., 1993). Another study found that the amount of medication was inversely related to positive ratings of the birth experience (Doering et al., 1975). Several studies document that epidurals are associated with less pain but also less satisfaction with the birth experience (Gennaro, 1988; Chamberlain et al., 1993). Of women who delivered vaginally with medication, 86% said they would not use medication the next time (Yarow, 1992). Several studies have shown that the major factor associated with birth satisfaction was the woman's ability to influence decisions (Humenick, 1981). Pressure from staff to take or not to take medication was perceived as a negative factor (Green, 1993). In a study by Lowe (1989), confidence in the ability to handle labor was the most significant predicator concerning pain perception in active labor (see Research Highlight).

RESEARCH HIGHLIGHT

Pain Perception in Active Labor

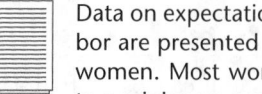 Data on expectations and experiences of pain in labor are presented from a prospective study of 710 women. Most women preferred to keep drug use to a minimum even though they expected labor to be "quite" or "very" painful. The goal of avoiding drugs was unrelated to education or social class. Women who wanted to avoid drugs were more likely to do so and were more satisfied with the birth overall than women who used drugs. In general, women tended to get what they expected. Breathing and relaxation exercises were widely used and were most successful for those who had expected them to be so. All these expectations also were associated with higher levels of satisfaction with the birth. Anxiety about the pain of labor was a strong predictor of negative experiences during labor, lack of satisfaction with the birth, and poor emotional well-being postpartum. Ten percent of the women felt under some pressure by staff to use drugs. Women who felt pressure by staff either to use or not to use drugs reported lower satisfaction with the birth than other women.

Critique: These findings reinforce the point made by the same authors in three previous studies: High expectations are not bad for women. On the contrary, they are associated with achieving the desired goal and with better psychological outcomes. In light of increased satisfaction if women do not feel under pressure from staff concerning drugs, staff need to discuss the issue with women in labor with sensitivity and respect for women's views on the subject. The data about prenatal anxiety about labor pain are very important. Further research is needed to discover more about this as improving outcomes could possibly occur by helping women cope with this specific anxiety.

Green, J. M. (1993). Expectations and experiences of pain in labor: Findings from a large prospective study. *Birth, 20*(2), 65–72.

NURSING GUIDELINES
Pain Relief Measures

- Use a variety of pain relief measures.
- Use pain relief measures *before* pain becomes severe. (It is easier to prevent severe pain and panic than to alleviate them once they occur.)
- Include pain relief measures that the client believes will be effective.
- Take into account the client's ability to be active or passive in the application of the pain relief measure.
- Regarding the potency of the pain relief measure needed, rely on the client's experience of the severity of pain rather than the known physical stimuli.
- If a pain relief measure is ineffective the first time it is used during a contraction, encourage the woman to try it at least one or two more times before abandoning it.

Many women said they could have avoided medication if they had more support (Korte et al., 1992). Nurses can provide support by actively assisting with coping strategies that help to boost the client's self-esteem (Humenick, 1992; Simkin, 1991). It is physically and emotionally challenging for nurses continually to learn new skills, update existing skills, and provide constant support to women in labor. However, the rewards are almost as great for the nurse as for the client.

Three Systems of Nonpharmacologic Pain Relief

The study of pain is a science, and nursing activities for decreasing pain should be based on research findings. Not enough well-controlled research has been done on noninvasive pain reduction strategies, especially during childbirth. However, nurses can perform and teach clients several nonpharmacologic techniques that can be categorized according to the three systems of pain theory described by Melzack (motivational-affective, cognitive-evaluative, or sensory-discriminative).

Motivational-Affective System

The motivational-affective system causes a fight-or-flight response to pain. Thus, none of the pain reduction techniques of the other systems will be as effective if this fight-or-flight response is not managed. The opposite is the physiologic relaxation response, which is a primary goal of pain management in labor.

Relaxation. Virtually every method of prepared childbirth heavily emphasizes muscle relaxation during labor. Muscle tension is a response to pain and anxiety. Relaxation relieves pain by interrupting the spiraling process of pain and anxiety. The behavioral response of relaxation, therefore, is incompatible with pain and anxiety responses.

How a person responds to pain may influence the perceived intensity of pain. For example, when clients observe themselves relaxed instead of tense, they may evaluate their pain as less intense. Another theory is that relaxation may reduce the pain signal input to the thalamus, limbic system, and cortex.

Relaxation undoubtedly provides pain relief for other reasons, depending on the individual person. For some women in labor, efforts to relax can be a distraction from pain. Of 1,761 women, 88% rated the effectiveness of relaxation as a "good" or "very good" method of pain relief in labor (Chamberlain et al., 1993). The teaching of relaxation is discussed in Chapter 19, and techniques for relaxation are presented in Appendix C.

When the nurse encounters a woman who has been trained in relaxation techniques, the nurse finds out how best to assist her. It is particularly helpful to identify cues that will encourage relaxation if the woman becomes tense. These cues may be verbal or tactile-kinesthetic, such as touching or moving the tense body part.

If the woman has not been trained in relaxation, the nurse explains that relaxing during a contraction is important because it can help the woman feel more calm and less stressed. The nurse may use simple techniques that can make a significant difference in the woman's relaxation level because they take advantage of conditioned responses. The quickest and easiest technique to promote relaxation is to instruct the woman to take a deep breath or yawn and then "go limp" or relax when she exhales. The nurse suggests that the woman try this technique at the beginning and end of contractions and any time during contractions when she feels the need to relax. (The client who chooses to yawn may find it becomes spontaneous and more frequent.) This relaxation technique may be enhanced by comfortably positioning and slightly flexing the extremities.

Jaw relaxation is an abbreviated form of progressive relaxation that is easy for the nurse to teach to the untrained or trained client. It works on the premise that if one area of the body is relaxed, other areas of the body will feel the effects. It is useful for brief, moderate to severe pain, such as in contractions. It is more effective if taught in the absence of severe pain and tension, that is, between contractions or during early labor (McCaffery et al., 1989). The Client Education: Jaw Relaxation lists the steps to use when teaching jaw relaxation.

The Cognitive-Evaluative System

The rationale for using cognitive-evaluative strategies is that learning new behavioral responses to pain and stress can give the woman a sense of control over pain and decrease negative emotions, thoughts, and judg-

---

CLIENT EDUCATION
Jaw Relaxation

Use the following steps to learn how to perform jaw relaxation:

1. Let your lower jaw drop slightly, as though you were starting a small yawn.
2. Keep your tongue quiet in the bottom of your mouth.
3. Let your lips get soft.
4. Breathe slowly, evenly, and rhythmically; inhale, exhale, and rest.
5. Allow yourself to stop forming words with your lips and stop thinking about words.

ments related to the pain. This, in turn, may reduce pain, suffering, and pain behavior (Turner et al., 1990).

Reviews of studies show that prepared childbirth techniques generally are associated with decreased use of pain medications and increased maternal satisfaction with the childbirth experience. Whether or not these techniques decrease pain is unclear. Although some investigators have reported that women who used prepared childbirth techniques rated their labor pain much less and another study, slightly less, two other studies have found no such relationship (Turner et al., 1990). The literature on the usefulness of cognitive coping strategies in pain control has been unclear.

Breathing Techniques. Minimal research has been done to document the effectiveness of breathing techniques as a coping strategy during labor and birth. However, when 57 primiparas were interviewed within 24 hours of birth, breathing was chosen as one of the most helpful during childbirth (Koehn, 1992).

Two researchers did not separate relaxation from breathing techniques when evaluating its effectiveness; 89% of women rated relaxation and breathing techniques as "good" to "very good" pain relief. (Of the same group, 93% rated the epidural as "good" to "very good" pain relief; Chamberlain et al., 1993.) Breathing and relaxation were rated as "very helpful" to "controlled pain completely" in 58% of multiparas and 48% of primiparas (Green, 1993).

Women who have taken childbirth education classes are easily identified by their use of specific breathing techniques. Although techniques may vary, the nurse should observe the various techniques used so that he or she can assist the woman later, if necessary, by breathing with her or by helping the labor support person to do so. (For a more complete description of Lamaze breathing techniques, see Chap. 19 and Appendix C.)

The untrained woman and her partner can usually be taught some simple breathing. (For more information on teaching untrained women breathing techniques, see Chap. 19.) Habituation can occur with breathing techniques, so changing to modified paced breathing can help (see Chap. 19).

Attention Focusing. Attention focusing can take several forms. Lamaze-trained women are taught to use either a focal point or imagery as an attention-focusing device during contractions. Laboratory research has suggested that attention focusing may be more effective in reducing pain than relaxation training (Turner et al., 1990).

A focal point is typically used when the woman wants to keep her eyes open during contractions. It can vary from something in the labor room to look at

to a specific picture or item the woman chooses to bring with her. If the woman wants to have her eyes closed during some or all of the contractions, she can use imagery.

Imagery is an activity that people actually do on and off during the day on a regular basis. It is a temporary shift away from the here and now, which some people may call *daydreaming* or *zoning out.* Unlike daydreaming, the conscious experience of imagery involves a certain level of discipline (Steffes, 1988).

The power of imagery is considered by some theorists to be the image's physiologic affect on the body that decreases pain by altering the physical cause of pain. Although the scientific basis of imagery is unknown, the professional literature refers to imagery as a useful technique that fits within the scope of nursing practice (McCaffery et al., 1989). Imagery has been shown to attenuate pain significantly (Fernandez et al., 1989; Wells, 1989). These findings contradict previous reviews that have not assigned prime importance to imagery. The nurse may want to find out if the couple have already chosen an image and if not, may teach them one to use.

The nurse also can assist untrained women to use this by verbally guiding them through the process using any of the "Imagery Exercises" in Appendix C. The nurse may want to perform the exercise between contractions initially and then move gradually to doing it during the woman's contractions. Coupled with relaxation and paced breathing, imagery can be a powerful adjunct to help women cope with labor. To break habituation, the woman can go back and forth periodically between a focal point and imagery.

Patterned Physical Movements. It is not unusual to see people in pain using patterned movement, such as rocking the body from side to side or rhythmic head motions. Women in labor also seem to benefit from patterned physical movement, such as walking or rocking in a chair. Many hospitals have moved rocking chairs into labor rooms and are encouraging women in labor to try them.

Music. Another simple strategy that has been effective during brief episodes of pain is listening to music. The client may bring a portable compact disc player or tape recorder and her favorite music to the hospital. Usually during the contraction, and between contractions if she wants, the woman listens to the preselected music through earphones. This provides a demanding auditory stimulus that is difficult to ignore. For visual input, she may focus on an object or close her eyes and imagine something suggested by the music. The woman may tap out the beat to the music to help increase her concentration on the distraction. She also may move her body or parts of her body in rhythm to the music.

A variety of types of music can be used to avoid habituation.

Verbal Coaching, Support, Information. From the beginning of labor, the woman needs to have someone with her at all times. The presence, actions, and words of this person can support the woman. This person may be the nurse, the father, a doula, or someone else. At times, the nurse's greatest contribution is to support the father so that he can support the mother.

Toward the end of the accelerated phase of labor or in transition, most couples need increasing support from the labor nurse. When a woman requests medication, she often is asking not necessarily for medication alone but for help. It is important to know that a woman who panics during a contraction often feels like she is drowning. The waves keep coming, there is no let up, and it is hard for her to catch her breath. Holding her hand and saying, "Relax; it's okay" will not offer much help. It is necessary for the nurse to know exactly what to do to be effective. The client's partner also can help by using the simple steps listed in the Client Education: The Take Charge Routine (Simkin, 1989).

As pain increases in intensity, the complexity of the stimuli should be increased. Try to provide stimuli through all the major sensory modalities, as follows:

- Auditory (throat breathing)
- Visual (face of partner)
- Tactile (hold her wrist or face)

CLIENT EDUCATION
The Take Charge Routine

Reserve this for any time in labor when your partner reacts in any of these ways:

- She hits an emotional low.
- She is in despair, weeps, or cries out.
- She wants to give up and feels she cannot go on.
- She is very tense and cannot relax.
- She is in a great deal of pain.

The take charge routine is exactly that. You move in close and do all you can to help her until she regains her inner strength. Usually her despair is brief; with your help she can pass through it and her spirits will rise.

Use whatever parts of the following seem appropriate:

- *Remain calm.* Your touch should be firm and confident. Your voice should remain calm and encouraging.
- *Stay close by her side, your face near hers.*
- *Anchor her.* Hold her shoulders or her head in your hands gently, confidently, and firmly, or hold her tightly in your arms.
- *Make eye contact.* Tell her to open her eyes and look at you. Say it loudly enough that she can hear you but calmly and kindly.
- *Change your ritual during contractions.* Try a different position. Try changing the breathing pattern. Breathe with her or pace her with your hand or voice.
- *Encourage her every breath;* guide her in the patterned breathing: "Breathe with me . . . BREATHE WITH ME . . . That's the way . . . just like that . . . Good . . . STAY WITH IT . . . just like that . . . LOOK AT ME . . . Stay with me . . . Good for you . . . It's going away . . . Good . . . Good . . . Good . . . Now just rest. That was so good." You can whisper these words or say them in a calm encouraging tone of voice. Sometimes you have to raise your voice to get her attention, but try to keep your tone calm and confident.
- *Talk to her between contractions.* Ask her if what you are doing is helping. Make suggestions; for example,

"With the next one, let me help you more. I want you to look at me the moment it starts. We will breathe together so it won't get ahead of us. Okay? Good. You're doing so well. We're really moving now..."

- *Repeat yourself.* She may not be able to continue what you tell her for more than a few seconds, but that's fine. Say the same things again and help her continue.
- *What if she says she can't or won't go on?*
  Don't give up on her. This is a difficult time for her. You cannot help her if you decide she cannot handle it. Acknowledge to her and to yourself that it is difficult but not impossible.
  Ask for help and reassurance. The nurse, midwife, or another support person can help a lot—measuring dilation, giving you advice, doing some of the coaching, trying something new, even reassuring you that your partner is okay and that this is normal.
  Remind her of the baby. It may seem surprising, but laboring women are so caught up in labor that they do not think much about their baby. It may help for her to remember why she is going through all this.
- *What about pain medications?* Do you call for them or not? It depends on:
  Her prior wishes. Did she want an unmedicated birth? How strongly did she feel about it?
  How rapidly she is progressing and how far she still has to go.
  How well she responds to your more active coaching.
  Whether she is asking for medications herself and how easily she can be talked out of them.

These factors help you decide what to do. It is sometimes difficult to balance present wishes against prior wishes. Try to stick with what she wanted before labor regarding medication use, but if in labor she insists on changing the plan, respect her wishes.

■ Kinesthetic (not mentioned by Simkin but could be having woman nod or tap out breathing rhythm)

McCaffery et al. mention, however, that with very high pain intensities, simpler distractions should be considered if the client has limited energy to concentrate.

When women were asked to rate helpful and unhelpful factors in the relief of pain other than pharmacologic and nonpharmacologic (eg, breathing, relaxation) methods, a companion in labor was rated as the most helpful, far above other choices (Chamberlain et al., 1993) (Fig. 23-3). Recent reports question whether labor nurses spend enough time in supporting activities with women in labor to be helpful companions (McNiven et al., 1992) and whether expectant fathers are really up to the challenge (Chapman, 1992). The **doula** is an old concept of a support person for the woman in labor. Doulas are women experienced in childbirth who provide continuous physical, emotional, and informational support to the woman. Throughout the United States, doulas are being trained by the National Association of Childbirth Assistants and Doulas of North America to assist women in labor. Klaus et al. (1993) describe the combined results of six randomized trials of 1,500 women, comparing groups of women who had a doula with groups who did not. The results for women who had a doula present include the following:

■ 50% reduction in the cesarean rate
■ 25% reduction in the length of labor
■ 40% reduction in the use of oxytocin
■ 30% reduction in the use of analgesics
■ 40% reduction in the need for forceps
■ 60% reduction in the request for epidurals

As mentioned previously, part of the uniqueness of labor pain is that the woman may possess anxiety-reducing knowledge. If the woman does not obtain

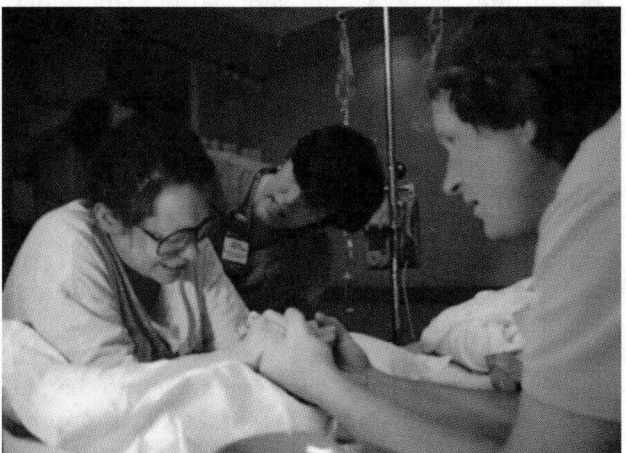

FIGURE 23–3 Having a supportive companion during labor is a very helpful factor in the relief of pain.

this information for herself, the nurse can supply it. For example, the nurse may tell the woman approximately how long it will be before the next contraction and how long that contraction will last. During intense contractions, the nurse may count down at 15-second intervals until the end of the contraction, telling the woman how long it will be until the contraction ends. The nurse may time the contraction to reassure the woman by telling her when the contraction has reached its peak and will begin to subside. Information about the progress of labor, such as cervical dilatation and descent of the fetus, also is important. It is a reminder that there is a purpose to labor, that labor does end, and that the end is getting closer.

Such information not only reduces anxiety, but may motivate the woman to tolerate pain. Especially toward the end of labor, when pain increases, the knowledge that labor is almost over may enable the woman to tolerate an intensity of pain that she would otherwise find unbearable. The nurse also should encourage the client to take one contraction at a time and not worry about the next one. The nurse should tell the woman that the contractions will not get stronger.

Knowing that she and her fetus are not in danger also reduces anxiety. Sometimes the woman finds the forces of labor so unexpectedly powerful that she is fearful of harm. The nurse should periodically reassure the woman that she and her fetus are doing well (provided, of course, that this is true). The nurse may say, for example, that the baby's heart is strong and regular. Remembering that discomfort is associated with a normal process and not a life-threatening illness may be helpful to the woman. Briefly and simply, the nurse can remind the woman of what is happening (eg, that each contraction enlarges the opening for the fetus).

Understanding what is happening during labor seems to increase the woman's sense of control over the event. Feelings of powerlessness can provoke anxiety, so it is important to enhance the client's feelings of control. This may be done through instructions and explanations that help the woman cooperate with examinations and with the process of labor, such as effective pushing. In particular, the woman's feelings of control can be strengthened by teaching her about pain relief measures as early as possible. When this teaching has not been done before the onset of labor, the nurse can begin in early labor to explain certain pain relief measures. The woman then knows that pain relief is available, that there are several possibilities, and that to some extent she may choose from among them.

Distraction. Various strategies people use to cope with pain have yet to be uncovered and understood fully. Some of the techniques discussed earlier in other frameworks also are useful as distracters. Research and clinical observations show that distraction strategies are powerful techniques for making even severe pain bearable for the client (McCaffery et al., 1989). Within the area of distraction, there are numerous approaches.

The nurse needs to be familiar with a variety of distractors that he or she may suggest to the woman. What is sufficiently distracting for one woman may not be for another. A woman may need assistance with distractors even if she has attended prepared childbirth classes. (A review of the information in Chap. 19 and Table 23-2 will assist the reader in the following discussion of these distractors.) Some techniques used in the various methods of prepared childbirth are extremely distracting but difficult to teach quickly once labor is in progress.

Many of the activities serve dual purposes. The breathing rhythms and purposeful thoughts undoubtedly are distractors, but maintenance of rhythmic breathing also is thought to relieve pain by providing adequate oxygenation of the uterus. Although relaxation decreases the fight-or-flight response, the woman may find that her concentrated efforts to relax provide a significant distraction. Changing positions and massaging the abdomen require motor and cognitive effort and therefore may be distracting. Keeping the eyes open and focused on a particular point is perhaps the purest and simplest distracter.

Whatever type of distracters the woman may choose during a contraction, the nurse and others must take care not to prevent her from using them. Early in labor, it may be a helpful distraction for the woman to have someone talk with her during a contraction. However, she may find this irritating later on because it interferes with other strategies for coping with pain. In any event, the nurse needs to find out from the woman what, if anything, she wants the nurse to do for her during a contraction.

When the nurse wants to assist the laboring woman with pain relief using distractors, it is reasonable to approach the woman between, not during, contractions. The nurse can describe briefly one or two possibilities. The woman should be asked to decide which one she would like to try first. It usually is most helpful if the nurse first demonstrates the activity and then has the woman do it. If a song or counting is to be used, it is often much easier for the woman if the nurse counts or sings for her during the first contraction in which the pattern is used. If the woman does not like any of the distracters, the nurse may creatively invent some others or simply ask the woman for suggestions.

When discomfort intensifies or possible habituation develops, a more powerful form of distraction is needed. The nurse may teach the woman the "modified or patterned paced breathing" of the Lamaze method. Again, more distraction may be added to these breathing patterns by incorporating one or more of the distracters of the Lamaze method, such as the concentration point, abdominal massage, or silent counting. Another effective and relatively easy distracter to use is finger tapping a rhythm to a song, coordinating the rhythm with breathing.

During transition, the woman's focus tends to become extremely narrow because of the increase in the intensity and frequency of contractions. Whereas earlier in labor, the distracters could be suggested and taught between contractions, there is little time now, and it is difficult for the woman to focus on anything but labor. Therefore, distracters used during transition should be more simple and must be taught prior to the onset of transition.

Hypnosis. **Hypnosis,** a temporary altered state of consciousness in which the person has increased suggestibility, was introduced into obstetrics early in the 19th century and has been used in obstetrics on a limited basis since that time. Hypnosis is used in two ways to alter pain perception during labor and birth: self-hypnosis and posthypnotic suggestion. Most hypnotherapists teach the woman self-hypnosis so she can enter a trance during labor to reduce awareness of pain. Rarely do hypnotherapists accompany the woman during labor. Other therapists use a posthypnotic suggestion that will allay the woman's fears about pain and modify her interpretation of and reaction to contractions. Most studies on the efficacy of hypnosis are uncontrolled and thus are subject to bias. One of the drawbacks to hypnosis is the amount of time required for adequate hypnosis preparation (Simkin, 1995).

The Sensory-Discriminative System

To decrease pain perception using the sensory-discriminative system, three peripheral receptors can be used: mechanoreceptors, thermorecptors, and chemoreceptors. All three receptors are supplied by nerve fibers that differ in their speed of conduction to the cortex. Pain perception is decreased because the sensory information reaches the brain before the pain information (Hilbers et al., 1986). Table 23-3 lists possible pain-reducing strategies the nurse can use to assist the laboring woman.

Positioning. In the last decade, professionals and parents have begun to understand the benefits of various positions a woman uses during labor. The findings of researchers concerning the benefits of being upright and mobile during labor have contributed to this understanding. Roberts et al. (1983) studied position changes, and the overall results indicated that changing positions is important for efficient uterine contrac-

(*text continues on page 592*)

TABLE 23-2
Summary of Pain Relief Measures Used During Labor

Approximate Progress of Labor	Position	Eye Focus	Breathing Patterns	Woman's Possible Thoughts	Labor Partner's Activities Through All Phases of Labor
Onset to 3 cm, or contractions 5–20 min apart	Supported with pillows sitting or lying on side; may walk between contractions; may stand and lean on object or person during contractions; may prefer rocking chair; should change positions at least hourly to facilitate labor and decrease pain	Eyes open and focused on one particular object or person's face ("concentration point," "focal point"), or eyes may be closed while doing imagery during contractions	Inhales deeply at beginning of each contraction and relaxes totally on exhalation; takes a deep breath at end of each contraction Slow-paced breathing (inhale through nose or mouth, exhale through nose or mouth) *Minimum* rate is half individual woman's resting respiration rate	On inhalation, "In, 1, 2," on exhalation, "Out, 1, 2" or Concentrates on imagery or Concentrates on music	Times frequency of contractions; tells woman when each contraction half over Helps woman get in comfortable positions, changing positions at least hourly As need arises, may do abdominal massage for her or rub her lower back Reminds her to urinate—a full bladder can slow labor progress Gives love, support, encouragement, hugs, holding
Dilates from 4–7 cm, or contractions 2–4 min apart	Same as above	Same as above	May continue slow-paced breathing or use modified paced breathing (may accelerate as contraction intensifies, decelerate as contraction subsides); modified paced breathing maximum rate is twice woman's resting respiration rate Breathing may be inhale nose, exhale nose; inhale nose, exhale mouth; or inhale mouth, exhale mouth Breathing may be in 4/4 or other rhythm Modified paced breathing used only to break habituation, then may be able to return to slow paced	Counts each breath in 4/4 rhythm, emphasizing count of 1 (eg, "*1*, 2, 3, 4, *1*, 2, 3, 4," or silently breathes to "Yankee Doodle," or any 4/4 rhythm song) Concentrates on imagery or Concentrates on music	Same as above plus the following: As need arises, may breathe with her; remind her of eye focus or imagery; reminds her to breathe deeply at end of contraction; may need "the take charge routine." If back labor or backache, may try deep counterpressure with heat or ice on lower back and use back labor positions

(continued)

TABLE 23-2 *(Continued)*
Summary of Pain Relief Measures Used During Labor

Approximate Progress of Labor	Position	Eye Focus	Breathing Patterns	Woman's Possible Thoughts	Labor Partner's Activities Through All Phases of Labor
Dilates from 8 to 10 cm, or contractions 1–2 min apart	Same as above, but most women prefer to be in bed now	Same as above, but focusing eyes on another person may be more helpful to some at this stage	Slow, modified, or patterned paced breathing through mouth or nose (rhythm of 1–6 breaths and then 1 blow; may accelerate and decelerate with intensity of contraction) breathing is maximum rate of twice woman's resting respiration rate If not allowed to push but feels urge to push, blows repeatedly If uncomfortable between contractions, uses slow-paced breathing	Counts each breath according to rhythm selected (eg, "1, 2, 3, 4, 5, 6, blow") or Concentrates on imagery or Concentrates on music	Between contractions offers encouragement; wipes face with cool, wet cloth; moistens lips and mouth with water, ice chips, mouthwash, or Chapstick May need "The Take Charge Routine"; keep environment safe and calm; other activities in previous phases Pressure on area of buttocks or squeeze buttocks together to make urge to push more tolerable
Birth (fully dilated)	For pushing in labor room, labor delivery room (LDR), may be sitting and holding legs to 90-degree angle with body, squatting holding bed rails, squat bar, or support from people or on all fours (to rotate posterior baby); or lying on side with back curved and top knee pulled up; if no progress in 20 min, change position For birth in delivery room, or LDR, semi-propped sitting position; if legs not in stirrups, may put feet on bed or may give birth on her side	For pushing may focus on mirror or perineum, if visible, to see results of pushing	For pushing; two deep breaths, inhale, hold breath, hold 5–7 sec bearing down, release breath; repeat inhalation and continue as before until contraction is over or until instructed to stop pushing Alternate method: two deep breaths, on third breath, blow out slowly and bear down; repeat as necessary Making grunting noises is OK	For pushing may visualize newborn slowly coming out of uterus and through birth canal	For pushing, may stand at woman's back to support her in pushing position if no back rest, help hold legs or support in squat Counts aloud 5–7 sec during each breath holding, tells her "exhale, take a deep breath, and hold it," then counts to 5–7 sec again Reminds her to relax pelvic floor or "bulge" pelvic floor or "open up" Helps her to change to other positions as necessary; if no progress in 20 min, change position Offers cold cloth, love, encouragement

TABLE 23-3
Using the Sensory-Discriminative System to Decrease Pain Perception in Labor

Receptors	Nerve Endings	Location in Body	Transmission	Activities to Try With Laboring Woman
Mechanore-ceptors	Merkel's disks (take physical stimuli and transform them into electrical energy that is transmitted to the brain)	Epidermis—most numerous in skin of the palms, soles of feet, and external genitalia	Well-mylelinated, fast-transmitting, large-diameter fibers. Do not habituate rapidly so techniques can be effective for long time. Lips and index finger have large interpretive area in the brain.	Pressure on lips by using Chapstick, kissing Pressure maintained over upper lip with index finger Partner holding her hands, she can sit on her hands Holding bed rails or squeeze hands or objects Standing or placing soles of feet on other hard surface (eg, a stool) Sitting on firm surface Warm baths
	Meissner's corpuscles	Fingertips and hairless skin	These also transmit faster than pain.	Moving her fingertips in circles on the sheets Feeling soft textures like velvet, fur Feeling her partner's face Effleurage with firm pressure Playing with her hair Slow, firm pressure along a tense area in the same direction as hair grows Warm shower
	Pacinian corpuscles	Deeper layer of skin	Detect deep, rapid pressure sensations and vibrations. These are largest and most widely distributed receptors in the body. They are slow to habituate so can be used over long periods.	Leaning against warm, vibrating clothes dryer Feet in devices that vibrate warm water Vibrating pillows or cordless vibrators Vibrating shower massage
	Tactile hair end organs	Base of each individual hair; fired by hair movement	Detect light touch. Stimulation can increase pain because they travel on some of same fibers as pain.	Avoid: Tickling Light moving touch *against* hair follicles (ie, rubbing someone the wrong way) for example light effleurage Some movements of sheets, clothing, and air may irritate
	Joint receptors	Found in joint capsules, ligaments, synovial membrane	Slow to habituate. Joint movement and pressure into joints will fire these receptors and decrease pain.	Frequent changes of position Standing, walking, hugging, rocking Gently shaking joints Pelvic rock on all fours Breathing techniques may cause rib cage movement Avoid: Lying quietly in bed with little joint movement

(continued)

TABLE 23-3 *(Continued)*
Using the Sensory-Discriminative System to Decrease Pain Perception in Labor

Receptors	Nerve Endings	Location in Body	Transmission	Activities to Try With Laboring Woman
Chemorecep-tors (trans-form chem-ical stimuli into energy transmitted to brain)	Olfactory	Upper part of each nostril	These are unmyeli-nated small-diame-ter fibers.	Familiar *positive* smells, (eg, her own pillow case, herbs, special foods, body odor of significant other)
	Taste	Mouth		Familiar *positive tastes,* (eg, own mouthwash, special teas)
Thermorecep-tors (trans-mit infor-mation about tem-perature to the brain)		Skin	Not as well under-stood as other re-ceptors. They rapidly habituate and respond greatly to temperature changes.	Alternating hot and cold packs* Ice in plastic bag* Socks if feet are cool Neutral body warmth may be calming* Warm showers, bath* Warm hair dryer*

*Do not apply heat or cold to anesthestized or ischemic areas because tissues may be damaged.
(Data from Hilbers, S., & Gennaro, S. [1986]. *Nonpharmaceutical pain relief. NAACOG Update Series, Vol. 5.* Princeton, NJ; Continuing Professional Center.)

tions. Diaz et al. (1988) found that 95% of the women chose to be sitting, standing, or walking when given the choice.

Standing or walking during labor contributes to shorter duration of labor with decreased pain and increased comfort levels (Diaz et al., 1988; Flynn et al., 1980; Mendez-Bauer et al., 1975). Flynn et al. found that ambulation during the first stage shortens labor by 30% and reduces the need for analgesia by the same amount. Roberts et al. (1983) found that women prefer sitting in the first half of labor and lying on their side in late labor. The nurse can encourage women to try getting out of bed and see if that helps.

Positioning is an especially important and effective pain relief measure when the woman experiences back labor (ie, when the occiput of the fetus presses on the woman's sacrum). A popular position for women experiencing back labor is the all-fours position. If the forces of gravity and buoyancy are sufficient, this position may even succeed in rotating the fetus' head to an anterior position. If the fetus' head is not in the posterior position, this position may still relieve pain, especially during transition, when labor is often felt in the back.

Unless there are complications, the woman should be allowed to choose the positions she finds most comfortable. If she wants to lie on her back, however, the head of the bed should be elevated enough to avoid supine hypotension and her thighs slightly flexed with pillows to aid in muscle relaxation. The

nurse should encourage frequent position changes to find those that are associated with less pain and more efficient labor (Table 23-4).

Cutaneous Stimulation. The underlying mechanisms of pain relief from various cutaneous stimulation are usually unknown. Stimulation of the skin may activate the large diameter fibers, which may cause an inhibition of the pain messages carried by the smaller fibers. Another possibility is that certain types of skin stimulation may increase the endorphin levels. The effectiveness of some methods of cutaneous stimulation may be related to therapeutic touch (McCaffery et al., 1989). Cutaneous stimulation usually reduces the intensity of pain or makes it more bearable.

Heat and Cold. For centuries, heat and cold have been used for pain relief, but the mechanisms that explain the effects are still largely a matter of speculation (McCaffery et al., 1989). The application of heat or cold may be especially comforting to the laboring woman.

Heat is good for decreasing tension and promoting overall relaxation. It dilates blood vessels and is usually recommended for low to moderate pain. Many hospitals have remodeled and have added showers, tubs, and sometimes whirlpools in their labor areas. The efficacy of warm water in reducing labor pain has not been evaluated by randomized clinical trials; however, the published empirical observations and the positive reactions of the women will likely ensure its

TABLE 23–4
Positions for First Stage

Position	Advantages	Disadvantages
Standing	▪ Takes advantage of gravity during and between contractions ▪ Contractions less painful and more productive ▪ Fetus well aligned with angle of pelvis ▪ Relieves backache ▪ May speed labor	▪ Tiring for long periods ▪ May be impossible with anesthesia
Standing and leaning forward	▪ Same as with standing ▪ May be more restful than standing	▪ Same as with standing
Walking	▪ Same as with standing ▪ Movement in pelvis encourages descent	▪ Tiring for long periods ▪ Difficult or impossible with anesthesia, analgesia, or electronic fetal monitoring
Sitting upright	▪ Good resting position ▪ Some gravity advantage ▪ Can be used with electronic fetal monitor	▪ May slow labor progress if used for long periods
Semisitting	▪ Same as with sitting upright ▪ Vaginal examinations possible	▪ Same as with sitting upright ▪ Increases back pain
Sitting, leaning forward with support	▪ Same as with sitting upright ▪ Relieves back pain ▪ Good position for back rub	▪ Same as with sitting upright
Hands and knees	▪ Helps relieve backache ▪ Assists rotation of baby from occiput posterior position ▪ Allows for pelvic rocking ▪ May be used when other positions cause a drop in fetal heart rate	▪ Vaginal examinations inconvenient for most caregivers ▪ Hands and knees may go to sleep or hurt after a while ▪ May interfere with external fetal monitor tracing ▪ May be tiring for long periods
Kneeling, leaning forward with support	▪ Same as on hands and knees ▪ Less strain on wrists and hands than in hands and knees position	▪ May interfere with external fetal monitor tracing ▪ May be tiring for long periods
Side-lying	▪ Very good resting position ▪ Convenient for many interventions ▪ Helps lower elevated blood pressure ▪ May promote progress of labor when alternated with walking ▪ Safe if pain medications have been used	▪ Contractions may be less effective and longer ▪ May be inconvenient for vaginal examinations
Squatting	▪ Takes advantage of gravity ▪ May be comfortable and relieve backache ▪ May enhance fetal alignment and descent within pelvis	▪ May not enhance descent of fetus if station is high ▪ Tiring for long periods ▪ Legs can go to sleep if used for long periods
Back-lying (supine)	▪ Convenient for caregiver for procedures and vaginal examinations ▪ May be restful ▪ Convenient for electronic fetal monitoring	▪ May cause supine hypotension and fetal distress ▪ May increase backache ▪ Psychologically vulnerable ▪ Labor contractions found to be longest, most painful, and least productive

Reproduced from *Pregnancy, Childbirth and the Newborn* by Simkin, Whalley and Keppler, with permission from the Childbirth Education Association of Seattle and Meadowbrook Press, Inc. 1991.

continued use. Many women and nurses working in the labor room present glowing reports about the pain relieving benefits of a warm tub bath or long warm showers during labor. For women in labor who do not have access to a tub or shower, the nurse can try a hot water bottle, heating pad, or hot washcloths on the women's lower abdomen, groin, back, perineum, or thighs.

Cold receptors in the skin far out number heat receptors. Cold numbs painful areas and constricts blood vessels. Cold also slows the pain impulse transmission along nerve pathways and is usually recommended for acute pain because it penetrates two to three times more deeply than heat. For severe back pain, cold may feel better than heat. The nurse can put ice in a glove to try on the clients' back or back of her neck. A cold washcloth also may feel good. Cold is usually applied for 20 to 30 minutes or longer. The minimal effective time is 5 to 10 minutes. If cold relieves the pain, it will likely work better than heat because cold relieves more pain at a faster rate. In addition, once it is removed, relief from pain lasts longer (McCaffery et al., 1989).

The nurse may encourage the woman to try alternating heat and cold or using either intermittently. Alternating heat and cold may be more effective with severe pain (McCaffery et al., 1989).

Massage. Another type of cutaneous stimulation, massage, may be used during labor and may be an effective pain relief measure. One common massage technique is **effleurage,** or abdominal massage. Figure 23-4 illustrates two types of effleurage. Rubbing the lower back also is common. Rubbing a painful body part is a universal means of relieving pain.

The previous methods are examples involving relatively moderate stimulation of cutaneous fibers. Mild to moderate stimulation is ordinarily more effective than intense stimulation. One notable exception, however, is the use of intense pressure over the sacrum during a contraction. The pressure may be applied with the knee or fist, or the mother may lean back in a semisitting position on a tennis ball or have pressure applied with a rolling pin.

Rubbing of any part of the body, even between contractions, possibly may contribute to pain relief. This not only encourages relaxation, but experimentation

with cutaneous stimulation shows that it may help long after its use. The painful area need not always be the area of stimulation (McCaffery et al., 1989). For example, if an external monitor prevents abdominal massage, the thighs may be massaged instead. Some mothers find that foot massage by the father or nurse brings considerable comfort. To reduce habituation, massage may be used intermittently or in different locations.

Transcutaneous Electric Nerve Stimulation. **Transcutaneous electric nerve stimulation** (TENS) is a form of cutaneous stimulation that has been used for pain relief during the first stage of labor. The mechanisms behind the effectiveness of TENS in relieving pain are unclear. Some types of TENS appear to relieve pain by increasing endorphins. Other types may act as a counterirritant, masking pain or activating a complex neural inhibiting system (Reed et al., 1992).

In TENS, a mild electric current is applied to the skin by way of electrodes connected to a battery-operated device with controls to regulate the sensation. The client is usually taught before labor how to control the unit herself, and she uses it in conjunction with prepared childbirth techniques. It has the advantage shared by all types of **patient-controlled analgesia** of increased consumer satisfaction. The client usually feels a buzzing, tingling, or vibrating sensation. In one study of labor pain, two pairs of electrodes were placed on either side of the spinal column over the sacral and thoracic regions. Low-intensity stimulation was provided continuously, and the woman increased the stimulation during a contraction. No complications occurred except that sacral stimulation interfered with fetal heart rate monitoring.

Several studies of TENS have been done. However, the results of the trials remain inconclusive regarding its efficacy for clinical use. When TENS is used, the nurse may be involved with placing and securing the electrodes, explaining the use of the controls to the woman, and evaluating the effectiveness of TENS in relieving pain.

Acupressure. **Acupressure** is another possible method of cutaneous stimulation to help decrease a woman's labor pain. It is an ancient oriental technique used to promote relaxation, increase energy, relieve pain, and aid homeostasis. It is related to acupuncture but uses touch instead of needles to achieve results. Some believe that acupressure may release endorphins and other neurotransmitters associated with pain relief.

Some pressure points have been used to induce labor. Although there is no evidence that pressure alone will induce labor, it is recommended that specific points be avoided during pregnancy. These include the "Hoku" point, located on the hands deep within the web of skin between the thumb and forefinger, and the "chih-yin" point, located $\frac{1}{10}$ in. behind the lateral corner

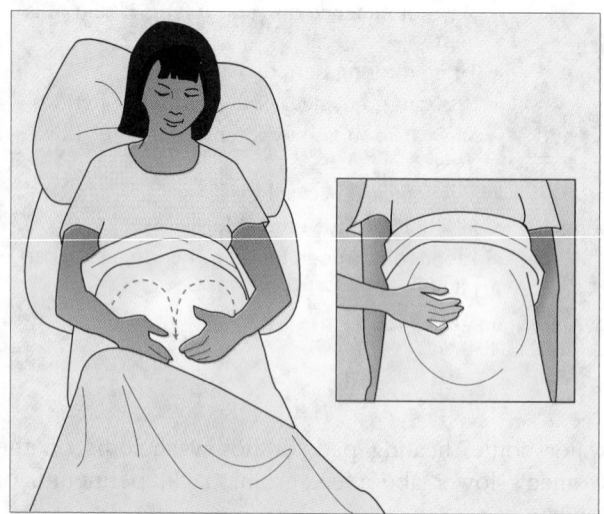

FIGURE 23–4 One- or two-handed effleurage, or abdominal massage.

of the smallest toenail. Other uterine stimulation points are located on the legs and for this reason, and because of major vessels, firm pressure should not be applied to the legs during pregnancy. In addition, pressure should not be applied to an area of infection; red, broken, or swollen skin; or major blood vessels (Jimenez, 1992). Formal evaluation of acupressure would be helpful to discover its usefulness in labor.

Therapeutic Touch. **Therapeutic touch** is based on the folk-healing practice known as *laying on of hands*. Healers place themselves in a meditative state, hold their hands just above the client, and transfer their energy to the client to relieve pain or other problems. Delores Krieger, Professor of Nursing at New York University, has taught the technique to thousands of health professionals. Therapeutic touch is one more method nurses trained in its use have to help their clients in labor (Lieberman, 1992).

Assistance With Change in Expectation and Goals

During the relatively brief and rapidly moving events of labor, any unexpected change in the parents' goals or expectations must be handled quickly. Otherwise, anxiety may persist or increase, resulting in an increased intensity of pain. Some items listed in the Assessment Guidelines are examples of areas in which a disturbing change may occur. Several examples of changes include the following:

- A physician unknown to the parents is in attendance at labor and delivery because of unforseen circumstances.
- The father is unable to attend the birth.
- Crowding of the labor section at this time limits use of planned facilities.
- Internal or external monitors may be used, which may signify complications or limit movement.
- Pain relief medications may be necessary.
- Complications involving labor or the fetus may arise.

When a situation occurs that disturbs the parents, the nurse should encourage them to express their feelings and indicate an appreciation of their disappointment. The nurse should explain the reasons for any rules, policies, or circumstances that prevent the parents from achieving their goals or expectations.

One difficult problem is assisting couples who are not able to achieve their ideal labor and birth. This ideal may vary greatly from one couple to another. Inability to achieve this ideal labor may cause profound feelings of failure in the parents. Also, the couple may refuse or be reluctant to accept measures incompatible with their ideal. Throughout childbirth, and particularly

when goals must change, the nurse praises the parents for their efforts and abilities to handle labor to promote feelings of success. For example, the woman may have the goal of an unmedicated labor, but she may find the pain intolerable and request medication. If medication is given, the nurse can say that she knows medication was not planned, allow the woman to express her feelings, and then praise the woman for the success of her efforts up to now and for the length of time medication was not necessary. The nurse may add that the woman's continuing effort may reduce the amount of medication required and stress to the father that his approval and support are extremely valuable.

Aftermath Assimilation

After anticipation of pain and the presence of pain, a third and final phase of the pain experience occurs: the aftermath. The pain experience does not end with the cessation of the painful sensations. The client does not necessarily immediately forget about the pain, especially if it was severe, frightening, or in any way disconcerting.

On the postpartum unit, women talk a great deal about their childbirth experiences. It is a frequent topic of conversation, regardless of whether the woman had an easy or difficult labor. Not only may the woman want to talk about the pain, but a variety of feelings resulting from the pain, such as nausea, vomiting, chills, anger, or embarrassment.

Clearly, at least some women need assistance during the aftermath phase of the pain experience. The most appropriate nursing action may be to assist the woman with the intellectual and emotional assimilation of her childbirth experience. In a sense, the nurse helps the woman relive her labor. The nurse can ask the woman questions that help her discuss her discomforts, emotions, thoughts, and overt responses and the reactions of others during her labor. The nurse needs to be particularly alert and responsive to the woman's needs for support, such as praise, confirmation that her perceptions of discomfort are believed by others, or reassurance that her behavior was acceptable. Some women need information to help them fill in memory gaps or to correct misunderstandings (McCaffery et al., 1989).

It is particularly important to encourage assimilation in women who may harbor feelings of failure about childbirth. Assimilation may help maintain or restore a positive self-concept for any woman and enhance her ability to deal with mothering and other impending tasks.

Most prepared childbirth instructors encourage the parents to write a "birth report" about their experiences during labor and birth. This writing is not only treasured for years to come, but is an excellent way for the couple to fill in the missing pieces and provide closure so they can move on to the new challenges of parenting (see Nursing Care Plan: The Woman in the Process of Aftermath Assimilation of Labor).

Evaluation

On-the-spot evaluation of pain reducing strategies will be necessary if the nurse is to be effective in helping the woman in labor. The woman should be encouraged to try any new strategies for several contractions before deciding whether it is helpful. After the same strategies are used for some time, the nurse will know that habituation may be likely, with a resultant increase in pain, and the nursing process begins anew.

Possible anticipated outcomes include the following:

- The client and partner demonstrate knowledge of pain relief measures.
- The client verbalizes relief of pain with methods chosen.
- The client adapts to changes in pain level, using a variety of relief measures.

- The client verbalizes control over the situation and makes appropriate informed choices.
- The client and partner verbalize feelings openly about their experiences.
- The client demonstrates a positive response to the labor and birth experience.

The Unique Nature of Obstetric Analgesia and Anesthesia

Few other surgical populations require such extensively coordinated, labor-intensive efforts by a broad range of healthcare providers. That is, the labor and delivery nurse, nurse anesthetist, anesthesiologist, nursery personnel, perinatologist, nurse midwife, and obstetrician may all be directly involved in client care activities requiring critical and differentiated skill. Ef-

NURSING CARE PLAN
The Woman in the Process of Aftermath Assimilation of Labor

Client Goals
1. Woman shares with nurse and others about how she felt when labor became too difficult to handle.
2. Woman understands reasons for increased pain beyond limits to realistically cope.
3. Woman expresses pride at ability to cope as well as she did.

Assessment	Potential Nursing Diagnoses	Nursing Planning/ Assessment	Evaluation
Encourage the woman to talk about all aspects of any discomfort experienced during labor Identify the presence of any feelings of guilt, lack of information, anxiety, or failure	Disturbance in Self Concept related to guilt about her perception that she was unable to use nonpharmacologic methods alone to handle pain during childbirth	Assist the woman to talk about those moments when she felt unable to be effective using breathing/relaxation *to provide catharsis* Praise her ability to resume use of breathing/relaxation techniques after she occasionally failed to use them to assist her to see how much perseverance she had	Woman shares with nurse and others how hard she worked at breathing, relaxation, etc. when pain increased Woman talks less about negative feelings related to handling pain during labor Woman expresses pride in how she handled labor
		Give information about reasons for increased pain at that time *to increase knowledge base* Point out positive attitude of others toward her efforts *to provide knowledge she may not have* Remind her that she successfully delivered a healthy baby *to help her see ultimate goal*	

fective communication between clinicians and a team approach to planning, decision making, and client monitoring to ensure optimal care are essential. Unlike the general surgical population, all decision making must take into account the effects nursing interventions will have on the woman and the fetus. This compels all nurses and other healthcare providers to have a detailed understanding of the extensive changes in maternal physiology at term, the chronology of fetal development, and the physiologic modes of adaptation to extrauterine life.

Two other factors about the unique requirements of the pregnant client are important to consider. First, maternal care usually involves extensive participation of family members throughout labor and delivery. Therefore, each healthcare team member must be able to direct and support the family member in ways that are productive to the client and that promote a successful course of labor and delivery. In addition, labor and delivery nurses should never fail to appreciate their role as a client advocate, because many women who have not had comprehensive prenatal care and teaching may feel inadequate or too uninformed to make competent decisions about their personal care or that of their fetus. Consequently, the nurse is a primary source of information and support in the decision-making process about analgesic modalities and communicates those needs and concerns to other providers who will be involved in the woman's care. Finally, obstetrics continues to be an area in which litigation concerning untoward maternal and fetal outcomes remains high, requiring all providers to be highly skilled in areas of decision making, family communication, chart documentation, and risk management techniques.

Within the last 2 decades, significant advances have been made in obstetric analgesia and anesthesia. Today, many healthcare facilities offer the full range of analgesic and anesthetic services provided by highly qualified advanced practice nurses specializing in anesthesia, certified registered nurse anesthetists (CRNAs), or physician anesthesiologists. These services range from administration of light sedation and systemic analgesics and narcotics, usually by the labor and delivery nurse, to regional anesthesia administered by the CRNA or anesthesiologist. Continuous lumbar epidural anesthesia has achieved great popularity in the last decade because it offers the woman a nearly pain-free labor and birth with minimal transplacental drug effects on the fetus.

Characteristics of Analgesia and Anesthesia

It is essential to define and differentiate the terms **analgesia** and **anesthesia.** This is a difficult distinction because analgesia and anesthesia represent two distinct poles of a continuum. Consequently, establishing a distinct demarcation between the two is difficult. Most anesthesia providers generally accept the notion that intravenously or intramuscularly administered analgesia represents a mild to moderate lessening or dulling of central nervous system function, thereby rendering the client conscious, but sedated, and experiencing a decreased level of pain. Lack of sensory perception of pain also may be achieved with epidural analgesia. Vital organ functions, such as ventilation, are not usually compromised, and protective airway reflexes remain intact. Clients should otherwise be able to respond to verbal command and have full, purposeful motor function. All regional block or conduction techniques are discussed under the category of anesthesia, although it is often considered an analgesic technique.

Anesthesia describes a total loss of sensory capability, whether imposed regionally to the pelvic area through regional anesthesia or centrally to the brain as in a general anesthesia, where consciousness is lost. Anesthesia usually implies that one or more vital organ functions are temporarily under partial or total control of the anesthesia provider. Analgesic techniques can rapidly and unexpectedly progress to an anesthetic state, such as in the case of inadvertent overdose or miscalculation of the mother's level of drug tolerance. In addition, it is well documented that the gravid client will require less medication than the nongravid client to achieve a similar therapeutic effect (Cheek et al., 1993). Although the exact mechanism as to why pregnant clients require less inhalational analgesia or anesthesia is uncertain, hormonal, serotogenic, and endogenous opiate changes during pregnancy may be responsible. The gravid client also requires less local anesthetic to produce the same level of spinal or epidural block because of acid–base changes in the cerebrospinal fluid or hormonal changes, such as high progesterone levels, which may increase nerve sensitivity to local anesthetics. Consequently, the nurse must be prepared to sustain vital functions of the mother or fetus should clients progress through planes of analgesia to anesthesia.

Role of the Labor and Delivery Nurse in Obstetric Analgesia and Anesthesia

For many reasons, labor and delivery nurses assume a professional role quite different from their counterpart in any other intensive care setting. The labor and delivery nurse must plan and implement most of the client care activities that incorporate a clear understanding of pain management techniques, including anatomic and physiologic mechanisms of pain, techniques of pain relief, drug administration, management of complications, client monitoring, and standards of anesthetic care.

The obstetric nurse is the single healthcare provider who is in constant attendance with the client. The nurse is the one clinician most familiar with assessing the client's need for pain relief, assessing levels of pain tolerance, observing the client's methods of adaptation or accommodation of painful stimuli, and monitoring the general course of labor as it relates to anesthetic interventions. These are all factors of paramount importance to the anesthesia provider when selecting, administering, managing, and assessing the effectiveness of anesthetic interventions.

Legal Implications of Practice in Anesthesia Care

The labor and delivery nurse is assuming increased responsibilities as a team member in providing analgesia and anesthesia to the obstetric client. There is great diversity among institutional policies that exist governing the scope of practice that labor and delivery nurses can assume when providing this care. It is incumbent on nurses to be aware of the locally determined limitations and the rights and privileges granted by their license to practice as a registered nurse.

Increasingly, it is the practice of state boards of nursing to broaden the scope of nursing practice so that there are fewer rather than more restrictions on clinical practice. Statutory stipulations for the practice of advanced nursing, however, often require formal training and credentialing that verifies to the public competence in the field (Simpson et al., 1992). Thus, nurses often find themselves in the dilemma of being encouraged to assume greater responsibilities, while having to deal with state statute or precedent that fails to define clearly the limits of the scope of practice. As the boundaries of nursing care are expanded, the legal authority for assumption of those rights will be less clear, at least until they become standards of practice.

This calls into question the issue of liability for the nurse if a negative client outcome results directly from a nurse's action that is not normally considered a traditional prerogative of a labor and delivery nurse. Even though the state board of nursing may tend to rule that such action is within the general scope of nursing practice, this does not necessarily mean that an insurance carrier or a court of law will agree. On the contrary, a nurse may be found negligent or practicing beyond the scope of authority as determined by common community practice and adequacy of educational preparation to assume new responsibilities. For instance, a nurse may be found liable in certain circumstances for a negative client outcome resulting from an independent decision to manipulate local anesthetic concentrations or rates of continuous infusions. The question is not whether the nurse is culpable for client harm or capable in the technical or judgmental skills to make the changes. Rather, the question is that the nurse lacks the publicly accepted or mandated authority to make such changes if they are not in concert with community practice standards and based on clear evidence that through credentialing or other educational preparation the nurse is qualified to manipulate the drug.

As nursing expands its practice and inevitably impinges on the traditional practice rights of medical and other specialized nursing personnel, competitive practice issues will most likely increase in the years ahead. These issues, not new to nursing, will continue to be discussed as long as the public expectation requires that nurses care for clients of increasing acuity and demonstrate increasing expertise with technologically advanced equipment and new therapeutic modalities. Resolution of these issues is a responsibility nursing must assume as a consequence of continued growth and sophistication as a profession. This requires effective communication within nursing and best efforts to protect the public interest and safety.

The labor and delivery nurse should understand not only the scope of professional responsibilities as they have been traditionally practiced, but also those gray areas in which practice is expanding and less well defined. These trends have a way of eventually finding their way into a more permanent practice pattern. However, until then, the nurse should be aware of hospital or departmental policy, state nurse practice acts, and professional and legal trends that will assist in providing a clearer definition of nursing practice in the challenging and dynamic field of obstetrics.

Analgesia for Labor and Vaginal Birth

Many different analgesic and anesthetic techniques and services are available to the client. Skillful obstetric anesthesia, including psychological and emotional support of the mother, may make birth less stressful for her and her newborn. Clearly, when the woman can make an informed decision regarding choice of analgesia or anesthesia and feels comfortable with that decision, her overall birth experience can be enhanced.

Techniques of Analgesia and Anesthesia

The woman has a variety of options available when selecting the particular type of analgesic support best suited for her labor and birth experience. Some of these techniques do not involve pharmacologic intervention. However, the nurse should make it clear to the client that no particular preference is irrevocable.

Many mothers may choose to use methods of natural childbirth. These clients need to understand that their decision to change from nonpharmacologic techniques to more direct means of pharmacologic intervention will be respected and supported by the nurse. Many women, for instance, will accept minimal doses of intramuscular (IM) or intravenous (IV) narcotics during labor. However, as cervical dilation proceeds, they often request placement of a lumbar epidural catheter for more complete pain relief. It also should be stressed that barring strict contraindications to a particular drug or technique, the choice should remain ultimately an independent one made by the woman in consultation with the nurse and the anesthesia provider.

There are four general categories of analgesia and anesthesia techniques:

1. Systemic medications using narcotics, sedatives, and tranquilizers, either by IV or IM routes
2. Inhalation anesthetics using subanesthetic concentrations of drugs
3. Regional anesthesia using continuous lumbar epidural analgesia and anesthesia, spinal anesthesia, sacral epidural anesthesia (caudal), or paracervical or pudendal block
4. General anesthesia

Selection of an Analgesic or Anesthetic

Several factors should be considered when planning and selecting the analgesic or anesthetic for labor and childbirth. Ideally, this process should begin early in the prenatal period, with information usually introduced by the obstetrician or office nurse or through prenatal classes conducted by qualified personnel. Obviously, these professionals must be well versed on all possible techniques and be able to provide answers to client questions. They also should be able to provide other resources, such as prepared reading material outlining the variety of options or early referrals to professional anesthesia providers. Too often, clients receive incomplete or inaccurate information that promotes certain unfounded biases or predispositions toward certain techniques and may not be in the best interest of the woman or fetus. For instance, clients may often say "I'm afraid of a needle in my back. It may paralyze me." Unfortunately, in this instance, the client may not have received sufficient information to make an informed decision concerning regional anesthesia, including the relative risks of the technique, the benefits of allowing more maternal participation in the delivery by avoiding systemic medications, and the level of profound pain relief to the mother and avoidance of depressant medication on the fetus.

Once the client is admitted to the labor and delivery suite, the CRNA or physician anesthesiologist should perform a history and physical and interview the client to assist her in determining which type of analgesic or anesthetic is best suited to her needs and those of the fetus. Even if a woman chooses not to use any type of analgesic or anesthetic for delivery, she should be interviewed by a qualified anesthesia provider early in the labor process in case circumstances arise that require immediate anesthetic intervention for the well-being of the client or fetus. Consent forms for anesthesia that delineate the type of anesthesia selected and alternative plans in case of emergency should be signed by the client at the time of the interview. An ideal analgesic or anesthetic experience should be tailored to the individual client, which is based on her personal physical and surgical history, prenatal course, and personal preferences.

Although no single modality of pain relief encompasses all desired outcomes, the following objectives should be kept in mind when helping a client select an analgesic or anesthetic:

- The woman should never be coerced into accepting a technique promoted only by the preferences or biases of the nurse, obstetrician, or anesthesia provider.
- The analgesic or anesthetic should provide satisfactory pain relief for the woman that will maximize her active participation and satisfaction with the process of labor and childbirth.
- The analgesic or anesthetic technique should promote client safety, not unduly interfere with the normal progression of labor and childbirth, and provide optimal surgical or delivery conditions.
- The analgesic or anesthetic should not be associated with undue risks to the woman or excessively depressant effects on the fetus.
- The analgesic or anesthetic should allow sufficient flexibility so that if emergent measures are required to deliver the fetus, induction can proceed smoothly with minimal time delays. In every instance, the woman should be informed of any alternative plans for anesthesia if they become necessary as a result of unexpected complications.

Nursing Considerations

The nurse plays an important role in the selection of analgesia and anesthesia and preparation of the client for delivery. The nurse should be conversant with the range of analgesia and anesthesia services available and provide appropriate information to the client. The nurse also should remember that pregnancy alters the normal physiologic state of clients and often exacerbates many preexisting diseases, so the client's normal homeostatic mechanisms or organ systems may be significantly compromised. Although pregnant clients are usually healthy young adults, and birth usually is a normal physiologic function, these clients can be at risk for complications during labor and delivery. If such complications arise, swift and deliberate nursing and medical interventions are required. The nurse must be knowledgeable of and prepared for such complications should the need arise.

Systemic Medications

Systemic medications are most often used to lessen pain and allay anxiety in the first stage of labor. In many instances, these drugs are the only pharmacologic intervention necessary for adequate pain relief during labor, especially when supplemented with paracervical or pudendal blocks administered close to or immediately prior to delivery. Systemic drugs are usually administered either by IV or IM routes. Brief mention is made, however, of analgesic techniques involving the use of nitrous oxide through inhalation.

The goal of systemic pain medication is to provide maximum pain relief to the woman while minimizing depressive effects on the fetus and uterine function. At the least, systemic medications have been found particularly useful in helping the woman relax sufficiently to regain control of breathing techniques and allow labor to proceed expeditiously. Titrated doses of systemic narcotics, for instance, are usually well tolerated by the woman and have little deleterious effect on the fetus because there is minimal placental drug transfer.

Systemic medications are beneficial in maintaining greater maternal physiologic homeostasis during labor. Endogenous catecholamines, such as epinephrine and norepinephrine, are elevated during labor and delivery, largely from the body's response to pain. These high levels of circulating catecholamines can cause uterine artery vasoconstriction, resulting in a decrease in uterine blood flow. Catecholamines also contribute to maternal metabolic acidosis, which may cause a shift of the oxygen dissociation curve, inhibiting the release of oxygen from hemoglobin and generally decreasing oxygen availability to the fetus. Maternal hyperventilation (ie, panting) in response to pain can produce maternal respiratory alkalosis, which compromises acid–base balance in the fetus. Administration of narcotics can effectively decrease these stress responses and return the client to a state of normoventilation, thus minimizing the possibility of compromised fetal perfusion and oxygenation.

Maternal overdose with systemic medications is possible because pregnant clients require less drug per weight than the nonpregnant client. IV drugs should always be titrated slowly to effect; that is, only what is required by the woman for a decrease in her discomfort or to afford sedation should be administered. Most drugs can be identified in colostrum, although in very small quantities, for up to 14 days after administration.

However, for breast-feeding clients, such effects appear to have minimal clinical relevance. For the client receiving systemic medications during labor, the nurse should monitor the client for the following:

- Loss of fetal variability and arrhythmias, most commonly atrial in origin
- Respiratory depression of newborn at birth if peak or cumulative effect of drug occurs with delivery
- Maternal nausea and vomiting
- Fetal hypotonus at delivery
- Maternal hypoventilation and hypotension
- Urinary retention from narcotics

Narcotics: Agents and Indications

Opioids remain the most commonly used and effective analgesic agents for the client in labor. These drugs affect the woman and fetus equally in terms of respiratory depression and sedation. However, none have been shown to have significant fetal effects, as demonstrated by neurobehavioral studies, or long-term effects on intelligence or subsequent development. Opioids cross the placenta rapidly, however, and may cause temporary postnatal ventilatory depression. Recording the last drug injection-to-delivery interval of any narcotic administered is crucial. This will avoid excessive neonatal depression at birth that coincides with the drug's peak effect.

Morphine may cause significant maternal and fetal ventilatory depression. Therefore, it is rarely given to the laboring woman. If morphine is indicated, it is usually given IV in doses of 1 to 2 mg titrated over several minutes. Onset of action occurs within 2 to 3 minutes, and the peak effect occurs in 1 to 2 hours (Shnider et al., 1994). Morphine also can be administered IM in doses of 5 to 10 mg.

Meperidine is commonly used for analgesia in the obstetric client and produces less ventilatory depression than morphine. Meperidine is administered IV in doses of 25 to 50 mg, repeated in smaller increments to achieve the desired level of analgesia. The drug also can be administered IM in somewhat higher doses. However, the rate of uptake is much less dependable, and onset is slower. Meperidine can precipitate maternal nausea and vomiting and cause decreases in fetal beat-to-beat variability and maternal tachycardia (Moore et al., 1992).

Other shorter acting synthetic narcotics, such as fentanyl and sufentanil, also are used in circumstances requiring short but intensive pain relief. Fentanyl and sufentanil can be used successfully when uterine manipulation is required to correct fetal presentation or when the need for forceps during childbirth is anticipated. Fentanyl is equianalgesic to morphine in the ratio of 100 μg:10 mg, respectively (Shnider et al., 1994).

IV fentanyl's duration of action is 30 to 60 minutes. The effects of sufentanil last somewhat longer. Both drugs should be used with extreme caution because of their high potency and ventilatory depressive properties. Fentanyl can be administered during labor for severe pain or as an adjunct to regional anesthesia for cesarean section. The dose is 25 to 100 μg IV and can be repeated hourly as needed (Schnider et al., 1993). Careful observation for signs of respiratory depression is essential.

Butorphanol (Stadol) and nalbuphine (Nubain), both agonist-antagonist non-narcotic analgesics, also have been used for labor. In theory, they maintain their analgesic effect yet demonstrate less ventilatory depression than the more traditional narcotics. The dose of butorphanol is 0.5 to 1 mg IV given in titrated doses and 2 mg IM every 4 hours. Nalbuphine doses are 3 to 5 mg IV or 10 to 20 mg IM.

Nursing Implications. Judicious use of narcotics in the first and early second stages of labor can be safe with minimal side effects to the woman or fetus. When administering these drugs intravenously, the nurse should be in constant attendance with the woman to assess ventilatory and cardiovascular effects. The client's blood pressure, pulse, and ventilatory rate should be taken every 5 minutes during titration and for 15 to 20 minutes (up to 1 hour) after administration to determine general client stability. When maternal pain has subsided in response to drug therapy, the nurse should be alert to signs and symptoms of hypotension and hypercarbia, which may occur from a reduction in endogenous catecholamines, drug-induced direct myocardial depression, and decreased peripheral vascular resistance. Continuous electronic fetal monitoring should always be used during maternal drug administration to detect any changes in fetal heart rate, pattern, or variability.

If required, the effects of all narcotic analgesics can be reversed with maternal administration of naloxone in incremental doses of 0.1 to 0.4 mg IV or 0.2 to 0.4 mg IM. Newborn doses should be initiated at 0.01 mg/kg (Levinson et al., 1993). Because the antagonistic effect is quick and complete, one should not attempt to reverse narcotic effects in the woman immediately prior to delivery, unless absolutely necessary. Narcotic antagonism will increase maternal pain and the risk for nausea and vomiting if other forms of pain relief, such as local anesthetics through infiltration or epidural, have not already been instituted. Extreme caution should be exercised when administering narcotic antagonists to mothers who have a documented history of drug abuse or methadone therapy because symptoms of withdrawal are likely to ensue in the woman and fetus. These same precautions should be applied to the use of the agonist-antagonist drugs.

Sedatives and Tranquilizers: Agents and Indications

Medications within the sedative and tranquilizer classifications are most often used for their anxiolytic properties, potentiation of narcotics, and promotion of sleep, especially when clients experience protracted initial stages of labor. They also are quite effective in lessening nausea and vomiting common during this period. Commonly used drugs are the benzodiazepines, phenothiazine derivatives, hydroxyzine, buterophenones, and to a lesser extent, barbiturates. Table 23-5 lists some commonly used sedatives and tranquilizers.

Nursing Implications. The primary untoward effect of sedative medication is possible overdose. Some women may exhibit **dysphoria** as an idiosyncratic reaction to the drug, becoming confused or agitated. If doses are too high, temporary amnesia may occur, interfering with the mother's ability to cooperate or manage her breathing techniques or pushing, when required. The normal progress of labor also may be slowed.

As with narcotics, equal caution should be used when administering sedative hypnotics or tranquilizers. The nurse should be in constant attendance during drug administration and record vital signs every 5 minutes during IV drug titration. Also, many of these drugs have a synergistic effect with narcotics, compounding respiratory depression if the woman has recently received narcotics. In this instance, it also is likely that the client may experience significant decreases in blood pressure. Maternal systolic blood pressure must be maintained above 100 mm Hg, otherwise fetal perfusion may be compromised. This critical perfusion pressure is for a healthy woman who does not suffer from chronic hypertension or eclampsia, in which case the critical systolic pressures for perfusion would be higher. As a general rule, blood pressure should not decrease 20% below the mother's normal, resting blood pressure for any significant time. When sustained hypotension occurs, the nurse may consider increasing IV infusion rates; placing the client in a head-down, left-lateral position; and administering oxygen. If hypotension does not resolve, pharmacologic intervention (such as ephedrine in an initial IV dose of 5 to 10 mg) may be required.

Inhalation Analgesia and Anesthesia: Agents and Indications

The inhalation method of analgesia for the client in labor is used less frequently, primarily because it has been supplanted by the increased acceptance and popularity of regional techniques. For clients who are fear-

TABLE 23–5
Sedatives and Tranquilizers

Drug	Indications	Considerations
Benzodiazepines, such as diazepam (Valium) and midazolam (Versed)	Reduction of maternal anxiety and narcotic requirements without prolonging labor IV bolus of diazepam usually reserved to treat convulsive disorders associated with eclampsia Midazolam, 1–2 mg IV helpful in decreasing maternal anxiety and aiding labor progression	Benzodiazepines exacerbate respiratory depression when given in combination with narcotics. Fetal drug effects generally manifested by decreased beat-to-beat variability; drug does not affect acid–base balance.
Phenothiazines, such as promethazine (Phenergan) and propiomazine (Largon)	Alleviation of anxiety, promotion of relaxation, emesis control, and prolongation of narcotic effect Normally given in conjunction with small doses of narcotics; when given alone, can produce confusion or delirium when the client is perceiving pain	Other phenothiazines, such as prochlorperazine (Compazine), are not recommended because of possibility of producing maternal hypotension.
Hydroxyzine hydrochloride (Vistaril)	Used in conjunction with IM narcotics to reduce the dosage of narcotic required Potent antihistaminic and antiemetic effects	This drug cannot be given intravenously.
Buterophenones such as droperidol (Inapsine)	Used in small, single doses of 0.625 mg IV to control or prevent nausea and vomiting	Dosages for sedation are not recommended. Higher dosages should be avoided to prevent possible hypotension.
Ketamine (Ketalar)	Used in low doses of 0.25–0.3 mg/kg of maternal body weight, permits analgesia while client remains conscious with reflexes intact Indicated for analgesia in special circumstances, such as in retained placenta or protracted repairs of cervical or vaginal tears or difficult low or midforceps delivery; can be a supplement to a pudendal block	This dissociative anesthetic should be used only by anesthesia providers. In small doses, it produces sedation and analgesia. This drug possibly produces dysphoria (feelings of unhappiness or being) and hallucinations. Quiet recovery is required. Midazolam (1–2 mg) given prior to ketamine limits or obtunds these episodes. This powerful amnestic possibly produces maternal memory loss for part or all of the labor and delivery.

ful of needles or complications associated with blocks or for those who arrive at the hospital with birth imminent, inhalation analgesia may be used. It is often used as a supplement to other analgesic techniques, particularly regional anesthesia, when the block is incomplete or waning. Most inhalation anesthetics can be administered at an analgesic concentration (subanesthetic concentration) sufficient to allow adequate pain relief, while allowing the woman to remain conscious during birth and able to take directions from her coach or delivery room personnel.

Nitrous oxide (N_2O) is perhaps the most widely used inhalation agent in obstetrics. It is administered during delivery from the anesthetic machine breathing circuit usually on an intermittent basis coinciding with the peak of contractions. It also can be used effectively during manual extraction of a placenta or minor repairs of the vagina or cervix or as an adjunct to pudendal block for episiotomy repair. Concentrations of the drug, usually between 30% and 50% administered with

oxygen, are adjusted according to the client's need, state of consciousness, and ability to push. N_2O has little deleterious effect on the fetus because the drug is rapidly cleared from maternal circulation through the pulmonary system. Other techniques of inhalation analgesia for childbirth include the combination of N_2O and subanesthetic concentrations of potent inhalation agents, such as enflurane and isoflurane. Analgesic concentrations of inhalation agents are usually relatively benign to the fetus and only cause transient depression after protracted maternal administration.

Nursing Implications

For decades, clients have chosen inhalation analgesia for childbirth. Historically, it has been known for its ease of application, low cost, reasonable effectiveness, and minimal complications. The primary problems of this technique of analgesia are those associated with depressant effects exerted on maternal airway reflexes, predisposing the client to vomiting and aspiration of gastric contents, loss of ability to swallow, and ventilatory depression. Loss of airway reflexes mandates endotracheal intubation of the client. Caution should always be used when inhalation agents are used because the loss of airway reflexes prior to establishing a patent airway could be disastrous. All inhalation agents should be administered by CRNAs or physicians appropriately credentialed to administer anesthesia.

Regional Blockade

Regional blockade, the use of a local anesthetic to interfere with a group of sensory nerve fibers, has become increasingly popular as the preferred form of pain relief for labor and vaginal birth. This technique allows the client to be awake and to participate in all facets of the birthing process. Additionally, this technique is not usually associated with the depressive effects of systemic agents, consequently allowing initiation with the bonding process and trials at breast-feeding. When properly administered, regional techniques provide a favorable physiologic environment for the fetus because drug uptake is minimal or of short duration and effect.

Regional blockade does not necessarily impede the normal progression of labor or the woman's ability to push the fetus down the birth canal. Pelvic muscle tone can be sustained so that fetal head rotation is possible. Because the client is awake, there is no concern for potential airway reflex obtundation, predisposing the woman to gastric aspiration. It also may be a preferred technique for clients with severe preexisting cardiac or pulmonary disease, such as asthma, when a general anesthetic would more likely compromise the preexisting condition. Perhaps the most compelling argument for the selection of regional blockade is that the quality of the block can afford near-complete pain relief in selected areas of the body yet not interfere with normal motor function unless an **intrathecal** (spinal) anesthetic is used (Fig. 23-5). This is in sharp contrast to systemic analgesic methods that although effective, provide pain relief by altering the perception clients have of pain to a more accommodating level of tolerance.

The most prevalent techniques of regional blockade include lumbar epidural blocks and spinal, caudal, pudendal, paracervical, and local infiltration of the perineum. Regardless of the type of regional technique selected, all necessary drugs and equipment required to treat respiratory or cardiovascular complications, including airways, endotracheal tubes, laryngoscope, an oxygen source, positive-pressure ventilation, and medications to treat arrhythmias and hypotension should be available. In spite of the benefits of regional blockade, there are some contraindications to the technique, including refusal by the woman, coagulation defects, skin lesions at the site of needle entry, or possibly pre-

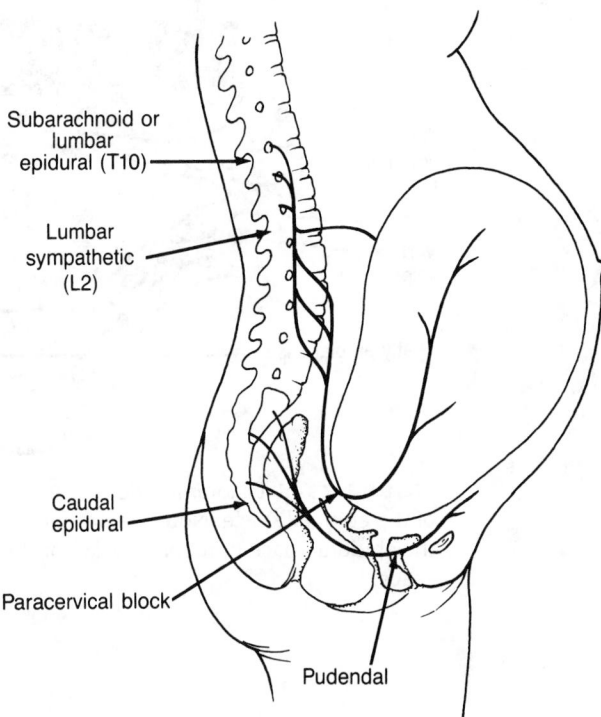

FIGURE 23–5 Pain pathways during labor and techniques of nerve block.

vious surgery for back injuries that altered normal spinal anatomy.

Lumbar Epidural Anesthesia

The primary objective of **epidural anesthesia** involves the placement of a volume of local anesthetic into the **epidural space.** This space, also called the potential space, is normally filled with segments of nerve roots from the spinal cord, fatty tissue, and an intricate networking of blood vessels. It is surrounded by a series of protective and supportive ligaments and the bony vertebral column. The space also is an outer covering to the several layers of dura, spinal fluid, and cord (Fig. 23-6). Through diffusion to surrounding nerve fibers, epidural anesthesia temporarily interrupts normal transmission of pain impulses from the pelvic area and provides an anesthetized state for dermatome areas preselected to block (Fig. 23-7). In carefully titrated doses, the client's motor function is usually uninterrupted, but sensory block is complete. After appropriate client teaching, signing procedure consent forms, and insertion of an IV infusion line, administration of the epidural can proceed when effective labor is established. The catheter can be placed earlier and a dose of local anesthetic administered if the woman is multiparous, not tolerating labor well, or an oxytocin drip has been instituted. The client should have received a minimum of approximately 1,000 mL of a crystalloid (balanced salt) IV solution, prior to the in-

(*text continues on page 606*)

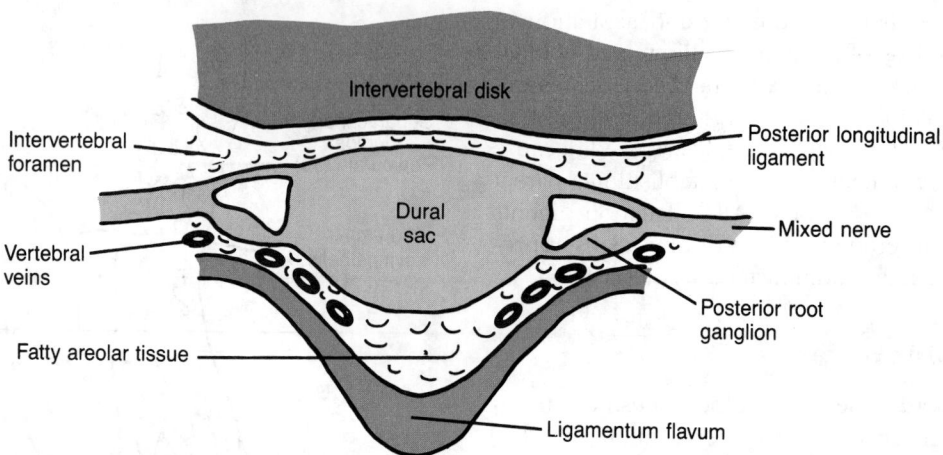

FIGURE 23–6 Diagrammatic cross-section of the vertebral canal showing the contents of the epidural space. Note the prominent epidural veins. Local anesthetic injected into the epidural space primarily blocks conduction of nerve roots as they traverse the epidural space.

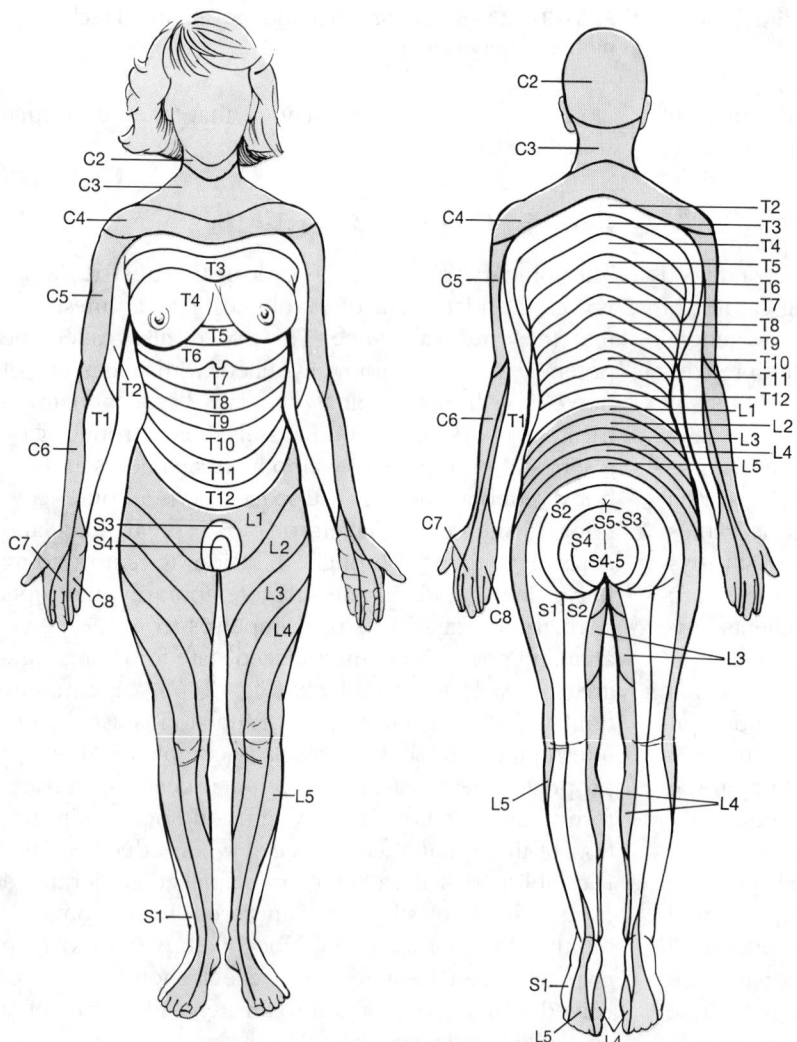

FIGURE 23–7 Dermatome levels. (Cousins, M. J., Bromage, P. R. [1988]. Epidural neural blockade. In M. J. Cousins & P. O. Bridenbaugh (Eds). Neural blockade in Clinical Anesthesia and Management of Pain p. 344, 2nd ed. Philadelphia: JB Lippincott, 1988)

TABLE 23–6
Local Anesthetics Commonly Used in Obstetrics

Local Anesthetic and Trade Name	Characteristics	Maximum Safe Initial Dose (mg)		Epidural	
		WITHOUT EPINEPHRINE	WITH EPINEPHRINE	DOSE* VAGINAL DELIVERY	DOSE* CESAREAN SECTION
2 chloroprocaine (Nesacaine)	Very low toxicity; most rapidly metabolized with little accumulation; rapid onset but poor spread	600	1,000	1%–2% 8–12 mL	3% 15–25 mL
Tetracaine (Pontocaine)	5 times toxicity but 10 times potency of procaine; today used only for spinal and topical; poor spread, very slow onset	100	200	Not available	
Lidocaine (Xylocaine)	Most versatile local anesthetic; moderate toxicity; rapid onset; moderate duration; excellent spread	300	500	1%–1½% 8–12 mL	1½%–2% 15–25 mL
Bupivacaine (Marcaine, Sensorcaine)	Slow onset; long duration; marked cardiac toxicity; low concentrations give excellent sensory and little motor block; ideal for obstetrics	175	225	¼%–½% 8–12 mL	½% 20–25mL

Block	Bilateral Pudendal Block		Hyperbaric Subarachnoid (Spinal)‡			Comments
			DOSES§			
DURATION† (MIN)	DOSE*	DURATION† (MIN)	VAGINAL DELIVERY	CESAREAN SECTION	DURATION‡ (MIN)	
30–60	1%–2% 10–20 mL	30–60	Not available			Large inadvertent subarachnoid injection associated with neurologic residual. Its rapid onset and metabolism make it an ideal drug for epidural in the obstetric client. Extremely low maternal and fetal toxicity.
	Not available		1% 6–8 mg	1% 8–12 mg	120–200	In past was used for epidural and local infiltration, but has been replaced by others owing to poor spread and slow onset. Now manufactured only for subarachnoid block.
60–90	1% 10–20 mL	60–90	1.5% or 5% 15–50 mg	5% 60–90 mg	60–120	Epidural use in past was thought to be associated with depressed neonatal muscle tone. Recent studies question this.
90–180	¼% 10–20 mL	180–720	0.75% 4–6 mg	0.75% 7–12 mg	100–150‖	Inadvertent intravascular injection associated with cardiovascular collapse.

*Doses are given as suggested concentration and milliliters required.

†Lower dose represents minimum duration without epinephrine; upper dose represents maximum duration using epinephrine.

‡All solutions described have a higher specific gravity than cerebrospinal fluid because they are weighted with local anesthetic and dextrose.

§Given as concentration of solution and milligrams of local anesthetic used. Note the low dose of local anesthetic required for subarachnoid block as compared with epidural block.

‖Addition of epinephrine to subarachnoid bupivacaine does not significantly prolong the duration of block.

jection of the drug into the epidural space to prevent hypotensive episodes secondary to sympathetic blockade and subsequent vasodilation.

The epidural catheter is inserted under sterile technique with the client in a sitting or lateral decubitus position with knees tucked to best expose the vertebrae to the anesthetist.

Once correct placement has been verified, the epidural catheter is guided through the needle to be left in the space and the needle pulled out over the catheter. Then the catheter is padded with a gauze sponge at the site of entry, taped to the woman's back, and brought over her shoulder for easy accessibility of the injection port. The client resumes a supine position with her head up slightly. Subsequent doses of local anesthetics can be administered as boluses through the catheter or connected to continuous infusion pumps to maintain a steady state of drug in the plasma, allowing lower concentrations of drug to be used.

Incremental dosing is used to achieve a sensory block to a level of approximately T10 (involving blockades of T10, T11, T12, and L1 segments) for the first stages of labor, eliminating the pain of uterine contractions and dilation of the cervix. During the second stage, the level of block can be elevated to alleviate pain from perineal stretching by blocking pudendal nerves at the S2, S3, and S4 segments. Dosing also can be increased to accommodate cesarean section when the level of block reaches T4. The most commonly used local anesthetics for epidural anesthesia are lidocaine 1% to 2%, bupivacaine 0.25% to 0.5%, and chloroprocaine 1.5% to 3% (Table 23-6).

Recently, the addition of small amounts of synthetic narcotics, such as fentanyl and butorphanol, which significantly decrease required doses of local anesthetics, has been incorporated into practice (Hughes, 1993; Table 23-7). Analgesia produced by narcotics, such as morphine, epidurally and intrathecally are segmental and effective for visceral pain but not usually effective for severe surgical or somatic pain, especially when used as the sole agent, without local anesthetics. Epidural and intrathecal narcotics are becoming more widely used even though there is a relatively high inci-

dence of pruritus and incidental nausea and vomiting. These effects can be diminished with a partial or total reversal of the narcotic with IV bolus or drip administration of antagonists, such as naloxone. These symptoms also can be treated with diphenhydramine (Benadryl) and appropriate antiemetics, such as droperidol, if reversal of analgesia is not desired (see Nursing Care Plan: Lumbar Epidural Anesthesia).

Subarachnoid Blockade

Subarachnoid blockade, also called spinal anesthesia, involves the injection of a local anesthetic into the subarachnoid space where the medication mixes with cerebrospinal fluid. It is used predominately for cesarean section when an epidural technique is not otherwise used. Because onset of the block takes only a few minutes to affect sensory and motor function, spinal anesthesia is not a viable option for labor. Selective spinal blockade, such as a saddle block, can be used for a forceps delivery or repair of an extensive episiotomy when spinal segments S1 through S5 are blocked. A spinal block, appropriate for a cesarean section, can be achieved when level T4 is affected. A disadvantage of spinal blockade is that only a single dose can be given because there is no catheter (as with the epidural) to allow redosing if initial levels are inadequate for surgical anesthesia. Continuous spinal anesthesia is rarely used because micropore spinal catheters have not been available since 1992.

The technique for administration of a spinal block is virtually the same as for an epidural, except that the dura is purposefully entered and local anesthetic injected directly into the spinal fluid. Injection of drugs for a spinal and epidural should not take place during uterine contractions because the level of the block may be pushed to unacceptably high levels. Lidocaine, bupivacaine, and tetracaine are the predominate local anesthetic agents used for spinal blockade. Lidocaine is effective for 1 hour, and bupivacaine and tetracaine are effective for 2 to 4 hours. 2-chloroprocaine is contraindicated because neurotoxic effects have been reported.

Combined Spinal-Epidural Technique

The combined spinal-epidural technique uses intrathecal (into the subarachnoid space) narcotics and epidural local anesthetics. This technique is advantageous because it provides the quick onset of spinal block analgesia with the ability to administer additional medication as needed through the epidural catheter. Some studies have shown that intrathecal sufentanil 10 μg provides profound analgesia for 1 to 3 hours (Camann et al., 1992; Honet et al., 1992; Sharkey et al., 1991). The desired pain relief from contractions is provided without affecting motor function, thereby en-

TABLE 23-7
Narcotic Doses (Bolus) for Epidural and Spinal Analgesia

Drug	Epidural	Spinal	Duration (h)
Morphine	3–4 mg	0.25–0.4 mg	12–24
Meperidine	50–100 mg	10–30 mg	4–16
Fentanyl	50–100 μg	20–25 μg	2–4
Sufentanil	20–30 μg	10 μg	2–5
Butorphanol	1–2 mg	—	2–3

NURSING CARE PLAN
Lumbar Epidural Anesthesia

A 24-year-old woman, gravida 3, para 2, is admitted to the labor and delivery suite in active labor. She is somewhat relaxed except during contractions and is actively attempting to establish appropriate breathing techniques. On physical examination, the cervix is found to be dilated to 3 cm. Vital signs of the mother and infant fetal monitoring strips indicate both are stable. The mother states a friend suggested she should have an epidural anesthetic and wants it administered as soon as possible.

Nursing Goals
1. To facilitate client understanding of analgesia options for labor and delivery
2. To prepare for implementation of the epidural procedure that will facilitate client compliance, understanding, and safety
3. To provide conditions during the anesthetic procedure to affect minimal disruption to the laboring process and maximize pain relief
4. To competently assess extent of pain relief from epidural anesthetic

Assessment	Nursing Diagnoses	Intervention/Rationale	Evaluation
Client and fetus stable/ early labor/request epidural/exhibits moderate pain	Knowledge Deficit relative to epidural procedure/unaware of other pain relief modalities	Explain other anesthesia alternatives/explain epidural procedure/ demonstration of epidural technique/nurse seeks anesthesia consult in order *to allay client concerns about the procedure*	Client understands alternatives/understands epidural benefits and risks/ signs procedural consent forms.
Establish extent of cervical dilation (5–6 cm)/assess state of client extracellular hydration/assess fetal condition and maternal stability via vital signs and electronic monitoring/assess degree of client discomfort, efficacy of coping mechanisms	Potential for Alterations in Maternal Ability to Cope with stress of labor and potential unfulfilled expectations of anesthesia	Acquire resuscitation equipment for possible emergency/have client empty bladder/establish IV line of nondextrose solution for preload in order *to prepare for undue emergencies,* take and record vital signs and fetal monitoring *to supply baseline data.*	Client communicates satisfaction and confidence with decision to have epidural anesthesia
Client exhibits acute pain/ active labor established	Potential for Alterations in Physical Regulation, Circulation, and Oxygenation	Position client in left lateral/knee/chest position/ continue fetal monitoring/ongoing communication with client *to answer questions and allay anxiety and provide information,* observe for signs of local anesthetic toxicity (tinnitus, hypotension, metallic taste in mouth, altered sensorium)/continue to coach client relative to breathing techniques *to expedite labor*/record vital signs every 5 minutes after block secure and pad epidural catheter *to optimize anesthetic*	Client exhibits stable vital signs/block is bilateral and provides pain relief/ fetus and mother are stable.

(continued)

NURSING CARE PLAN *(Continued)*
Lumbar Epidural Anesthesia

Assessment	Nursing Diagnoses	Intervention/Rationale	Evaluation
Client complains of continued pain in fundal area of uterus and predominance of right-sided pain relief in hip and thigh	Potential Alteration in Comfort	Take client vital signs/test motor function by having client move legs and feet/test sensory function by sequential pin prick from knees to upper abdomen *to identify level of dermatome blocked/* turn client to nonanesthetized side/lower head to facilitate cephalad movement of local anesthetic/check integrity of epidural catheter/seek anesthesia consult after preliminary interventions *to promote maximum health*	Block becomes bilateral/ client blood pressure returns to normal limits/ client states pain is becoming relieved

abling the client to move around freely, even ambulate during labor. Once the spinal needle is inserted and the dura mater is entered, the narcotic is administered. The spinal needle is withdrawn, and the epidural catheter is then threaded through the epidural needle into the epidural space. A cap is placed on the end of the catheter, which is securely taped to the client's back. When the client begins to feel contractions again, local anesthetics and additional narcotics can be infused through the epidural catheter. The side effects of this technique are the same as with other spinal or epidural narcotic techniques, primarily pruritus, nausea, and vomiting. Severe side effects can be treated by giving naloxone 0.4 mg IV or diphenhydramine 25 mg IV. The occurrence of spinal headaches following this technique is rare.

Pudendal and Paracervical Block

The **paracervical block** involves a submucosal injection of local anesthetic near uterine nerve fibers, at the vaginal fornix lateral to the cervix. It is most often administered by the midwife or obstetrician during the first stage of labor, obliterating visceral pain from the uterus, cervix, and upper vagina. It is accomplished transvaginally and requires only 1 to 2 minutes to execute. Neither hypotension nor loss of urge to push results. The block is somewhat less popular today than in the past because it has been associated with fetal distress in 10% to 40% of cases and poor neonatal outcome (Moore et al., 1992). Most assume that fetal ef-

fects result from the high concentration of local anesthetics in fetal blood or decreased uterine blood flow secondary to local anesthetic-mediated uterine vasoconstriction. All anesthetics except bupivacaine are used.

The **pudendal nerve block** involves interruption of sacral nerve transmission that supplies the vaginal vault, perineum, and rectum. Local anesthetic, usually 10 mL of 1% lidocaine, is administered transvaginally behind each sacrospinous ligament. The block is administered immediately prior to delivery and is ideal for episiotomy incision and repair or to facilitate a forceps delivery. Regional blockade can result in various complications. Table 23-8 describes these complications and possible nursing implications for each.

Nursing Implications

The labor and delivery nurse fulfills a series of important functions related to the administration and monitoring of an epidural or spinal block. These can be considered more easily when divided into three distinct time intervals: preblock preparation, block administration, and block maintenance. These implications for client care should be viewed primarily as effects or consequences that may occur secondary to the technique, not the technique itself.

Preblock Preparation. The nurse, in consultation with the anesthesia provider, will provide some or most of the primary teaching about the block and must be able to clarify expectations or concerns the client may have

TABLE 23-8
Complications of Regional Blockade

Complication	Cause	Nursing Implications
Maternal hypotension	Most frequently encountered complication resulting from sympathetic blockade causing profound vasodilation and venous pooling. Use of epinephrine with the local anesthetic may prolong the block and protracted hypotension.	Administer 1–2 L of an isotonic IV solution, such as Ringer's lactate, 30 min prior to block to expand vascular volume. Left uterine displacement is indicated.
	Hypovolemia, dehydration, or profound drug sensitivity may produce protracted or severe hypotension, which can compromise placental and fetal circulation.	Administer incremental doses of 5–10 mg of ephedrine IV and continue left uterine displacement.
		In severe cases, place the woman in Trendelenburg position and if necessary start a second IV line for rapid infusion of colloids or crystalloid.
Postdural or spinal headache	Mild to incapacitating headaches occur from inadvertent puncture of the dura mater while placing an epidural catheter, causing cerebrospinal fluid (CSF) leakage and allowing the brain stem to impinge on the cranial foramen.	Treat mild symptoms by having the woman lie flat or in a slight head-down position.
		Infuse ample crystalloid IV fluids or force oral fluids.
		When the woman sits up, have her wear a tight abdominal binder to increase pressure on the epidural space and slow CSF leakage.
	The severity of headache often depends on the gauge of the needle used and the resulting size of the dural tear.	After 24 hours, know that the anesthetist may administer an epidural blood patch by careful replacement at the site of puncture with 10–20 mL of the client's own, unclotted blood into the epidural space.
		Monitor closely; headache symptoms are eliminated rapidly following an epidural blood patch.
Nerve damage	Table leg supports and resulting pressure to peroneal or femoral nerves during lithotomy position. Regional anesthesia blocks the sensory feedback to the client so she is unable to protect herself from this injury.	Protect areas vulnerable to nerve injury, such as sides of the knees. Take the client out of lithotomy periodically to prevent focal compression neuropathies.
	Inadvertent injection of 2-chloroprocaine used in epidural block into the subarachnoid space can lead to permanent neurologic damage, including incontinence and foot drop.	Institute nursing care to treat foot drop and for incontinence.
		Provide psychological support.
High spinal or total spinal	Too large a volume of local anesthetic or excessive spread of local anesthetic may produce a regional anesthetic level high enough to interfere with voluntary breathing and produce profound hypotension. The level of block recedes over time. This also can occur when the dura is inadvertently punctured and a large volume of local anesthetic mixes with the CSF during epidural administration.	Maintain blood pressure and a patent airway. The anesthetist should intubate the client in respiratory or cardiac distress using a rapid sequence technique to prevent aspiration of gastric contents; 100% oxygen should be administered with controlled positive pressure ventilation.
		Place the woman in Trendelenburg position and left-lateral to facilitate venous return to the heart.
		Increase infusion of IV fluids and administer appropriate vasopressor therapy.
		Maintain reassuring verbal contact with the client, explaining the sudden changes required for proper care. The anesthetist may administer small doses of ketamine or midazolam for sedation.

(continued)

TABLE 23–8 (*Continued*)
Complications of Regional Blockade

Complication	Cause	Nursing Implications
Local anesthesia	Systemic concentrations of local anesthetics can reach toxic levels in the brain, leading to convulsions, which could result in fetal and maternal hypoxia, acidosis, and death.	Observe for warning signs that indicate toxicity and impending convulsions.
		Maintain continuous verbal contact with the client.
	High concentrations of local anesthetics often result when needle or catheter aspiration during block placement fails to reveal blood indicative of intravascular placement or the migrations of the epidural catheter into a vein.	Be alert for slurred speech or ringing in the ears, visual disturbances or other abnormal symptoms of the sensorium; the local anesthetic injection must be stopped if in progress; oxygen is applied, and vital signs are monitored.
		If convulsions ensue, maintain the airway; insert a bite block or oral airway. If the airway is unable to be maintained by these means, the anesthetist should insert an endotracheal tube. Thiopental 50–75 mg IV may be administered to abort the seizure followed by 5–10 mg of diazepam IV prophylactically.
		Have positive pressure ventilation and oral suction immediately available.
		Place the client in a supine and lateral position
		Administer IV fluids rapidly.
	Epidural catheter migration can occur during client movement. During pregnancy, veins in the epidural space are plentiful, dilated, and easily ruptured by the trauma of catheter migration.	Prior to the anesthetist redosing the epidural block, know that the epidural catheter position must be verified by aspiration for blood followed by careful titration of the dose of local anesthetic.

about the procedure. This includes a description of the procedure and associated risks and benefits to the woman and fetus. The nurse may be responsible for securing IV lines to administer crystalloid solution prior to the block, have necessary resuscitation equipment available, obtain preliminary vital signs prior to the procedure, and generally make the client as comfortable as possible prior to block administration.

Block Administration. The nurse will help position the client so that the block can be administered most effectively. The nurse may help communicate special instructions to the client from the anesthetist during the procedure and monitor fetal and maternal responses during intermittent epidural drug injections. The nurse should continue to monitor the client for signs of inadvertent intravascular injection and prodromal seizure behavior. The nurse will assess the extent of hypotension and subsequent hypoxia that may result from blockade of sympathetic nerve fibers following regional anesthesia. Nursing interventions include monitoring oxygen saturation by pulse oximetry, increasing IV fluids as indicated, and administering oxygen. The nurse also must begin to evaluate the quality of the block and the extent to which it is providing adequate pain relief.

Postblock Period. The nurse's primary responsibility is to determine the client's cardiovascular and ventilatory status by assessing vital signs intermittently. It may be necessary for the nurse to reposition the client side to side to ensure bilateral distribution of the local anesthetic and to prevent or treat signs of supine hypotensive syndrome. The nurse will monitor the integrity of the epidural catheter to make certain that the client's positional changes do not dislodge the catheter. When the client is receiving a continuous infusion of epidural local anesthetic or narcotics, the nurse must evaluate the dermatome level of the epidural. The client should be assisted to turn every hour. The nurse also should assess for a unilateral block, which may occur when the client remains on one side for an extended time. The client's ability to move her legs should be assessed regularly to ensure that the sensory blockade has not progressed to motor blockade. See Table 23–9 for a description of possible neurologic compromise. The nurse may have to discontinue continuous infusions of local anesthetics if the block level becomes too high or if the client's motor function is significantly impaired or signs of toxicity are observed. In these instances, the anesthesia provider should be notified immediately. All clients receiving epidural anesthesia or analgesia should be asked to empty their bladder regularly. Some clients will be unable to sense when their bladder is full because of sensory blockade to the pelvic area. Clients who are unable to void while receiving epidural anesthesia should be catheterized. After deliv-

TABLE 23-9
Neurologic Compromise Caused by Childbirth

Nerve	Root	Occurrence	Deficit
Lumbosacral	L4,L5	Most common in vaginal delivery; increased incidence with mid to high forceps delivery or platypellic pelvis	Hypoesthesia of lateral calf and foot; slight weakness of hip abductors; foot drop; slight weakness of quadriceps; usually unilateral involvement; resolves in 3 to 6 mo
Femoral nerve	L2–L4	Injured with retractors in cesarean delivery or with prolonged lithotomy positioning; with hyperacute hip flexion in lithotomy position (kinked where it passes under inguinal ligament)	Quadriceps paralysis (no knee extension); no patellar reflex; hypoesthesia of front of thigh and medial aspect of calf
Lateral femoral cutaneous nerve	L2–L3	Injured with retractors in cesarean delivery or lithotomy positioning (pressure with passage under inguinal ligament)	Numbness over anterolateral aspect of thigh; usually transient
Sciatic nerve	L4,L5 S1–S3	Uncommonly associated with delivery; associated with incorrect lithotomy positioning with knee extension or external rotation of hips	Classic symptom: pain in posterior gluteal region radiating to foot
Obturator nerve	L2–L4	Rarely involved in vaginal deliveries; lithotomy position	Inability to adduct leg; decreased sensation over medial thigh
Common peroneal	L4,L5 S1,S2	Lithotomy positioning with pressure on nerve over fibula	Equinovarus deformity; plantar flexion with inversion; loss of sensation over anterolateral aspect of calf and dorsum of foot and toes
Saphenous		Associated with lithotomy positioning (pressure on nerve over tibia)	Loss of sensation over medial aspect of foot and anteromedial aspect of lower leg

(Ostheimer, G. W. [1992]. Neurologic sequelae of childbirth and regional anesthesia. In G. W. Ostheimer (Ed.), *Manual of obstetric anesthesia* (2nd ed.) (p. 419). New York: Churchill Livingstone.)

ery, the nurse will remove the epidural catheter and check for patency of the entire length of the catheter and document findings on the client's medical record. If epidural narcotics are used, an apnea monitor may be indicated during postoperative recovery.

General Anesthesia

General anesthetics are rarely used for routine vaginal birth because the risks of complications, availability of regional and systemic techniques of pain relief, and the woman's desire to be awake for delivery do not justify its use. However, a general anesthetic is indicated in emergency situations, such as the need for uterine relaxation to relieve tetanic contractions, fetal manipulation for malpresentation, some footling and complete breech extractions, emergency hysterectomy for placenta accreta, reinversion of a prolapsed uterus, excessive hemorrhage from an abruptio placentae or placenta previa, precipitous fetal distress, and elective cesarean section. A general anesthetic is most often elected when regional anesthesia is contraindicated, rapid maternal physiologic control is required (such as in the case of hemorrhage), or when time limitations affect delivery (such as in imminent fetal demise).

Complications of general anesthesia occur infrequently because recent advances in monitoring modalities, including mass spectrometry, capnometry, and pulse oximetry, have greatly reduced anesthetic morbidity and mortality in all surgical populations. Gastric acid aspiration and failed intubation account for the highest number of maternal complications associated with the administration of general anesthesia (Shnider et al., 1993).

Nursing Implications

Nursing care for the pregnant client receiving general anesthesia is particularly critical when contrasted with the general surgical pupulation, because this client is at increased risk for aspiration of stomach contents. Approximately 35% of the clients who die from anesthesia during labor or delivery die from pulmonary aspiration (Moore et al., 1992). Even though food and fluids are withheld, the client is considered to have a full stomach because of delayed gastric emptying, which occurs during the late stages of pregnancy. An IV is established and IV fluids without dextrose, such as lactated Ringer's injection, are administered. A nonparticulate antacid, such as sodium citrate, is usually ordered to

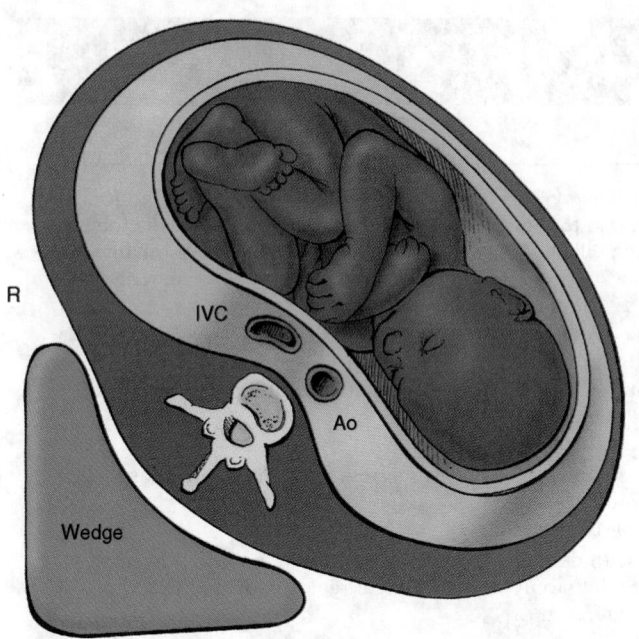

FIGURE 23-8 Lateral decubitus position with lateral pelvic tilt. (Stoelting, R. K., & Miller, R. D. [1989]. (*Basics of anesthesia.* [2nd ed.] p 372. New York, Churchill Livingstone.)

increase gastric pH. Prior to induction of anesthesia, a wedge is placed under the client's right hip to displace the uterus to the left, maximizing placental perfusion (Fig. 23-8). A rapid sequence induction technique is used to reduce the risk of aspiration further. The nurse may assist the anesthetist by applying cricoid pressure during induction and endotracheal intubation, which prevents the flow of any gastric contents into the tracheobronchial tree.

During recovery, the nurse maintains a patent airway and monitors the client's cardiopulmonary functions. Close monitoring of vaginal bleeding is essential to observe for any signs of impending hemorrhage. Routine postpartum care is performed.

Anesthesia for Cesarean Section

Cesarean delivery can be accomplished using spinal, epidural, or general anesthesia. Depending on the mother's desires and the circumstances for which the cesarean delivery is being performed, any technique has desirable attributes and will yield satisfactory outcomes.

Elective Cesarean Delivery

With an elective cesarean delivery, the obstetrician, the woman, and the woman's family have preplanned the birth of their newborn. Ideally, the woman will have learned of the procedure from her physician prior to admission or from the anesthesia provider during the preoperative interview in the hospital. Cesarean delivery accounts for as high as 20% to 25% of all births in the United States. This high number may be due in part to the malpractice crisis plaguing the obstetric field and the consequent defensive practice of medicine. Many obstetricians have been more inclined to deliver by cesarean at the first sign of failure to progress or of complications, rather than wait out the labor process, potentially exposing the woman and fetus to complications that can be avoided. More recent statistics show that this number may be decreasing in response to public and governmental inquiries regarding this unusually high incidence and the rising popularity and success of vaginal birth after cesarean delivery (VBAC).

Usual indications for elective cesarean delivery include cephalopelvic disproportion, failure to progress, malpresentation, previous uterine surgery, history of vaginal herpes, anticipation of hemorrhage (placental previa), fetal distress, or any other related fetal condition that questions the ability of the fetus to tolerate a vaginal delivery (Shnider et al., 1994). It is common practice in some institutions when multiple births are anticipated to allow the client a trial spontaneous vaginal delivery with the operating room supplies, equipment, and sterile procedures established and ready for an immediate cesarean delivery if complications arise with subsequent newborns. This same procedure is followed for women who have had previous cesarean deliveries and want a VBAC. It has been suggested that as many as 60% of the women who have had cesarean deliveries can deliver vaginally and uneventfully with proper precautions and equipment available in the delivery suite.

Epidural and Spinal Anesthesia

Spinal anesthesia remains the most popular anesthesia technique for cesarean delivery throughout the country, although medical facilities that maintain an active obstetric epidural service are using that technique almost exclusively. Spinal anesthesia has achieved widespread use because of its ease and rapidity of administration, usually within 5 minutes. Analgesia and motor block are profound. It has an induction to delivery time of 10 to 15 minutes if required. Many suggest that a spinal can be a likely alternative to general anesthesia for emergency cesarean delivery if there is a contraindication to the latter. Lidocaine 50 to 75 mg is the most widely used agent for the block, although bupivacaine 10 to 12 mg or tetracaine 8 to 12 mg can be used if a block of longer duration is required. Complete monitoring should be used, including electrocardiogram, precordial stethoscope, a blood pressure cuff, and a pulse oximeter to measure oxygen saturation.

The primary disadvantage of this technique is the sudden hypotension that can occur from the rapid onset of sympathetic neural blockade that results from the introduction of local anesthetic into the cerebrospinal fluid. Because maternal blood pressure should stay above 100 mm Hg systolic to ensure utero-placental perfusion, clients should receive at least 1 L, if not 2 L, of crystalloid solution intravenously prior to the procedure to minimize hypotension. Prophylactic use of ephedrine 25 to 50 mg IM or 10 mg IV after placement of the block and extracellular fluid enhancement can be effective therapy. In addition to these measures, lateral displacement of the uterus may be required after the block is set to alleviate hypotension. Although the block (spinal or epidural) is usually brought to the T4 level (nipple line), the client may still experience some uncomfortable pulling sensations when the surgeon surgically repairs and closes the uterus. If the client does not tolerate this procedure, the anesthetic can be supplemented with 5 to 10 mg IV of morphine or 50 to 100 μg IV of fentanyl to obtund these temporary sensations of discomfort.

Epidural anesthesia has the advantage of allowing a more controlled rise of the anesthetic and consequently less chance of encountering hypotensive problems from the sympathetic blockade. Drug administration can be titrated to the exact level required by the client. There also is a decreased chance of postspinal headache from dural tears. A labor epidural also can be used for a cesarean delivery by administering an additional dose of local anesthetic, often referred to as a "top up" dose. In this case, a larger volume of local anesthetic is administered epidurally prior to the surgical procedure to enhance the block. The larger volume has a faster onset of action. This allows the cesarean section to begin sooner. The normal time from initial administration of the epidural block to birth is 20 to 30 minutes. Chloroprocaine 3% or lidocaine 2% with epinephrine and sodium bicarbonate is the local anesthetic of choice in emergency situations in which fetal acidosis is suspected and rapid onset is required. Client monitoring is the same as for spinal anesthesia.

General Anesthesia

Prior to the induction of general anesthesia, the woman should receive nonparticulate antacids, such as 30 mL of sodium bicitrate, to increase the pH of gastric fluid. Particulate antacids should be avoided because aspiration of these products into the lung has been shown to cause more severe inflammatory changes in lung parenchyma (Gibbs et al., 1979). Clients should be monitored as described previously, including the use of capnometry or mass spectrometry (preferred) to evaluate the concentrations of all exhaled gases. Induction proceeds rapidly with the sequence including cricoid pressure applied by the circulating nurse or anesthesia assistant (Fig. 23-9), endotracheal tube insertion, balloon inflation, and auscultation of breath sounds to confirm proper placement of the endotracheal tube. Until the fetus is delivered, the woman

should receive 100% oxygen and a low concentration of a potent inhalation agent, such as isoflurane 0.5% to 0.75%. Isoflurane, halothane, and other volatile anesthetic agents in higher, anesthetic concentrations are avoided because they can cause uterine relaxation and promote bleeding. After delivery, anesthesia can be deepened by supplementing the anesthetic with nitrous oxide and narcotics, such as fentanyl, alfentanil, sufentanil, or morphine.

Emergency Cesarean Delivery

When fetal or maternal complications require immediate delivery, general anesthesia is usually the technique of choice. General anesthesia can be induced within 1 to 2 minutes after IV access is established. Emphasis is placed on maintaining basic anesthetic safety requirements and effective speed, affording the woman and fetus high concentrations of oxygen, and maintaining acceptable perfusion pressures in the brain and other vital organs. Regional techniques can be used if the anesthetist is adept at placement and time limitations are such that the level and intensity of the block are acceptable.

Postcesarean Delivery Pain Relief

In addition to traditional routes of IM and IV injection of narcotics for postoperative pain relief, the use of epidural injections of narcotics has become increasingly popular for control of pain after cesarean delivery. Clinicians report that 5 mg of a dilute solution of epidural morphine (Duramorph) is most effective. The therapeutic effects last 24 to 36 hours (Shnider et al., 1993). Fentanyl 50 to 100 μg also has proven to be effective, but the duration of action is only 2 to 4 hours.

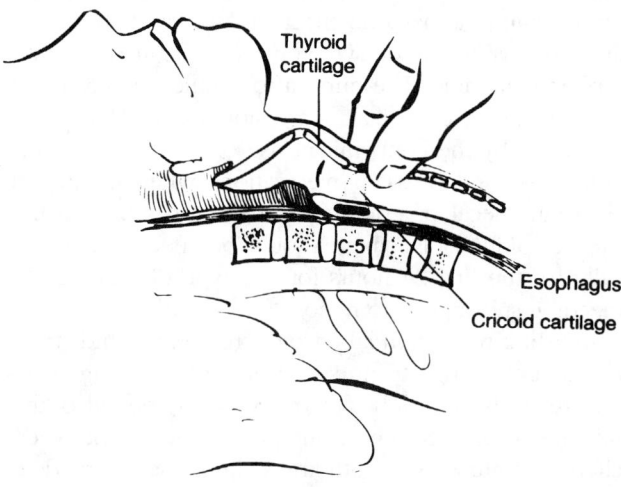

FIGURE 23-9 Technique of cricothyroid pressure (Sellick's maneuver).

These drugs are generally administered through the epidural catheter after delivery of the newborn. The epidural catheter is then removed.

Patient-controlled analgesia also has been used successfully in the postoperative period to control surgical pain. This mechanism allows the mother to self-administer, within preset limitations, small doses of narcotics through an IV access according to her own needs.

Nursing Implications

All clients who have undergone a cesarean delivery, whether by general or regional techniques, should recover in a similar fashion to other surgical clients. The labor and delivery nurse, therefore, must apply the same principles of client care that apply to any client in the postanesthesia care unit. After a general anesthetic, on the client's arrival to the recovery area, the nurse should obtain initial vital signs and continue to take them every 15 minutes for 2 hours or until the client is stable. The nurse should check the surgical incision for drainage and bleeding and make certain that the IV is patent. The client should receive oxygen administered through a face mask at a concentration of 40%. Oxygen saturation levels as measured by pulse oximetry should be recorded every 15 minutes. The nurse also should evaluate the client's need for further postoperative medication.

If a regional anesthetic has been used, vital signs should be taken as previously described. The extent of return of sensory and motor function should be documented by dermatome level. If epidural narcotics have been used for postoperative pain relief, the nurse should be especially vigilant in monitoring for respiratory depression. An apnea monitor can be used to observe ventilatory patterns.

A frequent side effect of epidural narcotic use is pruritus, which occurs in more than 60% of clients. IV administration of naloxone effectively controls this problem by reversing the narcotic effects. However, if continued analgesia is required, symptoms can be treated with diphenhydramine. The nurse also should keep in mind that respiratory or cardiac depression may be further exacerbated by the concomitant use of other central nervous system depressant medications when combined with intrathecal or epidural narcotics. In addition, the site of epidural placement should be checked periodically for the first 24 hours for any type of drainage or bleeding subsequent to removal of the catheter.

Assisting women in labor to decrease pain and stress is a real challenge to nurses. It is one that brings special rewards not only for the woman, but also the nurse. A special closeness and bond develops between client and nurse, and both know the nurse has made a difference. The woman's labor and birth experience can empower her and increase her self-esteem, and it is an event that she will always remember. The significance of the nurse's contribution to these outcomes can hardly be underestimated.

Summary Points

✔ Variability is the most striking feature of pain during labor. Some women report little or no pain, while others report severe pain. The average level of pain experienced by women in labor is probably very high.

✔ The nurse plays a vital role in the anesthesia care of the client because the nurse is the single healthcare provider in constant attendance with the client.

✔ The nurse is responsible for assessing the client's need for pain relief and her levels of pain tolerance. The nurse must plan and implement client care activities that incorporate pain management techniques based on knowledge and understanding of physiologic mechanisms of pain.

✔ The nurse is responsible for monitoring the vital signs of the client and fetus and assessing the effectiveness of anesthesia interventions.

✔ The nurse, in consultation with the anesthesia provider, manages the complications that may arise from analgesic and anesthetic medications and techniques.

✔ Although the obstetric nurse is not directly responsible for the administration of all analgesic and anesthetic techniques, expert client observational skills are essential. Continued observation of the client is required through the entire labor and birth process, including the postanesthesia period.

✔ The woman's ability to influence decisions about her care in labor, not pain management, may be the key to satisfaction with the birth experience.

✔ Many different psychological variables have been identified that influence client's reports about the experience of acute pain: fear and anxiety, expectancy, cognitive appraisal, self-efficacy, and perceived control.

✔ A wide variety of noninvasive coping strategies exist for women to use during childbirth, including relaxation, breathing, attention focusing, patterned physical movements, music, support person(s), distraction, positioning, and cutaneous stimulation. Few well-designed, controlled trials have been done to document the effectiveness of most of these strategies; however, they appear to be helpful, in varying degrees, to many women.

✔ A doula appears to have profound effects on the laboring woman and the labor process, including reducing the length of labor, cesarean birth rate, oxytocin use, analgesia use, forceps use, and requests for epidural anesthesia.

REFERENCES

Bacigalupo, G., Riese, S., Rosendal, H., & Saling, E. (1990). Quantitative relationships between pain intensities during labor and beta-endorphin and cortisol concentrations in plasma. Decline of the hormone concentrations in the early postpartum period. *Journal of Perinatal Medicine, 18,* 289–296.

Bandura, A. (1977). Self-efficacy: Toward a unifying theory of behavioral change. *Psychological Review, 84,* 191–215.

Bromage, P. R. (1993). Neurologic complications of regional anesthesia for obstetrics. In S. M. Shnider & G. Levinson (Eds.), *Anesthesia for obstetrics* (3rd ed.) (pp 433–453). Baltimore: Williams & Wilkins.

Byron, R., & Yonemoto, R., (1975). Pain and malignancy. In B. Crue Jr. (Ed.), *Pain research and treatment* (pp. 127–131). New York: Academic Press.

Camann, W. R., Denney, R. A., Holby, E. D., & Datta, S. (1992). A comparison of intrathecal, epidural and intravenous sufentanil for labor analgesia. *Anesthesiology, 77,* 884–887.

Caton, D. (1994). The obstetric patient. In R. R. Kirby & N. Gravenstein (Eds.), *Clinical anesthesia practice* (pp. 1082–1093). Philadelphia: W.B. Saunders.

Chalmers, I., Enkin, M., & Keirse, M. (Eds.) (1995). *Effective care in pregnancy and childbirth.* Oxford: Oxford Medical Publishers.

Chamberlain, G., Wraight, A., & Steer, P. (1993). *Pain and its relief in childbirth.* London: Churchill Livingstone.

Chapman, L. L. (1992). Expectant father's roles during labor and birth. *Journal of Obstetric, Gynecologic, and Neonatal Nursing, 21*(2), 114-120.

Cheek, T. G., & Gutsche, B. B. (1993). Maternal physiologic alterations during pregnancy. In S. M. Shnider & G. Levinson (Eds.), *Anesthesia for obstetrics* (3rd ed.) (pp. 3–17). Baltimore: Williams & Wilkins.

Davenport-Slack, B., & Boylan, C. (1974). Psychological correlates of childbirth and pain. *Psychosomatic Medicine, 36,* 215.

Diaz, A. G., Schwarez, R., & Fecina, R. (1988). Vertical position during first stage of the course of labor, and neonatal outcome. *European Journal of Obstetrics and Gynaecology, 11*(1).

Doering, S., & Entwistle, D. (1975). Preparation during pregnancy and ability to cope with labor and delivery. *American Journal of Orthopsychiatry, 45,* 825.

Fehder, W. P., & Gennaro, S. (1993). Recent trends in epidural analgesia for childbirth. *The Journal of Perinatal Education, 2*(2), 1–6.

Fernandez, E., Turk, D. C. (1989). The utility of cognitive strategies for altering pain perception: A meta-analysis. *Pain, 38,* 123–135.

Flynn, A. M., Kelly, J., & Hillins, G. (1980). The effect of ambulation in labor uterine action, analgesia and fetal well-being. *Gynecol Obstet, 512,* 981.

Frank, S. (1974). *The effect of the husbands presence at delivery and childbirth preparation classes on the experience of childbirth.* Dissert Abstr Int 34, 6208-B (Univ microfilm no 74-13895). East Lansing: Michigan State University.

Gennaro, S. (1988). The childbirth experience. In F. Nichols & S. Humenick (Eds.), *Childbirth education: Practice, research, and theory.* Philadelphia: W.B. Saunders.

Gibbs, C. P., Schwartz, D. J., Wynne, J. W. et al. (1979). Antacid pulmonary aspiration in the dog. *Anesthesiology, 51,* 380.

Green, J. M. (1993). Expectations and experiences of pain in labor: Findings from a large prospective study. *Birth, 20*(2), 65–72.

Hall, K., & Stride, E. (1954). The varying response to pain in psychiatric disorders: A study in abnormal psychology. *British Journal of Medical Psychology, 27,* 48–60.

Hilbers, S., & Gennaro, S. (1986). Nonpharmacological pain relief. *NAACOG Update Series, 5*(15).

Hill, H. F., Saeger, L. C., & Chapmam, C. R. (1986). Patient controlled analgesia after bone marrow transplantation for cancer. *Postgraduate Medicine,* 33–40.

Holyrod, K. A., Penzien, D. B., Hursey, K. G., Tobin, D. L., Rogers, L., Holm, J. E., Marcille, P. J., Hall, J. R., & Chila, A. G. (1984). Change mechanisms in EMG biofeedback training: Cognitive changes underlying improvement in tension headache. *Journal of Consulting and Clinical Psychology, 52,* 1039–1053.

Honet, J. E., Arkoosh, V. A., Norris, M. C., Huffnagle, H. J., Silverman, N. S., Leighton, B. L. (1992). Comparison among intrathecal fentanyl, meperidone, and sufentanil for labor analgesia. *Anesthesia and Analgesia, 75*(5), 734–739.

Hughes, S. C. (1993). Intraspinal opiates in obstetrics. In S. M. Shnider & G. Levinson (Eds.), *Anesthesia for obstetrics* (3rd ed.) (pp 157–191). Baltimore: Williams & Wilkins.

Humenick, S. (1981). Mastery: The key to childbirth satisfaction. A review. *Birth, 8,* 79.

Humenick, S. (1992). The empowering element of prepared childbirth. *The Journal of Perinatal Education, 1*(1), 64–65.

Jimenez, S. (1992). Teaching acupressure for pregnancy and birth. *The Journal of Perinatal Education, 1*(1), 58–63.

Kennell, J. H. (1994). The time has come to reassess delivery room routines. *Birth, 21*(1), 49–51.

Kimball, C. (1979). Do endorphin residues of betalipotrophin in hormone reinforce reproductive functions? *American Journal of Obstetrics and Gynecology, 134,* 127.

Klaus, M., Kennell, J., & Klaus, P. (1993). *Mothering the mother: How a doula can help you have a shorter, easier and healthier birth.* Boston: Harvard Common Press.

Koehn, M. (1992). Effectiveness of prepared childbirth and childbirth education. *The Journal of Perinatal Education, 1*(2), 35–43.

Korte, D. S. (1992). *A good birth: A safe birth.* Boston: Harvard Common Press.

Leighton, B. L. (1992). Comparison among intrathecal fentanyl, meperidine, and sufentanil for labor analgesia. *Anesthesia and Analgesia, 75,* 734–739.

Levinson, G., Shnider, S. M. (1992). Systemic medication for labor and delivery. In S. M. Shnider & G. Levinson (Eds.), *Anesthesia for obstetrics* (3rd ed.) (pp 115–133). Baltimore: Williams & Wilkins.

Lieberman, A. (1992). *Easing labor pain.* Garden City, NY: Doubleday.

Lowe, N. K. (1989). Explaining the pain of active labor: The importance of maternal confidence. *Research in Nursing and Health, 12,* 237–245.

Melzack, R., Taenzer, P., & Kinch, R. A. (1981). Labor pain: Nature of the experience and the role of prepared childbirth training. *Pain, 1*(Suppl.), S271.

Melzack, R., & Wall, P. D. (1965). Pain mechanisms: A new theory. *Science, 150,* 971–979.

Mendez-Bauer, C., Arroyo, J., & Ramos, C. (1975). Effects of standing position, spontaneous uterine contractility and other aspects of labor. *Journal of Perinatal Medicine, 3,* 89.

Moore, C. H. Blass, N. H., & Skerman, J. H. (1992). Obstetric anesthesia and analgesia. In W. R. Waugaman, S. D. Foster,

& B. M. Rigor (Eds.), *Principles and proactice of nurse anesthesia* (2nd ed.) (pp. 543–562). Norwalk, CT: Appleton and Lange.

Morgan, B., Bulpitt, C., Clifton, P., & Lewis, P. (1982). Effectiveness of pain relief in labor: Survey of 1000 mothers. *British Medical Journal, 285,* 689–690.

McCaffery, M., & Beebe, A. (1989). *Pain: Clinical manual for nursing practice.* St. Louis: C.V. Mosby.

McNiven, P., Hodnett, E., & O'Brien-Pallas, L. (1992). Supporting women in labor: A work sampling study of the activities of labor and delivery nurses. *Birth, 19*(1), 3–39.

Newham, J. (1984). A study of the relationship between beta-endorphin-like immunoreactivity and postpartum blues. *Clinical Endocrinology, 20,* 169.

Pittman, A. W., & Rudd, G. D. (1990). *Analgesic therapy, Part 2: Analgesia for severe pain.* Chapel Hill: Health Sciences Consortium 39.

Rayburn, W., Rathke, A., Leuschen, P. et al. (1989). Fentanyl citrate analgesia during labor. *American Journal of Obstetrics and Gynecology, 161,* 202.

Reed, L. B., & Edwards, W. T. (1992). Obstetric pain. In International Association for the Study of Pain-Task Force on Acute Pain (Eds.), *Management of acute pain: A practical guide.* Seattle: IASP Publications.

Reynolds, F. (1990). Commentaries: Pain relief in labor. *British Journal of Obstetrics and Gynecology, 97,* 757–759.

Roberts, J., Mendez-Bauer, C., & Wodell, D. (1983). The effects of maternal position on uterine contractility and efficiency. *Birth, 10,* 243.

Scott, D. B., & Hibbard, B. M. (1990). Serious nonfatal complications with extradural block in obstetric practice. *British Journal of Anaesthesia, 64,* 537–541.

Sepkoski, C., Lester, B., Ostheimer, G., & Brazelton, T. B. (1992). The effects of maternal epidural anesthesia on neonatal behavior during the first month. *Developmental Medicine and Child Neurology, 34,* 1072–1080.

Sharkey, S. J., Arkoosh, V. A., Norris, M. C., Honet, J. E., & Leighton, B. L. (1991). Comparison between intrathecal sufentanil and fentanyl for labor analgesia. *Anesthesiology, 74,* A841.

Shnider, S. M., & Levinson, G. (1994). Anesthesia for obstetrics. In R. D. Miller (Ed.), *Anesthesia* (4th ed.) (pp. 2031–2076). New York: Churchill Livingstone.

Shnider, S. M., & Levinson, G. (1993). In S. M. Shnider & G. Levinson (Eds.), *Anesthesia for obstetrics* (3rd ed.) (pp. 211–245). Baltimore: Williams & Wilkins.

Shnider, S. M., Levinson, G., & Cosmi, E. V. (1993). Obstetric anesthesia and uterine blood flow. In S. M. Shnider & G. Levinson (Eds.), *Anesthesia for obstetrics* (3rd ed.) (pp. 29–51). Baltimore: Williams & Wilkins.

Shnider, S. M., Levinson, G., & Ralston, D. H. (1993). Regional anesthesia for labor and delivery. In S. M. Shnider & G. Levinson (Eds.), *Anesthesia for obstetrics* (3rd ed.) (pp. 135–155). Baltimore: Williams & Wilkins.

Simkin, P. (1995). Non-pharmacological methods of pain relief during labor. In I. Chalmers, M. Enkin, & M. Keirse (Eds.), *Effective care in pregnancy and childbirth* (pp. 715–746). Oxford: Oxford Medical Publishers.

Simkin, P. (1991). Just another day in a women's life? Women's long-term perceptions of their first birth experience—Part I. *Birth, 18*(4), 203–210.

Simpson, J. S., & Foster, S. D. (1992). Legal and ethical aspects of nurse anesthesia practice. In W. R. Waugaman, S. D. Foster, & B. M. Rigor (Eds.), *Principles and practice of nurse anesthesia* (2nd ed.) (pp. 13–26). Norwalk, CT: Appleton & Lange.

Snyder, S. H. (1977). Opiate receptors and internal opiates. *Scientific American, 236,* 44–56.

Steffes, S. A. (1988). Relaxation: Imagery. In F. Nichols & S. Humenick (Eds.), *Childbirth education: Practice, research, and theory.* Philadelphia: W.B. Saunders.

Stoelting, R. K. (1991). *Pharmacology and physiology in anesthetic practice* (2nd ed.) (pp. 134–141). Philadelphia: J.B. Lippincott.

Terenius, L. (1981). Endorphins and pain. *Frontiers in Hormone Research, 8,* 162–177.

Thompson, S. C. (1981). Will it hurt less if I can control it? A complex answer to a simple question. *Psychological Bulletin, 90,* 89–101.

Thorp, J. A., Hu, D. H., Albin, R. M., McNitt, J., Meyer, B. A., Cohen, G. R., & Yeast, J. D. (1993). The effect of intrapartum epidural anesthesia on nulliparous labor: A randomized, controlled, prospective trail. *American Journal of Obstetrics and Gynecology, 169*(4), 851–858.

Turk, D. C., & Feldman, C. S. (1992). Noninvasive approaches to pain control in terminal illness: The contribution of psychological variables. In D. Truk & C. Feldman (Eds.), *Noninvasive approaches to pain management in the terminally ill.* New York: The Haworth Press.

Turner, G. A., Newnham, J. P., Johnson, C., & Westmore, M. (1991). Effects of extradural anesthesia on umbilical and uteroplacental arterial flow velocity waveforms. *British Journal of Anaesthesiology, 67,* 306–309.

Turner, J. A., & Romano, J. M. (1990). cognitive behavioral therapy. In J. Boncia (Ed.), *The management of pain* (Vol. II) (2nd ed.). Philadelphia: Lea and Febiger.

VanDalfsen, P. J., & Syrjala, K. L. (1990). Psychological strategies in acute pain management. *Critical Care Clinics, 6*(2), 421–431.

Vargo, M. M., Robinson, L. R., Nicholas, J. J., & Rulin, M. C. (1990). Postpartum femoral neuropathy: Relic of an earlier era? *Archives of Physical Medicine and Rehabilitation, 71,* 591–596.

Wells, N. (1989). Management of pain during abortion. *Journal of Advanced Nursing, 14,* 56–62.

West, A. (1981). Understanding endorphins: Our natural pain relief system. *Nursing, 81*(11), 50–53.

Wilmuth, L. (1973). Prepared childbirth and the concept of control. *Journal of Obstetric, Gynecologic, and Neonatal Nursing, 4,* 38.

Yarrow, l. (1992). Giving birth: 72,000 moms tell all. *Parents Magazine, November,* 149–159.

SUGGESTED READING

Klaus, M., Kennell, J., Klaus, P., (1993). *Mothering the mother: How a doula can help you have a shorter, easier and healthier birth.* Boston: Harvard Common Press.

Lieberman, A., (1992). *Easing labor pain.* Garden City, New York: Doubleday.

Melzack, R. (1984). The myth of painless childbirth. *Pain, 19,* 321–337.

McCaffery, M. (1990). Nursing approaches to Nonpharmacological pain control. *International Journal of Nursing Studies, 27*(1), 1–5.

Simkin, P. (1989). The birth partner: Everything you need to know to help a woman through childbirth. Boston: Harvard Common Press.

Shnider, S. M., & Levinson, G. (Eds.) (1993). *Anesthesia for obstetrics* (3rd ed.). Baltimore: Williams & Wilkins.

24

Immediate Care of the Newborn

Overview

Nursing Process:
Immediate Care
of the Newborn
Setting Goals
for Immediate Care
Assessment of the Newborn
Nursing Diagnoses
Intervention and Rationale
Evaluation

Objectives

- State the goals of nursing care in the immediate newborn period.
- Describe the various aspects of nursing assessment of the newborn in the first hour after birth.
- Discuss the methods of establishing the newborn's airway and maintaining respirations.
- Describe methods of maintaining a neutral thermal environment for the newborn immediately after birth.
- Discuss appropriate nursing interventions related to preventive measures performed soon after birth.
- Discuss ways to promote maternal-infant bonding during the first few hours of the newborn's life.

The moment of birth is a dynamic time that centers around the immediate needs of the newborn. The nurse is responsible for performing much of this immediate care. Although these needs have priority, the nurse should be aware of the emotional needs and questions of the parents and their desire to see and touch their newborn for the first time. The nurse should attempt to integrate these two aspects of the immediate postpartum experience. A description of a typical birth and the immediate care of a low-risk, full-term newborn in the hospital setting follows. Following this overview, each aspect of nursing care is explained in detail using the nursing process format.

Overview

The head passing through the vaginal opening initiates the beginning of several different activities that the birth attendant and nurse perform almost simultaneously. The birth attendant immediately suctions fluid and mucus from the newborn's mouth and nose with a bulb syringe to clear the air passages. At this point, the shoulders and the rest of the body can be delivered. The nurse notes the time of birth and the sex of the newborn and sets the 1-minute timer for the Apgar score. If the baby appears normal and is not in obvious respiratory distress, blood and body fluids are wiped away, a warm blanket is placed over the newborn, and the newborn may be placed on the mother's abdomen while the cord is being clamped and cut by the birth attendant. Sometimes, the father is permitted to cut the cord under close supervision. The physician or birth attendant may ask for a specimen of the cord blood to be saved for blood work. The change in environment and sudden stimulation usually cause vigorous crying in the newborn. The nurse should assess and record the newborn's 1-minute Apgar score and reset the timer for the 5-minute score.

As long as the 1-minute Apgar score is satisfactory, the newborn can remain on the mother's abdomen. The skin-to-skin contact helps to keep the newborn warm and promotes bonding between the mother and the newborn. The mother may want to attempt breast-feeding at this time.

At the appropriate time, the 5-minute Apgar score is performed; the mother helps the nurse wrap the newborn in a warm blanket. The nurse then places the newborn under the preheated radiant warmer to perform the assessment. After the Apgar score is completed, the nurse leaves the newborn uncovered and places a temperature probe on the abdomen to regulate radiant heat. At this time, the nurse performs a quick overall assessment, looking for any obvious abnormalities that should be brought to the physician's or birth attendant's attention. During this assessment, the nurse should suction the mouth and nose as needed.

A cord clamp is placed on the cord, and the excess is cut off with sterile scissors. Two completed identification bands are placed on the newborn's extremities, and one is placed on the mother's and father's wrists. Prophylactic eye care and vitamin K injection may be performed at this time. However, these procedures can be postponed for an hour or two so that the parents have time to bond with the newborn while he or she is in a quiet alert state.

When initial care of the newborn is completed, the nurse places a stockinette cap on the head, wraps the newborn in a warm blanket, and gives him or her back to the parents. If the newborn is to go to the nursery, assessment information and the newborn record are taken with the newborn. The nurse hands all the information to the nursery nurse and gives a verbal report. The delivery room nurse will check the newborn's identification bands with the nursery nurse. Some hospitals have labor, delivery, recovery, postpartum rooms. In this case, the newborn may receive all necessary care in the mother's room.

Most newborns easily adapt to extrauterine life. However, this transitional period can be hazardous, and nurses must be aware of and alert to potential problems and the newborn's changing condition. The nurse also must know exactly what to do to intervene appropriately if necessary, whether in the mother's room or in a traditional nursery.

Nursing Process: Immediate Care of the Newborn

Setting Goals for Immediate Care

Before any actual assessment or intervention is performed, the nurse must have certain goals in mind that will help to assist the newborn during the transition from intrauterine to extrauterine life. How the goals are accomplished may vary. It depends on the setting, agency policy, parents' wishes, and the condition of the mother and newborn. Goals for immediate care can include the following (see also the Nursing Care Plan: Immediate Care of the Newborn):

NURSING CARE PLAN
Immediate Care of the Newborn

Nursing Goals

1. Apgar score is between 7 and 10 at 1 and 5 minutes.
2. Vital signs remain within normal limits:
   (a) Apical pulse between 120 and 160 beats/min
   (b) Respiratory rate between 40 and 60 breaths per minute
3. Newborn's airway remains clear.
4. Newborn does not develop cold stress.
5. Newborn has appropriate identification (ie, band) before leaving birthing area.
6. Newborn does not develop ophthalmia neonatorum.
7. Newborn and parent demonstrate appropriate beginning attachment behaviors.

Assessment	Potential Nursing Diagnoses	Intervention/ Rationale	Evaluation

Apgar score
  Heart rate
  Respiratory effort
  Muscle tone
  Reflex irritability
  Color
	Ineffective Breathing Patterns related to alteration in response to extrauterine life	Have resuscitation equipment available and in good working order *to facilitate ease of use in an emergency.*
		Alert resuscitation team when problems are anticipated and summon when necessary.
		Place newborn in a modified Trendelenberg position *for drainage of mucus.*
			Newborn scores 7 to 10 at 1 and 5 minutes.

Ongoing general assessment of airway and responsiveness	Ineffective Airway Clearance related to excess mucus	Gently bulb suction mouth and nose *to remove fluid and mucus.* Use other suctioning methods as needed. Proceed with resuscitation measures if necessary.	Newborn breathes without difficulty.
	Impaired Gas Exchange	Gently rub body with towel *to stimulate breathing.* Use O$_2$ or resuscitation measures as needed *to promote gas exchange.*	Newborn is reactive, is pink, and cries lustily when stimulated.
Continuous temperature monitoring	Hypothermia related to newborn status	Dry head and body well *to minimize cooling by evaporation.* Place in radiant warmer on top of warm blanket *to provide warmth while allowing good visualization of newborn's breathing and color.* Tape temperature probe on abdomen *to regulate heat from radiant warmer.* Place stockinette cap on head when removing from warmer *to limit loss of heat.*	Newborn maintains stable temperature.

General status
  Size
  Maturation
		Weigh and measure length and head circumference *to obtain baseline data and to assess growth pattern.*	Newborn adapts to extrauterine life with minimal trauma.

(continued)

NURSING CARE PLAN *(Continued)*
Immediate Care of the Newborn

Assessment	Potential Nursing Diagnoses	Intervention/ Rationale	Evaluation
Normality of body systems Vital signs		Perform gestational age assessment *to assist in assessing newborn's need for any special care.* Examine body systems by thorough observation, inspection, auscultation, and palpation *to detect any anomalies.* Record, report as appropriate.	Newborn has good color and good muscle tone. Newborn remains free of trauma.
Recognition of needs of newborn	Risk for Infection related to immature immune system	Use good handwashing, aseptic technique, and appropriate glove use when caring for newborn *to help protect against infection.*	Newborn remains free of infection.
Protection from infection Protection from hypoprothrombinemia		Instill ophthalmic drops or ointment *to provide prophylaxis against ophthalmia neonatorum.*	Newborn does not develop eye infection.
		Administer vitamin K *to protect against hypoprothrombinemia.*	Newborn's clotting time is normal.
Proper identification		Apply matching identification bands to newborn, mother, and significant other *to ensure accurate identification of newborn.* Check numbers and information with mother *to reassure mother that newborn can be identified as hers.*	Mother has correct newborn.
Family interaction	Risk for Altered Parenting (maternal–newborn attachment process)	Encourage father or support person to be with mother *to promote family interaction.* Allow couple to hold and explore newborn as soon as possible *to promote bonding.* Point out newborn's features; explain normal variations *to assist parents in identifying newborn as theirs.* Observe for inappropriate maternal behaviors (eg, reluctance to touch newborn, lack of eye contact, inappropriate remarks) *to identify potential problems with bonding and allow for early intervention.*	Family interacts favorably.

- Establish and maintain an airway and respiratory effort.
- Provide warmth and prevent hypothermia.
- Provide a safe environment and routine preventive measures.
- Promote maternal-infant attachment.

Assessment of the Newborn

Accurate assessment of the newborn immediately after birth and continued observation during the first critical hours are vital. Information about the newborn's condition and responses that nurses gather at this time provides valuable baseline data for subsequent care. All immediate assessment and care should be well documented and reported to those who will assume care of the newborn.

Assessing Risk

Ongoing risk assessment is an important aspect of the newborn's care. It alerts healthcare professionals to potential problems and allows them time to prepare for these problems. A planned method of reporting and recording risk factor information for individual clients assists in ensuring that all information is transferred from one healthcare provider to another. Standardized risk assessment forms that contain information about the mother's prenatal and intrapartum course should be included in the newborn's chart to improve the continuity of care.

Most factors that cause the mother to be identified as high risk also place the fetus or newborn at increased risk. The mother's age, marital status, family history, and obstetric history are general factors to be considered. Factors that should be noted from the present pregnancy and intrapartum period are shown in Table 24-1. Examples are given of specific conditions or situations that would alert the nurse to the need to call a special resuscitation team or additional staff to assist with resuscitation.

Analgesia or anesthesia administered to the mother during the first and second stages of labor could have particular importance as a risk factor. How much medication was given and when may influence the newborn's immediate responses and responses that occur later. For example, newborns whose mothers have been heavily medicated may respond with excellent function and optimal Apgar scores at delivery. However, about 30 minutes later, these same newborns may be in a dangerously depressed respiratory state, requiring additional nursing care to help keep their airways clear of mucus.

Apgar Scoring System

The **Apgar system of scoring,** developed in 1953 by the late Dr. Virginia Apgar, provides an index for as-

sessing the newborn's condition at birth. The score should be determined for each newborn 1 and 5 minutes after birth. The 1-minute score has been found to be most predictive of immediate survival, while the 5-minute score may better predict long-term survival and neurologic damage (Jepson et al., 1991). The nurse often performs the assessment because the scores should be assigned by someone other than the birth attendant. All nurses who are responsible for the care of newborns should be familiar with the Apgar method of newborn assessment. This method provides a simple, accurate, and safe means of quickly appraising the newborn's condition.

The Apgar scoring system focuses attention on the following five signs of assessment that reflect the overall health status of the newborn. Each sign is evaluated according to the degree to which it is present and given a score of 0, 1, or 2 (Table 24-2). The scores of each of the signs are added to get a total score, with 10 being the maximum. In the assessment of specific problems in the newborn, the scores of individual assessment areas provide important information.

Heart Rate. The heart rate is the most important sign and will be present unless the newborn is in extremely poor condition. It may be evaluated by palpating the pulsation of the cord or by observing the pulsation where the cord joins the abdomen. Listening to the heart beat with a stethoscope is the most accurate method of ascertaining the beat. The newborn heart rate may range from 150 to 180 beats/min during the first few minutes of life. Within an hour after birth, it usually slows to between 130 and 140 beats/min. Crying or increased activity will increase the number of beats. A rate of 100 beats/min or less may indicate a need for resuscitation.

Respiratory Effort. A newborn who is responding well should cry vigorously and have no difficulty breathing. "Regular" respiration is usually established within a minute. Slow, irregular respiration or apnea indicates respiratory difficulty or depression. These signs should be reported immediately so that prompt treatment may be instituted.

Muscle Tone. A newborn with excellent muscle tone will keep the extremities flexed and resist efforts to extend them. A newborn who does not consistently keep the extremities flexed usually has only moderate tonus; one who is flaccid is in extremely poor condition.

Reflex Irritability. A gentle slap on the sole of the foot will usually cause the newborn who is in good condition to respond with a vigorous cry. This sign also can be observed when a newborn is suctioned for mucus by the way in which it resists the bulb syringe or catheter. A newborn is judged to have a poor response if it

TABLE 24–1
Perinatal Risk Assessment

Areas to be Assessed	Conditions Associated With Increased Risk
PRENATAL COURSE	
General prenatal information	Lack of prenatal care
	Weight gain ≤15 lb or ≥35 lb
Maternal health	Medical conditions:
	Diabetes: gestational; *insulin-dependent
	Heart disease
	Habits:
	Smoking
	Substance abuse
	Infections during pregnancy:
	Rubella
	Venereal disease
	Complications of pregnancy:
	Pregnancy-induced hypertension
	*Third-trimester bleeding
	Rh sensitization: moderate; *severe
	*Multiple fetuses
Results of prenatal tests	Estriol levels: ↓ or no ↑ after 36 wk
	Ultrasound: growth retardation ≥2 wk
	Amniocentesis:
	Bilirubin or meconium present
	L/S ratio <2:1
	Nonstress test: nonreactive
	Stress test: positive
INTRAPARTUM COURSE	
Length of pregnancy	≥37 wk; ≥42 wk; *<34 wk
Duration and character of labor	*Prolonged first or second stage
	Precipitous labor or delivery
	PROM >24 h
	*Difficult labor
	Cephalopelvic disproportion
Maternal conditions	Preexisting problems (see prenatal course)
	Progressive hypotension
	Progressive hypertension
	*Excessive bleeding
	Signs of infection, *severe
Fetal presentation and position	*Breech
	*Transverse lie
Events indicating possible fetal distress	Fetal monitoring
	*Persistent late decelerations
	*Severe variable decelerations
	Heart rate <120 or >160 for >30 min
	*Poor beat-to-beat variability
	*Scalp pH ≤7.25
	*Meconium-stained fluid
	*Prolapsed cord
Analgesia	Large or repeated doses of analgesia
	IM analgesia within 1 h of delivery
	IV analgesia within ½ h of delivery
Anesthesia	General anesthesia
	Conduction anesthesia with maternal hypotension
	*Cesarean delivery
Method of delivery	*Midforceps or high forceps delivery
	*Failed vacuum extraction

*Conditions usually requiring presence at delivery of someone skilled in resuscitation.

  L/S ratio = lecithin-sphingomyelin ratio; PROM = prolonged rupture of membranes; IM = intramuscular; IV = intravenous.

TABLE 24–2
Apgar Scoring Chart

Sign	Score		
	0	**1**	**2**
Heart rate	Absent	Slow (less than 100)	Over 100
Respiratory effort	Absent	Slow, irregular	Good, crying
Muscle tone	Flaccid	Some flexion of extremities	Active motion
Reflex irritability	No response	Weak cry or grimace	Vigorous cry
Color	Blue, pale	Body pink, extremities blue	Completely pink

cries weakly or merely makes a grimace. The newborn with a good deal of central nervous system depression may not respond at all.

Color. Cyanosis is seen in the majority of newborns at the moment of birth. As the fetal circulation changes to extrauterine circulation and breathing begins, a healthy newborn usually becomes pink within 3 minutes. **Acrocyanosis** (cyanosis of the extremities) is neither uncommon nor serious for a short while after birth. However, newborns who exhibit acrocyanosis will receive a 1 for this part of the evaluation.

Interpretation

Good Condition. An Apgar score of 7 to 10 implies that the newborn's condition is good. If the newborn breathes and cries (or coughs) seconds after delivery, no special procedures are usually necessary other than those of routine close observation, maintaining a clear airway, and supplying warmth.

Fair Condition. A score of 4 to 6 usually indicates that the newborn is in fair condition. There may be moderate central nervous system depression, some muscle flaccidity, cyanosis, and lack of readily established respiration. These newborns need their air passages cleared and require prompt administration of oxygen. Directing a stream of oxygen toward the newborn's face while suctioning the airway may be sufficient. However, oxygen is best administered by mask at a flow never exceeding 4 L/min. Gentle patting and rubbing with the receiving blanket to dry the newborn's body acts as an additional stimulus.

Poor Condition. A newborn who scores between 0 and 3 is in extremely poor condition. Resuscitation is needed immediately (see Chap. 41). If the newborn is obviously depressed at birth, resuscitative measures should begin even before the 1-minute evaluation. For a 5-minute Apgar score less than 7, the American Academy of Pediatrics suggests that additional scores be ob-

tained every 5 minutes for up to 20 minutes, unless there are two successive scores of 8 or greater (Freeman et al., 1992). Scores recorded at intervals will provide an index of recovery or continued problems.

General Assessment

A thorough physical examination is performed while the newborn is still in the hospital—within 24 to 48 hours of birth (see Chap. 28). However, a brief initial assessment should be done soon after birth to alert the physician or birth attendant to any problems. The following basic areas should be covered:

1. Inspection
   a. Head and face, anterior of body, posterior of body, and extremities: for any obvious defects or evidence of trauma
   b. Skin: for color, staining, peeling
   c. General appearance: for anything unusual
   d. Nostrils: for patency
   e. Cord: for three vessels
2. Auscultation
   a. Heart: for rate and quality of sounds
   b. Lungs on each side: for comparison and to evaluate efficiency of respiratory exchange
3. Palpation
   a. Liver: for enlargement
   b. Chest: for point of maximum impulse of heart

The cord should be checked for three vessels as soon as possible after it is cut, because the edges of the vessels are more difficult to see as the cord begins to dry. When first cut, the edges of the arteries are two white papular structures, which usually stand out slightly from the surface. The vein is larger, often gaping, so the lumen and thin wall are easily seen. The presence of only one artery suggests congenital abnormalities.

Prompt detection of congenital anomalies or other problems is essential in facilitating early treatment. Some congenital anomalies are obvious; others require close inspection and a knowledge of where and for what to look. If problems are ruled out, parents can be assured that their newborn is healthy.

Gestational Age Assessment

Estimation of gestational age during the prenatal period is usually based on the mother's expected date of delivery as calculated from her last menstrual period. After birth, a more accurate estimation can be made by physical examination of the newborn. The complete gestational age assessment is usually done in the nursery (see Chap. 28), but it is often helpful to use a shorter version during the immediate newborn period, especially if the newborn appears smaller or larger than expected from the mother's dates. Table 24-3 describes a method of rapid estimation of gestational age, including examination of sole creases, breast nodules, scalp hair, earlobes, and in the male newborn, testes and scrotum (Cunningham et al., 1993).

Nursing Diagnoses

Assessment of the newborn enables the nurse to work closely with other members of the healthcare team to identify problems and potential problems that require early intervention. During the immediate care of the newborn, the nurse should keep in mind certain potential nursing diagnoses. Problems that are possible during this early neonatal period include the following:

- Ineffective Breathing Patterns related to alteration in response to extrauterine life
- Ineffective Airway Clearance related to excess mucus
- Impaired Gas Exchange related to incomplete expansion of alveoli
- Hypothermia related to newborn status
- Risk for Infection related to immature immune system
- Risk for Altered Parenting (mother–newborn attachment process)

Intervention and Rationale

Nurses keep specific nursing diagnoses in mind while assessing the newborn. This will help them to plan interventions and implement nursing care. The nurse caring for a newborn is responsible for making sure that basic goals of immediate newborn care are met.

Establishing and Maintaining an Airway

At birth, newborns undergo profound and rapid physiologic changes as the fetoplacental circulation ceases to function. The newborn's survival depends on the rapidity and efficiency of these changes. The fluid-filled alveoli of the newborn's lungs must fill with air, and respiratory motion must occur to exchange that air.

As soon as the head of the newborn is born, measures are taken to promote a clear air passage. Mucus and fluid are wiped and suctioned from the newborn's mouth and nose to avoid aspiration of additional contents into the lungs with the first breath. It is important to suction the mouth first. Stimulation of the nasal passages may cause the newborn to gasp for breath, resulting in aspiration of mucus and fluid from the mouth. A **bulb syringe** is usually used for suctioning. Proper technique involves collapsing the bulb before placing it into the newborn's mouth. This will prevent the material in the oropharynx from being forced into the bronchi and lungs when the bulb is squeezed (Fig. 24-1). The bulb is then slowly allowed to inflate, which draws mucus and fluid up into the bulb. After suctioning the mouth and nose, the newborn is observed to make sure respiratory efforts begin and are main-

TABLE 24–3
Rapid Estimation of Gestational Age of the Newborn

Sites	Gestational Age		
	36 WK OR LESS	**37–38 WK**	**39 WK OR MORE**
Sole creases	Anterior transverse crease only	Occasional creases in anterior two-thirds	Sole covered with creases
Breast nodule diameter	2 mm	4 mm	7 mm
Scalp hair	Fine and fuzzy	Fine and fuzzy	Coarse and silky
Earlobe	Pliable, no cartilage	Some cartilage	Stiffened by thick cartilage
Testes and scrotum	Testes in lower canal, scrotum small, few rugae	Intermediate	Testes pendulous, scrotum full, extensive rugae

(Cunningham, F. G., MacDonald, P. C., Gant, N. F., Leveno, K. J., & Gilstrap, L. C. [1993]. *William's Obstetrics* [19th ed.]. Norwalk, CT: Appleton & Lange.)

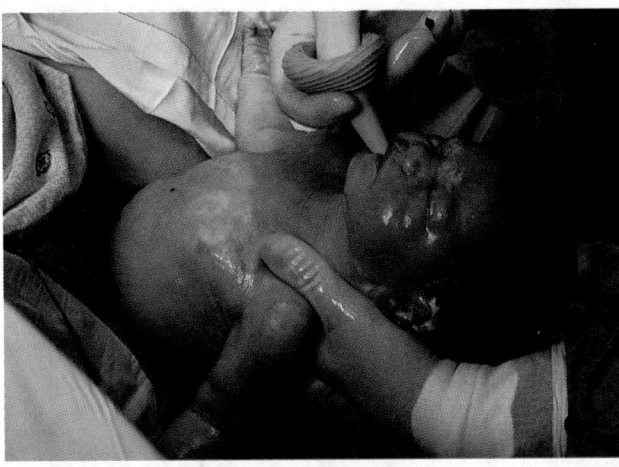

FIGURE 24–1 A bulb syringe is used to suction mucus and fluid from the newborn's mouth and nose.

tained. The first cry is eagerly awaited, because this is one way the newborn demonstrates respiratory effort. The newborn may not cry at once, but the removal of mucus and the stimulation provided by suctioning usually elicit a gasp or cry.

Some newborns cry very little but are alert, active, and breathing well. Others cry vigorously in an attempt to force mucus from the nose and throat. If it is necessary to stimulate the newborn to cry, it should be done with care. Drying the newborn with the blanket or gently rubbing the back or soles of the feet is usually sufficient stimulus to initiate crying. Spanking, forcible rubbing of the skin along the spine, alternate hot and cold tubbing, and dilatation of the anal sphincter are no longer done because they can be dangerous and shocking to the newborn.

The newborn should be placed in a modified Trendelenburg position to facilitate drainage of mucus. An exaggerated Trendelenburg position should be avoided, because the relatively large amount of abdominal contents will press against the diaphragm, and the partially expanded lungs and may impede the newborn's respiratory efforts. The bulb syringe should be used as needed. If the bulb syringe is not adequate to remove the mucus, an isolated DeLee suction device may be hooked up to mechanical suction. This device is rarely used orally anymore because of the potential danger of allowing mucus to enter the healthcare worker's mouth. The newborn must not be oversuctioned, because this may deprive him or her of oxygen by interfering with breathing. Deep, prolonged suctioning also can cause vagal stimulation, which can result in bradycardia (Freeman et al., 1992). Care should be taken not to traumatize the tissues of the oropharynx with the tip of the catheter, the bulb syringe, or forceful suction. If it is necessary to remove mucus through the nostrils, force should be avoided and the catheter should not be inserted far back. The catheter should be directed horizontally, as if passing over the roof of the mouth, instead of directed upward as for the adult client.

Emergency Resuscitation. For most normal newborns, there is little need for resuscitative measures beyond clearing the airway and gentle tactile stimulation. A small percentage of newborns do require assistance. For them, the immediate availability of assistance may be life-saving. Successful active resuscitation requires trained personnel; a warm, well-lighted, adequate work area; and appropriate equipment, including the means to deliver oxygen by positive pressure.

All birthing facilities should have a plan that can be immediately implemented when emergency resuscitation of a newborn is anticipated or needed (Freeman et al., 1992). Part of this plan should be a list of maternal and fetal conditions that would require someone specifically trained in newborn resuscitation to be present during the birth. The items starred in Table 24-1 are samples of conditions that might be included on the list. An additional item might be "request by the pediatrician or obstetrician."

Respiratory depression, the inability to initiate or sustain adequate respirations for sufficient gas exchange, is the most common cause of perinatal asphyxia. Maternal analgesia and anesthesia are among the most frequent contributors to respiratory depression, because they can reduce the responsiveness of the respiratory center in the brain of the newborn. Inadequate respirations that persist beyond 1 minute severely compromise the newborn by leading to a falling heart rate, decreased muscle tone, and greater possibility of acidosis (Maisels et al., 1992). A schematic approach for resuscitation is presented in Figure 24-2.

Before beginning resuscitative efforts with positive-pressure oxygen, the airway must be suctioned well. Oxygen delivered under pressure may force foreign material present in the airway deep into the newborn's lungs. A well-fitting mask is then placed over the newborn's mouth and nose, and oxygen is administered by **bag and mask ventilation** at a rate of 40 to 60 breaths per minute to deliver the oxygen into the bronchi. In most cases this procedure (*bagging*) is successful in stimulating breathing and correcting the evidence of hypoxia. When it is not, endotracheal intubation will be necessary (Maisels et al., 1992). Further details of resuscitative measures can be found in Chapter 41.

If resuscitative measures are used in the delivery room, the parents will usually be frightened and upset. They should not be ignored in the rush to resuscitate the newborn. The nurse should explain what is happening and assure the parents that although the newborn has a problem, measures are being taken to correct it.

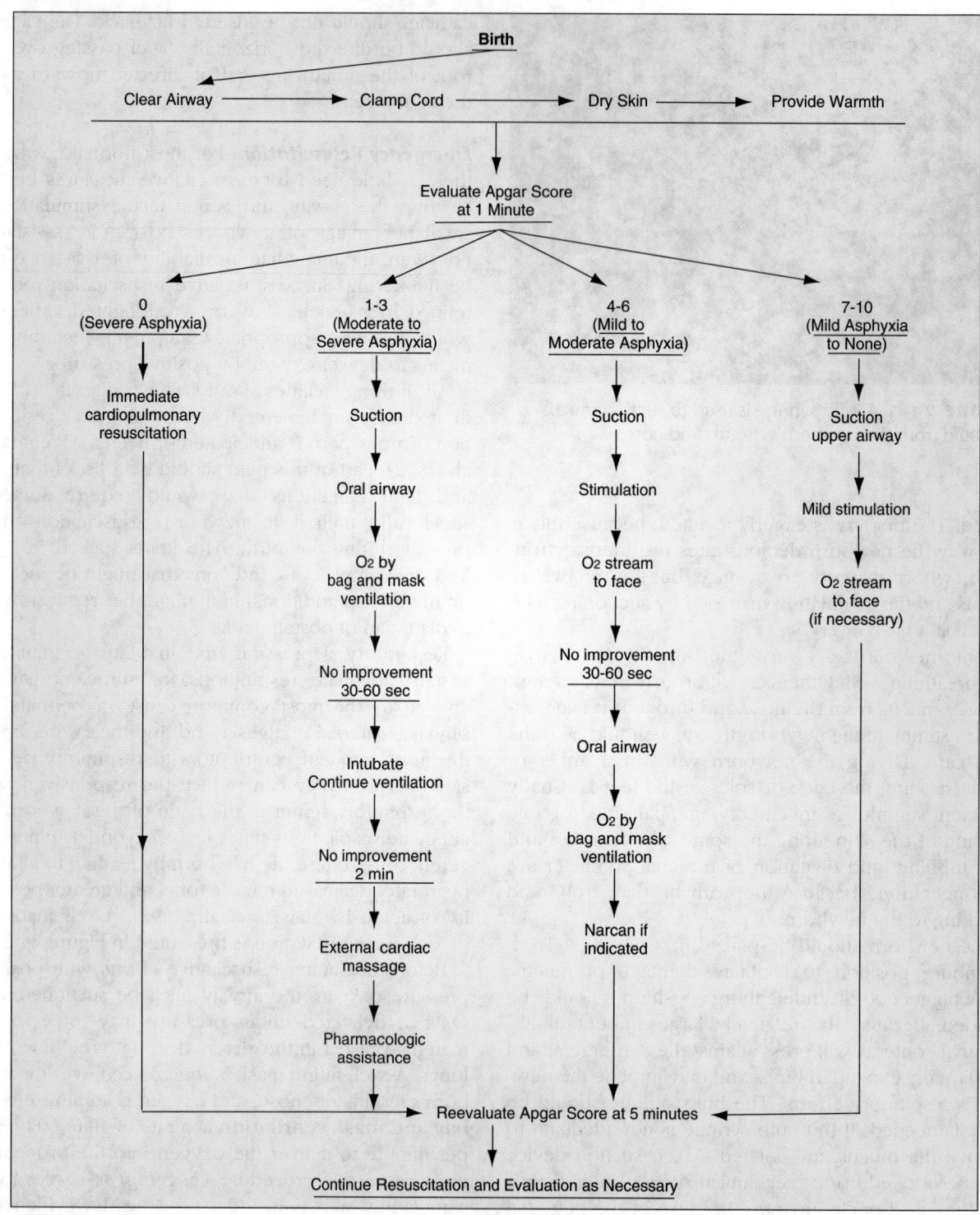

FIGURE 24–2 Schematic approach for resuscitation based on 1-minute Apgar score.

Providing Warmth and Preventing Hypothermia

Preventing hypothermia is another important aspect of immediate care of the newborn. The environmental temperature in the delivery room is much cooler than the intrauterine temperature. The newborn is also wet, which further increases the chilling effects of the transition to the outside world. Placing the newborn belly down on the mother's abdomen will provide warmth because the mother's body heat is transferred to the newborn. The amniotic fluid should be wiped from the newborn's head and body as soon as possible to minimize heat loss by evaporation. A cotton cap is often placed on the newborn's head to help prevent heat loss from this area. Using a radiant warmer, a prewarmed mattress, and warm instruments for the newborn's initial assessment provides a heat-gaining rather than a heat-losing environment.

Providing Routine Preventive Measures

Several important routine preventive measures must be implemented within the first few hours after the newborn's birth. The nurse will implement many of these or if not solely responsible, will work in collaboration with other members of the healthcare team. Included in this care is infection control, prophylactic treatments, and identification.

Infection Control. Infection control in the delivery room is not only important for the mother and newborn, but also for members of the healthcare team. Universal precautions should be observed by all members of the healthcare team. This includes thorough handwashing and putting on gloves before administering care to the mother or handling the newborn. Adherence to these measures will provide the healthcare worker with protection against blood- and body fluid-borne infectious diseases. It also will prevent the transmission of organisms that may be harmful to newborns because of their immature immune system.

A sterile environment should be implemented whenever possible when providing care to the mother and the newborn. Towels, sheets, and instruments should be replaced when soiled. Ill personnel should stay out of the delivery room. The umbilical cord stump is a potential portal of entry for infection, especially while still moist. Although it should be left uncovered, care should be taken that it is not contaminated. Further measures to prevent infection of the cord are implemented in the newborn nursery (see Chap. 29).

Prophylactic Eye Care. **Ophthalmia neonatorum,** infectious conjunctivitis, is a serious infection that can cause blindness in newborns. If the mother has a gonococcal or chlamydial infection, the newborn is at high risk for acquiring the infection during passage through the vagina. Newborns born by cesarean delivery also may be at risk of acquiring the infection due to ascending organisms (Freeman et al., 1992).

This infection is preventable. In the United States, the use of some form of prophylaxis against eye infections is required by law. Although 1% silver nitrate solution was used almost exclusively for years, erythromycin and tetracycline have replaced it in most areas of the country as the anti-infective agents of choice. Silver nitrate is rarely used anymore because it often causes a chemical conjunctivitis, and it is only effective against gonococcal, not chlamydial, infections (Freeman et al., 1992).

Recent studies have found that topical erythromycin and tetracycline alone may not be effective against chlamydial infections. Cunningham et al. (1993) recommend oral azithromycin as an alternative for preventing gonococcal and chlamydial infections. Others have recommended topical administration of these agents, along with systemic antibiotics.

Eye prophylaxis may be done in the delivery room or delayed until the newborn is taken to the nursery. Instilling drops or ointment may cause newborns to keep their eyes closed or may blur their vision. Therefore, delaying the procedure for a few hours allows the parents to get acquainted with their newborn while his or her eyes are open (see Procedure: Instillation of Eye Prophylaxis for guidelines and Fig. 24-3).

Prophylaxis Against Hypoprothrombinemia. A single 0.5- to 1-mg dose of phytonadione solution (Aquamephyton) is administered intramuscularly to the newborn in the delivery room or on admission to the nursery (Fig. 24-4). This water-soluble form of vitamin K_1 is a preventive measure against neonatal hemorrhagic disease. Amounts of the medication in excess of 1 mg may predispose to the development of hyperbilirubinemia and must be avoided (see Chap. 28 for discussion of hyperbilirubinemia).

Identification Methods. While the newborn is still in the delivery room, it is the nurse's responsibility to prepare and apply some form of identification. Most hospitals use flexible plastic bands that come in sets of three or four with identical numbers on them. The mother's name and admission number, the physician's name, the date, the time of birth, and the sex of the newborn are written on a special insert that is put into each band. Two bands are placed on the newborn, usually one on a wrist and one on an ankle, and another band is placed on the mother's wrist. In some hospitals, a fourth band is worn by the father or significant other so that this person can transport the newborn to and from the newborn nursery. The number on the bands should be entered on the newborn's record, and the information on the bands should be verified with the mother as soon as possible. The bands are checked with the nursery nurse when the newborn is admitted to the nursery and are rechecked with the mother's band each time the newborn is brought to her to make sure they match.

Newborn footprints and maternal fingerprints are sometimes used and have at times been required as methods of newborn identification. Although they are no longer recommended as a universal practice, many hospitals still use them.

The newborn's foot should be clean and dry and must be pressed firmly against the ink pad and then gently "walked on" the footprint form, beginning with the heel. Excess ink should be wiped from the newborn's feet. A less messy alternative to the ink pad is a disposable cardboard frame with squares of ink-coated plastic against which the newborn's feet and mother's

PROCEDURE 24-1
Instillation of Eye Prophylaxis

General Guidelines

1. Use agent prescribed by physician or by hospital policy: silver nitrate solution (1%), erythromycin (0.5%) ophthalmic ointment or drops, tetracycline (1%) ophthalmic ointment or drops.
2. Administer within 1 to 2 hours after birth.

Procedure for Instillation

Nursing Action	*Rationale*
Put on gloves. Clean eyelids and surrounding area with sterile cotton moistened with sterile water before manipulating eyelids.	This removes blood and body fluids left on skin following birth process and reduces the risk of transmitting hepatitis B virus or human immunodeficiency virus through the mucous membrane of the eye.
Stabilize newborn's head, and gently separate eyelids.	This allows drops or ointment to reach conjunctival sac.
Ophthalmic drops: Instill 2 drops in the conjunctival sac, and allow to run across the whole sac.	Instillation into conjunctival sac avoids direct contact with the cornea, which is very sensitive.
Ophthalmic ointment: Place a thin 1- to 2-cm line of ointment along the conjunctival sac, moving from the inner to the outer canthus. Be careful not to touch eyelid or eyeball with tip of tube.	Tip of tube could cause injury to newborn's eye or eyelid or carry infection from one eye to the other.
Carefully manipulate the lids to ensure the spread of the drops or ointment.	This promotes distribution of medication to all parts of conjuctiva.
Repeat in the other eye: For silver nitrate, use one ampule for each eye.	Using one ampule for each eye provides appropriate amount of medication.
For erythromycin, use one tube for each newborn.	Using a new tube avoids cross-contamination.
After 1 min, gently wipe excess solution or ointment from eyelids and surrounding skin with sterile water. Do not irrigate eyes.	Wiping helps avoid irritation of skin. Irrigation may decrease the effectiveness of the prophylactic agent.

thumb are pressed. The frame, with ink side down, is placed over the identification form on a clipboard. As with the ink pad method, the feet must be clean and dry, and each foot walked onto the form with gentle pressure, beginning at the heel. Nurses must be careful not to move the newborn's foot while pressing it down on the frame. Because the ink does not come in contact with the newborn's feet, clean up is not required. Other newer methods may also be available.

Promotion of Early Maternal–Newborn Attachment

The new mother should see and hold her newborn as soon as possible after birth. Many women will be eager to do this and will ask. Others may want to hold the newborn but will not know that it is permitted and may hesitate to ask. Still others may be too tired, too uncomfortable, or for some other reason may not be as eager for contact with the newborn. Although the reluctant mother should not be forced to hold her newborn, nurses may help to initiate the attachment process by bringing the newborn to the mother's side and showing it to her. If the condition of the mother and newborn are favorable, allowing the mother to breastfeed or have skin-to-skin contact with the newborn in the delivery room is an excellent way to promote attachment (Klaus et al., 1992). Allowing time for parents and newborn to be alone together, with the nurse near enough to provide assistance if needed, is another way of getting the new family off to a good start.

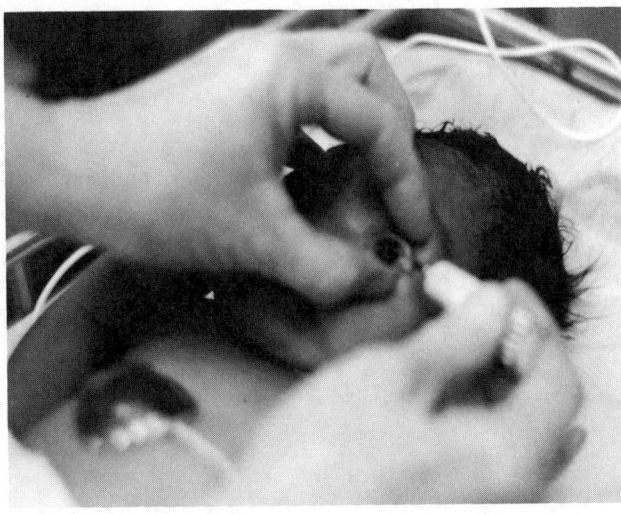

FIGURE 24-3 Ointment is applied to the eyes to prevent infection.

If the mother's or newborn's condition does not allow early contact, it is particularly important that the newborn be shown to the mother before being taken to the nursery. Furthermore, the mother must be given information about the newborn's condition on a regular basis and should be allowed to see her newborn whenever possible.

Special Consideration

Baptism of the Newborn. If the newborn is in imminent danger and may not live, the question of baptism should be raised with the parents. Baptism is a very important concept for people of the Christian faith, especially for those who consider themselves Roman

Catholic. It often means a great deal to the family of a critically ill newborn to have the nurse's assistance in making sure baptism is performed. If time allows, a member of the clergy should be called, but if this is not possible, anyone, preferably someone of the same faith or who has been baptized, may baptize the newborn. Nurses should be aware of their hospital's policies for baptism or other religious rites before the necessity arises. If baptism or another rite is performed, it should be recorded on the chart.

Evaluation

Nurses evaluate the effectiveness of their care of the newborn by monitoring the newborn and family for attainment of the evaluative criteria. Apgar scores of 7 to 10, vital signs within normal limits, absence of trauma or infection, completion of preventive measures, and evidence of good parent–newborn attachment all indicate that the early newborn period has been negotiated successfully. Identification of deviations from these criteria would lead to revisions in the nursing care plan to meet the needs of the individual newborn and family.

Summary Points

✔ Goals for immediate care of the newborn include establishing and maintaining respirations and respiratory effort, providing warmth and preventing hypothermia, providing routine preventive measures, and promoting maternal–newborn attachment.

✔ Nursing assessment of the newborn in the first hour after birth is directed toward assessing risk factors, obtaining Apgar scores, completing a brief general physical assessment, and making a rapid estimation of gestational age.

✔ Most newborns establish and maintain their airways with only mild stimulation and bulb syringe suctioning. For those having difficulty, active resuscitation may be needed using other methods of suctioning, giving oxygen, or by calling a specialized team to initiate other measures.

✔ A neutral thermal environment is provided by drying the newborn well, protecting him or her from drafts, and using a radiant warmer.

✔ Routine preventive measures consist of the use of universal precautions, prophylactic procedures, and methods of identification.

✔ Bonding between the parents and newborn is extremely important during the first few hours after birth and should be encouraged by the nurse.

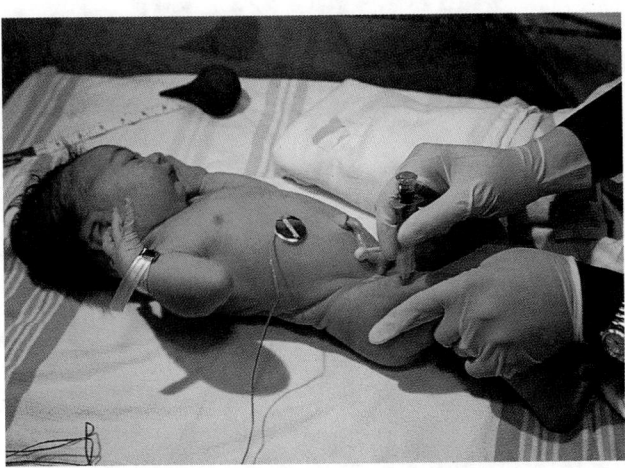

FIGURE 24-4 A single dose of the water-soluble form of vitamin K₁ is administered intramuscularly to the newborn as a prophylaxis against hypoprothrombinemia.

REFERENCES

Bryant, B. G. (1984). Unit dose erythromycin ophthalmic ointment for neonatal ocular prophylaxis. *Journal of Obstetric, Gynecologic, and Neonatal Nursing, 13,* 83–87.

Committee on Ophthalmia Neonatorum (1981). *Prevention and treatment of ophthalmia neonatorum.* New York: National Society to Prevent Blindness.

Cunningham, F. G., MacDonald, P. C., Gant, N. F., Leveno, K. J., & Gilstrap L. C., III. (1993). The newborn infant. In *Williams' obstetrics* (pp. 235–244) (19th ed.). Norwalk, CT: Appleton & Lange.

Freeman, R. K., & Poland, R. L. (Eds.) (1992). *Guidelines for perinatal care* (3rd ed.). Elk Grove Village, IL: American Academy of Pediatrics and American College of Obstetrics and Gynecology.

Jepson, H. A., Talashek, M. L., & Tichy, A. M. (1991). The Apgar score: Evolution, limitations, and scoring guidelines. *Birth, 22,* 83–92.

Klaus, M. H., & Kennell, J. H. (1992). Care of the mother, father and infant. In A. A. Fanaroff & R. J. Martin (Eds.), *Neonatal-perinatal medicine* (pp. 379–392) (5th ed.). St. Louis: Mosby Year Book.

Maisels, M. J., & Nelson, N. M. (1992). Peripartum considerations. In R. A. Hoekelman (Ed.), *Primary pediatric care* (pp. 436–444) (2nd ed.). St. Louis: Mosby Year Book.

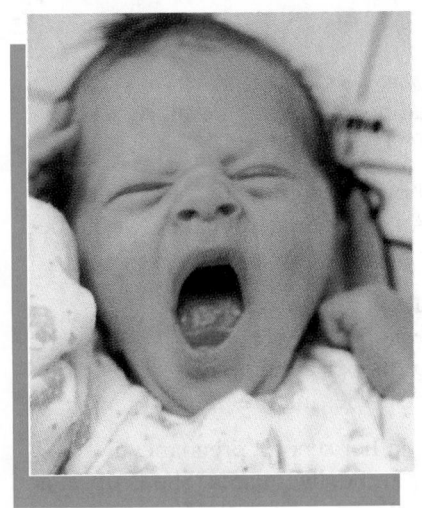

Assessment and Management in the Intrapartum Period

Critical Thinking Questions

1. Maria Devalia, age 25 and pregnant with her first child, comes to the clinic for a routine follow up appointment. During the visit, the client asks a lot of questions and expresses her concerns about labor. She says,"My sister had a breech delivery and my best friend had to have a cesarean delivery because the baby was too big. Is my baby breech? . . . Will my baby be able to fit through my body?"

    Using your knowledge about the passageway and passenger, design a teaching plan detailing the specific assessments that will help this client approach labor with confidence.

2. Kim DiNardo is progressing toward the transition phase of her labor. She and her partner have voiced a strong preference to avoid pain medication if possible. They have actively prepared for childbirth by practicing labor coping skills and comfort measures, attending childbirth classes and reading various books. The client is complaining of increased pain and discomfort. The couple continues breathing patterns but they don't seem to be helping. The partner seems overwhelmed and asks what else can they do? After assessing the client, you determine that the client is experiencing habituation.

    How would you help this couple to modify their current strategies for nonpharmacologic pain relief and propose acceptable options for pharmacologic pain relief.

3. You are caring for a mother in the recovery room who was heavily medicated immediately before delivery. She has her infant in bed with her.

    Explain the precautions necessary to promote safety of the client and neonate based on appropriate rationales that integrate your knowledge of obstetrical analgesia.

Multiple Choice Questions

1. The nurse is assessing a client. Which of the following findings would the nurse interpret as a premonitory sign of labor?

    A. Weight gain of 1 to 3 lbs
    B. Rupture of membranes
    C. Vaginal bleeding
    D. Cervical softening and effacement

2. The nurse determines that the client has completed the first stage of labor when:

    A. Contractions occur at 5-minute intervals
    B. Cervix is completely dilated
    C. Baby is delivered
    D. Cervix is dilated 3 to 4 cm

3. In the typical vertex presentation, the sequence of events by which the fetal head adapts to the birth canal during descent is:

    A. Flexion, external rotation, internal rotation , and extension
    B. External rotation, internal rotation, extension, and flexion
    C. Flexion, internal rotation, extension and external rotation
    D. External rotation, extension, flexion, and internal rotation.

4. The nurse determines a client has completed the second stage of labor when:

    A. Cervix is completely dilated
    B. Contractions occur at 2- to 3-minute intervals
    C. Baby is delivered
    D. Placenta is delivered

5. When developing a teaching plan for a client preparing for labor, the nurse anticipates dis-

cussing the possibility of an episiotomy. The nurse is correct in defining this as:

A. Surgical incision of the perineum during the end of the first stage
B. An opening into the cervical canal
C. Opening surgically into the vagina during the second stage of labor
D. A surgical incision of the perineum during the second stage of labor

6. Which of the following terms should the nurse use to document the condition when the baby's head settles into the brim of the true pelvis?

A. Engagement
B. Extension
C. Rotation
D. Quickening

7. When assessing the client's pelvic diameters, the pelvic inlet is considered of adequate size for childbirth if the diagonal conjugate is greater than:

A. 9.5 cm
B. 10 cm
C. 10.5 cm
D. 11.5 cm

8. A client comes to the labor and delivery area. The nurse notices fluid leading from the vagina and tests it with Nitrazine paper. When the paper turns blue green, the nurse may assume that the client has:

A. Ruptured membranes
B. Intact membranes
C. Vaginal secretions
D. Incontinence

9. A client is receiving systemic medication for pain relief. An appropriate outcome for this client is: The fetus will demonstrate signs of adequate tissue perfusion. To ensure this outcome, the nurse maintains the maternal systolic blood pressure above:

A. 100 mm Hg
B. 90 mm Hg
C. 80 mm Hg
D. 70 mm Hg

10. The nurse uses Leopold's maneuvers to:

A. Determine fetal well being
B. Evaluate cervical dilation
C. Evaluate fetal heart tones
D. Determine fetal position

11. During labor the nurse frequently assesses the fetal heart rate. An appropriate outcome would be: The fetal heart rate remains within:

A. 60 to 80 beats per minute
B. 80 to 120 beats per minute
C. 120 to 160 beats per minute
D. 160 to 200 beats per minute

12. A client who is in her second pregnancy is admitted to the labor and delivery area. She is upset and seems worried. "I was in labor the first time for over 30 hours." Which of the following nursing diagnoses would the nurse identify for this client?

A. Anxiety related to hospitalization
B. Fear related to difficult delivery
C. Pain related to contractions
D. Ineffective individual coping related to hospital environment

Study Questions

1. Name the four components that must be coordinated for labor to progress to delivery.

2. List the four main types of pelvises.

3. Name the three important A-P diameters of the fetal skull.

4. Define fetal presentation

5. Define crowning.

6. What is the normal duration of a uterine contraction?

7. Identify the normal fetal serum pH range during labor.

8. How often should vital signs be evaluated during labor?

9. List the prime causes of postpartal hemorrhage.

10. Identify six areas to be assessed during the fourth stage of labor.

11. Explain what is meant by the term pain tolerance.

12. List six cognitive evaluative strategies for pain relief.

13. Identify the five areas assessed by the Apgar score.

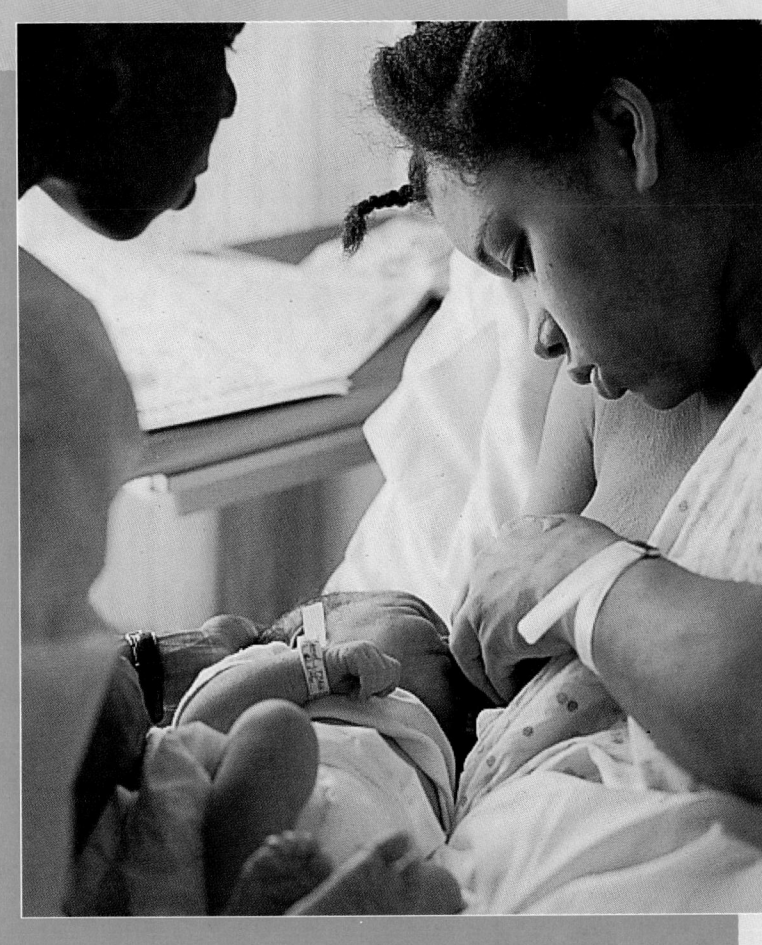

Assessment and Management in the Postpartum Period

VI

25

Biophysical Aspects of the Postpartum Period

Objectives

- Describe postpartum changes in the reproductive organs during the process of involution.
- Compare the characteristics of lochia during its three stages.
- Discuss changes in breasts in lactating and nonlactating women.
- Identify important hormone effects related to postpartum physiologic adaptations and return of fertility.
- Describe cardiovascular functional characteristics and blood constituents after giving birth.
- List respiratory and metabolic changes during the postpartum period.
- Discuss changes in renal function, urinary structures, and water metabolism after giving birth.
- Identify important changes in gastrointestinal, neuromuscular, and integumentary systems after giving birth.

The postpartum period encompasses the time between delivery until the reproductive organs have returned to their prepregnant state. Marked anatomic and physiologic changes occur during this period as the processes undergone during pregnancy are reversed (Table 25-1). Knowledge of the reproductive process in pregnancy and labor is a basis for understanding how the generative organs and the various systems of the human body adapt after the delivery.

The term **puerperium** (*puer*, a child, plus *parere*, to bring forth) refers to the 6-week period between the termination of labor and the return of the reproductive organs to their prepregnancy condition. The puer-

perium includes **progressive changes** in the breasts for lactation and **involution** ("pushing inward," or return to normal) of the internal reproductive organs. The changes brought about by involution are normal physiologic processes. However, except during the puerperium, such marked and rapid involution of tissues usually signals disease. Because postpartum changes are so profound, the quality of the mother's care at this time is important to ensure her immediate and future health. This chapter provides a basis for understanding postpartum changes. (The study summarized in the Research Highlight reveals that even though many biophysical processes have returned to prepregnancy states by the end of 6 weeks postpartum, it may take many months for the woman's functional status and role performance to return to "normal.") Chapter 27 covers postpartum nursing care.

Reproductive System Changes

Reproductive system changes during the puerperium occur in all the major internal reproductive organs (the uterus, the cervix, the vagina, the fallopian tubes) and in all the surrounding ligaments and musculature. Perineal tears or episiotomy also heal during the puerperium.

TABLE 25–1
Postpartum Physiologic Changes

Organ or System	Changes and Time Frame
Uterus	Undergoes involution at rate of 1 finger breadth per day; becomes pelvic organ in 9–10 d (nonpalpable); placental site heals by 6 wk
Cervix	Os closes to 1 cm by 1 wk; endocervical glands regress by day 4; edema remains 3–4 mo
Vagina	Rugae reappear by 3 wk; normal estrogen levels and lubrication return by 6–10 wk
Ovulation	Wide variation and affected by lactation: average first ovulation, 10–12 wk for nonlactating women, 12–36 wk for nursing mothers
Breasts	Secrete colostrum after delivery; milk produced in 3–4 d; may have transient engorgement
Cardiovascular system	Transient increase in blood volume after delivery, declines by day 3 and attains nonpregnant levels by week 4; increased cardiac output and stroke volume at delivery, decreases after 48 h with normal levels by week 3
Blood constituents	Early hemodilution followed by increased hematocrit days 3–7 and normal values by 4–5 wk; leukocytosis first 10–12 d that returns to normal by 2 wk; increased fibrinogen and clotting factors at delivery are normal by 3 wk; increased protein, lipids, and electrolytes return to normal by 2 wk
Respiratory system	Increased residual volume, resting capacity, and oxygen consumption; decreased inspiratory capacity, vital capacity, and maximum capacity; returns to nonpregnant pulmonary function by 6 mo
Urinary system	Diuresis in 12 h of delivery; output 3,000 mL for 4–5 d, return to nonpregnant renal function by 6 wk; bladder tone restored by end of 1 wk
Gastrointestinal system	Constipation and difficulty eliminating for 2–3 d; restored intestinal tone by end of 1 wk
Neuromuscular system	Numbness of thighs, fingers, or hands disappears in several days; backache improves in 6–8 wk

RESEARCH HIGHLIGHT

Changes in Functional Status After Childbirth

According to role theory, the woman's functional status in various aspects of life will change as the maternal role is assumed. This study explored changes in and variables associated with role performance, in the form of functional status, during the first 6 months following childbirth. Functional status was defined as the woman's readiness to assume infant care responsibilities and to resume usual household, social and community, self-care, and occupational activities.

A sample of 110 women was recruited from prepared childbirth classes and postpartum units (final n = 97). Subjects were married; English-speaking; older than 18 years; had delivered healthy, full-term newborns; had no major prenatal or postpartum complications; and had no medical problems. They were followed longitudinally, with data collected at 3 weeks, 6 weeks, 3 months, and 6 months postpartum. Research instruments included (1) Inventory of Functional Status After Childbirth, which tested various dimensions of function; (2) Postpartum Self-Evaluation Questionaire, which tested psychosocial variables; (3) Infant Characteristics Questionnaire, which measured infant temperament; and (4) background data sheets for health and demographic variables. Reliability and validity of the instruments were demonstrated.

The subjects were homogeneous; most were white, well-educated, and middle class. About half had professional or managerial positions. Slightly less than half were primi-

paras, and women with cesarean births were oversampled (40 of 97) for comparison purposes. Results revealed significant changes in total functional status during the 6 months following childbirth. By the traditional 6-week postpartum recovery period, less than 30% of women had fully resumed their usual levels of household or social and community activities. At this time, 25% still had not fully assumed their desired level of infant care responsibilities. In general, infant care responsibilities were fully assumed more rapidly than household, social and community, self-care, or occupational activities.

By 6 months postpartum, almost 20% of women had not fully resumed their usual level of household activities, and 30% had not fully resumed their usual level of social and community activities. None had fully assumed self-care activities by 3 weeks, and less than 20% had done so by 6 months. More than 60% of women who had returned to work by 6 months were not yet assuming full occupational activities. Variables most related to fuller functional status included energy level, vaginal delivery, increased parity, confidence in coping ability, father's support, and having an infant with predictable temperament. Recovery of functional status after childbirth takes at least 3 to 6 months.

Critique: Although adequate in design and sample size, subjects were from a select socioeconomic group. The findings indicating delayed resumption of full functioning may not be applicable to other populations.

(Tulman, L., Fawcett, J., Groblewski, L. et al. [1990]. Changes in functional status after childbirth. *Nursing Research,* 39[2], 70–75.)

Uterus

Immediately following delivery of the placenta, the uterus becomes an almost solid mass of tissue. Its thick anterior and posterior walls lie in close opposition, leaving the center cavity flattened. The uterus remains about the same size for the first 2 days after delivery but then rapidly decreases in size by involution. This is caused partly by the contraction of the uterus and the decrease in size of individual myometrial cells and partly by autolytic processes, in which some of the protein material of the uterine wall is broken down into simpler components that are then absorbed.

Placental Site

Immediately after the placenta and membranes are expelled, the placental site becomes an irregular, nodular, elevated area. Vascular constriction and thromboses occlude underlying blood vessels at the placental site. This accomplishes hemostasis (to control postpartum bleeding) and causes some endometrial necrosis. Invo-

lution occurs by the extension and downward growth of marginal endometrium and by endometrial regeneration from the glands and stroma in the decidua basalis. Except for the placental site, where involution is not complete until 6 to 7 weeks after delivery, the process is completed in the remainder of the uterine cavity by the end of the third postpartum week.

Afterpains

Afterpains are intermittent uterine contractions after delivery that are of varying intensity. These are most common in multiparas, whose uterine musculature does not sustain steady retraction because of decreased tone from prior childbearing. In primiparas, uterine tone is increased, and the musculature remains in a state of tonic contraction and retraction; thus, primiparas usually do not experience afterpains. However, if the uterus has been markedly distended, as with multiple pregnancy or polyhydramnios, intermittent contractions will occur, producing afterpains.

Afterpains frequently occur with breast-feeding, when the posterior pituitary releases oxytocin as a result of the newborn suckling. Oxytocin causes contractions of the lacteal ducts in the breasts, which express colostrum or milk, and causes the uterine muscles to contract. The sensation of afterpains can occur during active uterine contractions to expel blood clots from the uterine cavity.

Process of Involution

The separation of the placenta and the membranes from the uterine wall takes place in the outer portion of the spongy layer of the decidua. Remnants of this layer remain in the uterus to be partly cast off in a vaginal discharge called the *lochia.* Within 2 or 3 days after labor, this remaining portion of decidua becomes differentiated into two layers, leaving the deeper or unaltered layer attached to the muscular wall from which the new endometrial lining is generated. The layer adjoining the uterine cavity becomes necrotic and is cast off in the lochia. The process is like the healing of any surface: Blood oozes from the small vessels on this surface. The bleeding from the larger vessels is controlled by compression of the retracted uterine muscle fibers.

After involution, the uterus returns to normal size, although it is never as small as during its nulliparous state. Immediately following delivery, the uterus weighs approximately 1 kg (2 lb); at the end of the first week, about 500 g (1 lb); at the end of the second week, about 350 g (12 oz); and by the time involution is complete, about 40 to 60 g (1.5–2 oz; see Fig. 25-1).

Immediately after delivery of the placenta, the uterus sinks into the pelvis and the fundus is felt midway between the umbilicus and the symphysis. Within 2 to 4 hours after birth, it rises to the level of the umbilicus (12–14 cm or 5–5.5 inches above the symphysis pubis), and 12 hours later, it may be slightly higher (DeCherney

and Pernoll, 1994; see Fig. 27-2). Then fundal height decreases about 1 cm or one fingerbreadth per day. By the 10th day, it can no longer be palpated abdominally.

Lochia

Postdelivery uterine discharge is called **lochia,** and it occurs in three stages:

- **Lochia rubra**—This bright red discharge lasts 3 days and consists primarily of blood with small amounts of mucus, particles of decidua, and cellular debris from the placental site.
- **Lochia serosa**—The pinkish, watery discharge occurs as bleeding from the endometrium diminishes; it lasts until 10 days after birth and consists of old blood, serum, leukocytes, and tissue debris.
- **Lochia alba**—This thinner, scantier, whitish-tan discharge occurs after the 10th day and consists of leukocytes, epithelial cells, mucus, serum, and decidua. By the end of the third week, the discharge usually disappears, although a brownish mucoid discharge may persist for 6 weeks (Oppenheimer et al., 1986).

Lochia possesses a characteristic scent but should not have a foul odor. Standards for assessing lochia character and volume are described in Chapter 27.

Cervix

Immediately following delivery, the cervix collapses and has little tone; it appears soft and edematous and has multiple small lacerations. It can admit two fingers and is about 1 cm thick. Within 24 hours, it rapidly shortens and becomes firmer and thicker. The cervical os closes gradually, measuring 2 to 3 cm after a few days and 1 cm by 1 week. Histologic examination immediately after birth reveals almost universal edema and hemorrhage. The endocervical epithelium remains

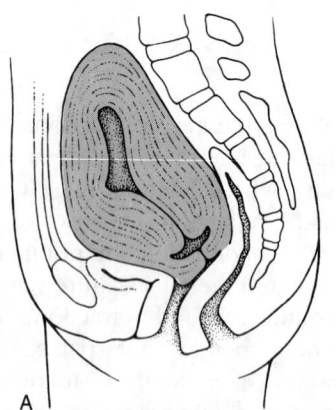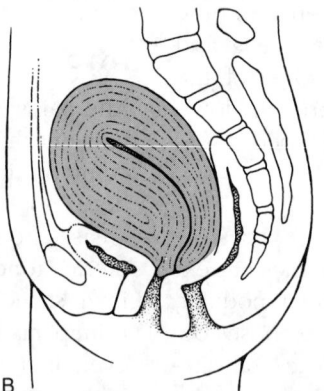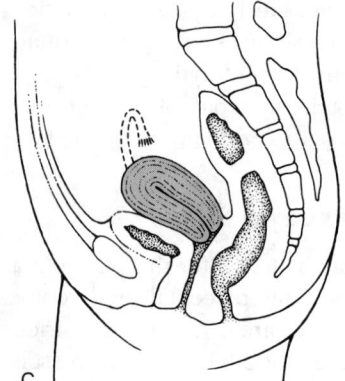

FIGURE 25-1 Changes in uterus size and shape following delivery. (**A**) Uterus after delivery. (**B**) Uterus at sixth day. (**C**) Nongravid uterus.

generally intact, with occasional areas of partial denudation. As early as the fourth day, the glandular hypertrophy and hyperplasia seen during pregnancy regress, and interstitial hemorrhage is reabsorbed. Cervical involution continues beyond 6 weeks, however, with edema and round cell infiltration persisting as long as 3 to 4 months.

Colposcopic examination of the cervix has demonstrated ulceration, laceration, bruising, and yellow areas within several days of delivery. These lesions, which are usually smaller than 4 mm, are seen more often in primiparas. Repeat examination 6 to 12 weeks later usually shows complete healing; this indicates rapid reepithelialization of the injured tissue. Cervical lacerations heal by proliferation of fibroblasts (DeCherney and Pernoll, 1994).

There is variable retraction of everted columnar epithelium (ectropion) beginning early in the postpartum period. As the cervix heals, there may be stellate scarring; the os is generally wider, shaped in a transverse slit, and may gape if lacerations occurred (Dunnihoo, 1992; Fig. 25-2).

Vagina and Perineum

The vagina is smooth and swollen and has poor tone following delivery. After 3 weeks, the vascularity, edema, and hypertrophy resulting from pregnancy and birth are markedly decreased. When vaginal cells are examined microscopically, the epithelium appears atrophic by the third to fourth week but regains its proper estrogen index by 6 to 10 weeks postpartum. This relative estrogen deficiency contributes to poor vaginal lubrication and decreased vasocongestion, which leads to a diminished sexual response in the weeks following delivery. The lower vagina usually has multiple superficial lacerations after birth; primiparas may have small tears of underlying fascia and musculature. Most of these are resolved by 6 weeks postpartum.

Vaginal rugae reappear by the fourth week postpartum, but many remain permanently flattened. After

birth, rugae are not as thick as in nulliparas. The vaginal mucosa thickens when ovarian function returns and often remains atrophic in lactating women until they begin to menstruate.

Immediately following delivery, the introitus is edematous and erythematous. If lacerations or an episiotomy is present, this condition may be exaggerated in the area of repair. In the absence of infections or hematomas, the perineum and introitus heal rapidly.

Most women are free of perineal pain by 1 month postpartum, although for some, discomfort may persist for up to 6 months. More than half of postpartum women have resumed sexual intercourse by 2 months, with the median time for comfortable intercourse about 3 months postpartum. A delay in restoration of perineal and introital integrity with persistent discomfort beyond median time periods is associated with vaginal lacerations, forceps delivery, perineal edema more than 4 days after birth, and vaginal infection (Abraham et al., 1990).

Fallopian Tubes and Ligaments

Histologic changes in the fallopian tubes reveal reduction in the size of secretory cells, decrease in the size and number of ciliated cells, and atrophy of the tubal epithelium. After 6 to 8 weeks, the epithelium reaches the condition of the early follicular phase of the menstrual cycle. Transient nonbacterial inflammation of the tubal lumina appears about the fourth day.

The *ligaments* that support the uterus, ovaries, and fallopian tubes, which have undergone great tension and stretching, are relaxed following delivery. It takes 2 to 3 months for them to return to their normal size and position.

Pelvic Muscular Support

The muscular and fascial support structures of the uterus and vagina may be injured during childbirth. This injury can lead to pelvic relaxation, which is weakening and lengthening of support structures for the uterus, vaginal wall, rectum, urethra, and bladder. Although relaxation of pelvic structures can occur in women who have not experienced childbirth or sexual activity, it is most often a delayed result of injuries during the birth process. Symptoms and signs of pelvic relaxation usually appear around menopause, when atrophic changes in fascia occur and the tonic effects of estrogens on pelvic tissues decrease.

The most common types of pelvic relaxation include rectocele, enterocele, uterine prolapse, urethrocele, and cystocele. These defects are due to distention and separation of muscle bundles, fascial lacerations, and stretching and tearing of support structures. They tend to worsen with time (see Chap. 10).

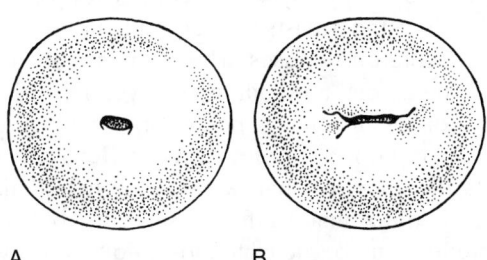

A   B

FIGURE 25-2 The perfectly round os of the nulliparous cervix becomes elongated after childbirth. The cervical os may gape if there have been significant lacerations during delivery. (**A**) Round os of nulliparous cervix. (**B**) Transverse slit of os in parous cervix.

The pelvic muscles are critical to maintenance of urinary continence when there is a sudden increase in intra-abdominal pressure, such as with coughing and sneezing. The various pelvic muscles, which are under voluntary control, combine with the smooth muscle of the urethra to maintain continence in women with intact muscle tone (Sampselle et al., 1990).

Repeated childbearing places women at increased risk of pelvic muscle relaxation. Women who have greater antepartum pelvic muscle strength tend to demonstrate greater strength following vaginal delivery. Women who practice postpartum pelvic muscle exercises show greater improvement in pelvic muscle strength than those who do not exercise (Sampselle et al., 1990; Dougherty et al., 1989). Exercises to aid restoration of pelvic and vaginal muscle tone recommended by Kegel may improve pelvic muscle support. Kegel exercises are often taught to clients as treatment for such pelvic support disorders as stress incontinence, cystocele, and uterine prolapse (Resnick, 1992; DeCherney and Pernoll, 1994).

Chapter 17 describes Kegel's exercises; approaches to teaching these exercises to postpartum clients are discussed in Chapter 27.

Abdominal Wall

The abdominal wall recovers partially from the overstretching but remains soft and flabby for some time. The skin eventually regains its elasticity, but the striae persist because of the rupture of the elastic fibers of the cutis. The striae become less conspicuous because of their silvery appearance. The process of involution in the abdominal structures requires at least 6 weeks. The abdominal walls regain their muscle tone and gradually return to their original condition, depending on prepregnancy tone, exercise, and amount of adipose tissue. However, if these muscles are overdistended or if they have lost their tone, there may be a marked separation or **diastasis** of the recti muscles so that the abdominal organs are not properly supported. Rest, diet, prescribed exercises, good body mechanics, and good posture may largely restore the tone of the abdominal wall muscles.

Breasts

Progressive changes occur in the breasts during pregnancy in preparation for lactation. The breast lobules develop under the stimulation of the estrogen and progesterone produced by the placenta, and the lactiferous ducts undergo further branching and elongation. Prolactin released from the anterior pituitary, cortisol from the maternal adrenal gland, human placental lactogen (hPL), and insulin, all of which appear in increasing amounts during gestation, also contribute to breast changes. Prolactin has a central role in the initiation of lactation, but its actions are inhibited during pregnancy as a result of high levels of estrogen and progesterone (Resnick, 1994).

In the last month of pregnancy, the parenchymal cells in the alveoli of the breasts hypertrophy and produce colostrum, a thin, yellow fluid. The abrupt drop in estrogen and progesterone levels at birth and expulsion of the placenta appear to initiate lactation.

Physiology of Lactation

At least six pituitary hormones play a role in mammary development and lactation: prolactin, adrenocorticotropic hormone, human growth hormone, thyroid-stimulating hormone, follicle-stimulation hormone (FSH), and luteinizing hormone (LH). In addition, human chorionic somatotropin, hPL, and steroid hormones secreted by the adrenal glands, ovaries, and placenta play a part, as does pancreatic insulin. Prolactin prepares the breasts for lactation through an increase in breast size and in the number and complexity of the ducts and alveoli during pregnancy. As pregnancy progresses, prolactin stimulates secretion by mammary alveolar cells, and estrogen and progesterone stimulate ductal and alveolar growth, but the latter two paradoxically inhibit milk secretion.

With expulsion of the placenta, the source of all hPL and most estrogen and progesterone during pregnancy is suddenly removed. The blood levels of these hormones fall rapidly, but the secretion of prolactin by the anterior pituitary gland continues. The appearance of milk after delivery has been demonstrated to coincide with falling estrogen and progesterone levels in the presence of elevated prolactin. The synthesis and secretion of milk are thus initiated when the inhibitory effects of estrogen and progesterone are removed and under the continuing effects of prolactin.

The secretion of milk begins at the base of the alveolar cells, where small droplets are formed and then migrate to the cell membrane; these are extruded into the alveolar ducts for storage. Milk ejection, or let down, is the process by which contraction of myoepithelial cells in the breasts propels milk along the ducts into the lactiferous sinuses. These sinuses are located beneath the areola, and milk is removed from them by the newborn's suckling. A neurohormonal reflex controls milk ejection, or the **let-down reflex**, and works through afferent nerve pathways to the hypothalamus. Suckling is the primary afferent stimulus, but the let-down reflex can be activated by auditory (newborn crying) and visual (seeing the newborn) stimuli. The efferent limb of this pathway is clearly hormonal, because oxytocin that is released from the posterior pituitary causes contraction of the myoepithelial cells of the breasts (Resnick, 1994).

The importance of higher cortical centers in the brain is demonstrated by the sensitivity of the let-down reflex to various noxious stimuli. Anxiety and tension, severe cold, and pain inhibit the let-down reflex and decrease milk ejection. This underlies the need for a comfortable, relaxed setting in which to breast-feed. Chronic stress in life situations also contributes to an ineffective lactation response.

Prolactin appears to be more critical for initiation of lactation than for its maintenance once it is established. With continued nursing, levels of prolactin released in response to suckling increase less dramatically than in the beginning. Eventually, prolactin levels may not rise at all with suckling. The pathways by which lactation and milk ejection are brought about are illustrated in Figure 25-3.

Colostrum

During late pregnancy, small amounts of colostrum may be secreted. After delivery, increased amounts of colostrum are produced for the first 3 to 4 days. Colostrum contains more protein and inorganic salts but less fat and carbohydrate than breast milk. Colostrum also provides immunoglobulin A, an important gastrointestinal antibody that the newborn lacks. Although the nutritive value of colostrum is lower than that of breast milk, it is particularly suited to the newborn's digestive system and provides important immunologic protection.

Lactation

On the third or fourth postpartum day, the breast milk usually "comes in." There is an obvious change in the color of the secretion from the nipples: It becomes bluish white, the usual color of normal breast milk. At this time, the breasts suddenly become larger, firmer, and more tender as lacteal secretion is established, causing the mother to experience throbbing pains in the breasts that extend into the axillae. This congestion, which usually subsides in 1 or 2 days, is caused in part by pressure from the increased amounts of milk in the lobules and the ducts but even more by the increased circulation of blood and lymph in the mammary gland, producing tension on the extremely sensitive surrounding tissues. This is called **primary engorgement** (see Chap. 30).

The efficiency and maintenance of milk production are controlled by the stimulus of repetitive nursing. The

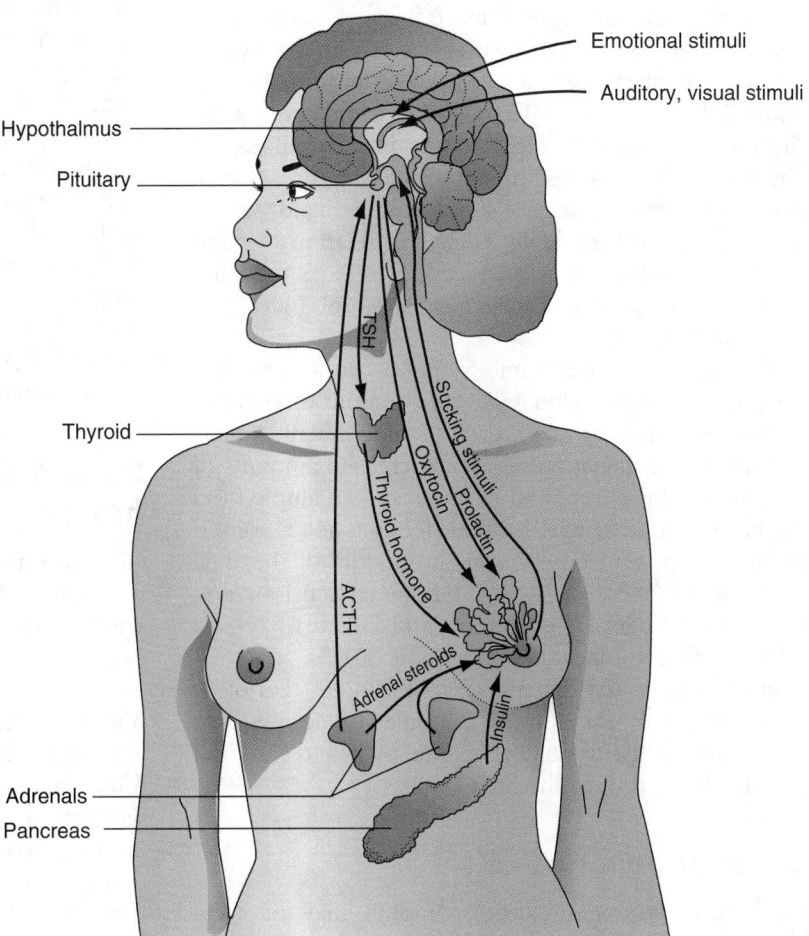

FIGURE 25-3 Neurohormonal pathways influencing lactation and the let-down reflex. (Redrawn from Hytten, F. E., & Leitch, I: [1971]. The physiology of human pregnancy [2nd ed.]. Oxford: Blackwell Scientific Publications.)

oxytocin released by suckling also stimulates uterine contractions, which explains the mild abdominal cramps often associated with the initiation of breast-feeding.

Breast milk contains proteins, minerals, vitamins, fats, and sugars needed for newborn nourishment. It has an abundance of hormones, neuropeptides, and natural opioids that may subtly shape the newborn's brain and behavior. The breasts extract potent hormones from the mother's blood and concentrate them in milk. Acting as an endocrine gland, breasts also generate some hormones, such as gonadotropin-releasing hormone and mammotrope-differentiating peptide (Angier, 1994).

Supply of Breast Milk

Breast milk varies markedly in its quality and quantity, not only in different people, but also in the same person at different times. In general, the amount of breast milk increases as the newborn's need for it increases. Nature seems to have carefully coordinated the mother's need for rest and the newborn's need for food during the first few days, when only colostrum is secreted. During this time, the newborn's suckling stimulates the lactation process. Although the secretion of breast milk would occur naturally, in the absence of suckling and complete emptying of the breasts, lactation would not continue for more than a few days.

If the newborn is put to breast consistently, by the end of the first week, a healthy mother usually has about 200 to 300 mL (6–10 oz) of breast milk a day. By the end of 4 weeks, this amount almost doubles, so she produces about 600 mL (20 oz) a day. Breast milk is produced on the basis of supply and demand (ie, the amount secreted gradually adjusts in relation to what the newborn takes at an average feeding). As the baby grows, the mother may have about 900 mL (30 oz) of breast milk a day.

The supply of breast milk depends on several factors, such as the mother's diet, the amount of exercise and rest she gets, and her level of contentment. An adequate diet for lactation requires increased amounts of protein, calcium, iron, and vitamins and an ample fluid intake. The mother who is breast-feeding needs a good night's sleep, a rest period in the middle of the day, and normal exercise. Worry, emotional tension, and too much activity (overexertion and fatigue) have an adverse effect on lactation (see Chap. 30).

For lactation, the actual size of the breast is not as important as the amount of glandular tissue, because the secreting tissues of the mammary gland, not the fatty tissues, produce the breast milk.

Lactation Suppression

The production and ejection of milk may be suppressed at the level of the breast, the pituitary, or the hypothalamus. The most simple, natural method is to avoid stimulation of the breast, which reduces the milk ejection reflex and decreases the stimulation of prolactin required for continued milk production. When the milk ejection reflex is inhibited for several days, the distended alveoli will suppress lactation. In about 60% to 70% of postpartum women, lactation can be suppressed by wearing a tight brassiere and avoiding stimulation of the nipples and breasts.

Some women experience engorged breasts with onset of lactation, causing discomfort. Engorgement usually resolves within 24 to 36 hours. Within 1 week, lactation ceases, and the breasts gradually return to their nonpregnant state. Prolactin secretion can be inhibited with synthetic ergot alkaloids, such as bromocriptine mesylate (Parlodel). This drug became unavailable in 1994, however. The administration of estrogens or androgens to suppress lactation is infrequently used because of the risk of thromboembolic or neoplastic disorders.

Endocrine System

Placental Hormones

After childbirth, plasma levels of hormones produced by the placenta decline rapidly. hPL cannot be detected within 24 hours, and human chorionic gonadotropin levels drop quickly. Estrogen levels fall 90% within 3 hours of birth and then continue decreasing slowly until 7 days postpartum when estrogen reaches its lowest level. Estrogen returns to follicular phase levels in about 3 weeks in nonlactating women. Return to normal estrogen levels is delayed in lactating women. Progesterone levels decline to below luteal phase levels by 3 days postpartum and cannot be detected by 7 days. Following the first ovulation, progesterone production begins again (see Table 25-2).

Hypothalamic-Pituitary-Ovarian Hormones

Gonadotropic hormones remain low after birth, until preparation for the first postdelivery ovulation begins with reactivation of the hypothalamic-pituitary-ovarian cycle. FSH and LH levels are low in postpartum women for 10 to 12 days. FSH increases to follicular phase concentrations by the third week. LH increases after the first ovulation. Ovulation and menstruation following childbirth are influenced by whether the woman is breast-feeding, as shown in Table 25-3. Nonlactating women may ovulate as early as 27 days after delivery (Resnick, 1994). Menses occurring within the first 6 weeks postpartum are rarely ovulatory. The first menses usually results from a cycle with inadequate

TABLE 25–2
Postpartum Endocrine Changes

Hormone	Changes After Birth: Time Frame
Human placental lactogen	Falls rapidly to undetectable levels in 24 h
Human chorionic gonadotropin	Falls rapidly after birth; remains low until ovulation occurs
Estrogen	Falls 90% in 3 h, lowest level in 7 d; returns to follicular levels in 3 wk
Progesterone	Falls in 3 d to below luteal levels, undetectable in 7 d; increases after ovulation
Follicle-stimulating hormone	Low for 10–12 d; reaches follicular levels in 3 wk
Luteinizing hormone	Low for 10–12 d; increases after ovulation
Prolactin	Nonlactating: falls to prepregnant levels in 2 wk
	Lactating: Rises with suckling, remains high for 6–12 mo, depending on frequency of nursing
Growth hormone	Remains low for several days
Thyroid hormone	Remains unchanged
Corticosteroids	Falls to nonpregnant levels by 1 wk
Renin, angiotensin II	Falls to nonpregnant levels by 2 h

corpus luteum function, in which LH and progesterone are low or absent (Scott et al., 1994). Once menstruation begins, the percentage of subsequent ovulatory menses rises rapidly.

Return of Fertility

The return of menstruation after delivery follows a linear pattern (see Table 25-3). In nonlactating women, the pattern is as follows:

- By 6 weeks postpartum, 40% menstruate.
- By 12 weeks postpartum, 65% to 70% menstruate.
- By 24 weeks postpartum, 80% to 90% menstruate.

In lactating women, the pattern is as follows:

- By 6 weeks postpartum, 15% menstruate.
- By 12 weeks postpartum, 45% menstruate.
- By 36 weeks postpartum, 55% to 75% menstruate.

TABLE 25–3
Return of Menstruation

	Average Time of First Ovulation (Weeks)	Average Time of First Menstruation (Weeks)
NONLACTATING WOMEN	10.2	7–9[‡]
LACTATING WOMEN	17.0*	30–36[§]
	28.0[†]	

*Lactating for 3 mo.
†Lactating for 6 mo.
‡First menses usually anovulatory.
§Depends on duration of lactation.

The time of first postdelivery ovulation varies considerably among lactating and nonlactating women. Differences in the strength of the suckling stimulus has a strong effect on return of ovulation in lactating women. Women who breast-feed for less than 1 month have a similar time for return of ovulation and menses as nonlactating women (Resnick, 1994). Partial weaning with use of formula supplementation and breast-feeding less than six times daily lead to earlier first ovulation, probably related to decreased prolactin levels.

Although gonadotropins return to normal levels whether or not the woman is lactating, return to normal estrogen levels is delayed by lactation. This is interpreted to mean that lactation causes a temporary refractory state of the ovaries to pituitary gonadotropins.

Other Endocrine Changes

Prolactin (a pituitary hormone) levels rise during pregnancy. After birth, prolactin decreases in nonlactating women and reaches nonpregnant levels within 2 weeks. In lactating women, prolactin rises sharply with suckling and remains elevated for months. Serum levels of prolactin are affected by extent of the suckling stimulus. In women who breast-feed one to three times per day, prolactin returns to normal baseline levels by 6 months. If breast-feeding occurs more than six times daily, high prolactin levels continue beyond 1 year.

Growth hormone levels are low through late pregnancy and early postpartum (about 3 days). In combination with other hormones (hPL, estrogens, cortisol) and the placental enzyme insulinase, which all drop after birth, the low growth hormone levels contribute to increased insulin availability early in the postpartum period. Women have low glucose levels during this time, and insulin-dependent diabetic mothers require less insulin after birth (see Chap. 31). Carbohydrate metabolism is altered, contributing to appetite changes observed following birth.

Thyroid hormone usually remains unchanged from late pregnancy. Values should not differ greatly from normal. Women who are unable to establish lactation or who experience delayed recovery from birth may have thyroid deficiencies. Fatigue is common after birth, probably related to rapid endocrine fluctuations and the energy expenditure and sleep deprivation accompanying labor and delivery. Continued fatigue for some weeks postpartum may be due to disrupted sleep because of the newborn's feeding and wake and sleep patterns.

Corticosteriods decrease after birth to nonpregnant levels by the end of the first week. Renin and angiotensin II decrease to nonpregnant levels by 2 hours after delivery. This indicates that the fetoplacental unit may supply renin found in maternal plasma during pregnancy.

Cardiovascular System

Most of the significant cardiovascular changes produced by pregnancy disappear by the end of the second postpartum week. Within a few days of delivery, blood pressure, heart rate, oxygen consumption, and total body fluids generally return to prepregnant levels. Other changes require several weeks to resolve.

Blood Volume

During pregnancy, blood volume increases 40% (by about 1,000 mL), attaining total volume of 5 to 6 L. Changes in blood volume after delivery are due to blood loss and postdelivery diuresis. The average blood loss for normal vaginal delivery is 400 to 500 mL; for cesarean delivery, it often exceeds 1,000 mL. Postpartum physiologic changes mediate the response to blood loss and exercise a protective effect. Loss of the endocrine functions of the placenta reduces vasodilation. The maternal vascular bed is reduced by 10% to 15% when uteroplacental circulation is eliminated, and extravascular fluid is mobilized for excretion by the kidneys.

Postpartum changes in blood volume occur rapidly. There is a transient 15% to 30% increase in circulating blood volume between 12 and 48 hours after delivery because of mobilization of extravascular fluid and diuresis. This produces a hemodilutional effect, with a decrease in hematocrit and increase in cardiac output. By the third postpartum day, blood volume has declined 16% from pregnancy-related increases (Resnick, 1994). Total blood volume decreases to nonpregnant levels of 4 L by the fourth postpartum week.

Cardiac Output

Cardiac output, which increases during labor, peaks immediately after placental separation as uterine contractions force a large volume of blood into the circulation (Laros, 1991). The increased stroke volume produced by pregnancy continues about 48 hours after delivery, due to increased venous return resulting from loss of placental circulation and reduced uterine blood flow. Postpartum diuresis causes a transient increase in blood volume. The combined effects of increased venous return and diuresis lead to cardiac output that is 35% greater in the early postdelivery period.

Within 2 weeks after delivery, cardiac output decreases by about 30% (Robson et al., 1987). Gradual reduction in blood volume occurs during the second to fourth postpartum weeks, permitting cardiac output to return to nonpregnant levels by about the third week postpartum (Cunningham, et al., 1993).

Blood Pressure and Heart Rate

Blood pressure undergoes little change under normal conditions. Orthostatic hypotension may occur in the first 48 hours after delivery because of splanchnic engorgement. After delivery, there often is transient physiologic bradycardia, lasting 24 to 48 hours, with heart rates of 40 to 50 beats/min. This results from hemodynamic changes, including increased stroke volume and cardiac output, and a vagal response to increased sympathetic nervous system activity during labor (Resnick, 1994). Milder bradycardia of 50 to 70 beats/min may continue for about 1 week. The heart rate returns to nonpregnant levels by about 3 months postpartum.

Blood Constituents

Red Blood Cells, Hematocrit, and Hemoglobin

Following early hemodilution caused by interstitial fluid mobilization, the hematocrit and hemoglobin rise in 3 to 7 days because of hemoconcentration that accompanies diuresis (greater loss of plasma volume than blood cells). The increased red blood cell (RBC) mass during pregnancy also contributes to increased hematocrit and hemoglobin. There is no RBC destruction during the postpartum period, but the RBC count gradually returns to normal levels as the increased RBCs of pregnancy reach the end of their life span. Hematocrit values return to prepregnant levels by the fourth or fifth postpartum week.

White Blood Cells

The white blood cell (WBC) count normally increases to 12,000/mm³ during pregnancy. A pronounced leukocytosis occurs during the first 10 to 12 days after delivery with values of 20,000 to 30,000/mm³. This leukocytosis is characterized by increased neutrophils and eosinophils and decreased lymphocytes. This shift to the left in the WBC count also is typical of infections, and combined with the increased erythrocyte sedimentation rate typical after delivery, it may make postpartum infection hard to identify.

Coagulation Factors

The increase in coagulation factors that occurs with pregnancy continues into the postpartum period. Clotting factors I, II, VIII, IX, and X are activated extensively after delivery. These decrease within a few days to prepregnant levels, but fibrinogen and thromboplastin remain elevated until the end of the third week postpartum. These increased clotting factors can interact with immobility, sepsis, or trauma to predispose women to postpartum thromboembolism.

Other Constituents

Effects of high estrogen levels during pregnancy on protein and fat synthesis result in increased production of fatty acids, cholesterol, triglycerides, lipoproteins, and clotting factors. These constituents return to prepregnant levels by 2 to 3 weeks postpartum. Serum electrolytes are altered after delivery, with a negative chloride balance resulting from rapid excretion of extracellular fluid during diuresis. Serum sodium rises in part because of falling steroid hormones and relatively greater loss of water than sodium. Increased serum potassium levels are probably caused by catabolism of tissues during involution. These changes are reversed by about 2 weeks postpartum.

Respiratory System

Changes in abdominal pressure and thoracic cage capacity after delivery result in rapid alterations of pulmonary function. Increases are found in residual volume, resting ventilation, and oxygen consumption. There are decreases in inspiratory capacity, vital capacity, and maximum breathing capacity. By 6 months postpartum, pulmonary functions return to nonpregnant levels. During this time, however, women have less efficient responses to exercise.

Acid–Base Balance

Acid–base balance changes during labor and in the early postpartum period. Progesterone during pregnancy creates a type of hyperventilation at the alveolar level, increasing oxygen saturation without changing respiratory rate. Pregnancy is characterized by respiratory alkalosis (caused by decreased carbon dioxide concentration in alveoli) and a compensated metabolic acidosis. During labor, these begin to change with rising blood lactate, falling pH, and hypocapnia (<30 mm Hg) toward the end of the first stage. These conditions continue into the early puerperium, but more normal nonpregnant values (PCO_2 35–40 mm Hg) appear within a few days. Falling progesterone levels affect this postpartum hypercapnia, which is accompanied by elevated base excess and plasma bicarbonate. Gradually, the pH and base excess increase until normal values are reached, about 3 weeks after delivery. The basic metabolic rate remains increased for 1 to 2 weeks following delivery.

Oxygen Saturation

Oxygen saturation and PO_2 are higher during pregnancy. In labor, women may experience decreases in oxygen saturation, especially when supine. This may be a result of decreased cardiac output in this position. Oxygen saturation rises rapidly after delivery, to 95% during the first postpartum day. An oxygen debt in the postdelivery period may occur, apparently related to the length and difficulty of the second stage of labor. There is increased resting oxygen consumption during this time, which also may be affected by lactation, anemia, and emotional and psychological factors.

Urinary System
Renal Function

During pregnancy, high levels of steroid hormones contribute to increased renal function. After childbirth, renal function is reduced partly due to decreased levels of steroid hormones. Hypotonia and dilation of urinary tract structures continue for up to 3 months (Cunningham et al., 1993). The ureters and renal pelvis of the kidneys remain dilated after delivery, returning to normal in 3 to 6 weeks, although this may occasionally take as long as 8 to 12 weeks. By 6 weeks postpartum, renal plasma flow, glomerular filtration rate (GFR), plasma creatinine, and nitrogen usually return to nonpregnant levels.

Bladder and Urethra

Passage of the fetus through the birth canal causes trauma to the urethra and bladder. The bladder mucosa following delivery shows varying degrees of edema and hyperemia, with diminished bladder tone. This results in less sensation of pressure and greater bladder capacity. The urethra and urinary meatus often are edematous. Tissue edema and hyperemia, combined with effects of analgesia, depress the urge to void.

Pelvic soreness adds to decreasing the voiding reflex. Postpartum diuresis may lead to rapid filling of the bladder. These factors often produce overdistention of the bladder with overflow incontinence and incomplete emptying of the bladder. Residual urine makes the bladder more susceptible to infection and interferes with normal voiding. Prolonged overdistention can result in atony of the bladder wall. With adequate emptying of the bladder, tone is usually restored within 5 to 7 days.

Water Metabolism

Reversal of the water metabolism of pregnancy results from decreased steroid hormones and postpartum involution. Catabolic processes contribute to elevated blood urea nitrogen (BUN), proteinuria, and occasionally acetonuria. Changes in blood volume and hormone levels affect postpartum diuresis, GFR, and serum electrolytes.

Diuresis

Profound diuresis occurs in the first 2 to 3 postpartum days. This removes the large amount of fluid retained during pregnancy. Renal plasma flow and GFR remain elevated during the first postpartum week and combined with increased blood volume, cause diuresis of up to 3,000 mL/d beginning within 12 hours of birth. Perspiration also increases during this time. Fluid is lost from the body tissues; combined with involutional changes, this causes weight loss of about 9 lb during the puerperium.

Urine Constituents

Glycosuria occurs early in the postpartum period in 20% of women but soon disappears. Lactosuria is normal in lactating women. Slight proteinuria (1+) occurs for 1 to 2 days in 50% of women due to postpartum catalysis. BUN is increased because of autolysis of uterine muscle (breakdown of excess muscle cells). Acetonuria may occur from changes in fat metabolism or dehydration.

Other Systems

Gastrointestinal System

The motility and tone of the gastrointestinal system usually returns to normal within 2 weeks after delivery. Most women are quite thirsty the first 2 to 3 days because of fluid shifts between interstitial spaces and circulation associated with diuresis. Fluid restriction during labor contributes to thirst. Most women are hungry

shortly after delivery and can enjoy a light meal and fluids. After recovery from the fatigue of labor and effects of analgesia and anesthesia, most mothers have a markedly increased appetite and will eat large portions of food. Changes in carbohydrate metabolism and energy expenditure during labor promote increased appetite.

Bowel Elimination

Constipation is common during the early postpartum period. This results from the relaxation of the intestines caused by pregnancy (adynamic ileus) and distended abdominal muscles that provide less assistance with elimination. These physiologic processes are exacerbated by the effects of food and fluid restriction during labor, predelivery enema (if given), and medications used during labor and delivery.

Bowel evacuation may be delayed for 2 to 3 days following delivery. Pain from hemorrhoids, episiotomy, or perineal lacerations, which commonly are present, further deters defecation. Most postpartum women are given stool softeners or laxatives, such as docusate sodium (DSS), bisacodyl (Dulcolax), or milk of magnesia, to aid elimination. The mother must reestablish regular bowel habits after bowel tone is restored.

Weight Loss

Weight loss immediately following delivery averages 12 lb and includes the weight of the fetus, placenta, amniotic fluid, and blood loss. Another 9 to 10 lb is lost during the first postpartum week due to uterine involution, lochia, perspiration, and diuresis. The mother's total weight loss related to delivery and postpartum processes ranges from 19 to 24 lb (Table 25-4). Many women gain 30 lb or more during pregnancy, and some of the weight not lost in the first weeks may be retained, especially during lactation (Brewer et al., 1989; Parham, 1990). Persistent weight increase and redistribution of adipose tissue are common after the first pregnancy (Smith et al., 1994).

Neuromuscular Systems

After delivery, neurologic adaptations caused by pregnancy are reversed. Discomforts resulting from nerve compression disappear as mechanical pressure from the enlarged uterus and pressure from fluid retention are relieved. Numbness of the thighs due to compression of nerves against the pelvic sidewall or beneath the inguinal ligament during pregnancy improves. Periodic numbness and tingling of the fingers, which affect 5% of pregnant women as a result of brachial plexus traction, are relieved. Elimination of edema and rever-

TABLE 25-4
Sources and Amount of Weight Loss During the Postpartum Period

Source of Weight Loss	Amount of Weight Loss	
	POUNDS	**KILOGRAMS**
Fetus and placenta; amniotic fluid and blood loss at delivery	12–13	5.5–6
Perspiration and diuresis during the first postpartum week	5–8	2.5–4
Uterine involution and lochia	2–3	1
Total weight loss	19–24	9–10

sal of physiologic changes in fascia, tendons, and connective tissue during pregnancy relieve pressure on the median nerve and improve carpal tunnel syndrome (pain, numbness, and tingling of sides of hands and fingers). Depending on their cause, leg cramps may improve after delivery.

Endocrine effects on fibrocartilage during pregnancy are gradually reversed during the postpartum period. The relative relaxation and increased mobility of pelvic articulations are restored to nonpregnant stability by about 6 to 8 weeks after delivery. This often relieves backache characteristic of pregnancy, although a new source of strain from lifting the newborn may confound symptomatic improvement. Postural changes caused by the enlarged uterus are reversed, improving lumbar lordosis and compensatory dorsal kyphosis. However, enlarged lactating breasts and weakened abdominal wall muscles may contribute to poor posture after delivery (Tulman et al., 1990).

Integumentary System

The increased melanin activity of pregnancy causing hyperpigmentation of nipples, areola, and linea nigra gradually decreases after delivery. Although darker coloration of these areas regresses, color may not return to prepregnant character, and some women have persistent darker pigment. Chloasma (mask of pregnancy) usually improves, although it may not disappear completely.

Vascular effects during pregnancy causing spider angiomas, darker nevi, palmar erythema, and epulis regress as estrogen levels decline rapidly following delivery. Spider angiomas, which occur in 10% to 15% of women, may be permanent, although smaller. Increased fine hair distribution seen in pregnancy usually disappears; coarse, bristly hair usually remains. Pruritus associated with hyperestrogen states improves postpartum.

Perspiration

Elimination of fluid and waste products through the skin is accelerated in the early puerperium, often to such a degree that the mother is drenched with perspiration. These episodes of **diaphoresis** (profuse sweating), which frequently occur at night, gradually subside. Diaphoresis is part of the reversal of water metabolism, in which excess fluid accumulated during pregnancy is eliminated.

Temperature

Slight rises in temperature may occur in the first 24 hours after delivery, but the mother's temperature should remain within normal limits during the puerperium (below 38°C or 100.4°F oral). When temperature exceeds this limit in any two consecutive 24-hour periods in the puerperium, the mother is febrile. Occasionally, fever for up to 12 hours may be caused by extreme vascular and lymphatic engorgement of the breasts.

Heart rate elevation accompanies significant fever. Slightly elevated temperature with a normal heart rate usually does not signify a complication. Any postpartum sustained rise in temperature with increased heart rate may indicate endometritis or other complications (see Chap. 38).

Summary Points

✔ Major postpartum changes occur in most body systems, restoring them to their normal prepregnant state.

✔ The uterus undergoes involution, with rapid decrease in size through reduction in cell numbers and size. The placental site heals by endometrial regeneration, as lochia progresses from rubra to serosa to alba.

✔ Breasts in lactating women secrete colostrum, increase in size, and begin producing milk within 3 to 4 days after birth. Lactation can be suppressed by avoiding breast stimulation and wearing tight support. Temporary engorgement is common in lactating and nonlactating women.

✔ Gonadotropic hormones, estrogen, progesterone, prolactin, corticosteroids, and other hormones undergo characteristic postpartum changes. Return of fertility is delayed by lactation, depending on the strength of the suckling stimulus.

✔ Early hemodilution, leukocytosis, and increased clotting factors occur postpartum. These and other cardiovascular functional changes return to normal prepregnant values in days to several weeks.

✔ Diuresis occurs in the 12 hours after delivery, with diaphoresis aiding in removal of excess tissue fluid and return to normal water metabolism.

✔ Decreased bladder sensitivity and tone, increased bladder capacity, and postpartum diuresis contribute to urinary distention and retention. Emptying the bladder and preventing distention promote return to normal voiding.

✔ Constipation is common in the puerperium due to decreased intestinal tone, limited fluids, and perineal discomfort. Intestinal tone is restored within 1 week.

✔ Neuromuscular discomforts from pregnancy fluid retention and postural changes improve within several days to weeks postpartum.

✔ Vital signs remain stable, with physiologic bradycardia and transient mild temperature elevation in the first few postpartum days.

REFERENCES

Abraham, S., Child, A., Ferry, J. et al. (1990). Recovery after childbirth: A preliminary prospective study. *Medical Journal of Australia, 152,* 9–12.

Angier, N. (1994). Mother's milk found to be potent cocktail of hormones. *The New York Times,* May 24.

Brewer, M. M. et al. (1989). Postpartum change in maternal weight and body fat deposits in lactating vs. non-lactating women. *American Journal of Clinical Nutrition, 49,* 259.

Cunningham, F. G., MacDonald, P. C., Gart, W. F., et al. (1993). *Williams' obstetrics* (19th ed.) Norwalk, CT: Appleton & Lange.

DeCherney, A. H. and Pernoll, M. L. (Eds.) (1994). *Current obstetric and gynecologic diagnosis and treatment* (8th ed.). Norwalk, CT: Appleton & Lange.

Dougherty, M. C., et al. (1989). The effect of exercise on the circumvaginal muscle in postpartum women. *Journal of Nurse Midwifery, 34,* 8.

Dunnihoo, D. R. (1992). *Fundamentals of gynecology and obstetrics* (2nd ed.). Philadelphia: J.B. Lippincott.

Laros, R. K. (1991). Physiology of normal pregnancy. In J. R. Willson & E. R. Carrington (Eds.), *Obstetrics and gynecology* (9th ed.). St. Louis: Mosby.

Oppenheimer, L. et al. (1986). The duration of lochia. *British Journal of Obstetrics and Gynaecology, 93*(7), 754–757.

Parham, E. S. (1990). The association of pregnancy weight gain with the mother's postpartum weight. *Journal of the American Diet Association, 90,* 550.

Resnick, R. (1994). The puerperium. In R. Creasey & R. Resnick (Eds.), *Maternal-fetal medicine: Principles and practice* (3rd ed.). Philadelphia: W.B. Saunders.

Resnick, N. M. (1992). Urinary incontinence in older adults. *Hospital Practice, Oct. 15,* 139.

Robson, S. et al. (1987). Haemodynamic changes during the early puerperium. *British Medical Journal, 294,* 106.

Sampselle, C. M., & Brink, C. A. (1990). Pelvic muscle relaxation: Assessment and management. *Journal of Nurse Midwifery, 35,* 127–132.

Scott, J. R., Disaia, P. J., Hemmond, C. B., Spellacy, W. N. (Eds.). (1991). *Danforth's obstetrics and gynecology* (8th ed.). Philadelphia: J.B. Lippincott.

Smith, D. E., Lewis, C. E., Caveny, J. L. et al. (1994). Longitudinal changes in adiposity associated with pregnancy: The CARDIA study. *Journal of the American Medical Association, 271,* 1747–1751.

Tulman, L., Fawcett, J. et al. (1990). Changes in of functional status after childbirth. *Nursing Research, 39*(2), 70–75.

26

Psychosocial Aspects of the Postpartum Period

Objectives

- Understand parenthood as a role transition.
- Assess behaviors that are appropriate to a successful transition and plan care that will support the parents' efforts in a healthy transition.
- Identify evidence of the reciprocal interaction that takes place between the parents and their newborn.
- Describe the importance of bonding and attachment for a successful transition to the parental role.
- Identify the tasks and behaviors that new parents must accomplish.
- Implement nursing care that supports the parents' efforts.
- Describe the process by which the maternal role is attained and identify the characteristics of maternal role competence.
- Develop expertise in using the nursing process to assess, plan, implement, and evaluate nursing care that supports and enhances the new parents' transition to parenthood.

Key Terms

Attachment   Maternal role
Bonding   attainment
En face position   Reciprocity
Engrossment

BOX 26–1
*Vital Areas in the Transition
to Parenthood*

- The needs of each person in the system as an individual
- The needs of the parents as a couple
- The influence of parent–child interaction over time

In Chapter 16 we make the point that pregnancy and parenthood can be considered role transitions. We note the tremendous change that comes with childbirth and the assumption of the new role together with the instability that can occur until new roles are assigned and the new member is integrated. In this chapter we continue the exploration of the psychosocial needs of the family that has recently added a new member.

Parenthood: A Continuing Process of Transition

The transition to parenthood as described in Chapter 16 is a process rather than a state; the process begins in pregnancy and flowers when parental responsibilities begin. This chapter continues that discussion and is based on the underlying assumption that the degree of ease and satisfaction with which people make the transition to parenthood depends mostly on how successfully they have defined and accepted their relationship with each other. If they have developed an ability to see each other as they are (not as they ought to be) and can allow for divergence of values and behaviors, work collaboratively toward a flexible power base for each, and develop norms that allow for mutual growth, then they are more likely to move smoothly into the new role (Gilliss et al. 1989; Feetham et al., 1993).

Assumptions About Parenthood

Much of the literature on parenting, particularly the early literature that relies heavily on a psychoanalytical orientation, singles out the content of the parent–child relationship or the parents' own childhood relationships as the primary determinants of the family's progression through this developmental phase. Such a focus neglects the needs of each person within the system, the needs of the parents, and the influence of the couple's (and the infant's) interaction over time (Box 26-1).

Considering these areas does not negate the importance of the parent–child relationship or the parents' own background, but it does focus some attention on the marital couple as an entity. In reality, the ultimate task of the new family is to balance the three areas of needs within the family. Moreover, the nurse must be aware of and respect these areas when working with families undergoing the transition to parenthood (Avant, 1988; Mercer et al., 1990).

Role Supplementation and Role Mastery

One integrative conceptual framework for the care and support of couples experiencing role transition to parenthood is role supplementation (Swendsen et al., 1978; Meleis, 1991). By using this framework, health providers can help the parents and their significant others gain the necessary information or experience to bring them to a full awareness of the anticipated behavior patterns, sensations, and goals involved in the complementary roles of mother and father. In essence, this approach assists the parents-to-be in moving to role mastery of parenthood. Chapter 16 described pregnancy as the anticipatory phase of the transition to parenthood. The impending role must be at least partly rehearsed, modeled, and clarified through a process of communication with significant others. In so doing, the role expectations become clearer, and the partners begins to put themselves into the role of parents (role take). As this is done, there is a better "fit" to the impending role, with increased confidence leading to role mastery. A schematic drawing of the role mastery process is shown in Figure 26-1. Ideally, this process should begin during pregnancy. A similar modified process, however, can be instituted or reinforced by the nurse in the important early postpartum period (see Research Highlight).

Other Conceptualizations of Parenthood

Parenthood as A Negative Change in the Quality of Life

Scholars in family research (Gilliss et al., 1989; Tulman et al., 1990; Fiese et al., 1993; Coffman et al., 1994) have pointed out that the majority of studies on the assump-

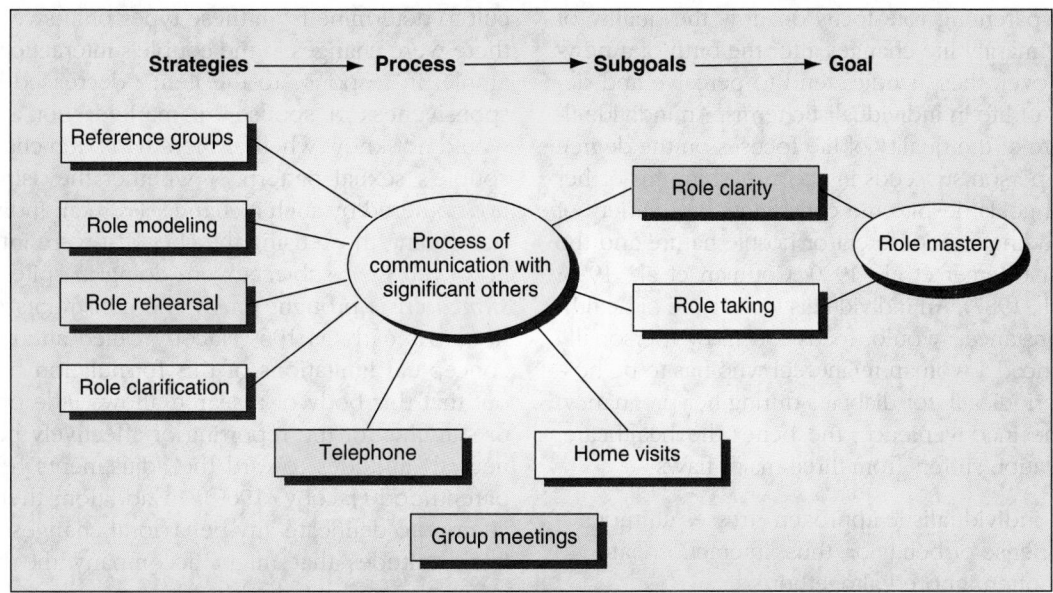

FIGURE 26-1 Conceptual framework of preventive role supplementation leading to role mastery. (After Swendsen, L. A., Meleis, A., & Jones, D. [1978]. Role supplementation for new parents: A role mastery plan. *MCN: American Journal of Maternal Child Nursing 3*(2), 84–91.)

RESEARCH HIGHLIGHT

Maternal Competence

One hundred twenty-one high-risk women (HRW) and 182 low-risk women (LRW) were studied postpartum in the hospital and at 1, 4 and 8 months postpartum to determine whether they would differ in the achievement of perceived maternal competence and whether predictors of maternal competence would differ for the two groups of women over time. (Maternal competence was considered by the author to consist of synchronous interaction with and caretaking of the infant.)

All subjects were recruited into a larger study during their 24th to 34th week of pregnancy. The authors do not reveal in this article how the sample was selected. The HRW and LRW groups had similar demographic characteristics, were 18 years or older, were fluent in English, and were planning to share parenting responsibilities with a male partner if they were not married.

The data were obtained by means of a variety of valid and reliable instruments. The authors carefully report the reliability measures and their findings in an understandable, logical manner.

The authors found no significant differences in the maternal role competence of the two groups of women or in the trajectory of change with time. Maternal role competence increased at 4 and 8 months over earlier levels. Selected variables explained from 33% to 52% of HRW's maternal competence and from 29% to 51% of the LRW's maternal competence over the four test periods. The two consistent predictors of maternal competence for both groups were self-esteem and mastery. State anxiety (ie, innate long-term anxiety) was a major predictor of maternal competence for both groups during the postpartum hospitalization. Fetal attachment was a predictor of maternal competence among the HRW only. Surprisingly, the authors found that perceived or received social support, partner relationships, family functioning, stress, maternal health status, and infant health status did not explain maternal competency at any test period.

Critique: This is another in a series of excellent substudies that explores the construct of maternal role attainment and the related construct of maternal role competence. The authors write in a clear concise way, briefly describing their theoretical framework that guides the study and the rationale for examining the problem. How the sample was selected (eg, convenience, random) was the only area that was left unaddressed. The sample size was appropriate for the statistics used. The authors conclude that given the surprising findings of the lack of prediction in the variables mentioned, further research on the variables and this construct is needed because about 50% of the variance is left unexplained. These conclusions are commensurate with the data. This article is timely and demonstrates the best characteristics of a program of research designed to explore and delineate important constructs that have relevance for the care of the childbearing family.

Mercer, R. T., & Ferketich, S. L. (1994). Predictors of maternal competence by risk status. *Nursing Research, 42*(1), 38–43.

tion of the parenting role focus on how the quality of personal or marital life changes after the birth of a newborn. Moreover, these studies tend to perceive and define quality of life in individualistic terms. An individualistic measure of the quality of life focuses on the degree to which a person succeeds in accomplishing his or her desires and goals despite the constraints of a variety of forces, including an indifferent or hostile nature and the social order (Mercer et al., 1990; Coffman et al., 1993; Cowan et al., 1987). An individualistic measure of healthcare, for instance, would focus on how personally inconvenienced a woman might feel who has to be hospitalized periodically for diabetes during her pregnancy. The less the inconvenience, the better the healthcare. This formulation suffers from three major flaws:

- First, the individualistic approach stresses attitudes at the expense of behavior; thus, interaction patterns are often ignored altogether.
- Second, the approach looks at the variable under study (eg, health, parenthood) as a "status" rather than a process and therefore fails to consider the reciprocal relationship between it and other aspects of the persons' lives.
- Third, the individualistic approach is laden with administrative bias that dictates that researchers must be more concerned with bureaucratic efficiency: if complaints can be reduced, then the best goal has been achieved (Rossa et al., 1990).

Parenthood as Crisis Versus Transition

Probably the best known series of studies on the assumption of the parenting role focuses on "parenthood as crisis." This line of research began with the Le Masters' article in 1957 and continued with Russell (1979), Dyer (1963), and the various reports of Hobbs et al. (1965, 1968, 1976, 1977). The principal question these studies pursued is, to what extent does becoming a parent constitute a "crisis"? It was assumed that this life change constituted a crisis (ie, extreme, incapacitating, negative change). With the exception of the Le Masters and Dyer articles, the only criterion for answering this question was a 23-item checklist originally developed by Hobbs (LeMasters, 1957; Dyer, 1963; Hobbs, 1965; Hobbs, 1968; Hobbs et al., 1976; Hobbs et al., 1977). Moreover, the checklist did not focus on the patterns (or changed patterns) of interaction between the couple; it stressed the coping ability of the parents. For instance, the parents were not asked if there was an interruption of routine, a change in their sex life and sleeping patterns, and the like. Instead, they were asked to indicate whether each item in the checklist bothered them by choosing from three choices: "not at all," "somewhat," and "very much." Thus, it was diffi-

cult to determine from these types of answers whether there were changes in the couple's interactions. For example, in response to the item, "decreased sexual responsiveness of spouse," if marked "not at all," one would not know whether there had been change in the couple's sexual pattern or whether they simply were not bothered by such a change. From an individualistic standpoint, those using the checklist were interested in how well their subjects were doing in spite of the *assumed* crisis brought on by the constraints of parenthood. As early as 1969, Jacoby called attention to the conceptual limitations of this formulation by pointing out that this body of research allows little opportunity or stimulus for the reporting of affectively positive (or neutral) attitudes toward the adjustments required by parenthood (Jacoby, 1969). In addition, there was no attempt to delineate any behavioral changes as distinct from attitudes that might accompany the behavioral changes. Interestingly, his critique appeared not to be taken seriously, and this criticism pertains today when researchers continue this line of investigation.

As pointed out in Chapter 16, there are many methodologic problems inherent in this research, which uses primarily small, skewed samples and lacks sophisticated analyses. Although this body of research has grave limitations and is essentially nonvalid, it was pioneering in a sense. Current difficulties arise when health providers accept these studies uncritically and proceed on the faulty assumption that parenthood for everyone is a time of crisis or extreme stress. In future research, greater attention must be paid to determining the social processes and patterns involved in the transition, and attitudes toward the phenomenon must be teased out. The importance of social networks and supports; the input of the newborn, including temperament; how couples define their stressors and resources; and how they communicate and modify their existing social roles are all important aspects to be considered.

Transition to Parenthood

Chapter 16 uses Rossi's (1968) formulation of phases in the process of role transition. Specifically, these are the anticipatory, honeymoon, plateau, and disengagement phases. In the puerperium, the honeymoon phase of the transition has the most bearing on the nursing care that the maternity nurse must provide. The anticipatory phase will also be reviewed, however, because we previously focused on its relevance to pregnancy rather than to parenthood.

Anticipatory Phase

Pregnancy is an anticipatory stage to becoming a parent, and parents need to accomplish certain tasks during this time. Decision making and expectations influence later parenting, as does the division of labor in the family. This becomes extremely crucial when the newborn arrives. Observing how the routine activities of family maintenance are carried out often indicates how well the parents accept their changing roles. This also gives a clue as to what role assignments the child may later assume in the family. The nurse should note whether there is any negotiation or flexibility between the couple when allocating and sharing tasks. If one partner unilaterally appoints the other to manage a responsibility or if there are rigid conceptions of "his work" and "her work," there may be subtle sabotage or task overload as responsibilities mount with the addition of the newborn (Avant, 1988; Mercer et al., 1990). How the family uses pregnancy to work out or rework their division of labor in the family has a large impact on their transition.

Couples in the anticipatory phase experience many intense feelings, challenges, and responsibilities. If used correctly, this can be an opportune time to test skills in preparing to accept and integrate the new family member into the system. The nurse can be helpful in aiding the couple to examine and understand what they are experiencing by providing accurate information and feedback of perceptions and offering validation of the dynamics that are emerging (Mercer et al., 1990; Pridham, 1993; Lamp, 1993).

Honeymoon Phase

The honeymoon phase refers to the postpartum period during which an attachment between the parents and infant is achieved through prolonged contact and intimacy (Rossi, 1968). This is a "psychic honeymoon" and not necessarily a time of romanticized peace and joy. Rather, it is an intense period when the mother and the father or partner explore their new family member and their relationships to the infant, who, in turn, is working out a complicated communication system with the parents so that his or her survival is assured. The couple's personal relationship is no less important, but most of their energies at this time are focused on developing the new relationship with the infant.

Reciprocal Interaction

The newer technology and sophisticated research on brain physiology and infant behavior have allowed a recognition of the amazing talents the newborn possesses for capturing the attention of the parents and holding them in real communicative interaction (Brazelton, 1986; Wilkie et al., 1986). The child learns to organize in response to positive stimuli and experiences. Overstimulation and noncontingent care (care that is not synchronized with the newborn's re-

sponses) hinder the organization of the newborn's central nervous system and development of a positive parent–newborn interaction (Brazelton, 1986; Wilkie et al., 1986; Koniak-Griffin et al., 1988a). Parents should be cautioned to avoid trying to do things strictly "by the book" or by schedules organized to expedite routines and procedures. Care for the newborn needs to be timed to the his or her activity and responses not to preordained schedules (Koniak-Griffin et al., 1988a; Koniak-Griffin et al., 1988b). Neonates have a repertoire of adaptive responses that enable them to survive and to capture the attention of the important adults around them. Research shows that newborns demonstrate a marked ability to habituate to different visual, auditory, and seminoxious stimuli. Research also shows definite auditory and visual orienting responses. For example, if a person talks and begins to play with the newborn, he or she responds by becoming alert and searching for a face. When the newborn finds the face, his or her expression softens, and as long as the face moves, the newborn follows it. If it becomes still, however, the newborn frowns and turns away.

Responses to auditory stimuli also demonstrate the ability of the neonate to make choices. When a man and woman stand on opposite sides of the newborn and begin to talk, the newborn will stop moving, and with face knit, the newborn will turn toward the female voice again and again. When presented with a nonhuman sound, newborns who are sucking will stop, then quickly resume; when hearing a human sound, newborns will stop sucking and then resume with a complex sucking pattern that researchers believe indicates a preference for the human sound. Newborns' ability to control and console themselves by such behaviors is a powerful reinforcer for parents who are ready to move beyond the initial bonding and continue their attachment (Brazelton, 1986; Morton et al., 1990).

Bonding and Attachment

Three major theoretical perspectives have contributed to attachment theory: psychoanalytical, ethologic, and learning theory. Psychoanalytical theory postulates that attachment arises from instinctual drives and object relations. From the ethologic standpoint, attachment consists of specific behaviors, such as imprinting, clinging when afraid, and crying, which promote physical closeness in humans. Learning theorists claim that attachment is formed through secondary drives when the mother meets the needs of the newborn, and the newborn associates need satisfaction with her.

In the 1970s, the concept of the "fourth stage of labor" developed. This time immediately after delivery was thought to be optimal for close contact between parents and child to initiate the process of bonding the trio together. Currently, the terms bonding and attachment are often used interchangeably to describe this process of parent–newborn affiliation (Mercer, 1982). Some believe there is a distinction between the terms and define **bonding** as the initial attraction and desire to get to know another person and **attachment** as the long, hard work of staying in love (Brazelton, 1986). Thus, bonding can be considered the initial step in a process in which the mutual attractiveness and response between parents and newborn develop and pave the way for the later development of love and affiliation.

Factors Associated With Attachment

Research has shed much light on the fascinating subject of how newborns and parents first develop their

---

BOX 26–2
Factors Associated With Attachment

1. Parents' emotional health, including ability to trust
2. Adequate social support system, including partner, family, and friends
3. A competent level of communication and ability to give care
4. At least partial parent and infant proximity; continuous proximity optimal
5. Parent–infant "fit," including satisfaction with sex of infant, compatibility of infant state with parents, and compatibility of temperament of all parties

Preconditions for "Attachment" Process

If these preconditions are not present or are distorted, intervention is needed.

- *Positive, reciprocal feedback*
  Includes verbal, nonverbal, and social real or perceived responses of infant to parent and parent to parent, which make the interactions mutually satisfying.
- *"Claiming behaviors," leading to identification of the newborn*
  The willingness to "claim" the newborn as theirs and identify with him or her gradually expands the newborn's identity; seeing infant as "like" them in some respects and "different" from them in others; allows for the infant's uniqueness and aids in the incorporation into the family's social system.
- *Mutuality in interaction*
  The newborn has and develops a repertoire of behaviors that calls forth corresponding behaviors in the parents, particularly the mother; these behaviors initiate and maintain contact with the parents. "Signaling behaviors" (crying, cooing, smiling) and "executive behaviors" (rooting, suckling, grasping) are crucial in bringing the parents near and maintaining contact.

(Source: Klaus et al., 1982; Mercer, 1982; Stainton, 1985; Brazelton, 1986; Wilkie et al., 1986.)

---

acquaintance (Brazelton, 1986; Mercer, 1986; Koniak-Griffin, 1993). Although much of the early findings were hampered by small, self-selected samples and many of the studies have undergone considerable revision, the initial research efforts did result in a much more flexible management of parental interaction during and after labor (Klaus et al., 1982; Korsch, 1983; Mercer, 1982; Mercer, 1994). Although definitive answers are still not available and some of the information must still be considered tentative, several important factors are associated with the process of attachment (Box 26-2).

Healthcare providers should be cautious when advising clients so as not to instill feelings of guilt in parents who cannot or do not participate in the birth process and who do not appear to bond immediately with the newborn. This attachment process varies from situation to situation and from culture to culture. The nurse must remember that attachment is a process, just as is the development of the parental role. It does not occur instantaneously at birth. This process takes time and can be impeded or facilitated by a variety of variables, some of which are discussed in Box 26-2. As the research continues in this area, more will be discovered about factors influencing this bonding process (Mercer et al., 1990).

Assumption of the Parental Role

The honeymoon phase continues as the parents continue in their transition. Certain behaviors become apparent. There is much more information on maternal behavior than on paternal behavior. As with attachment principles, these observations and findings should not be considered definitive.

Paternal Behavior

Although most researchers agree that more studies need to be done regarding paternal behavior, this type of research is still in the early stages. Early research in the 1970s concluded that there was no significant behavioral difference between fathers alone with their newborn and mothers alone with their newborn, but if the trio were together, the father tended to hold, touch, and vocalize more than the mother but smile significantly less (Park, 1978; Park et al., 1981). These and more recent findings establish that the father plays a far more active role than the passive cultural stereotype suggests (Jones et al., 1989a; Jones et al., 1989b; Pruett, 1987; Pruett, 1993; Garbarino, 1993; Mercer et al., 1990; Gamble et al., 1992; McAdoo, 1993).

Catalysts in the Attachment Process

Jordan (1990) has described several experiences during pregnancy and after the birth ("reality boosters") that are catalysts to aid the father in his attachment to his newborn and his transition to fatherhood (Box 26-3).

Fathers must work at the business of attachment. Grappling with the reality of the pregnancy and the child is central. The child becomes more real as the pregnancy progresses and through the first postpartum months. Like the mother, the father needs hands-on contact and interaction with the newborn during the first days and months to feel that the child is "real" and is theirs. Fathers must make strong efforts to become involved in the childbearing experience and in "fathering" to overcome society's obstacles that have previously excluded fathers from this process.

Recent research shows that in most instances, fathers bond to their offspring and are highly sensitive to their newborn's signals (Jones et al., 1989a; Jones et al., 1989b; Jordan, 1990; Mercer, 1990b). Fathers' responses after birth include perceiving the newborn as attractive, having a desire to hold and touch the newborn, and focusing attention on the newborn (Fig. 26-2). Observations of the father's behaviors with their newborns have documented a high degree of verbal and nonverbal interaction in the first several postpartum days (Jones et al., 1989a; Jordan, 1990; Mercer, 1990a). The term **engrossment** was coined by Greenberg and Morris (1974) to describe the behavior pattern noted in fathers when they are involved and interacting with their newborn and continues to be used today. This term refers to the absorption of the father

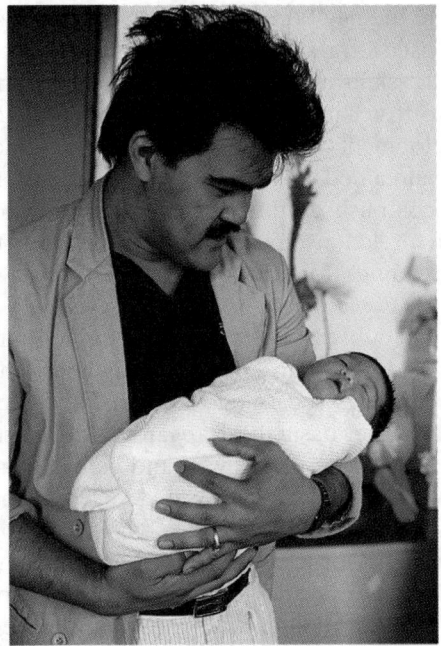

FIGURE 26–2 Paternal bonding.

in the interaction. Jones and Thomas (1989a), in a study monitoring cardiovascular changes in the father during engrossed infant interaction, found that fathers appeared highly sensitive to the stimuli of interacting with their newborns and responded in a complex manner to newborn signals. They conclude that there may be an autonomic balance that is situationally specific and may predict parental response just as other psychosocial measures do.

Controversies About Paternal Bonding

Some controversy exists as to whether maternal and paternal attachment behaviors should be considered separately or as "parental" behaviors. Similarities have been found between paternal and maternal interaction behaviors (Jones et al., 1989a; Jones et al., 1989b; Greenberg et al., 1974). As research accrues, however, it appears that differences and similarities continue to be noted (Jones et al., 1989a; Jordan, 1990). Rather than being compelled to define categories or list behaviors, it is appropriate to acknowledge these similarities and differences and design research to determine in what conditions they might pertain, particularly as society moves toward a more flexible masculine-feminine role definition.

Maternal Behavior

Reva Rubin, a pioneer in describing maternal behavior, focused on the mother and identified various phases of maternal behavior, particularly relating to maternal

---

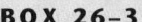

BOX 26–3
Experiences That Aid the Father in Attachment

During Pregnancy

1. The "theoretical" (idea of) pregnancy; the "official diagnosis"
2. Changes in the mother's body and behavior
3. Hearing the fetus' heartbeat; seeing the fetus on ultrasound
4. Feeling the fetus move; nicknaming
5. Telling others about the pregnancy
6. Nesting: getting things together in the home in preparation for the newborn

After Birth

1. Seeing and holding the newborn at birth
2. Telling others about the birth
3. Bringing the newborn into the home environment
4. Assuming responsibility for the newborn's care
5. Getting to know the newborn

touch and the newborn. She contended that mothering is composed of a set of interpersonal and production skills (eg, skills that produce events or things) designed to foster the emotional, intellectual, and physical development of the child (Rubin, 1961). Moreover, Rubin maintained that there were tasks that mothers must accomplish as they identify their newborn and establish a relationship with it (Box 26-4). See the suggested readings for more information about Rubin's work.

Although subsequent research has called into question the rigor of Rubin's methodology and sample size and her findings regarding touch and the time of its progression, her basic thesis regarding the existence of mothering tasks is still relevant and generally accepted today (Martel et al., 1984; Gay et al., 1988). Subsequent researchers have attributed the changes in observed maternal behavior to a changed philosophy surrounding maternity care and to changed hospital practices that involve the mother and parents in the newborn's care immediately and result in much shorter hospital stays. For instance, the slower progression of touch and the extreme dependency of the "taking-in phase" as described by Rubin are telescoped in modern hospitals (Gay et al., 1988; Hampson, 1989).

Maternal Role Attainment

There still remains a progression in mother–newborn interactions that facilitates bonding and attachment and leads ultimately to what Mercer (1986) has called "maternal role attainment." In Mercer's formulation, **maternal role attainment** is a process that occurs over 3 to 10 months that includes attachment to the infant through identifying, claiming, and interacting with him or her, thereby gaining gratification and competence in mothering behaviors and mother–infant interactions. Mercer also suggests that maternal attachment and adaptation may be delayed or hampered if the

woman's health status is less than optimal because of chronic illness and complications from childbirth.

Mother–infant interactions tend to be progressive but are less structured than previously described. Also, the surroundings can facilitate (or impede) interactions. In an environment where free interaction, holding, and nursing can proceed without restraint, the fingertip to enfolding progression of touch proceeds quickly as do the eye-to-eye contact and other interactive activities.

Phases of Maternal Role Attainment

In what is called an **introductory and acquaintance phase,** touching activities begin. Fingertip exploration, palmar contact, and gradual enfolding of the newborn are all noted. This may take minutes to hours (or even days if delay is experienced) depending on ease of interaction, physical proximity, clothing constraints, and physical condition of the mother and newborn. Culture and ethnic variations also can be noted. When the mother holds her newborn, she will move him or her around until she has eye contact and can gaze face to face. This is called the **en face position**.

The mother also uses sight, smell, and hearing to become acquainted and identify her newborn. Studies have found that the mother can distinguish her newborn's odor, and this aids in the claiming process (Hampson, 1989; Fig 26-3).

The mother's emotions also play a part as she begins to identify and incorporate similarities and dissimilarities of the newborn to her partner or husband, herself, and her family (Porter et al., 1985). As she becomes more acquainted with her newborn, she first identifies the newborn as her own and is interested in clarifying her emerging feelings for the child. She then relates the newborn's appearance and behavior to people and things that are familiar and have meaning for her. Finally, she interprets what the behavior and characteris-

---

BOX 26-4
Tasks and Behaviors of New Mothers

Tasks	Behaviors
Identifying the newborn	Taking-in phase: dependent; finger-tip touch of newborn; continued exploration; en face position to explore face; finally enfolding the newborn
Determining the relationship to the newborn	Taking-hold phase: independent and autonomous; concerned about her performance as a mother
Guiding and reconstructing the family constellation to include the newborn	Letting-go phase: becomes accomplished at mothering tasks; realizes physical separation of the newborn; relinquishes former role as "childless person"

(Rubin, R. (1961). Basic maternal behavior. Nursing Outlook, 11 *(11), 26–39.)*

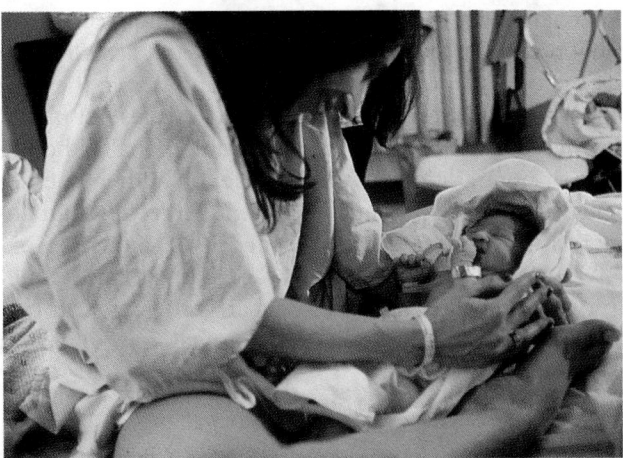

FIGURE 26–3 This mother is getting to know her newborn during the first few postpartum hours.

tics mean and will mean. She may anticipate that the curly hair will be wonderful for her girl or that the immediate rooting for food portends a hearty, robust nature (Censullo et al., 1985).

As attachment progresses, a mutual regulation and reciprocity phase can be seen. The newborn and mother develop a cuing system, which should result in the newborn's and mother's needs being met. The mother must become sensitive to the newborn's states, and the newborn must learn to send out signals and cues that can be interpreted by the mother. During this time of mutual adjustment, negative feelings may surface in the mother. She may feel that the newborn is too demanding, and his or her cues are not readable. Mutual regulation is never instantaneous and continues through infancy and to some degree, childhood. If the mother's feelings are denied by health providers and

family, the mother will feel inadequate and guilty, which will only intensify the negative feelings. The nurse's support during this time in acknowledging that these feelings are natural can be a great encouragement in the mother–newborn interaction (Censullo et al., 1985; Mercer et al., 1990a).

Researchers have described the concept of **reciprocity** as interactional cycles that occur simultaneously between the mother and newborn that are rhythmic and form the basis for communication. Several phases in the reciprocal–interactional cycles have been delineated (Brazelton, 1986; Censullo et al., 1985). They are summarized in Figure 26-4.

Postpartum Blues and Depression

As can be seen from the changes and stressors that accompany the birth process, the transition to parenthood can be a stressful time for the parents, particularly the mother. She is dealing not only with a role change, but also with her body's return to a prepregnant state, with all of its attendant physiologic and hormonal changes. She is often sleep deprived as well. Thus, in the early postpartum period, for no apparent reason (the mother thinks), she may feel let down and may have some or all of the following symptoms: irritability, tears, headache, anxiety, clouding of consciousness, mood lability, and feelings of inadequacy. Occasionally, appetite and sleep are disturbed. These symptoms are manifestations of the "baby blues" or "maternity blues" and are generally transient, lasting 1 to 10 days or a bit longer. At one time the blues were thought to be related substantially to the physiologic and hormonal changes the new mother underwent. However, research does not substantiate a primarily hormonal or

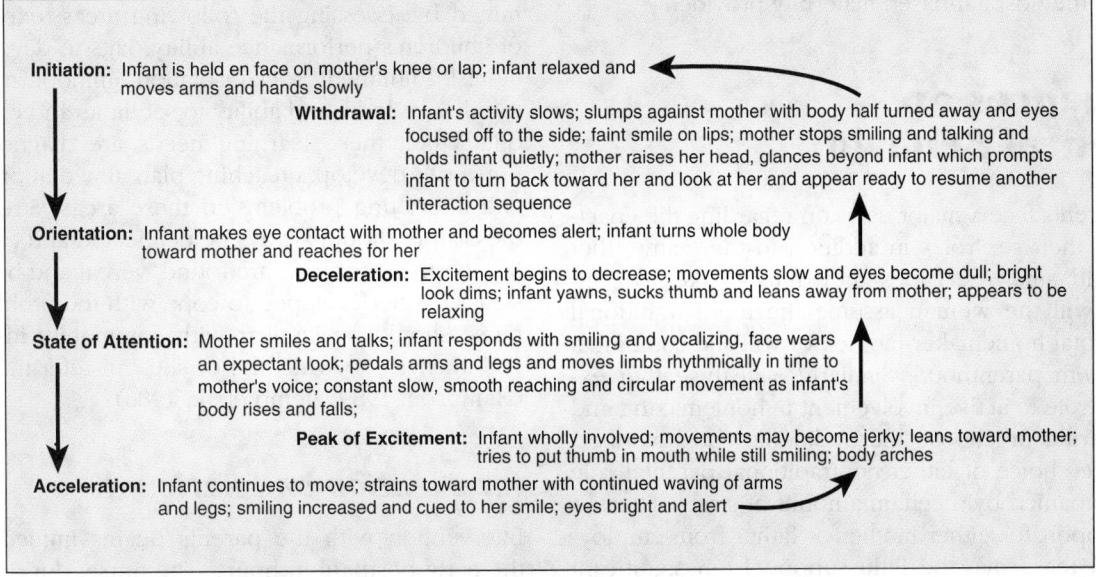

FIGURE 26–4 Phases in establishing maternal–infant reciprocity.

biologic etiology for the blues or postpartum depression (Affonso, 1992; Beck et al., 1992). Other causes, such as lack of social supports, and other ego and social adjustments accompanying this crucial role transition, together with discomfort, fatigue, and exhaustion, have been correlated to these conditions but have not been proven causative (Martell, 1990; Affonso, 1992; Beck et al., 1992; Beck, 1993). Crying often relieves the tension, and rest and support are extremely important. Anticipatory guidance and support by the nurse are important in helping the parents understand this condition as transitory (Lepper et al., 1994).

Occasionally, the woman experiences a true postpartum depression, which may begin in the first weeks after delivery and persist for months. The mother feels extremely fatigued (even with rest), inadequate, unable to cope, and gradually withdraws. This state may progress to a true psychosis. The symptoms mentioned are exacerbated and prolonged. Diagnosis and treatment are important; the nurse should be watchful for these symptoms and refer the mother if they persist (Martell, 1990; Lepper et al., 1994). This condition and its care are discussed more fully in Chapters 27 and 38.

Plateau and Disengagement Phases

The perinatal nurse does not often have the opportunity to observe the couple in the plateau phase of the transition to parenthood. This is the protracted middle period of a role cycle in which the role is fully exercised and the parents validate themselves as competent or not, depending on how well they and others perceive their parenting efforts (Rossi, 1968). Similarly, unless there is a perinatal or infant death, the disengagement-termination phase of the role cycle is not seen by the hospital-based maternity provider.

Influences on Parental Behavior

New parents face a major decision regarding the enactment of their sex roles in addition to the many other large and small decisions they must make. For instance, will the woman assume the more traditional role of total homemaker-mother, or will she combine a career with parenthood? Similarly, will the father extend his role to active involvement in homemaking and childbearing or choose the traditional "breadwinner" role? The choice of either nontraditional parental role is accompanied by a certain amount of stress. There is little support for either mother or father from employers, and there may be little support from significant others. On the other hand, assuming the traditional

parental roles can be stressful because this course of action may be thwarting the potential and actualization of the parents. Researchers have found that in the case of fathers' adjustment to parenthood, it does not matter so much whether they choose a traditional fathering role or nontraditional fathering role, but rather whether they assume the role in a consistent and coherent manner (Killien, 1993; Belsky et al., 1990; Stemp et al., 1986). More research on this fascinating topic should provide more insight into how care providers can better help the family make the parental role transition smoother.

Applying the Nursing Process to the Developing Family

Assessment and Nursing Diagnoses

Assessment and nursing diagnoses are based on careful observation and interviewing. Nurses should keep in mind that they are assisting with role supplementation that will lead to role mastery in the parents (see Fig. 26-1). Nurses can enhance the communication process for the parents and the parents' significant others by assessing and clarifying questions, concerns, and issues with them and encouraging them to use knowledgeable people in their networks. Apprising them of the availability of parenting support groups and the telephone for information purposes (eg, hot lines) and arranging home visits will contribute to role supplementation.

The nurse may find that Health Seeking Behaviors or Anxiety related to knowledge deficit may be primary diagnoses for the parents. Learning needs can be determined by assessing the following areas: expectations of children's performance ability, lags in developmental task fulfillment, social isolation, immobilization due to role overload, and ability to set limits and carry them out. When these learning needs are diagnosed, the nurse can develop a teaching plan aimed at preventing and alleviating problems in these areas. Strengths of the couple should always be delineated and enhanced. When other problems are found, verbal and behavioral skills can be developed to cope with the problem. The nurse should be familiar with community institutions and agencies to which he or she can refer the parents (Hampson, 1989; Stemp et al., 1986).

Intervention and Rationale

Intervention with the parents begins immediately in the early postpartum hours. The nurse, during the immediate and later postpartum periods, can be helpful to parents and facilitate bonding by pointing out and reinforcing parents' perceptions of their newborn's ability to interact with them. One reinforcer to attachment that can be shown to the mother and father is the manner of consoling the newborn. When a newborn is crying, even very loudly, he or she can be quieted by insistently saying "baby, baby, baby." Simply by using the voice, one can get the newborn to turn the head, put a fist into the mouth, and start looking for the speaker.

Another key element of nursing intervention with the expanding family is teaching parenting skills that promote the child's maturity, autonomy, and competence. If the parents have a realistic conception of the infant's needs and their resources, they need not expend all their energy on their parenting responsibilities at the expense of their own personal needs and growth. Nursing's involvement in the recent trend toward health maintenance and promotion has set the stage for classes that include information and skill development needed after the newborn arrives. Teaching styles and format for parenting classes resemble those in prenatal instruction. Nurses should be aware of what is available in their institution or the community so that they may make referrals when appropriate. It is impossible to teach all of the skills necessary for parenting. If nurses can help parents sort out problems, examine options and resources, and negotiate outcomes, however, they have accomplished a great deal and have been instrumental in this momentous role transition.

Evaluation

Nurses will know whether their nursing interventions have been successful if the mother and father or partner verbalize their questions and concerns and indicate appropriate solutions. If they verbalize realistic expectations for themselves and their newborns, manage their time successfully, and enlarge, maintain, and use their social supports, nurses will know that the role transition is proceeding in a healthy manner.

Summary Points

✔ Parenthood is a continuing process of role transition rather than a state. The phases of the role transition are the anticipatory phase, which was rehearsed during pregnancy, and the honeymoon phase, which occurs after childbirth and is the time when attachment between parents and newborn occurs through prolonged contact and intimacy. During the honeymoon phase, the parents continue their transition, and each has a series of tasks and behaviors appropriate to those tasks that help them attain the maternal and paternal roles. Much more is known about the tasks and behaviors related to the attainment of the maternal role than the paternal role. The latter topic is rich in research opportunities. The maternity nurse does not usually see the plateau and disengagement phases of the transition to parenthood. The plateau phase occurs over many years, and the parents validate themselves as competent or not depending on a variety of variables. Similarly, unless there is a perinatal or infant death, the maternity nurse does not see the disengagement phase.

✔ Alternate conceptualizations of parenthood include parenthood as a negative change in the quality of life and as a crisis. These last two orientations are not accepted by current researchers who view parenthood as a transitional process that may be accompanied by stressors but that leads to the development of competence in the maternal and paternal roles.

✔ After the birth, reciprocal interaction occurs between the parents and the newborn. The newborn has an amazing repertoire of adaptive responses to capture and hold the attention of adults and to survive. Bonding and attachment describe the parent–newborn affiliation process. Brazelton has made a distinction between the two terms: Bonding is the initial attraction and desire to get to know one another, while attachment is the long, hard work of staying in love.

✔ The mother must accomplish specific tasks during her role transition. These include identifying the newborn, determining her relationship to the child, and guiding and reconstructing the family constellation to include the new member. The tasks for the father are less well defined. However, research indicates that grappling with the "reality" of the newborn (ie, that the newborn is really here and he or she is really father's) is central to attaining the father role. Moreover, fathers must make strong efforts to become involved with the childbearing experience and to interact with and father the newborn to overcome society's tendency to exclude fathers from this process.

✔ The behaviors associated with maternal and paternal attachment have many similarities and differences. Rather than being compelled to define categories or list behaviors, further research is needed that can delineate under what conditions these differences and similarities emerge.

✔ Understanding the process of how the maternal role is attained and what constitutes maternal role "competence" has been clarified by the work of

Mercer et al. and Koniak-Griffin. Additional research is needed to advance the understanding of how the paternal role is attained.

REFERENCES

Affonso, D. D. (1992). Postpartum depression: A nursing perspective on women's health and behaviors. *IMAGE, 24*(3), 215–221.

Avant, K. (1988). Stressors on the childbearing family. *Journal of Obstetric, Gynecologic, and Neonatal Nursing, 17*(3), 179–184.

Beck, C. T., Reynolds, M. A., & Rutowski, P. (1992). Maternity blues and postpartum depression. *Journal of Obstetric, Gynecologic, and Neonatal Nursing, 21*(4), 287–293.

Beck, C. T. (1993). Teetering on the edge: A substantive theory of postpartum depression. *Nursing Research, 42*(1), 42–48.

Belsky, J., & Rovine, M. (1990). Patterns of marital change across the transition to parenthood: Pregnancy to three years postpartum. *Journal of Marriage and the Family, 52*(2), 5–19.

Brazelton, T. B. (1986). The behavioral competence of the newborn. In G. B. Avery (Ed.), *Neonatology: Pathophysiology and management of the newborn* (3rd ed.). Philadelphia: J.B. Lippincott.

Censullo, M., Lester, B., & Hoffman, J. (1985). Rhythmic patterning in mother-newborn interaction. *Nursing Research, 34*(3), 346–349.

Coffman, S., Levitt, M. J., & Guacci, N. (1993). Maternal stress and close relationships: Correlates with infant health status. *Pediatric Nursing, 19*(3), 135–140.

Coffman, S., Levitt, M. J., & Brown, L. (1994). Effects of clarification of support expectations in prenatal couples. *Nursing Research, 42*(2), 111–116.

Cowan, C., & Cowan, P. (1987). A preventive intervention for couples becoming parents. In C. F. Boukydis (Ed.), *Research on support for parents and infants in the postnatal period* (pp. 225–251). Norwood, NJ: Ablex Publishing..

Dyer, E. D. (1963). Parenthood as crisis: A re-study. *Marriage and Family Living, 25*(5), 196–201.

Feetham, S. L., Meister, S. B., Bell, J. M., & Gilliss, C. L. (1993). *The nursing of families: Theory/research/education/practice.* Newbury Park, CA: Sage Publications.

Fiese, B. H., Hooker, K. A., Kotary, L., & Scwagler, J. (1993). Family rituals in the early stages of parenthood. *Journal of Marriage and the Family, 55*, 633–642.

Fuller, S. A. (1986). Care of postpartum adolescents. *MCN: American Journal of Maternal Child Nursing, 11*(5), 398–403.

Gamble, D., & Morse, J. M. (1993). Fathers of breastfed infants: Postponing and types of involvement. *Journal of Obstetric, Gynecologic, and Neonatal Nursing, 32*(4), 358–365.

Garbarino, J. (1993). Reinventing fatherhood. *Families in Society: The Journal of Contemporary Human Services, 74*(1), 51–54.

Gay, J. T., Edgil, A. E., & Douglas, A. B. (1988). Reva Rubin revisited. *Journal of Obstetric, Gynecologic, and Neonatal Nursing, 17*(6), 395–399.

Gilliss, C. L., Highly, B. L., Roberts, B. M., & Martinson, I. M. (1989). *Toward a science of family nursing.* New York: Addison-Wesley.

Greenberg, M., & Morris, N. (1974). Engrossment: The newborn's impact on the father. *American Journal of Orthopsychiatry, 44*(7), 520–531.

Hampson, S. J. (1989). Nursing interventions for the first 3 postpartum months. *Journal of Obstetric, Gynecologic, and Neonatal Nursing, 18*(2), 116–122.

Hobbs, D. F. Jr. (1965). Parenthood as crisis: A third study. *Journal of Marriage and Family Living, 27*(9), 367–372.

Hobbs, D. F. Jr. (1968). Transition to parenthood: A replication and extension. *Journal of Marriage and Family Living, 30*(9), 413–417.

Hobbs, D. F. Jr., & Cole, S. P. (1976). Transition to parenthood: A decade of replication. *Journal of Marriage and the Family, 38*(11), 723–731.

Hobbs, D. F. Jr., & Wimbish, J. M. (1977). Transition to parenthood by black couples. *Journal of Marriage and the Family, 37*(11), 677–689.

Jacoby, A. P. (1969). Transition to parenthood: A reassessment. *Journal of Marriage and Family Living, 31*(11), 720–727.

Jones, C. L., & Lenz, E. R. (1989a). Father-newborn interaction: Effects of social competence and infant state. *Nursing Research, 35*(2), 149–153.

Jones, C. L., & Thomas, S. A. (1989b). Fathers blood pressure and heart rate in relationship to interaction their newborns. *Nursing Research, 38*(4), 237–241.

Jordan, L. (1990). Laboring for relevance: Expectant and new fatherhood. *Nursing Research, 39*(1), 11–16.

Keefe, M. R., & Froese-Fretz, A. (1991). Living with an irritable infant: Maternal perspectives. *MCN: American Journal of Maternal Child Nursing, 16*(5), 255–259.

Killien, M. G. (1993). Returning to work after childbirth: Considerations for health policy. *Nursing Outlook, 41*(2), 73–78.

Klaus, M. H., & Kennell, J. H. (1982). *Parent-infant bonding* (2nd ed.). St Louis: C.V. Mosby.

Koniak-Griffin, D., & Rummell, M. (1988a). Temperament in infancy: Stability, change and correlates. *Maternal Child Nursing Journal, 17*(2), 25–40.

Koniak-Griffin, D., & Ludington-Hoe, S. M. (1988b). Developmental and temperament outcomes of sensory stimulation in healthy infants. *Nursing Research, 37*(2), 70–76.

Koniak-Griffin, D. (1993). Maternal role attainment. *IMAGE, 25*(3), 257–262.

Korsch, B. M. (1983). More on parent-infant bonding. *Journal of Pediatrics, 102*(3), 249–252.

Lamp, J. M. (1993). Humor in postpartum education: Depicting a new mother's worst nightmare. *MCN: American Journal of Maternal Child Nursing, 17*(2), 83–85.

Le Masters, E. E. (1957). Parenthood as crisis. *Marriage and Family Living, 19*(11), 352–355.

Lepper, H. S., DiMatteo, M. R., & Tinsley, B. J. (1994). Postpartum depression: How much do obstetric nurses and obstetricians know? *BIRTH, 21*(3), 149–154.

Martel, L. K., & Mitchell, S. K. (1984). Rubin's "puerperal change" reconsidered. *Journal of Obstetric, Gynecologic, and Neonatal Nursing, 13*(3), 145–149.

Martell, L. K. (1990). Postpartum depression. *MCN: American Journal of Maternal Child Nursing, 15*(2), 90–93.

McAdoo, J. L. (1993). The roles of African American fathers: An ecological perspective. *Families in Society: The Journal of Contemporary Human Services, 74*(1), 28–35.

Meleis, A. I. (1991). *Theoretical nursing: Development and progress* (2nd ed.). Philadelphia: J.B. Lippincott.

Mercer, R. T. (1982). Parent-infant attachment. In L. J. Sonstegard et al. (Eds.), *Women's health, Vol. 2: Childbearing.* New York: Grune & Stratton.

Mercer, R. T. (1986). *First time motherhood: Experiences from teens to forties.* New York: Springer.

Mercer, R. T., & Ferketich, S. L. (1990a). Predictors of family functioning eight months following birth. *Nursing Research, 39*(72), 6–82.

Mercer, R. T., & Ferketich, S. L. (1990b). Predictors of parental attachment during early parenthood. *Journal of Advanced Nursing, 15*(3), 268–280.

Mercer, R. T., & Ferketich, S. L. (1994). Predictors of maternal role competence by risk status. *Nursing Research, 43*(1), 38–43.

Morton, J., Johnson, M. H., & Mauer, D. (1990). On the reasons for newborn's responses to faces. *Infant Behavior & Development, 13*(4), 99–103.

Park, R. (1978). The father's role in infancy: A reevaluation. *Birth and the Family, 5*(1), 211–213.

Park, R., & Tinsley, B. R. (1981). The father's role in infancy: Determinants of involvement in caregiving and play. In M. Lamb (Ed.), *The role of the father in child development* (pp. 429–457) (2nd ed.). New York: John Wiley.

Porter, R. H., Cernoch, J. M., & Perry, S. (1985). The importance of odors in maternal-infant interaction. *Nursing Research, 34*(3), 342–345.

Pridham, K. F. (1993). Anticipatory guidance of parents of new infants: Potential contribution of the internal working model construct. *IMAGE, 25*(1), 49–56.

Pruett, K. (1987). *The nurturing father.* New York: Warner Books.

Pruett, K. D. (1993). The paternal presence. *Families in Society: The Journal of Contemporary Human Services, 74*(1), 46–50

Rossa, M. W., & Beals, J. (1990). Measurement issues in family assessment: The case of the family environment scale. *Family Process, 29*(6), 191–198.

Rossi, A. (1968). Transition to parenthood. *Journal of Marriage and Family Living, 30*(2), 26–39.

Rubin, R. (1961). Basic maternal behavior. *Nursing Outlook, 11*(11), 683–686.

Russell, C. (1979). Circumplex model of family systems: III. Empirical evaluation with families. *Family Process, 18*(3), 29–43.

Stainton, M. C. (1985). The fetus: A growing member of the family. *Family Relations, 34*(7), 321–326.

Stemp, P. S., Turner, R. J., & Noh, S. (1986). Psychological distress in the postpartum period: The significance of social support. *Journal of Marriage and the Family, 48*(5), 271–277.

Swendsen, L. A., Meleis, A., & Jones, D. (1978). Role supplementation for new parents. *MCN: American Journal of Maternal Child Nursing, 3*(2), 84–91.

Tulman, L. (1986). Initial handling of newborn infants by vaginally and cesarean delivered mothers. *Nursing Research, 35*(2), 96–100.

Tulman, L., & Fawcett, J. (1990). Functional status during pregnancy and the postpartum: A framework for research. *IMAGE, 22*(3), 191–194.

Wilkie, C. F., & Ames, E. W. (1986). The relationship of infant crying to parental stress in the transition to parenthood. *Journal of Marriage and the Family, 48*(8), 545–550.

SUGGESTED READING

Alfonso, D. D., Lovett, S., & Paul, S. M. (1990). A standardized interview that differentiates pregnancy and postpartum symptoms from perinatal clinical depression. *BIRTH, 17*(9), 121–130.

Keefe, M. R., & Froese-Fretz, A. (1994). Living with an irritable infant: Maternal perspectives. *MCN: American Journal of Maternal Child Nursing, 16*(5), 255–259.

Lepper, H. S., DiMatteo, M. R., & Tinsley, B. J. (1994). Postpartum depression: How much do obstetric nurses and obstetricians know? *BIRTH, 21*(3), 149–154.

Maloni, J. A., McIndoe, J. E., & Rubenstein, G. (1987). Expectant grandparents class. *Journal of Obstetric, Gynecologic, and Neonatal Nursing, 16*(1), 26–29.

Mercer, R. T., Ferketich, S. L., & DeJoseph, J. (1988). Effect of stress on family functioning during pregnancy. *Nursing Research, 37*(5), 268–275.

Rubin, R. (1961). Basic maternal behavior. *Nursing Outlook, 11*(11), 683–686.

Rubin, R. (1961). Puerperal change. *Nursing Outlook, 12*(12), 753–751.

Tomlinson, P. S. (1990). Verbal behavior associated with indicators of maternal attachment with the neonate. *Journal of Obstetric, Gynecologic, and Neonatal Nursing, 19*(1), 76–77.

27

Nursing Care in the Postpartum Period

Objectives

- Identify normal physiologic changes and signs of potential danger to be assessed in the postpartum woman.
- Identify psychosocial adaptations to be assessed in the new mother or couple and family.
- Identify and describe cultural components of postpartum care.
- Identify nursing diagnoses, interventions, and evaluation of care for the postpartum woman, her partner, and the new family.
- Formulate teaching plans relevant to the postpartum woman and the new family.
- Identify strategies for follow-up care after discharge from the hospital or birth center.
- Develop a nursing care plan for the postpartum woman and the new family.

Key Terms

Afterpains
Engorgement
Involution
Lochia alba

Lochia rubra
Lochia serosa
Uterine atony

The postpartum period is a time of major physical and psychological transition for the new mother and the entire family. Parents and children (if any) must adapt to a new family structure, integrate the newborn into their family system, and develop different interactional patterns within the family unit. Because of the extensive adaptations required, there is increased family vulnerability during the postpartum period. Stress from a variety of sources can have a negative effect on family function and interactions because of its impact on physical and mental health (Mercer et al., 1990). In addition, numerous changes occur in the mother's physiologic status immediately after childbirth and up to 6 months after delivery (Tulman et al., 1990).

Nursing care during the postpartum period takes the physical and psychological needs of mothers and families into consideration. The nurse must accurately observe the mother's physiologic functioning and provide timely and focused nursing interventions. The mother's needs for emotional support must be met, anticipatory guidance and health teaching must be given according to the client's readiness to learn, and the developing relationship between parents, siblings, and newborn must be enhanced and nurtured.

Nurses make significant contributions to the care of the postpartum family because of their unique ability to respond to physical and psychosocial needs. Many clients opt for early discharge (within 24 hours after delivery) for personal and economic reasons. This trend has an impact on the nurse's opportunities for providing care, assessing the client's independent functioning with her newborn, and teaching in the hospital setting (McGregor, 1994). This trend suggests an expanded role for nurses in providing care and follow-up in the client's home environment. Care Path: Vaginal Birth provides a sample plan of care for the client who is in the hospital for up to 24 hours.

Postpartum Nursing Care

The goals of nursing care during the postpartum period are to assist the new mother and her family to adapt successfully to the transitions after childbirth and the requirements of parenthood. The emphasis of nursing care is on the assessment and modification of factors that affect the mother's recovery from labor and delivery, her ability to assume caretaking of the newborn, and the mother's and family's role transitions and functional abilities.

Nursing Assessment

Physiologic postpartum assessment focuses on the involution processes of the reproductive organs, biophysical changes of other body systems, and the initiation or suppression of lactation (see Chap. 25).

Observations are made and recorded according to a recommended schedule (Table 27-1). The nurse assesses the mother's comfort and well-being, including rest and sleep, appetite, ambulation, energy level, and elimination status.

Psychosocial assessment focuses on mother, newborn, and family interactions and adaptation. The mother's emotional state and response to the birth experience, interactions with the newborn, newborn feeding, adjustment to the caretaking role and to new family relationships, progress in learning self-care, and incorporation of the newborn into the family are assessed (see Chap. 26).

Although the greatest risk for postpartum complications is during the first 24 hours after delivery, potential problems can occur throughout the postpartum period. Assessment findings can identify signs of complications at an early stage and lead to prompt interventions (see Chap. 38).

Physiologic Assessment

Nursing assessment guidelines for the postpartum period are listed in the Assessment Guidelines: Postpartum Physiologic Status. Specific physiologic assessment measures are described below.

Immediate Postdelivery Assessment

Initial physiologic assessment after delivery includes the condition of the uterus, amount of bleeding, bladder and voiding, vital signs, and perineum. The fundus is palpated to ensure that it remains firm and well contracted. The nurse observes the amount of bleeding by inspecting the perineal pad and vaginal opening. Pulse and blood pressure are taken to assess for signs of deviations in cardiovascular function. The perineum is inspected for signs of hematoma, bleeding from lacerations, and edema. These observations are made every 15 minutes during the first hour after delivery. Temperature is taken at the end of the first postdelivery hour.

Hemorrhage is a major danger to the mother in the immediate postpartum period. Excessive bleeding from

CARE PATH
Vaginal Birth

Name _____

This care path is a guideline and is not intended to create a standard of care. This guideline may be modified based on individual client's needs.

Prob. #		*Intrapartum*	*0–4 Hours* Date:	*4–8 Hours* Date:	*8–12 Hours* Date:	*12–24 Hours* Date:
3	ADL	Bedrest or ambulation as tolerated	Bedrest or ambulation as tolerated	Up ad lib (assist PRN)	Up ad lib (assist PRN)	**Up ad lib (assist PRN)**
3	Assessment Monitor	Perinatal Unit admission assessment Ongoing assessments PRN	Immediate postpartum assessments VS Q 15″ until stable, then Q 4h VS are WNL	VS Q 4h, VS are WNL Postpartum checks Q 4h - are WNL Assess mother/infant attachment	**VS Q 4h, VS are WNL Postpartum checks Q 4h - are WNL Assess mother/infant attachment**	**VS Q 4h, VS are WNL Postpartum checks Q 4h - are WNL Assess mother/infant attachment**
1,2,4	Consults	Perinatal CNS Anesthesia PRN House officer PRN Resolve PRN NICU staff PRN	→ → → → →	Lactation consultant PRN Social Service PRN/WIC PRN	Lactation consultant PRN Social Service PRN/WIC	Lactation consultant PRN Social Service PRN/WIC
3	Procedures/ Tests	Hct PRN	Assess Rubella Titer status Assess need for Rhogam		Rhogam screen PRN	
1	Treatments	External EFM Internal EFM PRN	Ice to perineum Cath PRN	Ice to perineum Cath PRN Supportive bra PRN	Ice to perineum Cath PRN Supportive bra PRN Sitz bath PRN	Ice to perineum Supportive bra PRN Sitz bath PRN
1,2	Meds/IVs	Pain medication IV or IM PRN Alternative D$_5$LR/LR when in active labor PRN Epidural/Pudendal/ Pericervical Pitocin augmentation PRN	Pain medication PRN Tucks PRN Anusol PRN Pitocin 20u IV then D/C	Pain medication PRN Tucks PRN Anusol PRN Stool softener PRN	Pain medication PRN Tucks PRN Anusol PRN Stool softener PRN	Pain medication PRN Tucks PRN Anusol PRN Stool softener PRN Rhogam PRN Rubella vaccine PRN
1	Nutrition	Ice chips PRN	Tolerate PO fluids Regular diet	Adequate fluids Regular diet	Adequate fluids Regular diet	Adequate fluids Regular diet
2	Pt./Family Education	EFM Labor support coaching - encourage support person in role	Self peri care/safety issues Perineum care - comfort measures Mother/baby booklet Initiate bottle or breastfeeding Initiate infant care	Bath/cord care and baby care demo Self care reinforcement and demos Discuss normal involution, lochia, fatigue, activity levels, and nutritional needs	→ → →	Breast pump if indicated
2	Discharge Planning	Mother/baby teaching form	Determine LOS Begin discharge instructions	Continue discharge instructions	→	Assess parent/infant interaction Assess need for home health follow-up Discharge instructions reviewed with mother and S.O.
2,4	Spiritual/ Psycho/ Social/ Emotional Needs	Support client/S.O. Facilitate a positive childbirth experience	Assess maternal role strengths	Assist mother's transition through tasks of taking on maternal role	→	→

(continued)

CARE PATH
Vaginal Birth (Continued)

Name _____

This care path is a guideline and is not intended to create a standard of care. This guideline may be modified based on individual client's needs.

Prob. #		Intrapartum	0–4 Hours Date:	4–8 Hours Date:	8–12 Hours Date:	12–24 Hours Date:
	Multidisci- plinary Team Signatures	_____ _____ _____	_____ _____ _____	_____ _____ _____	_____ _____ _____	_____ _____ _____

Client Problems

1. *Discomfort/pain*
2. *Learning needs*
3. *Potential for instability - postpartum*
4. *Potential alteration in coping related to childbirth*

CLIENT IDENTIFICATION

---

the uterus or perineum is a frank sign of hemorrhage. Pulse rate of 90 to 100 beats/min, accompanied by low or falling blood pressure (systolic <100–110 mm Hg) can be signs of hemorrhage, shock, or embolism. Bleeding into the fundus or the presence of clots causes

TABLE 27–1
Schedule of Postpartum Physiologic Assessments

Area Assessed	Frequency
Temperature	1st h after delivery: once
	2nd–8th h: twice
	9th–24th h: every 4 h
	24th h to discharge: every 8 h
Pulse, respiration, blood pressure	1st h after delivery: every 15 min
	2nd–3rd h: every 30 min
	4th–24th h: every 4 h
	24th to discharge: every 8 h
Fundus, lochia, bladder	1st h after delivery: every 15 min
	2nd–3rd h: every 30 min
	4th–24th h: every 4 h
	24th h to discharge: every 8 h
Perineum	1st h after delivery: once
	2nd–24th h: every 4 h
	24th h to discharge: every 8 h
Breasts, legs	1st–8th h: once at end of 8 h
	9th–24th h: every 4 h
	24th h to discharge: every 8 h
Bowel elimination	9th h to discharge: daily stool

atony (relaxation) of the uterine musculature with a soft, large fundus often palpated above the umbilicus.

Bladder distention may occur, especially if intravenous fluids were administered during labor. A distended bladder can displace the uterus upward and to the site of the midline and interfere with its ability to contract, producing atony and increased bleeding (Fig. 27-1).

Family interactions are assessed in the immediate postdelivery period to establish baseline data regarding parent–newborn relationships (see Chap. 26). When there are no contraindications, the newborn is placed in the mother's arms, and the two, along with the father when present, are allowed to become acquainted. The nurse observes interactions, noting the influence of cultural factors. The mother's level of energy is assessed as is her readiness for relating to the newborn. Emotional states of mothers range from euphoria with high energy to fatigue and sleepiness immediately after birth. There is wide variation in women's responses during this time, influenced by many factors, such as the length and difficulty of labor, cultural patterns, family circumstances, condition of the newborn, and personality variables.

Vital Signs

Temperature is taken every 4 to 8 hours during the first few postpartum days because fever is usually the first symptom of infection. A temperature of 100.4°F (38°C) may be due to dehydration in the first 24 hours after delivery or the onset of lactation within 2 to 4 days.

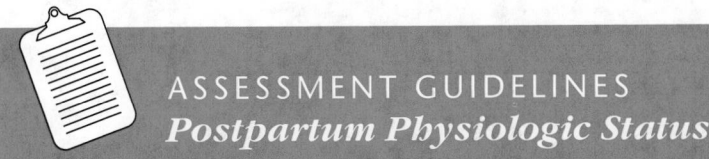

ASSESSMENT GUIDELINES
Postpartum Physiologic Status

Area Assessed	Expected Findings Day 1	Findings Days 2–3
Vital Signs		
Temperature	Elevated 100.4°F	Normal range
Pulse rate	40–70 beats/min	Bradycardia or normal
Blood pressure	Normal range	Normal range
Respiration	Normal range	Normal range
Involution		
Uterus	Fundus at umbilicus	Fundus 1–2 cm below umbilicus
Lochia	Rubra, moderate	Rubra to serosa, moderate
	Fleshy odor	Fleshy or absent odor
Abdomen	Soft, flabby	Soft, flabby
Perineum	Edematous, clean	Less edema, clean
Breasts		
Consistency	Soft, colostrum	Firmer, enlarged, warm
Nipples	Intact	May be reddened, sore
Lactation	Colostrum	Milk days 2–4
Legs	Pretibial/pedal edema, Homans' negative	Edema minimal, Homans' negative
Elimination		
Voiding	Up to 3,000 mL	Large, decreasing amounts
Defecation	None	Bowels move 2–3 d
Discomfort, pain	Perineal aching, hemorrhoid pain, generalized aches	Less perineal and hemorrhoid discomfort
Energy level	Fatigued, sleepy	Tired, moves slowly at first, energy returns but is variable
Appetite	Often thirsty	Very hungry, often voracious appetite
Emotional state	Euphoric, excited	Happy, contented to worried, concerned

Persistent or recurring fever above this level in the first 24 hours may signify infection.

Bradycardia is a normal physiologic change for 6 to 10 days postpartum with pulse rates of 40 to 70 beats/min. Rates above 100 (tachycardia) may indicate infection, hemorrhage, pain, or anxiety. A rapid, thready pulse associated with hypotension suggests hemorrhage, shock, or embolism.

Blood pressure generally remains within normal levels during pregnancy. Postpartum women can experience orthostatic hypotension because of diuresis and diaphoresis, which cause cardiovascular shifts in fluid volume. Persistent or severe hypotension may indicate shock or embolism. Elevated blood pressure suggests pregnancy-induced hypertension, which can first manifest in the postpartum period. Eclamptic seizures have been reported up to 10 days postpartum (Cunningham et al., 1993). Pulse and blood pressure are taken every 4 to 8 hours, unless deviations from normal require increased frequency.

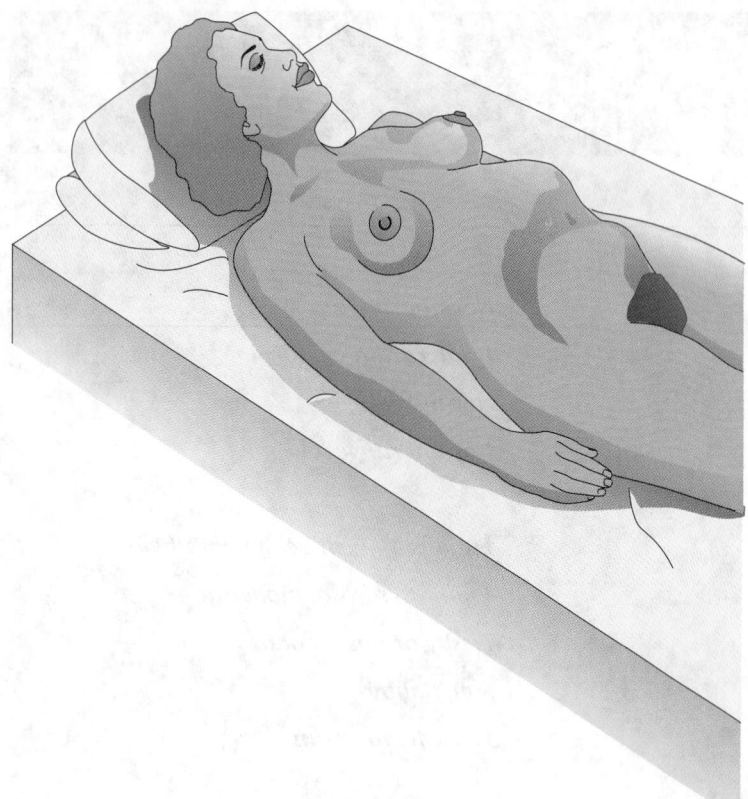

FIGURE 27–1 Full bladder displacing uterine fundus.

Involution

The progress of **involution**, the process by which the uterus returns to its prepregnancy size and condition, is determined by assessing the height and consistency of the uterine fundus (see Procedure 27-1: Fundal Massage and Expression) and the character and amount of lochia every 4 to 8 hours.

Fundus. The fundus may rise immediately following delivery and the first postpartum day, but it then decreases by about 1 cm (½ in) or 1 finger breadth per day (Fig. 27-2). By 10 days postpartum or sooner, the fundus can no longer be palpated abdominally. The consistency of the fundus should be firm, with a round, smooth shape. A soft or boggy fundus indicates atony or subinvolution. The bladder should be empty for accurate fundal assessment; a full bladder displaces the uterus and raises the height of the fundus.

Lochia. The character and amount of lochia indirectly indicate the progress of endometrial healing. In normal healing processes, the amount of lochia gradually diminishes with typical color changes that reflect decreasing blood components in the lochial flow. The quantity of lochia varies with individuals and is generally more profuse in multiparas. The amount of lochia may increase on early ambulation because of vaginal pooling and increased uterine contractions. Absor-

bency varies among brands of peripads. One study estimated that a peripad with more than a 6-in stain contained 50 to 80 mL of blood, while a peripad with less than a 4-in stain held 10 to 25 mL of blood (Luegenbiehl et al., 1990; Table 27-2 and Fig. 27-3).

Lochia is dark red (**lochia rubra**) in the first 1 to 3 days after delivery and is usually moderate in amount. About the fourth day, it becomes more serous and pink (**lochia serosa**) with a decrease in flow. After 1 week to 10 days, lochia becomes yellowish-white (**lochia alba**) with scant flow. Lochia alba persists until about 3 weeks postpartum and indicates normal progression of healing (Bond, 1993). The recurrence of fresh, red bleeding after lochia has progressed to serosa or alba may indicate infection or delayed hemorrhage.

Lochia smells similar to normal menstrual flow and should not have a foul or disagreeable odor. Heavy, persistent, and malodorous lochia rubra, especially if accompanied by fever, indicates a potential infection or retained placental fragments. If lochia serosa or alba continues beyond the normal time ranges and is accompanied by brownish malodorous discharge, fever, and abdominal pain, the woman may have endometritis.

Urinary Elimination

The woman is encouraged to void as soon as possible following delivery to avoid bladder distention. Even with a full bladder, the newly postpartum woman may

PROCEDURE 27–1
Fundal Massage and Expression

Nursing Assessment and Interventions	*Rationale*
Explain procedure and rationale; inform client it may be slightly uncomfortable; provide reassurance. Provide appropriate draping and privacy. Place clean peripad under client.	Increases cooperation and decreases anxiety
Have client empty her bladder.	Uterus displaced by distended bladder
Position client on back with feet together and knees apart. Put on gloves.	Relaxes abdominal muscles Standard infection precautions
Remove peripad; note time since last pad change and amount of saturation.	Blood loss estimated
With one hand supporting the lower fundus just above the symphysis pubis, cup the other hand around the fundus; rotate to massage gently until fundus is firm.	Locates fundus and determines height; avoids uterine inversion; stimulates contraction
When fundus is firm, squeeze fundus between hands. Expel any blood clots by firm downward pressure against supporting hand.	Expresses blood or clots collected in uterine cavity
Observe vulva for amount of bleeding, passage of clots; estimate amount.	Assesses extent of bleeding
Continue intermittent massage and observation of bleeding if fundus does not immediately contract.	Encourages uterine contraction and control of bleeding
Do not over massage the fundus.	Exhausts the muscle; increases uterine atony
Remove bloody pads; cleanse perineum; apply fresh perineal pads.	Promotes comfort and hygiene; reduces risk of infection
Discard pads and gloves according to agency policy.	Standard precautions
Record findings.	Communicates data to others
Notify physician if fundus fails to remain firm or bleeding continues to be excessive.	Additional measures, such as oxytocin, needed to prevent hemorrhage

not experience an urge to void. This decreased perception of bladder fullness is due to increased bladder capacity, resulting from reduced intra-abdominal pressure, edema of the trigone area at the base of the bladder resulting from trauma, and impaired transmission of afferent neural impulses due to regional anesthesia (Cunningham et al., 1993). The bladder may fill rapidly after delivery if the woman received intravenous fluids during labor and because of increased physiologic urinary output in the early postpartum period.

The nurse assesses the condition of the bladder by abdominal palpation, percussion, and observation. The contour of the abdomen, height and consistency of the fundus, and characteristics of the suprapubic area are assessed. Lochial flow is examined for increases in amount, which can be caused by a distended bladder and interferes with uterine contraction.

Bladder Distention. As the bladder fills with urine, it gradually protrudes above the symphysis pubis and

can be observed bulging in front of the uterus (see Fig. 27-1). If the bladder is markedly distended, the uterus may be pushed upward and to the side, and the fundus may become relaxed, leading to increased bleeding. When the hand is cupped over the fundus to massage it and bring it back to midline, the bladder protrudes further. When the hand is removed, the fundus returns to its displaced position. Other signs of bladder distention include an initial voiding of less than 300 mL, increased lochial flow, and a dull rather than hollow sound on percussion of the suprapubic area.

The most common cause of excessive uterine bleeding during the early postpartum period is uterine atony, which often is caused by bladder distention. Severe bladder distention leads to atony of the bladder musculature, which leads to inadequate emptying of the bladder and urinary retention. Urinary retention predisposes the woman to urinary tract infections. Early identification of bladder distention is important in

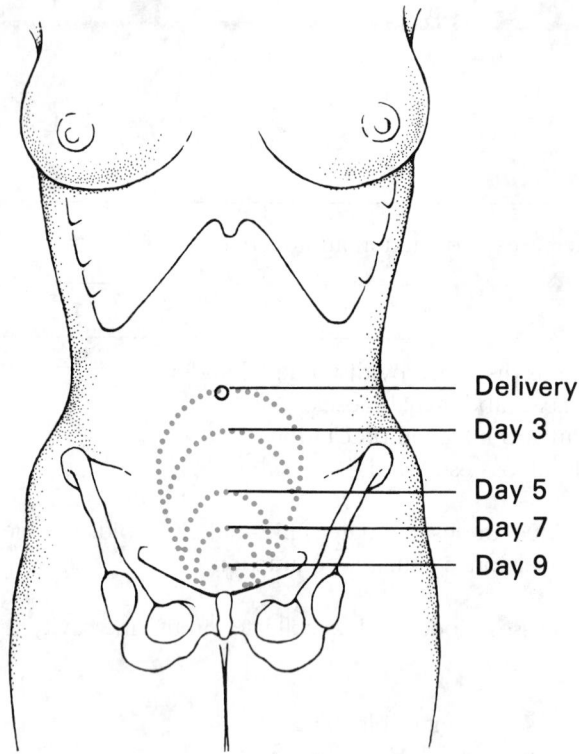

Delivery
Day 3
Day 5
Day 7
Day 9

FIGURE 27–2 Involution of the uterus.

preventing and minimizing these risks to the mother's health.

Perineum

The nurse makes frequent assessments of the perineum and perianal areas to identify normal characteristics and deviations from normal, such as hematomas, bruising (ecchymosis), edema, redness (erythema), and tenderness. The suture line, if present, is assessed for intactness, hematoma, bleeding, and signs of infection (redness, swelling, tenderness). The anal area is assessed for hemorrhoids and fissures. The woman is placed in Sims' lateral position to assess the perineum and perianal areas.

Perineal pain is common following repair of an episiotomy or lacerations. An edematous perineum adds tension to the suture line and increases pain. The amount of pain experienced is usually related to the extent of the surgical procedures and repair. Women who have spontaneous vaginal births without lacerations or episiotomies often experience less perineal pain.

Hemorrhoids appear as grapelike protrusions of the anus and are a frequent source of perianal pain. They result from pressure exerted on the pelvic floor by the presenting part during late pregnancy and labor and from straining during the expulsive phase of labor. They are most painful during the first 2 or 3 days after delivery; they gradually decrease in size and regress.

Intestinal Elimination

Constipation is commonly due to diminished intestinal tone and bowel motility from relaxation of the abdominal muscles and from the effects of progesterone on smooth muscles. The lack of food intake and dehydration during labor and delivery contribute to constipation. Assessment includes auscultation for bowel sounds, inspection and palpation for abdominal distention, inspection for presence of hemorrhoids and perineal swelling or ecchymosis, and inquiry about expelling flatus. The presence of bowel sounds indicates active intestinal processes.

Women with significant perineal pain often anticipate discomfort with defecation, which may inhibit spontaneous bowel movements. The first defecation usually occurs 2 to 3 days after delivery and is generally assisted by stool softeners or laxatives. Daily bowel movements are expected thereafter. An enema may be given if other measures are unsuccessful.

Lower Extremities

The lower extremities are observed to detect signs of postpartum thrombophlebitis, which is a serious complication. Women are predisposed to thrombosis in the lower extremities during pregnancy and the early postpartum period because of decreased venous return of blood from the legs and an increased tendency for coagulation. Prolonged compression of the large vessels

TABLE 27–2 *Characteristics of Lochia*		
Rubra	**Serosa**	**Alba**
Bright red, bloody, may have small clots	Pink to pink brown, serous, no clots	Cream to yellowish, may be brownish
Characteristic fleshy odor (animal-like scent)	Usually no odor (unless poor hygiene)	Usually no odor (unless poor hygiene)
1–3 d postpartum	4–7 d postpartum	1–3 wk postpartum
Heavy to moderate flow	Decrease in flow	Scant flow

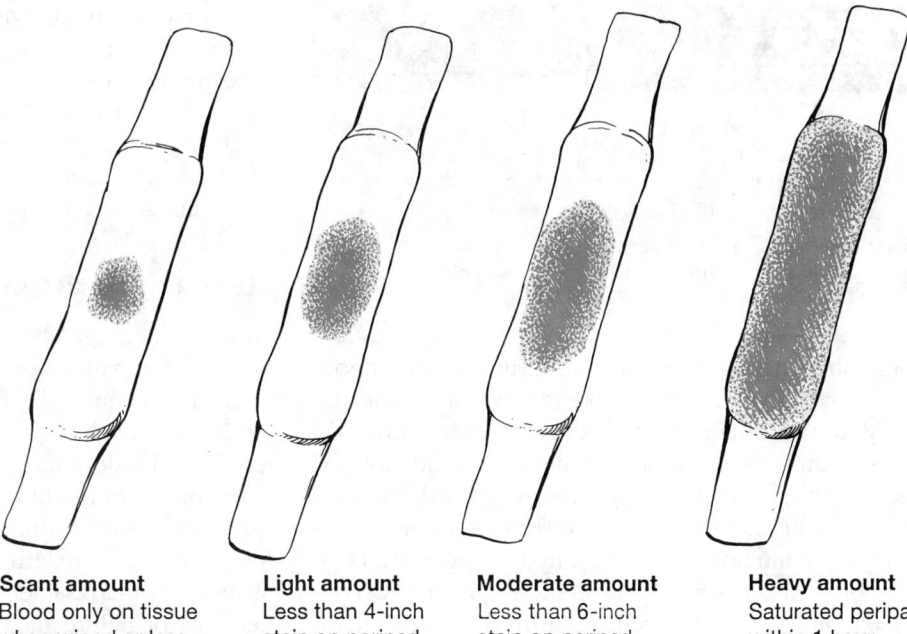

Scant amount	Light amount	Moderate amount	Heavy amount
Blood only on tissue when wiped or less than 1-inch stain on peripad.	Less than 4-inch stain on peripad.	Less than 6-inch stain on peripad.	Saturated peripad within 1 hour.

FIGURE 27-3 Assessing the volume of lochia by peripad saturation.

supplying the legs caused by pushing in the expulsive stage of labor also may contribute to thrombosis formation.

Postpartum assessment of the lower extremities includes inspection for size, shape, symmetry, color, edema, and varicosities. Temperature and swelling are felt by palpation. Signs of thrombophlebitis are unilateral swelling, redness, heat, and tenderness, usually in the calf. Femoral vein thrombosis causes pain and tenderness in the distal thigh and popliteal region. *Homans' sign*, the presence of calf pain with active dorsiflexion of the foot, is an unreliable test for thrombophlebitis (Way, 1994). Pulses in the lower extremities may be decreased or absent with thrombophlebitis. Clients who have delivered by cesarean may be more at risk for this complication due to increased bed rest prior to their first ambulation.

Breasts

Breast assessment during the postpartum period includes inspection of size, shape, color, and symmetry and palpation for consistency and tenderness to determine lactation status. In the first 1 to 2 days after delivery, the breasts undergo little change except for some secretion of colostrum. In breast-feeding mothers, as milk begins to be produced, the breasts become larger, firmer, and warmer and may feel lumpy or nodular. Women often experience discomfort with initial onset of lactation. In nonlactating mothers, these changes are less pronounced and regress over several days. Some women may experience marked **engorgement** with the onset of lactation. The breasts become quite large

and feel hard and tense, with taut, shiny skin and distended blue veins. They may be very painful, and the breasts may feel hot to the touch.

As breast-feeding is initiated, the nurse observes the breasts for changes, inspecting nipples and areola for redness and cracks, and asking the mother about tenderness. Full or engorged breasts should become softer and more comfortable after nursing.

Laboratory Tests

To assess for anemia, a complete blood count, hematocrit, or hemoglobin is done 24 to 48 hours after delivery. Blood values change postpartum (see Chap. 25) due to many physiologic adaptations as the woman returns to a nonpregnant state. With an average blood loss of 400 to 500 mL, a drop of 1 g in hemoglobin level or 3% in hematocrit value is within the expected range. Larger decreases in these values result from heavy bleeding at delivery, hemorrhage, or prenatal anemia (Table 27-3).

During the first 10 days postpartum, the white blood count may increase to $20,000/mm^3$ before returning to normal values (Bond, 1993). Because the cellular components of this leukocytosis are similar to those during an infection, this increase may conceal an infectious process unless the white blood count is higher than physiologic levels.

Identification of Risk Factors

Nursing assessment provides information about potential risk factors for development of complications, most

TABLE 27–3
Postpartum Hematologic Values

Blood Value	Normal Postpartum	Deviations From Expected
Hemoglobin	10.0–11.4 g/dL	<10.0 g/dL
Hematocrit	32%–36%	<30%
Leukocytes	14,000–30,000/mm³	>30,000/mm³

commonly hemorrhage and infection. Data about events that occurred during pregnancy, labor, and delivery can alert the nurse to clients at increased risk for postpartum complications. Multiparas tend toward heavier postpartum bleeding. Risk of hemorrhage is increased with excessive uterine distention during pregnancy from multiple pregnancy, hydramnios, or a large newborn (macrosomia). Lacerations of the cervix, vagina, and perineum predispose the woman to hemorrhage and infection. Prolonged labor resulting in maternal exhaustion and dehydration places the woman at increased risk of infection (Table 27-4).

High-risk pregnancy indicates that the client may be at increased risk for postpartum complications. Such conditions as anemia, suboptimal nutrition, substance abuse, and preexisting disease (diabetes, pregnancy-induced hypertension, cardiac disease, urinary and renal disease) are associated with a variety of postpartum problems.

Psychosocial Assessment

Assessment of emotional, behavioral, and social factors in the postpartum period allows the nurse to identify the mother's and family's needs for support, teaching, and anticipatory guidance; their response to the childbearing experience and postpartum care; and factors affecting the assumption of new parenting responsibilities. The nurse also assesses the mother's knowledge and abilities related to self-care, newborn care, and health maintenance and feelings about herself and her body image (see Chap. 26).

Reaction to the Childbirth Process

Most women need to review the birth experience during the postpartum period (Simkin, 1992). This allows them to integrate the experience and is a method of critical self-evaluation that is part of an important psychological task of the postpartum period. The woman's perceptions of the fit between her actual and expected or desired intrapartum behaviors provide indications of positive self-regard or potential problems in self-esteem. Embarrassment, apologies for behaviors, and feelings of failure may be expressed and are cues to decreased self-esteem.

Adaptations to Parenting and Caretaking

A number of maternal behaviors indicate adaptive responses to the newborn and caretaking responsibilities (see Chap. 26). New mothers who are relatively inexperienced may encounter some difficulties in caretaking. With practice, their abilities and self-esteem improve, supporting a positive emotional response to the newborn.

Parents with significant life stresses, socioeconomic difficulties, health problems, and pregnancy-related complications may not adapt as effectively to parenting as those without such stresses. Maladaptive behavior

TABLE 27–4
Postpartum Risk Factors

Risk Factor	Complication	Assessment Data
Uterine overdistention	Hemorrhage	Fundus boggy, atonic; excessive bleeding; low blood pressure; high pulse
Prolonged labor	Infection, dehydration	Fever, high pulse
Lacerations or episiotomy	Hemorrhage	Excessive bleeding, low blood pressure, high pulse
	Infection	Fever, high pulse, redness, edema
	Hematoma	Swelling, ecchymosis pain, dark mass
Premature rupture of membranes	Infection (endometritis)	Fever, high pulse, subinvolution
Prolonged second stage of labor	Thrombophlebitis	Unilateral calf pain, swelling, redness, positive Homans'
Retained placental fragments	Impaired urination (trigone edema)	Unable to void, small voiding, distended bladder
Breast-feeding	Delayed hemorrhage	Fresh red lochia, low blood pressure, high pulse
	Infection (mastitis)	Nipples red, sore; breasts hot, red, tender

occurs when parents respond ineffectively or inappropriately to their newborn's needs. Those who have not developed a sense of self-competence and feel little personal control in their lives often experience parenting difficulties (Turner et al., 1985).

Fathers also may exhibit adaptive or maladaptive responses to parenthood. Many of the same behaviors can be assessed to determine the level of paternal adaptation. The effects of different cultural practices on the parental and maternal roles must be considered (see Box 27-1).

Cultural Variations

Ethnic and cultural beliefs and practices influence parenting behaviors during the postpartum period

---

BOX 27-1
Cultural Beliefs and Practices in the Postpartum Period

Beliefs

Imbalance related to energy flows, hot-cold, yin-yang. Postpartum women are in a state of imbalance (decreased energy flows, cold state, excessive yin).

Practices

Rest and seclusion: Women need a long period of rest postpartum, avoiding physical activity and sex and limiting contact with others. Household responsibilities and newborn care often provided by female relatives

40 days—Mexican Americans, Southeast Asians (Laotian, Vietnamese, Cambodians)

1 month—Chinese, Japanese

2 weeks—Filipino

Avoid cold, maintain warmth: To restore balance postpartum, women must avoid chilling activities or foods or increase external heat.

Avoid bathing—Chinese, Mexican Americans, Southeast Asians, Japanese, Shinto (may shower, ritual bath at end of seclusion period)

Cannot wash hair—Chinese, Raza/Latina

Avoid exposure to breeze or wind—Chinese, Southern African Americans, Mexican Americans, Filipino, Southeast Asians

Add external heat—Hispanics, Filipinos, Asians (remain covered at all times, use extra blankets, slippers)

Dietary prescriptions or restrictions: Usually based on which foods are "hot" and "cold" by cultural definition

Chinese—Eat five to six meals daily, hot herbal teas, hot foods (rice, eggs, organ meats, chicken); cold foods avoided (water, raw and cold foods)

Hispanics—Avoid cold foods (fresh fruit and vegetables, sour, acidic, cold foods)

Hmong—Chicken and rice spiced with pepper, ideal postpartum foods

---

(see Chap. 4). The model of illness as resulting from body imbalances is common in nonwestern cultures. Balance may be perceived in terms of energy flow, hot and cold, or yin and yang (feminine-receptive and masculine-active principles). The postpartum woman is perceived to be in a state of imbalance and is vulnerable to illness unless she follows specific practices usually related to rest and seclusion, avoidance of cold, and diet (see Box 27-1; Bernstein et al., 1982; D'Avanzo, 1992; Monrroy, 1983; Pillsbury, 1982).

Some cultures may restrict the father's role in childbirth and postpartum experiences or establish specific types of parenting activities. Applying western expectations and methods of assessment of parental behaviors is inappropriate in these cultures.

Nursing Diagnoses

A careful assessment may produce a variety of actual and potential diagnoses, which include the following:

- Altered Bowel Elimination related to decreased bowel motility and abdominal muscle tone, dehydration, painful defecation
- Altered Patterns of Urinary Elimination related to postpartum diuresis and urinary retention from post-delivery edema
- Pain related to uterine contractions (afterpains), episiotomy, lacerations, hemorrhoids, breast engorgement, surgical incision
- Impaired Skin Integrity related to surgical incisions or lacerations
- Risk for Infection related to impaired skin integrity and tissue trauma from childbirth
- Fluid Volume Deficit related to decreased oral intake or blood loss
- Altered Nutrition: Less than body requirements related to increase need with lactation
- Sleep Pattern Disturbance related to physical discomforts or to the newborn's feeding needs
- Health Seeking Behaviors regarding self-care, newborn care, health maintenance, prevention of infections or complications
- Situational Low Self Esteem related to lack of knowledge about physiologic processes; self-care and newborn care; altered body image; emotional moodiness; and changes in personal and role identities
- Family Coping: Potential for Growth related to integration of the newborn into the family, family reorganization, altered role and lifestyle changes
- Altered Parenting related to fatigue, difficult labor, feelings of incompetence, or disappointment or conflict about the newborn
- Anxiety related to parenting responsibilities, mother's or newborn's condition, family adaptation

Nursing Planning and Intervention

Based on the assessment and diagnoses, plans are made to alter or alleviate actual or potential problems, and nursing interventions are implemented. Interventions include providing direct care, teaching, supporting the mother with self-care and newborn care, providing a supportive and health-promoting environment, coordinating care, working with family adaptations, and making referrals for other health or social services.

During the first hours after delivery, nursing care emphasizes rest and restoration. The new mother is assisted with basic activities (elimination, nutrition, ambulation, newborn care) so physiologic recovery can be maximized. Emotional support and reassurance about the birth experience and the transition to motherhood occur through attentive listening, clarification, providing information, positive reinforcement, and encouragement. All of these help to promote a positive self-concept and sense of competence in the woman.

Client teaching is a major postpartum nursing intervention directed toward meeting the mother's needs for knowledge and skills related to self-care, newborn care, postpartum processes, family adaptations, and health maintenance (see Client Teaching Guidelines: Postpartum Self-Care).

Each mother's understanding and ability in providing newborn care vary depending largely on her background and previous experiences. New mothers who have little experience with newborn care will need considerable instruction and support. Many new mothers are timid at first because they do not know what to expect of their newborn or are afraid of harming them. A mother who has had no previous experience with newborns needs some guided practice in changing diapers, dressing the newborn, feeding, and handling. Multiparas may feel uncertain about the response of an older child to the newborn and benefit from guidance in understanding and dealing with sibling rivalry. Many mothers need to know more about their own care; others need to know how to plan for family adjustments or prepare the home for the newborn. If the mother knows what she can expect and what to do, she usually can handle situations that might otherwise cause fear or apprehension.

The family may expect the mother to resume her usual activities immediately. It takes several weeks to months, however, before the mother is fully able to carry out functions in all areas, and the family needs guidance in setting realistic expectations and providing emotional and practical support to the mother.

The nurse's approach to postpartum teaching and counseling must respect various cultural perspectives and often will need modification according to cultural values and practices. In some cultures, the decision

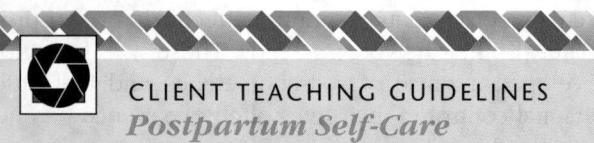

CLIENT TEACHING GUIDELINES
Postpartum Self-Care

Physical Self-Care

Involution (fundus, lochia, afterpains)
Bathing and showering
Perineal care (sitz bath, heat lamp, Tucks)
Breast care (breast support, cleansing, comfort measures, milk expression, ice packs)
Nutrition and hydration
Rest and sleep
Exercise (ambulation, Kegel and postpartum exercises)
Bowel and bladder elimination
Danger signs to report immediately

Psychosocial Self-Care

Emotional adjustments (birth review, self-image, blues)
Family adaptations to newborn
Role changes and alterations in lifestyle
Sexuality and contraception
Expectations of functional capacity
Dealing with visitors and friends
Community resources (mother's support groups, housekeepers, family service agencies, support for breastfeeding, community health agencies, parenting education)

Newborn Care

Feeding (breast, formula)
Positioning and handling
Bathing and hygiene
Cord and circumcision care
Diapering and clothing
Newborn behavior patterns (sleep, crying, elimination)
Newborn development (eyes, neuromuscular, interactional)
Temperature taking (use of thermometer)
Suctioning (bulb syringe)
Safety (infant car seat, nonflammable linens, clothing, never leave newborn alone on bed or table)
Signs of illness, when to call physician

makers are the extended family (D'Avanzo, 1992). Client teaching may need to include these decision makers and the parents to be effective in the areas of ambulation, nutrition, hydration, bathing, and newborn care. In providing psychosocial teaching and counseling, the nurse must be sensitive to the mother's and family's values. Clients from nonwestern cultures may consider it inappropriate to discuss postpartum sexuality, contraception, or psychological adjustments to parenthood.

Anticipatory guidance for discharge from the hospital or birth center focuses on assisting the client to prepare for stresses related to caring for the newborn at home and supporting optimal family adjustments. Because of the trend toward early discharge, the nurse must maximize each opportunity for client teaching and facilitate the mother's learning and sense of competence.

Although most new mothers are eager to go home, after discharge many women find themselves overwhelmed by the multiple demands of parenthood. New mothers often report feeling insecure in their ability to provide newborn care, concerned about their worth as a mother, and self-concept disturbances (Davis et al., 1985; Rutledge et al., 1987).

With limited time for providing intervention, as soon as the mother's physiological condition is stable and she has rested adequately, the nurse should encourage and assist the new mother to become active in her own and the newborns' care. Providing written materials, such as pamphlets about breast-feeding, newborn care and development, when to call the physician, and community referral sources, often helps the family at home. Approaches to postpartum teaching are further discussed in Chapter 19. Nursing interventions for potential complications and postpartum needs are described in the following sections.

Uterine Atony

When performing fundal assessments, the nurse may identify a boggy (atonic) fundus, particularly within the first 24 hours after delivery. This lack of uterine tone is known as **uterine atony**. The nurse should do intermittent fundal massage until the uterus becomes firm and maintains its tone (see Procedure 27-1: Fundal Massage and Expression and Fig. 27-4). During fundal massage, the nurse observes the vaginal orifice and notes the amount of bleeding. If fundal massage does not produce adequate contraction within a short time, the physician should be immediately notified. Oxytocic medications will usually be ordered to stimulate uterine contraction and control bleeding. If heavy bleeding continues despite a firmly contracted uterus, the nurse should notify the physician, because hemorrhage from a laceration or retained placental fragment is likely.

Postpartum women should be taught how to assess their own fundal height and firmness, because with early discharge, the progress of involution will need self-monitoring. Clients should be taught to recognize signs of deviation from the expected pattern, such as unchanged fundal height, boggy or tender fundus, persistent or new bright-red bleeding, and foul-smelling lochia. The importance of seeking medical attention for these deviations is explained and emphasized.

Afterpains

Uterine contractions similar to menstrual cramps, termed **afterpains,** often occur for about 2 days after delivery, primarily in multiparas and in women who have had an overdistended uterus. During breast-feeding, the mother experiences more severe afterpains because the newborn's suckling causes a release of oxytocin, which makes the uterus contract. Client teaching

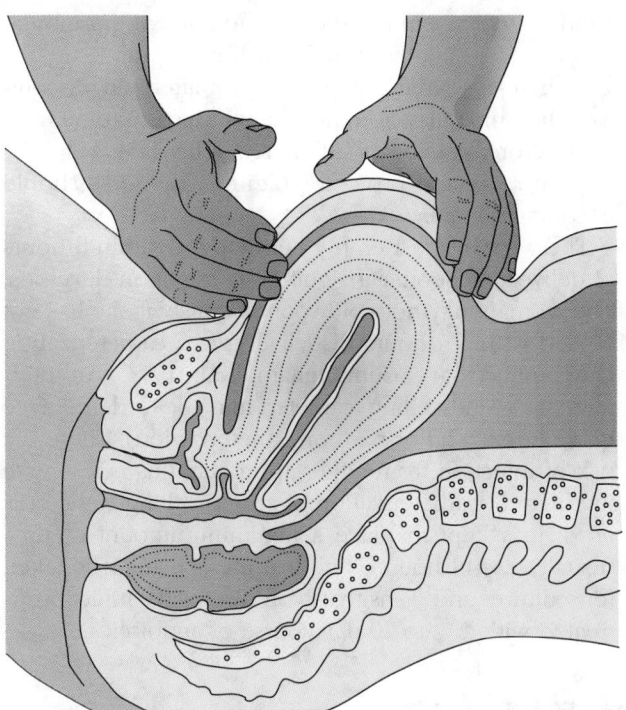

FIGURE 27–4 Fundal massage. With hands correctly positioned, gentle fundal massage stimulates the uterine muscles to contract, helping to restore normal tone and control bleeding.

includes an explanation of the cause and purpose of afterpains, with reassurance that they are helpful and will disappear in a short time. Self-care measures, such as regular emptying of the bladder, fundal massage, using a heating pad, lying prone, or doing leg-lift exercises, are taught. These actions increase circulation and uterine tone, which reduces discomfort. Analgesics may be ordered if afterpains are severe; the nurse can advise taking these about 30 minutes before breast-feeding and periodically as needed for comfort.

Bladder Distention

Some mothers have difficulty voiding after delivery and may develop a distended bladder if not assisted to void. Incomplete emptying of the bladder (voiding <300 mL) also can lead to distention and predispose to infection. To encourage spontaneous voiding, the nurse assesses the bladder frequently for fullness and explains the importance of regular voiding. The client is assisted to the bathroom or provided a bedpan and privacy. Running warm water or pouring warm water over the perineum often stimulates voiding. If voiding does occur, it is measured (subtracting the amount of water poured over the perineum) whenever possible; the bladder is assessed for any remaining fullness by determining the location of the uterus in relation to the midline of the abdomen. Application of firm pressure over the suprapubic area (client can do this with her hand) may assist in more complete emptying. Ambulation increases bladder tone, which is helpful.

If there is significant perineal or afterpain discomfort, the nurse may administer analgesics 15 to 30 minutes before voiding is attempted. This may help the woman relax and promote voiding. The nurse should encourage fluids.

The woman must empty her bladder within 8 hours of delivery or sooner if significant distention develops. The woman may not void spontaneously if she has not voided within 4 hours of delivery, and catheterization may be necessary (Cunningham et al., 1993). An intermittent or indwelling catheter may be ordered (see Procedure 27-2: Postpartum Catheterization). There is a risk of infection from either approach; this is less with intermittent catheterization. If an indwelling catheter is used, it is kept in place a minimum amount of time (usually 24–48 hours), and a urine specimen is taken for culture and sensitivity on removal. Infection is treated with a 7- to 10-day course of antibiotics.

Perineal Care

Some method of perineal cleansing frequently is used to promote comfort and reduce the risk of infection. The most common method is pouring a stream of warm water, often with antiseptic solution added, over the vulva and perineum after voiding and defecation. Equipment that directs a spray of warm water on the perineum may be available. The woman is instructed in self-administration of perineal care (see Client Teaching Guidelines: Perineal Self-Care). Instructions are provided, rationale explained, and techniques demonstrated, beginning with the first perineal care after delivery. This includes the technique for changing and disposing of perineal pads. When the nurse performs perineal care, gloves are used as part of standard precautions for exposure to blood and body fluids. Perineal pads should be placed in hazardous waste trash containers.

Cold and Heat Therapy

Cold therapy may be used immediately after delivery and for the first 24 to 48 hours when there has been significant perineal trauma or a large episiotomy. Cold therapy immediately after trauma effectively relieves pain and promotes vasoconstriction to decrease bleeding and edema, thus limiting the severity of the tissue trauma. For optimum benefit, an ice pack is applied to the perineum for 30 minutes, followed by a resting period of 30 to 60 minutes. Exposure to cold for longer than 1 hour triggers a protective secondary effect (Lewis reaction), in which the blood flow alternately

---

PROCEDURE 27–2
Postpartum Catheterization

Nursing Intervention	*Rationale*
Explain procedure and rationale; reassure about gentleness.	Increases cooperation, decreases anxiety
Have equipment positioned; put sterile gloves on.	Efficiency of procedure, reduces infection risk
Inform of each step in procedure; encourage deep breathing.	Reduces involuntary tension; encourages relaxation
Provide perineal care.	Cleanses perineum; promotes comfort; reduces infection risk
Gently separate vulva; cleanse vestibule.	Avoids tension on sutures; reduces infection risk
Place sterile cotton ball in introitus	Prevents lochia from draining out during procedure
Exposing urinary meatus, gently insert small-gauge flexible catheter until urine flows.	Provides for location of meatus, minimizes trauma
If bladder is markedly distended, pinch catheter after each 300 mL; wait 10–15 sec, then allow flow to continue.	Allows slow bladder deflation; encourages return of bladder tone
Withdraw catheter or inflate balloon if indwelling.	Indwelling catheter often ordered with severe distention
Replace perineal pad; help client reposition.	Promotes comfort and hygiene
Measure amount of urine; note color and character; record; send specimen to laboratory if ordered.	Ensures adequate emptying of bladder; assesses for infection
Remove gloves; discard bloody items in containers according to agency protocol.	Standard precautions

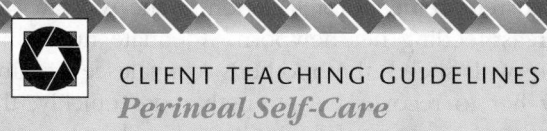

CLIENT TEACHING GUIDELINES
Perineal Self-Care

Procedure or Action	Rationale
Wash hands.	Reduces risk of infection by removing microorganisms
Remove used pad from front to back.	Reduces risk of transferring microorganisms from rectum to vagina
Without separating labia, pour or squeeze solution over vulva and perineum.	Rinses away lochia, cleanses vulva, reduces risk of transferring organisms from vulva to vagina
Pat dry with tissue from front to back.	Reduces friction, risk of transferring organisms from rectum to vagina
Apply Tucks, spray, or ointment as directed.	Promotes comfort
Apply fresh perineal pad from front to back; do not touch inner surface of pad; secure with sanitary belt or pantie.	Promotes comfort; reduces risk of infection and organism transfer; prevents pad from sliding
Wash hands.	As above

increases and decreases in the tissues being cooled to maintain tissue temperature above freezing and prevent tissue damage. Cold therapy continued longer than 24 to 48 hours may interfere with wound healing (Rhode et al., 1990).

Heat therapy may be used to relieve perineal discomfort and edema and to promote hygiene. Studies have not demonstrated, however, that heat therapy accelerates perineal healing (Rhode et al., 1990). Various types of sitz baths are a common form of moist-heat therapy. Continuous-flow sitz bathtubs and individual portable sitz basins are available. The woman sits in the sitz bath in water maintained at 38° to 41°C (100°–105°F) two to three times per day for 20 minutes. She is instructed in use of the sitz bath, and home approaches to continuing moist-heat therapy are discussed.

Dry-heat therapy also may be used. A heat lamp is positioned about 15 to 20 in from the perineum while the woman is lying down and draped for privacy and warmth. The lamp is used for 20 minutes three times per day. At home, mothers can use a desk lamp with a 40-watt bulb, being careful to keep it at a safe and comfortable distance of 20 in from the perineum.

Medication

Anesthetic sprays, ointments, or witch hazel pads (Tucks) may be applied directly to sutured areas on the perineum. These relieve pain and promote comfort. Analgesic medications are sometimes needed when pain is severe. Women with extensive perineal pain may need medication every 4 hours for the first 1 or 2 postpartum days. If medications are needed, they should be given about 30 to 40 minutes before the newborn's feeding period. This relieves the mother's pain and allows her to concentrate her energies and attention on the newborn.

Sitting

Mothers who have discomfort from perineal sutures usually find it uncomfortable to sit for the first few days. They may be observed sitting in a rigid position, bearing their weight on one side of the buttocks or the other, with obvious discomfort to the back and the perineum. The nurse can teach the mother how to sit comfortably with her body erect. The mother brings her buttocks together (hands may be used to push buttocks inward) and contracts pelvic floor muscles just before sitting, then holds this for a moment after letting her full weight down. This promotes comfort by reducing the tension and weight bearing of the perineal tissues.

Breast Care

The goals of breast care are prevention of infection, adequate breast support, and maternal comfort. The breasts should be handled gently and precautions taken to avoid rough rubbing or unnecessary pressure.

Hygiene and Comfort

The breast-feeding mother can cleanse her nipples with clear water. The best nipple care is provided by the body itself without outside interference (see Chap. 30). She should avoid soap, alcohol, or other drying agents. The nonlactating mother can use mild soap and water and bathe her breasts during her daily shower or bath. She needs to wear a tight-fitting brassiere or breast binder to suppress milk production.

Engorgement

Both lactating and nonlactating mothers may experience engorgement with throbbing pains in the breasts that extend into the axillae. Analgesic medications may provide pain relief until the condition subsides (1 or 2 days). The nonlactating mother should wear a tight brassiere or breast binder and may apply ice bags to the breasts and axillae to relieve pain. The application of heat, nipple stimulation, and removal of milk from the breast should be avoided. Lactating mothers can decrease the discomfort from engorgement by removing milk from the breast by putting the newborn to breast more frequently, using a breast pump, or massaging the breast.

Lactation Suppression

Mothers who are not breast-feeding may need measures to suppress lactation even in the absence of suckling. Mechanical measures include tight compression of the breasts with a breast binder or a tight-fitting support brassiere and application of ice packs. Fluids should not be restricted because these are important for postpartum recovery. The mother is instructed to avoid any stimulus to the breasts, such as suckling the newborn, expressing or pumping the breasts, or putting warm water on the breasts. Some women experience breast firmness, tenderness, and temporary engorgement. The postdelivery stimulus to lactation and discomfort from temporary engorgement usually decrease after 3 days.

Because of the increased risk of thromboembolism and the potential relationship to endometrial cancer, estrogen and androgen are rarely used today to suppress lactation. Bromocriptine mesylate (Parlodel) may only rarely be prescribed to stimulate the production of prolactin inhibitory factor, which suppresses lactation. The regimen is for 2.5 mg, one tablet twice a day with meals beginning at least 4 hours after delivery and continuing for 14 to 21 days. Occasionally, rebound breast secretion, congestion, and tenderness occur when the medication is discontinued. Hypertension, seizure, stroke, and myocardial infarction are serious but rare complications associated with this medication (Cunningham et al., 1993). The Maternal Health Advisory Committee of the Food and Drug Administration concluded in 1988 that routine medications should not be given to suppress postpartum lactation (Cunningham et al., 1993).

Health Maintenance
Nutrition

Shortly after the delivery, the woman may express a desire for something to eat or drink. Unless she has received a general anesthetic or is nauseated, there is usually no contraindication to giving her some nourishment. The postpartum diet should provide for balanced nutrition with enough calories to supply the additional requirements for lactation, if the woman will be breast-feeding her newborn. Adequate nutritional intake will speed the mother's convalescence and allow her to recover her strength more quickly; the quality and quantity of her milk also will improve. A well-nourished mother also may be better able to resist infections (Gutierrez, 1994). Mothers usually have good appetites and become hungry between meals, especially if breast-feeding. Between-meal snacks, including milk or milk products, will help to supply her with the additional milk requirements nursing mothers need (see Chap. 30). An increased intake of fluids is essential for lactating mothers.

Rest and Sleep

During the puerperium, the mother needs adequate rest and should be encouraged to relax and sleep whenever possible. Rest is facilitated by reducing worry and anxiety-producing situations and promoting comfort. Rest is especially significant for the mother who is breast-feeding because worry and fatigue inhibit milk supply. Fatigue magnifies worries about minor concerns, and emotional problems are often precipitated by sleeplessness and fatigue.

The nurse adjusts the hospital routine whenever possible to provide the mother with uninterrupted periods of rest. A formula-fed newborn may be fed occasionally by the nurse if the mother is sleeping. If the mother is unable to nap during the day, she can be encouraged to rest as quietly as possible at various times. The need for rest and sleep may need to be reinforced, especially during the "taking-hold" phase, when the mother is eager to assume care responsibilities.

Early Ambulation

The mother is encouraged to be out of bed as soon as possible following delivery unless there are contraindications. Early ambulation promotes circulation and reduces the risk of thrombophlebitis. Bladder and bowel functions are improved by ambulation, reducing the need for catheterization and decreasing abdominal distention and constipation.

Women who had local, epidural, or caudal anesthesia during delivery can ambulate as soon as they feel able. If the mother had intrathecal subarachnoid spinal anesthesia, she should remain flat in bed for at least 8 hours before ambulating. This helps to prevent leakage of spinal fluid through the needle puncture site in the dural membrane, reducing the incidence of postspinal headache. This recumbent position must be maintained while taking fluids and interacting with the newborn. The mother must remain flat and must not lift her head, so the nurse positions the newborn so the mother can look and touch without lifting her head.

The first time the mother gets up she should dangle her legs over the side of the bed for a few minutes. The nurse assesses her status, checking for dizziness or weakness. She is then assisted to stand, then walk a few steps to determine balance. The nurse accompanies her to the bathroom or chair and remains close at hand to give immediate assistance if the mother becomes weak or faint.

It is important that the nurse explain the purpose and value of early ambulation to the mother or other decision makers. Activity should be gradually increased according to the mother's strength.

Bathing

Postpartum women often have marked diaphoresis as interstitial fluids retained during pregnancy are excreted. Taking a shower is refreshing and promotes hygiene. Mothers with no complications are allowed to shower within a few hours of delivery. The first time the mother takes a shower, the nurse should remain nearby for safety. Tub baths usually are allowed in 2 weeks. In association with showers, the nurse provides self-care instructions for bathing and breast care.

Prevention of Constipation

Measures are generally instituted to prevent constipation, such as a stool softener or laxative the first few days after delivery. The nurse explains the purpose of these medications and encourages intake of fluids nd dietary roughage. The presence of bowel sounds indicates increasing bowel activity. Bowel sounds and the first stool are recorded by the nurse.

If a bowel evacuation has not occurred by the second or third day, a cleansing enema or rectal suppository may be prescribed. Should these measures not result in stool passage, an oil retention enema, followed some hours later by a cleansing enema, may be ordered.

The mother who is breast-feeding is advised to follow her physician's directions regarding use of laxatives, because some laxatives are excreted in breast milk and therefore affect the newborn (see Chap. 30). Client teaching for self-care emphasizes dietary approaches to encourage regular bowel elimination, such as good bowel habits, adequate fluid intake, and foods providing roughage. Prevention of constipation is discussed in Chapter 17.

Alleviation of Hemorrhoids

Hemorrhoids are a common problem for women during the postpartum period. They are most painful during the first 2 to 3 days after delivery, then gradually reduce in size and regress. Painful hemorrhoids are treated with sitz baths, anesthetic sprays or ointments, and cool astringent compresses (such as witch hazel).

Comfort is promoted by wearing perineal pads loosely and lying on the side in Sims' position while in bed. Prevention of constipation is the main measure to relieve ongoing difficulties with hemorrhoids.

Prevention of Infection

Thrombophlebitis. Postpartum women are instructed in measures to reduce the risk of thrombophlebitis. The importance of early and regular ambulation is emphasized, and the mother is advised to avoid leg-crossing at the knees and constricting garters or clothing that interferes with circulation. Signs of thrombosis and infection are described (severe unilateral calf or thigh pain, redness, swelling, heat), and the mother is instructed to report these immediately to the physician.

Perineal or Breast Infections. Proper techniques for applying and removing perineal pads and for wiping after voiding and defecating (front-to-back, single wipe, then discard tissue) are taught to reduce the risk of infection when an episiotomy or lacerations are present. Breast cleansing and support measures are discussed to minimize the potential for mastitis (see Chap. 38). The nurse teaches the client signs of infection (redness, heat, swelling, pain) and instructs her to report the presence of any signs to the physician immediately.

Postpartum Depression ("Blues")

Many mothers experience a transitory (hormone-related) depression beginning the second or third day after birth. Postpartum depression reduces the level of family functioning and may be related to the woman's lowered self-esteem. Symptoms of transitory depression include crying easily, feelings of despondency, loss of appetite, poor concentration, difficulty sleeping, feeling let down, and anxiety. These symptoms usually disappear within 1 to 2 weeks, although some women remain mildly depressed much longer. About one-fourth of women report high levels of depression 8 months postpartum (Mercer et al., 1990). Postpartum psychosis occurs in 1 to 2 per 1,000 births (Beck, 1992).

Mild postpartum blues usually respond to empathy, support, and acceptance by the nurse. The nurse can provide opportunities for the mother to express her anxiety, despondent feelings, and other concerns. Sharing these with an empathetic listener is often therapeutic. Helping the mother put her responses in perspective and explaining that this is a common experience can help alleviate the woman's concerns about having an inappropriate or abnormal reaction to childbirth. It also is helpful to encourage adequate rest and nutrition and to assist the mother to be successful in early mothering tasks. Seldom are psychotropic drugs necessary in transitory depression. Persistent and severe depression, however, may require psychotherapy or medications.

Postpartum Exercises

Postpartum exercises may be initiated to hasten recovery, prevent complications, and strengthen the muscles of the back, pelvic floor, and abdomen. By toning the muscles, these exercises assist the mother to restore her figure and can be psychologically and physiologically beneficial. Exercises can be started on the first postpartum day and increased gradually. The mother is counseled not to overexercise and to allow slow progression when adding to the routine. A new exercise can be added daily, with each done five to ten times per day for at least 6 weeks after delivery (see Appendix C for postpartum exercises).

Kegel exercises facilitate perineal healing and help restore vaginal, perineal, and pelvic muscle tone by increasing circulation and by isometric muscle activity. Kegel exercises consist of contracting the muscles of the perineum with enough force to stop a stream of urine. The contraction is held for a few seconds and then released. This exercise is repeated 50 to 100 times and can be done several times a day.

Kegel exercises strengthen the pubococcygeal muscle, which helps prevent urinary stress incontinence and pelvic relaxation and enhances orgasmic capacity. Postpartum women who do regular Kegel exercises show greater improvement in pelvic muscle strength than those who do not exercise (Samselle et al., 1990).

Sexuality and Contraception

Postpartum sexuality is affected by the degree of perineal trauma during birth and the decrease in the mother's steroid hormones, which is characteristic of the early postpartum period (see Chap. 9). Nurses must approach discussion of postpartum sexuality and contraception with sensitivity to cultural values and determine the appropriateness of counseling on an individual basis. Sexual adjustment after childbirth is a common concern of new parents and can be a source of conflict and confusion. The mother's interest in intercourse is usually less than her partner's in the first few months after delivery, and her physiologic responses are diminished because of low hormonal levels, the adjustment to the maternal role, and fatigue due to lack of sleep and rest. The nurse provides information about the normality of these responses, supports expression of concerns, and clarifies misunderstandings.

Lochia has generally ceased or progressed to the alba stage by 2 to 4 weeks postpartum, and the perineal area and episiotomy are well healed and not painful. Client teaching includes when to resume intercourse; the couple is advised that sex is appropriate after lochia has ceased and the perineum has healed to the point that intercourse is not painful, as long as there are no contraindicating factors, such as hematoma or infection. If intercourse causes discomfort, the couple should wait somewhat longer or use noncoital sexual practices if they find this acceptable. Positions for intercourse that avoid the penile shaft pressing posteriorly on the perineum also can alleviate discomfort.

For most couples, intercourse is resumed by the third postpartum week, so it is important to provide contraceptive information before the mother leaves the hospital. Although it is unlikely that she will ovulate and become fertile before 6 weeks, it is possible. Menses usually resume by about 9 weeks in the nonlactating woman and by 30 to 36 weeks in the lactating woman. The time of return of fertility, however, is unpredictable, and all postpartum women are counseled to use contraception if they want to avoid pregnancy (see Chaps. 9 and 25). Clients are encouraged to make an appointment for follow-up care with their provider, during which additional methods of contraception can be discussed.

Immunizations

During the postpartum period, rubella vaccine and Rho (D) immune globulin may be administered to the mother if indicated.

Rubella Vaccine

Postpartum women who are serologically negative for rubella (titer 1:8 or less) or who have a negative history for rubella immunization or disease infection are advised to have rubella vaccination before discharge. Titers of 1:16 or greater indicate immunity. Breast-feeding mothers can be vaccinated because the vaccine uses attenuated live virus and is not communicable. Women with hypersensitivity to egg protein may have allergic reactions. Pregnancy should be avoided for 3 months after vaccination because the rubella vaccine may be teratogenic to the fetus. The risk of fetal involvement from vaccination appears small, about 20% to 25% risk of a naturally acquired infection (Dunnihoo, 1992).

Rho (D) Immune Globulin

Rh-negative women who have not been previously sensitized receive Rho (D) immune globulin within 72 hours of delivery to prevent Rh-negative sensitization. Criteria for this immunization include an Rh-negative mother with a negative indirect Coombs' test (no Rh antibodies), an Rh-positive newborn, and a negative direct Coombs' test (no Rh antibodies) on cord blood. Women who meet these criteria receive 300 µg of cross-matched Rho (D) immune globulin. This dosage causes lysis of any fetal red blood cells that might have entered maternal circulation (fetomaternal transfusion) before the mother has time to build up antibodies against this foreign protein.

Discharge

The condition of the mother is confirmed before she is discharged from the hospital or birth center to determine satisfactory physiologic and psychosocial progress (see Nursing Guidelines: Evaluation for Discharge). Nursing assessments should include normal vital signs and normal findings relative to involution, perineal healing, elimination (bowel, bladder), lacta-

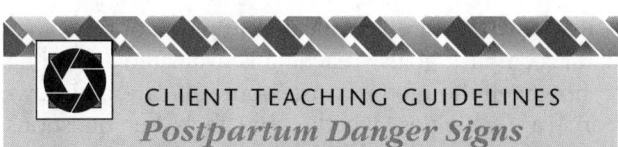

CLIENT TEACHING GUIDELINES
Postpartum Danger Signs

The following physical signs could indicate infection or hemorrhage and should be reported to the physician or primary care provider at once.

Heavy vaginal bleeding or bright-red lochia (after lochia has become dark red-brown or pale)
Fever (with or without chills)
Increased vaginal discharge, especially foul smelling
Swollen, tender, red, or hot area on one leg
Area of swelling or tender, red, hot area on breast
Burning or pain with urination, inability to void
Persistent perineal or pelvic pain

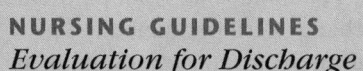

NURSING GUIDELINES
Evaluation for Discharge

Condition stable; no condition present that warrants observation
Blood loss not excessive; normal hemoglobin and hematocrit
All assessment findings within normal limits
Mother:
   Vital signs stable
   Fundus firm with lochia rubra or serosa; no clots
   Perineum intact, no hematoma
   Voiding in adequate amounts
   Taking fluids and foods without difficulty
   Homans' sign negative
   Ambulating without assistance
   No weakness or dizziness
   Postoperative:
      Incision clean, dry, intact
      Breath sounds clear
   Passing flatus and stool
Newborn:
   Appropriate weight for gestational age
   Normal cry, color, reflexes, activity
   Vital signs stable
   Mucus not excessive
   Sucking well at feedings
   Voiding and stooling normally
   Normal cord blood bilirubin
   Negative Coombs' test (if Rh incompatibility)
Caretaking:
   Signs of parental attachment
   Handles newborn competently
   Able to initiate feeding without difficulty
Client teaching for self and newborn care completed
   Accurate return demonstration of fundal check, perineal care, newborn care (feeding, diapering, cord care, suctioning)
   Verbal and written instructions provided for self-care and newborn care, limiting activities, family adjustments
   Accurate repeating of danger signs to report immediately
   Telephone numbers provided for obstetrician, pediatrician, or primary provider, hospital maternity unit, emergency services
Appointment made for office visit within 48–72 h or home visit scheduled by nurse within this time
Support people available

---

tion or lactation suppression, ambulation, laboratory tests, and immunization status.

The nurse assesses client knowledge and skill levels and reviews points for self-care and newborn care, return of ovulation and menstruation, contraception, resumption of sexual intercourse, prescribed medications, and danger signs to be reported immediately. The parents are assisted to identify support systems for household help with child care, cooking and cleaning, shopping, and other activities. The need for referral to community resources is assessed and recommendations made. Printed instruction sheets and brochures are helpful and should include danger signs and telephone numbers for assistance with questions or problems (see Client Teaching Guidelines: Postpartum Danger Signs). Follow-up care for mother and newborn is emphasized. After discharge, the mother and newborn may be seen within 48 to 72 hours in the physician's office, or a home visit is made by the nurse. The practice of providing the new mother with a hospital discharge formula pack should be evaluated in relation to her plans for newborn feeding. Howard reports that this practice decreases the time mothers exclusively breast-feed, decreases the chances mothers will be breast-feeding at all 4 months postpartum, and encourages mothers to introduce solid foods sooner into their newborn's diet (Howard et al., 1994).

Evaluation

Evaluation of the effectiveness of postpartum nursing care is a continuous process that feeds back into reassessment. The nurse uses specific outcomes to determine the success of interventions. Outcomes for physiologic care include achieving the purpose of the intervention, such as control of bleeding, relief of discomfort, initiation of voiding and defecation, successful ambulation, prevention of infection, normal progression of involution, and adequate nutrition and hydration.

Psychosocial care is evaluated in terms of outcomes that accomplish goals. Teaching is evaluated according to how well the mother carries out self-care and newborn care activities, whether she feels her questions have been adequately answered, and her ability to state knowledge (ie, danger signs, when to contact physician, resources available, newborn behavior, family adjustments to anticipate). Supportive care is evaluated by the mother's stated or apparent positive adaptations during the postpartum period, her ability to express feelings and share perceptions, and her sense of being in a caring environment.

When outcomes have not been met, the nurse reassesses the situation by gathering additional data, arrives at a new or modified nursing diagnosis, and develops additional plans to accomplish the goals of care. These plans are implemented through appropriate nursing interventions, which are reevaluated for accomplishment of their purposes in terms of outcomes for the client (see Nursing Care Plan).

First Weeks at Home

Challenges and stress arise from the process of integrating the newborn into the family and from the continued restoration of the mother's body. The trend toward earlier discharge means that some women may go home without their postbirthing needs being fully met (Williams, 1993). Many parents have limited contact with health providers following discharge, although they are contending with major changes and adjustments in what is often a new experience in their lives. Parents may find the first few weeks at home characterized by a disorganized household and greatly increased work related to diapers, feeding, and care of the newborn. The mother usually is coping with fatigue and physical discomforts and may feel frustrated trying to learn the newborn's patterns and ways of communicating.

Nursing Assessment

The new mother experiences a wide range of concerns in the first weeks postpartum. The most common concerns include changes in her figure, fatigue and lack of sleep, dealing with emotional changes related to hormones, newborn care and feeding, and changing roles and lifestyles. The nurse assesses the mother's and family's concerns and responses.

Changes in Body Image and Marital Relationship

A major concern and source of anxiety for the new mother is the return of her figure to normal. Although new mothers are initially delighted with their abdomen's decrease in size after delivery, this positive feeling turns to dismay when the abdominal wall remains soft and flabby and part of the weight gained during pregnancy is retained, making it impossible to wear clothes that fit before pregnancy. Frequently, the mother feels as though she is still several months pregnant.

Although mothers may want to lose weight and tighten up muscles, they often find that the newborn's demands and their own fatigue interfere with these attempts. A flabby postpartum figure and feeling unable to improve it can be depressing. The mother's partner is often disappointed because of the time it takes for the mother's figure to become slim. Both partners may fear that the figure changes are permanent.

Persistent discomforts from episiotomy pain, which may last 2 to 3 weeks; breast engorgement and nipple soreness; continued lochial discharge; fatigue; and the annoyance of leaking milk can decrease energy and affect the couple's relationship. Another concern is the lack of vaginal tone, which may affect the couple's sexual relationship (see Assessment Tool: Sexual History During Postpartum).

Fatigue and Lack of Sleep

Women have a deficit of energy and sleep postpartum due to the exhausting work of childbirth, the short hospital stay, poor sleep quality in the last weeks of pregnancy, and attending immediately to the needs of a newborn. Mulligan reports that fatigue is a major complaint of new mothers through 4 months postpartum and that mothers who have had cesarean deliveries experience greater fatigue than those who delivered vaginally (Mulligan et al., 1994). Gardner reports that fatigue levels increase by 2 weeks postpartum and decline by 6 weeks (Gardner et al., 1991).

To some degree sleep deprivation is a part of living for all new mothers, and it can be severe. The mother's sleep needs are curtailed by the newborn's needs for food and attention. It may be difficult for new mothers to obtain more than 30 to 45 minutes of uninterrupted sleep per night, particularly if other small children frequently need attention. Increased body tension as a result can lead to insomnia when there is the opportunity to sleep. Sleep deprivation can produce changes in mood and mental functioning, with the parents experiencing increased anxiety, irritability, illogical thought patterns, and mental confusion.

Newborn Care

Newborn behavior patterns vary, and parents must learn their newborn's particular patterns and ways of

(*text continues on page 686*)

NURSING CARE PLAN
Postpartum Care

Nursing Goals
The woman and family will experience a normal postpartum course that includes:
1. Normal progress of involution.
2. Effective healing and restoration of usual body functions.
3. Prevention or minimization of complications.
4. Optimal comfort, balanced rest and activity.
5. Appropriate nourishment for lactation and restoration.
6. Development of knowledge and skills for self and infant care.
7. Understanding of physiological and emotional changes.
8. Family adaptation and integration of the infant.

Assessment	Potential Nursing Diagnoses	Interventions/ Rationale	Evaluation
Physiologic Adaptations			
Conditions of fundus, lochia, vital signs, perineum Bladder and intestinal elimination Breasts and lactation Lower extremities Afterpains, perineal pain Ambulation and rest	Risk for Injury: uterine atony, hemorrhage, hematoma Fluid Volume Deficit related to excessive blood loss	Monitor vital signs, condition of fundus and perineum, and bleeding at scheduled frequencies *to identify if the client is bleeding.* Begin fundal message for atony, heavy bleeding *to firm the uterine muscle and stop hemorrhage.* Initiate emergency measures *to stop hemorrhage.*	Fundus contracted, lochia moderate, vital signs stable, perineum intact
	Altered Patterns of Urinary Elimination: urinary retention	Assess bladder regularly; encourage first void in 6–8 h; measure for adequacy; perform catheterization if indicated. *These steps prevent urinary retention and uterine atony.*	Voids within 6–8 h, adequate amount; continues urinary elimination without problems
	Constipation	Encourage fluids and roughage; assess for bowel sounds; administer stool softeners or laxatives *to aid ease of bowel evacuation.*	Bowel movement in 2–3 d, without significant discomfort
	Pain related to perineal trauma, engorgement	Apply comfort measures for pain (sitz baths, perineal care, ice packs, heat lamp, breast expression); administer pain medications *to reduce pain and discomfort.*	Adequate relief or absence of afterpains, perineal pain
	Impaired Skin Integrity: episiotomy, lacerations, nipple fissures Risk for Infection: mastitis, endometritis, cystitis	Monitor skin integrity; use preventive measures (nipple shield, cleansing, proper hygiene); teach infection prevention *to aid healing and prevent skin breakdown and infection.*	Skin intact; healing; no infection

(continued)

NURSING CARE PLAN *(Continued)*
Postpartum Care

Assessment	Potential Nursing Diagnoses	Interventions/ Rationale	Evaluation
Physiologic Adaptations		Identify and report early signs of infection *to start medical regimen for treatment*.	
	Altered Nutrition: Less than body requirements for lactation	Encourage frequent, nutritious meals and snacks, beverages; teach need for adequate nutrition *to meet body's caloric needs*.	Caloric intake correct for bodily needs; no excess weight loss or gain
	Risk for Injury: thrombophlebitis	Monitor condition of extremities *to identify signs and symptoms of thrombophlebitis*. Encourage ambulation *to reduce risk of developing condition*. Report early signs so medical treatment may start.	No signs of thrombophlebitis in legs
	Health Seeking Behaviors related to postpartum recovery	Explain physiologic changes; teach comfort measure techniques, infection prevention, and need for nutrition, activity, and rest *to promote and maintain health*.	Completes return demonstrations or states she understands information
Self-Care and Newborn Care Mother–newborn interactions Newborn caretaking knowledge and skills Self-care knowledge and skills Nutrition and hydration Understanding of physiologic and psychological changes Knowledge of signs of postpartum complications	Alterations in parenting related to fatigue, disappointment with newborn, feelings of incompetence Anxiety related to mother's or newborn's condition, parenting responsibilities, family adaptations	Encourage expression of feelings about newborn; promote rest; assist to acquire parenting skills *to enhance parenting skills*. Explain mother–newborn condition; reassure as appropriate; listen empathetically; teach and explore coping with caretaking and family adaptations *to reduce anxiety*.	Interacts frequently and affectionately with newborn; begins to identify behavior patterns, characteristics Performs newborn caretaking appropriately (bathing, feeding, diapering, handling, comforting)
	Self Esteem Disturbance related to body changes Situational Low Self Esteem: knowledge deficits, altered body image, emotional changes, role changes Knowledge Deficits: postpartal processes, self and newborn care, health maintenance, prevention of complications	Explain expected recovery of body shape and tone, self-care to aid recovery; teach parenting skills *to help mother be realistic with her expectations*. Provide information *to increase knowledge;* listen and discuss feelings; help normalize experiences; provide anticipatory guidance; provide information *to reduce specific deficits*.	Performs self-care appropriately (perineal care, sitz bath, heat lamp, perineal pad placement and removal, breast care, bathing) Mother's intake of nutrients and fluids adequate; hunger satisfied, reports feeling replenished Expresses understanding and acceptance of postpartum changes

(continued)

NURSING CARE PLAN *(Continued)*
Postpartum Care

Assessment	Potential Nursing Diagnoses	Interventions/ Rationale	Evaluation
Self-Care and Newborn Care			
	Bathing/Hygiene Self Care Deficit related to knowledge deficits, altered functional status	Assist with bathing and hygiene initially; encourage self-care when able *to promote comfort and good hygiene.*	Describes danger signs for postpartum complications, what to do if these occur
	Health Seeking Behaviors related to competence in self-care and newborn care, early identification of complications	Support and acknowledge development of competence in self-care and newborn care *to enhance positive self-esteem in the new role.* Teach and review danger signs to report immediately *to prevent further complications and to ensure prompt medical treatment.*	States plans for postpartum follow-up visit after discharge
Family Adaptation Planning for newborn care at home Integrating newborn into family Resources for assistance with home, newborn, child care Parents' reactions to newborn, caretaking Knowledge and concerns about sexuality Contraceptive needs and preferences Relationship between parents	Family Coping: Potential for Growth by integrating newborn Altered Parenting related to home and newborn care stresses Altered Family Processes related to stress of childbirth, newborn care, role and lifestyle changes	Support family incorporation of newborn through frequent parental caretaking and interaction *to enhance family coping.* Assist parents to identify stresses when newborn is home; develop plans for coping using available resources *to enhance parenting skills and family processes.*	Describe realistic plans for newborn care at home, have made appropriate preparations Interact positively with newborn, discuss changes in family structure and functioning with acceptance, no major problems
	Ineffective Individual Coping related to responses to family stresses, adjustment difficulties	Identify ineffective individual coping; provide teaching and support for more effective responses; refer if severe *to enhance individual coping.*	Reactions to newborn caretaking: effective coping, realistic understanding of stresses, concrete plans for dealing with difficulties Relationship between parents, mutually caring and supportive (within cultural contexts); no significant conflicts/ problems
	Altered Sexuality Patterns related to postpartum discomforts, decreased sexuality of mother, ineffective coping, fatigue	Teach parents expected alterations in sexuality, factors that affect postpartum sexual expression, when to resume sex *to enhance normalcy of sexual patterns.* Provide information *to reduce specific deficits.*	Express understanding and accepting of altered sexuality during postpartum State intention to use contraceptives, know method and how to use in first few weeks (if desire to avoid pregnancy)

ASSESSMENT TOOL
Sexual History During Postpartum

As part of postpartum nursing assessment, these questions about sexual experiences and concerns can be included. Several can be asked of both partners, and joint history taking is recommended.

1. How do you feel about the changes in appearance and emotions following birth?
2. How do you feel about each other's experience of the birth process?
3. How are you managing with the newborn's care at home?
4. Have you resumed sexual intercourse or other sexual activity?
5. Are you comfortable during intercourse, and has the episiotomy (if present) healed?
6. Do you have adequate vaginal lubrication during intercourse?
7. If breast-feeding, has this altered your sexual experiences or your relationship with your partner?
8. Are you using contraception? If not, are you concerned about getting pregnant again?
9. How has the newborn affected your sexual relationship and experiences?

communicating. Mothers are concerned about how normal these behaviors are, especially regarding weight gain, crying, bowel movements, feeding, and sleep patterns. Further confusion results from conflicting advice given to them about newborn care (eg, frequency of feedings, when to add solid foods, when to pick up a crying baby, dressing baby, who should visit).

The way a mother perceives and relates to her newborn has an impact on the child's subsequent growth and development and reflects the mother's satisfaction with her interaction with the newborn. If she feels satisfied, she has a more positive perception of the newborn and reinforcement of her own identity as a mother. This fosters a nurturing relationship.

About 25% to 30% of women who are breast-feeding when discharged have weaned their babies to a bottle by 1 month postpartum. The use of bottle supplementation in the hospital and lower satisfaction with breast-feeding are associated with problems in the early postpartum period (Kearney et al., 1990). Breast-feeding for more than 13 weeks has a protective effect against gastrointestinal and respiratory infections in the newborn (Howie et al., 1990).

Changing Roles and Lifestyles

Parents may not be completely prepared for the amount of adaptation required in their roles, relationships, and lifestyles as the newborn is integrated into the family. Many parents may actually "grieve" over the passing of former life patterns. The mother particularly may have to make major changes in career and other activities, although the gratifications of motherhood may be enough to compensate for these relinquishments. Alterations take place in the family constellation, and problems related to jealousy or rivalry among the other children may occur. Martial problems be-

tween spouses may arise from relative neglect of their relationship. With less time for each other and possible strain on their sexual relations, many couples report stress in their relationship following the birth of a new baby. Social isolation, lack of recreational activities, and financial concerns can compound family stresses.

Whether pregnancy was high risk or low risk, families experience changes in functioning during the transition to parenthood (see Research Highlight). More optimal family functioning appears related to less depression, greater social support, and less stress for negative life events during the year preceding pregnancy. At 8 months after birth, family functioning remains relatively disorganized, and incorporation of the newborn is not yet completely resolved. Among high-risk families, family functioning tends to reach its lowest point by 8 months after birth (Mercer et al., 1990).

Nursing Planning and Interventions

During the third trimester and immediate postpartum period, mothers have an increased interest in caretaking activities. Teaching about newborn care and behaviors is productive at this time. Pertinent topics include preparing other children for the newborn, exploring ways to meet the increased demands of a newborn for attention and continuous care, and considering sources of potential stress to the marital and family relations and ways of coping with these problems.

Reinforcing the importance of help with household tasks during the first few postpartum weeks at home may encourage the mother to make arrangements. This can help to alleviate fatigue and sleep deprivation. The mother will be more realistic in her expectations when she knows she will need time to regain her prepreg-

Family Functioning in the Months After Birth

The family undergoes significant adjustments after childbirth, with changes in its functional abilities. In addition to the stress posed by childbirth, other stresses can affect family functioning during the postpartum period. Negative life events and life changes have an impact on mental and physical health and predict postpartum illness and depression. Postpartum depression is associated with marital problems, less supportive spouses, and disrupted family relationships. Family dysfunction is related to abusive behavior and has negative effects on children's intellectual and language development. Greater social support and individual coping resources appear to mediate the effects of stress.

The study tested a theoretical causal model to determine the effects of stress on family functioning among low- and high-risk families for 8 months after birth. A group of well-tested instruments was used to measure some demographic variables and the variables of anxiety, depression, family functioning, stress from negative life events during the prior year, stress from childbearing risks, self-esteem, perception of health status, social support, sense of mastery, and parental competence.

The design was a comparative, longitudinal study with a sample of 593 subjects (parental pairs) recruited at 24 to 34 weeks of pregnancy; they were 18 years or older, fluent in English, and either married or planning to parent together. There were slightly more subjects in the low- than high-risk groups; 70% were white; most nonwhite were Asian and Hispanic. More than half were professionals, with 15% having unskilled or semiskilled positions. The study attrition rate was 40% over 1 year.

Data from the study support the concept that families, whether high or low risk, experience change in functioning during the transition to parenthood. Women and men from the low-risk group perceived family functioning as significantly less optimal at 8 months, indicating that family disorganization after birth and incorporation of the infant into the family were still unresolved. High-risk groups had reported less optimal family functioning during pregnancy, and this became worse postpartum.

Depression was the major explanatory variable in predicting reduced family functioning in high- and low-risk groups. Among high-risk women, more optimal family functioning was related to less depression, greater perceived support, less stress from negative life events, being younger, having more close friends, and being married. Among low-risk women, this was related to less depression, greater social support, less stress from negative life events, and lower parent–newborn attachment. This latter factor may indicate a relatively closer husband–wife relationship.

Among high-risk men, their own anxiety state and the stress of the partner's high-risk pregnancy were most predictive of decreased family functioning. It was hypothesized that the mother's involvement with a high-risk infant could have deprived the father of support she usually might offer. Better family functioning was associated among high-risk men with support at 1 month after birth, having medical treatment for a health problem during the pregnancy, and childhood relationships with their fathers. These men did not perceive as much decrease in family functioning as their partners. This might be due to changes in the mate relationship that is felt more acutely by the woman.

The theoretical model tested was supported better for the two groups of women than for the men. Stress from negative life events impacted the women's perceptions of family functioning, as was hypothesized, but not the men's. Social support, commonly identified as a mediator of stress, did fulfill this function for low-risk women only. Less self-esteem and self-mastery were major predictors of depression. Parents who felt good about themselves and in control perceived better postpartum family functioning. About one-fourth of both groups of women exhibited possible clinical depression, which persisted to 8 months after birth.

Critique: This study provides evidence for the importance of nursing care that assists parents to develop a sense of mastery related to self and newborn care. Interventions to support positive self-esteem should be a central focus of postpartum nursing care.

(Mercer, R. T., & Ferketich, S. L. (1990). Predictors of family functioning eight months following birth. *Nursing Research, 39*(2), 76–82.)

nant figure and to regain her energy level. Knowing that physical discomforts will exist for a while after delivery and knowing how to reduce these discomforts will prepare the mother and reduce stress from unrealistic expectations.

Nursing intervention is aimed at increasing the mother's sense of mastery and satisfaction in newborn care, thereby promoting healthier mother–newborn relationships and infant development. Mothers can be assisted to recognize and respond appropriately to their newborn's unique patterns, ways of communicating, and particular needs for stimulation, sleep, and feed-

ing. When able to respond more smoothly to her newborn, the mother's satisfactions are increased, and the development of a healthy relationship is encouraged.

Postpartum follow-up visits and telephone calls by nurses provide teaching and support for the new mother and family.

Evaluation

Nursing care is successful when the mother is able to cope adequately with self-care and newborn care during the first few weeks at home. Family adaptations that provide for the needs of other children, the parents, and the newborn are positive outcomes. The nurse may observe family functioning and maternal-newborn interactions during a home visit or may rely on the mother's reports by telephone or at an office visit. When difficulties arise, families who can identify and use appropriate resources have benefitted from nursing care.

Postpartum Follow-up Visit

A variety of home care and follow-up programs have emerged as "early" discharge has become the norm. However, the necessity of postpartum home care has not yet been validated through careful research analysis (Ghilarducci et al., 1993; Williams et al., 1993); it is also unclear on a national level the role of home follow-up care in maternal-child health services (Arnold et al., 1991).

When planning home follow-up care visits, it is important to have early postpartum contact with visits occurring within a few days of discharge (Arnold et al., 1991). Other visits may occur at intervals as needed during the 6- to 8-week postpartum period. The nursing process is used in home care visits to focus on the progress of involutional changes, the mother's physical condition and recovery, the family's adaptation to the newborn, the parents' sexual relations and need for contraception, and the newborn's growth and development.

Nursing Assessment

During the office follow-up visit, the weight and blood pressure are taken, and a urinalysis and complete blood count may be done (see Nursing Guidelines: Postpartum Follow-Up Visit). The condition of the abdominal wall is observed, and the breasts are inspected. If the mother is breast-feeding, the condition of the nipples and the degree of lacteal secretion are observed. If the mother is not breast-feeding, the breasts should be observed to see that lactation suppression has occurred.

A pelvic examination may be done to determine the condition of the uterus, the healing of the episiotomy or perineal lacerations, the tone of the pelvic floor muscles, and whether involution is complete. The presence, amount, and character of lochia are assessed. Questions about physiologic status are elicited and discussed. The newborn is assessed, and blood tests (bilirubin, phenylketonuria, screen for inborn errors of metabolism) may be obtained. The family's response to the newborn is discussed, and questions related to behavior, patterns of feeding, sleep and

> **NURSING GUIDELINES**
> *Postpartum Follow-up Visit*
>
> **Involution Status**
>
> Vital signs and weight
> Perineal examination
> Amount and character of lochia
> Condition of episiotomy or lacerations
> Condition of anus, hemorrhoids
> Pelvic examination
> Size and position of uterus and cervix
> Condition of vagina (musculature, lacerations)
> Pap smear
> Breast examination
> Condition of breasts and nipples
> Lactating or lactation suppression
>
> **Infant Development and Care**
>
> Growth and development of infant
> Infant behavior
> Patterns of feeding, sleep, and elimination
> Crying
> Weight gain
> Family response to newborn
> Reactions of siblings
> Relatives' and friends' visits or assistance
> Mother's response to caretaking, feeding, and reactions of others
>
> **Physical Recovery**
>
> Mother's physical condition and recovery
> Rest and exercise
> Weight loss
> Diet
> Energy level
> Recreation and activities
> Returning to work
> Physical discomforts and remedies
>
> **Sexuality and Contraception**
>
> Sexual relations
> Resumption of intercourse
> Concerns or difficulties
> Responses of mother and father
> Contraception
> Current contraceptive practice (if any)
> Desires for regulating fertility and family planning
> Contraceptive method selection and teaching

elimination, crying, weight gain, and so forth are explored (see Nursing Care Plan).

Nursing Planning and Intervention

Problems with healing or infection are treated, if present, and arrangements are made for further examinations and treatments as necessary. This return examination provides an opportunity to discuss any other problems or concerns relating to the birth experience. The mother's concerns about rest and exercise, weight, diet, her energy level, household tasks, relations with relatives and friends, sexual relations, and physical needs or discomforts are discussed. If weight continues to be a problem, a suitable weight reduction diet and exercise program can be started. If desired, the woman can resume full employment or activities at this time, if there are no complications and she feels psychologically ready. The need for further care or referrals is identified.

Contraception is discussed at this visit, and a suitable method is chosen if the parents wish to prevent another pregnancy. The method is instituted at this time, and the couple is instructed in its use and risks (see Chap. 9).

Evaluation

The effectiveness of nursing care is determined by outcomes for the mother and family. Physiologic outcomes, such as normal progression of lochia and healing of the episiotomy, can be observed. Satisfactory interaction between mother and newborn and development of mothering abilities signify effective outcomes in mother–newborn relationships. The mother, father, and family may describe effective adaptation to the newborn; new routines are developed and stabilized. Referrals and other sources of assistance are used and provide effective help. The mother and family believe their questions have been answered and feel capable of managing their new family processes.

Summary Points

✔ Although the postpartum period seems anticlimactic to the actual birth experience, women face major changes and adjustments that often leave them overwhelmed, fatigued, and frustrated. Nurses provide women and new families with expert knowledge, skills, and support, thus enhancing a smoother transition into the postpartum period.

✔ Assessment of fundal height and consistency and lochia changes provides information about uterine involution. Assessing for hemorrhage, bladder distention, infection, and psychosocial adaptations are key aspects of postpartum care.

✔ Cultural components and previous parenting experience must be identified and incorporated into the postpartum plan of care.

✔ Maternal discomforts arise from perineal sources (episiotomy, laceration, edema, hematoma), breasts (nipple soreness, engorgement), uterine cramping (afterpains), incisional pain, hemorrhoids, backache, and fatigue.

✔ Nursing care emphasizes monitoring physiologic, psychosocial, and family adaptations; providing rest

and comfort; supporting breast-feeding efforts; identifying and meeting educational needs; listening to the woman discuss and relive her birth experience; and providing immunizations (rubella vaccine, Rho [D] immune globin).

✔ Lactation suppression can be achieved with mechanical means (ice packs, brassiere, binder) or with medications, such as bromocriptine.

✔ Sexual intercourse may resume when lochia has ceased, the perineum is healed such that intercourse is not painful, and there are no contraindications, such as infection.

✔ Discharge from the hospital or birth center should not occur until the woman can demonstrate self-care measures and basic newborn care. Follow-up home visits and telephone calls provide additional support and teaching.

✔ Postpartum office visits are scheduled in 6 weeks after delivery to assess involution, physiologic restoration, newborn feeding and development, the family's adaptation, and contraception needs.

REFERENCES

Arnold, L. S., & Bakewell-Sach, S. (1991). Models of perinatal home follow-up. *Journal of perinatal and Neonatal Nursing, 5*(1), 18–26.

Beachy, P., & Deacon, J. (1992). Preventing neonatal kidnapping. *Journal of Obstetric, Gynecologic, and Neonatal Nursing, 21*(1), 12–16.

Beck, C. T. (1992). The lived experience of postpartum depression: A phenomenological study. *Nursing Research, 41*(3), 166–170.

Bernstein, G. L., & Kidd, Y. A. (1982). Childbearing in Japan. In M. A. Kay (Ed.), *Anthology of human birth.* Philadelphia: F.A. Davis.

Bond, L. (1993). Physiological changes. In S. Mattson & J. E. Smith (Eds.), *AWHONN: Core curriculum for maternal-newborn nursing.* Philadelphia: W.B. Saunders.

Cunningham, F. G., MacDonald, P. C., Gant, N. F., Leveno, K. J., & Gillstrap III, L. C. (1993). *Williams obstetrics* (19th ed.). Norwalk, CT: Appleton & Lange.

D'Avanzo, C. E. (1992). Bridging the gap with the southeast Asians. *American Journal of Maternal-Child Nursing, 17*(4), 104–208.

Davis, J., Brucker, M., & MacMullen, N. (1985). A study of mother's postpartum teaching priorities. *Maternal-Child Nursing Journal, 15,* 41–51.

Dunnihoo, D. R. (1992). *Fundamentals of gynecology and obstetrices,* 2nd edition. Philadelphia: J. B. Lippincott.

Gardner, D. L., & Campbell, B. (1991). Assessing postpartum fatigue. *American Journal of Maternal-Child Nursing, 16*(5), 264–266.

Ghilarducci, E., & McCool, W. (1993). The influence of home visits on clinic attendance. *Journal of Nursing-Midwifery, 38*(3), 152–158.

Gutierrez, Y. M. (1994). *Nutrition in health maintenance and health promotion.* Department of Family Health Care Nursing, VCSF School of Nursing, San Francisco.

Howard, C. R., & Howard, F. M. (1994). Infant formula distribution and advertising in pregnancy: A hospital study. *Birth, 21*(1), 14–19.

Howie, P. W., Forsyth, J. S., Ogston, S. A. et al. (1990). Protective effect of breast feeding against infection. *British Medical Journal, 300*(11).

Jacobson, J. (1985). A standard for assessing lochia volume. *American Journal of Maternal-Child Nursing, 10*(3), 174–175.

Kearney, M. H., Cronenwett, L. R., & Barrett, J. A. (1990). Breastfeeding problems inthe first week postpartum. *Nursing Research, 39*(2), 90–95.

Kunst-Wilson, W., & Cronenwett, L. R. (1981). Nursing care for the emerging family: Promoting paternal behavior. *Research in Nursing and Health, 4*(1), 201.

Luegenbiehl, D. L., Brophy, G. H., Artigue, G. S., & Phillips, K. E. (1990). Standardized assessment of blood loss. *American Journal of Maternal-Child Nursing, 15*(4), 241–244.

McGregor, L. A. (1994). Short, shorter, shortest: Improving the hospital stay for mothers and newborns. *American Journal of Maternal-Child Nursing, 19*(2), 91–96.

Mercer, T., & Ferketich, S. L. (1990). Predictors of family functioning eight months following birth. *Nursing Research, 39*(2), 76–82.

Monrroy, L. (1983). Nursing care of Raza/Latina patients. In M. Orque, B. Bloch, & L. Monrroy (Eds.), *Ethnic nursing care*. St. Louis: C.V. Mosby.

Mulligan, R. A., Pugh, L. C. (1994). Fatigue during childbearing period. In J. J. Fitzpatrick, J. S. Stevenson (Eds.). *Annual Review of Nursing Research, 12,* 33–49. NY: Springer Publishing.

Pillsbury, B. (1982). Doing the month: Confinement and convalescence of Chinese women after childbirth. In M. A. Kay (Ed.), *Anthropology of human birth*. Philadelphia: F.A. Davis.

Rhode, M. A., Barger, M. K. (1990). Perineal care: Then and now. *Journal of Nurse-Midwifery, 35*(4), 220–229.

Rutledge, D. L., & Pridham, K. F. K. (1987). Postpartum mother's perceptions of competence for infant care. *Journal of Obstetric, Gynecologic, and Neonatal Nursing, 16*(3), 185–194.

Samselle, C. M., & Brink, C. A. (1990). Pelvic muscle relaxation: Assessment and management. *Journal of Nurse-Midwifery, 35*(3), 127–132.

Simkin, P. (1992). Just another day in a woman's life? Part II: Nature and consistency of women's long-term memories of the first birth experience. *Birth, 19*(2), 64–81.

Tulman, L., Fawcet, J., Groblewski, L., & Silverman, L. (1990). Changes in functional status after childbirth. *Nursing Research, 39*(2), 70–75.

Turner, R. J., & Avison, W. R. (1985). Assessing risk factors for problem parenting: The significance of social support. *Journal of Marriage and Family, 47,* 881.

Way, L. W. (1994). *Current surgical diagnosis and treatment,* 10th edition. Norwalk, CT: Appleton & Lange.

Williams, L. R., & Cooper, M. K. (1993). Nurse-managed postpartum home care. *Journal of Obstetric, Gynecologic, and Neonatal Nursing, 22*(1), 25–31.

SUGGESTED READING

Atkinson, L. A., & Baxley, E. G. (1994). Postpartum fatigue. *American Family Physician, 50*(1), 113–118.

Collins, B. A., McCoy, S. A., Sale, S., & Weber, S. E. (1994). Descriptions of comfort by substance-using and nonusing postpartum women. *Journal of Obstetric, Gynecologic, and Neonatal Nursing, 23*(4), 293–300.

Dale, A., & Cornwell, S. (1994). The role of lavendar oil in relieving perineal discomfort following childbirth: A blind randomized clinical study. *Journal of Advanced Nursing, 19*(1), 89.

Donahue, D., Brooten, D., Roncoli, M., Arnold, L., Knapp, H., Borucki, L., & Cohen, A. (1994). Acute care visits and rehospitalization in women and infants after cesarean birth. *Journal of Perinatology, 14*(1), 36–40.

Fawcett, J., Pollio, N., Tully, A., Baron, M., Henklein, J., & Jones, R. C. (1993). Effects of information on adaptation to cesarean birth. *Nursing Research, 42*(1), 49–53.

Lentz, M. J., & Killien, M. G. (1991). Are you sleeping? Sleep patterns during postpartum hospitalization. *Journal of Perinatal and Neonatal Nursing, 4*(4), 30–38.

Ostgaard, H. C., & Anderson, G. B. T. (1992). Postpartum low back pain. *Spine, 17*(1), 53–55.

Thomas, L., Ptak, H., Giddings, L. S., Moore, L., & Oppermann, C. (1990). The effects of rocking, diet modifications, and antiflatulent medications on post cesarean section gas pain. *Journal of Perinatal and Neonatal Nursing, 4*(3), 12–24.

Tomlinson, P. S. (1987). Spousal differences in marital satisfaction during transition to parenthood. *Nursing Research, 36,* 239–243.

Walker, L. O. (1989). Stress process among mothers of infants: Preliminary model testing. *Nursing Research, 38*(1), 10–15.

Wilkerson, M. N., & Barrows, T. L. (1988). Synchronizing care with mother-baby rhythms. *American Journal of Maternal-Child Nursing, 13,* 264–269.

28

Assessment of the Newborn

Objectives

- Describe the physiologic changes that occur in the newborn during the transition period in the first few days of life.
- Discuss the importance of these changes and any deviations for the newborn's successful transition to extrauterine life.
- Describe the components and expected physical findings of a complete newborn physical assessment.
- Describe the expected findings of a neurologic assessment of the newborn regarding reflexes and other indicators of nervous system functioning.
- Identify physical characteristics used to determine gestational age.
- Discuss the usefulness to nurses of the assessment of behavioral states and responses of the newborn.

Key Terms

Apnea	Red reflex
Bilirubinometer	Respiratory acidosis
Brown fat	Rooting reflex
Grasp reflex	Scarf sign
Lanugo	Startle reflex
Meconium	Stepping reflex
Moro reflex	Sucking reflex
Neonatal Behavioral	Tonic neck reflex
Assessment Scale	Transitional
Periodic breathing	circulation
Periods of reactivity	Vernix caseosa
Physiologic	Witch's milk
jaundice	

In the immediate hours and days following birth, profound physiologic changes, critical for health and survival, occur in the newborn. In addition to these physiologic changes, the newborn must adapt in many different ways to a completely new environment. Therefore, knowledge of the physiologic basis for assessment and a complete assessment of the newborn during the initial hours and days following birth are crucial. A complete assessment will encompass several different areas that may overlap. These areas include physical, neurologic, gestational age, and behavioral assessment. Frequent physical assessments should be performed while the newborn is in the hospital or birth center. These are critical for determining if and how well the newborn is coping with the physiologic transition from intrauterine to extrauterine life. In addition, neurologic, gestational age, and behavioral assessments should be performed before the newborn leaves the hospital so that any actual or potential problems in these areas are discovered as early in the newborn's life as possible.

Registered nurses typically have the closest contact with newborns during the initial hours after birth. They are usually responsible for performing some or all of the newborn assessments. Therefore, nurses must possess the knowledge and skills necessary to evaluate comprehensively the newborn's status. Accurate early assessment is important due to the limited amount of time the newborn will remain in the hospital or birth center. During the time available, another important aspect of nursing care includes teaching the parents what to watch for throughout the first few days of their newborn's life.

Physiologic Basis for Assessment

As stated previously, the newborn undergoes profound physiologic changes. These complex changes must occur in an appropriate time frame for the newborn to survive and develop normally. The newborn passes through several phases during the adaptation to extrauterine life. Transition begins with labor when the fetus is stimulated by uterine contractions and pressure changes as a result of the rupture of the membranes. At birth, breathing must begin. This initiates profound changes and reorganization in the functioning of the organ systems and metabolic processes. Significant changes occur in the following areas:

- Respiration
- Circulation
- Immune system
- Temperature regulation: metabolism
- Neurologic system
- Gastrointestinal system
- Kidney function and urinary excretion
- Hepatic function

The final phase of the transition involves further reorganization of the metabolic processes to achieve a viable, steady state. This includes changes in blood oxygen saturation, reduction of enzymes, diminution in postnatal acidosis, and recovery of the neurologic tissues from the trauma of labor and delivery.

Respiratory Changes

Prior to birth, the oxygen needs of the fetus are met by the placenta; therefore, the fetal lungs do not need to function as organs of respiration. However, it has been confirmed in recent years that respiratory-like movements do occur. This "fetal breathing" may aid in the development of alveolar and bronchial structures and serve as practice for later breathing. Assessment of the frequency and character of fetal breathing contributes data about fetal well-being (Korones, 1986).

For the newborn to survive extrauterine life, adequate maturation of the lungs is essential. The lungs are in a continuous state of structural development throughout fetal life and early childhood. Canals begin to develop in the bronchial tree around the 17th week of gestation, and soon after, primitive air sacs begin to form. By 24 to 26 weeks' gestation, there is adequate vascularization and development of respiratory sacules. At this point, gas exchange is possible, and therefore independent survival also is possible. However, surface-active lipoproteins (surfactant) are not available at this time, and there is limited development of alveoli. Therefore, the fetus born this early is at high risk for respiratory problems and chances for long-term survival are decreased (Jobe, 1992). (See Chap. 41 for a discussion of respiratory problems in the preterm newborn.)

The normal, full-term fetus is ready to initiate effective breathing at the time of birth. Fetal respiratory movements have prepared the lungs for this activity, and the complex inter-relationships of swallowing and breathing have been developed. Although the fetus is prepared to breathe, it does not. Suggestions have been made as to why the fetus does not take real breaths before it is born. Inhibitory mechanisms have been identified in animal research and include facial immersion and the presence of fluid in the laryngeal area. It is important to clear fluid from the newborn's laryngeal area after birth to remove this inhibitory factor. Another suggestion for inhibition of "real" breathing in the fetus is that the fluid secreted by the alveolar cells in the deep respiratory tract, with which the fetal lungs are constantly filled, stimulates inhibitory stretch receptors.

Initiation of Respiration

Many factors are probably involved in stimulating the newborn's initial respirations. This would provide a margin of safety for the newborn. Physical, sensory, and chemical factors are involved, but it is not known precisely how each of these influences the other and to what degree. Some evidence suggests that the change in pressure from intrauterine to extrauterine life may produce enough physical stimulation to prompt respiration.

Cold, pain, touch, light, sound, and gravity are thought to play a role in initiation of respiration. Of these sensory stimuli, cold seems to play the most significant role. In animal studies, cold stimulation has induced breathing in fetal sheep (Korones, 1986). This does not mean that the newborn needs to be in a cold environment. Normal room air temperature is about 22°C (72°F). This is a decrease of more than 15°C (25°F) from the fetus' environmental temperature in utero. This 15°C drop in temperature may be sufficient to stimulate respiration.

Chemical changes that occur in the blood as a result of transient asphyxia during delivery also are powerful stimuli for the first breath. The changes include a lowered oxygen level, increased carbon dioxide level, and lowered pH, indicating **respiratory acidosis**. This presumably normal condition is characterized by the absence of metabolic acidosis. A vigorous newborn usually breathes within seconds and certainly within 1 minute after birth. If the asphyxia is prolonged, metabolic acidosis develops, depression (rather than stimulation) of the respiratory center occurs, and resuscitation is usually necessary (see Chap. 41) (Korones, 1986).

The newborn must put forth great effort to expand the lungs and fill the partially collapsed, fluid-filled alveoli. Surface tension in the respiratory tract and resistance in the lung tissue, thorax, diaphragm, and respiratory muscles must be overcome. In addition, any obstruction (eg, mucus) in the air passages must be cleared. The first active inspiration results from a powerful contraction of the diaphragm. This creates a high negative intrathoracic pressure, causing a marked retraction of the ribs because of the pliability of the newborn's thorax.

This first inspiration distends the alveolar spaces, replacing the fluid. On expiration, a residual volume of nearly 20 mL of air remains as molecules of pulmonary surfactant diminish surface tension. This allows for the second breath to occur with less effort. By this point, most of the small airways are open, and the third breath will occur with minimal effort. After several minutes of breathing, lung expansion is usually complete. Absorption of fluid from the lungs by drainage, swallowing, evaporation, and pulmonary, capillary, and lymphatic circulation is usually accomplished in the first hour (Nelson, 1992).

Characteristics of Neonatal Breathing

The first hour or so after birth has been described as the first period of reactivity (see the section entitled, "Behavioral Assessment"). At this time, respiration is rapid (reaching as high as 80 breaths per minute), and there may be transient flaring of the nostrils, retraction of the chest, and grunting. After this period, the neonatal respiratory rate usually ranges between 30 and 60 breaths per minute but continues to be irregular in rate and depth. Up to 20-second pauses in respiratory movement also may occur. This **periodic breathing** is normal. However, pauses of more than 20 seconds are considered **apnea** and are cause for concern (Rigatto, 1992).

Circulatory Changes

The anatomic changes that occur at birth are discussed in Chapter 7. The changes are rapid and consist of closure of several fetal structures and the redistribution of oxygenated blood to a circulation similar to that of an adult. Because all changes are not immediately complete, this time of conversion is called a period of **transitional circulation**.

Total Blood Volume

It is difficult to give accurate values for the total blood volume of the newborn because of the variables involved. These variables include time of clamping the umbilical cord, weight and gestational age of the newborn, type of delivery (vaginal or cesarean), and time after delivery the determination is made. Early or late clamping of the umbilical cord after delivery has been the subject of much study because when the cord is clamped may significantly influence the newborn's physiologic status.

For example, an additional 50 to 100 mL of blood may be added to the circulation if the newborn is placed below the level of the placenta and the clamping of the cord is delayed several minutes until the cord stops pulsating. It is unclear whether this placental transfusion that occurs with late clamping is advantageous for the newborn. The rapid increase in blood volume might stress the heart and pulmonary vasculature. However, according to some reports, the incidence of neonatal respiratory distress is decreased with delayed clamping (Shurin, 1992). Newborns who receive extra blood gain an increased storage supply of iron, resulting from the breakdown of the additional hemoglobin. This may contribute to hyperbilirubinemia during the first week of life. On the other hand, the extra iron stores may be used to good advantage later when iron is needed for rapid growth or when the dietary intake of iron is inadequate (Shurin, 1992).

Peripheral Circulation

Peripheral circulation in the newborn is somewhat sluggish. This may account for residual cyanosis of the newborn's hands, feet, and circumoral area. These areas often remain mildly cyanotic for 1 or 2 hours after delivery. The general circulatory lability probably accounts for the mottled appearance of the newborn's skin when it is exposed to air and for the "chilliness" of the newborn's hands and feet.

Pulse Rate

The pulse rate tends to be unstable and follows a pattern similar to that of respiration. When the respiration is rapid, the pulse tends to be rapid; similarly, when the respiration slows down, so does the pulse. Because the pulse is affected by internal and external stimuli, taking the *apical* pulse rate while the newborn is quiet provides a more accurate evaluation of the heart rate. The normal pulse rate is usually between 120 and 150 beats/min. Crying and intense activity may elevate the rate to 180 beats/min for short periods. During deep sleep, the rate may drop to 100 beats/min.

Blood Pressure

Accurate noninvasive assessment of arterial blood pressure is difficult in the newborn. Auscultation, palpation, and the color change (flush) method usually result in an imprecise systolic or (mean) pressure. Therefore, blood pressure has not always been checked routinely in the normal newborn. Invasive methods using an arterial catheter for direct recording of the blood pressure are usually limited to the sick newborn who has an arterial line in place for other reasons (see Chap. 41). However, the advent of the Doppler reflected ultrasound technique has made the estimation of systemic blood pressure more accurate, and taking the blood pressure is becoming a routine procedure in many normal newborn nurseries.

Blood pressure in the newborn is characteristically low, averaging 71/49 mm Hg at birth and rising slowly during the first week. Pressure varies according to the size and activity of the newborn. A small, preterm newborn will have a lower average, while a crying, active newborn will have a higher average. Causes for concern and further investigation in the term neonate include diastolic pressures lower than 25 mm Hg or higher than 60 mm Hg, and mean pressures of less than 30 mm Hg or greater than 70 mm Hg (Cabal et al., 1992).

Erythrocyte Count and Hemoglobin Concentration

The newborn has much higher erythrocyte, hemoglobin, and hematocrit levels than the adult. The erythrocyte level ranges between 5 million and 7 million/μl, the hemoglobin level is usually 15 to 20 g/dL of blood, and the hematocrit values average about 55% (Shurin, 1992). The following factors influence these values:

- Duration of gestation—During the final weeks of intrauterine life, hemoglobin concentration increases rapidly. The preterm newborn does not benefit from this increase and has a low concentration compared with the full-term newborn.
- Time of cord clamping—In newborns who receive additional blood as a result of delayed cord clamping, increased hemoglobin and hematocrit levels can be demonstrated for at least 3 or 4 days.
- Site of blood sample—In the first week of life, capillary blood samples usually show markedly higher hemoglobin and hematocrit values than venous samples drawn at the same time. This is due to peripheral venous stasis. Venous blood samples are considered to be more accurate. If only heel sticks are used for assessing blood values, anemia could go undetected. Warming the newborn's heel before the stick is suggested as a way to decrease the difference between the two values (Shurin, 1992).

Higher blood values are needed by the fetus in utero for adequate oxygenation. After birth, the need no longer exists because the lungs are functioning, so a gradual decrease takes place. Immediately after birth, the erythrocyte count is increased from cord blood levels because of a decrease in plasma volume. This reaches a maximum level 2 to 6 hours after birth. It then decreases to cord blood levels when the newborn is about 1 week old. Red blood cell production (erythropoiesis) is suppressed for several months after birth, and this, added to the increased blood volume caused by the newborn's rapid growth, results in a progressive decline in the hemoglobin concentration. A low point of 11 g/dL (±2.0) may be reached after 2 to 3 months. This may produce physiologic anemia that does not represent any abnormality or nutritional deficiency in the newborn and is not affected by giving iron or other hematinics. Active erythropoiesis resumes about this time, and if the iron supply is adequate, the hemoglobin concentration gradually increases to an average of 12.5 g/dL, where it stays during early childhood (Shurin, 1992).

Physiologic Jaundice

In the newborn period, the serum concentration of unconjugated bilirubin increases from approximately 2 mg/dL in cord blood to a mean peak of 6 mg/dL between 60 and 72 hours of age. This is usually followed by a rapid decline to 2 mg/dL by the fifth day of life and a slower decline to normal adult levels of less than 1 mg/dL by about the 10th day. Jaundice is the visible evidence of the rise in serum concentration of unconjugated bilirubin to levels of 5 to 7 mg/dL or above (Gartner et al., 1992). Approximately 40% to 60% of full-term newborns (and a higher number of preterm newborns) develop jaundice between the second and fourth days of life. In the absence of disease or specific causes, this has been called **physiologic jaundice**. Bilirubin levels greater than 5 mg/dL (or the appearance of jaundice) during the first 24 hours or bilirubin levels greater than 12 mg/dL at any time indicate that the condition might be pathologic jaundice. Further investigation is required (Gartner et al., 1992). (See Chap. 43 for a discussion of pathologic jaundice and its treatment.)

The etiology of physiologic jaundice is not fully understood. Possible mechanisms in the development of this condition are shown in Table 28-1. There seem to be some genetic and ethnic influences on the incidence of physiologic jaundice. Asian newborns and some other isolated groups have mean maximal serum unconjugated bilirubin levels between 10 and 14 mg/dL, which is approximately double that of non-Asian populations. Kernicterus also is significantly increased in Asian newborns. The increased levels may result from a genetic predisposition to slower maturation of hepatic bilirubin metabolism or a possible relationship to ethnic food or herbal medicines (Gartner et al., 1992).

Nurses should not be lulled into a false sense of security by the term physiologic. Any newborn who develops visible jaundice should be closely watched for symptoms of other potential problems. Parents of newborns who are discharged early should be instructed to observe their newborn for jaundice. If jaundice develops, the mother is usually instructed to bring the newborn in for a blood test. A portable **bilirubinometer** used for noninvasive home testing has been found to be a fairly accurate screening tool (Brucker et al., 1987).

Blood Coagulation

At birth, the vitamin K-dependent blood clotting factors (factors VII, IX, X, and prothrombin) are significantly decreased. The intestinal tract of the newborn does not harbor the bacteria necessary to help synthesize vitamin K. Thus, the newborn has a temporary deficiency in blood coagulation occurring between the second and fifth postnatal days. This deficiency is sometimes severe enough to cause clinical bleeding.

TABLE 28-1
Possible Mechanisms Related to Development of Physiologic Jaundice

Mechanism	Explanation
Increased production of bilirubin	The newborn's high erythrocyte count and shorter mean red blood cell life span lead to an increased breakdown of red blood cells, which contributes to the increased bilirubin load presented to the liver in the first days of life. Bilirubin from other sources, such as myoglobin, a protein found in muscle, also is produced in increased amounts in the newborn.
Decreased clearance of bilirubin by the liver	The unconjugated, fat-soluble form of bilirubin that is produced when hemoglobin is broken down is usually changed in the liver to the conjugated, water-soluble form that can be excreted. In the newborn, there is interference with this conjugation, possibly owing to inhibition of the activity of the enzyme glucuronyl transferase.
Immaturity of the liver	Uptake of bilirubin from the plasma by the liver cells may be decreased because of immaturity of the liver.
Recirculation of increased amounts of bilirubin from the intestine	Because of lack of intestinal bacterial flora in the newborn, bilirubin may be reabsorbed from the intestine and recirculated to the liver, rather than being excreted. Retention of meconium, which has a high bilirubin content, may add to the amount of bilirubin reabsorbed.

As a preventive measure, 0.5 to 1 mg of vitamin K is administered to the newborn during the first day of life (Shurin, 1992).

White Blood Cells

There is a wide range of normal for the leukocyte count at birth; the average is approximately 20,000 cells/μL. Neutrophils comprise about 70% of this total. During the first few days after delivery, there is a considerable decrease in the total count and a shift in the type of predominant cell. The neutrophils decrease, and the lymphocytes increase; by the end of the first week, the lymphocytes predominate and continue to do so until the child is 4 or 5 years old (Shurin, 1992).

Immune System Changes

The immune system begins to develop during fetal life but is still immature at birth. Nonspecific immunity is inadequate and differs in some ways from normal adult cell responses. Rigidity of leukocyte membranes is increased, and complement and bactericidal activity is deficient. The cells' ability to ingest particles (phagocytosis), however, is close to normal adult levels (Shurin, 1992).

Specific immunity also is limited at birth. Development of immunity to specific organisms requires exposure to the antigen by infection or immunization. In addition, the necessary ability to develop antibodies (immunocompetence) develops sequentially, beginning in fetal life and continuing for months or years after birth. Antibody responses of newborns, therefore, are limited compared with those of older children or adults (Yoder et al., 1992). The fetus who develops an infection in utero appears to develop immunoglobulin M (IgM) antibodies against the responsible agents. However, IgA and IgE are seldom found at birth. Some maternal antibodies cross the placenta. IgG is most frequently found, but which IgG antibodies the newborn receives depends on the mother's immune status. This passive immunity is transient. Because IgG has a half life of 20 to 30 days, the concentration falls rapidly and reaches its lowest level between the second and fourth months of life. Passive antibodies from placental transfer may interfere with active antibody formation; thus, early immunization or infection may not result in long-lasting immunity (Bellanti et al., 1994).

Temperature Regulation and Metabolic Changes

The newborn is born into an environment that is considerably cooler than the one encountered in the uterus. Because of this rapid change in environmental conditions, the newborn's temperature may drop several degrees after birth. In recent years, attention has been focused on the negative effects of hypothermia on the newborn. Increasing efforts have been made to prevent this temperature drop in the delivery room and in the nursery. Neonates are predisposed to heat transfer between themselves and the environment because they have a limited supply of subcutaneous fat and a large surface area in relation to body weight.

Heat Loss. Evaporation, conduction, convection, and radiation are four ways in which the newborn can lose body heat to the environment. Excessive loss by *evaporation* occurs most often in the delivery room when the newborn is wet (see Chap. 24), but it also can occur when the newborn is being bathed. Heat loss by evaporation may also occur from the lungs if the newborn has tachypnea or if the humidity is low. Heat loss by *conduction* involves the transfer of heat from a warm object to a cooler one by direct contact. This can occur when the newborn is placed on a cold surface or when cool blankets and clothing are used. Through *convection*, transference of heat is from a body to the surrounding air. The newborn's temperature is affected by air currents in the environment, such as those caused by air conditioners. The fourth mechanism, *radiation*, occurs when heat is transferred from a warm object to a cooler one when the objects are not in direct contact. This type of heat loss can occur in newborns if the walls of an incubator are cool or if the crib is placed close to a cool outside wall or window. Each of these mechanisms, with the exception of evaporation, also can be responsible for an increase in the newborn's temperature (Table 28-2).

Heat Production. To maintain a normal temperature when exposed to a cool environment, newborns increase their rate of heat production in an attempt to replace what is lost (see Table 28-2). Shivering is the most common mechanism of heat production in the adult. The neonate rarely shivers, but there may be an increase in voluntary muscular activity. The primary mechanism of heat production in the newborn is nonshivering thermogenesis. This consists of a chemical reaction occurring in brown fat that breaks down triglycerides into glycerol and fatty acids and thereby produces heat. **Brown fat** cells contain many small fat vacuoles in contrast to the single, large vacuole of white fat. These cells also have a richer blood supply, which helps to account for the darker color of the fat and aids in the distribution of the heat produced. Brown fat, usually not found in adults, accounts for approximately 1.5% of the total newborn body weight. Significant deposits of brown fat are found at the nape of the neck, in the axillae, around the kidneys and adrenals, between the scapulae, and in the mediastinum (Fig. 28-1; Korones, 1986).

TABLE 28-2
Thermal Regulation in the Newborn

MECHANISMS OF HEAT LOSS	PREVENTION
Evaporation—loss of heat to air by way of moisture from skin or lungs	Dry well after delivery, especially head; protect from exposure while wet during bath; avoid very low humidity.
Radiation—loss of heat to cool objects not in contact with newborn	Avoid placing newborn near cold outside walls or windows.
Conduction—loss of heat from newborn to cold surface	Do not place on cold surface; use warmed blankets in delivery room.
Convection—loss of heat to air by way of drafts	Keep newborn out of air flow currents.
MECHANISMS OF HEAT PRODUCTION AND CONSERVATION	**EFFECTS**
Nonshivering thermogenesis (metabolism of brown fat)	Increased metabolic consumption of calories
	Increased oxygen consumption
	Increased glucose consumption
Increase in voluntary muscular activity (shivering is rare in the newborn)	
Peripheral vasoconstriction	Conservation of heat for body core
	Hands and feet blue, mottled, or cold to touch
Assumption of fetal position	Decreased surface area for loss of heat

Heat Conservation. Conservation of body heat in the newborn occurs through peripheral vasoconstriction and assumption of a flexed or fetal position. This position decreases the surface area from which heat may be lost (see Table 28-2).

Effects of Cold Stress on the Newborn

The increased metabolic rate associated with nonshivering thermogenesis necessitates an increase in oxygen and calorie consumption. To replace the heat lost during a temperature drop of 3.5°C (6.3°F), newborns require a 100% increase in oxygen consumption for more than 1½ hours. Even vigorous full-term newborns may develop metabolic acidosis if hypothermia occurs. Prolonged cold stress may deplete brown fat stores, thus eliminating the newborn's ability to produce heat by this mechanism. Cold stress can be harmful or even fatal to a newborn who is having difficulty with metabolism or oxygenation. Efforts should be made to keep the newborn in a neutral thermal environment. In a neutral thermal environment, the newborn's metabolic rate, and therefore oxygen consumption, is minimal, but the body temperature remains within the normal range.

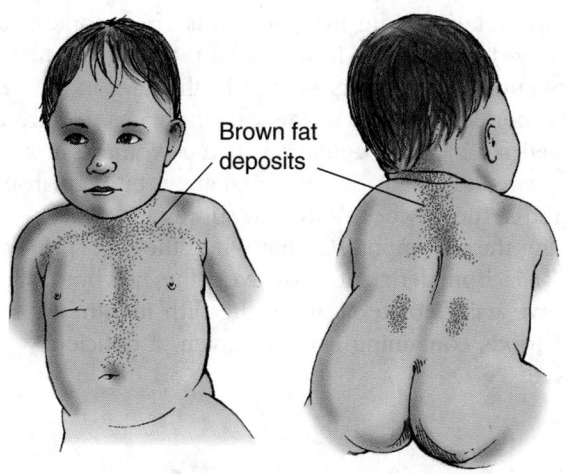

Brown fat deposits

FIGURE 28–1 Brown fat. Deposits of brown fat are found between the scapulae, at the nape of the neck, in the axillae, in the mediastinum, and surrounding the kidneys and adrenals. The skin overlying brown fat deposits feels slightly warmer to the touch. Brown fat reserves usually persist for several weeks after birth unless depleted for heat production required by cold stress.

Neurologic Changes

The nervous system of the newborn is neither anatomically nor physiologically developed fully. All neurons are present, but many remain immature for several months and some for years. Thus, newborns are uncoordinated in their movements, labile in their temperature regulation, and have poor control over their musculature—they "startle" easily, are subject to tremors of the extremities, and so on. However, during the neonatal period, development is rapid. As the various nerve pathways controlling the muscles are used, nerve fibers connect with one another. Gradually, more complex patterns of behavior emerge, and the higher cerebral levels begin to function.

Reflexes. The reflexes are important indices of the newborn's development. Their presence or absence at certain times reflects how well or normally the central nervous system is functioning. (Individual reflexes are discussed later in this chapter in the section entitled "Neurologic Assessment".)

Gastrointestinal Changes

During fetal life, the functions of the gastrointestinal tract are limited. The fetus does swallow amniotic fluid, and a fecal material called **meconium** is formed. However, the gastrointestinal tract is not responsible for the digestion or absorption of nutrients. By 36 to 38 weeks' gestation, the gastrointestinal system has matured enough to adapt readily to extrauterine life. The various enzymes necessary for digestion are active, and the muscular and reflex development provide the capability of transporting food (Bucuvalas et al., 1992).

Newborns do not have the ability to transfer food from the lips to the pharynx. For newborns to swallow, food must be placed well back on the tongue. Therefore, the nipple should be placed well inside the newborn's mouth. Sucking is facilitated by strong sucking muscles and ridges, or corrugations, in the anterior portion of the mouth. In addition, the sucking pads (deposits of fatty tissue in each cheek) prevent the collapse of the cheeks during nursing and make sucking more effective. This fatty tissue remains (even when fat is lost from the rest of the body) until sucking is no longer essential as a method of obtaining food. The salivary glands are immature at birth and manufacture little saliva until the infant is about 3 months old.

The newborn's intestinal tract is proportionately longer than that of an adult. Although it contains a large number of secretory glands and a large surface for absorption, its elastic tissue and supporting musculature are poor and not fully developed. This increases the likelihood of distention. Furthermore, nervous control is variable and inadequate. Nevertheless, the newborn digests and absorbs a tremendous amount of food in proportion to body weight. Most of the digestive enzymes seem to be present and adequate. Two exceptions are pancreatic amylase and lipase, which are somewhat deficient for several months but eventually reach a normal amount. Newborns can digest simple foods easily but have a difficult time with more complex starches. Protein and carbohydrates are easily absorbed, but fat absorption is poor.

Changes in Kidney Function and Urinary Excretion

The kidneys are functional during the greater part of fetal life. This is evidenced by the presence of urine in the bladder as early as the fourth month of gestation. Even at full term, however, the level of kidney function is low. All nephrons are present, but the surface area of the glomerular capillaries and the tubule length are about one-tenth of adult size (Spitzer et al., 1992).

Because of the relatively low rate of glomerular filtration at birth, excess water and solute cannot be disposed of rapidly and efficiently. There also are limitations in tubular reabsorption that may cause inappropriate substances from the glomerular filtrate, such as certain amino acids and bicarbonate, to appear in the urine (Spitzer et al., 1992). In the healthy neonate, these limitations do not have a detrimental effect, but they do restrict the ability of the newborn to respond to stress. As the kidneys grow and mature, function increases.

Within 24 hours of birth, 92% of healthy newborns void, but the first voiding may occur shortly after delivery and not be noticed. Voidings during the first days after birth may be scanty and somewhat infrequent unless the newborn was edematous at birth. As the fluid intake increases, so does the output. Frequency usually increases from two to six times on the first and second day to 5 to 20 times per 24 hours on subsequent days until the infant begins to develop bladder control and the number of voidings per day decreases. The urine of the newborn may appear cloudy owing to high mucus and urate content. With increased fluid intake, the urine becomes clear, straw colored, and nearly odorless. Uric acid crystals in the urine may cause a reddish "brick-dust" stain on the diaper that is sometimes confused with blood in the urine.

Changes in Hepatic Function

During fetal life, the liver performs an important role in blood formation. It is thought that this function continues to some degree after birth. Later in the neonatal period, the liver produces substances that are essential for blood coagulation. If the woman's iron intake was adequate during pregnancy, enough iron is stored in the newborn's liver to supply his or her needs during the first months of life when the diet (primarily milk) is iron deficient. However, the newborn's iron reserve will deplete at about the fifth month, and unless foods containing iron are given, a deficiency will ensue.

Physical Assessment

A physical assessment is an important part of newborn care. In recent years, many nurses have learned physical assessment skills, and in some hospitals, a pediatric nurse practitioner has the responsibility for part of the newborn physical examination. Although all nurses do not possess practitioner skills, those who work with newborns should be able to do a basic assessment and recognize deviations from normal.

Physical assessment of the neonate begins immediately after birth when the delivery room nurse observes the newborn to detect any anomalies or problems and assigns the Apgar score (see Chap. 24). The pertinent information that must be reported to the nurse when the newborn is brought to the nursery includes the following:

- The mother's prenatal history
- The course of labor and delivery
- The condition of the newborn at and following birth
- Any care given to the newborn in the delivery room

After confirming the report by looking at the newborn's record, the nursery nurse should perform an initial evaluation of the newborn's general condition (Table 28-3).

From this initial observation, the nurse can make a decision about whether the newborn needs immediate treatment, if time is needed for the temperature to stabilize, or if the assessment process can continue. Certain symptoms that might be cause for concern in an older child (eg, rapid rate and irregular rhythm of respirations) may represent normal physiology in a newborn (Table 28-4).

After the nurse performs an initial evaluation of the newborn's general condition, a newborn physical assessment can be performed. The Assessment Tool: Newborn Physical Assessment Guide can be used when learning to assess the newborn. The discussion of newborn characteristics that follows and Table 28-4 provide normal assessment findings and deviations from the norm and are helpful when using the assessment tool. Practice and experience also improve the nurse's ability to recognize the range of normal. Discussion of abnormalities is found in Chapters 41 to 43. The format of the Newborn Physical Assessment Guide

can be used for an admitting assessment or a later one. It is not intended to be a complete physical examination, but it should give the nurse a good idea of the newborn's status.

Methods used in physical examination are inspection, auscultation, palpation, and percussion, usually in that order. Percussion is not specifically used in the assessment tool. The examination is written for use in evaluating the newborn in a cephalocaudal (head to toe) direction. However, it may be best to begin with items such as auscultation of the chest, which requires the newborn to be quiet, before performing procedures that might cause the newborn to cry. Each examiner should establish a definite pattern and follow it each time so that nothing is missed. To avoid startling the newborn, it is helpful for the nurse to have warm hands, talk to the newborn quietly, and use slow, smooth movements. Having a pacifier available also can assist in quieting the newborn for parts of the examination.

When newborn assessments are performed, the parents should be included as much as possible. This is a good way for parents to get better acquainted with their newborn. The nurse must look at the newborn from the parent's viewpoint. The healthy newborn may have temporary characteristics that look unusual to the parents. The nurse should be ready to talk with the parents about their newborn, answer their questions, and reassure them that many unusual characteristics are normal and will dissapear in a few days. If the parents are not present for the examination, it should be discussed with them.

Assessment of the Head and Neck

Initially, the scalp, face, and neck should be observed carefully for any abrasions, contusions, or breaks in the skin. These can result from application of internal fetal

(*text continues on page 702*)

TABLE 28-3
Initial Evaluation of Newborn's General Condition

Action	Concerns
Observe the newborn's appearance.	Is the color ruddy, pale, cyanotic, or jaundiced? Is the color evenly distributed? The newborn usually is in a flexed position with good muscle tone. A "floppy" or very tense newborn needs careful observation.
Listen to the newborn's cry. This can be an indicator of general condition.	A lusty cry is usually a good sign; a weak or shrill cry can indicate central nervous system problems, and grunting sounds mean that the newborn is having to work hard to get oxygen.
Look for other signs of increased respiratory effort.	Are there substernal or intercostal retractions? Are respirations gasping? Are nostrils flaring? These can all indicate that the newborn is having to work hard to get sufficient oxygen.
Take the vital signs.	Are the vital signs within normal limits?

TABLE 28–4
Summary of Newborn Physical Assessment

Assessment Area	Usual Findings	Deviations
GENERAL OBSERVATIONS		
Muscle tone	Flexed position; good tone	"Floppy"; rigid or tense
Skin		
Color	Pink tone to ruddy when crying; appropriate to ethnic origin; acrocyanosis	Pallor, cyanosis, jaundice, ecchymosis, petechiae
Texture	Smooth; dryness with some peeling; lanugo on back; vernix	Excessive peeling or cracking; roughness
Rashes and pigmentation	Erythema toxicum; milia; mongolian spots	Impetigo, hemangiomas, nevus flammeus (port-wine stain)
Hydration	Skin pinch over abdomen immediately returns to original state	Skin maintains "tent" shape after pinch
Cry	Lusty	Shrill, weak, grunty
MEASUREMENTS		
Weight	2,700–4,000 g (6–9 lb)	
Length	48–53 cm (19–21 in)	
Head circumference	33–37 cm (13–14.5 in)	
Chest circumference	31–35 cm (12.5–14 in)	
VITAL SIGNS		
Temperature	Axillary (preferred method)—36.5°–37°C (97.7°–98.6°F)	Hypothermia, fever
	Rectal—36.5°–37.2°C (97.7°–99°F)	
Respirations	40–60 respirations/min; quiet and shallow; diaphragmatic; occasional periods of rapid breathing, alternating with short periods of apnea	Prolonged rapid breathing; apnea lasting longer than 10 sec; grunting; retractions; persistent slow rate
Heart rate (apical pulse)	120–160 beats/min; faster when crying (up to 180 beats/min); slower when sleeping (down to 100 beats/min)	Tachycardia—greater than 160 beats/min at rest Bradycardia—less than 120 beats/min when awake
HEAD	Vaginal delivery—elongated (molding)	Caput succedaneum, cephalhematoma, hydrocephaly, microcephaly
	Breech or cesarean birth—round, symmetrical	
	Size within normal range	
Fontanels	Flat, soft, firm	Bulging, sunken
Anterior	Diamond shaped; 2–3 cm wide; 3–4 cm long; smaller at birth with molding	Small, almost closed, closed (craniostenosis), widened
Posterior	Triangular shape, small, almost closed	Enlarged
Face	Small, round, symmetrical, fat pads in cheeks, receding chin	Asymmetrical, distorted
Eyes	Edematous lids, usually closed; blue or slate-gray; no tears; red reflex present; pupils equal, round, react to light	Elevation or ptosis of lids; epicanthal folds; absence of red reflex; unequal, dilated, or constricted pupils
	Common variations—subconjunctival hemorrhages, chemical conjunctivitis, occasional slight nystagmus or convergent strabismus	Purulent discharge; frequent nystagmus; constant, divergent, or unilateral strabismus
Mouth	Intact lips, gums, palate; epithelial pearls; "sucking blisters" on lips; tongue midline, mobile, appropriate size for mouth; can extend to alveolar ridge	Cleft lip or palate; white, cheesy patches on tongue, gums, or mucous membrane; large or protruding tongue
Nose	In midline; even placement in relation to eyes and mouth; nares patent; septum intact, midline	Flattened or bruised; unusual placement or configuration; obstructed nares; deviated or perforated septum
Ears	Well-formed cartilage; appropriate size for head; upper attachment on line extended through inner and outer canthus of eye; external auditory canal patent	Floppy, large, and protruding; malformed; low set; obstruction of canal

(continued)

TABLE 28–4 *(Continued)*
Summary of Newborn Physical Assessment

Assessment Area	Usual Findings	Deviations
NECK	Short, thick, full range of motion, no masses	Webbing, abnormal shortening, limitation of motion, torticollis, masses
CLAVICLES	Straight, smooth, intact	Knot or lump; decreased movement of extremity on one side
THORAX	Round, symmetrical, protruding xiphoid process	Asymmetrical, funnel chest
Breath sounds	Loud, bronchial, bilaterally equal	Decreased breath sounds; increased breath sounds; absent breath sounds
Heart sounds	Regular rate and rhythm; first and second sounds clear and distinct	Murmurs, arrhythmias
Breasts	Symmetrical; flat with erect nipples; engorgement second or third day not unusual	Redness and firmness around nipple
ABDOMEN	Symmetrical, slightly protuberant, no masses	Scaphoid or concave shape, distention, palpable masses, asymmetrical
Liver	Palpable 2–3 cm below right costal margin	Enlargement
Spleen	Tip may be palpable in left upper quadrant	Enlargement
Kidneys	May be palpable at level of umbilicus	Enlargement
Femoral pulses	Bilaterally equal	Unequal or absent
Umbilicus	No extensive protrusion or herniation; no signs of infection	Umbilical hernia, omphalocele, redness, induration, foul-smelling discharge
	Cord—bluish white, moist→black, dry; three vessels; no oozing or bleeding	Two vessels; bleeding or oozing from stump
GENITALIA	Appropriate for gender	Ambiguous genitalia
Female		
Labia	Edematous; labia majora cover labia minora; vernix in creases	Hematoma, lesions, fusion of labia
Vagina	Mucous discharge, possibly blood tinged	
Male		
Foreskin	Adherent to glans of penis	Opening below tip of penis (hypospadias)
Urethra	Opening at tip of penis	Opening above tip of penis (epispadias)
Testes	Palpable in each scrotal sac	Palpable in inguinal canal; not palpable
POSTERIOR OF BODY		
Spinal column	Straight, flexible; intact, no masses	Exaggerated curves, spina bifida, any masses, pilonidal cyst
Anus	Patent	Imperforate anus, anal fissures
EXTREMITIES	Symmetrical in size, shape, and movement	Unequal or abnormal size or shape; asymmetrical or limited movement of one or more extremities
Digits	Five on each hand and foot; appropriate size and shape	Missing digits, syndactyly (webbing), polydactyly (extra digits)
Hips	Even leg length, knee height, gluteal folds; no resistance or limitation to abduction	Uneven leg length, knee height, or gluteal folds; uneven or limited abduction; hip "click" or "clunk" on abduction
Feet	Straight, or postural deviation easily corrected with gentle pressure	Structural deformities—talipes equinovarus (clubfoot), metatarsus adductus
REFLEXES		
Rooting and sucking	Turns toward object touching cheek, lips, or corner of mouth; opens mouth; begins sucking movements; strong suck, pulls object into mouth	No rooting; weak, ineffective, or absent suck
	May be diminished or absent after eating	

(continued)

TABLE 28–4 *(Continued)*
Summary of Newborn Physical Assessment

Assessment Area	Usual Findings	Deviations
REFLEXES		
Grasp		
Palmar	Fingers grasp object when palm stimulated and hang on briefly	Weak or absent
Plantar	Toes curl downward when soles of feet are stimulated	Weak or absent
Moro	Symmetrical response to sudden stimulus—lateral extension of arms with opening of hands; formation of c-shape with thumb and forefinger; followed by flexion and adduction	Asymmetrical, absent, incomplete
Startle	Protective response to sudden loud noise or movement—abduction and flexion of all extremities accompanied by crying	Absent, incomplete
Stepping	Stepping movements when held upright with sole of foot touching surface	Asymmetrical or absent

monitor electrodes, forceps, or other instruments used in delivery. Any opening in the skin is a potential site for bacterial invasion and should be watched for signs of infection.

Head

The newborn's head is large, comprising about one-quarter of total body size. With cephalic presentation, it may initially appear asymmetrical because of the molding of the skull bones during labor. If there has been extended pressure on the head, caput succedaneum (a swelling of the soft tissues) or cephalhematoma (an accumulation of blood between the bone and the periosteum) might be present (see Chap. 43).

The suture lines between the skull bones and the anterior and posterior fontanels can usually be easily palpated. The fontanels should feel soft and should be neither bulging nor depressed. The diamond-shaped anterior fontanel is normally about 2 to 3 cm wide and 3 to 4 cm long at birth. It may feel smaller for the first day or two when there is marked overriding of the skull bones. Closure usually takes place by 12 to 18 months. The posterior fontanel is triangular and is located between the occipital and the parietal bones. It is smaller than the anterior fontanel, may be almost closed at birth, and is completely closed by the end of the second month.

The circumference of the head is measured by placing a nonstretchable tape measure just above the eyebrows and over the most prominent part of the occiput (Fig. 28-2). Normally, the head circumference is 2 cm larger than the chest circumference. However, an accurate measurement may not be obtained at first if molding is present. The normal range is 33 to 37 cm (13–

14½ in), depending on the general size of the newborn. The face is small and round, and the lower jaw appears to recede. Facial asymmetry, especially of the chin and mandible, is sometimes seen. This can be the result of posture in utero if the flexed head was tilted to one side and pressed against the shoulder. The nose also may be asymmetrical or have a deviated septum from intrauterine pressure. The nose must be free of obstruction because newborns are nose breathers and have difficulty breathing through their mouths.

Eyes

The eyes are closed much of the time but may open spontaneously if the newborn's head is lifted or rocked gently (this is important to remember when inspecting the eyes). A newborn has the ability to see and discriminate patterns as the basis for form perception. However, this capacity is limited by imperfect oculomotor coordination and an inability to accommodate for varying distances. In addition, the eye, the visual pathways, and the visual part of the brain are poorly developed at birth. Nevertheless, a good deal of visual experience is possible for the newborn.

Many mothers do not realize their newborn's visual capabilities and appreciate being informed of this. In addition, some mothers become anxious when they observe strabismus or nystagmus in their newborn. They should be reassured that this lack of coordination is normal during the first few months of life. Most newborns' eyes are blue or slate-gray at birth. At 3 months of age, the eyes have usually achieved their permanent color, although complete pigmentation of the iris does not occur until about 1 year of age. Newborns do not usually shed tears when they cry because the lacrimal

ASSESSMENT TOOL
Newborn Physical Assessment Guide

The examiner can use any system of notation that is helpful to fill in the spaces on the form. A suggestion is to use a check to indicate "within normal limits" and a plus or minus to indicate whether something is present or absent. When necessary, descriptions can be written in the spaces or under "comments."

Baby's name _____ Date and time of birth _____
Mother's name _____ Date and time of exam _____

Initial Evaluation

1. General appearance: Color _____ Muscle tone _____
2. Respiratory effort: Retractions _____ Gasping _____
   Grunting _____ Quality of cry _____
3. Temperature: _____
Comments: _____
_____

Assessment of Head and Neck

1. Observe and palpate the newborn's head for symmetry; note absence or presence of:
   Molding _____ Caput succedaneum _____ Cephalhematoma _____
2. Palpate the fontanels and sutures for: Fullness _____ Depression _____
   Overriding _____ Shape _____ Size _____
3. Measure circumference of head: _____
4. Evaluate ears: Position _____ Shape _____ Size _____
5. Evaluate symmetry of face: _____
6. Observe eyes for: Shape _____ Position _____ Size _____
   Appearance of pupils _____ Presence of hemorrhage _____ Red reflex _____
7. Evaluate mouth for: Clefts _____ Teeth _____ Frenulum linguae _____
8. Observe neck for: Length _____ Relationship to body _____
   Mobility _____ Presence of webbing or fat pad _____
9. Observe skin of scalp, face, and neck for: Abrasions or contusions _____
   Other breaks or marks _____
10. Observe nose for: Symmetry _____ Septum _____ Flaring _____
Comments: _____
_____
_____

Assessment of Body

General Appearance
1. Measurements: Weight _____ Length _____ Circumference of chest _____
2. Observe throughout evaluation for: General activity _____
   Posture _____ Responsiveness _____
3. Observe skin for: Lanugo _____ Vernix _____ Meconium staining _____
   Texture _____ Hydration _____ Color _____ Rashes _____
   Pigmentation _____
Comments: _____
_____

Thorax

1. Palpate clavicles for masses and intactness: _____
2. Inspect thorax for: Size _____ Symmetry _____ Shape _____

(continued)

ASSESSMENT TOOL *(Continued)*
Newborn Physical Assessment Guide

3. Auscultate for: Breath sounds _____ Heart sounds _____ Rhythm _____
4. Count: respiratory rate _____ Apical pulse _____
Comments: _____
_____

Abdomen

1. Inspect shape of abdomen: _____
2. Palpate: Liver _____ Spleen _____ Kidneys _____
3. Observe cord for number of vessels: _____
4. Palpate femoral pulses: _____
Comments: _____
_____

Genitals

1. Observe visible genitals for appropriateness with stated sex: _____
2. Observe female infant for: Maturation of labia _____ Vaginal discharge _____
3. Observe male infant for: Position of urethral opening _____
   Maturation of scrotum _____ Presence of testes _____
4. Note elimination: (should occur within 24 hours)
   Urine _____ Color _____ Amount/24 hours _____
   Stool _____ Color _____ Type _____ Number/24 hours _____
Comments: _____
_____

Posterior of Body

1. Palpate and inspect spinal column for: Masses _____
   Symmetry of vertebrae _____ Intactness _____
2. Determine patency of anus: _____
3. Observe pilonidal dimple for intactness: _____
Comments: _____
_____

Extremities

1. Note for all extremities: Symmetry _____ Abnormalities _____
   Ability to move _____
2. Count digits on: Hands _____ Feet _____
   Observe for polydactyly _____ Syndactyly _____
3. Evaluate rotation of hips: Abduct thighs to bed _____
   Rotate hips through full range of motion _____
   Observe leg length, front and back (Are they equal?) _____ Knee height _____
   Observe symmetry of leg creases _____
4. Note position of feet _____
   Can they passively be returned to normal? _____
Comments: _____
_____

Assessment of Neurologic Function and Reflexes—Elicit and Evaluate:

1. Rooting and sucking: _____
_____

(continued)

ASSESSMENT TOOL *(Continued)*
Newborn Physical Assessment Guide

2. Grasp: Palmar _____ Plantar _____

_____

3. Traction: (Pull to sitting position, note head and arm position) _____

_____

4. Moro: _____

_____

5. Stepping: _____

_____

Comments: _____

_____

_____

Items that require manipulation, such as palpation of the abdomen and abduction of the hips, require care in performance to avoid injury to the newborn and should not be attempted for the first time without supervision by a trained examiner.

(After NAACOG Technical Bulletin No. 2, "Physical Assessment of the Neonate.")

glands may not be functioning at birth. Tears may not appear for several weeks and sometimes for several months. If silver nitrate was used as a prophylactic, there may be some edema of the lids or purulent discharge. Small areas of subconjunctival hemorrhage, caused by changes of vascular tension in the eyes during delivery, may be present. These areas disappear spontaneously in 1 or 2 weeks and are not significant.

If an ophthalmoscope is used to examine the eyes, the pupil should appear as a small, red-orange circular spot when the light is directed at it. This is the **red reflex**. It is caused by light shining on the retina, and any opacities of the lens or other obstructions would be visible.

Ears and Hearing

The ears should be inspected for size, shape, position, malrotation, and anomaly. The point where the top of the ear is attached to the scalp should fall on or above an imaginary line drawn from the inner through the outer canthus of the eye (Fig. 28-3). Abnormal positioning of the ears is frequently associated with certain chromosomal abnormalities or kidney anomalies.

Otoscopic examination of the ear establishes the patency of the external auditory canal. The tympanic membranes are usually difficult to visualize for the first 2 or 3 days of life because of accumulated vernix caseosa. If an infection is suspected in the newborn, visualization should be attempted because otitis media can occur during the initial days of life (Phibbs, 1991). During the first few months, the light reflex is diffuse rather than its normal cone-shaped appearance.

The ear and nerve tracts for hearing are anatomically mature at birth. Newborns can hear after their first cry, and hearing apparently becomes acute within several days as the eustachian tubes become aerated and the mucus in the middle ear disappears. Hearing can be tested by sounding a bell or rattle near the newborn's head but out of eyesight. Hearing the sound causes blinking of the eyes, momentary cessation of activity, or a startle response. This is not an accurate test, but it may be helpful in alerting the examiner to a possible problem.

FIGURE 28-2 The circumference of the head is measured by placing a nonstretchable tape measure just above the eyebrows and over the most prominent part of the occiput.

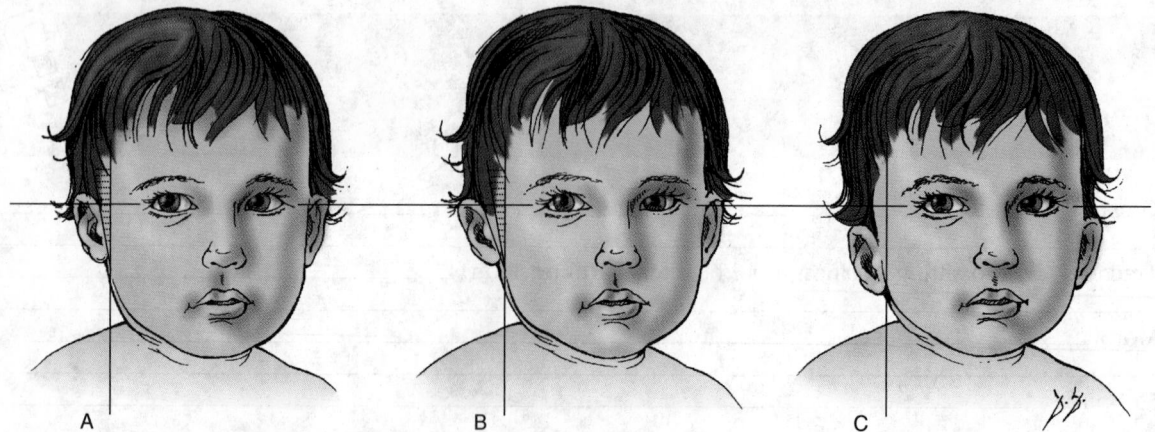

FIGURE 28-3 (A) Normal ear. **(B)** Abnormally angled ear. **(C)** Low-set ear.

Lips, Mouth, and Cheeks

The rounded, thickened areas often present on the lips (particularly on the center of the upper lip) are known as labial tubercles or "sucking blisters." They are not true blisters because there is no fluid in them. Sucking (fat) pads are usually present in the cheeks. The lips, gums, and palate should be examined to see that they are intact. Epstein's pearls, small white cysts that may be seen on the hard palate or gums, are not abnormal. Occasionally, a tooth is present, which may be pulled to avoid the possibility of its being aspirated. At this early age, the tongue does not extend far beyond the margin of the gums because the frenulum is normally short.

Neck

The newborn generally appears to have a short neck. This sometimes makes it difficult to tell if webbing or other problems are present. The head should be gently rotated to determine the range of motion of the neck, and the muscles should be palpated for any masses.

Assessment of the Body

General Appearance

The average full-term newborn weighs 3,500 g (7½ lb), and 95% weigh between 2,500 g (5½ lb) and 4,250 g (9½ lb). There is usually some weight loss in the first 3 to 5 days, possibly as much as 10% of the birth weight. This is usually regained by the 8th to 12th day.

Length also should be measured soon after birth to serve as a baseline from which to judge future growth. The average length of a full-term newborn at birth is 51 cm (20 in), with 95% between 46 and 56 cm (18 and 22 in; Fig. 28-4). Because the newborn usually assumes a somewhat flexed position, it can be difficult to get an accurate measurement from the top of the head to the heels. Measurement is more accurate when done on a firm surface, and it is helpful to have an assistant hold the head.

Color

The newborn's color should be assessed early in the examination. The color may be pink, reddish, or pale, becoming more ruddy with crying. The skin tends to be less pigmented in the neonatal period than later in

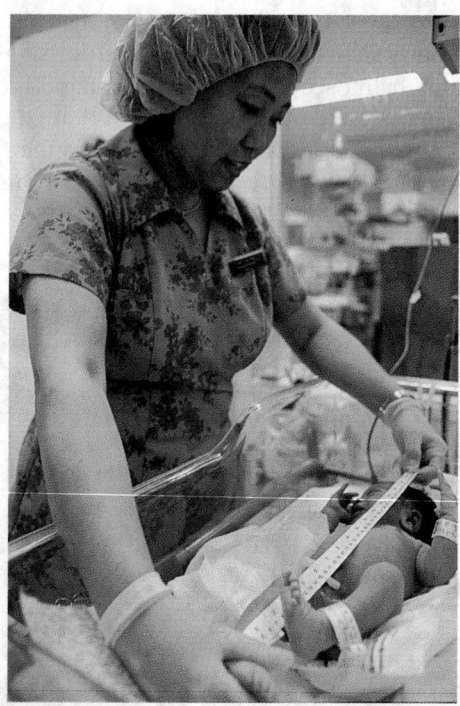

FIGURE 28-4 Length should be measured soon after birth to serve as a baseline from which to judge future growth.

life, so color changes may be noted even in darker-skinned newborns. Initially, the hands and feet are usually blue (acrocyanosis) owing to the sluggish peripheral vascular circulation. This cyanosis of the extremities is transient and often disappears in a few hours. If generalized cyanosis is present, the extent and circumstances of its appearance should be noted. The newborn who is cyanotic at rest and pink only when crying may have choanal atresia. Cardiac or pulmonary problems may be suspected if crying increases the cyanosis. The newborn who continues to be ruddy or plethoric even at rest should have a hematocrit done to rule out polycythemia. The very pale newborn should be checked for anemia or hypotension.

Frequent assessment of the newborn for jaundice is an important nursing responsibility that will help detect significant hyperbilirubinemia as early as possible. The red color of the blood or the pigment in the skin of dark-complected newborns sometimes hides the yellow of jaundice. The nurse should blanch the skin by pressing a finger on a bony area, such as the chest or forehead. This technique often allows any yellow to be seen before the newborn's normal skin color returns. The sclera and buccal mucosa also are good places to look for yellowing.

Skin

The skin of the normal full-term newborn is soft, velvety, and wrinkled. At birth, it is covered to varying degrees with **vernix caseosa**, a white, cheesy material made up of sebum and desquamating cells. The vernix protects the skin in utero and at term is found primarily in the body creases. After the vernix is removed or disappears, the skin is often dry and peeling. A fine, downy hair called **lanugo** may be found on the face, brow, and shoulders, especially in preterm newborns.

A variety of rashes, discolorations, and other "birthmarks" appear on the skin in the newborn period. Parents may mistake milia for "whiteheads" and may need to be warned not to squeeze them. Many are considered normal variations, and most fade with time; however, some can indicate genetic syndromes, and depending on their location, some can be disfiguring. Table 28-5 gives characteristics of several common rashes, discolorations, and birthmarks.

Thorax

The newborn's chest is round with a transverse diameter that is approximately equal to the anteroposterior diameter. The circumference, measured just above the nipple line, is slightly smaller than the head. The thorax is relatively short compared with the abdomen. The chest wall is thin with little musculature, and the rib cage is very soft and pliant. The tip of the xiphoid process often protrudes visibly. Engorgement of the breasts is common during the neonatal period in male and female newborns. Estrogen, which prepares the mother's breasts for lactation during pregnancy, passes through the placenta from the mother to the fetus. When estrogen is withdrawn after birth, the newborn's breasts may become engorged. Mammary engorgement in the newborn subsides without treatment but may persist for 2 or 3 weeks. Sometimes a small amount of fluid, called **witch's milk**, is secreted. The nurse should caution mothers against massaging the newborn's breasts or trying to squeeze out any fluid because this could lead to an infection, such as breast abscess or mastitis.

Respiration

The respiratory rate of the normal newborn ranges from 40 to 60 breaths per minute but is easily altered by internal and external stimuli. Respiration is normally quiet and shallow, and the chest and abdomen move together. Retractions, mild expiratory grunting, and nasal flaring may be considered normal during the first few minutes after birth. However, their presence after that time can indicate obstruction or abnormality.

Counting respirations in the newborn can be frustrating, because the newborn may have periods of rapid breathing alternating with short periods of apnea. Intermittent crying also may interfere with counting. Respirations should be counted for 1 full minute or longer if necessary. Because the newborn primarily uses diaphragmatic breathing, it is easier to count abdominal rather than chest excursions.

An alternate method is to count respirations by auscultation (Fig. 28-5). When auscultating the newborn's chest for breath sounds, it is best to use the bell or small diaphragm of the stethoscope, because the adult-sized diaphragm may not make complete contact with the newborn's small chest wall. Auscultation should be done with the newborn in both the upright and supine positions because breath sounds may be altered with changing positions. Bronchial breath sounds are normally heard over most of the chest and sound louder and harsher than in the adult because they are closer.

The nurse should watch for the sudden occurrence of dyspnea and cyanosis in a newborn who is breathing normally. This can occur even after the transition period is over. An episode of dyspnea or cyanosis may indicate some anomaly or other pathologic condition and should be reported promptly. The nurse should notify the physician if the respiratory rate is persistently below 40 respirations per minute or if it increases beyond 60 respirations per minute when the newborn is at rest.

TABLE 28–5

Common Newborn Skin Rashes, Discolorations, and Birthmarks

Type	Characteristics
Vascular nevi	
Telangiectic nevi (stork bites)	Tiny pink to red spots found commonly on nape of the neck, eyelids, and bridge of the nose; do blanch on pressure; usually disappear spontaneously during infancy, but some persist into adulthood.

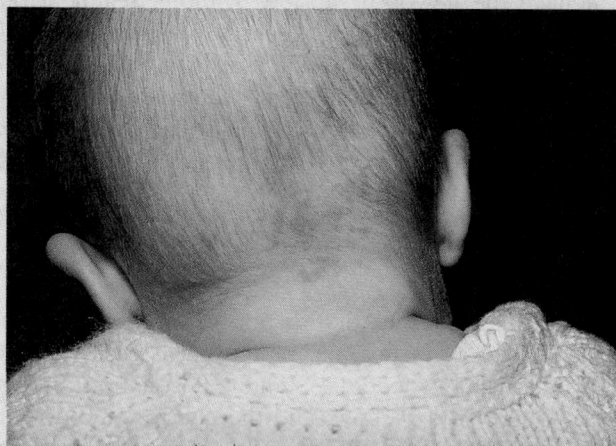

Stork bite

Nevus flammeus (port-wine stain)	Flat, purple-red, sharply demarcated areas, often found on the face (on African American newborns, they are deep purple-black); do not blanch on pressure, increase in size, or fade over time; disfigurement varies with size and placement.
	If the newborn also displays epileptic-like seizures, may indicate Sturge-Weber syndrome, a serious genetic disorder.
Nevus vasculosus (strawberry marks)	Dark red, rough-textured, sharply demarcated elevations usually found on head or face; continue to grow for several months, then shrink spontaneously and usually disappear by 7–10 y of age.

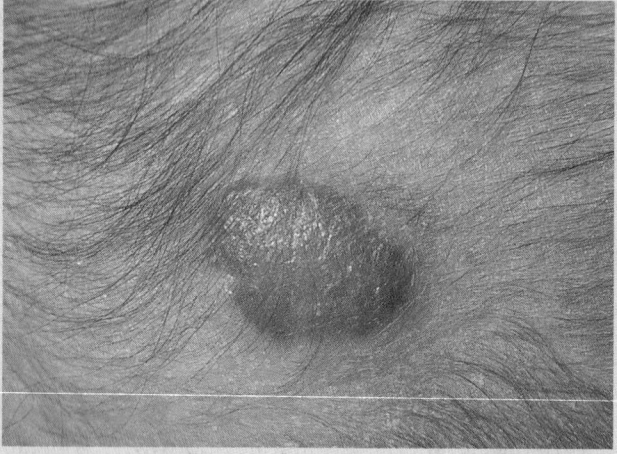

Strawberry mark

| Erythema Toxicum (newborn rash or fleabite dermatitis, although no fleas involved) | Blotchy, eryethematous rash with a small, blanched wheel in the center; develops most frequently on the back, shoulders, and buttocks; cause is obscure and no treatment is necessary; transient, likely to change within a few hours; and usually disappears entirely within a few days. |

(continued)

TABLE 28-5 *(Continued)*
Common Newborn Skin Rashes, Discolorations, and Birthmarks

Type	Characteristics
Pigmented nevi Mongolian spots	Gray-blue pigmented areas seen most often on lumbosacral region and buttocks of dark-skinned and Asian newborns; usually spontaneously disappear during late infancy or early childhood; have no relationship to mongolism.

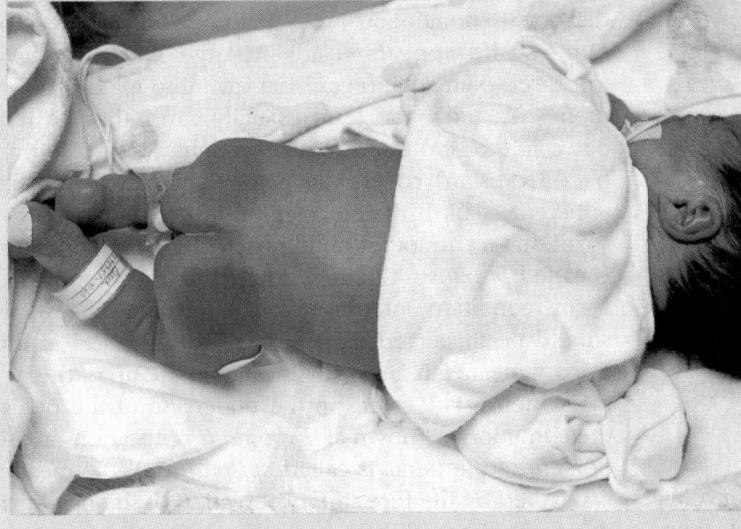

Mongolian spots

Café au lait spots	Patchy, flat, brown areas that are lighter in color than the surrounding skin; commonly found on the face, chest, arms, hands; usually of no significance; however, if spots are >1.5 cm long or more than six are present, they may indicate certain genetic syndromes (eg, Von Recklinghausen disease).
Milia	Pin-point sized, pearly white spots found commonly on the nose, forehead, or skull of the newborn; feel like tiny, firm seeds; result of sebaceous material retained within sebaceous glands; if left alone, will usually disappear.

Heart

The heart rate is determined by counting the apical pulse). It is normally between 120 and 160 beats/min and like the respiratory rate, changes with the newborn's activity. It beats faster with crying, increased activity, or rapid breathing and more slowly when the newborn is quiet, especially during the short periods of no breathing.

The first and second heart sounds should be clear and well defined. Murmurs may be present in the newborn period. They may be heard more easily with the bell of the stethoscope held lightly against the chest wall. During cardiac auscultation, murmurs are most likely to be heard at the right sternal border, the upper left sternal border, the lower left sternal border, and the apex. Any murmurs should be reported, recorded, and monitored. However, murmurs may be less significant in the newborn period than at other times because a closing ductus arteriosus may cause a temporary loud murmur. The nurse must be knowledgeable of other signs of cardiac problems because a serious heart anomaly may cause no murmur at all.

Early experiences in listening to the newborn's chest can be confusing because the heart rate and respirations are so much faster than an adult's and the newborn often wiggles and fusses. With practice, the student nurse will learn how to quiet the newborn and how to distinguish between the different sounds.

Abdomen

The abdomen is round and slightly protuberant because of the newborn's relatively large abdominal or-

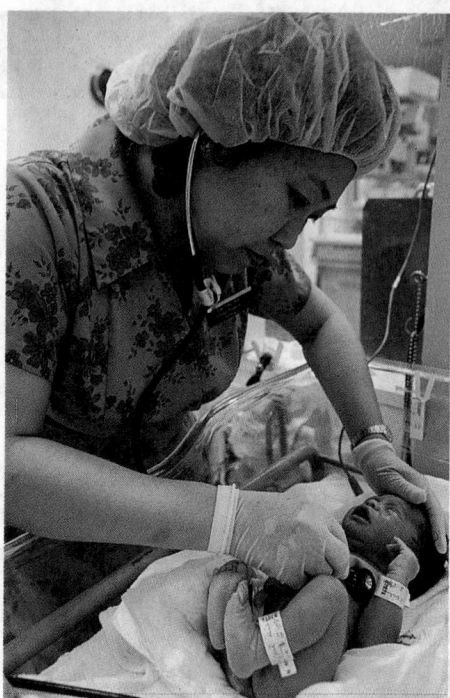

FIGURE 28–5 The newborn's respiratory rate can be determined by auscultation.

gans and weak muscular structures. Superficial veins are often visible. Observation can be a valuable part of the examination of the abdomen, because outlines of the anterior organs may sometimes be seen. An abdomen that is asymmetrical, scaphoid (sunken), or grossly distended suggests abnormalities and should be checked carefully.

Palpation should begin with gentle pressure or upward stroking of the abdomen, and then deeper palpation may be performed. The edge of the liver is usually palpable just below the right rib margin, but it is not sharp and may be missed if palpation is too high or forceful. The tip of the spleen may sometimes be palpated in the left upper quadrant. The kidneys can usually be palpated during the first 4 to 6 hours after birth, but they are more difficult to locate after this. If palpable, the lower edges are usually located approximately at the level of the umbilicus, about halfway between the newborn's side and midline.

The umbilical cord stump should be checked for bleeding or oozing, and the number of vessels should be noted if not already recorded (see Chap. 24). The umbilicus and surrounding area also should be inspected carefully. Redness, induration, skin warmth, and foul-smelling discharge are signs of infection that should be reported. Infection in this area is potentially dangerous in the newborn because it can spread up the open arteries into the peritoneum. Serous or serosanguineous discharge continuing after separation of the cord stump may indicate a granuloma. This has the appearance of a small, red button deep in the um-

bilicus. It can be cauterized by the physician with a silver nitrate stick.

Genitals

Female genitalia should be inspected for presence and size of the labia majora, labia minora, clitoris, and vaginal opening. Enlarged labia or vaginal discharge may be present due to in utero stimulation by maternal hormones. The discharge may be blood tinged, but this is not a cause for concern. The swelling and discharge disappear spontaneously. In male newborns, the scrotum usually appears relatively large and may have increased pigmentation at birth owing to maternal hormones. At term, the testes usually can either be palpated in the scrotum or easily brought down. The prepuce (foreskin) covers the glans penis and is usually adherent at birth. If the opening in the foreskin is so small that it cannot be pulled back at all, the condition is called *phimosis.* Circumcision may be recommended if the condition interferes with urination. The penis should be inspected to determine the location of the urinary meatus. It is usually located at the tip of the penis. When it is located on the underside of the penis, the condition is known as *hypospadias;* location on the dorsum of the penis is called *epispadias.* If the meatus is covered by the foreskin, observation of the newborn during voiding will help to determine its placement.

Posterior

The newborn should be placed in the prone position for inspection and palpation of the entire posterior surface of the body. Any masses or abnormal curvatures of the spine should be noted. Tufts of hair or small indentations, especially in the sacral area, may indicate spina bifida occulta. The perineal area should be inspected to determine the patency and location of the anus. A pilonidal "dimple," resulting from an irregular fold of skin, is sometimes seen in the midline over the sacrococcygeal area. It should be examined for intactness to make sure no sinus is present.

Extremities

Throughout the examination, the nurse observes the newborn's ability to move all four extremities. The limbs are compared according to their size, shape, and movement. Webbing (syndactyly) or extra digits (polydactyly) should be noted.

The newborn should be checked for congenital problems of the hip. This is done by placing him or her in the supine position with the legs flexed on the abdomen and abducted laterally toward the bed. Congenital dislocation of the hip may be manifested by uneven or limited abduction, uneven leg length or knee height, or a "hip click" (Fig. 28-6). Asymmetrical skin

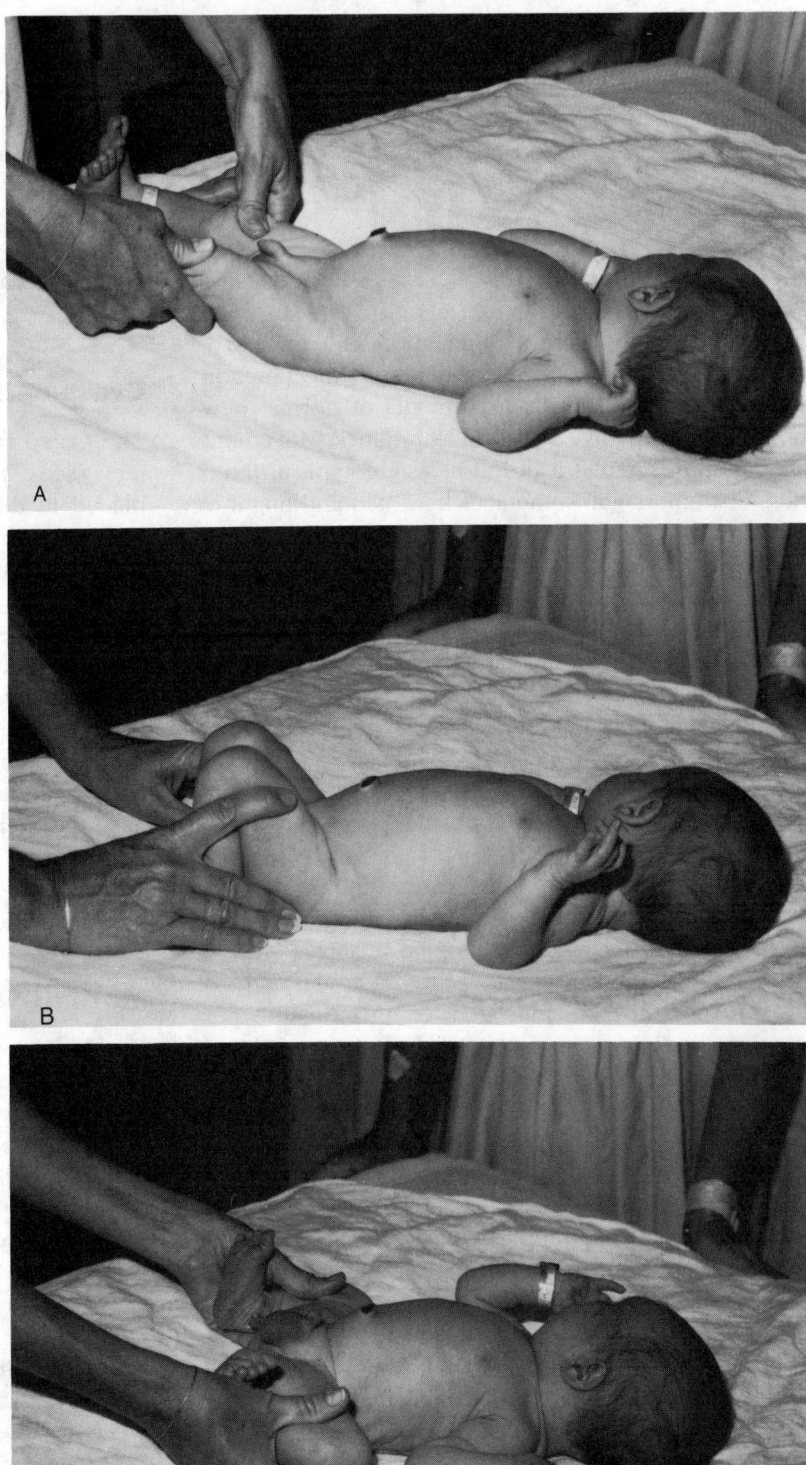

FIGURE 28–6 Assessment of the lower extremities. (**A**) Comparing the length of the legs. (**B**) Comparing the height of the knees. (**C**) Hip abduction.

folds on the posterior aspect of the thigh are not diagnostic but may alert the examiner to the present condition. Unusual positions of the feet can indicate congenital clubfoot or other foot and ankle deformities (see Chap. 42). If an unusually positioned foot can be moved to the normal position with ease, the condition may simply be due to intrauterine malposition.

Neurologic Assessment

The neurologic assessment helps to determine how well the newborn's nervous system is functioning. Some of the areas assessed during the physical, gestational age, and behavioral assessments also are indicators of nervous system functioning. For example, vital signs are part of the physical assessment but also could be included in the neurologic assessment because extreme lability of the temperature and blood pressure reflects immaturity of the autonomic neuromuscular mechanisms. This section focuses on the character of the newborn's movements and reflexes that are usually present at birth.

Movements

At the beginning of the examination, the newborn's movements should be observed before the newborn is touched. Spontaneous movements of normal newborns usually involve all of the extremities. Movements are random, symmetrical, but not stereotypical. Jitteriness or tremors will sometimes be noted and might be interpreted as seizures. It is important to differentiate between seizures and spontaneous movements because neonatal seizures are usually treatable, and brain damage might be avoided if they are identified early (Brann et al., 1992). Assessment Guidelines: Clinical Features Differentiating Tremors or Jitteriness From Seizures will help the nurse assess newborn movements.

Reflexes

Several reflexes should be assessed in the newborn at birth. These include rooting and sucking, grasp, Moro, startle, tonic neck, stepping, and protective. Most of these reflexes disappear within the first few months of life because they are indicators of an immature nervous system. However, some of the reflexes become highly developed or voluntary as the infant grows.

Rooting and Sucking

Gently stroking the newborn's cheek or corner of the mouth with a sterile nipple or clean finger causes the newborn to open his or her mouth and turn toward the stimulus (Fig. 28-7*A*). This is known as the **rooting reflex**. The **sucking reflex** can be evaluated by placing the nipple or finger in the newborn's mouth and noting the strength of the sucking response. These reflexes may not be strong if the newborn has eaten recently. However, a weak or absent response usually indicates prematurity, neurologic deficit or injury, or central nervous system (CNS) depression resulting from maternal drug use or medication during pregnancy.

Grasp Reflex

The **grasp reflex** is present at birth in the hands and feet (see Fig. 28-7*B*). Newborns grasp any object placed in their hands, cling briefly, and then let go. Even at birth they may be able to hold onto an adult's forefinger so securely that they can be lifted to a standing position. Although newborns cannot actually grasp with their feet, stroking the soles causes the toes to turn downward as though trying to grasp. These grasping movements are a reflex action at birth. However, with practice and experience, the hand grasp soon becomes voluntary and purposeful. A diminished grasp reflex response indicates prematurity. If the newborn has peripheral nerve damage or a fracture of the humerous, an asymmetrical grasp reflex of the hand will occur. No grasp response typically indicates severe neurologic deficit.

Moro or Startle Reflex

The **Moro** or **startle reflex** is a response to sudden stimuli or change in position. It indicates an awareness of equilibrium in newborns (see Fig. 28-7*C*). This reflex usually disappears by 3 months of age. The preferred method of eliciting this reflex is to hold the infant with head supported, then allow the head to drop backward or rapidly lower the whole body a short distance. Another way to test this reflex is to place the newborn in

ASSESSMENT GUIDELINES
Clinical Features Differentiating Tremors or Jitteriness From Seizures

Tremors or Jitteriness	Seizures
Rhythmic movements; equal in amplitude	Have fast and slow component
Provoked by external stimuli, such as noise or handling	Insensitive to stimuli
Examiner usually able to stop the movements by passively holding affected limb still	Are not stopped by manual restraint

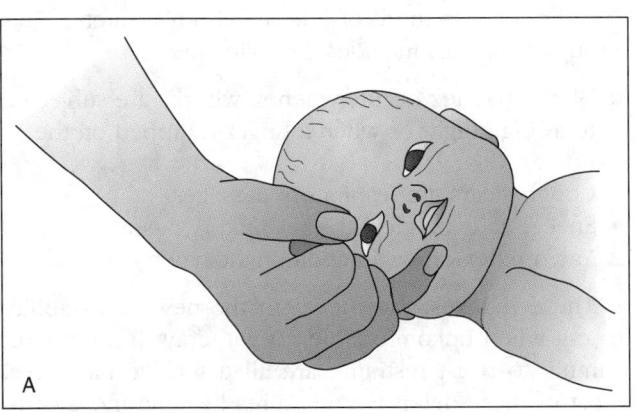

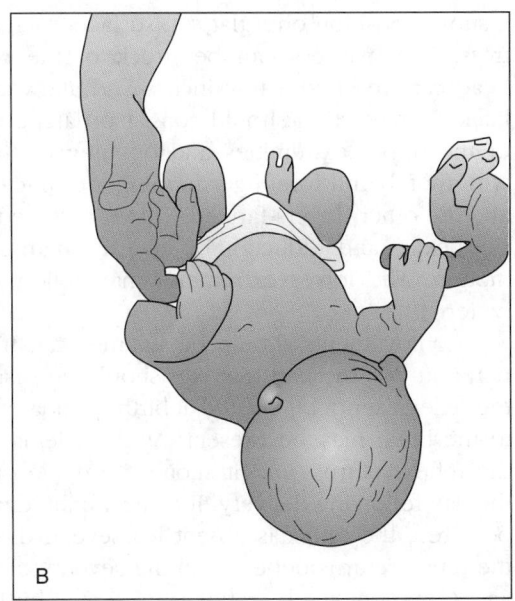

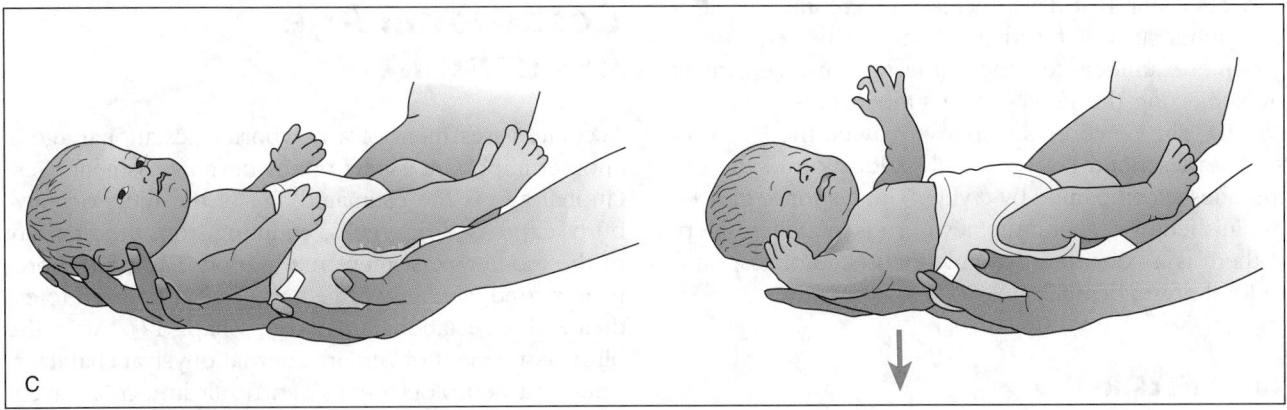

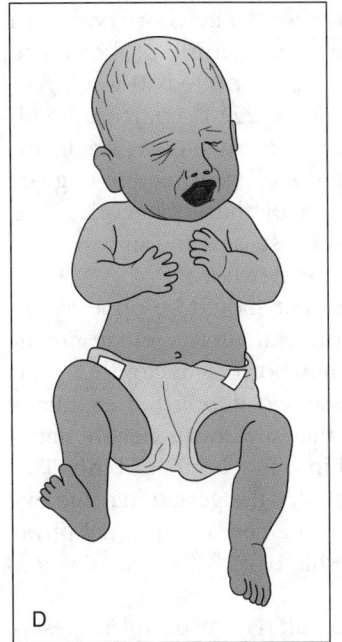

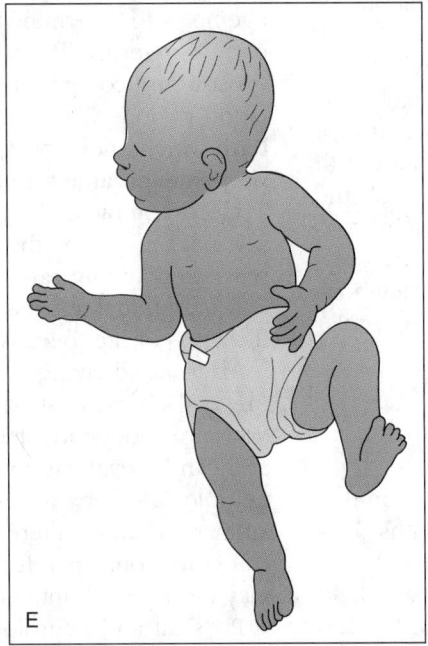

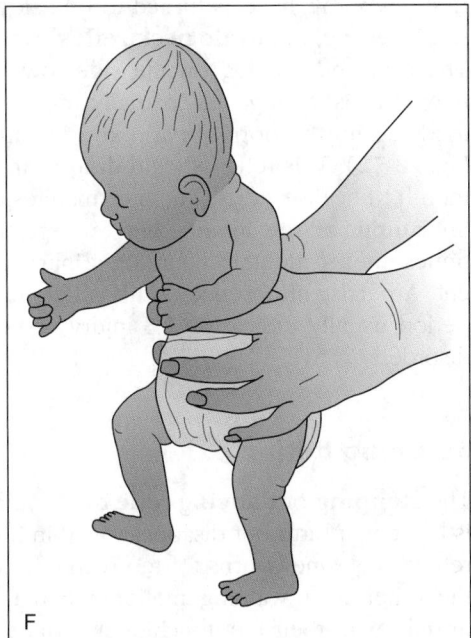

FIGURE 28-7 (**A**) Rooting reflex. (**B**) Grasp reflex. (**C**) Moro reflex. (**D**) Startle reflex. (**E**) Tonic neck reflex. (**F**) Stepping reflex.

a supine position on a flat soft surface, such as a mattress. The mattress can be struck or the newborn's head can be lifted a few inches and allowed to drop back. The reaction should consist of lateral extension of the upper extremities and opening of the hands, with thumb and forefinger forming a characteristic "C" and the other fingers fanned. This is followed by anterior flexion and adduction of the arms in an embracing motion. The lower extremities may follow a similar pattern.

The movements should be symmetrical. If they are not, injury to the part that lags should be suspected. If the reflex cannot be elicited at birth, edema of or injury to the brain may be present. As the edema subsides, the reflex returns, and it should be demonstrable on the day following delivery. If clinical brain damage has occurred, the reflex is absent for several days. When the reflex returns depends on the severity of the damage. Occasionally, the reflex is present at birth but disappears in the first days. Increasing cerebral edema or slow intracranial hemorrhage then is suspected.

Some examiners test the startle response separately by subjecting the newborn to sudden noise (see Fig. 28-7D). The newborn's response may be the Moro response described above or only adduction of the extremities accompanied by crying. The response may be diminished or absent if the newborn is in a deep sleep. If there is a consistent, complete absence of response to loud noise, deafness may be expected.

Tonic Neck Reflex

If a newborn's head is turned to one side while he or she is resting, the **tonic neck reflex** can be observed. The arm and the leg on the side toward which the newborn is facing are partially or completely extended, and the opposite arm and leg are flexed (see Fig. 28-7E). This reflex should disappear by the fourth month, because it is another manifestation of the immaturity of the infant's nervous system. If it continues after 4 months, neurologic injury may be present. A persistent absence of this reflex in the newborn period usually indicates CNS injury or neuromuscular disorders.

Stepping Reflex

The **stepping** or **dancing reflex** is another action that is present at birth but disappears within 2 months. This reflex causes newborns to step with one foot and then the other in a walking motion when they are held upright with their feet touching a surface (see Fig. 28-7F). An asymmetrical response may indicate CNS or peripheral nerve injury or fracture of the long bone of the leg.

Protective Reflexes

Protective reflexes are necessary and at times essential for the preservation of the newborn's safety. This group of reflexes includes the following:

- Blinking reflex occurs when newborns are subjected to a bright light or when a finger is tapped on the nose.
- Cough clears the respiratory passages.
- Sneeze reflexes clear the respiratory passages.
- Yawn reflex draws in additional oxygen.

These reflexes, together with the newborn's ability to cry when uncomfortable, to withdraw from painful stimuli, to resist restraint, are all defensive measures. Most of these defensive measures become more complex and highly developed as the infant grows and develops.

Gestational Age Assessment

Accurate assessment of a newborn's gestational age is another important aspect of newborn assessment. Gestational age is the estimated age of the fetus or newborn, expressed in weeks, counting from the first day of the mother's last menstrual period. During the prenatal period, a variety of techniques can be used to estimate the gestational age (see Chap. 17). After the birth, assessment of certain external physical characteristics and neurologic signs can result in a more accurate estimate. Knowing the approximate gestational age helps to determine whether the newborn was born early (preterm), born on time (term), or born late (post-term), compared with the expected 40-week gestation period. When gestational age is compared with birth weight, newborns can be designated as small, appropriate, or large for gestational age. Chapter 41 gives a more complete discussion of these categories, the potential problems they suggest, and the impact they have on planning care for the newborn.

A gestational age assessment should be done in the first days of life, because the extrauterine environment leads to rapid changes in newborn characteristics. The physical characteristics, assessed during the examination, are independent of the newborn's health status and can be evaluated within a few hours of birth. The neurologic criteria necessary for the gestational age examination can be altered by the newborn's initial physical condition. Therefore, this part of the examination may be deferred until later.

Physical and neurologic criteria are useful in gestational age assessment. Ballard and colleagues developed a system for assessing gestational age using seven physical and six neurologic signs. (see Assessment Tool: Estimation of Gestational Age by Maturity Rating; Ballard et al., 1979). Other combinations of criteria may be used in different settings. When learning to do the examination, it may be helpful at first to check only five of the criteria, such as the breasts, ears, genitalia, sole creases, and posture. As proficiency is achieved, the assessment can be expanded to include other areas (Sullivan et al., 1979).

Physical Characteristics

During the growth and development of the fetus, certain external physical characteristics develop in an orderly manner. The presence, absence, or degree of development of these characteristics at birth is used to help determine gestational age.

Skin and Vernix

The skin of premature newborns is thin, pink, smooth, almost transparent (with blood vessels visible), and thickly covered with vernix. The presence or absence of blood vessels is usually observed over the abdomen. With increasing age, the skin becomes thicker and more opaque. By 40 weeks, it is pale with few blood vessels visible and sparse vernix often occurring only in skin creases. The postmature newborn has no vernix and possibly has extensive desquamation and cracking of the skin (Fig. 28-8).

Lanugo

Fine lanugo hair covers the newborn's body at 20 weeks' gestation and begins to disappear first from the face, then the trunk, and then the extremities. If present in the term newborn, it tends to be located only over the shoulders.

Sole Creases

As gestational age increases, the soles of the feet become wrinkled first on the anterior portion and then in the area extending toward the heel by 37 weeks. At 32 weeks, one or two creases can be seen; they become more numerous, criss-crossed, and deeper, covering the anterior two-thirds of the sole. The entire sole, including the heel, is covered at 40 weeks (Fig. 28-9). In the post-term newborn, creases are deeper with possible desquamation of the soles.

Breast Tissue and Areola

The nipples are present early in gestation, but the areola is barely visible until 34 weeks. After this time, the areola becomes raised and hair follicles become evident. Newborns of less than 36 weeks' gestation have no breast tissue. At 36 weeks, a 1- to 2-mm nodule of breast tissue becomes palpable. This increases with gestational age under hormonal stimulation until it reaches 7 to 10 mm at 40 weeks.

Ear Form and Cartilage

Newborns less than 33 weeks' gestation have relatively flat ears. After 34 weeks, the upper pinnae begin to curve inward. By 38 weeks, the upper two-thirds of the pinnae are incurved; this extends to the earlobe by 39 to 40 weeks. Because ear form can vary widely from one individual to another, cartilage is more reliable than ear form when estimating gestational age. If the extremely premature newborn's ear is folded over, it remains in this position due to the absence of cartilage. Cartilage begins to appear at 32 weeks, this enables the ear to return slowly to its original position when folded over. By 36 weeks, the pinnae spring back when folded, and at term they are firm, with the ear standing erect away from the head. (See the ears in Fig. 28-10*A* and *B* for comparison.)

Genitalia

The characteristics of male and female genitalia change with gestational age. In the girl, the clitoris is prominent at 30 to 32 weeks' gestation, whereas the labia majora are small and widely separated. The labia majora increase in size and fullness with age, and at term they completely cover the labia minora and clitoris (Fig. 28-11*A–D*). In the boy, the testes are high in the inguinal canal at about 30 weeks, gradually descend to be felt high in the scrotal sac at 37 weeks, and are well descended into the lower scrotal sac by 40 weeks. Rugae first appear on the scrotum anteriorly at 36 weeks and extend to cover the entire sac by 40 weeks. The post-term newborn often has a pendulous scrotum covered with numerous rugae.

Hair

Strands of hair are very fine in early gestation and tend to mat together like wool, with small bunches sticking out from the head. The full-term newborn has silky hair that lies flat in single strands. In the post-term newborn, the hairline may recede. When using hair as an assessment criterion, it is important to make sure that it is free of vernix before it is assessed and to take into account racial variations in the texture and characteristics of hair.

Nails

At about 20 weeks, the nails appear and gradually grow to cover the nail bed. At term, the nails extend

ASSESSMENT TOOL
Estimation of Gestational Age by Maturity Rating

RACE _____ LENGTH _____

DATE/TIME OF BIRTH _____ HEAD CIRC. _____

DATE/TIME OF EXAM _____ EXAMINER _____

AGE WHEN EXAMINED _____

APGAR SCORE: 1 MINUTE _____ 5 MINUTES _____ 10 MINUTES _____

NEUROMUSCULAR MATURITY

NEUROMUSCULAR MATURITY SIGN	SCORE							RECORD SCORE HERE
	-1	0	1	2	3	4	5	
POSTURE								
SQUARE WINDOW (Wrist)	>90°	90°	60°	45°	30°	0°		
ARM RECOIL		180°	140°-180°	110°-140°	90°-110°	<90°		
POPLITEAL ANGLE	180°	160°	140°	120°	100°	90°	<90°	
SCARF SIGN								
HEEL TO EAR								

TOTAL NEUROMUSCULAR MATURITY SCORE

SCORE

Neuromuscular _____
Physical _____
Total _____

MATURITY RATING

score	weeks
-10	20
-5	22
0	24
5	26
10	28
15	30
20	32
25	34
30	36
35	38
40	40
45	42
50	44

GESTATIONAL AGE (weeks)

By dates _____
By ultrasound _____
By exam _____

PHYSICAL MATURITY

PHYSICAL MATURITY SIGN	SCORE							RECORD SCORE HERE
	-1	0	1	2	3	4	5	
SKIN	sticky friable transparent	gelatinous red translucent	smooth pink visible veins	superficial peeling &/or rash, few veins	cracking pale areas rare veins	parchment deep cracking no vessels	leathery cracked wrinkled	
LANUGO	none	sparse	abundant	thinning	bald areas	mostly bald		
PLANTAR SURFACE	heel-toe 40-50 mm:-1 <40 mm:-2	>50 mm no crease	faint red marks	anterior transverse crease only	creases ant. 2/3	creases over entire sole		
BREAST	imperceptible	barely perceptible	flat areola no bud	stippled areola 1-2 mm bud	raised areola 3-4 mm bud	full areola 5-10 mm bud		
EYE/EAR	lids fused loosely: -1 tightly: -2	lids open pinna flat stays folded	sl. curved pinna; soft; slow recoil	well-curved pinna; soft but ready recoil	formed & firm instant recoil	thick cartilage ear stiff		
GENITALS (Male)	scrotum flat, smooth	scrotum empty faint rugae	testes in upper canal rare rugae	testes descending few rugae	testes down good rugae	testes pendulous deep rugae		
GENITALS (Female)	clitoris prominent & labia flat	prominent clitoris & small labia minora	prominent clitoris & enlarging minora	majora & minora equally prominent	majora large minora small	majora cover clitoris & minora		

TOTAL PHYSICAL MATURITY SCORE

Reference
Ballard JL, Khoury JC, Wedig K, et al: New Ballard Score, expanded to include extremely premature infants. *J Pediatr* 1991; 119:417-423. Reprinted by permission of Dr Ballard and Mosby-Year Book, Inc.

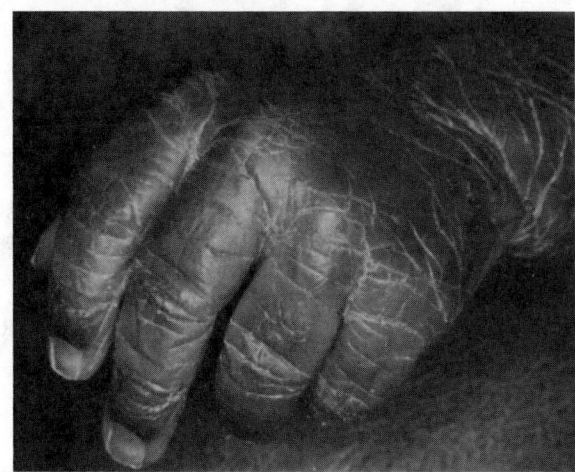

FIGURE 28-8 Post-term infant's hand. Note dry, peeling, cracked skin. (Sullivan R., Foster J., Schreiner R. L. (1979). Determining a newborn's gestational age. *MCN, American Journal of Maternal/Child Nursing,* January/February, 4:38–45)

slightly beyond the fingertips. Long nails well beyond the fingertips are characteristic of postmature newborns.

Skull Firmness

The preterm newborn has soft skull bones, particularly near the fontanels and sutures. The bones become firmer as gestation progresses, and at term, the sutures are not easily displaced.

Neuromuscular Development

Gestational age may be assessed according to a number of neuromuscular responses evident in the new-

born within the first few days of life. The newborn's posture, passive range of motion of certain parts, righting reactions, and various reflexes are evaluated. The development of muscle tone begins in the lower extremities and progresses in a cephalad direction.

The neuromuscular examination is best done when the newborn is in the quiet alert state, because certain reflexes are abolished during active (rapid eye movement) sleep and others during quiet sleep (Nelson, 1992). A shortened examination, including posture, tonicity, and recoil, may be done during the first few hours after birth, with the more extensive examination delayed. Charts and scoring systems are used for these parameters. Neuromuscular assessment items are included in gestational age scoring systems (see Assessment Tools: Dubowitz Scoring System and Estimation of Gestational Age by Maturity Rating).

Resting Posture and Extremity Recoil

The newborn's resting posture and extremity recoil in the first hour after birth provides a reasonable estimation of the newborn's neuromuscular development. The remainder of the neuromuscular examination is better carried out a day or two later to confirm the original findings. The resting posture of the premature newborn is characterized by little flexion of the upper extremities and only partial flexion of the lower. At about 30 weeks, there is slight flexion of the feet and knees. Flexion of the hips and thighs resulting in the characteristic frog position of the legs occurs at 34 weeks, but the arms are extended. At 36 to 38 weeks, the resting posture of the newborn is one of complete flexion of all four extremities (Fig. 28-12).

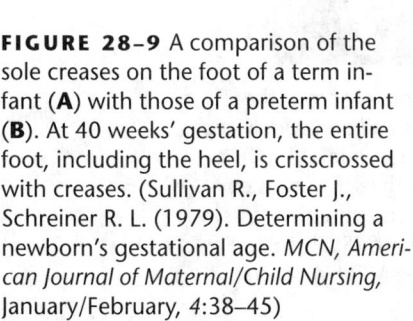

FIGURE 28-9 A comparison of the sole creases on the foot of a term infant (**A**) with those of a preterm infant (**B**). At 40 weeks' gestation, the entire foot, including the heel, is crisscrossed with creases. (Sullivan R., Foster J., Schreiner R. L. (1979). Determining a newborn's gestational age. *MCN, American Journal of Maternal/Child Nursing,* January/February, 4:38–45)

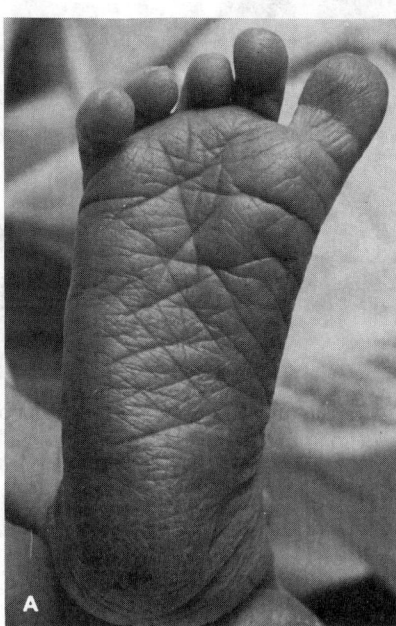

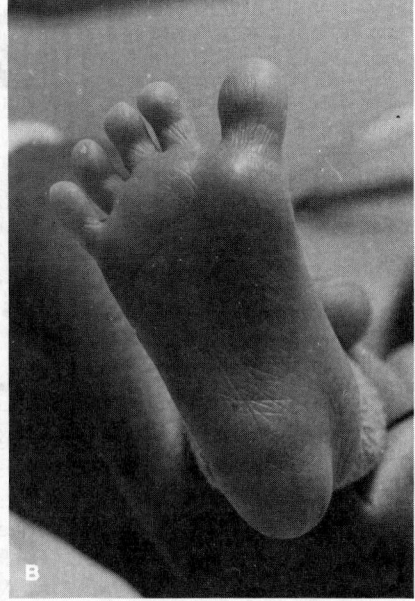

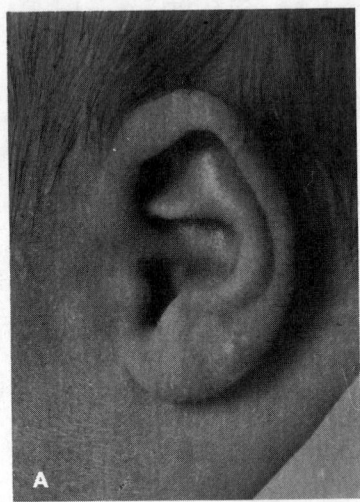
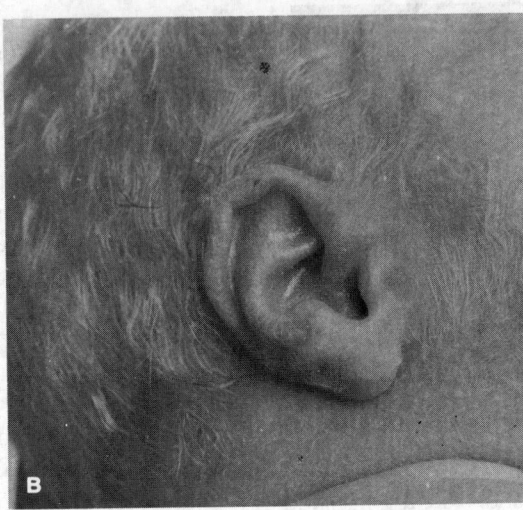

FIGURE 28-10 Cartilage is well developed in the term infant (**A**) and the ear is erect, away from the head, whereas the ears of the preterm infant (**B**) lie flat against the head. Also note the matted hair of the preterm infant. (Sullivan R., Foster J., Schreiner R. L. (1979). Determining a newborn's gestational age. *MCN, American Journal of Maternal/ Child Nursing,* January/February, 4:38–45)

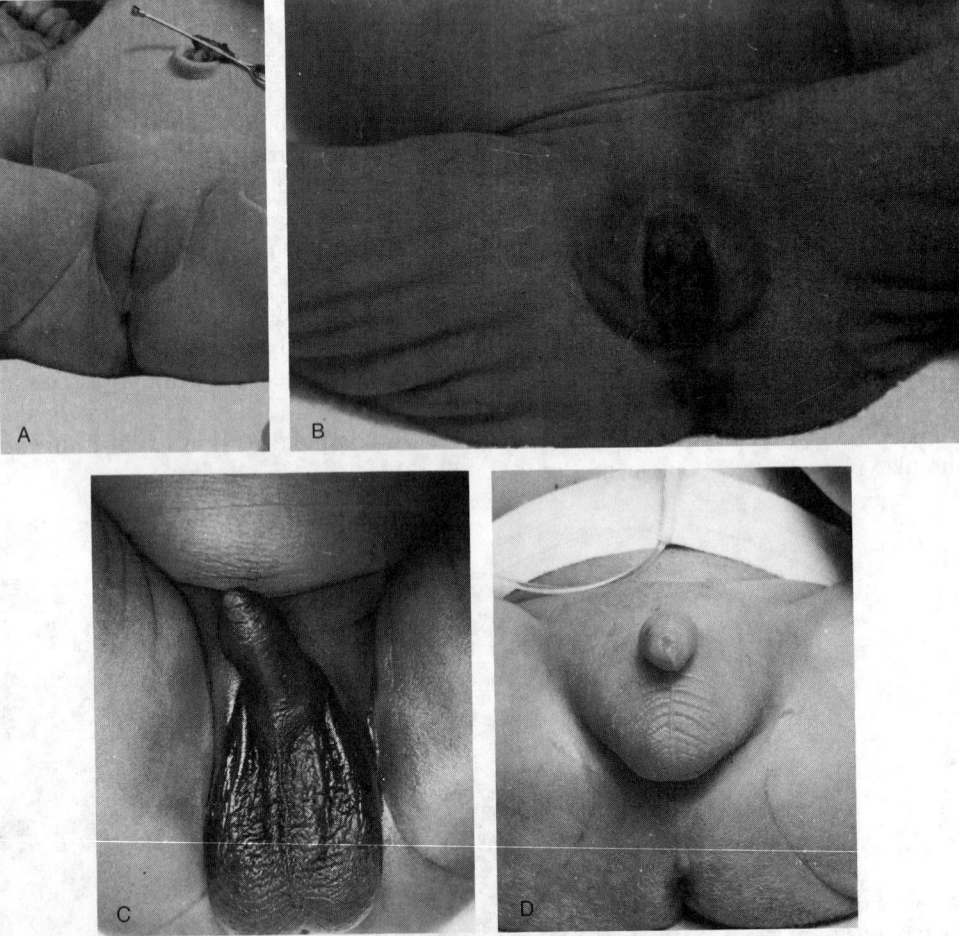

FIGURE 28-11 The labia majora of the term female infant (**A**) completely cover the labia minora and clitoris. However, in the preterm infant (**B**) they are small and widely separated. Also note the loose skin folds on the posterior thighs of the preterm infant. (**C**) In the male infant, the testes are well descended into the scrotal sac and the scrotum is covered with numerous rugae in the term infant, whereas (**D**) the testes remain high in the inguinal canal and the rugae are largely undeveloped in the preterm infant. (Sullivan R., Foster J., Schreiner R. L. (1979). Determining a newborn's gestational age. *MCN, American Journal of Maternal/Child Nursing,* January/February, 4:38–45)

Recoil of extremities lags behind flexion by about 2 weeks. To test recoil, the extremity should be flexed and held for 5 seconds, extended for 30 seconds, and then released. At 36 to 37 weeks, the extremities remain extended. Brisk return to the flexed position indicates a full-term newborn.

Ankle and Wrist Flexion

Pressure is applied to the foot to push it toward the anterior aspect of the leg. The resulting angle between the dorsum of the foot and the leg is then measured. In premature newborns, this angle is 45 to 90 degrees, whereas in full-term newborns the foot can be flexed until it touches the leg (Fig. 28-13*A* and *B*). Similarly, the wrist is flexed with enough pressure to bring the hand as close to the forearm as possible (square window). The angle between the hypothenar eminence of the wrist and the ventral aspect of the forearm is measured. During this test, care is taken not to rotate the wrist. In the premature newborn, the angle is 90 degrees. In the full-term newborn, the wrist can be flexed on the arm (see Fig. 28-13*C* and *D*).

Scarf Sign

The newborn's arms are drawn across the neck as far across the opposite shoulder as possible (like a scarf). In the premature newborn, there is less resistance and a greater draping (or scarf) effect. This maneuver is best carried out by lifting the elbow across the front of the body. Note how far across the chest the elbow will go. In the premature newborn, the elbow reaches near or across the midline, whereas in the full-term newborn, it does not reach the midline (Fig. 28-14).

Heel to Ear

With the newborn in the supine position with hips flat, the foot is drawn as close to the ear as possible without forcing it. In a premature newborn, there is very little resistance, the foot may almost touch the ear, and

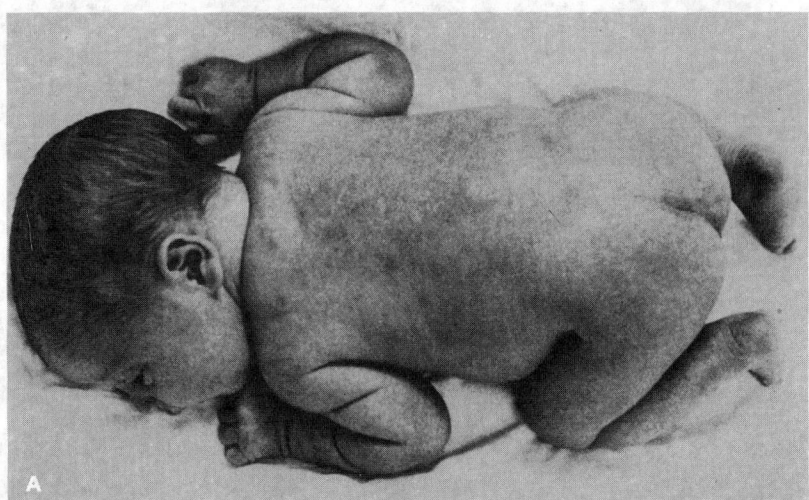

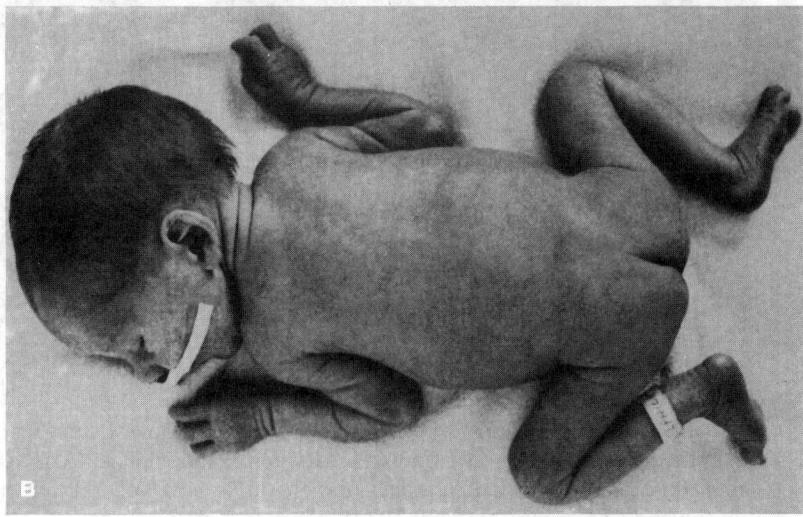

FIGURE 28–12 Resting posture (**A**). Note the flexion of the extremities in the term infant and (**B**) compare to the partial flexion in the preterm infant resulting in a froglike resting posture. (A clinical review of concepts and characteristics in infant development. In *Reflexes,* vol. 2. Evansville, IN: Mead Johnson and Company. Copyright 1974)

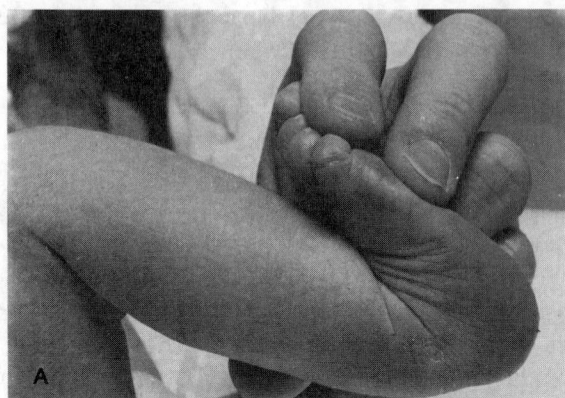
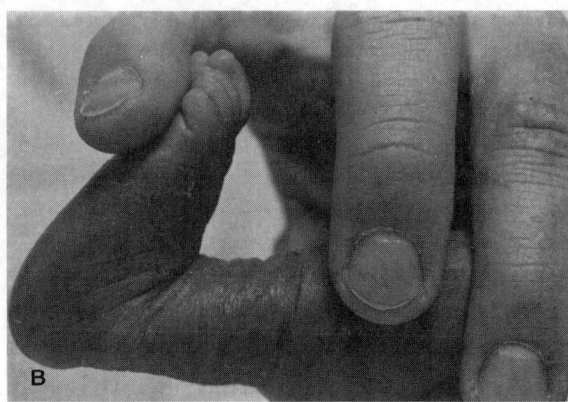
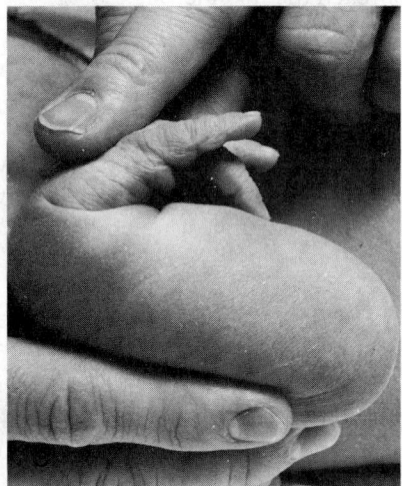
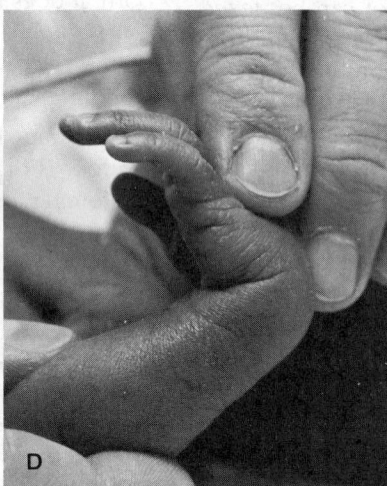

FIGURE 28–13 Dorsiflexion of the ankle—(**A**) In the term infant the foot can be flexed until it touches the leg. (**B**) In the preterm infant the foot can be flexed only to an angle of 45 to 90 degrees. Wrist flexion—(**C**) In the term infant, the wrist can be flexed onto the arm. (**D**) In the preterm infant, the wrist only can be flexed to an angle of about 90 degrees. (Sullivan R., Foster J., Schreiner R. L. (1979). Determining a newborn's gestational age. *MCN, American Journal of Maternal/Child Nursing,* January/February, 4:38–45)

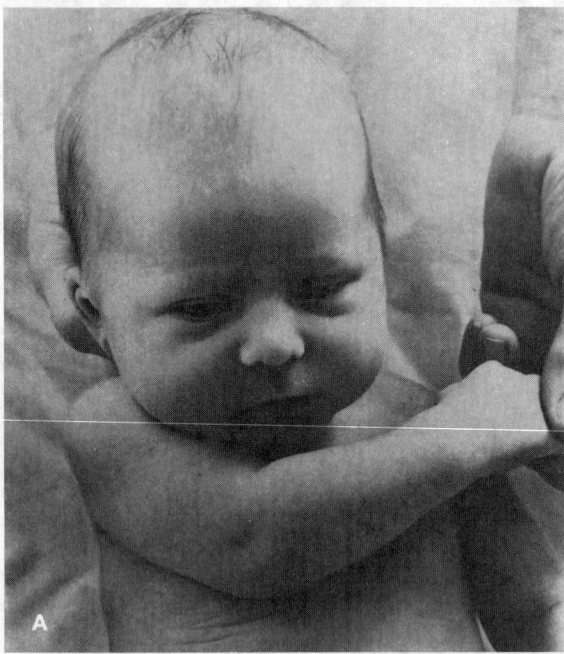
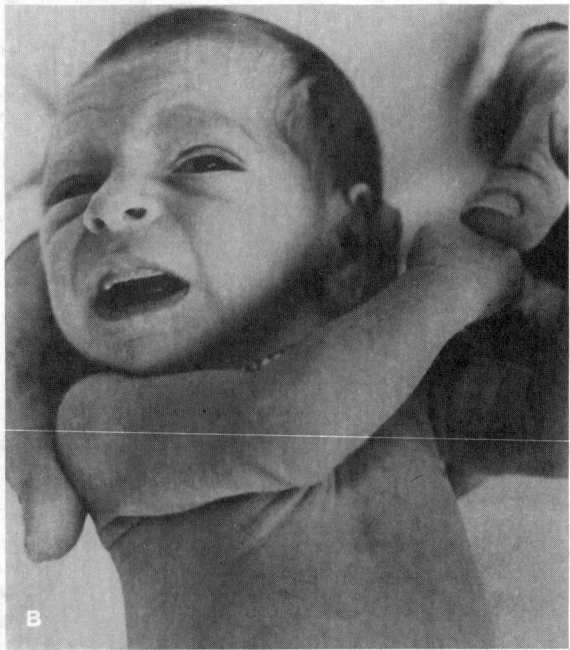

FIGURE 28–14 Scarf sign. (**A**) In the term infant, the elbow will not reach the midline. (**B**) In the preterm infant, the elbow will reach across the midline. (A clinical review of concepts and characteristics in infant development. In *Reflexes,* vol. 2. Evansville, IN: Mead Johnson and Company. Copyright 1974)

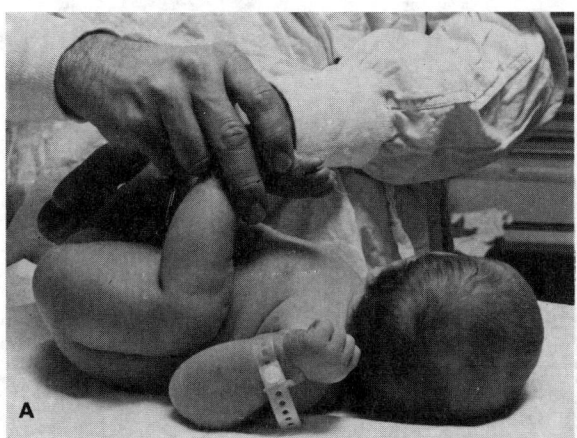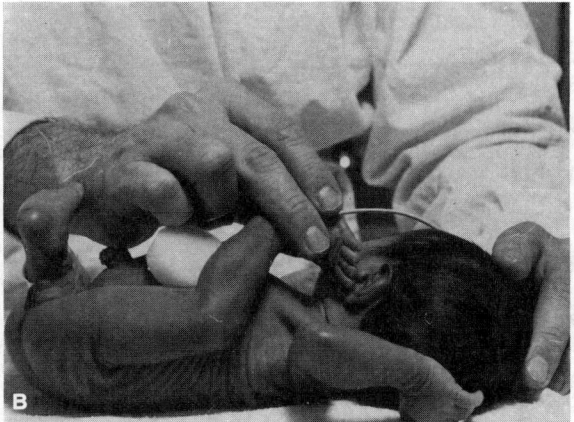

FIGURE 28–15 Heel to ear. (**A**) In the term infant, there is a marked resistance in the leg as the foot is gently drawn toward the ear. (**B**) In the preterm infant, very little resistance is noted. Note the difference in the popliteal angle. (Sullivan R., Foster J., Schreiner R. L. (1979). Determining a newborn's gestational age. *MCN, American Journal of Maternal/Child Nursing*, January/February, 4:38–45)

the leg is well extended. There is marked resistance in the full-term newborn; it is impossible to draw the foot to the ear, and the leg is not well extended (Fig. 28-15).

Popliteal Angle

Passive movement of the leg reveals an inverse relationship between muscle tone and popliteal angle. Thus, a smaller angle is associated with greater muscle tone. Premature newborns have larger popliteal angles than full-term newborns.

Ventral Suspension

The newborn is suspended in the prone position with the hand of the examiner supporting it under the chest (two hands may be used for a large newborn). The degree of extension of the back and head and the degree of flexion of the arms and legs are noted. The premature newborn hangs limply with arms and legs almost straight and back rounded. The full-term newborn extends the head, straightens the back, and flexes the arms and legs (Fig. 28-16).

Head Lag

With the newborn in a supine position, the hands or arms are grasped, and the newborn is pulled slowly to a sitting position. The position of the head should be observed in relation to the trunk. The premature newborn has no flexion of the neck. A gradual increase in flexion can be noted as gestation progresses. The full-term newborn holds the head erect while being pulled to a sitting position (Fig. 28-17).

Reflexes

Although there are differences in reflexes according to gestational age, these are not as age specific as the signs described previously and are less useful in determining gestational age. The reflexes of the normal newborn are discussed in the section "Neurologic Assessment." In the premature newborn, the rooting reflex is less developed, as evidenced by the slower response in turning the head toward the stimulus. The sucking reflex is weak or absent, depending on degree of prematurity and health condition. This reflex begins at about 34 weeks' gestation. The sucking reflex is of particular importance because it is related to the ability to take adequate nourishment with nipple feedings. The grasp reflex is weak, and the newborn cannot be lifted off the bed while grasping the examiner's finger. The Moro reflex also is weak, and the stepping reflex is often absent.

Behavioral Assessment

In addition to physiologic change, the newborn also demonstrates behavioral changes in the initial hours following birth. Periods of reactivity alternating with periods of sleep have been identified (Fig. 28-18). Observation of these changes in behavior and behavioral state provides clues to the newborn's well-being and adaptation to extrauterine life. Although most healthy newborns go through this period without difficulty, supportive care must be available in case appropriate adaptations do not occur. Nurses who care for newborns should be aware of the usual pattern of these changes to facilitate optimal care for the newborn and to provide information for the new parents.

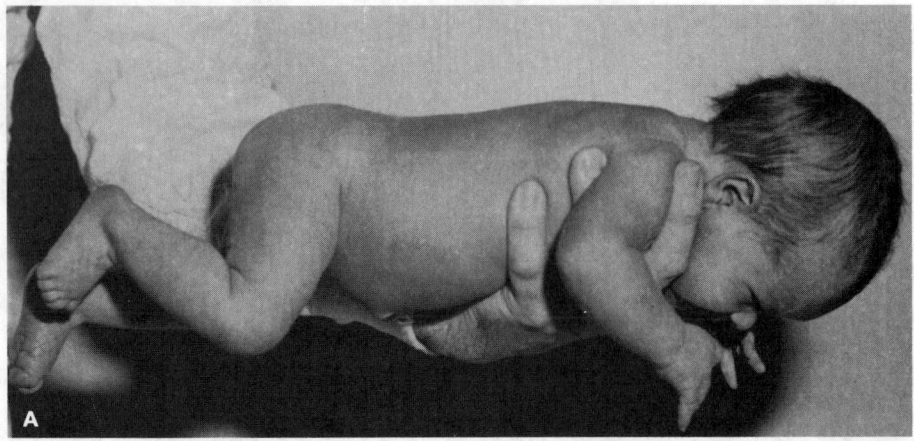

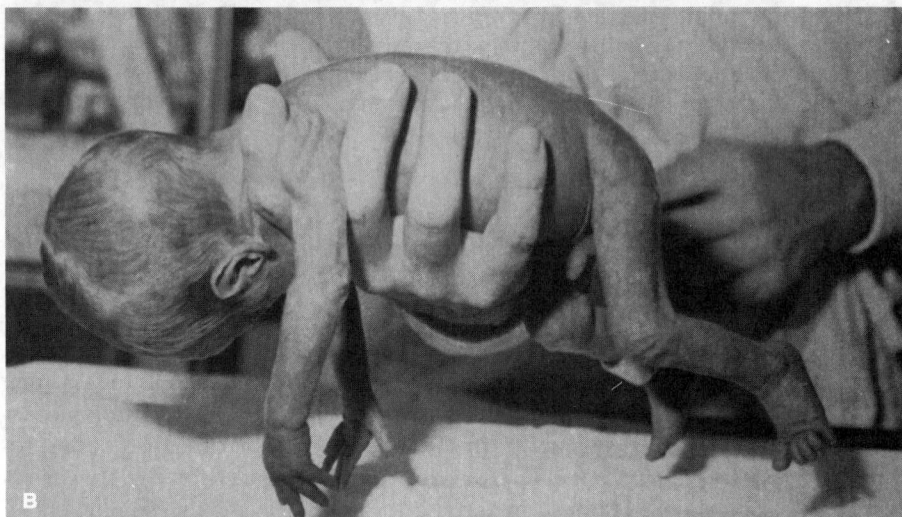

FIGURE 28-16 Ventral suspension. (**A**) When suspended in the prone position, the term infant's head extends, the back is straight, and the arms and legs flex. (**B**) However, the preterm infant hangs limply with the arms and legs almost straight. (Sullivan R., Foster J., Schreiner R. L. (1979). Determining a newborn's gestational age. *MCN, American Journal of Maternal/Child Nursing,* January/February, 4:38–45)

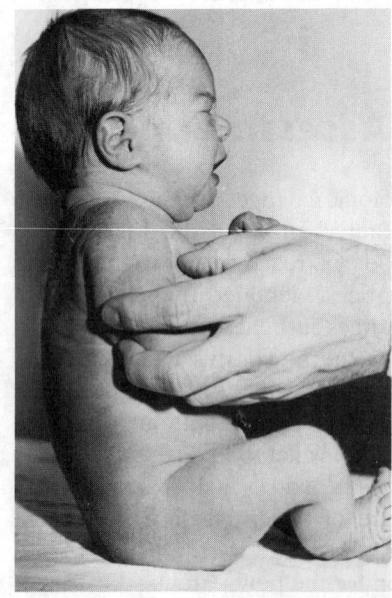

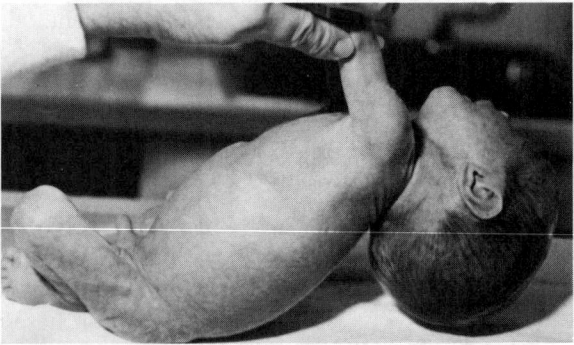

FIGURE 28-17 Head lag. (**A**) As the infant is slowly pulled from a supine to a sitting position, the term infant holds the head erect. (**B**) The preterm infant has no flexion in the neck. (Sullivan R., Foster J., Schreiner R. L. (1979). Determining a newborn's gestational age. *MCN, American Journal of Maternal/Child Nursing,* January/February, 4:38–45)

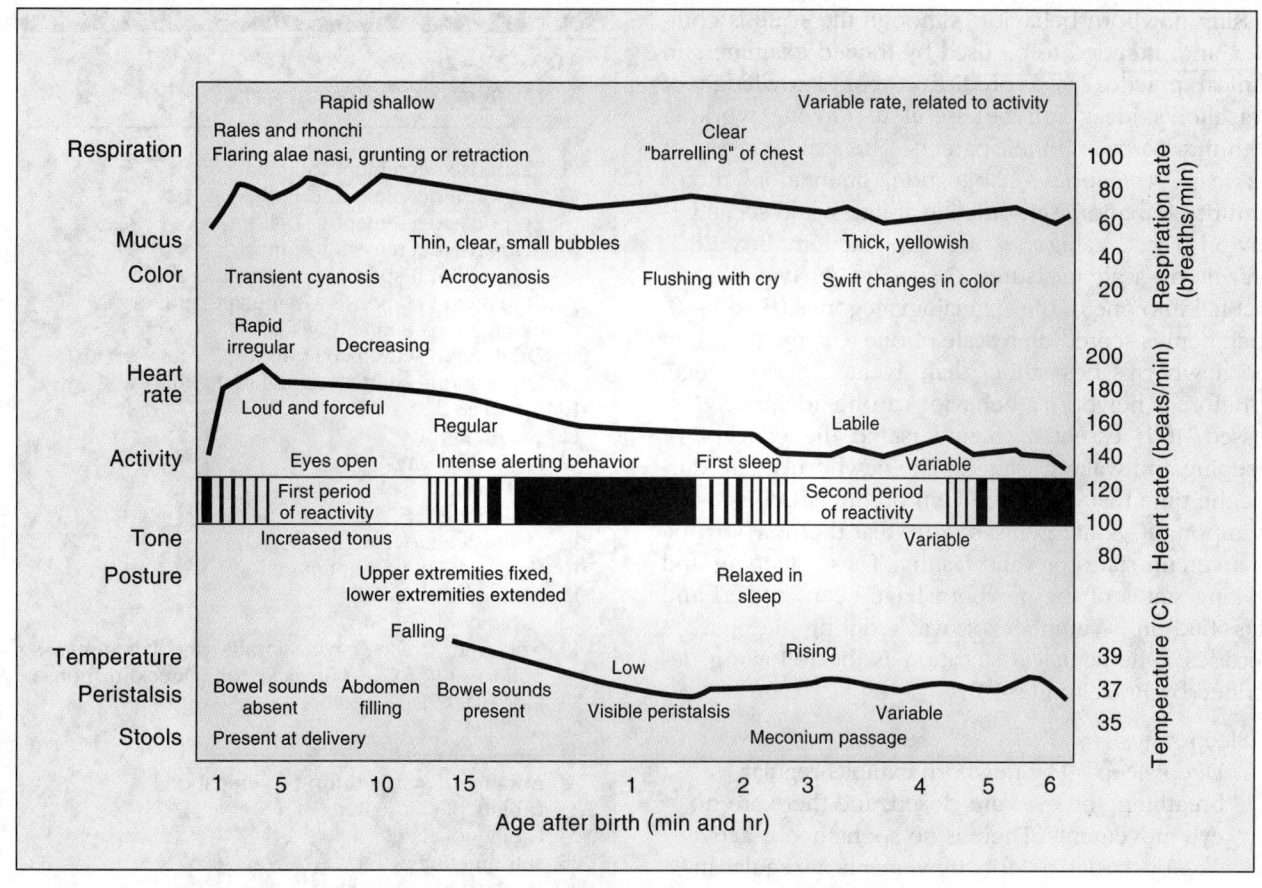

FIGURE 28-18 Periods of reactivity. (After Arnold, H. W., Putnam, N. J., Barnard, B. L., et al. [1965]. Transition to extrauterine life. *American Journal of Nursing, 65*(10), 78.)

Periods of Reactivity

A healthy newborn begins life with intense activity. This phase has been designated by some authorities as the first **period of reactivity**. In this phase, the newborn exhibits outbursts of diffuse, purposeless movements that alternate with periods of relative immobility in a quiet alert state. Vital signs may be unstable with rapid respirations and transient signs of increased respiratory effort, such as flaring of the nares and grunting.

Tachycardia may be present at times, and the heart rate may reach 180 beats/min in the first minutes of life, falling to an average of 120 to 140 beats/min soon after. Quiet times during this period are often ideal for initial breast-feeding or other interactions with the parents, as long as appropriate attention is paid to suctioning the newborn as necessary and keeping him or her warm.

After this initial responsive period, the newborn becomes relatively quiet and falls into a deep sleep during which there is no intense response to internal or external stimuli. This first sleep occurs, on average, about 2 hours after birth and may last a few minutes to several hours.

When next awake, the newborn is again hyper-responsive to stimuli. This has been termed the second period of reactivity. The newborn's color may change rapidly (from pink to moderately cyanotic), and the heart rate responds to stimulation and becomes rapid. Oral mucus may be a major problem in respiration during this period. The newborn may choke, gag, and regurgitate. A bulb syringe should be available for suctioning as needed. If mucus is excessive, appropriate intervention must be taken. Because the length of the second period of reactivity is variable, the newborn's caretaker should be alert to the possible occurrence of these problems during the first 12 to 18 hours of the newborn's life. However most healthy full-term newborns have achieved a state of behavioral equilibrium by about 6 to 8 hours after birth. Thus, the transition from intrauterine to extrauterine life has been successfully accomplished.

Behavioral Assessment Scales

Following the transition phase, newborns begin to exhibit unique behavioral competencies as they actively interact with their environment. Behavioral assessment by the nurse contributes important information about an individual neonate's behavioral responses.

The **Neonatal Behavioral Assessment Scale** (NBAS), developed by Brazelton (1973), is useful in assessing newborn behavior. Although the scale is complex and intended to be used by trained examiners in clinical practice as a predictive tool, knowledge of Brazelton's ideas can be useful to anyone working with newborns and their parents. The scale consists of six major categories—habituation, orientation, motor maturity, variation, self-quieting abilities, and social behavior. These categories are explained in Box 28-1. Brazelton's scale measures 27 specific behavioral items that fall into one of the six major categories (Box 28-2). Each item is scored on a scale of one to nine, based on the newborn's best rather than average performance.

Before a newborn's behavior can be adequately assessed, it is essential to understand the concept of sleeping and waking "states." The newborn's state during the time that any given item on the NBAS is tested is important. Some items *require* that the newborn be in a certain state for valid testing. These sleeping and waking states of the newborn have been studied and classified in a number of ways during the past 3 decades. One such classification is the following described by Brazelton (1973):

■ Sleep states:

Deep sleep—The newborn exhibits regular breathing; the eyes are closed, and there are no eye movements. There is no spontaneous activity except startles or jerky movements at regular intervals. External stimuli produce startles with some delay, and suppression of startles is rapid. Changes from this state are less likely than from other states.

BOX 28–2
Brazelton Scale Criteria

1. Response decrement to light
2. Response decrement to rattle
3. Response decrement to bell
4. Response decrement to pinprick
5. Orientation response—inanimate visual
6. Orientation response—inanimate auditory
7. Orientation—animate visual
8. Orientation—animate auditory
9. Orientation—animate visual and auditory
10. Alertness
11. General tonus
12. Motor maturity
13. Pull-to-sit
14. Cuddliness
15. Defensive movements
16. Consolability with intervention
17. Peak of excitement
18. Rapidity of buildup
19. Irritability (to aversive stimuli—uncover, undress, pull-to-sit, prone, pinprick, tonic neck response, Moro, defensive reaction)
20. Activity
21. Tremulousness
22. Amount of startle during examination
23. Lability of skin color
24. Lability of states
25. Self-quieting activity
26. Hand-to-mouth facility
27. Smiles

BOX 28–1
Brazelton Scale Criteria Categories

1. Habituation—How soon the neonate diminishes responses to specific repeated stimuli. Items tested are response to light, rattle, bell, and pinprick.
2. Orientation—How often and when the newborn attends to auditory and visual stimuli. Items include inanimate and animate visual and auditory stimuli.
3. Motor Maturity—Demonstrated by how well the newborn coordinates and controls motor activities as tested by items such as alertness, general tonus, and pull-to-sit.
4. Variation—Indicated by how often the newborn exhibits alertness, state changes, color changes, activity, and peaks of excitement.
5. Self-quieting abilities—How often, how soon, and how effectively the neonate can use his or her own resources to quiet and console himself or herself when upset or distressed. Behaviors tested include hand-to-mouth facility.
6. Social behaviors—Measured by how often and how much the newborn smiles and cuddles.

Light sleep—The eyes are closed, and rapid eye movements can be observed under closed lids. The newborn will exhibit a low activity level, with random movements and startles or startle equivalents. These movements are likely to be smoother and more monitored than in deep sleep. The newborn will respond to internal and external stimuli with startle equivalents, often with a resulting change of state. Irregular respirations and on–off sucking movements will be observed.

■ Awake states:

Drowsy or semidozing—The eyes may be open or closed, and the eyelids will flutter. The newborn's activity level is variable with interspersed, mild startles from time to time. The newborn is reactive to sensory stimuli, but the response is often delayed. A state change after stimulation is frequently noted. Movements are usually smooth.
Alert—The newborn is quiet and alert with a bright look. He or she seems to focus attention on a source of stimulation, such as an object to be sucked or a visual or auditory stimulus. Impinging stimuli may break through but with some delay in response. Motor activity is minimal.

Eyes open—The newborn will have considerable motor activity, with thrusting movements of the extremities and even a few spontaneous startles. The newborn is reactive to external stimulation, manifested by an increase in startles or motor activity. However, discrete reactions are difficult to distinguish because of general high activity level. Crying—This state is characterized by intense crying that is difficult to break through with stimulation.

Other sleeping and waking classifications include similar components but add transition states between sleeping and waking and within the sleep state (Thoman, 1990). There is great variation in the amount of time newborns spend in the various states and in the ease or difficulty with which they make the transition from one state to another. Sleep cycles generally lengthen with maturation of the CNS. Therefore, immature newborns are more likely to have shorter, less well-defined cycles (Brazelton, 1994).

How a newborn responds to being cuddled is one of the items that is assessed on the NBAS scale. The newborn is held in a cuddled position against the examiner's chest or shoulder. Their response is measured on a scale of 1 to 9. A 1 score indicates "actually resists being held, continuously pushes away, and thrashes or stiffens." On the other end of the scale, the 9 score indicates "molds into arms and relaxes, turns toward examiner's body when held horizontally, leans forward when held on the examiner's shoulder, and all of the body participates and baby grasps examiner to cling to him" (Brazelton, 1984).

Another item assessed on the scale is a newborn's ability to be consoled or to console himself or herself. This ability should be scored when the newborn is crying. Some newborns quiet down when they are dressed and left alone. Others need restraint to help them inhibit the startle reflex. These babies are the ones that usually do best when swaddled in a blanket.

Possible self-consoling activities that are counted in the assessment are hand-to-mouth efforts, sucking on fist or tongue, or using visual or auditory stimuli from the environment to quiet himself or herself. Discovering ways in which their newborn can console himself or herself or be consoled can be helpful to the parents.

Information from the NBAS can be used by the nurse as a guide for teaching parents what behaviors they can anticipate in their newborn. For example, they will be interested in knowing that most newborns focus on a bright red ball and follow it briefly when they are in the quiet alert state, that the newborn particularly likes to follow a moving human face or a high-pitched voice, and that responses are usually delayed when the newborn is in the drowsy state. Parents also would be interested to know that if they observe their newborn smiling, it may be a true social smile and not just a reflex or gas. According to Brazelton, he has seen close replicas of social smiles in the newborn period, and although it is difficult to tell whether or not these are "real" smiles, he feels confident that they are precursors of smiling behavior. As a result, parents should be encouraged to reinforce smiling behavior in their newborn (Brazelton, 1984).

Summary Points

✔ Many changes occur in the newborn during the transition period from fetal to extrauterine life. Knowledge of the necessary adaptations and expected changes assists the nurse in assessing and caring for newborns.

✔ Establishing adequate respiratory function in the neonatal period depends on maturity of the respiratory system, presence of stimuli to initiate respiration, and successful completion of the process of clearing fluid from the lungs and maintaining lung expansion.

✔ The change from fetal to neonatal circulation occurs shortly after birth in the normal term newborn and is essential to continuing adequate oxygenation of vital organs.

✔ Erythrocyte, hemoglobin, and hematocrit levels of newborns are high compared with those of adults; this is because of the fetal attempt to compensate for fetal circulation and to maintain adequate oxygenation.

✔ Thermoregulation is an important consideration during the newborn period because of the newborn's predisposition to lose heat. Nonshivering thermogenesis, the newborn's response to heat loss, results in increased consumption of oxygen and calories and may lead to metabolic acidosis.

✔ Physical assessment of the newborn begins at birth with the Apgar scoring and is done at intervals to identify the newborn's progress in adapting to extrauterine life and to detect deviations from normal.

✔ CNS functioning in the newborn period is assessed by observing the newborn's spontaneous movements for symmetry and smoothness; eliciting necessary reflexes, such as rooting, sucking, and blinking; and identifying the presence of other reflexes that are appropriate to the newborn period.

✔ Physical characteristics that are observed as part of the gestational age assessment include skin and vernix, lanugo, sole creases, breast tissue and areola, ear form and cartilage, and genitalia. Differences in neuromuscular development, such as resting posture and extremity recoil, ankle and wrist flexion, popliteal angle, scarf sign, heel to ear, ventral suspension, and head lag also are assessed and contribute to the assignment of a total score that helps determine the gestational age.

✔ Behavioral assessment not only contributes to the overall assessment of the newborn, but also is a valuable tool for the nurse in providing anticipatory guidance to the parents regarding ways of interacting with their newborn.

REFERENCES

Arnold, H. W., Putman, N. J., Barnard, B. L. et al. (1965). Transition to extrauterine life. American Journal of Nursing, 65(10), 77–80.

Ballard, J. et al. (1979). A simplified score for assessment of fetal maturation of newly born infants. *Journal of Pediatrics, 95,* 769–774.

Bellanti, J. A., Boner, A. L., & Valletta, E. (1994). Immunology of the fetus and newborn. In G. B. Avery, M. B. Fletcher, & M. G. Macdonald (Eds.), *Neonatology: Pathophysiology and management of the newborn* (pp. 1000–1028) (4th ed.). Philadelphia: J.B. Lippincott.

Brann, A. W., Jr., & Schwartz, J. F. (1992). Assessment of neonatal neurologic functioning. In A. A. Fanaroff & R. J. Martin (Eds.), *Neonatal-perinatal medicine* (pp. 691–699) (5th ed.). St. Louis: Mosby Year Book.

Brazelton, T. B. (1973). Neonatal behavioral assessment scale. *Clinics in Developmental Medicine, 50.*

Brazelton, T. B. (1994). Behavioral competence. In G. B. Avery, M. B. Fletcher, & M. G. Macdonald (Eds.), *Neonatology: Pathophysiology and management of the newborn* (pp. 289–300) (4th ed.). Philadelphia: J.B. Lippincott.

Brazelton, T. B. (1984). *The neonatal behavioral assessment scale* (2nd ed.). Philadelphia: J.B. Lippincott.

Brucker, M. C., & MacMullen, N. J. (1987). Neonatal jaundice in the home: Assessment with a noninvasive device. *Journal of Obstetric, Gynecologic, and Neonatal Nursing, 16,* 355–358.

Bucuvalas, J. C., & Balistreri, W. F. (1992). The neonatal gastrointestinal tract. In A. A. Fanaroff & R. J. Martin (Eds.), *Neonatal-perinatal medicine* (pp. 1019–1023) (5th ed.). St. Louis: Mosby Year Book.

Cabal, L. A., Siassi, B., & Hodgman, J. (1992). Neonatal clinical cardiopulmonary monitoring. In A. A. Fanaroff & R. J. Martin (Eds.), *Neonatal-perinatal medicine* (pp. 437–455) (5th ed.). St. Louis: Mosby Year Book.

Dubowitz, L. et al. (1970). Clinical assessment of gestational age in the newborn infant. *Journal of Pediatrics, 77,* 1–10.

Easterly, N. B., & Solomon, L. M. (1992). The skin. In A. A. Fanaroff & R. J. Martin (Eds.), *Neonatal-perinatal medicine* (pp. 1328–1358) (5th ed.). St. Louis: Mosby Year Book.

Gartner, L. M., & Lee, K. S. (1992). Jaundice and liver disease. In A. A. Fanaroff & R. J. Martin (Eds.), *Neonatal-perinatal medicine* (pp. 1075–1103) (5th ed.). St. Louis: Mosby Year Book.

Jobe, A. H. (1992). The developmental biology of the lung. In A. A. Fanaroff & R. J. Martin (Eds.), *Neonatal-perinatal medicine* (pp. 783–800) (5th ed.). St. Louis: Mosby Year Book.

Korones, S. B. (1986). *High-risk newborn infants: The basis for intensive nursing care* (pp. 209–210) (4th ed.). St. Louis: C.V. Mosby.

Nelson, N. (1992). Neonatal adaptations: Physiologic status of the healthy infant. In R. A. Hoekelman (Ed.), *Primary pediatric care* (pp. 436–467) (2nd ed.). St. Louis: Mosby Year Book.

Phibbs, R. H. (1991). The newborn infant. In A. M. Rudolph (Ed.), *Rudolph's pediatrics* (pp. 165–210) (19th ed.). Norwalk, CT: Appleton & Lange.

Rigatto, H. (1992). Fetal-neonatal respiration. In R. A. Polin & W. W. Fox (Eds.), *Fetal and neonatal physiology.* Philadelphia: W.B. Saunders.

Shurin, S. B. (1992). Hematologic problems of the fetus and neonate. In A. A. Fanaroff & R. J. Martin (Eds.), *Neonatal-perinatal medicine* (pp. 941–988) (5th ed.). St. Louis: Mosby Year Book.

Spitzer, A., Bernstein, J., Bolchis, H., & Edelman, C. M. Jr. (1992). The kidney and urinary tract. In A. A. Fanaroff & R. J. Martin (Eds.), *Neonatal-perinatal medicine* (pp. 1293–1327) (5th ed.). St. Louis: Mosby Year Book.

Sullivan, R., Foster, J., & Schreiner, R. L. (1979). Determining a newborn's gestational age. *MCN: American Journal of Maternal Child Nursing, 4,* 38–45.

Thoman, E. B. (1990). Sleeping and waking states in infants: A functional perspective. *Neuroscience Biobehavioral Review, 14,* 93–107.

Yoder, M. C., & Polin, R. A. (1992). Developmental Immunology. In A. A. Fanaroff & R. J. Martin (Eds.), *Neonatal-perinatal medicine* (pp. 587–618) (5th ed.). St. Louis: Mosby Year Book.

SUGGESTED READING

Anderson, C. (1986). Integration of the Brazelton neonatal behavioral assessment scale into routine neonatal nursing care. *Issues in Comprehensive Pediatric Nursing, 9,* 341–351.

Brazelton, T. B. (1984). *The Neonatal Behavioral Assessment Scale* (2nd ed.). Philadelphia: J.B. Lippincott.

Coen, R. W., Fanaroff, A. A., & Taylor, P. M. (1988). A fast, efficient newborn exam. *Patient Care, 22*(10), 192–207.

Coen, R. W., Fanaroff, A. A., & Taylor, P. M. (1988). The detailed newborn examination. *Patient Care, 22*(12), 90–112.

Keefe, M. R., Kotzer, A. M., Reuss, J. L. et al. (1989). Development of a system for monitoring infant state behavior. *Nursing Research, 38,* 344–347.

NAACOG (1990). *Neonatal thermoregulation. OGN Nursing Practice Resource.* Washington, DC: Author.

NAACOG (1991). *Physical assessment of the neonate. OGN Nursing Practice Resource.* Washington, DC: Author.

29

Nursing Care and Sensory Enrichment of the Normal Newborn

Objectives

- Discuss care of the newborn during the early transition to extrauterine life.
- State the important areas to address when protecting the newborn from injury and infection.
- Describe the various settings that are used to provide care for newborns.
- Summarize the elements of nursing care that are important in the continuing care of the newborn.
- Outline the components of basic child care information that parents need to be taught before discharge from the hospital.
- Contrast the pros and cons of neonatal circumcision.
- List the specific screening tests for inborn errors of metabolism that are most frequently required by state laws.
- State the major risk factors that are believed to be associated with sudden infant death syndrome.
- Discuss sensory enrichment for the newborn, including the rationale for its inclusion in newborn care and ways in which it can be implemented.
- Outline ways that maternity nursing is taking on an increased community focus.

Key Terms

Baby clean	Meconium
Colic	Mother-newborn
Couplet care	couple care
Cradle cap	Prickly heat
Hypertonic	Smegma
Inborn errors of	Thermistor
metablolism	Transitional stools

The care of the newborn presents an interesting challenge to those who work in maternity nursing. In a short time, the fetus, who has been completely dependent on the woman to supply all the physiologic needs, suddenly becomes an "independent" being. Although independent of the mother for vital functions, newborns still are very dependent in other ways. They could not survive long without a caretaker. In the immediate newborn period, this caretaker is often the nurse.

Because these first days and weeks are so critical, the care given by the nurse and the teaching provided for the parents are important. The nurse must use the utmost care when handling the newborns, keeping them warm and protecting them from exposure and injury, while making accurate observations and recording and reporting them. Communication and teaching skills contribute to the newborn's future well-being by helping the parents develop an understanding of their newborn's needs and acquire skill in his or her care. In this way, their concept of themselves as adequate parents is reinforced. The nurse also must be aware that some parents need assistance in developing healthy attitudes regarding child-rearing practices so that the newborn can make a satisfactory emotional and social adjustment. Opportunity must be provided in the hospital environment for the beginning development of a close parent–infant relationship. Also important is the maintenance of communication between the nurse and the parents.

This chapter describes the nursing care of the normal newborn. Using the nursing process as a framework, the essential aspects of care for the newborn during the transition period are presented. Different newborn care areas and measures to provide a safe environment are addressed. Continuing care of the normal newborn is discussed with an emphasis on parent teaching and discharge planning.

Nursing Care During the Transition Period

Shortly after birth, initial care is given to the newborn. During this time, any early problems are identified, and measures are instituted to deal with them (see Chap. 24). If the birthing room is not a labor, delivery, recovery, postpartum (LDRP) room where the newborn will remain until being released to go home, the newborn may initially be taken to the recovery room and remain with the mother and father for a while, go to a transitional nursery for initial care, or be admitted directly to the regular nursery. Of course, if the newborn has serious problems, admission to a special-care nursery is indicated.

The day of birth is the most hazardous time for the newborn; therefore, continuing observations must be made during the first 24 hours, with the first few hours being the most critical. A receiving or transitional nursery in the labor or nursery section provides an excellent physical environment for the extensive observations that are necessary. Care in a transitional nursery is similar to that of recovery room care for adults. A newborn whose mother has been heavily medicated during labor and delivery is particularly in need of this recovery care. If this kind of setup is not available, the newborn should be placed in an area of the regular nursery where close observation is possible. Newborns considered low risk, such as those whose mothers had little or no medication, can probably be safely left with their mothers under close supervision of a nurse. Where rooming-in is practiced, it may be delayed for several hours until the newborn is considered stable with no signs of respiratory or other problems.

Assessment During Transition

Ongoing early assessment of the newborn may occur in the LDRP room, recovery room, or nursery. When the newborn is admitted to the nursery, the nursery nurse receives a report from the delivery room nurse, checks identification bands according to hospital policy, and checks the newborn's record to note any additional important information. An initial assessment of the newborn follows (see Chap. 28). It is particularly important at this time to check the newborn's respiratory status and temperature and to observe for any congenital anomalies that might have been missed at birth but need immediate care.

Vital Signs

The vital signs should be checked every half hour until they are stable or as indicated by hospital policy. Apical heart rate and respirations should be counted for 1 full minute each. The pulse rate may vary with the newborn's activity, but a persistent rate below 120 beats/min or above 160 beats/min should be reported.

The newborn's temperature is checked on admission and then monitored until the axillary reading reaches about 36.6°C (97.8°F). The axillary route is preferred because it eliminates the potential danger of perforation of the rectum with the rectal thermometer (Fig. 29-1). In some settings, however, an initial rectal temperature is taken to determine rectal patency. Rectal temperature measures core temperature, while axillary temperature measures skin temperature. Skin temperature will decrease before core temperature. Therefore, the axillary reading is usually slightly lower than the rectal temperature. However, if the newborn has been chilled and brown fat stimulated, it may be higher (Bliss-Holtz, 1993). There has been some disagreement on the length of time needed to obtain an accurate temperature reading from the various sites, but several studies have concluded that 3 minutes is sufficient for a rectal temperature and 4 minutes for an axillary temperature (Bliss-Holtz, 1989). Electronic thermometers also provide accurate temperature readings. They beep when maximum temperature is reached, so timing is not an issue.

Color and Respiratory Pattern

The newborn's color and respiratory pattern are good indices of whether the newborn is experiencing respiratory insufficiency. Dyspnea (rapid respirations exceeding 50 breaths per minute), expiratory grunting, and persistent cyanosis should be reported. Because mucus in the nasopharynx often causes respiratory distress, the nurse should be particularly alert for its presence. Gagging, vomiting, breath holding, retraction of the head, choking, and cyanosis all may signify the presence of mucus, which is particularly prone to develop in the second period of reactivity following the first sleep period.

Breathing difficulties or excessive mucus may also indicate congenital anomalies, such as choanal atresia or tracheoesophageal fistula. Observing for the time

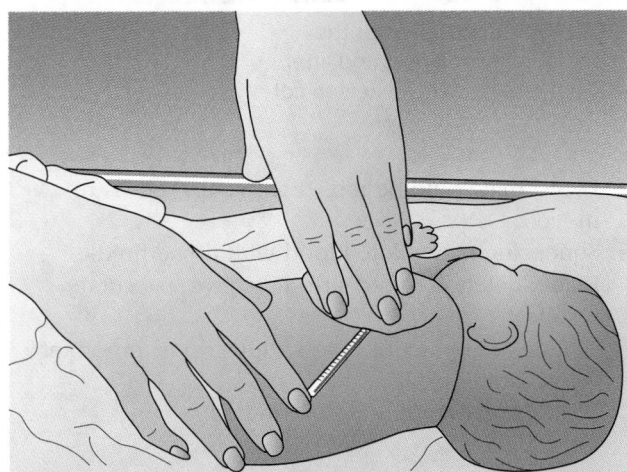

FIGURE 29–1 Taking an axillary temperature. The newborn's arm is held gently but firmly against his side while the thermometer is in place to ensure a more accurate temperature reading.

the breathing difficulties occur will help determine the cause. In some nurseries, especially those with high-risk populations, gastric contents are routinely aspirated to screen for anomalies of the gastrointestinal tract. Other nurseries do this only when there is evidence of a problem.

Cry and Activity

In a vigorous, normal newborn, the cry should be lusty, occurring especially when the newborn is handled or moved. If the newborn does not cry at all when disturbed or seems unusually sleepy or depressed or if the pulse and respiratory rate are slow, the condition should be reported. It may be necessary to stimulate the infant to cry periodically by rubbing the back, head, or feet or changing his or her position. Brief tremors and twitching are not unusual in the transition period, but if they are prolonged or occur frequently, they may indicate a problem, and the physician should be notified (see Chap. 28).

Blood Sugar Levels

Many newborns, including those who are preterm, are small for gestational age, or have diabetic mothers, are at risk for becoming hypoglycemic in the first few hours after birth (see Chaps. 41 and 43). Testing for this condition, using blood from a heel stick, is done routinely on all newborns in some nurseries. In other nurseries, it is done according to a protocol defining newborns most likely to become hypoglycemic soon after birth, such as those with diabetic mothers or who are large or small for gestational age. If routine testing is not done, the nurse should be aware that such central nervous system symptoms as poor muscle tone, weakness, tremors, eye rolling, high-pitched cry, and as a late symptom, convulsions may indicate low blood sugar levels. See Procedure 29-1 for more details on checking the newborn's blood sugar.

Elimination

The time of the newborn's first stool and voiding should be noted to indicate proper excretory function. Sometimes the nursery nurse must review the delivery record or check with the delivery room nurse to see whether the newborn voided or defecated before being brought to the nursery.

Condition of the Cord

The cord should be checked periodically. Any oozing or bleeding should be reported immediately. The cord should be reclamped or retied between the current clamp and the abdomen, as indicated.

PROCEDURE 29–1
Testing for Hypoglycemia

General Guidelines

- Surface blood flow can be improved by warming the newborn's foot by holding the heel in the palm of the nurse's hand or by wrapping the foot in a warm, moist compress for 3 to 5 minutes.
- Care should be taken not to squeeze the foot too vigorously when obtaining the sample, because this may dilute the blood with tissue fluid or cause hemolysis or soft-tissue damage.
- If the blood flow diminishes or stops before an

adequate amount is obtained, wiping the area with a sterile gauze square may result in increased blood flow.
- Positioning the newborn with the foot in a dependent position (lower than the body) also may increase blood flow.
- Use of an electronic glucose meter, such as a Glucometer, adds to the accuracy of timing the procedure and interpreting the results.

Nursing Action	*Rationale*
1. Hold the foot dorsiflexed against the shin, the thumb and forefinger encircling and exposing the heel and the other fingers stabilizing the ankle.	1. Holding the foot steady and preventing laceration or ineffective puncture decreases the chance of the newborn reflexly withdrawing from the painful stimulus.
2. Clean the heel with alcohol and allow to dry, or wipe with sterile gauze.	2. Alcohol does not enter the puncture wound.
3. Make a quick, clean stick in the outer surface of the heel with a disposable lancet (see Figure).	3. Tissue trauma is minimized.

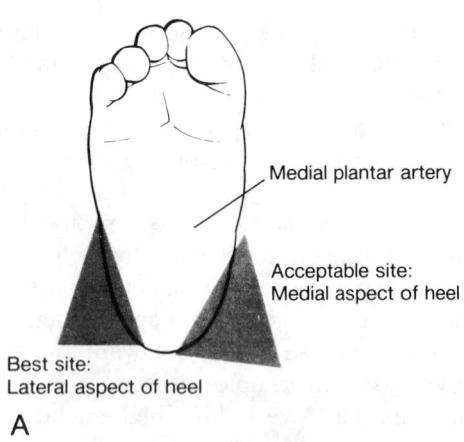

Medial plantar artery

Acceptable site:
Medial aspect of heel

Best site:
Lateral aspect of heel

A

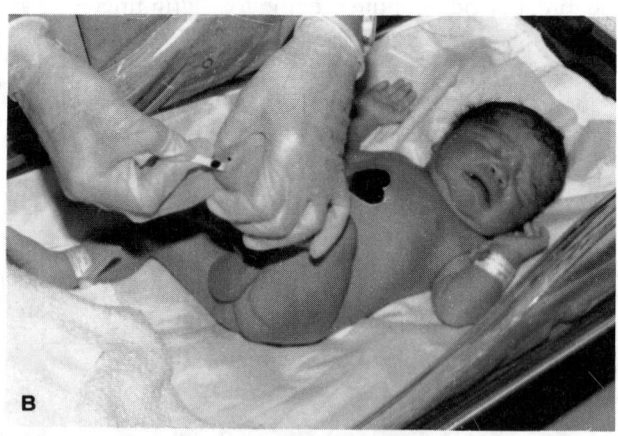

B

The heelstick procedure is used to test for blood glucose. (**A**) Appropriate sites for the heelstick procedure. (**B**) After the site is punctured with a pediatric microlancet and after elimination of the first drop of blood, the nurse holds the Dextrostix under the heel to collect the second drop of blood.

4. Wipe off first drop of blood with a sterile gauze square.	4. Blood that could be mixed with skin cells is removed.
5. When a second, large drop forms, without excessive squeezing, allow it to fall onto the Dextrostix strip to completely cover the sensitive area of strip.	5. Squeezing may dilute blood with tissue fluid. Inadequately covered strip may give inaccurate results.
6. Time for 60 seconds with timer or clock.*	6. Timing of contact of blood with strip is important for accurate results.
7. Wipe blood off strip with cotton ball, and place strip in Glucometer, following manufacturer's instructions, or compare strip with guide on bottle.	7. Blood sugar reading is determined.
8. Apply a small sterile bandage to heel.	8. Any bleeding is controlled.

Not all electronic glucose meters require the same directions for timing. Check the manufacturer's instructions for correct use.

Nursing Diagnoses

Initial assessment of the newborn, coupled with the nurse's knowledge of the expected physiologic status of the newborn, will lead to formulation of potential or actual nursing diagnoses. For a list of possible nursing diagnoses, see Box 29-1.

Planning and Intervention

Hospitals and birthing settings vary as to what is included in routine care during the transition period. Certain procedures, such as eye prophylaxis (see Chap. 24) and vitamin K injection (see Chap. 24), are done in the nursery if they are not included in the delivery room care. Equipment for suctioning and resuscitation must be on hand, and someone who is trained in its use should be immediately available. A bulb syringe should be in each newborn's bassinet.

The assessment findings noted in the previous section guide the planning and intervention for each newborn. The nurse will also monitor the newborn for potential complications that would lead to identification of problems requiring collaboration between the nurse and physician (see Care Path: Normal Newborn).

Preventing Hypothermia

Hypothermia is a major concern in the transition period (see Chap. 28). When a radiant warmer is used, the servocontrol should be set to maintain the abdominal skin temperature at 36.5°C. (97.7°F) The skin probe **thermistor** should be taped securely to the anterior abdominal wall and covered with an aluminum patch to shield it from the radiant heat source (Freeman et al., 1992).

The skin probe should be checked periodically to make sure it is in contact with the skin. A probe not touching the skin causes the warmer to misinterpret the newborn's temperature and continue to radiate heat after the desired temperature is reached. The newborn can become overheated or possibly burned. Hyperthermia, like hypothermia, increases the metabolic requirements and oxygen consumption (Hey, 1994). If an iso-

---

BOX 29–1
Nursing Diagnoses

- Ineffective Airway Clearance related to excessive oropharyngeal mucus
- Ineffective Thermoregulation related to newborn transition to extrauterine environment
- Risk for Infection related to maturational factors—immature immune system
- Risk for Injury related to maturational factors—unable to protect self

---

lette is being used as a warmer, its temperature should also be checked periodically, because it can rise higher than expected and cause overheating. For a description of a research study involving thermoregulation, see Research Highlight.

Initial Bath

Usually, the first bath is delayed until after the temperature has stabilized to around 36.6°C (97.8°F). Bathing is often done under the radiant warmer, because wetting the skin causes heat loss by evaporation. Some degree of temperature drop usually occurs, therefore the temperature is rechecked after the bath, and the newborn remains under the warmer until the temperature is stable again.

The type of initial bath given and the agents used depend on hospital policy. Warm water may be used with sterile cotton sponges to wash any blood, meconium, and amniotic fluid from the face, head, and body, or a mild soap can be used followed by careful rinsing (Freeman et al., 1992).

The vernix caseosa is usually removed from the newborn's skin during the bath, although there is no recognized need to remove it completely, unless it is stained with blood or meconium. There is some indication that the vernix serves a protective function and may be bactericidal (Coen et al., 1987). It usually disappears spontaneously in about 24 hours. If it remains in the creases and folds of the skin longer than 2 days or appears to cause irritation, gentle wiping will usually remove it. (For more information on infant bathing, see section entitled Bathing and Hygiene.)

Specific Prophylaxis Against Infection

Several procedures routinely done for the newborn are directed toward prevention of specific types of infection. Within the first few hours after birth, a prophylactic agent that is effective against gonorrhea and *Chlamydia* is placed in the eyes to prevent ophthalmia neonatorum (see Chap. 24). Initial skin and cord care helps prevent colonization of the skin and umbilical area with potentially pathogenic bacteria. When choosing an agent to cleanse the skin, the agent must not have an adverse effect on the skin, must not be toxic if absorbed, and must not give rise to new infection problems by altering the skin flora (Freeman et al., 1992).

If any invasive procedure, such as an injection, is done before the initial bath, the site should first be cleaned carefully to remove any amniotic fluid or blood to reduce potential contamination with organisms, such as hepatitis B virus, human immunodeficiency virus (HIV), or herpes simplex virus. For cord care, Triple Dye or an antimicrobial agent, such as bacitracin ointment, is

(*text continues on page 734*)

CARE PATH
Normal Newborn

Name _____

This care path is a guideline and is not intended to create a standard of care. This guideline may be modified based on individual client's needs.

Prob. #		Birth	0–4 Hours Date:	4–8 Hours Date:	8–12 Hours Date:	
1	ADL	Bedrest and position for holding	⟶	⟶	⟶	
1,3	Assessment Monitor	Apgars Newborn assessment	Newborn assessment on admission and Q 8h **VS, Respiratory status, skin color, and temp WNL** Observation: check for maternal hepatitis surface antigen	Temp PRN and Q shift	Newborn assessment Q 8h VS WNL	
1,2,3	Consults	**NICU Team in attendance PRN**	**Orthopedics PRN** **Genetics PRN** **Infectious disease PRN**	**Orthopedics PRN** **Genetics PRN** **Infectious disease PRN**	**Orthopedics PRN** **Genetics PRN** **Infectious disease PRN**	
1,2,3	Procedures/ Tests	Cord blood PRN	Chemstrips PRN BP PRN **O₂ sat PRN-O₂ sat WNL** Attach security sensor Assess hepatitis titer	Chemstrips PRN		
1–4	Treatments	Gastric lavage PRN	⟶ Initial Newborn bath Cord care	Cord care Cath PRN Ultrasounds PRN Circumcision PRN and circ care	Cord care Cath PRN Ultrasounds PRN Circumcision PRN and circ care	
3	Meds/IVs	Illotycin ointment	Vitamin K IM		Hepatitis vaccine PRN	
2	Nutrition	Initiate breastfeeding	Continue breastfeeding Initiate formula feeding	⟶ Continue formula feeding	⟶	
1–4	Pt./Family Education	See Maternal Care Path				
1–4	Discharge Planning	See Maternal Care Path				
1–4	Spiritual/ Psycho/ Social/ Emotional Needs	See Maternal Care Path				
	Multi-disciplinary Team Signatures	_____ _____ _____	_____ _____ _____	_____ _____ _____	_____ _____ _____	

Client Problems

1. *Alteration in body temperature*
2. *Alteration in nutritional requirements*
3. *Potential for infection*
4. *Alteration in skin integrity*

CLIENT IDENTIFICATION

12–24 Hours Date:	Day 2 Date:				
⟶	Bedrest and position for holding				
⟶	Temp PRN and Q shift VS WNL				
⟶					
Orthopedics PRN Genetics PRN Infectious disease PRN	**Orthopedics PRN Genetics PRN Infectious disease PRN**				
Metabolic screen					

Cord care
Ultrasounds PRN
Circumcision PRN and
  circ care
Discharge weight
	Cord care
	Ultrasounds PRN
	Circumcision PRN and
	  circ care
	Discharge weight				

⟶ ⟶	Continue breastfeeding Continue formula feeding				

Assess need for home
  health follow-up
	Assess need for home
	  health follow-up				

_____ _____ _____ _____	_____ _____ _____ _____				

RESEARCH HIGHLIGHT

Thermoregulation in the Newborn

Thermoregulation is an important topic in the newborn period, with emphasis on preventing hypothermia, especially during the first hours of life. Less attention is given to hyperthermia, but it has been suggested that higher environmental temperatures could cause an increase in the newborn's temperature. This study of 20 full-term, average for gestational age, well newborns more than 1 day old was designed to investigate the question of whether extra coverings and warm environments could elevate the newborn's temperature to a range that would cause clinical concern. Twelve infants were randomly assigned to the experimental group and eight to the control group. After a routine feeding, temperatures were measured by rectal probe for 2½ hours, with the experimental infants bundled in five blankets and a hat in a room temperature of 26.6°C (80°F) and the control group wrapped with one blanket in a room temperature of 24°C (75°F). To control for other factors that might raise the newborn's temperatures, they were not fed during the study period, and their state of arousal (sleeping, awake and alert, or crying) was rated every 15 minutes and recorded.

Body temperatures of the control group remained relatively stable during the study period, with the exception of two, which decreased. For the experimental group, however, body temperature continued to rise for all newborns during the entire study period, with the temperatures of two infants reaching 38°C (100.4°F).

Nursing implications of this study are related to its verification of previous perceptions that changes in environmental temperature impact on the newborn's body temperature. This can alert nurses to the importance of concern about overheating the newborn's environment. When a newborn has an elevated temperature, the room temperature and the amount of covering being used should be investigated before making the decision that the newborn has a fever. The results of this study can be helpful in client teaching to help parents avoid overheating their newborns.

Critique: A limitation of the study was the inability to observe the newborns for more than 2½ hours, because the newborns needed to be fed, and this would have changed the thermal environment. The results of this study cannot be extrapolated to reflect what would happen in other age groups or with other types of environmental conditions.

(Cheng, T. L., & Parridge, J. C. [1993]. Effect of bundling and high environmental temperature on neonatal body temperature. *Pediatrics, 42*[2] 238–240).

---

recommended to prevent colonization (Freeman et al., 1992). Alcohol, which has been used for years to care for the cord, hastens drying of the stump but is probably not very effective in preventing cord colonization or umbilical infection (Freeman et al., 1992).

The initial cord care may be done following the bath. For example, Triple Dye, usually a one-time treatment, is applied to the cord and over the junction between the cord stump and the skin (Fig. 29-2). It leaves a temporary purple stain on the abdomen that may last several days. This should be explained to the parents

so they do not worry about the stain. If an ointment such as bacitracin is used, it should not be applied until the newborn no longer needs to be under the radiant warmer. The oily substance tends to concentrate the heat and could cause a burn.

Evaluation

The nurse will evaluate his or her care by determining whether the nursing goals for the transition period have been met. Anticipated outcomes may include the following:

- The newborn maintains a clear airway.
- The newborn's vital signs remain within normal limits.
- The newborn remains free of injury.
- The newborn demonstrates appropriate progression and adaptation to extrauterine life, requiring less intensive observation.

If any goals are not met, the nurse reassesses the care plan to determine possible revisions to meet the newborn's needs.

Providing a Safe Environment

As in the immediate newborn period (see Chap. 24), protection from injury and infection continues to be a

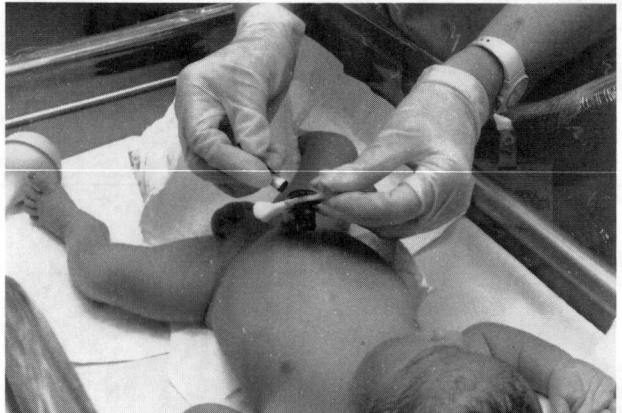

FIGURE 29-2 Initial cord care. Tripple-Dye is applied to the cord stump and approximately 1 inch of skin around the umbilicus.

major goal of nursing care throughout the newborn's hospital stay. Each newborn care setting formulates policies to provide safe, individualized care in a protective environment.

Preventing Infection

Prevention of infection is of paramount importance when caring for the newborn. Although the immune system begins to develop during fetal life, it is still very immature at birth (see Chap. 28). The neonate has emerged from a highly protected environment in utero to the outside world, where there is exposure to a wide variety of microorganisms. This contributes to the newborn's increased vulnerability to microbial attack during the first 6 weeks of life (Yoder et al., 1992). It is important, therefore, to attempt to limit the number of organisms to which the newborn is exposed in the early days of life.

Equally important, in light of current concerns about HIV and other diseases transmitted by blood and body fluids, is the use of standard precautions by those working with the neonates to protect themselves.

Minimizing Exposure to Organisms

Caretakers are the newborn's major source of exposure to organisms. Nurses and other staff members who care for newborns should be free from infectious diseases, such as respiratory or gastrointestinal infections and skin lesions, that could be transmitted to the neonates. Everyone who is in contact with the newborn, including parents and personnel, should assume responsibility for protecting the newborn from infection. Parents may need help in reminding family and friends to postpone their visits if they are not well.

Handwashing. The primary mechanism for preventing infection when handling the newborn is frequent, thorough handwashing with an antiseptic detergent or soap. Handwashing should be done at the beginning of a shift (see Nursing Guidelines: Handwashing at the Beginning of a Shift). After the initial wash, staff members should remember to wash their hands vigorously for 15 seconds before a feeding, after a diaper change, before going from one newborn to another, and after touching anything that is not clean, such as a cabinet door or their own face or hair (Freeman et al., 1992).

Personnel may need frequent reminders of the importance of handwashing in preventing hospital-acquired infections in neonates. Studies of handwashing behavior in hospitals have indicated that the frequency of handwashing between client contacts is very low (Larson, 1987). Parents also need instruction about the importance and technique of proper handwashing. Reinforcement should be given as necessary during the hospital stay.

NURSING GUIDELINES
Handwashing at the Beginning of a Shift

1. Remove watch and rings.
2. Wash hands (including between the fingers), wrists, forearms, and elbows thoroughly with antiseptic handwashing agent for approximately 2 minutes.
3. Clean fingernails with a plastic or orangewood stick.
4. Wash hands again, using a soft brush, soap pad, or vigorous friction.
5. Rinse thoroughly.
6. Dry with paper towels.

Gloving. With increasing concern about the potential transmission of infection from clients to healthcare providers, nonsterile gloves are recommended when caring for all newborns until amniotic fluid and blood are removed from their skin, usually during the first bath. It is also recommended that gloves be worn when changing the newborn's diapers. When wearing gloves for protection, to prevent cross-contamination, the gloves must be removed and the hands washed before going to a central area or giving care to another newborn (Freeman et al., 1992).

Nursery Dress Protocol. Protecting the newborn from infection has traditionally involved a dress protocol for those coming in contact with the newborn in the hospital. Most nursery nurses (and in many hospitals where rooming-in is practiced, the postpartum nurses as well) change to scrub suits or dresses when they come to work. These should be short sleeved so that hands, forearms, and elbows can be washed more readily. Scrub clothes can be changed easily when soiled, thus making the spread of infection from one newborn to another less likely. Hair should be worn short, or long hair should be pulled back to avoid allowing the hair to come in contact with the newborn or equipment. Caps, beard covers, and masks are no longer considered necessary for routine activities in the nursery (Freeman et al., 1992).

If circumstances necessitate masks, the mask should cover the nose and mouth, should be changed frequently, and when removed from the face, should be discarded, not pulled down around the neck. Masks can become a reservoir for bacteria when not applied properly or changed regularly. Other hospital personnel and visitors may be expected to put cover gowns on over their street clothes before coming into the nursery or into the mother's room if the newborn is there. If they are going to touch the newborn, they should wash their hands and arms before putting on the gown. The necessity of using cover gowns has been questioned in recent years, because some studies have shown that neonatal infection has not increased when cover gowns are not used (Rush et al., 1990).

Maternal Infection. Special problems are created when the mother has an infection. It is important to determine which maternal infections the newborn would be most likely to acquire if the two are not separated. Hospital policies vary in this matter. In many hospitals, the mother and newborn are routinely separated if the mother is febrile. Some of the suggestions offered in the guidelines from the American Academy of Pediatrics (AAP) and the American College of Obstetricians and Gynecologists are as follows (Freeman et al., 1992):

■ Maternal genital infections are rarely spread to the newborn after birth. A mother who is febrile without a specific diagnosed site of infection usually may handle and feed her newborn if she feels well enough and uses good handwashing technique. Additionally, she should wear a clean cover gown and be taught to protect the newborn from potentially contaminated items, such as her nightgown, bedclothes, and perineal pads.

■ When a respiratory infection is present, the mother should be informed that these infections can be spread by hands or contaminated articles. She should also be instructed in careful handwashing techniques and appropriate handling of tissues and other items contaminated by secretions. Wearing a mask may be helpful in reducing the droplet spread of infection.

■ A woman with a communicable disease that is in a stage that is likely to be transmitted to her newborn should be separated from the newborn until the disease is no longer communicable.

The mother who must be separated from her newborn needs special attention from the nurse. Making arrangements for the mother to see the newborn through the nursery window, bringing her frequent reports about the newborn, or providing a picture of the newborn taken with an instant camera can help ease the frustration of the separation. The mother who is breast-feeding may need assistance in pumping her breasts to ensure stimulation and continued milk supply until she is allowed to put the newborn to breast (see Chap. 30).

If the mother with an infection is allowed to care for her newborn and is instructed to wear a mask, the nurse should make certain that the mother understands how to use a mask most effectively (see Client Education: Instructions for Mother in Using a Mask).

Newborn Care Areas

Providing a safe environment also includes concern about the areas and equipment used for the newborn's

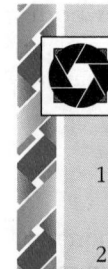

CLIENT EDUCATION
Instructions for Mother in Using a Mask

1. Prior to caring for your newborn, put the mask on so it is comfortable and you can see over it, and then wash your hands.
2. Avoid touching or adjusting the mask to avoid contaminating your hands.
3. Wash your hands if the mask is touched.
4. Wear a clean mask on each occasion that a mask is needed.
5. Change mask if it becomes moist.

care. Many hospitals today offer more than one setting for care of newborns. The newborn may be placed in a central nursery or together with the mother in the mother's room. Whichever setting is used, attention to the environmental aspects of safe care and to measures to ensure the security of the newborn is essential.

Mother and Newborn Care

Current interest in family-centered maternity care has led to having healthy newborns spend increasing amounts of time with their mothers and less time in central nurseries. In the free-standing birth centers or in hospitals with LDRP rooms, the mother and newborn usually are not separated. In these settings, initial newborn care is done in the birthing room, and the family may go home within a few hours after the birth. Some hospitals use newborn nurseries as admission nurseries, where the newborn goes for initial care and observation for a set time and then goes to the mother's room until discharge. This often is called **rooming-in.** It may be either optional or mandatory.

In each of these situations the father of the newborn, and quite often the siblings and other family members, are also involved. This family-centered approach to maternity care not only provides an environment that fosters a natural parent–child relationship from the beginning, but it also affords opportunities for both parents to learn about and practice newborn care (Fig. 29-3).

Staff responsibility for the newborn's care may vary depending on the situation. The nursery staff may still be responsible for meeting the rooming-in newborn's needs and for educating the parents about care. Alternatively, the newborn and mother may be cared for by the same nurse. This may be called **mother–newborn couple care** or **couplet care.** Nurses are prepared to provide this type of care by cross-training in nursery and postpartum. Having the same nurse care for the mother and newborn helps facilitate more flexible care

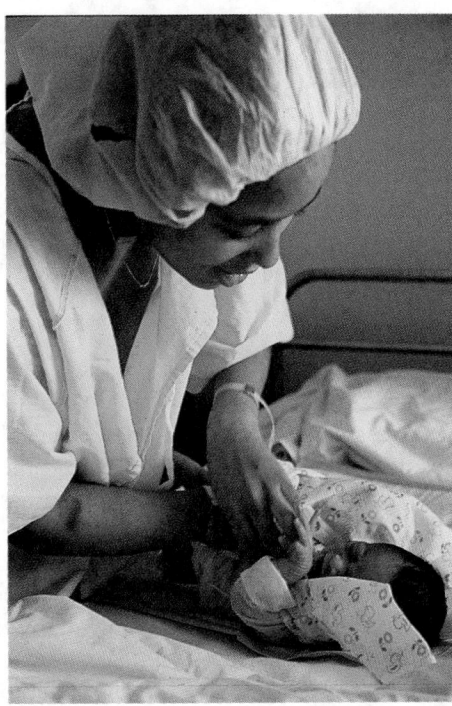

FIGURE 29-3 In the rooming-in unit, the new mother has an opportunity to bond with her newborn and practice dressing and wrapping her newborn.

routines and increased opportunities for parenting education (NAACOG, 1989).

Regardless of where they receive care, newborns must be protected from sources of infection. The same principles for asepsis used in the nursery must be followed when newborn care is provided in the mother's room. Plans for the safe care of newborns who are in the room with their mothers for extended periods need to include parental education about possible safety concerns. In addition to infection prevention, other areas to be addressed include use of the bulb syringe, positioning the newborn to avoid aspiration, keeping the newborn in the bassinet rather than on the mother's bed when not being held, and not leaving the newborn unattended in the room.

The Central Nursery

The central newborn nursery is designed for the care of a variable number of healthy newborns. When this system is in use, newborns are brought to their mothers at specified times during the day for feeding or visiting. The nursery staff assumes the responsibility for the major portion of newborn care. Some type of central nursery is found in most hospitals, if only for newborns whose mothers cannot care for them temporarily due to recovery from a cesarean birth or some other problem.

To ensure safe care for newborns in the central nursery, certain recommendations about lighting, equipment for emergency resuscitation, and distance between bassinets should be followed. Handwashing facilities and materials should be readily available. There should be one nursing staff member for each six to eight infants (Freeman et al., 1992). The precautions previously mentioned, such as handwashing, wearing scrub clothes, and following other aspects of nursery aseptic technique, afford additional protection.

There is a difference in nursery technique between what is considered to be nursery clean and what is considered to be **baby clean** (what is clean for an individual newborn). No common equipment, such as a common bath table, should be used to provide care for the newborns. There should be provisions in the nursery for individual technique to be followed. Each newborn should have his or her own crib and general supplies so that he or she can be given care, such as daily inspection bath, or be diapered or dressed in his or her own bed (Freeman et al., 1992).

The Newborn Requiring Isolation

Maternity units have varying policies for newborns who are suspected of or known to have infections. The infected neonate may be placed in a separate room in the nursery area, kept in the central nursery, allowed to room-in with the mother, or transferred to a pediatrics unit, depending on the type and manifestations of the infection, the staffing available, and hospital policy. Decisions are often made on an individual basis.

Nurses must be alert for newborns who show signs of or are at increased risk for developing an infection so that appropriate procedures can be implemented if necessary. Newborns who are born at home or on the way to the hospital should be bathed and observed for signs of infection. However, separate isolation facilities are not required (Freeman et al., 1992).

Isolettes are sometimes used for isolating newborns within the central nursery. This equipment may be helpful to keep the newborn separate and as a reminder of the isolation status, but it is not adequate isolation for infected neonates. Although the air coming into the incubator is filtered, the air being discharged into the nursery is not. Also, the surface and portholes of the incubator are easily contaminated with organisms from the infected newborn, so the hands and forearms of personnel are likely to be colonized (Freeman et al., 1992).

Isolated newborns may require closer observation and additional care related to the infection. However, they continue to need the usual care given to the healthy newborn. Also, their need for human contact, holding, and cuddling should not be forgotten.

Providing for Security

Abduction of newborns from hospitals is a subject of growing concern to many people. Although the number (12–18 in an average year) is not large compared with the number of births per year, it is a tragedy for the family and disastrous for the staff and hospital when it occurs. The National Center for Missing and Exploited Children (NCMEC), along with the Association of Women's Health, Obstetric, and Neonatal Nurses (AWHONN) and the National Association of Neonatal Nurses have developed a program for hospitals with guidelines on preventing these abductions. This program, called Safeguarding Their Tomorrows, includes written material, speakers, and a video (AWHONN, 1995).

Nurses and others responsible for the care of newborns in hospitals must be aware of the problem, know the security system that is in place in their hospital, and have knowledge about typical characteristics of an abductor (Box 29-2). Hospitals should have a written critical incidence response plan in case an abduction occurs or a person is observed acting suspiciously (NCMEC, 1991).

Many hospitals are taking additional steps, such as placing identification arm bands on fathers or other family members, employing security guards, and installing alarm systems.

BOX 29-2
The "Typical" Abductor

1. Female, 15 to 44 years old, often overweight
2. Most likely emotionally immature and compulsive
3. Frequently has lost a baby or incapable of having one
4. Often married or cohabitating; companion's desire for a child may be the motivation for the abduction
5. Considers the newborn her own once the abduction occurs
6. Usually lives in the community where the abduction takes place
7. In many cases, visits the nursery unit prior to the abduction; asks detailed questions about hospital procedures and the maternity floor layout
8. Plans the abduction but does not necessarily target a specific newborn; when an opportunity presents itself, simply a matter of "snatch and run"
9. Frequently impersonates a nurse or other hospital personnel
10. Often acquainted with hospital personnel and even the victim's parents

(From Safeguarding Their Tomorrows—A Resource by NAACOG, National Association of Neonatal Nurses and NCMEC. [1991]. Produced by Mead Johnson.)

Continuing Care and Parent Teaching

Following the transition period, the newborn needs continued care. The nurse is responsible for assessing, planning, and providing care for the newborn and the parental family unit while in the hospital or birth center; anticipatory guidance for infant care after the family returns home is also important.

Assessment

Ongoing assessment during the newborn's hospital stay varies according to hospital policy and the length of the stay. The nurse will be expected to assess the newborn's physical condition, behavioral patterns, interaction with the parents, and the parents' need for information about the newborn and his or her care (see Chap. 28). Early detection of problems in any of these areas is of primary concern.

Most nurseries use some type of flow sheet to record specific nursing assessments. These usually include the newborn's daily weight, vital signs, skin color and integrity, condition of cord, circumcision, activity level, intake, and elimination. These assessments usually are done at predetermined intervals. Nurses also should be alert for and report any changes that are noticed at any time while giving care. For example, subtle changes in the newborn's color, activity, posture, or vital signs can indicate beginning infection or potential problems.

Nursing Diagnoses

Awareness of potential nursing diagnoses, based on areas of assessment, will assist the nurse in planning care for the newborn. Ineffective Airway Clearance, Ineffective Thermoregulation, Risk for Infection, and Risk for Injury, as in the transition period, continue to be of concern. For a list of possible additional nursing diagnoses, see Box 29-3.

Planning and Intervention

During the newborn's hospital stay, the nurse is responsible for planning and providing care and involving the mother as much as possible to help her prepare to take over the responsibility when she gets home. This is easiest when mother and newborn receive care together, but it can also be arranged when a central nursery is used.

The trend is for shorter hospital stays. Currently, there is pressure from insurance providers and hospital administration to discharge mothers and newborns in the first 24 to 48 hours following uncomplicated vaginal births of normal full-term newborns. This increases the importance for the nurse to assess the mother's knowl-

- Risk for Impaired Skin Integrity related to moist umbilical cord stump
- Impaired Skin Integrity related to
  - Peeling and cracking of skin
  - Circumcision
- Knowledge Deficit related to
  - Lack of experience with newborn care
  - Proper newborn care and handling
- Risk for Altered Parenting related to
  - New parents' inexperience and feelings of incompetence
  - Lack of knowledge about newborn growth and development
- Risk for Altered Parent/Infant Attachment related to
  - Anxiety with parental role
  - Feelings of inadequacies about parenting
- Altered Urinary Elimination related to
  - Imperforate meatus
  - Insufficient fluid intake
- Family Coping: Potential for Growth related to positive adaptation to parental role

edge and skill in caring for her newborn and to develop a teaching plan with her. The plan should provide information about the basic principles or procedures related to newborn care to provide safe care for the newborn and any additional knowledge that is incomplete or incorrect. A written plan or checklist of the mother's learning needs and what teaching has been done is helpful to provide continuity between healthcare providers. The father or other family members should be included as much as possible. Consistency in what is taught is necessary to avoid confusing the parents.

If the parents' primary language is not English, the nurse must ensure that they are able to understand what is being said and if not, that an interpreter is present to assist them.

Written information should be at the parents' education level and in the language understood by the parents. The nurse also should be sensitive to cultural differences and make an effort to find out about any culturally specific newborn care customs that the family may practice.

The following discussion provides some guidelines for newborn care that can be helpful for the nurse. They also can be used for teaching the mother and father, if he is present.

Handling and Positioning the Newborn

Although they are small, newborns are not as fragile as they sometimes seem. They should be treated gently, of course, but firm, smooth handling helps them feel secure. There is no one right way of turning, lifting, or holding a newborn, but the following points should be kept in mind:

- The head and buttocks need to be supported.
- Newborns are wiggly and can push themselves out of your grasp.
- It is easier to pick a newborn up from the back-lying (supine) position than from the side-lying or face down (prone) position.

A suggested way to lift a newborn is to place one hand under the neck to support the head and shoulders and the other hand under the buttocks to grasp the opposite thigh (Fig. 29-4). The newborn can then be lifted up to a holding position or moved from one place to another.

A useful position for holding or carrying the newborn is the "football hold" (Fig. 29-5). Mothers appreciate learning about this position, because like the nurse, they often have times when they need to hold the newborn and still have one hand free.

Positioning in the crib is usually on the side with a blanket roll at the back extending from shoulder to hip for support. If the blanket roll is behind the head, it may push the head forward and cause the newborn to be uncomfortable. The sidelying position allows for drainage of secretions, such as mucus or regurgitation of milk.

An alternative position would be to place the newborn on his or her back. Although the backlying position does not facilitate drainage of secretions, recent studies demonstrate that there is little danger of aspiration when a healthy newborn sleeps in this position. Positioning the newborn on the abdomen is no longer recommended for sleep. Studies have linked the prone

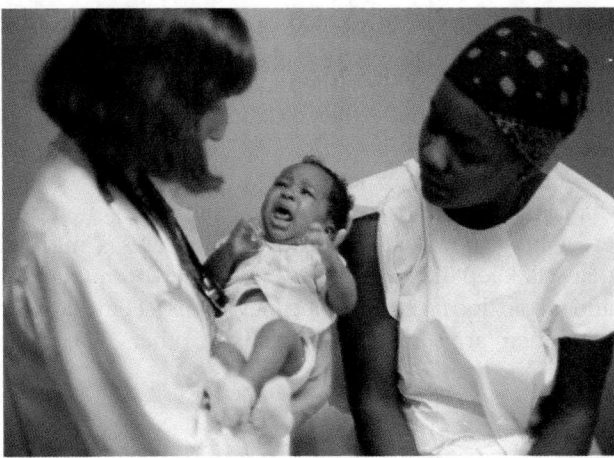

FIGURE 29-4 A good way to lift the newborn is to place one hand under the neck to support the head and shoulders and the other hand under the buttocks to grasp the opposite thigh.

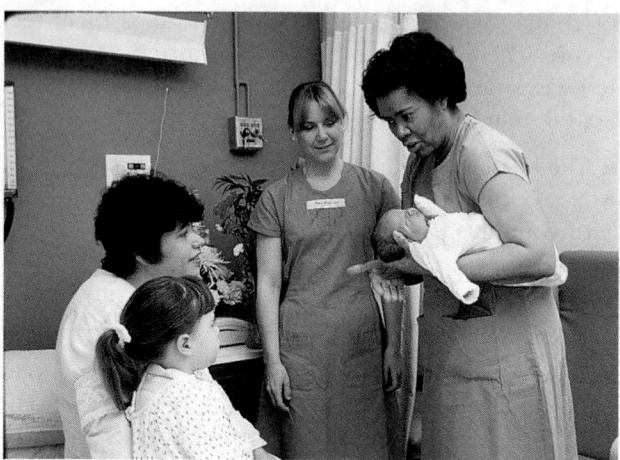

FIGURE 29–5 This nurse is demonstrating how to carry the newborn using the "football hold."

sleeping position with sudden infant death syndrome (SIDS; AAP Task Force, 1992).

Dressing, Diapering, and Wrapping

Confidence in dressing and undressing the newborn comes with practice. Putting on a shirt or gown should be done gently. Helpful hints include enlarging the neck opening to avoid dragging the garment over the face and reaching through the sleeve with your fingers from the outside when pulling the hand through to avoid snagging the fingers.

Diapering is fairly simple when disposable diapers that fasten with tapes are used. Concern about the adverse effect of disposable diapers on the environment, however, has led many hospitals and new parents to use cloth diapers. These can be held in place with pins or with diaper covers that have Velcro closures. If pins are used, they should be inserted pointing toward the back of the newborn so there is less danger of sticking the newborn if they open. The diaper should be folded down in front to below the umbilicus to allow for circulation of air around the cord stump, which assists in the drying process.

Wrapping the newborn snugly in a blanket (swaddling) makes him or her easier to handle and often quiets a fussy newborn. Figure 29-6 illustrates a method that will keep the blanket around the newborn securely and avoid loose ends. Some newborns seem happier with their arms inside the blanket; others like their arms free.

Bathing and Hygiene

Bath time is an excellent opportunity for making the observations of the newborn that are necessary during the immediate postnatal period. How frequently a bath is given and what materials are used may vary from in-

stitution to institution. Because most full-term newborns leave the nursery in less than 24 to 48 hours, the initial sponge bath may be the only one they receive while in the hospital.

Sponge Bath. A sponge bath should be given to the newborn until the umbilical cord and circumcision are healed. The newborn can be adequately cleaned by this method. It also is easier to keep the cord from getting wet. See Procedure 29-2 for a description of the proper procedure for a sponge bath.

When possible, parents should have an opportunity to observe or participate in a demonstration of a sponge bath before going home. If there is an opportunity for only one bath with the parents present, the nurse can combine the demonstration and return demonstration by discussing the bath with the parents first and then letting them do part of the bath, with the nurse there for moral support and assistance as necessary.

The basic principles of bathing should be conveyed to the parents. However, they should not be made to feel that there is only one way to bathe the newborn. Parents develop their own manner of bathing the newborn according to manual dexterity, size and activity of the newborn, and facilities available.

Nurses also should explore with the parents what equipment and facilities are available in the home and instruct them in how the use of these might differ from what is available in the hospital. Usually the necessities can be met without undue expenses or difficulty. For instance, a large counter or table that can be washed and padded adequately (and is a comfortable height) can be used as the bath area. A large pan or basin serves well for the bathtub in the early weeks; it should be kept only for the newborn's use. Thus, the extra expense of special equipment can be minimized. A soft towel and washcloth, for the newborn's use only, and a mild soap are also needed.

Some parents and newborns enjoy the bath as a daily routine, but others do not or cannot always find the time. For these, as long as the face, neck creases, and diaper area are washed as needed, giving a bath every other day should be sufficient. A sponge bath should continue to be the type of bath given until the cord stump has fallen off and the umbilicus has healed. After this time, the newborn can be introduced to tub baths gradually. Although infants usually grow to enjoy bathtime, not all like baths at first. A good way to begin is to start by washing the face and head as in a sponge bath, soap the body, and then use the tub for rinsing.

Skin Care. The newborn's skin is often dry and peeling within a few days after birth. Dry cracks may appear in the wrist and ankle areas. Sometimes, this is a cause of concern to parents, and they want to put oil or some

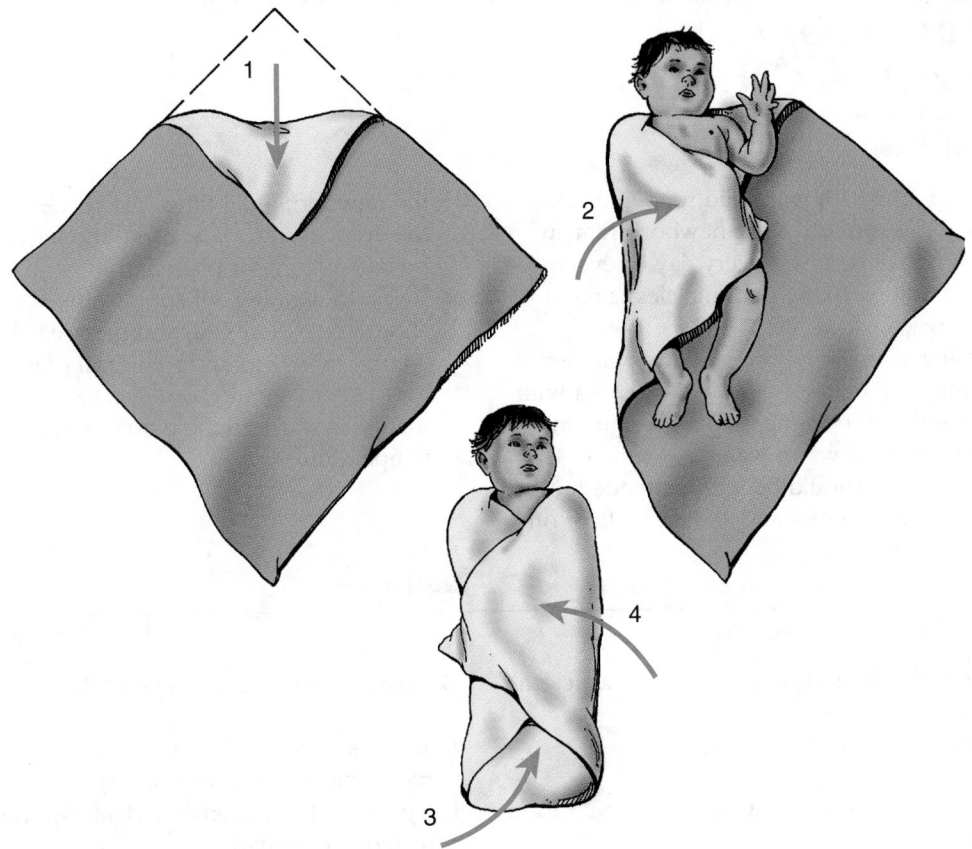

FIGURE 29–6 Swaddling an infant. 1. Fold down top corner of blanket, and place infant on blanket with neck near fold. 2. Bring corner of blanket around from infant's right side and tuck under left side. 3. Bring bottom corner up to chest. 4. Bring remaining corner around and tuck under right side. Wrap securely, but not too tightly—leave some room for infant to move.

other preparation on the skin to get rid of the dryness. They can be reassured that the flakiness and cracks will disappear in a few days and that oil and some lotions may make matters worse by causing a rash.

The skin is thin, delicate, extremely tender, and easily irritated. Because the skin is a protective covering, breaks in its surface may lead to infection. Skin disturbances can constitute an actual threat to the newborn's well-being.

The newborn does not usually perspire until after the first month. Warm weather or excessive clothing may cause the newborn to develop **prickly heat,** a closely grouped, pinhead-size rash of papules and vesicles, on the face, neck, and wherever skin surfaces touch. Fewer clothes and lower room temperature may help to relieve this problem.

Sometimes despite good care, a diaper rash may occur. This is usually an ammonia dermatitis, caused by the reaction of bacteria with the urea in the urine. The most important prophylaxis is to keep the diaper area clean and dry. Petroleum jelly, a bland protective ointment such as A and D, or a commercial ointment can be used to protect the area. Pastes may not be advised,

because they are much more adhesive than ointments and thus create cleansing problems.

A simple treatment that is often effective and can be used either in the hospital or at home is to expose the reddened buttocks to air and light several times a day, using care to keep the rest of the newborn covered.

Some mothers find that boiling the diapers is an effective measure, because this destroys the bacteria. Many of the detergents and conditioners used today have antibacterial agents in them. These may be effective in washing the diapers, although there is some evidence that nondetergent cleaning agents are gentler on the newborn's skin. Care should be taken to rinse the diapers thoroughly (at least twice) because the residue of the detergent or soap can be irritating. Diaper services are very effective in sterilizing diapers and preventing diaper rash and are a good solution for many mothers. Disposable diapers are also less likely to cause diaper rash, but some brands may contain substances that are irritating to some newborns. The expense of disposable diapers or diaper service needs to be considered when making the choice.

(*text continues on page 744*)

PROCEDURE 29-2
Sponge Bath

General Guidelines

- A complete sponge bath with mild soap and water is given on admission and if the newborn remains in the nursery, may be given every day or every other day in addition to the periodic cleansing of face and buttocks.
- Daily cleansing of the newborn's skin may be limited to washing the buttocks and perianal area with a mild soap and water during diaper changes and washing the face with warm water as needed.
- The newborn never should be left unattended, even on a large work area; one hand should be kept on the newborn at all times. If it is necessary to leave the area, even for a second, the newborn should be taken along or placed in the crib.
- Before beginning, all supplies needed for the bath should be assembled, and the area should be warm (75°–80°F) and free from drafts. The water for the bath should be about 98° to 100°F. Water that feels warm to the elbow is approximately that temperature.

Action	Rationale
Eyes: Use a clean cotton ball or clean area of the washcloth for each eye.	Contamination from one eye to the other is avoided.
Wipe from inner corner to outer corner.	Using this method of wiping avoids bringing contaminated material into contact with tear ducts.
Observe for any redness, swelling, or discharge; report and record.	Early signs of infection or inflammation can be detected and treated.
Face: Wash face first with clean water, using soft washcloth or cotton balls.	Using clean water avoids introducing any soap in water that could irritate skin or eyes.
Nose and Ears: Use a small twisted piece of cotton moistened with water if some dried mucus needs to be removed from the nose.	The nose usually does not need cleaning because the newborn sneezes to clear the nasal passages.
Twisted cotton or a soft washcloth can be used to clean the *outer* ear. Nothing should be put *inside* the ear or nose.	Cotton-tipped applicators should not be used to clean inside the nose or ears because the delicate tissues could be injured.
Head: Swaddle the newborn in a blanket or towel and hold in the football position.	Keeps newborn warm during procedure and makes him or her easier to hold.
Use the same soap that the newborn is bathed with or any brand of baby shampoo to lather scalp.	Gentle soap or shampoo avoids irritation of scalp.
Rinse head well with very wet washcloth or by holding newborn over basin and scooping water up with hand and dripping over head.	Rinsing off all soap will further prevent scalp irritation.
(In hospital nurseries the head is often rinsed under the faucet, but this is not advised for home use.)	(Home sinks are not designed to allow this to be done easily. Inexperienced parents also may have difficulty regulating the temperature and keeping the water out of the infant's ears and eyes.)
Dry immediately and thoroughly.	Complete drying helps minimize heat loss from a large surface area, such as the head.
Wash the head each time the newborn is bathed.	Frequent washings help prevent **cradle cap** (common dermatitis on infants consisting of thick, yellow, greasy scales on scalp).
Avoid putting oil on the hair.	Using oil may predispose to cradle cap.

(continued)

PROCEDURE 29–2 *(Continued)*
Sponge Bath

Action	Rationale

Body and Extremities:
Wash one area at a time with warm water and mild soap. Keep other areas covered.

Covering and exposing only one area at a time helps avoid chilling.

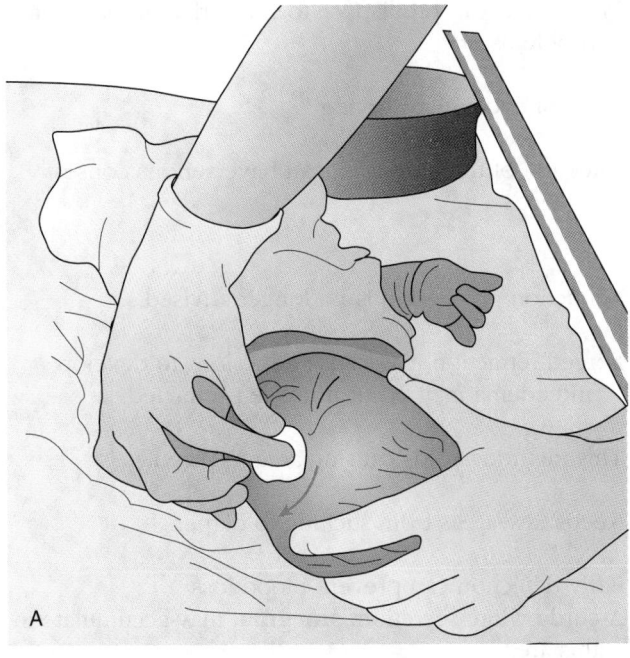

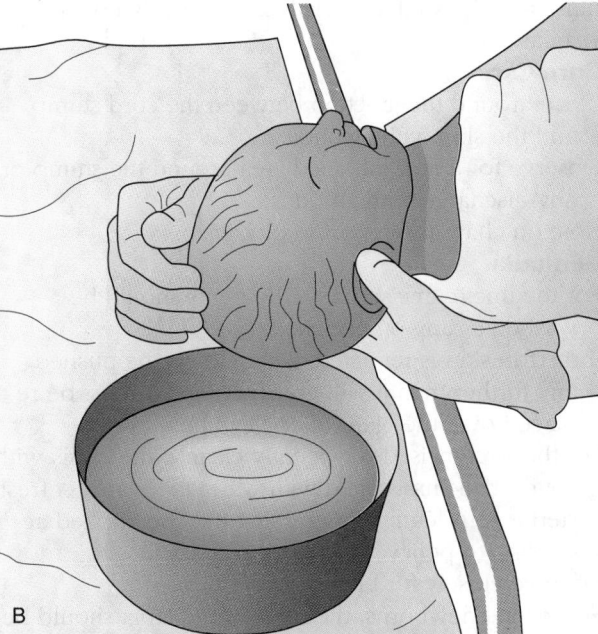

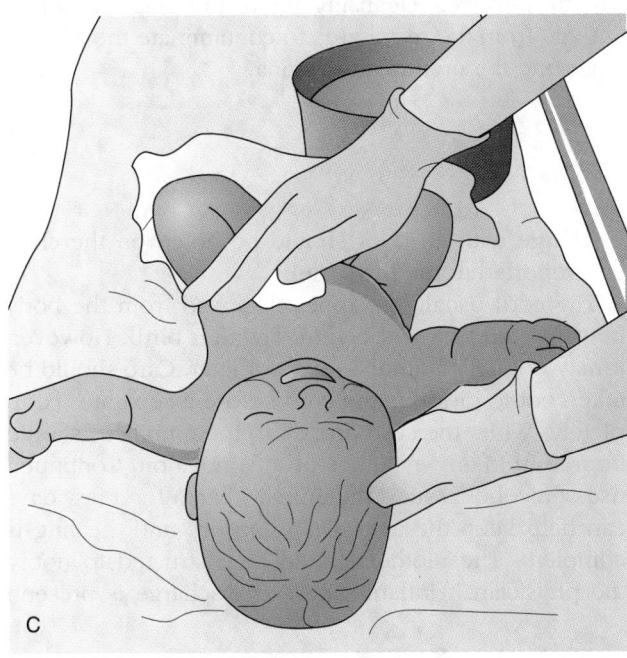

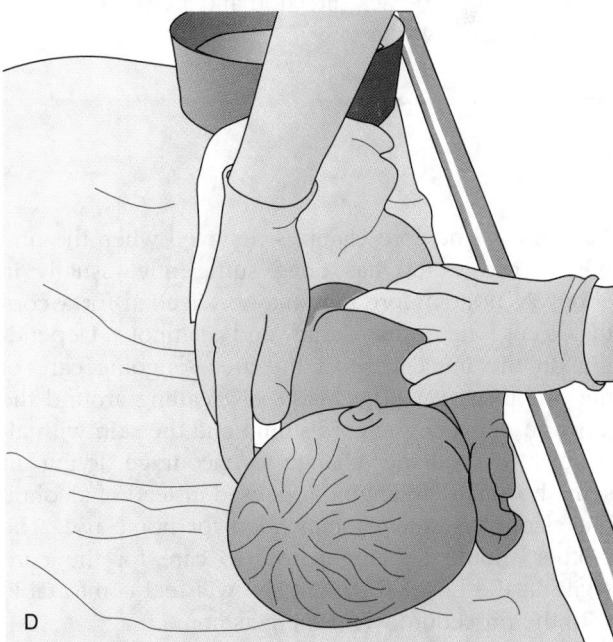

The cleanest areas of the newborn are bathed first (eyes [**A**], head [**B**]) before the chest (**C**) and back (**D**).

(continued)

PROCEDURE 29-2 *(Continued)*
Sponge Bath

Action	Rationale
Body and Extremities:	
Pay special attention to area under chin, palms of hands, between fingers and toes, and in other areas where skin surfaces come together.	Lint and body secretions can collect in these areas and cause skin irritation or odor.
Rinse and dry well, especially in previously noted areas.	Moist areas can predispose to skin irritation or other problems.
Cord Care:	
Clean around the junction between the cord stump and the skin with alcohol.	Alcohol encourages drying.
Observe for a red, inflamed area around the stump or any discharge with an odor.	Infection of the umbilicus can have serious consequences.
Note on chart and report to physician.	
Genitalia	
For the uncircumcised boy, the penis should be washed as any other part.	Retraction of foreskin is no longer advised.
If the foreskin is retracted, it should not be pushed any further than it will go easily, and it must be replaced over the glans after cleaning.	Forced retraction may cause adhesions to develop, and edema may occur if it is left retracted.
For the circumcised boy, gently cleanse the penis with cotton balls moistened with warm tap water. A fresh sterile petroleum jelly dressing may be applied according to policy.	This method avoids causing area to bleed. Keeps raw areas from sticking to diaper.
Observe closely for bleeding.	Early detection can prevent blood loss
For female newborns, the folds of the labia should be carefully cleansed with moistened cotton balls, using the front-to-back direction and a clean cotton ball for each stroke.	A curdy white secretion, **smegma,** may accumulate in this area. The front-to-back cleansing avoids bringing fecal material from the rectal area to contaminate the area around the urethra and vagina.

Cord Care. The cord clamp is removed when the umbilical cord stump has dried sufficiently, usually in about 24 hours. More time may be needed for a cord that is cut long or that is thick and gelatinous. Depending on the initial care of the area, ongoing care of the umbilicus usually consists of cleaning around the junction between the cord stump and the skin with alcohol at each diaper change to encourage drying. In some hospitals, an antibiotic is used instead of alcohol, but alcohol is still recommended for home use. The mother should be taught how to care for the cord while in the hospital so that she will feel comfortable with the procedure when she gets home.

To promote drying of the cord, newborns do not receive a tub bath until the cord has separated and the umbilicus has healed. A cord dressing is unnecessary because exposure to the air enhances drying of the cord. A red, inflamed area around the stump or any discharge with an odor should be noted on the chart and reported to the physician.

The cord usually becomes detached from the body between the fifth and eighth day after birth. However, it may not detach until 14 days or later. Care should be taken not to dislodge the cord before it separates completely. When the cord drops off, the umbilicus should be free from any evidence of inflammation. Continued use of alcohol around the umbilical area for a few days can help keep the area clean and dry until healing is complete. The mother should be instructed to notify the physician if inflammation or discharge is present.

Circumcision

Circumcision, the surgical excision of the end of the prepuce (foreskin) of the penis, is an elective procedure often performed in the neonatal period. For many years, it was almost routine in hospitals in the United States, but it is less frequent in other parts of the world. Since the statement by the Committee on Fetus and Newborn of the AAP in the 1970s that there is "no absolute medical indication for routine circumcision" (Committee on Fetus and Newborn, 1975), studies have shown that circumcision rates dropped from 85% in 1978 to about 60% by 1990 (Schoen, 1990).

The value of circumcision is controversial. Some of the advantages that have been stated by advocates of the procedure are that circumcision decreases the risk of urinary tract infection in male infants, promotes better hygiene, and decreases the incidence of inflammation, infection, and cancer of the penis. Those who are opposed to routine circumcision contend that good personal hygiene practices by uncircumcised boys also can prevent these problems. In addition, opponents of the procedure also list potential hazards, such as pain, hemorrhage, infection, and penile injury, as reasons for discouraging routine circumcision (Nelson et al., 1992).

This issue is still unresolved. In the late 1980s, a task force on neonatal circumcision considered evidence in support of circumcision's role in the prevention of urinary tract infections in male infants and sexually transmitted diseases in young men (AAP, 1989). In their report, evidence for and against circumcision was presented. It was recognized that there are potential medical benefits and advantages of circumcision as well as risks and disadvantages. More prospective studies are needed (Poland, 1990; Schoen, 1990).

Decision Making and Consent. The parents of the male newborn are asked to make the decision about circumcision. Traditional, cultural, and religious factors may be involved in deciding whether the procedure should be done. Studies have shown that major influences on the decision are the physician's opinion and whether fathers and older brothers of the newborn are circumcised. Some mothers are concerned about having to clean the penis and retract the foreskin if circumcision is not done, and they choose circumcision for that reason. Receiving information during the prenatal period about the pros and cons of circumcision and about cleaning the circumcised and uncircumcised penis can be helpful to parents and can give them more time to make an informed decision. If not already given to them, however, the information should be made available soon after the newborn's birth.

The decision concerning circumcision is becoming more of a dilemma for some parents. When it was a recommended procedure, parents found it easier to justify the possible risks and discomforts by saying, "It's the best thing to do." Now that the procedure is not encouraged by many physicians, the parents have to take more responsibility. The final decision is up to them, and a consent form must be signed by one parent before the circumcision is done. Informed consent

often means listening to a long list of possible undesirable side effects of the procedure. Some parents may feel guilty after deciding to have their newborn circumcised. The nurse must give the parents factual answers to their questions and then support them in their decision, whichever it may be.

Care During Circumcision. If the decision is made to circumcise the newborn, the procedure is usually delayed for 12 to 24 hours until the newborn has had time to stabilize. It also may be done on an outpatient basis after discharge from the hospital. Because the newborn will be restrained in a supine position for some time, it is best if he is not fed just prior to the circumcision to avoid regurgitation and potential aspiration. After checking to be sure the consent has been signed, the nurse prepares for the procedure by placing the newborn on the restraint board (Fig. 29-7) and setting out the sterile gloves, instruments, and drapes that the physician will use.

Several techniques have been devised for circumcising newborns. The most common methods are the Gomco (Yellen) clamp or the Plastibell. Further explanation of these techniques is given in Figures 29-8 and 29-9. The nurse should assess the newborn's condition periodically during the procedure and be alert for any changes.

Although studies of behavioral and physiologic responses of the newborn during circumcision indicate that he does feel pain, the procedure is usually performed without anesthesia. With increasing evidence of neonatal pain, more physicians are encouraging the

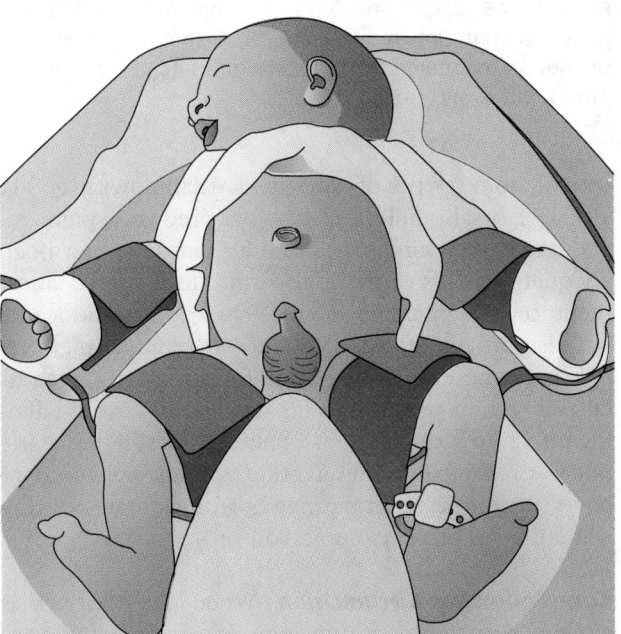

FIGURE 29-7 The newborn is placed on a plastic restraining form to restrict movements during the circumcision procedure.

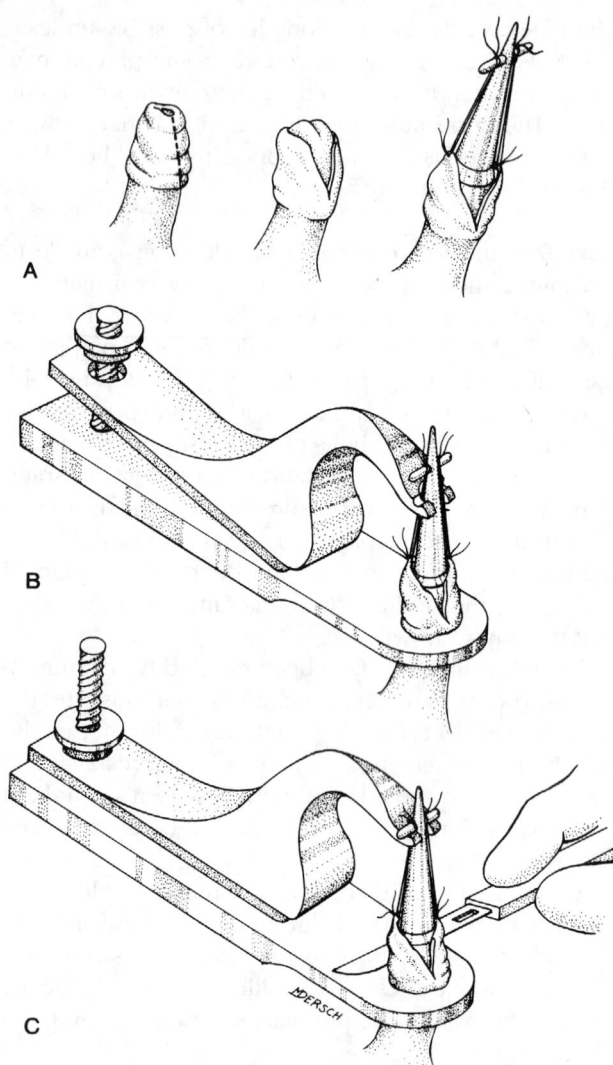

FIGURE 29-8 Circumcision using Gomco clamp. **(A)** Prepuce is slit and drawn over cone. **(B)** Clamp is applied and pressure is maintained for 3 to 5 minutes. **(C)** Excess prepuce is cut away.

use of some type of anesthetic (Rabinowitz et al., 1995). Dorsal-penile nerve block reduces pain responses during circumcision, but there have not been adequate studies of the long-term effects of this anesthetic on the infant (Schoen, 1990). Topical lidocaine has also proven effective with no noted adverse effects (Wetherstone et al., 1993). Comfort measures, such as talking to him or stroking his head, may have a calming effect. In a study by Marchette et al. (1989), playing music or a tape of intrauterine sounds appeared to have a positive effect on newborn heart rates during some phases of the circumcision procedure.

Care Following Circumcision. When the newborn is circumcised, the main principles of postoperative care are to keep the wound clean and observe it closely for bleeding. For the first 24 hours, the area is covered with a sterile gauze dressing to which a liberal amount

of sterile petroleum jelly has been added. If the circumcision is done with the Plastibell, no dressing or petroleum jelly is used.

Mothers are naturally anxious about their newborns at this time. Therefore, as soon as feasible after the circumcision, the nurse should take the newborn to his mother. It may be helpful to show her what the circumcision looks like and explain how it will look when healing so that she can recognize any deviations from normal; the nurse also should teach the mother how to care for it. With the Plastibell, the plastic ring and suture drop off with the foreskin in about 7 to 10 days. The newborn may be fed immediately after the circumcision, and mother and newborn seem to enjoy the comfort that the feeding and cuddling bring.

When changing the diaper, the ankles should be held with one hand so that he cannot kick against the operative area. Unless the physician orders otherwise, the circumcision dressing can be removed postoperatively when the newborn voids for the first time. Cleansing must be done gently, as often as necessary, with cotton balls moistened with warm tap water. A fresh sterile petroleum jelly dressing is usually applied to the penis each time the diaper is changed for the first day. The penis must be observed closely for bleeding and should be inspected every hour during the first 12 hours. If the newly circumcised infant is in the nursery, it is advisable to place the crib where he can be watched conveniently. To keep nursing personnel alerted to the recent procedure, some signal, such as a red tag, can be attached to the identification card on the crib. If bleeding occurs, it can usually be controlled with gentle pressure. If bleeding persists, the physician should be notified immediately.

Because the length of the maternity stay has been considerably shortened, circumcision may be done on

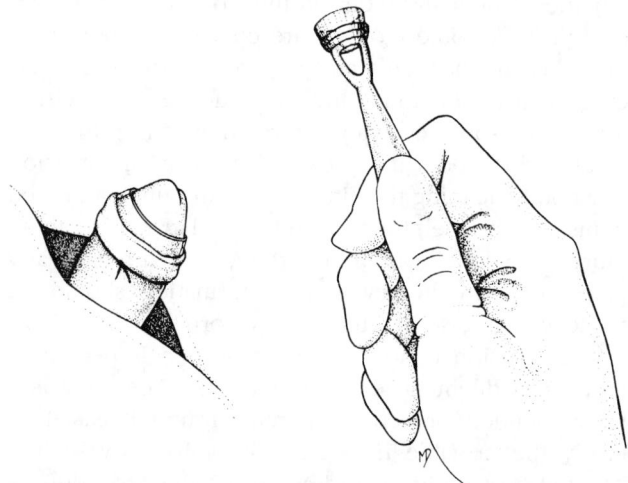

FIGURE 29-9 Circumcision using the Plastibell. The bell is fitted over the glands. Suture is tied around the rim of the bell. Excess prepuce is cut away. The plastic rim remains in place until it falls off, after healing has taken place.

the day of discharge; therefore, the nurse should ascertain the physician's wishes for aftercare and make certain that the mother knows how to care for her newly circumcised newborn. Generally, the care is the same as that described.

Care for the Uncircumcised Male. For the uncircumcised male newborn, in the past, it was recommended that the foreskin be retracted for cleansing purposes beginning a few days after birth. Some parents may still hold this belief. However, in most newborn boys, the still-developing prepuce is continuous with the epidermis of the glans and is therefore nonretractable (NAACOG, 1985). Forced retraction may cause adhesions to develop. If the foreskin is retracted, it should not be pushed any further than it will go easily, and it must be replaced over the glans after cleaning, or edema may occur.

Current recommendations are to wait until separation occurs naturally with further growth and development, sometime between 3 years and puberty, before trying to retract the foreskin (Poland, 1990). Most foreskins are retractable by 3 years of age and should be pushed back gently for cleaning about once a week. As the child learns to do more for himself, he should be taught to retract the foreskin and wash the penis, as he is taught to wash other areas of his body. As he gets older, cleaning should be done as part of his daily hygiene (Poland, 1990).

Weight

The newborn should be weighed on the day of birth and then daily or every other day while in the hospital. Newborns who remain in the hospital longer than 5 days should be weighed at intervals prescribed by the medical staff, and the weight should be recorded accurately.

During the first few days after birth, the infant may lose 5% to 10% of the birth weight. This is due partly to the minimal intake of nutrients and fluid and partly to the loss of excess fluid and brown fat (Brans, 1987). About the third or fourth day, the weight begins to increase, usually equaling the birth weight by the 10th day of life. Many infants regain their birth weight sooner. During the first 5 months, the weight gain should average 4 to 6 oz per week. After this time, the average gain is 2 to 4 oz per week. At 6 months of age, the infant has usually doubled the birth weight. By the first birthday, the infant has tripled the birthweight.

Keeping track of weight gain patterns is one way to note the newborn's condition and progress. When the newborn is not gaining weight at the expected rate, the physician should be notified. However, some newborns are slow gainers. This may not be cause for alarm if the newborn is otherwise healthy.

Sleeping

Newborns who are well and comfortable usually sleep much of the time. Although there are considerable variations, newborns may sleep as much as 20 hours a day. They wake and cry when they are hungry or uncomfortable. The sleep of a newborn is not the sound sleep of the adult. Rather, newborns move a good deal, stretch, and at intervals, awaken momentarily.

The sleeping position should be varied each time the newborn is returned to the crib. They can be placed on either side or on the back. Positioning on the right side immediately after a feeding allows gravity to promote emptying of the stomach. As they get older and learn to roll over, infants will assume the position that they like most for sleep.

Crying

After newborns are dressed and placed in a warm crib, they usually do not cry unless they are wet, hungry, ill, or uncomfortable for some reason or are moved. A caregiver can learn to distinguish a newborn's condition and needs from the character of the cry, which may be described as follows:

- A fretful, hungry cry, with fingers in the mouth and flexed, tense extremities is easily recognized as hunger.
- A fretful cry accompanied by green stools and passing of gas may indicate indigestion.
- A loud, insistent cry with drawing up and kicking of the legs usually denotes colicky pain.
- A whining cry is noticeable when the newborn is ill, premature, or very frail.
- A peculiar, shrill, sharp-sounding cry suggests injury, especially to the central nervous system.

This information about the ways in which newborns cry give clues to their condition or needs can be helpful to the mother. Newborns have only their posture and their voice at this time to communicate their needs, so it is essential that the mother learn to interpret her newborn's cues.

Hypertonic Newborns. Some newborns seem to be fussy from birth. They appear very active, startle easily, cry readily and more frequently (and apparently for no reason), are alert and awake much of the time, and generally do not fit the usual newborn activity pattern of sleeping and eating. These newborns may be described as **hypertonic** (ie, they do not seem to be able to relax as well as other newborns).

The parents of hypertonic newborns may find it difficult to adjust to their newborn. They may experience a great deal of anxiety until they are informed (or learn by trial and error) that this is "normal behavior" for this child. Too often they assume they must be doing something "wrong," because despite their efforts, their newborn remains fussy, tense, and crying. The nurse can help the parents by giving them anticipatory guidance about their newborn's behavior and helpful ways he or she can be soothed. Also, the physician should be informed of the nurse's observations and interventions so appropriate, consistent advice can be given to the parents.

These newborns usually respond favorably to being held securely. Thus, wrapping them snugly with a receiving blanket, cuddling them securely, and changing their position slowly and surely rather than quickly are ways to help allay undue tenseness.

An automatic swing with a music box or a bouncer chair with a vibrator may be soothing. A newborn can be placed in a swing for a short time when supported by pillows. Additional ways of lulling a fretful infant to sleep include recorded heartbeat sounds, various types of music, or a ride in the car. The parents should be encouraged to experiment to determine which sounds have the best effect on their newborn (see Client Education: Sensory Enrichment).

Any new activity or procedure should be introduced slowly to hypertonic newborns. For instance, when a tub bath is given for the first time, the newborn should be placed in a small amount of water very slowly. Each lower extremity should be immersed gradually so as not to frighten or startle the newborn too much. The parents should not consider an occasional evening out a luxury. It should be considered a necessary item in the care of their newborn. These infants do place greater demands on their parents than do infants of a more placid nature. A short time away can help restore the parents' perspective and good humor.

Some newborns who cry excessively have **colic,** which is defined as paroxysmal abdominal pain resulting in intense cries with legs pulled up against the abdomen. The cause of colic is not known, but it seems to be related to feeding patterns, such as swallowing too much air, overfeeding, or inadequate burping. Interventions to relieve stomach distress, such as feeding in a more upright position, burping more often, and placing in a prone position over the knee or a folded blanket while rubbing the back, are often helpful. Many newborns with colic will also respond favorably to the same strategies that help hypertonic newborns.

Urinary Elimination

Urinary activity of the fetus is evidenced by the presence of urine in the amniotic fluid. The newborn usually voids during delivery or immediately after birth. However, urinary function may be suppressed for several hours. If the newborn does not void within 24 hours, the condition should be reported to the physician. Urinary retention may be caused by an imperforate meatus.

After the first 2 or 3 days, the infant voids 10 to 15 times a day. When the urine is concentrated, red, or rusty, there may be uric acid crystals in the urine.

Intestinal Elimination

During fetal life, the content of the intestines is made up of greenish-black, tarlike material called **meconium.** It is composed of epithelial and epidermal cells and lanugo hair probably swallowed with the amniotic fluid. The color of the meconium is due to bile pigment. Before birth and for the first few hours after birth, the intestinal contents are sterile. Apparently, there is no peristalsis until after birth, because normally, there is no discoloration of the amniotic fluid indicating passage of meconium.

The newborn passes meconium stools for the first few days of life. After this time, the stools gradually begin to change to greenish brown and then to yellowish brown. These **transitional stools** are less sticky than meconium and contain some milk curds. Following the transitional stools, the characteristics depend on whether the infant is fed breast milk or formula. See Fig. 29-10 for a more detailed description.

Most newborns pass the first stool within 12 hours of birth. Nearly all have a stool in 24 hours. If a newborn has not passed a stool by this time, an imperforate anus or intestinal obstruction must be considered as a possible reason for the delay, and the newborn must be observed closely.

The daily number of stools on about the fifth day of life usually ranges from four to six. As the infant grows, this number decreases to one or two each day. The type of stool of the breast-fed baby may be influenced by the mother's diet. Slight variations from the normal may have little significance if the newborn appears to be comfortable and sleeps and nurses well. If the stools have a watery consistency, are green, contain much mucus, and have a foul odor and flatus is being passed, the condition may be evidence of some digestive or intestinal irritation or infection and should be reported to the physician. During the hospital stay, the number, color, and consistency of stools should be recorded daily on the newborn's record.

Screening for Inborn Errors of Metabolism

Certain disorders related to **inborn errors of metabolism** (hereditary deficiency of a specific enzyme or specific chemicals needed for normal metabolism) are detectable by blood tests soon after birth. Early detection and appropriate treatment can often prevent or decrease permanent defects resulting from these disorders. Although many tests have been developed, not all are used in mass screening. To be most useful, the

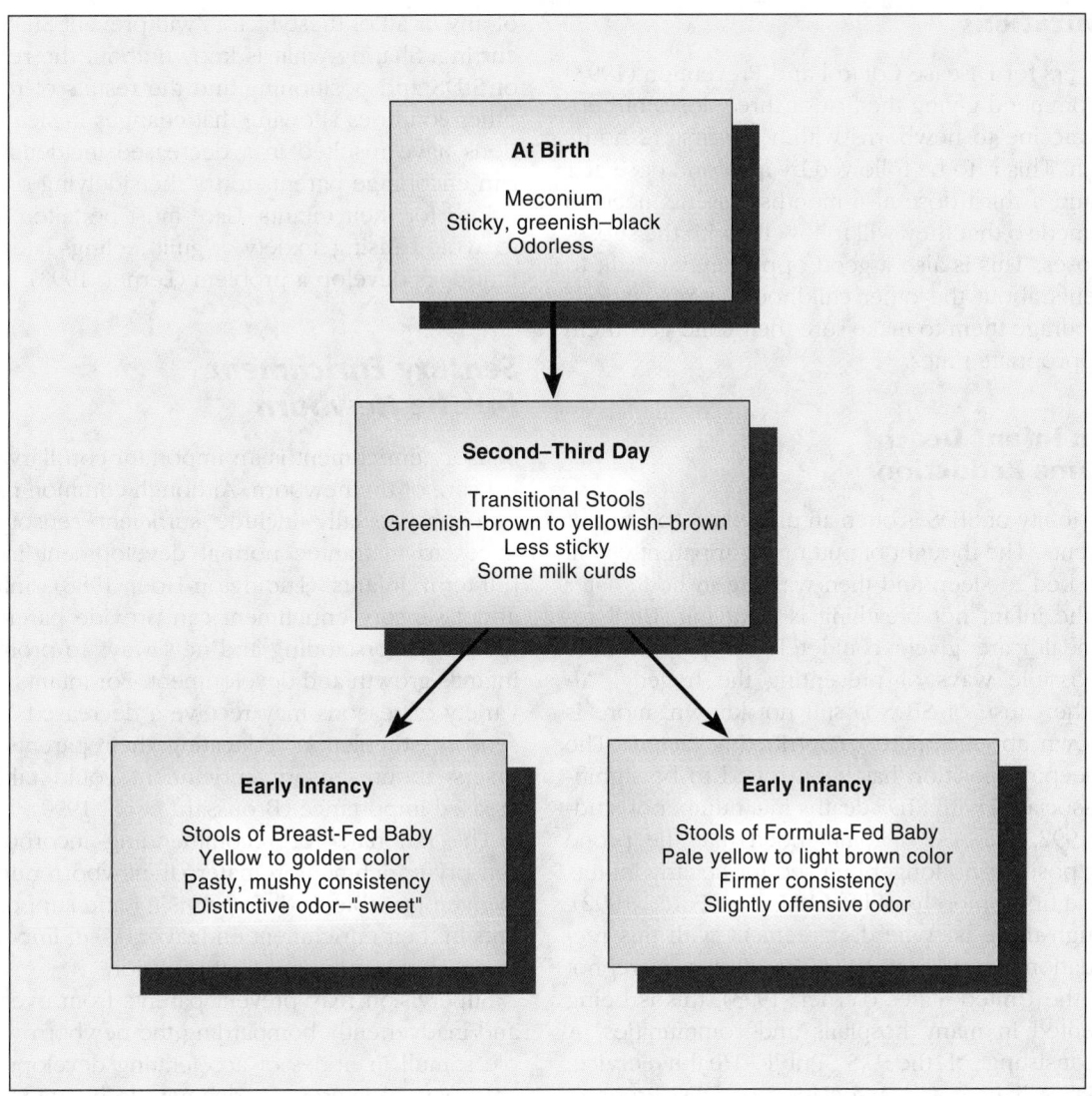

At Birth

Meconium
Sticky, greenish–black
Odorless

Second–Third Day

Transitional Stools
Greenish–brown to yellowish–brown
Less sticky
Some milk curds

Early Infancy

Stools of Breast-Fed Baby
Yellow to golden color
Pasty, mushy consistency
Distinctive odor–"sweet"

Early Infancy

Stools of Formula-Fed Baby
Pale yellow to light brown color
Firmer consistency
Slightly offensive odor

FIGURE 29–10 Stool cycle.

test should be sensitive and specific, and effective intervention should be available for those who have positive tests (Zinn, 1992).

Phenylketonuria (PKU), congenital hypothyroidism, and galactosemia meet these criteria and are the conditions most often tested for in government-funded neonatal screening programs. In some states, additional tests that are included in the testing programs are maple syrup urine disease and the hemoglobinopathies (sickle-cell anemia and thalassemia). Tests for other conditions may be done on the blood of newborns identified as at risk by family history.

Nurses often are responsible for obtaining the blood for the tests. This is usually done by heel stick, as described previously in this chapter. The way the blood is collected is important to the accuracy of the test. The blood is dropped on approved filter paper to saturate premarked circles completely and must be applied to one side only. After collection, the blood spots should be dried at room temperature and not subjected to ex-

cessive heat. Care should be taken to avoid handling the specimen, placing it on a wet surface, or allowing it to be contaminated by other substances (AAP Section on Endocrinology, 1993).

The blood sample for the tests should be obtained before the newborn leaves the hospital. The usual recommendation is to wait until 24 hours after birth. However, if the newborn is discharged before this time, it is better to obtain the blood early than to risk missing the tests altogether in case the mother does not bring the newborn back. Newborns initially screened before 24 hours of age should be rescreened for PKU by the third week of life for better reliability of this test. Because results are thought to be related to food intake by the newborn, early testing may miss some affected newborns (Freeman et al., 1992). Recent information, however, indicates that most newborns with PKU have an elevated blood phenylalanine concentration during the first day of life and probably will not be overlooked by early testing (Burton, 1993).

Immunizations

The Centers for Disease Control and Prevention (1993) now recommend giving the first of three doses of hepatitis B vaccine to newborns within the first 12 hours after birth. This is to be followed by a second dose at 1 month and a third dose at 6 months. Parents need to be informed so that they will follow up with the subsequent doses. This is also a good opportunity to talk to the parents about the other childhood immunizations and encourage them to make sure their child gets them at the appropriate times.

Sudden Infant Death Syndrome Reduction

The possibility of SIDS is often an unspoken concern of new parents. The thought of putting an apparently well infant in bed to sleep and then walking in hours later to find the infant not breathing is terrifying. Until recently, healthcare givers could tell the parents little about possible ways of preventing the tragedy. Although the cause of SIDS is still not known, more is now known about apparent contributing factors. The prone sleeping position has been found to be significantly associated with SIDS deaths in a number of studies. In 1992, the AAP recommended that the prone sleeping position no longer be used for healthy infants during the first 6 months of life (AAP Task Force, 1992).

Although there is some disagreement with this recommendation because most of the studies were not done in the United States (Lerner, 1993), this is being implemented in many hospitals and communities. A group consisting of the U.S. Public Health Service, AAP, SIDS Alliance, and Association of SIDS Program Professionals is promoting a "Back to Sleep" campaign through the distribution of literature for parents and professionals. In Norway, an intervention program designed to avoid prone sleeping for infants (Markestad et al., 1995) resulted in a 50% decrease in SIDS in the 3 years following the program, compared with the 3 years before the program in the same population.

Research is continuing on other factors that might relate to the increased incidence of SIDS in the prone position. Risk in the prone sleeping position was potentiated in one study by the use of a natural fiber mattress, swaddling, recent illness, or heating of the infant's room (Ponsonby et al., 1993). Infants sleeping prone also have an increase in sleep duration with fewer arousals (Kahn et al., 1993; Poets et al., 1995). Risks related to SIDS in other studies include lack of prenatal care, maternal smoking, and avoidance of breast-feeding (Lerner, 1993).

Nurses should provide new parents with information about the risk factors for SIDS. It is also important to let them know that there are no guarantees that avoidance of any or all of these factors will prevent SIDS from occurring. Sharing what is known about the relationship of SIDS and positioning and the results of research in other countries showing that changes in sleeping positions have resulted in a decreased incidence of SIDS can encourage parents to try the sidelying or back positions for their infants. Care must be taken, however, to avoid causing anxiety or guilt feelings later if the infant does develop a problem (Lerner, 1993).

Sensory Enrichment for the Newborn

Sensory enrichment is an important corollary to physical care of the newborn. Although common patterns of parenting usually include sufficient sensory experiences to guarantee normal development in healthy, full-term infants (Ludington-Hoe, 1988), information about sensory enrichment can provide parents with a greater understanding and new ways to promote their infant's growth and development. For infants who for a variety of reasons may receive a decreased amount of sensory stimulation, educating their parents or caregivers about sensory enrichment could take on increased importance (Broussard et al., 1990).

The rationale for recommending incorporation of sensory enrichment in maternal–newborn nursing care is given in Table 29-1. Supervising and supporting parents in their enrichment endeavors is an important maternal–newborn nursing intervention.

Supervision may prevent parents from overzealously and inadvertently bombarding the newborn with multiple stimuli in hopes of accelerating development. Parents may misinterpret enrichment to be an approach to increasing their child's intelligence. The overstimulated infant may withdraw, and benefits of sensory enrichment may be negated. Some children who have been "pushed" to improve their intelligence lose interest in learning or suffer emotional setbacks. Overstimulation and "pushing" an infant is always a potential risk when educating parents about sensory enrichment. To support the parent, the nurse must first have an understanding of the rationale for sensory enrichment, the development of the central nervous system, the effects of sensory enrichment, maternal and newborn assessments to prevent overstimulation, principles guiding active sensory enrichment interventions, and safe sensory enrichment interventions that can be incorporated into previously existing caregiving strategies with the newborn.

The newborn is capable of perceiving environmental events at birth. Some senses may be exquisitely sensitive at this time, such as the olfactory sense, and others may be relatively immature, such as the visual and auditory senses. However, even the immature senses perform well within their limitations.

TABLE 29-1
Rationale for Sensory Enrichment

Reason	Explanation
1. Sensory enrichment facilitates satisfaction with the maternal (parental) role.	Sensory enrichment offers the caregiver a repertoire of approaches that foster pleasure in the infant, an emotional response that the caregiver can then observe. When mother (parent) has knowledge of and ability to recognize her infant's cues, this positive feedback promotes satisfaction with the maternal (parental) experience.
2. Sensory enrichment promotes positive interactions between parent and infant.	Sensory enrichment fosters a positive interaction cycle. Infants actively participate in interactions. They initiate and regulate behavioral exchanges and communicate in accordance with certain rules, using gestures and prespeech movements and sounds. They begin with random movements at birth, and by 6 weeks of age, facial expressions and hand gesturing indicate "greeting" and withdrawal responses to people and objects. Mutually enjoyable interactions between caregiver and infant may constitute the foundation of optimum development. It is important for the parents to be aware that gratification and the beneficial effects of this interaction cycle can be disturbed if inappropriate or overstimulating activities occur.
3. Sensory enrichment is an integral force influencing infant development.	When infants reach a state of homeostatic control (physiologic balance and stability), they can then devote their energies to seeking social stimuli. This increases infants' availability to their world. Once available and interested in the environment, infants respond in such a way that they learn more about themselves and their world.

TABLE 29-2
Assessment of Infant Rhythms

Observe the newborn for rhythm of interaction when he or she is lying in crib in a quiet alert state with eyes open and an expression of interest on his or her face. At this time, newborns are most receptive to the presentation of sensory stimuli and will demonstrate the stages of their rhythm.

Stage	Observations
Presentation Stimulus is presented by softly calling infant's name.	Observe for alerting response and slight movements in the trunk, legs, and head as acknowledgment of the stimulus.
Orientation	Observe newborn's attempts to orient toward the stimulus by trunk straightening, slight head righting or raising, head turning toward the stimulus, and fanning motions of the fingers and toes.
Attentiveness	Observe length of time newborn is attentive as demonstrated by pupil dilation; slowing of heart rate, respiratory rate, and sucking rate; cessation of gross arm and leg movements; and quiet gazing.
Acceleration	Watch for acceleration of body movements, squirming then flailing of arms and legs, extending the fingers and toes, and twisting the torso.
Peak of excitement	Be aware of newborn's behaviors as he or she reaches a level at which no more input can be tolerated without jeopardizing physiologic status or behavioral balance. The only alternative left for this newborn is withdrawal if sensory enrichment continues rather than subsides.
Withdrawal	Observe newborn's attempt to shut out or get away from the sensory stimuli: turns head away, averts gaze, drowns out sound by wailing, or physically distancing from the source. It is often best to allow newborns to console themselves rather than adding to the sensory input with active consoling (cooing, rubbing, talking).
Refractory stage	This is a period of recovery that varies in duration for each newborn but lasts generally 10 to 20 seconds. Newborns need time to regroup their resources and organize themselves for another interaction. They will stop crying, slow their movements, regain their posture and flaccid expression, and eventually become alert as they gain control over their autonomic functions, motor movements, state of alertness, and interactional faculties. Sustained human presence accompanied by silence will facilitate rapid recovery, making the newborn available for another rhythmic interaction.

Highlighting these stages for the parent and family members will help them avoid overstimulating the newborn, and allow interactions to remain mutually gratifying. Most parents are relatively synchronous with their infant's rhythm within 3 months of birth.

Nursing Intervention and Client Education

Awareness of a newborn's characteristic rhythm of interaction (Table 29-2), maternal reciprocity, and signs of attention, habituation, fatigue, and engagement-disengagement cues ensures personalization of enrichment interventions and avoidance of overstimulation.

Influencing Principles. Each sense can be appropriately stimulated to use and expand sensory capabilities. Sensory stimulation may be actively and passively provided by the environment. Active provision means that deliberate efforts to stimulate each sense are being made; passive stimulation occurs spontaneously without conscious intent. Fortunately, the day-to-day passive stimulation provided by most caregivers ensures development within the normal range. These instinctual presentations of sensory stimuli are to be encouraged if they are in accordance with the principles of sensory enrichment. These principles are described briefly in Box 29-4.

When these principles are used to guide interventions, sensory enrichment becomes more beneficial to the infant. Because the nurse will not be able to provide continuity of enrichment once the newborn goes home, exposing the parents to sensory enrichment techniques and giving them opportunities to practice the techniques in the hospital are helpful.

Sensory enrichment techniques can be divided into six categories directed toward the individual senses: visual, auditory, tactile, vestibular, olfactory, and gustatory. Client Education: Sensory Enrichment provides information about newborns' preferences and capabilities and suggests strategies for enriching their sensory experience in each area.

Discharge Planning and Teaching

Discharge planning for the mother and newborn may begin in the prenatal class or clinic when discussions are held about planning for what happens after the newborn comes home. During the hospital stay, nurses continue to assess the family's needs for assistance in planning for care of the newborn at home. Early discharge (less than 24 hours after birth) for mothers and newborns without complications is a reality in many places, owing either to the parents' desire, hospital policy, or insurance limits. Observations and care traditionally done by hospital personnel are now the responsibility of the new parents. This increases the need for adequate instruction but decreases the time available for teaching. Use of a standardized checklist makes it easier to ensure that all necessary points are covered. While a checklist can be helpful, the nurse must individualize it for each client and adapt the teaching to each client's specific needs (Salam, 1995).

BOX 29-4
Principles Influencing Nursing Interventions

1. Newborns have *right-sided preferences* during the first 3 months. The newborn's right side is more sensitive to touch than the left; the right side conducts messages to the brain faster than the left; and newborns turn their heads to the right more reliably than to the left. Stimulating experiences encourage more newborn attention if they are begun on the right side, regardless of eventual handedness.
2. It is best to present the stimulus during *periods of alert inactivity* when newborns are awake with their eyes open but their legs and arms still if newborn attention or concentration is desired. During this restive phase, newborns can attend to and track stimuli with ease and sustained interest. The alert, inactive state characterizes the newborn for an hour or two immediately after birth and for 5 to 10 minutes before and after feedings.
3. Newborns become alert for longer periods if they are in *upright positions* and are *being held*. Sitting in this manner increases gazing by 70%. When newborns look around, they receive visual stimulation, which helps them learn how to relate to their environment.
4. *Avoid* stimulating a newborn to the *point of agitation,* because agitation increases heart rate and respiratory rate and prolongs inspiratory phases, which can induce aspiration. Some types of sensory stimulation will agitate some newborns and please others. Each newborn should be the guide, and his or her particular rhythm and readiness for stimulation, as manifested by engagement cues, should be respected.
5. A *latency to response time* occurs because of the newborn's neuromuscular immaturity. In the newborn period the time it takes for the brain to develop and send a message to the muscles and for the muscle activity to be organized and expressed as a discernible behavior in response to a sensory event is generally 15 to 75 seconds after the stimulus. For example, auditory responsivity is eyes brightening when mother's voice is heard; visual attentiveness tends to emerge slowly over 1 to 2 minutes.

As part of the plan for taking the newborn home, the nurse discusses with the parents their understanding of the need to use a car seat for the newborn. Car seats may be mandatory in most states but are not used consistently by many parents. Nurses should be well informed about the use of car seats and should take the opportunity to advocate their use whenever possible. New parents are usually receptive to information that will help them provide good care for their newborn, so discussing car seats is particularly appropriate at this time. A space on the discharge chart form to indicate the use of a car seat encourages staff members to include this in the discharge planning and teaching.

(*text continues on page 756*)

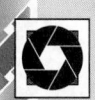

CLIENT EDUCATION
Sensory Enrichment

Sense	Preferences/Rationale	Strategies
Visual	Newborns prefer to gaze at items that provide contrast between figure and background.	Two big black dots on a white background, drawn on a paper plate and pasted on a popsicle stick (called a *popsicle face*), will appeal to newborns.
	Black against white offers the greatest contrast. Faces, especially eyes, are loved by newborns.	Black-and-white glossy photos of the mother's or father's face or Black-and-white schematic faces (next best thing in absence of real faces) can be placed within the newborn's field of vision.
	Moving objects are more fascinating to a newborn than stationary ones.	Black & white mobiles should have pattern facing down toward newborn and be placed 10 to 13 inches from the newborn's face.
	Circular items are preferred because of the newborn's immature ocular movement ability.	Cylinders and circles painted black and white, can be used as mobiles, or rattles.
	Black and white sharp images of geometric figures, such as cylinders and circles rather than rectangles and squares are best.	Eye-to-eye contact in the face-to-face position provides objects which are both circular and mobile.
	Newborns do not like to look at plain-colored walls or walls with little figures on them.	
	Animals and cartoon characters are inappropriate visual stimuli for the full-term newborn and are not appreciated until after the first year.	
	In the first 6 months of life, infants prefer to look at big geometric figures rather than small ones, with preference for increasing complexity and visual information processing. Stripes (especially good for the first 3–4 wk), black-and-white checkerboards, bull's eyes, dots, and triangles are appealing geometric shapes.	Cards depicting geometric shapes items can be used separately as stimuli or in mobiles and crib hangings. Black-and-white geometric-shaped mobiles may be made from other materials also (see Figure)

Sense	Preferences/Rationale	Speech Strategies
Auditory	The newborn has the capacity to hear all sounds greater than 55 dB, with slightly higher sensitivity to the lower frequencies. Newborns can learn to discriminate their mother's and father's voice from all others within the first 2 wk and have, at that time, a distinct reaction pattern established to the voice they hear.	Talking to infants is important. The more speech they hear, the sooner they will learn language. The more speech to which they are exposed, the more likely they are to reach their potential for mental skills. Gorski and coworkers have suggested that maternal speech is the most important aspect of the newborn's sensory environment, and desirable maternal speech can ameliorate anticipated delays and handicaps in high-risk infants.

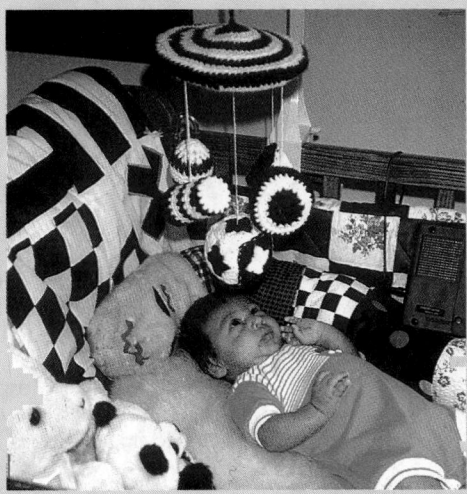

A mobile with black and white circles and cylinders provides good visual stimulation for the infant. (Courtesy of S. Ludington)

(continued)

CLIENT EDUCATION *(Continued)*
Sensory Enrichment

Sense	Preferences/Rationale	Strategies
Auditory	Although slightly more sensitive to the low-frequency male voice, newborn behavior suggests a preference for the female voice. Women tend to exhibit cooing behaviors, which are various-pitched musical sounds. Instinctual maternal speech uses exaggerated intonation. Higher-pitched sounds are attention-getting sounds, while low, bass sounds are consoling and quieting. Monotonous speech and monotone sounds are boring to the newborn, who prefers modulating auditory input. The newborn accustoms to monotone quickly and does not attend to it. Some fathers have a tendency to speak in bass, monotone speech patterns and should be encouraged to use more inflection and exaggerated tone. Slow speech, 55 words per minute or less, is easier for the newborn to discern than faster speech.	Approach infant in face-to-face orientation to provide non-verbal cues with the verbalization. Speak to newborns in slow melodic tones with inflection and exaggeration. Respond to vocalizations by the newborn. Vocalizations can be encouraged by asking questions and waiting for a response.
	Speech stimulates the development of the left hemisphere of the brain; music stimulates the right hemisphere. Newborns have demonstrated less agitation in the presence of classical music than rock and roll music. However, individual preference may be for the music to which the neonate was exposed while in utero. If the mother played jazz during her pregnancy, her newborn will probably enjoy jazz more than unfamiliar classical music. Mothers have much latitude in choice of music, but true, pure tones are preferred to synthesized music.	*Sound Strategies* Provide musical stimulation for infants. Start with the music the infant was exposed to while in utero, then slowly introduce new arrangements. Although not usually pure tones, music boxes are high-pitched and will often engage the fussy newborn's attention. Background music on a radio or tape recorder can lull a newborn to sleep.
Tactile	The skin is the largest sense organ in the newborn. Newborns are very sensitive to touch, especially around the mouth, in the palms, over the soles of the feet, and around the genitals. Tactile stimulation, or touching, is instrumental in helping the neonate adjust to life outside the womb. Neonates separated from their mother at birth were found to cry in a characteristic manner that stopped when they were placed skin-to-skin with their mother and did not occur with neonates who were placed with their mothers immediately after birth.	Skin-to-skin touch is to be encouraged.
	Skin-to-skin touch in a rhythmic, stroking pattern has been found to reduce weight loss from 10% of birth weight to 3% of birth weight. Newborns cannot be spoiled by too much caressing. The closer they are held and the more often they are patted, the more secure they become. Observe the power of touch on newborns: It can make them either quiescent or aroused. Reassuring parental touch makes crying subside, extremities flex, and the eyes open if the newborn does not fall asleep.	Provide skin-to-skin stroking. While stroking, give extra strokes of slightly more pressure to the most sensitive tactile areas, outlined previously. Stroking that is begun on the right should continue on the left to encourage midline awareness. Stroking the head is comforting to neonates, especially if stroking from the forehead to the occiput. Slow repetitive strokes over the top of the head can calm colicky infants, as do finger strokes across the forehead.

(continued)

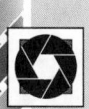

CLIENT EDUCATION *(Continued)*
Sensory Enrichment

Sense	Preferences/Rationale	Strategies
Tactile	Some newborns prefer being stroked in the head-to-toe direction—a pattern reminiscent of the process of nerve myelinization. Stroking at a slow pace, such as 12 to 16 times per minute, has been associated with reductions in apnea and irregular breathing in the neonate.	
	Many infants become quite fond of stroking and never tire of it. For these infants, it becomes a relaxation technique and is widely used in Australia and India. Touch is believed to help relieve the unspent tensions infants accumulate throughout the day and accelerate neuromuscular development.	The mother can collect swatches of different textures with which to stroke the infant. These tactile experiences wil be especially valuable if the texture is experienced within context (eg, fur on a panda bear, rough on daddy's face, smooth on the mirror). Caution should be exercised so that the infant is not assaulted by multiple sensations.
Vestibular	Vestibular stimulation refers to movement, and the term is derived from the vestibule of the ear, which perceives alterations in fluid pressure as movement occurs. Movement stimulation begins in utero as the fetus moves about in weightless space, stretching and rotating.	Following birth, newborns should have opportunities to move, stretch, pull, and push. These activities are best facilitated by "tummy time," being placed on the tummy in a safe place for self-initiated, unstructured movement. If infants are accustomed to sleeping on their side or back, tummy time may be upsetting. Having a parent on the floor in a face-to-face orientation may alleviate some of the stress of this new position. It is important to try to get a newborn to enjoy this position, because the freedom of movement afforded by it enables the child to crawl within normal time limits rather than significantly later.
	All newborns exhibit individual patterns of spontaneous activity; some are quite active and others calm. Activity patterns may be an early index of a child's temperament. Movement stimulation, especially rotary movements, has been associated with enhanced motor development.	Infant exercises provide opportunities for vestibular stimulation. Extension and flexion of all extremities followed by tummy tickles, pressure against the kicking foot, circular swinging of the well-supported infant, and relaxation techniques are possibilities.
		Some parents may inquire about the efficacy of gym classes for motor stimulation of infants. The American Academy of Pediatrics issued a policy statement indicating that exercise and swim classes had no known benefits and could overstress ligaments and immune systems, respectively, in the first year of life.
	Rocking is the most common vestibular stimulation that is passively given, providing excellent opportunities for vestibular sensations that aid in weight gain and neuromuscular coordination.	There is no recommended rate of rocking or frequency, but a little each day can be encouraged.
	Newborns like the movement provided by being carried. In fact, infants who are carried in a pouch while the mother is moving about, appear to fall into deep levels of sleep more smoothly, awaken less irritable, and show more secure attachment at 7 months of age.	Parents can provide vestibular stimulation by carrying infants in front carriers as they go about their daily tasks or go for walks.
Olfactory	Olfaction in the newborn is quite sensitive. Shortly after birth, newborns will change their breathing and activity rates in response to strong artificial odors. At 5 days of age, the newborn can differentiate the odor of the mother's breast pad from that of a stranger's. If mother's nipples have been smeared with	

(continued)

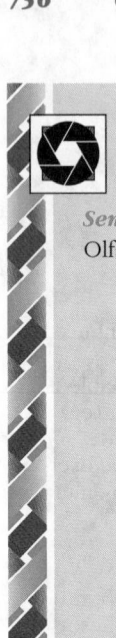

CLIENT EDUCATION *(Continued)*
Sensory Enrichment

Sense	Preferences/Rationale	Strategies
Olfactory	petroleum jelly, the neonate will violently refuse approaching the noxiously scented nipple. This ability to perceive maternal odor originates at birth, when the newborn is held close. By 2 weeks of age, newborns are able to recognize their mother's axillary odors. At this time, their olfactory sensitivity is instrumental to the bonding and parental recognition process and emotional development. The importance of olfactory markers for emotional development is revealed when one considers that olfaction is the only sense that is not mediated by the reticular activating system, going instead directly to the limbic center of the brain. The limbic center is the seat of emotions. The most potent stimulus is breast milk, followed only by the body scents of both parents.	Providing various smells, such as cherry juice, nutmeg, cinnamon, and honey, is not really necessary but may be enjoyable. The infant detects these scents when in the kitchen environment without special attention to them for the first 6 months of life. After that, smelling can become a stimulating game. Various "scratch and sniff" books are available in toy stores.
Gustatory	The most prevalent taste sensation to which the newborn is exposed is breast milk (or formula). As the nipple is compressed against the hard palate, the milk spurts onto the bitter receptors in the back of the tongue. With repetitive stimulation of the bitter receptors, the infant grows fond of the bitter-tasting foods. However, infants always like sweet tastes and can smile with sweet and frown with sour tastes. When infants require blood sampling and painful procedures, such as circumcision, administration of 12% sugar water immediately before the procedure acts as a powerful analgesic agent and cuts crying by half. Breast milk is the preferred gustatory stimulus for newborns.	Avoiding giving the infant sour tastes (eg, lemon juice, cranberry juice) so that the newborn does not associate the caregiver with unpleasant stimuli. During the first year of life, infants should not be given honey because of the high likelihood of developing botulism from this source.

Please see reference list at end of chapter for sources of information in this display.

Plans for healthcare follow-up of the newborn should be discussed with the mother. A follow-up appointment should be made with a private physician or at a well-baby clinic. Instructions about potential significant symptoms in the newborn that should be reported to the physician must be addressed (see Client Education: Events That Should Be Reported to the Primary Healthcare Provider). Most new mothers appreciate an opportunity to talk to the nurse regarding their concerns about taking the newborn home. Taking time for such a talk is well worth the nurse's effort, because it can help make those first few days at home less frightening and more enjoyable for the new parents.

The decreased length of stay in the hospital after the newborn's birth has given maternity nursing an increased community focus. Some ways maternity nurses have found to respond to this challenge include expanding their predischarge teaching to be more responsive to client needs, giving the parents a phone number they can call at any hour if they need help or further information after they get home, making postdischarge phone calls to all clients within the first 2 days after discharge, and in some cases, even making home visits (Williams et al., 1992). For some new mothers, especially the inexperienced, a referral to a community health or home health agency for home visits and continuing care may be appropriate for follow-up. Some families with financial problems also may need to be referred to a family service agency.

Evaluation

Before the newborn's discharge from the hospital, the nurse will evaluate the effectiveness of the newborn's care and the effectiveness of parent teaching. Possible anticipated outcomes may include the following:

- The newborn is free of infection or any other complication.
- The newborn maintains a stable temperature.

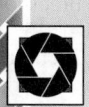

CLIENT EDUCATION
Events That Should Be Reported to the Primary Healthcare Provider

1. If the skin color changes:
    a. To blue (cyanosis), around the mouth or all over
    b. To yellow (jaundice)
2. Temperature above 38.4°C (101°F) or below 36.1°C (96°F)
3. Projectile vomiting two or more times
4. Refusal of two consecutive feedings
5. Periods of apnea (absence of breathing) longer than 15 seconds
6. Behavior changes, such as excessive crying, fussiness, lethargy, or difficulty in rousing the newborn
7. Elimination pattern changes, such as two or more green, watery stools; hard stools; or decreased number of wet diapers (less than five per day)
8. Local signs of bleeding or infection:
    a. Swelling, redness, or discharge from eyes
    b. Swelling, redness, discharge, or bleeding from umbilical cord stump
    c. Swelling, redness, discharge, or bleeding from circumcision

- The newborn takes nourishment well, whether breast or bottle.
- Appropriate parent–newborn attachment behaviors are observed.
- The parent(s) demonstrate or return demonstrate skills in newborn care, including handwashing, use of bulb syringe, assessment, and bathing.
- The parents are able to repeat instructions or answer questions related to response to emergency situations, danger signs or changes in the newborn requiring a call to the primary healthcare provider, follow-up visits to the healthcare provider, and newborn safety measures, including use of a car seat.

Any unmet goals would indicate a need for reassessment and further interventions, such as additional teaching or referrals.

Summary Points

✔ During the first hours of life, the newborn's ability to make the transition to extrauterine life is monitored closely. Assessment of respiratory status, safety, and regulation of temperature continue to be a high priority.

✔ Nursing care of the newborn after the transition period is most often given with the parents present

and will involve teaching them what they want to or will need to know about caring for the newborn.

✔ The newborn's immature immune system leads to increased vulnerability to infection, which necessitates protective measures, such as frequent handwashing, and adhering to dress protocols by nurses and other caregivers.

✔ The nurse needs to be knowledgeable about the current beliefs and practices regarding circumcision of newborn male infants. Information should be provided to the parents to assist them in making the decision if they have not already done so.

✔ Most states require that newborns be screened for specific inborn errors of metabolism. The tests most frequently required are for PKU, congenital hypothyroidism, and galactosemia.

✔ The cause of SIDS is still not known. The condition cannot be reliably prevented, but a strong relationship is associated with the newborn's prone sleeping position. Other associated risk factors include the use of soft mattresses, recent illness, overheating, and swaddling.

✔ Newborns are known to be much more competent at birth than was formerly believed. New parents, interested in their newborn's growth and development, usually appreciate receiving information about sensory capabilities and ways of providing sensory enrichment. Teaching them strategies related to the six senses can be helpful, but equally important is to teach them how to avoid overstimulating the newborn.

✔ Before discharge from the hospital, the parents need information about care of the newborn, including newborn characteristics, hygiene and clothing, feeding, safety, elimination, signs of illness, SIDS reduction, and sensory enrichment.

✔ Maternity nursing is taking on an increased community focus, as many new parents and their newborns are returning home in the first 24 to 48 hours after birth. Maternity nurses are responding, not only with expanded predischarge teaching, but also with follow-up through postdischarge telephone calls, home visits, and referrals to home health agencies.

REFERENCES

American Academy of Pediatrics Task Force on Infant Positioning and SIDS (1992). Positioning and SIDS. *Pediatrics*, *88*, 1120–1126.
American Academy of Pediatrics (1989). Report of the AAP Task Force on Circumcision. *Pediatrics*, *84*, 388–391.

American Academy of Pediatrics (1993). Newborn screening for congenital hypothyroidism: Recommended guidelines. *Pediatrics, 91*, 1203–1209.

Bliss-Holtz, J. (1989). Comparison of rectal, axillary, and inguinal temperatures in full-term newborn infants. *Nursing Research, 38*(2), 85–87.

Bliss-Holtz, J. (1993). Determination of thermoregulatory state in full-term infants. *Nursing Research, 42*, 204–207.

Brans, Y. W. (1987). *Neonatology in obstetrical practice.* Philadelphia: J.B. Lippincott.

Burton, B. K. (1993). Inherited metabolic disorders. In G. B. Avery, M. B. Fletcher, & M. G. Macdonald (Eds.), *Neonatology: Pathophysiology and management of the newborn* (4th ed.). Philadelphia: J.B. Lippincott.

Centers for Disease Control (1993). General recommendations on immunizations. *Morbidity and Mortality Weekly Report, 43*, 9.

Coen, R. W., & Koffler, H. (1987). *Primary care of the newborn.* Boston: Little, Brown.

Committee on Fetus and Newborn, American Academy of Pediatrics (1975). Report of the ad hoc task force on circumcision. *Pediatrics, 56*, 610–611.

Freeman, R. K., & Poland, R. L. (Eds.) (1992). *Guidelines for perinatal care* (3rd ed.). Elk Grove Village, IL: American Academy of Pediatrics and American College of Obstetricians and Gynecologists.

Hey, E. (1993). Thermoregulation in the newborn. In G. B. Avery, M. B. Fletcher, & M. G. Macdonald (Eds.), *Neonatology: Pathophysiology and management of the newborn* (4th ed.). Philadelphia: J.B. Lippincott.

Kahn, A., Grosswasser, J., Sottiaux, M., Rebuffat, E., Franco, P., & Dramaix, M. (1993). Prone or supine body position and sleep characteristics in infants. *Pediatrics, 91*, 1112–1115.

Larson, E. (1987). Rituals in infection control: What works in the newborn nursery? *Journal of Obstetric, Gynecologic, and Neonatal Nursing, 16*(6), 411–416.

Lerner, H. (1993). Sleep position of infants: Applying research to practice. *MCN: American Journal of Maternal Child Nursing, 18*, 275–277.

Marchette, L., Main, R., & Redick, E. (1989). Pain reduction during neonatal circumcision. *Pediatric Nursing, 15*(2), 207–210.

Markestad, T., Skadberg, B., Hordvik, E., Morild, I., & Irgens, L. M. (1995). Sleeping position and sudden infant death syndrome (SIDS): Effect of an intervention programme to avoid prone sleeping. *Acta Paediatrica, 84*, 375–378.

NAACOG Committee on Practice (1985). *Nurse's role in neonatal circumcision* (pamphlet). Washington, DC: Author.

NAACOG Committee on Practice (1989). *OGN nursing practice resource mother-baby care* (pamphlet). Washington, DC: Author.

NAACOG, National Association of Neonatal Nurses, and NCMEC (1991). *Safeguard their tomorrows: A resource to help prevent infant abductions in your hospital* (Program materials). Evanston, IN: Mead Johnson.

National Center for Missing and Expoited Children (1991). *Guidelines for preventing abduction of infants from the hospital* (2nd ed.). : Author.

Nelson, N. M., & Super, D. M. (1992). Neonatal adaptations: Establishment of equilibrium. In R. A. Hoekelman (Ed.), *Primary pediatric care* (pp. 462–464) (2nd ed.). St. Louis: Mosby-Year Book.

Poets, C. F., Rudolph, A., Neuber, K., Bach, U., & Von Der Hardt, H. (1995). Arterial oxygen saturation in infants at risk of sudden death: Influence of sleeping position. *Acta Paediatrica, 84*, 379–382.

Poland, R. L. (1990). The question of routine circumcision. *New England Journal of Medicine, 322*(18), 1311–1315.

Ponsonby, A. L., Dwyer, M. B., Gibbons, L. E., Cochrane, J. A., & Wang, Y. G. (1993). Factors potentiating the risk of sudden infant death syndrome associated with the prone position. *New England Journal of Medicine, 329*, 377–381.

Rabinowitz, R., & Hulbert, W. C. Jr. (1995). Newborn circumcision should not be performed without anesthesia (Commentary). *Birth, 22*, 45–46.

Rush, J., Chiovitti, R., Kaufman, K., & Mitchell, A. (1990). A randomized controlled trial of a nursery ritual: Wearing cover gowns to care for healthy newborns. *Birth, 17*(1), 25.

Salam, C. M. (1995). Mothers' perception of infant care and self-care competence after early postpartum discharge. *Internation Journal of Childbirth Education, 10*(2), 30–39.

Schoen, E. J. (1990). The status of circumcision of newborns. *New England Journal of Medicine, 322*(18), 1308–1311.

Wetherstone, K. B., Rasmussen, L. B., Erenberg, A., Jackson, E. M., Claflin, K. S., & Leff, R. D. (1993). Safety and efficacy of a topical anesthetic for neonatal circumcision. *Pediatrics, 92*, 710–714.

Williams, L. R., & Cooper, M. K. (1993). Nurse-managed home care. *Journal of Obstetric, Gynecologic, and Neonatal Nursing, 22*(1), 25–31.

Yoder, M. C., & Polin, R. A. (1992). Developmental Immunology. In A. A. Fanaroff & R. J. Martin (Eds.), *Neonatal-perinatal medicine* (pp. 587–618) (5th ed.). St. Louis: Mosby-Year Book.

Zinn, A. B. (1992). Inborn errors of metabolism. In A. A. Fanaroff & R. J. Martin (Eds.), *Neonatal-perinatal medicine* (pp. 1016–1048) (5th ed.). St. Louis: C.V. Mosby.

Broussard, A. B., & Rich, S. K. (1990). Incorporating infant stimulation concepts into prenatal classes. Journal of Obstetric, Gynecologic, and Neonatal Nursing, *19*, 381–387.

van der Meer, A. L. H., van der Weel, F. R., & Lee, D. N. (1995). The functional significance of arm movements in neonates. *Science, 267*, 693–695.

White-Traut, R. C., Nelson, M. N., Burns, K., & Cunningham, N. (1994). Environmental influences on the developing premature infant: Theoretical issues and applications to practice. *Journal of Obstetric, Gynecologic, and Neonatal Nursing, 23*, 393–401.

REFERENCES FOR CLIENT EDUCATION: SENSORY ENRICHMENT

Anisfeld, E., Wagner, D., Casper, V. et al. (1989). *The effects of a carrying intervention on the development of attachment in infants* (p. 126A). Kansas City, MO: Society for Research in Child Development Abstracts of the April 1989 Biennial Convention.

Apostolakis, E., & Cha, C. (1982). Visual preference of preterm and term neonates. *Journal of the California Perinatal Association, 11*(1), 62.

Blass, E. M., & Hoffmeyer, L. B. (1989). *Sucrose is an analgesic agent in 1–3-day-old human infants* (p. 129A). Kansas City, MO: Society for Research in Child Development Abstracts of the April 1989 Biennial Convention.

Cernoch, J. M., & Porter, R. H. (1985). Recognition of maternal axillary odors by infants. *Child Development, 56*, 1593–1598.

Christensson, K., Cabrera, T., Christensson, E., Uvnas-Moberg, K., & Winberg, J. (1995). Separation distress call in the human neonate in the absence of maternal body contact. *Acta Paediatrica, 84,* 468–473.

DeCasper, A. J., & Spence, M. J. (1986). Prenatal maternal speech influences newborns' perception of speech sounds. *Infant Behav Dev, 9,* 133–150.

Dunkle, T. (1982). The sound of silence. *Science, 82,* 48–51.

Eimas, P. D. (1985). The perception of speech in early infancy. *Scientific American, 25*(2), 46–52.

Engen, T. (1982). *The perception of odors.* New York: Academic Press.

Fantz, R. L., & Fagan, J. F. (1975). Visual attention to size and number of pattern details during the first 6 months. *Child Development, 46*(1), 3–18.

Fantz, R. L., & Miranda, S. B. (1975). Newborn infant attention to contour. *Child Development, 46,* 224.

Freeman, D. G. et al. (1979). *Effects of kinesthetic stimulation on weight gain and on smiling in premature infants.* Paper presented at the Annual Meeting of the American Orthopsychiatric Association, San Francisco, April 15.

Gorski, P. A., Davison, M. F., & Brazelton, T. B. (1979). Neurobehavioral organization of the high risk neonate. *Seminars in Perinatology, 3*(1), 61–72.

Haith, M. M. (1980). The response of the human newborn to movement. *Journal of Experimental Child Psychology, 31,* 235–243.

Kattwinkel, J., Nearman, H., Mars, H. et al. (1974). Apnea of prematurity and effects on CPAP, cutaneous stimulation and levels of urinary biogenic amines. *Pediatric Research, 8,* 468.

Kennell, J. H., & Klaus, M. H. (1983). Early events: Later effects on the infant. In J. D. Call, E. Galenson, & R. L. Tyson (Eds.), *Frontiers of infant psychiatry* (pp. 7–16). New York: Basic Books.

Klaus, M. M., & Fanaroff, A. A. (1976). Bach, Beethoven, or rock—and how much. *Journal of Pediatrics, 88,* 300.

Ludington, S. M. (1976). *Vaginal and cesarean infants' responses to extra tactile stimulation* (dissertation) (p. 74). Denton: Texas Woman's University.

Ludington-Hoe, S. M. (1983). What can newborns really see? *American Journal of Nursing,* 1286–1289.

Menzies, A. (1981). Effect of infant temperament and prone position on motor development. *Aust J Adv Nurs, 2*(1), 24–29.

Morse, P. A. (1972). The discrimination of speech and nonspeech stimuli in early infancy. *Journal of Experimental Child Psychology, 14,* 477–492.

Morton, J., Johnson, M. H., & Maurer, D. (1990). On the reasons for newborns' responses to faces. *Infant Behav Dev, 13,* 99–103.

Ottenbacher, K. J., & Petersen, P. (1983). The efficacy of vestibular stimulation as a form of specific sensory enrichment: Quantitative review of the literature. *Clinical Pediatrics, 23*(8), 428–433.

Porter, R. H., Cernoch, J. M., & Perry, S. (1983). The importance of odors in mother-infant interactions. *Maternal-Child Nursing Journal, 12*(3), 147–154.

Rice, R. D. (1979). The effects of sensorimotor infant stimulation treatment on the development of high risk infants. *Birth Defects, 15,* 7–26.

Werner, L. A., & Gillenwater, J. M. (1990). Pure-tone sensitivity of 2- to 5-week-old infants. *Infant Behav Dev, 13,* 355–375.

30

Nutritional Care of the Newborn

Objectives

- Identify factors to be considered when choosing the method of newborn feeding.
- Discuss advantages and contraindications for breast-feeding.
- Describe the physiologic mechanisms of lactation.
- Describe nursing assessments and interventions to assist the breast-feeding mother.
- Explain newborn sucking behavior and its influence on breast-feeding success.
- Discuss suggestions for addressing common breast-feeding concerns and problems.
- Compare breast milk and various commercial formulas regarding nutritional composition.
- Describe nursing assessments and interventions to assist the mother who is feeding her newborn formula.
- Describe methods of formula preparation.
- Discuss nutritional considerations during the infant's first year of life.

Key Terms

Bifidus factor   Let-down reflex
Colostrum   Nipple confusion
Inverted nipples

Nutrition is a key factor in preserving and promoting health throughout the life cycle. It is particularly important during the rapid growth phase of infancy.

According to Neumann et al. (1977), infant feeding is more than just "nutrient refueling"; it is also a "social, psychological and educational interaction between caretaker and baby." This concept of infant feeding has been gaining increased recognition. In addition, feeding practices in early infancy have undergone extensive study to determine possible long-term effects.

Because good nutrition is so vital to the overall health and development of the infant, the nurse who works with expectant women and new mothers must have knowledge of all aspects of the infant's nutritional needs. This chapter discusses the physiology and reflexes involved in infant feeding, energy requirements of the newborn, the choice of feeding method, various aspects of breast-feeding and formula feeding, common feeding concerns in the newborn, and nutritional considerations throughout the first year of life.

The Newborn's Ability to Handle Food

Until birth, the nutritional needs of the fetus are met through placental circulation. One of the major physiologic adaptations that the infant must make in the transition from intrauterine to extrauterine life is to adjust to the change in the source and mechanism of nourishment. The newborn must take food into the body orally, digest it, and assimilate it.

This is partially accomplished by a combination of several reflexes that should be present in the newborn at birth—sucking, swallowing, and rooting. These reflexes are usually very strong in the newborn. In fact, the swallowing reflex and peristaltic movements in the stomach become active during the last 2 months of fetal development. This is noted by the bits of vernix caseosa and lanugo that are found with other debris in the meconium stool. In the delivery room, the newborn will often swallow mucus and suck on anything that gets near his or her mouth.

The rooting reflex enables the newborn to locate the food source. Although human infants do not have to search for food, the rooting reflex causes the infant to turn toward anything that touches its cheeks or lips. This helps the infant latch onto the bottle or breast. Studies in Sweden have demonstrated that newborns not exposed to analgesics who are placed on their mother's chest in skin-to-skin contact will actively seek the breast. This is accomplished by arm and leg movements followed by mouthing and sucking movements that usually result in their taking the breast by their own efforts within the first hour after birth (Righard et al., 1990).

The newborn's gastrointestinal tract must suddenly begin to process a relatively large amount of food. Although the system is functional at birth and the necessary enzymes and digestive juices are present, the mucosa and musculature are somewhat immature (Fletcher, 1993). At birth, the newborn's stomach is small, but it can dilate considerably and may stretch to three or four times its resting capacity. The stomach may be distended not only by the food taken in, but also by air swallowed when sucking or crying.

The Newborn's Basic Energy Requirements

The energy requirement for a normal term newborn after the first day of life is 100 to 120 kcal/kg per day. This equals about 340 to 408 kcal/d for the average 3.4-kg (7.5-lb) newborn. Breast milk and most commercial formulas provide 20 kcal/oz (30 mL). Therefore, the infant taking eight feedings a day (every 3 hours) needs to average 2 to 2.5 oz per feeding. The breast-fed infant, nursing more frequently (every 2 hours), might average 1.5 oz per feeding. Many newborns will take in less than these amounts during the first few days. As their appetite increases, they will take larger amounts. The specific nutritional components of breast milk and formula are discussed later in this chapter.

Choosing the Method of Feeding

Choosing the method of infant feeding is an important decision for parents to make. The choice is influenced by physical, psychological, and social factors. Ideally, the subject of infant feeding is raised during the prenatal period. During this time, it is important for parents to explore their attitudes concerning feeding methods with the nurse. It is also important for the nurse to present the benefits and possible contraindications to the types of feeding methods and to answer any questions the parents may have. This provides an opportunity for the nurse to help the parents make the decision that is most suitable for them.

In the past, breast-feeding (by the mother or a "wet nurse") was essential for the survival of the infant. In some underdeveloped countries, this is still true to some extent. However, in most of the modern world, methods of artificial feeding have offered women an alternative. The production of infant formulas has become a big business, and formula feeding is safe for most infants and convenient for the mother. However, breast-feeding is still considered the preferred method of feeding for infants up to 4 to 6 months of age (Institute of Medicine, 1991).

Because breast-feeding is the preferred method of feeding, the nurse should be a positive influence on the mother's choice to breast-feed. Expectant parents should be informed about the advantages of breast-feeding to the mother and infant and the differences between human milk, cow's milk, and infant formula (Table 30-1). Many women are uninformed about the differences among these methods and may base their decision on how their mothers fed them or what a friend has said. For these women, information can be useful in helping them to make a decision based on facts. When nurses do not promote breast-feeding, the uninformed or undecided woman may not receive a

TABLE 30–1
*Composition of Mature Breast Milk, Cow's Milk, and a Routine Infant Formula**

Composition/dL	Mature Breast Milk	Cow's Milk	Routine Formula With Iron†
Calories	75.0	69.0	67.0
Protein (g)	1.1	3.5	1.5
Lactalbumin (%)	80	18	
Casein (%)	20	82	
Water (mL)	87.1	87.3	
Fat (g)	4.0	3.5	3.7
CHO (g)	9.5	4.9	7.0
Ash (g)	0.21	0.72	0.34
MINERALS			
Na (mg)	16.0	50.0	25.0
K (mg)	51.0	144.0	74.0
Ca (mg)	33.0	118.0	55.0
P (mg)	14.0	93.0	43.0
Mg (mg)	4.0	12.0	9.0
Fe (mg)	0.1	Tr.	1.2
Zn (mg)	0.15	0.1	0.42
VITAMINS			
A (IU)	240.0	140.0	158.6
C (mg)	5.0	1.0	5.3
D (IU)	2.2	1.4	42.3
E (IU)	0.18	0.04	0.83
Thiamine (mg)	0.01	0.03	0.04
Riboflavin (mg)	0.04	0.17	0.06
Niacin (mg)	0.2	0.1	0.7
Curd size	Soft	Firm	Mod. firm
	Flocculent	Large	Mod. large
pH	Alkaline	Acid	Acid
Anti-infective properties	+	±	–
Bacterial content	Sterile	Nonsterile	Sterile
Emptying time	More rapid		

*Composite of a number of sources.
†Enfamil.
(Fletcher, A. B. [1993]. Nutrition. In Avery, G. B., Fletcher, M. B., & MacDonald, M. G. [Eds.], *Neonatology* [4th ed.]. Philadelphia: J.B. Lippincott.)

strong enough motivation to breast-feed, and the breast-feeding mother may not get the support she needs (Jacobi et al., 1993).

However, it is important that nurses do not force breast-feeding on a mother who is strongly opposed to it. A mother should not be made to feel guilty about her decision to bottle feed. Women who choose not to (or cannot) breast-feed should be assured that formula feeding is safe and healthy for their baby.

Choosing to Breast-feed

There has been growing concern in recent years that many women are deterred from breast-feeding by publicity, free formula from formula companies, and lack of perceived support for breast-feeding by healthcare providers in hospitals. The World Health Organization-UNICEF Baby Friendly Hospital Initiative is part of a worldwide effort to increase the frequency and duration of breast-feeding by encouraging hospitals to adopt ten steps to successful breast-feeding (Box 30-1). Elimination of free formula provided to hospitals is part of this effort but is controversial in the United States (Young, 1995). An attempt to offer legislative support for breast-feeding was made by the state of Florida. A law was passed that endorses breast-feeding

---

BOX 30-1
Ten Steps to Successful Breast-feeding

The following list applies to every facility providing maternity services and care for newborns:

1. Have a written breast-feeding policy that is routinely communicated to all healthcare staff.
2. Train all healthcare staff in skills necessary to implement this policy.
3. Inform all pregnant women about the benefits and management of breast-feeding.
4. Help mothers initiate breast-feeding within ½ hour of birth.
5. Show mothers how to breast-feed and how to maintain lactation even if they should be separated from their infants.
6. Give newborns no food or drink other than breast milk, unless medically indicated.
7. Practice rooming-in; allow mothers and newborns to remain together 24 hours a day.
8. Encourage breast-feeding on demand.
9. Give no artificial teats or pacifiers (also called dummies or soothers) to breast-feeding infants.
10. Foster the establishment of breast-feeding support groups, and refer mothers to them on discharge from the hospital or clinic.

(From World Health Organization/Unicef. Protecting, promoting and supporting breast-feeding: The special role of maternity services. Geneva, Switzerland: World Health Organization.)

---

and allows the mother to breast-feed in any public or private location (Livingston, 1993).

Nurses play an important role in promoting lactation and breast-feeding throughout the reproductive cycle. During the prenatal period, nursing assessment of breast-feeding plans (whether or not the mother will breast-feed and for how long), beliefs about breast-feeding, and breast-feeding knowledge have been found to influence the decision to breast-feed. Throughout the assessment, the nurse should recognize that the mother's culture or socioeconomic situation also may influence her decision to breast-feed (O'Campo et al., 1992).

In the current atmosphere of breast-feeding promotion, research studies from many disciplines have focused increasing attention on favorable aspects of breast-feeding. Although knowledge is still incomplete, many advantages of breast-feeding have been identified. Many women will make their decision to breast-feed based on a combination of these advantages.

Biochemical and Nutritional Considerations

The composition of cow's milk and human milk is dissimilar in many ways. For example, the content of water and lactose is similar, but the amounts of protein differ. Human milk contains less than 1% protein, whereas cow's milk contains approximately 3.4%. Another difference is the ratio of whey protein (lactalbumins), which is more easily digestible, to casein (curds). The protein in human milk is 60% whey and 40% casein. Cow's milk has a 20% whey and 80% casein protein ratio (Lawrence, 1994). Thus, cow's milk is much more difficult for the infant's immature gastrointestinal system to digest. Infants today are seldom given unmodified cow's milk because of these and other reasons.

Commercial infant formula companies use nutrition and food scientists, physicians, and analytical chemists to develop formulas with increased similarities to the composition of human milk (Benson et al., 1992). However, despite the fact that the formula has been modified by altering the protein and fat and by adding vitamins and minerals in approximate amounts, the composition of formula and human milk still differs in many ways. The following are examples:

■ The forms of some nutrients are different in infant formula because they need to be stable over time; in contrast, the nutrient forms found in human milk are relatively unstable because they are intended for immediate consumption.
■ Certain nutrients in human milk, such as water-soluble vitamins, vary according to maternal diet; they are always the same in formula.

■ There are differences in the bioavailabiltiy of certain nutrients, such as zinc and iron, from human milk and infant formula: Adding certain substances to formula can necessitate the addition of other substances in increased amounts. For example, iron is antagonistic to zinc and copper; therefore, in iron-fortified formula, these trace elements must be added in greater concentrations than found in human milk (Benson et al., 1992).

Another difference of unknown consequence is the rigidly consistent composition of formula compared with the variability of mother's milk. Besides the changes that occur in the progression from **colostrum** to mature milk (discussed later in this chapter), the composition of mother's milk varies within each period of nursing. The foremilk, which accumulates in the alveoli between feedings, is relatively dilute and low in fat. The hindmilk, which is secreted during the nursing period, is higher in fat and protein (Lawrence, 1994). Other differences in composition of breast milk relate to the time of day the infant nurses and long-term changes that occur as the infant gets older.

Brain Growth and Intellectual Development Factors

Differences in human milk that may influence brain growth and intellectual development have been the topic of recent study. Lucas et al. (1992) studied 300 preterm infants with birth weights of less than 1,850 g; some of the mothers provided breast milk for them, and others did not. Children were tested at 18 months and again at 7½ to 8 years of age. Those who received breast milk had significantly higher IQs, even when other factors, such as social class and mother's educational level, were controlled. Lawrence (1992) hypothesizes that cholesterol, a basic constituent of brain tissue, and omega-3 fatty acids might be involved in the result of this study because they are present in human milk but not in formula. Another study (Kallio et al., 1992) found that serum cholesterol levels rose significantly faster in infants who were exclusively breast-fed during the first year of life than in those who were weaned to formula in the early months. Temboury et al. (1994) tested a group of healthy full-term infants between 18 and 29 months of age using the Bayley Scales Index of Mental Development. Lower scores were associated with bottle feeding.

Immunologic and Antiallergenic Factors

Many studies have shown that breast milk, including colostrum, is rich in defense factors, such as immunoglobulins, lactoferrin, enzymes, macrophages, lymphocytes, and ***bifidus factor*** (a growth enhancer of lactobacilli not found in the milk of other mammalian species). These factors contribute unique antibacterial, antiviral, antiprotozoan, and anti-inflammatory properties (Lawrence, 1994; Riordan, 1993b).

Recent research in a variety of populations has indicated that breast-feeding offers effective protection against diarrhea. This protection is apparently related to the difference in intestinal flora of breast-fed infants compared with those on formula. The intestinal flora of breast-fed babies consists mainly of lactobacilli and bifidobacteria. These organisms are nonpathogenic and produce feces with a low pH, which in turn inhibits growth of many pathogenic bacteria (Riordan, 1993b; Lawrence, 1994). In addition, a study by Duncan et al. (1993) demonstrated a protective effect against otitis media.

One known advantage of the immunoglobulin secretory IgA, which is present in human milk, is the protective antiabsorptive effect it has in keeping protein molecules from passing through the intestinal walls. During the first 6 months of life, foreign proteins are more likely than in later life to be absorbed through the intestinal wall. This can lead to allergies. Cow milk protein is one of the most common food allergens encountered in infancy. Human milk proteins, on the other hand, are virtually nonallergenic to humans (Lawrence, 1994).

Psychological Factors

Psychological advantages of breast-feeding are not as easily documented as the physical advantages. Breast-feeding may more positively influence the quality of the mother–child interaction because it establishes a more direct, intimate biologic relationship. Some studies have demonstrated that the increase in oxytocin and prolactin levels during lactation plays a role in inducing mothering behavior. Also, the delay in return of the menstrual cycle that occurs with unrestricted breast-feeding has been shown to result in a more even mood cycle for the lactating woman (Lawrence, 1994).

Other Factors

Benefits for the infant include the following:

■ Breast milk is safer because it cannot be incorrectly mixed and is less likely to be contaminated.
■ The infant does not have to wait to eat; if the mother is nearby, milk is always available at the right temperature.
■ The action of sucking at the breast is different from sucking on a bottle and may promote better development of the mouth and jaw (see Fig. 30-4).

Benefits for the mother include the following:

- Uterine involution is stimulated by the release of oxytocin when the infant sucks.
- Breast-feeding offers the convenience of not having to prepare bottles or incur the added expense of buying formula.
- A woman who breast-feeds is less likely to conceive again during the first 8 to 10 months of lactation. This is not as reliable as other contraceptive measures, yet exclusive breast-feeding does delay ovulation. This can be helpful for those who cannot afford, or do not accept, artificial contraception (Lethbridge, 1988; Lawrence, 1994).

See the references and suggested readings lists for a more complete discussion of the advantages of breast-feeding.

Choosing to Formula Feed

Today, formula feeding offers a safe alternative to breast-feeding, and women often choose this method of feeding for personal and medical reasons. If a woman makes a knowledgeable decision to formula feed her infant, the nurse should support her decision and give her guidance.

Personal Factors

Some feel that breast-feeding is tiring, confining, or simply distasteful. Some are afraid that it will disfigure their breasts; others fear they will fail to successfully breast-feed, especially if previous attempts to breast-feed were unsuccessful.

Social pressure associated with the mother's culture, socioeconomic class, and peer group greatly influences the choice of feeding method. For example, bottle feeding may be the accepted practice in the community or neighborhood. In addition, relatives, friends, and others who are against breast-feeding can sway the mother's choice. On the other hand, pressure from those who are overly enthusiastic about breast-feeding can turn the mother against it. Plans for early return to employment can be a significant factor in choosing to bottle feed, especially if the mother perceives that too much effort is required to continue breast-feeding after going back to work.

Contraindications to Breast-feeding

Although there are few absolute contraindications to breast-feeding, there are several reasons a woman may not be able to breast-feed, at least temporarily. These reasons include conditions of the infant, diseases or infections of the mother, certain medications the mother is taking, breast infection and painful nipples, or pregnancy.

Galactosemia, a serious disorder in the infant caused by a lack of the enzyme necessary for proper metabolism of galactose, is a contraindication to breast-feeding. Infants with this condition must have a galactose-free diet, and breast milk is rich in lactose, a precursor of galactose (Riordan, 1993b; Lawrence, 1994). Other conditions in the infant, including phenylketonuria, maple syrup urine disease, breast milk jaundice, and cleft lip or palate, might also necessitate permanent or temporary avoidance of breast-feeding.

Mothers with certain diseases or infections may not be able to breast-feed. The American Academy of Pediatrics and American Association of Obstetricians and Gynecologists recommend that mothers with certain diseases or infections, such as active untreated pulmonary tuberculosis, cytomegalovirus infection, chronic hepatitis B virus (until the infant is immunized), and human immunodeficiency virus, should be counseled not to breast-feed their infants (Freeman et al., 1992). However, these might not be considered absolute contraindications in some situations when the benefits of the breast milk might outweigh the danger of the disease (Lawrence, 1994). Active herpes simplex virus infections are not contraindications to breast-feeding unless there are vesicular lesions in the breast area (Freeman, 1992). Certain maternal medications that are known to be detrimental to breast-feeding infants may lead to recommendations to avoid breast-feeding either temporarily or permanently (see Appendix E).

Breast infection or painful, cracked, or fissured nipples might require changes in the breast-feeding routine and discontinuance of sucking on the affected breast for a while. However, the breast should continue to be emptied by some means. Becoming pregnant might be an indication for weaning because of the physiologic strain that it places on the mother. However, some women in developing countries do breast-feed through a subsequent pregnancy, and in many parts of the world, this is not uncommon. Increased food intake to adjust to increasing demands is probably necessary to support the growth of the fetus (Riordan et al., 1993).

Generally when conditions are present that pose a potential problem for mother or infant, the decision about the feeding method can be made on an individual basis. In many cases, if the mother is determined to breast-feed, she can pump her breasts and keep up her milk supply until it is possible for her to begin nursing.

Breast-feeding

If the new mother chooses to breast-feed, the degree to which she perseveres in this endeavor is often influenced by her care in the hospital. A consistent approach to assisting with breast-feeding is important.

The development of breast-feeding protocols in hospital settings can help to standardize teaching and minimize contradictory information. Most women leave the hospital with their newborn before they have had time to establish lactation. Therefore, the nurse should explain the mechanisms of lactation to increase the mother's understanding of the process. It is also important for nurses to gain the mother's trust, give anticipatory guidance about initiation of breast-feeding, and teach ways to prevent or deal with possible problems. The nurse must also be aware that the mother's culture may influence how she will breast-feed. There are cultural variations concerning whether colostrum should be fed to newborns, how much exposure or manipulation of the breast is appropriate, and what rituals are thought to be necessary to promote a good milk supply. These variations should be considered as the nurse teaches the mother about breast-feeding (Fig. 30-1).

Mechanisms of Lactation

The nurse should have a working knowledge of how the breasts function in the lactation process to give guidance to new breast-feeding mothers. Figure 30-2 reviews the anatomic structures of the breast, and the lactation process is discussed briefly below. For a thorough discussion of the anatomy of the breasts and the physiology of lactation, the reader is referred to Chapter 25. Two major mechanisms are involved in lactation: the secretion of milk and the milk-ejection reflex (see Fig. 25-4).

Secretion of Milk

The secretion of milk is a prerequisite for successful breast-feeding. During pregnancy, major changes occur in the mammary glands in preparation for milk production. From the second trimester on, a secretion with fairly stable composition (precolostrum) can be found in the breasts. When the infant is born and the placenta is expelled, the secretion undergoes a transition. Precolostrum becomes colostrum, which changes during the following 10 days to a month to mature milk. Changes in mammary secretion after birth are believed to be influenced by decreased levels of estrogen and progesterone and relatively increased levels of the hormone prolactin (Worthington-Roberts, 1993). The release of prolactin from the anterior pituitary is essential to milk production. It is released in response to stimulation of afferent nerves in the nipple when the infant suckles at the breast (Riordan, 1993a).

Colostrum is higher in protein and lower in fat and lactose than mature milk. It also contains greater amounts of other substances, such as sodium chloride and zinc, and is rich in antibodies. Besides its nutrient purpose and anti-infective function, colostrum also may

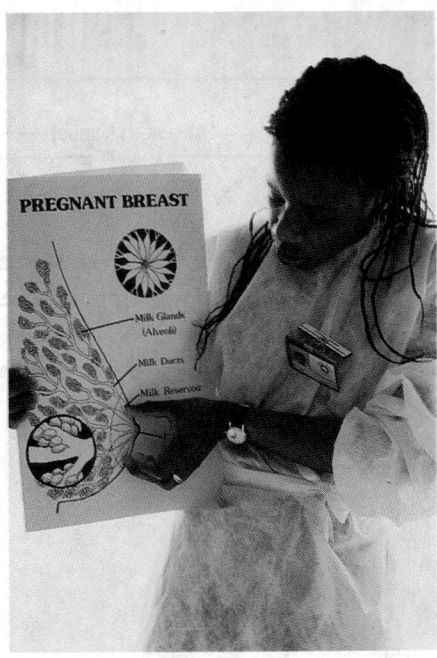

FIGURE 30-1 Teaching about the lactation process, anticipatory guidance about the initiation of breast-feeding, and ways to prevent or deal with possible problems is an important component of nursing care.

act as a laxative in facilitating the passage of meconium (Lawrence, 1994). As the prolactin levels continue to increase and the estrogen and progesterone levels drop, newly secreted milk is progressively mixed with the colostrum until the mature milk stage is reached. During this time, there is a decrease in the concentration of immunoglobulins and total protein and an increase in lactose, fat, and total calories (Lawrence, 1994).

In the early stages of lactation, milk secretion can be stimulated by having the infant nurse from both breasts at each feeding and by increasing the frequency of the feedings. Milk production begins slowly in some mothers, but it can be stimulated by allowing the infant to nurse both breasts every 2 to 3 hours. Although prolactin stimulates the synthesis and secretion of milk into the alveolar spaces, it is thought that the amount of milk produced is regulated by the amount left in the alveolar spaces after a feeding. Therefore, frequent emptying of the breasts is important, especially in the early stages of lactation. The production of milk and the quantity produced depend on frequent and complete emptying of the breasts. If the breasts are not entirely emptied, back pressure in the alveoli and possibly an inhibitory factor in the milk cause milk secretion to decrease and eventually stop (Lawrence, 1994).

Milk-Ejection Reflex

The second mechanism involved in lactation is the milk-ejection or **let-down reflex**. Oxytocin, released from the posterior pituitary in response to the infant's

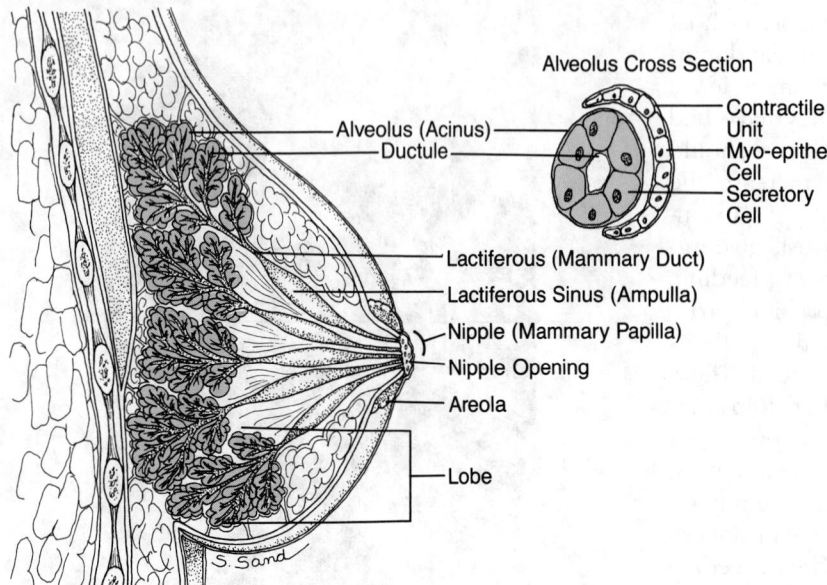

Alveolus Cross Section

Alveolus (Acinus)
Ductule
Contractile Unit
Myo-epithelial Cell
Secretory Cell

Lactiferous (Mammary Duct)
Lactiferous Sinus (Ampulla)
Nipple (Mammary Papilla)
Nipple Opening
Areola
Lobe

S. Sand

FIGURE 30–2 Schematic diagram of the breast. (Redrawn from Riordan, J., & Countryman, B. A. [1980]. Basics of breast-feeding, part II: The anatomy and psychophysiology of lactation. *Journal of Obstetric, Gynecologic, and Neonatal Nursing, 9*[4],210.)

sucking, stimulates the myoepithelial cells in the alveoli to contract and eject the milk through the ducts into the lactiferous sinuses. This reflex affects the quantity of milk the infant is able to obtain because the milk has to be in the sinuses before it can be removed by the infant's sucking. The quality of milk is also affected because the infant does not receive the fat-containing hindmilk until the foremilk is removed. Failure of the let-down reflex may be a direct or indirect cause of early termination of breast-feeding in many women (Box 30-2).

Nursing Process: Breast-feeding

The nursing process can be a good method to use when helping the mother and infant establish or continue breast-feeding. The nurse should assess the mother and her infant, formulate nursing diagnoses, and plan interventions that are individualized according to the needs of the mother and infant.

Assessment

A complete assessment is essential to determine the mother's level of knowledge and to detect any actual or potential problems. Assessment tools or checklists can be helpful (see Assessment Tool: Breast-feeding).

It is important to ask the mother whether she has previously breast-fed and what this experience was like. If the mother has other children, it is sometimes falsely assumed that she must have nursed before and therefore does not need help. However, there are a number of reasons why a mother might not have nursed her previous infant(s) and why, even if she did, nursing this baby might be different. The nurse should assess the interaction between mother and infant. The mother's questions and the way she handles the newborn give the nurse clues to possible or potential problems.

BOX 30–2
Possible Consequences of an Inadequate Let-Down Reflex

1. Let-down reflex does not occur. (Mother may be tense, nervous, in pain, and so forth.)

2. Milk is not propelled into ducts by contraction of myoepithelial cells.

3. Insufficient milk is available to infant = hungry infant.

4. Mother is afraid she does not have enough milk → further inhibits let-down → gives infant formula → less sucking stimulation → decreased milk production.

5. Engorgement due to inadequate emptying of breasts → more difficult for infant to suck → may lead to infection from stasis of milk.

6. Breast-feeding is terminated—reasons given:
   "I didn't have enough milk."
   "My breasts were too sore."
   "My breasts were infected, so the doctor told me to stop."

ASSESSMENT TOOL
Breast-Feeding

Assessment Before Breast-Feeding:

1. Mother's previous experience with breast-feeding:
   Has she breast-fed before? _____
   If yes, what was her experience with it? _____
   If no, has she had close contact with anyone who was breast-feeding? _____
2. Mother's knowledge about breast-feeding:
   Has she taken prenatal classes? _____
   Has she attended La Leche meetings or other breast-feeding classes? _____
   What books has she read about breast-feeding? _____
   Pamphlets? _____
   Other sources of information? _____
3. Assessment of mother's current condition:
   Number of hours postdelivery? _____
   Type of delivery? _____
   Apparent mood: anxious, eager, uncomfortable, tired, cheerful? _____
   Breasts: soft, firm, engorged, large, small _____
   Nipples: size, protractility _____ .
4. Assessment of infant's current condition:
   Size: appropriate for gestational age? _____ Term _____ Preterm _____
   Physical condition: _____
   State: alert, sleepy, crying, sucking on fist _____
5. Maternal–infant interaction:
   Position in which mother holds infant spontaneously: _____
   Confidence mother demonstrates in handling infant: _____

Assessment of Breast-Feeding Behavior:

1. Positioning
   a. Mother finds comfortable position for herself.
   b. Mother holds infant correctly: supports head and body, brings infant in close, supports breast with other hand using "C" hold.
   c. Mother makes sure infant has mouth open wide and brings infant to breast, rather than breast to infant.
2. Timing
   a. Mother feeds infant at least every 2 to 3 hours.
   b. Sucking time is not limited. Sufficient time is allowed for emptying of breast after let-down.
3. Breasts and nipples
   a. Engorgement of breast? _____ Areola? _____
   b. Appearance: bruises, cracks, abrasions
   c. Sensation: tenderness or pain

Assessment of the infant's role during the breast-feeding experience is also important. Shrago et al. (1990) developed an assessment tool, the Systematic Assessment of the Newborn at Breast, to assist the nurse in identifying the infant's contribution to breast-feeding. The tool assesses four areas of infant behavior: 1) alignment, 2) areolar grasp, 3) areolar compression, and 4) audible swallowing. The authors suggest that an initial breast-feeding assessment should be done within the first 12 hours after birth. Walker also advocates early assessment of the breast-feeding newborn and stresses the importance of the nurse actually observing the feeding and not relying solely on the mother's report (Walker, 1989). Even after the newborn appears to be nursing well, periodic observation of a feeding is important to reassess the newborn's behaviors and detect any possible problems.

ASSESSMENT TOOL
Systematic Assessment of the Newborn at Breast

1. Alignment

   Infant is in flexed position, relaxed, and with no muscular rigidity.

   Infant's head and body are at breast level.

   Infant's head is aligned with trunk and is not turned laterally, hyperextended, or hyperflexed.

   Correct alignment of infant's body is confirmed by an imaginary line from ear to shoulder to iliac crest.

   Mother's breast is supported with cupped hand during first 2 weeks of breast-feeding.

2. Areolar grasp

   Mouth is open wide; lips are not pursed.

   Lips are visible and flanged outward.

   Complete seal and strong vacuum are formed by infant's mouth.

   Approximately one-half inch of areolar tissue behind the nipple is centered in infant's mouth.

   Tongue covers lower alveolar ridge.

   Tongue is troughed (curved) around and below areola.

   No clicking or smacking sounds are heard during sucking.

   No drawing in (dimpling) of cheek pad is observed during sucking.

3. Areolar compression

   Mandible moves in a rhythmic motion.

   If indicated, a digital suck assessment reveals a wavelike motion of the tongue from the anterior mouth toward the oropharynx (a digital suck assessment is not routinely performed).

4. Audible swallowing

   Quiet sound of swallowing is heard.

   Swallowing may be preceded by several sucking motions.

   Swallowing may increase in frequency and consistency after milk ejection reflex occurs.

(Shrago, L., & Bocar, D. [1990]. The infant's contribution to breastfeeding. Journal of Obstetric, Gynecologic, and Neonatal Nursing, *19[3], 211.)*

Nursing Diagnoses

Nursing diagnoses concerning situations that may cause problems or concerns for the mother should be based on observation and assessment of the mother's ability to feed the infant and of her knowledge pertaining to her own and her newborn's anatomy. The diagnosis Knowledge Deficit about breast-feeding related to lack of experience (or lack of information) can be more specific by including the areas in which the new mother needs help (ie, Knowledge Deficit about positioning infant for breast-feeding related to lack of experience with breast-feeding after a cesarean delivery).

The North American Nursing Diagnosis Association lists specific diagnoses related to breast-feeding. These include Ineffective Breastfeeding, Effective Breast-feeding, and Interrupted Breast-feeding. Carpenito (1995) suggests that Potential for Enhanced Breast-feeding also be added as a wellness diagnosis.

If problems are detected during the assessment, specific nursing diagnoses can be related to the particular problems. For the mother, a diagnosis might be Pain related to sore nipples; for the infant, a diagnosis might

be Altered Nutrition: Less than body requirements related to ineffective sucking technique.

Planning and Intervention

After gathering information about the mother and newborn and formulating nursing diagnoses, the nurse can plan individualized interventions. The following sections provide information to be used in the planning and implementation process (see Nursing Care Plan: Newborn and Mother Who Are Breast-feeding).

Initiation of Breast-feeding

The first hours after birth are generally an excellent time for the initiation of breast-feeding. The newborn usually is awake and alert for the first hour or so and often tries to suck on his or her fist. Taking advantage of this heightened sucking reflex gives an opportunity for a successful initial breast-feeding experience (Auerbach et al., 1993). In their Guidelines for Perinatal Care, the American Academy of Pediatrics and the American College of Obstetricians and Gyne-

NURSING CARE PLAN
Newborn and Mother Who Are Breast-Feeding

Nursing Goals

1. Mother verbalizes understanding of
   Breast-feeding processes
   Positioning of self and infant
   Self-care during lactation
2. Mother demonstrates appropriate positioning of self and infant and handling of infant.
3. Mother does not develop nipple or breast problems.
4. Infant "latches on" to breast, sucks, and swallows milk.
5. Infant maintains hydration and good nutritional status.

Assessment	Potential Nursing Diagnoses	Intervention/ Rationale	Evaluation
Mother's experiences with breast-feeding	Knowledge Deficit about breast-feeding related to lack of information and experience	Review with mother her prenatal preparation for breast-feeding *to determine her level of knowledge.*	Mother expresses understanding of breast-feeding process.
		Provide information *to supplement her knowledge, regarding*	
Mother's knowledge of self-care		*Lactation process Let-down reflex Breast care Nutrition for lactation Adequate sleep and rest*	Mother demonstrates appropriate hygiene, adequate intake, and adequate rest.
Mother's —position during breast-feeding —handling and positioning of infant		Assist mother with breast-feeding techniques *to increase ability to breast-feed:* Achieving comfortable position	Mother assumes comfortable position, and infant "latches on" to breast without difficulty.
Infant's reflexes (rooting, sucking, swallowing) and responsiveness	Altered Nutrition: Less than body requirements related to infant's lack of efficient breast-feeding efforts or lack of responsiveness	Demonstrate newborn reflexes. Teach how to arouse sleepy infant. Encourage frequent (every 2–3 h) feeding. Teach ways of determining adequate intake: Six to eight wet diapers per day Sleeping well Gaining weight	Infant experiences minimal weight loss.
Infant's skin turgor, sleeping, and elimination	Fluid Volume Deficit related to inadequate fluid intake	Check infant's hydration.	Infant remains well hydrated and sleeps well.
Infant's sucking effectiveness, latch-on response, interest in nursing; mother's positioning of infant	Ineffective Breast-feeding related to poor infant sucking reflex	Teach mother how to assist infant in latching on to the breast and how to check for proper placement of mouth and tongue on the breast *to assist infant in developing an effective suck.* Discourage use of supplemental feedings *so infant will be hungrier and more eager to nurse.*	Infant latches on to breast and sucks effectively.

(continued)

NURSING CARE PLAN *(Continued)*
Newborn and Mother Who Are Breast-Feeding

Assessment	Potential Nursing Diagnoses	Intervention/ Rationale	Evaluation
Mother's nipples and breasts: tenderness, cracking, engorgement	Ineffective Breast-feeding related to sore nipples Pain related to infant sucking on nipple	Provide information about breast and nipple care *to alleviate discomfort, which may allow longer nursing periods and more adequate emptying of breasts to prevent further problems.* Provide comfort measures and analgesics as needed. Teach about manual expression or breast pumps if necessary *to empty breasts adequately and prevent engorgement.* Refer to support groups or lactation consultant as indicated *when mother's support system is inadequate or problems are overwhelming.*	Tenderness of nipples resolves, and mother does not develop breast engorgement or cracked nipples.
Maternal–infant interaction and breast-feeding behaviors	Effective Breast-feeding as evidenced by —Infant is eager to nurse, latching on well, and appears content after nursing. —Mother verbalizes satisfaction with the breast-feeding process.	Assess, reinforce, and add to knowledge base regarding breast-feeding. Provide information about resources available after leaving hospital.	Breast-feeding continues without difficulty and with continuing satisfaction of mother and infant until natural weaning occurs at time desired by mother and infant.

cologists recommend that breast-feeding should begin as soon as possible after delivery (Freeman et al., 1992). If the mother has been heavily medicated or the labor has been long or difficult, the mother and newborn may be sleepy and will need close supervision during the breast-feeding attempt. Even if the newborn is too sleepy to nurse well at this time, the closeness to the mother and the contact with the nipple may still be enough to stimulate release of oxytocin and prolactin.

Some hospital policies require that the newborn must receive a water feeding before beginning to breast-feed. This is done to help clear out excess mucus, assess pharyngeal coordination, and detect congenital anomalies, such as tracheoesophageal (TE) fistula. However, Lawrence (1994) points out that colostrum can serve the same purpose as water and because it is a physiologic secretion, is not irritating and can be absorbed by the respiratory tract in case of aspiration. Also, if signs of possible TE fistula, such as polyhydramnios or excessive mucus, are noted, the

presence or absence of the condition can be confirmed by passing a tube into the stomach to determine if the esophagus is patent.

Initial Supervision

An interested and experienced nurse should be immediately available to mothers during their first feeding experiences. Many of the problems associated with unsuccessful breast-feeding can be prevented or solved through purposeful nursing action.

When assisting the new mother with initial breast-feeding experiences, it is important to remember that the mother and newborn must learn how to work as a team during the breast-feeding process. Hence, practice is essential. Even though the mother may have breast-fed before, infants display a wide range of nursing behaviors, and the experience of breast-feeding each infant can be somewhat "new." The mother needs to learn how to handle the newborn appropriately, how to interpret cues of hunger and satiety, and how to help the newborn grasp the nipple to withdraw the milk. The newborn must learn to associate the nipple with food and to coordinate grasping of the nipple with sucking and swallowing to get food successfully. It is not surprising that it takes the mother and newborn a few days to become adept at this process.

Preparations for early breast-feeding experiences should begin before the newborn is hungry and fussy. Instructions should be given about handwashing, handling the newborn, and any other activities associated with feeding. Information about the feeding reflexes of the newborn and how they are used during the feeding experience also may be helpful to the mother. During the actual nursing period, the nurse can reinforce this information and show the mother how to elicit the responses. It is essential for the mother to gain confidence in her ability to handle the newborn during the short time she is in the hospital. It is a learning process that may take time. Although it may be difficult for the nurse to watch the inexperienced mother learn to breast-feed her newborn, the nurse must avoid taking over and interrupting the learning process.

The nurse who assists the mother with the first feeding experience should record the type of instruction given, the response of the mother and newborn to the experience, and whether the feeding took place in the delivery room, recovery room, or in the mother's room. This information can help other staff members working with the mother to provide assistance and consistency.

Positioning the Mother

The nurse should assist new mothers in experimenting with various positions during breast-feeding. An inexperienced mother may be unaware of the options and should be given an opportunity to try various positions while help is available. If the mother is shown only one position, she may think there is only one "right" way to do it.

The best positions for any mother and infant depend on several factors, including the size and shape of the breast, the size of the infant, and the condition of the mother, who may have a sore perineum or tender incisional area from a cesarean section. The mother should be encouraged to avoid using the same position at every feeding at first. Varying the nursing position changes the position of the infant's mouth on the nipple and promotes more complete emptying of the breast. This can assist in preventing the nipples from becoming tender and the ducts from becoming plugged.

If the mother wants to lie down to breast-feed, the nurse can suggest that she be on her side with her arm raised and her head comfortably supported. The newborn lies on his or her side flat on the bed or supported so that he or she can grasp the breast easily.

Tucking the baby's feet close to the mother's body allows for room to breathe.

The mother who prefers to sit up to breast-feed may be most comfortable in a chair with a stool to support her feet. If she stays in bed, the high Fowler's position is probably best. After a cesarean birth, the mother may be more comfortable if her knees are bent and abducted, with pillows to support them on each side. It is often helpful to place a pillow under the arm that is supporting the newborn to reduce the tension on the muscles or to place a pillow under the newborn to raise him or her to a sufficient height to reach the breast easily. An alternate position consists of the infant facing the breast, positioned under the mother's arm in the football hold, and supported by a pillow. This is especially helpful for the mother who has delivered by cesarean section or who wants to nurse twins simultaneously.

Some mothers improvise positions that work well for them and their newborn, but other mothers may need help finding a comfortable position. Often, in their eagerness to get the newborn on the breast, mothers become tense and assume uncomfortable positions (although they assure the nurse that they are comfortable). The nurse should encourage the mother to relax and take her time discovering what positions work best.

Positioning the Newborn

After the mother has found a comfortable position, the nurse can assist her in positioning the newborn to latch on to the breast correctly (Fig. 30-3). To nurse satisfactorily, the newborn needs to be held properly by the mother. Although some mothers know how to support an infant at the breast, many are awkward and need definite instructions. The following are some helpful teaching points:

- Mother and infant must be comfortable.
- The infant should be at the level of the breast so that the body weight does not pull on the breast.
- The infant must be able to grasp the nipple and most of the areola. If only the nipple is grasped, the infant is not able to draw out the milk because the milk sinuses are not compressed. The result might be damage to the nipple and pain to the mother.

Client Education: Positioning the Newborn on the Breast provides guidelines for the new mother. These guidelines will help her position the newborn and prevent or decrease nipple soreness (Auerbach et al., 1993).

Some women may use their second and third fingers to "shape" and introduce the nipple into the infant's mouth. This is an alternate technique that used to be taught and may be more natural for some mothers (Lawrence, 1994). However, some find it to be counter-

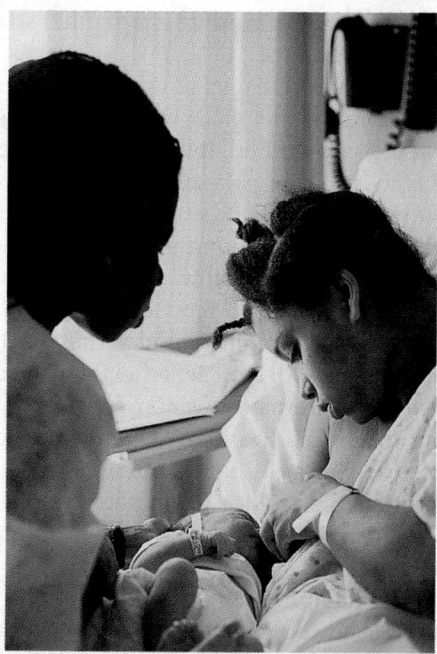

FIGURE 30–3 After the mother has found a comfortable position, the nurse can assist her in positioning the infant to latch onto the breast correctly.

productive because the mother's fingers are frequently placed on the areola, where the infant's gums should be. This prevents the infant from getting enough of the areola into his or her mouth.

Advice to get the entire areola into the infant's mouth is misleading and often impossible to follow, because many areolae are too large to fit. The infant simply needs enough of the areola in the mouth to allow his or her jaws to compress the sinuses, which are behind the nipple and under the areola.

The mother may need assistance in determining whether the infant's mouth is correctly positioned on the breast. When the infant latches on correctly, the mouth is opened wide and the lips are flared outward. The tongue forms a trough under the nipple and areola and extends beyond the lower gum. If there is a question about tongue placement, it can be observed by gently pulling down on the infant's lower lip (Shrago et al., 1990). Incorrect placement of tongue or lips can cause nipple damage and ineffective sucking.

Instructions About Sucking Behavior

Because the inside of the mouth cannot be directly visualized, it is difficult to determine what is happening while the infant is sucking at the breast. The sucking behavior of infants has been the subject of much study throughout the last few decades. Observation, x-rays, and ultrasound have been used in an attempt to visualize the process (Minchin, 1989). There is still not complete agreement on what happens during the sucking

process, but the following description provides an idea of how the infant's mouth interacts with the mother's breast to obtain milk.

To extract milk from the breast, the infant needs to use more than just suction. The nipple is drawn well back into the mouth, the lips close to form a seal around the areola, the sinuses are compressed and emptied by up and down movements of the jaw, and the milk is then swept into the back of the infant's mouth with regular undulations of the tongue. Creation of a vacuum may also be involved in drawing the milk from the breast (Smith et al., 1988). Swallowing occurs when enough milk has been obtained to induce the reflex. This activity is carried on rhythmically, at about one suck per second interspaced with periods of rest, until the infant is satisfied (Fig. 30-4).

If the infant has a good grasp on the breast, the jaws move up and down regularly, and swallowing movements can be seen in the infant's throat. The mother should be instructed to listen for quiet swallowing sounds (Shrago et al., 1990). If the grasp is poor, clicking or smacking sounds may be heard, and the infant's cheeks may draw in with each suck. Ineffective sucking should not be allowed to continue. The infant should be removed from the breast and repositioned to start again with a better grasp. Early correction of a faulty sucking technique can significantly improve chances for successful breast-feeding (Righard et al., 1992).

Breast tissue pressing against the infant's nose may obstruct breathing and cause the infant to stop suck-

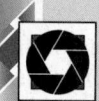

CLIENT EDUCATION
Positioning the Newborn on the Breast

Place the baby's head in the bend of your arm with his buttocks or upper thigh cradled in your hand.

Position the baby well over on his side, completely turned toward you.

Pull the baby tightly against your body (tummy to tummy). His lower arm should be around your waist. Make sure the baby's shoulder and hip are in alignment.

Make sure the baby's mouth is at the level of your nipple.

Help the baby grasp your nipple by supporting your breast with your hand, four fingers below and thumb above, with all fingers behind the areola.

Tickle the baby's lips gently with your nipple, wait for the baby to open his mouth *wide,* center your nipple, and bring the baby close to your body so that his lower lip is flanged outward, the baby's nose and chin just touch your breast and your nipple is in his mouth, past the gums.

ing. Pulling in the infant's buttocks and legs closer to the mother's body may help by changing the head position slightly and allowing more air space. Lifting the breast slightly to allow more air space is another suggestion. Depressing the breast tissue with the thumb or index finger is more likely to dislodge the breast from the mouth (Lawrence, 1994).

Sometimes the let-down reflex is so active that the milk literally streams out of the nipple. The baby may have to temporarily stop sucking and may have difficulty swallowing fast enough to keep up with the stream. The infant may have to nurse a bit, stop, and continue as he or she learns to cope with the increased flow. Temporarily placing the infant in a more upright position may help him or her be able to handle the milk and prevent choking.

Any time the infant is removed from the breast, the mother must first break the suction. Failure to do this can result in pain or trauma to the nipple. To break the suction, a clean little finger can be placed in the corner of the infant's mouth or the infant's chin can be pulled down. Sometimes the mother needs to pull away a little at the same time so the infant does not grasp the nipple again.

Individual Differences. Newborns exhibit a wide variety of sucking behaviors. Some, after finding the nipple, suck vigorously without stopping until they are satisfied. Others suck vigorously for a time, appear to sleep or to rest, and then resume sucking. Some infants mouth the nipple before actually sucking but eventually nurse well. Others seem rather disinterested in nursing. However, even initially disinterested infants usually begin to nurse better as the mother's milk comes in.

The important point is that individual differences exist. Therefore, care must be taken to allow for these differences. Trying to force a style or speed on an infant that is not natural to him or her only results in frustration for the infant and the mother. The nursing period should be adapted to the infant, not the infant to the nursing period. Mothers appreciate learning about these variations, because they often do not realize that infants have different eating behaviors and often think there is only one right way to nurse. Giving mothers anticipatory guidance and instruction in this aspect of nursing is an important component of nursing care.

The nurse can suggest methods that the mother can use to encourage her newborn to breast-feed. In newborns who seem disinterested or less adept at nursing, introducing the nipple into the mouth and expressing a few drops of colostrum or milk often encourage sucking. If the infant falls asleep instead of sucking, removal from the breast followed by gentle stimulation (eg, singing, playing with the infant's hands) may arouse the infant and initiate sucking. If it does not, the mother should be reassured that the infant will nurse when hungry. The infant should be left at the mother's bedside, so she is available when her newborn is ready to eat. If taken to the nursery, the newborn should be brought to the mother as soon as he or she awakens. A formula feeding should not be given in the nursery.

Nipple Confusion. If breast-feeding was not initiated early and the infant has had experience with a rubber nipple, **nipple confusion** may result. The sucking behavior required to obtain milk from the bottle is different from the sucking behavior of breast-feeding. Milk from the bottle comes into the infant's mouth with little effort. The infant does not use his or her tongue to extract milk, instead the tongue must be thrust forward to control the flow of milk (see Fig. 30-4*F*). It is not surprising that many infants have some difficulty switching from bottle to breast. Avoiding rubber nipples for the first 4 to 6 weeks is thought to be the best way to avoid this problem. However, if it occurs, most infants can be retrained to breast-feed with a little time and patience. It is helpful for the mother to know about these sucking differences so that she will not become frustrated and will be able to seek assistance if necessary.

Nursing Assistance and Support

Once the infant has taken the breast without difficulty and has been sucking well for several minutes, the nurse probably does not need to remain in constant attendance at the bedside. Allowing the mother some opportunity to feel that she can manage on her own will help to instill confidence in her ability to manage breast-feeding. However, she should never be left without adequate instruction and reassurance that the nurse is readily available.

When a newborn has some initial difficulties with latching on to the breast, the nurse may need to remind the mother that the first few days are a learning period for mother and newborn. Many mothers feel that all newborns know how to suck at the breast. Therefore, she thinks that she must be doing something wrong if her newborn does not latch on immediately. Other mothers may feel rejected and may state "The baby doesn't like me," or "The baby doesn't want my milk." The nurse can help the mother understand the infant's behavior by explaining that taking milk from the breast is more than just a simple act of sucking, and some infants need help in learning how. This knowledge may help the mother to stop blaming herself and allow her to enjoy the nursing experience.

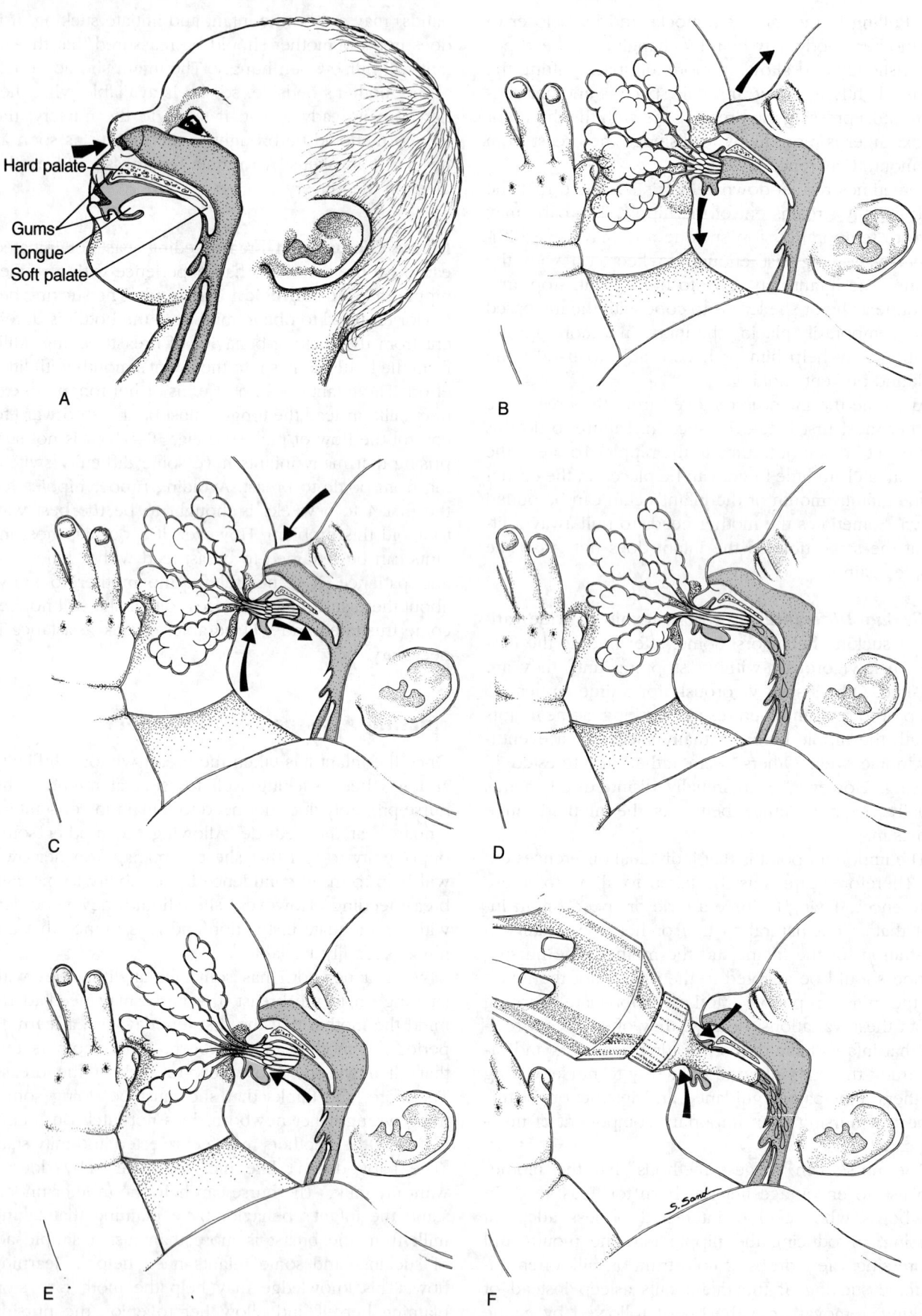

Hard palate

Gums

Tongue

Soft palate

A

B

C

D

E

F

S. Sand

Feeding Schedule

A self-regulatory or self-demand schedule is the usual accepted practice today, especially for breast-fed babies (ie, the baby is fed when he or she indicates hunger). When a set schedule is used and the infant is made to wait until it is "time" for a feeding, he or she may not nurse well. The infant may be over-hungry and exhibit frantic behavior, may be exhausted from crying, or may have lost the feeling of hunger by the time he or she is fed. Similarly, an infant in a deep sleep state will be difficult to arouse and probably will not feed well.

Mothers can be taught to observe their infants for behavioral feeding cues (Walker, 1989). Clues to a lighter sleep state would include rapid eye movements under closed eye lids, startles, and sucking movements (see Chap. 28). When mothers and babies are together most of the time, as in a rooming-in situation, problems can be avoided because the mother knows when the newborn is awake and can feed as needed. She also has the opportunity to learn to recognize the cry and behavior that indicate that her baby is hungry.

Self-demand feeding does not mean that a newborn should be allowed to go for long periods of time without eating. Although most breast-fed babies want to nurse every 2 to 3 hours at first and may go as long as 5 hours for one period each day; some babies cry very little, do not give typical hunger cues, and may go much longer between feedings. Mothers of these infants may need to be encouraged to feed them before they actually seem hungry. Frequent nursing is helpful in stimulating milk production, ensuring adequate intake, and satisfying the infant's sucking needs. Each time the infant has a growth spurt, he or she wants to nurse more frequently for a few days until the supply catches up with the increased demand. Infants gradually go longer between feedings, and their eating patterns become less varied. This is encouraging news for the mother who may feel that the newborn is nursing all the time.

Length of Nursing Time

Limiting sucking time during the initial stages of breast-feeding as a means of preventing sore nipples is no longer considered necessary according to most sources. If positioning and attachment are correct, unlimited nursing has not been found to increase nipple soreness (Moon et al., 1989).

Time limitations can actually cause some problems for the breast-feeding mother. With severe limitation, such as starting with 1 or 2 minutes on each breast per feeding, the let-down reflex does not have a chance to function before the newborn is removed from the breast. Even with 4 or 5 minutes per side, there may be increased incidence of breast engorgement and reduction in the infant's fluid intake. Millard (1990) points out that the clock is a central part of our culture and that pediatric advice focusing on timing the breast-feeding experience may make it difficult for the new mother to relax and follow the infant's cues.

Offering both breasts at each feeding, especially at first, provides maximum stimulation for the mother and an adequate supply of milk for the infant. Nursing should begin on the side used last during the previous feeding. Using a safety pin on the bra strap may help the mother remember on which breast to start feeding. The mother may need some guidelines on the amount of time to expect the infant to nurse. She should be told that a minimum of 5 to 7 minutes on each side is needed to allow time for the let-down reflex to occur and the ducts to be emptied. As the infant's thirst and hunger increase, he or she may want to nurse 10 to 15 minutes on the first breast and a little less on the second.

If the mother develops severe nipple problems, she might need to shorten the time on the affected breast and complete the emptying by expressing the milk. If the breasts are full and the let-down reflex is functioning well, the infant usually gets most of the milk in the first 5 to 10 minutes of sucking. Therefore, the mother should not worry that the infant is not getting enough

---

FIGURE 30–4 Differences between breast and bottle sucking behavior. (**A**) Normal breathing for a young infant is through the nose; the back of the mouth is closed by contact of tongue and palate. (**B**) Infant opens mouth wide to receive the breast, the tongue comes forward over the lower gum to form a trough under the nipple and areola, and the nipple is pulled far back into the mouth. (**C**) Undulations of the tongue from front to back press nipple against hard palate, squeezing milk out of sinuses. Note how lips form a seal around areola. (**D**) When milk reaches the back of the throat, the swallowing reflex is initiated. (**E**) The gums open, allowing sinuses to refill, followed by closure of the gums, and the cycle is repeated. Enough suction is maintained to keep nipple back in the mouth, and the infant continues to breathe through the nose, one breath to one or two swallows. (**F**) Rubber nipple is less pliable, maintains its shape, and may strike soft palate, interfering with normal tongue action and sometimes causing gagging. Milk comes more freely, and tongue may be thrust against gums to control overflow.

milk if she has to limit nursing time for a short period due to nipple soreness.

Supplementary Feedings

The subject of whether to give supplementary feedings to newborns has long been controversial. Many proponents of breast-feeding feel that giving the infant any artificial feedings is detrimental to establishing and maintaining lactation and interferes with breast-feeding success. Others feel that there are legitimate indications for occasional or regular artificial feedings. One study found that giving one bottle a day after the second week did not increase breast-feeding problems (Cronenwett et al., 1992). However, others say that regular supplementation this early could create problems for many breast-feeding couples. If possible, it is usually recommended that no supplements be used for the first 6 weeks.

Supplements are usually given by bottle either after breast-feeding or instead of breast-feeding. Expressed breast milk can also be given by bottle when the mother is unable to feed the infant herself. To avoid nipple confusion when supplements are necessary, alternates to use of a bottle are suggested. Feedings can be placed in the infant's mouth by dropper, syringe, or spoon. If the mother can put the infant to breast but needs to supplement her milk or encourage the infant to suck, a special supplementation device can be used. The device consists of a pouch that delivers milk to the infant through a tube that enters the infant's mouth next to the mother's nipple (Fig. 30-5; Walker et al., 1993).

Care of the Nipples

To facilitate breast-feeding, it is important to discuss nipple care with the new mother. Cleanliness is important in breast-feeding, but it is the hands that need washing, not the nipples. A natural antisepsis is provided in the oils secreted by the nipple and by enzymes in the milk. Washing the breasts with plain water at the time of the daily bath or shower is thought to be enough. Soap should be avoided because it is drying and can lead to cracking.

Keeping the nipples dry is another important aspect of their care. Air drying after each nursing period and leaving the bra flaps down for 15 to 30 minutes several times a day are recommended. The warm air from an electric hair dryer on low setting, held 6 to 8 inches away for 2 to 3 minutes can increase comfort (Lawrence, 1994). Milk left around the nipple after the baby nurses should be allowed to dry on the breast rather than being wiped away, because it is soothing and healing (Lawrence, 1994). Plastic liners in the bra should be removed because they hold in moisture.

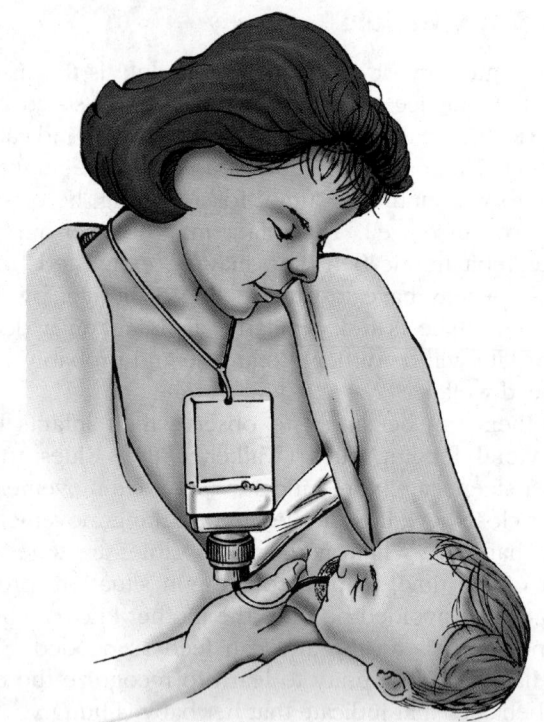

FIGURE 30–5 The supplemental nutrition system allows the mother to continue breast-feeding while providing supplementary formula to the infant through a tube placed next to her nipple.

Many women experience milk leakage, especially as the milk comes in. Something absorbent, such as a breast pad or a clean, folded handkerchief, can be used to keep the nipple drier and prevent milk from leaking through to the outer layer of clothes. They should be changed frequently when they get damp.

Routine use of nipple ointments and creams is not advisable. If used, the substance should be safe for mother and infant and not have to be washed off before the infant is fed (Box 30-3). If the mother has extremely dry skin or application of some substance is recommended for a specific reason, it should be used after breast-feeding, applied in small amounts, and rubbed in well so that air circulation is not obstructed and the ducts in the nipple and areola do not become plugged.

Continuing Support

Because short hospital stays allow less time for nurses to provide assistance to the breast-feeding mother, many women need additional support after leaving the hospital. The father or other family members may fill this need if they are available, but if family members are absent or information is lacking, additional support is often needed.

Hospital- or community-based nurses may provide follow-up care after the woman has returned home.

BOX 30-3
Agents Used for Sore Nipples

Caution: Although these are for *external* use by the mother, anything placed on the nipple will be taken *internally* by the infant, unless washed off well before nursing.

A & D ointment—For external use only. This contains anhydrous lanolin but no vitamins.

Mammol ointment—Directions are to wash and dry nipples before and after use. This contains Bismuth subnitrate, which can be reduced to nitrate by bacteria in infant's bowel and can cause methemoglobinemia.

Massé cream—Instructions are to clean breasts before and after nursing. This contains a few potentially problematic ingredients. Peanut oil can be aspirated to cause bronchitis or can be an allergen.

Moist towelettes—These are not advertised for use on nipples, but some hospitals suggest for mothers to use them before nursing. They are meant for external use only.

Hydrous lanolin—This is highly allergenic for those allergic to wool and may contain pesticide residue.

Anhydrous lanolin—Modified lanolin is hypoallergenic; no cautions are advised concerning ingestion or use on wounds.

(From Auerbach, K. G. et al. [1993]. Breastfeeding and human lactation.)

Some hospitals encourage mothers to call the nursery or obstetric unit if they need support or help with problems. Although many mothers are reluctant to call, they welcome the chance to ask questions if the nurse calls or visits them at home. Some hospitals and private doctors hire nurses to make follow-up home visits. The mother may also be referred to a public health or home health agency.

Nursing mothers' groups, which exist in most communities, also offer education and support. One well-known group is La Leche League International, which holds breast-feeding classes for women before and after the infant is born and publishes books and pamphlets about breast-feeding. In many communities, there are 24-hour phone numbers that nursing mothers may call if they are having problems with breast-feeding.

Another source of help for the nursing mother is the lactation educator or consultant. These individuals have special training and experience in the area of assisting mothers with breast-feeding. The lactation educator presents prenatal classes specifically on breast-feeding and is available to the mother for counseling and advice after the newborn arrives. The lactation consultant is a health professional who has additional training and experience, is prepared to assist mothers

with more serious breast-feeding problems, and usually works in a clinic setting or in private practice.

Addressing Common Concerns and Problems of Breast-feeding

Inverted Nipples. Retracted or **inverted nipples** should be identified during prenatal assessments, and remedial interventions should be started prior to the birth. When the nipple does not protrude beyond the areola or is slightly retracted, many women are concerned that they have inverted nipples. How the nipple looks when it is not in the infant's mouth is not a good indication of how it will function when the infant sucks on it. When gentle pressure is used to compress the area behind the nipple, the normal flat nipple will come out, but the inverted or "tied" nipple will retract further (Lawrence, 1994). Wearing breast shells and using a breast pump before each feeding can make it easier for the infant to grasp the nipple (Riordan et al., 1993; Table 30-2).

Painful Nipples. Nipple pain is frequently a reason for discontinuing breast-feeding. Although it may not be possible to prevent or eliminate this problem completely, it can be minimized with good care. Measures to prevent nipple trauma include the following:

- Make sure the infant's mouth is positioned correctly on the breast so that he or she is not chewing on the nipple.
- Change nursing positions with each feeding so that different areas of the nipple are subjected to the greatest stress from sucking.
- Do not allow the breasts to become engorged so that the infant has difficulty grasping the breast.
- Feed the infant on demand so that he or she does not become overly hungry, causing him to suck the nipple too vigorously.
- Start each feeding on alternate breasts so that both breasts are subjected to the vigorous sucking that occurs at the beginning of the feeding.

The mother should also avoid allowing the infant to suck on empty ducts. Before the let-down reflex is established, she can manually express a few drops of colostrum or milk to fill the ducts before allowing the infant to begin nursing.

The mother can probably benefit from anticipatory guidance about nipple soreness. She needs to know that it is not unusual and is usually self-limiting. The discomfort is often most noticeable as the infant begins to suck but diminishes rapidly as the let-down reflex occurs. The discomfort with the first few sucks can last for several days or weeks and does not mean that anything is wrong.

TABLE 30–2
Breast-Feeding Aids

Item	Uses	Comments
Breast cups	Treat inverted nipples Keep milk from leaking onto clothing Relieve engorgement Protect sore nipples from sticking to bra or pad	Vary in size, shape, comfort, and ability to be sterilized
Nipple shields	Protect sore nipples Help baby who does not accept breast easily	Use with caution: 　May cause preference for rubber nipple 　Lack mouth-to-breast contact; interfere with stimulation of milk production 　Interfere with areolar compression and infant's ability to extract milk; frequent weight check of infant required
Breast pads	Absorb milk leakage and help protect clothes	Can use disposable paper pad, washable cotton pads, folded men's handkerchiefs, or cut-up soft used diapers Caution: Use of pads with plastic or waterproof liners possible contribution to nipple soreness or breast infection by keeping area moist
Feeding tube devices (Supplemental Nutrition System, LactAid)	Provide additional source of nourishment while stimulating lactation for adoptive nursing, relactation, reluctant nursers, infants with suckling problems, or those who are ill or handicapped	Deliver milk to suckling infant at the breast; plastic bag or bottle containing milk suspended around mother's neck; thin flexible tubing, placed in infant's mouth with mother's nipple
Breast pumps	Aid in expression of milk: 　To stimulate lactation when infant cannot be put to breast or is not sucking well 　To obtain milk and maintain milk supply when mother is absent (eg, working)	Vary in type and efficiency. Two types of suction: 1) Draw and hold—pressure increased, held while milk flows, released, then build up again. 2) One pump per second—continuous rhythm of pump-release at 1-second intervals
Electric		Come in various sizes; best for frequent and long-term use; may be expensive, but can be rented and insurance may pay; hand-pump conversions
Battery operated		Less expensive and more portable, but may not be very long lasting or consistent; added cost of batteries unless electric plug adaptor or rechargeable pack available
Manual		Many varieties; least expensive and most portable, but take more effort and both hands to operate; suction created by drawing a piston through a cylinder, rubber bulb, trigger handle, running water from a faucet, or the mother sucking on a tube; amount of pressure controllable with care, but can be traumatic to breast and nipple tissue

When choosing a pump, mothers also should consider safety (UL Approval), ease of cleaning, and how the breast cup fits or can be adapted to their breast size. Some pumps work better for some women than others. Childbirth educators, the La Leche League, lactation educators, or lactation consultants are good sources for information about breast pump features and availability.

Most studies conducted on various methods used to relieve nipple soreness have not demonstrated their effectiveness (Ziemer et al., 1990). Some methods seem to create, rather than solve, problems (Auerbach et al., 1993; see Box 30-4). However, one study (Buchko et al., 1994; also see Research Highlight) found that mothers using warm water compresses reported relief of pain.

Nipple trauma can occur with or without nipple pain. Fissures, erosions, or blisters on the nipples can be entry-ways for bacteria and possible infection. The nurse should teach the mother how to assess for signs

Comfort Measures for Nipple Soreness

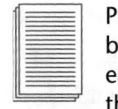 Postpartum nipple pain is a frequent concern of breast-feeding mothers and sometimes leads to early weaning. This study was designed to look at three comfort measures and evaluate the extent to which they alleviate nipple soreness.

Seventy-three primiparous, breast-feeding women were randomly assigned to four groups, each using a different method of nipple care: 1) warm moist tea bag compress, 2) warm water compress, 3) expressed milk massaged into the nipple and areola and air dried, and 4) no specific care (control group). All women were given verbal and written instructions about breast-feeding that included massaging the breasts and expressing a few drops of colostrum before each feeding; positioning the infant for proper latching on, sucking, and comfort; and varying the nursing positions several times a day. After the initial interview and instruction, the women were asked to complete a questionnaire in the hospital on the first day and for the next 6 days at home. Questions were related to pain intensity, pain effect or unpleasantness, strength of the infant's suck, and other aspects of their breast-feeding experience.

Results of the study indicated that the highest mean scores for pain intensity occurred on day 3; the highest mean scores for pain effect or unpleasantness were on day 4. There was no correlation between sucking strength and either of the pain measures on any day of the study. A comparison of the four groups showed that the warm water compress group had the lowest scores on both of the pain measures throughout the week.

Critique: The results of this study can be useful to nurses in several ways. Nurses who teach women about breast-feeding in the prenatal and postpartum periods can provide anticipatory guidance to prepare new mothers for the nipple discomfort most women experience, especially on the third and fourth day after the infant's birth. Also, information about warm water compresses may provide the women with an inexpensive and relatively easy way to relieve nipple discomfort. Suggestions for future studies would be to use a larger sample, continue the study into the second week to find out at what point nipple discomfort is no longer a problem, and further investigate the relationship between treatment group and cracked or bleeding nipples.

(Buchko, B. et al. [1994]. Comfort measures in breastfeeding, primiparous women. *Journal of Obstetric, Gynecologic, and Neonatal Nursing*, Vol. 23, pp 46–52.)

of trauma and how to minimize risk of infection if they occur. Good handwashing and avoidance of handling the nipples are important. Interventions to prevent nipple pain can also help prevent nipple trauma or minimize damage after its occurrence.

If symptoms of mastitis or breast abscess develop, such as localized increased warmth, tenderness, or redness, the physician should be consulted so that treatment can be started immediately. Because these problems usually occur after the woman has left the hospital, she should be given some guidance before discharge and instructed to observe her breasts for signs of infection. Antibiotics are usually the treatment of choice. Most physicians feel that it is best for the woman to continue breast-feeding even when these difficulties develop (Lawrence, 1994; see Chap. 38).

Engorgement. When the milk comes in, usually 2 to 3 days postpartum, the breasts suddenly become larger and firmer, with varying degrees of tenderness. Lymphatic and venous engorgement are usually transitory. Ideally, painful engorgement does not occur if the infant sucks early and frequently, the let-down reflex is established, and the alveoli are emptied periodically.

If clinical engorgement does occur, prompt treatment is important, not only for the mother's comfort but also to prevent the condition from progressing and interfering with the lactation process (Table 30-3).

Prevention of engorgement is preferable to treatment and is generally possible with good management. Early and regular nursing is considered by many to be the best preventive measure. When the mother and newborn are together around the clock, as in rooming-in, engorgement tends to occur less often because the newborn can nurse in response to the mother's needs and his or her own. If rooming-in is not available, the infant can be taken to the mother as soon as her breasts begin to fill and as often thereafter as is necessary to maintain her comfort.

Not Enough Milk. Insufficient milk supply is one of the most frequently reported reasons for early introduction of formula or termination of breast-feeding (Hill, 1991; Henly et al., 1995). In many instances, the milk supply is not deficient, but for various reasons, the mother perceives it to be. A primary reason for a mother's perception that her milk supply is insufficient is the infant's fussiness after a feeding (Hill, 1991). Assessment of mother and infant can help determine whether the problem is actually insufficient milk, if the mother's knowledge about breast-feeding and infant responses is insufficient, or if there is another problem.

Many mothers worry that they do not have enough milk. The mother can be assured that the infant is probably getting an adequate amount of milk if he or she is wetting at least six to eight diapers a day, having at least one stool, sleeping fairly well, and steadily gaining weight. Audible swallowing during nursing is another indication that the infant is getting milk. Crying and weight gain are not the most reliable indicators, because colicky babies cry for reasons other than hunger and usually gain well. Some breast-fed babies are slow weight gainers, despite an adequate milk supply. If the mother thinks her infant is not getting enough milk, she can usually increase the supply by putting the infant to her breast more often and not lim-

TABLE 30–3
Engorgement in the Lactating Woman: Prevention and Treatment

Changes in Breasts and Surrounding Tissues	Cause	Prevention or Treatment
Breasts are larger, firmer, and more tender.	Venous and lymphatic congestion and filling of the alveolar cells with milk.	Early, frequent sucking by the infant; establishment of the let-down reflex; and periodic emptying of the alveoli are preventive measures.
Skin appears shiny.	Emptying of the breasts is delayed.	Move the milk from alveoli to the sinuses where infant can obtain it by prefeeding massage or alternate massage during feeding.
Tissue surrounding nipple becomes taut.	Continued distention makes emptying difficult, leading to further engorgement.	
Nipple retracts, making it extremely difficult for the infant to grasp nipple and areola adequately.		Use an oxytocin nasal spray to stimulate let-down reflex.
Breasts may be reddened and warm to the touch.		Use hot packs or a hot shower before nursing to improve flow of milk.
Severe engorgement: Breasts are painful when touched or moved. Throbbing pains extend into axilla.	Progressive engorgement: Ducts become occluded by surrounding congested tissues and the thick, tenacious character of the retained secretions.	Relieve discomfort: Apply ice packs between nursing periods.
Secondary lymphatic and venous stasis occur.	Milk cannot be emptied.	Use a bra for good uplift support. Analgesics such as aspirin, acetaminophen, or codeine are used for pain relief, timed for mother's comfort during nursing periods.

iting the sucking time. It is also helpful for the mother to understand the concept of supply and demand—the more milk the infant takes from the breast, the more the mother produces. Sometimes women mistakenly think that they can "save" their milk and have more for the next feeding if they give the baby a bottle at one feeding. Getting more rest and increasing fluid and protein intake may help increase the milk supply.

Some mothers fear that they are losing their milk when engorgement subsides because their breasts go back to a more normal size and feel less full. The nurse should tell the mother that this might happen and that it simply means that the swelling, not the milk supply, has gone down.

If the mother's breasts feel full but the infant does not seem to be getting enough milk, there could be a problem with the let-down reflex. It may be helpful for the mother to learn how to recognize when the let-down reflex is occurring. Mothers usually feel the let-down as a kind of tingling or drawing sensation in the nipple, followed by a fuller, heavier feeling of the breasts. Because let-down occurs bilaterally, another sign is dripping of milk from one breast while the infant is sucking on the other. In addition, there is often a change in the infant's sucking as the milk begins to flow more freely and he or she does not have to work as hard.

The let-down reflex can be influenced profoundly by psychological factors and the mother's emotions. If let-down is not occurring, the nurse can help the mother determine and eliminate disturbing factors. The mother may need to lie down, have a warm drink, or discover other ways of relaxing before feeding. A relaxed atmosphere, adequate assistance, effective pain relief, and a supportive attitude on the part of the nurse and family are important to the establishment of the let-down reflex.

Sometimes mothers are concerned that their milk is not rich enough because they compare the thin, bluish white breast milk with the creamy color of cow's milk. Explaining the differences, including color, between cow's milk and human milk can be helpful.

In some cases, the mother may truly have an insufficient milk supply. If the mother is receiving guidance and support, has tried all of the usual ways to increase the milk supply, and the infant is still showing signs of not doing well, other causes for the problem should be sought, and supplementation may need to begin.

Maternal risk factors for insufficient lactation include the following:

- Women who have had augmentation or reduction mammoplasty (Neifert et al., 1990)
- Women who had minimal breast enlargement during pregnancy (Neifert et al., 1990)
- Maternal anemia (Henly et al., 1995)
- Anything that causes the infant to provide an inadequate, irregular, or ineffective sucking stimulus

Early intervention in cases of lactation insufficiency is important before the infant loses too much weight and the mother gets discouraged. Depending on the cause of the problem, breast-feeding may be stopped, and supplementation may be needed while solutions to the problems are pursued. In other cases, the mother may be able to continue partial breast-feeding with supplementation.

Instruction for Mother's Self-Care

The lactating mother may concentrate solely on her infant's needs and neglect her own health. How much rest the mother is getting, her diet, any medications she is taking, and possible exposure to contaminants may affect the quantity and/or quality of her breast milk. The mother should be aware of these factors and do everything possible to make sure her infant receives adequate amounts of safe, nutrient-filled breast milk.

Rest. Rest is one of the most important considerations for the lactating mother. The detrimental effects of fatigue and worry already have been discussed. In the hospital, the nurse is able to act as a buffer between the mother and some of these problems. When she leaves the hospital, she leaves this somewhat protected environment. Thus, the nurse should make sure that parents understand the importance of rest for the mother and that they have made adequate plans to provide for it. The mother's main energies should be directed to the care of the infant and other family members. Housekeeping chores should be simplified, and activity must be restricted so that the mother gets sufficient rest. If it is at all possible, the mother should have help at home. Because her sleep is broken at night, naps during the day become particularly essential; they should not be considered a luxury. If the mother does not get adequate rest, her milk supply will decrease. Active women may need help realizing the importance of naps and rest periods. It is helpful if visitors (including relatives) are restricted at first. Frequent visitors can become fatiguing to the mother, and they may be a source of potential infection in the newborn.

Diet. The daily diet of the lactating mother is similar to that recommended during pregnancy (see Chap. 18). However, according to the Food and Nutrition Board of the National Research Council, the need for calories, vitamin A, vitamin C, niacin, riboflavin, and iodine is greater than during pregnancy. Hopefully, the new mother has become more aware of good nutrition during her pregnancy and will be able to incorporate the proper foods into her diet to meet these increased needs. The nurse should discuss the recommendations with her, assess her knowledge, and give instruction as necessary.

If the mother's diet was adequate during pregnancy, additions rather than changes are all that is necessary. Nursing mothers, not realizing that their nutritional needs increase even over the needs of pregnancy, may go back to their prepregnant diet or limit their intake in the hope of losing weight. Dieting should be discouraged during lactation. Any limitation of maternal nutrient intake during lactation can interfere with the quantity of milk produced and if the limitation is severe, with the composition of the milk.

Individual caloric needs vary with the body size of the woman and with the quantity of breast milk produced. According to the recommended dietary allowances (National Research Council, 1989), approximately 85 kcal is required for each 100 mL of milk produced. The average milk secretion is 750 mL/d during the first 6 months and 600 mL/d during the second 6 months. Based on these figures, the average lactating woman requires an extra 500 kcal/d over that recommended for a nonpregnant woman. Fat stores from pregnancy are assumed to provide some calories for the woman during the first few months. Additional calories are necessary for women whose pregnancy weight gain was below normal or whose weight during lactation falls below the standard for their age and height (National Research Council, 1989).

Women who are producing more milk, for example, mothers of large infants or twins, will likely require additional calories. The mother's weight is one of the best criteria in determining adequate caloric intake; it should remain relatively stationary. Wide fluctuations require that the diet be adjusted, most likely in the amount of carbohydrates and fats consumed, assuming that protein intake is adequate.

Increasing the daily milk intake to at least 1½ qt fulfills the additional protein, thiamine, riboflavin, calcium, phosphorus, and niacin needs. Supplementing the citrus fruit recommendations in pregnancy with generous servings of other fruits and vegetables fulfills the vitamin C requirements. To ensure optimum vitamin and mineral intake, many physicians prescribe that the vitamin supplement capsules taken during pregnancy be continued.

A high fluid intake also is necessary for milk production. Fluid intake between 2,500 and 3,000 mL is recommended for the mother engaged in normal activity under mild environmental conditions. More fluid may be required in hot weather or with physical exertion. Concentrated urine or constipation may be indications of inadequate fluid intake. The fluid intake should include a good deal of water and other beverages. Many mothers find that drinking a beverage before nursing facilitates the let-down reflex.

Mothers may have heard that certain foods should be avoided during lactation. Although some infants may be bothered by specific foods that their mothers eat, this is not universally true. Most mothers can eat any nutritious food without causing the infant distress. However, because many infants seem to be upset after the mother eats large quantities of certain foods, such as chocolate or cabbage, moderation should be the rule when eating these foods. If the mother is bothered by a particular food, she should avoid it because it could also have an effect on the infant. In addition, some infants seem to have more sensitive taste buds and will object to certain flavors in the milk by being reluctant to nurse.

Drugs. Most drugs ingested by the mother while she is lactating are secreted in the milk. How much is secreted in the milk, and what effect the drug has on the baby are variable. The concentration of the drug in breast milk depends on several factors, including the concentration in the mother's blood, the lipid solubility of the drug, the degree of ionization, and the composition of the milk.

Usually the amount of drug in the milk is small, but the cumulative effect over a 24-hour period may give the infant a fairly large dose. Some drugs seem to have highest concentrations shortly after they are ingested. Therefore, taking them after breast-feeding rather than before might help to minimize the infant's exposure (Lawrence, 1994). Delayed excretion or inactivation of drugs due to the immaturity of the infant's renal and hepatic functions can be a factor in the concentration of the drug in the infant's body. Decreased renal function in the mother also can lead to increased concentrations of drugs in the milk.

Interpreting the data concerning concentration of drugs in breast milk is hampered by the fragmentary and contradictory nature of the information available. Most drug companies give a warning in their inserts that says "safety in pregnancy and lactation has not been established and the benefits of the drug must be weighed against possible risks." When drugs are prescribed for a nursing mother, she should remind her physician that she is breast-feeding. If she is taking drugs for a chronic condition, she should discuss with her physician the possible effects on the infant before she decides on the method of feeding her infant. Certain drugs have adverse effects on the nursing infant and are therefore contraindicated during lactation. Other drugs should be used with caution. (See Appendix E for further information on drugs in breast-milk.) If these drugs are given to the mother, the infant should be observed closely for signs of reactions to the drugs. Many drugs that are considered safe when taken in single doses can cause problems in the infant if taken regularly and frequently. Long-acting forms of drugs should be avoided (Lawrence, 1994).

Some nonprescription medications also contain substances that can be harmful to the infant when passed through the breast milk. For example, Bromo-Seltzer and some over-the-counter sleeping aids, both of which contain bromides, and migraine headache remedies that contain ergot should not be used because bromides and ergot are contraindicated during breast-feeding. Also, some laxatives, such as cascara, can cause diarrhea in the infant. Mothers need to be warned to read the labels of any medications they plan to take to determine the presence of potentially harmful components.

Contaminants in Breast Milk. Ever since investigators first discovered DDT in breast milk in the 1950s, people have been asking if breast milk is still safe for infants. Many different contaminants are present in breast milk. These include other pesticides and toxic chemicals, such as polychlorinated biphenyls (PCBs) and polybrominated biphenyls. These contaminants are stored in maternal body fat from which they are mobilized and transferred to the infant through the milk fat. Damaging effects of these chemicals in infants as a result of ingestion from their mother's milk have not been proven. However, evidence from animal studies shows that heavy dosages can adversely affect the nursing infant. In addition, prenatal effects of PCBs were seen in Japanese newborns of mothers with heavy contamination during pregnancy (Lawrence, 1994). Lead has also been found in human milk, but it is found in larger amounts in other forms of milk.

More research is needed to determine the possible long-term effects of contaminants in breast milk. The benefits of breast-feeding still seem to outweigh the possible dangers in most cases. Women who have had excessive exposure to contaminants should be encouraged to have their milk analyzed to aid them in making a decision about the method of feeding. Nurses should join with others in attempts to rid the environment of pollutants as a more permanent solution to the problem.

Expression of Milk

In some instances, the mother wants to feed her infant with breast milk, but the infant cannot be fed at the breast. In these cases, articificial means are necessary. In other situations, the breast-fed infant is not able to empty the breast completely. At such times, it becomes necessary to empty the breasts of milk by artificial means. This is important because if the breasts are not completely emptied and this condition persists for several days, lacteal secretion is inhibited, and future milk supply may be jeopardized.

Two methods of expressing milk from the breasts include manual expression and breast pump expression. Before attempting to empty the breast using the chosen method, the mother may find it helpful to use measures to facilitate the let-down reflex, such as taking a warm shower, having a warm drink, or gently massaging the breasts.

Manual Expression. It is helpful if a woman learns the technique of manual expression before the newborn arrives, although it can be taught afterward if necessary. The mother should have the opportunity to try it in the hospital, where she can practice under the supervision of the nurse. This will enable her to do it with more confidence when she returns home.

A sterile glass or wide-mouthed container should be ready before beginning, and if the milk is to be fed to the infant, a sterile bottle and cap also are needed. It may be desirable to massage the breast for a few seconds to stimulate the flow of milk, as described in the section concerning breast engorgement.

Prior to expression of milk, the hands should be washed thoroughly with warm water and soap and dried with a clean towel. Because daily breast care is designed to maintain cleanliness, the same cleansing ritual required before putting the infant to breast should be used. Steps to manually express milk are listed in Client Teaching Guidelines: Expressing Breast Milk (also see Fig. 30–6).

CLIENT TEACHING GUIDELINES
Expressing Breast Milk

1. One hand is used to support the breast and to express the milk; the other is used to hold the container that receives the milk. Although some authorities advocate that the right hand be used to milk the left breast, the decision as to which hand is used should depend on how the mother can accomplish this with the greatest ease.
2. The forefinger is placed below and the thumb above the outer edge of the areola. The first action is gentle but firm pressure toward the chest wall, and the second is movement of the finger and thumb toward each other, drawing forward with a slight milking motion. The forefinger is kept straight so that pressure can be exerted between the middle of this finger and the ball of the thumb. As the finger and thumb are alternately brought together and released, compressing the area of the lactiferous sinuses between them, milk is forced out in a stream (see Fig. 30-6).
3. The fingers should not slide forward on the areola or the nipple during the milking process. It is of paramount importance to avoid pulling, pinching, or squeezing movements, because these can bruise and damage the breast tissue.
4. The position of the thumb and forefinger should be changed as the sinuses are emptied, moving in a clockwise direction, so that milk can be removed from all the sinuses.

Many authorities advocate this method of emptying the breast rather than using the breast pump, because the action more nearly simulates the action of the infant's jaws during nursing. Furthermore, because no mechanical equipment is required, it can be readily used when necessary after the mother is discharged from the hospital.

Breast Pump Expression. For many women, a breast pump is the preferred way to express milk. Many types of pumps are available, including electric, battery operated, and hand pumps (see Table 30-2). Which pump to use and whether to buy or rent depend on factors such as the length of time it will be needed and the reason for its use. When a pump is used, there is always the potential danger of traumatizing the breast tissue. Average sucking pressure for the normal newborn has been found to range from –50 to –155 mm Hg, with a maximum of up to –220 mm Hg/in^2 (Lawrence, 1994). Some pumps can exert pressure greater than this and are more likely to cause damage. Information about maximum pressure of specific pumps should be checked with the manufacturer.

When assisting a new mother to use an electric breast pump in the hospital, the mother should be given explanations about why the pump is used, how it works, and how to use it. This helps reduce the mother's anxiety, which could interfere with the milk-ejection reflex. The nurse should stay with the mother and assist her the first few times until she feels confident enough to use the pump alone. Measuring and recording the amount of breast milk obtained gives the mother evidence that she is increasing or keeping up her milk supply. If the milk is to be fed to the infant, it can be poured into a sterile nursing bottle; labeled with the infant's name, the time, and date; and refrigerated immediately. After use, the pump should be washed with soap or detergent, and the removable parts, such as the bottle and cap, breast funnel, and rubber connection tubing, should be washed thoroughly, wrapped, and autoclaved.

Guidance for Working Mothers

An increasing number of women are choosing to breast-feed even though they plan to return to work. The new mother may ask the nurse for an opinion of whether it is possible to breast-feed if she must return to work soon after the newborn arrives. Many factors are involved in the decision and eventual outcome for the individual mother. The nurse can use the questions listed in Nursing Guidelines: Questions to Ask the Working Mother to assess what information the mother needs in her decision-making process.

Ideally the nursing infant will be in close proximity to the workplace and can be brought to the mother for

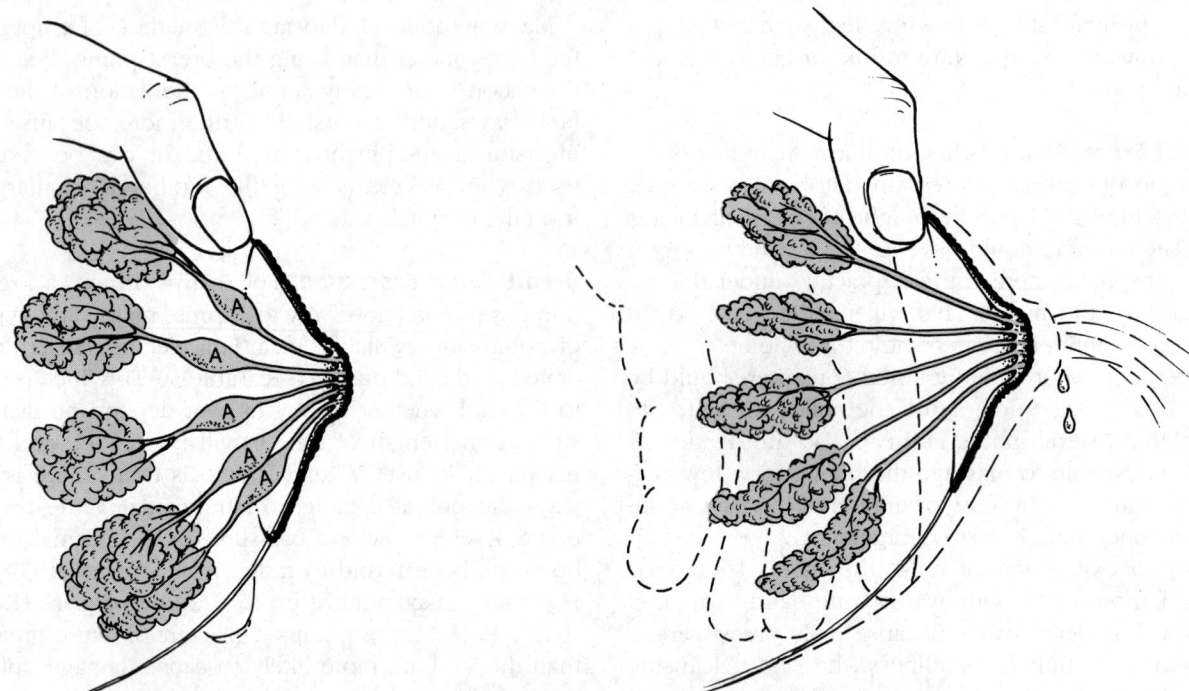

FIGURE 30–6 A lateral view of the left breast showing the method of expressing milk from the breast. The thumb and forefinger are placed on opposite sides of the breast just behind the areola. The lactiferous sinuses (ampulla, *A*) are compressed, and milk is forced out as the thumb and forefinger are brought together. See "Client Teaching Guidelines: Expressing Breast Milk."

nursing, or the mother can go to the infant during breaks. In reality, the average working mother will probably be away from the baby during the entire working day. Her breasts will continue to fill at the regular feeding times when she first goes back to work. The mother can empty them by hand expression

NURSING GUIDELINES
Questions to Ask the Working Mother

■ How soon will she start working?
  Waiting at least 6 weeks until breast-feeding is well established is preferable. Returning to work prior to 2 months postpartum has been found to increase breast-feeding problems and shorten the duration (Kearney et al., 1991).
■ How flexible is her job? Can she come home to feed during the day or have the baby brought to her? If not, is there time and a place to pump her breasts at work?
  The answers to these questions determine the arrangements she needs to make before starting work.
■ How much support does she have? Are family and friends supportive? Is her employer or supervisor supportive?
  Support from those around her will make it easier for her to continue with her dual roles.

or breast pump to keep up the supply and have breast milk fed to the baby when she is not there; instead, she can allow the daytime milk supply to dwindle by not pumping and have formula fed to the infant during the day. She should be aware that those who pump their breasts during the day can usually keep the milk supply at a higher level than those whose breasts are only emptied by the infant in the morning and evening (Auerbach, 1984).

Before going back to work, the mother should make her decisions and practice the method of expression she chooses. She also needs to arrange for refrigeration facilities if she is going to express milk at work. Employers vary in the amount of support offered to breast-feeding mothers. Some employers provide an electric breast pump, a place to pump, and facilities for storage. However, many employers do not have any policy that actively supports the lactating woman.

Some mothers find that their milk supply diminishes when they first return to work. Factors involved may be inadequate rest, reduction of intake of food and fluids, and temporary inhibition of the let-down reflex related to the tension involved with starting back to work. These tensions are emotional and physical, and letting mothers know that they should not expect to be very productive during the first few days back to work may make this time less stressful (Auerbach, 1993).

The working, breast-feeding mother has to pay particular attention to obtaining enough food, fluids, and rest. Studies have shown that most mothers who breast-fed their babies after returning to work felt it was worthwhile and would do it again. They often reported how much they enjoyed the special closeness that breast-feeding promoted between them and the infant, even though they did not have a lot of time to spend with the infant (Auerbach, 1984).

Counseling Concerning Weaning

When it comes to initiating breast-feeding, many mothers receive advice and counseling. However, little is said about how or when they should stop nursing. Although abruptly stopping at the time set by the physician is sometimes the accepted method of weaning from the breast, this can be uncomfortable and distressing to mother and infant. The most recent professional advice advocates that the infant be weaned slowly at a time chosen by the mother or infant. The mother should be helped from the beginning to feel comfortable with any length of time she chooses, even if it is considerably longer or shorter than usual.

The mother can begin to wean her infant by omitting the feeding in which the infant is least interested or the one that is least convenient for her. She can offer the infant a substitute for the omitted feeding, such as rocking, cuddling, going for a walk, or having a drink of juice from a bottle or cup. Anywhere from 1 week to 1 month later, when mother and infant are ready, another feeding may be dropped. This can be continued until the child is completely off the breast. Feedings should not be dropped when there are stressful situations in the family, such as illness, traveling, or guests.

The child can be weaned to a cup or a bottle depending on age and sucking needs. Slow weaning gives the mother and infant an opportunity to adapt to the changes and is less likely to cause emotional trauma. However, the end of a satisfying experience often is felt as a loss to the mother and the infant, even when approached slowly.

Sudden weaning is seldom necessary because the mother can express milk for a short time if she and the infant must be separated due to illness or absence for some other reason. Untimely weaning, stopping breast-feeding before the mother is prepared to stop, is as likely to be traumatic to the mother as it is to the infant, especially if nursing has been a satisfying experience. Lorick (1993) suggests that the mother may go through a grieving period that may be compounded by guilt. The nurse can help the mother understand that the grieving process is not unusual under these circumstances. She should discuss ways that the mother can continue the nurturing relationship with her child. Support from the father or another significant person is

also important to help guide her through this difficult time.

If the mother has physical discomforts during this time, a good supportive bra and mild analgesics will probably be helpful. Other suggestions are to allow warm water from the shower to run over the breasts and to express or pump small amounts of milk to relieve breast fullness (Riordan, 1993).

Evaluation

The nurse's interest and assistance can play a major role in the successful outcome of the breast-feeding experience for the new mother and infant. To increase the effectiveness of her interventions, the nurse should evaluate these outcomes and implement additional interventions when indicated. After a teaching session, the nurse evaluates whether the mother verbalizes understanding of the breast-feeding process, assumes a comfortable position, and uses the suggested techniques for positioning the infant on the breast.

The infant's weight and hydration also may be used as criteria for evaluation. The infant has at least six to eight wet diapers a day, has good skin turgor, and begins to regain birth weight by 1 week of age. Other evaluations are made depending on the situation. If the criteria are not met, the nurse might need to assess for further problems or provide the mother with additional information or demonstrations.

Formula Feeding

The mother who chooses to bottle feed her infant may have as many concerns about feeding as the breast-feeding mother, especially if this is her first child. She may not know how to feed an infant or prepare the formula. She also may feel a little uncertain about her choice of feeding method and may wonder if the formula will agree with her infant. By keeping up to date on the latest information about infant nutrition, the nurse can help allay the mother's fears about the adequacy of formulas, instruct her in safe preparation, and give guidance about when to seek medical assistance.

Comparison of Formulas

To provide adequate nutrition for an infant, a formula must meet the following criteria: It must have an appropriate distribution of calories from protein, fat, and carbohydrate; it must meet the infant's need for water, energy, vitamins, and minerals; and it must be readily digestible. The Infant Formula Act of 1980, which was amended in 1986, partly governs the composition of infant formula by stating a maximum concentration for nine nutrients and a minimum concentration for 22 nutrients (Benson et al., 1992).

The model usually used in the composition of a formula is human milk. Companies that manufacture infant formula make frequent adjustments to match new discoveries concerning the composition of human milk (Table 30-4). Many ingredients and processes are used in an effort to make commercial formulas meet the nutritional standards and come as close as possible to the composition of human milk. Formulas generally use a nonfat cow's milk base with added vegetable oil and carbohydrate. Most also attempt to duplicate the 60-40 whey-casein ratio of human milk by using dialyzed whey. The dialysis removes electrolytes, bringing the formula closer to the lower electrolyte human milk.

TABLE 30-4
Composition of Frequently Used Milks and Formulas

Milk or formula	Cal/dL	Percentage Composition			mmol/dL		mg/dL		Type of Carbohydrate	Type of Protein	Remarks
		PRO	FAT	CHO	NA	K	CA	P			
Human milk	74	1.1	4.5	6.8	0.7	1.3	34	121	Lactose	Human	
Cow's milk	67	3.5	3.7	4.9	2.2	3.5	117	92	Lactose	Cow	
Goat's milk	67	3.2	4.0	4.6	1.5	4.5	129	106	Lactose	Goat	Insufficient folate
Enfamil	67	1.5	3.7	7.0	1.2	1.8	55	56	Lactose	Cow	
Enfamil With Iron	67	1.5	3.7	7.0	1.2	1.8	55	46	Lactose	Cow	
Similac	67	1.6	3.6	7.2	1.1*	2.0*	51	39	Lactose	Cow	
Similac With Iron	67	1.6	3.6	7.2	1.1*	2.0*	51	39	Lactose	Cow	
Similac PM 60/40	67	1.6	3.5	7.6	0.7	1.5	40	20	Lactose	Casein, whey	60/40 lactalbumin; casein
S-M-A	67	1.5	3.6	7.2	0.6	1.4	44	33	Lactose	Whey from cow, cow	60/40 lactalbumin; casein
Advance	54	2.0	2.7	5.5	1.3	2.2	51	39	Corn syrup, lactose	Cow, soy	16 cal/oz
Isomil	67	2.0	3.6	6.8	1.3	1.8	70	50	Corn syrup, sucrose, corn starch	Soy, methionine	
Soyalac-i	67	2.1	3.8	6.7	1.4	1.9	63	52	Sucrose, tapioca	Soy, methionine	
Nursoy	67	2.3	3.6	6.8	0.9	1.9	64	44	Sucrose	Soy, methionine	
ProSobee	67	2.5	3.4	6.8	1.8	1.9	79	53	Corn syrup solids	Soy, methionine	
Soyalac	69	2.2	3.8	6.6	1.5	2.0	63	52	Dextrose, maltose, sucrose	Soy, methionine	
Meat base	67	2.8	3.3	6.3	0.8	1.0	99	66	Sucrose, tapioca	Beef	High protein, low sodium
Nutramigen	67	2.2	2.6	8.8	1.4	1.7	63	47	Corn syrup solids	Casein hydrolysate	
Pregestimil	67	1.9	2.7	9.1	1.4	1.8	63	42	Corn syrup, tapioca	Casein hydrolysate, cystine, tyrosine, tryptophan	

*Slightly higher if made from powder.
(After Avery, G. B, Fletcher, M. B., & MacDonald, M. G. [Eds.] [1993]. *Neonatology* [4th ed.]. Philadelphia: J.B. Lippincott.)

Formula is available in various sized cans in ready-to-use, concentrated, or powdered form. In the hospital nursery, the infant usually receives ready-to-feed formula in a disposable bottle. However, because formula in disposable bottles is expensive, one of the other packaging methods will probably be recommended for home use (Table 30-5). Some infants are not able to tolerate formulas based on cow's milk. Many formulas have been developed to try to meet the nutritional needs of these infants. Soybean-derived products are commonly used as the protein source in these artificial formulas. Soy protein isolate has a lower biologic value than casein and whey, so slightly larger amounts are needed to meet the infant's nutritional needs. Soy protein also can cause sensitization in some infants. Formulas such as Nutramigen and Pregestimil, which use casein hydrolysate as a protein source, are expensive but are recommended for infants with true milk allergy (Fletcher, 1993).

For the non–breast-fed baby, formula is the recommended food for at least the first 6 months and preferably for the first year of life (Fig. 30-7). In weight-conscious American society, it might seem that nonfat milk would be a good choice for an infant who is gaining weight too rapidly. In addition, nonfat dry milk may seem desirable for economic reasons. However, nonfat milk is not recommended for infants younger than 1 year because it provides an excessive intake of protein with inadequate calories. This can cause the mobilization of body fat for energy requirements and growth needs. The infant may look healthy but have little reserve for illness. Nonfat milk also lacks an adequate content of iron, ascorbic acid, and essential fatty acids. Low-fat (2%) milk is midway between nonfat and whole milk in fat content but probably would not meet all the infant's energy needs. Commercial milk substitutes, such as filled milk and imitation milk, also do not meet the infant's nutritional requirements and are not

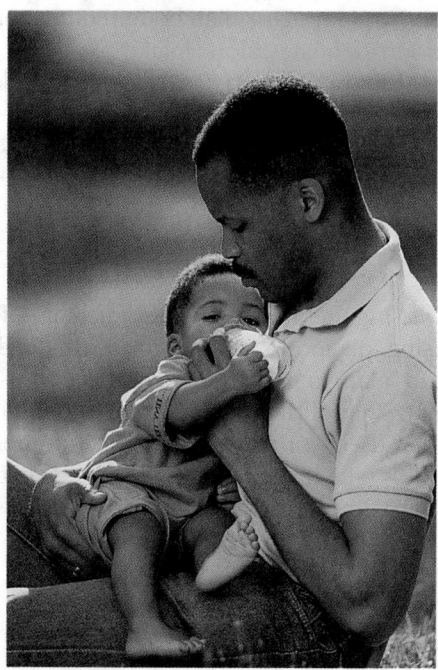

FIGURE 30-7 For the non–breast fed baby, formula is the recommended food for at least the first 6 months, and preferably the first year, of life.

recommended for infant feeding (California Department of Health Services, 1990).

Nursing Process: Formula Feeding

The nurse can use the nursing process format to ensure that the needs of the mother who is formula feeding are met. Through assessment, diagnoses, and interventions, individualized nursing care can be provided.

Assessment

Assessing maternal concerns and knowledge about infant feeding techniques and formula is an important part of nursing care, especially for the first-time mother. The nurse should talk with the mother to assess her level of knowledge and her experience with infant feeding. The nurse also should observe the mother and infant during feeding to assess the mother's handling of the infant and the infant's feeding reflexes, responsiveness, and amount of intake.

Nursing Diagnoses

Possible nursing diagnoses related to formula feeding include the following:

■ Knowledge Deficit (maternal) related to lack of information or experience with infant feeding

TABLE 30–5 *Types of Formula*		
Type	Packaging Available	Comments
Ready to feed	Small cans, large cans, bottles	Most convenient; most expensive; should not be diluted
Concentrate	Large or small cans	Less expensive; must be diluted 1:1 with water from safe source
Powder	Large cans	Least expensive; simple to prepare individual bottles with warm water from safe source; sometimes difficult to dissolve

- Altered Nutrition: Less than body requirements related to inadequate caloric intake
- Risk for Fluid Volume Deficit related to inadequate fluid intake
- Altered Nutrition: More than body requirements related to excessive caloric intake

Planning and Intervention

After assessing the mother and her infant and formulating nursing diagnoses related to bottle feeding, the nurse can plan interventions specific to this mother and infant. The following sections provide information that can be used during the planning and implementation process (see the Nursing Care Plan: Newborn and Mother Who Are Bottle Feeding).

Feeding in the Hospital

Bottle-fed newborns are typically given water for their first feeding. Many hospitals have a routine for when the bottle-fed newborn receives the first water feeding and when the formula feedings start. In some hospitals, the nurse must give the first water in the nursery. Other hospitals allow the mother to give the first water. If this is the case, the nurse should be present to observe the newborn's response to the water. She should also teach the mother how to use the bulb syringe because water often causes the newborn to bring up mucus.

The first feeding experiences are important for the mother and newborn. The mother begins to learn how the newborn communicates wants and needs. In addition, the newborn learns to coordinate feeding behaviors and begins to find out how the discomfort from hunger is relieved and who provides the relief. The nurse can encourage this process between the mother and newborn by being available during initial feeding periods to observe their behaviors, assess their interaction, and intervene with suggestions or demonstrations as necessary. If the nurse must intervene, he or she should be careful not to make the mother feel as though she is incompetent or inadequate.

The mother should be helped to find a comfortable position for feeding her newborn. She may want to sit up in a chair instead of in the bed. Holding the newborn in a semireclining position allows any air that is swallowed to rise to the top of the newborn's stomach, where it is more easily expelled. To minimize the amount of air swallowed, the bottle should be tilted enough to keep the nipple filled with milk (Procedure 30-1).

Infants have many different feeding behaviors, some of which may not correspond to the mother's expectations. Identifying the infant's individual behavior patterns and interpreting this individuality to the mother can help avert potential problems.

If the mother is concerned that her newborn is not taking enough milk, she should be assured that newborns are often sleepy the first few days after birth. In addition, full-term newborns do not need many calories until the second or third day because they have reserves of fat and water. The bottle-fed infant, like the breast-fed infant, should have the opportunity to be on a self-demand schedule. Bottle-fed infants average a longer period between feedings than breast-fed babies due to the larger curd of the formula. However, this varies greatly among infants. Some are hungry every 2 to 3 hours; others wait 4 or more hours between feedings.

Anticipatory Guidance for Formula Feeding

Before the mother and newborn leave the hospital, the mother should be given information about the nutritional needs of the newborn, the usual amounts of formula that the newborn will take, the types of available bottles and nipples, and how to prepare the formula.

Nutritional Needs and Typical Amount of Feeding. It is important for the mother to know that the newborn's stomach is small at birth, so the newborn should not be expected to take the entire 4 oz in the bottle during the first few weeks. As the infant grows and the stomach capacity and energy needs increase, formula consumption will also increase. At times of particularly fast growth, the infant will want to eat more at each feeding or eat more frequently.

The average formula-fed newborn will take approximately 20 oz of formula per day, increasing to about 32 ounces by the age of 4 to 6 months (California Department of Health Services, 1990). Again, the reminder should be given that each infant is an individual and that infants of the same age and weight may have different needs.

Bottles and Nipples. A wide variety of bottles and nipples is available. Bottle types include glass bottles with plastic nipple caps; boilable, nonbreakable plastic bottles; and plastic bottles that are bent at an angle to help ensure that the nipple is always full of milk. There are also kits that consist of a hollow plastic holder that suspends a disposable plastic bag containing the milk. This type of bottle is supposed to lessen the amount of air that is swallowed because the bag collapses, rather than filling with air, when the milk is sucked out. However, the infant can still swallow air around the nipple.

Nipples also come in several shapes and sizes. Some nipples supposedly resemble the mother's breast in ap-

NURSING CARE PLAN
Newborn and Mother Who Are Bottle-Feeding

Nursing Goals
1. Mother verbalizes understanding of
    Feeding process
    Positioning of infant while feeding
2. Mother demonstrates appropriate positioning and handling of infant.
3. Infant receives appropriate amount of formula.
4. Infant maintains hydration and good nutritional status.

Assessment	Potential Nursing Diagnoses	Intervention/ Rationale	Evaluation

Infant's nutritional status: weight gain, skin turgor, sleeping patterns	Knowledge Deficit about infant feeding related to lack of information and experience	Provide information as needed regarding
		  Newborn sucking reflexes
		  Handling infant during feeding
		Assist mother with feeding processes:
		  Comfortable positioning of mother and infant
		  Placing nipple in infant's mouth
		  Checking flow of milk
		  Keeping nipple full
			Mother expresses understanding of infant feeding process and handles infant appropriately.
			
			Mother demonstrates appropriate feeding techniques.

Mother's knowledge of formula preparation and feeding practices	Altered Nutrition: Less than body requirements related to inadequate caloric intake
	Altered nutrition: More than body requirements related to excess nutrient intake
	Risk for Fluid Volume Deficit related to inadequate fluid intake
		Provide anticipatory guidance:
		  How much formula infant needs
		  Types of formula, bottles, nipples
		  Preparation of formula
		Answer mother's questions regarding
		  Hunger cries
		  Bubbling (burping)
		  Regurgitation
		  Hiccups
		  Constipation
		  Introduction of solid foods
		Provide literature as appropriate
			Infant receives appropriate amount of formula at appropriate rate with minimal amount of air.
			Infant's weight gain is appropriate.
			Infant is well hydrated and well nourished.

pearance, some are supposed to elicit sucking responses more like the breast, and some come in three, color-coded thicknesses to be used for milk, water, or juice. The number of bottles and nipples needed depends on the method of preparation.

Methods of Formula Preparation. Strict sterilization procedures for preparing formulas at home are no longer considered necessary if an uncontaminated water source and good refrigeration are available and the hands and equipment are cleaned properly. Studies

have shown that there is no higher incidence of illness or infection in infants who were fed formula prepared by the clean technique compared with those who were fed formula prepared by a strict sterilization technique (Hughes et al., 1987).

However, there may be specific instances when sterilization is recommended. Therefore, all four basic methods of formula preparation are given in Table 30-6. The following points are common to all methods of preparation:

■ Hands should be washed well before starting.

PROCEDURE 30-1
Tips for Bottle Feeding

Action	Rationale
Have milk at temperature preferred by infant. Warm refrigerated formula by placing in container of warm water or holding under running warm water from faucet. Shake to distribute warmth. Check temperature by shaking a few drops on wrist.	Infants demonstrate preferences for formula temperature: from cool to room temperature to comfortably warm.
Avoid using a microwave oven to warm bottles.	Temperature of formula may be underestimated because bottle feels cool on outside. Heat may destroy some vitamins. Hot spots in formula may burn infant's mouth. Bottle may explode.
Hold infant in a semireclining position for the feeding.	Provides opportunity for closeness and nurturing interactions with the infant. Allows opportunity to observe infant's feeding behavior, prevent choking.
Gently stroke the infant's lips with the nipple.	This may help encourage the infant to open its mouth.
Make sure the nipple is placed correctly on top of the tongue.	Some infants elevate their tongue when opening their mouths, and the nipple gets placed under the tongue.
The infant should be stimulated to open its mouth wide enough so that the tongue can be seen.	This usually helps in placing the nipple in the right position.
Do not push the nipple too far into the mouth.	This may cause gagging if it strikes the soft palate.
Hold bottle in tilted position to keep nipple constantly filled with liquid.	This helps prevent swallowing of air.
Watch for rising air bubbles as the baby sucks.	This indicates that the infant is getting milk.
Check milk flow from nipples: Is it too fast? (Nipple hole is too large.) Is it too slow? (Nipple hole is too small.)	If the milk comes too fast, the infant does not get enough sucking, and the risk of aspiration is increased. If the milk doesn't come easily, the infant may tire from sucking before getting enough milk.
Nipple holes can be checked by holding the bottle upside down. The milk should drop freely but not run in a stream.	
Occasionally remove nipple from infant's mouth during feeding.	This will prevent the infant from sucking on a collapsed nipple.
A normal feeding time is between 15 and 20 minutes if the milk is coming at the right speed.	If the feeding takes longer, the infant may get too tired. If the feeding is much shorter, the infant may not meet his or her sucking needs.
Do not force the infant to finish a full bottle—put in the bottle the amount the infant is expected to take.	Overfeeding or refusal of bottle can result from forcing an infant to eat more.
Discard milk left in bottle at end of feeding.	Milk or formula is a good place for bacteria to grow. It may spoil or sour if left at room temperature.
Avoid putting the infant to bed with the bottle propped.	This increases risk of choking, ear infection, and tooth decay. The infant may get too much or too little milk, resulting in inappropriate weight gain or loss. Also, infant may become dependent on the bottle.
Meet the infant's nutritional needs for the first 4–6 months by the following: ■ Giving infant formula and occasional water	These are sufficient to meet nutritional needs during this time.

(continued)

PROCEDURE 30–1 *(Continued)*
Tips for Bottle Feeding

Action	Rationale
■ Avoiding sweetened drinks, sugar water, soda, gelatin water, corn syrup, honey, use of bottle to introduce solid foods (mixing pureed foods, cereal in bottles)	These may satisfy appetite without providing nutrients, and increase the risk of tooth decay. Honey may lead to infant botulism. Prior to 4–6 months, formula is sufficient food for infant, and "extrusion reflex" is present, which interferes with infant's ability to take solid food from a spoon. When solid foods are needed, giving them in a bottle interferes with infant's experience of individual textures and flavors, infant's active participation in feeding experience, and development of facial muscles used in speech.

■ If canned milk is used, the top of the can should be washed with soap and water using friction and rinsed thoroughly. Hot water can be poured over the top just before opening.

■ All equipment should be washed thoroughly in warm soapy water. A bottle and nipple brush should be used, and water should be squeezed through the nipple to make sure no milk particles or residue remain. Equipment should be rinsed thoroughly so all soap or detergent is gone.

■ Opened cans of formula or milk should be covered with fresh foil or plastic wrap, placed in the refrigerator, and used within 48 hours.

Table 30-6 describes formula preparation for concentrated formula. For other types of formula, such as ready to feed, and powdered, the one-bottle method is most practical. With ready-to-feed formula, the desired amount is simply poured into the bottle. Powdered formula is also prepared one bottle at a time by placing

TABLE 30–6
Formula Preparation Using Concentrated Formula

One-Bottle Method	Clean Method	Aseptic Method	Terminal Sterilization
1. Open can of concentrated formula; pour ½ of total amount desired into bottle. 2. Add equal amount of fresh tap water from safe source. 3. Feed within 30 min of preparation. 4. Discard if not used within 1 h.	1. Same as one-bottle method, but prepare day's supply at one time. 2. Refrigerate immediately after preparation.	1. Equipment includes glass or enamel pitcher, measuring cup and spoons, mixing spoons, funnel, can opener, tongs. 2. Sterilize bottles, nipples, nipple caps, and equipment by boiling for 10 min in pan or sterilizer half full of water. 3. Mix formula in pitcher. 4. Pour into bottles. 5. Put on nipples and caps. Refrigerate until needed.	1. Prepare as in clean method. 2. Apply nipples and caps loosely. 3. Place in sterilizer with water in bottom, and cover with tight-fitting lid. 4. Boil for 25 min. 5. Tighten nipple collars. 6. Refrigerate until needed.

For all methods, start by washing hands, formula can top, bottles, nipples, and equipment well.
Ready-to-feed and powdered formula can be prepared by any of the above methods.
Ready-to-feed formula needs no water or mixing.
For powdered formula, follow directions on can for proportions.

the powder in a clean bottle, then adding the water just before use. Once prepared, the formula should either be fed to the infant within 30 minutes or refrigerated. Formula should be discarded if it is not used within 1 hour or kept refrigerated.

Evaluation

Evaluating the nursing care of the formula-fed infant includes asking the mother to verbalize her understanding of the infant feeding process and observing how she holds the infant for feeding and assumes a comfortable position. The infant's response to feeding should also be evaluated. This includes verifying that the infant receives an appropriate amount of formula at an appropriate rate without swallowing a large amount of air. The nurse should evaluate nursing interventions by making sure that the mother is knowledgeable about her infant's nutritional needs, the typical amount of formula that the infant will take during a feeding, the types of available bottles and nipples, and the methods of preparing formula.

Common Concerns Related to Newborn Feeding

Several topics related to infant feeding are of concern to the new mother regardless of the method of feeding. Common areas of concern typically include hunger, bubbling (burping), regurgitation, and constipation.

Hunger

The mother may wonder how she will be able to tell if her infant is hungry and how she will know that her infant is getting enough to eat. The nurse can tell her that most infants, when awakened from sleep by hunger "pains," fuss and cry and make sucking movements with their mouths. However, infants may have difficulty distinguishing between hunger and other discomforts at first. If the infant awakens a short time after a feeding, the mother should try other comfort measures before assuming that the infant is hungry. These include holding the infant, changing the diaper, and bubbling. Occasionally, an infant appears hungry when he or she is only thirsty. A small amount of water will satisfy this infant. An infant who is frequently hungry and crying, refuses water with apparent disgust, and seizes the nipple ravenously and nurses with great vigor when a feeding is offered may either need to eat more frequently for a while if breast-fed or be offered more formula at each feeding if bottle fed.

Bubbling (Burping)

A baby should be bubbled after about 5 minutes of feeding or in the middle and at the end of each feeding. The bubbling technique consists of holding the infant in an upright position and gently patting or stroking the back. The infant should not be pounded on the back; this is neither effective nor conducive to his or her well-being. The change in position (from semireclining to upright) is an important factor in eliciting a bubble. Often, holding the infant upright and pressing him or her against the breast is all that is necessary.

An alternate position is for the mother to sit the infant up on her lap, with his or her chest resting on her hand and chin supported by her thumb and index finger, while she pats the infant with her other hand. A third position is to place the infant prone over the knees; the knee nearest the infant's head should be slightly elevated. The last two positions are sometimes preferred by nurses in the newborn nursery because they keep the infant away from the nurse's face and hair, which avoids cross-contamination from nurse to infant.

If the infant is being placed in his crib and the mother is in doubt about whether the infant has brought up all the air, the infant should be placed on his right side for a short time. This will help bring up the air and prevent the infant from choking on any milk that might be regurgitated with the air (Fig. 30-8).

Regurgitation

Regurgitation occurs because the newborn's gastrointestinal tract is unstable, so milk may be brought up with the gas bubbles. A cloth diaper is usually kept in front of the infant while he or she is being bubbled in case this occurs. Regurgitation, which is merely an overflow and often occurs after nursing, should not be

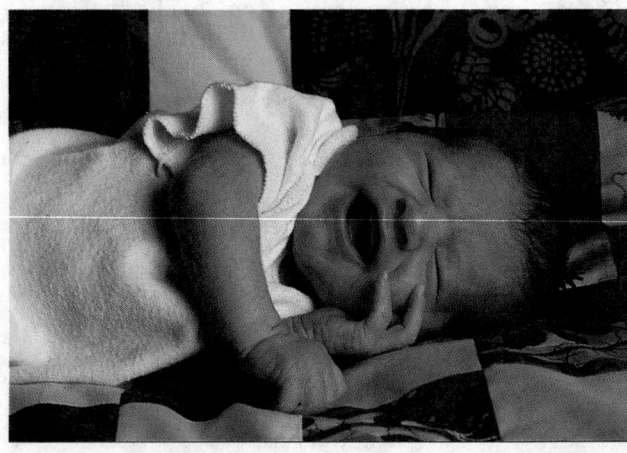

FIGURE 30-8 Placing infants on their side will help bring up any excess air and prevent the infant from choking on any milk that might be regurgitated with the air.

confused with vomiting. Vomiting may occur at any time, is accompanied by other symptoms, and usually involves a more complete emptying of the stomach. Regurgitation is simply a means of relieving the distended stomach. It usually indicates that the infant either has taken too much food or has taken it too rapidly.

Hiccups

Hiccups are not unusual for infants and do not seem to bother them. If the mother is disturbed, she can try giving the infant a few sips of water. However, hiccups will go away without treatment.

Constipation

Constipation is almost nonexistent in breast-fed infants and is uncommon in those fed commercially prepared formulas. However, mothers frequently express concern about possible constipation. Many parents believe that an infant is constipated if he or she does not have a bowel movement once a day. The nurse can explain that the consistency, not frequency, of the stool indicates the presence of constipation. Constipated stools are hard, formed, and difficult to pass.

Nutritional Considerations Throughout the First Year

During the first year of life, the infant's growth exceeds that of any future period. In the first 4 months, the birth weight usually doubles, and by 1 year, it may triple. However, the infant's caloric needs per unit of body weight are relatively constant during the first year. This is because as he or she becomes more physically active from the fourth month on, the rate of growth is slowing, and energy is relocated from growth to activity.

Introduction of Solid Foods

When solid foods should be added to the infant's diet has been the subject of much debate. Recommendations in the literature and actual practice often differ markedly. A breast-fed or formula-fed infant receives an adequate amount of all essential nutrients during the first 6 months without the addition of solid food. However, many infants in the United States receive solid foods at an earlier age. This early feeding often occurs because the parents think it helps their infant sleep through the night, or they consider it a sign that their infant is more advanced than infants who are only taking milk.

Many reasons are suggested for delaying the introduction of solids until the infant is 4 to 6 months old. First, the infant is not developmentally ready to deal with nonliquid foods until about the end of the third month; before this time, nonliquid food is usually pushed out of the mouth. Also, large protein molecules from solid foods may pass through the mucosa of the infant's immature gastrointestinal tract and become antigens. These antigens will sensitize the infant and cause allergic reactions. After 6 months, the gastrointestinal system is more mature, and the infant's antibody production has reached a more desirable level. In the breast-fed infant, early introduction of solid foods may interfere with the desire for breast milk, decrease the infant's sucking, and subsequently decrease the milk supply. Other drawbacks to early feeding of solids are the potential for not supplying the infant's nutritional needs, the relatively high cost of the food, and the possibility of overfeeding.

Infantile Obesity

Infantile obesity has become a growing concern in recent years because of its possible relation to adult obesity. Studies have shown mixed results in answering the question of the effect of infantile obesity (or the infant's diet) on adult obesity. There is evidence, however, that breast-feeding and late introduction of solid foods protects the infant from obesity, at least in the early years (Lawrence, 1994).

The nurse can provide the parents with some suggestions for avoiding obesity in their infant:

- Use factors other than weight gain to evaluate your role as parents.
- Discover your infant's satiety behavior, and avoid encouraging your infant to finish the last drop or bite.
- Recognize that not all your infant's needs are nutritional. Non-nutritive cuddling is important and can be implemented when the infant is not truly hungry.
- Promote physical activity in your infant. Infants should have freedom of movement as much as possible instead of being constantly restricted in infant carriers or swaddling.
- Avoid early introduction of solid food.

Nutritional Supplements

Vitamins

It is generally believed that breast milk and commercial formulas contain adequate vitamins for normal infants and that routine supplementation is unnecessary (Lawrence, 1994). However, some sources recommend a vitamin D supplement of 400 IU/d, just to be on the safe side. Breast-fed infants with dark skin or infants with little possibility of significant exposure to sunlight may be more likely to need vitamin D supplementation (Freeman et al., 1992). If the infant is fed a formula made of fresh or evaporated cow's milk, vitamin C, folic acid, and iron supplementation is necessary (California Department of Health Services, 1990).

Iron

Iron deficiency anemia is the most common nutritional deficiency encountered in infants and children between the ages of 6 and 30 months. Those from lower socioeconomic groups are particularly vulnerable. However, the incidence of iron deficiency has decreased since the introduction of iron-fortified formula (Bradley et al., 1993). Breast-fed infants rarely have iron deficiency anemia, and most authorities do not recommend iron supplementation until 4 to 6 months of age. At this age, iron-fortified infant cereal can be added to the infant's diet (Lawrence, 1994). For formula-fed infants, formula fortified at a level of 10 to 12 mg/dL of elemental iron is recommended beginning at birth and continuing until the infant is 12 months old (Freeman et al., 1992). Formula fortified with 7.5 mg/dL also results in adequate iron status (Bradley et al., 1994). These sources of iron should be adequate as long as they continue to be available to the infant.

Iron deficiency anemia often results because many infants are switched to fresh cow's milk by the time they are 6 months old. This causes two problems with the infant's iron levels. First, cow's milk is low in iron. Second, there is evidence that drinking fresh cow's milk during infancy is associated with microscopic blood loss from the intestine, which contributes to iron deficiency anemia (Lawrence, 1994).

Fluoride

Supplementation with fluoride for all breast-fed infants has been recommended in the past, because fluoride is found in only trace amounts in human milk. Current recommendations are to supplement with 0.25 mg beginning the first 2 weeks after birth, only if the local water supply has a fluoride concentration of less than 0.3 ppm. Bottle-fed infants would be supplemented according to the same recommendations (California Department of Health Services, 1990).

Summary Points

✔ The infant's basic nutritional needs can be met by either breast milk or commercial formula based on cow's milk and modified to approximate human milk.

✔ Breast milk contains vitamins and minerals in bioavailable forms and provides factors that are antibacterial, antiviral, antiprotozoan, anti-inflammatory, and antiallergenic.

✔ The nurse can play an important role in promoting lactation by encouraging early initiation of breast-feeding, assisting in positioning the mother and infant, and teaching the mother how to help the infant latch on to the breast and how to break suction at the end of the feeding.

✔ Infants who are breast-feeding may need to nurse every 2 hours or more at first, because colostrum and breast milk are more easily digested than formula, so the infant may be hungry sooner. This frequent stimulation also promotes the production of milk on a supply and demand basis.

✔ The sucking movements needed to remove milk from a bottle are different than those used to suckle from the breast, and changing from one to the other can be confusing for the infant.

✔ Anticipatory guidance from the nurse about common problems, such as nipple soreness and breast engorgement, can prevent or minimize many problems and promote a longer duration of breast-feeding.

✔ Mothers who are formula feeding their infants also need assistance with feeding techniques and information about the formulas available and how to prepare them correctly.

✔ Breast milk or iron-fortified formula are recommended as the infant's only food for the first 4 to 6 months of life and as the milk of choice for the first year.

✔ Breast milk and commercial formula are considered to be nutritionally adequate; however, vitamin D, iron, and fluoride supplements are sometimes given.

✔ Solid foods are added to the infant's diet between 4 to 6 months, when the infant's system is mature enough to handle nonliquid food. Iron-fortified cereal is an important source of iron at this time.

REFERENCES

Auerbach, K. G. (1984). Employed breastfeeding mothers: Problems they encounter. *BIRTH, 11*(1), 17–20.
Auerbach, K. G., Riordan, J., & Countryman, B. A. (1993). The breastfeeding process. In J. Riordan & K. G. Auerbach (Eds.), *Breastfeeding and human lactation* (pp. 215–252). Boston: Jones and Bartlett.

Benson, J. D., & MacLean, W. C., Jr. (1992). Composition of infant formula: Infusion of new knowledge. In M. F. Picciano & B. Lonnerdal (Eds.), *Mechanisms regulating lactation and infant nutrient utilization.* New York: Wiley-Liss.

Bradley, C. K., Hillman, L., Sherman, A. R., Leedy, D., & Cordano, A. (1993). Evaluation of two iron-fortified, milk-based formulas during infancy. *Pediatrics, 91,* 908–914.

Buchko, B., Puch, L. C., Bishop, B. A., Cochran, J. F., Smith, L. R., & Lerew, D. J. (1994). Comfort measures in breastfeeding, primiparous women. *Journal of Obstetric, Gynecologic, and Neonatal Nursing, 23,* 46–52.

California Department of Health Services-Maternal and Child Health Branch (1990). *Nutrition during pregnancy and the postpartum period: A manual for health care professionals.* Sacramento: Author.

Carpenito, L. J. (1995). *Nursing diagnosis: Application to clinical practice* (6th ed.). Philadelphia: J.B. Lippincott.

Cronenwett, L., Stukel, T., Kearney, M., Barrett, J., Covington, C., Del Monte, K., Reinhardt, R., & Rippe, L. (1992). Single daily bottle use in the early weeks postpartum and breastfeeding outcomes. *Pediatrics, 90,* 750–766.

Duncan, B., Ey, J., Holberg, C. J., Wright, A. L., Martinez, F. D., & Taussig, L. M. (1993). Exclusive breast-feeding for at least 4 months protects against otitis media. *Pediatrics, 91,* 867–872.

Fletcher, A. B. (1993). Nutrition. In G. B. Avery, M. B. Fletcher, & M. G. Macdonald (Eds.), *Neonatology: Pathophysiology and management of the newborn* (pp. 330–356) (4th ed.). Philadelphia: J.B. Lippincott.

Freeman, R. K., & Poland, R. L. (Eds.) (1992). *Guidelines for perinatal care* (3rd ed.). Elk Grove Village, IL: American Academy of Pediatrics and American College of Obstetricians and Gynecologists.

Henly, S. J., Anderson, C. M., Avery, M. D., Hills-Bonczyk, S. G. Potter, S., & Duckett, L. J. (1995). Anemia and insufficient milk in first-time mothers. *Birth, 22*(2), 87–95.

Henrikson, M., Wall, G., Lethbridge, D., & McClurg, V. (1992). Nursing diagnosis and obstetric, gynecologic, and neonatal nursing: Breastfeeding as an example. *Journal of Obstetric, Gynecologic, and Neonatal Nursing, 21,* 446–456.

Hill, P. D. (1991). The enigma of insufficient milk supply. *MCN: American Journal of Maternal Child Nursing, 16,* 312–316.

Hughes, R. B., Sauvain, K. J., Blanton, L. H. et al. (1987). Outcome of teaching clean vs terminal methods of formula preparation. *Pediatric Nursing, 13*(4), 275–276.

Institute of Medicine, National Academy of Sciences, Food and Nutrition Board (1991). *Nutrition during lactation.* Washington, DC: National Academy Press.

Jacobi, A. M., & Levin, M. (1993). Promotion and support of breastfeeding. In B. S. Worthington-Roberts & S. R. Williams (Eds.), *Nutrition in pregnancy and lactation* (pp. 402–461) (5th ed.). St. Louis: C.V. Mosby.

Kallio, M. J. T., Salmenpera, L., Siimes, M. A., Perheentupa, J., & Miettinen, T. A. (1992). Exclusive breast-feeding and weaning: Effect on serum cholesterol and lipoprotein concentrations in infants during the first year of life. *Pediatrics, 89,* 663–666.

Kearney, M. H., & Cronenwett, L. (1991). Breastfeeding and employment. *Journal of Obstetric, Gynecologic, and Neonatal Nursing, 20,* 471–480.

Lawrence, R. A. (1992). Can we expect greater intelligence from human milk feedings? *BIRTH, 19,* 105–106.

Lawrence, R. A. (1994). *Breastfeeding—A guide for the medical profession* (4th ed.). St. Louis: C.V. Mosby.

Lethbridge, D. J. (1988). The use of breastfeeding as a contraceptive. *Journal of Obstetric, Gynecologic, and Neonatal Nursing, 17*(1), 31–37.

Lethbridge, D. J., McClurg, V., Henrikson, M., & Wall, G. (1993). Validation of the nursing diagnosis of ineffective breastfeeding. *Journal of Obstetric, Gynecologic, and Neonatal Nursing, 22,* 57–63.

Livingston, C. (1993). From the editor. *International Journal of Childbirth Education, 8*(2), 2.

Lorick, G. (1993). Untimely weaning: Assisting the mother who may grieve. *International Journal of Childbirth Education, 8*(2), 41.

Lucas, A., Morley, R., Cole, T. J., Lister, G., & Leeson-Payne, C. (1992). Breast milk and subsequent intelligence quotient in children born preterm. *Lancet, 339,* 261–264.

Mennella, J. A., & Beuchamp, G. K. (1991). Maternal diet alters the sensory qualities of human milk and the nursling's behavior. *Pediatrics, 88,* 737.

Millard, A. V. (1990). The place of the clock in pediatric advice: Rationales, culture themes, and impediments to breastfeeding. *Soc Sci Med, 31*(2), 211–221.

Minchin, M. K. (1989). Positioning for breastfeeding. *BIRTH, 16*(2), 67–73, 76–80.

Moon, J. L., & Humenick, S. S. (1989). Breast engorgement: Contributing variables and variables amenable to nursing intervention. *Journal of Obstetric, Gynecologic, and Neonatal Nursing, 18,* 309–315.

National Research Council, Subcommittee on the Tenth Edition of the RDAs (1989). *Recommended dietary allowances.* Washington, DC: National Academy Press.

Neifert, M., DeMarzo, S., Seacat, J. et al. (1990). The influence of breast surgery, breast appearance, and pregnancy-induced breast changes on lactation sufficiency as measured by infant weight gain. *BIRTH, 17*(1), 31–38.

Neumann, C. C., & Jelliffe, D. B. (1977). Foreword: Symposium on Nutrition in Pediatrics. *Pediatric Clinics of North America, 24*(1), 1.

O'Campo, P., Faden, R. R., Gielen, A. C., & Wang, M. C. (1992). Prenatal factors associated with breastfeeding duration: Recommendations for prenatal interventions. *BIRTH, 19,* 195–201.

Righard, L., & Alade, M. O. (1990). Effect of delivery room routines on success of first breast-feed. *Lancet, 336,* 1105–1107.

Righard, L., & Alade, M. O. (1992). Sucking technique and its effect on success of breastfeeding. *BIRTH, 19,* 185–189.

Riordan, J. (1993a). Anatomy and psychophysiology of lactation. In J. Riordan & K. G. Auerbach (Eds.), *Breastfeeding and human lactation* (pp. 81–103). Boston: Jones and Bartlett.

Riordan, J. (1993b). The biologic specificity of breastmilk. In J. Riordan & K. G. Auerbach (Eds.), *Breastfeeding and human lactation* (pp. 105–134). Boston: Jones and Bartlett.

Riordan, J. (1993c). Child health. In J. Riordan & K. G. Auerbach (Eds.), *Breastfeeding and human lactation* (pp. 459–484). Boston: Jones and Bartlett.

Riordan, J. (1993d). The cultural context of breastfeeding. In J. Riordan & K. G. Auerbach (Eds.), *Breastfeeding and human lactation* (pp. 27–48). Boston: Jones and Bartlett.

Riordan, J. (1993e). The ill breastfeeding child. In J. Riordan & K. G. Auerbach (Eds.), *Breastfeeding and human lactation* (pp. 485–513). Boston: Jones and Bartlett.

Riordan, J., & Auerbach, K. G. (1993a). Breast related problems. In J. Riordan & K. G. Auerbach (Eds.), *Breastfeeding and human lactation* (pp. 379–400). Boston: Jones and Bartlett.

Riordan, J., & Auerbach, K. G. (1993b). Maternal Health. In J. Riordan & K. G. Auerbach (Eds.), *Breastfeeding and human lactation* (pp. 349–377). Boston: Jones and Bartlett.

Shrago, L., & Bocar, D. (1990). The infant's contribution to breastfeeding. *Journal of Obstetric, Gynecologic, and Neonatal Nursing, 19*(3), 209–215.

Smith, W. L., Erenberg, A., & Nowak, A. (1994). Imaging evaluation of the human nipple during breast-feeding. *AJDC, 142*, 76–78.

Temboury, M. C., Otero, A., Polanco, I., & Arribas, E. (1994). Influence of breast-feeding on the infant's intellectual development. *Journal of Pediatric Gastroenterology and Nutrition, 18*, 32–36.

Walker, M. (1989). Functional assessment of infant breast-feeding patterns. *BIRTH, 16*(3), 140–147.

Walker, M., & Auerbach, K. G. (1993). Breast pumps and other technologies. In J. Riordan & K. G. Auerbach (Eds.), *Breastfeeding and human lactation* (pp. 279–332). Boston: Jones and Bartlett.

Worthington-Roberts, B. S. (1993). Lactation: Basic considerations. In B. S. Worthington-Roberts & S. R. Williams (Eds.), *Nutrition in pregnancy and lactation* (pp. 316–346) (5th ed.). St. Louis: C.V. Mosby.

Young, D. (1995). Baby-friendly expert work group in the United States: Blowing the whistle (editorial). *BIRTH, 22*, 59–62.

Ziemer, M. M., Paone, J. P., Schupay, J., & Cole, E. (1990). Methods to prevent and manage nipple pain in breastfeeding women. *Western Journal of Nursing Research, 12*, 732–744.

SUGGESTED READINGS

Briggs, G. G., Freeman, R. K., & Yaffe, S. J. (1994). *Drugs in pregnancy and lactation* (4th ed.). Baltimore: Williams & Wilkins.

Brown, L. P., Arnold, L., Allison, D., Klein, M. E., & Jacobsen, B. (1993). Incidence and pattern of jaundice in healthy breast-fed infants during the first month of life. *Nursing Research, 42*, 106–110.

Cunningham, A. S., Jelliffe, D. B., & Jelliffe, E. F. P. (1991). Breast-feeding and health in the 1980s: A global epidemiologic review. *The Journal of Pediatrics, 118*, 659–665.

Janke, R. R. (1994). Development of the breast-feeding attrition prediction tool. *Nursing Research, 43*, 100–104.

Jensen, D., Wallace, S., & Kelsay, P. (1994). LATCH: A breastfeeding charting system and documentation tool. *Journal of Obstetric, Gynecologic, and Neonatal Nursing, 23*, 27–32.

Kearney, M. H., Cronenwett, L. R., & Barrett, J. A. (1990). Breast-feeding problems in the first week postpartum. *Nursing Research, 39*(2), 90–95.

Walker, M., & Driscoll, J. W. (1989). Sore nipples: The new mother's nemesis. *MCN: American Journal of Maternal Child Nursing, 14*, 260–265.

Ziegler, E. E. (1992). Growth and body composition of breast-fed and formula-fed infants: Inferences regarding nutrient intakes. In M. F. Picciano & B. Lonnerdal (Eds.), *Mechanisms regulating lactation and infant nutrient utilization*. New York: Wiley-Liss.

Ziemer, M. M., & Pigeon, J. G. (1993). Skin changes and pain in the nipple during the 1st week of lactation. *Journal of Obstetric, Gynecologic, and Neonatal Nursing, 22*, 247–256.

Assessment and Management in the Postpartum Period

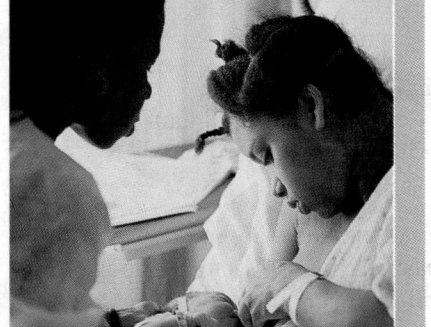

Critical Thinking Exercises

1. You are teaching a group of postpartum clients about physiologic changes that they may be experiencing during this time. Develop a teaching plan that addresses each of these changes, relating the specific physiologic adaptations that have occurred in pregnancy.

2. Mark and Linda Placito are preparing to take their first baby home. They are excited but anxious about all the changes that will be occurring. The husband has taken 2 weeks vacation from work to spend time with his wife and the new baby. The couple's parents live nearby and are planning to visit frequently.

   How would you counsel this couple in making a successful role transition to parenthood?

3. Lisa Webster states that she wants to breast-feed her infant but is concerned because she has such small breasts and is afraid that the infant won't get enough milk. "My sister had to stop breast-feeding because of this."

   What aspects would you address with this client and how would you counsel her so that she has a positive experience.

4. Leslie and Bill Jackson are taking their newborn son, Will, home. They have read and heard a lot about the importance of infant stimulation. They are concerned about how to provide the appropriate type and amount of stimulation to enrich their son's growth and development.

   What topics would you address with this couple and how would you instruct them; be sure to include specific suggestions for appropriate activities and toys.

Multiple Choice Questions

1. Based on the nurse's knowledge about after pains, the nurse would anticipate that afterpains are most likely to occur in a:

A. Primigravid client
B. Multigravid client
C. Client who is bottle feeding
D. Client who had a cesarean delivery

2. Following a normal vaginal delivery approximately 24 hours ago, the nurse assesses the uterus to be approximately 1 fingerbreadth below the umbilicus. The nurse should:

A. Massage the fundus
B. Assess for a full bladder
C. Continue routine monitoring
D. Notify the physician

3. A client who has decided to bottle feed her infant is experiencing breast engorgement. The nurse instructs the client to do which of the following?

A. Apply warm soaks every 2 to 3 hours
B. Manually express the milk
C. Wear a tight brassiere
D. Restrict oral fluids

4. The nurse instructs a client who has decided to breast-feed about proper nipple care. Which of the following statements indicates effective teaching?

A. "I will wash my nipples with soap and water before each feeding"
B. "I will keep my nipples clean and dry"
C. "I will use plastic breast shields to protect my nipples"
D. "I will use an antiseptic solution four times a day"

5. Immediately after delivery, a client with a mediolateral episiotomy complains of perineal discomfort. An appropriate nursing intervention would be to:

A. Administer bromocriptine mesylate
B. Apply heat
C. Apply ice
D. Administer oxytocin

6. When instructing the mother in breast-feeding, the nurse recommends that the mother allow the infant to nurse at each breast for at least:

   A. 2 to 3 minutes
   B. 3 to 5 minutes
   C. 5 to 7 minutes
   D. 10 to 15 minutes

7. Approximately 8 hours after delivery, the nurse notes that the client's temperature is elevated to 100° F. Heart rate is within normal limits. The nurse identifies the nursing diagnosis of hyperthermia related to:

   A. Postpartal diuresis
   B. Bladder distention
   C. Vaginal infection
   D. Uterine infection

8. Following a vaginal delivery, the nurse instructs the client about how to perform Kegel exercises. The statement that best illustrates the client's understanding about the rational for these exercises is:

   A. "These exercises will help improve my breathing"
   B. "These exercises will help strengthen my perineal muscles"
   C. "These exercises will help strengthen my calf muscles"
   D. "These exercises will help tone up my abdomen"

9. The nurse is preparing a teaching plan for a client who delivered approximately 24 hours ago. Which of the following should the nurse include as a danger sign to report?

   A. Bright red lochia and increased flow
   B. Fatigue and weight loss
   C. Vaginal dryness when sexual activity is resumed
   D. Uterus no longer palpable after 2 weeks

10. While assessing a 6 hour old neonate, the nurse identifies which of the following as problematic?

    A. Anterior fontanel open
    B. Irregular abdominal respirations
    C. Dusky color
    D. Not yet passed meconium

11. A client who breast fed her first child plans to bottle feed her new infant. The nurse should instruct the mother that the stools of her bottle fed infant will be:

    A. Looser and lighter green in color
    B. Same as those of her breast fed infant
    C. Thicker and darker yellow in color
    D. Passed more frequently

12. A new mother asks the nurse about how she will know if her breast fed infant is getting enough to eat. Which of the following outcomes identified on the teaching plan would be appropriate?

    A. The neonate will wet 4 to 6 diapers within 24 hours
    B. The neonate will feed every 4 hours
    C. The neonate will exhibit steady weight gain
    D. The neonate will burp after each feeding

13. Postpartally, the client begins to show acceptance of the neonate as a individual. The nurse interprets that this client is in which phase of maternal adaptation?

    A. Taking in
    B. Taking hold
    C. Dependent
    D. Letting go

Study Questions

1. Define involution.

2. Name the three stages of lochia.

3. Explain the physiologic basis for constipation in the postpartum period.

4. List the preconditions necessary for attachment.

5. By what postpartal day should the fundus no longer be palpable?

6. Identify four mechanisms the neonates uses to conserve and produce heat.

7. Define Epstein's pearls.

8. Explain the physiologic basis for breast engorgement in the neonate.

9. Identify the physical characteristics assessed as part of a gestational age assessment.

10. List the six categories in Brazelton's behavioral assessment.

11. Name the hormone involved with the let down reflex.

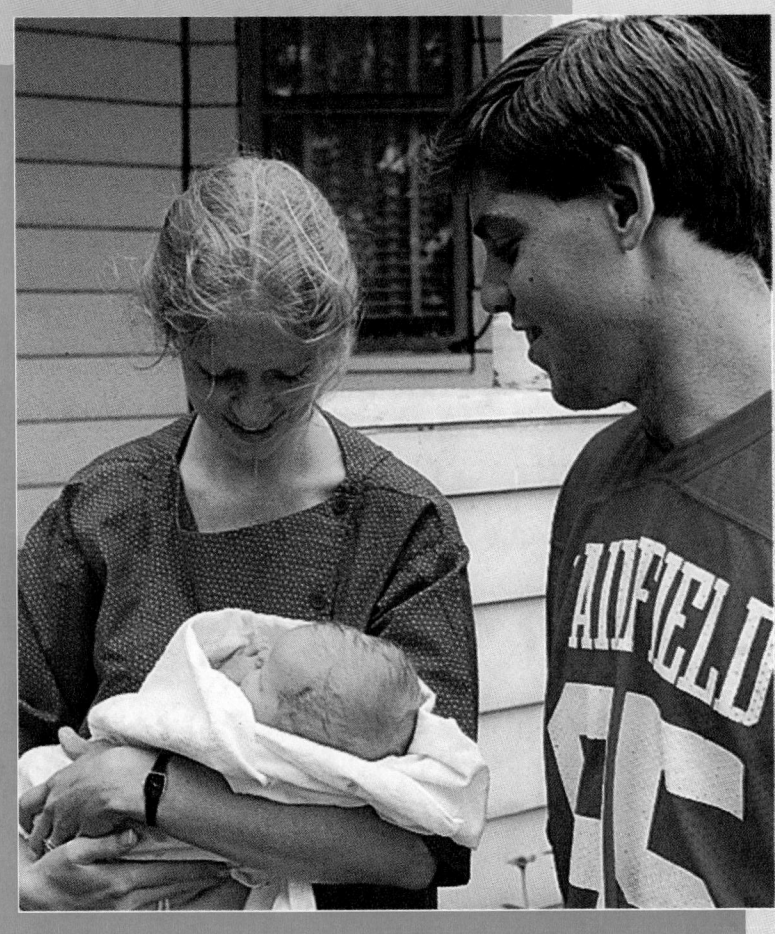

Assessment and Management of High-Risk Maternal Conditions

VII

31

Gestational Related Complications

Objectives

- Define hyperemesis gravidarum, and explain the underlying pregnancy changes that might cause this condition.
- Identify the three most common causes of bleeding in early pregnancy.
- Discuss the management of the client experiencing bleeding early in pregnancy.
- Compare and contrast placenta previa and abruptio placentae.
- Describe the pathophysiology of disseminated intravascular coagulation.
- List the classifications for hypertensive disorders in pregnancy, including the main differentiating characteristic.
- Discuss the current therapeutic regimen for mild and severe preeclampsia and eclampsia.
- Identify the major pathologic problems involved with hemolysis, elevated liver enzymes, and low platelets syndrome.

Childbearing is usually considered a normal process. However, problems can occur during the pregnancy that alter its normal course. Therefore, early and frequent health surveillance is necessary to determine any significant threats to maternal and fetal well-being, allowing for timely intervention and the achievement of a good outcome for the woman and fetus.

Complications associated with pregnancy can be divided into two broad categories: those related solely to pregnancy and concurrent disorders and conditions existing prior to or occuring suddenly during pregnancy. Such non–pregnancy-induced conditions are described in Chapter 32.

Although there are only a few major complications exclusively related to pregnancy, they may present serious health hazards. These complications, which are discussed in this chapter, include the following: hyperemesis gravidarum, hemorrhagic complications of early pregnancy, hemorrhagic complications of late pregnancy, and hypertensive disorders of pregnancy.

Hyperemesis Gravidarum

Mild nausea and vomiting are common and normal early pregnancy. However, when it become excessive, pathologic effects may result. **Hyperemesis gravidarum** or **pernicious vomiting** refers to excessive nausea and vomiting that results in fluid and electrolyte imbalance, marked weight loss, acetonuria, and nutritional deficits. Although mild nausea and vomiting between the 5th and 12th weeks affect 50% to 80% of pregnant women, hyperemesis gravidarum occurs in only approximately 1% to 2% of pregnancies (Blackburn et al., 1992).

Manifestations and Causes

The pregnant woman with hyperemesis gravidarum displays a diversity of signs and symptoms. Although the exact cause is unknown, various factors, such as hormonal and psychological factors, have been associated with the development of this condition.

Clinical Picture

In the clinical picture of the pregnant woman suffering from mild nausea, the first symptom occurs during her first trimester and is usually most pronounced when arising in the morning, hence the term "morning sickness." However, it also may occur at other times of the day. Normally, this pattern persists for a few weeks and then suddenly ceases.

A small number of women who have morning sickness develop persistent vomiting that lasts for 4 to 8 weeks or longer. These women vomit several times a day and may be unable to retain any liquid or solid foods, resulting in possible dehydration and starvation. Diminished urinary output and dryness of the skin are symptoms of dehydration. Hypovolemia with associated hypotension may result if dehydration is not corrected.

Starvation, which is regularly present, manifests itself in a number of ways. Weight loss may vary from 5 lb to as much as 20 or 30 lb, depending on the duration and severity of the condition. In these clinical situations, digestion and absorption of carbohydrates and other nutrients have been so inadequate that the body has been forced to burn its reserve stores of fat to maintain body heat and energy. When carbohydrates are not available, fat is burned for energy. However, the process of combustion is not completed. Consequently, certain incompletely burned by-products of fat metabolism appear in the blood and the urine (eg, ketosis [presence of excessive ketones]). In severe cases, considerable changes associated with starvation and dehydration become evident in the blood chemistry, including an increase in the nonprotein nitrogen, uric acid, and urea and a moderate decrease in the chlorides. Vitamin starvation is typically present, and in extreme cases, when marked vitamin B deficiency exists, polyneuritis occasionally develops, resulting in disturbances of the peripheral nerves.

Causes

The exact cause of hyperemesis gravidarum is unknown; however, certain organic processes underlie all cases of vomiting, regardless of whether the symptoms are mild or severe. The endocrine imbalance created by a high level of chorionic gonadotropins and estrogens, metabolic changes of normal gestation, fragments of chorionic villi entering the maternal circulation, and the diminished motility of the stomach are believed to cause the clinical symptoms (Blackburn et al., 1992).

Because of the absence of a demonstrable pathologic explanation for the problem, some believe there is a psychological basis for excessive vomiting. Some theorists have proposed that hyperemesis gravidarum is related to the woman's ambivalence and difficulty in psychologically adjusting to pregnancy and the mothering role.

Medical Diagnosis and Prognosis

The technical definition of hyperemesis gravidarum is intractable vomiting beginning before the 20th week of pregnancy and resulting in disturbed nutritional status. Altered electrolyte balance, dehydration, weight loss of 5% or more of prepregnancy weight, ketosis, and acetonuria provide clinical evidence of altered nutritional state (Long et al., 1993).

Appropriate diagnostic testing should be performed to detect underlying causes of nausea and vomiting, such as gastroenteritis, hepatitis, cholecystitis, or peptic ulcer, which may contribute to the hyperemetic status of the pregnant woman.

Perinatal outcome may be improved through early treatment to prevent significant maternal weight loss. Studies have shown that the incidence of fetal growth retardation was significantly greater in patients with hyperemesis who had lost more than 5% of their prepregnant weight (Gross et al., 1989). Serious cases of hyperemesis gravidarum are rare, and recovery is usually rapid once fluid and electrolyte balance is restored.

Medical Management

Medical management is directed toward preventing significant weight loss, correcting fluid and electrolyte imbalance, and treating acidosis or alkalosis. The goals of intervention follow:

- To treat the dehydration by liberal administration of parenteral fluids (approximately 3,000 mL in 24 hours)
- To reverse starvation by administering intravenous (IV) glucose and thiamine chloride subcutaneously and, if necessary, by feeding a high-caloric, high-vitamin fluid diet enterally (nasogastric tube) or by the parenteral hyperalimentation method
- To stop vomiting by administering antiemetics

- To treat the emotional component with an understanding attitude (supportive measures)

Ideally, the client can be treated at home with frequent, small feedings; avoidance of spicy food and symptom-provoking stimuli; and prescribed medications of antiemetics or antihistamines, such as pyridoxine (vitamin B_6) 10 to 30 mg/d and chlorpromazine (Thorazine) 10 to 25 mg every 4 to 6 hours. If electrolyte disturbances are present or outpatient treatment fails, hospitalization is required. IV hydration with a low-dose infusion of promethazine (Phenergan) can be used in doses of 10 to 25 mg/L five to six times per day for more than 48 hours after vomiting. In refractory patients with persistent weight loss and ketosis, enteral and parenteral hyperalimentation may be necessary. Oral intake of fluids is restricted until the nausea and vomiting subside.

Initially, IV therapy may be tried in an outpatient setting to correct mild to moderate dehydration. A solution of dextrose with saline is commonly used. Potassium and vitamins are added if vomiting has been prolonged. If weight gain is inadequate, supplemental nutritional treatment is crucial to prevent severe fat and protein depletion. Supplemental nurtrition can be administered either enterally or parentally, depending on the patient's condition. Total parenteral nutrition (TPN) may be prescribed peripherally or using a central venous line if extensive long-term nutritional needs exist. Occassionally, the woman with hyperemesis may be unable to respond successfully to treatment (Long et al., 1993).

Nursing Assessment

During the initial contact with the woman with hyperemesis, the nurse should assess the client's pattern of nausea and vomiting, including onset, duration, frequency, and predictability. Results of laboratory studies should be carefully reviewed for evidence of hemoconcentration (elevated hemoglobin and hematocrit), fluid and electrolyte imbalances (decreased sodium, potassium, and chloride), and vitamin deficiency (B and folate). Electrolyte imbalances and vitamin deficiencies should be corrected with IV fluids and parenteral vitamins before the client receives TPN (Long et al., 1993).

The client's current weight should be measured and compared with her nonpregnant weight. Questions should focus on the client's activities for daily living, lifestyle, and attitudes about herself and the pregnancy. A detailed nutritional history, including dietary habits, should be obtained. This information is then compared with findings on physical examination, such as changes in skin turgor, energy level, and color of mucous membranes, which indicate dehydration.

Nursing Diagnosis

Assessment of the client with signs and symptoms of hyperemesis gravidarum may lead the nurse to specific nursing diagnoses. For a list of possible nursing diagnoses, see Box 31-1.

Nursing Intervention

The nurse must carefully monitor the client's intake and output during the course of hospitalization. Generally, oral intake is restricted; however, once vomiting ceases, oral feedings are started. Various approaches are used to restore oral intake. Small quantities of dry food (eg, crackers or toast) may be given hourly, alternating with small quantities (1 oz) of water. This is followed by a progression to clear liquids. If clear liquids and dry food are tolerated well, the client may advance slowly to a soft diet and finally, to a normal diet. When preparing solid foods, the nurse should arrange the portions attractively and in small amounts. The nurse also should be aware of the effects that food odors have on the woman and work with the client to eliminate offending odors.

The nurse should obtain daily weights to evaluate the client's progress. Together with other members of the healthcare team, daily calorie requirements are determined, based on ideal body weight with the addition of 300 nonprotein calories per day to meet energy requirements for pregnancy. Weight gain is considered the most important indication of maternal nutrition and fetal growth. Glucose tolerance should be checked by daily serum glucose levels or bedside finger stick blood glucose monitoring every 4 to 6 hours (Wolk et al., 1991).

If the client is receiving IV fluid replacement or parenteral nutrition, care and monitoring of the infusion are essential. Because a major side effect of peripheral parenteral nutrition is phlebitis, occurring in 5% of all patients, IV catheter sites should be monitored closely for pain, redness, or edema. IV tubing should be changed daily, or at least every 48 hours, and IV sites changed according to agency protocol.

A hygienic environment is important for the client. Quick removal of emesis from the client's room and use of room deodorizers will decrease noxious odors that may disturb appetite and diminish food appeal.

Psychological support is most effectively provided by the nurse who demonstrates an understanding and empathetic manner. A calm and nonjudgmental attitude may facilitate the client's verbalizations of any psychological conflicts concerning family, financial, or social difficulties (see Nursing Care Plan: Hyperemesis Gravidarum).

Nursing Evaluation

Anticipated outcomes of nursing care include the following:

- The client verbalizes the effects of hyperemesis gravidarum on perinatal outcome and of treatment to prevent complications.
- The client responds to oral or peripheral nutrition or TPN and ceases vomiting.
- The client shows a positive weight gain.
- The client maintains skin integrity.
- The client verbalizes positive coping mechanisms.

Hemorrhagic Complication of Early Pregnancy

The causes of bleeding in pregnancy are usually considered in relation to the stage of gestation in which they are most likely to cause complications. Frequent causes of bleeding during the first half of pregnancy include abortion, ectopic pregnancy, and hydatidiform mole. The two most common causes of hemorrhage in the latter half of pregnancy are placenta previa and abruptio placentae.

Abortion

Abortion refers to the termination of pregnancy by any means before the fetus is sufficiently developed to

---

BOX 31–1
Nursing Diagnoses—Hyperemesis Gravidarum

- Maternal-fetal fluid volume deficit related to the following:
    - Excessive fluid losses from vomiting
    - Inadequate fluid intake
- Altered Nutrition: Less than body requirements related to persistent nausea and vomiting
- Risk for Activity Intolerance related to weakness from inadequate nutrition and increased energy demands of pregnancy
- Knowledge Deficit related to the condition, etiology, and treatment
- Anxiety related to effects of hyperemesis on fetal well-being
- Risk for Impaired Skin Integrity related to dehydration from excessive vomiting
- Ineffective Individual Coping related to difficulty accepting the pregnancy
- Ineffective Family Coping: Compromised related to client's illness and separation during hospitalization

NURSING CARE PLAN
Hyperemesis Gravidarum

Nursing Goals

The woman with pernicious vomiting (hyperemesis gravidarum) will maintain nutritional health of self and fetus throughout pregnancy as evidenced by:
1. Reducing and eliminating nausea and vomiting.
2. Restoring circulatory volume and fluid and electrolyte balance.
3. Preserving skin integrity.
4. Coping with the psychological tasks of pregnancy and motherhood.
5. Continuing fetal growth and development.

Assessment	Potential Nursing Diagnoses	Intervention/ Rationale	Evaluation

History
  Onset, duration, and
    frequency of vomiting
    episodes
  Prepregnancy weight
  Current weight
  Previous eating disorder
Laboratory
  Blood
    Electrolytes
      (decreased)
    Hemoglobin and
      hematocrit
      (elevated)
    *p*H (acidosis, alkalosis)
    BUN (increased)
AST (elevated)
  Urine
    Ketones (present)
    Specific gravity
      (elevated)
	Altered Nutrition: Less than body requirements related to pernicious vomiting	Restrict or limit oral intake until vomiting ceases *to maintain electrolyte balance and prevent further vomiting.*
		Offer antiemetic medications as ordered, eg, low-dose Phenergan infusion—10–25 mg/L for 5–6 days and at least 48 h after vomiting *to maintain electrolyte balance and prevent further vomiting.*
		Initiate and maintain IV therapy *to correct hypovolemia and electrolyte imbalance*
		Record intake and output, including emesis *to assess hydration*
		Record daily weights *to assess loss of undue weight.*
			Client responds to restricted intake by ending her vomiting
			Client's electrolyte imbalances and hypovolemia are corrected
			
			Client's urine output remains greater than 30 mL/h
			Client ceases weight loss and begins to gain weight

Other diagnostic tests
  Liver function
  Renal function
  Gastric function
		Initiate total parenteral nutrition (TPN) if unable to establish oral feedings for prolonged period *to maintain nutritional balance*
		Advance diet slowly to clear liquids, soft foods, and solid foods, respectively (if client tolerates oral feedings); arrange food attractively in small quantities *to return client to normal oral intake and prevent exacerbation of vomiting.*
			Client receives TPN as needed
			
			Client consumes diet that adequately meets nutritional demands of pregnancy

Integrity of skin
  Pressure sores
  Turgor
  Color (jaundice, pallor)
  Dryness
  Thinness
		Inspect mouth for irritation or lesions *to insure oral mucosal integrity*
		Assist with oral and personal hygiene and offer frequent mouthwashes *to insure oral mucosal integrity*
			Client's mouth remains free of irritation and lesions

(continued)

NURSING CARE PLAN (Continued)
Hyperemesis Gravidarum

Assessment	Potential Nursing Diagnoses	Intervention/Rationale	Evaluation

Integrity of oral cavity
  Tenderness
  Redness
  Lesions
		Explain effects of condition on skin integrity and oral cavity; emphasize importance of preventive intervention *to provide information to client to insure skin/mucosal integrity*	Client maintains good personal and oral hygiene
			Client's skin retains its integrity

History
  Planned vs. unplanned pregnancy
  Financial difficulties
  Interpersonal conflicts in family
Communication patterns
  Ability to verbalize feelings
  Maintenance of eye contact
  Nonverbal behaviors
Achievement of the psychological tasks of pregnancy
	Ineffective Coping with the psychological tasks of pregnancy and motherhood	Control environment by restricting or limiting visitors as necessary *to allay anxiety*
		
		Assist client in achieving the psychological tasks of pregnancy *to insure psychological integrity*
		Offer psychological support *to allay anxiety and promote trust*
		Provide positive reinforcement for concerns expressed about pregnancy and fetal well-being *to promote psychological well being*
		Refer for mental health services if necessary *to promote mental health*
		Refer to social worker for socioeconomic assistance if necessary *to promote social well being*
			Client relaxes and remains calm
			
			Client begins achieving the psychological tasks of pregnancy
			
			Client indicates her trust in the nurse
			
			Client verbalizes feeling about pregnancy and fetal well-being
			
			Client accepts referral sources of assistance

Pregnancy test positive High level of hCG Fetal heart tones (Doppler) Fundal height	Altered Fetal Nutrition related to maternal malnourishment	Explain purposes and prepare for diagnostic tests as indicated (eg, sonography) *to allay anxiety and promote compliance* Monitor fetal heart tones, fetal movement (if present), fundal height, *to assess fetal well being*	Client indicates her understanding of diagnostic tests and follows instructions Fetus retains normal fetal heart tones Fetal movement is present Client shows growth in fundal height

survive. In the United States, this definition is confined to the period before the 20th week of the pregnancy or the delivery of a fetus weighing <500 g (about 1 lb, which is 454 g; Cunningham et al., 1993). The term *miscarriage* is commonly used by lay people to denote an abortion that has occurred spontaneously, rather than one that has been medically induced. Spontaneous abortions occur in 10% to 15% of all pregnancies (Bennett, 1992).

A birth classified as an abortion is not the same as a preterm birth. **Preterm birth** refers to the termination of pregnancy, spontaneously or therapeutically, after the fetus is viable but before it has attained full term, that is before the end of 37 weeks' gestation (Mattson et al., 1993).

Types of Abortion

The term abortion may be subdivided into two main groups: spontaneous and induced. In **spontaneous abortion**, the process starts of its own accord through natural causes. An **induced abortion** is artificially induced, whether for therapeutic or other reasons. Induced abortion is discussed in Chapter 12. Spontaneous abortions can be further subdivided based on the signs and symptoms presented. These subdivisions include *threatened, inevitable, complete, missed, recurrent, and illegal* (Box 31-2).

Manifestations and Causes

Several studies have shown that if a live, appropriately grown fetus is present at 8 weeks' gestation, the fetal loss rate at less than 28 weeks is 2% if the woman is older than 30 years and is 5% to 10% if the woman is older than 40 years (Bennett, 1992). Spontaneous abortions generally occur 1 to 3 weeks after the death of the embryo or fetus.

Clinical Picture. Almost invariably the first symptom is bleeding due to the separation of the fertilized ovum from its uterine attachment. The bleeding is often slight at the beginning and possibly persists for days before uterine cramps occur, or the bleeding may be followed immediately by cramps. Occasionally, slight bleeding may persist for weeks. The uterine contractions soften and dilate the cervix and lead to either complete or incomplete expulsion of the products of conception.

Causes. The etiology of spontaneous abortion is varied and often is nature's way of extinguishing imperfect embryos. Microscopic study of the material passed in these cases shows that the most common cause of spontaneous abortion is an inherent defect in the products of conception. This defect may express itself in an abnormal embryo, an abnormal trophoblast, or both.

In first-trimester abortions, 80% are associated with some defect of the embryo or trophoblast that is either incompatible with life or would result in a grossly deformed child. The incidence of abnormalities due to chromosomal errors in the second trimester is about 53% (Cunningham et al., 1993). It is usually difficult, if not impossible, to determine whether the germ plasma of the spermatozoon or the ovum is at fault in these cases. Abortions of this sort are not preventable.

Spontaneous abortions may result from causes other than defects in the products of conception. Severe acute infections, such as pneumonia, pyelitis, and typhoid fever, often lead to abortion. Endocrine disorders affecting progesterone and estrogen levels may alter

---

BOX 31-2
Types of Abortions and Related Symptoms

Threatened abortion	Vaginal bleeding or spotting occurring in early pregnancy that may or may not be associated with mild cramps; closed cervix; the process may abate or result in an abortion.
Inevitable abortion	The above process has progressed such that termination of the pregnancy cannot be prevented; bleeding is moderate to copious; uterine cramping is moderate to severe; the membranes may or may not have ruptured; the cervical canal is dilating.
Incomplete abortion	Part of the products of conception has been passed, but part (usually the placenta) is retained in the uterus; heavy bleeding usually persists until the retained products of conception have been passed; uterine cramping is severe; the cervix is open, with tissue present.
Complete abortion	All of the products of conception have been expelled; bleeding is slight; uterine cramping is mild.
Missed abortion	The fetus dies in utero but is retained; regression in uterine growth and breast changes are present; if 6 weeks or more elapse between fetal death and expulsion, degenerative changes occur (eg, maceration [general softening], mummification [drying up into a leather-like structure] and, rarely, lithopedion formation [stony material]); symptoms, except for amenorrhea, are usually lacking; malaise, headache, and anorexia are occasionally present; hypofibrinogenemia may result; the condition may be discovered because fundal height fails to increase, or fetal heart tones are absent.
Recurrent abortion	Spontaneous abortion occurs in successive pregnancies (three or more).
Illegal abortion	Termination of pregnancy outside of appropriate medical facilities (eg, hospitals or clinics), generally by nonphysician abortionists; the frequency of such abortions is not precisely known but has dropped precipitously in the United States because of legalized abortion; the method may involve ingestion of drugs, such as quinine or castor oil, or the placement of a foreign body, such as a urethral catheter, into the uterus with or without the instillation of toxic substances; severe infection, often with shock and renal failure, may result.

the endometrial lining of the uterus and result in abortion. Occasionally, abnormalities of the genital tract, such as a congenitally short cervix or uterine malformations, can result in an abortion. Abortion also is common in women whose mothers were treated with diethylstilbestrol during pregnancy. Retroposition of the uterus rarely causes abortion, as was formerly believed.

Many women explain abortion as a result of an injury or excessive activity. Women exhibit the greatest variation in this respect. In some women, pregnancy may continue despite falls, automobile accidents, and different trauma. In others, a trivial fall, anxiety, or overfatigue may be related to abortion, but there is no way to determine a cause and effect relationship.

Medical Diagnosis and Prognosis

Determining the cause of vaginal bleeding in early pregnancy is essential for accurate diagnosis. The vagina and cervix are carefully inspected to ascertain possible causes of the bleeding and to determine if the cervix is dilated.

Ultrasound can be used to differentiate between a live fetus and a pregnancy that will end in spontaneous abortion. Prognosis is evaluated by ultrasound markers that can explain bleeding and distinguish between harmless and ominous blood loss. The accompanying clinical symptoms of pelvic cramping and low back pain suggest spontaneous abortion.

Current prognostic opinions are based on the results of studies done during the last decade. One interesting study revealed that in women with scant bleeding that lasts less than 3 days and with a normal obstetric ultrasound, the risk of pregnancy failure is lower than in women who bleed for 3 days or more and have at least one abnormality on ultrasound examination (Mantoni, 1985). However, other studies have shown that threatened abortion was significantly correlated with the risk of spontaneous premature birth or the term delivery of a low–birth-weight newborn (Hert et al., 1985). Additional associated maternal complications include preeclampsia, placenta previa, abruptio placentae, and breech delivery.

Medical Management

The pregnant woman should contact her physician or midwife whenever bleeding occurs during pregnancy. The client may be kept at home, and bed rest and sexual abstinence may be prescribed. Occasionally, sedatives are ordered to promote relaxation. If bleeding becomes copious and is accompanied by cramps or uterine contractions, hospitalization may be recommended. IV therapy for fluid replacement or blood transfusions are prescribed as necessary.

In cases of **incomplete abortion**, when only part of the products of conception have been passed, efforts are made to aid the uterus in emptying its contents. Because there is a danger of maternal hemorrhage, oxytocin may be administered. If this is ineffective, surgical removal of the retained products of conception should be done promptly. Many times the tissue is loose in the cervical canal and can simply be lifted out with ovum forceps; otherwise, *dilatation and curettage* (D&C) of the uterine cavity or vacuum extraction may be necessary.

In cases of **missed abortion**, when the fetus has died but is retained, the products of conception are often spontaneously expelled within 4 to 5 weeks of fetal death. If this does not occur, surgical removal of the abortus is necessary. If symptoms of infection (eg, fever, foul discharge) are present, evacuation of the uterus should be delayed only long enough to obtain appropriate studies (especially smears and cultures) and to initiate antibiotic therapy. Such prompt and aggressive management effectively reduces the incidence of more serious complications, such as septic shock, thrombophlebitis, renal failure. Rh_o (D) immune globulin (RhoGAM) should be administered within 72 hours after any abortion for Rh-negative women who have not been previously sensitized.

Nursing Assessment

Bleeding in the first half of pregnancy, no matter how slight, must be considered a possible *threatened abortion*. The nurse must first obtain a detailed, accurate history, including length of gestation; source of prenatal supervision; onset, duration, and intensity of the bleeding episode; and any changes in bleeding with activity levels. The client should be asked to describe the quantity of bleeding in amounts to which she can relate (eg, a teaspoon, one-half cup). Characteristics of the blood loss (eg, bright red or dark brown, with or without tissue fragments or mucus, malodorous, steady trickling, or intermittent spotting) must similarly be assessed and if the bleeding has increased or decreased since its onset. The presence, nature, and location of accompanying discomforts, such as cramping, dull or sharp pain, and dizziness, also are evaluated.

Assessment of blood loss for hospitalized women often includes weighing perineal pads before and after use and then subtracting to find the difference (see Research Highlight). When tissue is present on the pad, it is useful to examine the pad for products of conception to ascertain whether the abortion is complete. Frequent assessment for symptoms of hypovolemia, such as syncope, should be done. Appropriate safeguards for syncopal episodes, such as no unaccompanied ambulation, should be in place until the bleeding is controlled. When blood loss is a slow "trickle" and occurs

RESEARCH HIGHLIGHT

Estimating Blood Loss

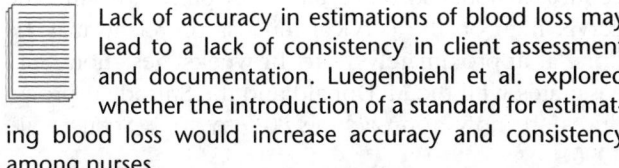 Lack of accuracy in estimations of blood loss may lead to a lack of consistency in client assessment and documentation. Luegenbiehl et al. explored whether the introduction of a standard for estimating blood loss would increase accuracy and consistency among nurses.

A sample of 42 staff members and student nurse volunteers from the obstetric, gynecologic, and neonatal units were asked to estimate blood loss from predetermined measured amounts on 24 peripads, 12 from brand C and 12 from brand G. Each participant completed a data sheet with demographic information, a list of common blood loss descriptors, and a section to record a descriptive term and cubic centimeter amount for each blood-saturated peripad. On the second test day, an educational program was given to the participants regarding guidelines to describe and estimate amounts of blood loss consistently. Following the program, the participants were asked to estimate the amount of blood loss on the same 24 peripads. Accuracy and consistency increased when using cubic centimeters to estimate blood loss on peripads. Consistency increased but accuracy did not when estimations were given using descriptive terms. The researchers also found that accuracy was influenced by the pad brand or type.

Critique: These results suggest that nursing can improve the validity of statements regarding blood loss by using a consistent standard for estimation. By accurately estimating blood loss, assessments will improve, leading to timely intervention for the bleeder. Consistency among the nursing staff in estimating blood loss should enable each nurse to assess the total blood loss and report accurate findings to the physician. Valid nursing assessment leads to optimal patient care and increases trust between nurses and physicians.

Luegenbiehl D. L., Brophy G. H., Artique G. S., et al. (1990). Standardized assessment of blood loss. *MCN: American Journal of Maternal Child Nursing, 15,* 241–244.

over several hours, its culmulative effect can surprise the unsuspecting client and nurse.

Nursing Diagnosis

As a result of the comprehensive assessment of the woman with a spontaneous abortion, nursing diagnoses are formulated. Examples of possible nursing diagnoses are listed in Box 31-3.

Nursing Intervention

Interventions are based on the type of abortion, prognosis, and identified nursing diagnoses. If the client is at home, she is generally placed on restricted activity. If she is having only slight vaginal bleeding or even

BOX 31-3
Nursing Diagnoses—
Spontaneous Abortion

- Anxiety related to uncertainty of pregnancy outcome
- Fluid Volume Deficit related to excessive blood loss from spontaneous abortion
- Anticipatory Grieving related to actual or threatened loss of pregnancy
- Pain related to uterine contractions
- Risk for Infection related to retained products of conception
- Situational Low Self Esteem related to inability to carry pregnancy to term successfully

spotting without pain, she should be instructed to stay in bed and eat a well-balanced diet. However, some midwives and physicians may not recommend restricted activity, based on the concept that the uterus is well insulated from outside influences. The client should be instructed to save for inspection all perineal pads and all tissue and clots passed. If the bleeding disappears within 48 hours after instituting bed rest, the woman may get out of bed but should be instructed to limit her activities for the next several days. The nurse also should instruct the client to avoid coitus for 2 weeks following the last incidence of bleeding or as otherwise recommended by the physician.

If the client requires hospitalization, nursing care focuses on stabilizing the client. The nurse plays a primary role in reinforcing explanations given by the physician or midwife; monitoring the client's status, including vital signs, amount of bleeding, and comfort level; facilitating diagnositic tests, such as complete blood count, type, and cross-match; and preparing the patient for ultrasound or procedures such as D&C or vacuum extraction as necessary.

Psychosocial support is of prime importance because bleeding episodes are frightening and anxiety producing for all pregnant women. Emotional reactions of shock and disbelief are normal regardless of the type of abortion. The woman often searches for answers regarding the cause of her condition. She may express guilt and blame herself for behaviors that she feels may have contributed to the situation. Verbalization of feelings should be encouraged among all family members. The nurse should respond to concerns by offering accurate information on the cause of most spontaneous abortions and any facts specifically related to the actual case. False reassurance that "everything will be all right" should be avoided because the client may lose her pregnancy.

Particular consideration is given to the special needs of the client experiencing **recurrent abortion** (three or more consecutive first-trimester spontaneous losses). Her prognosis for carrying a pregnancy to term decreases with each abortion. A complete diagnostic workup is necessary to determine the cause and treatments indicated.

Nursing Evaluation

The anticipated outcomes for the client with a spontaneous abortion include the following:

- The client verbalizes the physiologic changes occurring with her condition and related treatment.
- The client exhibits no signs or symptoms of fluid volume deficit.
- The client experiences no complications.
- The client is able to retain pregnancy if bleeding is not excessive or no other contraindications to pregnancy exist.
- The client discusses the impact of the loss on her family, progresing appropriately through the grieving process.

Incompetent Cervix

An **incompetent cervix** is a mechanical defect in the cervix. The defect causes the cervical os to dilate prematurely during the midtrimester of pregnancy, resulting in late habitual recurrent abortion or **preterm labor.** This may be caused by congenital anomalies of the uterus or cervix or prior trauma. The symptoms include painless dilatation, presence of bloody show, and bulging of the membranes.

Medical Diagnosis

The diagnosis of incompetent cervix is usually made when a second-trimester pregnancy is lost, with a clinical picture of sudden, unexpected rupture of the membranes followed by painless expulsion of the products of conception. An anatomically incompetent cervix will accept a Hegar number 8 cervical dilator without any prior dilatation required and is much wider than usual on hysterography (Bennett, 1992).

Management

When repeated termination of pregnancy in the second trimester is due to an anatomic factor, a surgical treatment known as **cerclage** (suturing the cervix) may be performed to prevent relaxation and dilation of the cervix. A modified *Shirodkar technique* or the *McDonald technique* are the most common procedures. With the Shirodkar technique, the vaginal mucous membrane is elevated. A band of homologous fascia or a narrow strip of some material, such as Mersilene, is

then carried around the internal os and tied. The vaginal mucosa is then restored to its original position and sutured. With the McDonald technique, a simpler procedure, a nonabsorbable suture is placed around the cervix high on the cervical mucosa. Cerclage may be done at approximately 12 to 14 weeks' gestation. Success rates with the McDonald and the Shirodkar procedures are now approaching 80% to 90% (Scott et al., 1990).

After cerclage, the main concerns are monitoring fetal heart rate and observing for signs of rupture of the membranes or uterine contractions. If the membranes rupture, the suture is removed, and the uterus is usually emptied because of the risk of infection. However, in some selected pregnancies, increased doses of antibiotics are used after membranes rupture to maintain the pregnancy. If contractions begin, the client should be placed on bed rest, and a tocolytic agent, such as ritodrine hydrochloride, may be given in an effort to control the contractions.

The cerclage usually is removed after week 37 of gestation. This is often followed by the onset of labor and a relatively rapid delivery. In some situations, cesarean delivery may be elected to preserve the suture for future pregnancies.

Ectopic Pregnancy

An **ectopic pregnancy** refers to any gestation that is implanted outside the uterine cavity. Most ectopic pregnancies are tubal gestations located most frequently in the ampullar portion of the fallopian tube; the isthmus portion is the next most frequent site (Fig. 31-1). Other types, which make up about 5% of all ectopic pregnancies, are interstitial (in the interstitial portion of the tube), cornual (in a rudimentary horn of a uterus), cervical, abdominal, and ovarian gestations.

The rate of ectopic pregnancy in the United States from 1970 to 1987 increased from 4.5 to 16.8 per 1,000 pregnancies in women between 15 and 44 years of age (Centers for Disease Control [CDC], 1989). Although the actual number of deaths from ectopic pregnancies has declined during this period, the percentage of all maternal deaths attributed to this condition has increased. Ectopic pregnancies are now the second leading cause of maternal mortality in this country (Cunningham et al., 1993). Reported rates of ectopic pregnancies are 40% higher among African American and other minority women than among white women (CDC, 1989). The incidence of the disease is particularly high in women between 35 and 44 years of age. Studies done more than 1 decade ago revealed that the chances of a woman having a repeat ectopic pregnancy are between 5% and 20% (Kitchin et al., 1979; Romney et al., 1981).

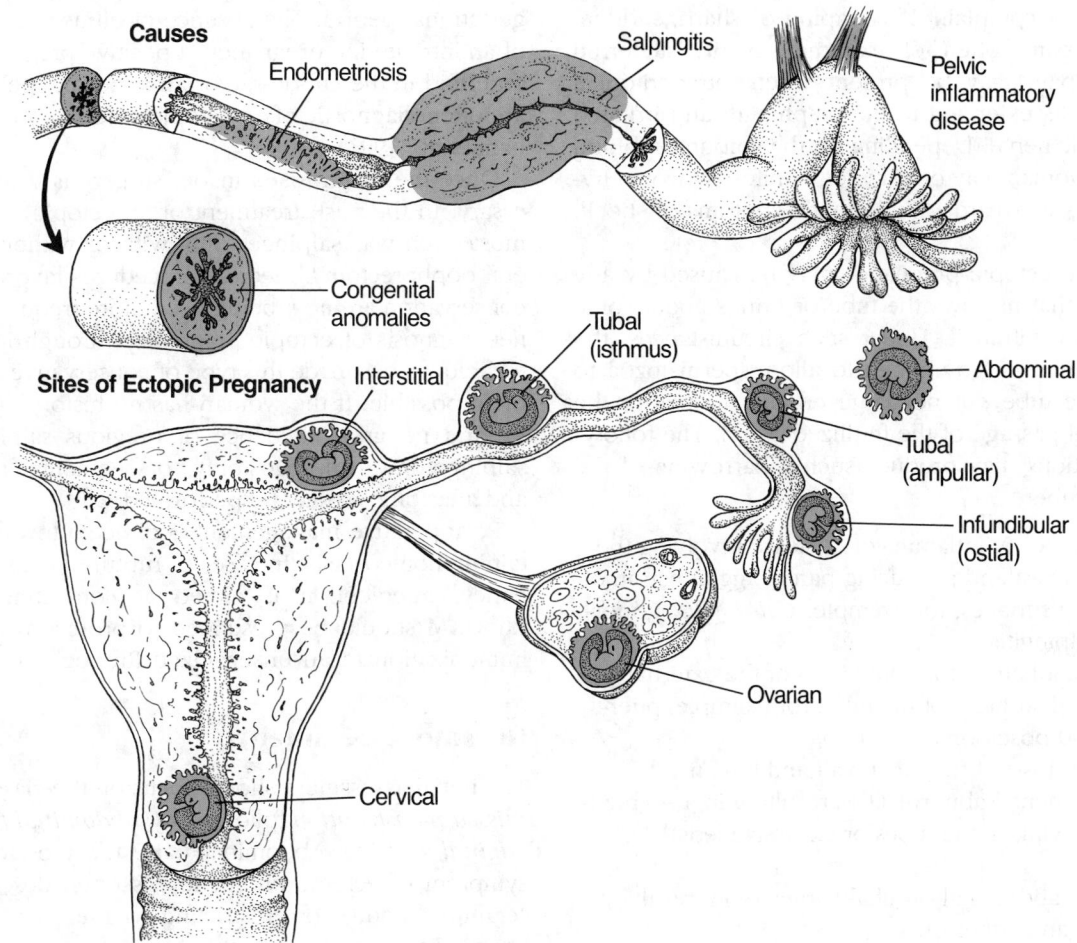

Causes

Endometriosis

Salpingitis

Pelvic inflammatory disease

Congenital anomalies

Sites of Ectopic Pregnancy

Interstitial

Tubal (isthmus)

Abdominal

Tubal (ampullar)

Infundibular (ostial)

Ovarian

Cervical

FIGURE 31-1 Causes and sites of ectopic pregnancy.

About once in every 200 pregnancies, the fertilized ovum, instead of traveling the length of the fallopian tube to reach the uterine cavity, becomes implanted within the walls of the fallopian tube. Because the wall of the tube is not sufficiently elastic to allow the fertilized ovum to grow and develop there, rupture of the tubal wall into the tubal lumen or peritoneal cavity inevitably results.

Within the first 12 weeks of pregnancy, rupture most frequently occurs into the tubal lumen, and the products of conception with much blood pass out the fimbriated end of the tube and into the peritoneal cavity, a *tubal abortion.* Rupture may occur through the peritoneal surface of the tube directly into the peritoneal cavity; again, there is an outpouring of blood into the abdomen from vessels at the site of rupture.

Occasionally, an ectopic pregnancy may develop in the portion of the tube that passes through the uterine wall; this is known as **interstitial pregnancy.** In rare instances, the products of conception, after rupturing through the tubal wall, may become implanted on the peritoneum. This extraordinary occurrence, known as an **abdominal pregnancy,** may in some cases result in delivery of a live infant through an abdominal incision.

Manifestations and Causes

Most ectopic pregnancies result from abnormalities that interfere or prevent the normal passage of the ovum through the fallopian tube. In an early ectopic pregnancy, there often are no signs and symptoms. Once the ectopic pregnancy ruptures, however, classic manifestations are present.

Clinical Picture. The clinical picture of a woman with an ectopic pregnancy varies, depending on the site of implantation. In cases of unruptured ectopic pregnancy, vague and variable discomforts may develop. At first, the woman exhibits the usual early signs and symptoms of pregnancy and regards her pregnancy as normal. Vaginal bleeding, which occurs when the embryo dies and the decidua begins to slough, often appears scant and dark brown. Within 3 to 5 weeks after a missed menstrual period, abdominal pain often develops. The nature, duration, and intensity of pain vary considerably with the length of gestation, site of implantation, and extent of blood loss. Pain is the predominant symptom of tubal rupture and may be localized on one side or felt over the entire abdomen. The woman may complain of cramping or sharp, sudden, knifelike pain, often of extreme severity. Referred shoulder pain may be present when intraperitoneal bleeding has extended to the diaphragm and irritated the phrenic nerve. Depending on the amount of blood loss, the woman may or may not manifest syncope, hypotension, tachycardia, and other symptoms of shock.

Causes. An ectopic pregnancy may be caused by any condition that narrows the tube or brings about some constriction within it. Under such circumstances, the tubal lumen is large enough to allow spermatozoa to ascend the tube but not large enough to permit the downward passage of the fertilized ovum. The following conditions may produce such a narrowing of the fallopian tube:

- Previous pelvic inflammatory disease involving the tubal mucosa and producing partial agglutination of opposing surfaces, for example, *Chlamydia,* gonorrheal salpingitis
- Previous inflammatory processes of the external peritoneal surfaces of the tube, for example, puerperal and postabortal infections
- Endometriosis of the tubal wall and lumen
- Developmental abnormalities resulting in a segmental narrowing of the tubes or excessive length or kinking
- Previous abdominal or tubal surgery with resultant scarring and adhesions
- Previous tubal sterilization
- Use of low-dose progesterone oral contraceptives

Other factors that may potentially contribute to ectopic pregnancies have been suggested in several important studies conducted during the last decade. Research has revealed that *smoking* causes an increased incidence of ectopic pregnancies (Chow et al., 1988; Handler et al., 1989). A study by Edelin (1983) showed that women who became pregnant while using an *intrauterine device* (IUD) were 10 times more likely to have an ectopic pregnancy than if the device were not being used. Although an association between *prior induced abortions* and increased risk of ectopic pregnancies has been suggested, little evidence supports this claim in women without postabortion complications (Chung et al., 1982; Holt et al., 1989).

Medical Management

The therapeutic goal of medical management is early diagnosis of ectopic pregnancy based on a detailed health history, physical examination, and selected diagnostic tests. The diagnostic procedures include tests for human chorionic gonadotropin (hCG), culdocentesis, curettage, laparoscopy, and ultrasonography. Hormonal levels of hCG are usually lower in ectopic pregnancies than in uterine pregnancies of the same

gestational period. The absence of ultrasonic evidence of an intrauterine pregnancy, a positive pregnancy test, and fluid in the cul-de-sac or an abnormal pelvic mass are often diagnostic of an ectopic pregnancy (Cunningham et al., 1993).

Once the diagnosis is made, surgery is usually necessary. In the past, treatment of an ectopic pregnancy most often was salpingectomy with or without ipsilateral oophorectomy. Medical procedures favoring tubal conservation are now being used more frequently. Earlier diagnosis of ectopic pregnancy through improved techniques has made this type of conservative management possible. If the woman has no history of infertility and no gross evidence of previous salpingitis, a salpingotomy, salpingostomy, or segmental resection and anastomosis may be performed.

Postoperative management is directed toward maintaining homeostasis. In cases of ruptured ectopic pregnancy, intervention is aimed at combating shock. RhoGAM should be prescribed to protect against isoimmunization in an unsensitized Rh-negative woman.

Nursing Assessment

The initial assessment should focus on the classic triad: *missed menstruation* followed by *abdominal pain* and *vaginal spotting.* Abdominal pain, the most common symptom of ectopic pregnancy, is often described as "crampy," "dull," or "restricting to the shoulder and back." The patient also should be questioned about any contraceptive methods, particularly the use of an IUD. A history of previous tubal damage caused by disease or developmental problems further supports the likelihood of a tubal pregnancy.

Vital signs are assessed; however, these may not differ markedly from normal values unless tubal rupture and internal bleeding have occurred. During the pelvic examination, the patient is assessed for fullness in the cul-de-sac, cervical pain, and adnexal tenderness. The uterus is generally not enlarged beyond the size of 8 weeks' gestation. Laboratory analysis frequently reveals falling hematocrit and hemoglobin levels and leukocytosis.

The amount of bleeding evident may be a poor indicator of the severity of the situation, because blood loss may be concealed in the pelvic cavity. Extensive blood loss leading to hypovolemic shock may be manifested by a rapid, thready pulse; tachypnea; and hypotension. The umbilicus may display a blue tinge (**Cullen's sign**), indicating bleeding in the peritoneal cavity.

Nursing Diagnosis

Based on the nursing assessment and differential medical findings, nursing diagnoses are identified. A list of possible nursing diagnoses is shown in Box 31-4.

BOX 31–4
Nursing Diagnoses—Ectopic Pregnancy

- Fluid Volume Deficit related to the following:
  Bleeding from rupture at implantation site
  Excessive fluid loss from surgery
- Anticipatory Grieving related to loss of pregnancy
- Pain related to tubal rupture—peritonitis, intraperitoneal bleeding
- Knowledge Deficit related to lack of information about treatment and possible complications

Nursing Intervention

For the patient with a suspected ectopic pregnancy, the nurse should explain the various diagnostic tests and provide support. When acute rupture of a fallopian tube occurs, the situation presents a surgical emergency requiring nursing care aimed at combating shock. An IV infusion is maintained so that blood or plasma expanders can be administered as needed to replace losses from the hemorrhage and surgery.

Postoperatively, vital signs should be carefully monitored, fluid replacement administered, and intake and output recorded. Oral intake of foods and fluids should be avoided until bowel function has returned to normal. Early ambulation is encouraged. The nurse must accurately record and assess vaginal bleeding and the perineal pad count, continously monitoring the client for signs and symptoms of hemorrhage. The surgical site may require special care and dressings. Patients are often given broad-spectrum antibiotics prophylactically. Steroids are administered to decrease the postoperative inflammation that can contribute to the development of adhesions.

Emotional care is directed toward facilitating effective coping by encouraging the patient and her family to verbalize their feelings, allowing them privacy to grieve the death of the fetus, and listening to their concerns about future chances for a successful pregnancy. Information about the causes of ectopic pregnancy may assist them in resolving feelings of guilt and self-blame.

Nursing Evaluation

The following are anticipated outcomes of nursing care:

- The client verbalizes the pathophysiology of her condition and treatment alternatives.
- The client demonstrates no signs or symptoms of complications.
- The client discusses the impact of the loss on her and her family, progressing appropriately through the grieving process.

Hydatidiform Mole

Hydatidiform mole (molar pregnancy) is a gestational trophoblastic neoplasm that arises from the chorion. There are two types of molar growth: *partial* and *complete*. Each one has a distinct cytogenic origin, pathologic characteristics, and clinical manifestation.

The *complete* mole is characterized by a large amount of edematous enlarged villi without a fetus or fetal membranes. The mole has a grapelike appearance with clusters of vesicles on all or part of the decidual lining of the uterus (Fig. 31-2). The chromosomal composition most often is 46XX, with the chromosomes completely of paternal origin. This phenomenon, called **androgenesis**, could occur in one of two ways: One ovum with an inactive nucleus is fertilized by two sperm, and subsequent growth results in two sets of paternal genomes; one ovum is fertilized by a haploid sperm that reproduces itself. The exclusive presence of the paternal genes, which are required for the successful development of the extraembryonic components of the conceptus, explains the excessive abnormal villi development and absence of fetus with the molar pregnancy. This is because the embryonic components are less dependent on paternal genes (Surani, 1986).

The *partial mole* is characterized by normal villi intermingled with **hydropic** (swollen) villi and some fetal material or an amnionic sac. It is usually associated

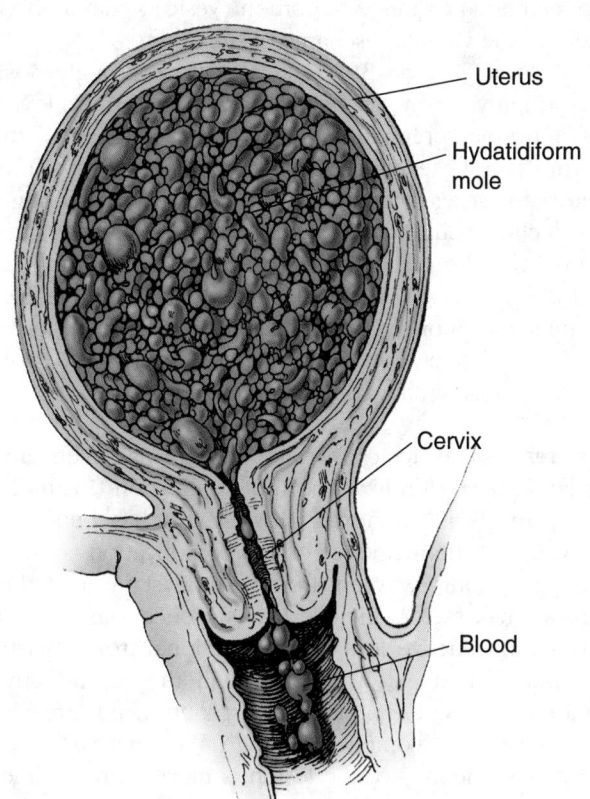

FIGURE 31-2 Hydatidiform mole.

Uterus
Hydatidiform mole
Cervix
Blood

with one haploid maternal and two haploid paternal sets of chromosomes (triploid karyotype).

Hydatidiform mole is an uncommon condition, occurring about once in every 1,500 to 2,000 pregnancies in the United States and Europe. According to an epidemiologic study completed several years ago, the estimated ratio of partial to complete moles is 2:1 (Buckley, 1984).

Manifestations and Causes

A hydatidiform mole is a placental tumor that develops once pregnancy has occurred. For unknown reasons, the embryo dies in utero, but the placenta continues to develop. In the early stages of the disease, the manifestations are difficult to distinquish from those of a normal pregnancy. Genetic abnormalities occurring at the time of fertilization appear to be responsible for the disease.

Clinical Picture. The pregnancy appears to be normal at first, although in about one-third to one-half of women with complete moles, the uterus is larger than expected for gestational dates. Bleeding is a common symptom and may vary from brownish-red spotting to heavy, bright red bleeding. Vomiting in a rather severe form may appear early. Fetal heart tones are absent in the presence of other signs of pregnancy. Preeclampsia may appear before the 20th week of gestation. Women with partial moles typically have a clinical diagnosis of spontaneous or missed abortion. Vesicles may be evident in the vaginal discharge of the abortus.

A blood or urine β-hCG level will be strongly positive (highly elevated when compared with those levels of a normal pregnancy). In a molar pregnancy, the serum β-hCG levels are still very high 100 days after the last menses, when the level normally would begin to decline (Cunningham et al., 1993). However, this value must be carefully evaluated, because highly elevated levels also may be associated with multiple gestations with more than one placenta. Initial hCG levels may be relatively lower in patients with a partial mole than in those with a complete mole.

Causes. The exact cause of the abnormal ovum and spermatozoic fertilization and replication in molar pregnancies is unknown. However, it has been observed that the incidence of this complication is much higher among women from southeast Asia. Other known risk factors include low socioeconomic status, prior reproductive loss, prior gestational trophoblastic neoplasia, and extremes of age in the reproductive years (Grimes, 1984). The most pronounced effect of age is seen in women older than 45 years, when the relative frequency of the lesion is more than 10 times greater than at ages 20 to 40 years (Cunningham et al., 1993).

Medical Diagnosis and Prognosis

Diagnosis is obtained from the characteristic ultrasound appearance of the hydatidiform mole. The image typically is one of multiple echogenic (dense) regions within the uterus, corresponding to hydropic villi and focal intrauterine hemorrhage, without any fetus detected.

With appropriate therapy, hydatidiform mole is generally not associated with maternal mortality. However, clients with complete hydatidiform moles have a higher incidence of **choriocarcinoma**, a malignant sequelae (10%–30%), when compared with patients with partial moles (<10%; Scott et al., 1990). Other complications associated with moles include thecalutein cysts, trophoblastic embolization of the lung, and **disseminated intravascular coagulation** (DIC). Blood loss commonly leads to iron-deficiency anemia.

Medical Management

The first phase of medical management for hydatidiform mole consists of emptying the uterus. D&C is the usual procedure in almost all clients. Primary hysterectomy is an alternative treatment in clients who have completed childbearing and desire sterilization. The tissue obtained must be carefully evaluated by the pathologist, because although a mole is a benign process, choriocarcinoma, an extremely malignant tumor, sometimes complicates the picture.

The second phase of medical management is β-hCG level surveillance by radioimmunoassay to detect any changes that suggest trophoblastic malignancy. The usual protocol consists of weekly measurements of hCG levels until they are normal for 3 weeks, then monthly measurements until they are normal for 6 months, followed by measurements every 2 months for the next 6 months. Negative β-hCG levels should be evident within 6 weeks after evacuation. Physical and pelvic examinations are performed at 2-week intervals until complete remission has occurred, and a chest x-ray is obtained to detect metastases. Avoidance of pregnancy is recommended during the period of follow-up to avoid confusion with rising β-hCG levels.

Because the use of prophylactic chemotherapy is controversial and may produce several adverse effects, it is generally not recommended in women with uncomplicated hydatidiform mole. Women receiving chemotherapy should be observed closely for blood dyscrasias and renal complications.

Nursing Assessment

A thorough history and physical examination are essential. Assessment of fundal height provides basic data about expected gestational age, which, in the case of hydatidiform mole, is beyond that expected by menstrual history but may suggest multiple gestation. Careful auscultation for fetal heart sounds reveals no findings, whereas the pregnancy tests remain highly positive (owing to unusually high levels of hCG) beyond the time of usual decline in hCG levels. The client also may report intense nausea and vomiting, which result from the rising hCG levels.

Vital signs, especially blood pressure (BP), which may reveal hypertension before the 20th week of pregnancy, should be evaluated. Bleeding, which often develops during the second trimester, should be carefully assessed for clear, filled vesicles. Results of laboratory studies often reveal falling hemoglobin and hematocrit levels and proteinuria.

Nursing Diagnosis

After completing the nursing assessment, the nurse develops appropriate nursing diagnoses. For a list of possible nursing diagnoses, see Box 31-5.

Nursing Intervention

Once the diagnoses are made, the nurse assists with client preparation for evacuating the uterus. Preoperative and postoperative nursing care will vary, depending on the type of medical procedure required.

During client teaching, the nurse must emphasize the need for follow-up surveillance of hCG levels for an entire year. In addition, family planning counseling should be offered to assist the woman in selecting a desirable contraceptive. The nurse should advise the client to avoid pregnancy for at least 1 year, after which time conception is permitted if hCG levels are within normal limits.

Psychosocial support also is an important component of nursing care for the woman with a hydatidiform mole. Although the woman may never have experienced a "true pregnancy," her reactions after treatment frequently resemble those of women who have had a spontaneous abortion or an ectopic pregnancy. Further anxiety and despair may be created by the postponement of future pregnancies and the risk of

---

BOX 31–5
Nursing Diagnoses—Hydatidiform Mole

- Fluid Volume Deficit related to uterine bleeding
- Anticipatory Grieving related to loss of pregnancy
- Altered Tissue Perfusion related to pregnancy-induced hypertension
- Altered Nutrition: Less than body requirements related to nausea and vomiting
- Knowledge Deficit related to the need for follow-up
- Fear related to the possibility of malignancy

---

potential neoplasms. The nurse should provide opportunities for the client to express her varying reactions to the situation, including extreme remorse, anger, and fear. Much understanding and guidance are required by the client and her family to work through grief reactions and assess future plans (see Nursing Care Plan: Hemorrhagic Complications of Early Pregnancy).

Nursing Evaluation

The following are anticipated outcomes of nursing care:

- The client verbalizes the pathophysiologic changes occurring in her reproductive system and the need for immediate treatment and follow-up procedures.
- The client exhibits no signs or symptoms of complications.
- The client returns to her previous level of functioning after the operative procedure (evacuation).
- The client discusses the impact of the loss on her and her family, progressing appropriately through the grieving process.
- The client verbalizes the need for continued follow-up for at least 1 year.

Choriocarcinoma

Choriocarcinoma is a highly malignant trophoblastic neoplasm that develops during or shortly after some forms of pregnancy. Approximately one-third to one-half of choriocarcinomas are preceded by hydatidiform mole. The characteristic progression of this disease involves a rapidly growing mass that invades uterine muscle and blood vessels and causes hemorrhage and necrosis. The chorionic villi of hydatidiform moles are absent. Metastases to the lungs, vagina, brain, and blood vessels are early complications, often occurring before the presentation of the primary disease symptoms.

Trophoblastic neoplasia is suspected in the presence of persistent or rising titers of hCG when pregnancy is absent. Modern treatment of choriocarcinoma has greatly improved the prognosis. In the past, hysterectomy offered the only possible cure. Currently, drugs such as methotrexate and dactinomycin offer much promise as successful chemotherapeutic agents that may be used alone or in combination with irradiation. If the disease is treated early, an overall cure rate of about 85% can be achieved (Scott et al., 1990).

Hemorrhagic Complications of Late Pregnancy

Bleeding and possible hemorrhage during late pregnancy are emergency situations. They may seriously

(*text continues on page 820*)

NURSING CARE PLAN
Hemorrhagic Complications of Early Pregnancy

Nursing Goals

The woman with hemorrhagic complications of early pregnancy will carry fetus to term or terminate the pregnancy without complications as evidenced by:
1. Identifying signs of early antepartal bleeding.
2. Seeking appropriate medical interventions to support/terminate pregnancy.
3. Complying with restrictions prescribed to save the pregnancy.
4. Maintaining health without signs of hypovolemic shock and/or infection.
5. Expressing feelings of fear, grief, and anger to effectively cope with threatened/actual loss.

Assessment	Potential Nursing Diagnoses	Intervention/ Rationale	Evaluation
History Previous spontaneous abortions Multiple therapeutic abortions Pelvic inflammatory disease or previous tubal damage Previous ectopic pregnancy Current pregnancy confirmed Nausea and vomiting Lower abdominal pain or knifelike pain in lower quadrant (suggestive of ectopic pregnancy) Uterine cramping or contractions Previous bleeding coagulation problems Contraceptive use, especially IUD	Knowledge Deficit related to physiological alterations in the reproductive system	Instruct client about "danger signals" in early pregnancy and appropriate actions indicated *to alert client to take appropriate measures* Maintain bedrest or limited physical activity *to insure well being of mother and fetus* Monitor vital signs and fetal heart tones if indicated *to assess fetal well being* Explain diagnostic ultrasound (or other prescribed procedures) and prepare for testing *to insure maternal compliance and allay anxiety* Provide client education on pathophysiology of condition and management *to provide information*	Client repeats danger signals in early pregnancy and what actions to take Client complies with limited activity Client's vital signs remain stable Client acknowledges understanding of procedures Client repeats accurate description of her condition
Physical examination Spotting or active bleeding (color, quantity, consistency) Relaxed or dilated cervix Fundal height (higher than expected with hydatidiform mole) Tenderness in adnexa Lower abdominal pain (right or left side) Blood pressure (elevated with hydatidiform mole) Vital signs		Instruct client to increase fluid intake and to eat a well-balanced diet *to insure appropriate nutrition*	Client increases fluid intake and eats a well-balanced diet
Laboratory Complete blood count Rh factor Hemoglobin, hematocrit Ultrasound to determine cause of bleeding Ectopic pregnancy			

(continued)

NURSING CARE PLAN *(Continued)*
Hemorrhagic Complications of Early Pregnancy

Assessment	Potential Nursing Diagnoses	Intervention/Rationale	Evaluation

Threatened abortion
Incomplete abortion
Hydatidiform mole
Signs and symptoms of shock
  Rapid, thready pulse
  Tachypnea
  Pallor, clammy skin
  Decreased blood pressure
  Restlessness
  Decreased urine output
  Decreased level of consciousness
Laboratory screening for coagulation defect
	Fluid Volume Deficit related to bleeding complications of early pregnancy	Draw blood, type, and crossmatch *to insure blood compatibility*
		
		Record pad count; note quantity, quality, and constituents of drainage *to assess blood loss*
		
		Start and maintain IV infusion for administration of blood, antibiotics, or other medications as prescribed (use large-bore cannula) *to prepare for shock/prevent infection*
		
		Replace IV fluids as prescribed *to insure electrolyte balance*
		
		Monitor intake and output (insert Foley catheter, if necessary) *to assess hydration*
		
		Observe for signs and symptoms of shock; frequently assess vital functions, state of consciousness *to prevent shock*
		
		Replace fibrinogen, if indicated *to enhance clotting*
		
		Institute nursing interventions for treatment of shock, if necessary; administer oxygen *to stabilize blood pressure*
		
		Explain potential medical or surgical procedures that may be necessary (eg, dilation and curettage, laparoscopy, salpingectomy, induction) *to prepare client and provide appropriate information*
		
		Administer RhoGAM to Rh-negative client who aborts pregnancy *to prevent Rh disease*
			Client receives IV infusions and medications as ordered
			
			Client's fluid and electrolyte balance is maintained
			
			Client has her intake and output monitored
			
			Client does not show signs of hypovolemic shock
			
			Client is stabilized
			
			Client demonstrates her knowledge of potential medical and surgical procedures in discussions
			
			Client receives RhoGAM if Rh negative

(continued)

NURSING CARE PLAN *(Continued)*
Hemorrhagic Complications of Early Pregnancy

Assessment	Potential Nursing Diagnoses	Intervention/ Rationale	Evaluation

Physical examination
  Fever
  Local tenderness
  Malodorous vaginal
   discharge
  Pain in lower abdomen,
   adnexa
	Risk for Infection related to excessive fluid volume deficit	Provide client education on
		  Perineal hygiene (eg,
		   wipe perineal area from
		   front to back after void-
		   ing) *to prevent infection*
		Avoidance of tampons to
		  control bleeding *to pre-
		  vent infection/TSS*
			Client demonstrates proper cleansing technique after voiding

History
  Large amount of ante-
   partal bleeding
  Illegal abortion
		Observe for symptoms of
		  infection
		   Tenderness
		   Swelling
		   Redness
		   Pain
			Client remains free of signs and symptoms of infection

		Encourage fluid intake or
		  administer parental fluids
		  as ordered *to maintain
		  fluid balance*
			Client takes adequate amounts of fluids

		Administer antibiotics and
		  pain medication as pre-
		  scribed *to prevent infec-
		  tion and insure client
		  comfort*
			Client receives antibiotics and pain medications as prescribed

Signs and symptoms of
  anxiety
   Jitteriness
   Restlessness
   Crying
   Nail biting
Expresses
  "Why me"
  Fear of losing baby
  Anger
	Grieving related to actual or threatened loss of pregnancy	Provide opportunities for
		  expressions of grief,
		  anger, self-blame *to sup-
		  port grieving process*
			Client expresses feelings of grief, anger, and self-blame

		Allow client to be with sup-
		  portive family members
		  to support client
			Family members offer each other mutual support

		Provide factual information
		  about abortion (or ec-
		  topic pregnancy, hyda-
		  tidiform mole) and possi-
		  ble future reproductive
		  capacities *to provide ap-
		  propriate information*
			Client demonstrates under-standing of potential loss of pregnancy

		Initiate referral for genetic
		  counseling if appropriate
		  *to provide for appropri-
		  ate decisions concerning
		  future pregnancies*
			Client complies with refer-ral suggestions

jeopardize fetal well-being and maternal health, increasing maternal and perinatal morbidity and mortality. Bleeding late in the pregnancy is commonly associated with placental disorders. Problems that develop may have originated early or late in pregnancy as the placenta matures and becomes more vascular. The most common cause of bleeding and hemorrhage (blood loss of 500 mL or more) during the later months of pregnancy is placenta previa. Premature separation of the placenta (abruptio placentae) is an-other potentially serious condition associated with third-trimester bleeding. These conditions are compared in Table 31-1.

Placenta Previa

Normally, the placenta is implanted in the fundus (upper portion) of the uterus. In **placenta previa** the placenta is implanted in the lower uterine segment so that it wholly or partially covers the internal cervical os.

TABLE 31-1
A Comparative Overview of Placenta Previa and Abruptio Placentae

	Placenta Previa	Abruptio Placentae
ETIOLOGY	Unknown	Unknown
ASSOCIATED RISK FACTORS	Multiparity, multiple gestation, advancing age (especially over age 35), uterine incisions, previous cesarean birth, breech presentation	Maternal hypertension, grand multiparity, multiple gestation, hydramnios, external trauma (rare), short umbilical cord (rare), cocaine use
INCIDENCE	1:167 deliveries	1:77–1:200 deliveries
MANIFESTATIONS	Painless bleeding appearing at the end of the second trimester or in the third trimester; minimal to severe (usually bright red)	Bleeding—may or may not be external (often dark brown)
	Uterus soft, normal tone	Uterus rigid and tender; tetanic, persistent uterine contractions (severe abruptio)
	Observed blood loss comparable to signs of shock	Shock out of proportion to blood loss
PROGNOSIS	Maternal mortality 0.1%	Maternal mortality 0.5%–5%
	Major problem: prematurity	Major problem: prematurity
		Perinatal mortality 15%
ULTRASONOGRAPHIC FINDINGS	Abnormal placental implantation—lower uterine segment	Normal placental implantation—upper uterine segment
RECURRENCE	1:17	1:6–1:18
COMPLICATIONS	Hemorrhage	Hemorrhage
	Hypovolemic shock	Hypovolemic shock
	Thrombocytopenia	Coagulation defects (eg, hypofibrinogenemia)
	Anemia	
	Premature rupture of membranes and labor	Renal failure
	Fetal malposition	Anemia
	Air embolism	
	Postpartum hemorrhage	
	Uterine rupture	

Placenta previa is classified as total, partial, or low implantation by the location of the placenta in the lower uterine segment and the degree to which the internal cervical os is covered (Fig. 31-3). *Total placenta previa* occurs when the placenta completely covers the internal cervical os. *Partial placenta previa* occurs when the placenta partially covers the internal cervical os. *Low implantation of the placenta* occurs when the placenta encroaches on the region of the internal cervical os so that it can be palpated by the physician on digital exploration around the cervix but does not extend beyond the margin of the internal os.

Manifestations and Causes

During the later months of pregnancy, changes occurring in the lower uterine segment cause varying degrees of placental separation from its site of attachment. This separation opens up the underlying blood sinuses of the uterus from which the bleeding occurs.

Clinical Picture. The main sign in the woman presenting with placenta previa is painless, bright-red vaginal bleeding during the second or third trimester. The bleeding may begin as spotting, or it may start with profuse hemorrhage. Most commonly, uncontrolled bleeding does not occur with the first episode. In fact, there may be several episodes of bleeding before there is sufficient blood loss to necessitate aggressive intervention and pregnancy termination. The uterus usually remains soft in women with placenta previa.

Causes. There is no known cause of placenta previa. However, certain risk factors have been associated with

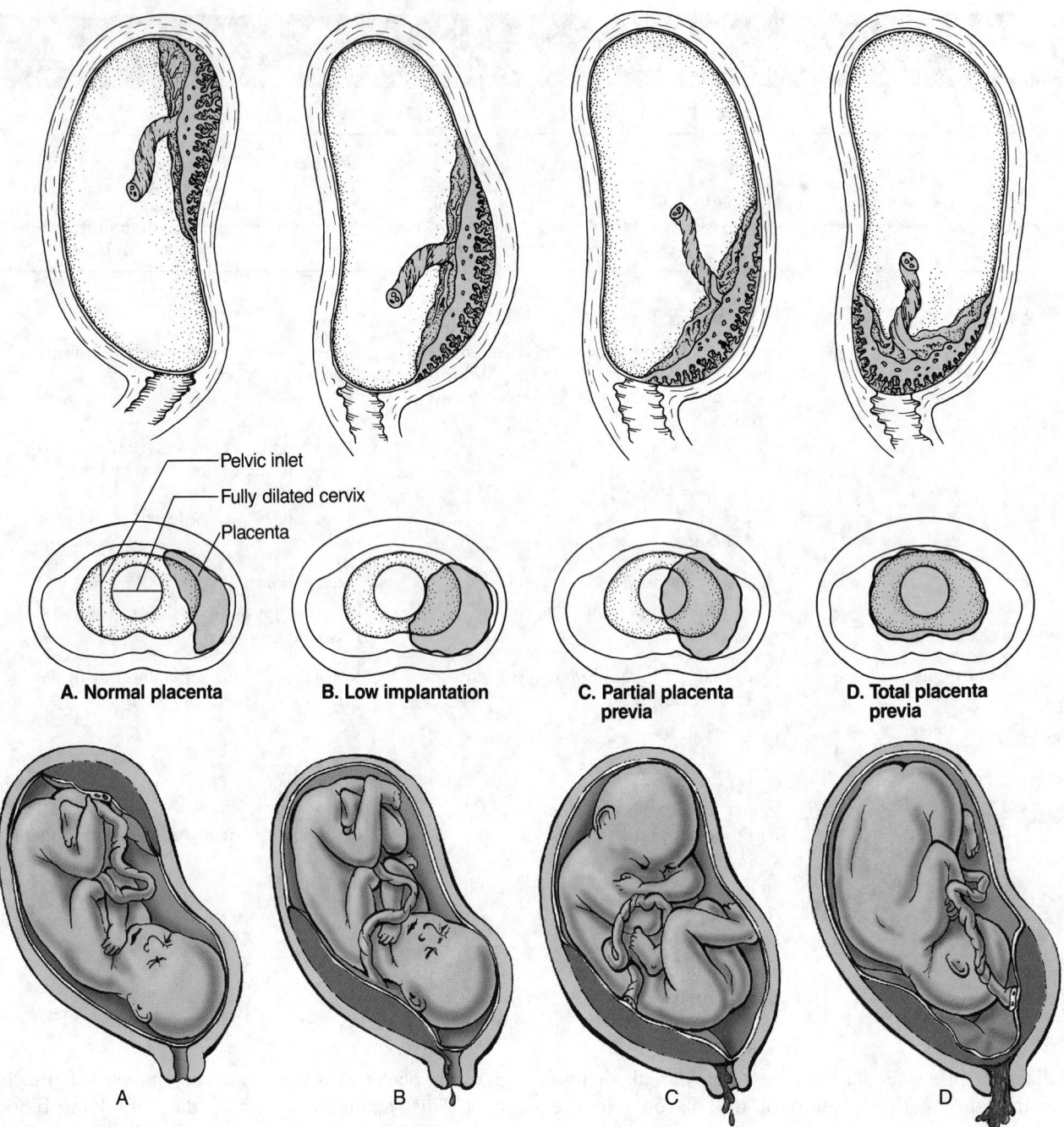

Pelvic inlet
Fully dilated cervix
Placenta

A. Normal placenta **B. Low implantation** **C. Partial placenta previa** **D. Total placenta previa**

A   B   C   D

FIGURE 31–3 Placenta previa. (**A**) Normal. (**B**) Low implantation. (**C**) Partial placenta previa. (**D**) Total placenta previa.

the increased risk of developing placenta previa. These include multiparity, advancing maternal age, multiple gestation, previous cesarean birth, and uterine incisions.

Medical Diagnosis and Prognosis

The possibility of placenta previa should always be suspected in women with uterine bleeding during the latter half of pregnancy. Diagnosis can be established clearly and simply by using sonographic techniques to locate the placenta. Placental localization by ultrasound scanning offers 95% accuracy. Patients found to have low-lying placenta or placenta previa are now being followed by serial ultrasound examinations to observe changes in placental position. Many of the early placenta previas appear to migrate away from the cervix as pregnancy progresses because of formation of the lower uterine segment (Ancona et al., 1990).

In unusual circumstances when the diagnosis of placenta previa cannot be confirmed with ultrasound, a physical examination of the cervix may be performed in the operating room under a **double set-up**. This means preparations, including personnel and equipment, for a sterile vaginal examination and an immediate vaginal or cesarean delivery are available in case severe hemorrhage results from mild manipulation.

Until recent years, placenta previa was associated with a maternal mortality rate of approximately 10%. Early diagnosis and modern methods of management have reduced this figure considerably. However, placenta previa still creates problems for the client and fetus. Two main problems for the woman include bleeding and obstruction of the birth canal. The woman also is at increased risk for postpartum hemorrhage, anemia, and infection. For the fetus, the most significant concern is prematurity. In utero, the fetus may be compromised because of hypoxia created by the decreased oxygen supply with placental separation. Intrauterine growth retardation may occur as a consequence of decreased circulation to the fetus.

Medical Management

Medical interventions are determined by the location of the placenta, the amount of bleeding, and the gestational age of the fetus. The goal of medical management is to ensure the birth of a mature neonate without complications to the client or fetus. Conservative management is appropriate when the fetus is not mature (by weight or dates <36 weeks) and the bleeding is not excessive. Under such circumstances, bed rest and close observation of maternal and fetal well-being often result in cessation of the bleeding and provide valuable time for the fetus to mature. To prolong gestation in patients with third-trimester bleeding and preterm labor, tocolysis with magnesium sulfate, terbutaline, or ritodrine may be used. Delivery is planned when fetal maturity by amniocentesis is confirmed, usually 36 to 37 weeks' gestation. If the fetus is at term by size and dates, if labor has begun, or if bleeding is sufficient to threaten the well-being of the woman or fetus, delivery is initiated. Under emergency situations, delivery must be performed regardless of gestational age.

In all instances of total previa or greater than 30% partial previa, cesarean birth is the delivery of choice. The procedure is preferably performed under light, general inhalation anesthesia. Vaginal delivery sometimes may be accomplished with low implantation of the placenta, especially if the baby is small and the cervix is partially dilated. Under these circumstances, the obstetrician may elect to rupture the membranes in the hope that the presenting part may enter the pelvis and control the bleeding by compressing the area of placenta that has separated.

Nursing Assessment

Assessment of the woman with placenta previa is similar in many ways to the approach used for the woman with a spontaneous abortion, discussed previously in the chapter.

Initial evaluation of the client by the nurse should include assessment of baseline vital signs; bleeding; uterine activity and condition (size, contour, irritability, and relaxation); pain or tenderness, especially in the abdomen; fetal heart tones and activity; and level of consciousness. The client must be typed and cross-matched so that blood is available in case transfusion is necessary. All perineal pads should be saved and carefully examined by the nurse for blood loss. The perineal pads also should be weighed to help estimate the amount of blood loss (1 g = 1 mL; Schmidt, 1993). The client also should be instructed to report if she feels any fluid escaping from her vagina. Initially and periodically, the uterus should be gently palpated to detect contractions, suggesting the onset of labor.

Because bleeding is from the uterine decidua, the amount of actual visible blood loss may be deceiving. The client should be assessed for signs of shock, such as pallor, coldness and tachycardia, and fetal hypoxia secondary to inadequate oxygenation. Fetal heart tones and pattern are evaluated initially and then continuously through application of an external monitoring system. Hemoglobin and hematocrit also may be measured daily to assess blood loss. During the observation period, serial fundal height measurements (by placing mark on abdomen) might be able to demonstrate an increasing uterine distension secondary to occult bleeding.

Nursing Diagnosis

From the assessment, the nurse formulates nursing diagnoses for the woman with placenta previa. For a list of possible nursing diagnoses, see Box 31-6.

BOX 31–6
Nursing Diagnoses—Placenta Previa

- Fluid Volume Deficit related to the following:
    Excessive blood loss from abnormal placental implantation
    Risk of separation with cervical dilation
- Altered Tissue Perfusion: Peripheral related to hypovolemia
- Risk of infection related to the following:
    Hemorrhage
    Placenta previa
- Anxiety related to risk to fetal well-being
- Knowledge Deficit related to treatment regimen
- Impaired Home Maintenance Management related to bed rest and activity restrictions
- Risk for Altered Parent/Infant Attachment related to possible special care needs of infant
- Self Esteem Disturbance related to complication of pregnancy

Nursing Intervention

Plans for nursing intervention vary, depending on whether conservative or active medical management is prescribed. However, continuous close monitoring of maternal and fetal status is essential.

The client who is being managed at home or who is being discharged after an initial bleeding episode may require a referral for homemaking services and child care. Assistance in these areas is likely to facilitate client compliance with bed rest or restricted activities.

Ongoing assessments of maternal and perinatal status should be performed by the nurse to detect changes. Any indication of compromise to the client or the fetus should be reported immediately. The nurse also should be alert for the possiblity of infection and continued bleeding after delivery. Client education should focus on preoperative teaching to prepare the woman for a probable cesarean delivery and preparation of the family for a possible premature infant with special-care needs.

The client experiencing an excessive blood loss prior to or during delivery often requires this loss to be replaced. Packed red blood cells, fresh frozen plasma, platelets, and cryoprecipitate are the most commonly used blood products. Packed red blood cell transfusions increase oxygen delivery, whereas fresh frozen plasma may be given to replace clotting factor deficiencies (Dorman, 1989). It also may be necessary to administer oxygen to prevent maternal and fetal hypoxia.

The nurse should help the woman with a diagnosis of placenta previa to maintain her self-esteem by listening to her concerns and offering clear explanations about the situation and management approach. It is natural for the woman and her family to have many fears about the fetus' well-being, maternal dangers, and a possible cesarean delivery.

Nursing Evaluation

The following are anticipated outcomes of nursing care:

- The client verbalizes the effects of placenta previa on perinatal outcome and treatment to prevent complications.
- The client follows the prescribed treatment protocols.
- The client maintains adequate tissue perfusion and oxygen to the maternal–fetal unit.
- The client delivers a healthy newborn at or near term.
- The client returns to her previous level of functioning following delivery (generally cesarean section) without complications.

Abruptio Placentae

Abruptio placentae is the premature separation of a normally implanted placenta from the uterine wall. It is a serious complication; it is the most common cause of intrapartum fetal death and accounts for nearly 15% of perinatal mortality. It occurs in about 0.5% to 1.5% of all pregnancies (Ricci, 1992).

Manifestations and Causes

The causative mechanism of abruptio placentae is not known. However, it may be due to an inherent weakness or anomaly in the spiral arterioles, and certain conditions are believed to be contributing factors. The degree of placental separation and direction of the bleed (upward toward the fundus versus downward toward the cervix) determine the signs and symptoms exhibited by the client with abruptio placentae. The separation may be marginal, partial, or complete, and the bleeding may or may not be visible.

Clinical Picture. The clinical picture will vary, depending on the type of premature separation present (Fig. 31-4). **Covert abruptio placentae,** also called *concealed* abruptio placentae, is characterized by central separation that entraps lost blood between the uterine wall and the placenta. In this situation, a concealed hemorrhage often masks the seriousness of the problem. When a separation occurs at the margin, blood passes between the uterine wall and fetal membranes, creating an *external* hemorrhage. This type is called **overt** or revealed **abruptio placentae**. Blood also may infiltrate the myometrium, causing a blue discoloration of the uterus, known as a **Couvelaire uterus**.

Abruptio placentae also may be classified by degree of placental separation, in terms of *partial* or *complete* separation, or by grading (grade 1–3) according to clinical and laboratory findings related to the degree of separation. The three clinical findings used are external or occult uterine bleeding, uterine hypertonus or hyperactivity, and fetal distress or fetal death. The primary laboratory findings analyzed are serial maternal hematocrits (evaluated every 2–3 hours; maintained ≥ 30%) and the fibrinogen level, which is 450 mg/dL in the third trimester of normal pregnancy. If it falls below 300 mg/dL, significant coagulation abnormalities are usually present (Benedetti, 1991; Table 31-2).

The effects on the fetus depend mainly on the degree of disruption at the uteroplacental interface. Marginal separation may have no clinically apparent effect. Intermediate degrees of separation produce variable effects, while complete abruption usually causes fetal death from anoxia (Scott, 1994b). Understanding these variable effects comes from knowledge of the normal uteroplacental physiology. The amount of oxygen delivered to the fetus depends on uterine blood flow, the amount of blood diverted away from the intervillous space, the diffusion capacity of the placenta, the consumption of oxygen by the placenta, and the oxygen-carrying capacity of maternal and fetal blood.

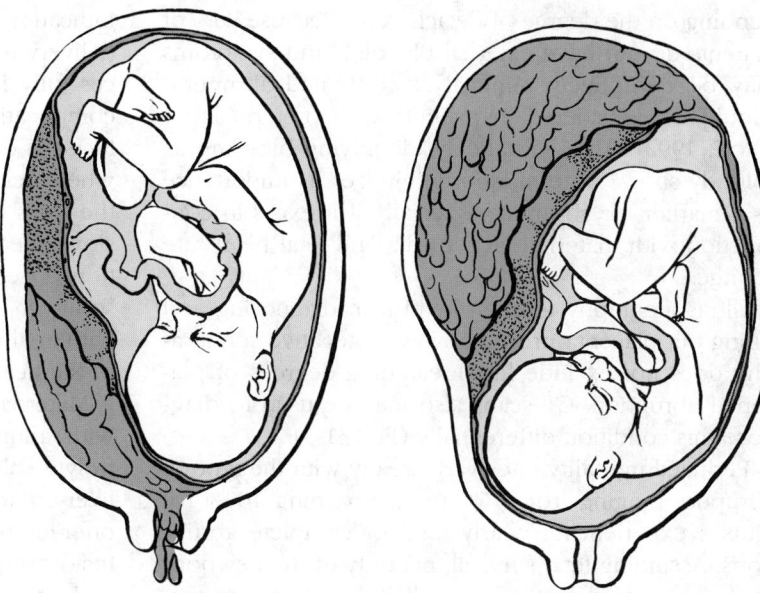

FIGURE 31–4 Abruptio placentae at various separation sites. Partial abruptio, external hemorrhage (*left*). Complete abruptio, concealed hemorrhage (*right*).

Based on data gathered from experimental studies on sheep, fetal oxygen consumption is well maintained by increases in fetal oxygen extraction until oxygen delivery is reduced by approximately 50%. The clinical dilemma is that the severtiy of the placental separation may progress rapidly, especially after abdominal trauma. Therefore, even mild abruption should be observed closely with continuous external fetal heart rate monitoring for at least 4 to 6 hours or until signs and symptoms have subsided (Scott, 1994b).

The manisfestations of an abruption are dark vaginal bleeding (if overt abruptio); abdominal pain, often sudden, severe, and "knifelike"; and a firm, tender uterus. The pain is produced by the accumulation of blood behind the placenta, with subsequent distention of the uterus. Because of the almost woody hardness of the uterine wall, fetal parts may be difficult to palpate. The contraction pattern typical of an abruptio placentae is frequent, low-amplitude contractions with an increase in resting tone. Shock is often out of proportion to visible blood loss, as manifested by a rapid pulse, dyspnea, yawning, restlessness, pallor, syncope, and cold, clammy perspiration.

Causes. The precise cause of the condition is unknown. It is frequently associated with maternal hypertension, grand multiparity (five or more pregnancies), short umbilical cord, and occasionally, automobile accidents and trauma. Other possible contributing factors include multiple gestation and hydramnios.

Medical Diagnosis and Prognosis

The diagnosis of abruptio placentae is determined by the client's history, physical examination, and diagnostic tests. The presenting symptoms vary greatly de-

---

TABLE 31–2
Grading of Abruptio Placentae by Degree of Placental Separation

Grade	Concealed Hemorrhage	Uterine Tenderness	Maternal Shock	Coagulopathy Overt	Fetal Distress	Comments
0	No	No	Absent	No	No	A retrospective diagnosis by examination of the placenta; no symptoms
1	No	No	Absent	No	No	Includes the diagnosis of "marginal sinus rupture"; blood loss variable
2	Yes	Yes	Absent	Rare	Yes	Will usually progress to grade 3 unless delivery is effected promptly
3	Yes	Yes	Present	Common	Fetal Death	Major maternal complication (eg, renal cortical necrosis)

Green, J. [1989]. Placenta previa and abruptio placenta. In R. Creasy & R. Resnik [Eds.], *Maternal-fetal medicine; Principles and practice*. [2nd ed.] [p. 601]. Philadelphia: W.B. Saunders.

pending on the degree of detachment. Because 20% of patients do not have external bleeding and symptoms may be deceptively minimal, a concealed abruption should be considered in patients with preterm labor (Ricci, 1992). Also, mistakenly identifying bleeding as "bloody show" of term labor minimizes its importance as a marker for abruptio, especially if it exists in conjunction with maternal tachycardia and fetal heart rate changes.

Ultrasonography is often helpful in diagnosing and ruling out placenta previa; however, negative sonography does not exclude life-threatening degrees of placental abruption. CT scans also may be used to diagnose this condition differentially (Fig. 31-5).

Perinatal mortality rates vary greatly with the type of abruptio, ranging from 15% to approaching 100% for fetuses experiencing nearly total or complete abruptions. Assuming fetal survival, maturity of the newborn at the time of delivery also will influence prognosis. Maternal mortality from abruptions has declined significantly and is now uncommon, although morbidity may be severe in some cases (Cunningham et al., 1993). Some of the complications of an abruption include hypovolemic shock, coagulopathy, and DIC.

Medical Management

Treatment depends on the condition of the fetus and the woman at the time the diagnosis is made. If the fetus is alive and at or near term, prompt delivery by cesarean birth (unless vaginal delivery can be accomplished quickly) is used for moderate to severe abruptions. If the fetus has already succumbed, usually an indication of an extensive placental separation, vaginal delivery is preferred unless hemorrhage cannot be successfully handled with blood replacement or if other complications arise. The risk of serious coagulation defects, as described subsequently, is likely to be greater when delivery is performed transabdominally. When the fetus is immature and blood loss is occurring at a slow rate, delivery may be delayed. Ongoing evaluation of fetal viability should be performed with ultrasonic Doppler devices to hear the fetal heart tones and with real-time ultrasound, which allows visualization of the heart movements.

Maternal hypovolemia and anemia may be corrected with administration of fresh whole blood and electrolyte solution either prior to or during labor and delivery. Packed red cells and lactated Ringer's solution offer alternative replacements that may minimize transfusion requirements while increasing oxygen delivery and circulating volume.

A central venous pressure (CVP) line or arterial line is inserted and maintained for hemodynamic monitoring of critically ill women. An indwelling urinary catheter (Foley) is used to assess fluid status and urinary output accurately.

If Couvelaire uterus occurs, the uterus is not able to contract well after delivery because the muscle is filled with blood. The uterus feels hard and boardlike on palpation. Treatment consists of complete evacuation of the uterus and stimulation of contractions with IV oxytocin.

Nursing Assessment

Nursing assessment of the woman with abruptio placentae includes all of the components described for patients with spontaneous abortion and placenta previa. Initial and ongoing assessments of maternal and fetal status are essential. Initial laboratory studies should include hemoglobin, hematocrit, fibrinogen levels, fibrin degradation products (FDP), thrombin time, prothrombin time, and partial thromboplastin time. These clients should be typed and cross-matched for several units of packed red blood cells because of the potential for a serious hemorrhage.

Nursing Diagnosis

Assessment of the client for signs and symptoms of abruptio placentae leads the nurse to specific nursing diagnoses (Box 31-7).

Nursing Intervention

Nursing interventions should be based on the presenting symptomatology and appropriate nursing diagnoses, in conjunction with any additional workups or

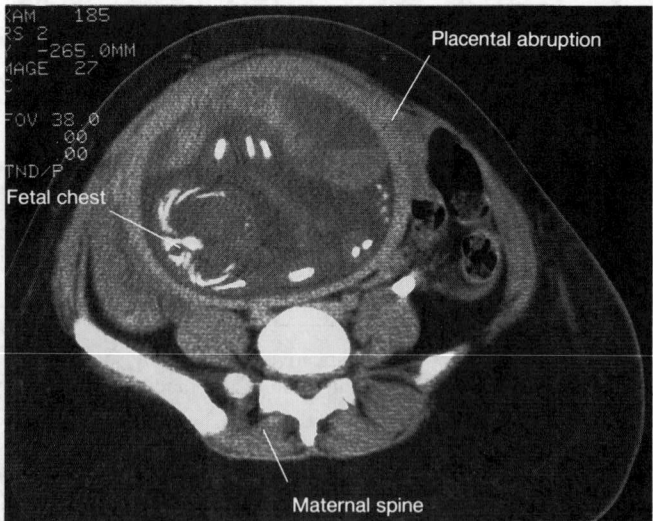

FIGURE 31–5 Computed tomography scan of placental abruption at 28 weeks with fetal demise resulting from an automobile accident. The maternal spine and fetal chest are visible. (Courtesy of Val A. Catanzarite, MD, PhD, and Cindy Maida, BS, RDMS, Sharp Perinatal Center, San Diego, California.)

BOX 31-7
Nursing Diagnoses—Abruptio Placentae

- Pain related to bleeding from premature separation of placenta
- Fluid Volume Deficit related to excessive blood loss (overt or concealed)
- Anxiety related to uncertainty of pregnancy outcome
- Altered Tissue Perfusion: Peripheral related to hypovolemia
- Risk for Injury (fetal) related to impaired placental perfusion
- Knowledge Deficit related to treatments and procedures

---

therapies ordered by the physician. If the abruption is mild and the fetus is immature, careful and continuous nursing observation is necessary to detect evidence of progressive maternal blood loss or changes in fetal status, such as ominous decelerations or bradycardia. In some women, the supine position can cause the heavy gravid uterus to compress the major maternal blood vessels, leading to decreased placental perfusion. If this occurs, use of the lateral recumbent position can relieve the compression and increase uteroplacental exchange. Because the major vessels run along the right side of the spine in about 25% of women, the left lateral position may be more effective in some women. Independent turning to her right side or back can be allowed in most women, if there is adequate perfusion confirmed by a reassuring fetal heart tracing and normal maternal BP. Restricting maternal movement to only one position needs to be justified, because discomfort from fatigue of certain supporting muscle groups can occur, especially for those on long-term bed rest.

In more acute situations, hourly intake and output should be recorded. An output of 30 to 60 mL/h is desired. Oxygen may be administered by face mask at 8 to 10 L/min to prevent or minimize fetal hypoxia. If a CVP line is in place, readings must be carefully obtained, recorded, and reported. Normal range during pregnancy is 5 to 12 mm Hg. Occasionally, pulmonary artery wedge pressure monitoring with the Swan-Ganz catheter may be done. Normal range for pulmonary artery (PA) pressure is 10 to 20 mm Hg; the normal range for pulmonary wedge pressure (PWP) is <6 to 8 mm Hg (Schmidt, 1993).

Observations should be made for signs and symptoms of maternal hypovolemia and hypoxemia, such as tachycardia and shortness of breath. It also is essential for the nurse to assess the client for adverse reactions to blood transfusions. Administering more than 10 U is considered massive transfusion; after administering 4 to 6 U, clotting studies and potassium level should be reevaluated (Schmidt, 1993).

In cases of moderate to severe abruption and a live fetus, the nurse should provide preoperative teaching about the possibility of a cesarean delivery and birth of a preterm infant. A realistic attitude about the client's health situation and honest factual information are important aspects of the psychological support offered by the nurse to the family.

Following delivery, the nurse should continue assessing fluid-volume balance and vital signs. The uterus should be palpated frequently for atony. The client should be evaluated for signs of excessive blood loss.

Nursing Evaluation

Anticipated outcomes of nursing care for the woman with abruptio placentae are similar to those for the woman with placenta previa. Additional anticipated outcomes follow:

- The fetus demonstrates adequate tissue perfusion and oxygenation.
- The client discusses the impact of fetal or neonatal loss on her and her family, progressing appropriately through the grieving process.

Other Problems Associated With Bleeding

Bleeding may lead to hypovolemia and hemorrhagic shock unless vigorous treatment is implemented to control bleeding and replace blood loss. In most emergency situations, the uterus must be expeditiously emptied of all contents. Delay may result in complications, such as hypofibrinogenemia and DIC.

Hypofibrinogenemia

Hypofibrinogenemia, a deficiency of fibrinogen in the blood, occurs in the childbearing woman who has depleted her blood fibrinogen in an attempt to control bleeding by clot formation. For example, following an abruptio placentae, thromboplastin enters the circulation, causing small fibrin clots to form in the capillaries. As the level of fibrinogen decreases in the circulating blood, normal clotting mechanisms are impaired. This complication also is seen in other entities, such as amniotic fluid embolus, prolonged retention of a dead fetus, and septic abortion. Because of the danger of this complication, fibrinogen levels (normal, 300–500 mg/dL) should be obtained. The nurse also can perform a simple *clot observation test* by placing a small amount of fresh blood in a test tube and watching how quickly a clot is formed. A firm clot should form in 4 to 12 minutes.

Medical Management

Treatment for hypofibrinogenemia involves replacement of blood and fibrinogen and termination of the pregnancy. The administration of cryoprecipitate generally is effective in raising the fibrinogen concentration of plasma.

Disseminated Intravascular Coagulation

Consumptive coagulopathy, or DIC, is a paradoxic disorder with anticoagulation and procoagulation effects existing simultaneously. In DIC, clotting is overstimulated throughout the circulatory system. The most frequent initiating event is an abruption; however, other obstetric complications, such as **pregnancy-induced hypertension** (PIH), retained products of conception, infection, trauma, saline abortion, or amniotic fluid embolism, may be causative factors. These pathologic conditions act on either the intrinsic or the extrinsic pathways, creating increased formation of thrombin. The thrombin interacts with fibrinogen, resulting in formation of clots. Eventually the body's clotting fac-

tors are depleted, and severe hemorrhage occurs (Cunningham et al., 1993).

Pathophysiology

Because of the failure of the normal checks and balances of blood coagulation, DIC results in a system-wide, rather than a local, generation of thrombin and plasmin. (For a review of the normal coagulation pathways, see Fig. 31-6.) Excess thrombin leads to **thrombosis** (clot formation), depletion of clotting factors, and platelets <100,000 (**thrombocytopenia**). The excess plasmin generated has three damaging effects: It degrades fibrinogen as it circulates in the bloodstream (Weiner, 1991); it inactivates several clotting factors (V, VIII, IX, XI), adding to the anticoagulation effect; and it activates the first and third complement components, which trigger cell lysis, immunoadherence, and other immune phenomena (Fig. 31-6).

Anticoagulation also occurs because of the presence of the FDPs, or fibrin split products (FSPs), from the breakdown of fibrin and fibrinogen. FSP binds the soluble fibrin monomers and prevents their polymerization. Thrombocytopenia results not only from in-

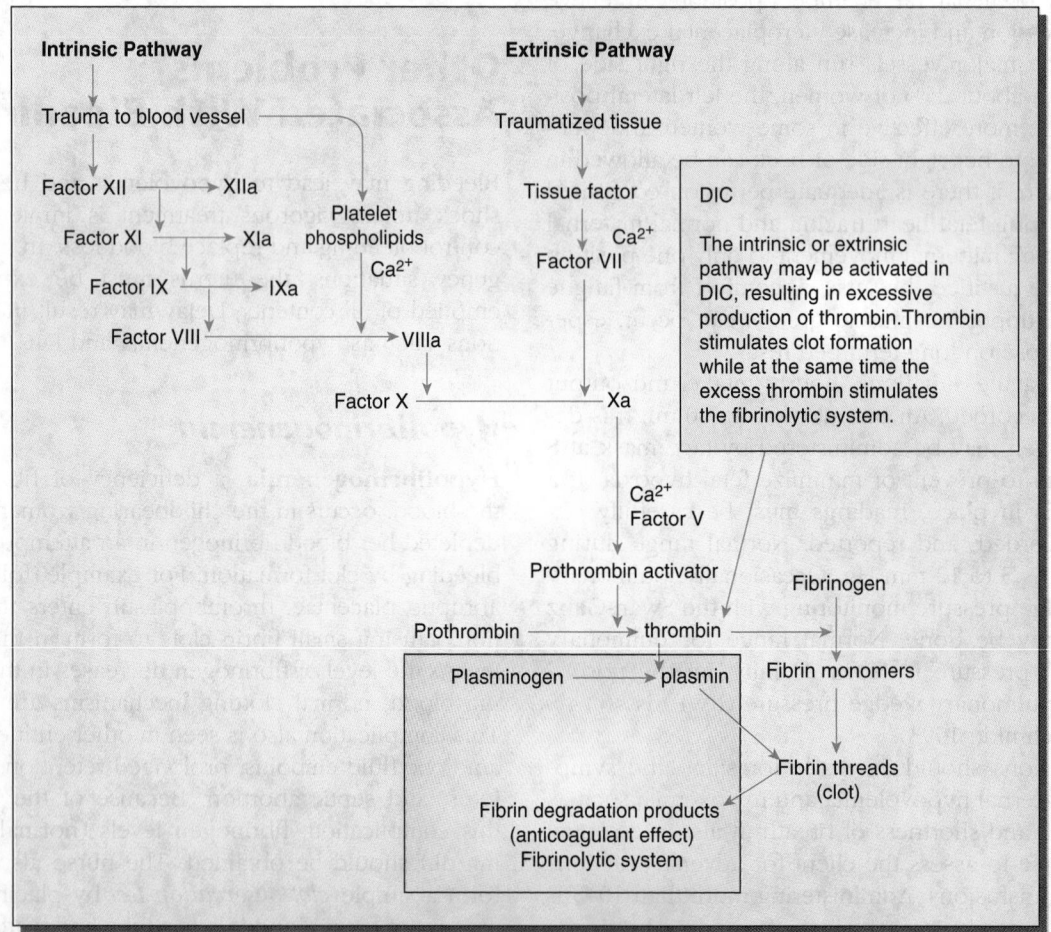

FIGURE 31-6 Normal blood coagulation pathways, the fibrinolytic system, and disseminated intravascular coagulation.

creased consumption, but also from increased clearance secondary to the FSPs coating the platelets. The inability to clot leads to hemorrhage from at least three sites at once, such as hematuria, epistaxis, and oozing from puncture wounds (Weiner, 1991).

The fibrin monomers that do polymerize are filtered out within the microvasculature. These fibrin plugs restrict flow, resulting in tissue hypoxia, which produces multiorgan cellular destruction. Endothelial damage enhances platelet activation and alters the vessel's ability to respond to endogenous vasoactive substances. The kidneys are frequently affected, developing acute tubular necrosis and subsequent renal failure (Dorman, 1989). Contact between fibrin and red blood cells (RBCs) within the blocked microvasculature results in RBC breakdown (hemolysis). The subsequent release of intracellular material from the hemolysis propagates the DIC cycle (Weiner, 1991).

Medical Diagnosis

Antithrombin III (AT III), a glycoprotein and major in vivo inhibitor of thrombin generation, is presently the most sensitive laboratory parameter for the diagnosis of DIC. AT III binds to activated factors XII, XI, IX, and X, causing thrombin inactivation. In combination with heparin, the thrombin inactivation is rapidly accelerated (Sisson, 1992). Abnormal consumption of this inhibitor by thrombin or another activated serine protein must occur if DIC is present. The concentration of AT III declines when consumption exceeds production (Weiner, 1991).

The results of common laboratory assessments reveal several abnormalities. These are presented in Table 31-3. Plasma fibrinogen and platelets are decreased; FDPs, thrombin time, prothrombin time, and partial thromboplastin time are increased in more than 50% of patients with acute DIC. In 15% of patients, the FDP level is normal, possibly because the FDP are degraded past the point detectable (Bick, 1978).

Medical Management

Current medical intervention for DIC is directed toward four main strategies as outlined in Box 31-8: removal of the triggering event, replacement of clotting factors and platelets, anticoagulant therapy, and inhibition of residual fibrinolysis (only if first three steps did not stop bleeding).

TABLE 31-3
Laboratory Tests for Disseminated Intravascular Coagulation (DIC)

Test	Nonpregnant Values	Normal Pregnancy	Result in DIC
Antithrombin III		Normal	Increased consumption (>70%); decreased concentration
Clotting time	6–12 min	Normal	Normal
Clot retraction	Good	Good	Poor (lyses in 15–60 min)
Fibrinogen	200–400 mg/dL	300–500 mg/dL	Usually depressed
Thrombin time	12–18 s	Shortened	Usually prolonged
Prothrombin time	11–13 s	Shortened	Usually prolonged
Partial thromboplastin time or activated partial thromboplastin time	40–60 s / 25–45 s	Shortened / Shortened	Usually prolonged / Usually prolonged
Factor assays		Normal	V, VIII, XIII reduced
Platelets	150,000–400,000/mm^3	Normal	Usually decreased
Red blood cell morphology		Normal	Often abnormal (eg, schistocytes)
Fibrin split products		Usually absent	Present
Euglobulin clot lysis		Normal	Usually shortened
Plasminogen		Normal	Usually depressed
Plasma protamine paracoagulation		Fibrin monomer absent	Fibrin monomer present
Ethanol gelation		Fibrin monomer absent	Fibrin monomer present
Protamine sulfate precipitation		Fibrin monomer absent	Fibrin monomer present
Staphylococcal clumping		Fibrin monomer absent	Fibrin monomer present

(Cavanagh, D. et al. [1982]. *Obstetric emergencies*. Philadelphia: Harper & Row. Weiner, C. [1991]. *Critical care obstetrics*. Boston: Blackwell Scientific Publications.)

BOX 31-8
Therapy for Acute Disseminated Intravascular Coagulation (DIC)

■ Removal of the triggering event
   Volume replacement and expansion (crystalloid, plasmanate, albumin)
   Evacuation of uterus (if indicated)
   Antibiotics (if indicated)
■ Replacement of clotting factors and platelets (component therapy)
   Fresh frozen plasma
   Prothrombin complex
   Platelets
   packed red cells (in the face of hemorrhage)
■ Anticoagulant therapy
   Low-dose heparin (2500–5000 U q8–12 h) if AT III activity exceeds 70%
   AT III concentrates (if unavailable, fresh frozen plasma)
   Antiplatelet drugs (for chronic DIC)
■ Inhibition of residual fibrinolysis (only after first three steps undertaken and client continues to bleed): epsilon-aminocaproic acid

(Weiner, C. [1991]. Disseminated intravascular coagulopathy associated with pregnancy. In S. Clark, D. Cotton, G. Hankins, & J. Phelan [Eds.] Critical care obstetrics [2nd ed.]. Boston: Blackwell Scientific.)

Nursing Management

The nurse must perform careful assessment of women at risk for early signs of DIC. Clinical manifestations may be difficult to assess in the early stage but become more obvious as the severity of the disease progresses. Symptoms include bleeding from the gums and injection sites, petechiae and purpura on the skin, restlessness, anxiety, and tachycardia.

Continuous electronic fetal heart rate monitoring and uterine activity are necessary to assess fetal well-being. The presence of late decelerations, tachycardia, and loss of variablility may indicate impaired fetal gas exchange and indicate a need to expedite delivery. An indwelling urinary catheter is inserted to evaluate urinary output carefully. Output should be maintained at 30 mL/h to ensure adequate renal perfusion. Need for fluid replacement also is assessed by urine-specific gravity, hematocrit, and central hemodynamic monitoring by CVP, PA, and PWP. As with other hemorrhagic disorders, ongoing assessments about the quantity of actual blood loss are necessary. Serial assessment of maternal vital signs is necessary to assess adequacy of peripheral perfusion. The nurse should be alert to signs of alterations in mental status (confusion), pulmonary dysfunction (dyspnea, tachypnea, and cyanosis), and liver dysfunction (jaundice, nausea), which indicate overall multiorgan status. Pulse oximetry and measurements of arterial blood gases may be useful to evaluate the client's oxygen saturation (Sisson, 1992).

Hypertensive Disorders of Pregnancy

Hypertensive disorders include a variety of vascular disturbances that antedate pregnancy or occur as a complication during gestation or the early postpartum period. Because of the many cardiovascular alterations, pregnancy may induce hypertension in women who have been normotensive prior to gestation or may aggravate existing hypertensive conditions.

Classification

Hypertension is defined as a BP of 140/90 mm Hg or higher or a rise of 30 mm Hg or more in systolic pressure or 15 mm Hg or more in diastolic pressure above baseline. For diagnosis of hypertension, the BP elevations must be present on two occassions at least 6 hours apart.

The classification system and definition of the hypertensive disorders of pregnancy originally developed in 1972 by Hughes (Hughes, 1972) was modified in 1986 by the American College of Obstetricians and Gynecologists (ACOG, 1986; Cunningham et al., 1993). Four basic categories of hypertensive disorders complicate pregnancy: PIH, chronic hyperpertension, chronic hypertension with superimposed PIH (coincidental hypertension), and late or transient hypertension (see Assessment Guidelines: Hypertensive Disorders of Pregnancy).

The term PIH covers specific conditions that develop as a direct result of pregnancy. Until recently, **toxemia** was the term used to describe hypertension with onset during pregnancy. This condition was believed to be caused by toxins derived from the products of conception circulating in the blood. However, because these "toxins" have never been identified, the current diagnostic label is PIH. It is used to describe this syndrome of hypertension, edema, and proteinuria, with the later two not always present. If hypertension includes proteinuria or pathologic edema (nondependent, involving face and hands and persisting after rising), the diagnosis of **preeclampsia** should be made. This distinction between PIH and preeclampsia, however, is regional, because in America, the terms are used synonymously; in Europe, they are not (Fukashima, 1995). If seizures occur in conjunction with proteinuria, pathologic edema, or hypertension, the diagnosis of **eclampsia** should be made.

Preeclampsia is further divided into mild and severe depending on the manifestations present. This distinc-

ASSESSMENT GUIDELINES
Hypertensive Disorders of Pregnancy

A. Pregnancy-induced hypertension (PIH)
1. Preeclampsia—hypertension with proteinuria or edema developing after the 20th week of gestation
   a. Symptoms may occur earlier with hydatidiform mole
   b. Occurs almost exclusively in primigravidas
   c. Affects women at extremes of reproductive age (less than 20 y or more than 35 y)
   d. May be seen in multigravidas with the following:
      (1) Uterine overdistention as with twins or hydramnios
      (2) Vascular disease, including essential chronic hypertension and diabetes mellitus
      (3) Chronic renal disease
   Hypertension: 140/90 or an increase of 30 mm Hg systolic or 15 mm Hg diastolic over baseline; observation of these criteria on at least two occasions 6 h or more apart
   Edema: a weight gain of 3 lb or greater in 1 wk or an accumulation of fluid greater than 1+ pitting edema after 12 h of bed rest
   Proteinuria: 3 g/L or greater of protein in a 24-h urine collection (2+ by dipstick)
   Severe preeclampsia:
   When one or more of the following are present:
   ■ Systolic blood pressure of 160 mm Hg or diastolic of 110 mm Hg on two occasions at least 6 h apart while the client is on bed rest
   ■ Proteinuria of at least 4 g/24 h or 3+ to 4+ by semiquantitative analysis
   ■ Cerebral or visual disturbances, such as altered consciousness, headache, scotomata, or blurred vision
   ■ Pulmonary edema or cyanosis
   Signs of advancing disease:
   ■ Epigastric or upper quadrant pain
   ■ Thrombocytopenia or impaired liver function

2. Eclampsia—extension of preeclampsia with grand mal seizure
   ■ One-half the cases occur before labor.
   ■ One-fourth of the cases occur during labor.
   ■ One-fourth of the cases occur within 48 h postpartum.
B. Chronic hypertension
   1. Blood pressure of 140/90 before pregnancy
   2. Blood pressure of 140/90 before 20th week gestation or persisting indefinitely following delivery
   3. For differential diagnosis after the 20th week of gestation:
      a. Hemorrhage and exudates seen on funduscopic examination
      b. Plasma urea nitrogen: ≥20 mg/dL
      c. Plasma creatinine levels: ≥1 mg/dL
      d. Presence of chronic disease, such as diabetes mellitus or connective tissue diseases
C. Chronic hypertension with superimposed preeclampsia—often a quick progression to eclampsia, which may develop before the 30th week of gestation
   1. Documented evidence of chronic hypertension
   2. Evidence of a superimposed, acute process
      a. Elevation of systolic blood pressure 30 mm Hg or of diastolic blood pressure 15–20 mm Hg above baseline on two occasions at least 6 h apart
      b. Development of proteinuria
      c. Edema as observed in women with preeclampsia
D. Late or transient hypertension—transient elevations of blood pressure are observed during labor or in early postpartum period, returning to normal within 10 d postpartum

(Cunningham, G. et al. [1993]. Williams obstetrics [pp. 764–784]. Norwalk, CT: Appleton & Lange.)

tion is crucial because a severe condition means an immediate delivery is indicated (except in selected very premature cases as discussed later). Severe preeclampsia is indicated by the presence of more serious symptoms occurring in isolation or together. Two of the most characteristic are a diastolic BP >110 mm Hg or persistent proteinuria 3+ or more.

Hemolysis, elevated liver enzymes, low platelets (HELLP) syndrome reflects the severity of the disease process. The presence of multiorgan swelling and tissue damage is reflected in various possible symptomatology: Hepatocellular necrosis and edema cause epigastric pain and elevated liver enzymes (aspartate aminotranaminase [AST] and alanine aminotransaminase [ALT]); pulmonary edema causes shortness of breath; renal lesions lead to persistent proteinuria of >1+, oliguria, or elevated serum creatinine; severe vasospasms can lead to microangiopathic hemolysis, evidenced by hemoglobinemia, hemoglobinuria, hyperbilirubinemia, and decreased placental perfusion, causing fetal growth retardation; cerebral edema causes headache and visual disturbances (Cunningham et al., 1993; ACOG, 1986).

The term **gestational hypertension** refers to a relatively benign condition of elevated BP during pregnancy without the signs of proteinuria and edema. There is no evidence of preeclampsia or previous hypertension. Following delivery, the BP returns to normal prepregnancy values. If hypertension develops without edema or proteinuria during labor or in the early postpartum period and then returns to normal within 10 days following delivery, it is described as **late or transient hypertension.**

The term **chronic hypertension** is used when the client has a coincidental hypertensive vascular disorder that is unrelated to pregnancy and was evident prior to gestation or persists postpartum. If the pregnant patient with chronic hypertension or renal disease develops the complication of preeclampsia or eclampsia, the condition is called pregnancy-aggravated hypertension and includes **superimposed preeclampsia** or **superimposed eclampsia.**

Pregnancy-Induced Hypertension

In the United States, the overall incidence of PIH is commonly cited to be about 5%. The prevalence of the disease may be much higher among certain groups, including primigravidas younger than 20 years, women with chronic hypertension, women from low socioeconomic backgrounds, and women older than 35 years. The recurrence rate is correlated to the severity of the prior pregnancy condition. Mild PIH usually does not recur; however, severe preeclampsia tends to recur in 30% to 50% of the women (Harvey et al., 1992; Scott, 1994). The risk for eclampsia in twin pregnancies is two to three times than that of single pregnancy. The working woman, who may lack sufficient bed rest, has a twofold increase in the development of preeclampsia (Zuspan 1994).

Fetal death rates are related to the severity of the hypertension and to the development of the HELLP syndrome. The mortality rate associated with HELLP syndrome ranges between 2% and 24% for the woman and 7.7% and 60% for the fetus, depending on the study referenced (Harvey et al., 1992). The loss of maternal and infant lives to pregnancy-related hypertension can most often be prevented. With improved prenatal care and a rational approach to management, dramatic declines in maternal mortality have been reported. It is now believed that in general, eclampsia is preventable and fortunately has become less common in the United States (Cunningham et al., 1993). Long-term outcome for children of term preeclamptic women is usually good if they are not born hypoxic or acidotic (Cunningham et al., 1993). However, in preterm infants, a slight delay in growth up to 1.5 years has been noted (Martikainen, 1989).

Pathophysiology

Arteriolar vasoconstriction, systemic vasospasms, and vascular damage characterize PIH. Arterial circulation is disrupted by alternating segments of constriction and dilation. The vasospastic action damages the blood vessels by decreasing their blood supply and stretching them in areas where segment dilation is occurring. The endothelium is injured; platelets, fibrinogen, and other blood products may be released into the interendothelium. The vascular damage leads to increased albumin permeability and resultant fluid shifts from intravascular to extravascular space (third spacing) seen clinically as edema. Fig. 31-7 summarizes the events associated with this form of PIH, known as "dry" PIH, and its resulting signs and symptoms. Edema also may be from the other form of PIH, known as "wet" PIH, in which increased vascular volume is due to water retention secondary to decreased glomerular function (Box 31-9).

Preeclampsia

The pathophysiologic changes associated with preeclampsia result in the typical triad of signs and symptoms, including hypertension, proteinuria, and edema.

Manifestations. Preeclampsia is characterized by elevated BP, proteinuria, or edema after the 20th week of pregnancy in a gravida who previously has been normal in these respects. Unless the preeclamptic process is halted by treatment or delivery, eclampsia is likely to ensue.

Hypertension may occur suddenly, or it may be gradual and insidious. The absolute BP level is probably of less significance than the relationship it bears to previous determinations and the time in gestation when these determinations are recorded. The healthy client's BP decreases to a nadir during the second trimester and early third trimester and rises thereafter. A sustained rise of 30 mm Hg systolic or 15 mm Hg diastolic may indicate an abnormality, most likely preeclampsia (Cunningham et al., 1993).

The next most constant sign of preeclampsia is sudden excessive weight gain, which is largely due to an accumulation of water in the tissues. Such weight gain

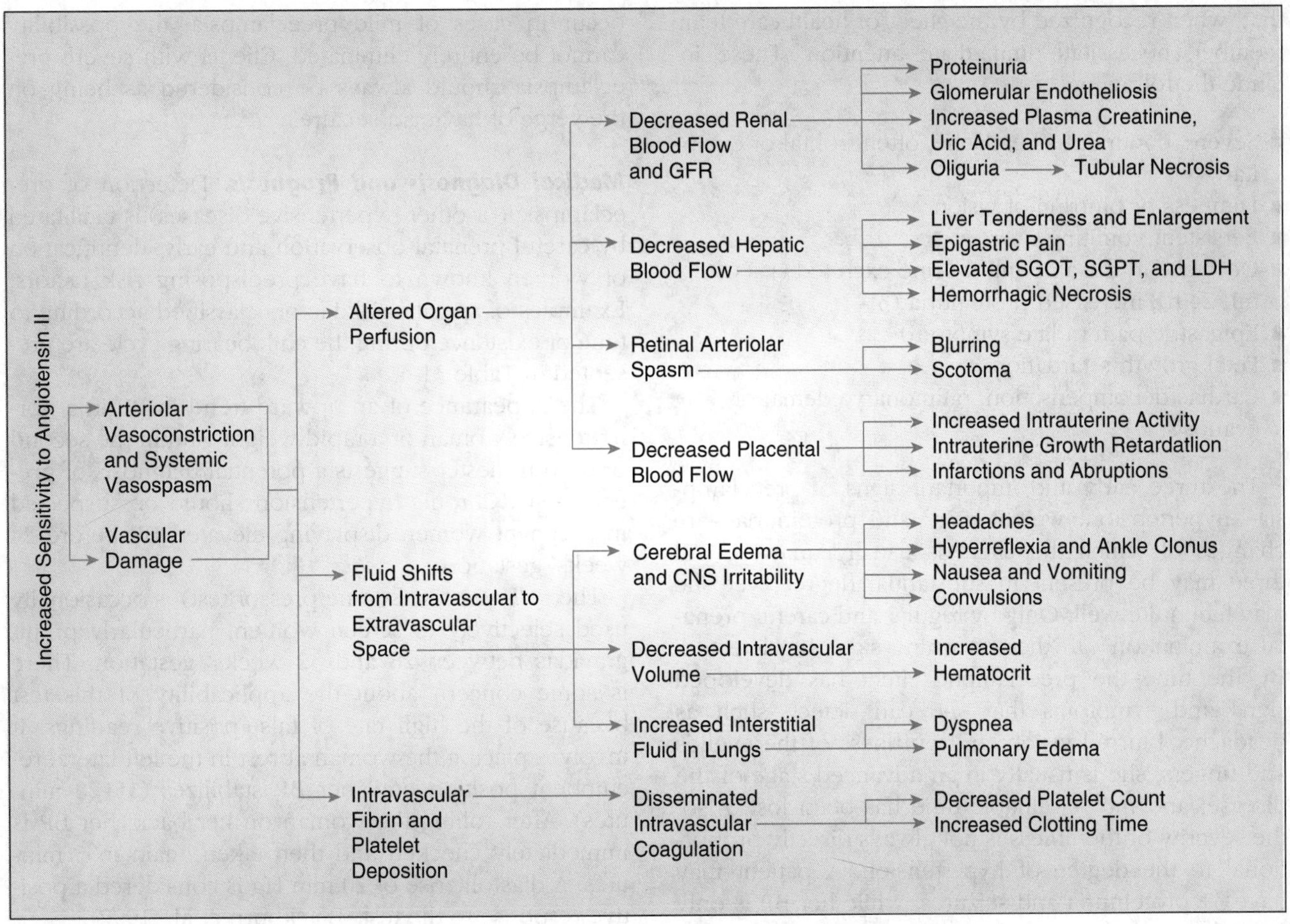

Increased Sensitivity to Angiotensin II

Arteriolar Vasoconstriction and Systemic Vasospasm

Vascular Damage

↓

Altered Organ Perfusion

Decreased Renal Blood Flow and GFR
→ Proteinuria
→ Glomerular Endotheliosis
→ Increased Plasma Creatinine, Uric Acid, and Urea
→ Oliguria → Tubular Necrosis

Decreased Hepatic Blood Flow
→ Liver Tenderness and Enlargement
→ Epigastric Pain
→ Elevated SGOT, SGPT, and LDH
→ Hemorrhagic Necrosis

Retinal Arteriolar Spasm
→ Blurring
→ Scotoma

Decreased Placental Blood Flow
→ Increased Intrauterine Activity
→ Intrauterine Growth Retardatlion
→ Infarctions and Abruptions

Fluid Shifts from Intravascular to Extravascular Space

Cerebral Edema and CNS Irritability
→ Headaches
→ Hyperreflexia and Ankle Clonus
→ Nausea and Vomiting
→ Convulsions

Decreased Intravascular Volume
→ Increased Hematocrit

Increased Interstitial Fluid in Lungs
→ Dyspnea
→ Pulmonary Edema

Intravascular Fibrin and Platelet Deposition

Disseminated Intravascular Coagulation
→ Decreased Platelet Count
→ Increased Clotting Time

FIGURE 31–7 Pathophysiologic alterations occurring in severe PIH. Key: PIH, pregnancy-induced hypertension; CNS, central nervous system; GFR, glomerular filtration rate; SGOT, serum glutamic-oxaloacetic transaminase; SGPT, serum glutamic-pyruvic transaminase; LDH, lactate dehydrogenase. (Modified from Gilbert, E. S., & Harmon, J. S. [1992]. *High-risk pregnancy and delivery: Nursing perspectives* [2nd ed.]. St. Louis: C. V. Mosby.)

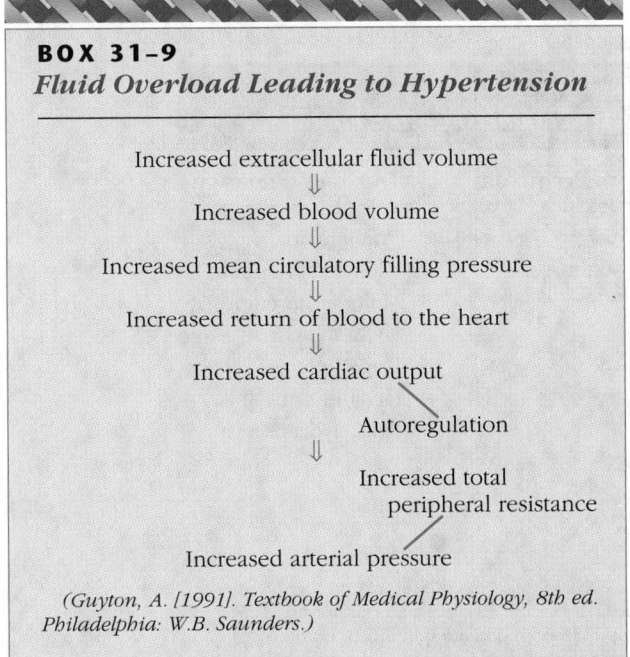

BOX 31–9
Fluid Overload Leading to Hypertension

Increased extracellular fluid volume
⇓
Increased blood volume
⇓
Increased mean circulatory filling pressure
⇓
Increased return of blood to the heart
⇓
Increased cardiac output
Autoregulation
⇓
Increased total peripheral resistance
Increased arterial pressure

(Guyton, A. [1991]. Textbook of Medical Physiology, 8th ed. Philadelphia: W.B. Saunders.)

represents occult edema and almost always precedes the visible face and finger edema characteristic of the advanced stages of the disease. A weight increase of 1 lb/wk is normal, but if the woman gains more than 2 lb in any week or 6 lb in 1 month, preeclampsia should be suspected (Cunningham et al., 1993).

The sudden appearance of protein in the urine, with or without other findings, should always be regarded as a sign of preeclampsia. Because the degree of proteinuria can vary from hour to hour due to the vasospastic nature of this illness, a 24-hour urine collection and complete urinalysis, including a microscopic examination, is more accurate than a one-time dip stick. This also helps to exclude infection as a cause of proteinuria. Because proteinuria usually develops later than the hypertension and the weight gain, it may indicate progression of the disease process.

More than 300 mg/dL or >1+ on a dip stick sampling of random urine is considered abnormal (Scott, 1994).

As mentioned previously, there also are other multi-organ clinical manifestations of **severe preeclampsia** that, when recognized by the client or healthcare team member, necessitate immediate attention. These include the following:

- Severe, continuous headache, often frontal or occipital
- Dimness or blurring of vision
- Persistent vomiting
- Decrease in the amount of urine excreted (<400 mL/24 h); increased proteinuria (3+–4+)
- Epigastric pain (a late symptom)
- Fetal growth retardation
- Cardiac decompensation, pulmonary edema, or cyanosis

The three early and important signs of preeclampsia—hypertension, weight gain, and proteinuria—are changes of which the client is usually unaware. All three may be present in substantial degree, yet she may feel quite well. Only by regular and careful prenatal examination can these warning signs be detected. By the time the preeclamptic client has developed signs and symptoms that she can detect, such as headache, blurred vision, and puffiness of the eyelids and fingers, she is usually in an advanced stage of the disease, and much valuable time has been lost. Also, the severity of the illness is not always directly proportional to the degree of hypertension. A patient may have 3+ proteinuria and seizures, while her BP is only 140/85 (Cunningham et al., 1993).

Headaches are rarely observed in the milder cases but are encountered more frequently as the disease progresses. In general, clients who develop eclampsia often experience severe headache as a forerunner of the first seizure. The visual disturbances range from a slight blurring of vision to various degrees of temporary blindness. Although seizures are less likely to occur in cases of mild preeclampsia, the possibility cannot be entirely eliminated. Clients with severe preeclampsia should always be considered as being on the verge of having a seizure.

Medical Diagnosis and Prognosis. Detection of preeclampsia (or other hypertensive diseases) is facilitated by careful prenatal observation and early identification of women known to have predisposing risk factors. Examples of specific risk factors classified according to time of existence during the childbearing cycle are presented in Table 31-4.

The appearance of an upward trend in BP in a normotensive woman or a rapid weight gain in the second or third trimester suggests a potential diagnosis of preeclampsia. Chronic hypertension should be suspected in pregnant women displaying elevated BP before 24 weeks' gestation.

The *roll-over test* (supine pressor test) is occasionally used selectively to screen women, particularly primigravidas between 28 and 32 weeks' gestation. There is some concern about the applicability of this test because of the high rate of false-positive readings. It involves placing the woman at rest in the left lateral recumbent position until her BP stabilizes (15–20 minutes). After rolling the woman on her back, her BP is immediately checked and then taken again in 5 minutes. A diastolic rise of 20 mm Hg is considered a positive response to the test (Blackburn et al., 1992).

Determination of mean arterial pressure (MAP) also may be useful in predicting risk for developing hypertensive disease, because it reflects the resistance against which the heart works. The calculation of the MAP follows:

$$MAP = \frac{\text{Systolic BP} + 2\,(\text{diastolic BP})}{3}$$

TABLE 31–4
Pregnancy-Induced Hypertension (PIH): Recognizing Risk Factors

Before Pregnancy	Possibly Before Pregnancy	During Pregnancy
Nulligravida	Diabetes mellitus*	Primigravida
Age extemes	Preexisting hypertensive, vascular, or renal disease	Glomerulonephritis
≤20 y		Multiple gestation
≥35 y*		Hydramnios
Underweight		Large fetus
Obesity		Hydatidiform mole
Dietary deficiencies		Fetal hydrops
Family history of hypertension-vascular disease*		
Diagnosis of severe PIH in previous pregnancy		

*Predisposes to chronic hypertension and PIH.
(Scott, J. [1994]. Hypertension disorders of pregnancy. In J. Scott, P. DiSaia, C. Hammond, & W. Spellacy [Eds.], *Danforth's obstetrics and gynecology* [pp. 351–365]. Philadelphia: J. B. Lippincott.)

An increase of 20 mm Hg in MAP is considered ominous.

The prognosis for women with preeclampsia depends on the maternal effects of hypertension on the body systems (eg, cardiovascular, central nervous system, renal) and the ability to prevent or control the disease before eclampsia develops. The combination of proteinuria and hypertension dramatically increases the risk of perinatal mortality and morbidity. The only definitive cure for preeclampsia is delivery.

Some maternal complications may occur as a result of severe preeclampsia. These include eclampsia, pulmonary edema, cerebral hemorrhage (massive or disseminated), congestive heart failure, arrhythmias, myocardial infarction, DIC, HELLP, adult respiratory distress syndrome, and intravascular endothelial damage. The fetus is at risk for placental abruption (2%–10% of cases), intrauterine growth retardation, acute hypoxia, intrauterine death, and prematurity.

Medical Management. Medical management is directed toward prevention and early detection of the development of preeclampsia through early and regular prenatal care. Women with recognized risks for hypertensive disease should have prenatal health supervision scheduled at more frequent intervals, especially during the third trimester. Every pregnant woman should be assessed every 2 weeks during the first 2 months of the third trimester and then each week during the last month of pregnancy. The importance of frequent and regular BP readings cannot be emphasized too strongly.

The results of innovative studies have suggested that low-dose aspirin therapy protects against the appearance of preeclampsia in high-risk pregnant women (Beaufils et al., 1985; Wallenburg et al., 1986; Wallenburg et al., 1987). However, in a recent multicenter, double-blind clinical trial, the incidence of preeclampsia following aspirin therapy was not significantly less, and an increased incidence of placental abruption was found in women who received low-dose aspirin prophylaxis (Sibai et al., 1993).

If mild symptoms of the disease develop (eg, minor elevation of BP with minimal or no signs of edema and proteinuria), the client may remain at home and be examined at least twice a week. The treatment plan includes the following:

- Restriction of activities, including bed rest during the greater part of the day, and sexual abstinence
- Administration of prescribed sedative drugs as necessary to encourage rest and relaxation
- Ingestion of a well-balanced diet with ample protein, particularly lean meat, fish, and eggs; sometimes a "no added salt" restriction

If the client's condition does not respond promptly to restricted activity at home, hospitalization may be recommended. Medical care of the hospitalized mild preeclamptic woman is directed toward the following:

- Protecting the client from the effects of high BP (eg, cerebral hemorrhage)
- Preventing the occurrence of eclamptic seizures and improving uteroplacental blood flow to decrease fetal risks
- Delivering the fetus as close to maturity as possible with the safest method

With severe preeclampsia, delivery is always the appropriate therapy for the woman.

The dilemma is in regard to the fetus; when the gestational age is less than 25 to 30 weeks, the risks of premature birth are great for the fetus. Conservative management is controversial and appropriate only with meticulous observation of the maternal and fetal condition with no evidence of fetal distress, fetal growth retardation, or progression of the disease to a more serious stage (Scott et al. 1990).

The woman with severe preeclampsia should be admitted to the labor and delivery suite or the maternal-fetal intensive care unit where continuous observations and emergency drugs and supplies are available. The nature of drug therapy prescribed by the physician depends on the client's condition. In mild preeclampsia, medications may or may not be ordered. When severe preeclampsia develops, however, immediate and intensive therapy is imperative.

Anticonvulsant therapy is of major importance to prevent and control seizures. The dosage of drugs used should be regulated so that drowsiness and sleep, from which the client can be easily awakened, is achieved. Sedation also suppresses the client's hyperactive reflexes. Magnesium sulfate ($MgSO_4$) is the drug of choice in the United States to prevent and control maternal eclamptic seizures. Because Mg^{2+} is a calcium channel blocker, it has the dual effect of inhibiting cerebral neurotransmitter release (slowing nerve impulses) and decreasing the excitability of muscle fibers to direct stimulation, thereby relaxing smooth muscles (vasodilatation and decreased uterine contractions). A complete assessment of the client's reflexes should be performed prior to and during the administration of $MgSO_4$ to monitor the level of nervous system effect and verify adequate conductivity to maintain respiratory effort (see "Nursing Assessment").

When $MgSO_4$ is being used for prevention of potential seizures, a loading dose of 4 to 6 g to be given over 15 to 20 minutes is recommended, because rapid IV injection causes an uncomfortable feeling of warmth due to vasodilatation (see "Eclampsia" for initial rate used to stop a seizure; Perinatal Advisory Council of Los Angeles Communities, 1991). IV administration of $MgSO_4$ allows titration and more careful regulation of the medication. The maintainance dose can be prepared by adding 40 g of $MgSO_4$ to 1,000 mL of 5% dextrose in lactated Ringer's solution. This yields 2 g MgSO$_4$ per 50 mL of solution for a 2 g/h maintainance dose; this dose should be adjusted later based on patellar reflexes, urine output, and therapeutic serum magnesium therapeutic level (4–8 mg/dL; Scott, 1994).

MgSO$_4$ also may be given intramuscularly in doses of 10 to 20 mL of a 50% solution (5–10 g). The dose is divided, half injected into each buttock. Often 0.5 mL of 1% procaine is added to each injection to minimize discomfort. The injections should be given deeply into the upper quadrant of each buttock and followed by massage. Intramuscular injection is painful but requires less IV fluid. A repeat dose of MgSO$_4$ should not be given unless the reflexes and respiratory rate are normal, because it depresses both.

Other sedatives, such as phenobarbital, have long been used for mild preeclampsia when agitation is associated with the hospitalization, with dosing of 15 to 30 mg given three to four times per day (Zuspan, 1994). Although some clinicians use morphine in the management of severe preeclampsia, it is best reserved for clients with the added stimulus of pain (ie, labor). Minimizing this stimulus certainly reduces the likelihood of a seizure. Another drug that is an effective anticonvulsant is diazepam (Valium) in 5- to 10-mg doses intramuscularly. If the situation warrants, it may be given intravenously. Diazepam is usually reserved for severe cases and is discussed further in the management of eclampsia.

Current medical management for hypertension in mild to moderate preeclampsia is nonpharmacologic, because commonly used antihypertensive agents, such as beta blockers, decrease placental perfusion and may have an untoward effect on the fetus (Redman, 1991). Several clinical trials have concluded that that drug treatment was not mandatory for a good pregnancy outcome in cases of mild to moderate hypertension (Hogstedt et al. 1985; Collins et al., 1989).

In cases of severe preeclampsia and eclampsia, when the diastolic BP exceeds 100 to 110 mm Hg, drugs may be administered as a temporary measure. Antihypertensive therapy with pharmacologic agents is directed toward reducing peripheral BP, decreasing the left ventricular workload, and increasing blood flow to the uterus and renal system. The risk of a cerebrovascular accident also may be reduced.

When pharmacologic agents are used for clients, the goal is to reduce the diastolic pressure to between 90 and 100 mm Hg. For years the drug of choice has been hydralazine hydrochloride (Apresoline), but as of July 1993, the parenteral form is no longer produced (Zuspan, 1994). It may still be used if an oral form is available and appropriate. This potent vasodilator acts by an unknown cellular mechanism to directly relax arterial smooth muscle, causing decreased systemic vascular resistance, particularly in the cerebral, coronary,

splanchnic, and renal circulations. In experimental animals, hydralazine administration caused release of vasodilator prostaglandins and decreased responsiveness to sympathetic nerve stimulation (Wingard et al., 1991).

Alternative drugs now include alpha and beta blockers used intravenously in 20-mg intervals, or nifedipine, a calcium channel blocker, given orally in 10-mg increments. The drugs should be titrated to achieve the desired BP (Zuspan, 1994). The maternal BP must be monitored every 2 to 3 minutes after the initial dose, then every 5 to 10 minutes until the hypertensive crisis is stabilized. Labetalol hydrochloride (Normodyne) is an adrenergic blocker that acts on alpha and beta receptors to cause vasodilatation. The standard dose is 20 to 50 mg intravenously (Scott, 1994). Unlike most beta blockers, labetalol increases, rather than decreases, uteroplacental perfusion (Clark et al., 1994).

Other antihypertensive agents are administered to treat severe preeclampsia. However, their use in pregnancy is controversial because of potentially adverse maternal or fetal effects. Diazoxide, a nondiuretic thiazide, is a potent vasodilator that decreases vascular resistance and increases cardiac output and heart rate. When titrated in small 30- to 60-mg boluses, rather than the standard nonpregnant 300-mg bolus dose, it was shown to be safer (Cunningham et al., 1993). Nitroprusside sodium (Nipride), an arteriolar and venous vascular smooth-muscle dilator, has been associated with fetal cyanide toxicity; therefore, it is limited to postpartum use (Harvey et al., 1992).

Conflicting medical opinions exist as to whether diuretics should be administered to treat PIH, because these drugs may further deplete the intravascular volume and worsen vasospasm. Studies have shown conflicting results regarding the benefits of diuretics. It is believed that this may be due to the new finding that there are two kinds of PIH, the "wet" form and the "dry" form (Fukashima, 1995). The dry form is related to decreased intravascular volume secondary to capillary leakage from vascular damage. With this dry form of PIH, the use of diuretics was shown more than 20 years ago to be contraindicated, because they further reduce the renal and uteroplacental perfusion (Gant et al., 1975).

However, with the wet form of PIH, diuretics have proven useful. The wet form involves increased vascular volume, with resultant increased capillary pressure, causing water leakage into the interstitial space. One of the prinicipal causes of PIH is the thickening of the glomerular membranes, which reduces the rate of fluid filtration from the glomeruli into the renal tubules and results in water and sodium retention (fluid overload; Guyton, 1991).

According to a model developed by Guyton (1991), this fluid overload leads to hypertension and edema (see Box 31-9). With invasive hemodynamic monitoring, this fluid overload is identified as **preload** (the amount of blood in the ventricles at end diastole) and is approximated clinically as pulmonary capillary wedge pressure (PCWP). A fluid overload condition during pregnancy will show as a markedly elevated PCWP (>15 mm Hg; normal, 8 ± 2) or noninvasively by a pulse wave contour that is shifted to the right, indicating increased peripheral resistance. The oliguria that is present may be the first sign of incipient pulmonary edema. These clients respond well to aggressive afterload reduction and diuresis (Clark et al., 1994). Afterload (systemic vascular resistance) can be reduced by bed rest in the left lateral position and administration of antihypertensive drugs. Use of furosemide (Lasix) in conjunction with fluid restriction to 50 to 80 mL/h have been used with success in clients with wet PIH (Fukashima, 1995). Furosemide acts within the renal tubule by decreasing active resorption of sodium and chloride in the ascending limb of the loop of Henle. These solutes then act as osmotic agents to prevent water resorption (Guyton, 1991).

In the presence of oliguria, the need for volume replacement in the client with severe preeclampsia can be carefully assessed and managed through pulmonary artery catheterization. If the PCWP is low, the oliguria is considered secondary to the depleted intravascular volume, and these patients respond well to further volume replacement, either colloid or crystalloid solutions (Burke, 1989).

Fetal well-being is of continuous concern in the medical management of the client with preeclampsia. Various prenatal assessment tests are used to ascertain adequacy of fetal oxygenation and placental functioning. These include the nonstress test, performed weekly or more often if indicated; the contraction stress test (CST); biophysical profiles; and occasionally biweekly or daily serum estriol determinations. If nonstress tests are unsatisfactory on two or more occasions and other indices of fetal well-being (such as CSTs) indicate potential fetal compromise, the pregnancy may not be allowed to continue. Amniocentesis is usually performed to determine fetal lung maturity prior to planned delivery. In such situations, induction of labor may be most desirable for the welfare of the woman and fetus. If conditions for induction of labor are not favorable, cesarean delivery may be the procedure of choice. This most often occurs when preeclampsia is severe and fulminating. The signs and symptoms of preeclampsia usually abate rapidly after delivery, but the danger of seizures does not pass until 48 hours postpartum. Therefore, continuation of previously prescribed sedation throughout this interval may be indicated. In most cases, the elevated BP and the other derangements return to normal within 10 days to 2 weeks.

Nursing Assessment. The objective of nursing assessment is to recognize symptoms before they become obvious to the client or to identify any changes in the client with PIH that suggest disease progression. The early symptoms and manifestations related to more severe preeclampsia, such as persistent headache, blurred vision, spots or flashes of light before the eyes, epigastric pain, vomiting, torpor (sluggishness), or muscular twitchings, are all important. Data collected in relation to these symptoms, in addition to nutritional status, fluid intake and elimination, and attitudes about pregnancy, when accurately recorded, can be of great assistance in planning the course of therapy.

During the first prenatal examination, it is particularly important to assess the woman for predisposing risk factors associated with hypertensive disease in pregnancy. Prepregnancy weight should be recorded and compared with current weight.

Subsequently, the pattern of weight gain should be carefully followed and recorded by the nurse. Weight gain of approximately 1 lb/wk is regarded as normal. Sudden gains of more than 2 lb/wk should be viewed with suspicion and gains of more than 3 lb/wk viewed with alarm. Weight increases of the latter magnitude call for more frequent BP determinations, and if these also are abnormal, stricter medical management may be indicated.

Because finger edema is a frequent forerunner of preeclampsia, which may precede the hypertension by several weeks, it is a most valuable warning signal for assessment. In investigating suspected edema, it is important to ask the client if her ring is becoming tight. It also is essential to observe for edema of the hands, arms (ulnar surface and wrist), and face. Facial edema, which generally does not become apparent in early disease states, is characterized by swelling of the eyelids and a marked coarseness of features.

If the client is hospitalized, initial assessment should include all of the parameters described previously plus several other components. Body weight should be obtained on admission and daily at the same time of day thereafter. Vital signs and BP readings should be assessed every 2 to 4 hours, more frequently if indicated by the woman's condition or by medications. Clients with severe preeclampsia or hypertensive crisis require continuous assessment of the BP and MAP. The lungs should be auscultated for signs of pulmonary edema. Evaluations are made daily, or at more frequent intervals if indicated, for fluid intake and output (hourly for women with severe preeclamptic or hypertensive crisis). Urinary output should be at least 30 mL/h. Urine specimens also should be checked for protein, specific gravity, and cast analysis. The retinal arterioles and nail beds should be examined for evidence of vasospasm, which may be seen in clients with severe PIH etiology.

Hemodynamic monitoring using a pulmonary artery catheter (also known as a Swan-Ganz catheter) provides a valuable assessment tool for continuously measuring CVP and pulmonary artery pressure in cases of severe preeclampsia. Pulmonary capillary wedge pressure may be measured intermittently. These assessments reveal variable results, as discussed previously, depending on the subset type of PIH (wet versus dry; see Chap. 32 for normal hemodynamic values in pregnancy; Clark et al., 1989). Recent evidence suggests that hemodynamic monitoring with a CVP line is insufficient because there may be a large disparity in the function of the right and left ventricles in severe preeclamptic clients (Cotton et al., 1985).

Results of laboratory studies, such as type and cross-match; complete blood count; DIC profile; blood urea nitrogen (BUN), creatinine, and uric acid levels; arterial blood gases; and serum estriol determinations, should be assessed for baseline values and changes reflecting altered organ functioning. The effects of preeclampsia on the kidneys, liver, and fetoplacental unit and in some cases, the presence of hematologic abnormalities may be evidenced through laboratory changes. In severe preeclampsia, serum creatinine, BUN, and uric acid levels are elevated; creatinine clearance and proteinuria are decreased; and arterial blood gases and urinary sediment are changed. Liver pathology may be revealed through marked elevations in AST, ALT, and **lactate dehydrogenase** (LDH).

One of the most significant elements of the nurse's physical examination is assessment of reflexes, because abnormal findings may indicate central nervous system pathology. Signs of excessive nervous system irritability generally precede the onset of seizures in preeclamptic women. Assessment of deep tendon reflexes is performed, most often in the patellar tendon of the quadriceps muscle. However, a comprehensive examination also should include the brachioradialis, Achilles, biceps, and triceps reflexes. Selected information on testing of deep tendon reflexes is presented in Assessment Guidelines: Assessing Deep Tendon Reflexes. The nurse must remember to observe the symmetry of the reflexes from one side of the body to the other. **Clonus,** rapid alternating contraction and relaxation of a muscle group, should be assessed by briskly dorsiflexing the foot while slightly flexing the knee. Involuntary oscillations may be seen between flexion and extension when continuous pressure is applied to the sole of the foot in the hyper-reflexic client. If difficulty is encountered in producing muscle stretch reflexes, the nurse may find certain reinforcement techniques helpful, such as instructing the client to contract muscles other than the ones being evaluated.

It is particularly important for the nurse to observe the client with moderate to severe preeclampsia for changes in level of consciousness and any signs of impending seizure. Clinical appraisal includes assessing the client's awareness of external stimuli and internal state or mood, alertness, and emotional expression. Observations are made for disturbances in orientation and attention span.

Nursing Diagnosis. The complexity of this disorder creates many potential associated nursing problems. Focus should be placed on diagnoses related to alterations in tissue perfusion. For a list of possible nursing diagnoses, see Box 31-10.

Nursing Intervention. During the prenatal period, the nurse should instruct all women about the importance of maintaining a well-balanced diet high in protein intake. It is believed that the development of preeclampsia may be related to poor nutritional status. Therefore, dietary counseling is a significant component of client education. In addition, all pregnant women should be informed, both orally and in writing, about the warning signs of preeclampsia, which they should immediately report to the nurse or physician. The nurse should perform ongoing assessments of maternal and fetal status.

The woman manifesting early symptoms of preeclampsia who is managed at home on modified activity or bed rest should be encouraged to position herself frequently in the left lateral position. Lateral positioning has been shown to decrease BP, increase uterine and renal blood flow, return extravascular fluid into the vascular space, and decrease endogenous catecholamine production (Doany et al., 1987; Zuspan, 1994). The nurse should teach clients about prescribed sedatives or antihypertensive agents. BP should be monitored regularly by the community health nurse or a trained family member.

If symptoms of preeclampsia remain evident or progress, the client is likely to be admitted to the hospital. In establishing a therapeutic hospital atmosphere, the nurse should see that the environment is as comfortable and pleasant as possible. The client should be in a single room, free from noise and strong lights. Every effort should be made to relieve the client's anxiety, which sometimes is brought about by apprehension regarding her illness or which may be due to concern for the welfare of her family at home. The client with severe preeclampsia or hypertensive crisis requires a 1:1 nurse-client ratio.

The nurse should see that the equipment necessary for safe and efficient care of the client is immediately available in the client's room and is in good working order. An oral airway (or padded tongue blade) always should be available at the bedside to prevent the client from biting her tongue if a seizure develops. Equipment for catheterization and administration of appropriate medications should be readily available. The

ASSESSMENT GUIDELINES
Assessing Deep Tendon Reflexes

A. Assess deep tendon reflexes hourly (patellar [knee jerk], biceps, and radial reflexes).

1. To test reflexes, strike the tendon, and observe for contraction of the appropriate muscle. The muscle must simply contract.

2. Absence of or decrease in the patellar reflex indicates that a toxic blood level (>10 mEq/L of Mg) has been reached.

3. Promote relaxation for proper testing, because these reflexes are difficult to elicit when the client is tense.

4. Compare symmetry of reflexes and record using the following scale:
   0 = Reflex absent
   +1 = Reflex hypoactive
   +2 = Normal reflex
   +3 = Reflex hyperactive
   +4 = Clonus

B. Test the muscle reflex by stimulating the tendon; the reflex is involuntary. A sensory impulse is initiated when a stimulus is applied to the tendon, and in return, a motor response is elicited.

1. When testing reflexes on a client who has recently received epidural or spinal anesthesia, motor responses will be diminished. An accurate response will not be elicited if the knee jerk is used. The biceps or radial reflex will have to be used.

C. Assess the knee jerk reflex or patellar tendon reflex.

1. The knee should be positioned halfway between the longest and shortest positions.

2. Support is given under the knee with the foot off the bed (45-degree angle).

3. The patellar tendon is struck (tapped) just below the patella, and the quadriceps muscle group should be observed for contraction (slight movement). The lower leg should extend in response.

D. Assess the biceps reflex.

1. The forearm should be resting on the client's trunk.

2. Place the thumb firmly on the client's biceps tendon (antecubital space) and strike the thumbnail briskly with the reflex hammer.

3. The biceps muscle will respond by slight movement. The lower arm should flex in response.

E. Assess the radial reflex.

1. The client's hand and forearm should be resting on her trunk. Place a finger over the tendon, and gently tap the finger with the reflex hammer.

2. The brachioradial tendon is located on the lateral surface of the lower end of the radius. If the tendon cannot be felt, tap the lateral surface of the lower end of the radius. The brachioradial muscle will respond by a slight movement. The response consists of the hand jerking.

F. Use techniques for relaxation.

1. If the client is having difficulty relaxing, two techniques can be tried.

a. Testing the knee jerk—Have the client lock her fingers together and pull in opposite directions (monkey grip). This technique will help the client relax her leg by having her concentrate on a physical activity.

b. Testing the biceps or radial reflexes—Have the client bite down hard. This technique will help the client relax her arm by having her concentrate on doing something else.

2. *Clonus* is the sudden stretching of a hypertonic muscle, producing reflex contraction. If the stretch is maintained during subsequent relaxation, further reflex contraction occurs, and this may continue almost indefinitely, unless the stretch stimulus is released. It is demonstrated by dorsiflexion of the foot or by sharply moving the patella downward, but it may be present at any joint. Clonus represents an increase in reflex excitability and may be present in an extremely tense client.

---

nurse must ensure proper drainage of the indwelling urinary catheter at all times and monitor the client's urinary output carefully.

Other necessary supplies for the care of the preeclamptic woman may include padded side rails, suction apparatus for aspirating mucus, and equipment for administering oxygen, in case cyanosis or depressed respiration indicate the need. An emergency medication tray should be immediately accessible, including items such as $MgSO_4$, calcium gluconate ($MgSO_4$ antagonist), sodium bicarbonate, hydralazine, and epinephrine.

BOX 31-10
Nursing Diagnoses—Preeclampsia

- Altered Tissue Perfusion related to vasospasm from preeclampsia
- Risk for Injury (fetal) related to inadequate placental perfusion
- Risk for Injury (maternal) related to effects of preeclampsia, its treatment, or complications
- Knowledge Deficit related to lack of information about PIH and its treatment
- Anxiety related to possible effects of PIH on self and fetus
- Intravascular Fluid Volume Deficit related to fluid shift to interstitial space—"dry" PIH condition
- Fluid Volume Overload related to fluid retention—"wet" PIH condition
- Social Isolation related to bed rest or hospitalization
- Impaired Home Maintenance Management related to bed rest or hospitalization

---

When any treatment is ordered, the procedure is best carried out after sedation has been administered. If the client is not in labor, the nurse must be alert to watch for signs of labor, particularly after sedation has been given.

Regardless of the severity of the preeclampsia, certain responsibilities are carried out by the nurse. Complete bed rest is essential. Because rest and relaxation are major considerations in the care of the preeclamptic woman, the nurse should plan a schedule of activities so that the client is disturbed as little as possible.

The hospitalized client is encouraged to eat the prescribed diet, which is ample in protein and calories. Sodium is usually neither restricted nor forced but held to normal recommended dietary allowances of 2.5 to 7 g of salt per day. The client should be instructed not to add salt to food and to avoid foods high in sodium. Patients on IV therapy for acute prenatal or intrapartum fluid maintenance need restricted total fluid intake to prevent further multiorgan swelling, especially cerebral edema (Benedetti et al., 1980). The maintainance rate should be 75 mL/h, rather than the usual 125 mL/h given during normal labor. One liter of normal saline can cause a 12% decrease in colloid osmotic pressure for up to 3 to 5 days after delivery (Harvey et al., 1992).

Frequent observations are made for progressive symptoms or changes in condition, with special attention to visual disturbances, headaches, and epigastric pain. Urine should be tested for protein, using a clean-catch, midstream specimen. A 2⁺ reading of proteinuria is considered significant for mild preeclampsia and 3⁺ - 4⁺ for severe preeclampsia.

Because serious side effects may occur with $MgSO_4$ administration, it is essential for the nurse to monitor urinary output, deep tendon reflexes, and respiratory rate prior to, during, and after $MgSO_4$ administration. Mg^{2+} serum levels are drawn every 6 hours (see Nursing Guidelines: Administering Magnesium Sulfate [$MgSO_4$]).

The fetal heart rate should be assessed through external continuous electronic monitoring because many of the prescribed drugs may affect the fetus. The nurse also must remember to assess the client for vaginal bleeding or uterine rigidity.

Nursing Evaluation. Anticipated outcomes of nursing care include the following:

- The client identifies the signs and symptoms of disease progression and reports them promptly.
- The client verbalizes the effects of her disease on perinatal outcome, the treatment plan, and potential complications.
- The client demonstrates compliance with the prescribed treatment plan.
- The client maintains adequate tissue perfusion and oxygen to the maternal-fetal unit.
- The client delivers a healthy newborn at or near term.

Eclampsia

Eclampsia is the progression of a more severe form of preeclampsia in which generalized seizures or coma occurs. A seizure results when there is an excessive synchronous electrical discharge (ie, depolarization) of neurons within the central nervous system (Volpe, 1995). The incidence of eclampsia is about 0.2% of all deliveries (Scott, 1994). Eclampsia is one of the gravest complications of pregnancy, with the maternal mortality rate ranging from 0% to 14% and perinatal mortality ranging from 14% to 27% (Clark et al., 1994).

Eclampsia is usually preceded by headache; excitability or hyper-reflexia; visual disturbances, such as blurring or temporary blindness (amaurosis); epigastric pain; and hemoconcentration. However, as many mistakenly believe, it is not directly proportional to the severity of the hypertension or proteinuria (Cunningham et al., 1993; Clark et al., 1994; Scott, 1994). According to Zuspan (1994), 20% of women have eclampsia with BPs of <140/90 and no proteinuria.

An eclamptic episode is most likely to occur as term approaches. It is rarely seen prior to the last 3 months. In general, eclampsia is preventable. It has become less common in the United States because most women now receive prenatal care. The precise cause of seizures in eclampsia remains unknown, but proposed etiologic factors are hypertensive encephalopa-

---

NURSING GUIDELINES
Administering Magnesium Sulfate (MgSO$_4$)

Preparation of the MgSO$_4$

A. IV dose*
Administer MgSO$_4$ therapy IV through Buretol and IV controller

1. Use 1,000 mL D$_5$ ¼ NS and withdraw 80 mL.
2. Add 80 mL MgSO$_4$ 50% solution, making 40 g/L or 1 g/25 mL.
3. Give 4-g loading bolus. (Note: If given to stop seizure in progress, may give 4–6 g MgSO$_4$ 10% in 100–150 mL over 10–15 min or 3–5 min depending on situation but *no* faster than 1 g/min.)
   a. Fill Buretrol with 2 g MgSO$_4$ (50 mL) and add 2 g (4 mL) MgSO$_4$ 50% solution to total 4 g MgSO$_4$ (54 mL).
   b. Infuse the 4 g loading dose of MgSO$_4$ over 15–20 min.
   c. Assess vital signs every 5–15 min during loading dose, and record in nursing notes.
4. Following bolus, MgSO$_4$ therapy is to run between 1 and 2 g/h or as ordered by physician.

B. IM dose
MgSO$_4$, 10 g or 5 g
1. 10 g of MgSO$_4$ in 20 mL of a 50% solution.
2. Divide into two doses, 10 mL in two syringes.
3. Add 0.5 mL of lidocaine to each 10 mL of MgSO$_4$ in the syringe.

Nursing Assessment of Client Receiving MgSO$_4$

A. Assess for signs of MgSO$_4$ intoxication (hypermagnesemia).
1. Early signs:
   a. Hot all over
   b. Flushing
   c. Thirsty
   d. Sweating
   e. Depression of reflexes
   f. Hypotension
   g. Flaccidity
2. Later signs:
   a. Central nervous system depression
   b. Respiratory paralysis
   c. Hypocalcemia
   d. Cardiac dysrhythmias
   e. Circulatory collapse
   f. Fetal bradycardia

B. Assess deep tendon reflexes every 1–4 h if the client is receiving continuous IV infusion or before each dose if intermittent therapy is administered. Disappearance of the patellar reflex is one of the most important clinical signs to detect increasing hypermagnesemia. If the client has received regional anesthesia (epidural), however, the biceps or radial reflex will have to be tested.

C. Assess central nervous system depression, which is at first characterized by anxiety. This changes to drowsiness, lethargy, slight slurring of speech, ataxic gait, and a tendency to fall sideward while standing erect. Constantly evaluate the client's orientation to person, place, and time.

D. Monitor intake and output hourly. Specific gravity should be obtained. Urine should be checked for proteinuria, color, and volume (30 mL or more per hour).

E. Assess blood pressure (BP) and temperature-pulse-respiration (TPR) at least every 15–30 min if the client is receiving an IV infusion. For the client on intermittent therapy of MgSO$_4$, BP and TPR should be taken before and after each administration.
1. Do not administer MgSO$_4$ if the client's respirations are less than 12–14 per minute or there is a drop in pulse rate, BP, or any other sign of fetal distress.

F. Draw Mg level every 6 h or as indicated by deep tendon reflexes, respiratory status, and level of consciousness.

Normal	1.5–2.5 mEq/L
Therapeutic	4.0–7.5 mEq/L
Absence of reflexes	≥10 mEq/L
Respiratory arrest	≥15 mEq/L
Cardiac arrest	≥25 mEq/L

G. Assess for signs and symptoms.
1. Assess complaints about headache, malaise, nausea, and vomiting to determine whether these signs are due to progression of toxemia or drug therapy.
2. Assess for complaints of pain at the site of the injection if receiving MgSO$_4$ intramuscularly.

H. Calcium gluconate (10% solution) is kept at the client's bedside.
1. This is the antidote for magnesium intoxication (usually reverses respiratory depression and heart block). The dosage should be 5–10 mEq (10–20 mL) given intravenously over a 3-min period.

*Used at the University of California, Los Angeles Medical Center

---

thy, vasospasm, hemorrhage, ischemia, and edema of the cerebral hemisphere (Clark et al., 1994).

Manifestations. The onset of eclampsia is often sudden. Typically, the seizure continues for only 60 to 75 seconds. Normally, the seizure begins with the *stage of invasion*, which lasts only a few seconds. During this stage, the client's eyes roll to one side and stare fixedly into space. Immediately, twitching of the facial muscles

ensues. The next phase is the *stage of contraction,* which lasts 15 or 20 seconds and is characterized by generalized tonic muscular contraction. The face is distorted, the eyes protrude, the arms are flexed, the hands are clenched, and the legs are inverted.

Suddenly the jaws and eyelids begin to open and close violently. The other facial muscles and then all the muscles of the body alternately contract and relax in rapid succession. The muscular movements are so forceful that the unprotected client may injure herself by falling or biting her tongue. Foam, which is often blood tinged, exudes from the mouth; the face is congested and purple, and the eyes are bloodshot. This phase in which the muscles alternately contract and relax is called the *stage of seizure*. It may last a minute or so. Gradually, the muscular movements become milder and farther apart, and finally the client lies motionless.

Throughout the seizure, the diaphragm remains fixed, with respiration halted. For a few seconds, the client appears to be dying of respiratory arrest, but just when this outcome seems almost inevitable, she usually takes a long, deep, stertorous inhalation, and breathing is resumed. Then the postictal state follows, and the client may be tired but coherent, semicomatose, or comatose. The client does not remember anything about the seizure or in all probability, events immediately before and after.

The postictal state may last from a few minutes to several hours, and then the client may become conscious, or this may be followed by another seizure. The seizures may recur during coma, they may recur only after an interval of consciousness, they may never recur, or as stated previously, they may rapidly recur. Mild cases of eclampsia involve one or two seizures; in severe cases, there may be 100 seizures (Cunningham et al., 1993). Seizures may start before the onset of labor (prenatal), during labor (intrapartum), or anytime within the first 48 hours after delivery (postpartum). About 20% of the cases develop postpartally, generally within 24 hours of delivery (Clark et al., 1994).

On physical examination, the findings of eclampsia are similar to those in preeclampsia but are highly variable. Edema may be marked but sometimes is clinically absent. Oliguria, or diminution of urinary excretion, is common and may progress to complete anuria. Fever is present in about half of these women.

In some eclamptic women, 1 or 2 days are required for clear consciousness to be regained. During this period, clients are often in an obstreperous, resistant mood and may be exceedingly difficult to manage. A few women develop actual psychoses. In unfavorable cases, the coma deepens, urinary excretion diminishes, the pulse becomes more rapid, the temperature rises, and pulmonary edema develops. The last is a serious symptom and usually is interpreted as a sign of cardiovascular failure. Pulmonary edema is readily recognizable by noisy, gurgling respirations; shortness of breath (dyspnea); and the large quantity of frothy mucus that exudes from the mouth and nose. Toward the end, seizures cease altogether, and the final picture is one of vascular collapse, falling BP, and overwhelming pulmonary edema.

Although it is difficult to forecast the outcome, the following are unfavorable signs: oliguria, prolonged coma, a sustained pulse rate of more than 120 beats/min, temperature of more than 39.5°C (103°F),

more than 10 seizures, proteinuria >10 g/L in 24 hours (normal, 0.3 g/L in 24 hours), systolic BP of more than 200 mm Hg, and pulmonary edema. If none of these signs is present, the outlook for recovery is good; if two or more are present, the prognosis is definitely serious.

Medical Management. It is important to differentiate eclampsia from epilepsy, encephalitis, and other central nervous system diseases during late pregnancy. This may be of special concern in situations of absent prenatal care. Until another cause can be identified, *all pregnant women having seizures should be considered eclamptic* (Cunningham et al., 1993).

Whether or not an anticonvulsant should be given to arrest the seizure has been controversial. Sibai and Anderson (1991) contend that no anticonvulsant should be given because rapid dosing of agents such as diazepam may lead to apnea or cardiac arrest or both. However, they also contend that if seizures recur, there is some degree of consciousness after each seizure and respirations resume at a rapid rate. Cunningham et al. (1993), however, have observed that in rare cases, seizures can recur so rapidly that the woman appears to be in a prolonged, almost continutous seizure that can lead to death. They have observed that $MgSO_4$ "will practically always arrest eclamptic seizures and prevent their reoccurence," so they recommend that as soon as the seizure is identified, the $MgSO_4$ should be administered (Cunningham et al., 1993).

The general principles followed for client management are comparable among institutions. They include prevention, termination of pregnancy, sedation, and follow-up. Because eclampsia is largely preventable, it is essential to provide comprehensive and regular prenatal care and education directed toward early detection and treatment of PIH. In almost all instances of eclampsia, efforts to effect delivery should be undertaken as soon as the client is stabilized. This involves control of seizures and hyper-reflexia by using adequate doses of anticonvulsants and initiating diuresis. It is often helpful to initiate hemodynamic monitoring using a pulmonary artery catheter or CVP line, in addition to assessing urinary output in an attempt to optimize fluid balance.

Usually, efforts to accomplish delivery before the client is stabilized may result in increased maternal morbidity and mortality (Cunningham et al., 1993). The exception to this is if the woman is in cardiac arrest and cardiopulmonary resuscitation (CPR) is being used. The gravid uterus in the supine position obstructs venous return and cardiac output. If the left lateral position is used, the torso rolls, and part of the force of compression is lost; chest compressions yield only 30% of normal cardiac output. Therefore, if optimal cardiac output cannot be restored with CPR in late pregnancy, delivery should commence promptly (Satin et al., 1991). The method of delivery should be by the most expeditious route. Prolonged attempts at induction in the face of an unripe cervix are not indicated.

Anticonvulsants are used to depress excessive neuronal firing and thereby stop seizures. The most commonly used drugs and their specific anticonvulsant dosing include the following:

- Magnesium sulfate—This drug is probably the most common drug used in eclamptic women. A standard protocol for stopping an eclamptic seizure is to administer 4 to 6 g of $MgSO_4$ 10% solution IV in 100 to 150 mL over 10 to 15 minutes, followed by a 2 g/h maintainance dose. This dose is adjusted later based on patellar reflexes, urine output, and serum magnesium therapeutic level (4–8 mg/dL; Scott, 1994). There is some variation in the literature on the time period for administration, with a more rapid period of 3 to 5 minutes recommended by Zuspan (1994) and a slower administration period of 20 minutes recommended by Clark et al. (1994). The actions, alternate routes of administration, doses, and precautions are discussed previously in this chapter.

- Diazepam IV for seizure control—Generally, 40 mg is diluted in 500 mL of 5% dextrose in water, and this is administered at a rate of 30 drops per minute. Diazepam can cause fetal depression if more than 30 mg is used within 15 to 20 hours before delivery. For this reason, $MgSO_4$ remains the anticonvulsant of choice.

Because a large percentage of women with severe preeclampsia develop hypertensive disease in subsequent pregnancies, careful, prolonged follow-up is imperative.

Nursing Assessment. Immediate assessments must be made and recorded by the nurse. Events preceding the seizures, the exact time of onset, and the duration of each convulsive phase should be noted. When the client stops thrashing, the nurse must check maternal vital signs and fetal heart tones (usually continuously monitored). This assessment is repeated every 5 minutes until the client stabilizes and then every 15 minutes. The depth and duration of postictal stage following seizures are observed. The chest should be auscultated to detect any signs of pulmonary edema or cardiac failure. Urinary output and parenteral fluid intake also should be carefully monitored.

For more comprehensive assessment, hemodynamic measurements may be obtained by an appropriately trained physician inserting a Swan-Ganz catheter. Data should be collected on central volume status, including pulmonary capillary wedge pressure, cardiac output, and MAP.

Amid all of the demands of this acute situation, it also is important for the nurse to remember to assess for signs of labor or abruption in the unconscious and the conscious prenatal client. In eclampsia, labor or placental separation may proceed with few external signs, and occasionally the birth is precipitous. The nurse should be suspicious when the client grunts or groans or moves about at regular intervals, every 5 minutes or so. If this occurs, the consistency, texture, and height of the uterus should be assessed and observations made for bloody show and bulging of the membranes or bleeding. Seizures that occur during labor may speed up the labor process, and more rapid preparation for delivery should be made.

Respirations may cease during the seizure, and close attention to their return is essential. Usually it does return, and respiratory activity after an eclamptic seizure is often rapid (> 50 breaths per minute) in response to hypercarbia. A temperature of 39°C (102.2°F) or more is probably the result of central nervous system damage (Cunningham et al., 1993).

As a consequence of maternal hypoxemia caused by the seizures, fetal bradycardia might follow it. The fetal heart rate usually recovers within 3 to 5 minutes; if fetal bradycardia persists more than 10 minutes, another cause should be considered, such as placental abruption.

Nursing Diagnosis. Assessment of the eclamptic woman may lead the nurse to formulate appropriate nursing diagnoses similar to those for the client with preeclampsia. Early recognition of these diagnoses provides a basis for appropriately planning nursing interventions. For a list of possible additional diagnoses, see Box 31-11.

Nursing Intervention. If eclampsia develops, the nurse must intervene immediately to protect the client from self-injury and further physiologic decompensation. Nursing management is coordinated with medical therapy. If a physician is not immediately available to give the anticonvulsant $MgSO_4$, then this becomes the nurse's responsibility under her hospital's protocol for emergency treatment of eclampsia.

BOX 31–11
Nursing Diagnoses—Eclampsia

- Risk for Injury related to the following:
  Seizure activity
  Adverse effects of medication
  Altered level of consciousness
  Respiratory or cardiac arrest with rapidly recurring seizures
  Abruptio placentae
- Impaired Gas Exchange related to pulmonary edema
- Ineffective Airway Clearance related to seizure activity
- Fear related to uncertain outcome

The eclamptic woman must never be left alone. To prevent injury, the side rails of the bed should be padded or cushioned with pillows, and some device, such as airway or padded tongue blade, that can be inserted between the jaws at the onset of a seizure should be kept within easy reach.

Turning the client's head and body to the side when the seizure begins aids circulation to the uteroplacental unit and may prevent aspiration. Prompt administration of oxygen by mask should be initiated (Scott, 1994). Eclamptic women must never be given fluids by mouth unless they are thoroughly conscious.

Because loud noises, bright lights, jarring of the bed, or sudden drafts may be enough to precipitate a seizure, the nurse must protect the eclamptic woman from all extraneous stimuli. The room should be darkened, but the light should be sufficient to permit observations of changes in condition. Only conversation that is absolutely necessary should be carried out in the room, and this should be in the lowest tone possible.

During the postictal stage that follows cessation of the seizure, care must be taken to see that the client does not aspirate vomitus or mucus. An oral airway may be inserted into the client's mouth. Her nasopharynx should be suctioned. Oxygen administration is initiated during or immediately following the seizure to prevent or treat maternal-fetal hypoxia. The client should be positioned in bed to promote drainage of secretions to maintain a patent airway. It may be necessary to raise the foot of the bed of the comatose client a few inches to promote drainage of secretions from the respiratory tract. When this measure must be used, it is particularly important to watch for signs of pulmonary edema, which would be aggravated by this position. If pulmonary edema develops, the foot of the bed should be lowered and the head of the bed elevated to relieve dyspnea.

Although the nurse is not directly responsible for decisions related to pregnancy termination, her role encompasses direct intrapartum care and prenatal preparation of the client for labor and delivery. Therefore, it is essential for the nurse to understand the guidelines for decision making used by the obstetrician. Careful and continuous monitoring of maternal and fetal status and direct interventions to support and educate the client and answer questions may prevent further aggravation of the client's hypertensive state and may promote a more positive perinatal outcome.

Nursing Evaluation. Anticipated outcomes of nursing care include the following:

- The client remains free of injury.
- The client verbalizes the effects of her disease on perinatal outcome, the treatment plan, and potential complications.

- The client demonstrates compliance with the prescribed treatment plan.
- The client maintains adequate tissue perfusion and oxygen to the maternal-fetal unit until delivery.
- The client delivers a healthy newborn at or near term.

HELLP Syndrome

A variant of severe preeclampsia, HELLP syndrome affects 4% to 12% of clients with preeclampsia (Dildy et al., 1991). HELLP is an acronym for the major pathologic problems seen: hemolysis, elevated liver enzymes, and low platelet count. It was first described by Weinstein (1987) as a unique set of findings present in some severe preeclampsia clients.

Manifestations and Causes

Typically, the client with HELLP presents with general flulike symptoms that begin gradually. The manifestations can appear as early as the 17th week of gestation to the first postpartum week. The initial signs and symptoms usually are seen early in the third trimester. Commonly, epigastric or upper quadrant pain resulting from liver distention is present. The client often has other nonspecific signs and symptoms, such as nausea, malaise, edema, or diffuse abdominal pain. Clinically, many clients with HELLP do not meet the standard hypertension criteria for severe preeclampsia, and some (15%) have a diastolic of ≤90 mm Hg (Dildy et al., 1991). Proteinuria is uncommon; however, it may occur late in the disease.

The exact cause of the syndrome is unknown. Some have thought that platelet deposition at the sites of endothelial damage caused by intense vasospasms may be the explanation for depleted platelet levels (thrombocytopenia; Cunningham et al., 1993).

Medical Diagnosis and Management. The presence of fragmentation hemolysis strongly suggests this syndrome. Blood analysis reveals **microangiopathic hemolytic anemia**, also known as traumatic hemolytic anemia. When exposed to excessive shear or turbulence in the circulation, odd-shaped RBC fragments appear in the peripheral blood (Berkow, 1992). Evidence of RBC injury may be identified directly by finding **schistocytes** (RBC fragments or portions of disrupted cells) and **echinocytes** (contracted RBCs with spiny projections; also known as burr cells). These erythrocyte types were originally identified as a component of severe preeclampsia more than 1 decade ago by Cunningham and associates using the scanning electron microscope (Cunningham et al., 1985). Treatment for hemolysis is directed toward the underlying process, the intense vasospasms, because significant anemia is uncommon.

Hemolysis also can be measured by increased serum levels of lactate dehydrogenase (LDH), a key intracellular enzyme involved in glucose metabolism. Under normal circumstances, this enzyme remains intracellular, with only a low level in the extracellular serum (45–90 IV/L). A high serum level (>600 IV/L) indicates significant cell lysis (Sibai et al., 1991), but because LDH is present in many other types of cells, such as liver, heart, and brain, LDH measurements lack specificity for which organ has been damaged. LDH evaluations also are used clinically in conjunction with other liver enzymes to evaluate liver damage.

Two other liver enzymes that are measured in the blood serum are aspartate transaminase (AST) and alanine transaminase (ALT). The aminotransferases are the key enzymes that catalyze intracellular protein metabolism and normally occur only in small quantities in the extracellular serum (AST = 7–27 IV/L; AST = 1–21 IV/L; Berkow, 1992). Significantly elevated serum AST (>72 IV/L) may occur when liver ischemia causes hepatocyte lysis, or necrosis. However, AST also is present inside heart, skeletal muscle, brain, and kidney cells; therefore, its elevation is not a specific marker only for liver damage. The comarker ALT is useful because it is found primarily in liver cells and therefore has greater specificity for liver disease (Berkow, 1992).

When the liver fails to function normally in its role of hemoglobin degradation, it also is possible to have a build up of bilirubin, known as hyperbilirubinemia, which causes jaundice. Hepatic infarction may lead to intrahepatic hemorrhage and subcapsular hematoma. If it ruptures into the peritoneal cavity, it could result in shock and death. If liver rupture is suspected, a laparotomy is required.

The third component, low platelets or **thrombocytopenia,** is defined as a serum platelet level <100,000/mL (normal, 150,000–350,000/mL) This is an ominous sign, and delivery is usually indicated (Cunningham et al., 1993). This decrease indicates that an abnormal change is taking place but is not diagnostic of a bleeding risk until a moderate thrombocytopenia level of <50,000/mL is reached (Guyton, 1991). Platelet transfusion is usually necessary at this level for clients requiring cesarean delivery but is not necessary until <10,000/mL in nonsurgical clients (Clark et al., 1994).

The decision regarding whether or not immediate delivery is indicated for clients diagnosed with HELLP is controversial, due to the risks related to fetal immaturity. Some clinicians favor a compromise, using a conservative approach for pregnancies with very immature fetuses. They believe that in the absence of DIC and fetal lung maturity, the client may be given two doses of steroids to accelerate fetal lung maturity and then deliver 24 hours after the last dose (Sibai et al., 1991). During this time, maternal and fetal conditions should be monitored closely. Nonstress testing and biophysical profile can be used to assess fetal well-being.

The mode of delivery depends on the cervix. A prolonged induction is not indicated because of the increased risk of maternal morbidity. Continued monitoring of the client and newborn after delivery is crucial, because the major laboratory findings may not appear until 48 to 72 hours postpartum.

Chronic Hypertension (With and Without Superimposed Pregnancy-Induced Hypertension)

Chronic hypertension is characterized by the presence of high BP ($\geq$140/90 mm Hg) prior to pregnancy or by its appearance prior to the 20th week of gestation or when high BP persists beyond 6 weeks postpartum. The etiology of this hypertension is usually related to vascular or renal disease. Most often women with chronic hypertension are multipara and usually older than 30 years.

Difficulty is encountered in establishing a diagnosis of chronic hypertension because many women are not seen between pregnancies, and BPs are not recorded. Also, BP normally decreases during the second trimester, which could mask a preexisting hypertension if the client does not report for care until the fourth or fifth month of gestation. The presence of diabetes mellitus, renal disease, collagen vascular disease, and a variety of clinical findings (eg, plasma urea nitrogen concentration >20 mg/dL, plasma creatinine concentration >1 mg/dL, retinal hemorrhages, and exudates) suggest that hypertension is chronic.

At least 75% of women with chronic hypertension are able to complete their pregnancies successfully. Fifteen percent develop superimposed preeclampsia, which carries an ominous fetal prognosis (20% mortality) and an increase in maternal mortality. Chronic hypertension is associated with an increase in perinatal morbidity and mortality; with each rise of 5 mm Hg in the MAP, there is a progressive increase in the number of perinatal deaths (Page et al., 1976).

Medical Management

The treatment for most pregnant women with chronic hypertension is no different from treatment for the nonpregnant woman. Prepregnancy antihypertensive and diuretic medications are continued. Thiazides are the drugs of choice despite reports of neonatal thrombocytopenia. The antihypertensive drug most often recommended is oral hydralazine hydrochloride and methyldopa (Aldomet). Methyldopa is classified as a centrally acting sympatholytic. Sympatholytics with central actions decrease BP by causing a reduced sympathetic nerve firing rate; the locus of their action is within the central nervous system. A potential site of action for methyldopa is in the nucleus tractus solitarius of the brain stem. This region contains interneurons that relay inhibitory information from the baroreceptor terminals to excitatory vasomotor regions in the rostral ventral medulla. Activation of presynaptic alpha$_2$ adrenergic receptors in these interneurons inhibits sympathetic discharge. All medications should be titrated to the lowest possible effective dose.

The pregnancy is allowed to run its normal course unless gestation aggravates the existing hypertension. When the gravida with this chronic process develops a further elevation of BP (systolic BP 30 mm Hg or diastolic BP 15–20 mm Hg above baseline), significant proteinuria, or edema, the condition is called *superimposed preeclampsia.*

In superimposed preeclampsia, after 24 to 48 hours of intensive medical therapy, pregnancy termination is generally indicated. Even though the fetus may be preterm, its chances for survival under these circumstances are generally better outside the uterus.

In a small number of women, the hypertension will be so severe with evidence of kidney involvement, severe retinal changes, or cardiac involvement that therapeutic abortion might be considered in the first trimester. It also is important to consider the advisability of postpartum tubal ligation in this group of women, who are generally older, with established families, and for whom additional pregnancies may represent a serious health hazard. This can be only a recommendation; the final decision rests with the client.

Summary Points

✔ Hyperemesis gravidarum is extreme nausea and vomiting during pregnancy. The underlying pregnancy changes that cause the clinical symptoms associated with this condition are believed to be the following:

■ The endocrine imbalance created by a high level of chorionic gonadotropins and estrogens
■ Metabolic changes of normal gestation
■ Fragments of chorionic villi entering the maternal circulation
■ Diminished motility of the stomach

✔ The three most common causes of bleeding in the first trimester are abortion (miscarriage), ectopic pregnancy (tubal pregnancy), and hydatidiform mole (molar pregnancy).

✔ Placenta previa and abruptio placentae have several features in common and major differences:

■ With placenta previa, the implantation of the placenta is always near the cervical os: Complete previa covers the cervical os; partial previa partially covers the cervical os; and low-lying previa is next to the cervical os. Abruptio placentae is the premature separation of the placenta prior to the birth of the fetus. It can be partial or complete, with apparent or concealed hemorrhage.
■ Both placental abnormalities can cause significant third-trimester bleeding and can be diagnosed by ultrasonography localization. They differ in that in abruptio placentae, the implantation can be anywhere in the uterus; with placenta previa, the placenta may or may not prematurely separate. The necessitiy for a cesarean delivery depends on the severity of the condition. Complete previa and abruption always require operative delivery.

✔ The pathophysiology of DIC is explained by the fact that DIC represents a failure of the normal checks and balances of coagulation, resulting in a system-wide, rather than a local, generation of thrombin and plasmin.

■ Excess thrombin leads to excess clot formation (thrombosis) and depletion of clotting factors and platelets (thrombocytopenia, <100,000).
■ The excess plasmin generated has three damaging effects:
   Degrades fibrinogen as it circulates in the blood stream
   Inactivates several clotting factors (V, VIII, IX, XI), adding to the anticoagulation effect
   Activates the first and third complement components, which trigger cell lysis, immunoadherence, and other immune phenomena

✔ There are four basic categories of hypertensive disorders complicating pregnancy:

■ PIH
■ Chronic hyperpertension
■ Chronic hypertension with superimposed PIH
■ Late or transitional hypertension

✔ The main differentiating characteristic is the time of onset, with PIH occuring after 20 weeks and chronic hypertension occurring before 20 weeks' gestation.

✔ The current therapeutic regimen for mild and severe preeclampsia and eclampsia depends on the severity of the disease. Once symptoms of severe preeclampsia or eclampsia present, the client needs immediate delivery, regardless of gestational age, because it can be lethal to the woman and fetus. Mild preeclampsia can be treated at home antepartally with intermittent bed rest and serial NSTs;

once labor starts, fluids should be limited. IV MgSO4 and a quiet environment should be used to prevent seizures. Diastolic BP >110 should be treated with an antihypertensive agent.

✔ HELLP syndrome is a serious variant of severe pre-eclampsia. It involves hemolysis, elevated liver enzymes, and low platelets.

REFERENCES

American College of Obstetricians and Gynecologists (1986). Management of preeclampsia. *Technical Bulletin,* No. 91.

Ancona, S., Chatterjee, M., Rhee, I. et al. (1990). The mid-trimester placenta previa: A prospective follow-up. *European Journal of Radiology, 10,* 215–216.

Beaufils, M., Uzan, S., Donsimoni, R., & Colau, J. (1985). Prevention of preeclampsia by early antiplatelet therapy. *Lancet, 1,* 840.

Benedetti, T. (1991). Obstetric hemorrhage. In S. Gabbe, J. Niebyl, & J. Simpson (Eds.), *Obstetrics: Normal and problem pregnanies* (2nd ed.) (pp. 573–606). New York: Churchill & Livingstone.

Benedetti, T., & Quilligan, E. (1980). Cerebral edema in severe pregnancy induced hypertension. *American Journal of Obstetrics and Gynecology, 137,* 860.

Bennett, M. (1992). Abortions. In N. Hacker & J. G. Moore (Eds.), *Essentials of Obstetrics and Gynecology* (2nd ed.) (pp. 415–424). Philadelphia: W.B.Saunders.

Berkow, R. (1992). *Merck manual of diagnosis and therapy.* Rahway, NJ: Merck Research Laboratories.

Bick, R. (1978). Disseminated intravascular coagulation and related syndromes: Etiology, pathophysiology, diagnosis, and management. *American Journal of Hematology, 5,* 265.

Blackburn, S., & Loper, D. (1992). *Maternal, fetal, and neonatal physiology: A clinical perspective.* Philadelphia: W.B. Saunders.

Buckley, J. (1984). The epidemiology of molar pregnancy and choriocarcinoma. *Clinical Obstetrics and Gynecology, 27,* 153–159.

Burke, M. (1989). Hypertensive crisis and the perinatal period. *Journal of Perinatal Neonatal Nursing, 3,* 33–47.

Centers for Disease Control (1989). Ectopic pregnancy: United States. *39,* 401–404.

Chow, W., Weiss, D. J. N. et al. (1988). Smoking and tubal pregnancy. *Obstetrics and Gynecology, 71,* 167–170.

Chung, C., Smith, R., Steinhoff, P. et al. (1982). Induced abortion and ectopic pregnancy in subsequent pregnancies. *American Journal of Epidemiology, 115,* 879–887.

Clark, S., Cotton, D., Hankins, G., & Phelan, J. (1994). *Handbook of Critical Care Obstetrics.* Boston: Blackwell Scientific Publications.

Clark, S., Cotton, D., Lee, W. et al. (1989). Central hemodynamic assessment of normal term pregnancy. *American Journal of Obstetrics and Gynecology, 161,* 1439.

Collins, R., & Wallenburg, H. (1989). Pharmacological prevention and treatment of hypertensive disorders in pregnancy. In I. Chalmers, M. Enkin, & M. Keirse (Eds.), *Effective care in pregnancy and childbirth* (p. 512). Oxford: Oxford University Press.

Cotton, D., Gonick, B., Dorman, K. et al. (1985). Cardiovascular alterations in severe pregnancy-induced hypertension: Relationship of central venous pressure to pulmonary capillary wedge pressure. *American Journal of Obstetrics and Gynecology, 151*(6), 762–764.

Cunningham, F., Lowe, T., Guss, S., & Mason, R. (1985). Erythrocyte morphology in women with severe preeclampsia and eclampsia. *American Journal of Obstetrics and Gynecology, 153,* 358.

Cunningham, G., MacDonald, P., Gant, N., Leveno, K. et al. (1993). *Williams obstetrics.* Norwalk, CT: Appleton & Lange.

Dildy, G., Phelan, J., & Cotton, D. (1991). Complications of pregnancy-induced hypertension. In S. Clark, D. Cotton, G. Hankins, & J. Phelan (Eds.), *Critical care obstetrics* (2nd ed.) (pp. 251–288) Boston: Blackwell Scientific Publications.

Doany, W., & Brinkman, C. (1987). Antihypertensive drugs in pregnancy. *Clinical Perinatology, 14,* 783–805.

Dorman, K. (1989). Hemorrhagic emergencies in obstetrics. *Journal of Perinatal Neonatal Nursing, 3,* 23–32.

Edelin, K. (1983). Evaluation of female pelvic pain. *Hospital Medicine, 19,* 37–67.

Fukashima, T. (1995). *Pregnancy hypertension: A new look at an old problem.* Obstetrics Grand Rounds, UCLA School of Medicine.

Gant, N., Madden, J., Siiteri, P., & MacDonald, P. (1975). The metabolic clearance rate of dehydroisoandrosterone sulfate, III. The clearance rate of thiazide diuretics in normal and future preeclamptic pregnancies. *American Journal of Obstetrics and Gynecology, 123,* 159.

Grimes, D. (1984). Epidemiology of gestational trophoblastic disease. *American Journal of Obstetrics and Gynecology, 150,* 309.

Gross, S., Librach, C., & Cecutti, A. (1989). Maternal weight loss associated with hyperemesis gravidarum: A predictor of fetal outcome. *American Journal of Obstetrics and Gynecology, 160,* 906–909.

Guyton, A. (1991). *Textbook of medical physiology.* Philadelphia: W.B. Saunders.

Handler, A., Davis, F., Ferre, C., & Yeko, T. (1989). The relationship of smoking and ectopic pregnancy. *American Journal of Public Health, 79*(9), 1239–1242.

Harvey, C., & Burke, M. (1992). Hypertensive disorders in pregnancy. In L. Mandeville & N. Troiano (Eds.), *High-risk intrapartum nursing* (pp. 147–164). Philadelphia: J.B. Lippincott.

Hert, J., & Heisterberg, I. (1985). The outcome of pregnancy after threatened abortion. *Acta Obstetrics and Gynecology of Scandinavia, 64,* 151–156.

Hogstedt, S., Lideberg, S., Axelsson, O., Lindmark, G. et al. (1985). A prospective controlled trial of hetoprolol-hydralazine treatment in hypertension during pregnancy. *Acta Obstetrics and Gynecology of Scandinavia, 64,* 505.

Holt, V., Daling, J., Voigt, L. et al. (1989). Induced abortion and the risk of subsequent ectopic pregnancy. *American Journal of Public Health, 79*(9), 1234–1238.

Hughes, E. (1972). *Obstetric-gynecologic terminology.* Philadelphia: F.A. Davis.

Kitchin, J., Wein, R., Nunley, W. et al. (1979). Ectopic pregnancy: Current clinical trends. *American Journal of Obstetrics and Gynecology, 134,* 870–876.

Long, P., & Russell, L. (1993). Hyperemesis gravidarum. *Journal of Perinatal Neonatal Nursing, 6*(4), 21–28.

Mantoni, M. (1985). Ultrasound signs in threatened abortion and their prognostic significance. *Obstetrics and Gynecology, 65*(4), 471–475.

Martikainen, A. (1989). Growth and development at the age of 1.5 yrs in children with maternal hypertension. *Journal of Perinatal Medicine, 17,* 259.

Mattson, S., Chritoff, B., & Zukowsky, K. (1993). Risks associated with gestational age and birth weight. In S. Mattson &

J. Smith (Eds.), *NAACOG core curriculum for maternal-newborn nursing* (pp. 659–681). Philadelphia: W.B. Saunders.

Perinatal Advisory Council of Los Angeles Communities (1991). *Prenatal and intrapartum protocols.* Los Angeles

Page, E., & Christianson, R. (1976). The impact of mean arterial pressure in the middle trimester upon the outcome of pregnancy. *American Journal of Obstetrics and Gynecology, 125,* 740–746.

Redman, C. (1991). Controlled trials of antihypertensive drugs in pregnancy. *American Journal of Kidney Disease, 17,* 149.

Ricci, J. (1992). Antepartum hemorrhage. In N. Hacker & J. G. Moore (Eds.), *Essentials of obstetrics and gynecology* (2nd ed.) (pp. 154–162). Philadelphia: W.B. Saunders.

Richardson, B. (1989). Fetal adaptive responses to asphyxia. In F. Manning (Ed.), *Fetal monitoring* (pp. 595–611). Philadelphia: W.B.Saunders.

Romney, S., Gray, M., Little, A. et al. (1981). *Gynecology and obstetrics: The health care of women.* New York: McGraw-Hill.

Satin, A., & Hankins, G. (1991). Cardiopulmonary resuscitation in pregnancy. In S. Clark, D. Cotton, G. Hankins, & J. Phelan (Eds.), *Critical care obstetrics* (2nd ed) (pp. 579–598). Boston: Blackwell Scientific Publications.

Schmidt, J. (1993). Hemorrhagic disorders. In S. Mattson & J. Smith (Eds.), *Core curriculum for maternal-newborn nursing* (pp. 465–483). Philadelphia: W.B. Saunders.

Scott, J. (1994a). Hypertension disorders of pregnancy. In J. Scott, P. Disaia, C. Hammond, & W. Spellacy (Eds.), *Danforth's obstetrics and gynecology* (7th ed.) (pp. 351–365). Philadelphia: J.B. Lippincott.

Scott, J. (1994b). Placenta previa and placental abruption. In J. Scott, P. Disaia, C. Hammond, & W. Spellacy (Eds.), *Danforth's obstetrics and gynecology* (7th ed.) (pp. 489–500). Philadelphia: J.B. Lippincott.

Scott, J., DiSaia, P., Hammond, C. et al. (1990). *Danforth's obstetrics and gynecology.* Philadelphia: J.B. Lippincott.

Sibai, B., & Anderson, G. (1991). Hypertension. In S. Gabbe, J. Niebyl, & J. Simpson (Eds.), *Obstetrics: Normal and problem pregnancies* (2nd ed.) (pp. 993–1056). New York: Churchill Livingstone.

Sibai, B., Caritis, S., Phillips, E., Lebanoff, M. et al. (1993). *Prevention of preeclampsia: Low-dose aspirin in nulli-parous women: A Multi-center double-blind placebo controlled trial.* San Francisco: Society of Perinatal Obstetricians.

Sisson, M. (1992). Disseminated intravascular coagulation. In L. Mandeville & N. Troiano (Eds.), *High-risk intrapartum nursing* (pp. 225–235). Philadelphia: J.B. Lippincott & NAACOG.

Surani, M. (1986). Evidences and consequesnces of difference between maternal and paternal genomes during embryogenesis in the mouse. In J. Rossant & R. Pedersen (Eds.), *Experimental approaches in mammalian embryonic development* (p. 401). New York: Cambridge University.

Volpe, J. (1995). *Neurology of the newborn.* Philadelphia: W.B. Saunders.

Wallenburg, H., Dekker, G., Makovitz, J. et al. (1986). Low-dose aspirin prevents pregnancy-induced hypertension and preeclampsia in angiotensin-sensitive gravidas. *Lancet, 1,* 1–3.

Wallenburg, H., & Rotman, N. (1987). Prevention of recurrent idiopathic fetal growth retardation by lowdose aspirin and dipyridamole. *American Journal of Obstetrics and Gynecology, 157,* 1230–1235.

Weiner, C. (1991). Disseminated intravascular coagulation associated with pregnancy. In S. Clark, D. Cotton, G. Hankins, & J. Phelan (Eds.), *Critical care obstetrics* (2nd ed.) (pp. 180–198). Boston: Blackwell Scientific Publications.

Weinstein, L. (1987). The HELLP syndrome: A severe consequence of hypertension in pregnancy. *Journal of Perinatology, 6,* 316.

Wingard, L., Brody, T., Larner, J., & Schwartz, A. (1991). *Human pharmacology: Molecular to clinical.* St. Louis: Mosby Year Book.

Wolk, R., & Rayburn, W. (1991). Parental nutrition in obstetric patients. *Nutrition in Clinical Practice, 5,* 139–152.

Young, B. (1990). Placental regulation of fetal oxygenation and acid-base balance. In R. Eden & F. Boehm (Eds.), *Assessment and care of the fetus: Physiological, clinical and medicolegal principles* (pp. 171–177). Norwalk, CT: Appleton & Lange.

Zuspan, F. (1994). Preeclampsia: Acute hypertension. In F. Zuspan & E. Quilligan (Eds.), *Current therapy in obstetrics and gynecology* (4th ed.) (pp. 279–281). Philadelphia: W.B. Saunders.

32

Concurrent Medical Complications of Pregnancy

Objectives

- Describe the effects of pregnancy on diabetes.
- Describe the effects of diabetes on pregnancy.
- Identify two methods for classifying diabetes during pregnancy.
- Present five nursing interventions appropriate for the care of the pregnant diabetic.
- Discuss the effects of pregnancy on cardiac disease.
- Discuss the effects of cardiac disease on pregnancy.
- Describe nursing care needs of a pregnant woman with cardiac disease.
- Differentiate between the etiologies, medical therapy, and nursing management of iron deficiency anemia, folic acid deficiency, and sickle cell diseases.
- Discuss the effects of thyroid and chronic renal disease on pregnancy and related nursing care.
- Describe the effects of asthma on pregnancy, including nursing implications.
- Discuss the nursing care of the pregnant woman experiencing minor and major trauma.

Pregnancy may be complicated by a variety of disorders and conditions that can profoundly affect the client and her fetus. Some of these disorders, such as cardiac disease, may exist prior to the client becoming pregnant. Some conditions, such as abdominal trauma, may occur suddenly during the pregnancy. Others, such as diabetes, may begin with the pregnancy or be present prior to conception. The pathophysiology of many disorders may adversely affect pregnancy. Similarly, the physiologic changes may modify the clinical course of some disorders and their management.

This chapter describes the most common metabolic, cardiac, hematologic, pulmonary, and traumatic conditions that may complicate pregnancy. Management of these conditions is discussed, emphasizing the nursing process to meet the physical, psychological, and sociocultural needs. Infectious conditions that may occur during pregnancy, such as sexually transmitted diseases and urinary tract infections (UTIs), are discussed more completely in Chapter 11.

Diabetes Mellitus

Diabetes mellitus, the most common metabolic complication of pregnancy, illustrates the interaction between the physiologic changes of pregnancy and the pathophysiology of disease. There is a significant change in the course of diabetes when pregnancy occurs. At the same time, diabetes profoundly affects the course of pregnancy and the fetus.

Diabetes mellitus is a disorder of carbohydrate metabolism resulting from a deficiency in insulin production by the pancreatic cells of the islets of Langerhans. Insulin is an essential hormone required for glucose

transfer into the muscle and adipose tissue cells. When glucose is unable to enter body cells because of inadequate insulin, fat and protein metabolism are altered. To review the pathophysiologic events of diabetes mellitus, see Box 32-1.

In recent years, the incidence of diabetes during pregnancy in the United States has increased to approximately 180,000 pregnancies per year (Langer, 1990). Diabetics are now able to conceive and maintain pregnancies because of the advances in management and there has been an increased recognition of the milder forms of **gestational diabetes** (glucose intolerance first identified during pregnancy). Gestational diabetes occurs in 1% to 3% of pregnancies, and **pregestational diabetes**, diabetes that existed prior to conception, occurs in 0.1% to 0.2%. (Coustan, 1991).

Effect of Pregnancy on Diabetes

Pregnancy is considered a *diabetogenic condition*, one in which the balance of maternal glucose production and use is stressed by the growing fetus, who derives energy solely from maternal glucose stores. This coupled with the physiologic adaptations that normally occur in pregnancy may greatly affect diabetes by altering insulin and carbohydrate metabolism.

During the first trimester, maternal insulin needs decrease because of the low levels of **human placental lactogen** (hPL), an insulin antagonist produced by the placenta that promotes lipolysis to increase the amount of circulating free fatty acids for maternal metabolic use. Presumably, glucose is spared for fetal use.

Also, during the first trimester, rising levels of *estrogen* and *progesterone* significantly influence the woman's metabolic status by stimulating the pancreatic beta cells to increase insulin secretion and release. Large quantities of glucose and amino acids are transported to the fetus, and lower glucose levels result. As pregnancy progresses, maternal hyperinsulinemia continues but with increased tissue resistance to insulin (Harvey, 1992).

During the second and third trimesters, rising levels of hPL, estrogen, progesterone, cortisol, prolactin, and **insulinase** (an enzyme that accelerates insulin degradation) increase **insulin resistance**, a glucose sparing mechanism that allows for an abundant supply of glucose for fetal use. During this time, maternal insulin requirements increase, often dramatically.

At birth, with placental expulsion, there is a sudden drop in placental hormone levels, cortisol, and insulinase. This leads to an abrupt decrease in insulin requirements and a return to prepregnancy sensitivity to insulin.

The physiologic changes in the kidney associated with pregnancy also affect diabetes. The glomerular filtration rate of glucose is increased, while tubular glucose reabsorption is decreased. Consequently, the re-

BOX 32-1
Pathophysiologic Events of Diabetes Mellitus

The pathophysiologic events occurring with diabetes are outlined below. Each of these events ultimately leads to the classic signs and symptoms associated with diabetes.

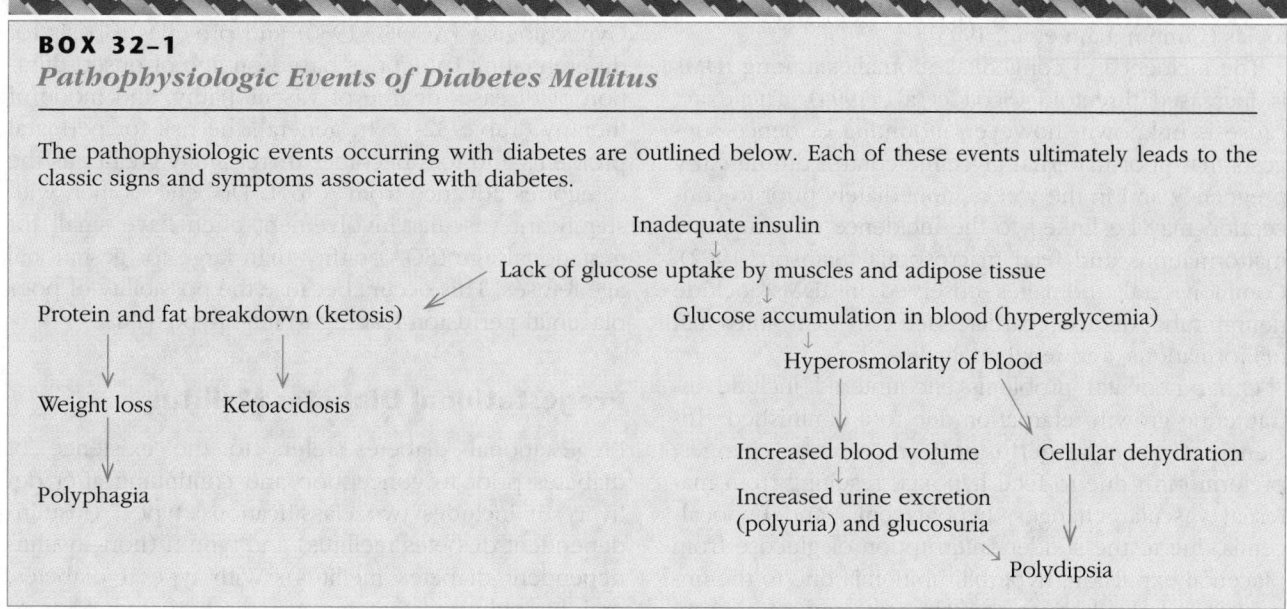

nal threshold for glucose is reduced from prepregnancy levels. Ketone clearance also is reduced because of the decline in peripheral tissue uptake of glucose.

Caloric intake may be decreased because of diminished appetite, anorexia, or vomiting during the first trimester. Concomitantly, there is a significant transfer of glucose and glucogenic amino acids to the embryo or fetus. These factors place the pregnant diabetic at risk for **hypoglycemia** or starvation ketosis.

Hyperglycemia may develop in the second half of pregnancy due to the progressive increasing insulin antagonist factors and rising insulin requirements. This condition can lead to **diabetic ketoacidosis** (DKA), which is an acute emergency characterized by blood glucose levels >350 mg/dL, ketonemia (with plasma ketone levels >5 mmol/L), and acidosis (with plasma bicarbonate levels <9 mEq/L; Vignati et al., 1985). Pregestational, or type I, diabetics are at the greatest risk for developing DKA. Development of DKA also has been associated with beta-agonist tocolytics used for the treatment of preterm labor (Harvey, 1992). Elevated rates of perinatal and fetal mortality continue to occur with DKA.

Vascular diseases occurring secondary to diabetes may progress during pregnancy. Meticulous management of the pregnant diabetic may prevent or minimize the development of diabetic nephropathy and retinopathy.

Effect of Diabetes on Pregnancy

Despite great gains achieved in modern obstetric management, perinatal mortality and morbidity remain significantly higher in diabetic pregnancies than in normal (nondiabetic) pregnancies. Reported perinatal mortality rates vary from 2% to 5% in major treatment centers (Heppard et al., 1992). The risk factor for maternal-fetal complications is increased for women with a longer duration of diabetes, especially if there is a history of poor control prior to conception. The major factors affecting pregnancy outcome appear to be the degree of glycemic control and the severity of underlying vascular disease.

Diabetes can have a deleterious effect on pregnancy. Pregnant diabetics are at increased risk for hyperglycemia, infection, *pregnancy-induced hypertension* (PIH), and *hydramnios*. The infant of a diabetic mother (IDM) is at high risk for **macrosomia** (excessive fetal growth) and congenital anomalies.

Hyperglycemia and possibly DKA can result from an increase in ketones released from the breakdown of fatty acids. DKA in the pregnant woman often results from the stress of an infection.

Infection, especially genitourinary tract infection, is more common and more serious. The presence of glycosuria places the pregnant diabetic at risk for monilial vaginitis, which may in some cases become intractable.

The overall incidence of PIH increases fourfold even with no associated preexisting vascular disease. If diabetic vascular changes are present, then the risk is even greater.

The incidence of **hydramnios** is increased. The exact cause is unknown; however, it is believed to be related to osmotic pressure, hypersecretion of amniotic fluid, and diuresis from fetal hyperglycemia. If coupled with fetal macrosomia, hydramnios can cause cardiopulmonary symptoms.

Prolonged fetal hyperinsulinism and hyperglycemia lead to macrosomia. If this occurs, the possibility of a difficult vaginal delivery and postpartum hemorrhage is increased. The rate of cesarean section deliveries is increased, primarily due to fetal compromise and dystocias (Cunningham et al., 1993).

The incidence of congenital anomalies among IDMs is increased threefold (Scott et al., 1994). The exact cause is unknown; however, mounting evidence suggests that poor maternal glycemic control during early pregnancy and in the weeks immediately prior to conception may be linked to the incidence of congenital malformations and fetal macrosomia (Samson, 1992). Common fetal anomalies observed in IDMs include neural tube defects, cardiac defects, gastrointestinal malformations, and renal anomalies.

Other neonatal problems encountered include intrauterine growth retardation due to a diminished efficiency of placental perfusion from vascular changes; preterm birth due to fetal hypoxia, resulting from maternal vascular changes; hypoglycemia and hypocalcemia due to the sudden interruption of glucose from placental expulsion; hyperbilirubinemia due to the immaturity of the liver for metabolism; and respiratory distress syndrome from the inhibition of fetal enzymes necessary for surfactant production by high fetal insulin levels. The IDM inherits a predisposition to diabetes. These and other conditions are discussed in Chapter 43.

Classification

Several methods for classifying diabetes are available in clinical practice. White (1978) developed a classification system for identifying risk categories among pregnant diabetics. This widely applied system was modified by the American College of Obstetricians and Gynecologists (ACOG, 1986) and provides a basis for differentiating categories based on age of onset, duration of disease, degree of vasculopathy, and mode of therapy (Table 32-1). In general, the risk for perinatal problems and loss becomes increasingly greater as the categories advance from A to T. Diabetic women with significant vascular involvement often have small for gestational age (SGA) rather than large for gestational age fetuses. This occurs because the possibility of poor placental perfusion leading to fetal hypoxia.

Pregestational Diabetes Mellitus

Pregestational diabetes refers to the existence of diabetes prior to conception and continuing after delivery. It includes two classifications: type I (insulin-dependent diabetes mellitus) and type II (non–insulin-dependent diabetes mellitus). With type II diabetes, oral hypoglycemic agents are discontinued prior to conception, if possible, or as soon as pregnancy is diagnosed to prevent the possibility of teratogenic effects on the fetus. Usually, women with type II diabetes taking oral hypoglycemic agents for glucose control require insulin during pregnancy. Therefore, most women with pregestational diabetes are insulin dependent.

Gestational Diabetes Mellitus

Gestational diabetes mellitus (GDM) refers to a "genetically and clinically heterogeneous group of disor-

---

TABLE 32–1
Classification of Diabetes in Pregnancy

Pregestational Diabetes

Class	Age of Onset	Duration (Years)	Vascular Disease	Therapy
A	Any	Any	None	A-1, diet only
B	Over 20 y	Less than 10	None	Diet and insulin
C	10–19 y	10–19	None	Diet and insulin
D	Before 10 y	More than 20	Benign retinopathy	Diet and insulin
F	Any	Any	Nephropathy	Diet and insulin
R	Any	Any	Proliferative retinopathy	Diet and insulin
H	Any	Any	Heart disease	Diet and insulin
T	Any	Any	Renal transplant	Diet and insulin

Gestational Diabetes

Class	Fasting Plasma Glucose		Postprandial Plasma Glucose	Therapy
A-1	Less than 105 mg/dL	*and*	Less than 120 mg/dL	Diet only
A-2	More than 105 mg/dL	*and/or*	More than 120 mg/dL	Insulin

Modified from *The American College of Obstetricians and Gynecologists*. (1986). *Classification of diabetes in pregnancy*. Technical Bulletin No. 92. Washington, DC: ACOG

ders that share carbohydrate intolerance in common" and are diagnosed during pregnancy (Hollingsworth, 1992). Women with no personal history of glucose intolerance who demonstrate hyperglycemia first diagnosed during pregnancy are considered gestational diabetics. Typically, the diagnosis of GDM is made in the second half of pregnancy. Fetal nutrient demands increase, maternal glucose levels increase from increased maternal nutrient ingestion, and maternal insulin resistance increases during this period.

The ACOG classification of gestational diabetes includes two subgroups that are differentiated based on fasting blood glucose values (see Table 32-1). The degree of clinical manifestations presenting with GDM may vary widely. Most women in class A1 are asymptomatic and managed by diet alone; those in class A2 are often insulin dependent. Concern about early diagnosis and careful monitoring of GDM arises from the observed increased risk for perinatal and maternal morbidity and mortality (Coustan, 1991). However, with appropriate management, the perinatal outcomes excluding congenital abnormalities approximate those of the normal obstetric population (Landon, 1991). Conditions associated with GDM include an increased incidence of intrauterine fetal death, macrosomia, perinatal asphyxia, shoulder dystocia, birth trauma, operative deliveries, neonatal respiratory distress syndrome, hypoglycemia, hyperbilirubinemia, hypocalcemia, and polycythemia. The likelihood of stillbirth in the woman with appropriately managed GDM is no different than for the general population (Cunningham et al., 1993).

Most women with GDM can be managed by diet alone. If the glucose levels cannot be normalized with this management, then insulin treatment or exercise protocols need to be added. Vaginal deliveries are most often the method of birth. The woman diagnosed with GDM usually finds that her condition regresses completely following delivery. However, a majority of women with GDM will later develop overt diabetes.

Diagnosis and Screening

Numerous laboratory tests are performed to help diagnose and screen for diabetes. Current standards of prenatal care include screening all women for GDM between 24 and 28 weeks' gestation, except those with confirmed diabetes. Any woman with one or more risk factors for diabetes (Box 32-2) should be screened during the first prenatal visit. The screening procedure involves ingestion of 50 g of oral glucose without regard to time of day or oral intake. Blood is drawn 1 hour following glucose ingestion for evaluation of plasma glucose level. A threshold value of 140 mg/dL is considered a positive screen result and should be followed

---

BOX 32–2
Risk Factors for Development of Gestational Diabetes Mellitus

- Previous large newborn (9 lb or more)
- Family history of diabetes mellitus
- Glucosuria on two successive occasions
- Obesity—weight > 200 lb
- Unexplained pregnancy wastage (spontaneous abortions, stillbirths)
- Multiparity
- Presence of hydramnios
- Previous newborn with a congenital anomaly
- Hypertension

---

by a standard 3-hour glucose tolerance test (GTT; Fig. 32-1). Factors known to affect values include nausea and vomiting, smoking, eating, exercise, and caffeine (Howard, 1992). If GDM is suspected late in pregnancy because fetal size is greater than indicated by estimated date of delivery or **glycosuria** (glucose in the urine) appears, rescreening is recommended.

During a normal pregnancy, glucose may appear in the urine with blood sugars as low as 100 mg/dL due to a lowered renal threshold to glucose excretion. The pregnant woman's urine is tested for glucose at the initial prenatal visit and again on subsequent visits. Urine also is tested for ketones. Both tests are administered routinely to pregnant women with diabetes.

Although glucosuria does not necessarily indicate high blood glucose levels, any woman exhibiting glycosuria should be suspected of having GDM. The diagnosis should be established or ruled out by evaluation of blood glucose levels with the GTT.

The oral GTT (100 g) is preferred to the intravenous (25 g) test because it appears to be more sensitive and assesses the gastrointestinal factors involved in insulin secretion (Gabbe et al., 1991). The client should be instructed to ingest a carbohydrate load of 150 to 300 g/dL for 3 days prior to the test and to have nothing by mouth (except water) after midnight before the test (Howard, 1992). A fasting blood glucose is drawn the next morning. The woman is then given a carbohydrate load, and 1-, 2-, and 3-hour postprandial venous blood samples are taken for glucose. An oral GTT is considered abnormal if two of the woman's blood glucose values are elevated or if one blood glucose value is exceeded in two successive tests.

For the pregestational diabetic, **glycosylated hemoglobin** (HbA$_{1c}$) levels, which measure the percentage of hemoglobin with glucose attached, are performed to evaluate overall glycemic control. These levels are usually obtained prior to conception, at the first prenatal visit, and at least once every trimester. In addition, fast-

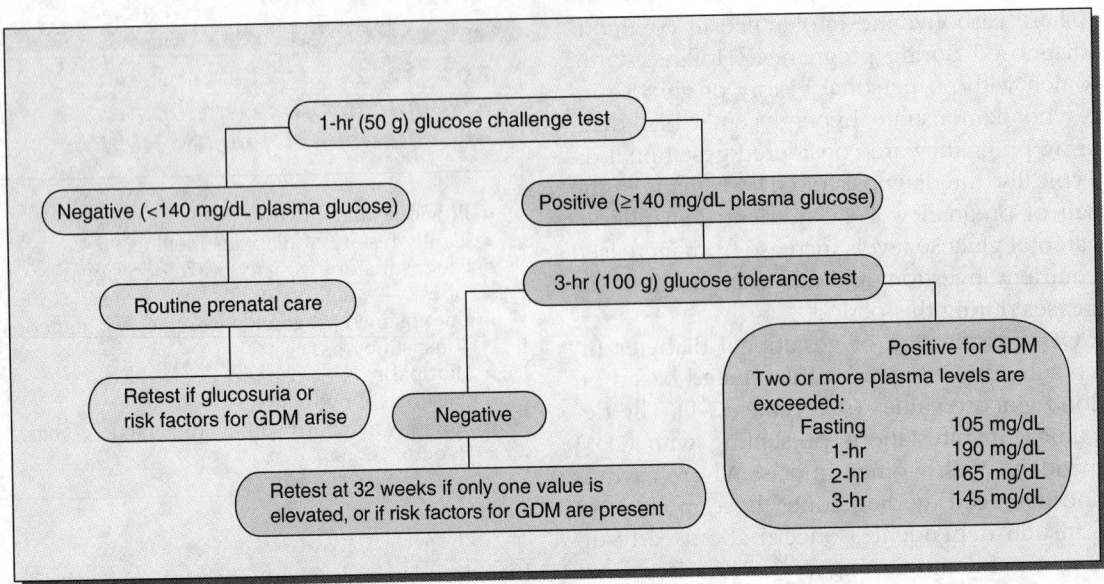

FIGURE 32–1 Screening for gestational diabetes mellitus. Modified from American Diabetes Association, 1990; Gabbe, 1993.

ing blood glucose and postprandial blood glucose levels may be ordered.

Nursing Process

A multidisciplinary approach to managing diabetes during pregnancy should be used. A variety of specialists, including perinatologists, obstetricians, endocrinologists, nurses, midwives, diabetic and perinatal clinical nurse specialists, nutritionists, and social workers, may be needed to ensure client understanding of the disease process, medical management, and self-care activities. Within the perinatal team, the nurse assumes a key role in providing client with education and anticipatory guidance and alleviating anxiety. The following are the major objectives of nursing care:

- Identification of women at risk for gestational diabetes
- Provision of appropriate perinatal care
- Maintenance and control of blood glucose levels
- Provision of adequate client education and counseling
- Prevention or early detection of potential maternal and fetal complications
- Promotion of a positive psychosocial adjustment to a high-risk pregnancy

The plan of nursing care is developed in cooperation with the client (see Nursing Care Plan: The Pregnant Diabetic Woman). With intensive diabetic care prior to and during pregnancy, perinatal morbidity and mortality rates are reduced (Cunningham et al., 1993; see Research Highlight). All diabetic women of reproductive age should receive preconceptual counseling regarding the effects of diabetes on pregnancy and the fetus and the effects of pregnancy on diabetic control and com-

plications. Improvements in ambulatory self-monitoring and community-based care have reduced the need for inpatient hospital education of pregestational diabetic women without compromising maternal and neonatal outcomes. Hospitalization is recommended for women who have had poor glucose control prior to conception to reeducate and reestablish metabolic control and decrease frequent visits to the hospital during pregnancy (Hollingsworth, 1992). Class A1 diabetics should have weekly fasting blood sugars (FBS) done and begin contraction stress tests (CSTs) weekly starting at 4 weeks' gestation. Class A2 and B diabetics should have weekly FBS in the office, home glucose monitoring after meals and at bedtime, and CSTs and nonstress tests (NSTs) weekly starting at 32 weeks every 3 to 4 days (Heppard et al., 1992). More frequent monitoring is often necessary for class C through T diabetics.

Nursing Assessment

Prenatal assessment should include observations for any previously identified signs and symptoms of diabetes in all pregnant women. The client's family and prenatal history should be carefully obtained and reviewed for predisposing factors. The previously described screening protocols for diagnosis should be followed.

In clients with pregestational and GDM, knowledge of disease and normal physiologic and psychological changes of pregnancy are assessed. As part of the comprehensive and ongoing prenatal care, the nurse or another member of the perinatal health team also should perform the various assessments initially and throughout the pregnancy. See Assessment Guidelines: Diabetic Client for information about specific areas to assess.

(text continues on page 860)

NURSING CARE PLAN
The Pregnant Diabetic Woman

Nursing Goals

The pregnant diabetic woman will successfully maintain pregnancy without perinatal complications as evidenced by:

1. Maintaining blood glucose levels of fasting blood sugar <90 mg/dL and 2-h post-prandial <145 mg/dL.
2. Complying with self-management instructions (eg, diet, exercise, monitoring blood sugar, insulin management) as ordered.
3. Expressing fears, griefs, and concerns regarding self-care and effects on the fetus.
4. Delivering a healthy term infant without signs of distress and/or hypoglycemia.

Assessment	Potential Nursing Diagnoses	Intervention/ Rationale	Evaluation

Maternal factors
  Previous large infant (9 lb or greater)
  Family history of diabetes mellitus
  Glucosuria
  Obesity
  Unexplained pregnancy wastage (previous habitual spontaneous abortions or unexplained stillbirth)
  Previous birth of infant with congenital abnormality
  Multiparity
	Alteration in Carbohydrate Metabolism related to diabetes	Screen for predisposing factors for diabetes *to identify early women at risk for GDM*	Client at risk for GDM is identified.

		Assist in preparing for 2-h postprandial or oral glucose tolerance test (GTT) *to diagnose GDM.*	Client understands the purpose of testing and follows instructions.
		Determine blood glucose levels using a glucose meter. Metabolic control is assessed by blood glucose levels. *During pregnancy insulin requirements fluctuate widely, affecting carbohydrate, fat and protein metabolism.*	Client has blood glucose levels accurately monitored.
		Observe for signs and symptoms of hypoglycemia and hyperglycemia *to provide early treatment.*	No signs and symptoms of hypoglycemia or hyperglycemia are evident.
		Administer 4 oz orange juice for symptomatic hypoglycemia *to rapidly raise blood glucose level and prevent tissue damage from glucose depletion.*	Signs of hypoglycemia are rapidly relieved.
		Administer prescribed amount of regular insulin and document *to restore normal metabolism of carbohydrates, protein, and fats.*	Client receives prescribed insulin and displays no adverse reaction.

Fetal–newborn factors
  Hydramnios
  Low-gestation-age infant
Signs of diabetes
  Polyuria
  Polydipsia
  Polyphagia
  Weight loss
		Chart blood glucose levels, treatments, and insulin administration *to improve communication and diabetic management by members of the health team.*	Accurate records are maintained in the medical chart.

(continued)

NURSING CARE PLAN *(Continued)*
The Pregnant Diabetic Woman

Assessment	Potential Nursing Diagnoses	Intervention/ Rationale	Evaluation
Physical examination, including assessment of optic fundi, cardiovascular system, vital signs, blood pressure, fundal height Glucose tolerance test 24-h diet recall Past experience managing diabetes (eg, self-administration of insulin) Exercise schedule (predictability, length)	Knowledge Deficit related to diabetic self-care during pregnancy		
		Explain changes in insulin regulation throughout childbearing cycle. Pregnancy is a diabetogenic condition that may cause fluctuations in insulin requirements; *the client needs to understand insulin control for appropriate self-care.*	Changes in insulin requirements throughout pregnancy are explained by the client.
		Request nutritional consultation to *provide in-depth dietary counseling to meet individual needs and preferences.*	Individualized nutritional counseling is provided to client.
Knowledge of complications of diabetes		Review prescribed dietary plan (exchange lists) and assess understanding *to promote fetal growth and normalize blood glucose levels.*	Client understands and follows prescribed diet and gains optimum amount of weight.
		Instruct newly diagnosed insulin-dependent diabetic on the techniques for insulin preparation, administration, and storage *to prepare the client for self-administration of insulin.*	Client demonstrates safe procedure in preparation, self-administration, and storage of insulin.
		Instruct in blood glucose monitoring (BGM) and importance of maintaining fasting blood sugar between 60 and 120 mg/dL; *BGM helps to determine insulin needs; maintaining euglycemia improves maternal and fetal outcomes.*	Client shows proper technique in return demonstration of BGM.
		Instruct in fractional urine testing for acetone levels *to indicate development of DKA.*	Urine acetone levels are correctly checked.
		Provide specific information on signs and symptoms of diabetic complications (eg, DKA, insulin	Signs and symptoms of diabetic complications during pregnancy are identified by client.

(continued)

NURSING CARE PLAN *(Continued)*
The Pregnant Diabetic Woman

Assessment	Potential Nursing Diagnoses	Intervention/ Rationale	Evaluation
		shock, hypertensive disorders of pregnancy, UTI) *to help client intervene appropriately at home and prevent maternal and fetal injuries.*	
		Discuss activities for daily living and the benefits of daily exercise *to prevent hypoglycemia and decrease insulin needs.*	Client maintains safe level of activities and avoids hypoglycemia.
Response to diabetes Expectations about pregnancy Achievement of maternal tasks of pregnancy	Self Concept Disturbance related to complication of pregnancy	Allow client to ventilate feelings regarding high-risk pregnancy *to promote adaptation to high-risk pregnancy by alleviating anxiety.*	Fears, griefs, and concerns are expressed.
		Assess family adjustment to high-risk pregnancy and identify possible stressors; *family support decreases client stress and improves compliance.*	Client identifies stressors in family, and family adjustment is evaluated.
		Identify resources in family and community to help client adapt to high-risk pregnancy *to provide needed support following discharge.*	Potential resources in family and community are identified.
		Involve supportive family member(s) in education of diabetes management *to reinforce diabetic self-care at home.*	Family members demonstrate understanding of condition and provide support.
Fetal factors Heart rate Activity (e.g., kicking) Periodic changes, variability on electronic fetal monitor Prenatal diagnostic tests Lecithin-sphingomyelin ratio Nonstress test Oxytocin challenge test Sonography Estriol levels	Altered Tissue Perfusion: uteroplacental, related to diabetes in pregnancy	Perform electronic monitoring of fetal heart rate (FHR)(continuous or q 2–4 h, if stable) while in hospital and report nonreassuring pattern; *baseline FHR, variability and pattern are obtained, and potential fetal problems may be identified.*	Reassuring FHR pattern is maintained.
		Instruct client to maintain fetal movement (FM) count and report significant changes in fetal activity; *FM is correlated with well-being and a decrease in movement may occur with impending labor.*	Fetus remains active.

(continued)

NURSING CARE PLAN *(Continued)*
The Pregnant Diabetic Woman

Assessment	Potential Nursing Diagnoses	Intervention/ Rationale	Evaluation
		Prepare for prenatal diagnostic tests and explain rationale for them (eg, nonstress tests [NST], sonography, biophysical profile, amniocentesis). *Compliance is increased when client understands purpose of test; NST detects nonreassuring FHR and uterine activity; sonography assesses fetal growth; biophysical profiles identify fetal compromise; fetal lung maturity is determined by PG levels in amniotic fluid.*	Client remains relaxed during testing and understands reasons for procedures. Appointments are maintained.
		Place client in left lateral position during bedrest. *Uteroplacental perfusion is increased in the left lateral position, and supine hypotension may be prevented.*	Client remains on left side while in bed

RESEARCH HIGHLIGHT

Management of Gestational Diabetes

This prospective study was designed to test the hypothesis that intensified management of gestational diabetes (GD) would reduce adverse outcomes. Subjects in the intensified management group (*n* = 1145) were compared with those receiving conventional management (*n* = 1316) and to a contemporaneous randomized control group (nondiabetic, *n* = 4922). The intensified management group did self-monitoring of blood glucose seven times a day (fasting, preprandial, 2-hour postprandial, and at bedtime) using memory reflectance meters, whereas the conventional group was seen at the clinic weekly for glucose assessment with weekly fasting and 2-hour postprandial evaluation and self-monitoring with glucose strip determinations four times daily (fasting and 2 hours after meals). Both groups were treated by diet alone or with diet and insulin. Results showed that the intensified management group had rates of macrosomia, cesarean section, metabolic complications, shoulder dystocia, stillbirth, neonatal intensive care unit days, and respiratory complications lower than those in the conventional management group and comparable to those of the nondiabetic controls. Other maternal complication rates were comparable for the three groups. The level of glycemia was clearly related to pregnancy outcome in GD.

Critique: The researchers conclude that the intensified management approach is significantly associated with improved perinatal outcomes. This conclusion must be considered in relation to the study's limitations. Subjects were not randomly assigned to groups but were designated based on availability of the memory reflectance meters. The sample was composed predominantly of Hispanics and may not be representative of other populations. Despite these weaknesses, the findings support the importance of nurses educating clients about maintenance of near normoglycemic blood glucose levels.

Langer, O., Rodriguez, D. A., Xenakis, M. J., McFarland, M. B., Berkus, M. D., & Arredondo, F. (1994). Intensified versus conventional management of gestational diabetes. *American Journal of Obstetrics and Gynecology, 170,* 1036–1046.

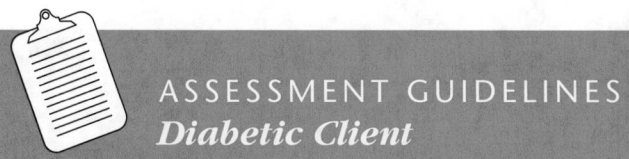

ASSESSMENT GUIDELINES
Diabetic Client

Areas Assessed	Scientific "Rationale"
Baseline vital signs, height, and weight	Initial findings can be compared with subsequent findings to identify potential problems; for example, a steady rise in blood pressure or sudden increase in weight may be a sign of pregnancy-induced hypertension, a frequent complication associated with diabetes.
Gestational age	Adequate determination of gestational age assists in managing pregnancy and planning timing and method of delivery.
Uterine size, fetal activity, and fetal heart rate	These evaluations reflect fetal status and well-being and aid in the prevention of possible complications.
Urinalysis, culture, and sensitivity	These tests help to detect asymptomatic bacteriuria, a precursor to overt pyelonephritis, to which the diabetic is especially prone.
Optic fundi examination, initially and subsequently at least once a trimester	Examination of optic fundi helps to detect any vascular changes accompanying diabetes.
Client knowledge base about self-monitoring	Information about the client's understanding allows the development of an appropriate teaching plan to ensure compliance and minimize risk of complications.
Psychosocial, economic factors with special considerations to the potential stress evoked by a high-risk pregnancy	Research has shown that gestational diabetics experience more stressful responses than pregestational diabetics for all aspects of the medical regimen.
Support systems and services	Because of the high risk of the pregnancy, available resources need to be evaluated so that necessary support systems and assistance can be obtained.
Serum alpha-fetoprotein screening at 16 to 18 weeks	Elevated levels are associated with neural tube defects; if elevated, a follow-up ultrasound is indicated.
Glycosylated hemoglobin levels (A1 or A1c)	These levels reflect the average serum glucose concentration over the last 4 to 12 weeks. Results of studies have shown that an elevation in pregnancy is associated with an increased incidence of complications.
Ultrasound examination at 16 to 18 weeks	Ultrasound examination at this time confirms gestation age and surveys the fetus for congenital anomalies.
Serial ultrasounds during the second and third trimesters	Serial ultrasounds help determine appropriate growth pattern of fetus.

(continued)

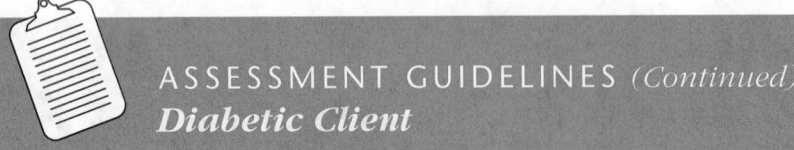

ASSESSMENT GUIDELINES *(Continued)*
Diabetic Client

Areas Assessed	Scientific "Rationale"
Nonstress tests (NSTs) weekly or more frequently beginning at 30 to 32 weeks	NST provides important information about fetal well-being.
Other fetal assessment techniques, such as contraction stress tests, fetal movement counts, biophysical profile, amniocentesis, and estriol levels	Valuable information about fetal well-being can be obtained from these tests.
Common complications, such as infections, nephropathy, hydramnios, and cardiovascular problems	Pregestational and gestational diabetics may experience a higher incidence of adverse outcomes with poor glycemic control.

Nursing Diagnoses

As a result of the nursing assessment, several potential nursing diagnoses may be identified that focus on alterations in the life processes of the pregnant diabetic. Box 32-3 lists some examples of possible nursing diagnoses.

BOX 32–3
Nursing Diagnoses: Diabetes

■ Altered Nutrition: Less or more than body requirements related to interaction between diabetes and pregnancy
■ Knowledge Deficit related to:
  - Diabetic self-care during pregnancy
  - Interaction between diabetes and pregnancy
  - Signs and symptoms of complications associated with diabetes
■ Body Image Disturbance related to complications of pregnancy
■ Altered Tissue Perfusion related to vascular changes associated with diabetes
■ Risk for Injury to fetus related to uteroplacental insufficiency
■ Risk for Injury to mother related to complications associated with diabetes
■ Risk for Infection related to increased susceptibility associated with diabetes
■ Risk for Impaired Skin Integrity related to skin stretching from hydramnios
■ Ineffective Management of Therapeutic Regimen related to:
  - Lack of understanding about diabetes and pregnancy
  - Inadequate support services

Nursing Intervention

Adequate control of pregnant women with GDM or pregestational diabetes is of primary concern when planning nursing interventions to prevent or lessen the incidence of perinatal mortality and morbidity. Major components of direct nursing care and client education relate to nutrition management, insulin administration, blood glucose monitoring, and exercise. Nurses assume an important responsibility in promoting appropriate self-management of diabetes by ensuring that clients have a sound knowledge base about these aspects of care and providing client teaching about all aspects of care (see Client Teaching Guidelines: Diabetes and Pregnancy) There are several obstetric considerations of which the nurse also must be aware when implementing care.

Nutrition. Ideally, diabetic women who anticipate pregnancy will follow a prescribed well-balanced dietary regimen before conception and will be in a state of good metabolic control. The caloric requirement for the normal-weight client is 35 calories per kilogram of ideal weight per day or approximately 2,000 to 2,500 calories. Of the total calories, 40% to 50% should be in the form of carbohydrates, particularly complex carbohydrates and soluble fiber; 30% to 35% should come from fat, ideally <35% unsaturated fats; and 20% to 25% should come from protein (Sweet Success, 1992). The exact caloric intake is based on the client's prepregnant weight and daily activities. For obese women with GDM, the caloric intake should be 1,500 to 1,800 kcal/d, no less than 25 kcal/kg of the ideal prepregnancy body weight, with a lower pregnancy weight gain of 15 to 20 lb (Hollingsworth, 1992). It is difficult to decrease caloric intake below 1,800 calo-

CLIENT TEACHING GUIDELINES
Diabetes and Pregnancy

Each of the following areas listed below should be addressed with the pregnant diabetic client. Use them as a guide for developing an appropriate client teaching plan.

Effects of diabetes on pregnancy and vice versa

Nutritional requirements (eg, regular intake at prescribed times; prescribed diet, weight gain)

Signs and symptoms of hypoglycemia and hyperglycemia and appropriate management (eg, half glass of orange juice if glucose level <60 mg/dL)

Home blood glucose monitoring using prescribed glucose meter and regular recording of blood glucose levels

Prescribed insulin (eg, action, dose, route, timing, storage, sliding scale doses if ordered, changing needs during pregnancy, intrapartum, and postpartum)

Technique for administration of insulin (eg, drawing medication, rotating injection sites, method of administration, use of continuous insulin pump if prescribed)

Antepartum evaluation procedures (eg, fetal movement counts, ultrasound, amniocentesis, nonstress test, contraction stress test, biophysical profile)

Exercise during pregnancy (eg, appropriate exercises, timing of exercise, preventing hypoglycemia)

Signs of developing infections (eg, urinary tract infections, upper respiratory infections)

Self-care activities that decrease risk of contracting infections (eg, avoiding contact with infected individuals, wearing cotton-crotch underwear, drinking at least six to eight glasses of water per day, drinking cranberry juice, urinating frequently and after sexual intercourse, completing prescribed course of antibiotics, using appropriate technique [front to back wiping] to clean perineum)

Signs and symptoms of diabetic ketoacidosis

Anticipatory guidance regarding labor and delivery (eg, timing, method of delivery, glucose monitoring and insulin administration if appropriate, analgesia and anesthesia)

Technique for testing urine for ketones

---

ries and maintain adequate protein and carbohydrate intake; therefore, weight reduction even for overweight women is generally not recommended. The following guidelines should be considered in nutritional counseling:

- At least 30 g/d more protein is recommended in the second and third trimesters than in the nonpregnant state. Clients with nephropathy and proteinuria require additional protein.

- Complex carbohydrates should be included in each meal to delay absorption of glucose.

- Adequate fat consumption should be encouraged to delay gastric emptying and prevent hyperglycemia. Diabetic women with deficient intake of carbohydrates are at risk for acidosis and ketonemia.

- The caloric requirement should be evenly distributed (three meals and three snacks) throughout the day.

- A weight gain of 22 to 27 lb at term is desirable for most pregnant women.

- An evening snack consisting of a complex carbohydrate and protein is effective in preventing hypoglycemic episodes during the night.

- Concentrated sweets should be avoided because they are likely to produce marked swings in blood glucose.

Insulin Administration. The goal of treatment with insulin is **euglycemia,** blood glucose levels as near the normal range as possible. The incidence of maternal, fetal, and neonatal complications during diabetic pregnancy is directly correlated with the degree of maternal glycemic control maintained (Jovanovic et al., 1981; Landon et al., 1988; Mandeville, 1991). Maintaining optimal blood glucose levels requires meticulous regulation of medication, adherence to the prescribed diet, and carefully planned activity.

Progressive insulin resistance is characteristic of pregnancy. It is not unusual for insulin requirements to increase as much as twofold to threefold. During the latter half of pregnancy, the effective half-life of insulin is reduced because of increased placenta degradation. This often necessitates the use of evening and morning doses of insulin to achieve good control in the insulin-dependent diabetic.

Adjustment of insulin dosage is individualized according to the clinical picture and the results of blood glucose analysis. It is recommended that all pregnant clients requiring insulin use human-derived insulin, which is less antigenic than porcine insulin. Porcine insulin should be used with clients on tight control who do not experience hypoglycemic episodes and with blood sugars less than 60 mg/dL to prevent symptomatic hypoglycemia (Hollingsworth, 1992). The daily dosage of insulin is frequently split, with about two-thirds being administered in the morning and about one-third after dinner. A small amount of fast-acting insulin is often added to each dose of intermediate-acting insulin to control the 4- to 6-hour interval before the intermediate insulin begins to have a significant effect on blood glucose level. The combined insulins are administered approximately one-half hour before meals. In some clients, more frequent, small dosages of regular insulin may have to be administered throughout the day in response to fasting and postprandial blood sugar levels (Engel, 1989).

The nurse must instruct the client about time interval peaks for insulin. As this information is discussed, it should be related to the signs and symptoms of hypoglycemia and hyperglycemia (Box 32-4). All clients and their families should be informed about the use of Glucagon (1 mg subcutaneously or intramuscularly) for treatment of serious hypoglycemia.

If the diabetic woman is unable to regulate her plasma glucose levels adequately by intermittent insulin injections, a portable insulin pump may be used to improve metabolic control. Implanted into the subcutaneous tissue of the woman's abdomen by way of a small-gauge needle, these electromechanical devices continuously deliver a fixed small amount of insulin. The dosage of insulin delivered by the pump is based on capillary blood sample levels drawn by the client or nurse. A bolus of insulin may be self-administered by the client before meals. This type of system does not include an integral glucose sensor or feedback mechanism and is called an open-loop system.

All insulin-dependent diabetics should be counseled about changes in their insulin demands because of pregnancy. Counseling sessions provide excellent opportunities to reinforce the client's acquired skills in self-management and to allay fears concerning new interventions.

The gestational diabetic may occasionally require insulin therapy despite nutritional management. Oral hypoglycemics are not recommended during pregnancy because of the possibility of teratogenic effects on the fetus. The client should be taught about proper technique for injection, rotation of sites, storage of medication, and skin care.

Blood Glucose Monitoring. Control of diabetes is now assessed by home blood glucose monitoring. Many different machines are available, such as the Accu-Chek Easy and One-Touch, which are available for use with blood glucose reagent strips (see Procedure 32-1). Recent advances in technology allow some devices to store 2 weeks to 3 months of glucose data that can be rapidly analyzed by the computer to measure glucose control by the hour, day, week, and month. Measurements of blood glucose levels are usually obtained four times a day (when rising in the morning and then before lunch, dinner, and at bedtime) or more frequently as indicated by metabolic control (Cunningham et al., 1993). Some clinicians recommend that daily determinations include a blood glucose reading 1 hour after a major meal. The goals of therapy are fasting glucose levels of less than 95 mg/dL and 2-hour postprandial levels less than 120 mg/dL; however, this degree of rigid control should not be demanded in clients having frequent hypoglycemic reactions.

Client education should focus on specific guidelines for using the machine, when to test blood glucose, how to perform the finger stick, and how to record the results. The client should enter all blood glucose levels

---

BOX 32-4

Signs and Symptoms of Hypoglycemia, Hyperglycemia, and Diabetic Ketoacidosis

Hypoglycemia	*Hyperglycemia*	*Ketoacidosis*
Hunger	Increased appetite	Hunger
Nausea	Nausea	Nausea and vomiting
Headache	Headache	Headache
Sweating	Polyuria	Polyuria
Nervousness	Polydipsia	Polydipsia
Tremulousness	Dry mouth	Dry mouth
Weakness and fatigue	Fatigue	Weight loss
Shallow respirations	Tachypnea	Rapid respirations (Kussmaul respirations)
Pallor; cold, clammy skin	Flushed, hot skin	Shortness of breath
Blurred vision	Abdominal cramps and rigidity	Malaise
Numbness around lips and tongue	Drowsiness	Fatigue
Disorientation, irritability	Odor of acetone on breath	Weakness
Stupor	Stupor	Severe dehydration
Loss of consciousness	Coma	Mental disorientation
Coma	Oliguria or anuria	Fluid and electrolyte imbalances
Seizures	Depressed reflexes	

PROCEDURE 32–1
*Glucose Testing Using the Accu-Chek Easy™ Glucose Meter**

Objective: To accurately determine maternal blood glucose level with a minimum of trauma.

Nursing Action	Rationale
1. Gather equipment in area near client (eg, glucose meter, test strips [with valid expiration date], disposable lancet, alcohol swabs or antiseptic wipes, sterile gauze squares [if needed], small Band-Aids, sharps needle container, disposable gloves).	Gathering all equipment in advance prevents delays in collecting the blood sample and interruptions in the testing procedure.
2. Wash hands and apply gloves.	Handwashing is an important aspect of standard precautions and prevents spread of nosocomial infections.
3. Prepare for specimen collection: Warm client's fingers with warm water or compress. Instruct client to lower or dangle hand below heart level. Massage client's hand and finger before cleaning and lancing.	Warming the fingers causes vasodilation. Dangling the hand below the level of the heart slows venous return and increases blood flow to the targeted area. Massage produces local heat, which aids vasodilation.
4. Check the code number on the display to be sure it matches the code on the test vial label. When a flashing drop appears over the strip symbol, the monitor is ready for a test.	Checking codes ensures reliability and validity of test results.
5. Remove a test strip from the vial. Compare the colors on the test strip to the "unused" pad printed on the vial label. The colors should match.	Color matching before testing ensures that the results obtained are accurate.
6. Select finger (not thumb) to be used. Select a site on the lateral aspect, palm side of the fingertip.	Early site selection prevents interruptions during the testing procedure.
7. Rub and cleanse fingertip with alcohol or antiseptic wipe for 15 seconds. Allow skin to dry thoroughly.	Use of alcohol or other antiseptic decreases the possibility of contamination. Evaporation of the alcohol minimizes its irritating effects on injured tissue and may decrease possible hemolysis.
8. Insert lancet into lance device in locked position ("click" is heard), and twist off protective cover.	
9. Grasp client's finger gently to stabilize. Gently hold lance device against fingertip and use thumb to press the pen's "trigger" to puncture the lateral aspect of palm side of the client's fingertip. Note: Do not use venous blood.	The ends of the fingers contain more pain sensitive nerves than the palm side of the finger.
10. Withdraw device and hold fingertip downward to allow blood droplet to form.	Holding the finger downward increases blood loss through the puncture site.
11. Apply one drop of blood to the target area of the test strip, completely covering the area.	Uncovered portions of the reagent strip may be read as low glucose.
12. Within 30 seconds, insert the test strip into the monitor with the target area facing the dark red dot on the monitor. Be sure to push the strip all the way in, as far as it will go.	To ensure reliability of test results, the directions must be followed for timing and use of equipment. False results may occur if blood is left on the reagent strip too long.

(continued)

PROCEDURE 32–1 *(continued)*
Glucose Testing Using the Accu-Chek Easy™ Glucose Meter*

Nursing Action	Rationale

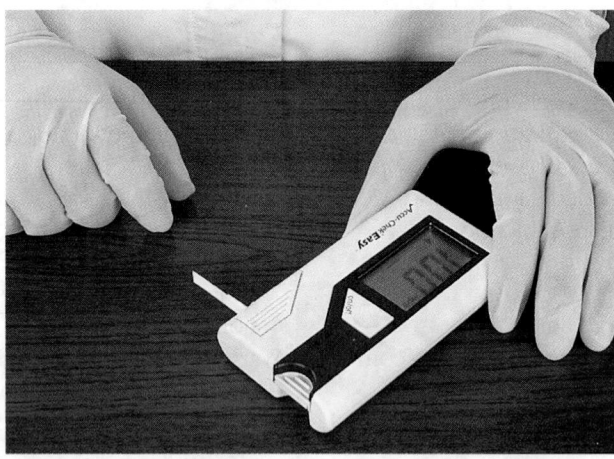

Example of a blood glucose monitor.

Nursing Action	Rationale
13. Small arrows will flash in the corner of the display. In 15–60 seconds, the blood glucose will appear.	Flashing arrows indicate that the machine is functioning properly.
14. While meter is reading strip, press swab or gauze square against client's fingertip to stop bleeding.	Pressure on the puncture site stops bleeding.
15. After results appear on screen, remove the test strip from the monitor and compare the back of the test strip with the color chart on the test strip vial label. The visual result and the monitor's result should agree.	Visually checking the test strip validates results obtained by the machine.
16. Record test results. Notify physician or nurse midwife immediately for abnormal results.	Regular recording of blood glucose levels aids management of diabetes and helps to identify possible complications.
17. Discard the used test strip in a biohazard container and the used lancet directly into the sharps needle container. Cleanse meter and door with antiseptic wipe.	Proper disposal and cleaning minimizes the risk of infection transmission and cross-contamination.
18. Remove gloves and wash hands.	

*Note: The procedure for use of this system is similar to the "One-Touch" Glucose Meter manufactured by Life Scan. Adapted with permission from Tokos Clinical Services Corporation.

in the home record keeping system, which also includes insulin doses, weight, and diet. Additional teaching about when to notify the healthcare team also should be provided.

Exercise. Although pregnancy is not an optimum time to begin vigorous exercise, low- to moderate-intensity exercise is believed to be safe and beneficial. With regular exercise, hypoglycemia is less likely (Rosas et al., 1992). During exercise, there is an increased affinity for and binding of glucose, which enhances glucose use

(Artal et al., 1985). The effects of exercise may last up to 12 hours. Research findings suggest that pregnant women in supervised diet and cardiovascular exercise programs have lower levels of glycemia than those managed on a regimen of diet alone (Jovanovic-Peterson et al., 1989). Furthermore, exercise in combination with diet is an effective alternative to insulin for controlling GDM (Rosas et al., 1992).

Exercise prescriptions should be individualized and carefully supervised by members of the healthcare team. Exercise following a meal may be helpful in preventing meal-related blood glucose elevations. Women should be counseled to avoid exercising during peak periods of insulin action and to keep a fast-acting carbohydrate source nearby. Well-controlled diabetic women who regularly engage in exercise may continue exercise during pregnancy. They should be reminded to eat a snack consisting of carbohydrate or protein before the activity. The client should be encouraged to follow a consistent and structured program of activity rather than an irregular and unpredictable schedule. If signs of hypertensive complications arise, exercise programs should be discontinued.

Obstetric Considerations. Pregnant women with diabetes are at risk for developing infections (eg, urinary tract and vaginal infections) that predispose them to preterm labor and birth. The use of magnesium sulfate is recommended for treatment of preterm labor because β-sympathomimetic tocolytics may cause DKA.

Under optimum circumstances, the diabetic woman should deliver near term, usually between 38 and 40 weeks' gestation. Assessment of the phosphatidylglycerol (PG) content in amniotic fluid is often performed to verify fetal lung maturity prior to delivery unless gestational age dating has been well established. The amniotic PG test is a more accurate predictor of fetal lung maturation than the L/S ratio. When PG is present, delivery is planned. Vaginal delivery is usually possible for diabetic women who have maintained well-controlled plasma glucose levels. Oxytocin induction may be attempted when labor does not begin spontaneously by 40 weeks' gestation, the cervix is considered favorable, and the fetus is not macrosomic. Cesarean section is indicated for cases of fetal compromise, macrosomia, or an unfavorable cervix. Cousins (1987) examined the results of 24 investigations on pregnancy complications among diabetics. His findings revealed that primary, repeat, and total cesarean section rates increase step-wise from nondiabetic to gestational to class B and C to class D, F, and R diabetics. Early delivery is necessary only for deteriorating fetal condition or in selected cases of maternal vascular disease, hypertension, and previous stillbirth.

During labor and delivery, an intravenous infusion of regular insulin and glucose using a calibrated pump is used to control maternal glucose in insulin-dependent diabetics. If an elective induction is planned, the regular morning insulin dose is withheld. Gabbe and associates (1991) recommend 10 U of regular insulin be added to 1,000 mL of solution containing 5% dextrose. In most cases, an infusion rate of 100 to 125 mL/h results in acceptable glucose control following these protocols. Glucose levels are monitored hourly with a glucose meter. A heparin lock may be inserted to avoid the repeated finger sticks necessary for close blood glucose surveillance. Because neonatal hypoglycemia is related directly to intrapartum maternal glucose levels and to the degree of antepartum metabolic control, it is important to maintain maternal plasma glucose levels at approximately 100 mg/dL during labor (Gabbe et al., 1991). Uterine activity and fetal heart rate (using scalp electrode with ruptured membranes) are monitored continuously. Following delivery, insulin is administered as indicated by blood glucose monitoring, and the client is closely observed for insulin reactions.

During the postpartum period, family planning counseling should be provided to diabetic women. Special areas for consideration include the need to use safe barrier methods of contraception (oral contraceptives may have adverse effects, particularly among overt diabetics), family size and spacing in relation to disease progression, and the risk of developing gestational or overt diabetes in the future. Another family planning option is the progestin implant system (Norplant), which reportedly has minimal effects on carbohydrate metabolism (Cunningham et al., 1993).

Nursing Evaluation

Successful management of the pregnant diabetic involves the client and all members of the healthcare team. Anticipated outcomes of nursing care include the following:

- The client verbalizes the effects of her disease on pregnancy, labor, and birth and perinatal outcomes.
- The client identifies the signs and symptoms of disease progression and possible complications.
- The client implements the prescribed treatment plan and self-care activities.
- The client demonstrates adequate tissue perfusion and oxygenation to the maternal-fetal unit as evidenced by diagnostic testing.
- The client gives birth to a healthy newborn at or near term.

Cardiac Disease

Approximately 1% of all pregnant women have some type of cardiac disorder (Gabbe et al., 1991). In the past the most common type of heart disease seen in pregnancy was **rheumatic heart disease** resulting from episodes of rheumatic fever causing recurrent inflammation and valvular scarring. With this disease, the mitral valve was most often affected, with stenosis resulting in approximately 90% of the cases. Recognition of the role of streptococcal infection and its appropriate therapy has greatly reduced the frequency of the cardiac consequences of rheumatic fever.

Congenital heart disease present at birth is now becoming the most common cardiac problem encountered in pregnancy. Another new population of women with uncorrected, partially corrected, or totally corrected congenital heart defects is challenging healthcare professionals. The most common defects found in pregnancy are atrial septal defect (ASD), ventricular septal defect (VSD), patent ductus arteriosus (PDA), pulmonary stenosis, aortic stenosis, coarctation of the aorta, and tetralogy of Fallot (Elkayam et al., 1990). These clients have an assortment of defects and vary in their **functional capacity** (ability to function) during pregnancy. In general, women who have no symptoms and who do not have cyanotic heart disease tolerate pregnancy well (Kirkland, 1992). Although coronary artery disease and myocardial infarction in pregnancy are rare, older childbearing women may be at increased risk for these conditions.

About 6% to 10% of women of childbearing age are affected by a cardiac condition known as **mitral valve prolapse** (MVP; Scott et al., 1994). The underlying pathology involves prolapse of the mitral valve leaflets into the left atrium during ventricular systole, causing some backflow of blood. A midsystolic click and late systolic murmur are characteristic of the syndrome. Most women with MVP are asymptomatic and are able to tolerate pregnancy well.

Parenteral substance abusers represent a growing number of pregnant women at high risk for acquiring **bacterial endocarditis**, an inflammation of the inner lining of the heart, usually involving the heart valves. The tricuspid valve is most often infected in this population. Bacteria may be introduced directly by injection of contaminated materials, such as using toilet water from public restrooms for injection and infected syringes, or indirectly when the user injects intravenously or "skin pops" subcutaneously, becoming contaminated with her own skin flora. The most common offending microorganism is *Staphylococcus aureus*. Common symptoms of endocarditis in the substance abuser before hospitalization include fever for about 2 weeks, pleuritic chest pain, urinary symptoms, dyspnea (on exertion, orthopnea, paroxysmal, nocturnal), and a cardiac murmur (may have a late onset).

Peripartum cardiomyopathy, congestive failure with cardiomyopathy, is a relatively rare condition that may cause devastating problems. This disease occurs between the last trimester of pregnancy and the first 5 postpartum months without obvious cause or history of cardiac disease (Cruikshank, 1994). The main pathologic features are reduced left ventricular ejection fraction and impaired ventricular contractile power. The prognosis of this disease is directly related to the duration of the illness. Clinical manifestations include breathlessness, tachycardia, arrhythmias, cardiomegaly, and edema.

Eisenmenger's syndrome develops when progressive pulmonary hypertension leads to a shunt reversal in women with a congenital left-to right shunt. This syndrome is most likely to arise with a VSD or PDA because of the high pressure and high flow associated with these defects. Decreased systemic vascular resistance associated with pregnancy increases the occurrence of right-to-left shunting, causing decreased pulmonary perfusion and hypoxemia for the woman and fetus (Drummond, 1992).

The risks of perinatal mortality and maternal morbidity and mortality for women with a cardiac disorder during pregnancy depend on three factors: the underlying cardiac lesion; the functional derangement produced by the lesion; and the development of pregnancy-related complications, such as PIH, hemorrhage, and infection. The quality of health services rendered and the client's psychosocial capabilities also influence outcome (Cunningham et al., 1993). For most types of heart disease, the major threat imposed by pregnancy is that the increasing blood volume will precipitate congestive heart failure. Overall, maternal-fetal prognosis for pregnancies complicated by cardiac disease is steadily improving.

Effect of Pregnancy on the Cardiovascular System

The cardiovascular changes normally occurring in pregnancy are comprehensively described in Chapter 15. Box 32-5 highlights some of these changes.

Some of the normal cardiovascular changes of pregnancy also may be observed in heart disease. Therefore, they should be carefully considered when the cardiac status of the pregnant woman is evaluated. The healthy woman has the ability to adapt to the stresses that pregnancy superimposes on the cardiovascular system; however, the woman with heart disease may not have the cardiac reserve to adjust to these new demands.

BOX 32–5
Cardiovascular Changes of Pregnancy

- Increased cardiac output (30–50% more than prepregnancy level)
- Increased stroke volume
- Increased heart rate (10 beats/min)
- Expanding blood volume
- Decreased vascular resistance and blood pressure
- Functional systolic murmurs (splitting S_1, audible S_3)
- Upward displacement of diaphragm (false impression of cardiac enlargement)
- Accentuated breathing effort similar to dyspnea
- Lower extremity edema
- Increased venous return with contractions and subsequent increase in cardiac output
- Increased mean arterial pressure during contractions

Effect of Cardiac Disease on Pregnancy

The pathophysiology of cardiac disease evident in pregnancy depends on the type of cardiac disorder present. For most types of heart disease, the major threat imposed by pregnancy is that the increasing blood volume will precipitate congestive heart failure. If maternal blood flow is severely compromised, signs and symptoms of right-sided, left-sided, or total failure may develop in the woman. Placental circulation also may diminish, resulting in a higher risk of prematurity and low birth weight. Pregnant women who have successfully undergone surgical repair and have no residual effects of heart disease generally experience pregnancy without complication. Unlike these women, clients with cyanotic heart disease are at greater risk for perinatal morbidity and mortality. The incidence of congestive heart failure increases in women older than 30 years and is further aggravated by parity.

Cardiac disease is the most common indirect cause of maternal mortality in the United States; following hypertension, hemorrhage, and infections, it is the fourth most common direct cause (Gilstrap, 1989). Mitral stenosis is the most frequent valvular defect associated with maternal death in pregnancy (Austin et al., 1991). A system of identifying the risk of maternal mortality associated with specific cardiac lesions during pregnancy has been developed by Clark (1991; Box 32-6).

A major problem in managing clients with artificial cardiac valves (eg, ball valves, tilted disk valves, and bileaflet valves) is coagulation. Women with biosynthetic tissue valves (eg, porcine valves) usually do not require anticoagulants, unless they are experiencing other cardiac complications. Reports have revealed that such pregnancies are relatively uneventful; however, in women who receive heparin during pregnancy, the incidence of fetal loss is 13%, and the incidence of preterm delivery is 20% (Kulb, 1990). This finding may be partially related to the fact that pregnant women with a prosthetic heart valve have a relatively fixed cardiac output. They demonstrate a suboptimal increase in cardiac output and stroke volume compared with that usually seen during pregnancy and particularly in labor (McColgin et al., 1989). Newer mechanical valves have reduced this problem to some extent. Pregnancy exposes women who have had previous valvuloplasty to three common complications: thromboembolism, infective endocarditis, and cardiac decompensation. Several factors contribute to the risk of thromboembolism from either the valve site or the periphery: thrombogenicity of the valve, trauma to the formed elements of blood, increased clotting factors, and venous stasis (Chyun, 1985). The danger is increased if the pregnant woman discontinues anticoagu-

> **BOX 32-6**
> *Mortality Risk Associated With Cardiac Disease During Pregnancy*
>
> ---
>
> **Group I: Mortality <1%**
>
> Atrial septal defect*
> Ventricular septal defect*
> Patent ductus arteriosus
> Pulmonary and tricuspid disease
> Corrected tetralogy of Fallot
> Biosynthetic valve prosthesis (porcine and human allo- graft)
> Mitral stenosis, New York Heart Association (NYHA) class I and II
>
> **Group II: Mortality 5%–15%**
>
> Mitral stenosis with atrial fibrillation
> Mechanical valve prosthesis
> Mitral stenosis, NYHA class III and IV
> Aortic stenosis
> Coarctation of aorta*
> Uncorrected tetralogy of Fallot
> Previous myocardial infarction
> Marfan's syndrome with normal aorta
>
> **Group III: Mortality 25%–50%**
>
> Pulmonary hypertension
> Coarctation of aorta, complicated
> Marfan's syndrome with aortic involvement
>
> *Uncomplicated.*
> *From Clark, S. L. (1991). Structural cardiac disease in pregnancy. In S. L. Clark, D. B. Cotton, G. D. V. Hankins, & J. Phelan (Eds.), Critical care obstetrics (2nd ed.). Boston: Blackwell Scientific Publications.*

lants to protect the fetus from teratogenic effects (as experienced with sodium warfarin and related drugs).

Other common complications associated with cardiac disease include arrhythmias and shunt reversal. Maternal conditions, such as obesity, smoking, and anemia, contribute to the severity of the effects of cardiac disease during pregnancy. Women with heart conditions that reduce cardiac output (eg, mitral valvular disease) are at risk for intrauterine growth retardation. The incidence of spontaneous abortion, preterm labor, and stillbirth also is higher, particularly among women with cyanotic congenital cardiac disease. The fetus of women with congenital heart disease is at risk for congenital cardiac anomalies; the reported incidence ranges from 1.1% to as high as 14% (Shime et al., 1987).

Classification

The American Heart Association has developed a classification system for heart disease based on the woman's functional capacity (Table 32-2). This taxonomy is used as a guide for therapy by members of the healthcare team. With appropriate management, women in classes I and II generally are able to experience a normal pregnancy with no or few problems, whereas women in classes III and IV are at higher risk of significant hemodynamic morbidity and mortality. Maternal mortality rates have been classified by ACOG (1992; Drummond, 1992) into three groups based on specific cardiac lesions (see Box 32-3). Whenever possible, class III and IV women with correctable lesions should be counseled to undergo cardiac surgery before conception. The development of other specific pregnancy-related complications that produce cardiovascular stress (eg, PIH, anemia, hemorrhage, infection) can alter a woman's functional classification.

Diagnosis

The most useful criteria in establishing a diagnosis of heart disease in pregnancy include the following:

- Cyanosis
- Clubbing of fingers
- Persistent neck vein distension
- Diastolic, presystolic, or continuous heart murmur
- Unequivocal cardiac enlargement
- Harsh systolic murmur associated with a thrill
- Sustained cardiac arrhythmia
- Persistent split second sound
- Criteria for pulmonary hypertension (Cunningham et al., 1993)

TABLE 32-2
Classification of Heart Disease

Class	Description
I	Cardiac disease with *no* limitation of physical activity. Absence of symptoms of cardiac insufficiency and anginal pain.
II	Cardiac disease with *slight* limitation of physical activity. Comfortable at rest. Fatigue, palpitation, dyspnea, or anginal pain with *ordinary* physical activity.
III	Cardiac disease with *moderate* to *marked* limitation of physical activity. Comfortable at rest. Excessive fatigue, palpitation, dyspnea, or anginal pain with *less* than ordinary physical activity.
IV	Cardiac disease with *inability* to perform any physical activity without discomfort. Symptoms of cardiac insufficiency or of the anginal syndrome may occur *at rest* and with *any* physical activity.

(Criteria Committee of New York State Heart Association. [1964]. *Nomenclature and criteria for diagnosis of diseases of the heart and blood vessels* [6th ed.]. Boston: Little, Brown.)

Serious heart disease is usually absent in pregnant women who do not fulfill the above criteria.

Nursing Process

An interdisciplinary team effort is needed to care for the pregnant woman with cardiac disease. The nurse works closely in collaboration with the obstetrician, cardiologist, nutritionist, clinical nurse specialist, anesthesiologist, and social worker. Nursing care is determined to a considerable extent by the functional capacity of the client.

Nursing Assessment

The pregnant woman with cardiac disease needs to be assessed thoroughly to ensure the most optimal outcome. A detailed assessment provides valuable information to help the client and her fetus achieve this outcome.

A thorough history should be obtained on all women with heart disease. The client's ability to perform various types of physical activity before and during pregnancy and any complaints of associated cardiovascular effects, such as dyspnea on exertion, palpitations, chest pain, fatigue, coughing, and cyanosis, need to be evaluated. Under optimum conditions, preconception evaluation is performed to determine baseline cardiac function and functional capacity.

A complete physical examination, with special attention to auscultation of the heart for abnormal heart sounds and breath sounds, is essential. The onset of atrial fibrillation in pregnancy or the puerperium is particularly ominous, because the condition is often associated with various types of heart failure and pulmonary emboli.

The extremities and more central body surfaces should be observed carefully for edema and tenderness. Baseline maternal vital signs, blood pressure, hemoglobin oxygen saturation, and fetal heart rate are obtained at the initial assessment and then compared frequently with subsequent readings. Capillary filling time and venous distention are assessed with each visit.

The pattern of weight gain, complaints of any discomforts of pregnancy, and side effects and interactions of any prescribed medications are assessed continuously. Any deviations need to be evaluated to ascertain whether they indicate complications or just the normal physiologic changes of pregnancy.

The client needs careful observation for signs and symptoms of cardiac decompensation that may be evidenced with congestive heart failure and other complications; these symptoms may appear suddenly or develop gradually and are presented in Box 32-7.

BOX 32-7
*Signs and Symptoms
of Cardiac Decompensation*

Dyspnea
Palpitations
Chest pain
Cough
Pulse irregularity
Sweating
Orthopnea
Weakness
Progressive, generalized edema
Rales at the base of the lungs
Pallor

The following routine diagnostic tests are done initially to establish a baseline for comparison with subsequent tests:

- Electrocardiogram
- Chest x-ray
- Hemoglobin and hematocrit
- White blood cell count
- Urinalysis
- Prothrombin, partial thromboplastin, thrombin clotting times, and heparin assay if the client is receiving anticoagulant therapy

Other diagnostic tests, such as echocardiography, and pulse oximetry, may be indicated by the client's status. Fetal well-being is evaluated by fetal ultrasound, fetal movement studies, or NSTs, as necessary.

Hemodynamic monitoring may be implemented during the antepartum or intrapartum period to provide valuable information about the cardiac status of the acutely ill pregnant woman (predominantly functional classes III or IV). The Swan-Ganz flow-directed pulmonary artery catheter allows continuous measurement of right atrial pressure, pulmonary artery pressure, pulmonary capillary wedge pressure, and central venous pressure. It can be used effectively to assess cardiac output and to administer fluids or drugs. In clients without hemodynamic monitoring, vital signs may be assessed as frequently as every 10 to 30 minutes during labor. If the pulse rate increases above 100 beats/min, the physician should be notified.

Nursing Diagnoses

As is true of all concurrent diseases of pregnancy, nursing assessment is an essential step in formulating nursing diagnoses. Examples of nursing diagnoses that

specifically apply to the woman with a pregnancy complicated by heart disease are shown in Box 32-8.

Nursing Intervention

Nursing intervention is directed toward assisting the client to minimize the workload on the cardiovascular system and reduce the risks of complications developing during pregnancy and the postpartum period. Information obtained from preconception cardiac assessment of the woman with congenital heart disease is particularly helpful in managing nursing and medical care. The nurse should review the signs and symptoms of cardiac decompensation and other complications (eg, PIH, preterm labor) with all clients.

Nursing care for the pregnant client with cardiac disease focuses on activity and rest, nutrition, medications, and prevention of infection. The nurse also must be aware of specific obstetric considerations throughout the pregnancy.

Stress, Rest, and Activity. Regardless of cardiac classification level, all women with heart disease should have a minimum of stress and obtain additional rest during pregnancy. A minimum of 10 hours of sleep per night and additional morning and afternoon rest periods are recommended. Based on knowledge of the client's functional capacity, the nurse and client should explore the need for modifying and adjusting activity level during pregnancy (eg, limiting housework, shopping). Some women may need to terminate employment. Complete bed rest in the second half of pregnancy is

BOX 32-8
Nursing Diagnoses: Cardiac Disease

- Knowledge Deficit related to:
  - Effects of cardiac disease on pregnancy
  - Signs and symptoms of complications
- Activity Intolerance related to increased metabolic needs of pregnancy in presence of impaired cardiac function
- Altered Tissue Perfusion, cardiopulmonary, related to:
  - Increased preload or afterload
  - Demands of pregnancy on the cardiac workload
  - Maternal cardiac decompensation
- Risk for Infection related to bacterial invasion, pulmonary congestion, or invasive procedures
- Altered Protection related to thromboembolism secondary to valvular defects, decreased venous return, or hypercoagulability of pregnancy
- Anxiety related to fears of uncertainty of pregnancy outcome
- Risk for Injury to the fetus and preterm labor related to intrauterine hypoxia

necessary for certain cardiac disorders. It is required for all class IV women. Custom-fitted support stockings are beneficial to all cardiac clients in the latter half of pregnancy and should definitely be worn when bedridden. They reduce hemodynamic fluctuations that accompany changes in maternal posture and increase venous return by improving muscle function (Cruikshank, 1994).

Nutrition. The pregnant woman with cardiac disease should adhere to the following nutritional guidelines:

- Eat a well-balanced nutritional diet (approximately 2,200 calories) with large amounts of high-quality protein and iron.
- Do not add salt to food (2 g/d of sodium permitted); sodium-rich foods may need to be restricted (1–1.5 g/d) if complications arise or the disease is severe.
- Follow prescriptions for use of supplementary iron to prevent anemia.
- Avoid or limit foods and beverages containing caffeine.
- Eliminate foods high in vitamin K (eg, raw, deep-green, leafy vegetables) if receiving heparin.
- Gain between 22 and 27 lb because excess weight gain places additional strain on the heart and circulatory system.

Medications. Various medications may be used during pregnancy for the client with cardiac disease. The client may have been receiving medication prior to conception, or she may be placed on the medication during the pregnancy.

Women who were receiving digitalis prior to pregnancy must continue use of the drug throughout the childbearing cycle. Changes in the cardiovascular system also may necessitate digitalis treatment for previously nonmedicated women. Maternal and fetal heart rate are slowed by digitalis, which crosses the placental barrier. If arrhythmias develop during pregnancy, cardioversion may be accomplished safely with quinidine.

Diuretic therapy is generally not recommended for class I and II women during pregnancy; however, it may be prescribed for class III and IV women. Thiazides, such as chlorothiazide, and hydrochlorothiazide are the commonly prescribed diuretics. The woman on diuretic therapy should be observed for potassium depletion and postural hypotension. Neonatal thrombocytopenia, electrolyte imbalance, and SGA fetuses have been observed in fetuses whose mothers used thiazide diuretics in pregnancy (Sibai et al., 1991).

Propranolol (Inderal) may occasionally be administered to clients who develop symptoms such as palpitations, chest pain, and dyspnea with conditions such as mitral valve prolapse.

Sodium warfarin (Coumadin) used as an anticoagulant for women who have had valve replacements is associated with an increased risk of spontaneous abortion and congenital anomalies, such as nasal hypoplasia, dwarfism, intrauterine growth retardation, and ophthalmologic abnormalities. The use of this drug and other oral anticoagulants is contraindicated during pregnancy (Cruikshank, 1994).

Heparin, an alternative anticoagulant that does not cross the placental barrier, may be prescribed prior to conception and during early pregnancy. The drug is administered in two to three subcutaneous boluses or continuously through an infusion pump. The nurse should provide specific information about the actions, side effects, and self-administration of heparin to all women beginning therapy. The nurse also should be aware that use of this drug increases the risk for maternal hemorrhage, preterm birth, and stillbirth (Cunningham et al., 1993).

Antibiotic therapy is prescribed for women diagnosed with bacterial endocarditis. The choice of antibiotic is determined by the identified causative organism from culture and sensitivity tests. Penicillins and cephalosporins cross the placenta and are well tolerated by the fetus. Prophylactic antibody therapy is recommended for intravenous substance abusers who are at risk for developing bacterial endocarditis (Biswas et al., 1991). Just prior to delivery, some physicians similarly prescribe a prophylactic antibiotic for women with valvular heart disease and congenital defects because of their high susceptibility to subacute bacterial endocarditis.

Prevention of Infection. Febrile episodes increase cardiac demands and are often associated with tachycardia. Spread of the infectious organism may cause direct damage to the heart. Therefore, the nurse should caution the pregnant woman with cardiac disease against contact with people suffering from respiratory infections or other contagious diseases. An early dental examination and treatment of all caries (with antibiotic prophylaxis) are encouraged. Proper perineal care should be emphasized as a means of preventing UTIs and pyelonephritis. The nurse should stress the need to report signs of potential infections immediately and to follow prescribed treatment protocols (see Chap. 11).

Obstetric Considerations. Prior to conception, the client with cardiac disease should be counseled about the risks she and her fetus may experience during pregnancy. Additionally, those with congenital heart disease must be advised about the danger of their child inheriting a congenital heart lesion. Most of these lesions follow a polygenic **multifactorial** (a combination of genetic and environmental factors) mode of inheritance with a 2% to 5% risk of recurrence (Gianopoulos, 1989).

During the prenatal period, clients with cardiac disease are often monitored more frequently than healthy, pregnant women. Prenatal visits may be scheduled as often as every 2 weeks in the first half of pregnancy and every week thereafter to detect and promptly treat complications. The nurse should assist the client and her family to understand the disease process and its relationship to pregnancy. Because the risk for premature labor and delivery is increased, pregnant women with cardiac disease should be instructed on the presenting signs and symptoms. Ultrasound examinations are often performed to establish gestational age, rule out congenital defects, and follow growth throughout the pregnancy. Other types of prenatal fetal surveillance evaluations may include the NST, CST, biophysical profile, and Doppler velocimetry.

Intrapartum management is directed toward controlling or manipulating intravascular volume, heart rate, and vascular resistance to prevent or minimize the hemodynamic effects of the birth process and events that may occur during labor and birth (Kirkland, 1992). Women with heart disease are usually allowed to go into spontaneous labor and have a vaginal delivery unless obstetric indications indicate the need for a cesarean section.

During the intrapartum period, women with congenital conditions must have an intravenous access that permits the administration of fluid and plasma expanders and vasoactive medications (Kirkland, 1992). It is essential that the laboring woman with cardiac disease be relieved of discomfort and anxiety. Effective intrapartum pain relief may reduce cardiac workload by as much as 20% (Scott et al., 1994). Systemic analgesics combined with sedatives may be administered early in the first stage of labor. Caudal or epidural anesthesia may be initiated as labor advances or for delivery. Hypotension, a common side effect of epidural anesthesia, may be avoided by keeping the laboring woman in the lateral recumbent position and carefully administering intravenous fluids. The nurse can help the client and her family to relax by maintaining a calm manner and keeping them informed about intrapartum progress. To improve cardiac circulation and maximize oxygenation, the client is placed in a side-lying position with her head and shoulders elevated. Oxygen may be administered if pulmonary complications arise. Intake and output are assessed frequently and fetal heart rate is monitored continuously.

The degree of intrapartum monitoring necessary is based on the client's functional status, underlying disease, and secondary complications. During labor, many clients with cardiac disease require continuous electrocardiogram surveillance; some also need hemodynamic monitoring for blood gas and blood pressure measurements. Invasive hemodynamic monitoring is most often used in women with class III and IV cardiac disease, sepsis, pulmonary edema, heart failure, intraoperative or intrapartum cardiovascular decompensation, massive fluid loss or replacement, shock, or coronary artery disease (CAD) (Troiano, 1992; ACOG, 1988). A pulmonary artery catheter is indicated when a complete hemodynamic profile is required for management (Kirkland, 1992). Pulse oximetry may be useful as an indicator of hypoxemia in less severe cases. During initiation of invasive hemodynamic monitoring, the nurse is responsible for assisting the physician in gathering and preparing the equipment and supporting the client. Following insertion of the catheter, the nurse regularly assesses the laboring woman's hemodynamic status. Normal hemodynamic values during pregnancy and changes associated with uterine contractions are presented in Box 32-9.

BOX 32-9

Normal Hemodynamic Values in Pregnancy and Changes With Uterine Contractions

Parameter	Value and Standard Deviation	Parameter	Effects
Pregnancy		*Intrapartum With Uterine Contractions*	
Cardiac output (L/min)	6.2 ± 1.0	Intravascular blood volume	↑ by 300–500 mL
Systemic vascular resistance (dyne/sec/cm^{-5})	1210 ± 266	Cardiac output	↑ by 30–50%*
Pulmonary vascular resistance (dyne/sec/cm^{-5})	78 ± 22	Heart rate	Variable
Mean pulmonary artery pressure (mm Hg)	13 ± 2	Blood pressure	↑ systolic and diastolic
Pulmonary capillary wedge pressure (mm Hg)	7.5 ± 1.8	Oxygen consumption	↑ dramatically
Central venous pressure (mm Hg)	3.6 ± 2.5		
Left ventricular stroke work index (g/m/m^{-2})	48 ± 6		

Postpartum—5 minutes cardiac output ↑ 65%; postpartum—60 minutes ↑ 40%

For clients with prosthetic valves, anticoagulants should be discontinued during labor and delivery and resumed 6 to 12 hours after delivery. Risk of intrapartum hemorrhage is related to the coagulation status of the woman and fetus. The American Heart Association recommends antibiotic prophylaxis only for women with prosthetic heart valves or grafts to prevent infective endocarditis associated with birth. However, antibiotic therapy for women with congenital heart disease and those undergoing cesarean section, induction of labor, or forceps delivery is a common practice in many medical centers because of the serious morbidity and mortality associated with endocarditis and bacteremia (Clark, 1991; Kirkland, 1992; Pitkin, 1990).

In the second stage of labor, forceps or a vacuum extractor are commonly used to avoid the stress of increased abdominal pressure created by maternal pushing. Delivery may be accomplished in the lateral or a supine position with the client tilted to the left to decrease the risk of supine hypotension. High stirrups should not be used for women with cardiac disease because they compress the popliteal veins and increase blood volume in the chest and trunk from the effects of gravity. Drugs containing ergot should not be administered because of resulting increases in blood pressure.

Nursing care in the postpartum period is similar to that for other clients, with special consideration given to the possible need for limited activity and additional rest. Stool softeners may be prescribed to prevent straining on defecation. Discharge planning is particularly important for clients with cardiac disease. The nurse should refer the family to community agencies if assistance is needed with newborn care or household responsibilities.

Nursing Evaluation

Anticipated outcomes of nursing care are that the pregnant woman with cardiac disease does the following:

- Verbalizes the effects of her disease on pregnancy, labor and delivery, and perinatal outcome
- Identifies signs and symptoms of cardiac decompensation and obstetric complications and reports them promptly
- Implements the established treatment plan (eg, limited activity and increased rest, prescribed diet and medications, avoidance of contact with infected people) and prevents potential complications
- Maintains adequate cardiac output to meet maternal and fetal needs
- Maintains adequate tissue perfusion and oxygenation to the maternal-fetal unit
- Exhibits no signs or symptoms of thromboembolism or infection

- Delivers a healthy newborn at or near term
- Secures the needed additional resources to assist with child care, household, and other responsibilities

Hematologic Disorders

Although a variety of hematologic disorders may affect the pregnant woman, 75% to 90% of diagnosed cases are classified as Iron Deficiency Anemia (IDA). The remaining cases encompass a variety of acquired and hereditary anemias, such as folic acid deficiency, and the hemoglobinopathies (sickle cell disorders). The existence of a hematologic abnormality increases the pregnant woman's risk for developing other complications, such as infection.

Iron Deficiency Anemia

Iron deficiency anemia (IDA) is the most common hematologic disorder in pregnancy. It affects approximately 15% to 25% of pregnant women, depending on the ethnic and socioeconomic groups being studied (Scott et al., 1994). Pregnancy can affect a client's risk for IDA; IDA also can affect the pregnancy.

Effects of Pregnancy on Iron Deficiency Anemia

Several physiologic changes occurring in pregnancy contribute to the risk for developing IDA. There is a pronounced increase in maternal plasma volume and a relatively lower increase in total red blood cell volume and hemoglobin mass. These alterations increase the nutrient-carrying capacity of the plasma but reduce the viscosity of whole blood. The disproportionate rise in blood constituents causes hemodilution with a resultant fall in hemoglobin concentration unless the need is met by augmented hematopoiesis. These changes are unrelated to the pregnant woman's iron status; they occur whether the client is or is not receiving iron supplementation.

The fetus' iron requirement must be secured from the woman. Iron requirements dramatically increase in the second half of pregnancy, when the fetus receives almost all of the iron transported to it. Because many women have depleted iron stores as a result of regular menstrual blood loss, these added demands often result in the total depletion of stored iron and the development of overt anemia during pregnancy. Women with a history of poor nutritional status, close spacing of pregnancies, twin gestation, or excessive vaginal bleeding may be at risk of developing IDA during pregnancy (Hoffman, 1993).

Effects of Iron Deficiency Anemia on Pregnancy

In most clients with mild to moderate anemia, the signs and symptoms, such as fatigue and exercise intolerance, are few and often indistinguishable from the normal discomforts of pregnancy. In such women, anemia may be detected by frequent prenatal hemoglobin or hematocrit determinations. IDA renders the pregnant woman particularly susceptible to infection and complications of blood loss with or after birth. Severely anemic women, those with hemoglobin <8 g/dL, are usually symptomatic, and in the most severe cases, these women can even develop heart failure as a result of the anemia.

Chronic anemia limits the amount of oxygen available for fetal exchange, putting the client at an increased risk for abortion and premature birth. Severe anemia also is associated with an increased frequency of SGA newborns. However, maternal IDA does not lead to reduced iron stores in the fetus.

Diagnosis

Diagnosis of IDA is based on laboratory test values. A hemoglobin level below 10 g/dL or a hematocrit of less than 30% in the pregnant woman generally suggests IDA (Scott et al., 1994), and further evaluation is indicated to determine the reasons for the condition. Erythrocyte indexes aid in assessing the cause of the low hemoglobin level. With IDA, the red blood cells are characteristically **microcytic** (immature) and **hypochromic** (insufficient hemoglobin). The mean corpuscular volume (size of the erythrocyte) and mean corpuscular hemoglobin (quantity of hemoglobin in the erythrocyte) are decreased; however, these findings are less prominent in pregnant women compared with nonpregnant women. Serum ferritin may be used to provide a more precise measurement of available iron stores. Ferritin levels <10 mg/L are diagnostic of IDA.

Nursing Management

The pregnant woman with IDA requires comprehensive nursing care in collaboration with other healthcare team members. A thorough assessment, including nutritional history, is essential. Client education, nutritional counseling, and possible referrals for supplemental food programs are key elements of nursing care.

All pregnant women should have a complete blood count, including hemoglobin, hematocrit, and red blood cell indices, early in the prenatal period. Oral administration of iron is commonly prescribed to prevent or treat iron deficiency. Approximately 3 to 5 mg/d of iron is needed to supply the needs of the woman and fetus, with demands for iron increasing in the last 5 months of pregnancy to as much as 3 to 7 mg/d (Cunningham et al., 1993). Many oral preparations of organic and inorganic iron are available for treatment. The most common compounds include ferrous sulfate (200–300 mg two to three times daily) and ferrous gluconate (320 mg two to three times daily). These drugs may be ingested after meals to decrease gastrointestinal side effects. Injectable iron therapy (iron dextran [Imferon]) is rarely required, unless the client cannot tolerate oral preparations or is noncompliant with therapy. More often, a failure to respond to oral iron therapy is the result of failure to take the medication (iron tends to produce gastrointestinal symptoms) or a concurrent folic acid deficiency. It is important to assess the existence of side effects in all pregnant women receiving iron supplementation. The client should be instructed about dietary measures to minimize the gastrointestinal side effects of iron therapy. Constipation may be a particularly troublesome side effect; it can be relieved by ingestion of prescribed stool softeners, such as docusate sodium (Colace), and by increasing fiber and fluids in the diet. The nurse also should inform the client that unabsorbed iron is excreted in feces, causing the stool to turn green or black.

Serum ferritin levels should be obtained after the 20th week of gestation and repeated at 6- to 8-week intervals in women being given replacement iron therapy. Response to iron supplementation in IDA occurs quickly. A rise in hematocrit and hemoglobin values should be noted 2 weeks after onset of therapy.

A comprehensive 7-day diet history is taken to evaluate the pregnant woman's general nutritional status and the quantity of iron available through nutritional sources. Other factors to consider are the woman's financial and social situation; use of community resources, such as Women's, Infant's and Children's Supplemental Food Program; and eating habits. An iron-rich diet is recommended for all pregnant women. The nutritional counselor or nurse should provide instruction about dietary sources of iron. Dietary sources include fortified cereals; liver; beets; raisins; leafy, green vegetables; red meat; eggs; legumes; dried fruits; and whole grains (Hollingsworth, 1992). Ideally, an extra 1,000 mg of iron should be added to the daily diet. Although there is no need to prescribe ascorbic acid with iron compounds, clients should be advised to eat foods rich in vitamin C, such as fruit juices and dark green vegetables, because this vitamin is needed for optimal absorption of iron. Clients also should be informed that iron absorption may be reduced due to phosphates in milk and eggs, phylates in cereals, bicarbonate, tea, and some food preservatives (Hoffman, 1993).

The client should be cautioned about using antacids, which also block iron absorption.

Folic Acid Deficiency

Folic acid deficiency can produce severe anemia, usually of the megaloblastic type in pregnancy. **Megaloblastic anemia**, characterized by immature red blood cells failing to divide that becoming enlarged and fewer in number, is much less common than IDA, occurring in fewer than 3% of pregnant women (there is a higher prevalence in twin gestations). In its full-blown form, hemoglobin may be as low as 3 to 5 g/dL, white blood cells and platelets are reduced, and the mean corpuscular volume is elevated. Symptoms of this type of anemia include glossitis, sore tongue, and anorexia. Perinatal outcome may be seriously threatened by folic acid deficiency, which is reportedly associated with a higher incidence of early abortion, UTIs, and abruptio placentae.

Treatment consists of oral administration of 1 mg folic acid daily and ingestion of a diet that contains foods high in folic acid. Sources include fresh green vegetables, especially asparagus, broccoli, spinach, lima beans, and lettuce; fresh fruits, such as bananas and melons; peanuts; red meats, such as liver and kidneys; fish; and poultry. The pregnant client should be instructed to prepare vegetables by steaming them in small quantities of water to decrease folic acid loss. Prevention is achieved with prenatal vitamin-mineral supplements, which include 0.5 to 1 mg folic acid.

Hemoglobinopathies

Hemoglobinopathies present special problems in pregnancy. The most commonly encountered of these are sickle cell anemia (SS disease), sickle cell-hemoglobin C disease (SC disease), and sickle cell β-thalassemia disease (S-thalassemia disease). These are recessively inherited diseases seen principally in the African American population. They are invariably associated with an increased perinatal morbidity and mortality (eg, increased rate of spontaneous abortion). Susceptibility to some infections is increased because of impaired immune system function.

Detailed counseling is required in the management of hemoglobinopathies. Important considerations include the impact of pregnancy in precipitating crises, the genetic implications of childbearing, and the limited life expectancy of women with certain conditions, such as SS disease.

Sickle Cell Anemia (SS Disease)

Sickle cell anemia occurs when the gene for the production of S hemoglobin is inherited from both parents. When S hemoglobin is transmitted from one parent but not the other, the person has the sickle cell trait but does not exhibit frank anemia. About 1 in 12 African Americans has sickle cell trait and is heterozygous, whereas 1 in every 576 African American women has the disease (Cunningham et al., 1993). The actual incidence of sickle cell anemia in pregnancy is about one-third as high as in the general population, probably because many affected people do not survive to childbearing age or elect not to carry their pregnancies to term. Pregnant women with sickle cell trait have a predisposition to UTIs and hematuria but are otherwise normal.

People affected by sickle cell anemia have inherited a defect in the hemoglobin molecule that causes erythrocytes to become elongated and crescent shaped (sickle), particularly when they are exposed to temperature variations, lowered blood pH, or increased blood viscosity. Decreases in circulating oxygen levels resulting from infections, acid–base imbalance, dehydration, trauma, hemorrhage, exercise, anesthesia, high altitudes, alcohol and drug abuse, and air pollution also may cause sickling crises (Clark et al., 1994). Clinically, the hallmark of sickling episodes are times during which there is ischemia and infarction within various organs, causing acute pain (Cunningham et al., 1993).

Sickle cell anemia has great impact throughout the childbearing cycle. The anemia is exacerbated during pregnancy, and life-threatening hemolytic crises can occur at a more frequent rate than in the nonpregnant state. In the past, maternal mortality rates were reportedly as high as 10% to 20%; however, meticulous medical and obstetric care can greatly reduce the frequency of complications. Major problems encountered in women with sickle cell anemia include pulmonary complications, infection, congestive heart failure, and hypertension. Other complications reported are severe anemia, pyelonephritis, pneumonia, and PIH. The rates are higher for spontaneous abortion, intrauterine growth retardation, premature labor, stillbirth, and neonatal death.

Sickle Cell-Hemoglobin C Disease (SC Disease)

Sickle cell-hemoglobin C disease (SC disease) occurs when the gene for the production of hemoglobin C is inherited along with that for hemoglobin S. It is much less common (1 in 2,000 pregnant African American women) and certainly less serious in the nonpregnant state (Cunningham et al., 1993). During pregnancy and the puerperium, however, a marked increase in symptoms occurs. In contrast to sickle cell anemia, the perinatal mortality is increased only slightly. Because some women with SC disease are not diagnosed until pregnancy, all African American women should have a screening test for the presence of sickle hemoglobin at the first prenatal visit. If the screen is positive, hemoglobin electrophoresis is performed. The pregnancies of women with SC disease are managed the same as pregnancies in clients with sickle cell anemia.

Sickle Cell β-Thalassemia Disease (S Thalassemia Disease)

Sickle cell-thalassemia disease results from the inheritance of the gene for hemoglobin S from one parent and the allelic gene for thalassemia from the other parent. Perinatal mortality and morbidity of this disease appear to follow an intermediate course between those with sickle cell anemia and hemoglobin SC disease and those with sickle cell trait (Scott et al., 1994). Although thalassemia has been reported among all populations, it is most common in people from the Mediterranean region, with a significant prevalence among African Americans and Southeast Asians from Cambodia, Laos, and Vietnam. The pregnancy of a woman with sickle cell-thalassemia is managed the same as the pregnancy of a woman with sickle cell anemia.

Nursing Management

The nurse plays an important role in caring for the pregnant client with sickle cell disease. Women with diagnosed sickle cell anemia require the most meticulous prenatal care. The main goal of therapy is to prevent conditions that cause sickling and to minimize the complications of sickling when it occurs.

All African American pregnant women not previously tested should be screened for sickle cell anemia at the time of their first prenatal visit. Frequent prenatal visits are strongly recommended, usually biweekly until 20 weeks' gestation and then weekly thereafter. Hemoglobin levels are frequently assessed for rapid decreases, which suggest sickle cell crisis. Regular screening of urine is recommended for early diagnosis of asymptomatic bacteriuria. Intensive fetal surveillance is required, beginning with ultrasounds early in the pregnancy to determine gestational age and then serially to monitor fetal growth. Biweekly NSTs and amniotic fluid volume assessments begin at 30 weeks' gestation.

Throughout pregnancy, the diet of women with sickle cell anemia should be supplemented with folic acid because of the rapid destruction of red blood cells. Fluid intake should be well maintained to prevent dehydration. It is not unusual for pregnant women with sickle cell disease to have hemoglobin levels in the range of 6 to 9 g/dL. Multiple prophylactic transfusions of packed red cells are sometimes used to suppress the client's bone marrow from forming abnormal cells. At the same time, it permits the client to exist on transfused cells during the period of risk. Delivery should be scheduled as soon after 36 weeks when fetal lung maturity can be demonstrated, unless fetal compromise requires earlier delivery (Scott et al.,

1994). Intrapartum management is similar to that for cardiac disease.

The nurse plays an essential role in educating women with sickle cell anemia about their disease and early signs of complications. Nutritional counseling is important, particularly about the need for iron and folic acid intake. Information about the nature and purpose of the antepartum diagnostic tests being performed should be provided. Ongoing assessments should include questions about symptoms of infection and other health problems. All clients with sickle cell disease should be advised to avoid contact with people suffering from infectious diseases. Following delivery, counseling about family planning methods is necessary. Sterilization is often the preferred contraceptive method because of the complications caused by pregnancy and the expected shortened life span of women with this disease.

Chronic Renal Disease

Women with chronic renal disease and renal transplants are now living long enough to bear children. If renal function is under control, the chance for a surviving newborn is greater than 85% (Samuels, 1991). However, as renal impairment worsens, so do the chances of pregnancy complications. A potentially deleterious effect of pregnancy in women with underlying renal disease is the tendency of pregnancy to cause hypertension, which can further decrease renal function by causing an increase in glomerular capillary pressure (Ferris, 1990). Combined renal disease and hypertension may be associated with fetal growth retardation, preterm birth, and increased perinatal mortality. Therefore, an important goal of management is to prevent elevations in blood pressure.

Pregnant women who have had renal transplants may be treated with corticosteroids, such as prednisone. The prognosis for pregnancy after transplantation is good if the woman's general health is optimum, blood pressure is normal, and there are no signs of graft reaction. During pregnancy, hemodialysis may be performed if renal function fails. Newborns born to mothers on immunosuppressive therapy are prone to hyperglycemia at birth from suppression of fetal insulin activity by corticosteroids.

All pregnant women with chronic renal disease should have baseline renal function studies, such as blood urea nitrogen, creatinine, electrolytes, creatinine clearance, and total protein excretion performed, and serial measurements if indicated. The nurse should obtain regular urine cultures because the potential for renal infection is a major concern. Pregnant women should be instructed about the signs of a UTI and preventive measures, including personal hygiene, voiding after intercourse, and drinking cranberry juice and six to eight glasses of water per day (see Chap. 11). Careful fetal surveillance is indicated when hypertension complicates renal disease.

Thyroid Disease

Anatomically and physiologically, the thyroid gland is substantially affected by pregnancy. The thyroid gland moderately enlarges as a result of glandular hyperplastic and increased vascularity. The effects of placental estrogen cause physiologic changes, such as an increase in the thyroxine (T_4)-binding globulin concentration and as a direct consequence, an increase in serum levels of T_4 and T_3. There is an increase in basal metabolic rate and oxygen consumption, heat intolerance, emotional lability, and amenorrhea.

Hyperthyroidism (Maternal Thyrotoxicosis)

Approximately 1 in 1,000 to 1,500 pregnancies is complicated by hyperthyroid disease (Cunningham et al., 1993). Most commonly, hyperthyroidism during pregnancy is caused by Graves' disease, an organ-specific autoimmune process usually associated with thyroid-stimulating antibodies. Although a woman with uncontrolled hyperthyroidism is likely to be anovulatory and thus unable to conceive, many women with milder disease do conceive. In some cases, the hyperthyroidism is first diagnosed during pregnancy. If the condition is not detected and treated properly, maternal complications, such as spontaneous abortion, PIH, perinatal death, premature labor, and postpartum hemorrhage, may occur. There also is a greater risk for delivering an SGA newborn and for neonatal thyrotoxicosis.

Women with exophthalmic goiter produce a long-acting thyroid stimulator, which is an immunoglobulin G (IgG). This crosses the placenta and can cause hyperthyroidism in the newborn.

Signs of hyperthyroidism during pregnancy are tachycardia that exceeds the increase caused by normal pregnancy, a high pulse rate while sleeping, an enlarged thyroid gland, **exophthalmos** (abnormal protrusion of the eye), weakness, sweating, and failure to gain weight in spite of normal intake of food (Cunningham et al., 1993).

Findings of diagnostic laboratory studies may be confusing, especially in milder cases, because pregnancy and hyperthyroidism are hypermetabolic states with increased protein binding of thyroid hormone (Blackburn et al., 1992). This results in higher values for studies such as the protein-bound iodine and total thyroxine, with lower triiodothyronine uptake. Multiple thyroid function studies and the use of newer radioimmunoassays for thyroid-stimulating hormone

may prove useful in diagnosis. A total serum T_4 above approximately 15 mg/dL should suggest the possibility of hyperthyroidism.

Surgical treatment (subtotal thyroidectomy) is seldom indicated during pregnancy, except in noncompliant clients and those hypersensitive to antithyroid drugs. The problem with medical therapy is that the preferred antithyroid drug (propylthiouracil [PTU]) crosses the placenta, and if doses are excessive, the fetal thyroid can be suppressed, leading to fetal goiter or even cretinism. This is best avoided if the woman is maintained in a euthyroid or very mildly hyperthyroid state using the lowest possible dose of PTU (Cunningham et al., 1993).

A major complication of hyperthyroidism is the rare occurrence of thyroid storm during pregnancy and the puerperium. This condition is manifested by high fever, tachycardia, sweating, severe dehydration, and occasional cardiac decompensation. Treatment consists of early recognition followed by hospitalization. Large doses of PTU, potassium iodide, and possibly intravenous steroids are administered.

Severe Hypothyroidism

Severe hypothyroidism is rare during pregnancy because the condition is usually associated with amenorrhea and anovulation. However, women with mild hypothyroidism may conceive. Although the results of some studies show that women with hypothyroidism may be at greater risk for spontaneous abortion, abruptio placenta, stillbirth, low birth weight, and developmentally delayed infants, more recent findings suggest that perinatal morbidity is minimally increased, and perinatal mortality is not affected (Scott et al., 1994). In general, newborns of women with hypothyroidism appear healthy and without evidence of thyroid dysfunction. In some cases, newborns born to women with more severe hypothyroidism may be similarly afflicted.

Hypothyroidism is characterized by easy fatigability, anorexia, cold intolerance, lethargy, constipation, dry skin, headache, thin nails, and delayed deep tendon reflexes. An elevated thyroid-stimulating hormone level in association with low T_3 and T_4 levels and a reduced T_4 index establish the diagnosis of hypothyroidism. Levothyroxine (Synthroid) replacement (0.15–0.30 mg/d) is usually required to treat this condition (Scott et al., 1994).

Systemic Lupus Erythematosus

Systemic lupus erythematosus (SLE) is a chronic, multisystem autoimmune disorder that primarily affects the connective tissue. The disease is characterized by exacerbations and remissions. Preeclampsia is a common condition associated with SLE, and differentiation between SLE and severe preeclampsia may be difficult depending on the degree of vascular, renal, and central nervous system involvement (Cunningham et al., 1993). African American, Asian American, and Native American women are disproportionately affected by SLE compared with white Americans (Sala, 1993). The incidence of SLE in pregnancy may vary from 1 in 1,660 to 1 in 2,952 births (Montoro, 1987). The clinical manifestations are numerous and may vary widely among individuals.

The etiology of SLE is believed to be multifactorial. The prognosis is related to the systems involved. The symptoms of this disease imitate those of other disorders and depend on the system being affected. Pregnancy can bring about exacerbations of SLE commonly affecting the renal system, the central nervous system, and the placenta (Sala, 1993). It has been suggested that most exacerbations of lupus nephropathy during pregnancy represent the adverse effect of hypertension or superimposed PIH (Ferris, 1990). Clients who have been in complete remission for 6 months before conception have the least complicated pregnancies and best perinatal outcomes (Cunningham et al., 1993). The overall risk of spontaneous abortion in clients with SLE is increased (25%–35% incidence), with recurrent spontaneous abortions common. SLE during pregnancy most often affects the renal system, the central nervous system, and the placenta. The placental vasculature may be affected by lesions and immunoglobulin deposits, which can lead to stillbirths, intrauterine growth retardation, and other perinatal complications. Maternal SLE also is associated with fetal cardiac abnormalities, most frequently complete heart block (Troiano, 1992).

Diagnosis

The diagnosis of SLE is based on criteria established by the American Rheumatism Association in 1982. It includes the presence of four or more of the following criteria:

- Malar rash (fixed erythema, flat or raised)
- Discoid rash (raised erythematous patches with scales)
- Photosensitivity
- Oral or nasal ulcers
- Arthritis
- Serositis
- Renal disorder (persistent proteinuria)
- Neurologic disorder (seizures or psychotic symptoms)
- Hematologic disorder (hemolysis, leukopenia, or thrombocytopenia)
- Immunologic disorder (positive lupus erythematosus preparation, anti-deoxyribonucleic acid, anti-SM, or false-positive serologic tests for syphilis)
- Antinuclear antibody (Clark et al., 1994)

Nursing Management

Treatment of the disease involves corticosteroids and immunosuppressive agents. Additional supplementation with low-dose aspirin (about 75 mg) has improved perinatal outcomes in women who have suffered excessive reproductive losses associated with the lupus anticoagulant (an IgG or IgM; Scott et al., 1994). Infection control is particularly important during steroid therapy.

Intrapartum nursing care should include the following:

- Meticulous handwashing
- Limiting the number of vaginal examinations
- Hourly or more frequent blood pressure and vital sign monitoring
- Hourly monitoring of output and urinary protein
- Assessing deep tendon reflexes
- Examining for clonus and edema
- Continuous electronic fetal monitoring
- Using strict sterile technique for all invasive procedures (Sala, 1993)

Because exacerbations of the disease commonly occur after delivery, careful observation during the postpartum period is critical. This includes assessing for potential thrombotic insults, monitoring vital signs, and observing for signs and symptoms of potential infection.

Asthma

Asthma is the most common disease affecting the lungs during pregnancy. Asthma is a chronic lung disease characterized by reversible airway obstruction; airway inflammation; and increased airway responsiveness to a variety of stimuli (National Asthma Education Program Expert Panel Report, 1991).

Two major classifications of asthma exist: 1) extrinsic asthma, which tends to run in families, have an onset in childhood, and be related to allergies and 2) intrinsic asthma, which is nonallergic in origin and often begins in adult life without family history of atopy or allergies. Pregnancy may or may not impact the course of asthma in any woman. Results of the large retrospective studies published to date demonstrate roughly equal numbers of women experience improvements in their asthma, remain unchanged, or observe worsening disease (Clark et al., 1994). Women tend to repeat the same pattern of response to each pregnancy; those who experience worsening of asthma in one pregnancy are likely to do so in subsequent pregnancies. There is little evidence of any effect of asthma on pregnancy unless the condition is serious and hypoxia results. In such cases, there is an increase in abortion, fetal growth retardation, premature labor, and stillbirth (Cruikshank, 1994).

Nursing Management

Management of asthma during pregnancy is similar to that in the nonpregnant state. Pregnant asthmatics should be followed closely during the prenatal period to ensure appropriate maternal and fetal assessment. The nurse accurately assesses the woman's history of the disease and may assist in administering pulmonary function tests. Monitoring of peak expiratory flow rates, an objective measurement of the degree of airway openness, can provide the pregnant woman and nurse with critical information about asthma management (Geiger-Bronsky, 1993).

For many asthmatics, no drug treatment is prescribed. For those receiving medication, client instruction regarding use of prescribed drugs is an important nursing role. Acute episodes of asthma are treated with the inhalation of sympathomimetic agents, such as albuterol (Ventolin) or terbutaline, used two to three times per day. Hospitalization may become necessary for acute episodes of asthma. In these situations, intravenous theophylline and corticosteroid therapy may be administered for continued respiratory difficulty. Oxygen therapy is used to prevent fetal hypoxia. Frequent blood gas analysis is necessary to prevent maternal respiratory alkalosis and subsequent fetal hypoxia and identify impending respiratory failure. For maintenance therapy, an aerosol bronchodilator is often prescribed. Women receiving glucocorticoid inhalers require blood glucose level monitoring.

Pregnant asthmatics should be counseled about the need to prevent dehydration and respiratory infections and avoid hyperventilation, excessive physical activity, and environmental allergens. Upper respiratory infections are managed aggressively with appropriate antibiotics and physiotherapy. Prenatal fetal surveillance is indicated to assess growth and development. Early ultrasonography for gestational dating and serial follow-up, along with NSTs, are commonly performed. Pregnancy is usually allowed to proceed to term unless the maternal condition deteriorates or fetal compromise occurs. In labor, regional analgesia (epidural) is preferred to narcotic agents, which release histamine and may provoke asthma and depress respirations. Continuous fetal monitoring and maternal pulse oximetry also are important components of care (Beischer et al., 1992).

Trauma in the Pregnant Woman

Physical trauma occurs in 1 in every 12 pregnancies, and its consequences may be serious to the woman, fetus, or both (ACOG, 1991; Pearlman et al., 1989; see Research Highlight). Motor vehicle accidents are the leading cause of trauma during pregnancy, followed by falls and direct assaults of the abdomen from battering in physical abuse situations (Goodwin et al., 1990; Pearlman et al., 1990). The rate of emergency department visits for trauma during pregnancy is about 24 per 1,000 deliveries; major abdominal trauma occurs in 0.62 of 1,000 pregnancies (Williams et al., 1990).

Factors Determining Risk in Trauma

The severity, frequency, and time of onset of these complications are related to the type and location of injury, gestational age, and severity of the injury. Trauma during pregnancy is associated with an increased risk of spontaneous abortion, preterm labor, abruptio placentae, stillbirth, and fetomaternal transfusion (Pearlman et al., 1990). Uterine rupture and direct fetal injury are infrequent but life-threatening complications of trauma.

Abdominal trauma can be fatal to the woman and fetus or may primarily affect the fetus. Direct blows to the maternal abdomen without overt maternal injury, as a result of motor vehicle accidents, falls, or assaults, may have little consequence to the woman but may have great significance for fetal well-being and survival.

When pregnancy is less than 16 weeks' gestation, the fetus is located deep in the pelvis, and the risk of abruption from trauma is reduced. At later gestational ages, the fetus and placenta are higher in the abdomen and more susceptible to the effects of trauma. Even relatively minor forces against the abdomen appear sufficient to shear the placental attachments away from the decidua basalis. Adverse effects are always possible from abdominal trauma, regardless of gestational age.

Minor Trauma

Most trauma (approximately 75%–85%) experienced by pregnant women is minor. Minor trauma involves limited bruising, lacerations, and contusions, usually from falls or blows to the abdomen and occasionally from motor vehicle accidents. Even when maternal injury is minor, placental and fetal injuries may result in fetal demise.

The incidence of minor trauma increases with gestational age, with 80% of falls occurring after the

RESEARCH HIGHLIGHT

Pregnancy Outcomes After Trauma

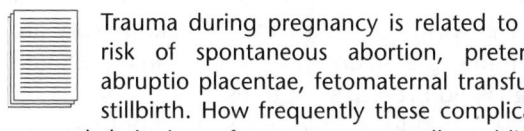 Trauma during pregnancy is related to increased risk of spontaneous abortion, preterm labor, abruptio placentae, fetomaternal transfusion, and stillbirth. How frequently these complications occur and their time of onset are not well established. This controlled, prospective cohort study compared 85 women with varying degrees of trauma during pregnancy to a control group of 85 pregnant women matched for gestational age. The purpose of this study was to compare pregnancy outcomes between women experiencing trauma and uninjured pregnant women serving as controls.

Women beyond 12 weeks' gestation with trauma to the head and central body were included. Those beyond 20 weeks had at least 4 hours of cardiotocographic monitoring, ultrasound evaluation, and an acid elution assay to estimate volume of fetomaternal transfusion. History included type of injury, classified as motor vehicle accident with use of restraints noted; fall to horizontal or from height; or direct blow to the abdomen (kick, punch). There were no significant differences in demographic and obstetric variables between the study and control groups.

Motor vehicle accidents were the most common type of injury (52%), followed by falls (26%) and direct blows to abdomen (14%). Of all the trauma victims, 88% had minor or no injuries on clinical examination (minor bruising, lacerations, contusions), 9% had moderate injuries (broken long bones, fractured ribs, extensive bruising), and 2.4% were critically ill. Immediate adverse outcomes occurred in 20% and included abruptio placentae, ruptured membranes, onset of labor, or fetal death. Abruptio placentae occurred more frequently among those less severely injured; neither the less severe injury nor the minimal physical findings ruled out immediate adverse effects.

The rate of fetomaternal transfusion was 31% in the trauma group and 8% in the control group—a highly significant difference. The volume of transfusion also was greater in women with trauma. Anterior location of the placenta and uterine tenderness were the only physical signs associated with fetomaternal transfusion. Trauma subjects using restraints during motor vehicle accidents had a nonsignificant tendency to more frequent transfusions than those not wearing restraints.

Nearly two-thirds of subjects had contractions every 2 to 5 minutes during the first hour of monitoring; only 6.7% had no uterine activity during 4 hours of monitoring. Contractions stopped in 90% of women without tocolysis. Ultrasonography accurately predicted abruptio placentae in 40% of the cases. When immediate adverse effects were excluded, women with minor to moderate trauma had no differences in pregnancy outcomes from the control group in terms of birth weight, gestational age at delivery, or Apgar score.

Critique: The strengths of this study include its prospective design, comparability of groups, and applicability of findings to clinical practice. The results suggest that it is appropriate for nurses to allay fears of pregnant women and their families after trauma has been carefully evaluated, which includes at least 4 hours of cardiotocographic monitoring.

Pearlman, M. D., Tintinalli, J. E., & Lorenz, R. P. (1990). A prospective study of outcome after trauma during pregnancy. *American Journal of Obstetrics and Gynecology, 162*(6), 1502–1507.

32nd week of pregnancy (Rosenfeld, 1990). Pregnant women experience falls more frequently during the third trimester due to the protuberant abdomen, which affects balance, fatigue, hypotension, hyperventilation, and loosening of pelvic joints. Trauma from assaults (blows to the abdomen) is less frequent after 36 weeks' gestation, probably due to the social stigma associated with striking an obviously pregnant woman (Williams et al., 1990).

Major Trauma

Moderate to major trauma involves broken long bones, fractured ribs, and extensive bruising, lacerations, and contusions. About 9% to 10% of injuries to pregnant women involve moderate trauma, while 2% to 3% involve major trauma and critical condition (Pearlman et al., 1990). Women suffering major trauma often are critically ill on arrival at the hospital emergency room. Maternal death is usually caused by head and chest injuries rather than abdominal trauma. The leading cause of fetal death from trauma is maternal death. Most fetal deaths in which the woman survives trauma are due to abruptio placentae resulting from maternal shock or damage to the placenta or uterus (Rosenfeld, 1990; Kettel et al., 1988).

Preterm labor is a common problem, occurring in about 20% of pregnant women suffering moderate to major trauma (Williams et al., 1990). It is not unusual for contractions to occur after trauma, resulting from uterine contusion with extravasation of blood from myometrial capillaries and subsequent irritability. As the extravasated blood is reabsorbed, uterine irritability diminishes. In about 90% of women, contractions stop without **tocolysis**, medications used to stop preterm labor (Pearlman et al., 1990). However, tocolysis may actually mask uterine activity resulting from abruptio placentae, presenting an increased threat to fetal survival.

Fetomaternal transfusion occurs in about 30% of major abdominal injuries during pregnancy, particularly when the placenta is located anteriorly. Ruptured membranes and abnormalities in fetal heart tracings also may occur, frequently in combination with preterm labor or abruptio placentae.

Gunshot Wounds in Pregnancy

The incidence of gunshot wounds in the U.S. population is increasing. Pregnant women are being seen more frequently in emergency rooms after sustaining gunshot wounds to the abdomen.

As the uterus enlarges during pregnancy, it is more susceptible to injury from a gunshot. The musculature of the pregnant uterus is relatively dense, so most of the energy of a missile is transmitted to the muscle. Injury to other organs is relatively rare. Maternal morbidity and mortality from gunshot wounds are low.

The ratio of fetus to amniotic fluid increases with advancing gestation, and the fetus presents a larger target. The incidence of fetal injuries, which can range from minor to lethal, is between 60% and 90%, half of which are serious. In addition to direct injury to the fetus, the bullet may injure the cord, membranes, or placenta. Perinatal mortality resulting from gunshot wounds during pregnancy ranges between 47% and 70% (Franger et al., 1989). Subsequent perinatal mortality varies from 41% to 71%, compared with maternal mortality, which accounts for less than 5% of the cases of penetrating trauma.

After gunshot injury to the pregnant uterus, abdominal tenderness often appears later than it would in the nonpregnant state. Guarding and rigidity are often diminished or absent. Vital sign changes may not appear until a reduction of 35% (as much as 1,500 mL at term) of maternal blood volume has occurred, due to the normal hypervolemia of pregnancy. The risk to the fetus can be severe, because homeostasis is maintained in the woman at the expense of the fetus by reducing uteroplacental blood flow.

Nursing Process

The maternity nurse often is involved in assessment and treatment of pregnant women with abdominal trauma. The management of the injured pregnant woman usually occurs initially in the emergency room. The maternity nurse and obstetrician should be involved in treatment at an early point (see Nursing Care Plan: The Woman with Abdominal Trauma During Pregnancy).

Nursing Assessment

As for all types of serious trauma, initial assessments focus on adequacy of airway, presence of breathing, cardiovascular status, and extent of the injury. Fetal status, including heart rate pattern and fetal move-

ments, is assessed to evaluate for hypoxia. Uterine tenderness, tone, contractions, and vaginal bleeding or fluid leakage also are assessed. Information about the circumstances of the injury is obtained to the extent possible. The woman's health and prenatal history are included in the assessment to aid correct interpretation of vital signs and present symptoms.

The nurse carefully should assess for abruptio placentae. Initial signs and symptoms of abruption may be minimal. When abruption results from trauma, bleeding is less common than in other causes. Vaginal bleeding was found as a presenting sign in only 20% of fetal deaths due to trauma-related abruption (Kettel et al., 1988). In a number of reported cases, fetal distress was the initial presenting symptom of abruption rather than usual symptoms of vaginal bleeding, abdominal pain, uterine tenderness, or maternal hypovolemia.

Altered pain location patterns may result from the pushing of the abdominal viscera upward by the enlarging uterus. The normal response to peritoneal irritation is altered by stretching of the abdominal wall. As a result, muscle guarding and rebound can be blunted despite significant injury to the abdominal organs (Neufeld, 1993). Ultrasound examination, not widely used in blunt trauma, may be useful for fetal assessment. Maternal intraperitoneal injury can be safely detected in any trimester with diagnostic peritoneal lavage (DPL) by open technique above the uterus (Cunningham et al., 1993). Computed tomography and magnetic resonance imaging should be used as a complement to DPL and ultrasound when evaluating abdominal trauma in pregnancy because they have the potential to identify specific organ damage.

Nursing Diagnoses

As a result of the nursing assessment, several nursing diagnoses may be identified. For all pregnant women experiencing abdominal trauma, risk for injury is an important nursing diagnosis. Injury can be related to tissue hypoxia, hemorrhage, cardiovascular collapse, brain damage, or tissue damage. Box 32-10 lists some examples of other frequent nursing diagnoses.

Nursing Intervention

Minor to Moderate Trauma. With a previable fetus, treatment is focused on the woman's safety and pain reduction. In pregnancies greater than 20 weeks' gestation, 4 to 24 hours of monitoring are recommended to assess for abruptio placentae (Pearlman et al., 1990; Rosenfeld, 1990). Even if there are no signs of fetal distress or injury, a period of monitoring is important, because abruption can be delayed by several hours to as late as 4 to 5 days (Pearlman et al., 1990). With a reassuring fetal heart rate pattern and no evidence of

(*text continues on page 884*)

NURSING CARE PLAN
The Woman With Abdominal Trauma During Pregnancy

Nursing Goals
1. Woman receives immediate life support and emergency care to control effects of trauma.
2. Adequate oxygenation is maintained and bleeding is controlled to ensure fetal well-being.
3. Woman obtains adequate pain relief.
4. Potential complications are identified early, and appropriate treatment is initiated.
5. Woman and family understand and accept the effects of trauma on her and the fetus.
6. Woman and family express feelings about effects of trauma and grieve losses.

Assessment	Potential Nursing Diagnoses	Intervention/ Rationale	Evaluation

Adequacy of airway, presence of breathing
Cardiovascular status (blood pressure, pulse, perfusion, hemorrhage)
Extent of injury (minor, moderate, severe)
Areas involved in injury
Potential fractures (extremiteis vertebra, pelvis, head)
Fetal status
  Fetal heart rate and pattern
  Fetal movements
Uteroplacental status
  Tenderness, tone, contractions (frequency, intensity, duration)
  Vaginal bleeding or fluid leakage
Circumstances of injury
  Type (motor vehicle, fall, blow to abdomen)
  Location (home, street, other building, outdoors, and so forth)
  Persons present and immediate first aid
Health and prenatal history
  Significant chronic illness or health problems
  Prenatal problems and treatment
  Current medications, activity restrictions
  Alcohol and street drug use
Reactions of woman and family
  Orientation, mentation
  Emotional responses (fear, anger, anxiety, grief)
  Capacity for information and understanding
	Risk for Injury related to tissue hypoxia, hemorrhage, cardiovascular collapse, brain damage, and tissue damage
	Alteration in Fluid Volume related to blood loss (hemorrhage)
		Assist with emergency life support measures *to maintain airway patency, restore breathing, and promote circulation.*
		Ensure patent airway
		Control bleeding; *hemorrhage may be masked by hypervolemic state during pregnancy.*
		Immobilize fractured extremities, vertebra, and pelvis *to prevent further damage.*
		Obtain IV access (large-bore catheter)
		Administer IV fluids and blood replacement *to restore circulating blood volume.*
		Give cardiovascular resuscitation with lateral uterine displacement, if necessary.
		Monitor vital signs q 5–10 min (BP, pulse and respirations—rate & quality); auscultate breathe sounds *to detect symptoms of hypovolemic shock; altered breath sounds may indicate pneumo- or hemothorax.*
		Monitor fetal heart rate (baseline, variability, decelerations, accelerations), uterine activity, and fetal movement for 4 h or more (external monitor); *the fetus may suffer injury when the mother experiences minor or major*
			Client maintains patent airway and circulation.
			
			Bleeding, shock, and hemorrhage are controlled.
			
			Vital signs are stabilized.
			
			Fetal heart rate pattern remains reassuring, and movement is present. Uterine contractions are absent.

(continued)

NURSING CARE PLAN *(Continued)*
The Woman With Abdominal Trauma During Pregnancy

Assessment	Potential Nursing Diagnoses	Intervention/ Rationale	Evaluation
		trauma; manifestations include alterations in FHR and bleeding. Preterm labor may occur but not be recognized.	
		Inspect perineum for presence of bleeding or amniotic fluid; *vaginal bleeding may be a symptom of injury to the uterus, placenta, or fetus; premature rupture of the membranes may also occur.*	Client has no evidence of bleeding or amniotic fluid leakage on inspection.
		Perform vaginal examination (VE) *to determine cervical status, vaginal bleeding and amniotic fluid leakage.*	VE reveals closed cervix.
		Monitor neurologic status (eg, level of consciousness, Glascow coma score); *alterations in neurologic status may indicate head injury or progressive shock.*	Client maintains normal circulatory volume.
		Administer oxygen at 10–12 L/min via face mask for hypotension, nonreassuring FHR pattern, or dyspnea; *maternal hypovolemia or respiratory distress decreases available oxygen to mother and fetus.*	
		Assess for external and internal bleeding; *vaginal bleeding is a symptom of abruptio placentae resulting from abdominal trauma.*	Symptoms of abruptio placentae are absent.
		Obtain arterial blood gases (ABGs) as ordered *to provide a measure of acid-base balance, O_2 saturation, CO_2 level, and so forth.*	ABG measures remain normal. Client's skin color remains normal for racial or ethnic group.
		Observe skin color; *pallor indicates poor tissue perfusion.*	
		Type and crossmatch; *identification of blood type and group is needed for possible transfusion.*	
		Perform ultrasound and nonstress test (NST) *to*	Results of the ultrasound and NST are normal.

(continued)

NURSING CARE PLAN *(Continued)*
The Woman With Abdominal Trauma During Pregnancy

Assessment	Potential Nursing Diagnoses	Intervention/ Rationale	Evaluation
		look for evidence of abruptio placentae, fetal trauma, and preterm labor.	
		Displace uterus laterally and avoid supine positioning *to reduce vena cava compression and promote fetoplacental oxygenation.*	Client remains on side.
		Maintain strict intake and output (I&O) every hour *to assess fluid balance.*	Hourly I & O is recorded.
		Monitor lab studies, especially CBC; *blood loss can be estimated by Hgb and Hct levels; may lose 30% to 35% of blood volume before shock is evident.*	Normal Hgb and Hct values are obtained on CBC.
		Prepare for emergency cesarean delivery, if needed; *fetal trauma, abruptio placentae and preterm labor may require emergency delivery.*	
	Alteration in Comfort: acute pain related to effects of trauma.	Determine most effective method of analgesic administration; continuous infusion versus intermittent IV push versus IM injection; *narcotic administration should be given via the safest and most effective method for the client's condition.*	Client receives adequate pain control.
		Observe for symptoms of abruptio placentae (eg, pain, uterine tenderness, irritability and rigidity, uterine contractions, increasing fundal height); *although abdominal pain is a symptom of abruptio placentae it may not be evident after trauma; the height of the uterus increases as it fills with blood.*	Evidence of abruptio placentae is absent.
		Position to maximize comfort *to enhance comfort.*	Client comfort is maintained.
		Splint trauma site (eg, abdomen) with pillow, whenever possible *to increase comfort.*	

(continued)

NURSING CARE PLAN (*Continued*)
The Woman With Abdominal Trauma During Pregnancy

Assessment	Potential Nursing Diagnoses	Intervention/ Rationale	Evaluation
	Anxiety related to possible injury to self and fetus.	Identify support person(s) and involve them whenever possible *to decrease client stress.*	Appropriate support is provided to client.
		Provide an environment where concerns about injuries to self and fetus may be expressed *to improve coping and decrease anxiety.*	Client and family express feelings and concern and resolve fears about subsequent effects on mother or fetus.
		Answer questions simply and directly *because client understanding may be decreased due to trauma and anxiety.*	
		Remain calm, use reassuring manner, assure that all is being done to protect mother and fetus *to decrease client anxiety and increase confidence in care-giving.*	Pregnancy continues and the mother successfully delivers a healthy, term infant.
		Support initial grieving if fetal loss occurs; *grieving is a normal adaptation to loss that must occur prior to acceptance of the loss.*	When fetal death occurs parents grieve effectively and move toward acceptance and integration of loss.

abruptio placentae or preterm labor, women with minor trauma can be discharged within a few hours.

Women who are Rh negative with a gestation of 12 or more weeks may be evaluated for fetomaternal hemorrhage. The frequency and volume of the hemorrhage are not necessarily related to the severity of the blunt trauma or the gestational age of the fetus (Pearlman et al., 1990; Rose et al., 1985). Administration of

Rh immune globulin (300 mg) prophylactically is recommended (Williams et al., 1990; Pearlman et al., 1990).

Nursing care includes keeping the client and family informed about the condition of the woman and fetus, the treatment plan, and the expected course and outcomes. Clear, simple explanations are necessary because the high levels of anxiety and fear reduce the family's capacity to process information. Emotional support and reassurance to the extent possible are important. After the immediate crisis has passed, the nurse should encourage the client and family to express feelings and relive the events to assist with integrating and accepting the experience. If fetal risk or loss occurs, the nurse supports the parents through the grieving process (see Chap. 42).

Prior to hospital discharge, the nurse should instruct all pregnant women who have experienced trauma about the signs and symptoms of preterm labor, rupture of membranes, abruption, and fetal death. The method for self-monitoring of fetal movement using daily records also should be reviewed. If less than four

BOX 32–10
Nursing Diagnoses: Trauma

- Pain related to effects of trauma
- Anxiety related to danger to self and fetus
- Knowledge Deficit related to extent of injuries and necessary procedures
- Impaired Tissue Integrity related to mechanical destruction, pressure, or shearing
- Fluid Volume Deficit related to abnormal fluid loss from hemorrhage

movements per monitored hour are noted, the woman should call her obstetrician or nurse midwife immediately, and an NST should be performed.

Major Trauma. Immediate nursing care priorities for the pregnant woman are the same as those for the nonpregnant trauma victim:

- Securing and maintaining an airway
- Ensuring adequate breathing
- Maintaining an adequate circulatory volume (replacement of lost blood)
- Controlling bleeding
- Immobilizing fractured extremities, vertebrae, and pelvis to reduce blood loss in the surrounding tissues

Two large-bore (14–16 gauge) intravenous lines are required in most seriously injured trauma clients. Early intravenous access for volume resuscitation is vital for the fetus. Vasoconstriction during early maternal hypovolemia can reduce blood flow to the fetus by 10% to 20% before maternal blood pressure is affected. Thus, it is possible for the fetus to be in shock while the woman is not (Lee et al., 1990; Morkovin, 1986). Supplemental oxygen may be needed to obtain a hemoglobin saturation of 90% or greater.

The care of the pregnant woman experiencing major trauma differs from that of the nonpregnant woman because of physiologic changes of pregnancy and the need to care for a second client, the fetus. Blood volume is increased during pregnancy; therefore, blood replacement should be generous. If blood is not immediately available, fluid replacement should be substituted until it is. The pregnant woman maintains her vital signs longer in the face of excessive hemorrhage than does the nonpregnant woman. Pulse and blood pressure may be sustained at virtually normal levels until almost immediately before vascular collapse. Failure to recognize and treat the difference in pregnancy can lead to sudden collapse and irreversible shock.

In late pregnancy, when the woman is lying supine, the weight of the uterus and its contents creates pressure on the vena cava. The resulting reduction in venous return to the heart reduces cardiac output, maternal blood pressure, and placental blood flow. It also may increase venous pressure in the lower half of the body, producing more bleeding if the extremities are injured. The pregnant woman should be placed on her left side whenever feasible. This allows the uterus to fall forward, relieving vena cava pressure.

All women suffering major trauma to the uterus in middle to late pregnancy must be evaluated for signs of abruptio placentae and preterm labor. Electronic fetal monitoring is used to obtain an NST and to rule out premature labor. Ultrasonography may be used to evaluate the condition and placement of the placenta. The fetus must be monitored closely by the maternity nurse to detect early signs of fetal distress and to initiate appropriate action.

Assessment of fetal viability is an important part of the management of the pregnant trauma victim. When the fetus is not viable, fetal monitoring is usually not required, and the primary consideration is the woman's safety. In the event of premature labor with a viable fetus, preparation should be made to care for the premature newborn on delivery. In some circumstances, a cesarean delivery may be necessary. In cases of severe trauma, if there is no response to advanced cardiac life support within a few minutes, maternal cardiopulmonary resuscitation should be continued, and an emergency cesarean section should be performed for a viable fetus. During the procedure, closed or open heart massage without aortic cross clamping is continued on the woman (Neufeld, 1993).

Gunshot Wounds. Nursing management of a pregnant client with a gunshot wound is individualized according to the type and extent of injuries and maternal and fetal condition. It is not necessary to explore the abdomen surgically in every case. Selective observation can often be used when the woman's condition is stable. If the entrance of the wound is below the fundus and the bullet can be seen on x-ray in the uterine muscle, less than 20% of clients require surgical management of a visceral wound. The bullet can be removed without an associated cesarean operation. The risk of precipitating labor is low if surgical procedures are carefully done. Cesarean delivery is necessary when the size of the uterus prohibits adequate exploration or repair of maternal injuries or if the fetus is mature and is suspected of having sustained an injury. With a fetal death, delivery can await spontaneous labor or can be induced, depending on maternal condition and indications (Franger et al., 1989).

Prevention of Abdominal Trauma During Pregnancy. The nurse plays a key role in educating the pregnant client about measures to prevent trauma (see Client Education: Preventing Accidental Trauma). The use of seatbelts during pregnancy and proper placement should be reviewed with every pregnant woman by the maternity nurse. As term approaches, seatbelts become increasingly uncomfortable, and the woman is less inclined to use them. Proper placement of seatbelts is critical during later pregnancy. Belts with shoulder harnesses are best; the lower belt should be worn encircling the pelvis below the protruding abdomen (see Chap. 17). In a collision, the sudden deceleration that occurs on impact delivers substantially more force to the lower abdomen when a seatbelt is across it, with risk of contusion and compression. In pregnancies beyond 20 weeks, the sudden increase in

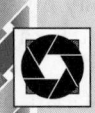

CLIENT EDUCATION
Preventing Accidental Trauma

- Wear shoulder harness seatbelts 100% of the time; position lap belt across pelvis below abdomen.
- When driving an automobile, be sure you are seated comfortably, have good visibility, and can readily control the car.
- As pregnancy progresses, stay aware of changes in body posture and in your center of gravity.
- Avoid climbing ladders, fences, trees, and onto counters because this upsets your balance and can lead to falls.
- Avoid stretching to reach objects on high shelves because this can upset your balance and lead to falls.
- Lift objects carefully, using good body mechanics (keep back straight, bend knees, and use thigh muscles); don't lift very heavy objects.
- Bathe and shower with care in late pregnancy; if your tub has a high edge, have assistance when you get in and out; use tub and shower mats to prevent slipping on wet surfaces.
- Remove obstacles in areas of routine traffic, throw rugs that might slip out from under you, sharp protruding corners.
- Wear comfortable, low-heeled shoes that provide good support and traction.
- Avoid dangerous situations for violence; do not provoke arguments; do not walk alone at night or frequent places where fights or arguments might occur.

intrauterine pressure directed upward through the amniotic fluid can result in abruptio placentae. When seatbelts are not worn, maternal deaths due to head trauma and internal injuries associated with motor vehicle accidents significantly increase.

Home safety and avoidance of falls are other important preventive measures. The nurse should review sources of household hazards and plan with the woman to reduce or eliminate these. The woman is taught how to move, sit, stoop, and carry objects as pregnancy progresses toward term to avoid losing balance and falling. Factors that increase risk for family violence can be assessed and reviewed with the woman (see Chap. 33).

Evaluation

Immediate intervention is effective when the pregnant trauma victim's vital signs stabilize, and immediate risks of hemorrhage, shock, cardiac arrest, and further complications are controlled. Further success can be measured by early detection and management of complications, such as preterm labor, abruptio placentae,

and fetomaternal transfusion. The optimal outcome is full recovery and health of the woman and fetus; the fetal condition is good, and pregnancy continues without adverse effects.

Psychosocial interventions are effective when parents can express their feelings and concerns, resolve fears about subsequent effects on mother and newborn, and express understanding of the events related to the trauma and its treatment. Parents who can accept the injury, understand factors connected with its occurrence, and plan for reducing risks of future injuries have benefitted from nursing intervention. When fetal death occurs, parents are able to grieve effectively and move toward acceptance and integration of this loss.

Summary Points

✔ Diabetes mellitus is a metabolic disorder that may have a pregestational or gestational onset. The placental hormones create resistance to insulin in body cells and cause changes in insulin needs during pregnancy.

✔ Screening for diabetes is performed at 24 to 28 weeks' gestation unless a diagnosis of diabetes exists prior to pregnancy.

✔ Pregnant diabetics are at risk for hypoglycemia, hyperglycemia, vascular disease, maternal infection, preeclampsia or eclampsia, and hydramnios. The fetus is at higher risk for congenital anomalies, macrosomia, and neonatal hypoglycemia.

✔ Unlike preexisting diabetes, gestational diabetes is often manageable by diet and exercise, without the need for insulin administration.

✔ Two major categories of heart disease are seen in pregnancy: rheumatic and congenital heart disease. Common congenital lesions include ASD, VSD, PDA, pulmonary stenosis, aortic stenosis, coarctation of the aorta, and tetralogy of Fallot.

✔ The cardiovascular changes occurring during pregnancy place women with heart disease at risk for cardiac decompensation and congestive heart failure.

✔ Pregnancy exposes women who have had previous valvuloplasty to three common complications: thromboembolism, infective endocarditis, and myocardial decompensation.

✔ Nursing interventions for pregnant women with heart disease include counseling regarding reducing stress, balancing rest and activity, obtaining adequate nutrition, properly administering medications, preventing infection, and recognizing symptoms of complications.

✔ The most common hematologic disorder of pregnancy is IDA, which often occurs because of depleted iron stores and the added demand for iron during gestation.

✔ Exacerbations of sickle cell anemia frequently occur during pregnancy; a major goal is to prevent sickle cell crisis.

✔ Chronic renal disease may increase the risk for hypertensive disease and infection during pregnancy.

✔ Thyroid disease involves either hyperthyroidism or hypothyroidism. The symptoms and management of these disorders vary markedly.

✔ Pregnant asthmatics may experience little or no effects during pregnancy, or their illness may be exacerbated. Close prenatal supervision is required to maintain optimum peak expiratory flow rates and to prevent maternal hypoxia, which can adversely affect the fetus.

✔ Trauma occurs frequently in pregnancy and is most often due to motor vehicle accidents, followed by falls and direct assaults to the abdomen. The risks associated with trauma include spontaneous abortion, preterm labor, abruptio placentae, stillbirth, and fetomaternal transfusion. The maternal prognosis relates to the degree of trauma (major versus minor). Placental and fetal injuries may occur even when maternal injury is minor.

✔ Airway, breathing, and circulation are the immediate priorities for the pregnant woman experiencing major trauma. However, the physiologic changes of pregnancy and the presence of a second client, the fetus, require additional nursing care measures.

REFERENCES

American College of Obstetricians and Gynecologists (1991). Technical Bulletin Number 161. Trauma during pregnancy. *International Journal of Gynecology and Obstetrics, 40,* 165–170.

Biswas, M. K., & Perloff, D. (1991). Cardiac, hematologic, pulmonary, renal and urinary tract disorders in pregnancy. In M. L. Pernoll (Ed.), *Current obstetric and gynecologic diagnosis and treatment.* Norwalk, CT: Appleton & Lange.

Blackburn, S. T., & Loper, D. L. (1992). Maternal, fetal and neonatal physiology. Philadelphia: W.B. Saunders.

Chyun, D. A. (1985). Pregnancy and cardiac valvular prostheses. *Journal of Obstetric, Gynecologic, and Neonatal Nursing, 14,* 38–44.

Clark, S. I., Cotton, D. B., Hankins, G. D. V., & Phelan, J. P. (Eds.) (1994). *Handbook of critical care obstetrics.* Boston: Blackwell Scientific Publications.

Cousins, L. (1987). Pregnancy complications among diabetic women: Review 1965–1985. *Obstetrical and Gynecological Survey, 42,* 140–149.

Cruikshank, D. P. (1994). Cardiovascular, pulmonary, renal, and hematologic diseases in pregnancy. In J. R. Scott, P. J. DiSaia, C. B. Hammond, & Spellacy (Eds.), *Danforth's obstetrics and gynecology* (7th ed.). Philadelphia: J.B. Lippincott.

Engel, N. S. (1989). Insulin therapy in pregnancy. *MCN: American Journal of Maternal Child Nursing, 14,* 19.

Ferris, T. F. (1990). Pregnancy complicated by hypertension and renal disease. *Advances in Internal Medicine, 35,* 269–288.

Franger, A. L., Buchsbaum, H. J., & Peaceman, A. M. (1989). Abdominal gunshot wounds in pregnancy, Part 1. *American Journal of Obstetrics and Gynecology, 160*(5), 125–1127.

Gianopoulos, J. G. (1989). Cardiac disease in pregnancy. *Medical Clinics of North America, 73,* 639–651.

Harvey, M. G. (1992). Diabetic ketoacidosis during pregnancy. *Journal of Perinatal and Neonatal Nursing, 6,* 1–13.

Heppard, M. C., & Garite, T. J. (1992). *Acute obstetrics: A practical guide.* St. Louis: Mosby Year Book.

Kulb, N. W. (1990). Cardiac disorders. In K. Buckley & N. W. Kulb (Eds.), *High risk maternity nursing manual.* Baltimore: Williams & Wilkins.

Landon, M. B. (1991). Diabetes mellitus and other endocrine diseases. In S. G. Gabbe, J. R. Niebyl, & J. L. Simpson (Eds.), *Obstetrics: Normal and problem pregnancies.* New York: Churchill Livingstone.

Langer, O. (1990). Critical issues in diabetes and pregnancy: Early identification, metabolic control, and prevention of adverse outcome. In I. R. Merkatz, J. E. Thompson, P. D. & Mullen, R. D. Goldenberg (Eds.), *New perspectives on prenatal care* (pp. 445–459). New York: Elsevier.

Langer, O., Rodriguez, D. A., Xenakis, M. J., McFarland, M. B., Berkus, M. D., & Arredondo, F. O. (1994). Intensified versus conventional management of gestational diabetes. *American Journal of Obstetrics and Gynecology, 170,* 1036–1046.

McColgin, S. W., Martin, J. N., & Morrison, J. C. (1989). Pregnant women with prosthetic heart valves. *Clinical Obstetrics and Gynecology, 32,* 76–88.

National Diabetes Data Group (1979). Classification of diabetes mellitus and other categories of glucose intolerance. *Diabetes, 28,* 1039.

Niebyl, J. R. (1991). Drugs in pregnancy and lactation. In S. G. Gabbe, J. R. Niebyl, & J. L. Simpson (Eds.), *Obstetrics: Normal and problem pregnancies.* New York: Churchill Livingstone.

Samuels, P. (1991). Renal disease. In S. G. Gabbe, J. R. Niebyl, & J. L. Simpson (Eds.), *Obstetrics: Normal and problem pregnancies.* New York: Churchill Livingstone.

Scott, J. R., & Branch, D. W. (1994). Immunologic disorders in pregnancy. In J. R. Scott, P. J. DiSaia, C. B. Hammond, & Spellacy (Eds.), *Danforth's obstetrics and gynecology* (7th ed.). Philadelphia: J.B. Lippincott.

Sibai, B. M., & Anderson, G. D. (1991). Hypertension. In S. G. Gabbe, J. R. Niebyl, & J. L. Simpson (Eds.), *Obstetrics: Normal and problem pregnancies.* New York: Churchill Livingstone.

Troiano, N. (1992). Cardiac diseases in pregnancy. In L. K. Mandeville & N. H. Troiano (Eds.), *High-risk intrapartum nursing.* Philadelphia: J.B. Lippincott.

White, P. L. (1978). Classification of obstetric diabetes. *American Journal of Obstetrics and Gynecology, 130,* 228–239.

SUGGESTED READING

Algert, S., Shragg, P., & Hollingsworth, D. R. (1985). Moderate caloric restriction in obese women with gestational diabetes. *Obstetrics and Gynecology, 65,* 487–91.

American College of Obstetricians and Gynecologists (1986). Management of diabetes mellitus in pregnancy. Technical bulletin no. 92.

Artal, R., Wiswell, R., & Romen, Y. (1985). Hormonal response to exercise in diabetic nondiabetic patients. *Diabetes, 39*(Suppl 2), 78–80.

Austin, D. A., & Davis, P. A. (1991). Valvular disease in pregnancy. *Journal of Perinatal and Neonatal Nursing, 5,* 13–24.

Beischer, N. A., & Mackay, E. V. (1992). *Obstetrics and the newborn*. Philadelphia: W.B. Saunders.

Clark, S. L. (1991). Structural cardiac disease in pregnancy. In S. L. Clark, D. B. Cotton, G. D. Hankins, & J. P. Phelan (Eds.), *Critical care obstetrics* (pp. 114–135). Oradell, NJ: Medical Economics Books.

Coustan, D. R. (1991). A guide for managing gestational diabetes. *Contemporary Ob/Gyn, 6,* 19–32.

Cunningham, F. G., MacDonald, P. C., & Gant, N. F. (1993). *Williams obstetrics* (19th ed.). Norwalk, CT: Appleton & Lange.

Drummond, S. B. (1992). Cardiac disease in pregnancy. *Critical Care Nursing Clinics of North America, 4,* 659–665.

Elkayam, U., Cobb, T., & Gleicher, N. (1990). Congenital heart disease and pregnancy. In U. Elkayam & N. Gleicher (Eds.), *Cardiac problems in pregnancy* (pp. 73–98). New York: Alan R. Liss.

Gabbe, S. G., Niebyl, J. R., & Simpson, J. L. (Eds.) (1991). *Obstetrics: Normal and problem pregnancies*. New York: Churchill Livingstone.

Geiger-Bronsky, M. J. (1992). Asthma and pregnancy: Opportunities for enhancing outcomes. *Journal of Perinatal and Neonatal Nursing, 6,* 35–45.

Gilstrap, L. C. (1989). Heart disease during pregnancy. *Clinical Obstetrics and Gynecology, 32,* 1.

Golde, S. H. (1991). Diabetic ketoacidosis in pregnancy. In S. I. Clark, D. B. Cotton, G. D. V. Hankins, & J. P. Phelan (Eds.), *Critical care obstetrics* (2nd ed.). Boston: Blackwell Scientific Publications.

Goodwin, T. M., & Breen, M. T. (1990). Pregnancy outcome and fetomaternal hemorrhage after noncatastrophic trauma. *American Journal of Obstetrics and Gynecology, 162,* 665–671.

Hoffman, J. A. (1993). Iron deficiency anemia: An update. *Journal of Perinatal and Neonatal Nursing, 6* 13–20.

Hollingsworth, D. R. (1992). *Diabetes and birth* (2nd ed.). Baltimore: Williams & Wilkins.

Howard, E. D. (1992). Gestational diabetes mellitus screening tests: A review of current recommendations. *Journal of Perinatal and Neonatal Nursing, 6,* 37–42.

Jovanovic, L., Druzin, M., & Peterson, C. M. (1981). Effect of euglycemia on the outcome of pregnancy in insulin-dependent women as compared with normal control subjects. *American Journal of Medicine, 71,* 921–927.

Jovanovic-Peterson, L., Durak, E. P., Peterson, C. M. (1989). Randomized trial of diet versus diet plus cardiovascular conditioning on glucose levels in gestational diabetes. *American Journal of Obstetrics and Gynecology, 161* (2), 415–419.

Kettel, L. M., Branch D. W., & Scott, J. R. (1988). Occult placental abruption after maternal trauma, Part 2. *Obstetrics and Gynecology, 71,* 449–453.

Kirkland, C. J. (1992). The impact of pregnancy on the woman with congenital heart disease: Considerations for intrapartum nursing care. *NAACOG Clinical Issues in Perinatal and Women's Health Nursing, 3*(3), 429–442.

Landon, M. B., & Gabbe, S. G. (1988). Diabetes and pregnancy. *Medical Clinics of North America, 72,* 1493–1511.

Lee, R. B., Wudel, J. H., & Morris, J. A. (1990). Trauma in pregnancy. *Journal of the Tennessee Medical Association, 83,* 74–76.

Mandeville, L. K. (1991). Diabetes mellitus in pregnancy. In C. J. Harvey (Ed.), *Critical care obstetrical nursing* (pp. 161–169). Gaithersburg, MD: Aspen Publishers.

Maternal & Child Health Branch, Department of Health Services (1992). *Sweet success, California diabetes and pregnancy program. Guidelines for care.* CA.

Montoro, M. (1987). Systemic lupus erythematosus during pregnancy. In S. L. Clark, J. P. Phelan, & D. B. Cotton (Eds.), *Critical care obstetrics*. Oradell, NJ: Medical Economics.

Morkovin, V. (1986). Trauma in pregnancy. In. R. G. Farrel (Ed.), *Ob/Gyn emergencies*. Rockville, MD: Aspen Publishers.

National Asthma Education Program Expert Panel Report (1991). *Guidelines for the diagnosis and management of asthma*. Bethesda, Md: U.S. Department of Health and Human Services, Public Health Service, National Institutes of Health.

Neufeld, J. D. (1993). Trauma in pregnancy, what if . . .? *Emergency Medicine Clinics of North America, 11,* 207–221.

Pearlman, M. D., Tintinalli, J. E., & Lorenz, R. P. (1989). Blunt trauma during pregnancy. *New England Journal of Medicine, 323,* 1609–1613.

Pearlman, M. D., Tintinalli, J. E., & Lorenz, R. P. (1990). A prospective study of outcome after trauma during pregnancy. *American Journal of Obstetrics and Gynecology, 162*(6), 1502–1507.

Pitkin, R. M. (1990). Pregnancy and congenital heart disease. *Annals of Internal Medicine, 112,* 445–454.

Rosas, T., & Constantino, N. (1992). Exercise as a treatment modality to maintain normoglycemia in gestational diabetes. *Journal of Perinatal and Neonatal Nursing, 6,* 14–24.

Rose, P. G., Strohm, P. L., & Zuspan, F. P. (1985). Fetomaternal hemorrhage following trauma. *American Journal of Obstetrics and Gynecology, 153,* 844–847.

Rosenfeld, J. A. (1990). Abnormal trauma in pregnancy. *Postgraduate Medicine, 88*(6), 89–94.

Rothenberger, D., Quattlebaum, F. W., Perry, J. F. Jr., Zabel, J., & Fischer, R. P. (1978). Blunt maternal trauma: A review of 103 cases. *The Journal of Trauma, 18,* 173–179.

Sala, D. J. (1993). Effects of systemic lupus erythematosus on pregnancy and the neonate. *Journal of Perinatal and Neonatal nursing, 7,* 39-48.

Samson, L. F. (1992). Infants of diabetic mothers: Current perspectives. *Journal of Perinatal and Neonatal Nursing, 6,* 61–70.

Shime, J., Mocarski, E. J. M., Hastings, D., Webb, G. D., & McLaughlin, P. (1987). Congenital heart disease in pregnancy: Short- and long-term implications. *American Journal of Obstetrics and Gynecology, 156,* 313–322.

Vignati, L., Asmmal, A. C., Black, W. L., Brink, S. J., & Hare, J. W. (1985). Coma in diabetes. In A. Marble, L. P. Krall, R. F. Bradley, A. R. Christlieb, & J. S. Soeldner (Eds.), *Joslins's diabetes mellitus*. Philadelphia: Lea & Febiger.

Williams, J. K, McClain L., Rosemurgy A. S., & Colorado, N. M. (1990). Evaluation of blunt abdominal trauma in the third trimester of pregnancy: Maternal and fetal considerations. *Obstetrics and Gynecology, 75,* 33–37.

33

Violence Toward Women in the Childbearing Years

Objectives

- Describe social and psychological factors associated with battery, rape, and sexual abuse of women.
- Explain the cycle of domestic violence, and discuss appropriate nursing care through the cycle.
- Analyze factors that make abuse more frequent during pregnancy.
- Compare the types of rape and contrast sexual, and aggressive aspects of each.
- Describe nursing care of the woman in each phase of the rape trauma syndrome.
- Develop immediate nursing care plans for women experiencing battery, rape, and sexual abuse.
- Outline procedures for examination and collection of evidence in suspected rape or sexual assault.
- Identify ways the nurse can assist the abused woman to become more empowered.

Key Terms

Abuse	Sexual abuse
Battery	Sexual assault
Incest	Rape trauma syndrome
Rape	Violent retaliation

Violence is a problem of great magnitude in the United States. Consider the following statistics:

- It is estimated that one woman is beaten every 18 seconds. Reports of assaults against women have increased by nearly 50% over the past 20 years (Senate Judiciary Committee, 1990).
- An estimated 25 million wives are abused by their husbands every year (Witkin-Lanoil, 1987).
- Over a lifetime, about one-third of all women will experience sexual violence (Sampselle, 1991). For as many as half of these, sexual abuse occurs before their 18th birthday (Bagley, 1991; Brown et al., 1990; Wyatt et al., 1990).
- It is estimated that a woman is raped every 6 minutes, with a rate of about 73 rapes per 100,000 women (Senate Judiciary Committee, 1990). This statistic becomes even more frightening when realizing that less than 10% of rape victims report the attack (Gibbs, 1991).

Most of this violence occurs *within* the home; women are the most likely victims, and their assailants are often not strangers but men known to them. Some researchers have estimated that domestic violence may occur in as many as half of all American families (Stenchever et al., 1991). Pregnancy can increase the risk of domestic **abuse,** which makes this problem of great importance to maternity nurses. Battering episodes increase during pregnancy, with a reported incidence of 40% to 70% (Helton et al., 1987; Parker et al., 1991; Torres, 1991).

This chapter addresses domestic violence, sexual abuse, and rape and explores the nursing role in helping to prevent and address violence against women. Box 33-1 describes the types of violence discussed in this chapter, most of which have specific (and often legal) meanings.

Domestic Violence

Family violence, spouse abuse, and battering are social problems found in all cultures and in every stratum of society. These are the most common but least reported forms of violence in the United States. **Battery** is a

leading cause of injury to women. Up to 25% of women seen in the emergency department are there because of domestic violence. The serious immediate effects of battering include severe injury or death. About one-fourth of all murders are domestic; 50% are spouse killings. About one-third of female homicide victims are killed by their husbands or boyfriends; fewer men are killed in domestic violence (Brasseur, 1994). Incidents of wife abuse frequently include child abuse. Long-term effects include continued neglect or abuse of children, perpetuation of patterns of family violence, serious psychopathology, and family disruption.

The abused woman is often repeatedly subjected to physical force, threat of harm, or psychological manipulation. Physical violence usually refers to hitting, punching, or shoving. Nonphysical abuse can include verbal attacks and insults, emotional deprivation, social isolation, economic deprivation, intellectual ridicule, sexual exploitation, and home imprisonment. The abusive man intends to cause injury and pain and does not expect retaliation. The woman usually is afraid of the man's greater strength and ability to inflict injury and has no effective way of defending herself (Walker, 1984a).

Factors Contributing to Abuse and Battery

Personal, cultural, social, and political factors contribute to abusive behavior patterns. Some of these include the following:

- Abusive family patterns
- Sex role stereotyping
- Societal devaluation of women
- Imbalance of power or status in families
- Culturally approved aggression
- Psychopathology

Children who witness or experience battering are more likely to become involved in abusive relationships. The cycle of family violence is transmitted from generation to generation. Children learn that it is acceptable in an intimate relationship to respond violently when feeling strong emotions, such as anger, frustration, and stress. They learn that violence is normal in families and that loving and hurting are not incompatible. Abusive people usually have low self-esteem, are possessive, and have strong feelings of jealousy (Chez, 1994).

Dysfunctional family systems contribute to abuse through the methods children learn to handle power, intimacy, and loyalty. When the husband's and wife's status in the family are out of balance (ie, overadequate wife, inadequate husband), children develop distorted perceptions. Internalization of shame by boys in this family model can lead to rage to cover up for

BOX 33-1
Legal Definitions of Violence

Different types of violence toward women include the following:

- *Battery:* Acts of physical violence, which can include hitting, beating, burning, twisting body parts, shaking, or slapping
- *Abuse:* Behaviors intended to hurt or harm, which can be physical, psychological, emotional, sexual, or economic
- *Assault:* Violent or aggressive acts, which include all forms of physical violence as battery; also may include use of dangerous weapons, such as knives, guns, rods, and others
- *Sexual assault:* Violent or aggressive acts that involve sexual contact without the victim's consent
- *Rape:* Sexual contact without consent; using force, threat or deception; involving some degree of vaginal penetration (Some states include oral and anal sexual contact also.)
- *Incest:* Sexual abuse by a parent, step-parent, or significantly older sibling

shame. When rage is used as a defense against shame, it may later erupt into violence or abuse when the person acquires a position of power (Bradshaw, 1988).

Feminist theory views abuse of women as an expression of male domination manifested within the family that is reinforced by social institutions, economic structures, and sexist division of labor. Relationships of female submission and male control are fostered by this socialization process. Patriarchal social values encourage "machismo," providing cultural support for male violence precipitated by stress and frustration. The root cause of physical violence is the batterer's need for dominance and control, which is central in the oppression of women (Breines et al., 1983; Campbell et al., 1984).

Devaluation of women remains an underlying cause of violence. The cultural view of women as property or possessions of men resulted from a perceived need to control female sexuality (eg, reproduction) and thus ensure paternity. Women are still emerging from a long era of dehumanization, during which they had no personal freedom, civil rights, legal protection, or control over their bodies and lives (Miles, 1989; Yyllo et al., 1988). Residual effects still impacting women can be seen in current economic discrimination, sexist attitudes, career opportunity limitations, child care difficulties, sensualized advertising, and amount of violence against women.

Other factors that contribute to domestic violence include cultural tolerance based on beliefs in the privacy of the family, institutional indifference with little legal action against batterers, women's economic insecurity due to fewer educational and job opportunities, and religious traditions that support women's inferiority and uphold men's rights to exercise control over the family.

Characteristics of Victims and Abusers

Battered women (victims) often attribute their abuse to personal deficiencies. With traditional family and sex role perspectives, they value family unity and believe it is their responsibility to keep the man happy and make the relationship work. If this does not happen, they feel they have failed as women and deserve to be punished. They begin to believe the man's accusations that they are bad wives, girlfriends, or lovers or inadequate mothers. After years of being given this message, they internalize it into their low self-esteem and feelings of worthlessness. Believing they deserve beating, they become hopeless and depressed.

Battering men come from all racial, ethnic, religious, and socioeconomic groups and represent all occupations and professions. They usually have a pattern of using violence to solve problems. They have an underlying sense of inadequacy, inferiority, and insecurity; frequently, they also have lower educational and occupational levels than their wives. Assumptions fostered by the culture about male superiority are contradicted by their inability to handle frustrations at work or home, feelings of socioeconomic inferiority, and sense that they cannot achieve their goals. Many men feel undeserving of their wives, yet they blame and punish them. This ambivalence is expressed by alternating episodes of violent eruptions and remorse, contrition and attention. Although they accept the machismo image and often have underlying rage, these men seem childlike, dependent, and needy of nurturing when not angry.

The pattern of abuse is repetitious, with deliberate use of severe violence that may result in injuries. Many people cannot comprehend why a battered woman would stay in an abusive relationship. Women stay because they may perceive no other options, are economically dependent, have traumatic bonding with the man (with elements of loyalty, deserving beating, and learned helplessness), or hope that he will change. Family violence may have been the woman's experience growing up; thus, it is an expected part of life. The woman may fear rejection if she brings abuse to the attention of friends or social agencies (Pahl, 1985). Characteristics of victims and abusers are summarized in Box 33-2. Some myths about battering relationships are discussed in Box 33-3.

Cycles of Domestic Violence

Domestic violence generally follows cycles, which occur over weeks or months (Fig. 33-1). Tension builds over minor conflicts or disagreements, with the woman

BOX 33–2
Characteristics of Abused and Abuser

Abused (Victim)

FAMILY INFLUENCES
- Violence in family
- Weak religious affiliation
- May have lower socioeconomic status (but not necessarily)
- Traditional sex roles (submissive, passive woman)
- Dysfunctional family system (internalized guilt)

PERSONALITY TRAITS
- Low self-esteem
- Learned helplessness
- Feel responsible for being abused
- Low frustration tolerance (complaining)
- Multiple symptoms and health problems
- Guilt, worthlessness
- Critical, aloof, distant
- Untrusting, fearful
- Deny abuse, anger, fear

LIFESTYLE INFLUENCES
- Alcohol abuse
- Verbal disputes
- Financial dependence on man
- Isolation from sources of support (friends, family, groups)

Abuser (Assailant)

FAMILY INFLUENCES
- Violence in family
- Weak religious affiliation
- May have lower socioeconomic status (but not necessarily)
- Traditional sex roles (dominant, aggressive man)
- Dysfunctional family system (internalized shame)

PERSONALITY TRAITS
- Sense of inadequacy, inferiority (overcompensated)
- Blame others for own actions
- Excessively jealous, possessive
- Overreactive, behavior extremes
- Concealed self-loathing
- Emotionally immature, aggressive
- Poor impulse control
- Disrespect for women

LIFESTYLE INFLUENCES
- Alcohol abuse
- Verbal disputes
- Work difficulties
- Restricts woman's freedom, limits mobility, contact with others

becoming compliant, passive, or withdrawn to avoid or deflect the man's anger. The man senses her anger and interprets lack of action as weakness, which further exacerbates his aggressiveness. Tension continues to build over incidents, eventually exploding into acute battering that often is triggered by an unrelated event. Common precipitants are arguments about spending money, jealousy by the husband over slights, sexual problems, drinking or drug use, conflicts over childrearing, the husband's unemployment, or pregnancy. The battering phase usually lasts 2 to 24 hours, although it could be a week or more. After severe beating, the woman usually does not seek care at once, experiencing a state of shock or disbelief and minimizing the injuries. Fear and helplessness may prevent the woman from seeking help. In the final phase, both feel relief, and the man often expresses extreme love and kindness and is contrite about his behavior. He may promise it will never happen again and may give her gifts. The woman wants to believe him and thinks that this is his real nature and that he will change his abusive behavior (Griffith-Kennedy, 1986). The cycle repeats itself over the years. Violence usually begins early in marriage, and many women remain for 6 to 7 years in a violent home situation, especially if they have small children. Most women leave the man two to four times and return before they permanently end the relationship. The longer the woman waits to take action,

the more entrenched the family dynamics become. Unhealthy interaction patterns are reinforced, with each partner knowing how to hurt the other emotionally. With time, the phases of building tension and acute battering get longer, and the relief and reconciliation phase gets shorter or may disappear (Walker, 1984b).

As months and years pass, the woman may withdraw from relatives, friends, and neighbors. She is reluctant to be seen with injuries and is fearful or embarrassed to talk about the beatings, and the husband is possessive and jealous of all outside relations. Social isolation increases with growing helplessness and powerlessness. Accepting abuse and pain as a part of life, the woman often develops serious emotional and somatic problems, such as paralyzing anxiety, nightmares, depression, tremors, sweating, alcohol and drug abuse, hypertension, ulcers, and paranoia.

Violence During Pregnancy

Battering often begins or increases during pregnancy. In a battering relationship, pregnancy leads to increased violent episodes. Many women are first beaten when their husbands learn about the pregnancy (Walker, 1984a). Some estimate that between 40% and 60% of women have been battered while pregnant (Parker et al., 1991). Pregnancy, with its physical changes and psychological stresses, adds coping de-

BOX 33–3
Myths About Battering Relationships

Myths	*Facts*
Battering occurs only in a small percentage of couples.	Battering occurs in 50%–60% of marriages; only 10% of women report abuse.
Battering occurs only in lower socioeconomic groups.	Spouse abuse occurs in middle- and upper-class families, all age and racial groups; lower class families have a higher incidence of abuse.
Battered women invite or provoke abuse.	Abuse is triggered by trivial events, silence or distancing by women, alcohol and drug use, and the batterer's loss of control. Women are terrified and try to avoid confrontation.
Alcohol and drug use cause battering.	Abuse is associated with alcohol or drugs, but these are excuses for violence or ways to shift the blame—they reduce inhibitions and impulse control and enhance violent tendencies.
Battered women can leave abusive relationships if they so choose.	Women often are financially dependent, value marriage, and feel responsible; believe family problems are their fault; think their children need a father; are isolated from family and friends; fear more violent retaliation if they leave; have no place to go and few resources.
Batterers and battered women cannot change.	Both can learn new behaviors and ways of coping with appropriate help; women can develop self-worth and assertion and relate to men in adaptive ways; men can rechannel aggression, verbalize feelings, restructure their views of women to respect their rights.
Battering men are uneducated and unable to cope in the world.	Many battering men are well educated, successful professionals.

mands to an already strained relationship. The man often is jealous of the fetus, fearing that attention will be taken away from him and resenting this intrusion into his relationship with the woman. With immature personality development and inadequate coping skills, the man becomes angry and frustrated. This leads to violence, sometimes with a conscious or subconscious intent to end the pregnancy (Hillard, 1986).

Physical violence is directed toward the woman's abdomen, breasts, and genitals. Blows to the face and

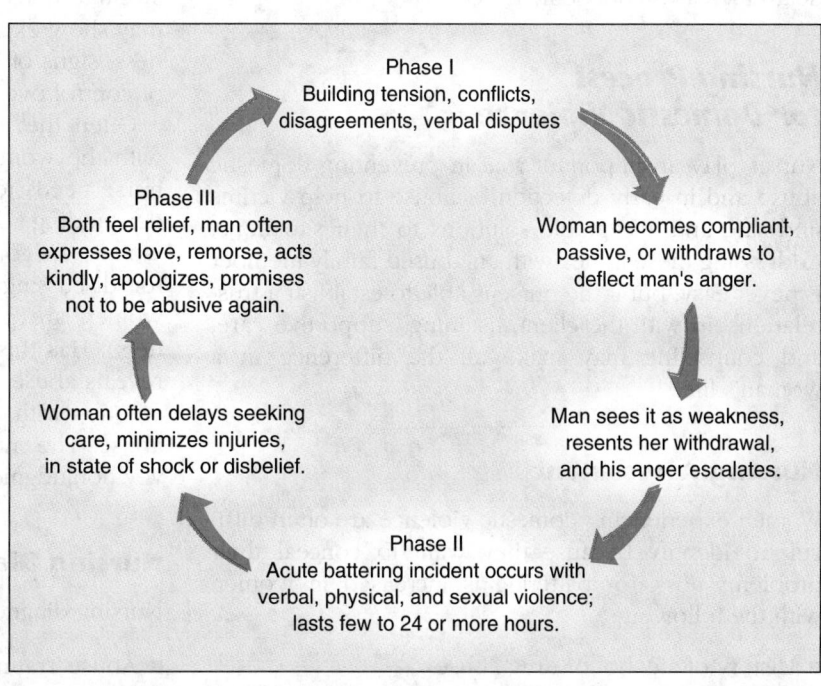

FIGURE 33–1 Cycles of domestic violence.

...ttery during pregnancy leads ...m labor, fetal injury, fetal death ...ck et al., 1989; Satin, 1991) and ... newborns. The battered pregnant ...nsidered high risk, and she may have a ... of physical and psychological complaints ...ne prenatal period. Her social and psychologi- ...eeds require careful assessment and specific inter- ...entions to prevent injury to the woman and fetus and to ensure a positive outcome of pregnancy.

During the postpartum period, the battered woman may be psychologically and physically exhausted. Her confusion, fear, and self-involvement may increase her risk for postpartum depression and make bonding with the newborn difficult. Ambivalence may arise from conflicts between the husband's and newborn's needs, which can adversely affect many aspects of mothering. She is at risk for being an abusive mother, even if she leaves the relationship. If she stays, she will face continued battering, and there is a 50% risk that the man also will abuse the child (deLang, 1986).

Violent Retaliation

Women who do leave abusive relationships may be at risk for **violent retaliation**, even years afterwards. Approximately 1,400 women are killed each year by their husbands, ex-husbands, or boyfriends (Ingrassia et al., 1994). Most physical assaults against women are committed by men with whom they were intimately involved, and the majority of men who kill their wives were living apart from them at the time of the murder (Koss et al., 1994). Leaving or staying in the relationship both may be dangerous for the women. With each violent attack, the likelihood of serious injury and death increases (Brasseur, 1994).

Nursing Process for Domestic Violence

Nurses play an important role in preventing domestic abuse and in early detection of abuse to help victims find safe and acceptable solutions to their situations. Addressing these issues with an abused family member is never easy, but if the nurse is able to establish a trust relationship with the client, listening, supportive care, and counseling may make all the difference in a woman's life.

Nursing Assessment

Women experiencing domestic violence are often difficult to identify because they want to conceal their problems. Risk for battering is increased in women with the following:

- History of alcohol or drug abuse

- History of child abuse
- Spouse abuse in a previous marriage

Battering might be suspected in women with the following:

- Neglected grooming and appearance
- Depression manifest by fatigue and hopelessness
- Repeated somatic complaints
- Voiced expression of helplessness and powerlessness
- Power inequity (authoritarian male, submissive, passive female) in their spousal relationship
- Social isolation (do not have a network of relatives and friends whom they see regularly and from whom they receive support).

During examination, a woman with injuries may present certain cues to abuse. She may have an inappropriate explanation for the injury (fell down stairs, ran into the door). The site and types of injuries tend to be typical, including bruises, abrasions, or contusions of the head, eyes, back of neck, throat, chest, breasts, abdomen, or genitals. Usually the injuries are multiple, in contrast to single or dual sites on extremities (ankles, wrists, feet, hands) in nonabusive injuries. A period of time (days to weeks) may have elapsed before injuries are reported, whereas nonabusive injuries usually are reported promptly. The abused woman is often hesitant, evasive, or inconsistent in providing details on how the injury occurred, and her affect may be inappropriate (avoiding eye contact, embarrassment, fright, disorientation, depression). If her husband is present, she may appear anxious and glance at him or seek approval to answer questions. He may be reluctant to leave her alone with the nurse, may interject answers to questions, or may demand to be present. She may show expressions of hopelessness and powerlessness, signs of clinical depression, or feelings of a lack of control over her life.

Often the nurse must build a trusting relationship with the woman before abuse can be disclosed. The nurse needs to convey unconditional acceptance, understanding, sensitivity, and positive regard for the woman. A conditional statement may open the door for discussing abuse, with the nurse saying, "Many women are physically hurt by their husbands (partners). Has this ever happened to you?" If the woman reveals abuse, this may be accompanied by a flood of emotion with crying and pouring out details of years of abuse. The nurse must listen empathetically and convey nonjudgmental emotional support.

Nursing Diagnosis

Nursing diagnoses may include the following:

- Abuse Trauma related to family violence

- Ineffective Family Coping (with destructive behavior)
- Fear related to threat of injury or death
- Powerlessness related to personal and interpersonal characteristics
- Ineffective Individual Coping related to family violence anxiety
- Self Esteem Disturbance related to abusive dynamics
- Social Isolation related to extreme anxiety, depression, or paranoia
- Rape-Trauma Syndrome (wife rape)
- Risk for Injury related to the physical trauma

Planning and Intervention

Nurses use supportive counseling, reassurance, and education in the care of battered or abused women. Empathetic listening and acceptance provide the environment in which the woman can express, examine, and work through her situation (see Nursing Guidelines: Establishing Therapeutic Relationships With Abused Women). The basic objective is empowerment. She will be facing choices among "unacceptable" alternatives, none of which seems to be a perfect solution. The nurse must be understanding of the woman's ambivalence toward the abuser; the woman would not remain in a cycle of violence unless there were powerful ties to

---

NURSING GUIDELINES
Establishing Therapeutic Relationships With Abused Women

Helpful Responses

- Ask directly about abuse; identify abusive behaviors.
- Accept the woman's perception of abuse.
- Support seriousness of abuse and that woman does not deserve it.
- Assist the woman to identify her alternatives clearly.
- Assist the woman to seek her strengths and clarify values.
- Identify specific community resources (eg, shelters, legal aid, financial aid, home assistance, employment agencies).
- Recommend women's support groups, networks for abused women.
- Warn the man that abuse is a crime and must be stopped.
- Convey acceptance and respect for the woman's choices.

Inhibitive Responses

- Lack of acknowledgment when abuse is disclosed.
- Disbelieving the woman's perception of abuse.
- Blaming the woman for abuse (support of abuser).
- Expressing opinions about what she should do.
- Advising her to leave the relationship.
- Becoming frustrated with her indecision or choice.
- Becoming caught up in her hopelessness.

---

her spouse or partner. During this process, the nurse clarifies misunderstandings and supports the woman's capacity to change, to make and follow through with decisions, and to clarify her values and beliefs. This helps the woman increase self-esteem and explore self-beliefs that keep her caught in the cycle of violence, such as guilt, powerlessness, and self-blame.

The abused woman has three basic alternatives:

1. Leave the relationship (with threat of homicide, child custody battles, loss of material support).
2. Stay and hope that the man will change through counseling, therapy, or legal intervention (change is slow, and risk of abuse or death continues).
3. Stay and resign herself to no change (risk of abuse or death continues).

No alternative seems perfect, yet the woman must make her own decision. Nurses can become frustrated at indecision or the choice to remain in the relationship. They need to assess their own feelings about the process of helping abused women (see Assessment Guidelines: Self-Assessment of Feelings About Helping Abused Women). Rescuing the abused woman is impossible, and the cycle will not stop until she is empowered to take the initiative. The woman needs to reestablish a sense of control over her life and feel safe enough to function. The nurse assists this process by building a trusting relationship, allowing expression of fear, providing empathy no matter how terrible the story becomes, extending dignity by exhibiting a regard for the woman's worth, and attempting to facilitate her decision-making abilities.

The nurse informs abused women of community services, such as women's shelters and safe houses. Physical safety is a central concern. The woman is informed of her legal rights and how law enforcement can protect her from battering. Legal options vary in each state. If she decides to leave, she is advised to take the children (if any) to protect them from abuse and facilitate obtaining custody. She needs to bring extra clothing, important documents, money, and emergency supplies. If the woman decides not to leave, she needs encouragement to use available resources, and reassurance of the nurse's continued respect and support.

Nursing intervention may include care for the abusive man. Group therapy for couples with violent relationships is becoming more available. These groups focus on helping the couple to appreciate similarities between their concerns and problems, obtain feedback on adaptive and maladaptive behaviors, learn and practice new behaviors, and improve self-esteem. Because of the diverse factors associated with family violence, each partner may need to be treated separately in the initial phases.

Couple therapy may be effective when the woman is protected from further violence (often by living apart) and the man is motivated to seek help. Because both

ASSESSMENT GUIDELINES
Self-Assessment of Feelings About Helping Abused Women

Nurses may need to assess their own feelings and attitudes concerning their approaches to intervening with abused women, by asking themselves these questions:

- To what extent am I meeting my own needs rather than those of my clients?
- Are some of my feelings inappropriate, such as pity, fear, or helplessness?
- Am I attempting to cope with my own feelings about the woman's process by withdrawing,

blaming her, prematurely confronting her, or pressuring her inappropriately to make a decision?

- Do I believe that the woman has the resources, strengths, interests, and abilities necessary to cope constructively with her difficulties?

---

are involved in creating and sustaining their relationship, couple therapy allows exploration of relationship dynamics and roles. Therapeutic strategies focus on control of the abuser's anger, cessation of violence, and learning nonfighting techniques for handling conflict (Fig. 33-2). Couples learn to control their violent interactions, using new adaptive behaviors. Patterns of violence resist change without modification of socioeconomic or educational factors, which may be difficult.

When the abusive man refuses therapy or when couple or group therapy is unsuccessful, the woman again must face the choice of leaving or staying in the abusive relationship. Breaking the symbiosis with the abusive man is often extremely difficult. The nurse works toward empowerment through use of "I am" statements, values clarification, grief therapy, and support for independent decisions. The woman identifies and builds on her strengths and resources. Support groups, individual counseling, and psychotherapy can be recommended. The nurse must remember that leaving a violent family situation is a long process, taking an av-

erage of 4 to 7 years. Most women who enter a shelter return home. Abused women often need rehabilitation that takes years, as they slowly gain ego strength and self-esteem. The nurse contributes to this process by effective counseling and support at every contact with an abused woman (See Nursing Care Plan).

Evaluation

Recovery from the trauma of abuse takes time, with periods of backsliding. Signs of progress are seeking safety, acknowledging need for help, and expressing fears. The woman is able to identify her strengths and available support systems, clarify her values and beliefs, feel deserving of respect, and understand and pursue her legal rights. Physical injuries are treated without delay. When the woman is pregnant, the fetus and other children are protected from abuse. She makes choices from alternatives and follows through with her decisions. As she progresses through these steps, she establishes a sense of increased control over her life and feels safe enough to function.

Sexual Abuse and Assault

Sexual assault is motivated by the intention to do harm, exert dominance or punish by physical means involving sexual contact, rather than by sexual desire. Victims feel frightened, helpless, violated, and disempowered (Botash, Braen, Gilchrist, 1994). **Sexual abuse** involves sexual contact without consent, often with the intent of hurting; physical violence is not always present in sexual abuse, but emotional or psychological violence usually is part of the process.

Childhood sexual abuse occurs when caretakers (parents, relatives, babysitters) have sexual contact with children younger than 18 years, and at least a 3-

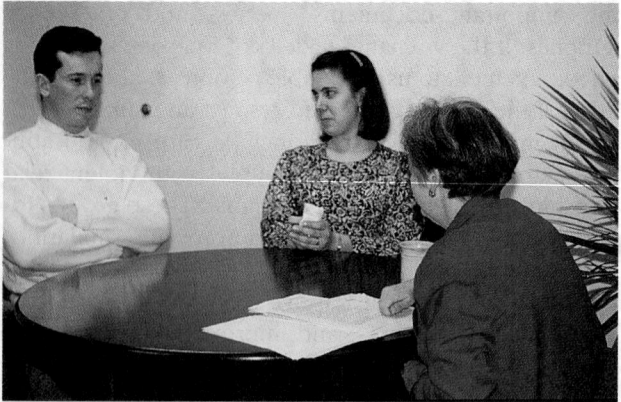

FIGURE 33-2 Therapy is an option for couples in an abusive relationship, if the male partner is willing to seek help in making changes in his behavior.

NURSING CARE PLAN
The Battered Woman

Nursing Goals
1. Abused/battered woman is identified early.
2. Woman obtains care for injuries promptly.
3. Woman understands her options and knows the available community resources.
4. Woman understands the cycle of violence and develops methods of avoiding recurrence.
5. Safety of the woman and her children is assured.

Assessment	Potential Nursing Diagnoses	Intervention/ Rationale	Evaluation
Physical injuries (bruises, cuts, scratches, broken bones)	Risk for Injury	Treat injuries *to prevent complications and aid healing.*	Injuries heal without complication.
		Provide comfort measures *to relieve pain.*	Woman is comfortable.
Emotional responses (fear, hopelessness, depression)	Fear, Anxiety, Hopelessness, Powerlessness	Develop trust, offer acceptance and positive regard *to build relationships.*	Trusting relationship develops.
		Assist to understand choices/options *for empowerment.*	She undersatnds her choices.
Confusion, indecision	Decisional Conflict	Assist to clarify her values and self-beliefs *to arrive at best decision.*	She makes the best decision for herself.
Risk for continued battering	Risk for Injury	Assist her to determine extent of risk for more violence (self and children) *to prevent further injuries.*	She clearly describes extent of continued risk.
		Encourage her to seek shelter care for self and children if risk is great.	Woman seeks shelter. Further injuries are prevented.
Family coping patterns	Ineffective Family Coping	Assist her to examine family coping patterns, identify possible ways to change these, refer to family counseling *to develop more effective coping.*	Family uses coping methods that avoid violence.
Level of self-esteem	Self Esteem Disturbance	Build self-esteem by acceptance, supporting strengths, empowering with information *to change negative self-beliefs.*	She expresses more positive self-regard and belief in her abilities.

year age difference exists between victim and perpetrator (Hunter, 1991). **Incest** involves sexual abuse by the father, mother, step-parent, or older sibling. If children are abused sexually by a stranger, this is considered sexual assault. The peak age for occurrence of childhood sexual abuse is 7 to 12 years (Koop, 1985; Hunter, 1991; Tower, 1988). The Child Abuse Prevention and Treatment Act (1974) and the women's movement have helped focus attention on this problem, increasing public awareness and underscoring the fre-

quency of a history of childhood abuse among women (Hurley, 1991).

Victims of childhood sexual abuse often suffer long-lasting consequences. They avoid revealing their experiences because of guilt, shame, and repression (Kinzl et al., 1991). Psychological and behavioral difficulties, such as depression, suicidal ideation, eating disorders, and personality disorders, are common. Incest survivors may have difficulty with interpersonal relationships, avoid intimacy, and have low self-esteem, sexual dysfunctions, and antimale feelings (Coker, 1990; Brown et al., 1990). Post-traumatic stress disorder may occur, with symptoms of recurrent nightmares or recollection of the event, anxiety, numbing of responses, and withdrawal from the external world (Pettit, 1991).

Sexual Assault in Pregnancy

Sexual assault occurs less often than physical violence during pregnancy. Sexual assaults tend to occur in early pregnancy (mean gestational age, 15 weeks). The type of sexual contact is primarily vulvar and vaginal, followed by oral and anal contact. Physical trauma occurs less often in pregnant victims, with injuries directed more toward the head, neck, and extremities than to the abdomen, chest, or back. Spontaneous abortion within 4 weeks of sexual assault appears infrequent and low–birth-weight newborns and preterm births are common (Satin, 1991).

Nursing Assessment

Victims of sexual abuse or assault may be in acute psychological disorganization if seen shortly after the event, appearing fearful, anxious, crying, or distraught. Some may appear emotionless and calm. Others may not provide direct signs if the abuse occurred at an earlier time. Possible signs of sexual abuse include the following:

- Self-inflicted injuries (cuts, nail biting, hair pulling)
- Broken bones, both old and new injuries
- Genital and breast injuries
- Recurrent nightmares
- Withdrawal, disengagement
- Substance abuse
- Mental illness or depression
- Chronic interpersonal difficulties, especially with men
- Low self-esteem, self-blaming

Physical examination focuses on signs of trauma, such as bruises and abrasions, genital pain or bleeding, oral cavity injury (torn frenulum, broken teeth, split lip), petechiae of face and conjunctiva (from choking), loss of scalp hair, and fingernails bitten to the quick. In the pelvic examination, signs of recent injury include labial swelling and erythema, fourchette tears, abrasions or bruises of vulva, vaginal wall lacerations, and anal erythema, fissures, or tears. Physical signs usually are absent when abuse occurred in the past, unless there are healed scars or fractures.

Laboratory and diagnostic tests may include vaginal smears or cultures for sexually transmitted diseases (STDs); blood tests for STDs, including human immunodeficiency virus (HIV), and for substance use; and x-rays of fractures.

Nursing Diagnosis and Intervention

Nursing diagnoses may include the following:

- Risk for Injury (from self or other)
- Anxiety or Fear
- Self Esteem Disturbance
- Abuse Trauma related to sexual abuse or assault
- Sleep Pattern Disturbance
- Sexual Dysfunction
- Ineffective Individual Coping

Care following acute assault initially focuses on controlling hemorrhage, shock, or respiratory distress. The nurse reassures the woman that she is now safe and acknowledges the traumatic nature of the assault. Speaking and moving slowly, touching gently, and explaining everything that is happening are important. Believe the woman's description of what happened, and assure her that someone will remain with her. When evidence will be collected, follow the specific protocols for rape and assault victims.

Longer term interventions have the goals of supporting the woman in acknowledging that sexual abuse has occurred, openly discussing and sharing her experiences, and initiating personal growth to overcome residual psychological effects. Group therapy has been effective in decreasing depression, anger, and guilt; reducing isolation; improving self-esteem; and promoting effective coping among sexually abused women and incest survivors (Axelroth, 1991; Coker, 1990; Pettit, 1991). Writing in a diary can be a safe, private way to describe the abuse experience and explore its impact on the woman's life. Repressed feelings often are brought up, examined, and released this way.

Women's support groups can aid exploring power and gender issues, handling and expressing anger, and developing assertiveness. Confronting the perpetrator is necessary in some form for complete recovery from childhood sexual abuse. This allows anger to be directed appropriately and enhances a sense of power. The goals of the confrontation must focus on the woman's own growth, however; expecting an apology from the perpetrator leads to disappointment (Coker, 1990; Kinzl et al., 1991).

Evaluation

Care is effective when the abuse or assault victim receives immediate care for injuries and recovers physically and emotionally. For longer term problems, effective care results in identifying and expressing the sexual abuse experience, participating in therapeutic processes to work through feelings and develop effective coping, and expressing a positive outlook. Having satisfying relationships, a healthy self-concept, and the ability to function well denote full recovery from sexual abuse.

Rape

Rape is the fastest growing reported violent crime in the United States. The National Center for the Prevention and Control of Rape estimates that one out of three women may be raped in her lifetime; many victims will not report it or seek assistance. Rapes of women from 6 months to 93 years old have been documented. In 75% of rapes, the assailant is known to the woman (Newsweek, 1990; Dennis, 1988; Burge, 1989).

Legal definitions of rape vary by state. The key features include some form of sexual contact and the absence of consent. The use of force, deception, or coercion must be present when the victims are competent adults. Consent is considered impossible for victims who are drugged, unconscious, mentally retarded, physically unable to move, or of minor age (statutory rape). Eleven states still have laws defining rape as nonconsenting sexual intercourse committed by a man "with a woman not his wife" (Weingourt, 1990). Definitions of the types of rape are provided in Box 33-4.

Social and Psychological Factors in Rape

The United States has a higher incidence of rape than many other countries: 4 times more than Germany, 13 times more than England, and 20 times more than Japan (Newsweek, 1990). Rape is more common in large metropolitan areas, although it is increasing rapidly in midsize cities. More rapes occur during the summer. While young African American women are victims most often, women of all ages and races are at risk.

Men who commit rape have varied backgrounds. More than half of these men are young (younger than 25 years), and about 60% are married with apparently normal sexuality. More than one-third of these men were sexually abused as children (Groth et al., 1977). Victims tend to be the same race and often are a friend or casual acquaintance.

Rape is not a crime of passion or lust; it is an act of aggression. Power, control, and dominance are the underlying motives. In a largely patriarchal system, as in the United States, rape occurs more frequently because physical aggression is accepted as a means to implement the societal norm for maintaining male power and control (Stets, 1991; Sampselle, 1991). This use of force is justified by the following common (and convenient) male myths:

- Women secretly desire to be raped (overcome by male sexual power).

> **BOX 33-4**
> *Types of Rape*
>
> *Acquaintance or confidence rape.* Victim has a previous nonviolent relationship with assailant, but he uses deception or coercion to gain access or obtain sex.
>
> *Date rape.* Assailant usually has planned sex during the date and will do whatever is necessary to obtain it. Men justify rape more when the woman initiated the date, the man paid expenses, or they went to the man's residence.
>
> *Wife rape.* Assailant uses force or coercion to obtain sexual contact with his wife (by marriage or common law), without her consent. In some states, wife rape is legally impossible because wives are excluded from statute.
>
> *Stranger or blitz rape.* Victim and assailant are strangers; rape is sudden and unexpected; use of weapons and threats of violence are frequent.
>
> *Power rape.* Assailant uses sexual intercourse to dominate victim and put her in a powerless position; sexual conquest fulfills his fantasy of strength and potency; he believes the woman enjoys the rape and uses only enough force to subdue the victim.
>
> *Anger rape.* Assailant uses sexual contact to express feelings of rage, often motivated by revenge to symbolically punish a significant woman in his life. Attacks on older women often are anger rape, which is characterized by brutality and degradation.
>
> *Sadistic rape.* Sadism characterizes assailant's relationships, with aggression being eroticized. He uses abuse and torture, becoming aroused by victim's struggles. While the rape often is planned, the victim is a stranger. These types of rape may end in murder, and although infrequent, they capture much media attention.

- Women provoke rape by their seductive behavior (dress, appearance, being in a secluded area).
- Women cannot actually be raped without implicit consent (disregarding fear of harm or death).

Box 33-5 details these and other commonly held myths about rape.

The male proclivity toward rape is surprisingly persistent and common. Around 1980, male college students were asked whether they would rape a woman if they could be certain they would not be caught and punished. About 35% said they might do it (Malamuth, 1981). Ten years later, another survey of college-age men found that 51% would rape a woman if they thought they would not be punished. Most also thought the woman would enjoy it (Sampselle, 1991). Men tend to justify date rape more when the woman initiated the date, the man paid the expenses, or they went to the man's residence (Muchlenhard, 1988).

Strong sociocultural forces promote and perpetuate violent behavior. The United States has powerful social

---

BOX 33-5
Myths About Rape

Myths	*Facts*
Rape results from uncontrolled sexual desire.	Rape is a violent assault, using sex as a weapon.
	Most rapists have access to consensual sex.
Rape is impulsive, one-time, due to momentary lack of judgment.	Most rapes are planned; most convicted rapists commit 15–20 rapes before they are caught.
Women cannot really be raped against their will.	Most women resist rape or feel resistance puts their life in danger. Lack of resistance does not imply consent.
Rapists are strangers.	In about 50% of rapes the victim and assailant know each other.
Women actually enjoy rape.	Victims report being terrified, degraded, humiliated, and hurt.
Women provoke rape by their dress or being in unsafe areas.	Appearance does not justify acts of violence, nor does location. Over half of all rapes occur in the victim's or assailant's home.
Most rapists are African American, and most victims are white.	In 90% of rapes, victim and assailant are the same race, but rapes by African Americans are reported more often.
Women report rape falsely.	False reports of rape are about 2%; only 1 in 10–20 rapes is reported to police.

---

norms that support competition, aggression, use of force to attain goals, and overt and covert violence. Studies of primitive tribal societies have shown that rape is not integral to maleness but is a method used by men programmed for violence to express their sexual identity (Garrison, 1983). In the United States, part of the man's sexual identity is having control and dominance over women.

Rape Trauma Syndrome

Rape is a physical and psychological crisis. The **rape trauma syndrome** is experienced by most victims of sexual assault and has characteristic symptoms, beginning with confusion and disorganization of reactions, proceding through an intermediate adjustment phase, and concluding with a long-term reorganization process (Burgess et al., 1979; Golan, 1978). It is similar to *post-traumatic stress disorder,* in which physiologic or behavioral signs and symptoms develop following a psychologically traumatic event that is outside the usual range of human experience. These unusual traumatic events may be natural disasters, serious accidents, or damaging intentional actions (McLeer, 1988). The phases of the rape trauma syndrome are discussed in the following sections.

Confusion and Disorganization

The acute phase begins during the rape and may last for several days to 3 weeks. The woman experiences fear, shock, disbelief, and possibly denial. She may be embarrassed, humiliated, and helpless. Often she feels guilty and self-blaming, alternating anger with the desire for revenge. Feelings of powerlessness and helplessness are common. Women may douche or bathe to cleanse themselves, even though they know this will destroy evidence.

The rape victim's affect varies from crying to seeming calm, composed, and subdued. Physiologic reactions may include flushing, perspiration, sighing respirations, hyperventilation, dizziness, abdominal pain, nausea, diarrhea, or urinary frequency. Mentally there may be impaired attention, difficulty concentrating, or poor memory. Most women relive the scene repeatedly, searching for what they should have done differently.

Intermediate Adjustment Phase

After the acute phase, the woman resumes her usual activities and appears composed and outwardly adjusted. She is coping by using denial and suppression, which are necessary for her to gain a sense of control over her life. She may institute security measures (install locks, have an unlisted telephone number, carry a self-defense device) or move to a different location. Some women take self-defense courses or obtain a weapon. The emotional trauma is not resolved by these actions, however, and her coping mechanisms begin to deteriorate. Friends may be less supportive, because they perceive that the trauma is over.

Reorganization Phase

As the rape victim's suppression of feelings and emotions deteriorates, she becomes depressed and anxious. Fears begin to surface, especially fear of being alone or in places similar to where the rape occurred. She may experience sleep disturbances, sexual dysfunctions, menstrual problems, or eating disorders. The need to express and integrate these experiences usually leads to seeking help. Individual therapy or support groups offer specific assistance to rape survivors. Gradually, the rape experience is integrated and accepted.

The last phase of reorganization is recovery; it may take weeks to years before the woman returns to full functioning. Successful recovery is a growth process, bringing the woman to a higher level of self-acceptance and wisdom. She has progressed through recovery when physical symptoms have abated, reliving the rape has diminished and lost its power, and experiences in work and interpersonal relationships are satisfying.

Nursing Assessment

Care for the rape victim includes responding sensitively to the woman's experience, keeping in mind the need to preserve evidence for possible criminal prosecution. Each hospital or clinic has specific protocols for collecting rape evidence (see Assessment Guidelines: Collecting Evidence in Suspected Rape). Usually evidence must be collected within 72 hours to be useful. The history includes the following:

- Date of last normal menstrual period
- Date of last instance of voluntary sexual intercourse
- Number, dates, and outcomes of pregnancies
- Current contraceptive use
- Recent STDs and treatment
- Recent gynecologic surgery
- Use of tampons and douches, last date of use
- Current medications, allergies, immunizations
- Health problems and conditions
- Description of the assault, including vaginal, oral, or anal penile penetration; if assailant had orgasm; whether a condom was worn; other types of sexual contact
- Activity since the rape, including urination, defecation, douching, bathing, brushing teeth, gargling, taking medication or alcohol, changing or repairing clothing

The physical examination includes inspecting clothing for tears or stains and physical or pelvic examination. Typical physical injuries are bruises of the head, neck, and upper extremities. Scratches and lacerations may be present. Oral cavity injuries may include torn frenulum, broken teeth, or split lip. Common genital injuries include tears of the fourchette, abrasions, bruises, vaginal lacerations, or vulval swelling. Anal injuries include erythema, bleeding, mucosal tears, hematoma, or sphincter laxity or spasm. Signs of trauma are documented by a traumagram (drawing) or photograph if possible.

Laboratory Tests and Specimens. Specimens to document the assault and aid identification of the assailant are collected according to specific institutional proto-

ASSESSMENT GUIDELINES
Collecting Evidence in Suspected Rape

Specimens are collected to document the assault and aid in identification of the assailant. All slides, test tubes, envelopes, and packaging materials are labeled personally by the examining healthcare provider, with the woman's name, date and time, and site of specimen. All transactions are witnessed and signed by the giving and receiving parties (obtaining, packaging, and labeling specimens, giving specimens to laboratory or police). All clothing is removed and placed in a sealed bag. Specimens to be obtained include the following:

- Foreign material on victim's clothes or body (eg, dirt, sand, fibers, leaves, semen)
- Fingernail clippings and scrapings (bits of assailant's skin, hair, blood)
- Oral swab around teeth for semen (if fellatio reported)
- Scalp and pubic hair combed onto sterile sheet (for hair samples from assailant)

- Swabs from upper thighs and perineum for semen
- Aspiration of vaginal secretions (for sperm, acid phosphatase, and blood group antigens)
- Pap smear (may reveal intact sperm several days after assault)
- Anal washings or swabs (if anal penetration reported)

cols. For the victim's health and safety, tests are done for pregnancy and STD. Pregnancy caused by rape occurs in 1% of victims who are not sterile (Botash et al., 1994). To determine if pregnancy prophylaxis is necessary, estimate time of ovulation (95% of conceptions after a single act of intercourse occur between 5 days before and 10 hours after ovulation). The beta-human chorionic gonadotropin pregnancy test will detect pregnancy 5 days after implantation; if positive during the acute evaluation, the victim was pregnant at time of the rape.

STD tests may include the following:

- Oral, vaginal, cervical, and rectal specimens for gonorrhea and *Chlamydia*
- Vaginal smears for trichomoniasis, bacterial vaginosis, and candidiasis
- Labial, vaginal, or cervical specimens for herpes simplex or cytomegalovirus
- Serologic test for syphilis
- Blood tests (antigen, antibody) for hepatitis B and HIV

Nursing Diagnosis and Intervention

Nursing diagnoses in the *acute phase* may include the following:

- Fear or Anxiety related to the rape experience
- Fear or Anxiety related to procedures for evidence and interactions with health professionals and police
- Risk for Injury (immediate trauma, infection, pregnancy)
- Pain related to trauma from assault or later examination
- Self Esteem Disturbance
- Rape-Trauma Syndrome (disorganized phase)
- Decisional Conflict related to informing family and friends

Nursing diagnoses in the *intermediate and reorganization phases* may include the following:

- Risk for Infection (STD)
- Decisional Conflict related to pregnancy (if occurs)
- Self Esteem disturbance
- Rape-Trauma Syndrome (intermediate and late effects)
- Sexual Dysfunction
- Altered Family Processes
- Impaired Adjustment
- Sleep Pattern Disturbance

During the *acute phase*, nursing care focuses on providing support for the woman during examination and evidence collection. Reassurance is provided that she is now safe, and the traumatic experience is acknowledged. The nurse's actions are gentle and slow, with a nonjudgmental and accepting attitude. Explanations are provided for each step in the examination and process of evidence collection. The woman is never left alone. Treatment is provided for physical injuries, including pain relief. Family or friends are kept informed, reassured that the victim is safe, and given emotional support.

Pregnancy Prevention. If there is risk of pregnancy and the rape occurred within 24 to 72 hours, hormone therapy is prescribed if the woman desires. These regimens are 98% effective in preventing pregnancy (Table 33-1). The nurse explains that nausea commonly occurs with these drugs; antinausea medication usually is prescribed. There may be breast tenderness, headache, and irregular bleeding. Withdrawal bleeding usually occurs several days after taking the hormones. The woman is apprised of the teratogenic effects of high estrogen doses and advised regarding abortion options if pregnancy occurs despite prophylaxis.

Sexually Transmitted Disease Prevention. Rape victims are offered prophylaxis against gonorrhea and *Chlamydia* infection. About half will require treatment for vaginitis or STDs if they do not receive prophylaxis (Botash et al., 1994). Some regimens also include treatment for syphilis (Table 33-2).

If the assailant is thought to be homosexual or an intravenous drug user, hepatitis B prophylaxis is indicated unless the victim has already been immunized. This is especially important when vaginal or anal assault causes bleeding. Blood is drawn for hepatitis B antigen and antibody tests; the woman is then given hepatitis B immune globulin with a repeat dose in 1 month if the blood test is negative.

Treatment with zidovudine (Retrovir) for potential exposure to HIV is not proven effective. The decision to use this treatment should be based on risk assess-

TABLE 33–1
Pregnancy Prevention for Rape Victims

Regimen	Dosage
Norgestrel/ethinyl estradiol (Ovral)	Two tablets initially, then two tablets 12 h later
Diethylstilbestrol	25 mg orally bid for 5 d
Conjugated estrogens (Premarin)	50 mg/d IV for 2 d or 30 mg/d orally for 5 d

Note: Hormone therapy must be started within 24–72 h of the rape. These regimens are not FDA approved for this purpose.

TABLE 33–2
Sexually Transmitted Disease Prevention for Rape Victims

Regimen	Dosage
Ceftriaxone (Rocephin) plus	250 mg IM (for penicillin-resistant gonorrhea and syphilis)
doxycycline hyclate or	100 mg orally bid for 7 d (for *Chlamydia*)
azithromycin (Zithromax)	1 g orally (for *Chlamydia*)
Spectinomycin HC1 (Trobicin) or	2 g IM (for gonorrhea when ceftriaxone cannot be used)
ciprofloxacin HC1 (Cipro) plus	500 mg orally (do not use if younger than 18 y or pregnant)
Doxycycline or azithromycin	As above
erythromycin	500 mg orally qid for 7 d (for *Chlamydia* and gonorrhea in pregnancy)
Penicillin G procaine plus probenecid (Benemid)	4.8 million U IM (two sites)
	1 g orally (for gonorrhea and syphilis)

ment, considering the assailant's HIV status, the type of exposure, and nature of physical injuries.

During the *intermediate and reorganization phases,* care focuses on emotional support, therapy, and physical follow-up. While using suppression to cope, the woman may not feel the need for counseling. The nurse respects this and keeps communication open for future needs. The family may be more receptive to counseling and can be referred. As the woman's needs for resolving the experience increase, the nurse becomes an accepting listener and suggests resources for therapy or counseling. Initially, the woman identifies, expresses, and explores feelings. Acceptance is key to therapeutic progress. Next, the woman seeks understanding, examining the sources and reasons for her feelings. Attitudes and beliefs that diminish self-esteem and behaviors that are nonadaptive can be clarified. Strategies are developed for more effective behaviors and attitudes. In the last phase, the woman implements changes and evaluates their effects on her functioning and satisfaction.

Follow-up occurs in 1 to 2 weeks with repeat gonorrhea and *Chlamydia* cultures, assessment of injury healing, and response to hormone pregnancy prophylaxis; pregnancy testing often is indicated. At 6 to 8 weeks, tests for HIV, hepatitis B, and syphilis may be done or repeated. Further HIV testing may be recommended at 3 and 6 months.

Evaluation

Nursing care is effective when the woman experiencing rape receives immediate and sensitive evaluation, treatment for injuries, and collection of evidence ac-

cording to legal specifications. During each phase, the woman feels accepted and supported.

Summary Points

✔ Violence directed toward women is a major problem in the United States today; most of this violence occurs within the home.

✔ Battery and sexual abuse are more common experiences among woman than statistics reveal. Many episodes are not reported due to limited mobility and fear of repercussions or rejection.

✔ In a battering relationship, the incidence of violent events increases during pregnancy because of increased psychological stresses in a strained coping situation.

✔ Patterns of childhood abuse are often found in men who commit battery and sexual assault. Women who remain in abusive relationships often experienced childhood abuse.

✔ Cycles of domestic violence tend to be repeated over months and years, becoming closer together and more violent.

✔ Women remain in battering and abusive relationships because they cannot perceive that other choices are available to them. Helping women develop inner strength, self-respect, and psychosocial resources can eventually lead to perception of other choices.

✔ Rape occurs more frequently in the United States than other developed countries, which is related to sociocultural norms that support violence and aggression to attain goals.

✔ Rape trauma syndrome has characteristic phases from shock, disbelief, and denial to intermediate adjustment and finally to reorganization.

REFERENCES

Axelroth, E. (1991). Retrospective incest group therapy for university women. *J College Stud Psychotherapy, 5*(2), 81.

Bagley, C. (1991). The prevalence and mental health sequels of child sexual abuse in a community sample of women aged 18 to 27. *Canadian Journal of Community Mental Health, 10*(1), 103.

Bohn, D. K. (1990). Domestic violence and pregnancy: Implications for practice. *Journal of Nurse-Midwifery, 35,* 86.

Botash, A. S., Braen, G. R., & Gilchrist, V. J. (1994). Acute care for sexual assault victims. *Patient Care, 28*(13), 112–137.

Bradshaw, J. (1988). *Healing the shame that binds you.* Deerfield Beach, FL: Health Communications.

Brasseur, J. W. (1994). The battered woman: Identification and intervention. *Clinician Reviews, April 9,* 45–74.

Breines, W., & Gordon, L. (1983). The new scholarship on family violence. *Signs, 8*(3), 490–531.

Brown, B., & Garrison, C. (1990). Patterns of symptomatology of adult women incest survivors. *Western Journal of Nursing Research, 12*(5), 587.

Bullock, L., & McFarlane, J. (1989). Birthweight/battering connection. *American Journal of Nursing, 5*(9), 153.

Burge, S. K. (1989). Violence against women as a health care issue. *Family Medicine, 21,* 368.

Burgess, A. W., & Holmstrom, L. L. (1979). *Rape crisis and recovery.* Englewood Cliffs, NJ: Prentice-Hall.

Campbell, J., & Humphreys, J. (1984). *Nursing care of victims of family violence.* Reston, VA: Prentice Hall.

Chez, N. (1994). Helping the victim of domestic violence. *American Journal of Nursing, 94*(7), 33–37.

Coker, L. (1990). A therapeutic recovery model for the female adult incest survivor. *Issues in Mental Health Nursing, 11,* 109.

deLang, C. (1986). The family place: Children's therapeutic program. *Children Today, March/April,* 12.

Dennis, L. I. (1988). Adolscent rape: The role of nursing. *Issues in Comprehensive Pediatric Nursing, 11,* 59.

Garrison, J. (1983). *Research on rapists: Response to violence in the family and sexual assault* (Vol. 6, No. 2.). Rockville, MD: National Center for the Prevention and Control of Rape.

Gibbs, N. (1991). When is it rape? *Time, June 3,* 48.

Golan, N. (1978). *Treatment in crisis situations.* New York: Free Press.

Griffith-Kennedy, J. (1986). Abuse and battering. In J. Griffith-Kennedy (Ed.), *Contemporary women's health: A nursing advocacy approach.* Menlo Park, CA: Addison-Wesley.

Groth, A. N., & Burgess, A. W. (1977). Sexual dysfunction during rape. *New England Journal of Medicine, 297*(14), 764.

Helton, A., McFarlane, J., & Anderson, E. (1987). Battered and pregnant: A prevalence study. *American Journal of Public Health, 77*(10), 1337.

Hillard, P. J. (1986). Physical abuse and pregnancy. *Family Practice Recertif, 8*(9), 89.

Hunter, J. (1991). A comparison of the psychological maladjustment of adult males and females sexually molested as children. *Journal of International Violence, 6*(2), 205.

Hurley, D. (1991). Women, alcohol, and incest: An analytical review. *J Studies Alcohol, 52*(3), 253.

Ingrassia, M., & Beck, M. (1994). Patterns of abuse. *Newsweek, July 4,* 26–33.

Kinzl, J., & Biebl, W. (1991). Sexual abuse of girls: Aspects of the genesis of mental disorders and therapeutic implications. *Acta Psychiatr Scand, 83,* 427.

Koop, C. (1985). *Surgeon general's workshop on violence and public health report.* Washington, DC: U.S Dept. of Health and Human Services.

Koss, M., Goodman, L. A., Fitzgerald, L. F. et al. (1994). *No safe haven.* Hyattsville, MD: American Psychological Association.

Levinson, D. (1989). *Family violence in a cross cultural perspective.* Newbury Park, CA: Sage.

Malamuth, N. (1981). Rape proclivity among males. *J Soc Issues, 37,* 138.

Miles, R. (1989). *Women of the world.* Topsfield, MA: Salem House.

Muchlenhard, C. L. (1988). Misinterpreted dating behaviors and the risk of date rape. *J Soc Clin Psychol, 6*(1), 20.

(1990). The mind of the rapist. *Newsweek, July 23,* 46.

Parker, B., & McFarlane, J. (1991). Identifying and helping battered pregnant women. *MCN: American Journal of Maternal Child Nursing, 16,* 161.

Pahl, J. (Ed) (1985). *Private violence and public policy.* London: Routledge & Kegan Paul.

Pettit, M. (1991). Recognizing post-traumatic stress. *RN, 54,* p. 15.

Pitts, D. (1990). Women and violence. *Crossroads, 3*(1), 1–2.

Sampselle, C. (1991). The role of nursing in preventing violence against women. *Journal of Obstetric, Gynecologic, and Neonatal Nursing, 20*(6), 481.

Satin, A. (1991). Sexual assault in pregnancy. *Obstetrics and Gynecol, 77*(5), 710.

Senate Judiciary Committee (1990). *Report.* Washington, DC: United States Senate.

Stenchever, M., & Stenchever, D. (1991). Abuse of women: An overview. *WHI, 1*(4), 187.

Stets, J. (1991). Psychological aggression in dating relationships: The role of interpersonal control. *Journal of Family Violence, 6*(1), 97.

Torres, S. (1991). A comparison of wife abuse between two cultures: Perceptions, attitudes, nature and extent. *Issues in Mental Health Nursing, 12*(1), 113.

Tower, C. (1988). *Secret scars: A guide for survivors of child sexual abuse.* New York: Penguin Books.

Walker, L. E. (1984a). Battered women, psychology, and public policy. *Am Psychol, 39*(10), 1178–1182.

Walker, L. E. (1984b). *The battered woman syndrome* (Vol. 6). New York: Springer.

Weingourt, R. (1990). Wife rape in a sample of psychiatric patients. *Journal of Nursing Sch, 22*(3), 144.

Witkin-Lanoil, G. (1987). Too close to home. *Health, January,* 6.

Wyatt, G., & Newcomb, M. (1990). Internal and external mediators of women's sexual abuse in childhood. *Journal of Consult Clin Psychol, 58*(6), 758.

Yyllo, K., & Bogard, M. (Eds.) (1988). *Feminist perspectives on wife abuse.* London: Sage.

Zdanuk, J. M., Harris, C. C., & Wisian, N. L. (1987). Adolescent pregnancy and incest: The nurse's role as counselor. *Journal of Obstetric, Gynecologic, and Neonatal Nursing, 16*(2), 99.

34

Addictive Disorders in Pregnancy

Objectives

- Increase knowledge of the incidence and prevalence of smoking, problem drinking and alcoholism, and drug abuse in the childbearing population.
- Increase knowledge of the pathophysiology of smoking, drinking, and drug use on the mother and infant, including pregnancy outcomes and fetal and perinatal effects.
- Develop knowledge and expertise in taking accurate smoking, drinking, and drug use histories and making appropriate referrals when necessary.
- Develop knowledge and expertise in applying the nursing process to the childbearing woman who smokes or uses or abuses other substances including alcohol.
- Develop knowledge regarding Quit Smoking programs for the pregnant woman and expertise in counseling the childbearing woman regarding smoking cessation.
- Develop knowledge regarding alcohol and other substance abuse rehabilitation programs and expertise in counseling the childbearing woman regarding using these programs.

Key Terms

Al-Anon	Ethanol
Cocaine	Fetal alcohol syndrome
Crack	Nicotine

The United States is continuing to experience an unprecedented surge of addictive behaviors in its population. All levels of society are besieged with the consequences of these behaviors, some of which include grave health problems, time lost from work, unemployment, reproductive wastage, family disorganization, homicide, and suicide. A curious dichotomy has appeared in the United States. There has been a rise in health consciousness, and people are implementing preventive health behaviors, such as attention to a healthy diet, moderate drinking, quitting smoking, and exercise. However, at the same time, more Americans are being immersed in the addictions of smoking, alcohol, and other chemical abuse. When these addictions go unchecked, they lead to the destruction of the person's health, life, and often, their family structure.

The impact of substance abuse on the fetus is serious. Animal and human studies throughout the last decade have indicated the adverse effects of perinatal exposure to numerous pharmacologic substances in pregnancy outcomes, fetal characteristics, and infant development. Such substances include tobacco, cannabis, caffeine, alcohol, amphetamines, barbiturates, and a variety of illegal drugs, including heroin and cocaine. The dangers of smoking and drinking during pregnancy have been known for many years, as have the problems of newborns of heroin-addicted mothers. However, the increasingly large numbers of newborns of mothers abusing crack and cocaine have heightened public awareness and concern about the overall problem of substance abuse in pregnant women (Adams et al., 1988; Hamilton, 1990). This chapter discusses the major categories of addictive disorders, the implications of these addictions for perinatal outcomes, and nursing interventions for addictive disorders.

Smoking

Tobacco smoking has not historically been classified as an addiction. However, research indicates that at least one substance found in cigarettes, **nicotine**, is a powerful addictive agent. A person who is addicted to nicotine has an extremely difficult time giving up cigarettes, particularly because tobacco is a legal, easily

obtained substance (Warner, 1989; Council on Scientific Affairs, 1990; Gilpin et al., 1994). The recent legislative hearings on the manipulations of the tobacco industry to make their product more addictive and the protestations of that industry that their cigarettes are not addictive underline the real health and social problems inherent in using tobacco.

An estimated 20% to 30% of American women of childbearing age smoke. Even more disturbing is that perhaps as many as 50% of pregnant women smoke despite clear and consistent evidence that smoking has adverse effects on the mother, the fetus, and the infant (Aaronson et al., 1989; Floyd et al., 1991; Windsor et al., 1993a). A recent national telephone survey found that an estimated 39% of women who had smoked before pregnancy quit smoking while pregnant, and 27% of them quit as soon as they found out they were pregnant. Women who had less education (less than 12 years) and who were heavy smokers (more than one pack a day) were significantly less likely to quit. Of the women who quit, 70% resumed smoking within 1 year of delivery (Fingerhut et al., 1990). These findings suggest that the health of the fetus is a strong influence on women's smoking habits. However, these findings also suggest that women may be less aware of the deleterious effects on their infant when they resume smoking and expose their infant to a smoke-filled environment (Bauman et al., 1991).

Effects on the Maternal-Fetal System

Effects on the Mother

Cigarette smoke contains more than 2,000 pharmacologically active substances. Most of these chemical agents are in the gas phase of the smoke and include carbon monoxide, nitrous oxide, cyanide, and other compounds. Only a small number of these compounds, such as nicotine and hydrocarbon products, are found in the minute particles of cigarette smoke (Surgeon General's Report, 1979; Cook et al., 1990; Council on Scientific Affairs, 1990).

Physiologic Effects. Nicotine is the most researched substance in cigarettes. This compound is readily absorbed by the lungs and is considered to be primarily responsible for the pharmacologic and physiologic effects of smoking. Blood nicotine levels vary according to the duration and intensity of inhalation, number of inhalations per cigarette, brand of cigarette, and presence or absence of filters (Cook et al., 1990; Warner, 1989). Nicotine is known to cross the placenta, but its effects on the fetus are primarily indirect through maternal vasoconstriction and reduced oxygen availability due to the release of catecholamines from peripheral nerve cells and adrenal glands (Kleinman et al., 1987; Floyd et al., 1991).

Smoking has been implicated in cardiovascular disease (Warner, 1989; Surgeon General's Report, 1979). The vasoconstrictors, norepinephrine and epinephrine, are increased within 2.5 minutes of smoking one cigarette. This is reflected in an increase in maternal pulse and blood pressure, followed by an increase in fetal heart rate. Cigarette smoke also contains carbon monoxide, which combines with hemoglobin to form carboxyhemoglobin. Levels of this substance may be three to eight times higher than normal in smokers, impairing oxygenation in the woman and the fetus. Noxious by-products of smoke also are transmitted through breast-feeding (Lieberman et al., 1994; Floyd et al., 1991; Fingerhut et al., 1990; Fox et al., 1990).

In addition to vasoconstriction and reduced oxygen availability, smoking interferes with the metabolism of several minerals, including calcium; a variety of vitamins; hormones; glucose; fatty acids; and amino acids. Malabsorption of these is reflected in the mother's nutritional status and eventually in her fetus (Aronson et al., 1989).

Pregnancy Outcomes. The literature reflects a heightened awareness of the substantial effects of smoking on pregnancy. Most of the studies deal with the effect on the fetus and infant rather than on the mother. Research has shown that the duration of pregnancy is shorter when the mother is a smoker. Up to 14% of all preterm deliveries in the United States may be attributable to maternal smoking. Also, an increase in the level of smoking is associated with an increase in the frequency of early fetal and neonatal death due to premature delivery. In turn, these deaths are associated with smoking-related increases in the incidence of bleeding during pregnancy, abruptio placentae, placenta previa, and premature and prolonged rupture of membranes (Adams et al., 1988; Floyd et al., 1991).

Placental abnormality and dysfunction also have been associated with smoking. There is evidence that smoking reduces placental blood flow and plasma volume and leads to artificially elevated hematocrit. The intervillous spaces of the placenta are larger in smokers, and serum concentrations of human placental lactogen, which is an indicator of the metabolic activity of the placenta, are lower in smokers. Toxicity and placental ischemia also occur as consequences of nicotine-induced constriction of the uterine vessels (Aaronson et al., 1989; Adams et al., 1988; Fried et al., 1990; Dicker et al., 1994).

A relationship has been shown between maternal smoking during pregnancy and the risk of spontaneous abortion. However, this relationship is less clear and has received much less study than that of smoking and intrauterine growth retardation (IUGR). In addition, the relationship of gestation to abortion is unclear (Kleinman et al., 1987; Cook et al., 1990; Lieberman et al., 1994).

Research indicates that all the associations with smoking cannot be related solely to intrauterine exposure. The data, although not definitive, suggest that the effect of smoking may be cumulative (ie, if a woman does not smoke in a current pregnancy but did at previous times in her life and in other pregnancies, the current fetus may still be affected; Kleinman et al., 1987; Zuckerman, 1988; Albrecht et al., 1994; Box 34-1).

Effects on the Infant

Recent evidence, based on prospective studies and other well-designed research, has substantiated the fact that fetal size, growth, and mortality are related to maternal cigarette smoking.

Stillbirth. According to the U.S. Public Health Service, approximately 4,600 stillbirths each year in the United States are attributable to smoking. Research indicates that there is a 30% higher rate of stillbirths among women who smoke than among those who do not. These women also have a 26% higher rate of perinatal mortality. Quitting during pregnancy improves the rate significantly. However, for previous heavy smokers, the rate is still not as good as for nonsmokers (Adams et al., 1988; Zuckerman, 1988; Fox et al., 1990; Floyd et al., 1991).

Low Birth Weight. A positive association between maternal cigarette smoking and reduced newborn birth weight (in the range of 150–200 g) emerges from every study of these two characteristics. The hypothesis that the relationship between smoking and weight reduc-

---

BOX 34–1
Effects of Smoking on Mother and Infant

Mother	Infant
Addiction to nicotine	Low birth weight
Vasoconstriction	Stillbirth
Catecholamine release	Sudden infant death syndrome
Cardiovascular disease	
Vitamin and mineral interference	Congenital malformations
	Allergies
Placental dysfunction	Respiratory morbidity
Contamination of breast milk	Growth, cognitive, and language deficits

tion in the newborn is one of cause and effect is supported by several types of evidence. For instance, this relationship has been consistently observed in a wide variety of populations differing by geographic location, race, and socioeconomic circumstances. Furthermore, there is an inverse relationship between mean birth weights and the number of cigarettes smoked during pregnancy, an evident dose-response effect (Kleinman et al., 1987; Surgeon General's Report, 1979; Fox et al., 1990). Studies suggest that the reduction in birth weight of newborns of smokers is due primarily to a decrease in the lean body mass of the newborn and that the deposition of subcutaneous fat is relatively unaffected. Studies also have shown that newborns of smokers have decreased birth length and decreased head circumference (Zuckerman, 1988; Fingerhut et al., 1990; Lieberman et al., 1994).

Sudden Infant Death Syndrome. Several studies have documented that maternal smoking significantly increases the likelihood of sudden infant death syndrome (SIDS; Aronson et al., 1989; Cook et al., 1990). Haglund et al. (1990) found that smoking doubled the risk of SIDS in his sample and seemed to influence the time of death because infants of smokers died at an earlier age than SIDS infants of nonsmokers.

Congenital Malformations. There is no clear-cut evidence of a relationship between smoking and congenital malformations. However, several studies have found persistent associations for congenital heart conditions, central nervous system (CNS) malformations, hypospadias, inguinal hernia, and eye and ear malformations (Aronson et al., 1989; Fried et al., 1990; Cook et al., 1990).

Respiratory Morbidity. There is growing evidence that children who were exposed prenatally to cigarette smoke are significantly more prone to allergies and bronchitis. Infants and children who share a household with smokers, particularly when the mother smokes, also suffer from a significantly higher rate of allergies, bronchitis, and other respiratory ailments (Rush et al., 1989; Neuspiel et al., 1989; Chassin et al., 1992). Girls suffer from more of these ailments than boys when the mother smokes. It is thought that this finding may be due to the possibility that mothers and female children share more activities in closer proximity (Moessinger, 1989; Bauman et al., 1991; Kandel et al., 1994).

Growth and Development. The growth and development of newborns and infants may be affected by smoking. Although some studies are not controlled for the effects of other addictive substances, such as alcohol and drugs, investigators have found that newborns of smokers performed less well on the Brazelton Neonatal Behavioral Assessment Scale than newborns of nonsmokers (Flynn et al., 1992; Floyd et al., 1991). Fox et al. (1990) found that height and weight deficits of newborns of smokers were not overcome by 3 years of age, and the children of smokers who had quit smoking during pregnancy performed significantly better on the McCarthy Scales of Children's Abilities than did the children of mothers who continued smoking during their pregnancy. After controlling for a variety of confounding variables, Fried et al. (1990) found significant associations with poorer language development and lower cognitive scores at 36 and 48 months for children exposed to prenatal smoking.

The consistent weight of evidence indicates that maternal smoking during pregnancy increases the newborn's perinatal morbidity and mortality risk. Moreover, it interferes with maternal metabolism and the mother's cardiovascular system, which, in turn, affects the fetus. This risk increases directly with the number of cigarettes smoked, irrespective of the use of "reduced" tar and nicotine brands. In addition, the presence of other risk factors increases considerably the risks related to smoking.

Gillies et al. (1989) found that the main reasons pregnant women gave for smoking included those related to mood control (to relax, calm themselves, provide enjoyment, dispel boredom) and addiction. Older women admitted that addiction was the main reason for their smoking. Younger women who were single (especially divorced or separated), came from unskilled or semiskilled occupations, or had a husband or partner who was unemployed indicated that mood control was their main reason for smoking.

Nursing Process

The nurse can use the nursing process framework to assess the pregnant woman who smokes. Once a thorough assessment is performed, nursing diagnoses can be made. This information will help the nurse plan interventions that are specific to the woman's individual situation.

Assessment

A thorough lifestyle history must be included in the medical and obstetric history. This should include how long the woman has smoked, how many cigarettes a day she smokes, and any physical effects of smoking (eg, respiratory disease, cancer). The nurse also should ask the woman her reasons for smoking, if other members of her household smoke where she usually smokes, and if her smoking is associated with any specific behavior(s). The nurse should assess the woman's knowledge of the negative effects of smoking on herself and her growing fetus (Duncan et al., 1991).

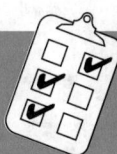

	Why Do You Smoke?				
	Always	Frequently	Occasionally	Seldom	Never
A. I smoke cigarettes to keep from slowing down.	5	4	3	2	1
B. Handling a cigarette is part of the enjoyment of smoking it.	5	4	3	2	1
C. Smoking cigarettes is pleasant and relaxing.	5	4	3	2	1
D. I light up a cigarette when I feel angry about something.	5	4	3	2	1
E. When I run out of cigarettes I find it almost unbearable until I can get them.	5	4	3	2	1
F. I smoke cigarettes automatically without even being aware of it.	5	4	3	2	1
G. I smoke cigarettes to stimulate me, to perk myself up.	5	4	3	2	1
H. Part of the enjoyment of smoking a cigarette comes from the steps I take to light up.	5	4	3	2	1
I. I find cigarettes pleasurable.	5	4	3	2	1
J. When I feel uncomfortable or upset about something, I light up a cigarette.	5	4	3	2	1
K. I am very much aware of the fact when I am not smoking a cigarette.	5	4	3	2	1
L. I light up a cigarette without realizing I still have one burning in the ashtray.	5	4	3	2	1
M. I smoke cigarettes to give me a "lift."	5	4	3	2	1
N. When I smoke a cigarette, part of the enjoyment is watching the smoke as I exhale it.	5	4	3	2	1
O. I want a cigarette most when I am comfortable and relaxed.	5	4	3	2	1
P. When I feel "blue" or want to take my mind off cares and worries, I smoke cigarettes.	5	4	3	2	1
Q. I get a real gnawing hunger for a cigarette when I haven't smoked for a while.	5	4	3	2	1
R. I've found a cigarette in my mouth and didn't remember putting it there.	5	4	3	2	1

How to Score

1. Write the number you have circled after each statement in the corresponding space below.
2. Total the scores in each column. For example, the sum of your scores A, G, M gives you your score for the first column.

A_____ B_____ C_____ D_____ E_____ F_____

G_____ H_____ I_____ J_____ K_____ L_____

M_____ N_____ O_____ P_____ Q_____ R_____

Column Totals   (1)_____ (2)_____ (3)_____ (4)_____ (5)_____ (6)_____

In this test examining reasons why you smoke, a score of 11 or above on any factor indicates that it is an important source of satisfaction for you. The higher you score (15 is the highest), the more important a particular factor is in your smoking. A low score on all the factors usually indicates that you do not smoke much or have not been smoking for many years. If so, giving up smoking—and staying off—should be easier.

1. Stimulation:

If you score high or fairly high on this factor, it means that you are one of those smokers who is stimulated by the cigarette—you feel that it helps wake you up, organize your energies, and keep you going. If you try to give up smoking, you may want a safe substitute, a brisk walk or moderate exercise, for example, when you feel the urge to smoke.

2. Handling:

Handling things can be satisfying, but there are many ways to keep hands busy without lighting up or playing with a cigarette. Substitute a favorite pen, piece of jewelry, or some other harmless object.

(continued)

ASSESSMENT TOOL (Continued)
Analysis of Smoking Behavior

How to Score

3. Accentuation of Pleasure—Pleasurable Relaxation:

Those who do get real pleasure out of smoking often find that an honest consideration of the harmful effects of their habit is enough to help them quit. They substitute social and physical activities and find that they do not seriously miss their cigarettes.

4. Reduction of Negative Feelings, or "Crutch":

Many smokers use the cigarette as a kind of "crutch" in moments of stress or discomfort. But the heavy smoker, the person who tries to handle severe personal problems by smoking many times a day, is apt to discover that cigarettes do not help in dealing with problems effectively. Stress management strategies are often helpful for this type of smoker, as are physical exertion and social activities.

5. Craving or Dependence:

Quitting smoking is difficult for the person who scores high on this factor. Going "cold turkey" usually works better for this type of smoker. Aversion strategies are often helpful for they serve to create negative mental images of smoking.

6. Habit:

If you are smoking out of habit, you no longer get much satisfaction from your cigarettes. Gradual reduction may be an effective strategy. The key to success is becoming aware of each cigarette smoked and asking, "Do I really want this cigarette?"

Government document. Reprinted with permission from U.S. Department of Health and Human Services. Oct. 1983 (revised). *A Self-Test for Smokers*. DHEW Publication No. (CDC) 75-8716. Washington, DC: U.S. Government Printing Office.

Nursing Diagnoses

Possible nursing diagnoses may include the following:

- Knowledge Deficit related to physiologic effects of smoking on self and fetus
- Risk for Injury related to effects of smoking

Planning and Intervention

The nurse should counsel the client at the first visit, particularly in the case of mothers with other risk factors. Health education is an essential part of prenatal care. Smoking is one behavior that is preventable and can be stopped (see Nursing Care Plan: The Pregnant Smoker). The nurse can be an appropriate role model for the mother and father or partner by not smoking, providing a smoke-free environment, and encouraging the mother to participate in a smoking cessation program (Flynn et al., 1992; Flewelling et al., 1992; Perry et al., 1992).

Smoking Cessation Programs for Pregnant Women.
Studies have found that smoking cessation programs tailored for the participant have the best "quit-and-stay-quit" rates. Gritz et al. (1988) evaluated self-help

smoking cessation programs geared toward nurses. They concluded that when nurses were given pamphlets that specifically addressed concerns nurses had (eg, weight control, managing break time, use of a "buddy support" system) in addition to other self-help materials and counseling, cessation rates compared favorably with other targeted self-help programs. Other researchers have found televised cessation programs, mass media, and saturation school programs to be effective. Cessation programs tailored specifically for the pregnant woman have been effective (Flynn et al., 1992; Perry et al., 1992; Warnecke et al, 1992; Windsor et al., 1993a; Windsor et al., 1993b).

Windsor (1985) found that including *The Pregnant Woman's Self-Help Guide to Quit Smoking* together with a 10-minute counseling session on health education skills and *Because You Love Your Baby* brought a much better quit rate in their clients than a general "how to stop smoking" manual.

Alexander (1987) outlined several factors the nurse should consider when suggesting a smoking cessation program for pregnant women.

- Analysis of smoking behavior as illustrated in the Assessment Tool: Analysis of Smoking Behavior also helps to educate the mother

NURSING CARE PLAN
The Pregnant Smoker

Nursing Goals

The pregnant smoker will stop smoking, at least for the duration of the pregnancy, as evidenced by the following:
1. Performing self-help activities to quit smoking
2. Securing needed resources for meeting support needs
3. Maintaining own health and health of fetus
4. Delivering a healthy term newborn without perinatal complications

Assessment	Potential Nursing Diagnoses	Rationale/ Intervention	Evaluation
Complete lifestyle history Analysis of smoking behaviors (see Assessment Tool) Social support, including spouse, family, and friends	Knowledge Deficit about the hazards of smoking for fetus and infant	Counsel regarding the benefits to fetus and infant with cessation of smoking (include second-hand smoke effects to the infant) *to increase knowledge base*.	Client states benefits of smoking cessation for the fetus and infant.
		Instruct regarding the effects of smoking on health *to increase knowledge base*.	Client states effects of smoking on health.
		Refer to smoking cessation programs to *support stopping smoking*.	Client attends smoking cessation program or implements a stop-smoking plan of her own.
		Counsel regarding hunger control, managing break time, avoiding smoking environments, brushing teeth after eating, changing routines, exercise *to increase knowledge and support client's efforts to quit*.	Client changes behaviors to assist with cessation of smoking.
		Refer to smoking cessation program or self-help program *to support quitting efforts*.	Client takes steps to stop smoking.
Vital signs Fetal heart tones Fundal height Baseline weight and weight gain or loss during pregnancy	Altered Placental Tissue Perfusion related to smoking	Record and closely follow blood pressure, pulse, fetal heart tones, fundal height, and weight *to monitor progress of pregnancy*.	Blood pressure and pulse remain within normal limits. Fetal heart tones remain within normal limits. Fundal height shows appropriate growth for gestational age. Client has adequate weight gain.
Glucose, amino acids, hematocrit, and hemoglobin		Follow glucose levels, amino acids, hematocrit, and hemoglobin.	Glucose levels, amino acids, hematocrit, and hemoglobin remain within normal limits.
		Follow ultrasound results for possible intrauterine growth retardation.	Fetus shows appropriate growth for gestational age.
Fetal heart tone and reactivity	Risk for Injury to fetus related to smoking effects	Record fetal heart tones *to monitor pregnancy progress*.	Fetal heart tones remain within normal limits.

(continued)

NURSING CARE PLAN *(Continued)*
The Pregnant Smoker

Assessment	Potential Nursing Diagnoses	Rationale/ Intervention	Evaluation
Vaginal bleeding or leaking fluid		Counsel regarding signs and symptoms of spontaneous abortion, preterm labor, premature rupture of membranes, abruptio placentae, and placenta previa *to increase knowledge base.*	Client describes signs and symptoms of spontaneous abortion, preterm labor, premature rupture of membranes, abruptio placentae, and placenta previa.
Presence of preterm uterine contractions Fetal movement		Instruct client regarding counting fetal movements, palpation and timing uterine contractions, determining leaking membranes or vaginal bleeding, knowing when to call the doctor *to increase knowledge base and promote self-care behaviors.*	Client counts fetal movements, palpates and times contractions, observes for leaking membranes or vaginal bleeding, and calls the doctor when appropriate.

- Elicitation of social support by means of a buddy system or spousal and family support
- Self-help efforts as described in reading material targeted to pregnant women
- Stimulus control components, such as avoiding or leaving an environment where smoking takes place, brushing teeth after eating, changing routines, exercising
- Gradual reduction in smoking; questionable for some people; best option for most people, quit "cold turkey"

Evaluation

Cessation of smoking in the pregnant client is the goal of nursing intervention. However, the nurse should not be discouraged if the client does not quit cold turkey or has relapses after stopping initially. Nursing interventions also are successful if the client keeps her prenatal appointments and reduces the number of cigarettes smoked per day. The client's knowledge of the harmful effects of smoking on the maternal and fetal systems should be evaluated. Whether the client has social support also should be determined. The nurse should evaluate to what extent the client has participated in a smoking cessation program and whether or not the client has implemented

any behavioral changes that were formerly associated with smoking.

Alcohol Abuse

Concern about the effects of parental alcohol consumption at the time of conception and during pregnancy is not new. Epidemiologic and experimental research on maternal drinking and perinatal outcomes accumulated in the 1900s. However, Prohibition in the 1920s caused a virtual shutdown of research activity, and the early studies that were not lost or destroyed were rejected as too primitive. In 1968, Lemoine et al. first described a syndrome that occurred in the infants of alcoholic women. In 1973, Jones and Smith coined the term **fetal alcohol syndrome** (FAS) to define a pattern of prenatal and infant growth deficiency, developmental delay or mental retardation, microcephaly, fine motor dysfunction, and a characteristic facial dysmorphology in infants of mothers who drank heavily (Jones et al., 1973; Box 34-2). Since that time, the thousands of clinical, epidemiologic, and experimental studies on the topic have shown that ethanol and its metabolites have the potential to alter the growth and development of the embryo and fetus (Weiner et al., 1988; Jessup, 1990; Cook et al., 1990). As research evidence continues to grow, the terms *fetal alcohol effects* (FAE) and *alcohol-related birth defects* (ARBD) have been coined to differentiate the syndromes more specifically (Jessup, 1990).

Although the minimum dose of alcohol that produces FAS is still unclear, a woman does not have to be an alcoholic to place her newborn at risk for FAS. Defining what constitutes alcoholism and alcoholics is often a problem because amount and frequency of drinking are not the only criteria. Many investigators and clinicians believe that the way alcohol affects the person, both physiologically and affectively, irrespective of the amount or timing of drinking, is an essential additional criterion (Jessup, 1990; Healy, 1986; Pietran-

toni et al., 1991). However, women who are chronic alcoholics run a much higher risk of having defective newborns. Researchers have found that women who drink 2 to 4 oz of hard liquor per day run a 10% risk of having an abnormal child. Women who drink 4 oz or more per day have a 19% risk. Even if the average daily consumption is less than 2 oz, risk is still present (Fig. 34-1; Chasnoff, 1986; Pietrantoni et al., 1991).

There is little conclusive evidence regarding the effects of paternal drinking on childbearing, although the research is not well developed. The evidence is also inconclusive for other types of drug use, although evidence is accumulating slowly as better studies are being designed.

Effects on the Maternal–Placental–Fetal System

Effects on the Mother

The effects of **ethanol** on humans are well known. For those who are not alcoholics, there is a feeling of general CNS stimulation, relaxation, mild euphoria, vasodilation, and well-being when alcohol is taken in small to moderate amounts. However, alcohol is a CNS depressant, and the initial effects soon wear off and may be replaced with symptoms associated with CNS depression. Judgment is impaired even in the euphoria stage, and if drinking continues, motor responses and other physiologic responses, such as loss of concentration, mood alteration, nausea, headache, and sleepiness, can occur. Stupor, coma, and death may occur if dosage is sufficient. For chronic alcoholics and even for people who drink moderate amounts on a daily basis, there can be adverse nutritional effects, impulsive

FIGURE 34–1 Growth retardation and maternal drinking patterns. Growth retardation occurred among newborns of women who drank heavily throughout pregnancy significantly more frequently than among newborns of rare and moderate drinkers. No significant difference was found between newborns of moderate drinkers as compared with those of women who drank rarely. Neonates born to women who drank heavily early in pregnancy and reduced consumption before the third trimester were comparable to those born to rare and moderate drinkers. Similar findings were observed in the incidence of length and head circumference below the 10th percentile. Abnormalities were identified more frequently among newborns of women who continued drinking heavily. These associations were independent of the eight variables thought to influence fetal growth and development: maternal age, parity, ethnicity, cigarette smoking, marijuana use, prepregnancy weight, baby's sex, and gestational age.

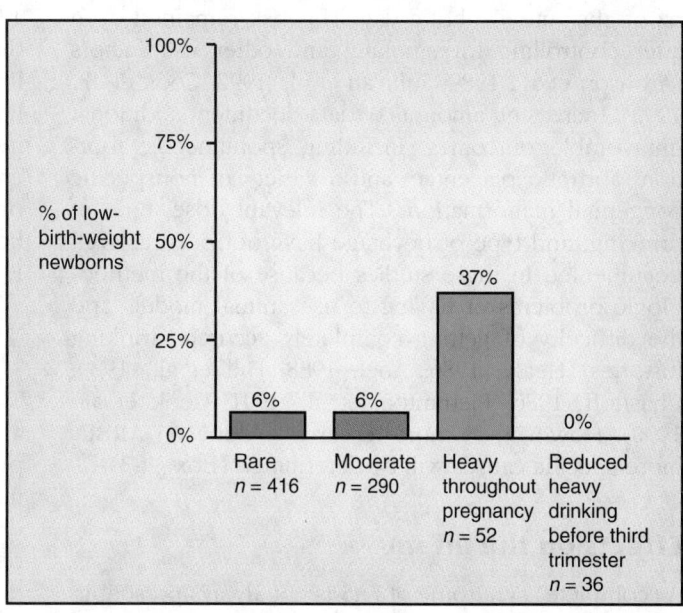

behavior, impaired judgment, and family, occupational, and social problems (Healy, 1986; Eward et al., 1986; Chasnoff, 1986; Pietrantoni et al., 1991).

Physiologic Effects. Ethanol alters maternal physiology, directly and indirectly affects the maternal–placental–fetal system, and causes detrimental effects on fetal growth development. Vitamin transport and absorption and carbohydrate, protein, and lipid metabolism are disrupted. Ethanol is toxic to the cells of the brain, liver, pancreas, and other organs. The central nervous, cardiovascular, and gastrointestinal systems are placed at particular risk. Cognitive and affective functions also suffer due to the toxicity and destruction alcohol produces in the CNS (Chasnoff, 1986; Pietrantoni et al., 1991).

It is difficult to discuss effects on the mother without considering the impact on the fetus. Ethanol and its metabolite, acetaldehyde, are transported across the placenta where ethanol's biochemical and pathophysiologic effects alter fetal development by disrupting cell differentiation and growth. Alcohol-induced alterations in maternal physiology and in the intermediate metabolism of carbohydrates, proteins, and fats can alter the environment in which the fetus develops. Chronic exposure to high doses of alcohol interferes with the passage of amino acids across the placenta and their incorporation into proteins. FAS results from the cumulative actions of high blood alcohol concentration on the maternal–placental–fetal systems throughout pregnancy (Weiner et al., 1988; Pietrantoni et al., 1991).

Pregnancy Outcomes. Additional pregnancy outcomes besides FAS result from consuming alcohol. Several studies have reported increased stillbirths, low–birth-weight newborns, and lower placental weights for newborns of mothers who consumed greater than 1.6 oz of absolute alcohol a day. This risk remained even after controlling for smoking and other risk factors (Aronson et al., 1989; Sullivan et al., 1992; Cook et al., 1990). Increasing amounts of data document additional unfavorable outcomes, including spontaneous abortion, abruptio placentae, and a variety of nonspecific congenital malformations. The relevant dose, time of drinking, and type of beverage have not been as well documented in these studies because of the methodologic problems of having to use animal models and the difficulty of getting completely accurate drinking histories (Healy, 1986; Abel, 1988; Hill et al., 1989; Chasnoff, 1986; Pietrantoni et al., 1991; Cook et al., 1990). However, as more research is done on ARBD, more specific causes will be determined (Box 34-3).

Effects on the Infant

A "complete" syndrome of FAS is not always present in infants. Children whose mothers drank only occasion-

---

BOX 34–3
Effects of Alcohol on Mother and Infant

Mother	*Infant*
Possible alcohol addiction	Low birth weight
Interference with carbohydrate, fat, and protein metabolism	Disruption of cell growth and differentiation
Spontaneous abortion	Nonspecific abnormalities
Placental abnormalities and dysfunction: low weight, abruptio, previa	Fetal alcohol syndrome

---

ally, drank intermitently during pregnancy, or drank only "small amounts" (<2 oz/d) daily may be born with only one or a few of the conditions associated with FAS (Weiner et al., 1988; Chasnoff, 1986; Hill et al., 1989; Pietrantoni et al., 1991). These children would be diagnosed as having FAE or ARBD.

Variability also occurs in the extent of the abnormalities seen in children exposed as fetuses. An estimated 2% to 10% of alcohol-complicated pregnancies produce children with FAS; another 30% to 40% of these children have some effects. Differences appear due to the mediating factors of dose levels, chronicity of alcohol use, gestational age, duration of exposure, and sensitivity of fetal tissue (Weiner et al., 1988; Box 34-4).

Abel (1988) conducted a retrospective study of the clinical literature on siblings of FAS clients and found that the disorder was present in 170 of 1,000 older siblings; however, it was found in 771 of 1,000 younger siblings. The risk for FAS in the general population is 1.9 per 1,000 births; therefore, these findings clearly indicate the high risk of FAS among siblings if one sibling is diagnosed with FAS. In addition, subsequent siblings had increasingly greater numbers of symptoms, indicating that the mother continued and probably increased her drinking irrespective of the known effect on her children. This reinforces the point that alcoholism is a chronic, progressive disease (Abel, 1988; Hill et al., 1989).

Assessment and Management

The family and others around the problem drinker or alcoholic, called codependents, may have their own problems of attempting to control the situation and may lose their sense of self amidst the problems of the drinker (Jessup, 1990). Health professionals also can be codependent, ignore the signs and symptoms of the disease, and minimize the seriousness of the client's drinking problem (Healy, 1986; Smith, 1992; Yates et

BOX 34-4
Mediating Factors in Type and Extent of Infant Abnormalities

Dose

- Alcohol passes through placental membranes easily in both directions dependent on blood alcohol concentration (BAC) gradient of the mother.
- Fetal alcohol metabolism depends on mother's ability to metabolize alcohol.
- With continuous drinking and steady maternal BAC, difference between maternal and fetal BAC is small.
- Dose–response relationship: greatest risk (multiple deformities and disorders) = >3 oz absolute alcohol per day (six standard drinks).
- Dose *plus* chronicity of drinking = most severely affected.

Gestational Age

- Organ systems are most vulnerable at the time of their most rapid cell division.
- First trimester: high concentrations disturb cell membranes and migration, causing morphologic abnormalities.
- Throughout pregnancy: disturbance of carbohydrate, lipid, and protein metabolism and RNA and DNA synthesis causes retardation of cell growth and division.
- Third trimester: disturbs rapid brain growth and neurophysiologic organization, causing impaired central nervous system growth and development and limiting future intellectual and behavioral capacities.

Genetic Susceptibility

- Genotype partially determines growth and morphology's susceptibility to alcohol effects.
- Some (undetermined in humans) genotypes appear more affected (ie, fraternal twins = both affected by heavy daily maternal drinking, but one much more markedly).

(Weiner, L., & Morse, B. D. [1988]. Fetal alcohol syndrome: Clinical perspectives and prevention. In I. J. Chasnoff (Ed.), Drugs, alcohol, pregnancy and parenting. Boston: Kluwer Academic Publishers.)

al., 1994). At least 8 to 10 out of every 100 women of childbearing age have an alcohol problem. Therefore, knowledge of the disease and awareness of the possibility of the health provider's own codependency issues will help to clarify clinical standards of practice (Midanik et al., 1994; Robbins et al., 1993). A nurse who has the disease in his or her own family may find that working with the alcoholic person arouses feelings of anxiety, fear, or anger. **Al-Anon**, the self-help group for friends and family of people who have drinking problems, is an appropriate resource for the nurse who is dealing with these feelings (Jessup, 1990; Hinderliter et al., 1993; Smith, 1992).

Nursing Process

As with other clients, the nurse uses the nursing process to assess, plan, and implement care for mothers who may be drinking. It is particularly important that the assessment and diagnosis stages be carried out meticulously. If a woman is suspected or proven to be a problem drinker or alcoholic, counseling and referral are a large part of the planning and intervention stages.

Assessment

If the nurse suspects or discovers that the client has a drinking problem or drinks moderately but consistently, the nurse must explore the client's reasons for drinking. At times, the client's age or lifestyle may be such that social drinking is expected. In this case, the woman may not realize the impact of her behavior on her fetus, especially if the woman is young or emerging from adolescence (Huselif et al., 1992). The effects of FAS should be clearly explained, and various counseling and assistance avenues can be used.

Alcohol problems in a family have been conceptualized as intrafamilial stressful events. The application of the McCubbin Double ABX model, described in Chapter 16, is useful in helping the nurse to make an assessment of family functioning (Captain, 1993).

The Ten-Question Drinking History (TQDH), developed and incorporated into Boston City Hospital's prenatal clinic records, has excellent test and retest reliability and provides a short, efficient tool for reliable assessment (see Assessment Guidelines: Ten-Question Drinking History; Weiner et al., 1988). Weiner et al. (1988) recommend that separate, direct questions be asked about the amounts of consumption in the three categories (TQDH). When the questions are asked in a direct, nonjudgmental fashion, most clients accept the nurse's concern and respond as honestly as they can. Clients who answer evasively should be calmly and firmly engaged in further discussion. Defensive reactions often indicate an alcohol problem.

The TQDH is not the only instrument developed to assess drinking behavior accurately, nor is a structured tool the only way to obtain a drinking history. Open-ended, probing questions also are extremely helpful. However, they require more time per interview, and the interviewer must be skilled in interviewing techniques.

Box 34-5 provides signs and symptoms for the nurse to observe. This and the TQDH or a similar tool can form the backbone of thorough assessment and provide a basis for diagnoses. Jessup (1990) suggests that the indicators for alcohol abuse or dependence also can be used to help make the mother aware of some of her own behaviors.

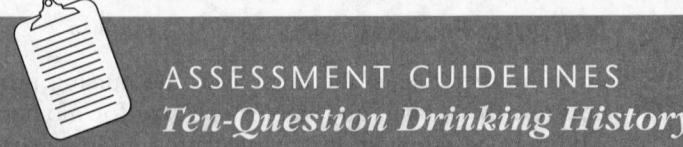

ASSESSMENT GUIDELINES
Ten-Question Drinking History

Beer	How many times per week?
	How many glasses each time?
	Ever drink more?
Wine	How many times per week?
	How many glasses each time?
	Ever drink more?
Liquor	How many times per week?
	How many glasses each time?
	Ever drink more?

Has your drinking habit changed during the past year?

(Weiner, L., & Morse, B. A. [1988]. Fetal alcohol syndrome: Clinical perspectives and prevention. In I. J. Chasnoff [Ed.], Drugs, alcohol, pregnancy and parenting. *Boston: Kluwer Academic Publishers.)*

Nursing Diagnoses

Nursing diagnoses are based on the information elicited during the assessment. Possible nursing diagnoses may include the following:

- Altered Family Process: Alcoholism
- Altered Health Maintenance
- Risk for Violence: Self-directed or directed at others
- Knowledge Deficit concerning the effects of alcohol on self and fetus
- Risk for Injury related to alcohol use
- Risk for Trauma related to alcohol use

Planning, Intervention, and Rationale

Intervention for the problem drinker or alcoholic is a process whereby the drinking woman is no longer supported to drink, but is supported to begin recovery. Female alcoholics tend to drink in isolation and deny they have a problem. When open and honest discussion of the alcohol problem occurs between the nurse and the client, the "conspiracy of silence" is challenged, and the client and healthcare team can address the problem appropriately (Jessup, 1990). After the problem is admitted and confronted, the nurse and the client should classify the drinking problem and plan treatment strategies appropriate to the classification (see Nursing Guidelines: Intervention Process for Problem Drinking and Dependence).

Weiner et al. (1988) suggest a three-phase classification of problem drinking, which has been helpful in

designing treatment strategies. The classification is based on motivating factors, rather than on quantity or frequency of drinking (see Client Teaching Guidelines: Classification of Problem Drinking). Although the phases are not invariably progressive, most clients move from one to the next if help is not received. This is because alcohol addiction is progressive. Not all clinicians, particularly those whose specialty is treatment of addictive behaviors, would classify the problem drinker differently from the alcoholic. However, this classification method is a useful treatment strategy to help the nurse refer and counsel.

Treatment and Rehabilitation Programs. Treatment of alcoholism and problem drinking consists of extensive assessment, counseling, and participation in an outpatient, inpatient, or residential program and involvement in self-help, 12-step programs (eg, Alcoholics Anonymous, Al-Anon, Al-Ateen). Involvement in self-help, 12-step programs can create a sober support system for the recovering alcoholic mother and provide her with ongoing role models, particularly after she has received institutional and professional help (Jessup, 1990; Robbins et al., 1993; Weiner et al., 1988).

Evaluation

When the woman returns for subsequent visits, the nurse should ask her questions to determine how she is progressing. Using the TQDH (or similar tool) and the indicators of alcohol abuse or dependence chart

BOX 34–5
Indicators of Alcohol Abuse and/or Dependence

Medical Indicators

Liver disease

Pancreatitis

Hypertension

Gastritis, esophagitis

Hematologic disorders

Poor nutritional status

Cardiac arrhythmias, other cardiac disease

Alcoholic myopathy

Ketoacidosis

Neurologic disorders

Intrauterine growth retardation

Historical Indicators

Depressive disorder

Psychiatric treatment or hospitalization

Reference to alcohol (or other drug)-abusing partner

Physician prescription or other procurement of psychoactive drugs

Multiple emergency room visits

Complicated perinatal history

Low birth weight

Prematurity

Fetal alcohol syndrome or fetal alcohol effects

Foster or other caretaker placement of another child

Learning disability or hyperactivity in another child

Behavioral Indicators

Smell of alcohol on breath

Mood swings

Memory lapses or losses

Difficulty concentrating

Blackouts

Inappropriateness

Irritability or agitation

Depression

Slurry speech

Staggering gait

Bizarre behavior

Loss of job

Decreased job performance

Suicidal feelings, gestures, or attempts

Sexual dysfunction

Conflicts with spouse, family, or friends

Domestic violence

Child abuse and neglect

Automobile accidents or citation arrests

Children with scholastic or behavioral problems

Secretiveness or vagueness about personal or medical history

(Jessup, M., & Green, J. [1987]. Treatment of the pregnant alcohol-dependent woman. Journal of Psychoactive Drugs, 19*(2), 16.)*

NURSING GUIDELINES
Intervention Process for Problem Drinking and Dependence

1. Expression of concern
   - Discuss concern about continued drinking in a nonjudgmental manner.
2. Presentation of consequences
   - Make use of the powerful motivator of mother's sense of responsibility for a new life.
   - Present consequences of drinking and options open to the mother in as positive terms as possible. Women respond positively to a hopeful message of potential benefits of drinking cessation. Avoid provoking guilt and self-criticism because these can result in increased alcohol consumption.
3. Referral for treatment
   - Use inpatient and outpatient detox and rehabilitation programs.
   - Use self-help, 12-step programs (Alcoholics Anonymous, Al Anon).

may be helpful. Abstinence indicates successful counseling. Strong indicators of continued drinking include failure to return for follow-up visits and evasiveness about drinking activity. However, if the woman is attending a 12-step program, she may be influenced in her drinking patterns and become sober eventually. The nurse should use all means available for follow-up.

Drug Abuse

Drug use during pregnancy is associated with devastating effects on the mother and the infant. Health professionals, social services, and public health agencies are inundated with infants showing the effects of their mother's drug use (Chasnoff, 1988; Day et al., 1991; Lake et al., 1992). Health professionals must realize that when dealing with a drug-addicted mother, they will eventually be dealing with either a drug-exposed or a drug-addicted infant (Dicker et al., 1994; Evans et

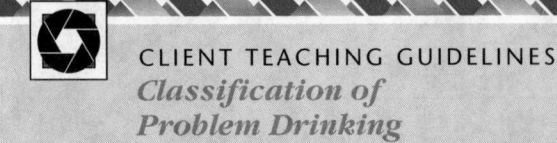

CLIENT TEACHING GUIDELINES
Classification of Problem Drinking

Social problem drinking: an essential ingredient in marriage and social life. Social networks pressure to drink. Alcohol used to alleviate boredom. Brief, supportive counseling and information help stop drinking at least for pregnancy. Referral to agencies and self-help, 12-step groups most important.

Symptom problem drinking: alcohol used to relieve wide range of psychological symptoms (fear, anger, depression, confusion, self-blame) and to alter mood and perception. Pregnancy activates fears, conflicts, and ambivalence about self and ability to mother. Realistic discussion of fears and conflicts with repetition of information about pregnancy and the birth process is needed. These women need extensive counseling and support regarding social problems and pregnancy and referral to self-help, 12-step programs.

Alcohol dependence (alcoholism): physiologic and psychological tolerance and dependence has developed (addiction). Medical complications are apparent. Extensive assistance needed with medical problems and child care and social problems. Alcohol treatment centers, halfway houses, and Alcoholics Anonymous are absolutely essential for therapy and support.

(Weiner, L., & Morse, B. A. [1988]. Fetal alcohol syndrome: Clinical perspectives and prevention. In I. J. Chasnoff [Ed.], Drugs, alcohol, pregnancy and parenting. Boston: Kluwer Academic Publishers.)

al., 1991). In addition, the rising incidence of human immunodeficiency virus infection in women and infants is strongly associated with maternal and paternal drug use. All of these negative effects on the fetus caused by the woman's drug use have initiated legal cases concerning fetal abuse.

Despite the growing incidence of drug use during pregnancy, the effects on the mother and the infant, and the legal cases concerning fetal abuse, no professional group has become an advocate for this special population of substance abusers. Nurses are in an ideal position to assume this role.

Over-the-Counter and Prescription Drugs

Studies in the late 1970s evaluating drug use by women during pregnancy revealed that as many as 50% to 60% of women used some analgesic, and approximately 25% used sedative drugs during pregnancy. These women were receiving prenatal care, and the use of illicit drugs was rarely considered (Kaul et al., 1978; Chasnoff et al., 1984). In the early 1980s, Chasnoff et al. (1984) found that 3% of their mater-

nity clients at Prentice Women's Hospital and Maternity Center who were screened for routine prenatal care had sedative-hypnotics in their urine. However, women who abuse prescription and over-the-counter (OTC) drugs tend to mix these with illegal drugs. Therefore, it is difficult to get true prevalence figures. In addition, women who use drugs are likely to mix them with cigarettes, alcohol, and caffeine, all of which have known noxious effects on the woman and fetus (Aronson et al., 1989; Sobatka, 1989). The nurse should remember that many women feel that taking their "prescribed" drugs is really not abuse. They feel that because the doctor gave the drugs to them, they are safe and legal. However, many women who abuse prescription drugs shop physicians, hoard medications, and self-medicate (Isacson et al., 1988; Joffee et al., 1994).

Teratogenic effects are possible with any OTC or prescribed drugs under certain conditions. This is especially true if the woman who is abusing OTC or prescribed drugs is taking several combinations of drugs or drugs known to have teratogenic effects on the fetus (Bologna et al., 1990). Box 34-6 lists drugs and chemicals commonly used by pregnant women, and Table 34-1 lists common OTC and prescribed drugs known to have teratogenic effects on the fetus (Swonger et al., 1991; Koran, 1990a; Fig. 34-2).

Illegal Substances and Street Drugs

Women who use street drugs often have no idea what drugs they are taking. This is because street drugs are often mixed with substitute substances. Caffeine, pseudoephedrine, and phenylpropanolamine are often sold as amphetamine. Valium is passed off as methaqualone (Quaalude), and street tetrahydrocannabinol is almost always phencyclidine (PCP). PCP is a common substitute because it is widespread and inexpensive. Many street drugs also contain hazardous, inert contami-

BOX 34-6
Drugs and Chemicals Commonly Used by Pregnant Women

Antibiotics	Hair cosmetics	Sugar substitutes
Analgesic and anti-inflammatories	Antihistamines	Anthelmintics
Paints or solvents	Pediculocides	Laxatives
Cold medications	Psychotropics	Antiemetics
Pesticides	Corticosteroids	
	Contraceptives	

(Koran, G. [1990]. Teratogenic drugs and chemicals in humans. In G. Koran (Ed.), Maternal-fetal toxicology: A clinician's guide. New York: Marcel Dekker.)

TABLE 34–1
Some Potentially or Positively Teratogenic Drugs

Drug	Teratism
Accutane (isotretinoin)	Use is associated with congenital anomalies.
Alcohol	Regular use during pregnancy is associated with fetal alcohol syndrome and withdrawal syndromes at birth.
Androgens	Prolonged therapy with high doses during first 12 wk causes masculinization of the female fetus.
Antiepileptics	Phenytoin (Dilantin) may cause cleft palate and congenital heart anomalies. Teratogenicity also has been reported for phenobarbital, trimethadione, and primidone. Risk of teratogenicity has to be weighed against risk to fetus if woman has a seizure during pregnancy. Antiepileptics also cause vitamin K deficiency in fetus.
Antimicrobials	Tetracyclines compete with calcium in the developing fetal skeleton. They should not be used from the middle to the end of pregnancy. Ototoxic antimicrobials, such as gentamicin, streptomycin, and kanamycin, cross the placenta and may damage the fetal labyrinth. The fetal liver cannot metabolize chloramphenicol, and therefore its use in the mother can cause a "gray-baby syndrome." Sulfonamides given near term may cause jaundice in the neonate, but when given earlier in pregnancy, the fetus is protected from this effect by placental metabolism of bilirubin. Other teratogenic antimicrobials include isoniazid, novobiocin, quinine, chloroquine, and nitrofurantoin.
Antineoplastics	Methotrexate, mercaptopurine, cytosine arabinoside, and others have been noted to cause teratogenic effects, most frequently when used during the first trimester.
Antithyroid drugs	Hypothyroidism occurs in fetus.
Anxiolytics	No teratogenicity was found in a large study, but there have been isolated reports. Food and Drug Administration requires warning that use of anxiolytics (meprobamate and benzodiazepines) during the first trimester of pregnancy may increase risk of congenital malformations.
Digitoxin	This is harmful late in pregnancy.
Estrogens	Female offspring have higher risk of adenocarcinoma if exposed to estrogens in utero.
Glucocorticoids	Fetal abnormalities occur when given in large doses during pregnancy.
Iodide 131	This can destroy thyroid of fetus.
Magnesium sulfate	This drug, often used in preeclampsia, causes respiratory depression if used close to time of delivery.
Narcotics	Addiction in mother causes a withdrawal syndrome in the newborn at birth. Use near the time of delivery causes difficulty in initiating neonatal respiration that can be alleviated by administering a narcotic antagonist to the newborn.
Oral anticoagulants	Coumarins cross the placenta freely and may cause bleeding in the fetus. Coumarins given during the first trimester have been associated with fetal anomalies. Heparin can be used safely.
Oral hypoglycemics	These can cause profound hypoglycemia in the fetus. Should not be used during pregnancy. Insulin can be used instead because it does not cross the placenta.
Oxidant drugs	May cause hemolysis if fetus has G6PD* deficiency. Oxidant drugs include primaquine, nitrofurantoin, naphthalene, sulfonamides; chloramphenicol, and vitamin K.
Phenothiazines	These accumulate in the eye of the fetus and cause retinopathy.
Piperazine antihistamines	Meclizine and cyclizine are teratogenic, at least in animal studies.
Progesterone	Use by the mother during the first 12 wk may be associated with congenital anomalies or masculinization of the female genitalia.
Reserpine	This causes norepinephrine depletion, leading to respiratory distress, lethargy, bradycardia, and nasal stuffiness.
Ribavirin	Inhalation of vapor is associated with congenital anomalies.
Salicylates	Given late in pregnancy, salicylates may cause hypoprothrombinemia and fetal or neonatal hemorrhage. Salicylates compete with bilirubin for protein binding sites and may cause kernicterus.
Thiazide diuretics	Thiazides cross the placenta and are not recommended for routine use in pregnancy. The risks are unknown.
Tobacco	Use during pregnancy is associated with decreased birth weight and increased spontaneous abortions.
Vaccines	Live vaccines should be avoided during pregnancy because fetal infection may occur.
Vitamin C	Megadose may cause withdrawal scurvy in the newborn at birth.

*G6PD = glucose-6-phosphate dehydrogenase.

(From Swonger, A., & Matejski, N. [1991]. *Nursing pharmacology: An integrated approach to drug therapy and nursing practice* [2nd ed.]. Philadelphia: J.B. Lippincott; with permission.)

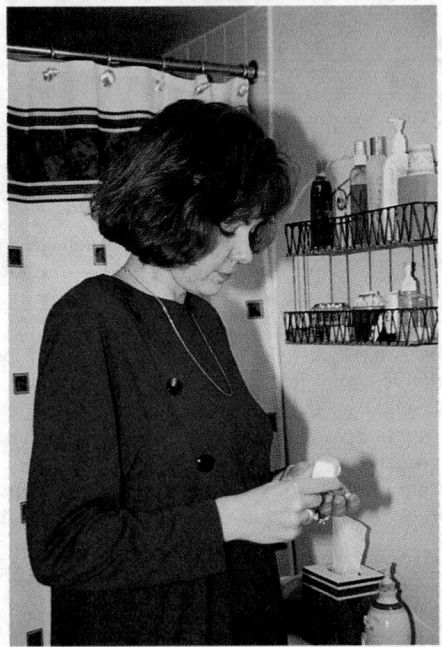

FIGURE 34-2 Pregnant women who use or abuse prescription or OTC drugs may be putting their fetus at serious risk. Teratogenic effects are possible with any prescribed or OTC drugs under certain conditions.

nants, such as sugar and talcum powder. Substitute drugs and contaminants are often teratogenic in their own right, cause teratogenic interactions, and pose difficult problems in getting accurate drug histories (Schnoll, 1986; Hoegerman et al., 1991).

One of the most addicting, dangerous drugs on the streets today is **cocaine**. This drug is widely used because it can be smoked, snorted, or injected. Crack, a derivative of cocaine, has become the nation's top drug concern (Jones, 1991; Kelleher et al., 1994). Cocaine has similar effects as other street drugs, and users appear to have similar characteristics. In a study comparing cocaine and heroin users, Hasin et al. (1988) found that cocaine-dependence indicators did not differ from heroin-dependence indicators among regular users. These abusers tended to be abusers of many drugs, in addition to alcohol, caffeine, and cigarettes. In addition, many pharmacologic, physiologic, and social effects were the same. Therefore, because it would be impossible to describe all of the effects of all abused drugs, cocaine will be used as the benchmark drug to describe the physiologic effects of drugs on the woman and subsequently, the fetus.

Effects on the Maternal–Placental–Fetal System

Effects on The Mother

The physiologic changes associated with pregnancy may significantly affect the way the body handles drugs. Therefore, pregnant women who use drugs put themselves and their fetus at risk.

Physiologic Effects. Two principal groups of changes characterize pregnancy and drug disposition:

■ Alterations in kinetics due to maternal changes
■ The effects of the placental–fetal compartment

Other important determinants of drug transport across the placenta are water and lipid solubility, molecular weight of the drug, and the surface area available for diffusion. The increase in maternal renal function and blood volume results in a decrease in protein binding because of the decrease in serum albumin concentration. This allows for easier passage of drugs across the placental–fetal compartment (Koran, 1990b).

The alkaloid cocaine, an odorless, crystalline powder, is readily absorbed through the mucous membranes and is a powerful, short-acting CNS stimulant similar to amphetamines. Cocaine reaches the brain and the neurons of the sympathetic nervous system in 3 minutes after being snorted, 15 seconds after intravenous administration, and 7 seconds after being smoked in a free base form (**crack**). Euphoria is rapid but short-lived (30 minutes; Lynch et al., 1990; Chasnoff, 1991).

Cocaine blocks presynaptic reuptake of norepinephrine and dopamine, producing an excess of these neurotransmitters at the postsynaptic receptor sites. This flood of neurotransmitters, combined with reduced reuptake in the cerebrocortex, hypothalamus, and cerebellum, results in a hyperaroused, extremely euphoric state equivalent to electric stimulation of the reward centers of the brain. Cocaine is highly addictive, and dependence is extremely difficult to break because the stimulation is so pleasurable. Because there is little physiologic withdrawal, there are many misconceptions about the drug, especially among young people. The initial euphoric rush soon tapers off and is replaced by dysphoria, irritability, impatience, pessimism, fatigue, and a strong desire for additional use of cocaine and other drugs (Lynch et al., 1990; Lindenberg et al., 1993).

Figure 34-3 summarizes the process by which cocaine affects the woman and fetus. Although other drugs use the same process with similar actions and effects, cocaine's extreme euphoric effect surpasses other substances (Lynch et al., 1990; Smith, 1988; Keith et al., 1989).

Pregnancy Outcomes. Many different pregnancy complications occur in mothers who use drugs, even drugs that are prescribed. As mentioned previously, many abusers are poly-abusers. Therefore, specific outcomes for specific drugs may be difficult to determine, even if the research is directed toward users of a specific substance. In general, research has shown a significant incidence of spontaneous abortion; maternal anorexia, with consequent fetal malnutrition; uteroplacental in-

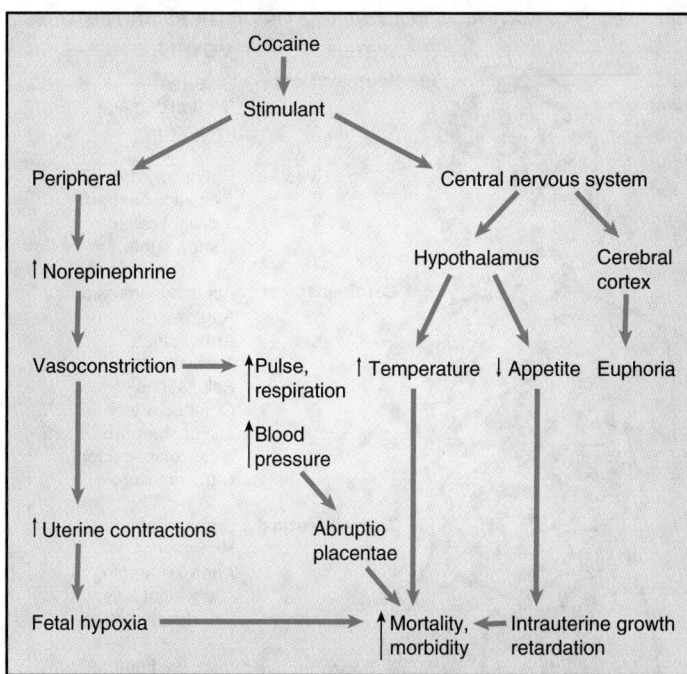

FIGURE 34–3 Physiologic effects of cocaine on the maternal–placental–fetal system. (Weiner, L., & Morse, B. A. [1988]. Fetal alcohol syndrome. Clinical perspectives and prevention. In I. J. Chasnoff (Ed.), *Drugs, alcohol, pregnancy, and parenting* [p. 138]. Boston: Kluwer Academic Publishers.)

sufficiency; intrauterine growth retardation; premature separation of the placenta and other placental abnormalities; hyperirritability of the uterus, leading to premature labor; and chorioamnionitis (Keith et al., 1989). Figure 34-4 illustrates the outcomes of cocaine abuse on the mother, fetus, and infant (Bologna et al., 1990; Fried et al., 1990).

Effects on the Infant

As with the mother, poly-abuse results in a variety of poor fetal outcomes. The mother's use affects multiple organ systems and consequent growth and development, including intellectual and learning ability. Low birth weight, CNS dysfunction, hyperirritability, developmental delay, SIDS, and learning disabilities are all associated with drug use by the mother (Hasin et al., 1988; Keith et al., 1989; Wilson, 1989; Jones, 1991; Bateman et al., 1993 (see Figure 34-4).

Assessment and Management

Along with causing physical and psychological harm to the woman and her fetus, substance use in pregnancy raises difficult ethical and legal questions. How can health professionals provide a safe intrauterine environment for the fetus and simultaneously respect the woman's right to privacy? Should infants and children be allowed to live with known substance users (Collins et al., 1994; Chavkin et al., 1991; Nyamathi, 1991; Campinha-Bacote et al., 1993).

Typically, a person's privacy was considered more important than the protection of the fetus. However, in a recent case in Illinois, two cocaine-using mothers

were held responsible for their infants' death and morbidity. The mother whose infant died due to cocaine-induced oxygen deprivation was charged with involuntary manslaughter. The other infant was removed from the mother's custody, and this mother was charged with child abuse and neglect. These cases represent a turn from the trend to protect the person's privacy to efforts to protect the fetus. The issues are volatile and are reviewed in most settings on a case-by-case basis. Nursing interventions require cautious, cooperative decision making (Lynch et al., 1990; Keith et al., 1989; Sullivan et al., 1993). The article by Pollitt listed in the suggested readings section at the end of this chapter provides an interesting perspective on these emerging dilemmas.

Perinatal nurses need to work with their institution's legal departments to develop policies that delineate each health provider's responsibilities when caring for women involved in substance abuse. Communication networks among health providers, especially nurses, need to be established so that expertise in dealing with these clients can be kept current and at maximum efficiency (Lynch et al., 1990; Chavkin et al., 1991).

Nursing Process

Assessment

The assessment and diagnosis stages must done carefully and thoroughly. The steps outlined for care of the alcoholic pertain to the drug user as well, because both are in the throes of an addictive, progressive disease.

A detailed drug and alcohol use history should be obtained, even if the mother does not exhibit the gross signs of substance abuse. Box 34-7 illustrates charac-

EFFECTS OF MATERNAL COCAINE USE ON MOTHERS AND FETUSES/BABIES

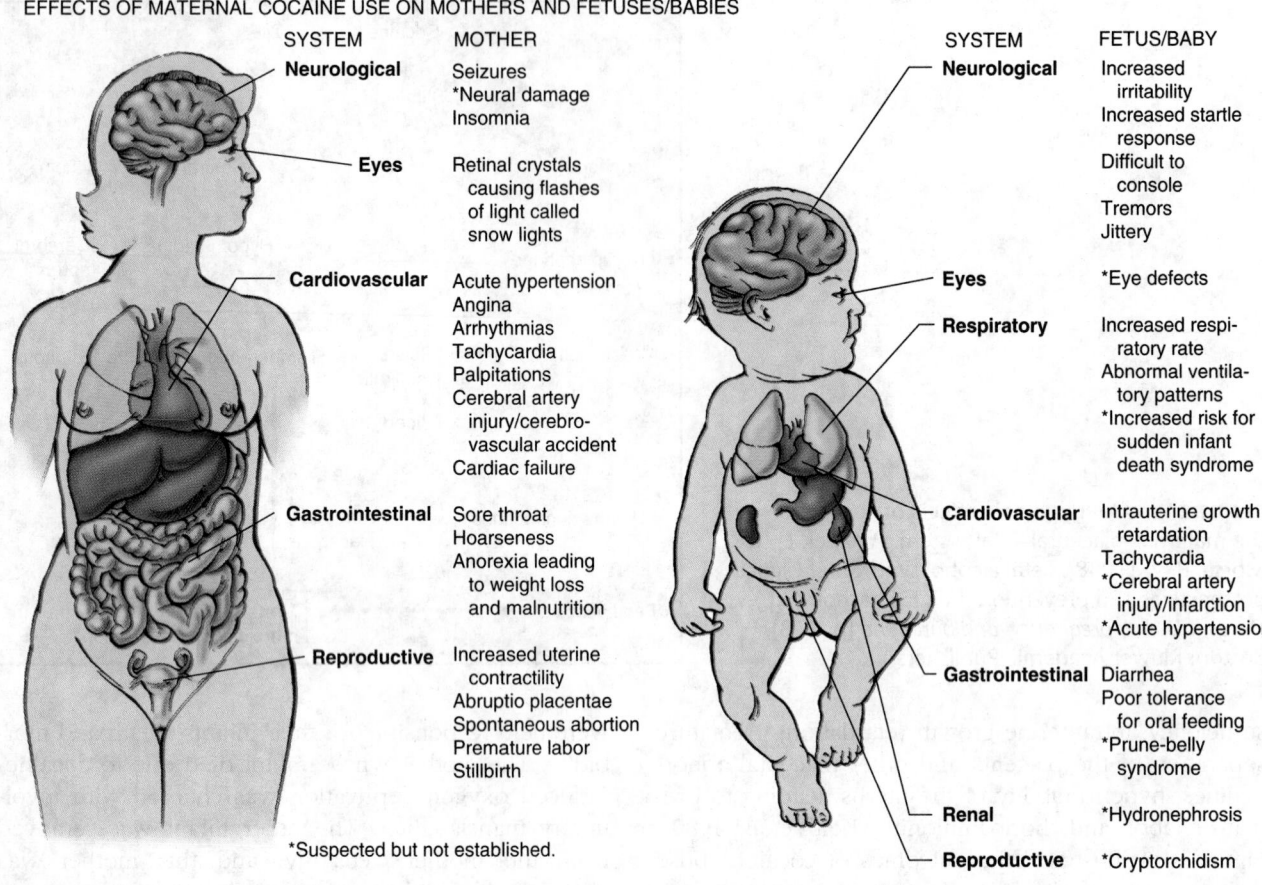

SYSTEM	MOTHER
Neurological	Seizures *Neural damage Insomnia
Eyes	Retinal crystals causing flashes of light called snow lights
Cardiovascular	Acute hypertension Angina Arrhythmias Tachycardia Palpitations Cerebral artery injury/cerebro- vascular accident Cardiac failure
Gastrointestinal	Sore throat Hoarseness Anorexia leading to weight loss and malnutrition
Reproductive	Increased uterine contractility Abruptio placentae Spontaneous abortion Premature labor Stillbirth

SYSTEM	FETUS/BABY
Neurological	Increased irritability Increased startle response Difficult to console Tremors Jittery
Eyes	*Eye defects
Respiratory	Increased respi- ratory rate Abnormal ventila- tory patterns *Increased risk for sudden infant death syndrome
Cardiovascular	Intrauterine growth retardation Tachycardia *Cerebral artery injury/infarction *Acute hypertension
Gastrointestinal	Diarrhea Poor tolerance for oral feeding *Prune-belly syndrome
Renal	*Hydronephrosis
Reproductive	*Cryptorchidism

*Suspected but not established.

FIGURE 34–4 Outcomes of cocaine abuse on mother, fetus, and infant.

BOX 34–7
Identifying Characteristics of the Substance Abuser

Physical Appearance and Demeanor

Client looks physically exhausted.

Pupils are extremely dilated or constricted.

Appearance of pregnancy fails to coincide with stated getational age.

Track marks, abscesses, or edema is visible in upper or lower extremities.

Nasal mucosae are inflamed or indurated.

Client is not well oriented.

Medical History

Acquired immunodeficiency syndrome

Cellulitis

Cirrhosis

Endocarditis

Hepatitis

Pancreatitis

Pneumonia

Obstetric History in Prior Pregnancies

Abruptio placentae

Fetal death

Low–birth-weight newborn

Meconium staining

Premature labor

Premature rupture of membranes

Sexually transmitted disease

Spontaneous abortion

In Current Pregnancy

Early contractions

Inactive or hyperactive fetus

Poor weight gain

Sexually transmitted disease

Spotting or vaginal bleeding

(Lynch, M., & McKeon, V. A. [1990]. Cocaine use during pregnancy. Journal of Obstetric, Gynecologic, and Neonatal Nursing, 19, *285–289.)*

teristics that indicate moderate to heavy substance abuse. The article by Hinderliter et al. (1993) in the suggested readings list provides effective assessment tools to identify alcohol and drug use in pregnant women in the prenatal care setting.

Because the use of illegal drugs is a legal problem, the nurse may have a judgmental attitude toward these clients. A concerned, nonjudgmental approach may enable the mother to feel more comfortable discussing her use of drugs. This information will then allow the nurse to make accurate diagnoses and plan appropriate interventions.

The nurse should remember that the mother does not have to be using "street drugs" to inflict harm on her infant. The client who is dependent on OTC and prescription drugs is also an addict; her use can have harmful effects on the maternal–placental–fetal system as well.

Nursing Diagnoses

Potential nursing diagnoses may include the following:

- Risk for Injury related to drug use
- Risk for Trauma related to drug use
- Knowledge Deficit related to effects of drug use on self and fetus
- Risk for Violence: Self-directed or directed at others

Intervention and Rationale

Most drug-using clients do not have early prenatal care. In fact, most of these clients delay seeing a healthcare professional until they feel that they are ready to deliver. They do this to avoid a long labor without drugs and to satisfy their need for a last "fix" before submitting to the confinement of the hospital. As a result, there is evidence that a substantial proportion of drug-abusing women deliver at home, in the ambulance, or on the stretcher (Silver et al., 1987; von Windeguth et al., 1989). If the mother is delivering in the hospital, however, the nurse should prepare immediately for high-risk conditions because the labor, birth, and newborn are all considered high risk. Addicts also tend to make considerable efforts to nourish their addiction during enforced periods of hospital confinement. A portion of these clients supplement their supply with barbiturates, tranquilizers, or cocaine (Lake et al., 1992; Reichett et al., 1990).

The nurse should remember that because many of these women are truly addicts and deteriorated, they may have lost nearly all of their material necessities. In addition, their moral sense, judgment, and cognitive functioning are often blunted or nonoperational. Care of these clients requires a multidisciplinary team, including a member who is skilled in identifying and treating the

medical problems frequently found in substance-abusing women (Lynch et al., 1990; Silver et al., 1987).

Therapy entails supporting the woman to start the recovery process while she is pregnant (Box 34-8). The nurse should meet with the mother on an ongoing basis whenever possible for prenatal checkups and to help the mother plan for labor and delivery. Written material should be used liberally because memory is often impaired, and advice and instructions may be quickly forgotten. Every effort should be made to determine, support, enhance, and teach parenting skills. Clear, concrete directions are necessary, and as with the alcoholic, reinforcement and reiteration regarding all phases of child care are necessary (see Nursing Care Plan: The Pregnant Substance Abuser).

Treatment and Rehabilitation Programs. If the woman seeks prenatal care, it is vital to refer her to a 12-step program (Narcotics Anonymous; Cocaine Anonymous). This is as crucial for the drug addict as for the alcoholic. Alcoholics Anonymous accepts drug-addicted clients because many recovering drug addicts have an alcohol addiction problem and vice versa. It is also important to get pregnant women started on withdrawal medications or therapy to limit any further complications. This may include using methadone treatment for heroin addicts. Although this treatment is controversial and may cause similar physiologic effects on the mother and the fetus, other risk factors associated with heroin use (including

---

BOX 34–8
National Resources for Drug Treatment

American Council for Drug Education
204 Monroe Street
Rockville, MD 20850

National Association for Perinatal Addiction Research and Education
11 E. Hubbard Street, Suite 200
Chicago, IL 60611

National Council for Drug and Alcohol Information
P.O. Box 2340
Rockville, MD 20857

National Institute on Drug Abuse
5600 Fishers Lane
Rockville, MD 20857

National Perinatal Association and Parent Care, Inc.
101½ South Union Street
Alexandria, VA 22314-3323

Office for Substance Abuse Prevention
Parklawn/Rockwall II
5600 Fishers Lane, 9th Floor
Rockville, MD 20857

NURSING CARE PLAN
The Pregnant Substance Abuser

Nursing Goals

The pregnant substance abuser completely stops all substance use for the duration of the pregnancy and thereafter as evidenced by the following:

1. Performing self-help activities to stop substance use
2. Securing needed resources for meeting support needs
3. Keeping medical appointments throughout pregnancy and for newborn after delivery
4. Delivering a healthy term newborn without perinatal complications
5. Maintaining her own health and health of fetus

Assessment	*Potential Nursing Diagnoses*	*Rationale/ Intervention*	*Evaluation*
Physical appearance and demeanor (see Boxes 34-5 & 34-7)	Knowledge Deficit related to effects of substance abuse on self, fetus, and infant	Establish a trusting, therapeutic relationship with the client, remaining non-judgmental *to encourage client receptiveness.*	Client discloses drug use and keeps medical appointments.
Medical history for opportunistic diseases (see Boxes 34-5 & 34-7)		Counsel regarding the benefits to the fetus, infant, and self with cessation of substance abuse *to increase knowledge base and support recovery.*	Client states benefits of cessation of substance abuse for fetus or infant and self and takes steps to stop substance abuse.
Obstetric history (see Boxes 34-5 & 34-7)			
Current problems of contractions, spotting, bleeding			
Weight gain or loss		Instruct regarding the effects of substance abuse on health *to increase knowledge base.*	Client states effects of substance abuse on health.
Sexually transmitted diseases			
Drinking history using 10-question drinking history (TQDH)		Refer to 12-step program *to support recovery.*	Client attends 12-step program.
Medications taken		Refer to inpatient and outpatient detox and rehabilitation programs as needed *to support recovery.*	Client admits herself to inpatient or outpatient detox or rehabilitation programs as needed.
Illicit drug use			
Support systems, including spouse, family, and friends			
		Encourage use of positive support systems *to assist the client to stop substance abuse and support recovery.*	Client uses positive support systems to stop substance abuse.
			Toxicology screens remain negative.
History of substance abuse (See Boxes 34-5 & 34-7 and TQDH)	Altered Parenting related to substance abuse	Refer to 12-step program or other rehabilitation group *to support recovery.*	Client attends and continues to participate in self-help programs.
Involvement and success of self-help programs		Involve spouse, family, and friends in infant care *to support mother in parenting skills.*	Support systems are actively involved in infant care.
Toxicology screening results			
Spousal, family, friends support		Encourage attendance at childbirth and infant care classes *to increase knowledge base and increase parenting skills.*	Client attends childbirth and infant care classes.
Current physical and emotional state		Counsel regarding withdrawal behaviors of infants and comfort measures to be used *to increase knowledge and prepare mother.*	Client recognizes withdrawal behaviors in infant and takes appropriate measures to comfort.
Involvement in prenatal care and childbirth classes			

(continued)

NURSING CARE PLAN *(Continued)*
The Pregnant Substance Abuser

Assessment	Potential Nursing Diagnoses	Rationale/ Intervention	Evaluation
Perception of parenting role		Discuss passage of drugs/alcohol through breast milk.	Client remains drug and alcohol free.
Desire for having and keeping the infant		Instruct regarding infant care *to increase parenting skills.*	Client gives appropriate care for the infant.
Knowledge of infant care			
		Refer to home health nurse for follow-up visits after birth *to monitor infant's progress.*	Home health nurse finds infant well cared for.
History of substance abuse (see Boxes 34-5 & 34-7 and TQDH)	Risk for Injury to fetus related to substance abuse effects	Refer to 12-step program.	Client participates in self-help program.
Involvement and success of self-help programs		Record fetal heart tones *to monitor fetal progress.*	Fetal heart tones remain within normal limits.
Toxicology screening results		Counsel regarding signs and symptoms of spontaneous abortion, preterm labor, premature rupture of membranes, abruptio placentae, and placenta previa *to increase knowledge.*	Client describes signs and symptoms of spontaneous abortion, preterm labor, premature rupture of membranes, abruptio placentae, and placenta previa.
Fetal heart tones and reactivity			
Presence of preterm uterine contractions			
Vaginal bleeding or leaking fluid			
Fetal activity			
Results of ultrasound			

malnutrition, sexually transmitted diseases, acquired immunodeficiency syndrome, abuse, and trauma) may be decreased because the woman is given a legal oral drug.

When a drug-addicted pregnant woman enters the hospital, withdrawal medication may be needed, and the client needs to be referred to appropriate inpatient and detoxification units. Box 34-9 summarizes the laboratory screens that are ordered for the mother. Many tertiary care hospitals have alcohol and drug abuse units. However, many are reluctant to take pregnant women because there are no perinatal care experts on staff routinely (Michaels et al., 1988; Lake et al., 1992). Hence, the nurse must be thorough in his or her referral, and the perinatal team must be aware of all options.

If the woman is in labor and drug use is recent, the goal is to stabilize the woman and fetus. The woman is placed in the left lateral recumbent position, given oxygen, and closely monitored. Seizure precautions and neurologic assessments are required if the woman is experiencing a cocaine-induced hypertensive episode. The nurse should maintain ongoing assessment of vital signs to detect any respiratory or cardiovascular impairment (Lynch et al., 1990; Smith, 1988; Michaels

et al., 1988) The use of the fetal monitor is imperative for these clients because they are extremely high risk. As stated previously, a high-risk addicted newborn is expected, and all necessary precautions are taken for his or her safety.

After a drug-addicted mother has given birth, it is important to encourage participation in self-help recovery groups. Inpatient treatment, when necessary, is also crucial. Participation in these programs may help to ensure the health, safety, and well-being of the mother and her newborn.

Evaluation

Reduction and cessation of drug use are indicators of successful intervention. However, recovery is a long process, and spectacular results are not readily seen. The nurse should not be discouraged if clients do not seem to respond dramatically. Often, an excellent indicator that the nurse is making an impact is if the woman keeps her prenatal appointments. For many addicts, a critical "bottoming out" must occur before she can accept her disease and begin recovery.

BOX 34–9
Laboratory Screening of the Pregnant Addict

Blood Work

Complete blood count with indices

α-Fetoprotein (if between 16 and 18 weeks' gestation)

Rubella titer

Blood type

Rh determination

Coombs' test

Sickle-cell preparation, if indicated

Urine Tests

Urinalysis

Culture

Toxicology

Screening for Infection

Chest x-ray

Tuberculin skin test

Hepatitis B antigen and antibody

Serology

Venereal disease reaction level

Fluorescent treponemal antibody (lues) test

Cervical culture for *Chlamydia trachomatis*

Human immunodeficiency virus antibody screen

Cervical-rectal cultures for *Neisseria gonorrhoeae*

Obstetric Screening

Ultrasound scan to confirm pregnancy after 6 weeks' gestation and serial scans for fetal measurement between 20 and 38 weeks' gestation

Cervical Pap smear

(I. J. Chasnoff [Ed.] [1986]. Drug use in pregnancy (pp. 7–16). Boston: MIP Press Limited.)

Summary Points

✔ The far-reaching impact of the addictive disorders of smoking, drinking, and drug abuse is staggering in terms of wasted human potential. Nurses need to develop methodologies and protocols to identify all substance abuse in the pregnant client and to establish protocols for primary, secondary, and tertiary intervention for the mother and her newborn.

✔ It is estimated that as many as 50% of pregnant women smoke (20%–30% of all childbearing women smoke) despite clear warnings of the adverse effects on themselves and their infants.

✔ Smoking during pregnancy has many adverse outcomes, including preterm delivery, intrauterine growth retardation, placental abnormality and dysfunction, premature rupture of the membranes, increased frequency of early fetal and neonatal death, and spontaneous abortion.

✔ Smoking also affects the infant adversely. Fetal size, growth, and mortality are all related to maternal cigarette smoking. Women who smoke have a 30% higher rate of stillbirths than their nonsmoking counterparts, and quitting during pregnancy improves the rate significantly. The positive association between maternal cigarette smoking and low birth weight is conclusive, irrespective of economic circumstances, social class, ethnicity, and education.

✔ The methodology for a smoking cessation program designed for pregnant women should include analysis of smoking behavior, elicitation of social support, self-help efforts, and exploration of gradual reduction versus total abstinence.

✔ Epidemiologic and experimental research on prenatal drinking and perinatal outcomes began accumulating in the 1900s and has culminated in the delineation of a syndrome of prenatal and infant growth deficiency, developmental delay, mental deficiency, and a characteristic facial dysmorphology, which has become known as FAS.

✔ Adverse pregnancy outcomes related to alcohol use and drug abuse include increased stillbirths, low–birth-weight newborns, lower placental weights, a higher incidence of spontaneous abortion and abruptio placentae, and a variety of nonspecific congenital anomalies.

✔ Research indicates that as many as 50% to 60% of pregnant women use some sort of analgesic, and 25% use sedatives during pregnancy. Street drugs and other illicit substances do greater damage to the woman and her fetus. Women who use drugs tend to be poly-abusers, often starting with prescribed drugs.

✔ Drug use (even if prescribed) during pregnancy causes a variety of adverse pregnancy complications, including an increased incidence of spontaneous abortion, maternal anorexia with fetal malnutrition, uteroplacental insufficiency, intrauterine growth retardation, premature separation of the placenta and other placental abnormalities, chorioamnionitis, and hyperirritability of the uterus, leading to premature labor.

✔ Adverse effects on the newborn include low birth weight, CNS dysfunction, hyperirritability, developmental delay, SIDS, impaired intellectual ability, and a variety of learning disabilities.

REFERENCES

Aaronson, L. S., & MacNee, C. L. (1989). Tobacco, alcohol and caffeine use during pregnancy. *Journal of Obstetric, Gynecologic, and Neonatal Nursing, 18*(4), 279–287.

Abel, E. L. (1988). Fetal alcohol syndrome in families. *Neurotoxicology and Teratology, 10,* 1–2.

Adams, E. H., Gfroerer, J. C., & Rouse, B. A. (1988). Epidemiology of substance abuse including alcohol and cigarette smoking. *Annals of the New York Academy of Science, 562*(6), 14–20.

Albrecht, S. A., Rosella, J. D., & Patrick, T. (1994). Smoking among low-income, pregnant women: Prevalence rates, cessation interventions, and clinical implications. *BIRTH, 31*(3), 155–162.

Alexander, L. (1987). The pregnant smoker: Nursing implications. *Journal of Obstetric, Gynecologic, and Neonatal Nursing, 16*(5), 167–173.

Bailey, S. L. (1992). Adolescents' multisubstance use patterns: The role of heavy alcohol and cigarette use. *American Journal of Public Health, 82*(9), 1220–1224.

Bateman, D. A., Ng, S. K. C., Hansen, A., & Heagarty, M. C. (1993). The effects of interuterine cocaine exposure in newborns. *American Journal of Public Health, 83*(2), 190–193.

Bauman, K. E., Strecher, V. J., Keyes, L. L., Glover, L. H., Haley, N. J., Stedman, H. C., & Loda, F. A. (1991). Passive smoking during the first year of life. *American Journal of Public Health, 81*(7), 850–853.

Bologna, M., Koren, G., & Jones, M. (1990). Drugs and chemicals most commonly used by pregnant women. In G. Koren (Ed.), *Maternal-fetal toxicology: A clinician's guide.* New York: Marcel Dekker.

Burton, R. (1906). *Causes of melancholy, Vol I, Part I, Section 2. The Anatomy of Melancholy.* London: William Tegg.

Campinha-Bacote, J., & Bragg, E. J. (1993). Chemical assessment in maternity care. *MCN: American Journal of Maternal Child Nursing, 18*(1), 24–28.

Captain, C. (1993). Family recovery from alcoholism: Mediating family factors. In G. D. Wegner & R. J. Alexander (Ed.), *Readings in family nursing* (pp. 368–382). Philadelphia: J.B. Lippincott.

Chasnoff, I. J., Schnoll, S. H., & Dunn, J. (1984). Maternal substance abuse during pregnancy: Effects on infant development. *Toxicology Teratology, 6*(6), 277–280.

Chasnoff, I. J. (1986). Alcohol use in pregnancy. In I. J. Chasnoff (Ed.), *Drug use in pregnancy* (pp. 75–80). Boston: MTP Press Limited.

Chasnoff, I. J. (1988). The interfaces of perinatal addiction. In I. J. Chasnoff (Ed.), *Drugs, alcohol, pregnancy and parenting.* Boston: Kluwer Academic Publishers.

Chasnoff, I. J. (1991). Cocaine and pregnancy: Clinical and methodologic issues. In I. J. Chasnoff (Ed.), *Clinics in perinatology: Substance abuse and pregnancy* (pp. 113–124). Philadelphia: W.B. Saunders.

Chassin, L., Presson, C. C., Sherman, S. J., & Edwards, D. A. (1992). The natural history of cigarette smoking and young adult social roles. *The Journal of Health and Social Behavior, 33*(4), 328–347.

Chavkin, W., Allen, M. H., & Oberman, M. (1991). Drug abuse and pregnancy: Some questions on public policy, clinical management, and maternal and fetal rights. *BIRTH, 18*(2), 107–112.

Collins, B. A., McCoy, S. A., Sale, S., & Weber, S. E. (1994). Descriptions of comfort by substance-using and nonusing postpartum women. *Journal of Obstetric, Gynecologic, and Neonatal Nursing, 23*(4), 293–300.

Cook, P. S., Petersen, R. C., & Moore, D. T. (1990). In T. B. Haase (Ed.), *Alcohol, tobacco, and other drugs may harm the unborn.* Rockville, MD: U.S. Department of Health and Human Services, Public Health Service.

Council on Scientific Affairs (1990). Council reports: The worldwide smoking epidemic: Tobacco trade, use, and control. *Journal of the American Medical Association, 263*(24), 3312–3318.

Day, N. L., & Richardson, G. A. (1991). Prenatal Marijuana use: Epidemiology, methodologic issues, and infant outcomes. In I. J. Chasnoff (Ed.), *Clinics in perinatology: Substance abuse and pregnancy* (pp. 77–92). Philadelphia: W.B. Saunders.

Dicker, M., & Leighton, E. A. (1994). Trends in the US prevalence of drug-using parturient women and drug-affected newborns, 1979–1990. *American Journal of Public Health, 84*(9), 1433–1438.

DiFranza, J. R., & Brown, L. J. (1992). The Tobacco Institute's "It's the Law" campaign: Has it halted illegal sales of tobacco to children? *American Journal of Public Health, 82*(9), 1271–1272.

Duncan, C., Stein, M. J., & Cummings, S. R. (1991). Staff involvement and special follow-up time increase physicians' counseling about smoking cessation: A controlled trial. *American Journal of Public Health, 81*(7), 899–901.

Evans, A. T., & Gillogley, K. (1991). Drug use in pregnancy: Obstetric perspectives. In I. J. Chasnoff (Ed.), *Clinics in perinatology: Chemical dependency and pregnancy* (pp. 23–32). Philadelphia: W.B. Saunders.

Eward, A. M., Wolfe, R., & Moll, P. (1986). Psychosocial and behavioral factors differentiating past drinkers and lifelong abstainers. *American Journal of Public Health, 76*(1), 68–70.

Fingerhut, L., Kleinman, J. C., & Kendrick, J. S. (1990). Smoking before, during and after pregnancy. *American Journal of Public Health, 8*(5), 541–544.

Flewelling, R. L., Kenney, E., Elder, J. P., Pierce, J., Johnson, M., & Bal, D. G. (1992). First-year impact of the 1989 California cigarette tax increase on cigarette consumption. *American Journal of Public Health, 82*(6), 867–876.

Floyd, R. L., Zahniser, S. C., Gunter, E. P., & Kendrick, J. S. (1991). Smoking during pregnancy: Prevalence, effects, and intervention strategies. *BIRTH, 18*(1), 48–53.

Flynn, B. S., Worden, J. K., Secker-Walker, R. H., Badger, G. J., Geller, B. M., & Costanza, M. C. (1992). Prevention of cigarette smoking through mass media intervention and school programs. *American Journal of Public Health, 82*(6), 827–834.

Fox, N. L., Sexton, M., & Hebel, J. R. (1990). Prenatal exposure to tobacco: I & II: Effects on physical growth at age three. *International Journal of Epidemiology, 19*(3), 66–77.

Fried, P. A., & Watkinson, B. (1990). 36 and 48 month neurobehavioral follow up of children prenatally exposed to marijuana, cigarettes and alcohol. *Developmental and Behavioral Pediatrics, 2*(4), 49–58.

Gillies, P. A., Madeley, R. J., & Power, F. L. (1989). Why do pregnant women smoke? *Public Health Reports, 103*(9), 337–343.

Gilpin, E. A., Pierce, J. P., Cavin, S. W., Gerry, C. C., Evans, N. J., Johnson, M., & Bal, D. G. (1994). Estimates of population smoking prevalence: Self-vs proxy reports of smoking status. *American Journal of Public Health, 84*(10), 1576–1579.

Gritz, E. R., Marcus, A. C., Reeder, S. J., & Berman, B. A. (1988). Evaluation of a worksite self-help smoking cessation program for registered nurses. *American Journal of Health Promotion, 3*(3), 26–35.

Haglund, B., & Cnattingius, S. (1990). Cigarette smoking as a risk factor for sudden infant death syndrome: A population based study. *American Journal of Public Health, 80*(1), 29–32.

Hamilton, D. (1990). Crack's children grow up. *Los Angeles Times, 1A*(ff), August 24.

Hasin, D. S., & Grant, B. F. (1988). Cocaine and heroin dependence compound in poly-abusers. *American Journal of Public Health, 78*(5), 567–573.

Healy, J. M. (1986). Reducing the destructive impact of alcohol: The search for acceptable strategies continues. *American Journal of Public Health, 76*(7), 749–750.

Hill, R. M., Hegemeur, S., Tennyson, L. M. (1989). The fetal alcohol syndrome: A multihandicapped child. *Neurotoxicology, 10,* 585–596.

Hinderliter, S. A., & Zelenak, J. P. (1993). A simple method to identify alcohol and other drug use in pregnant adults in a prenatal care setting. *Journal of Perinatology, 13*(2), 93–102.

Hoegerman, G., & Schnoll, S. (1991). Narcotic use in pregnancy. *Clinics in perinatology: Chemical dependency and pregnancy* (pp. 51–76). Philadelphia: W.B. Saunders.

Huselif, R. F., & Cooper, M. L. (1992). Gender roles as mediators of sex differences in adolescent alcohol use and abuse. *The Journal of Health and Social Behavior, 33*(4), 348–352.

Isacson, D., & Smedby, B. (1988). Defining heavy use of prescription drugs. *Medical Care, 26*(11), 1103–1110.

Jessup, M. (1990). Fetal alcohol syndrome: Prevention and intervention for the nurse. *California Nurse, 84*(2), 12–13.

Joffee, G. M., & Kasnic, T. (1994). Medical prescription of dextroamphetamine during pregnancy. *Journal of Perinatology, 14*(4), 301–303.

Jones, K. L., & Smith, D. W. (1973). Recognition of the fetal alcohol syndrome in early infancy. *Lancet, 2*(112), 999–1001.

Jones, K. L. (1991). Developmental pathogenesis of defects associated with prenatal cocaine exposure: Fetal vascular disruption. *Clinics in perinatology: Chemical depencency and pregnancy* (pp. 139–146). Philadelphia: W.B. Saunders.

Kabat, G. C., Marabia, A., & Wynder, E. L. (1991). Comparison of smoking habits of blacks and whites in a case-control study. *American Journal of Public Health, 81*(11), 1483–1497.

Kandel, D. B., Wu, P., & Davies, M. (1994). Maternal smoking during pregnancy and smoking by adolescent daughters. *American Journal of Public Health, 84*(9), 1407–1413.

Kaul, A. F., & Harsfield, J. C. (1978). Prospective analysis of analgesics and sedative hypnotics in hospitalized obstetric and gynecologic patients. *Drug Intelligence Clinical Pharmacologia, 12*(5), 95–99.

Keith, L. G., McGregor, S., & Frank, A. (1989). Substance abuse in pregnant women: Recent experience at the Perinatal Center for Chemical-Dependence of Northwestern Memorial Hospital. *Obstetrics and Gynecology, 73*(5), 715–720.

Kelleher, K., Chaffin, M., Hollenverg, J., & Fischer, E. (1994). Alcohol and drug disorders among physically abusive and neglectful parents in a community-based sample. *American Journal of Public Health, 84*(10), 1586–1590.

Kleinman, J., & Kopstein, A. (1987). Smoking during pregnancy. *American Journal of Public Health, 77*(7), 823–825.

Koran, G. (1990a). Teratogenic drugs and chemicals in humans. In G. Koran (Ed.), *Maternal-fetal toxicology: A clinician's guide.* New York: Marcel Dekker.

Koran, G. (1990b). Changes in drug disposition in pregnancy and their clinical implications. In G. Koran (Ed.), *Maternal-fetal toxicology: A clinician's guide* (pp. 3–13). New York: Marcel Dekker.

Lake, M. F., Angel, J. L., Murphy, J. M., & Poekert, G. (1992). Patterns of illicit drug use at the time of labor in a private and public hospital. *Journal of Perinatology, 12*(2), 135–151.

Lieberman, E., Gramy, I., Lang, J. M., & Cohen, A. P. (1994). Low birthweight at term and the timing of fetal exposure to maternal smoking. *American Journal of Public Health, 84*(7), 1127–1113.

Lindenberg, C. S., Gendrop, S. C., Nencioli, M., & Adames, Z. (1993). Substance abuse among inner-city Hispanic women: Exploring resiliency. *Journal of Obstetric, Gynecologic, and Neonatal Nursing, 23*(7), 609–616.

Lynch, M., & McKeon, V. A. (1990). Cocaine use during pregnancy. *Journal of Obstetric, Gynecologic, and Neonatal Nursing, 19*(4), 285–289.

Michaels, B., Noonan, M., & Hoffman, S. (1988). A treatment model and nursing care for pregnant chemical abusers. In I. J. Chasnoff (Ed.), *Drugs, alcohol, pregnancy and parenting* (pp. 47–57). Boston: Kluwer Academic Publishers.

Midanik, L. T., & Clark, W. B. (1994). The demographic distribution of US drinking patterns in 1990: Description and trends from 1984. *The American Journal of Public Health, 84*(8), 1218–1228.

Moessinger, A. A. (1989). Mothers who smoke and the lungs of their offspring. In D. E. Hutchings (Ed.), *Annals of the New York Academy of Science, 562*(June 30), 101–104.

Neuspiel, D. R., Cereen. S., & Andrews, P. (1989). Parental smoking and post-infancy wheezing in children: A prospective cohort study. *American Journal of Public Health, 79*(2), 168–171.

Nyamathi, A. M. (1991). Relationship of resources to emotional distress, somatic complaints, and high-risk behaviors in drug recovery and homeless minority women. *Research in Nursing & Health, 14*(2), 269–277.

Obstetric Advisory Committee of Perinatal Advisory Council of Los Angeles Communities (1988). Perinatal protocol: Maternal substance use and neonatal drug withdrawal. *Journal of Perinatology, 8*(4), 387–392.

Perry, C. L., Kelder, S. H., Murray, D. M., & Klepp, K. I. (1992). communitywide smoking prevention: Long-term outcomes of the Minnesota heart health program and the Class of 1989 study. *American Journal of Public Health, 82*(9), 1210–1216.

Peters, H., & Theorell, C. J. (1991). Fetal and neonatal effects of maternal cocaine use. *Journal of Obstetric, Gynecologic, and Neonatal Nursing, 20*(2), 121–126.

Pietrantoni, M., & Knuppel, R. A. (1991). Alcohol use in pregnancy. In I. J. Chasnoff (Ed.), *Clinics in Perinatology: Substance Abuse in Pregnancy.* Philadelphia: W.B. Saunders.

Reichett, S., & Christensen, B. (1990). Reflections during a study on family therapy with drug addicts. *Family Process, 29*(9), 273–287.

Robbins, C. A., & Martin, S. S. (1993). Gender, styles of deviance, and drinking problems. *Journal of Health and Social Behavior, 34*(12), 302–321.

Romano, P. S., Bloom, J., & Syme, S. L. (1991). Smoking, social support and hassles in an urban African-American community. *American Journal of Public Health, 81*(11), 1415–1422.

Rovner, J. (1990). House Subcommittee Approves strong antitobacco measure. *The Nation's Health, October,* 3.

Rush, D., & Callahan, K. R. (1989). Exposure to passive cigarette smoking and child development. In D. E. Hutchings (Ed.), *Annals of the New York Academy of Sciences, 562*(June 30), 74–100.

Sampson, P. D., Bookstein, F. L., Barr, H. M., & Streissguth, A. P. (1994). Prenatal alcohol exposure, birthweight and measures of child size from birth to age 14 years. *American Journal of Public Health, 84–89,* 1421–1428.

Schnoll, S. H. (1986). Pharmacologic basis of perinatal addiction. In I. J. Chasnoff (Ed.), *Drug use in pregnancy* (pp. 7–16). Boston: MTP Press Limited.

Sobatka, T. J. (1989). Neurobehavioral effects of prenatal caffeine. In D. E. Hutchings (Ed.), *Annals of the New York Academy of Science. 562*(6), 327–339.

Silver, H., Wapner, R., & Lorz-Vega, M. (1987). Addiction in pregnancy: High risk intrapartum management and outcome. *Journal of Perinatology, 7*(3), 178–184.

Smith, J. (1988). The dangers of prenatal cocaine use. *MCN: American Journal of Maternal Child Nursing, 13*(3), 174–179.

Smith, G. B. (1992). Attitudes of nurse managers and assistant nurse managers toward chemically impaired colleagues. *IMAGE, 24*(4), 295–300.

Sullivan, W. P., Wolk, J. L., & Hartman, D. J. (1992). Case management in alcohol and drug treatment: Improving client outcomes. *Families in Society: The Journal of Contemporary Human Services, 73*(2), 195–203.

Sullivan, J., Boudreaux, M., & Keller, P. (1993). Can we help the substance abusing mother and infant? *MCN: American Journal of Maternal Child Nursing, 18*(3), 153–157.

Surgeon General's Report (1979). *A Report of the Surgeon General, Publication No. (PHS) 79-50066.* Washington, DC: Public Health Service, Office of Smoking and Health, U.S. Department of Health, Education and Welfare.

Swonger, A., & Molejski, N. (1991). *Nursing pharmacology: An integrated approach to drug therapy and nursing practice* (2nd ed.). Philadelphia: J.B. Lippincott.

von Windeguth, B. J., & Urbano, M. T. (1989). Cocaine abusing mothers and their infants: A new morbidity brings challenges for nursing care. *Journal of Community Health Nursing, 6*(2), 147–153.

Warnecke, R. B., Langenberg, P., Wong, S. C., Flay, B. R., & Cook, T. D. (1992). The second Chicago televised smoking cessation program: A 24 month follow up. *American Journal of Public Health, 82*(6), 835–840.

Warner, K. E. (1989). Smoking and health. *American Journal of Public Health, 79*(2), 141–143.

Warner, K. E. (1991). Tobacco industry scientific advisors: Serving society or selling cigarettes? *American Journal of Public Health, 8*(7), 839–842.

Weiner, L., & Morse, B. A. (1988). FAS: Clinical perspectives and prevention. In I. J. Chasnoff (Ed.), *Drugs, alcohol, pregnancy and parenting.* Boston: Kluwer Academic Publishers.

Wilson, G. S. (1989). Clinical studies of infants and children exposed prenatally to heroin. In D. E. Hutchings (Ed.), *Annals of the New York Academy of Science, 562*(6), 183–193.

Windsor, R. A., Cutter, G., & Morris, J. (1985). Effectiveness of smoking cessation methods for smokers in a public health maternity clinic: A randomized trial. *American Journal of Public Health, 75*(12), 1389–1392

Windsor, R. A., Li, C. Q., Lowe, J. B., Perkins, L., Ershoff, D., & Glynn, T. (1993a). The dissemination of smoking cessation methods for pregnant women: Achieving the Year 2000 objectives. *American Journal of Public Health, 83*(2), 173–178.

Windsor, R. A., Lowe, J. B., Perkins, L. L., Smith-Yoder, D., Artz, L., Crawford, M., Amburgy, K., & Boyd, N. R. Jr. (1993b). Health education for pregnant smokers: Its behavioral impact and cost benefit. *American Journal of Public Health, 83*(2), 201–206.

Yates, J. G., & McDaniel, J. L. (1994). Are you losing yourself in codependency? *American Journal of Nursing, 94*(4), 32–36.

Zuckerman, B. (1988). Marijuana and cigarette smoking during pregnancy: Neonatal effects. In I. J. Chasnoff (Ed.), *Drugs, alcohol, pregnancy and parenting.* Boston: Kluwer Academic Publishing.

SUGGESTED READINGS

Casey, D. (1993). The greatest gift of all. *The American Journal of Nursing, 93*(9), 46–47.

Eliason, M. J., & Williams, J. K. (1990). Fetal alcohol syndrome and the neonate. *Journal of Perinatal and Neonatal Nursing, 3*(4), 64–72.

Farley, P. B., & Hendrix, M. J. (1993). Impaired and nonimpaired nurses during childhood and adolescence. *Nursing Outlook, 41*(1), 25–31.

Fost, N. (1989). Maternal-fetal conflicts: Ethical and legal considerations. In D. E. Hutchings (Ed.), *Annals of the New York Academy of Science, 562*(6), 248–254.

Hickner, J., Cousineau, A., & Messimer, S. (1990). Smoking cessation during pregnancy: Strategies used by Michigan family physicians. *Journal of the Board of Family Practice, 3*(1), 39–42.

House, M. A. (1990). Cocaine. *American Journal of Nursing, 90*(5), 41–45.

McCormick, M. C., Brooks-Gunn, J., & Shorter, T. (1990). Factors associated with smoking in low-income pregnant women: Relationship to birth weight, stressful life events, social support, health behaviors and mental distress. *Journal of Clinical Epidemiology, 43*(3), 441–448.

Polk, D., Glendon, K., & DeVore, C. (1993). The chemically dependent student nurse: Guidelines for policy development. *Nursing Outlook, 41*(4), 166–170.

Pollitt, K. (1990). A new assault on feminism. *The Nation, 250*(12), 409–418.

Robins, L. N., & Mills, J. L. (Eds.) (1993). Effects of in utero exposure to street drugs. *American Journal of Public Health, 83*(Supp.), 9–32.

35

Adolescent Sexuality, Pregnancy, and Childrearing

Objectives

- Describe the effects of adolescent pregnancy and parent-hood on the mother, infant, family, and society.
- Explain how an unplanned pregnancy affects adolescent development.
- Identify the four steps or decisions the adolescent con-sciously or unconsciously makes that lead to parenthood.
- Discuss the nurse's role in primary, secondary, and tertiary prevention of adolescent pregnancy.

Adolescence is the developmental period that bridges the gap between childhood and adulthood. In this stage, the person must adapt and adjust childhood behaviors to the culturally acceptable norms of society. Important in this process are the tasks of ego (identity) development, achievement of personal independence, and attainment of higher cognitive skills. Biologic changes occur rapidly during this period; primary and secondary changes in sexual characteristics are described in Chapter 6. The degree of physical change prompts others to alter their expectations for behavior, and the adolescent's self-image may be modified. All of these changes impact on the person's cognitive, social, and personal development.

During adolescence, boys and girls experiment with a variety of adult roles and attempt to develop a realistic sense of self (Marcia, 1980; Havighurst, 1972). This is the appropriate time to acquire the education, training, and skills necessary to function in society and to learn other, non–work-related adult activities and skills. Adolescents frequently experiment with a variety of new activities, many potentially harmful, such as unsafe sexual encounters, substance abuse, and violence. The increasing mortality of adolescents during the last 25 years, as compared with other age groups in the United States, reflects this risk-taking behavior (Greydanus, 1987). Violence (accidents, suicides, and homicides) contributes to more than 75% of adolescent deaths (U.S. Department of Commerce, Bureau of the Census, 1993).

Substance abuse while driving partially accounts for the high automobile fatality rate among adolescents, who also are the victims of violence, exploitation, and abuse. Sexual experimentation may lead to unplanned pregnancy or sexually transmitted diseases (STDs). Most adolescent pregnancies are unintentional and result from a combination of risk-taking behavior, inadequate reproductive knowledge, and general belief in invulnerability ("It won't happen to me;" Howe, 1986).

This chapter introduces the student to the developmental process of adolescence; trends and issues in adolescent sexuality, pregnancy, and childbearing; and the antecedents and consequences of these phenomena. Approaches to nursing care are described as they relate to primary, secondary, and tertiary prevention. The importance of directing intervention toward preventing unintended adolescent pregnancy is emphasized. The student will identify applications of the nursing process that promote optimum health, social, and developmental outcomes for childbearing and childrearing adolescents and their offspring.

Theoretical Views of Adolescence

According to Erikson's (1959) theory of psychosocial development, adolescence is a particularly decisive period for forming an identity. Adolescents must become people in their own right—individuals who are in charge of their lives and know who they are. The major developmental task of adolescence is to resolve the conflict between **identity achievement** and identity diffusion. The adolescent either develops a solid sense of self with plans for the future or is unable to develop a firm personal or vocational identity. Personality formation during adolescence is influenced by how the previous stages of development were completed (Erikson, 1959). For example, adolescents who failed to establish a sense of trust during early childhood may continue to mistrust others. Similarly, those who did not develop a sense of initiative during the preschool years may lack the confidence needed to experiment with different identities and to become comfortable with their own individuality.

The adolescent faces the challenge of developing a vocational and sexual identity necessary for establishing a career and intimate relationships in adulthood. If the identity confusion crisis is resolved with reasonable success during adolescence, the person advances into the adult stages of development and their corresponding crises with a firm identity. If the ego-identity crisis is not resolved successfully, an altered development of the ego occurs, and the person is less likely to resolve the crises of adulthood.

Marcia (1966, 1967, 1980) refined Erikson's conceptualization of adolescent identity formation by viewing identity as a continually changing organization of attitudes, values, and beliefs. A well-developed identity enables a person to be aware of personal strengths and uniqueness. A less well-developed identity results in the inability to define strengths and weaknesses and a lack of a well-articulated sense of self. Four identity statuses are described by Marcia; these individual styles of coping with the identity crisis are described below:

■ **Identity achievers** have experienced a period of decision making and are now committed to an occupation and to a set of ideologic values, all primarily self-chosen. They have strength in their belief system and are adaptive and well adjusted.

- People in the **foreclosure** status are similar to identity achievers, but some of their choices have been determined by parents or others and are not self-selected.
- Individuals with the status of **identity diffusion** demonstrate no commitment to an occupation or ideologic system.
- **Moratoriums** are characterized by the presence of struggle and attempts to make commitments about occupational or ideologic decisions (Marcia, 1980, 1966, 1967).

Cognitive Development

Piaget (1971) contends that adolescence is a qualitatively unique period, set apart from childhood by the person's expanding cognitive abilities (Piaget, 1971). Young adolescents have not yet entered the stage of formal cognitive operations. This stage, attained by most adolescents between 15 and 20 years of age, is individually influenced by social and school experiences and neurologic development. The thought processes of adolescents in the stage of concrete operations or only partial formal operations are somewhat egocentric. Consequently, they may have difficulty planning for the future and implementing behavior change. Older adolescents are capable of abstract thinking (**formal operational thought**), which enables them to understand the thought processes of others and to interact with the environment in new ways.

Developmental Tasks

Developmental tasks are physical or cognitive skills that a person must accomplish during a particular age

to continue developing. Havighurst (1972) proposed eight developmental tasks for the adolescent years (Box 35-1). The first four, which assume central importance during early adolescence, depend more on physical maturity and biologic changes than those of later adolescence. According to Havighurst (1972), the developmental tasks through which the person must proceed may differ from culture to culture; however, *biologically determined tasks* (steps 1–3) are more likely to be culturally universal than are *tasks having a strong cultural component* (steps 5–8). Successful mastery of the developmental tasks promotes the adolescent's emergence into adulthood as a well-adjusted person, competent and capable of adapting to future demands of development.

Growth during adolescence is divided into three substages: early, middle, and late. The characteristics of each period are described in Box 35-2. Pregnancy during any substage of adolescence makes the normal developmental issues of this period more difficult to resolve. Concerns about changing body image, increasing dependence on family members for emotional and financial support, and the normal physiologic and psychological changes of pregnancy create internal stress, with which the adolescent is often unprepared to cope. To further complicate this situation, the adolescent faces many potential conflicts between the de-

---

BOX 35-1
Developmental Tasks of Adolescence

Task 1	Achieving more mature relations with age mates of both sexes
Task 2	Achieving a masculine or feminine social role
Task 3	Accepting one's physique and using the body effectively
Task 4	Achieving emotional independence from parents and other adults
Task 5	Preparing for marriage and family life
Task 6	Preparing for an economic career
Task 7	Acquiring a set of values and an ethical system as a guide to behavior; developing an ideology
Task 8	Desiring and achieving socially responsible behavior

(Havighurst, R. J. [1972]. Developmental tasks and education. New York: David McKay.)

BOX 35-2
Characteristics of the Stages of Adolescence

Early Adolescence (Pubescence to 15 Years)

- Rapid physical growth and development
- Beginning assertion of independence, with movement away from parents
- Increasing emphasis on close peer relationships
- Concrete thinking with some effort toward abstract problem solving
- Egocentricism
- Present orientation

Middle Adolescence (16 to 17 Years)

- Development of formal abstract thinking abilities
- Introspection
- Increasing future orientation
- Preoccupation with sexual exploration
- More formal separation from parents
- Testing of limits and a preference for peer activities

Late Adolescence (18 to 20 Years)

- Establishment of a secure body image and gender identity
- Maintenance of stable relationships
- Behaviors oriented toward others and self
- Realistic problem-solving skills
- Concerns with emotional intimacy and career planning

TABLE 35-1

Developmental Tasks of Adolescence and Parenthood and Related Conflicting Behaviors

Adolescence	Parenthood	Conflicting Behaviors
Narcissism and egocentrism; focus on self and needs	Forming an empathic and mutualistic relationship with newborn	Competition between adolescent and newborn for attention of mate, family, friends; unable to differentiate own feelings from newborn's feelings
Identity formation: develop peer relationships, participate in role experimentation, need for period of moratorium	Maternal identification and role differentiation	Reluctance to assume parenting responsibilities; resentment toward newborn
Body image formation and sexual identity formation	Acceptance of body image changes of pregnancy, labor and delivery, and postpartum	Rejection of body image changes; refusal to breast-feed
Emancipation from family	Family role reassignments	Resentment of dependence on family for support and financial assistance; conflict with mother about childrearing
Cognitive development: transition from concrete to formal operations	Decision making and future planning regarding childrearing	Difficulty understanding general principles of child development, infant play, and safety

(Modified from Sadler, L. S. & Catrone, C. [1983]. The adolescent parent: A dual developmental crisis. *Journal of Adolescent Health Care, 4,* 100–105.)

velopmental tasks of adolescence and the tasks of parenthood. Sadler et al. (1983) identified five major areas of conflict (Table 35-1).

An unplanned and early pregnancy requires the adolescent to shift her energies from the task of internalizing an identity to generativity in rearing the next generation, often without having mastered a true sense of intimacy. As a parent, the adolescent must attempt to meet the daily care needs of a newborn by providing a safe environment, adequate caregiving, and nurturing. Because the adolescent mother must prematurely assume an adult role, she may be forced to remain in the developmental stage of foreclosure (Sadler et al., 1983).

Similar psychological risks may exist for the adolescent father, whose developmental tasks also are likely to be interrupted by an early, unplanned pregnancy. The young father may feel isolated, alone, and over-whelmed. A variety of stressors may impact his life and influence his future plans (eg, potential interruption of education, lack of family support, and financial difficulties).

Pathways to Adolescent Pregnancy

The pathway to pregnancy and childbearing for the adolescent encompasses a series of choices in the area of sexuality. Flick (1986) identified four steps or decisions the adolescent consciously or unconsciously makes that can lead to parenthood (Table 35-2). Unfortunately, responsible decision making regarding sexual activity and parenthood requires certain skills that adolescents often lack. These include the following abilities:

TABLE 35-2

Decision Points Leading to Parenthood

Decision 1	Sexual activity	To become sexually active or to remain sexually inactive
Decision 2	Contraception	To use or not to use contraceptives appropriately
Decision 3	Pregnancy resolution	To deliver or to abort
Decision 4	Parenthood	To rear the child or to place the child formally or informally for adoption

(Modified from Flick, L. H. [1986]. Paths to adolescent parenthood: Implications for prevention. *Public Health Reports, 101*(2), 132–147.)

- Understanding the factual information that applies to them (cognition)
- Incorporating their sexual identity into their evolving value structure in the presence of peer pressure (socialization)
- Evaluating the many variables that influence them on a daily basis and change from day to day (situation-specific behavior; Juhasz et al., 1980)

Sexual Activity

National survey data suggest that adolescent sexual behavior has risen dramatically (Leigh et al., 1994). Of all 18-year-olds, 71% reportedly are sexually experienced (Alan Guttmacher Institute, 1994). Sex is much less common among younger teenagers; 30% of those 15 years or younger report having had intercourse. While minority populations have been found to have higher rates of sexual activity, the greatest increase during the 1980s occurred among white and nonpoor teens. The change in attitudes toward adolescent sexuality, which became evident in the 1960s, has resulted in the gap between boys' and girls' sexual behavior narrowing as more girls have become sexually active (Alan Guttmacher Institute, 1994). Because an increasing number of unmarried girls in all segments of society in the United States are having intercourse at an earlier age, the period of exposure to unintended adolescent pregnancy has expanded. The younger the adolescent, the more sporadic and infrequent is the level of sexual activity.

The statistics show that in each successive age group, a higher percent of women have had intercourse in each age category. In addition, age appears to be the most important factor in determining whether an adolescent is sexually experienced (Alan Guttmacher Institute, 1994). Other research findings have demonstrated several additional factors associated with adolescent sexual activity (eg, low socioeconomic status [SES], poor educational achievement, large family size or single-parent household, perceived sexual activity of peers, partner pressure, and lack of sex education; Hofferth et al., 1987; Hogan et al., 1985; Brooks-Gunn et al., 1989). Sex is more common among adolescent men than women and among African American teenagers than among white or Hispanic youth (Leigh et al., 1994; Alan Guttmacher Institute, 1994). Increasing evidence reveals that for some young women, having sex is not a voluntary choice but a result of coercion or force.

Contraception

Adolescents considering or engaging in sexual activity face decisions regarding contraception. Although the use of contraceptive techniques among adolescents may be erratic and limited, data suggest that contraceptive use, particularly condom use, increased consider-

ably from the early to the late 1980s (Forrest et al., 1990; Leigh et al., 1994). Two-thirds of adolescents report using some method of contraception the first time they have sexual intercourse (Forest et al., 1990). Nonuse or inadequate use of contraceptives by adolescents has been found to be associated with low SES, low educational achievement, little communication with parents, and lack of knowledge of siblings' or parents' birth control experience (Flick, 1986; Brooks-Gunn et al., 1989; Abrahamse et al., 1988; Maynard et al., 1994). Peer influences include having friends who are parents. A positive relationship has been found between age at first intercourse and effective contraceptive use (Flick, 1986; Brooks-Gunn et al., 1989; Abrahamse et al., 1988); older adolescents are much more likely to use contraceptives than are younger ones. Adolescent girls who have more contacts with school-based family planning programs have been found to use contraceptives more consistently than those with fewer contacts (Brindis et al., 1994). Sachs (1986) demonstrated that cognitive development in adolescents predicts contraceptive choices. Although some data suggest that knowledge of contraceptive methods increases adolescents' use of contraceptives, case studies by the Alan Guttmacher Institute (1981a) indicate that adolescents are exposed to mixed messages about contraception. Furthermore, birth control services are not effectively delivered to American youth (Trussele, 1988; Jones et al., 1985; Macdonald, 1987).

Pregnancy Resolution

Half of all first pregnancies occur in the 6 months after the first intercourse and one-fifth in the first month (Zabin et al., 1979; Marsiglio et al., 1986). Adolescents who become pregnant due to ineffective use or nonuse of contraceptive methods face the decision of whether to terminate their pregnancies voluntarily. Results of some studies indicate that the decision to deliver rather than to abort is more likely for older adolescents, high school dropouts and those with poor school performance, members of large or single-parent families, and those who had a sister who was pregnant as an adolescent (Brooks-Gunn et al., 1989; Friede et al., 1986; Abrahamse et al., 1988). The adolescents most likely to terminate an unwanted pregnancy are affluent, white, well educated, and those whose parents have more education (Alan Guttmacher Institute, 1981, 1994; Kafka, 1988; Neilsen, 1987). Nearly 60% of white adolescents whose pregnancies are unintended choose abortion, compared with fewer than 50% of African American and Hispanic adolescents (Henshaw, 1992). Teenagers who have abortions most often cite their young age, concern about how having a baby would change their lives, and low income as reasons for making that decision (Facts in Brief, 1994; Torres et al., 1988).

Parenthood

Less data exist about adolescents who choose adoption, because the likelihood that an adolescent will place her baby for adoption has declined dramatically in recent years, particularly among white women. Between 1982 and 1988, only 3% of unmarried, non-Hispanic, white women relinquished their newborns (Alan Guttmacher Institute, 1994). The limited published studies suggest that adolescents who make adoption plans are more similar to those who choose abortion than to those who become parents (Resnick, 1984; McLaughlin et al., 1988). Few negative consequences have been found for adolescents who relinquish their newborns compared with those who keep them (McLaughlin et al., 1988). Adolescents who relinquish their newborn tend to have a higher SES, while adolescents who keep their newborn tend to be younger, from single-parent families, and express less approval of abortion as an alternative to childbirth.

Incidence of Adolescent Pregnancy, Abortion, and Birth

Each year, more than 1 million teenagers become pregnant. In 1991, the birth rate was 62 births per 1,000 girls 15 to 19 years old (531,591 actual births according to the Centers for Disease Control and Prevention [CDC]). This represents a rise in birth rates of 27% for younger adolescents and 19% for older adolescents over a 5-year period (1986–1991). While births to white girls account for more than two-thirds of all teenage births, the incidence of adolescent pregnancies and births is much higher among minority groups. For example, more than 40% of first births among African Americans are to adolescents, compared with 20% of those among white girls. The Hispanic adolescent birthrate is slightly lower than the African American and higher than the white birthrates; however, a dramatic increase in births to young Hispanic women has been observed in recent years (Table 35-3).

The number of nonmarital births to adolescents has quadrupled since 1960, while the number of marital teenage births has declined significantly (Facts at a Glance, 1994). First births to unwed teenagers has risen dramatically to 81% (Alan Guttmacher Institute, 1994). The incidence of nonmarital childbearing is twice as high among African Americans as among white people, although in the last 15 years the rate of adolescent births has risen more rapidly among young unmarried white girls (National Center for Health Statistics, 1988). Most pregnant adolescents are single, and 85% have an unintended pregnancy (Alan Guttmacher Institute, 1994).

Thirty-five percent of the estimated pregnancies among women 19 years and younger in 1990 were terminated by elective abortion, and another 14% ended in miscarriage (Henshaw, 1993). Since the late 1970s, the abortion rate has declined among sexually experienced teenagers. In 1990, adolescents accounted for less than one-third of all abortions in the United States.

Impact of Adolescent Pregnancy and Childrearing on Society, the Family, and the Individual

Despite the increasing effort to reduce its incidence, adolescent pregnancy and parenthood remain major national concerns because of the potentially adverse consequences for society, the family, and the individual. The National Research Council's Panel on Adolescent Pregnancy and Childbearing published an extensive review of the literature documenting the public and private costs of early childbearing (Hofferth et al., 1987). Since that report's publication, additional data on the association between adolescent parenthood and

TABLE 35–3
Adolescent Birth Rates By Ethnicity or Race Between 1980 and 1991

Race or Ethnicity	Birth Rate per 1,000 Girls 15–19 Years Old				
	1980	1986	1989	1990	1991
Hispanics	82	80	91	100	107
Non-Hispanic African Americans	105	104	112	116	118
Non-Hispanic whites	41	36	40	43	43

Note: 1980 data are reported for 22 states, accounting for 90% of Hispanic births; 1986 data are for 30 states and DC; 1989 data are for 47 states and DC; 1990 data are for 48 states and DC; 1991 data are for 49 states and DC. Source: Child Trends, Inc., Facts at a Glance, January 1994.

long-term welfare dependence have indicated that early childbearing may have an important relationship in the intergenerational transmission of disadvantage (Duncan et al., 1990; Furstenberg et al., 1990).

Social Costs

The cost associated with adolescent childbearing in the United States in 1989 was estimated at $21.5 billion; with the rising teenage birthrate and the upward trend in actual spending on families begun by teenagers, this amount is likely to have increased considerably in recent years (Caldas, 1994). This estimate was based on the costs of Aid to Families with Dependent Children (AFDC), Medicaid, and food stamp payments only; it *excluded* housing subsidies, special education, child protective services, day care, and other special service programs. If every birth to an adolescent mother in 1990 had been delayed until the woman were in her 20s, the federal government would have saved 40% of the calculated expenditures, or $10 billion (Center for Population Options, 1992). As teenage mothers grow older, many become independent and move off public assistance; however, women who become mothers as adolescents are more likely to be on public assistance than those who first give birth at 20 to 24 years (Alan Guttmacher Institute, 1994). Hoffman et al. (1993) demonstrated that aside from the effect of background factors, such as poverty, there are still statistically significant and quantitatively important negative effects of early childbearing on economic well-being of adolescent mothers. Nearly 60% of teenage families live in poverty, compared with 13.5% of the total population (Gold et al., 1991).

Effects on the Family

The family of the adolescent is greatly affected by an unplanned pregnancy. Many parents initially react with anger and hurt to the news of their child's pregnancy; however, they may become more supportive at the birth of a grandchild and offer assistance to their daughter in need. The majority of pregnant and parenting adolescents choose to remain single and live within the context of their nuclear or extended family. Furstenberg et al. (1978) found that 88% of adolescents remained in this arrangement 1 year after their baby's birth, and 5 years later, 70% of never-married mothers still lived with their families of origin. The roles of family members shift when grandparents and significant others assume additional financial and child care responsibilities. The developmental stage of the adolescent mother influences her level of dependence on family members and the family adaptation required. Economic and social support increase the adolescent's potential for psychological development and emo-

tional satisfaction in the role of "mother" (Friedman et al., 1983).

Effects on the Adolescent Mother

The age at which the adolescent conceives greatly influences the effect the pregnancy will have on her life. An unplanned pregnancy has different implications for the 18- or 19-year-old high school graduate than for the 13- or 14-year-old junior high school student. In general, adolescent parents are less likely to complete high school, attend college, find stable employment, or be self-supporting than later childbearers (Hayes, 1987; Hofferth et al., 1987). As more schools offer a wide variety of special programs for pregnant minors and young mothers, teenage pregnancy is becoming less a factor in determining whether an adolescent graduates from high school (Males, 1993; Fig. 35-1). However, premature parenthood often causes delays in school completion, changes the young mother's choices of routes toward school completion, and often thwarts her plans for postsecondary education (Pittman, 1990).

Thirty-one percent of adolescents who become mothers before 17 years and 24% of those who are 18 to 19 years old when they first give birth have a second child within 2 years (Facts at a Glance, 1994). The percentage of first births to unmarried teenagers has increased sharply since the early 1960s—from 33% to 81% (Facts at a Glance, 1994). Although few adolescent mothers marry the fathers of their newborns, many may maintain regular or sporadic contact. Early marriage to the child's father does not seem to improve the course of events; adolescent mothers who stay single are more likely than those who marry to finish high school and to avoid another pregnancy. Nearly one-third of first marriages among adolescents end in divorce within 5 years compared with 15% among cou-

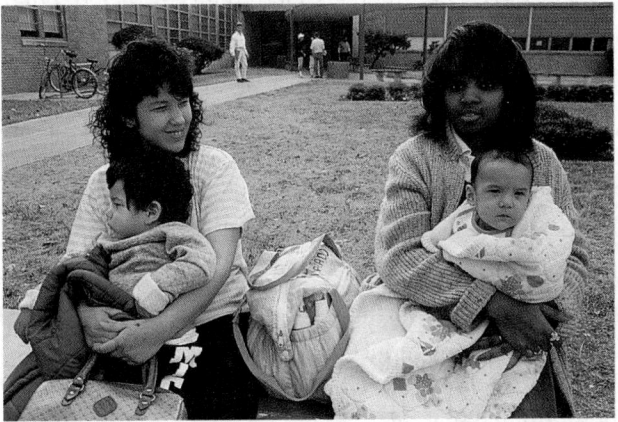

FIGURE 35-1 Schools may offer special programs for pregnant minors and young mothers to enable them to graduate from high school.

ples who delay marriage until they are 23 to 29 years old (Alan Guttmacher Institute, 1994).

Effects on the Father

In general, adolescent fathers tend to be less adversely affected by early parenthood than adolescent mothers; however, they are at risk for lower educational achievement and associated decreased vocational and economic attainment (Marsiglio et al., 1986; Elster et al., 1987). High school dropout rates are higher for adolescent fathers than for other young men and are not influenced by marital status. The results of studies suggest that the effects of adolescent parenthood on school completion are graver for white and Hispanic boys than for African American boys (Marsiglio et al., 1986; Hardy et al., 1988). Recent data from the Alan Guttmacher Institute indicate that about one in five fathers of babies born to adolescents are not themselves adolescents. Nearly one-third of the fathers of babies born to 15-year-old mothers are 6 or more years older than the mother (Facts at a Glance, 1994).

Risks of Pregnancy and Childbearing During Adolescence

Childbearing at any age is a momentous event. For the adolescent, however, it is often accompanied by a different set of problems from those experienced by adult mothers. Perinatal risks, including low birth weight (LBW) and STDs, infant health risks, and psychosocial risks for the adolescent parent and child, are foremost among these.

Perinatal Risks

Older adolescent mothers and their expected child face minimal biomedical risk compared with younger adolescents, for whom rates of maternal and neonatal deaths are disproportionately high (Committee on Adolescence, 1989). Nonwhite adolescents are at greatest risk for adverse outcomes. For the mother who is younger than 15 years, there is a greater probability that her infant will be stillborn or premature, be LBW, or have increased morbidity or mortality during the first year of life. In addition, the mother is at greater risk for decreased weight gain, urinary tract infections, STDs, pregnancy-induced hypertension (PIH), iron deficiency anemia, cephalopelvic disproportion (CPD), and prolonged labor.

It is difficult to isolate and identify the independent effect of maternal age on perinatal complications because most adolescents who become pregnant are poor, have limited access to and use of healthcare, and

display a variety of behaviors known to have a negative influence on pregnancy outcomes (Spivak et al., 1987). Available data indicate that early, regular, comprehensive prenatal care and adequate nutrition decrease the risks of perinatal complications for pregnant adolescents and their children (Spivak et al., 1987; Gale et al., 1989).

Sexually Transmitted Diseases

The incidence of STDs, especially acquired immunodeficiency syndrome (AIDS), among adolescents has risen dramatically in recent years. Approximately 3 million adolescent women and men acquire an STD annually, accounting for 25% of all new STDs each year (Alan Guttmacher Institute, 1994). *Chlamydia,* trichomoniasis, gonorrhea, human papillomavirus, genital herpes, hepatitis B, syphilis, and human immunodeficiency virus (HIV) are among the most common STDs. The rising incidence of AIDS in 20- to 29-year-olds is of major concern, because many of these cases are likely to have originated in the late adolescent years (CDC, 1993). If the proportion of reported cases increases in the heterosexual population as projected in the years ahead, adolescents will be at even higher risk for the infection (see Chap. 11). The consequences of untreated STDs may include perinatal transmission of the disease to an offspring, pelvic inflammatory disease, ectopic pregnancy, and infertility.

Low Birth Weight

The increased risk of LBW is one of the most important medical aspects of adolescent pregnancy. A birth weight of 2,500 g or less is considered to be LBW. The younger the pregnant adolescent is, the more likely she is to bear LBW infants. Compared with white teenagers, African American teenagers have a substantially higher incidence of LBW babies (National Center for Health Statistics, 1993). When considering this neonatal risk, it is important to recognize that findings from studies, when adjusted for socioeconomic factors and prenatal care, indicate that the percentages of LBW newborns and rates of infant mortality are fairly similar for the babies of adults and adolescents (McAnarney, 1987). (LBW is discussed further in Chap. 41.)

Newborn Health Risks

Newborns of adolescent mothers are more likely than those born to older women to have health problems during childhood and to be hospitalized (Alan Guttmacher Institute, 1994). A variety of health problems contribute to increased infant morbidity and mortality, particularly in offspring of younger and African American adolescent mothers; these include LBW, hypoglycemia, respiratory distress syndrome, pneumonia, seizures, apnea, necrotizing enterocolitis, and sudden infant death syndrome (Alan Guttmacher Institute, 1981; Miller et al., 1985). Additionally, infants of adolescent mothers experience an increased mortality in infancy from external events, such as accidents, violence, and infection (CDC, 1992). Many factors are believed to be responsible for the increased morbidity and mortality in infants of adolescent mothers, such as child spacing, SES, race, educational attainment, prenatal healthcare availability and use, health habits (smoking, alcohol use, drug use, personal hygiene), low gynecologic age, and acute and chronic medical problems. Use of early prenatal healthcare and avoidance of detrimental health habits are the most significant factors in limiting mortality, LBW, and prematurity (Zuckerman et al., 1986). Nurses play an important role in helping adolescents to recognize the need for early and regular prenatal care as a vital step toward promoting physical and psychological well-being during the prenatal period.

Psychosocial Risks for the Adolescent Parent and Child

The psychosocial consequences of adolescent parenting may be disturbing and appear to increase with socioeconomic disadvantage and decreasing age of adolescent parents. The findings of several studies suggest that adolescent mothers have poorer patterns of interaction with their infants and toddlers, spend less time talking to them, maintain less eye contact, and use less praise and more punishment than adult women (Spivak et al., 1987; Brooks-Gunn et al., 1986; Mercer, 1990). Maternal psychological distress, often evidenced as depression, has been observed to predict child behavior problems from 2 to 3 years but may be buffered by emotional support from maternal grandmothers and friends (Leadbeater et al., 1994). Older adolescents often view childrearing problems more realistically than younger ones because of their more advanced cognitive skills, greater psychosocial assets, and larger support networks. Young adolescent mothers tend to show aggressive behaviors toward the baby (as would a jealous sibling), use teasing, and relate to the child as a plaything to meet their needs. Inconsistencies in parenting behaviors are often displayed by middle adolescents, who sometimes are able to respond appropriately to their baby's needs and at other times are not interested in the child.

Although the literature is inconclusive, there appears to be more neglectful parenting and a higher incidence of poor intellectual, developmental, and educational outcomes in children of adolescent mothers compared with those of older mothers (Furstenberg et al., 1990; Brooks-Gunn et al., 1986). Many of these differences become more pronounced as the children develop, with boys being more affected than girls, at least in the early years. By the high school years, educational failure and juvenile delinquency become major problems for the offspring of adolescent parents (Furstenberg et al., 1987).

The results of many studies suggest that low SES, poor education of parents, and higher incidence of family instability with multiple caregivers are associated factors, perhaps more important than the specific age of the mother (Spivak et al., 1987; Gale et al., 1989; Coll et al., 1986). Changes in maternal life course (eg, moving off welfare after the child's preschool years, entering into a stable marriage) may significantly influence the child's outcome.

The Nursing Process and the Well Adolescent (Primary Prevention)

Nursing care of the well adolescent is directed toward optimizing health status, preventing illness, and interrupting the sequence of steps leading to parenthood. Although this section focuses on the latter area, secondary emphasis must be placed on the importance of appraising the adolescent's physical, cognitive, and psychosocial development. Particular consideration is given to assessment of health history, physical examination, and identification of health risks related to growth during adolescence (eg, eating disorders, iron deficiency anemia, STDs, skin lesions, sports-related trauma, and dental caries). (See Assessment Tool: Physical Examination for STDs in Chap. 11.) Development of secondary sex characteristics, menstrual history, and concerns about body image should be carefully assessed. Specific laboratory tests are often included in the health evaluation (eg, hemoglobin and hematocrit, urinalysis, sickle cell screening for African American adolescents, very low-density lipoprotein [VDRL]).

A major nursing goal in **primary prevention** is to avert conception, either through promotion of abstinence or by regular use of effective methods of birth control. Nurses employed in hospitals, community agencies, and schools can provide education, counseling, and family planning services to prevent premature parenthood. A particularly important area for nursing involvement is in active outreach activities, especially to young, sexually active adolescents. To provide effective care, the nurse must create an environment in which adolescents feel comfortable seeking help for their health concerns. Adolescents are particularly interested in the issue of confidentiality, which, if not carefully considered, may be a significant access barrier to healthcare (Thompson, 1989). Providers, adolescents, and their parents need to be aware of the nature and effect of laws and regulations in their jurisdictions requiring notification or consent, because these may place constraints on relationships.

Family Life and Sex Education

The need for sex education is foremost in the area of primary prevention. This ideally should cover anatomy, human sexuality, and contraception methods. Many adolescents do not comprehend the potential consequences of their sexual activity or specifically, the risks of pregnancy with unprotected intercourse. The principal theme of the "just say later" model is abstinence from sexual activity during adolescence. The "safe sex" model advocates prevention strategies and assumes that most adolescents will be sexually active. Both models incorporate sex education and counseling designed to increase the adolescent's knowledge and decision-making skills. Results of many sex education studies indicate that increasing an adolescent's sexual knowledge does not increase his or her sexual activity and that adolescents not receiving sex education may have little opportunity to acquire information regarding sexuality from reliable sources (Howard et al., 1990; Brooks-Gunn et al., 1989; Marsiglio et al., 1986).

Results of a recent CDC study (Kirby et al., 1994) of published evaluations of school-based pregnancy and STD prevention programs revealed that few were able to decrease unprotected intercourse, either through delaying sex or increasing contraceptive use. The following components were found to characterize successful programs:

- Application of social learning theories
- A narrow focus on reducing specific sexual risk-taking behaviors that may lead to HIV and STD infection or unintended pregnancy
- Reinforcement of age- and experience-appropriate values against unprotected sex
- Modeling and practice in communication and negotiation skills to prevent unprotected sex

Sex education should begin as soon as the child expresses curiosity about sex and related matters and can comprehend accurate explanations. By the beginning of adolescence, the child should have a clear understanding of how fertilization occurs and the events from fertilization through delivery and the postpartum periods, including the biologic and the social consequences of pregnancy. A variety of other topics may be included in sex education programs, such as the types of contraception available, the effects of childbearing on the adolescent's life and future life course, and rational decision making. The importance of making conscious decisions regarding life options needs to be emphasized, because many adolescents have difficulty delaying gratification and planning for the future. By strengthening the value of competing goals (such as school achievement and employment opportunities) and by providing alternative strategies (such as intimacy without sexual behavior or with regular contraceptive use), the adolescent's motivational constructs may be changed (Brooks-Gunn et al., 1989). Adolescents often require assistance to recognize when they want to say no and to develop the skills to do so effectively.

The exact nature and scope of sex education courses may be partially determined by the sponsoring organization, the age of participants, the community involved, and available resources. The nurse may function in the role of consultant, instructor, or guest speaker. Teaching methods need to be concrete, providing frequent reinforcement of content because of the wide variation in abstract thinking abilities among adolescents. Role play may assist adolescents to cope with issues related to peer pressure and to explore individual decision making.

Contraception

Recent data indicate that most teenagers who use contraceptives rely on over-the-counter methods for a considerable period before they consult a healthcare provider. Only 40% of sexually experienced teenage women visit a healthcare provider for contraceptives within 12 months of initiating intercourse. The majority of sexually experienced adolescent women and their partners do use a contraceptive, primarily the condom or the birth control pill (Alan Guttmacher Institute, 1994). However, at any time, 75% of teenage women who have had sex are at risk of unintended pregnancy (Forrest et al., 1990). Most at-risk adolescents use contraceptives but may not adhere to the steps required for effective protection (Alan Guttmacher Institute, 1994). Family planning services that provide education, counseling, contraceptives, and basic laboratory testing need to be accessible and available to all adolescents. A comprehensive history and physical examination should precede the recommendation or prescription of contraception. (Further information on specific contraceptive methods is found in Chap. 9.)

Because contraceptive behavior may be influenced by many factors, it is important to identify and discuss the adolescent's concerns about side effects of various techniques. Individual counseling about the actions, effectiveness, and safety of selected methods helps allay anxieties and ensure matching of the adolescent and an appropriate contraceptive method. Actual behavior may not always be predicted by personal attitudes toward contraception. The adolescent's motivation to control fertility needs to be appraised. The sexually active adolescent who is not using or is ineffectively using contraceptives must be aided to recognize a compelling reason for use of contraception, or there will be no change in behavior. For the adolescent who is not sexually active, counseling is directed toward reinforcing the choice of abstinence and supporting feelings of comfort with that decision.

The Nursing Process and the Pregnant Adolescent (Secondary Prevention)

Nursing care in the area of **secondary prevention** encompasses assessment, diagnosis, planning and intervention, and evaluation to support the adolescent and her family from conception through childbirth. The scope of secondary prevention differs depending on whether the decision is made to abort or to carry the fetus to term. The following essential components of intervention programs for pregnant and childbearing adolescents, their families, and male partners have been identified by the Office of Adolescent Pregnancy Programs in the Department of Health and Human Services:

- Pregnancy testing
- Maternity counseling
- Family planning counseling and service
- Primary and preventive healthcare
- Nutrition counseling, education, and services
- Venereal disease counseling, testing, and treatment
- Family life education
- Adoption counseling and referral
- Pediatric care

A well-planned and coordinated interdisciplinary effort is necessary to meet effectively the healthcare needs of pregnant and parenting adolescents. The nurse is an essential member of the multidisciplinary team, often composed of physicians, social workers, nutritionists, psychologists, and other health professionals.

Early entry of the pregnant adolescent into the healthcare system is of crucial importance in secondary prevention, because delayed onset of prenatal care or fewer prenatal visits increases the risk for poor obstetric outcome. A variety of factors may contribute to the pregnant adolescent's failure to seek adequate prenatal care (eg, lack of knowledge, lack of motivation, lack of financial resources, fear of consequences of exposure of the pregnancy, embarrassment, and fear of the healthcare delivery system).

Assessment

The goal of assessment is to obtain the necessary data to plan interventions to promote optimal health and development for the pregnant and parenting adolescent, her child, and family. The nurse's assessment of the adolescent includes direct questions and clinical observations. Demonstration of genuine interest and the ability to be a good listener are essential for an accurate nursing assessment. Mercer (1983) identified four major areas of nursing assessment, including the adolescent's developmental level, health status, knowledge base, and social support system.

Developmental Level

The nurse should assess the adolescent's *developmental level* carefully, because it may differ from her chronologic age. Developmental level will have an influence on how the adolescent reacts to the physiologic changes of pregnancy and ultimately, the adolescent's feelings about the newborn and mother-infant interactions later on. Examples of questions that should be considered are provided in the Assessment Tool: Assessing Adolescent Developmental Level.

Health Status

The nurse's assessment of the pregnant adolescent's health status includes a comprehensive nursing history, physical examination, and selected laboratory tests. (A detailed discussion of the health status assessment and examples of prenatal assessment tools are contained in Chap. 17). The nurse must devote particular attention to selected components of the assessment, including the sexual history, substance abuse history, nutritional status, immunization status, and pelvic examination.

Many adolescents are sensitive about their sexual history and may be embarrassed to respond to selected questions. The nurse should demonstrate a nonjudgmental attitude and reassure the adolescent that information related to initiation of coital activity and frequency, sexual partners, previous use of contraceptive methods, prior conceptions and abortions, and history of STDs will be kept confidential. The history of substance abuse includes questions related to past and current use of caffeine, nicotine, alcohol, and over-the-counter and recreational drugs.

The adequacy of the adolescent's dietary intake is determined using a comprehensive nutritional assessment tool (see Chap. 18). Young adolescents are at higher risk for nutritional deprivation during pregnancy because they often have lower nutrient stores at the time of conception. Their nutrition during pregnancy may not accommodate their own growth needs plus those of the fetus. In addition to diet history (dietary habits, likes, and dislikes), the nurse should assess who in the adolescent's family is responsible for making major dietary choices (selecting, purchasing, preparing, and serving food). Because the adolescent is at risk for anemia, hemoglobin and hematocrit values are assessed.

Baseline weight and blood pressure measurements are significant components of the physical assessment

ASSESSMENT TOOL
Assessing Adolescent Developmental Level

Developmental Stage

- Have the major developmental tasks of adolescence been achieved?
- What personal values does the adolescent express?
- Does she demonstrate increasing independence from her parents and development of a strong sense of personal identity?
- Is the adolescent attending school or employed?
- How does she spend her free time and with whom?
- Does she keep her scheduled appointments for prenatal care and arrive on time?
- Is she able to express herself freely to members of the health team?
- What are her major goals and plans for the future?
- Is the adolescent in the cognitive stage of concrete thinking or formal operations? If she is able to present her situation logically and consider her problems in the situation realistically, she is at the formal operations level of cognitive functioning (Piaget, 1971). Younger adolescents functioning at the concrete level are not capable of solving complex problems or understanding abstractions.

Reaction to the Psychological Changes of Pregnancy

- Do the adolescent's verbal expressions reflect a positive or negative attitude about being pregnant?

- Is she depressed about the pregnancy?
- Does she feel frightened or alone?
- What does this pregnancy represent to the adolescent?
- Does she verbally or nonverbally express negative feelings about her changing body image?
- What does the nurse observe about the adolescent's appearance (appropriateness of dress, posture, eye contact)?

Prenatal and Postnatal Feelings About the Quality of Mother-Newborn Interactions

- What does the adolescent verbally and emotionally express about her fetus and newborn during the prenatal and postnatal periods (positive or negative statements, complaining remarks, facial gestures)?
- Are her self-care activities consistent with these expressions?
- Does the newborn meet the mother's expectations? Who does she think the newborn looks like?
- How does the young mother handle her newborn (use of touch, stroking, verbalizations)?
- Does she avoid eye contact with her newborn or seem tense during interaction?
- What is the mother's response to her newborn's cries?

---

because pregnancy-induced hypertension is a common medical complication of adolescent pregnancy. Current status of immunizations is assessed (diphtheria, tetanus, polio, measles, mumps, and rubella), and tuberculosis screening is performed. Vision and dental evaluations may be given if necessary.

Because the pelvic examination may be anxiety-inducing for the adolescent, the nurse prepares her for this assessment by carefully explaining each step of the procedure in relation to reproductive anatomy. Demonstration of relaxation techniques may be helpful. Some adolescents benefit from observing the examination in a mirror or by assisting in insertion of the speculum. Clinical pelvimetry is performed using a gentle technique to determine spatial capacity and risk

for CPD. Cervical cytology is done to rule out dysplasia and carcinoma in situ. Additional gonococcal cultures and wet preps for *Candida, Chlamydia, Trichomonas, Gardnerella,* and gonorrhea may be collected because of the increased incidence of STDs in adolescents (see Chap. 11).

When assessing health status, consideration also should be given to the influence of cultural and religious practices on the belief system of the pregnant adolescent. For example, many immigrants from Haiti living in areas such as New York and Miami are followers of voodoo (Gustafson, 1989). Their belief system may include consultation with the root doctor and certain prescribed healing ceremonies. Hispanic pregnant adolescents may seek healthcare from *curanderas* in their communities, who may offer folk remedies and general advice (Clark, 1979).

Knowledge Base

The nurse identifies the learning needs of the adolescent by assessing her knowledge base and determining her immediate and future concerns. Several important areas for assessment are described in the Assessment Guidelines: Adolescents' Knowledge and Attitudes.

Social Support

The assessment of social support encompasses four types of supportive acts as defined by House (1981): emotional support (empathy, caring, love, and trust), instrumental support (eg, assistance with finances, child care), informational support (information for problem solving), and appraisal support (information for self-evaluation). The nurse may use the Assessment Tool: Social Support to help in gathering the relevant information.

Nursing Diagnoses

Nursing diagnoses are based largely on psychosocial and physical data obtained during assessment. Adolescents are likely to possess knowledge deficits in several areas. Initially, these deficits may be related to pregnancy options available and related care needs. Later, they relate to physiologic, psychological, and social implications of early childbearing; self-care needs during pregnancy; signs and symptoms of pregnancy

complications; preparation for childbirth; infant growth and development; parenting skills; and family planning. Examples of specific diagnoses include the following:

- Altered Nutrition: Less than body requirements related to lack of knowledge of adequate nutrition or lack of availability of quality food
- Body Image Disturbance related to pregnancy weight gain and altered body dimensions
- Altered Comfort related to physiologic changes of pregnancy
- Altered Family Processes related to the stress of adolescent pregnancy and parenting
- Self Esteem Disturbance related to conflict between the maternal role and identity formation
- Altered Parenting related to impaired parent-infant attachment (bonding), adolescent egocentrism, inadequate support systems, or unrealistic expectations of the infant

Planning and Intervention

The adolescent's specific healthcare plan depends on the stage of adolescence, her level of cognitive development, and her ability to achieve the tasks of adolescence (Mercer, 1983). In general, nursing interventions are directed toward the following goals:

- Establish a trusting relationship with the client. To achieve this goal, the nurse must be knowledgeable about normal adolescent growth and development, be aware of personal feelings about adolescent sexuality and pregnancy, and demonstrate a nonjudg-

ASSESSMENT GUIDELINES
Adolescents' Knowledge and Attitudes

Knowledge

- Sexual functioning
- Reproduction
- Pregnancy and childbirth
    Anatomy and physiology of pregnancy, labor and delivery, and postpartum
    Medications and anesthesia
    Breathing and relaxation techniques
- Infant growth and development
    Nutritional needs
    Developmental milestones
    Behavioral cues
- Parenting skills
    Bathing

    Diapering
    Feeding
    Mother-infant communication
- Family planning
    Past experiences and preferences

Attitude and Feelings

- Preparations for newborn
- Level of interest in learning about newborn
- Discipline techniques and strategies
- Mother-infant interaction (during feeding and caretaking)

ASSESSMENT TOOL
Social Support

Questions to Ask the Adolescent Mother

- With whom does the adolescent live?
- How does she feel about these people?
- Does the socioeconomic status of the family place the pregnant adolescent at risk?
- What is the nature of her relationship with the newborn's father and his family (marital or nonmarital relationship and quality of relationship)?
- What types of support does the pregnant adolescent receive from family members, her partner, and friends (eg, information, financial)?
- Other than the pregnancy, are there significant family or marital problems in the adolescent's life?
- Who will help the young mother care for her baby when she returns to school or work?
- How long will this assistance be available?
- Are agencies available in the community to assist her with financial problems, child care, and educational and vocational needs?

Questions to Ask Other Family Members, Such as the Adolescent's Mother

- Do they plan to provide the aid the adolescent expects?
- How does the adolescent interact with members of the family?
- Are the living conditions safe for a pregnant adolescent and infant (overcrowding, violence in neighborhood, pollutants)?
- Is transportation available to and from the prenatal care setting?

The nurse also should assess the specific needs of the adolescent father. Panzarine and Elster (1982) identified areas of potential psychosocial stresses that may be experienced by prospective adolescent fathers; these relate to the role and responsibilities of fatherhood, the relationship with his partner, changes in usual sources of support, the health of mother and newborn, and anxiety regarding labor and delivery (see Assessment Tool).

Questions to Ask the Prospective Adolescent Father

- What are the young man's concerns regarding his role as father?
- Is he experiencing any self-doubts about his capabilities to be a parent?
- Does he express feelings of "being trapped," or does he feel committed to the relationship and the newborn?
- What is the reaction of the adolescent father's family and friends to the pregnancy?
- Is he interested in learning more about childbirth and child care?
- What are his anxieties about labor and delivery and his role during this event?

Financial responsibilities and anticipated changes in vocational or educational plans may be of particular concern. Although many adolescent fathers do not have the skills necessary for securing a well-paying job, they may feel obligated to compromise school plans because of financial necessities (Panzarine & Elster, 1982). The adolescent father's perceptions about his relationship with his partner may differ from those of the pregnant adolescent.

---

mental attitude and effective interpersonal communication skills.
- Secure a safe pregnancy outcome for the adolescent and her fetus or a safe termination of pregnancy.
- Promote the adolescent's self-care activities during pregnancy, labor, delivery, and the puerperium (eg, personal hygiene, exercise, nutrition, postpartum family planning, and follow-up).
- Assist the adolescent to secure resources for meeting her support needs (emotional, instrumental, informational, and appraisal support).
- Facilitate the adolescent's attainment of the maternal role by demonstrating effective parenting skills and attachment behaviors.

- Enhance the adolescent's self-esteem and maturation.

(See Nursing Care Plan: The Pregnant Adolescent).

Pregnancy Care

To meet the previously described goals most effectively, the adolescent should be assigned to a primary care nurse who is regularly responsible for her prenatal nursing care. The nurse must emphasize the importance of initiating care early in pregnancy, keeping prenatal appointments, and communicating significant symptoms and problems to members of the healthcare

NURSING CARE PLAN
The Pregnant Adolescent

Nursing Goals

The pregnant adolescent will demonstrate physiological and psychological adaptation to the stressors of adolescence and pregnancy as evidenced by:
1. Establishing a trusting relationship with the healthcare team.
2. Performing self-care activities during pregnancy, labor and delivery, and the puerperium
3. Delivering a healthy term infant without perinatal complications
4. Securing needed resources for meeting support needs
5. Demonstrating attainment of the maternal role
6. Manifesting increased self-esteem and maturation

Assessment	Potential Nursing Diagnoses	Intervention/ Rationale	Evaluation
Developmental and cognitive level Relationship with peers and family Planned versus unplanned pregnancy	Self Concept Disturbance related to conflict between the maternal role and identity formation	Assist in development of problem-solving techniques and provide positive reinforcement for use of existing effective ones *to improve self-concept.*	New problem-solving skills are developed while existing effective ones are maintained.
Attitude toward pregnancy		Assist in achievement of the psychological tasks of pregnancy *to aid in maternal role acquisition.*	Client progressively achieves the psychological tasks of pregnancy.
Achievement of the psychological tasks of pregnancy Problem-solving skills Goals and values		Discuss potential areas of conflict between pregnancy and adolescence while offering psychological support for these conflicts (eg, peer and family relationships, education and personal goals) *to promote adaptation to the pregnancy as well as the maternal role*	Client is able to cope with the conflicts between pregnancy and adolescence and develops future plans for self and infant (eg, child care, continued education, and employment).
		Refer client to adolescent pregnancy support group *to provide needed support and an environment in which the adolescent feels secure and able to express her feelings*	Client participates in an adolescent pregnancy support group.
Concerns with body image Prepregnancy weight and weight gain during pregnancy	Body Image Disturbance related to body changes in pregnancy	Encourage expression of feelings regarding body changes during pregnancy *to promote adaptation and provide nurse with information about distressful changes*	Client openly discusses feelings regarding body changes during pregnancy.
Self-concept Developmental level		Counsel client regarding normal body changes during pregnancy; *accurate and realistic information about body changes during pregnancy is provided via counseling*	Client is able to describe the normal body changes during pregnancy and accepts these alterations.

(continued)

NURSING CARE PLAN *(Continued)*
The Pregnant Adolescent

Assessment	Potential Nursing Diagnoses	Intervention/ Rationale	Evaluation
Baseline weight and weight gain or loss during pregnancy Hgb and Hct	Altered Nutrition: Less than body requirement related to lack of knowledge of adequate nutrition	Explain relationship between weight gain, nutritional intake, and infant development *to improve self-care capabilities*	Client gains adequate weight (25 to 30 pounds).
		Instruct client on proper selection of foods from the four basic food groups or food pyramid *to improve diet*	Client follows healthy diet using food from four basic food groups on food pyramid.
Nutritional intake Nausea, vomiting, anorexia		Instruct client to keep a 24-hour food diary and analyze it with her *to assess client's diet and to reinforce proper selection of foods*	Client records 24-hour food diary and brings it in for analysis with the healthcare provider.
Who is the primary meal preparer?		Collaborate with primary meal provider regarding food selection *to assist adolescent in maintaining self-care*	Primary meal provider prepares nutritional food.
Use of prescribed vitamins and iron		Instruct client on purpose, side effects, and administration of prenatal vitamins and iron *to enhance compliance*	Client takes prenatal vitamins and iron as prescribed.
Financial constraints influencing dietary intake		Assess financial ability and management to attain proper nutrition *to increase ability to purchase proper foods*	Client effectively budgets finances in order to purchase nutritional foods.
Maternal–infant attachment	Altered Parenting related to impaired parent–infant attachment, adolescent egocentrism, inadequate support systems, or unrealistic expectations of the infant	Discuss parenting skills and infant care *to provide adolescent with information and allow for clarification of questions*	Client demonstrates appropriate parenting skills and infant care.
		Refer client to parenting and infant care classes; *acquisition of parenting and infant care skills may be enhanced in a group*	Client attends parenting and infant care classes.
Clients expectations of infant behavior Developmental level		Discuss expectations of infant behavior and parenting role *to provide anticipatory guidance for adolescent*	Client relates probable infant behavior with proper parenting response.
		Explain importance of parent–infant attachment and provide information on methods to enhance it *to promote a positive parent–infant relationship*	Client seeks interactions with infant and uses methods to promote attachment.

(continued)

NURSING CARE PLAN (Continued)
The Pregnant Adolescent

Assessment	Potential Nursing Diagnoses	Intervention/ Rationale	Evaluation
Client's relationship with family members, especially mother	Altered Family Processes related to the stress of adolescent pregnancy and parenting	Encourage communication of expectations between family members and client *to facilitate family adaptation*	Client and family members communicate expectations.
		Encourage discussion of future plans for client, infant, and family *to allow family to problem solve*	Client makes future plans for self, infant, and family.
Extent of involvement of the baby's father		Encourage involvement of infant's father, if both partners agree *to broaden support to client and promote adaptation*	Infant's father is present and involved.

team. Using a nonauthoritarian manner when relating information is likely to improve nurse-client communications and to increase satisfaction with services and client compliance. Active involvement of the adolescent in the various components of her prenatal care (such as self-care activities and prenatal education) should be encouraged as an approach to promoting personal responsibility and autonomy. The adolescent's sense of control may be enhanced if she is allowed to test her urine, weigh herself, plan her diet, and listen to fetal heart tones (Mercer, 1983).

Prenatal Education. One of the most important aspects of nursing care is prenatal education. Instructional programs for pregnant adolescents may include information on the basic anatomy and physiology of pregnancy, labor, delivery, and the postpartum period; body mechanics and exercise during pregnancy; nutritional intake for pregnancy and lactation; signs of true versus false labor; breathing and relaxation techniques; breast-feeding; and family planning. To promote maternal role acquisition, anticipatory guidance should be provided about normal infant growth and development, child care, and mother-infant communication styles.

Prenatal classes may be offered in a variety of settings, such as hospitals, churches, and other community agencies. Instructional programs are frequently divided into weekly sessions that last from 30 minutes to 2 hours. Several teaching methods may be used, including lecture, discussion, demonstration, and role play. Active participation helps the adolescent to integrate her personal experiences with theoretical knowledge (Ruszala-Herbst, 1984). Examples of role play sit-

uations include how to schedule follow-up well baby care; what to do when a child has a fever, diarrhea, or a diaper rash; and what to do when an infant does not stop crying in the middle of the night.

The nurse is likely to discover that giving demonstrations and having the adolescent perform selected caretaking tasks (such as taking the infant's temperature, cleaning the cord, and burping) are more effective than didactic approaches. Audiovisual presentations and written materials should be used to stimulate interest and to reinforce learning. Opportunities should be available for exploration of individual concerns and discussion of conflicts between information taught in class and practices in the home.

Nutritional Counseling. Nutritional counseling is provided on an individual basis. The four food groups or the food pyramid is reviewed in relation to fetal growth and development. The nurse should provide examples of foods rich in iron and folate, because inadequate intake of these nutrients and low body stores place the pregnant adolescent at a distinct risk for development of anemia (Worthington-Roberts, 1993). The distribution of additional weight to the baby, placenta, breasts, and body fluids should be fully explained to allay possible anxieties about excessive weight gain during pregnancy. Opportunities are provided for the adolescent to plan meals with consideration to age-related and cultural preferences.

The nurse should initiate a referral to the nutritionist for follow-up services if the adolescent is at nutritional risk because of poor weight gain, eating disorders, iron deficiency anemia, or slow fundal growth. The Special Supplemental Food Program for Women, Infants, and

Children (WIC) is an additional source of nutritional assistance for some pregnant adolescents (see Chap. 18).

Promoting Problem-Solving Skills. Nursing intervention also is designed to assist the adolescent in developing effective problem-solving skills. The adolescent must learn how to do the following:

- Identify the problem and the goal.
- Obtain appropriate data.
- Generate and weigh options.
- Decide on one option.
- Implement the option and evaluate potential outcomes.

Sachs (1986) recommends that adolescents be assisted with practice decision making in groups possessing similar cognitive skills.

Inclusion of Family Member. The family system of the pregnant adolescent must be considered when planning and implementing nursing care. A variety of family forms may exist; however, pregnant adolescents most frequently live with one or both parents or with another member of the family. The father of the infant also may be considered an important member of the unmarried adolescent's family. The nurse should facilitate effective family communications whenever possible by encouraging the adolescent to involve her family in the childbearing experience (eg, attendance at prenatal classes and birth). Parental support is particularly important, because it increases the potential for dealing with the adolescent's problems on a continuing basis (Hartman, 1989). Because the adolescent may have difficulty accepting help from others and trusting that others will help her, the nurse may need to provide counseling on how to secure a supportive environment.

It is important for the nurse to be considerate of the adolescent father, because his needs are often ignored by healthcare professionals. Before interacting with these young men, the nurse must carefully appraise whether any biased attitudes exist toward them. It is commonly assumed that adolescent fathers are uninterested in becoming involved in their partner's pregnancies or the rearing of their children; however, the results of several studies indicate that many young fathers become deeply involved when permitted (Hardy et al., 1989; Redmond, 1985; Robinson et al., 1986; Fig. 35-2). The nurse can assist the prospective father to cope with the stresses of pregnancy by several interventions. Including him in the decision-making process is particularly helpful, because it may allay his fears, decrease his sense of helplessness and alienation, and provide him with an opportunity to function in an adult role (Barret et al., 1986). Counseling

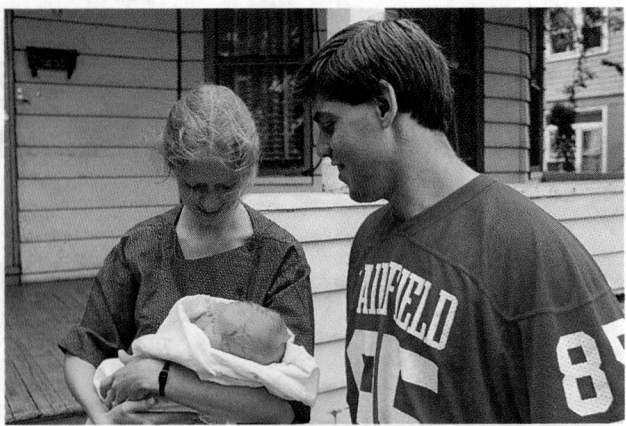

FIGURE 35-2 The nurse should not assume that adolescent fathers are uninterested in their partner's pregnancies or in rearing their child. Many young fathers become deeply involved when permitted.

is provided early in the prenatal period whenever possible, regarding the psychological and physiologic changes occurring during pregnancy and how these may impact on the couple's relationship. Accurate information about the childbirth process and healthcare services needs to be included. The prospective father should be invited to attend routine prenatal visits and to participate by listening to fetal heart tones and palpating fetal movements. Anticipatory guidance is offered regarding issues specific to adolescent fatherhood (eg, the father's role in labor and delivery, future financial responsibilities, sources of support, and legal rights). The couple should be encouraged to verbalize their feelings about the pregnancy and expectations of each other during the phases of childbearing and childrearing.

Labor and Delivery Care

Optimal intrapartum care for adolescents should include all of the features of nursing care described in Chapter 22. Adolescents have a particularly great need for adequate support during labor because they may be afraid of the hospital and have fears related to lack of accurate knowledge of the birthing process. Adequate intrapartum support has been associated with a decreased need for analgesia and anesthesia, lower pain, more enjoyment, and greater satisfaction with the birth experience (Hodnett et al., 1989). Unfortunately, many adolescents do not have supportive family members, mates, or friends present during the intrapartum period. Therefore, supportive nursing interventions are particularly needed and beneficial; these may include information about the labor and delivery process, demonstration of relaxation and breathing techniques to cope with contractions, provision of physical comfort measures, and encouragement and reassurance.

Continuous primary care from the same nurse is beneficial.

If the fetus' father is present and interested in supporting the laboring adolescent, his active participation in the birth process should be encouraged. The nurse may need to support the father in his efforts to assist his partner, to interact with the newborn after delivery, and to cope with his new parenting role. The initiation and maintenance of early newborn contact after delivery is especially important for adolescent parents. The nurse may assist the new parents in getting acquainted with their newborn by encouraging touch, verbalization, proximity, and caretaking behaviors.

Puerperium Care

The adolescent mother requires the same physical nursing care in the postpartum period as an adult woman (see Chap. 27). However, her developmental and cognitive level may necessitate further focus on self-care (perineal and breast care, sleep and rest, comfort measures) and selected psychosocial aspects of the puerperium. In particular, nursing care should be planned and implemented to promote the adolescent's maternal role acquisition. The nurse should provide the following:

- Opportunities for extended contact with the newborn. Rooming-in or mother–newborn units allow the adolescent mother to receive more instruction, promote satisfaction with care, and may increase attachment to the infant (Winkelstein et al., 1987; Fig. 35-3).
- Instruction and counseling regarding safe and effective parenting skills, such as feeding (techniques, timing, positioning, intake), bathing, diapering, and dressing. Content on "how to care for the sick baby"

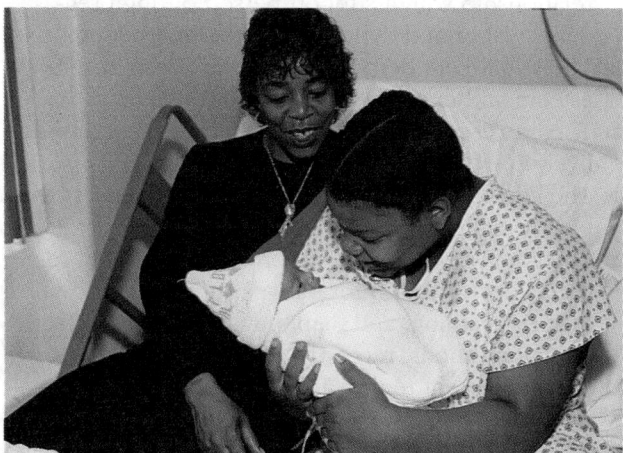

FIGURE 35–3 Adolescent mothers should be given every opportunity to bond with their newborns.

and "protecting the infant from accidents" were identified as most important informational needs in a survey of postpartum adolescents (Howard et al., 1985). Other instructional areas include the stages of infant and child growth and development, methods to enhance the infant's cognitive and social development through maternal verbalizations and sensory stimulation (see Chap. 29), infant supplies, alternative methods of child care, and immunizations.

- Positive reinforcement of self-care activities and effective mothering skills. Whenever desired maternal behaviors are demonstrated, the nurse should praise the client, because this reinforcement can enhance her self-esteem and promote learning.

The developmental level and cognitive abilities of the adolescent need to be considered in client teaching and counseling. Younger mothers may prefer short sessions of individualized instruction rather than formal classes that remind them of school. "Hands-on" teaching sessions are particularly effective with adolescents whose thinking is still fairly concrete (Fullar, 1986). To maximize learning with group instruction, classes should be brief and conducted among a small group of peers. Media such as videocassettes, film, and closed-circuit hospital television may be useful for instruction, because many adolescents are familiar and comfortable with these techniques. Written materials should be appropriate for the adolescent's developmental and reading level.

The nurse may assist the adolescent to make decisions about family planning by first asking about her knowledge of contraception and her experience with various methods. Misconceptions about actions and side effects of specific contraceptive methods should be clarified. Regardless of the preferred method, the nurse must determine how the adolescent will obtain and pay for the contraceptive. If medical supervision is required, the adolescent should be aware of sources of follow-up healthcare.

When providing postpartum care, the nurse must remember that the adolescent's normal egocentrism may require the nurse first to concentrate care on the mother and her immediate concerns. Feelings about the labor and delivery experience and her current physical status often need to be discussed before newborn caretaking. Some young mothers appear excessively demanding of the nurse's attention and time because of fears related to their lack of experience with newborn care and hospitalization. Others seem passive and afraid to initiate interactions with their newborn until the nurse or a close family member is present. Older adolescents may demonstrate effective problem-solving skills and the ability to communicate their needs clearly.

Several interventions may facilitate interpersonal communications with adolescent mothers who often have difficulty spontaneously speaking with adults (Fullar, 1986). The nurse should avoid open-ended questions and long silences that may increase the adolescent's anxiety. Gentle inquiries and supportive statements may help to relax the adolescent (eg, "Young mothers are often concerned about..."). A checklist approach to assessment should be avoided.

Early discharge planning is of prime importance in the care of postpartum adolescents, their newborns, and their families. Optimally, plans for follow-up care begin during pregnancy and are a component of the comprehensive adolescent healthcare service. When this type of assistance is unavailable or the adolescent has received no prenatal care, the nurse may need to initiate a referral to the social worker for additional support (eg, housing, financial aid, temporary foster care for the newborn, WIC, or alternative schools with child care). The adolescent should be referred to the community health nurse if continued assessment and instruction are required for self-care or educational needs. Research indicates that most adolescent mothers and fathers benefit from parenting education programs offered during early childrearing (Glanville et al., 1990; Heifer, 1987). A variety of programs may be available in local schools and community facilities. The nurse may provide valuable assistance by discussing the advantages of these programs and giving the adolescent mother current information on the types and locations of adolescent parenting groups.

Abortion Care

The physical and psychosocial nursing care needs of adolescents considering voluntary termination of pregnancy are similar to those of adult women (see Chap. 12). The procedure to be used for an abortion is determined by the length of pregnancy. Before counseling a pregnant adolescent about abortion as an alternative option to childbearing, the nurse must be knowledgeable about state laws regarding abortion for minors. A minor woman has a constitutional right to consent to an abortion; however, states may impose parental notification requirements consistent with constitutional principles. Parental approval or notification is not required unless the state has enacted such a requirement (Henshaw, 1992). In states having no such legal requirement, informing a parent of the adolescent's intent to have an abortion without her permission may subject the nurse to liability for breach of client confidentiality.

The adolescent receiving abortion counseling is likely to have had little or no experience with an unplanned pregnancy or abortion decision. She may experience confusion, isolation, or fear related to being judged by healthcare professionals. Multiple or conflicting goals may make the decision to abort complex (eg, the desire to please her parents and her partner, affirm her own values and ethics, and balance a career and motherhood goals; Brown, 1983). Through reflective listening, the nurse can help the adolescent to clarify the conflicts she may be experiencing between her needs and the needs of her partner and family. Other issues surrounding the adolescent's abortion decision that may need to be addressed include how to inform her partner and parents about the pregnancy; secure funds for the abortion procedure; and explain absence from school or work.

Evaluation

Evaluation of nursing care is conducted through a variety of techniques. Records are maintained on the adolescent's attendance at prenatal visits. Learning outcomes in prenatal classes may be evaluated by written multiple choice tests, verbal questions, and problem-solving exercises. Logs containing descriptions of the adolescent's behavior observed by nurses in the labor and delivery and postpartum units also are helpful. The health and growth of the newborn may be evaluated by progression of height and weight, immunization status, incidence of illness, emergency room visits, and hospitalizations.

Other examples of specific outcome criteria include the following:

- The adolescent initiates early prenatal care and returns for regular prenatal care.
- The adolescent implements appropriate self-care activities during pregnancy (adequate nutrition, exercise, personal hygiene, attendance at prenatal classes).
- The adolescent establishes and maintains a positive relationship with a support person during pregnancy, labor and delivery, and the puerperium.
- The adolescent demonstrates an increase in self-esteem and maturity level during pregnancy.
- The adolescent effectively copes with labor and delivery.
- The adolescent delivers a healthy, term newborn of birth weight within normal limits.
- The adolescent acquires appropriate maternal role behaviors (affection for baby; appropriate and safe feeding, bathing, and diapering techniques; effective communications, recognition of illness).
- The adolescent returns for scheduled family planning follow-up care and well-baby care.
- The adolescent expresses gratification in the maternal role.

■ The adolescent secures needed assistance for continued schooling or employment and other needs through appropriate use of community resources.

The Nursing Process and the Childrearing Adolescent (Tertiary Prevention)

Tertiary prevention emphasizes the return of the client to a maximum state of health and functioning. The objectives of tertiary prevention for the childbearing adolescent follow:

■ To enhance the ability of the adolescent mother and her family to assume useful, satisfying, and self-sufficient roles in society
■ To optimize the physical, psychosocial, and intellectual development of the adolescent's child
■ To prevent recidivism (rapid, repeat, unplanned pregnancy)

Most repeat adolescent pregnancies are unplanned and unwanted. The younger the adolescent is at the time of her first pregnancy, the more likely she will conceive again as an adolescent. Data from the National Longitudinal Survey of Youth reveal that approximately 25% of teenage mothers have a second child within 24 months of their first birth (Kalmuss et al., 1994). In this large study, adolescent characteristics before the first birth (such as race or ethnicity and parents' level of education) and at the time of the first birth (eg, schooling completed and desire for pregnancy) affected whether they had a close second birth. Young mothers who had more educated parents and those who obtained additional schooling after their first birth were found to be *less* likely to have a closely spaced second birth, while those who married were more likely to have another child. Repeat pregnancies during adolescence are of concern because there is greater morbidity and mortality for the subsequent children born to adolescents and because of spiraling psychosocial problems.

Tertiary prevention programs use a multidisciplinary team that may consist of nurses, case managers, nutritionists, counselors, physicians, social workers, and teachers. Services available are individualized for the needs and stage of development of each parent, the newborn, and family. A variety of specialized services may be offered:

■ Family planning and reproductive health services
■ Pediatric care: well baby care and emergency care for young children
■ Parenting education
■ Life skills training (consumer education, budgeting, household financial management, homemaking skills)
■ Alternative school programs
■ Employment training and counseling
■ Referral to community support services (eg, WIC, AFDC, child care)

The role of the nurse in tertiary prevention programs varies greatly. In some programs, the nurse assumes broad responsibilities as the case manager accountable for coordination of services; in others, the nurse's role is narrower in scope (eg, family planning, parenting instruction, support group leadership). Opportunities exist in many tertiary prevention programs for an ongoing relationship between the nurse and the adolescent mother. The nurse may assist the young mother to improve parenting behaviors by applying the following strategies:

■ Respecting and acknowledging her positive efforts, achievements, and role development
■ Creating an environment conducive to learning (eg, showing empathy, using praise)
■ Providing anticipatory guidance focusing on normal developmental behavior and change (eg, newborn cues)
■ Describing and modeling effective mothering techniques
■ Reinforcing that learning to be a parent is a gradual process
■ Minimizing "rules" of parenting behaviors
■ Focusing on varied positive outcomes rather than negative behaviors, such as missed appointments
■ Avoiding making assumptions about the mother's motivations (Fleming et al., 1993)

The nurse should encourage involvement of the adolescent's family system in supporting her efforts to gain the education and skills that optimize her life choices and to rear her infant in a nurturing and stimulating environment. Research findings indicate that African American grandmothers, in particular, provide valuable support that ensures that adolescents develop in their mothering roles and prepares them for the full responsibility of infant care (Flaherty, 1988). However, in some families, residing with grandmothers may have negative consequences on the quality of adolescent mothers' and especially grandmothers' parenting (Chase-Lansdale et al., 1994). The newborn's father also may have an important impact on how the adolescent mother adapts to parenthood. The nurse may assist the father by helping him to perceive his parental role realistically and by facilitating communications with his newborn's mother. Promoting mutual responsibility for the well-being of the child is one of the major challenges nurses face in caring for adolescent parents.

Summary Points

✔ The incidence of adolescent pregnancy has increased in recent years and has become a major social concern. Mounting economic costs are associated with supporting families started by teenage mothers (eg, AFDC, food stamps).

✔ The developmental tasks of adolescence (eg, achieving emotional independence from parents, preparing for an economic career) are interrupted by an unplanned pregnancy, which causes the young mother to move prematurely into the stage of generativity before internalizing an identity.

✔ The four steps leading to adolescent parenthood include decisions to become sexually active or remain sexually inactive, use or not use contraceptive(s) appropriately, deliver or abort, and rear or relinquish the child.

✔ Examples of maternal health problems during adolescent pregnancy include nutritional deficiencies, STDs, PIH, substance use, CPD, and preterm labor. The children of adolescent mothers are at risk for LBW, morbidity and mortality during infancy, and later academic and behavioral problems.

✔ The adolescent father often experiences isolation and may be adversely affected by having his education interrupted, achieving poorer vocational outcomes, lacking family support, and suffering financial difficulties.

✔ Primary prevention includes nursing interventions to avert conception either through promotion of abstinence or regular use of effective contraceptives in sexually active adolescents.

✔ Nursing care in the area of secondary prevention includes assessment, diagnosis, planning, intervention, and evaluation aimed at supporting the adolescent and her family from conception through childbirth. The nurse should assess the pregnant adolescent's developmental level, health status, knowledge base, and support system.

✔ In the area of tertiary prevention, the nurse applies the nursing process to enhance health, social, and developmental outcomes of the adolescent mother and her family and to prevent repeat, unplanned pregnancy.

REFERENCES

Abrahamse, A. F., Morrison, P. A., & Waite, L. J. (1988). *Beyond stereotypes: Who becomes a single teenage mother?* New York: Rand.

Alan Guttmacher Institute (1994). *Sex and America's teenagers*. New York: Author.

Alan Guttmacher Institute (1981a). *Teenage pregnancy: The problem that hasn't gone away*. New York: Author.

Alan Guttmacher Institute (1981b). *Factbook on teenage pregnancy*. New York: Author.

Barret, R. L., & Robinson, B. E. (1986). Adolescent fathers: Often forgotten parents. *Pediatric Nursing, 12,* 273–277.

Brindis, C., Starbuck-Morales, S., Wolfe, A. L., & McCarter, V. (1994). Characteristics associated with contraceptive use among adolescent females in school-based family planning programs. *Family Planning Perspectives, 26,* 160–164.

Brooks-Gunn, J., & Furstenberg, F. F. (1989). Adolescent sexual behavior. *American Psychologist, 44*(2), 249–257.

Brooks-Gunn, J., & Furstenberg, F. F. (1986). The children of adolescent mothers: Physical, academic, and psychological outcomes. *Developmental Review, 6,* 224–251.

Brown, M. A. (1983). Adolescent and abortion: A theoretical framework for decision making. *Journal of Obstetric, Gynecologic, and Neonatal Nursing, 12,* 241–247.

Caldas, S. J. (1994). Teen pregnancy: Why it remains a serious social, economic, and educational problem in the U.S. *Phi Delta Kappan, 75,* 402–406.

Centers for Disease Control, U.S. Dept of Health and Human Services (1992). *Monthly vital statistics reports, 40,* 12.

Centers for Disease Control and Prevention, Division of STD/HIV Prevention (1993). *1992 annual report.* Atlanta: Author.

Center for Population Options (1992). *Teenage pregnancy and too early childbearing: Public costs personal consequences.* Washington, DC: Author.

Chase-Lansdale, P. L., Brooks-Gunn, J., & Zamsky, E. S. (1994). Young African-American multigenerational families in poverty: Quality of mothering and grandmothering. *Child Development, 65,* 373–393.

Clark, A. L. (1979). *Culture/childbearing/health professionals.* Philadelphia: F.A. Davis.

Coll, C. G., Vohr, B. R., Hoffman, J. et al. (1986). Maternal and environmental factors affecting developmental outcome of infants of adolescent mothers. *Journal of Developmental & Behavioral Pediatrics, 7*(4), 230–236.

Committee on Adolescence (1989). Care of adolescent parents and their children. *Pediatrics, 83*(1), 138–140.

Duncan, G. J., & Hoffman, S. D. (1990). Teenage welfare receipt and subsequent dependence among black adolescent mothers. *Family Planning Perspectives, 22,* 16–20.

Elster, A. B., Lamb, M. E., & Tavare, J. (1987). Association between behavioral and school problems and fatherhood in a national sample of adolescent youths. *Journal of Pediatrics, 111*(6), 932–936.

Erikson, E. H. (1959). Identity and the life cycle (monograph). *Psychological Issues, 1*(1), 1–171.

(1994). *Facts at a glance.* Washington, DC: Child Trends.

(1994). *Facts in brief.* New York: The Alan Guttmacher Institute.

Flaherty, M. J. (1988). Seven caring functions of black grandmothers in adolescent mothering. *Maternal-Child Nursing Journal, 17*(3), 191–207.

Fleming, B. W., Munton, M. T., Clarke, B., & Strauss, S. S. (1993). Assessing and promoting positive parenting in adolescent mothers. *MCN: American Journal of Maternal Child Nursing, 18,* 32–37.

Flick, L. H. (1986). Paths to adolescent parenthood: Implications for prevention. *Public Health Reports, 101*(2), 132–147.

Forrest, J. D., & Singh, S. (1990). The sexual and reproductive behavior of American women, 1982-1988. *Family Planning Perspectives, 22,* 206–214.

Friede, A. F., Hogue, C. J. R., Doyle, L. L. et al. (1986). Do the sisters of childbearing teenagers have increased rates of childbearing? *American Journal of Public Health, 76*(10), 1221–1224.

Friedman, S. B., & Phillips, S. (1983). Psychosocial risk to mother and child as a consequence of adolescent pregnancy. In E. R. McAnarney (Ed.), *Premature adolescent pregnancy and parenthood* (pp. 269–277). New York: Grune & Stratton.

Fullar, S. A. (1986). Care of postpartum adolescents. *MCN: American Journal of Maternal Child Nursing, 11,* 398–403.

Furstenberg, F. F., Levine, J. A., & Brooks-Gunn, J. (1990). The children of teenage mothers: Patterns of early childbearing in two generations. *Family Planning Perspectives, 22*(2), 54–61.

Furstenberg, F. F., Brooks-Gunn, J., & Morgan, P. (1987). *Adolescent mothers in later life.* New York: Cambridge University Press.

Furstenberg, F. F., & Crawford, A. (1978). Family support, helping teenage mothers to cope. *Family Planning Perspectives, 8,* 148–164.

Gale, R., Seidman, D. S., Dollberg, S. et al. (1989). Is teenage pregnancy a neonatal risk factor? *Journal of Adolescent Health Care, 10*(5), 404–408.

Glanville, C. L., & Tiller, C. M. (1990). Implementing negotiating strategies into teen parenting programs. *Journal of the National Black Nurses Association, 4*(1), 45–54.

Gold, R. B., Kenney, A., & Singh, S. (1990). *Poverty in the United States: 1990.* Washington, DC: U.S. Bureau of the Census, Current Population Reports, Series P-60, No. 175, 1991.

Greydanus, D. E. (1987). Risk-taking behaviors in adolescence. *Journal of the American Medical Association, 258*(15), 2110.

Gustafson, M. B. (1989). Western voodoo: Providing mental health care to Haitian refugees. *Journal of Psychosocial Nursing and Mental Health Services, 27*(12), 22–25.

Hardy, J. B., Duggan, A. K., Masnyk, K. et al. (1989). Fathers of children born to young urban mothers. *Family Planning Perspectives, 21*(4), 159–163.

Hardy, J. B., & Duggan, A. K. (1988). Teenage fathers and the fathers of infants of urban, teenage mothers. *American Journal of Public Health, 78*(8), 919–922.

Hartman, K. (Ed.) (1989). Joint statement on adolescent health care. *NAACOG Newsletter, 16*(4), 5–16.

Havighurst, R. J. (1972). *Developmental tasks and education.* New York: D McKay.

Hayes, C. D. (Ed.) (1987). *Risking the future: Adolescent sexuality, pregnancy and childbearing* (Vol. I). Washington, DC: National Academy Press.

Heifer, R. E. (1987). The perinatal period, a window of opportunity for enhancing parent–infant communication: An approach to prevention. *Child Abuse and Neglect, 11*(4), 565–579.

Henshaw, S. K. (1993). Abortion trends in 1987 and 1988: Age and race. *Family Planning Perspectives, 24,* 85–86.

Henshaw, S. K. (1992). The accessibility of abortion services in the United States. *Family Planning Perspectives, 23,* 246–252, 253.

Hodnett, D. E., & Osborn, R. W. (1989). A randomized trial of the effects of montrice support during labor: Mothers' views two to four weeks postpartum. *Birth, 16*(4), 177–183.

Hofferth, S. L., & Hayes, C. D. (Eds.) (1987). *Risking the future: Adolescent sexuality, pregnancy, and childbearing* (Vol. II). Washington, DC: National Academy Press.

Hoffman, S. D., Foster, E. M., & Furstenberg, F. F. Jr. (1993). Reevaluating the costs of teenage childbearing: Responses to Geronimus and Korenman. *Demography, 30,* 291–296.

Hogan, P., & Kitagawa, E. (1985). The impact of social status, family structure and neighborhood on the fertility of black adolescents. *American Journal of Sociology, 90,* 825–855.

House, J. S. (1981). *Work stress and social support.* Reading, MA: Addison-Wesley.

Howard, M., & McCabe, J. B. (1990). Helping teenagers postpone sexual involvement. *Family Planning Perspectives, 22*(4), 21–26.

Howard, J. S., & Sater, J. (1985). Adolescent mothers: Self-perceived health education needs. *Journal of Obstetric, Gynecologic, and Neonatal Nursing, 14,* 399–404.

Howe, C. L. (1986). Developmental theory and adolescent sexual behavior. *Nurse Practitioner, 11*(2), 65–71.

Jones, E. F., Forrest, J. D., Goldman, N. et al. (1985). Teenage pregnancy in developed countries: Determinants and policy implications. *Family Planning Perspectives, 17*(2), 53–63.

Juhasz, A. M., & Sonnenshein-Schneider, M. (1980). Adolescent sexual decision-making: Components and skills. *Adolescence, 15,* 743–750.

Kafka, D. (Ed.) (1988). NYC teenagers who are young, white or unmarried are the most likely to end unwanted pregnancies. *Family Planning Perspectives, 20*(5), 240–241.

Kalmuss, D. S., & Namerow, P. B. (1994). Subsequent childbearing among teenage mothers: The determinants of a closely spaced second birth. *Family Planning Perspectives, 26,* 149–153.

Kirby, D., Short, L., Collins, J., Rugg, D., Kolbe, L., Howard, M. et al. (1994). School-based programs to reduce sexual risk behaviors: A review of effectiveness. *Public Health Reports, 109,* 339–360.

Leadbeater, B. J., & Bishop S. J. (1994). Predictors of behavior problems in preschool children of inner-city Afro-American and Puerto Rican adolescent mothers. *Child Development, 65,* 638–648.

Leigh, B. C., Morrison, D. M., Trocki, K., & Temple, M. T. (1994). Sexual behavior of American adolescents: Results from a U.S. national survey. *Journal of Adolescent Health, 15,* 117–125.

Macdonald, D. I. (1987). An approach to the problem of teenage pregnancy. *Public Health Reports, 102*(4), 377–385.

Males, M. (1993). Schools, society, and "Teen" pregnancy. *Phi Delta Kappan, 75,* 566–568

Marcia, J. E. (1966). Development and validation of ego identity status. *Journal of Personality and Social Psychology, 3,* 551–558.

Marcia, J. E. (1967). Ego identity status: Relationship to change in self-esteem, "general maladjustment," and authoritarianism. *Journal of Personality, 35,* 119–133.

Marcia, J. E. (1980). Identity in adolescence. In J. Adelson (Ed.), *Handbook of adolescent psychology* (pp. 159–187). New York: Wiley & Sons.

Marsiglio, W., & Mott, F. L. (1986). Impact of sex education on sexual activity, contraceptive use and premarital pregnancy. *Family Planning Perspectives, 18*(4), 151–162.

adolescent mothers. *MCN: American Journal of Maternal Child Nursing, 18,* 32–37.

Flick, L. H. (1986). Paths to adolescent parenthood: Implications for prevention. *Public Health Reports, 101*(2), 132–147.

Forrest, J. D., & Singh, S. (1990). The sexual and reproductive behavior of American women, 1982-1988. *Family Planning Perspectives, 22,* 206–214.

Friede, A. F., Hogue, C. J. R., Doyle, L. L. et al. (1986). Do the sisters of childbearing teenagers have increased rates of childbearing? *American Journal of Public Health, 76*(10), 1221–1224.

Friedman, S. B., & Phillips, S. (1983). Psychosocial risk to mother and child as a consequence of adolescent pregnancy. In E. R. McAnarney (Ed.), *Premature adolescent pregnancy and parenthood* (pp. 269–277). New York: Grune & Stratton.

Fullar, S. A. (1986). Care of postpartum adolescents. *MCN: American Journal of Maternal Child Nursing, 11,* 398–403.

Furstenberg, F. F., Levine, J. A., & Brooks-Gunn, J. (1990). The children of teenage mothers: Patterns of early childbearing in two generations. *Family Planning Perspectives, 22*(2), 54–61.

Furstenberg, F. F., Brooks-Gunn, J., & Morgan, P. (1987). *Adolescent mothers in later life.* New York: Cambridge University Press.

Furstenberg, F. F., & Crawford, A. (1978). Family support, helping teenage mothers to cope. *Family Planning Perspectives, 8,* 148–164.

Gale, R., Seidman, D. S., Dollberg, S. et al. (1989). Is teenage pregnancy a neonatal risk factor? *Journal of Adolescent Health Care, 10*(5), 404–408.

Glanville, C. L., & Tiller, C. M. (1990). Implementing negotiating strategies into teen parenting programs. *Journal of the National Black Nurses Association, 4*(1), 45–54.

Gold, R. B., Kenney, A., & Singh, S. (1990). *Poverty in the United States: 1990.* Washington, DC: U.S. Bureau of the Census, Current Population Reports, Series P-60, No. 175, 1991.

Greydanus, D. E. (1987). Risk-taking behaviors in adolescence. *Journal of the American Medical Association, 258*(15), 2110.

Gustafson, M. B. (1989). Western voodoo: Providing mental health care to Haitian refugees. *Journal of Psychosocial Nursing and Mental Health Services, 27*(12), 22–25.

Hardy, J. B., Duggan, A. K., Masnyk, K. et al. (1989). Fathers of children born to young urban mothers. *Family Planning Perspectives, 21*(4), 159–163.

Hardy, J. B., & Duggan, A. K. (1988). Teenage fathers and the fathers of infants of urban, teenage mothers. *American Journal of Public Health, 78*(8), 919–922.

Hartman, K. (Ed.) (1989). Joint statement on adolescent health care. *NAACOG Newsletter, 16*(4), 5–16.

Havighurst, R. J. (1972). *Developmental tasks and education.* New York: D McKay.

Hayes, C. D. (Ed.) (1987). *Risking the future: Adolescent sexuality, pregnancy and childbearing* (Vol. I). Washington, DC: National Academy Press.

Heifer, R. E. (1987). The perinatal period, a window of opportunity for enhancing parent–infant communication: An approach to prevention. *Child Abuse and Neglect, 11*(4), 565–579.

Henshaw, S. K. (1993). Abortion trends in 1987 and 1988: Age and race. *Family Planning Perspectives, 24,* 85–86.

Henshaw, S. K. (1992). The accessibility of abortion services in the United States. *Family Planning Perspectives, 23,* 246–252, 253.

Hodnett, D. E., & Osborn, R. W. (1989). A randomized trial of the effects of montrice support during labor: Mothers' views two to four weeks postpartum. *Birth, 16*(4), 177–183.

Hofferth, S. L., & Hayes, C. D. (Eds.) (1987). *Risking the future: Adolescent sexuality, pregnancy, and childbearing* (Vol. II). Washington, DC: National Academy Press.

Hoffman, S. D., Foster, E. M., & Furstenberg, F. F. Jr. (1993). Reevaluating the costs of teenage childbearing: Responses to Geronimus and Korenman. *Demography, 30,* 291–296.

Hogan, P., & Kitagawa, E. (1985). The impact of social status, family structure and neighborhood on the fertility of black adolescents. *American Journal of Sociology, 90,* 825–855.

House, J. S. (1981). *Work stress and social support.* Reading, MA: Addison-Wesley.

36

Complications of Labor

Objectives

- List the most common causes of dystocia as they relate to the mechanics of labor, known as the "four P's" of the birthing process.
- State the three defining characteristics of preterm labor.
- During the waiting time for induction of a post-term pregnancy, what can be done to gain reassurance of fetal well-being?
- Identify three ways to induce labor.
- Discuss the goal of shock management and four main therapies used to accomplish this goal.
- Describe the management for prolapsed cord.
- List the three primary clinical characteristics and four aims of medical management of fluid embolism.
- Discuss multiple gestation, including the unique aspects of vaginal delivery of twins.

Key Terms

Amnioinfusion
Amniotic fluid
  embolism
Amniotomy
Arrest of descent
Basal tone
Brow presentation
Cephalopelvic
  disproportion
Cervical ripening
Compound
  presentation
Contracted pelvis
Cystocele
Dysfunctional labor
Dystocia
Face presentation
Failure to progress
Failure of descent
Hypertonic uterine
  dysfunction
Induction
Inversion of the uterus

Molding
Multiple pregnancy
Pathologic retraction
  ring
Persistent occiput
  posterior
Placenta accreta
Post-term pregnancy
Preterm labor
Prolonged deceleration
  phase
Protracted descent
Protracted active phase
  dilation
Protraction disorders
Rectocele
Secondary arrest of
  dilation
Shoulder dystocia
Shoulder presentation
Stripping the
  membranes
Transverse arrests

For most women, childbirth is a normal, healthy process for which women have been uniquely designed. However, in about 25% of pregnancies, a deviation from normal presents a threat to maternal and fetal well-being (Hobel, 1992).

This chapter looks at perinatal complications, known as *intrapartum problems*, that involve labor and delivery. Some deviation from normal exists in either the maternal-fetal unit or the supportive system: the uterus, pelvis, placenta, umbilical cord, or amniotic fluid. The complications addressed in this chapter include dystocia, preterm labor and birth, post-term pregnancy, hemorrhagic complications, umbilical cord prolapse, amniotic fluid embolism, and multiple gestation.

Dystocia

Dystocia refers to the abnormal progress of labor. The labor is longer, more painful, or abnormal because of problems with the mechanics of labor, powers, passageway, passenger, or psyche. Dystocia is the most common indication for primary cesarean section, accounting for 50% of surgical deliveries (Sokol et al., 1994).

Causes

Causes of dystocia can be described in terms of the "three P's" of labor: the powers, passageway, and passenger (discussed in Chaps. 20 and 21). A fourth "P," the person or psyche, is often added to the list because certain aspects of maternal response to labor can affect the length of labor. Abnormal labor may be related to problems occurring in any of these four aspects of the birth process:

- **Powers**: Uterine contractions may not be sufficiently strong or appropriately coordinated during the first stage of labor to cause cervical dilatation and effacement. During the second stage, voluntary pushing combined with uterine contractions may not be sufficient to cause descent and expulsion of the fetus.
- **Passageway**: Variations in the size and shape of the bony pelvis, such as contractures of the pelvic diameter, or other abnormalities of the reproductive tract, such as immature pelvic size or deformities, can interfere with engagement, descent, or expulsion of the fetus.
- **Passenger**: Malpresentation or malposition, unusual size, or abnormal development of the fetus can prevent entrance into or passage through the birth canal.
- **Psyche**: Maternal factors, such as anxiety, lack of preparation, and fear, can interact with the other factors, or sometimes operate alone, to prolong labor.

For labor to progress and result in a timely birth, the forces, or *powers,* including uterine contractions and maternal "bearing down" in the second stage, must be coordinated and of adequate strength to propel an irregular object, the fetus, or *passenger*, through the birth canal, or *passageway*. The passenger must be of appropriate size and shape and be able to undergo the necessary maneuvers to pass through the different dimensions of the birth canal. The passageway also must be of normal size and configuration and not present undue obstacles to the descent, rotation, and expulsion of the fetus.

Problems With the Powers— Uterine Dysfunction

Problems with the *powers* of labor involve the forces of labor, uterine contractions, and bearing down efforts. **Dysfunctional labor** is a term commonly used to describe abnormal uterine contractions that interfere with the normal progress of labor. Uterine dysfunction with prolonged labor can result in maternal and fetal complications. Intrauterine infection, a common maternal complication, especially if the membranes have been ruptured for a prolonged period, can result in fetal and neonatal infection and death, even if antibiotics are used to treat the woman (Cunningham et al., 1993). Maternal exhaustion and dehydration also may occur if labor is allowed to become prolonged.

Classification

Attempts have been made to classify labors that do not follow the usual pattern so that the problems may be more easily identified and managed. One method of classification is according to the *quality* of uterine contractions. Ineffectual contractions can be described as hypotonic or incoordinate (hypertonic; Cunningham et al., 1993). A second classification is by *time of onset*. Primary inertia (dysfunction) occurs at the beginning of labor. Secondary inertia develops after labor is established.

Dysfunctional labor also has been classified by the *pattern and timing* of the disruption of progress. According to the classic work done by Friedman (1978), dysfunction could be classified by the length of the phases of labor, rather than by the quality of the contractions. Friedman plotted cervical dilatation and degree of descent against lapsed time on a graph, demonstrating the normal labor pattern as an S-shaped curve (see Chap. 21 and Fig. 21-1 for a discussion of the phenomenon of labor). Categories of delayed progression, according to Friedman, are prolonged latent phase, protraction disorders, and arrest disorders (Fig. 36-1; Friedman, 1978).

There is some overlapping between these classifications. Hypertonic uterine dysfunction, primary inertia, and prolonged latent phase all occur in early labor and are most common in the **nullipara** (no prior births). Hypotonic uterine dysfunction, secondary inertia, and protraction or arrest of the active phase all occur later in labor and tend to be more common in the **multipara** (one or more prior births). Often clinically, "**primipara**" is used to identify a woman during the first birth experience. Technically it does not apply until *after* she has delivered. Nullipara is more accurate *before* or *during* the first labor experience and therefore is the term used in this discussion if the first birth has not occurred yet.

Friedman divided the first stage of labor into two phases: latent and active. His use of curves to plot dilatation and descent has been useful in detecting and estimating the severity of dysfunctional labor. The "**Friedman labor curve**" is the most common **partogram**, or graph, used to assess *normal progress*: adequate dilatation and descent during parturition (process of giving birth; Bashore, 1992).

The latent phase has a mean duration of 8.6 hours in nulliparas and 5.3 hours in multiparas. This phase is considered prolonged if it lasts longer than 20 hours in the nullipara or 14 hours in the multipara. The active phase, or clinically apparent labor (active labor), be-

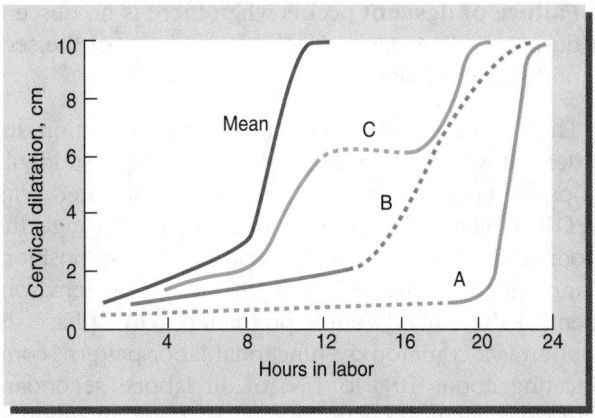

FIGURE 36–1 The major labor aberrations shown in comparison with the mean cervical dilatation time curve for nulliparas. A = prolonged latent phase, B = protracted active phase dilation, and C = secondary arrest of dilation. (Friedman, E. [1965]. *Greenhill obstetrics* [13th ed.] Philadelphia: W.B. Saunders.)

gins when the cervix is dilated 3 to 4 cm. It is briefer than the latent phase and has a mean duration 5 hours in nulliparas and 2.2 hours in multiparas (Zlatnik, 1994a). During the active phase of labor, the two types of abnormal labor patterns that can occur are protraction disorders and arrest disorders.

Protraction Disorders. **Protraction disorders** are characterized by a slower than normal rate of cervical dilation (**protracted active phase dilation**) and by delayed descent of the fetal head in the active phase of labor (**protracted descent**). The diagnostic criteria for the limits for abnormality of cervical dilation is 1.2 cm/h for nulliparas and 1.5 cm/h for multiparas. For protracted descent, the criteria are less than 1.0 cm/h for nulliparas and less than 2.0 cm/h for multiparas (Sokol et al., 1994). A slowing of progress can indicate cephalopelvic disproportion (CPD), especially in a nullipara. However, most clients with protraction disorders, when given supportive fluids, reassurance, and minimum sedation, go on to dilate fully, although this occurs at a slower rate than usual.

Arrest Disorders. Arrest disorders occur during active labor (unless otherwise specified) and are defined by the following criteria (Sokol et al., 1994):

- **Prolonged deceleration phase:** The deceleration phase is more than 3 hours in a nullipara and more than 1 hour in a multipara.
- **Secondary arrest of dilation:** No progress in cervical dilation occurs for more than 2 hours.
- **Arrest of descent:** The fetal head does not descend for more than 1 hour in a nullipara and more than 0.5 hours for a multipara.

■ **Failure of descent** occurs when there is no descent during the first stage, deceleration phase, or the second stage of labor.

These disorders may occur following protraction disorders or when a normally progressing labor suddenly stops. Arrest disorders are frequently associated with CPD (inability of the fetus' head to pass through the woman's pelvis because of shape, size, or position; Cunningham et al., 1993). In the inner city environment of the United States, protracted active-phase dilatation is a common dysfunctional labor pattern, complicating about 10% to 15% of all labors; secondary arrest of dilatation occurs in 5% to 10% of all reported labors (Sokol et al., 1994).

Failure to Progress. When the rate of progress in active labor falls below the Friedman curve but there is normal uterine activity and no CPD, labor may fail to progress due to inability of the cervix to dilate normally. This is called **failure to progress** (Curet, 1994). However, in clinical practice, failure to progess is frequently defined more broadly. It often is used as a "catch all" indication for cesarean section when the exact etiology for lack of progress is unknown or when the presenting uterine dysfunction pattern or type of arrest disorder has not been identified.

When failure to progress occurs in early labor despite the presence of uterine contractions, a factor to consider is whether the client is actually in labor. It is not unusual for a woman in late pregnancy to experience Braxton Hicks contractions; progressive cervical changes must take place to signify true labor. Appearance of **bloody show** (the blood-tinged mucous plug from the cervical os) aids in the diagnosis of labor, particularly when it accompanies cervical changes. Without signs of progress to confirm labor, uncomfortable uterine contractions signify false labor. For the diagnosis of dystocia, cervical changes must have occurred and progressed, only to have the progression slowed or halted at some point.

Etiologic Factors in Dysfunction

Uterine dysfunction can occur when there is a disturbance of any factor that promotes uterine contractility, such as lack of stimuli or strong inhibition. Alterations in the intracellular control of the muscle fiber may be present.

The most common causes of uterine dysfunction are moderate degrees of **pelvic contractures** and fetal malposition of even a small degree. If the uterine activity has previously been normal in active labor and then fades, CPD should be ruled out as a possible cause of uterine fatigue prior to pharmacologic stimulation of the uterus. In more than 50% of the cases, the cause for uterine dysfunction is not apparent clinically. However, the following physical and pharmacologic factors have been shown to contribute to uterine dysfunction (Cunningham et al., 1993):

■ Uterine overdistention, due to a large fetus, multiple gestation, or polyhydramnios
■ Cervical rigidity associated with cervical fibrosis and an elderly nullipara
■ Massively obese clients (associated with slower and more discordant labor)
■ Advanced maternal age (hardening of the connective tissue junctions between the pelvic bone components associated with increased length of second stage)
■ Pathologic retraction ring (treated by uterine relaxation and cesarean section)
■ Excessive analgesics (prolong latent phase [not predictive of later dystocia])
■ Epidural anesthesia (associated with transient decrease in contractility for 10–30 minutes)

Hypertonic Contraction Pattern

A normal contraction is characterized by fundal dominance in duration and onset of the contractile segmental response. The contraction starts at the uppermost region of the uterus (superior aspect) and proceeds downward toward the cervix (inferior aspect). In comparison, **hypertonic uterine dysfunction** (incoordinate dysfunction) involves a distortion of this *pressure gradient* (the comparative difference in pressure or force exerted by various regions of the uterine muscle) (Fig. 36-2A). The midsegment may contract with more force than the fundus (top of uterus), or there could be a complete asynchronism of the impulses originating in each cornu (upper corner region of the uterus). Along with the decreased coordination, there can be an increased frequency or elevated **basal tone** (resting tone) more than 15 mm Hg (Cunningham et al., 1993; Curet, 1994).

This dysfunction normally occurs during the latent phase of labor, often associated with a prolonged latent phase. Some researches have theorized that multiple pacemaker sites may be the cause of this dysfunctional pattern, finding it more common with uterine overdistension and fetal malpresentation (Sokol et al., 1994). Other factors associated with the length of the latent phase include how low in the pelvis the fetal presenting part is at the onset of labor and the degree of cervical dilatation at the onset of the latent phase. These two factors quantify the additional progress that is needed to accomplish the delivery.

Although hypertonic contractions are ineffective in accomplishing dilatation, the increased uterine tone usually results in maternal discomfort. These contractions are often described as "colicky" and extremely painful. The uterus may be tender to palpation, even

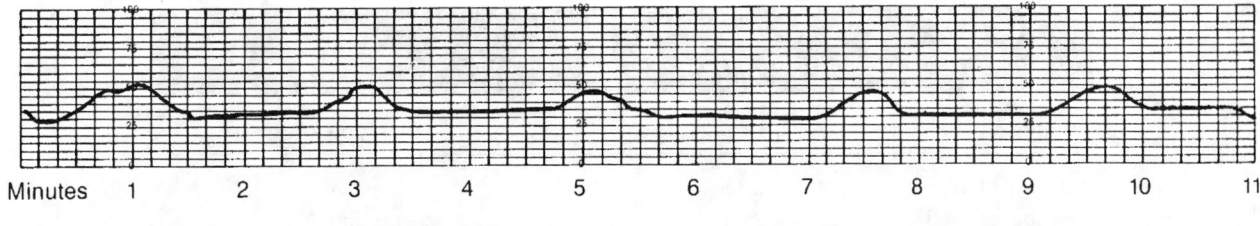

A

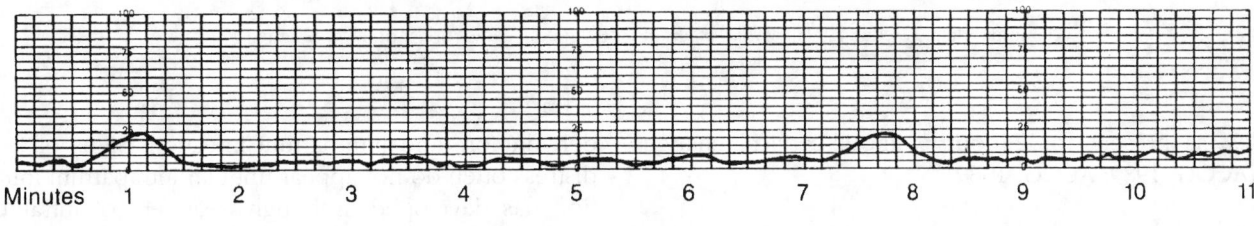

B

FIGURE 36-2 (**A**) Hypertonic uterine activity (noted elevated basal tone). (**B**) Hypotonic uterine activity (note decreased frequency of contractions and insufficient rise in pressure).

between contractions. It is important to rule out abruptio placentae as a cause (Cunningham et al., 1993).

Management. Treatment for hypertonic contractions and consequent prolonged latent phase usually is rest and administration of fluids. When medication is indicated, an injection of 10 to 15 mg of morphine intramuscularly may be prescribed because it inhibits the abnormal excitability and resulting uncoordinated contractions pattern (Curet, 1994; Bashore, 1992).

A short-acting barbiturate also may be administered to help promote rest. Intravenous (IV) fluids are used to maintain hydration and electrolyte balance. In clients who are sedated to stop their labor during the latent phase, about 90% resume normal labor when the sedation has disappeared (Sokol et al., 1994). **Tocolytic** agents, such as ritodrine, have been used with some success (Cunningham et al., 1993).

Oxytocin is usually contraindicated when treating this type of dysfunction (Calderyo-Barcia, 1957; Bashore, 1992). With the uterus in a constant state of increased muscle tone, oxytocin presents the danger of causing an even greater resting tension, which might interfere with fetal oxygenation. Also, it may not correct the uncoordinated action of the two segments, which underlies this problem. Occasionally, the contractions remain uncoordinated and ineffective even after the client has rested. In these cases, cesarean delivery is usually the choice, especially if signs of fetal distress are evident.

Complications. Fetal distress tends to appear early in labor when hypertonic dysfunction exists. The constant increase in uterine tone predisposes the fetal hypoxia. Occasionally, prolonged rupture of membranes may accompany this condition and can lead to intrapartum infection.

Hypotonic Contraction Pattern

Hypotonic uterine dysfunction occurs in approximately 4% of all labors (Curet, 1994). When uterine contractions have no basal tone, they are less frequent and their slight rise in pressure is insufficient to dilate the cervix at a satisfactory rate, and hypotonic uterine dysfunction occurs (Fig. 36-2*B*). Even at the acme of a contraction, the uterus can be indented with palpation. This condition usually occurs in the active phase, but contractions also may become hypotonic during the second stage of labor (Table 36-1). Hypotonic contractions are diagnosed as a pattern of uterine activity that is less than the "adequate labor" pattern. Adequate labor has been defined in terms of the *Montevideo unit*, which is the product of the average contraction peak in mm Hg (increase above the baseline) multiplied by the number of contractions in 10 minutes (frequency; Calderyo-Barcia, 1957). Using this unit, the latest American College of Obstetricians and Gynecologists (ACOG) definition of adequate labor describes a wide range of uterine activities: The amplitude of each contraction varies from 25 to 75 mm Hg, and contractions occur over a total of 2 to 4.5 minutes in every 10-minute window, achieving 95 to 395 Montevideo units. Because 95% of women at the first evidence of cervical dilatation have three to five contractions every 10 minutes that are greater than 25 mm Hg above the baseline, the criterion for an arrest of active labor is when a uterine contraction pattern of 200 Montevideo units or

TABLE 36-1
Criteria for Differentiating Dysfunctional Labor

Criteria	Hypertonic	Hypotonic
Phase of labor	Latent	Active
Symptoms	Painful	Painless
Fetal distress	Common	Rarely
Medication		
Oxytocin	Unfavorable reaction	Favorable reaction
Sedation	Helpful	Little value

(Cunningham, F., et al. [1993]. *Williams obstetrics* [19th ed.]. New York: Appleton & Lange.)

less is present for 2 hours without cervical change (ACOG, 1989; ACOG, 1989).

Management. To allow for timely diagnosis and intervention, it is recommended that clients have vaginal examinations at least every 2 hours (Sokol et al., 1994). Uterine dysfunction is often a protection against some degree of pelvic contraction or abnormality of fetal size or presentation (Cunningham et al., 1993). This is especially true if it is a secondary arrest of dilatation. If a marked degree of disproportion exists or if there is an uncorrectable malposition or marked fetal distress, a cesarean delivery is used. Once these are ruled out, augmentation of contractions can be done by amniotomy or oxytocin administration. If the woman is becoming fatigued or dehydrated, rest and fluids may be tried first.

If membranes are intact, initial treatment may be an amniotomy, artificial rupture of the membranes (AROM). When the head is the presenting part and engaged, cord prolapse is rare. Therefore, a longstanding recommendation has been that AROM not be done in nonvertex presentations or when the head is high. Another factor to consider is that when the head is high, the intact membranes actually provide a better wedge against the cervix than a high presenting part after rupture (Sokol et al., 1994). Amniotomy alone may stimulate effective contractions. However, it must be used judiciously because it is a commitment to deliver the fetus within a reasonable time because of the risk of infection with prolonged rupture. (See the section "Post-term Management" for further discussion on AROM.)

An enema also may stimulate labor, and if effective, improvement should occur within 2 hours. If strong, regular contractions with progressive cervical effacement and dilatation or fetal descent fail to occur, oxytocin augmentation of labor is believed to be the most effective therapy (Curet, 1994).

Complications. Untreated hypotonic uterine dysfunction exposes the woman to the dangers of exhaustion,

dehydration, and intrapartum infection. Signs of fetal distress often do not appear until an intrapartum infection has developed. Although treatment of intrauterine infection with antibiotics offers protection for the woman, it appears to be of little value in protecting the fetus (Cunningham et al., 1993).

Other Problems With Expulsive Forces

Problems other than those associated with uterine contractions can interfere with labor. These problems include inadequate voluntary expulsive force and pathologic retraction and constriction rings.

Inadequate Voluntary Expulsive Forces. When the cervix is fully dilated, most women cannot resist the urge to push or bear down during a uterine contraction. The combined force of the maternal abdominal musculature and the contraction of the uterus helps propel the fetus down the vagina and through the vaginal outlet. Such factors as anesthesia and heavy sedation can interfere with the urge and ability to push. Fatigue or intensification of pain during pushing also can cause the woman to push less effectively. In rare instances, a physical problem, such as a spinal cord injury, may be the reason for insufficient expulsive efforts.

Management is usually related to the cause. Careful selection and timing of analgesia and anesthesia can help prevent the problem. If continuous epidural anesthesia is used, it may be necessary to allow the effects to wear off sufficiently for the woman to be able to push. If the woman is "holding back" because of pain, analgesia may be needed. In any event, appropriate encouragement, support, instruction, and positioning can be helpful (Cunningham et al., 1993).

Pathologic Retraction and Constriction Rings. Localized rings or constrictions of the uterus sometimes occur in association with prolonged rupture of the membranes or long labors. The **pathologic retraction ring,** also called Bandl's ring, is the most common. It is an exaggeration of the normal physiologic retraction ring, which occurs at the junction of the upper and lower uterine segments (Fig. 36-3; see Chap. 21). The uterus above the ring becomes thicker, whereas the lower uterine segment thins out and ruptures unless the obstruction is relieved or delivery is accomplished by cesarean delivery (Sokol et al., 1994). **Constriction rings** are rare and not well understood. They usually conform to a depression in the fetus, such as the neck or abdomen, and do not go all the way around. The area of spasm is thick, but the lower uterine segment does not become stretched or thinned out. Cesarean birth, using an anesthetic that relaxes the uterus, is usually the treatment of choice.

Assessment

Nursing assessment is an essential component in the care of the client with uterine dysfunction to aid in detecting the condition, assist in decisions about the course of treatment, and monitor maternal and fetal well-being during attempts to promote more effective contractions. The nurse in the labor area often is the first to detect deviations from the normal labor pattern. An internal or external electronic fetal monitor is helpful to the nurse in assessing the length and frequency of contractions. However, the external monitor does not accurately portray the strength of the contraction. The nurse must be able to evaluate the intensity of labor contractions by palpation, without relying exclusively on the electronic monitor (see Chap. 22 for assessment of uterine contractions). Subjective statements of pain and related behavior, such as crying and moaning, are often not reliable indicators of the strength of contractions. These should be evaluated in light of objective data from uterine palpation and the electronic monitor.

Assessing the condition of the fetus is important. The nurse needs to watch the monitor for changes in the fetal heart rate and baseline variability. The nurse also should be alert for other signs of fetal distress, such as meconium-stained amniotic fluid and increased fetal activity. Maternal vital signs should be checked frequently (blood pressure and pulse should be monitored every 2 hours and temperature every 4 hours if the client is afebrile, more frequently if febrile). Elevation of maternal temperature and increased pulse rate are clinical signs that may alert the nurse to the onset of secondary complications, such as infection. Urine should be checked for acetone. Acetonuria is a sign of exhaustion and dehydration. A record of intake and output also is helpful in assessing hydration.

Nursing Diagnoses

From the assessment, the nurse assists with recognizing the medical diagnosis of dysfunctional labor. The nurse also can identify a number of potential nursing diagnoses, which could become actual depending on the progress of the situation. For a list of possible nursing diagnoses see Box 36-1.

Planning and Intervention

The nurse plans interventions based on the assessment, nursing diagnoses, and medical plan of treatment. Care includes comfort measures, emotional support, and explanations of what is happening; the nurse

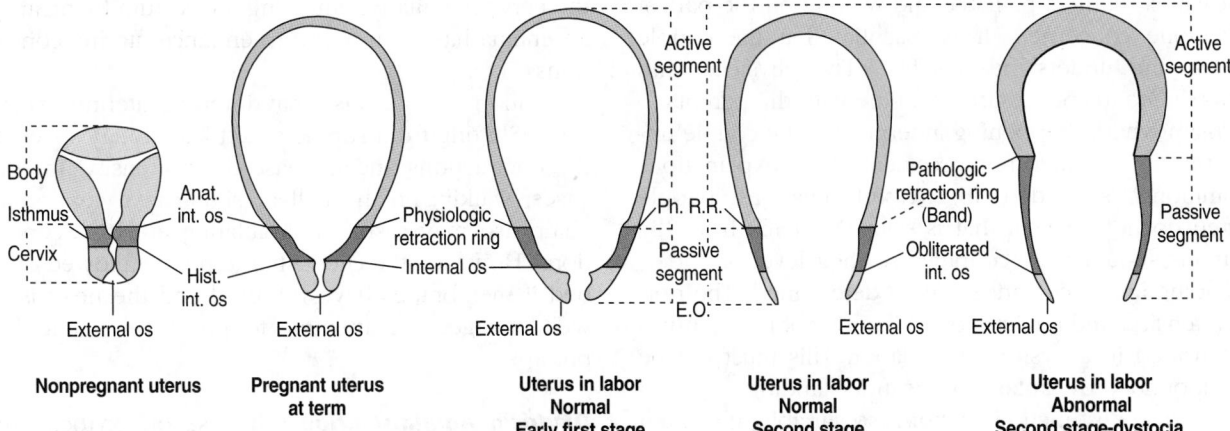

FIGURE 36–3 Sequence of development of the segments and rings in the uterus in pregnant women at term and in labor. Note comparison of the uterus of a nonpregnant woman, the uterus at term, and the uterus during labor. The passive lower segment of the uterine body is derived from the isthmus; the physiologic retraction ring develops at the junction of the upper and lower uterine segments. The pathologic retraction ring develops from the physiologic ring. (Anat. Int. Os, anatomic internal os; Hist. Int. Os, histologic internal os; Ph. R. R., physiologic retraction ring; E.O., external os) (After Cunningham, F., et al. [1993]. *Williams obstetrics* [19th ed.] New York: Appleton & Lange.)

> **BOX 36–1**
> *Nursing Diagnoses: Dystocia*
>
> ■ Risk for Fluid Volume Deficit related to
>   - Prolonged labor and restricted fluid intake
>   - Increased insensible fluid loss during prolonged labor
> ■ Fluid Volume Excess related to oxytocin therapy
> ■ Risk for Infection related to
>   - Prolonged rupture of membranes
>   - Invasive monitoring
> ■ Pain related to
>   - Intense uterine contractions
>   - Prolonged labor
>   - Ineffective contractions
> ■ Fatigue related to prolonged labor
> ■ Anxiety related to unexpected length of labor
> ■ Fear related to length of labor and uncertainty of outcome
> ■ Ineffective Individual Coping related to
>   - Fatigue
>   - Fear
>   - Lack of adequate support
> ■ Situational Low Self Esteem related to inability to complete labor and delivery as planned
> ■ Knowledge Deficit related to dystocia, treatment, and care
> ■ Risk for Injury (maternal) related to soft-tissue damage from difficult labor and delivery

also should administer and monitor effects of ordered medications.

Emotional Support. Dysfunctional labor can be extremely discouraging for the parents. The diagnostic procedures and treatment take time. Carrying out these measures requires patience and waiting on the part of everyone concerned. It is essential that the couple know and understand this fact. The physician and nurse need to spend sufficient time with the parents to explain what is happening in terms that the couple understands. Repeated reinforcement of the explanations commonly is needed. In stressful situations, people often do not hear all that is said. Feedback from the parents should be encouraged so their level of understanding and acceptance can be determined. The normal tension and anxiety found in any labor certainly is intensified in a dysfunctional labor. This must not be compounded by fantasy or misunderstanding.

Because dysfunctional labor is so variable, it is often impossible (and unwise) to give the parents any definite reassurances as to when effective labor will commence or when the birth will occur. However, some kind of boundaries must be identified about when this ineffective phase will end and progress will begin so that the mother has some goal toward which to work. Therefore, it is important to reassure the client,

reminding her that her case is not unique (after many hours, clients think that theirs is the longest labor in obstetric history), that certain specific measures are known and can be taken to help effective labor begin, and that competent medical and nursing care will be given throughout labor. An explanation of the plan for treatment enables the parents to anticipate more realistically what is in store, reassuring them that certain definite measures are available and are being used.

Comfort Measures. Comfort measures that promote relaxation should be used. Sponge baths, changes in position, soothing back rubs, quiet conversation, reading or other diversionary activities, clean linen, and a quiet, restful environment are all appropriate. Unless she is actually sleeping, isolating the client in a dark room on the premise that she needs sleep or rest only contributes to her fear. Frequent observations are needed to see when she awakens. Human contact is one of the most important aspects of care with complicated labor and should never be neglected. The presence of the same person, nurse, or physician is helpful for the reasons mentioned in Chapter 22. Allowing the client to have a significant or familiar person of her choice, such as partner or mother, also is important. Coaching the client in breathing patterns and relaxation techniques also can be comforting and helps to conserve her strength.

Certain comfort measures aid in correction of some dysfunctional labor patterns. For example, an overdistended bladder may not be noticed by the client but may add to her discomfort. Emptying of the bladder often speeds cervical dilatation, possibly by allowing the fetal head to descend further with better proximity to the cervix. Similarly, emptying the rectum by means of an enema has been found to enhance uterine contractions.

Position changes also may improve uterine contractions. Shifting from supine to left lateral may space out the contractions and increase their intensity. In some cases, walking in the hall or sitting in a comfortable chair also may assist in stimulating effective contractions. However, the client should not be allowed out of bed if membranes have ruptured and the head is not well engaged, in attempts to prevent possible cord prolapse.

Oxytocin Administration. The use of oxytocin infusion has become more common in the last decade in modern obstetrics, with about 25% of all hospital births in the United States being either induced or augmented. Thus nurses working with clients in labor and delivery must have a thorough understanding of this uterine stimulant. Synthetic oxytocin (Pitocin or syntocinon developed in 1953) is as effective as the natural substance, is chemically pure, eliminates the danger of reaction to animal protein, and is the product used in obstetrics today (Ross et al., 1992). Oxytocin may be used to initiate (induce) labor contractions or to augment contractions that are weak and ineffective. (Use of oxytocin to treat postpartum uterine atony is discussed later in the Chapter.)

The following are usually considered to be *absolute contraindications* to the use of oxytocin for either augmentation or induction (ACOG, 1991a):

- Any obstruction that would interfere with descent of the fetus, such as malpresentation, CPD, or anomaly of the birth canal. If the presenting part is above the pelvic inlet, oxytocin should not be started.
- Hypertonic or incoordinate uterine contractions. Oxytocin makes the condition worse, leading to formation of a constriction ring (Bandl's ring).
- Fetal distress. Contractions interfere with uteroplacental blood flow, which may add to the distress.
- Any contraindication for vaginal birth, such as placenta previa, classic uterine incision, active vaginal herpes, or invasive cervical carcinoma

Relative contraindications occur when there is an increased risk of complications, but the drug may be used judiciously in selected clients under close surveillance. Relative contraindications include conditions that would increase the danger of uterine rupture, such as grand multiparity (more than four) or overdistention of the uterus (twins, hydramnios; O'Brien et al., 1991; Pozaic, 1992).

Previously, the use of oxytocin in clients with a history of uterine surgery was thought to be an absolute contraindication. However, recent studies have shown it can be used safely with close supervision in selected cases of vaginal birth after cesarean (VBAC). In one multicenter study involving 581 clients with a trial of labor in which oxytocin was given, the rate of successful births was 64%. However, two cases of uterine rupture were reported (Flamm et al., 1987). In a later study, it was found that oxytocin did not increase the risk of rupture in clients undergoing VBAC (Rosen et al., 1991). If the decision is made to use oxytocin, strict management criteria, including using internal electronic fetal monitoring and intrauterine pressure catheters and limiting the total dose of oxytocin, have been recommended by several investigators who reviewed the use of oxytocin during VBAC (Clark et al., 1994; Paul et al., 1985; Cunningham et al., 1993).

The amount and rate of oxytocin administration must be carefully controlled; this can be done effectively only by use of the IV route, using an infusion pump to help provide a consistent and precise rate. Types of solution, amount of oxytocin added, and rate of infusion vary according to agency protocols or physician preference. Oxytocin is commercially available as 10 U/mL and is added to a balanced salt solution, such as normal saline (0.9% NaCl) or lactated Ringer's solution, that will not exacerbate the water-retention properties of oxytocin.

A piggyback system, using two containers of the same IV salt solution, one containing oxytocin and the other without, is recommended. The oxytocin may be discontinued if necessary while still keeping the IV line open. If the IV tubing injection port closest to the IV catheter insertion site is used for the piggyback line, there is less oxytocin in the tubing in case it becomes necessary to discontinue the oxytocin. Fetal oxygenation status must be assessed every 15 minutes to ensure that the increased contraction pattern is not interfering with uteroplacental perfusion (American Academy of Pediatrics and ACOG, 1992). If there was significant interference with perfusion, the fetus would show signs of fetal distress, such as the fetal heart rate pattern of late decelerations.

The ACOG current recommendation for oxytocin induction is an initial dose of 1 to 2 mU. For augmentation, the initial dosing should be smaller, 0.5 to 1.0 mU/min. The dosing should be increased 1 to 2 mU/min incrementally until an adequate dilatation rate of 1 cm/h or a contraction pattern is reached: Contractions should be of moderate to strong intensity, occurring every 2 to 3 minutes, lasting no more than 45 to 60 seconds, and with at least a 30-second rest between contractions. Once effective labor has been established with these criteria, it may be possible to decrease the dose of oxytocin. Also, repositioning the client to left lateral may be the only corrective measure necessary for hyperstimulation, because in the supine position, contractions may become more frequent, although less intense and consequently less painful. The maximum recommended dose is 20 mU/min, because when the infusion rate approaches 40 mU for prolonged periods, there is a dramatic drop in urinary output, which creates the possibility of water intoxication (ACOG, 1991a; Pozaic, 1992; Sokol et al., 1994).

Ideally, the contractions stimulated by oxytocin mimic natural labor as closely as possible. External or internal electronic fetal monitoring is mandatory when oxytocin is used during labor. Internal monitoring is advantageous because it provides a more accurate picture of the intensity of the contractions than external monitoring.

Extreme caution is necessary, especially at the beginning of the oxytocin infusion, because of the unpredictability of the individual's response. Sensitivity to oxytocin varies widely from client to client and from time to time in the same client depending on a variety of influencing factors. Increased sensitivity is associated with ruptured membranes, term gestation, high parity, favorable cervix (soft, effacing, dilating, and anterior), and irritable uterus. Sensitivity of the client should be assessed carefully by beginning with small amounts (see Procedure 36-1).

Oxytocin is potentially dangerous to the woman and fetus. These dangers can be minimized by carefully monitoring the drug administration, the character of the contractions, and the condition of the fetus. When the contractions increase in frequency, strength, and length above normal levels, the fetal and placental circulation may be impaired, and fetal distress may result. Birth injuries from being propelled too rapidly through the birth canal or being forced through a pelvis that is too small are possible. Tetanic and tumultuous contractions can result in abruptio placentae or rupture of the uterus, adversely affecting the woman and fetus. Cervical lacerations from too rapid passage of the fetus through the pelvis and amniotic fluid embolism are additional dangers for the woman (Williams, 1993).

Oxytocin infusion also may have some maternal side effects. Hypertension with frontal headache may develop. Both of these effects disappear when the drug is discontinued. Oxytocin has antidiuretic properties that can lead to water intoxication when used in large amounts. This problem can be decreased by using an electrolyte solution rather than dextrose in water for the infusion, avoiding infusion of a large volume of fluid, or using high doses of oxytocin (>20 mU/min) for prolonged periods.

Evaluation

Anticipated outcomes of care may include the following:

- The client maintains fluid and electrolyte balance.
- The client remains free of signs of infection or other complications.
- The fetus does not demonstrate signs of fetal distress.
- The client's labor progresses to the birth of a healthy newborn.
- The client verbalizes fears and concerns, understanding of the disruption of the labor progress and planned interventions, and experience of minimal pain and discomfort.
- The client demonstrates positive coping strategies.

Problems With the Passageway

The second major category of factors causing dystocia is related to variations or abnormalities of the maternal reproductive tract, especially the pelvis. These problems interfere with engagement, descent, or expulsion of the fetus.

Contracted Pelvis

In a **contracted pelvis**, there is sufficient reduction in one or more of its major diameters to interfere with the progress of labor. The pelvis may be contracted at the inlet, the midpelvis, or the outlet. A contracted pelvis is the most frequent cause of a disproportion between the size of the fetus and the size of the birth canal.

With an *inlet contraction*, the anteroposterior diameter of the inlet is decreased to 10 cm or less, or the greatest transverse diameter is 12 cm or less. Either of these contractions results in an increase in obstetric difficulties. The incidence of difficult labors is increased even more when both diameters are contracted (Cunningham et al., 1993). Contraction of the inlet may be the result of rickets or generally poor development. A woman who is small is more likely to have a pelvis that is small in all dimensions, but she also is more likely to have a small baby. Effects of a contracted pelvic inlet on the fetus include failure of the presenting part to engage, increased incidence of malpositions and deflexed attitudes, and extreme molding of the presenting part. Because the presenting part does not fit well in the inlet, prolapsed umbilical cord also is more likely.

Midpelvic contraction is less defined than contraction of the inlet or outlet. However, the midpelvis is considered contracted when the distance between the ischial spines is less than 9.0 cm (normal is 10.5) or when the sum of the interspinous and the posterior sagittal distance is less than 13.5 cm (normal is 15.0–15.5 cm). Contraction of the midpelvis is a fairly frequent cause of dystocia. Because the presenting part is able to engage in the pelvis, this condition is harder to recognize than inlet contraction, making management more difficult. As labor progresses, molding and caput succedaneum formation (edema occurring under the fetal scalp during labor) may give the impression that the head is lower than it actually is, resulting in a difficult forceps delivery. Transverse arrest of the head also may occur, in which the long axis of the fetal head is blocked by a contracture in the transverse plane of the inlet.

An *outlet contraction* is identified when the distance between the ischial tuberosities is less than 8 cm. Other dimensions of the outlet are important in determining the degree of difficulty caused by the outlet contraction. The incidence of perineal tears and the need for forceps are increased, but cesarean section is rarely necessary. If dystocia is severe, usually there is a midpelvic contraction.

Variations In Pelvic Shape

The shape of the pelvis may be equally or more important than its size, although these factors may complement each other. For example, large size may compensate for a shape that is not optimal. The normal female or *gynecoid* pelvis has the best dimensions in all planes for the passage of the fetus. The other three pelvic variations adversely influence the prognosis for a vaginal delivery. (See Chap. 20 for discussion of pelvic types.)

PROCEDURE 36-1
Oxytocin (Pitocin) Induction and Augmentation

Intervention	*Rationale and Comments*

1. Explain procedure and rationale to client.
2. Apply fetal monitor and monitor the fetal heart rate (FHR) to establish a baseline tracing.
3. Start an IV infusion (primary line) using an electrolyte solution.
4. Prepare a second IV (secondary line), and add the prescribed amount of oxytocin. The IV tubing is inserted into the infusion controller (or pump) and primed to clear air from the line.
5. "Piggyback" the secondary line into the primary line at the port closest to the needle insertion site and then turn on at the prescribed rate of infusion.

6. Turn on oxytocin infusion pump at prescribed rate.

7. Monitor FHR, uterine resting tone, frequency, duration and intensity of contractions, blood pressure, and pulse, and record at intervals comparable to the *dosage regimen* (ie, at 30- to 60-min intervals) when the dosage is evaluated for maintenance, increased, or decreased. Evidence of maternal and fetal surveillance should be documented. All observations and increases or decreases in oxytocin are documented on the fetal heart tracing and the woman's chart.
8. Once the desired frequency of contractions has been reached and labor has progressed to 5–6 cm dilatation, oxytocin may be reduced by similar increments (or as prescribed by physician).
9. If hyperstimulation of the uterus occurs (less than 2 min between contractions and lasting longer than 60 s) or a nonreassuring FHR pattern occurs, the following actions are taken:
   a. Turn off oxytocin infusion.
   b. Speed up primary infusion.
   c. Change position; may turn to left side.
   d. Give oxygen 6–8 L/min by face mask.
   e. Notify charge nurse (supervisor) and physician STAT.
   f. Provide support to parents.
   g. Document on monitor strip and client's chart.
   h. Document effectiveness of interventions.
10. Notify the physician of hypertonic or hypotonic contractions or failure to progress.

1. An informed client is less anxious and fearful.
2. Ensures fetal reactivity.

3. An electrolyte solution minimizes the risk of water intoxication.
4. Oxytocin must be administered with an infusion pump (or controller) to ensure accurate dose administration.

5. The secondary line contains the oxytocin. If there is an indication to stop the oxytocin infusion, it can be done without affecting the infusion of the primary line, and fluid volume can be maintained.
6. No other medications should be given through the oxytocin (secondary) line, because it is given at prescribed rates and may be turned off if contractions are too close, hypertonus occurs, or the FHR pattern indicates fetal distress.
7. If uterus becomes hyperstimulated, blood flow to uteroplacental site is decreased, and fetus will suffer from hypoxia.

8. Sensitivity to oxytocin increases as labor progresses. If stable pattern is achieved, need for oxytocin decreases.

9. Intrauterine resuscitation is initiated when there is significant interruption of oxygenation due to decrease or cessation of uteroplacental perfusion.

10. Clients may vary in their individual responsiveness to oxytocin. Some may require more; some may require less.

(*continued*)

PROCEDURE 36–1 *(continued)*
Oxytocin (Pitocin) Induction and Augmentation

Intervention	Rationale and Comments
11. Continue to assess client's progress, both physically and emotionally (care for the client, not the monitor).	11. Induced or augmented labor is stressful to couple. The nurse is attuned to their responses and intervenes as indicated. They need to know that progress is occurring.
12. Notify the physician to evaluate client when oxytocin infusion is 10 mU/min. *Note.* A client seldom requires more than 20–40 mU/min of oxytocin to achieve progressive cervical dilation; 90% of clients respond to 16 mU or less.	12. Assesses client's response to oxytocin.
13. Accurately record fluid intake and output every 2 h.	13. This ensures proper hydration and rules out fluid retention due to antidiuretic action of oxytocin.

(Adapted from American College of Obstetricians and Gynecologists [1991]. Induction/augmentation of labor. Technical Bulletin # 157. Washington, DC: ACOG.)

Cephalopelvic Disproportion

Cephalopelvic disproportion implies a relationship between the size of the fetal head and the size of the pelvis. This indicates that the problem could originate with the passageway, the passenger, or a combination of the two. CPD (or fetopelvic disproportion if the head is not the presenting part) can be absolute or relative. When the fetus cannot pass safely through the birth canal under any circumstances, it is considered absolute. In many cases, however, whether the fetus can be delivered vaginally depends on the efficiency of the uterine contractions; the stretchability of the maternal soft tissues; the attitude, presentation, and position of the fetus; and the moldability of the fetal head.

Management

Extreme degrees of pelvic contraction or problems with the fetus often can be detected during prenatal care. A decision can then be made about the advisability of cesarean delivery. In doubtful cases, the client may be given a **trial of labor** (labor attempted) for 4 to 6 hours to determine whether with adequate contractions, the head can pass through the pelvis. For these women, labor may be even more anxiety provoking than usual, depending partly on the support and information they have received. If cesarean delivery is the outcome, there may be a great deal of disappointment and perhaps even a feeling of failure. The warm, empathic attitude of the nurse is particularly needed for these clients. Frequent reports on the progress of labor should not be overlooked, whether or not the progress is favorable.

Problems With the Passenger

The position and presentation of the fetus at the beginning of labor can greatly influence the progress of labor. Even slight deviations can affect uterine contractions adversely or prevent the fetus from passing through the birth canal.

Persistent Occiput Posterior and Transverse Arrest

The fetal head usually enters the pelvic inlet transversely and therefore must travel an arc of 90 degrees during internal rotation to the direct occiput anterior position (see Chap. 20 and Fig 20-2). In about one-fourth of all labors, however, the head enters the pelvis with the occiput directed diagonally posterior, that is, in either the right occiput posterior or the left occiput posterior position. Under these circumstances, the head must rotate through an arc of 135 degrees in the process of internal rotation (Fig. 36-4*A–D*).

With good contractions, adequate flexion, and a fetus of average size, the majority of cases of occiput posterior position undergo spontaneous rotation through the 135-degree arc as soon as the head reaches the pelvic floor. This is a normal mechanism of labor.

In approximately 10% of cases, rotation may be incomplete (Cunningham et al., 1993), or the head may rotate through a 45-degree arc to the direct occiput posterior position, a condition known as **persistent occiput posterior** (see Fig. 36-4*E–F*). If rotation is incomplete, the head becomes arrested in the transverse position, a condition known as **transverse arrest**.

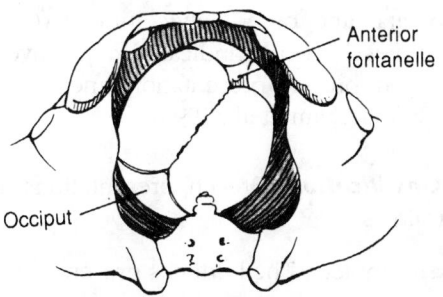

A. Right occiput posterior

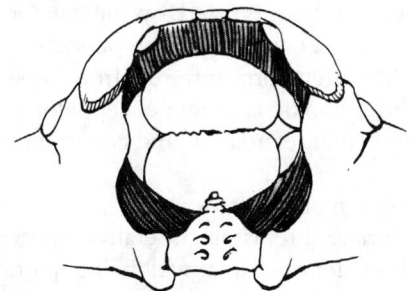

B. Internal rotation: ROP to ROT

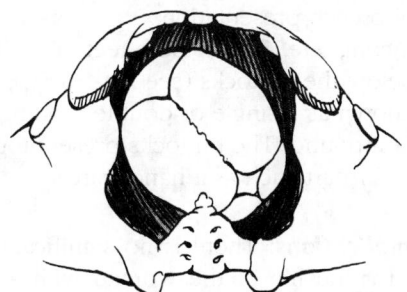

C. Internal rotation: ROT to ROA

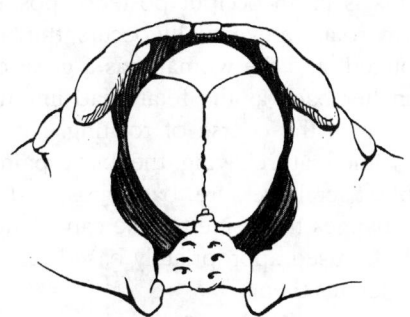

D. Internal rotation: ROA to OA

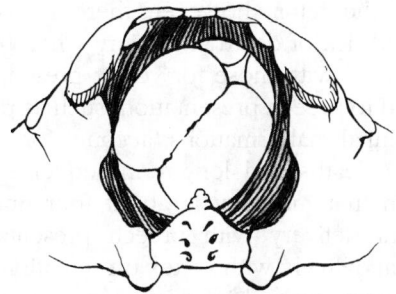

E. Right occiput posterior

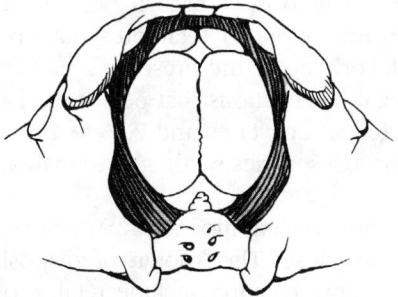

F. Internal rotation: ROP to OP

FIGURE 36–4 Occiput posterior. (**A** through **D**) Long arc rotation from right occipito-posterior (ROP) to occipitoanterior (OA) position. (**A**) ROP. (**B**) Internal rotation: ROP to right occipitotransverse (ROT). (**C**) Internal rotation: ROT to right occipitoanterior (ROA). (**D**) Internal rotation: ROA to OA (**E** and **F**) Short arc rotation from ROP to occipitoposterior (OP) position. (**E**) ROP. (**F**) Internal rotation: ROP to OP.

Both transverse arrest and persistent occiput posterior position represent deviations from the normal mechanisms of labor. Narrowing of the midpelvis may play a role in the etiology.

Management. Some controversy exists about the management of persistent occiput posterior. Although first and second stages tend to be prolonged in nulliparas, management is the same as for occiput anterior positions, resulting in no increased risk to the fetus, as long as no other existing maternal or fetal complications are present. If there is a borderline, nonreassuring fetal heart rate pattern during entry into the second stage in a nullipara with persistent occiput posterior, a decision about the mode of delivery should be made. The likelihood of a prolonged second stage with its increased duration of pressure on the fetal head should be considered in this decision. A cesarean section is the less risky option. This set of circumstances occurred recently in a California malpractice case regarding perinatal brain damage. The plaintiff was awarded $49 million. The jury held the hospital liable for not performing as a client advocate when a physician failed to perform a timely cesarean delivery in the presence of severe fetal distress not recognized by the doctor or nurse, during a 3-hour second stage with persistent occiput posterior. The newborn suffered from a skull fracture and severe hypoxic-ischemic encephalopathy, leading to severe mental retardation and cerebral palsy (Halle, 1993).

However, an overly aggressive surgical approach also is not appropriate. Premature operative intervention in cases with evidence of fetal well-being, particularly if the station is high, seems contraindicated. Forceps rotation on the perineum is appropriate to reduce lacerations if this can be easily accomplished (Cunningham et al., 1993).

When the fetus is in an occiput posterior position, regardless of how rotation eventually occurs, the labor is usually prolonged, and the woman has a great deal of discomfort in her back as the fetal head impinges against the sacrum in the course of rotating. Nursing intervention is aimed at relieving the back pain as much as possible. Sacral pressure, back rubs, and frequent position changes from side to side can be helpful. They should be used appropriately based on how well the client tolerates them.

Breech Presentation

Because fetal lie often changes spontaneously as gestation progresses, it is important to wait until after the 33rd week for the diagnosis of breech presentation. **Breech presentation** refers to fetal presentation in which the buttocks or feet are the presenting part. The incidence of breech presentations that persist until delivery is only 4% for all deliveries and 20% to 25% for preterm newborns (this varies with gestational age; Dierker, 1994).

In those that do not convert, more than 50% of cases have no identifiable cause. The known predisposing factors for a breech presentation include fetal anomalies, uterine anomalies, uterine overdistention, high parity, and pelvic obstruction by placenta previa, my-omata, and other pelvic tumors (Cruikshank, 1994). Studies have not indicated a positive correlation between breech presentation and a contracted pelvis (Cunningham et al., 1993).

Classification. Breech presentations are classified as follows:

■ Complete. The buttocks present with the feet and legs flexed on the thighs and the thighs flexed on the abdomen (Fig. 36-5*A*).
■ Frank. The buttocks present with the hips flexed and the legs extended against the abdomen and chest (see Fig. 36-5*B*); this is the most common type of breech presentation.
■ Incomplete. One or both feet or the knees extend below the buttocks (see Fig. 36-5*C*); this is also known as a single or double footling breech.
■ Compound. The buttocks present together with another part such as a hand (rare).

Complications. There is no significant increased danger for the life of the woman with a fetus in breech presentation. However, there is an increased incidence of lacerations of the birth canal, episiotomy extensions, cesarean deliveries, and postpartum infections. Labor is not prolonged, contrary to previous belief (Cunningham et al., 1993).

For the fetus, however, there is considerable increased risk of death and injury when breech data are compared with those for vertex presentations. Factors related to breech presentation, such as prematurity and congenital malformations, account for a good number of the deaths and long-term sequelae. Research has shown that mortality is about four times greater for vaginal delivery with breech presentation than for vaginal delivery with vertex presentation; 64% is due to malformations and infection, with approximately one-third due to the potentially preventable factors of trauma and asphyxia (Kaupilla, 1975).

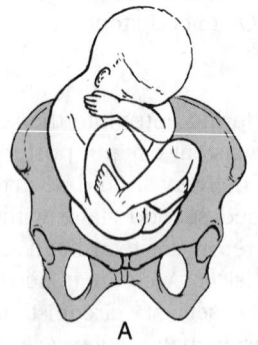 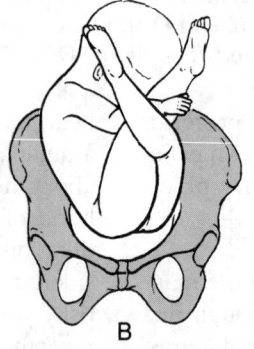 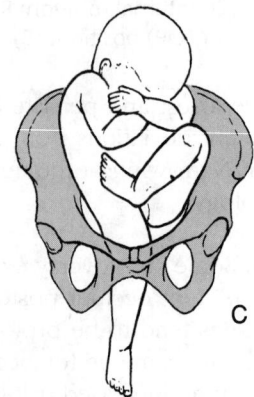

A   B   C

FIGURE 36-5 Breech presentation may be (**A**) complete breech, (**B**) frank breech, or (**C**) incomplete or footling breech.

Trauma to the head is a significant risk to term and preterm newborns, regardless of route of delivery. With prematurity, the fetal body may deliver through an incompletely dilated cervix, which then entraps the fetal head. This entrapment also can happen with cesarean delivery if the incision is inadequate or suboptimal uterine relaxation occurs, which also entraps the fetal head causing tentorial tears and cerebral hemorrhage during delivery of the aftercoming head (Cruikshank, 1994).

Other factors related to death or damage of the newborn include asphyxia from cord prolapse, aspiration of amniotic fluid due to breathing before the head is born, and injury, such as fractures, resulting from manipulation and possible rough handling during the delivery.

External Version. With the increasing use of cesarean delivery for breech presentation, many obstetricians are taking a new look at **external version** (manipulation to turn the fetus from a breech presentation to a vertex) as a way to prevent breech deliveries. This may be attempted if labor has not begun and the fetus is more than 36 weeks. Success is not guaranteed with version. Only about 50% to 75% can be turned to vertex. Several fetuses do return to the breech position after version (Shields et al., 1992; Dierker, 1994).

Relative contraindications for using **external cephalic version** include uterine anomaly, classical cesarean scar (vertical uterine incision), oligohydramnios, and nonreactive fetal testing (Dierker, 1994). Opinions differ concerning the degree of risk with this procedure and whether the results are worth the major risks of cord compression or abruptio placentae (Shields et al., 1992). Fetal-maternal hemorrhage also has been reported and led to the recommendation of giving anti-*D* globulin to Rh-negative women before attempting external version.

Prior to starting, the client receives nothing by mouth for 8 hours and has a nonstress test (NST) and an ultrasound to confirm presentation. To promote uterine relaxation during the procedure, the client receives terbutaline or a continuous infusion of a tocolytic, such as ritodrine. During the procedure, the fetus is manipulated transabdominally under ultrasound guidance, attempting to elevate the breech out of the maternal pelvis, while guiding the fetal head into the pelvis. An NST is performed again prior to discharge, and the mother is instructed to count fetal movements (for 1 hour after a meal) to ensure fetal well-being (Shields et al., 1992; Dierker, 1994).

Delivery Methods. Choosing the route of delivery in the breech presentation is the subject of much debate. Because breech presentation has resulted in a threefold to tenfold excess of perinatal morbidity and mortality compared with cephalic presentation, the inci-

dence of cesarean delivery for breech presentation has increased substantially in the last few decades (Gimovsky et al., 1982; Dierker, 1994).

Because cesarean delivery carries a greater risk for maternal morbidity and mortality, the policy of universal cesarean delivery for all fetuses in breech presentation has come into question. Data have shown that with proper selection, nearly half of fetuses in breech presentation can be delivered safely through the vaginal route (Cruikshank, 1994).

An interesting study was done by Gimovsky in the early 1980s, which is still used as a guide for care. A randomized, prospective investigation was done with clients having term, *nonfrank* breech presentations. Rigid criteria were used for pelvic adequacy, which eliminated 33% of clients originally randomized to trial of labor. Of those remaining, 44% accomplished a vaginal delivery and showed less maternal morbidity and comparable cord blood gases, better Apgar scores, less birth injury, and shorter hospital stays than the comparative cesarean section group. The conclusion of this study was that a trial of labor under *carefully selected conditions* is a reasonable alternative to cesarean delivery for the term nonfrank breech presentation (Gimovsky et al., 1983).

Several scoring systems have been developed to evaluate the feasibility of vaginal delivery in breech presentations. The Zatuchni-Andros Prognostic Index (Table 36-2) is an example. These systems are designed to be a guide in deciding on the route of delivery. The recommendation is that a score of three or less is a good indication for a cesarean birth, a score of four requires further observation and subsequent evaluation, and a score of five or more will hopefully result in a successful vaginal delivery (Cunningham et al., 1993).

The scoring system does not take into account all of the important factors that must be considered. Therefore, it should not take the place of the obstetrician's clinical judgment for each woman (Box 36-2).

Of the breech presentations, frank breech is usually considered most favorable for vaginal delivery. Because the buttocks fit into the pelvis more evenly, the incidence of cord prolapse is only 0.4% when compared with 5% for complete breech and 10% for incomplete breech. Also the frank breech presentation dilates the cervix better than other breech presentations (Cruikshank, 1994).

It would seem that the small preterm fetus might be easy to deliver vaginally in a breech position. However, these fetuses are apt to have proportionately larger heads. Although the cervix dilates sufficiently for the breech to pass, the head may become trapped by the cervix. The deflexed head (extended backward rather than flexed forward) represents another situation in which a fetus' head may become trapped but this time, by the bony pelvis. Therefore, it is not rec-

TABLE 36–2
Zatuchni-Andros Prognostic Index

	Points		
	0	**1**	**2**
Parity	Primigravida	Multipara	
Gestational age	39 weeks or more	38 weeks	37 weeks or less
Estimated fetal weight	8 lb (3,630 g)	7–7 ¹⁵/₁₆ lb (3176–3629 g)	<7 lb (3,173 g)
Previous breech*	0	1	2 or more
Dilation†	2 cm	3 cm	4 cm or more
Station†	−3 or higher	−2	−1 or lower

*Greater than 2,500 g.
†Determined by vaginal examination on admission.
(Zatuchni, G. I., Andros, G. J. [1967]. Prognostic index for vaginal delivery in breech presentation.
American Journal of Obstetrics and Gynecology, 98, 854.)

ommended to allow a vaginal delivery with estimated fetal weight less than 1,500 g (Cruikshank, 1994).

A most important consideration in the delivery decision is the obstetrician's knowledge of and skill in vaginal breech deliveries. This can be a problem because the trend toward cesarean delivery for breech presentation does not allow opportunity for much practice in breech vaginal delivery.

The mechanism of labor in breech vaginal delivery is comparable to that for vertex presentations. The steps are shown in Figure 36-6. Initially descent is slower, but among women of similar parity, dilatation, and effacement, it is approximately the same for breech and vertex presentations.

Spontaneous breech deliveries sometimes occur, but usually some degree of assistance is necessary. Most often assistance is needed for delivery of the aftercoming head. This may be accomplished by the application of Piper forceps (see Chap. 37) or by one of several maneuvers, such as the Mauriceau-Smellie-Veit maneu-

BOX 36–2
Factors Used in Clinical Decisions Related to Delivery Method for Breech Presentations

Circumstances Considered Indications for Cesarean Delivery

Estimated fetal weight < 1,500 g

Estimated fetal weight > 3,850 g

Any degree of contraction or unfavorable shape of the pelvis

A hyperextended head

Maternal or fetal indications for delivery but not in labor

Complications of labor, such as acute fetal distress, placenta previa, abrutio placentae, prolapsed cord, or uterine dysfunction

An apparently healthy preterm fetus of 26 or more weeks' gestation; woman in active labor or in need of delivery

Severe fetal growth retardation

Previous pregnancies resulting in perinatal death or birth trauma

A firm request for sterilization

Footling presentation

Previous cesarean

Fetal anomalies

Circumstances Usually Favorable for Vaginal Delivery

Gestational age between 36 and 38 weeks

Estimated fetal weight between 6 and 7 lb

Presenting part at the beginning of labor at 0 station or below

Soft, effaced cervix, dilated to 3 cm or more

Ample pelvis with expectation of head entering in direct occiput anterior position

Obstetric history of breech delivery of newborn weighing greater than 7 lb, or vertex delivery of newborn weighing greater than 8 lb

Frank breech presentation

Cunningham, F., et al. (1993), Williams Obstetrics *(19th ed.). New York: Appleton and Lange.*

ver (Fig. 36-7). Maintaining head flexion is important. Suprapubic pressure by the obstetrician or an assistant is usually needed (Cruikshank, 1994).

Many physicians prefer local or pudendal anesthesia for vaginal breech deliveries because it does not interfere with labor and allows the woman to participate actively. Epidural anesthesia also is preferred for the same reasons, and it permits more comfortable intravaginal manipulation and extractions. For difficult breech deliveries, a general anesthetic, such as halothane, might be used because these agents inhibit uterine contractions and make intravaginal manipulation easier.

Assessment. Through assessment of the woman in labor, the nurse may be the one who initially identifies signs that the fetus is in a breech presentation. Findings might include palpating the head in the fundus when doing Leopold's maneuvers, locating the fetal heart tones slightly above the umbilicus, feeling the buttocks when doing a vaginal examination, and noting the passage of meconium after the membranes have ruptured.

When breech presentation is confirmed by ultrasound, the nurse continues to monitor the condition of the woman and fetus while the decision of delivery method is being made. Information provided by the nurse often plays an important role in this decision. Continuous assessment of fetal well-being is particularly important because of the increased possibility of cord prolapse with a breech presentation. Use of an electronic fetal monitor is helpful.

Nursing Diagnoses. Based on the assessment, the nurse identifies appropriate nursing diagnoses. For a list of possible nursing diagnoses, see Box 36-3.

Planning and Intervention. Based on assessment, nursing diagnoses, and the medical treatment plan for the client, the nurse plans specific nursing interventions. Interventions would include initiating monitoring techniques; reporting maternal and fetal condition and any changes in condition; preparing the client for the selected type of delivery, whether vaginal or cesarean; and explaining to the client and her family what is happening. Explanation and appropriate reassurance are important for women who have breech presentations because many have heard frightening stories of what may happen if the fetus is breech. Anxiety and fear may interfere with the woman's ability to work effectively with her labor (see Nursing Care Plan: Woman with Breech Presentation).

Evaluation. Possible anticipated outcomes include the following:

■ The woman and fetus remain free of signs of distress or complications.

■ The client demonstrates an understanding of the delivery method chosen.
■ The client gives birth to a healthy newborn.
■ The client demonstrates less anxiety and fear as evidenced by her facial expressions and improved relaxation.
■ The client demonstrates positive coping strategies.

Other Malpresentations

Other abnormal fetal presentations can affect the normal progress of labor. These may include shoulder, face, brow, and compound presentation.

Shoulder Presentation. **Shoulder presentation**, or "transverse lie," occurs when the fetus lies crosswise in the uterus instead of longitudinally. The shoulder is usually the fetal part in the brim of the inlet. Sometimes, however, it is the back, abdomen, ribs, or flank, depending on how the fetus is positioned. Studies have shown that this complication occurs once in 300 to 500 cases, and it is seen most often in multiparas, resulting from abdominal wall relaxation. Other common etiologic factors include prematurity, placenta previa, and contracted pelvis (Cunningham et al., 1993).

Shoulder presentation is a serious complication that increases the hazards of delivery for the woman and even more so for the fetus. Frequently, an arm prolapses into the vagina, making delivery even more difficult. If neglected, this presentation results in uterine rupture and death to the woman and fetus.

External version in late pregnancy or early labor is occasionally successful, especially in the multipara. **Internal version** (realigning the fetus by internal manipulation) and extraction are hazardous procedures frequently associated with rupture of the uterus. It is rarely justified except in the case of a twin. Generally, transverse lie with the woman in active labor is an indication for cesarean delivery.

Face Presentation. **Face presentations,** in which the face (chin) enters the pelvic inlet first, are seen in about one of 600 clients. Factors that favor extension of the head and prevent flexion are implicated in these presentations, a contracted pelvis being paramount among these. These fetuses may deliver spontaneously if labor is effective, and the pelvis is adequate. The face comes through the vulva with the chin anterior.

If there is indication that the pelvis is contracted or that there is fetal distress, a cesarean delivery is indicated. Because edema of the scalp is common in vertex presentations, facial edema often is present to the extent that the landmarks resemble a breech presentation. The edema and purplish discoloration disappear within a few days, but the newborn's appearance gives the parents a great deal of concern. The nurse can be

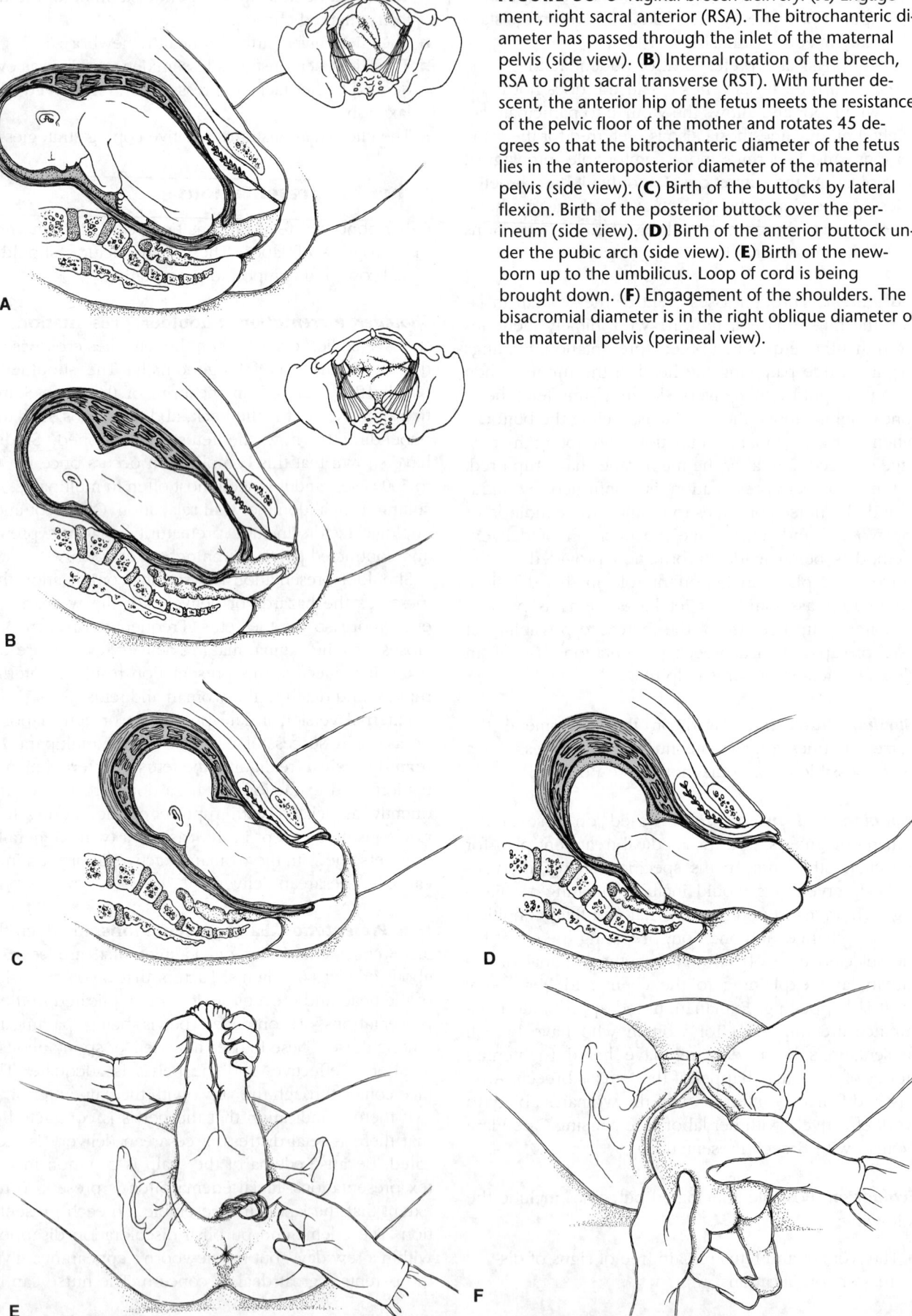

FIGURE 36–6 Vaginal breech delivery. (**A**) Engagement, right sacral anterior (RSA). The bitrochanteric diameter has passed through the inlet of the maternal pelvis (side view). (**B**) Internal rotation of the breech, RSA to right sacral transverse (RST). With further descent, the anterior hip of the fetus meets the resistance of the pelvic floor of the mother and rotates 45 degrees so that the bitrochanteric diameter of the fetus lies in the anteroposterior diameter of the maternal pelvis (side view). (**C**) Birth of the buttocks by lateral flexion. Birth of the posterior buttock over the perineum (side view). (**D**) Birth of the anterior buttock under the pubic arch (side view). (**E**) Birth of the newborn up to the umbilicus. Loop of cord is being brought down. (**F**) Engagement of the shoulders. The bisacromial diameter is in the right oblique diameter of the maternal pelvis (perineal view).

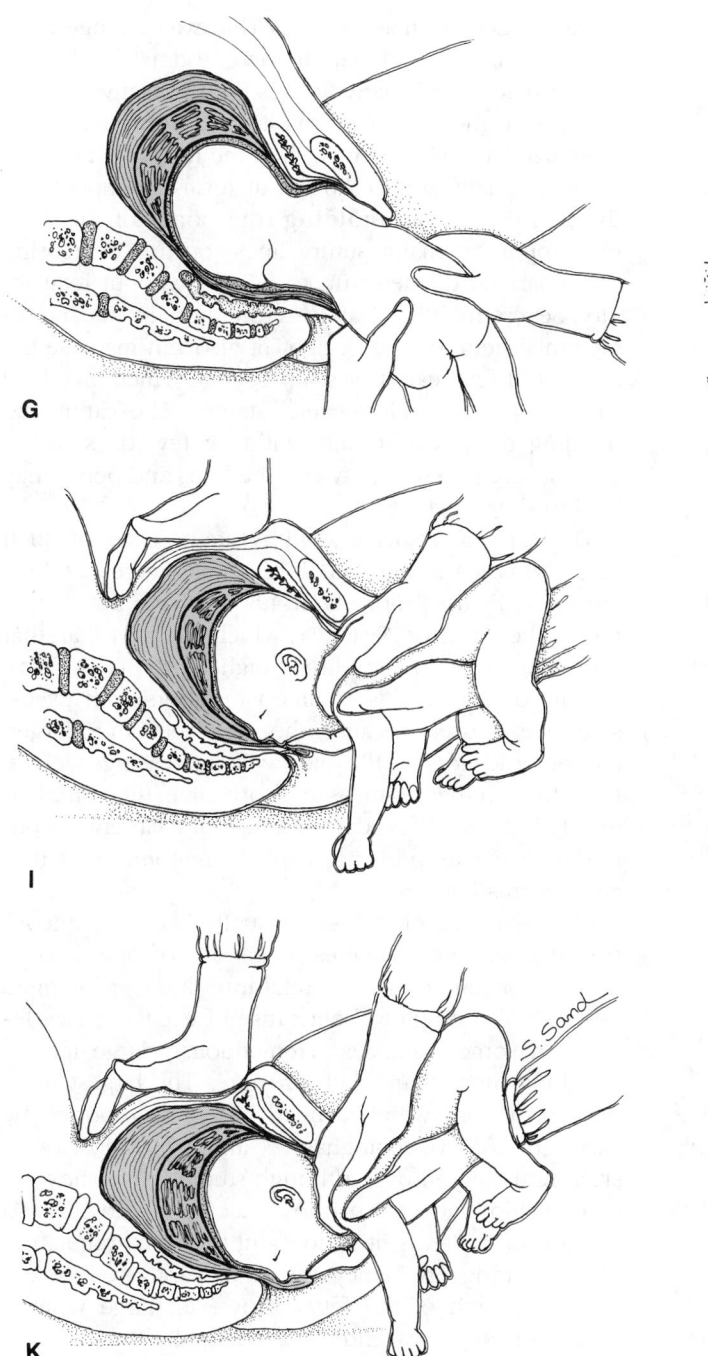

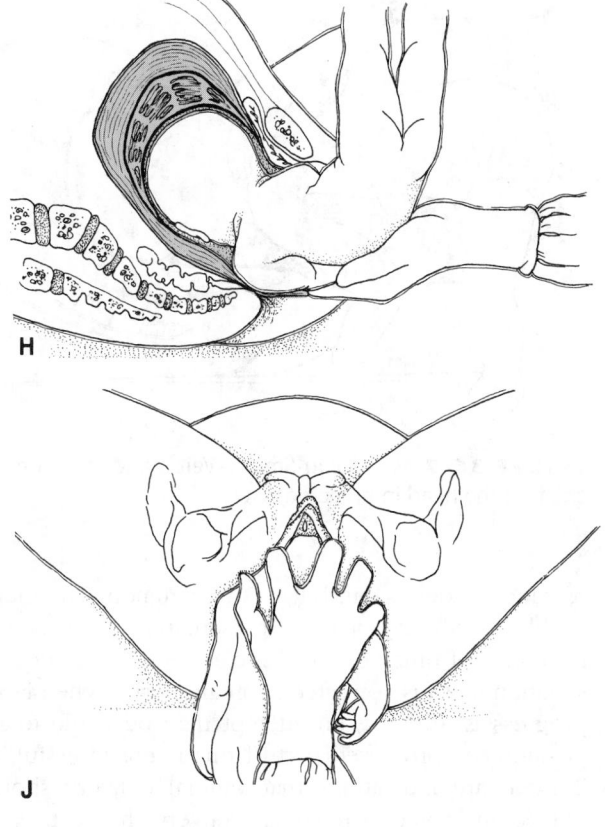

FIGURE 36-6 *Continued.* (**G**) Delivery of the anterior shoulder under the pubic arch (side view). (**H**) Delivery of the posterior shoulder over the perineum (side view). (**I**) Mauriceau-Smellie-Veit maneuver (with an assistant). The occiput is directly under the symphysis pubis. The assistant applies suprapubic pressure (side view). (**J**) Delivery of the head is attempted after the hairline is visible at the introitus (perineal view). (**K**) Mauriceau-Smellie-Veit maneuver continuing. Delivery of the head by flexion upward over the perineum with continuous suprapubic pressure (side view).

helpful in reassuring the parents that the condition is temporary and will resolve without sequelae.

Brow Presentation. In **brow presentation,** the largest diameter of the fetal head, the occipitomental, presents at the pelvic inlet. The fetus is impossible to deliver as long as brow presentation persists, unless the fetus is small and the pelvis is large. However, this is an unstable presentation and often spontaneously converts to an occiput or face presentation.

Brow presentations are somewhat more rare than all of the other malpresentations. The same etiologic factors that underlie a face presentation pertain here. The principles of treatment are the same as for face presentations. If the labor is progressing not unduly vigorously without fetal distress in the closely monitored fetus, no intervention is necessary. If labor does become hyperactive, or more likely erratic, prompt cesarean section is indicated (Cunningham et al., 1993).

Compound Presentation. **Compound presentations** are present when an extremity prolapses alongside and enters the pelvis at the same time as the presenting part. The most common combination is for an upper extremity to prolapse alongside the head. Prolapse of a leg in cephalic presentations or an arm in breech pre-

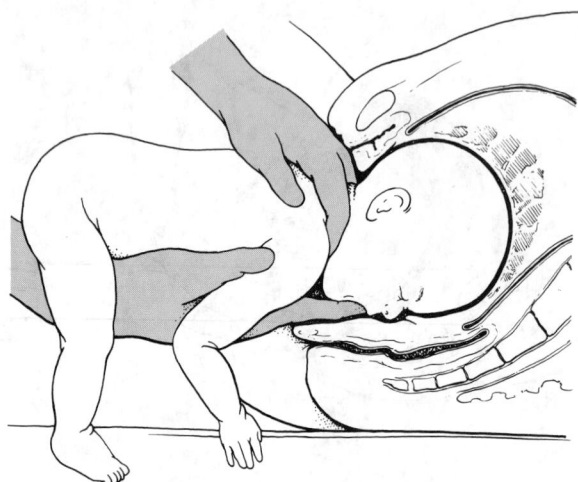

FIGURE 36-7 Mauriceau-Smellie-Veit maneuver for extracting the head in breech delivery.

sentations does occur, but it is uncommon. The major problem with any of these presentations is increased incidence of umbilical cord prolapse. If left alone, the situation often is corrected spontaneously. When labor progress is arrested, an attempt may be made to reposition the prolapsed part. If this is unsuccessful, or if there are indications that vaginal delivery should not be attempted, a cesarean delivery should be performed.

Macrosomia

Macrosomia, or excessive size of the fetus, is defined as fetal weight more than 4,500 g (9.9 lb; ACOG, 1991b). About 1% of deliveries involve a macrosomic fetus of more than 4,500 g, whereas 10% of fetuses delivered are more than 4,000 g (8.8 lb; Sokol et al., 1994). Previously, fetal weights of more than 4,000 g

---

were defined as macrosomic. This was changed because it was believed that the lower estimate will result in the inclusion of many fetuses with a relatively small increase in the risk of morbidity as a consequence of their size (ACOG, 1991b). When the fetal biparietal diameter, usually 9.5 to 9.8 cm at term, attempts to fit through the pelvis, **molding** (the bones of the skull overlapping at major suture lines) occurs, decreasing the biparietal diameter up to 0.5 cm without fetal injury. Severe molding may lead to tentorial tears and intracranial hemorrhage. A tight fit also can increase the amount of fetal caput or scalp edema, which may lead to errors in determining fetal station. The caput and molding disappear usually within a few days. However, severe pressure between the fetus and pelvis may lead to skull fracture.

The trauma associated with the passage of such large fetuses through the birth canal increases fetal mortality. Fetuses more than 4,500 g have a mortality rate in the range of 2% to 3%, which is higher than that for controls of lower birth weights (ACOG, 1991b). Uterine dysfunction is common in labors with excessive size fetuses because the head becomes larger, harder, and less malleable with increasing weight. Even though these fetuses are born alive, they often do poorly in the first few days because of a variety of conditions, such as bruising, cephalhematoma, and brachial plexus injuries.

Excessive size of the fetus usually is due to uncontrolled gestational diabetes, large size of one or both parents, or multiparity. Postmaturity due to prolonged gestation is thought to be a cause of excessive size fetuses in some instances. Tremendously large fetuses weighing more than 11 lb are rare. The largest newborn on record weighed nearly 24 lb as reported by Beach in 1879 (Cunningham et al., 1993). Most oversized fetuses are boys. Although studies have shown a relationship between maternal diet and growth and survival of the fetus, it is doubtful that strict regulation of diet during pregnancy can significantly reduce excessive growth of the fetus. However, large women who are heavy may tend to have large babies.

Shoulder Dystocia. One major complication of an oversized fetus is **shoulder dystocia**, in which the shoulders arrest at either the pelvic brim or the outlet. The incidence of shoulder dystocia in newborns weighing more than 4,500 g is reportedly 8% to 20%. Approximately 15% to 30% of macrosomic fetuses experiencing shoulder dystocia will sustain some recognizable injury to the brachial plexus, but 70% to 80% of brachial plexus injuries recognized at birth resolve within 12 months (ACOG, 1991b). The time between delivery of the head and delivery of the body must be as short as possible to decrease fetal compromise.

A large mediolateral episiotomy and adequate anesthesia are mandatory in preparation for delivery of the

---

BOX 36-3
Nursing Diagnoses: Breech Delivery

- Risk for Injury (fetal) related to possibility of cord prolapse
- Risk for Injury (maternal) related to
  - Cesarean delivery
  - Invasive monitoring
- Anxiety related to concern about possible cesarean delivery
- Knowledge Deficit related to
  - Breech presentation, treatment, complications, and care
  - Care following cesarean delivery
- Situational Low Self Esteem related to problematic labor
- Fear related to perceived threat to self and fetus

NURSING CARE PLAN
Woman With Breech Presentation

Nursing Goals
1. Client verbalizes understanding of breech birth and possible cesarean delivery.
2. Mother has minimal discomfort and does not develop complications.
3. Fetal distress does not develop.
4. Infant is born without complications.

Assessment	Potential Nursing Diagnoses	Intervention/ Rationale	Evaluation
Signs of breech presentation Leopold's maneuver: head in fundus; breech in pelvis Vaginal examination: breech presenting Passage of meconium		Check for fetal presentation and position; report and record findings	
Progress of labor	Risk for Alteration in Labor Progress related to abnormal fetal presentation	Monitor uterine contractions *to assess labor progress* Monitor changes in cervical dilatation and effacement and in fetal presentation and position *to assess labor progress*	Client progresses in labor
Condition of fetus Fetal heart rate and pattern Fetal movement	Risk for Fetal Distress related to increased risk of prolapsed cord	Monitor fetal heart rate tracing for changes, particularly variable decelerations; check for increased fetal movement; *to assess onset of fetal distress*	Fetus remains free of distress
Indications for cesarean delivery Fetal distress Position other than frank breech (complete or footling breech position) Evidence of CPD	Knowledge Deficit related to breech birth Anxiety and fear related to concern about possible cesarean section	Gather data to assist in decision concerning route of delivery Keep client and family informed of progress of labor and plan of treatment *to allay anxiety* Reassure as appropriate Prepare for surgery, if decision made for cesarean; do preoperative and postoperative teaching *to maximize outcomes and allay anxiety*	Client verbalizes understanding of breech birth and cesarean delivery Client verbalizes relief from anxiety and fear Infant is born in good condition

body. The newborn's mouth and nose should be cleared to prevent aspiration. A number of methods or techniques have been developed to free the anterior shoulder from beneath the symphysis to facilitate delivery. Figure 36-8 illustrates one such technique. Other methods include suprapubic pressure, combined with downward pressure on the fetal head or delivery of the posterior arm first, then rotating the fetus to deliver the anterior shoulder. The McRoberts technique involves sharply flexing the maternal thighs against the maternal abdomen to reduce the angle between the

sacrum and spine, thus freeing the impacted shoulder (Bashore, 1992). Care must be taken not to apply too vigorous traction on the head or neck and not to rotate the body excessively. Occasionally, deliberate fracture of the clavicle is necessary to save the newborn's life (Cunningham et al., 1993).

Fetal Anomalies

Any fetal anomaly that increases the size of a fetal part or parts can be a cause of dystocia. This occasionally

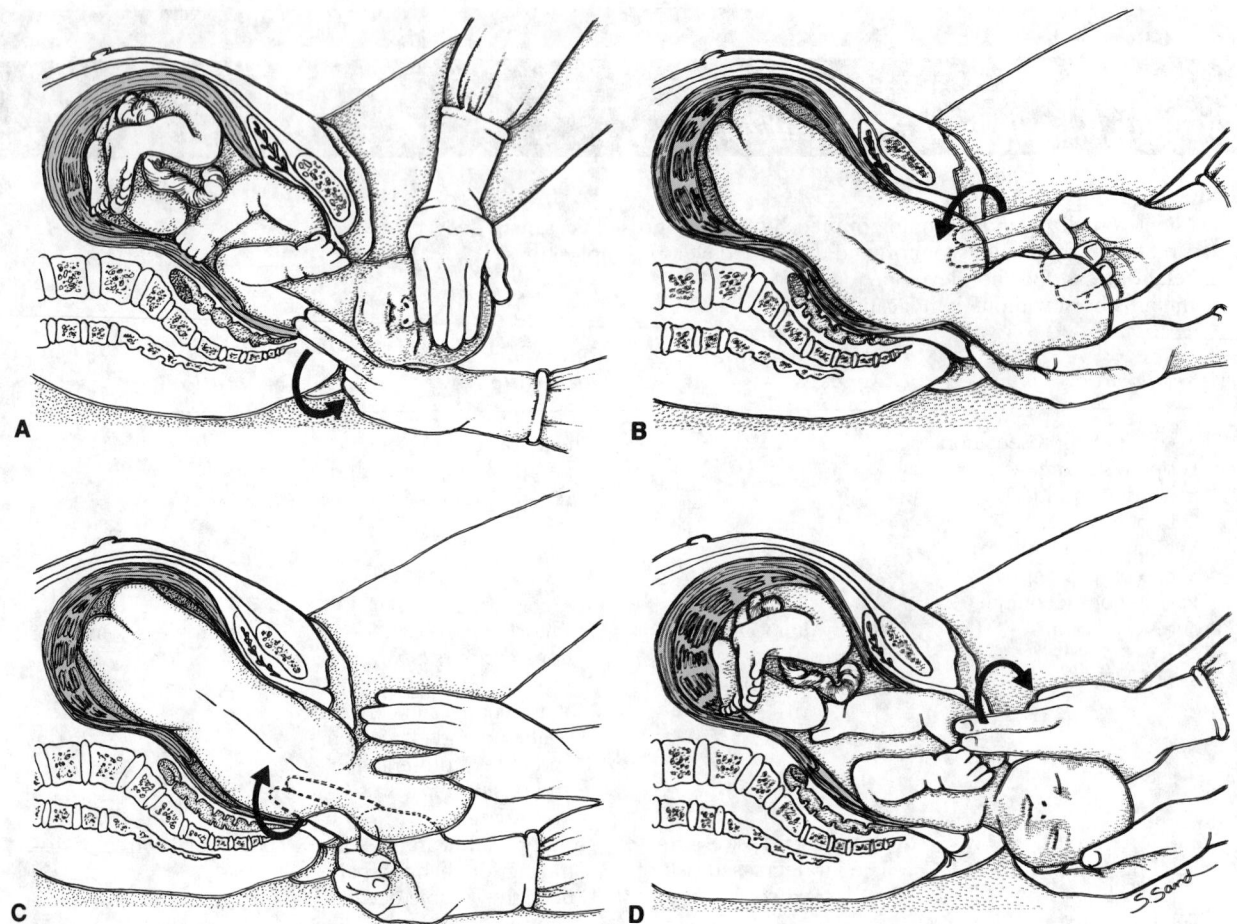

FIGURE 36–8 Maneuvers to relieve shoulder dystocia. (**A**) First phase beginning. The posterior shoulder is rotated 180 degrees. (**B**) First phase is completed. Former anterior shoulder is now posterior, and former posterior shoulder is now anterior. An attempt is made to deliver the shoulders normally at this time. If the attempt fails, the physician proceeds to the second phase. (**C**) Second phase beginning. The newly posterior shoulder is rotated 180 degrees. (**D**) Second phase is completed. Original anterior shoulder is now anterior once again, and the original posterior shoulder is now posterior once again. The remainder of the delivery is performed in the usual way.

occurs as the result of a large fetal abdomen from a greatly distended bladder or enlargement of the kidneys or liver. Another rare cause of problems is incomplete twinning, resulting in conjoined ("Siamese") twins.

Hydrocephalus. The most common fetal anomaly causing dystocia is **hydrocephalus**, or an excessive accumulation of cerebrospinal fluid in the ventricles of the brain with consequent enlargement of the cranium. This condition is encountered in approximately 1 in 2,000 fetuses and accounts for approximately 12% of all malformations at birth (Cunningham et al., 1993). Associated defects, such as spina bifida (present in about one-third of the cases), are common. Varying degrees of cranial enlargement are produced, and frequently the circumference of the head exceeds 50 cm,

sometimes reaching 80 cm. The amount of fluid present is usually between 500 and 1,500 mL, but as much as 5 L has been reported. Because the distended cranium is too large to fit into the pelvic inlet, breech presentations are exceedingly common and are observed in about one-third of such cases.

Whatever the presentation, there is gross disproportion between the size of the head and that of the pelvis. Serious dystocia is the usual consequence (Fig. 36-9). The woman is in danger of an obstructed labor, resulting in uterine rupture, especially when the condition is undetected. Hydrocephalus may be suspected when the enlarged fetal head is palpated as a large symmetrical mass in the fundus or above the symphysis pubis. The condition is often accompanied by hydramnios, excessive amniotic fluid, which makes abdominal palpation of the enlarged head more difficult.

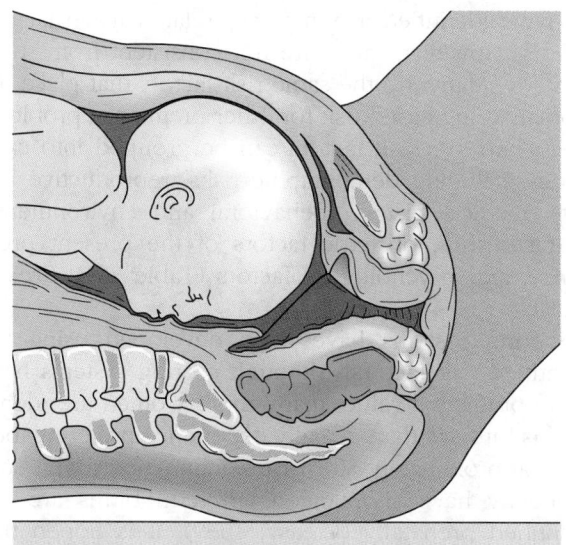

FIGURE 36–9 Severe dystocia from hydrocephalus, cephalic presentation. Note the disparity between the small size of the face and the rest of the cranium.

Ultrasound is useful in making this diagnosis, because the width of the ventricles can be assessed, the thickness of the cerebral cortex can be evaluated, and the size of the head can be compared with that of the thorax and abdomen. By vaginal examination, large fontanels, wide suture lines, and an indentable, thin cranium may be palpated.

Sometimes the obstetrician may find it necessary to puncture the cranial vault and aspirate some of the cerebrospinal fluid to reduce the head to a size that can pass through the birth canal or to circumvent dangerous extensions of a low transverse incision. With a cephalic presentation, the ventricle is tapped transvaginally after the cervix is dilated to about 3 cm; for a breech presentation, it is done at the base of the skull after the breech and trunk are delivered. When this type of aspiration is necessary, fetal death is common. Therefore, only fetuses with severe associated abnormalities receive this treatment. All others should be delivered by cesarean.

When hydrocephalus is diagnosed early through the use of ultrasound, a shunt may be inserted in utero to minimize fetal brain damage and to delay delivery until the fetus is more mature. With the increasing success of fetal surgery, there is hope for the future. Labor and birth with a hydrocephalic fetus are difficult for all concerned. The woman must undergo a difficult labor with increased danger to herself and high probability of death for the fetus. The family is stressed by the high-risk situation. The physician and nurse must cope with a grave crisis and a poor prognosis. In this situation, the nurse must exercise nursing skill during the labor and after the delivery. The components of care

that are useful in helping the parents in such a crisis are discussed in Chapter 42.

Problems With the Psyche

The client's psyche may exert considerable influence on the duration and character of labor. The woman who is fearful, anxious, or even extremely excited may become tense and have difficulty working with her contractions. These women may have longer, more uncomfortable labors. The release of catecholamines in response to stress is thought to lead to uterine dysfunction. Increased tension also leads to fatigue. Childbirth preparation classes, in many instances, help to prevent these problems. Supportive nursing care during labor also can aid the woman in relaxation.

Management Options

The holistic view of physiology attempts to integrate the mind–body interplay into therapies. Dystocia may be caused by the inhibitory neurogenic factors of uterine sympathetic nerve stimulation (β_1 adrenergic receptors), adrenal release of catecholamines, and central nervous system release of endorphins. Holistic approach practitioners initially may use the following options prior to pharmacologic interventions (Wray, 1993):

- Modification of the environment to decrease maternal stress
- Discussion with the woman to detect any underlying fears or concerns for herself or as they relate to the fetus or delivery
- Correction of maternal exhaustion and dehydration with rest and fluid intake
- Ambulation or possibly a shower or jacuzzi

Preterm Labor and Birth

Preterm labor is defined as labor occurring prior to the completion of 37 weeks of gestation. Prevention and management of preterm labor is a major focus of perinatology because prematurity is the main cause of neonatal morbidity and mortality, accounting for about 75% of all neonatal deaths. Inspite of the introduction of new diagnostic and therapeutic technologies during the last 4 decades in the United States, the rate of preterm delivery has remained unchanged, affecting approximately 1 in 10 births (ACOG, 1995).

Prediction

The ability to predict which woman is most likely to experience spontaneous preterm labor and delivery is a difficult task because the causes of preterm labor are not well understood. In most cases, the cause of preterm labor is unknown. However, several studies in the last 15 years have demonstrated certain conditions to be associated with the initiation of preterm labor (Newton et al., 1979; Mamelle et al., 1984; Romero et al., 1989; Klein et al., 1990):

■ Uterine overdistention by conditions such as poly-hydramnios and twins
■ Uterine anomalies
■ History of uterine surgery
■ Previous or present early uterine activity
■ Fetal anomalies
■ Maternal infections, such as asymptomatic bacteri-uria (almost twice the risk of entering preterm labor as women without bacteria in their urine)
■ Cocaine (four times normal incidence of preterm labor)
■ Smoking
■ Psychological stress, long employment hours, and fatigue

In an effort to predict which women are at increased risk for spontaneous preterm labor and delivery, stud-

ies have identified a number of related maternal risk factors. However, these are not consistent from study to study. Many are the same risk factors that place the woman at increased risk for other pregnancy problems (see Chap. 6). Risk factors can be grouped into categories including demographic risks, reproductive history, medical history, behavioral and environmental characteristics, obstetric factors of the present pregnancy, and psychological factors (Table 36-3; Creasy, 1989).

Scoring systems have been developed using the identified risk factors. Although scoring systems have some predictive value, many more women are identified as "at risk" than actually experience preterm labor. Also, approximately 50% of pregnant clients who subsequently have spontaneous preterm births are not identified prenatally (Creasy, 1989). It is hoped that eventually biochemical and biophysical measurements to be used with the scoring systems will improve the accuracy of predicting women at risk. Indicators, such as weekly monitoring showing increased uterine irritabiltity from baseline or identification of fetal fibronectin from cervicovaginal secrections as a marker of

TABLE 36-3
Risk Factors Associated With Preterm Labor

DEMOGRAPHIC FACTORS	MEDICAL HISTORY AND STATUS	MAJOR RISK FACTORS*
Nonwhite	Heart disease	Multiple gestation
Unmarried	Anemia	Hydramnios
Two children at home	Third trimester urinary tract infection	Abdominal surgery during pregnancy
Low socioeconomic status	DES exposure in utero	Cervix dilated >1 cm at 32 wk
Maternal age <20 y or >40 y	**BEHAVIORAL AND ENVIRONMENTAL**	Cervical shortening <1 cm at 32 wk
Single parent	**CHARACTERISTICS**	Uterine irritability
Height <150 cm	Poor nutrition	
Weight <45 kg	Smoking (more than 10 cigarettes per day)	**PSYCHOLOGICAL FACTORS**
	Use of alcohol or illicit drugs	Stress
PAST REPRODUCTIVE HISTORY	Exposure to toxins	Psychic trauma
Prior induced abortions	Working outside home	Negative attitude toward pregnancy
Prior low–birth-weight newborn	Heavy or stressful work	
Prior preterm delivery	Long, tiring trip or commute	
Prior second trimester spontaneous abortion	Unusual fatigue	
Less than 1 y since last birth		
	OBSTETRIC FACTORS IN PRESENT	
MAJOR RISK FACTORS	**PREGNANCY**	
Previous preterm delivery	Lack of or late prenatal care	
Previous preterm labor, term delivery	Low prepregnancy weight	
Uterine anomaly	Weight gain <5 kg by 32 wk	
History of cone biopsy	Engagement of head at 32 wk	
Two second-trimester abortions	Development of pregnancy complications, such as febrile illness	
More than two first-trimester abortions		
History of pyelonephritis		

(Adapted from Kulb, N. W. [1990]. Preterm labor. In K. Buckley & N. W. Kulb [Eds.], *High risk maternity nursing manual.* Baltimore: Williams & Wilkins; and Creasy, R. K. [1989]. Disorders of parturition. Preterm labor and delivery. In R. K. Creasy & R. Resnick [Eds.], *Maternal-fetal medicine: Principles and practice* [2nd ed.]. Philadelphia: W.B. Saunders.)

decidual disruption, could prove useful in the future once they are fully validated (ACOG, 1995).

Prevention

Efforts to prevent preterm labor are directed toward prevention or detection of risk factors and treatment of these factors as appropriate. Although cervical change is technically necessary for a diagnosis of preterm labor, uterine activity may signal treatment to start to prevent the expected cervical change. If it is only false labor, delivery will not occur even if no therapy is given, so any therapy will give excellent results.

The anticipated success rate depends on the stage of labor at which treatments are administered. The earlier in labor they are begun, the better the success rate. Various definitions of success have been used, including delay of labor for 48 hours, delay of labor for 7 days, and delay of labor until fetus is 2,500 g in birth weight or 37 weeks of gestation (Parsons et al., 1994).

In early labor, when the cervix is dilated 2 to 3 cm, bed rest, hydration, and sedation achieve a 50% success rate in stopping uterine activity. These measures increase the intravascular volume and uterine blood flow and reduce fetal head pressure on the cervix. The addition of tocolytic therapy improves this success rate to 75% (Main et al., 1985; Bennett et al., 1989; Parsons et al., 1994).

Some researchers suspect that bacterial infection of the lower genital tract contributes to the onset of preterm labor. One study demonstrated an incidence of 18.7% in clients with Group B-streptococcus (GBS) colonization compared with 5.5% in clients negative for GBS (McDonald et al., 1989). Therefore, some experts have recommended that a screening GBS urine and cervical culture be done at 22 weeks' gestation; if these are positive, the client needs appropriate antibiotic and follow-up cultures to test for cure (Parsons et al., 1994)). However, because the prevalence of GBS colonization of the lower urogenital tract is high (15%–40%) and the attack rate among fetuses of colonized women is low (1%–2%), routine screening of all pregnant women is not the standard of care, and chemoprophylaxis for all colonized women is not perceived as justifiably beneficial or cost effective in the United States (ACOG, 1995).

Avoiding intercourse also has been suggested as a preventive measure in clients susceptible to preterm labor, both for reducing the risk of infection and because the prostaglandins in seminal fluid are thought possibly to stimulate uterine contractions. Although coitus and orgasm have been linked to prematurity in some studies, it has not been linked in all studies. Also, no prospective studies support sexual abstinence routinely in all pregnancies for prevention of preterm labor (ACOG, 1995). Cervical cerclage has sometimes been suggested as a method of preventing preterm la-

bor and birth, but there is some evidence that placement of the cerclage may promote uterine contractions (Parisi, 1989).

There have been some efforts to use pharmacologic methods prophylactically. Use of progesterone to prevent preterm labor has shown mixed results. Possible teratogenic effects, such as cardiac defects, have resulted in a ban on the use of progestins during pregnancy by the U.S. Food and Drug Administration. The efficacy of prophylactic β-adrenergic therapy, such as oral terbutaline (Brethine), also is unclear after several studies. The most probable reason for their failure is that the blood concentration of the drug seldom achieves therapeutic levels (Parsons et al., 1994; ACOG, 1995).

Early Diagnosis

Prevention of preterm birth through early detection and treatment of preterm labor has become more possible since the discovery of new, more effective tocolytic agents to arrest labor. Preterm labor must be detected early if tocolytic agents are to be used, because their effectiveness decreases with the advance of labor. In some studies, client education and frequent evaluation of the cervix of high-risk clients have proven effective in early identification of preterm labor (Klein et al., 1990).

Home uterine activity monitoring, which had previously been shown by several nonrandomized trials to contribute to earlier detection and treatment of preterm labor, has been used as part of many preterm prevention projects and by some private physicians (Morrison et al., 1987; Koehl et al., 1989; Chibber et al., 1990). However, the initial enthusiasm for this modality has waned because in several recent randomized trials, the efficacy of home uterine monitoring has not proven to be useful (Blondel et al., 1992; Grimes et al., 1992). However, daily nurse contact has shown some benefit, although no additional benefit of the monitor was shown (Dyson et al., 1991). Therefore, ACOG has endorsed home uterine monitoring for preventing preterm delivery (Parsons et al., 1994).

Diagnosis of preterm labor in time to prevent preterm birth is often difficult. Possible early signs and symptoms, including abdominal, intestinal, or menstrual-like cramps; pelvic pressure; diarrhea; low backache; and increased vaginal discharge, are difficult to differentiate from false labor or common discomforts of advancing pregnancy (Kulb, 1990). Even the presence of regular uterine contractions does not always mean true labor has begun. Rupture of the membranes accompanied by regular uterine contractions establishes the diagnosis, but attempting to stop the labor at this point is problematic. Research has shown that awaiting progressive cervical effacement and dilatation to establish the diagnosis does not compromise efficacy of tocolysis, as long as dilatation is less than 3 cm (Utter et al., 1990).

Management and Nursing Care

Before deciding to attempt to inhibit labor, assessment of the condition of woman and fetus must be made to determine whether continuation of the pregnancy would be detrimental to the woman and whether the fetus would have a better chance of survival inside or outside the uterus. Actually only 25% of all preterm labor clients are candidates for treatment, because of the frequent coexistence of one or more of the following three categories of exclusion factors (Parsons et al., 1994):

■ Premature rupture of membrane (PROM) occurs in 25% to 40% of clients.
■ Serious maternal or fetal distress, such as abruption, chorioamnionitis, preeclampsia or HELLP syndrome (Hemolysis, Elevated Liver enzymes, Low Platelets), and major congenital anomalies incompatible with life occurs in 10% to 20% of clients.
■ Advanced cervical dilatation (>6 cm) occurs.

Indications for inhibition of labor include factors that prove the necessity for prolonging the in utero time. Because fetal lung maturity usually occurs by 36 weeks, the borderline preterm newborn between 36 and 38 weeks (>2,500 g) will usually not need pulmonary support after birth. Because tocolytic therapy may be associated with some maternal risks, instituting therapy for fetuses more than 35 weeks does not meet the risk to benefit ratio criteria for good clinical judgment. The following conditions indicate the need for tocolytic therapy (Malinowski, 1989; Sala et al., 1990):

■ Diagnosis of preterm labor
■ Gestational age greater than 20 weeks, but less than 36 weeks
■ Estimated fetal weight less than 2,500 g
■ Immature fetal lung profile (inadequate alveolar surfactants): lecithin-sphingomyelin (LS) ratio less than 2:1; phosphatidylglycerol (PG) absent

If the decision is made to attempt to halt the labor, a combination of supportive and pharmacologic interventions will probably be implemented.

General Measures

One major nonpharmacologic technique to quiet the uterus is to increase uterine blood flow by bed rest on the left lateral position and increased hydration. A common protocol is to start an IV with a balanced salt solution, such as Ringer's lactate, and give a bolus of 500 to 1,000 mL over a 30- to 60-minute period, followed by a maintenance dose of 125 mL/h (Parsons et al., 1994). The resultant increased plasma volume is thought to decrease the release of the antidiuretic hormone vasopressin and reduce oxytocin secretion from the posterior pituitary gland.

If urinary tract infection is suspected (burning on urination, urinary frequency), treatment should be initiated before culture results are obtained. Unnecessary vaginal manipulation should be avoided.

Tocolytic Agents

β-adrenergic agonists are synthetic pharmacologic agents that are β-adrenergic receptor specific. Because β_2 receptor activation reduces intracellular free calcium and resulting uterine contractility, timely use of these drugs can potentially stop contractions. This group of drugs includes ritodrine (Yutopar), terbutaline, and others that are used in other countries. Although ritodrine is the only drug approved by the U.S. Food and Drug Administration for use in inhibiting preterm labor, terbutaline is commonly used based on years of published clinical obstetric research (Parsons et al., 1994).

The efficacy of magnesium sulfate ($MgSO_4$) as a tocolytic agent is controversial, because a high dose is required to alter myometrial contractility through its role as a calcium antagonist. The optimal therapeutic range of 6 to 8 mEq/L is higher than that required for treatment of preeclampsia (4–7 mEq/L; Parsons et al., 1994). One study that showed a success rate equal to ritodrine used an infusion dose that averaged the high rate of 4.5 g/h (Hollander et al., 1987). Other studies with more commonly used doses (4 g loading; 2 g/h maintenance; mean serum Mg^{++} levels of 5.5 mEq/L) show conflicting results. Cox, in a study with methodology that offered more control (prospective, randomized design), identified little difference between $MgSO_4$ and normal saline infusion for 156 women in preterm labor with intact membranes (Cox et al., 1990).

Prostaglandin synthetase inhibitors are another class of drugs that have been shown to reduce uterine activity. Indomethacin and aspirin are in this category, because they inhibit synthesis of prostaglandin E_2 (PGE_2) and PGF_{2a}, which are believed to play a pathogenic role in preterm labor. PGE_2 and PGF_{2a} are produced in the membrane of uterine cells, are synthesized rapidly, have a short half-life, and act as hormones to increase gap junctions and improve coordination of uterine contractions. Indomethacin and aspirin inhibit the production of prostaglandins by blocking a key enzyme, cyclo-oxygenase, necessary for the conversion of arachidonic acid into prostaglandin (Zuckerman et al., 1974; Ulmsten, 1989).

Although some studies have shown indomethacin to be effective, because of the potential danger of premature closure of the ductus arteriosus in the fetus, it is not recommended for gestations more than 33 weeks.

Nifedipine, a *calcium antagonist*, is another tocolytic agent that has been evaluated clinically. One trial showed it to be more effective than ritodrine in stopping uterine contractions by blocking the influx of calcium through calcium channels in the cell membrane (Read et al., 1986).

Other agents being investigated have included *oxytocin antagonists, aminophyline,* and *diazoxide.* The oxytocin analog inhibitors can block vasopressin receptors and may have an adverse effect on maternal water secretion (Parsons et al., 1994). Further studies are needed to establish the safety and effectiveness of these agents. Table 36-4 summarizes the major tocolytic agents used.

Steroids

Respiratory distress syndrome (RDS) is the most common cause of morbidity and mortality in preterm newborns. This condition is related to a deficiency of surfactant in the immature lungs. According to the latest ACOG guidelines, corticosteroids should be considered for the induction of fetal lung maturity in 24- to 34-week gestations. Optimal benefits begin 24 hours after initiation of therapy and last 7 days. However, because several studies suggest an increased risk of infection with steroid use in women with preterm PROM without a reduction in the rate or severity of RDS, ACOG's latest official opinion warns that further research is needed to evaluate the risks and benefits of using corticosteroids. Because ruptured membranes accelerate lung maturity, many clinicians delay labor for 48 hours with PROM and borderline fetal lung maturity (ACOG, 1994; Garite et al., 1994).

Preterm Birth

Because therapy fails in about 25% of clients, preparations should made to allow the delivery to take place in a center with a neonatal intensive care unit. The short-term objective of postponing labor temporarily for 48 hours or more allows time for maternal transfer to occur if necessary and to begin fetal therapies to promote maturation of the fetal lungs (Parsons et al., 1994).

Management of preterm birth is focused on careful, continuous observation of fetal status. Systemic analgesics and anesthetics given to the woman during labor might depress the newborn at birth and should be avoided. The cervix does not have to reach 10 cm to stretch over the fetal head, so the second stage can begin earlier than with a term birth. It usually proceeds rapidly because passage down the birth canal offers less resistance to a smaller presenting part. Because these fetuses are more susceptible to intracranial hemorrhage, generous episiotomies, delivery of the head

between contractions, use of forceps, and cesarean deliveries or breech presentation are interventions used to protect the preterm fetus' head during the birth process (Klein et al., 1990).

Assessment

Initial assessment of the woman who is thought to be in labor before 37 weeks' gestation includes basic information about her health and obstetric history plus evaluation of her current condition. The nurse can assist in determining the presence of true labor by monitoring the frequency, intensity, and duration of contractions; checking for cervical effacement and dilatation; and observing for other signs of labor, such as rupture of membranes and bloody show. Assessment of the fetus for approximate size (fundal height at term is usually 36 cm), lung maturity profile (at term is L-S $\geq$ 2.0 and PG positive), and signs of fetal distress also is important. Prenatal history for date of first examination, ultrasound, and history of any complications also must be reviewed.

Once treatment is begun, the nurse evaluates maternal and fetal responses to therapies and reports any serious abnormalities promptly, ready to discontinue therapy as appropriate.

Nursing Diagnosis

Preterm labor is an alteration in the childbearing process. The nurse is an active participant with the physician in making and interpreting the assessment data to make the diagnosis of preterm labor and arrive at decisions for interventions. Specific nursing diagnoses might be made during this time to guide the nurse in providing appropriate nursing care. For a list of possible nursing diagnoses see Box 36-4.

Planning and Intervention

The woman with preterm labor and her family can be expected to have a high level of anxiety. This is understandable, because they are usually not prepared for the labor physically or emotionally and may be fearful that the fetus will not survive. Support from a primary nurse who can be with them through the admission process and provide information about what is and will be happening can be helpful in allaying their anxiety. Bed rest in the side-lying position and adequate hydration, either orally or intravenously, are usually instituted while the decision on further treatment is being made. An intake and output record should be kept. Comfort measures as with any labor should be used (see Chap. 22), and analgesic medications should be

(*text continues on page 985*)

TABLE 36-4
Drugs Used for Preterm Labor

TOCOLYTIC AGENTS

General indications for use:
- Signs of preterm labor
- Gestational age >20 wk but <36 wk
- Estimated fetal weight >500 g but <2,500 g
- No contraindications to continuation of pregnancy

General contraindications:
- Pregnancy <20 wk
- Ruptured membranes, especially with signs of infection
- Active uterine bleeding
- Maternal medical complications, such as diabetes mellitus or severe preeclampsia
- Acute or chronic fetal distress
- Major fetal anomalies
- Intrauterine fetal death
- Any maternal or fetal condition contraindicating the continuation of pregnancy
- Advanced labor with cervical dilatation beyond 4 cm

Drug	Action	Additional Contraindications	Side Effects and Complications	Dosage and Route	Remarks
ß-ADRENERGIC AGONISTS Ritodrine (Yutopar)	Exerts preferential effect on ß₂ receptors in smooth muscle of uterus, inhibiting contractility; in blood vessels causing vasodilation	Maternal cardiac disease, renal disease, diabetes, or hyperthyroidism Known hypersensitivity to drug	Maternal: Cardiovascular: Increased heart rate Widening pulse pressure: Slightly increased systolic BP Decreased diastolic BP Increased cardiac output Hyperglycemia Hypokalemia Fluid retention Pulmonary edema Subjective reactions Palpitations Tremors Nausea and vomiting	Intravenous infusion: 150 mg ritodrine to 500 mL of solution = 0.3 mg/mL Begin at 0.05 mg to 0.1 mg/min; increase by 0.05 mg/min every 10 min until UCs stop, side effects are unacceptable or maximum recommended dose of 0.35 mg/min is reached; continue IV 12 h after labor	Only drug approved by FDA for treatment of preterm labor Risk of pulmonary edema increased when given concurrently with corticosteroids Nurse should be alert for signs of pulmonary edema

Drug	Action	Contraindications	Side Effects	Dosage	Nursing Considerations
			Headache Nervousness Restlessness Anxiety Chest tightness or pain Dyspnea Fetal: tachycardia Neonatal: hypoglycemia	ceases; 30 min before discontinuing IV, start ritodrine PO Oral: Ritodrine 10 mg every 2 h for 24 h, then 10–20 mg every 4–6 h for maintenance	Not approved by FDA for tocolytic use Advantages over ritodrine: less expensive; may be given subcutaneously
Terbutaline (Brethine, Bricanyl)		Client taking terbutaline for asthma Others same as ritodrine	Similar to ritodrine	IV infusion: 0.01 mg/min, increase to 0.085 mg/min maximum Oral maintenance dose: 2.5–5 mg every 4–6 h Subcutaneous injections: 0.25 mg q 20–60 min Subcutaneous pump: Basal rate 0.05–0.1 mg/h Bolus of 0.25 mg/h (maximum of 7/d)	
ß-ADRENERGIC AGONISTS					
MAGNESIUM SULFATE	Exact mode of action unknown—depresses uterine activity when maternal serum magnesium levels 6–8 mEq/L	CNS depression Cardiac dysfunction Renal pathology	Maternal Related to increasing serum magnesium levels: hypotension, respiratory depression, hypotonus Magnesium toxicity: Respiratory arrest Circulatory collapse Cardiac arrest Fetal: distress in response to woman's symptoms Neonatal: respiratory depression, hypotonus	IV infusion: Loading dose: 4–6 g by slow IV push or over 30 min by infusion Maintenance: 2 g/h until UCs stop or signs of toxicity appear	Not approved by FDA for tocolytic use Nursing responsibilities: Monitor VS q 5 min during loading dose and q 15 min during maintenance Stop infusion and report if: BP is ≤90/60, respiration is ≤12/min; there is no patellar reflex; urine output is ≤30 mL/h Keep calcium gluconate at bedside

(continued)

TABLE 36–4 (Continued)
Drugs Used for Preterm Labor

DRUGS USED TO PREVENT RESPIRATORY DISTRESS SYNDROME

Drug	Action	Indications	Contraindications	Side Effects/ Complications	Dosage and Route	Remarks
CORTICOSTEROIDS Betamethasone (Celestone) Dexamethasone	Increased production of surfactant in fetal lungs	Preterm labor at gestational age of 24–34 wk L:S ratio not known or <2:1 Fetal membranes intact Possibility of delaying delivery for 48 h after initiation of therapy without undue risk to woman or fetus	Inability or contraindications to delaying delivery Gestational age >34 wk L:S ratio ≥2	Maternal: May increase adverse effects of diabetes or preeclampsia Increased risk of infection Delayed wound healing if cesarean birth Fetal/neonatal: No reports of serious side effects, but long-term effects not known	12 mg IM, repeat in 12–24 h × 1; 6 mg IM, repeat in 12–24 h × 1; repeat weekly 6 mg IM until L:S ratio 2:1/34 wk Effects seem to be transitory, peak at 48 h and last approximately 1 wk	Not approved by FDA for this use; controversy exists about effectiveness and potential dangers Use with tocolytic agent appears to increase risk of pulmonary edema

BP, blood pressure; UC, uterine contractions; FDA, Food and Drug Administration; VS, vital signs; CNS, central nervous system.

Nursing Diagnoses: Preterm labor

- Altered Cardiopulmonary Tissue Perfusion related to effects of tocolytic agents
- Fear related to uncertainty of outcome and effects of preterm labor on fetus
- Impaired Gas Exchange (neonatal) related to lung immaturity
- Pain related to uterine contractions
- Ineffective Management of Therapeutic Regimen related to lack of knowledge and complexity of therapy for preterm labor
- Diversional Activity Deficit related to imposed bed rest
- Constipation related to
  - Decreased gastrointestinal motility from prolonged bed rest
  - Adverse effects of tocolytic agents
- Altered Family Process related to effects of therapy on family
- Situational Low Self Esteem related to feelings of inadequacy from preterm labor complication
- Knowledge Deficit related to
  - Condition and treatment of preterm labor
  - Signs and symptoms of true labor
  - Tocolytic therapy

avoided or kept to a minimum. (See Nursing Care Plan: The Client at Risk for Preterm Labor)

Care of the Woman Receiving Tocolytic Therapy. The nurse plays an important role in the care of the client receiving a tocolytic agent by IV infusion. The nurse helps determine whether the client understands the nature of the treatment and possible side effects and provides information when needed. The client should be helped to maintain the left lateral position in bed to minimize the risk of supine hypotension. This is more easily accomplished when the client understands the rationale. Baseline data, including fetal heart rate, uterine activity, and maternal vital signs, should be obtained before the infusion is started. Also, the physician usually orders baseline laboratory studies, including complete blood count with differential, blood glucose, serum electrolytes, urinalysis and urine culture (to check for latent urinary tract infection), and a baseline electrocardiogram. These baseline data are needed to verify the current status in terms of the uterine activity and fetal well-being and to check for any physiologic contraindications to the medication, such as hypoglycemia, hypokalemia, or cardiac arrhythmias.

The nurse is usually responsible for starting the IV and preparing the infusion. The protocol varies with the institution, the doctor's orders, and the drug to be used. A large-gauge IV catheter usually is used (number 18 angiocath allows blood transfusion if needed).

The solution should be administered with the use of an infusion pump so the dosage can be carefully titrated. The usual initial dosage of ritodrine is 50 to 100 mg/min with the infusion rate being increased by increments of 50 mg/min every 10 minutes until uterine activity ceases or significant side effects develop. The usual effective dosage range is 150 to 350 mg/min (Malinowski, 1989; Neal et al., 1992).

Although the side effects for the different β-adrenergic agonists vary somewhat, ritodrine is fairly typical and is used in this example. While the infusion rate of the ritodrine is being increased, the maternal pulse, respirations, and blood pressure are taken as often as every 10 minutes. After the infusion rate is stabilized, they are monitored every 30 minutes until 1 hour after the infusion is discontinued.

Significant side effects to be reported include maternal pulse rate greater than 140 beats/min, chest tightness or pain, dyspnea, blood pressure less than 90/60 or a significant decrease from the client's baseline, or fetal tachycardia greater than 180 beats/min. These symptoms may require decreasing the IV rate or discontinuing the therapy. Milder symptoms, such as headache, restlessness, or nausea, may respond to a slight decrease in the dosage. Intake and output should be recorded, and the 24-hour intake should be limited to 1,500 to 2,000 mL to avoid fluid overload, which could lead to pulmonary edema.

If uterine contractions are successfully inhibited, the woman may be put on oral maintenance therapy. The initial oral dose should be given 30 minutes before the IV ritodrine is discontinued. Vital signs should be taken every 2 hours for the first 24 hours, then every 4 hours. Uterine activity and side effects also should be monitored. The side effects of the oral drug can sometimes be minimized by taking it with food.

Women on tocolytic therapy need emotional and physical support. Not only are they concerned about the outcome for themselves and their fetus, but they may be uncomfortable from the side effects of the drug and from the enforced bed rest. Helpful hints include the following:

- Suggesting use of a mattress pad or "egg-crate" mattress to help alleviate the hip discomfort from the side-lying position
- Encouraging use of pillows from home to provide comfort and brighten the room
- Assisting with personal hygiene, such as brushing teeth and washing hair
- Providing passive range of motion or isometric exercises to assist in maintaining muscle tone
- Assisting with finding activities that can be accomplished while in bed
- Providing comfort measures, such as back rubs

(*text continues on page 988*)

NURSING CARE PLAN
The Client at Risk for Preterm Labor

Nursing Goals

1. Client is able to identify factors that put her at risk for preterm labor.
2. Client takes steps to change behavior and reduce risks.
3. Client identifies early signs of preterm labor and seeks appropriate medical care.
4. Client undergoes tocolytic treatment:
   - Verbalizes understanding of condition, treatment, and instructions for self-care
   - Verbalizes concerns and subsequent reduction in fear and anxiety
   - Experiences minimal side effects
   - Copes effectively with situation.
5. Fetus does not develop signs of distress, or signs of distress are detected early and minimized.
6. Client undergoing preterm birth:
   - Verbalizes understanding of situation
   - Progresses in labor with minimal discomfort and without complications
   - Fetus/neonate has minimal distress and is born in good condition.

Assessment	*Potential Nursing Diagnoses*	*Intervention/ Rationale*	*Evaluation*
Risk factors associated with preterm labor: Maternal age < 18 or > 40 years Low socioeconomic status Poor nutritional status Employment outside of home Heavy cigarette smoking Alcohol or drug abuse Previous reproductive loss Previous low-birth-weight or preterm infant Maternal disease or infection Present pregnancy: Bleeding, overdistention of uterus, premature rupture of membranes	Knowledge Deficit regarding factors related to risk of preterm labor	Take history at first antepartum visit *to determine presence of risk factors;* reassess at each antepartum visit *to assess progress* Teach client to identify risk factors *to prevent negative outcomes* Teach methods of possible risk reduction: Improve nutrition Decrease or stop smoking Avoid alcohol and drugs Reduce stress *to maximize positive outcomes of pregnancy*	Clients at risk are identified Client identifies risk factors Client takes steps to reduce risks
Signs of labor Contractions q 10 min lasting 30 s or more Cervical change, Effacement = 80% Dilatation = 2 cm	Knowledge Deficit regarding signs of preterm labor	Provide information about signs of preterm labor to clients at risk: menstrual-type cramps, lower abdominal tightening or pressure, intermittent back ache, bloody show, watery vaginal discharge *to teach clients to recognize negative symptoms* Provide information about when and how to contact healthcare provider and come to hospital *to expedite entrance to hospital*	Client describes signs of preterm labor Client seeks medical care appropriately
Labor progress Continued cervical changes	Anxiety and fear related to unexpected early labor	On admission to labor unit: observe for signs of labor and progressive changes;	Client responds positively to care aspects

(continued)

NURSING CARE PLAN *(Continued)*
The Client at Risk for Preterm Labor

Assessment	Potential Nursing Diagnoses	Intervention/ Rationale	Evaluation
Frequency, intensity, and duration of uterine contractions Rupture of membranes or leaking amniotic fluid Bloody show		obtain laboratory values—CBC, urinalysis; test vaginal discharge with nitrazine paper for presence of amniotic fluid Encourage left side-lying position *to enhance fetal oxygenation* Provide oral or intravenous fluids *to maintain hydration*—initial 200 mL to 500 mL bolus as ordered Monitor and record intake and output	
Maternal emotional status		Provide appropriate, factual information to client and family about progress of labor and plan of care *to allay anxiety and keep patient informed*	Family understands client's condition and plan of care
		Allow partner or other person of client's choice to be present as desired *to support client*	Client acknowledges reduction of fear
Gestational age EDD Height of fundus Ultrasound		Assist in estimation of gestational age *to help determine choice of treatment*	
Fetal well-being Fetal heart rate, baseline, periodic changes, variability Fetal movement Tests of fetal maturity, L/S ratio, ultrasound		Apply external fetal monitor and observe for fetal status *to assess fetal well-being* Prepare client for ultrasound or amniocentesis if ordered *to provide information* Explain all procedures and their purposes	Fetal distress is detected early, and appropriate measures are instituted
Response to tocolytic treatment Uterine contractions Side effects (depending on agent used): Maternal vital signs: changes in heart or respiratory rate, blood pressure, or temperature Fetal heart rate		Explain procedures to client *to allay anxiety and keep client informed* Follow agency protocol for starting and monitoring infusion Monitor vital signs, fetal heart rate, uterine activity, maternal subjective reactions *to assess labor progress* Report side effects or complications *to ensure positive outcome* Provide physical and emotional support	Client understands procedure

(continued)

NURSING CARE PLAN *(Continued)*
The Client at Risk for Preterm Labor

Assessment	Potential Nursing Diagnoses	Intervention/ Rationale	Evaluation
Maternal subjective reactions: tremors, palpitations, nausea and vomiting, restlessness, chest tightness or pain, dyspnea	Alteration in Comfort related to unpleasant side effects and prolonged bedrest	Provide comfort measures, additional pillows for positioning, back rub, assistance with personal hygiene, restful atmosphere *to enhance client comfort*	Client responds to comfort measures
Contraindications to tocolytic treatment: Pregnancy < 20 weeks or > 36 weeks Active uterine bleeding Maternal illness Fetal distress or intrauterine death Advanced labor—cervical dilatation > 4 cm Ruptured membranes	Fear for self and fetus related to imminent preterm delivery	Keep client and family informed concerning progress of labor, plan of treatment, status of fetus *to provide information* Provide physical and emotional support, avoid leaving her alone *to ensure emotional stability* Monitor signs of progress of labor and fetal well-being *to pick up complications*	Client and family are knowledgeable about situation Client affirms that her fear has been minimized Infant receives prompt and efficient resuscitation as needed

Home Monitoring and Care. Nurses play a significant role in monitoring and caring for the client who is at risk for or experiencing preterm labor and is being monitored or treated at home. Studies of the effectiveness of home uterine monitoring have frequently raised the question of whether the positive results are related to the monitor or to the increased nurse–client interaction. When a client is being monitored at home, nursing responsibilities include daily evaluation and reporting of uterine activity, responses to treatment, and general health. The client is given a schedule for when to attach her monitor and transmit electronically the information, enabling the nursing service to "observe" her uterine activity at various points throughout the day. If they see increased uterine activity, they contact her physician regarding appropriate orders for tocolysis or the need for an office or hospital examination.

The nurse also educates the client about monitoring, pregnancy, nutrition, and stress management. The home care nursing service usually is available by telephone 24 hours a day.

When the home care includes use of a portable subcutaneous terbutaline pump, the nurse must have knowledge of the pump, the medication being used, and its side effects. The client is usually hospitalized at the beginning of therapy for stabilization and for instruction in self-administration of terbutaline using the pump. When she returns home, the nurse continues assessment of her condition and her ability to use the pump effectively (Sala et al., 1990)

Evaluation

For the woman at risk for preterm labor, effective nursing care is demonstrated by the identification and provision of appropriate intervention, considering that sometimes tocolysis is contraindicated. Possible anticipated outcomes include the following:

- The client demonstrates a decrease in signs and symptoms of preterm labor.
- The client is able to postpone birth at least 48 hours for prophylactic steroid therapy and hopefully until near term.
- The client demonstrates knowledge of signs and symptoms of preterm labor.
- The client initiates steps to decrease risk and seeks appropiate care if preterm labor begins.
- The client verbalizes understanding of her condition.
- The client demonstrates positive coping strategies to deal with the prolonged bed rest or hospitalization.
- The client and family experience minimal disruptions in family function.

Post-term Pregnancy

Post-term pregnancy, one of the most common complications of pregnancy, occurs when labor fails to start spontaneously in a pregnancy of 42 weeks or more. Depending on the accuracy of the estimated of gestational age, through use of early ultrasound and known conception dating, this delay occurs in about 3% to 14% of all pregnancies (Asrat et al., 1994). The more accurate the estimated gestational age, the lower the frequency of prolonged gestation.

In a true post-term pregnancy, the fetus is in substantial jeopardy. The degree of risk is positively correlated with the duration of the delay. After 42 weeks, the incidence of fetal and neonatal morbidity is 25%. The perinatal mortality rate doubles between 42 and 43 weeks' gestation and then increases fourfold to sixfold at 44 weeks and beyond (Asrat et al., 1994).

The cause of postdate gestation is unknown. It has been theorized to be related to alterations in hormonal regulation of labor onset. Possible risk factors include lack of the normal increase in estrogen near term due to fetal pituitary or adrenal gland insufficiency (as seen in anencephaly), deficiency of placental sulfatase (necessary for the production of estrogen), or decreased adrenocortical function leading to reduction in cortisol levels (cortisol reduces progesterone levels and promotes formation of estrogen precursors; Blackburn et al., 1992). Also, 50% of the women who have had a previous post-term pregnancy have a recurrence with the next pregnancy (Asrat et al., 1994).

The nature of the fetal risk is related to the progressive, degenerative placental changes. As the placenta ages, structural changes, such as increased syncytial degradation, fibrin deposits, fibrotic villi, villous necrosis with hemorrhage, and infarcts can occur. These changes can adversely alter the oxygen, nutrient, and water diffusion across the placental membrane. Oligohydramnios also can result, making the umbilical cord vulnerable to compression (Phelan, 1989; Blackburn et al., 1992; Lake, 1992) .

Although the placenta is able to maintain normal function, the risk continues to increase because the fetus continues to grow. Fetal macrosomia has been associated with uterine overdistension and dysfunction, CPD, shoulder dystocia, and postpartum hemorrhage (Lake, 1992).

Fetal Diagnostic Testing

Because it is known that prolonged gestation can compromise uteroplacental circulation, it is common practice to begin biweekly diagnostic surveillance during the 41st week to provide reassurance of fetal well-being (Freeman et al., 1991). Especially when pregnancy dating is unsure, there is a risk of fetal lung immaturity, or the cervix is uninducible (not physiologically ready to efface or dilate), antepartum testing provides a safer waiting period by using the following tests (see Chap. 39; Halle, 1993; Asrat et al., 1994):

■ NST: Fetal heart rate accelerations (reactivity) show normal brain stem function and an adequate fetal arterial blood gas of pH ≥ 7.20.

■ Contraction stress test: presence of late decelerations shows inadequate fetal oxygenation less than PaO_2 20, as sensed by peripheral chemoreceptors.
■ Amniotic fluid index (AFI): Using the semiquantitative four-quadrant ultrasound technique, AFI ≤ 5 shows decreased uteroplacental perfusion of oxygen and water or inadequate fetal kidney or esophageal function at more than 35 weeks' gestation.

Management and Nursing Care

Management for a post-term pregnancy involves the use of labor induction and cervical ripening. Throughout, the nurse plays an important role in assisting with these methods and closely monitoring the woman and fetus.

Readiness for Labor

Induction of labor means the artificial initiation of labor after the period of viability. In the well-dated pregnancy past 41 weeks' gestation, induction of labor provides the safest alternative for the woman and fetus to reduce the potential for fetal compromise and decrease the incidence of fetal macrosomia (Asrat et al., 1994). Other complications of pregnancy that may require induction include pregnancy-induced hypertension, diabetes, hemolytic disease, and postmaturity (see Chaps. 31 and 32).

Before induction is attempted, the physiologic readiness of the woman and fetus is evaluated. Tests for fetal maturity are usually done before induction. These may include evaluation of accuracy of dating, gestational age assessment by ultrasound, or fetal lung maturity assessment (see Chap. 39; ACOG, 1990).

Maternal readiness refers to the condition of the cervix and the likelihood that induction will be successful. More than 30 years ago, Bishop developed a pelvic scoring system to predict inducibility by evaluating the position of the cervix as it relates to the vagina; the cervical consistency, dilatation, and effacement; and the station of the fetal presenting part (Bishop, 1964). The higher the score, the more favorable the cervix, with a clinical trial showing a score of 9 or more associated with 100% successful inductions (Friedman et al., 1966). The current ACOG recommendation is to use the Bishop score to predict the likelihood of a vaginal delivery in the multiparous client (ACOG, 1991a; Table 36-5).

Cervical Ripening

Because about 80% of post-term clients have an unripe cervix (Freeman et al., 1991), methods to ripen the cervix are necessary to prepare the client for labor. **Cervical ripening** refers to the maturational process of softening and effacement of the cervix, which nor-

TABLE 36–5
Bishop Scoring System

Criteria	Score			
	0	1	2	3
Dilation (cm)	0	1–2	3–4	5–6
Effacement (%)	0–30	40–50	60–70	80
Station	−3	−2	−1–2	+1, +2
Consistency	Firm	Medium	Soft	—
Position	Posterior	Midposition	Anterior	—

(ACOG Technical Bulletin # 157, July 1991)

mally happens near term. It is believed to involve connective tissue changes, with a scattering of the previously dense collagen fibers. This scattering is caused by altered fibroblast activity under the regulation of a variety of hormones, including prostaglandins.

Prostaglandin, primarily PGE_2, is produced by the cervix and trophoblast from precursor phospholipids stored in the cell membrane (Lake, 1992). When needed, these phospholipids are converted to arachidonic acid, which is then acted on by the enzyme cyclo-oxygenase to become prostaglandin. This is a clinically important biochemical pathway, not only because of uterine and cervical effects, but also because prostaglandins have an effect on the fetal cardiac vasculature. In the fetus, the ductus arteriosus is kept open by the local (vascular endothelium) and systemic (placental) synthesis of vasodilating PGE_2 and PGI_2 (prostacyclin; Arnold-Aldea et al., 1990). This allows oygenated fetal blood to bypass the immature lungs, going directly from the pulmonary artery into the aorta through the ductus arteriosus. Because aspirin-like drugs inactivate cyclo-oxygenase, inhibiting prostaglandin synthesis, ingestion of large amounts of aspirin or use of indomethacin as a tocolytic after 34 weeks' gestation may cause an in utero closure of the ductus arteriosis and lead to fetal death (Carsten, 1992).

Prostaglandin E₂. Synthetic PGE_2 gel applied locally is the most successful and widely used agent to ripen the cervix. It works by stimulating fibroblast activity to dissociate collagen fibers and other biochemical changes that lead to softening, effacement, and dilatation. Although these changes can occur without contractions, it also may enhance myometrial sensitivity to oxytocin and accelerate gap junction formation, leading to more coordinated contractions.

The PGE_2 gel is now commercially available as Pepidil for 0.5 mg dosing by intracervical administration (Bredow et al., 1990). The protocol for use involves applying the gel in the afternoon or evening before the scheduled induction. Before administration, a reassuring fetal heart rate and uterine activity pattern should be obtained. Some protocols do not advise using the gel if abnormalities are noted, if there are prolonged or frequent uterine contractions, or if the membranes are ruptured. After gel insertion, continued monitoring for 2 to 4 hours or until contractions subside is recommended. To avoid hyperstimulation, oxytocin should not be administered for at least 4 hours after the last gel administration; some protocols recommend waiting until the next morning (Freeman et al., 1991; Sokol et al., 1994).

Laminaria Tents. *Laminaria* tents are a specific type of seaweed that is dried, compressed, shaped, and sterilized. *Laminaria* tents are most commonly used for therapeutic abortion and rarely for labor induction. Synthetic *Laminaria* also is available. When inserted in the cervical os, the smooth, rounded stem absorbs moisture and swells to three to five times its original size. When inserted the night before induction, the *Laminaria* causes gradual softening and dilatation of the cervix by morning. This dilatation can cause mild to moderate cramping, and the client should be advised of this possibility (Blumenthal et al., 1990).

Serial Induction With Oxytocin. Oxytocin may be given as an IV infusion for a specific time daily for 2 to 3 days. This is sometimes called serial induction. The oxytocin-induced contractions often bring the fetal head down into the pelvis and assist in ripening the cervix. The infusion is usually stopped at night so the client can eat and rest.

Methods of Induction

Three methods are currently used to initiate labor safely. These include stripping the membranes, AROM, and oxytocin infusion.

Stripping of Membranes. The manual separation of the chorioamniotic membranes from the lower uterine segment is known as **stripping the membranes.** It is done to initiate labor by triggering the endogenous release of local prostaglandins and stimulate an autonomic neural reflex that results in the maternal pituitary release of oxytocin (Lake, 1992). It is done as an outpatient prenatal procedure by the obstetrician and has variable results.

Artificial Rupture of Membranes. **Amniotomy**, or AROM, is a common method of enhancing labor that also has been used to induce labor. When the client is near term and the cervix is favorable, amniotomy is almost always followed by labor within a few hours. Because the intact membranes form a barrier against bacterial invasion of the uterus, delivery should be accomplished as quickly and safely as possible. Twenty-four hours with ruptured membranes is usually considered the maximum safe time period. After this time, amnionitis may occur.

Besides the danger of infection, amniotomy also increases the risk of cord prolapse and fetal head or cord compression. Amniotomy is contraindicated when the presenting part is high in the pelvis or if the fetus is in the breech or transverse position.

In post-term pregnancy, amniotomy is recommended as soon as it is safely feasible. This allows for early placement of a scalp electrode and intrauterine pressure catheter and examination of the amniotic fluid for evidence of meconium staining (Asrat et al., 1994). Meconium staining is four times more common in post-term pregnancies than it is in term pregnancies. This occurs either because of the activation of the mature vagal system with excretion of meconium or the increased likelihood of hypoxia-induced bowel relaxation (Freeman et al., 1991).

To perform an amniotomy, the obstetrician inserts the first two fingers of one hand into the cervix until the membranes are encountered. A long hook, usually an Allis clamp or a plastic Amnihook, is inserted into the vagina and the membranes are simply hooked and torn by the tip of the sharp instrument. Initially, the fluid may gush out, or it may leak out slowly. Leaking of amniotic fluid from the vagina usually continues throughout labor. The color, odor, and consistency of the amniotic fluid should be noted and monitored throughout the labor and delivery period. Usually it is clear and almost odorless. Any deviation can indicate problems. For example, brownish or greenish discoloration is a sign that the fetus has passed meconium in utero, and a foul odor is a sign of infection.

When minimal fluid is encountered at the time of rupture, thick meconium should be suspected. Severe hypoxia has been associated with decreased amniotic fluid production and bowel relaxation, so often they occur simultaneously. If this is the case, **amnioinfusion** (vaginal infusion to increase in utero fluid level) can be used to dilute the meconium. Instillation of normal saline solution through an intrauterine pressure catheter can be helpful in reducing the variable decel-

erations caused by cord compression (see Chap. 40; Freeman et al., 1991).

Assessment is an ongoing part of the nurse's responsibility when an amniotomy is performed. The condition of the woman and fetus is assessed before, during, and after the procedure, and any changes are reported to the physician. The nurse should be aware of of the possibility of the following: risk for infection related to rupture of membranes, pain related to increasing strength of uterine contractions, or anxiety or fear related to an unfamiliar procedure.

Nursing planning and intervention involve preparing the client for the procedure and carrying out the necessary assessments. The nurse should explain the procedure to the client, reassure her that it is no more uncomfortable than a vaginal examination, and describe the warm, wet sensations that she will probably experience. Expectations for increased strength of uterine contractions also should be explained.

Before the procedure, the nurse can assist the client in assuming a supine position, with knees flexed and relaxed. Antiseptic preparation of the vulva is accomplished according to hospital policy. Fetal heart tones should be monitored before, during, and after the procedure, or continuously with electronic fetal monitor. Cord compression or prolapse are clearly evident in changing electronic fetal monitor patterns. The time of amniotomy should be marked on the monitor strip. Time of procedures and the color, character, and amount of amniotic fluid are noted in the client's chart. The client's comfort is maintained by providing fresh bed linens and underpads as needed, because the amniotic fluid continues to leak during the ensuing labor.

Oxytocin Infusion. An efficient and safe method of induction is IV administration of oxytocin. The properties of this drug and its use have been addressed earlier in the section on dystocia management (see the section "Planning and Intervention: Oxytocin Administration" on page 962).

Hemorrhagic Complications

Hemorrhage is the fourth leading cause of maternal mortality in the United States. Even though there has been a dramatic decrease in maternal deaths, from 462 per 1,000 in 1935 to 7.9 per 1,000 in 1989 (Kochenour, 1994), obstetric hemorrhage remains significant, accounting for 11% of deaths (Clark et al., 1994).

Obstetric hemorrhage has been technically defined as blood loss of 500 mL or more. However many practitioners prefer to use a blood loss of 1,000 mL or more as the more clinically significant definition (Zlatnik, 1994b). Because normal maternal blood volume expansion is about 1,500 mL, most women can tolerate a blood loss equivalent to their additional volume without compromise (Hauth, 1994). The amount usually is measured visually using a reasonable approximation. However it can be measured by weighing items, with 1 g equal to 1 mL blood volume.

The major causes of hemorrhage associated with childbearing are placenta previa, abruptio placentae, and uterine atony. However, the nurse also must be alert to the possibility of other causes of bleeding related to the uterus, placenta, membranes, and umbilical cord during the intrapartum and early postpartum period.

Intrapartum Hemorrhage

Slight bleeding through the vagina is expected during the first stage of labor as a consequence of cervical effacement and dilatation. Heavy bleeding or bleeding from above the cervix can result from a number of causes and is reason for concern (Cunningham et al., 1993).

Disorders of Placental Attachment

Important causes of bleeding associated with labor are those related to the placenta and its membranes. Placenta previa and abruptio placentae have been discussed previously as complications of pregnancy (see Chap. 31) and are described only briefly here in relation to their role in labor and delivery.

Placenta Previa. The cardinal sign of placenta previa is painless, bright red vaginal bleeding. If bleeding has not been identified until after labor begins, contractions and bloody show may confuse the situation. Identification depends on accurate assessment of the extent of vaginal bleeding. Overt hemorrhage with huge blood loss is not difficult to diagnose, but it requires astute judgment to decide when bloody vaginal discharge ceases to be heavy "show" and becomes potential hemorrhage.

Prenatal history of ultrasound for placental location, episodes of vaginal bleeding, and any signs and symptoms of intrapartum hypovolemia, such as maternal-fetal tachycardia, can help with the identification. Any vaginal bleeding that the nurse believes to be excessive should be reported to the physician. Vaginal examination in these clients should be avoided. A speculum examination can help to identify the source of the bleeding.

Abruptio Placentae. Abruptio placentae can be a true obstetric emergency if the area of separation is extensive (>50%). The signs, in order of frequency, include the following (Hurd et al., 1983):

- Vaginal bleeding (80%)

- Uterine tenderness or back pain (68%)
- Fetal distress (60%)
- Abnormal uterine contractions (34%): high frequency or hypertonus
- Idiopathic preterm labor (22%)
- Fetal demise (15%)

Marginal sinus rupture was formerly treated as a separate clinical entity. It is now believed to be a mild type of abruptio placentae in which slight separation occurs at the edge of the placenta. The marginal sinus, located under the edge of the placenta, is one of the large maternal sinuses bathing the placental villi. If the placenta separates at a point along its margin, this maternal sinus is disrupted, and bleeding occurs. There is usually no increased pain or uterine tension, and the amount of vaginal bleeding may vary considerably. If the area of separation is small, as it usually is in marginal sinus rupture, there is no danger of hypoxia to the fetus. Generally there are no changes in fetal heart rate. When vaginal bleeding during labor is excessive, and placenta previa and abruptio placentae have been ruled out, the most probable cause is a small marginal separation of the placenta. Nursing care is the same as for other hemorrhagic conditions.

Placenta Accreta. At times, the attachment of the placenta to the uterus is so firm that the placenta does not separate spontaneously. **Placenta accreta** describes any implantation of the placenta in which this abnormally firm adherence to the uterine wall exists. This condition is usually the result of partial or total absence of the decidua basalis, which allows the placental villi to attach to the myometrium. When deeper penetration of the villi occurs, other terms may be used: *placenta increta* when the villi invade the myometrium and *placenta percreta* when they penetrate the myometrium. The abnormal adherence may be total, partial, or focal, depending on the number of cotyledons involved (Cunningham et al., 1993).

Predisposing factors to placenta accreta include implantations where decidual formation may be defective, such as in the lower uterine segment (placenta previa), over a previous cesarean section scar, or after uterine curettage. The reported incidence shows it is a rare occurence with about 1 per 2,562 deliveries. Conditions with which it has been associated (Read et al., 1980) include placenta previa, previous cesarean section or curettage, and grandmultiparity. The condition is usually not recognized until the third stage of labor when the placenta does not separate. Maternal hemorrhage may be profuse, and hysterectomy is often necessary.

Other Placental Anomalies

Some placental abnormalities are not identified until a problem arises during labor or until they are visualized after delivery. **Succenturiate placenta** (Fig. 36-10*A*) is an anomaly in which one or more small accessory lobes of the placenta develop in the membranes at a distance from the main placenta. The vessels connecting the lobe to the main placenta are supported only by membranes and may tear during delivery or when the membranes rupture. A succenturiate lobe may be retained in the uterus after expulsion of the placenta and result in maternal postpartum hemorrhage.

A **circumvallate placenta** (see Fig. 36-10*B*) is one in which the membranes are folded back on the fetal surface of the placenta, exposing a ring of the fetal surface around the umbilical cord. There is increased risk of repeated, small prenatal hemorrhages resulting in preterm birth. There also is an increased risk of retained placenta leading to postpartum hemorrhage.

With a **velamentous placenta** of the cord (see Fig 36-10*C*), blood vessels course unprotected for long distances through the membranes to insert into the margin of the placenta. If they pass over the internal cervical os as they course through the membranes, they are in a position to be compressed by the presenting fetal part or torn at the time of rupture of the membranes. These events may be a disaster for the fetus (Toot et al., 1992).

A **battledore placenta** (see Fig 36-10*D*) is when the cord inserts at the placental margin (eccentric insertion), rather than in the center of the placenta as with a normal insertion. It is not considered a clinically significant structural variation (Toot et al., 1992).

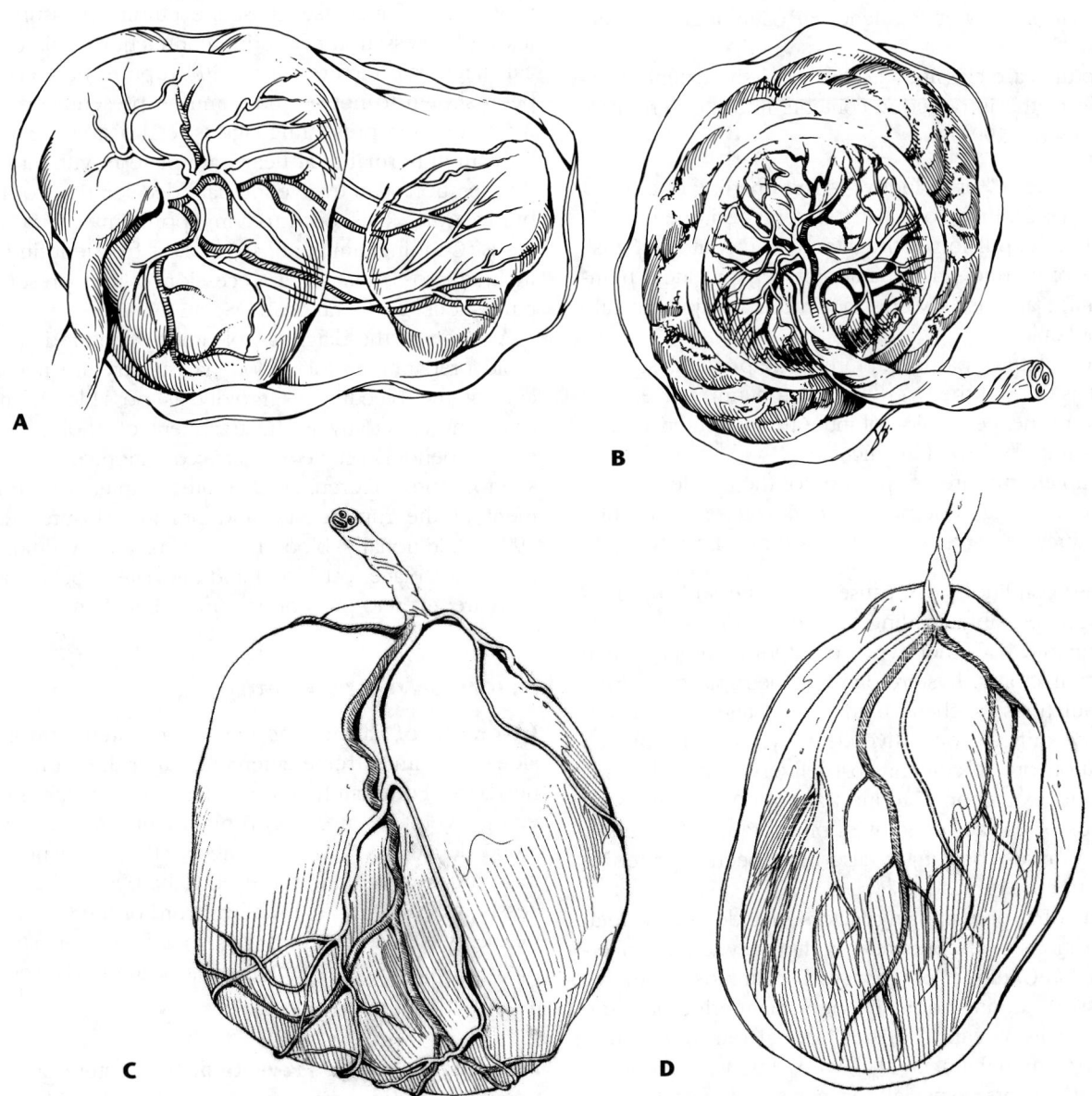

A

B

C

D

FIGURE 36-10 Placental anomalies. (**A**) Succenturiate placenta. (**B**) Circumvallate placenta. (**C**) Velamentous placenta. (**D**) Battledore placenta.

Rupture of the Uterus

The overall incidence of uterine rupture is generally quoted by most authors as being approximately 1 in 2,000, based on several multiyear surveys (Zuspan et al., 1988). Although the incidence has not changed to any degree in the last several decades, the etiology has changed, and the outcome has improved significantly.

Today, the most common cause is attributed to rupture of the scar from a previous cesarean delivery. A recent large study of 159,456 births delivered in almost 10 years (January 1983–June 1992), showed an overall incidence of 0.87%, or 1 in 113, in clients planning VBAC. It also showed an incidence three times higher for clients with two previous cesareans (2.3%) compared with those with one previous cesarean (0.64%; Leung et al., 1993). The probability of rupture of a classical scar (vertical uterine scar), is several times greater than that of a lower segment scar (Cunningham et al., 1993).

Ruptures are classified according to the extent of extrusion of the intrauterine contents into the peritoneal cavity (Scott, 1994):

- "Dehiscence" or "window"—The opening of the scar has an intact overlying visceral peritoneum with no expulsion of the intrauterine contents. This type of uterine scar separation rarely produces hemorrhage and usually does not cause a major clinical problem.
- Incomplete or partial rupture—The previous scar opens but not the overlying peritoneum, and extraperitoneal extrusion of intrauterine contents occurs into the broad ligament.
- Complete rupture—Separation of the previous scar and overlying peritoneum occurs with extrusion of intrauterine contents into the peritoneal cavity.

Other conditions can cause a weakness of the uterine wall, possibly leading to rupture. These include incision due to other types of uterine surgery, such as myomectomy, hysterotomy, or metroplasty; uterine manipulations, such as uterine curretage or perforation; or difficult operative delivery, such as breech extraction or difficult forceps delivery, especially version and extraction. Uterine trauma due to gun shot wounds or car accidents with blunt trauma to the abdomen or seat belt injury also have been reported to cause uterine rupture.

Additional predisposing factors include certain fetal malpositions or abnormalities, multiparity, uterine overdistension (multiple pregnancy, hydramnios, excessive fetal size), uterine anomaly, vigorous uterine pressure during delivery, and difficult manual removal of placenta (Cunningham et al., 1993). Injudicious use of oxytoxic agents, especially in parous women (associated with a significant number of cases of rupture and lower segment rupture due to neglected obstructed labor) fortunately is now rare in developed countries (Cunningham et al., 1993; Scott, 1994). As with any risk prediction, there can be an additive effect if more than one risk factor exists in any client. In other words, to allow a client with a prior cesarean delivery who currently has an overdistended uterus to experience a trial of labor with oxytocin augmentation is creating a high-risk situation.

Management. The signs and symptoms of uterine rupture depend on the severity of the rupture. Pain usually but not always precedes the definitive tear and then frequently lessens after the rupture occurs. Depending on the location of the rupture, bleeding may be scant or heavy, and some of the blood may escape vaginally (Scott, 1994). Although a few cases exhibit premonitory signs of increased baseline uterine pressure followed by cessation of uterine contractions, this classical diagnostic picture for uterine rupture has recently been shown to not be the common presentation. The most common presenting sign is fetal distress, particularly an abnormal fetal heart rate pattern with variable decelerations that evolve into late decelerations or fetal bradycardia. This occurred in approximately 80% of cases (Cunningham et al., 1993). Less frequent findings include gross hematuria, recession of the presenting part, shock, and fetal death (Scott, 1994).

As soon as the diagnosis of uterine rupture is made, rapid preparations for abdominal surgery are made to control the bleeding as rapidly as possible. In most cases, hysterectomy is the treatment of choice. However, depending on the woman's condition, age, and desire for more children, an alternate treatment is débridement of the rupture site and primary closure (Ricci, 1992). Additionally, blood transfusions and IV fluids are given to replace lost blood and alleviate shock. Antibiotics are given to prevent or combat infection.

Inversion of the Uterus

Inversion of the uterus, where the uterus turns inside out, is an extreme emergency after the birth of the newborn. Fortunately, the incidence of this life-threatening event is rare, occurring about once in every 2,000 deliveries. It is associated with a placenta that has fundal implantation. It used to be believed that excessive traction on the umbilical cord or the Credé maneuver were causative factors, but follow-up studies have failed to document this association (Benedetti, 1991).

Early Diagnosis and Prevention. With astute observational skills, inversion can sometime be identified promptly and corrected immediately without serious consequences. In an effort to deliver the placenta, traction on the cord leads to its advancement, but the client experiences a great deal of pain. If with continued traction on the cord, the placenta delivers attached to a *bluish gray mass* that fills the vaginal outlet, diagnosis of inversion can be made promptly and replacement accomplished quickly. In this situation, the client will remain in good condition, and bleeding will not be excessive.

A much more serious condition occurs once the placenta already has delivered, following a difficult extraction by fundal pressure and traction on the umbilical cord. In this situation, profuse vaginal bleeding is noted. The uterus cannot be palpated abdominally, and the cervix cannot be located. Instead, a grayish mass, oozing blood, fills the vagina. Rapid diagnosis and deinversion of the uterus will avoid blood loss, trauma, and shock.

Management. Several steps in treatment must be taken promptly and simultaneously. Two IV infusion systems are started, one with lactated Ringer's solution and one with whole blood. These are given promptly to refill the intravascular compartment and support cardiac output. An anesthesiologist administers a general anesthetic, usually halothane, to relax the uterus. The placenta is left in place until the infusions are working and uterine relaxation has been accomplished. If the placenta is removed prematurely, the risk of hemorrhage is increased. Attempts are made to replace the uterus in the vagina. The palm of the hand is placed on the center of the fundus with the fingers extended to identify the cervical margins. The fundus is pushed up through the cervix. When the uterus is returned to its normal shape, anesthesia is discontinued and oxytocin is begun to help the uterus remain contracted. Bimanual compression also aids in this. Until normal tone is ensured, the uterus is monitored transvaginally to detect any possible recurrence.

If the uterus cannot be replaced from below because of a constriction ring, a laparotomy is performed so that the uterus can be pulled up simultaneously from above and pushed up from below. The constriction ring may be incised. A traction suture in the fundus aids in repositioning. Treatment continues as previously described. Subsequent inversion is unlikely (Bowes, 1989).

Prophylaxis. The main method to prevent uterine inversion is not to attempt to deliver the placenta until it has separated. It has been known for several years that separation of the placenta before replacement of the uterus will only increase blood loss. Routine exploration of the postpartum uterus should be done, because it will detect a uterine inversion in its incomplete stage, before it has descended through the vaginal in-

troitus, preventing the possibility of a complete inversion (Benedetti, 1991).

Early Postpartum Hemorrhage

Hemorrhage during the postpartum period is the most common cause of serious blood loss associated with pregnancy, and it causes about one-third of all maternal deaths from hemorrhagic complications (Hauth, 1994). The debilitation and lowered resistance that often accompany the hemorrhage are related to postpartum infections, another leading cause of maternal death. To a large extent, death from postpartum hemorrhage is preventable if the condition is diagnosed early and treated aggressively.

Incidence

Approximately 5% of women who deliver vaginally lose more than 1,000 mL of blood. In cesarean deliveries, more than 50% of clients have a blood loss of 1,000 mL. As mentioned previously, up to 1,000 mL blood loss should be well tolerated. The diagnosis of clinically significant hemorrhage is therefore confirmed by evidence of continued vaginal bleeding in combination with severe anemia; maternal hemodynamic changes, such as hypotension or tachycardia; oliguria; or need for maternal blood replacement (Hauth, 1994). Postpartum hemorrhage is a fairly common complication of labor and one with which the nurse should be familiar. Nurses are expected to assume an important role in its prevention, detection, and treatment.

Causes

The three immediate causes of postpartum hemorrhage are, in order of frequency, uterine atony, lacerations of the birth canal (perineum, vagina, and cervix), and retained placental fragments. Clotting defects, uterine tumors, infections, and obstetric accidents, such as inversion of the uterus, also can be classified as causes of postpartum hemorrhage, but they are less common and of a more indirect nature.

Uterine Atony. Uterine atony is the most common cause of postpartum hemorrhage. The uterus contains huge blood vessels within its muscle fibers, and those at the placental site are open and gaping. Maternal blood flow to the placenta in late pregnancy is approximately 500 mL/min. If after placental separation from the uterine wall, the myometrium does not effectively contract, significant blood loss can occur quickly (Zlatnik, 1994b). The uterus must stay tightly contracted down, because continuous, slight relaxation gives rise to continuous oozing of blood, one of the most treacherous forms of postpartum hemorrhage.

Lacerations. Lacerations of the perineum, vagina, and cervix are more common after operative delivery. Tears of the cervix are particularly likely to cause serious hemorrhage. Bright red arterial bleeding in the presence of a hard, firmly contracted uterus (no uterine atony) suggests hemorrhage from a cervical laceration. The physician establishes the diagnosis by actual inspection of the cervix (retractors are necessary) and after locating the source of bleeding, repairs the laceration.

Perineal and vaginal tears also contribute to postpartum blood loss. In addition, perineal tears may do great damage in destroying the integrity of the perineum and in weakening the supports of the uterus, bladder, and rectum. Unless these lacerations are repaired properly, the resultant weakness may cause prolapse of the uterus, **cystocele** (a pouching downward of the bladder), or **rectocele** (a pouching forward of the rectum) later. These conditions, which often originate from perineal lacerations at childbirth, give rise to many discomforts and often necessitate operative treatment. Lacerations of the birth canal sometimes occur during the process of normal delivery and may be unavoidable even in the most skilled hands.

Retained Placental Fragments. Small, partially separated fragments of placenta may cause postpartum hemorrhage by interfering with proper uterine contraction. Routinely at delivery, the placenta should be inspected carefully to determine whether a piece is missing. If a portion is missing, exploration of the uterus is indicated to remove the placental fragment. In the case of continued postpartum bleeding, retention of placental fragments is generally ruled out by manual exploration. However, this is rarely a cause of immediate postpartum hemorrhage. More commonly, it is implicated in late hemorrhage in which profuse bleeding occurs suddenly 1 week or more after delivery.

Predisposing Factors

Certain factors predispose a client to early postpartum hemorrhage. In most cases, it may be anticipated in advance. Hemorrhage due to uterine atony can be anticipated following labors with overdistention of the uterus (large fetus, twins, hydramnios), oxytocin-stimulated labors, amnionitis, general anesthesia with halothane, and prolonged use of $MgSO_4$ (Benedetti, 1991).

Delivery of a large newborn, midforceps or forceps rotation, intrauterine manipulation, and cesarean delivery are examples of situations in which trauma is likely to lead to postpartum hemorrhage. This probably is a result of lacerations in the uterus or birth canal. A small woman may not withstand blood loss as well as a woman of average size or larger, because she is more likely to have a smaller blood volume.

Clinical Picture

Excessive bleeding resulting from trauma to the birth canal or a retained placenta may begin during the third stage of labor. More commonly, hemorrhage is noted at some point after expulsion of the placenta. Although this early hemorrhage involves expulsion of large amounts of blood and clots, the nurse must be aware that it also may be evidenced as a continuous trickle. These small constant trickles are not alarming in appearance and may not arouse concern or action. If the bleeding continues, signs and symptoms of hypovolemic shock develop.

Medical Management

Medical interventions for the woman experiencing an early postpartum hemorrhage depend on the cause of the hemorrhage. Early postpartum hemorrhage due to uterine atony usually is treated with fundal massage and oxytocic agents. If the hemorrhage is the result of lacerations or retained placental fragments, the client may be returned to the delivery room for repair of the laceration or uterine evacuation of placental fragments.

Persistent bleeding from a flaccid uterus can be treated by bimanual compression of the uterus. A fist is placed in the anterior vaginal fornix and pushed against the anterior wall of the uterus. With the other hand, the practitioner catches the posterior wall of the uterus through the abdominal wall. This bimanual compression often controls the flow until additional administration of oxytocics results in effective myometrial contraction. Refractory uterine atony may respond to 0.25 mg IM of 15-methyl-prostaglandin F_{2a} (Zlatnik, 1994b; Table 36-6). This provides the most efficient means of compressing the site of bleeding. Packing the uterus with gauze, a procedure once considered valuable to promote hemostasis in such cases, is seldom used today.

In some instances, surgical intervention may become necessary. Ligation of the uterine or hypogastric arteries often is attempted before resorting to hysterectomy to prevent continuing and potentially fatal blood loss (Gonik, 1989). Measures to prevent and treat shock are used concurrently with efforts to control the bleeding.

Hemorrhage and Shock

Shock can be defined as a disparity between the circulating blood volume and the capacity of the vascular bed (Clark et al., 1994). In hemorrhage shock, this disparity is a result of blood loss, which initially leads to hypotension. In response to this fall in blood pressure, the adrenal glands release catecholamines, which cause blood to be shunted away from nonvital areas, such as the skin, kidney, gut, muscles, and uterus by

TABLE 36-6
Pharmacologic Methods Used to Control Uterine Atony

Agent	Dose	Route
Oxytocin	10–20 U	IV drip,* IM, intramyometrial (multiple sites)
Methylergonovine	0.2 mg	IM
Prostaglandin F_{2a}	1 mg	Intramyometrial
Prostaglandin 15 methyl	0.25 mg	IM, intramyometrial (multiple sites)

(Zlatnik, F. [1994]. The normal and abnormal puerperium. In J. Scott, P. DiSaia, C. Hammond, & W. Spellacy [Eds.], *Danforth's obstetrics and gynecology* [pp. 163–173]. Philadelphia: J.B. Lippincott.)

vasoconstriction, and diverted to the brain and heart. Such redistribution may result in fetal hypoxia even *before the woman becomes overtly hypotensive.* Therefore, significant maternal shock is highly unlikely in the presence of a reassuring fetal heart rate tracing (Clark et al., 1994).

The normally expanded blood volume of the pregnant woman may allow for a larger absolute blood loss to occur before the appearance of clinical evidence of shock (Gonik, 1989). The pulse and blood pressure may not change significantly until large amounts of blood have been lost. The condition and size of the client also help determine the amount of blood loss that can be tolerated. Exhaustion from prolonged labor, preexisting anemia, or chronic disease reduces the ability of the body to compensate. When hemorrhage has been profuse enough, compensatory mechanisms, are activated and signs and symptoms of shock ensue.

Signs and symptoms of shock are related to the compensatory mechanisms. Initially, the pulse becomes rapid, the skin is pale and cool, and the respirations may be rapid and deep. In response to further vasoconstriction, the pulse rate continues to increase and becomes thready; the skin is cool, pale, and clammy; blood pressure falls; the respirations become more rapid and shallow; and urinary output decreases. Nausea and vomiting and increasing restlessness also may occur. As shock deepens, changes occur in level of consciousness from mental cloudiness, to lethargy, coma, and death (see Table 36-7).

Management of Shock

Identification and definitive treatment of the cause of the hemorrhage is a primary step in the prevention and treatment of hypovolemic shock. Other measures are

TABLE 36-7
Symptoms of Shock Related to Volume of Blood Loss

	Mild (20%–25% Loss)	Moderate (25%–35% loss)	Severe (>35% loss)	Irreversible
Respirations	Rapid, deep	Rapid, becoming shallow	Rapid, shallow, may be irregular	Irregular or barely perceptible
Pulse	<100 beats/min	100–120 beats/min	>120 beats/min	Irregular apical pulse
	Rapid; tone normal	Rapid; tone may be normal but is becoming weaker	Very rapid; easily collapsible; may be irregular	
Blood pressure	Normal or hypertensive	80–100 mm Hg systolic	<60 mm Hg systolic	None palpable
Skin	Cold and pale			
	Peripheral vasoconstriction	Cool, pale, moist; knees cyanotic	Cold, clammy; cyanosis of lips and fingernails	Cold, clammy, cyanotic
Urinary output	No change	Decreasing to 10–22 mL/h	Oliguric (<10 mL) to anuric	Anuric
Level of consciousness	Alert, oriented; diffuse anxiety	Oriented, mental cloudiness, or increasing restlessness	Lethargy; reacts to noxious stimuli; comatose	Does not respond to noxious stimuli
Central venous pressure	May be normal	3 cm H_2O	0–3 cm H_2O	

directed toward the body's responses to the blood loss. An important aspect of the management of serious hemorrhage is *fluid replacement* to combat hypovolemia. In early shock, there is a tendency to draw fluid from the interstitial space into the capillary bed. However, as shock continues, damage to the capillary bed causes increased capillary permeability, accentuating the loss of the intravascular volume. Clinically, this is reflected by the disproportionately large volume of fluid necessary to resuscitate clients in severe shock. Sometimes two to three times the amount indicated by calculation of blood loss is required (Clark et al., 1994).

Establishing two large-bore IV lines allows for more rapid volume expansion. It is recommended that lactated Ringer's solution be given in the amount and proportion necessary to maintain a systolic pressure of more than 90 mm Hg and urine output more than 25 mL/min. If initial vigorous fluid replacement therapy does not restore urine flow, insertion of a central venous catheter to obtain *central venous pressure* readings or a Swan-Ganz catheter to obtain *pulmonary wedge pressure* provides important information about fluid balance and needs. It also can aid in preventing circulatory overload (Gonik, 1989; Clark et al., 1994).

Blood transfusion plays an important role in preventing serious shock. The blood groups of all maternity clients should be known before labor, and cross-matched blood should be available for those in whom hemorrhage is anticipated or appears imminent. Seeing that the blood typing is carried out, ordering and calling for the cross-match, and making sure that the blood is sent to the unit are usually nursing responsibilities. Time is of the essence for these clients. Therefore, the nurse must preplan and establish priorities rapidly. For best results, sufficient blood replacement should be given to maintain the hematocrit at 30% (Gonik, 1989).

The body's oxygen-carrying capacity is diminished by blood loss. Therefore, oxygen administration by mask is usually ordered to increase the amount of oxygen in the circulating blood. Increasing the partial pressure of oxygen across the pulmonary capillary membrane by giving oxygen 6 to 8 L/min may forestall the onset of tissue hypoxia (Clark et al., 1994).

Additionally, elevating the lower extremities increases perfusion to vital organs until sufficient blood and fluid volume replacement can be accomplished. Some sources recommend using the Trendelenburg position, whereas others suggest that it be avoided because it may interfere with cerebral circulation and respiratory exchange (Bottoms et al., 1990).

Assessment

The nurse plays a primary role in the prevention, detection, and treatment of hemorrhage, especially that caused by uterine atony. Routine nursing assessment of vital signs, condition of the uterus, and amount of bleeding in the early postpartum period is directed toward detecting uterine atony and subsequent increased bleeding. Assessment should include review of the chart to identify any factors that would place the client at risk for hemorrhage. For the client at risk or any client with increased bleeding, vital signs, fundus, and amount of bleeding should be checked more frequently than routine. The client also should be monitored for other signs of impending shock, such as changes in skin color and temperature, decreased urinary output, or changes in level of consciousness.

Laboratory assessment of hemoglobin (Hgb) and hematocrit (Hct) are preferrably done on the second postpartum day to allow compensatory time for effects of hemodilution, but in severe bleeding cases, rough estimates of loss can be taken from an Hgb/Hct done immediately (1 g Hgb = 500 mL whole blood) compared with prehemorrhage values. Because many clients are discharged on the first postpartum day, this test is often run earlier, and the interpretation needs to be adjusted accordingly.

Nursing Diagnosis

Assessment of the client for signs and symptoms of hemorrhage may lead the nurse to identify nursing diagnoses. For a list of possible nursing diagnoses, see Box 36-5.

Planning And Intervention

If the nurse suspects that a woman may be hemorrhaging, it is important to remain with her constantly. The fundus should be checked immediately. The physician needs to be notified, and emergency equipment, including IV tray with large-bore (#18) needles, retention catheter, oxygen, suction, blood pressure, and central venous pressure apparatus, must be easily accessible.

BOX 36–5
Nursing Diagnoses: Hemorrhage

- Altered Fetal Tissue Perfusion related to decreased placental circulation
- Fluid Volume Deficit related to excessive blood loss
- Risk for Infection related to decreased resistance and compensatory mechanisms
- Fear related to
  - Uncertainty of outcome
  - Need for additional treatments and procedures
- Anxiety related to lack of knowledge of complications and treatments
- Situational Low Self Esteem related to complication of labor

Fundal Massage

The uterus should be located immediately and massaged gently but firmly. The lower uterine segment is supported with the edge of the hand a little above the mother's symphysis, while the fundus is massaged with the other hand (see Fig. 22-14). Thus, the uterus is cupped between the two hands and is supported as it is massaged, in an effort to prevent uterine inversion. Massage should be continued until the uterus assumes a woody hardness; if the slightest relaxation occurs, the massage must be restarted. In many cases, the uterus stays contracted most of the time, but occasionally it relaxes. It is crucial to monitor the fundus constantly for 1 full hour after bleeding has subsided. When the uterus is well contracted, care should be taken to avoid overmassage, because such practice contributes to muscle fatigue, which further encourages uterine relaxation and excessive bleeding.

Sometimes relaxation occurs 2 or more hours after delivery. In these cases, the uterus may balloon with blood, with little escaping externally. Accordingly, the consistency, size, and height of the uterine fundus (in reference to finger breadths above or below the umbilicus; eg, "1 below") should be checked frequently until several hours have elapsed. Ordinarily, the height of the fundus after delivery is about at the level of the umbilicus. If the uterus becomes distended with blood or if the bladder becomes full and presses upward against the uterus causing it to rise in the abdomen, the fundus can be palpated several centimeters above the umbilicus. When properly contracted, the uterus should feel about the size and consistency of a small, firm grapefruit.

Frequently, a large, boggy, relaxed uterus is difficult to outline through the abdominal wall. It may be necessary to push the hand well posteriorly toward the region of the sacral promontory to reach it. The fact that the uterus is hard to identify often means that it is relaxed, but palpation and massage usually cause it to become firm.

Allaying Anxiety

The frequent massage and deep palpation may be painful to the mother. They are disturbing, because they come at a time when she wants nothing more than to rest and sleep after her great effort. If she is awake and alert, the continued attention and scrutiny may increase her anxiety. It must be remembered that apprehension naturally accompanies hemorrhage and shock. Quick and efficient nursing observations and appropriate explanation and reassurance help allay the concerns of the mother and her partner.

If the mother or father expresses concern and questions the activity, the nurse can simply say, "The uterus has a tendency to relax and must be massaged so that it contracts to prevent bleeding." Usually, such a statement suffices. The mother may drift off to sleep between the nurse's observations. The nurse can gently rouse her by speaking her name before commencing massage so that the mother is not awakened abruptly to the painful sensation of someone compressing her abdomen.

Other Measures. Vital signs must be checked every 5 to 15 minutes, depending on the client's condition. Any abnormal variation should be reported promptly. Skin condition, level of consciousness, and urinary output also are monitored. A perineal pad count is kept to monitor blood loss. A record is kept of the number of pads saturated, how fully they are saturated, and the time it took for the saturation to occur. Thus, the nurse's documentation might read: "two pads saturated in 20 minutes." This type of report is more helpful to the physician than a more general, vague statement, such as, "saturating perineal pads quickly."

Evaluation

The effectiveness of nursing interventions related to hemorrhage and shock is evaluated first on the basis of prevention of the conditions and if they occur, on the responsiveness to treatment. Possible anticipated outcomes may include the following:

- Intrapartum or postpartum period demonstrates appropriate response.
- The client's vital signs return to and remain within normal limits.
- The client's blood loss decreases to minimal amounts.
- The client's output is approximately equal to her intake.
- The client remains free of infection.
- The client verbalizes understanding of her condition and treatment.
- The client's uterus remains contracted after delivery.

For intrapartum hemorrhage, the condition of the fetus also would be of concern with effectiveness of treatment focusing on the fetus' well-being before and after birth.

Prolapse of Umbilical Cord

During labor, the umbilical cord sometimes prolapses alongside or in front of the presenting part. Fortunately, this is a rare complication, affecting less than 0.5% of births overall, increasing to 1.5% with PROM (Garite, 1990). Factors predisposing a client to cord prolapse do so by preventing proper adaptation of the presenting part to the maternal pelvis. They include breech presentation (especially footling), transverse lie, unengaged presenting part, twin gestation, hydramnios, or a small fetus. When cord prolapse occurs, it is a potentially grave complication for the fetus, because if the cord is compressed between the presenting part and the bony pelvis, the fetal circulation may be shut off.

Manifestations

When prolapse occurs, a common time is after rupture of the membranes, when the presenting part (head, breech, or shoulder) is not engaged and is therefore not sufficiently down in the pelvis to prevent the cord from being washed past it in the sudden gush of amniotic fluid. The prolapse may be apparent (Fig. 36-11*C*), with the cord visibly protruding from the vagina, or it may be concealed (see Fig. 36-11*B*), with the diagnosis being made when the cord is felt during vaginal examination. Fetal distress, detected by heart rate changes, is sometimes the first indication, especially of occult cord prolapse (not protruding through the cervix; see Fig. 36-11*A*).

Management

The immediate treatment of cord prolapse is any method that reduces the pressure of the presenting part on the umbilical cord in an effort to prevent or minimize impairment of fetal circulation. Position changes, such as tilting the mother's body to place her head and shoulders lower than her hips, as in Trende-lenburg position, knee–chest position, or elevating the hips with a pillow allows the presenting part to move out of the pelvis and relieve the pressure on the cord (Fig. 36-12). Alternately or additionally, the presenting part may be pushed upward by pressure from a sterile gloved hand in the vagina (Fig. 36-13). This pressure needs to be maintained until preparations are made to deliver the fetus. If the cord has prolapsed outside the vagina, no attempt should be made to reposition it in the vagina. To avoid cooling and drying of the cord, it may be covered with sterile towels and moistened with warm sterile saline.

The goal of therapy is to deliver the fetus as soon as possible. If dilatation is incomplete, immediate cesarean delivery yields the best results for fetal survival. In occasional, carefully selected cases, prolapsed cord in vertex presentations with nearly complete dilatation can be delivered with minimal trauma to mother and newborn using vacuum extraction or forceps.

Assessment

When conditions exist that predispose a client to cord prolapse, more frequent vaginal examinations and closer attention to fetal heart rate changes can assist in early detection. An important routine practice after rupture of the membranes is to listen to and record the fetal heart rate immediately after the rupture and again in 10 to 15 minutes to detect decreased rate or irregularities if the cord has prolapsed. When fetal heart tones are electronically monitored, the cord compression from a cord prolapse usually is manifested by moderate to severe variable decelerations.

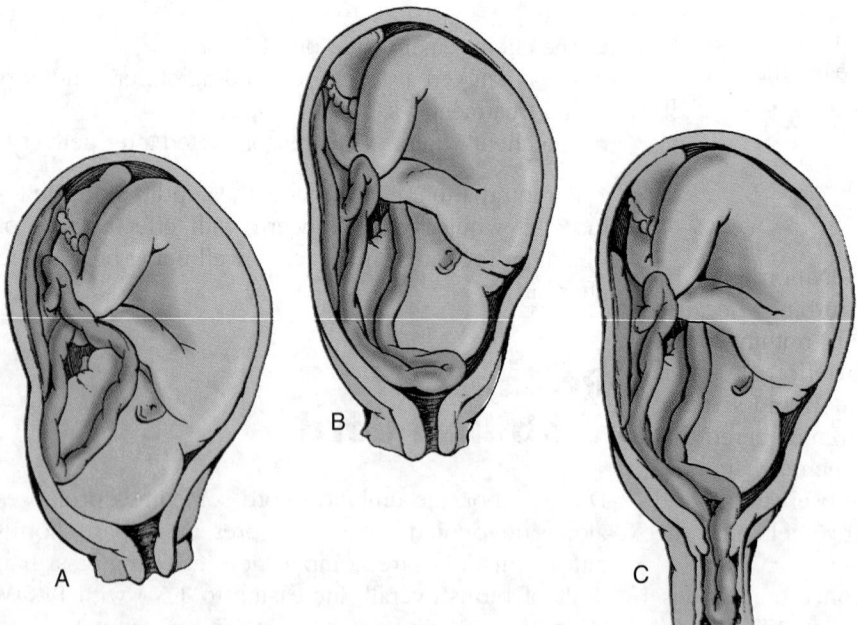

FIGURE 36–11 Prolapse of the cord. As the head comes down, the compression of the cord between the fetal skull and the pelvic brim will shut off its circulation completely. **(A)** Occult prolapse. **(B)** Cord prolapsed in front of head. **(C)** Cord prolapsed into vagina.

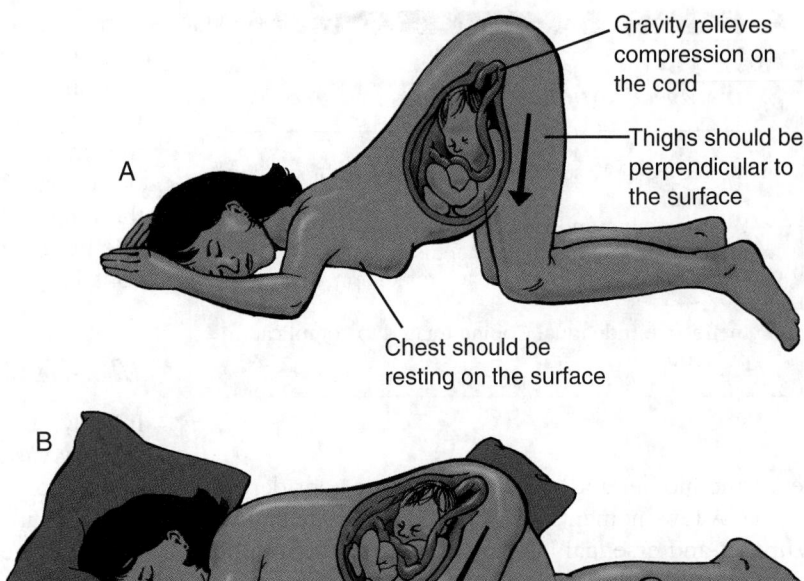

FIGURE 36-12 Prolapsed cord: Positioning to reduce cord compression. (**A**) Knee–chest position and (**B**) lateral Sims' position reduce cord compression and help to maintain umbilical cord circulation. Positioning should be combined with administration of oxygen to the woman.

Gravity relieves compression on the cord

Thighs should be perpendicular to the surface

Chest should be resting on the surface

Nursing Diagnosis

Following assessment, the nurse can identify possible nursing diagnoses. For a list of possible nursing diagnosis, see Box 36-6.

Planning and Intervention

The nurse is often the first to detect signs of a prolapsed cord. The nurse needs to act quickly to institute emergency procedures, such as positioning the woman and administering oxygen, alerting the physician and other staff, and preparing for cesarean delivery, if nec-

essary. Although the woman is not in physical danger or discomfort from the prolapsed cord, she usually senses that something is wrong from the heightened tension and the interventions being rapidly used. Calmness, warmth, and efficiency from the nurse are needed to reassure the woman that all possible measures are being taken to bring the situation under control.

The nurse should never leave the client unattended. Her partner (if present) should be treated with consideration. It is sometimes difficult when a crisis occurs to deal with the relatives of the woman with appropriate thoughtfulness, because most of the energy is directed toward meeting the demands of the situation. How-

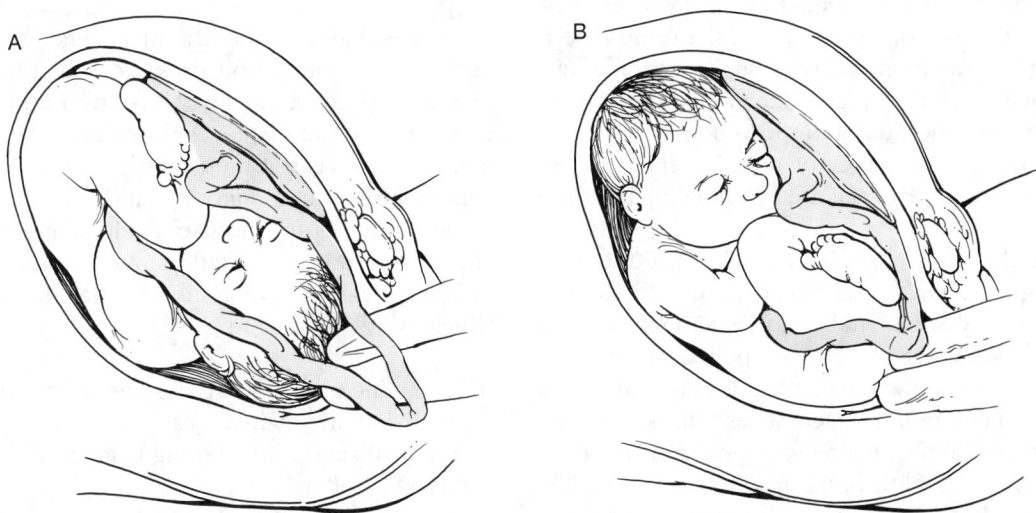

FIGURE 36-13 Prolapsed cord. Reduction of cord compression using gloved examiner's hand in vagina to elevate presenting part, (**A**) vertex or (**B**) breech.

> **BOX 36-6**
> *Nursing Diagnoses: Prolapsed Cord*
>
> ■ Altered Fetal Tissue Perfusion related to blood flow occlusion
> ■ Fear related to uncertainty of outcome
> ■ Anxiety related to danger to fetus
> ■ Knowledge Deficit related to condition, treatment, and care
> ■ Ineffective Individual Coping related to complication of labor

ever, the mother and her family must be considered as a unit. A few moments spent providing the family with support and essential information enable them to help support the mother.

Evaluation

Effectiveness of nursing interventions when a prolapsed cord occurs can be evaluated on the basis of fetal and maternal outcome. Possible anticipated outcomes of effective nursing care include the following:

■ The fetal heart rate remains within normal limits.
■ The client delivers a healthy newborn.
■ The client understands what is happening.
■ The client verbalizes a decrease in anxiety.
■ The client demonstrates positive coping strategies.

Amniotic Fluid Embolism

Amniotic fluid embolism is a life-threatening condition that develops when amniotic fluid enters the maternal circulation and subsequently reaches the pulmonary capillaries. For this to occur, there must be a tear through the amnion and chorion, an opening into the maternal circulation, and increased intrauterine pressure to force the fluid into the venous circulation. The most likely sites of entry are the endocervical veins and the uteroplacental area (Cunningham et al., 1993).

Amniotic fluid embolism is rare (1 in 3,500 to 1 in 80,000 pregnancies) but has a high maternal mortality rate, reported by some studies to be as high as 85% (Morgan, 1994). This along with pulmonary thromboembolism have now become the leading causes of maternal mortality in the United States (Morgan, 1994).

Amniotic fluid embolism most typically occurs during or just after the birth of the newborn, after a difficult labor, or after a labor in which oxytocin induction or augmentation was used. Other predisposing factors associated with amniotic fluid embolism include multiparity, advanced maternal age, large fetus, intrauterine fetal death, and meconium in the amniotic fluid.

Amniotic fluid invariably contains small particles of matter, such as vernix caseosa, lanugo, and sometimes meconium. These form multiple tiny emboli, causing occlusion of the pulmonary capillaries when reaching the lungs. The lethality of intravenously infused amniotic fluid varies depending on the particulate matter it contains.

Manifestations

Initially, there is a transient phase of intense pulmonary vasospasm, leading to acute right heart failure and hypoxemia. This may account for the 25% to 50% mortality in the first few hours (Gonik, 1989). There also may be an anaphylactic reaction to fetal debris, acting as matter foreign to the woman's body. Hemorrhage is another major concern, with thromboplastic materials in the amniotic fluid triggering a sequence of events leading to disseminated intravascular coagulation (Anderson, 1989).

The clinical characteristics typically include cyanosis, hypotension, and signs of acute respiratory distress, such as dyspnea, tachypnea, and chest pain. In 15% of clients, seizures signify the clinical presentation. Pulmonary edema occurs in up to 70% of clients who survive the initial cardiovascular insult; 40% of those subsequently develop a coagulopathy, which may present as a postpartum hemorrhage. Diagnostic workup includes arterial blood gases, complete blood count, and disseminated intravascular coagulation profile (platelet count, prothrombin time, partial thromboplastin time, and fibrin degradation products; Morgan, 1994).

Management

The general aims of medical management are to maintain oxygenation, blood pressure, and cardiac output and manage coagulopathy. More specifically, treatment may include intubation and mechanical ventilation with 100% oxygen if the client is unconscious. Central venous pressure monitoring and blood transfusions may be used as appropriate. IV fluids in normotensive clients should be restricted to avoid pulmonary edema. Pharmacologic interventions may include the following (Buckley, 1990; Morgan, 1994):

■ Dopamine (2–20 mg/kg per minute) to treat hypotension and maintain cardiac output.
■ IV digitalization (0.1–1.0 mg lanoxin in divided doses)
■ PGF_{2a} for postpartum hemorrhage
■ Morphine to decrease anxiety
■ Aminophylline to relieve bronchospasm

■ Hydrocortisone to decrease pulmonary edema and help overcome the overwhelming stress

Nursing Intervention

The nurse's role in the event of amniotic fluid embolism includes responsibility for monitoring client responses, anticipating possible therapies, and providing supportive care for the client and her family. The client should be placed in Fowler's position. Oxygen, medication, and blood products should be administered as ordered. Intake and output should be monitored closely. The client should not be left alone. If the fetus is undelivered, monitoring the fetal heart rate pattern and preparing for emergency delivery are additional nursing activities (Buckley, 1990). Because there is such a high incidence of maternal death with this condition, the nurse also may need to help the family through the grieving process.

Multiple Pregnancy

When two or more embryos develop in the uterus at the same time, the condition is known as **multiple pregnancy.** These are considered complicated pregnancies because there is an appreciable increase in morbidity and mortality. Although the incidence of twin gestation is only about 1% of all births, they contribute 12% to the perinatal mortality rate of 10 per 1,000 in the United States (Spellacy, 1994). Factors influencing incidence of multiple pregnancy and a description of types of twins are presented in Chap. 7.

Diagnosis

Early diagnosis of multiple pregnancy is an important factor in improving the perinatal outcome, because monozygotic twins can have serious growth discordance, and uterine overdistension can trigger premature labor (Cunningham et al., 1993). Detection late in pregnancy or at delivery correlates with increased risk for perinatal morbidity and mortality. Early diagnosis allows time for the woman and her family to be informed of the differences involved in multiple pregnancy and what can be done to improve the outcome. Referral to a perinatal center also can be made at a more optimum time.

Twins are suspected whenever uterine size is greater than ordinarily expected for any point in the pregnancy (discrepancy of more than 2 size-date comparisons, eg, 36 cm at 32 weeks). In addition, the palpation of three or four large parts in the uterus, the auscultation of two fetal heart tones of differing frequencies, or the history of twins "running in the family" all alert the obstetrician or nurse to the possibility of a multiple pregnancy.

Ultrasound can aid in the diagnosis of multiple pregnancy. Routine ultrasound screening of all pregnancies before the 20th week is practiced in some areas. There is no biochemical test that clearly differentiates between multiple and single pregnancies. Although human chorionic gonadotropin levels are usually higher in multiple pregnancies, they are not high enough to allow a definitive diagnosis (Cunningham et al., 1993).

High-Risk Problems

Several high-risk conditions are associated with multiple pregnancy (Table 36-8). In addition, monozygotic twins are less hardy than dizygotic twins. Weight differences are more pronounced, and they have a higher incidence of congenital anomalies and neonatal mortality.

Management and Nursing Care

Because of the prenatal and perinatal risk, the mother needs to be monitored carefully during the prenatal period. She is asked to see the obstetrician more frequently, at least every 2 weeks in the second trimester and at least weekly in the third trimester if there are no complications. If maternal hypertension or other problems that increase the risk for the fetuses occur, serial fetal surveillance should be done, usually with weekly NSTs on each fetus starting after 28 weeks and serial ultrasounds to verify adequate growth rates for each fetus and amniotic fluid volume (Spellacy, 1994). Frequent rest periods using the side-lying position may be prescribed.

TABLE 36–8
Maternal Complications With Twin Pregnancies

Problems	Increased Likelihood Over Singleton Pregnancy
Preterm labor	7–10
Hypertension	2–5
Abruption	3
Anemia	2–3
Hydramnios	3–5
Urinary tract infection	1–4
Postpartum hemorrhage	2–4
Cesarean section	2

(Spellacy, W. [1994]. Multiple pregnancies. In J. Scott, P. DiSaia, C. Hammond, & W. Spellacy [Eds.], *Danforth's obstetrics and gynecology* [7th ed.] [p. 335]. Philadelphia: J.B. Lippincott.)

Diet is regulated to allow for adequate weight gain. An increase of 300 kcal/d in the diet is recommended, beyond the 2,500 kcal total for a normal pregnancy. Protein intake is supervised (≥60 g), as are iron (60–100 mg/d) and folic acid (1 mg/d) intake. Sodium restriction has not been found to be beneficial (National Research Council 1989; Cunningham et al., 1993).

The latter weeks of a multiple pregnancy are likely to be associated with heaviness of the lower abdomen, back pains, and swelling of the feet and ankles. Abdominal distention makes sleeping difficult; therefore, the physician may prescribe a hypnotic. A well-fitting maternity girdle makes daytime more comfortable. Because of the excessive abdominal size, the mother may find that frequent, small meals are more suitable than the usual three larger meals a day. The nurse can be helpful in giving the woman anticipatory guidance regarding these matters during the prenatal period. Travel is curtailed because labor may begin at any time without warning, and delivery in strange surroundings may be hazardous. As with any client, she needs to be taught signs and symptoms of preterm labor.

Labor and Delivery

If not already hospitalized, the mother should come to the hospital at the first sign of labor. When labor is confirmed, a decision about the route of delivery must be made. It should take into account the presentation of the fetuses, the presence of any maternal or fetal complications, the gestational age, and the availability of anesthesia, an experienced obstetrician, and neonatal intensive care. During labor, steps are taken to ensure a successful outcome for the woman and fetuses.

A qualified perinatal team member should be present at all times. The nurse can be invaluable. Fetal heart rates must be monitored continuously, and maternal vital signs must be recorded. A combination of external and internal fetal monitoring after the membranes have ruptured usually proves satisfactory. Two units of cross-matched blood or its equivalent in blood fractions must be available. In addition, an IV infusion system capable of delivering blood is started (#18 lumen angiocath). Lactated Ringer's solution alternated with a 5% dextrose solution at 60 to 120 mL/h has been found to be satisfactory in the absence of hemorrhage or metabolic disturbance during labor (Cunningham et al., 1993).

It is recommended that two obstetricians be available and scrubbed for the delivery and that an anesthesiologist be in attendance, especially for the contingency of a cesarean delivery. Two staff members, with at least one skilled in resuscitation, are needed for each fetus at the time of delivery.

The decision for appropriate analgesia depends on the coexisting problems in the client. Use of narcotics, sedatives, and tranquilizers may lead to undue fetal depression if the fetuses are premature. For vaginal delivery, a pudendal block administered along with nitrous oxide and oxygen provides effective pain relief while minimizing the effect of anesthetic on the fetuses (Cunningham et al., 1993). One study showed that 130 women using epidural analgesia for vaginal delivery of twins had a significantly prolonged interval from complete dilatation until delivery (90 minutes compared with 30 minutes without an epidural; Crawford, 1987). For cesarean delivery of twins, either general anesthesia or epidural has proven satisfactory.

To accomplish the vaginal delivery of twins, the first twin is delivered either by vertex or assisted breech delivery. If the twins are monozygotic, the first fetus' cord must be clamped to prevent the second twin from bleeding through it. The cords should be labeled. The position of the second twin is ascertained, and it is brought into position by a combination of vaginal and abdominal manipulation. If there is a second sac, it is carefully ruptured to allow a slow loss of fluid and to guard against cord prolapse. A spontaneous or a prophylactic forceps vertex delivery is preferred. If the breech presents, the physician may have to assist in the extraction. If descent does not come about, version and extraction may be required. These require astute management on the part of the obstetrician and the anesthesiologist (Cunningham et al., 1993).

Routine use of oxytocin is delayed until after the delivery of the second twin. Then it is added to the IV infusion. The uterus is not massaged until after the placenta(s) are expelled. Massage then continues until the uterus remains firm and contracted (15–30 minutes). Ergonovine or methergine may be given intramuscularly after expulsion of the placenta(s) if the mother is not hypertensive, because methergine has been associated with aggravating hypertension.

As with any delivery, the nurse has the responsibility for supporting the mother and assisting the physician in whatever activities are indicated. Because these newborns are apt to be small (premature), oxygen or resuscitative measures may be necessary. The care is similar to that for any premature newborn (see Chap. 41). Sufficient supplies and equipment for resuscitation for each newborn should be procured early in the delivery and kept in readiness. Maternal vital signs and the fetal heart rate should be checked frequently.

Internal Version. Most useful in cases of multiple gestation, **internal version** (also called **internal podalic version**) is a maneuver designed to change any fetal presentation to a breech to facilitate delivery (Fig. 36-14). It is used when the delivery of the second twin is delayed or when the fetus is in a transverse lie.

When cervical dilatation is complete, the entire hand of the operator is introduced high into the uterus. One or both of the fetus' feet are grasped and pulled downward in the direction of the birth canal. With the exter-

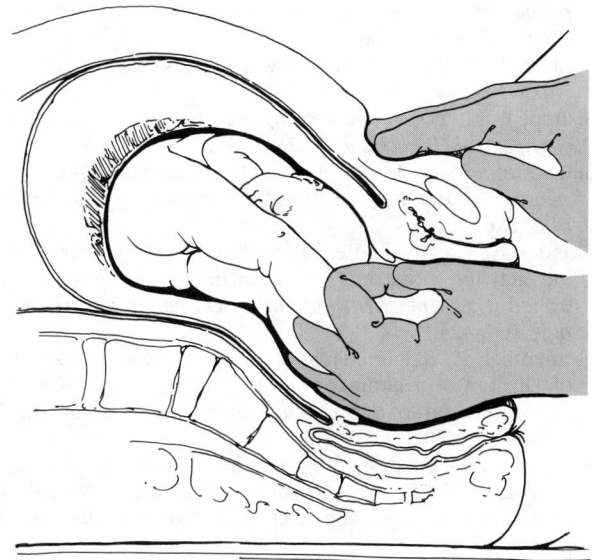

FIGURE 36–14 Internal version.

nal hand, the obstetrician may expedite the turning by pushing the head upward. The version is followed by breech extraction.

Postpartum

Physically, the care required by the mother depends on her general condition and the type of delivery. Complications are the same as those after single births, but the frequency of complications, such as uterine atony, may be increased due to the overdistention of the uterus.

The birth of more than one newborn can be a psychological shock to the parents, even if expected. One additional newborn may be desired and acceptable; two may impose an emotional or financial burden. The parents may wonder if they can manage the care of two newborns simultaneously. Problems may be compounded in feeding, especially if the mother plans to breast-feed, and in providing two of everything.

Parents need anticipatory guidance and support during the initial adjustment period. Some may need referral to a social worker or public health nurse to assist with plans for the multiple births. Many also appreciate information about special clubs for mothers of twins or introduction to other mothers who have successfully coped with the first few months after the birth of twins. If the newborns are small, the parents need the same type of extra support given to other parents of preterm newborns (see Chap. 41).

Summary Points

✔ Dystocia means "abnormal labor progress." Three possible categories include:

- Protraction disorders: protracted active phase dilation and protracted descent
- Arrest disorders: prolonged deceleration phase, secondary arrest of dilation, and arrest of descent
- Failure to progress is a diagnosis often used to identify lack of dilatation for any reason. Technically it refers only to cases in which the cervix fails to dilate in the presence of normal uterine activity and no CPD.

✔ Dystocia is caused by problems associated with the four mechanical aspects of labor:

- Powers: uterine dysfunction, either hypotonic or hypertonic and problems with expulsive forces
- Passageway: contracted pelvis, CPD, and variations in pelvic shape
- Passenger: occiput posterior, breech, other malpresentations, macrosomia, and fetal anomalies
- Psyche: stress response inhibiting normal contractility

✔ Preterm labor has three defining characteristics: onset of labor after 20 weeks and before 37 weeks, regular uterine contractions occurring once or more every 10 minutes for 1 hour, and cervical change.

✔ With preterm labor, the earlier treatment begins, the better the success rate of tocolytic agents, such as ritodrine and magnesium sulfate. If delivery can at least be delayed by a few days, this may help to avoid neonatal RDS, a serious complication of prematurity.

✔ Management and nursing care of preterm labor involve the use of bed rest, hydration, treatment of any infections, and possible administration of tocolytic agents.

✔ Post-term means that spontaneous labor has not started by 42 weeks after the first day of the last menstrual period. The pathophysiology caused by this delay involves placental degradation, leading to uteroplacental insufficiency of oxygen, nutrients and water, oligohydramnios, and possible umbilical cord compression.

✔ Management of post-term labor may include the use of induction, such as stripping the membranes, AROM, oxytocin induction, and amnioinfusion to minimize variable decelerations and dilute thick meconium.

✔ Hemorrhagic complications can be divided into two overall categories based on time of occurrence:

- Intrapartum hemorrhages: disorders of placental attachment, other placental anomalies, rupture of the uterus, and inversion of the uterus
- Early postpartum hemorrhages: uterine atony, lacerations, and retained placental fragments

✔ If uterine atony is suspected, fundal massage or oxytocic agents can help contract the myometrium and constrict the large uterine arteries. Therapy for shock is directed toward *fluid replacement* to combat hypovolemia and blood transfusions, oxygen administration, and positioning with legs elevated to improve oxygenation.

✔ Amniotic fluid embolism develops when amniotic fluid enters the maternal circulation. Manifestations typically include cyanosis, hypotension, and signs of acute respiratory distress, such as dyspnea, tachypnea, and chest pain.

✔ Multiple pregnancy occurs when two or more embryos develop in the uterus at the same time. To accomplish the vaginal delivery of twins, the first twin is delivered either by vertex or assisted breech delivery. If the twins are monozygotic, the first newborn's cord must be clamped to prevent the second twin from bleeding through it.

REFERENCES

American Academy of Pediatrics and American College of Obstetricians and Gynecologists (1992). *Guidelines for perinatal care*. Elk Grove Village; IL: Author.

American College of Obstetricians and Gynecologists (1989). *Dystocia*. Washington, DC: Author.

American College of Obstetricians and Gynecologists (1989). *Dystocia*. Washington, DC: Author.

American College of Obstetricians and Gynecologists (1990). *Assessment of fetal maturity prior to repeat cesarean delivery or elective induction of labor: Opinion No. 77*. Washington, DC: Author.

American College of Obstetricians and Gynecologists (1991a). *Induction and augmentation of labor: Technical Bulletin No. 157*. Washington, DC: Author.

American College of Obstetricians and Gynecologists (1991b). *Fetal macrosomia: Technical Bulletin No. 159*. Washington, DC: Author.

American College of Obstetricians and Gynecologists (1994). *Antenatal corticosteroid therapy for fetal maturation: Committee Opinion # 147*. Washington, DC: Author.

American College of Obstetricians and Gynecologists (1995). *Preterm Labor: Technical Bulletin No. 206*. Washington, DC: Author.

Anderson, H. (1989). Maternal hematologic disorders. In R. Creasy & R. Resnik (Eds.), *Maternal-fetal medicine: Principles and practice* (2nd ed.) (pp. 890–924). Philadelphia: W.B. Saunders

Arnold-Aldea, S., & Parer, J. (1990). Fetal cardiovascular physiology. In R. Eden & F. Boehm (Eds.), *Assessment and care of the fetus: Physiological, clinical, and medicolegal principles* (pp. 29–42). Norwalk, CT: Appleton & Lange.

Asrat, T., & Quilligan, E. (1994). Postterm pregnancy. In F. Zuspan & E. Quilligan (Eds.), *Current therapy in obstetrics and gynecology* (4th ed.) (pp. 275–277). Philadelphia: W.B. Saunders.

Bashore, R. (1992). Dystocia. In N. Hacker & J. G. Moore (Eds.), *Essentials of obstetrics and gynecology* (2nd ed.) (pp. 261–269). Philadelphia: W.B. Saunders.

Benedetti, T. (1991). Obstetric hemorrhage. In S. Gabbe, J. Niebyl, & J. Simpson (Eds.), *Obstetrics: Normal and problem pregnancies* (2nd ed.) (pp. 573–605). New York: Churchill Livingstone.

Bennett, N., Botti, J. (1989). New strategies for preterm labor. *Nurse Practice, 14*(4), 27–38.

Bishop, E. (1964). Pelvic scoring for elective induction. *Obstetrics and Gynecolgy, 24*(2), 266–268.

Blackburn, S., & Loper, D. (1992). *Maternal, fetal, and neonatal physiology: A clinical perspective*. Philadelphia: W.B. Saunders.

Blondel, B., Breart, G., Berthooz, Y. et al. (1992). Home uterine activity monitoring in France: A randomized, controlled trial. *American Journal of Obstetrics and Gynecology, 167*, 424.

Blumenthal, P., & Ramanauskos, R. (1990). Randomized trial of Dilapan and laminaria as cervical ripening agents before induction of labor. *Obstetrics and Gynecology, 75*, 365–368.

Bottoms, S., & Scott, J. (1990). Transfusions and shock. In J. Scott, P. DiSaia, C. Hammond et al. (Eds.), *Danforth's obstetrics and gynecology* (6th ed.). Philadelphia: J.B. Lippincott.

Bowes, W. (1989). Clinical aspects of normal and abnormal labor. In R. Creasy & R. Resnik (Eds.), *Maternal-fetal medicine: Principles and practice* (2nd ed.). Philadelphia: W.B. Saunders.

Bredow, V., Straube, W., & Goretzlehner, G. (1990). Experiences with labor induction at term with a PGE2 get (Prepidil gel). *Geburtshilfe and Frauenheilkunde, 50*(11), 865–869.

Buckley, K. (1990). Pulmonary disorders. In K. Buckley & N. Kulb (Eds.), *High risk maternity nursing manual*. Philadelphia: W.B. Saunders.

Calderyo-Barcia, R. (1957). *Oxytocin and pregnant human uterus*. Buenos Aires: 4th Pan-American Congress on Endocrinology.

Carsten, M. (1992). Endocrinology of pregnancy and parturition. In N. Hacker & J. G. Moore (Eds.), *Essentials of obstetrics and gynecology* (2nd ed.) (pp. 52–60). Philadelphia: W.B. Saunders.

Chibber, G., Cohen, A., Lindenbaum, C. et al. (1990). Patient attitude toward home uterine activity monitoring. *Obstetrics and Gynecology, 76*(Supp.), 90S–-92S.

Clark, S., Cotton, D., Hankins, G., & Phelan, J. (1994). *Handbook of critical care obstetrics*. Boston: Blackwell Scientific Publication.

Cox, S., Sherman, M., & Leveno, K. (1990). Randomized investigation of magnesium sulfate for prevention of preterm birth. *American Journal of Obstetrics and Gynecology, 163*, 767.

Crawford, J. (1987). A prospective study of 200 consecutive twin deliveries. *Anesthesia, 42*, 33.

Creasy, R. (1989). Preterm labor and delivery. In R. Creasy & R. Resnik (Eds.), *Maternal-fetal medicine: Principles and practice* (2nd ed.). Philadelphia: W.B. Saunders.

Cruikshank, D. (1994). Malpresentations and umbilical cord complications. In J. Scott, P. DiSaia, C. Hammond, & W. Spellacy (Eds.), *Danforth's obstetrics and gynecology* (7th ed.) (pp. 501–519). Philadelphia: J.B. Lippincott.

Cunningham, F., Mac Donald, P., Gant, N., Leveno, K. et al. (1993). *Williams obstetrics*. Norwalk, CT: Appleton & Lange.

Curet, L. (1994). Dysfunctional labor. In F. Zuspan & E. Quilligan (Eds.), *Current therapy in obstetrics and gynecology* (pp. 243–245). Philadelphia: W.B. Saunders.

Dierker, L. (1994). Breech delivery. In F. Zuspan & E. Quilligan (Eds.), *Current therapy in obstetrics and gynecology* (pp. 223–224). Philadelphia: W.B. Saunders.

Dyson, D., Crites, Y., Ray, D., & Armstrong M. (1991). Prevention of preterm birth in high-risk patients: The role of education and provider contact versus home uterine monitoring. *American Journal of Obstetrics and Gynecology, 164,* 756–762.

Flamm, B., Goings, J., Fuelberth, N., Fischermann, E. et al. (1987). Oxytocin during labor after previous cesarean section: Results of a multicenter study. *Obstetrics and Gynecology, 70,* 709.

Freeman, R., & Lagrew, D. (1991). Prolonged pregnancy. In S. Gabbe, J. Niebyl, & J. Simpson (Eds.), *Obstetrics: Normal and problem pregnancies* (2nd ed.) (pp. 945–956). New York: Churchill Livingstone.

Friedman, E. (1978). *Labor, evaluation and management.* New York: Appleton-Century-Crofts.

Friedman, E., Niswander, K., Bayonet-Rivera, N., & Sachtleben, M. (1966). Relation of prelabor evaluation to inducibility and the course of labor. *Obstetrics and Gynecology, 28*(4), 495–501.

Garite, T. (1990). Premature rupture of the membranes. In R. Eden, F. Boehm, M. Haire, & H. Jonas (Eds.), *Assessment and care of the fetus* (pp. 631–641). Norwalk, CT: Appleton & Lange.

Garite, T., & Spellacy, W. (1994). Premature rupture of membranes. In J. Scott, P. DiSaia, C. Hammond, & W. Spellacy (Eds.), *Danforth's obstetrics and gynecology* (7th ed.) (pp. 305–315). Philadelphia: J.B. Lippincott.

Gimovsky, M., & Paul, R. (1982). Singleton breech presentation in labor: Experience in 1980. *American Journal of Obstetrics and Gynecology, 143*(7), 733–739.

Gimovsky, M., Wallace, R., Schiffrin, B., & Paul, R. (1983). Randomized management of the nonfrank breech presentation at term: A preliminary report. *American Journal of Obstetrics and Gynecology, 146,* 34.

Gonik, B. (1989). Intensive care monitoring of the critically ill pregnant patient. In R. Creasy & R. Resnik (Eds.), *Maternal-fetal medicine: Principles and practice* (pp. 845–874). Philadelphia: W.B. Saunders.

Grimes, D., & Schulz, K. (1992). Randomized controlled trials of home uterine activity monitoring. A review and critique. *Obstetrics and Gynecology, 79,* 137.

Halle, J. (1993). *Campbell v. Centinella Hospital.* Superior Court, Los Angeles County.

Halle, J. (1993). Diagnostic evaluation of high-risk pregnancy. In S. Mattson & J. Smith (Eds.), *NAACOG core curriculum for maternal- newborn nursing* (pp. 157–185). Philadelphia: W.B. Saunders.

Hauth, J. (1994). Postpartum hemorrage. In F. Zuspan & E. Quilligan (Eds.), *Current therapy in obstetrics and gynecology* (pp. 272–274). Philadelphia: W.B. Saunders.

Hobel, C. (1992). Prenatal care. In N. Hacker & J. G. Moore (Eds.), *Essentials of obstetrics and gynecology* (2nd ed.) (pp. 82–92). Philadelphia: W.B. Saunders.

Hollander, D., Nagey, D., & Pupkin, M. (1987). Magnesium sulfate and ritodrine hydrochloride: A randomized comparison. *Obstetrics and Gynecology, 156*(3), 631–637.

Hurd, W., Miodovnik, M., Hertzberg, V., & Lavin, J. (1983). Selective management of abruptio placenta: a prospective study. *Obstetrics and Gynecology, 61,* 467.

Kaupilla, O. (1975). The perinatal mortality in breech deliveries and observations on affecting factors: A retrospective study of 2,227 cases. *Acta Obstetrics and Gynecology of Scandinavia, 39*(Suppl.), 1.

Klein, L., & Goldenberg, R. (Eds.) (1990). *Prenatal care and its effect on preterm birth and low birth weight. New perspectives on prenatal care.* New York: Elsevier.

Kochenour, N. (1994). Normal pregnancy and prenatal care. In R. Sokol, B. Brindley, & M. Dombrowski (Eds.), *Danforth's obstetrics and gynecology* (7th ed.) (p. 68). Philadelphia: J.B. Lippincott.

Koehl, L., & Wheeler, D. (1989). Monitoring uterine activity at home. *American Journal of Nursing, 89,* 200–203.

Kulb, N. (1990). Preterm labor. In K. Buckley & N. Kulb (Eds.), *High risk maternity nursing manual.* Baltimore: Williams & Wilkins.

Lake, M. (1992). Prolonged pregnancy. In L. Mandeville & N. Troiano (Eds.), *High-risk intrapartum nursing* (pp. 83–99). Philadelphia: J.B. Lippincott.

Leung, A., Leung, E., & Paul, R. (1993). Uterine rupture after previous cesarean delivery: Maternal and fetal consequences. *American Journal of Obstetrics and Gynecology, 169,* 945–950.

Main, D., Gable, S., Richardson (1985). Can preterm deliveries be prevented? *American Journal of Obstetrics and Gynecology, 151,* 892–898.

Malinowski, J. (1989). Fetal well-being in preterm and postterm gestation. In J. Malinowski, C. Pedigo, & C. Phillips (Eds.), *Nursing care during the labor process* (3rd ed.). Philadelphia: F.A. Davis.

Malinowski, J. (1989). Labor stimulation. In J. Malinowski, C. Pedigo, & C. Phillips (Eds.), *Nursing care during the labor process* (3rd ed.). Philadelphia: F.A. Davis.

Manelle, N., Lauman, B., Lazar, P. (1984). Prematurity and occupational activity during pregnancy. *American Journal of Epidemiology, 119,* 309.

McDonald, H., Vigneswaran, R., & O'Loughlin, J. (1989). Group B Streptococcal colonization and preterm labor. *Australian-New Zealand Obstetrics and Gynecology, 29,* 291.

Morgan, M. (1994). Amniotic fluid embolism. In F. Zuspan & E. Quilligan (Eds.), *Current therapy in obstetrics and gynecology* (pp. 210–211). Philadelphia: W.B. Saunders.

Morrison, J., Martin, R. (1987). Prevention of preterm birth by ambulatory assessment of uterine activity: a randomized study. *American Journal of Obstetrics and Gynecology, 156,* 536–543.

National Research Council (1989). *Recommended dietary allowances.* Bethesda, MD: National Academy Press.

Neal, A., & Bockman, V. (1992). Preterm labor and premature rupture of membranes. In L. Mandeville & N. Troiano (Eds.), *High-risk intrapartum nursing* (pp. 57–81). Philadelphia: J.B. Lippincott.

Newton, R., Webster, P., Binu P. (1979). Psychological stress in pregnancy and its relation to onset of premature labor. *British Medical Journal, 2:* 411.

O'Brien, W., & Cefalo, R. (1991). Labor and delivery. In S. Gabbe, J. Niebyl, & J. Simpson (Eds.), *Obstetrics: Normal and problem pregnancies* (2nd ed.). New York: Churchill Livingstone.

Parisi, V. (1989). Cervical incompetence. In R. Creasy & R. Resnik (Eds.), *Maternal-fetal medicine: Principles and practice* (2nd ed.). Philadelphia: W.B. Saunders.

Parsons, M., & Spellacy, W. (Eds.) (1994). *Danforth's obstetrics and gynecology.* Philadelphia: J.B. Lippincott.

Paul, R., Phelan, J., & Yeh, S. (1985). Trial of labor in the patient with a prior cesarean birth. *American Journal of Obstetrics and Gynecology, 151,* 297.

Phelan, J. (1989). The postdate pregnancy: An overview. *American Journal of Obstetrics and Gynecology, 32,* 219.

Pozaic, S. (1992). Induction and augmentation of labor. In L. Mandeville & N. Troiano (Eds.), *NAACOG high-risk intrapartum nursing* (pp. 101–114). Philadelphia: J.B. Lippincott.

Read, W., & Welby, D. (1986). The use of calcium antagonist (nifedipine) to suppress labor. *British Journal of Obstetrics and Gynecology, 93*, 933–937.

Ricci, J. (1992). Antepartum hemorrhage. In N. Hacker & J. G. Moore (Eds.), *Essentials of obstetrics* (2nd ed.) (pp. 154–162). Philadelphia: W.B. Saunders.

Romero, R., Oyarzum, E., Mazor, M. et al. (1989). Meta analysis of the relationship between asymptomatic bacteriuria and preterm delivery/low birth weight. *Obstetrics and Gynecology, 73*, 576.

Rosen, M., Dickinson, H., & Westhoff, C. (1991). Vaginal birth after cesarean: A meta-analysis of morbidity and mortality. *Obstetrics and Gynecology, 77*, 465.

Ross, M., & Hobel, C. (1992). Normal labor, delivery, and the puerperium. In N. Hacker & J. Moore (Eds.), *Essentials of obstetrics and gynecology* (2nd ed.) (pp. 119–133). Philadelphia: W.B. Saunders.

Sala, D., & Moise, K. (1990). The treatment of preterm labor using a portable subcutaneous terbutaline pump. *Journal of Obstetric, Gynecologic, and Neonatal Nursing, 19*, 108–115.

Scott, J. (1994). Cesarean section. In J. Scott, P. DiSaia, C. Hammond, & W. Spellacy (Eds.), *Danforth's obstetrics and gynecology* (pp. 563–576). Philadelphia: J.B. Lippincott.

Shields, J., & Medearis, A. (1992). Fetal malpresentations. In N. Hacker & J. G. Moore (Eds.), *Essentials of obstetrics and gynecology* (2nd ed.) (pp. 230–240). Philadelphia: W.B. Saunders.

Sokol, R., Brindley, B., & Dombrowski, M. (Eds.) (1994). *Danforth's obstetrics and gynecology.* Philadelphia: J. B. Lippincott.

Spellacy, W. (1994). Multiple pregnancies. In J. Scott, P. Disaia, C. Hammond, & W. Spellacy (Eds.), *Danforth's obstet-rics and gynecology* (pp. 333–341). Philadelphia: J.B. Lippincott.

Toot, P., Surrey, E., & Lu, J. (1992). Menstrual cycle, ovulation, fertilization, implantation and placenta. In N. Hacker & G. Moore (Eds.), *Essentials of obstetrics and gyneocology* (2nd ed.) (pp. 36–51). Philadelphia: W.B. Saunders.

Ulmsten, U. (1989). Prostaglandins in high risk obstetrics. In S. Brody & K. Ueland (Eds.), *Endocrine disorders in pregnancy.* Englewood Cliffs, NJ: Appleton-Lange.

Utter, G., Dooley, S., Tamura, R., & Socol, M. (1990). Awaiting cervical change for the diagnosis of preterm labor does not compromise the efficacy of ritodrine tocolysis. *American Journal of Obstetrics and Gynecology, 163*, 882–886.

Williams, J. (1993). Prolonged pregnancy and disorders of uterine action. In V. R. Bennett & L. Brown (Eds.), *Myles textbook for midwives* (12 ed.) (pp. 386–403). London: Churchhill Livingstone.

Wray, S. (1993). Uterine contractions and physiological mechanisms of modulation. *American Journal of Physiology, 264*, C1–C18.

Zlatnik, F. (1994a). Normal labor and delivery. In J. Scott, P. DiSaia, C. Hammond, & W. Spellacy (Eds.), *Danforth's obstetrics and gynecology* (pp. 105–128). Philadelphia: J.B. Lippincott.

Zlatnik, F. (1994b). The normal and abnormal puerperium. In J. Scott, P. DiSaia, C. Hammond, & W. Spellacy (Eds.), *Danforth's obstetrics and gynecology* (pp. 163–173). Philadelphia: J.B. Lippincott.

Zuckerman, H., Reiss, U., & Rubenstein, I. (1974). Inhibition of human preterm labor by indomethacin. *Obstetrics and Gynecology, 44*, 787–792.

Zuspan, F., & Quilligan, E. (1988). *Douglas-Stromme operative obstetrics.* Norwalk, CT: Appleton & Lange.

37

Operative Obstetrics

Objectives

- State the purpose of operative obstetrics and medical indications for instrument delivery and cesarean delivery.
- State the criteria used to classify types of obstetric forceps applications; list the types and delineation of those criteria for each.
- Describe the possible maternal and fetal complications from forceps and vacuum extractor use.
- Identify the three types of cesarean sections, stating which is the most common and why.
- List the components of routine preoperative nursing care for a cesarean delivery.
- Identify the main risk of vaginal birth after cesarean delivery (VBAC).
- Discuss the nurse's responsibility when caring for the client undergoing VBAC.

Key Terms

Cesarean delivery   Operative obstetrics
Dystocia   Vacuum extractor
Fenestrum

One of the main goals of obstetric care is the safe delivery of a healthy newborn. Should circumstances arise that threaten this goal, the obstetrician has several methods to expedite the delivery and prevent harm to the newborn and mother. The methods used are collectively called **operative obstetrics.** They include assisted delivery using forceps or a vacuum extractor and cesarean birth. The nurse's role is to collaborate with the physician in identifying clients in need of an expedited delivery and to assist with the preparation or procedure. Today many labor and delivery units include a surgical suite with nurses trained to circulate or scrub for surgery. Nurses are responsible for providing the necessary equipment and supplies, so their understanding of why and when a procedure is done, the types of instrumentation, and how they are used is essential to their supporting role.

Instrument-Assisted Vaginal Delivery

During the second stage of labor, it may become necessary to use instruments to assist with the delivery. Maternal indications for instrument delivery include the inability of the woman to push due to regional anesthesia (eg, epidural), maternal exhaustion, heart disease, or any health condition adversely affecting the woman that is likely to be improved by delivery. The chief fetal indications for assisted delivery include fetal distress, as suggested by decreasing fetal heart rate, or disadvantageous fetal positions, such as occiput posterior or occiput transverse.

Forceps Delivery

Obstetric forceps are used to provide traction, rotation, or both to the fetal head when the unaided expulsive efforts of the woman are insufficient. To accomplish this safely, eight main requirements must be fulfilled (Newnham et al., 1992):

1. Delivery must be mechanically feasible, as demonstrated by engagement of the head, deter-

mination of level of presenting part, and adequacy of maternal pelvis.
2. Presenting part must be either vertex, face with anterior chin, or aftercoming head in vaginal breech.
3. The position of the head must be known.
4. Uterine contractions must be present.
5. Membranes must have ruptured.
6. Cervix must be fully dilated.
7. Anesthesia must be adequate (pudendal and local are acceptable for low forceps, epidural or spinal for Kielland's forceps).
8. Bladder must be empty (if necessary, bladder can be drained by urinary catheterization prior to forceps delivery).

Types of Forceps

Some of the common types of obstetric forceps are illustrated in Figure 37-1. The instrument consists of two steel parts that cross each other like a pair of scissors and lock at the intersection. The lock may be of a sliding type, as in the first three types shown, or a screw type, as in the Tarnier instrument.

Each part consists of a handle, a lock, a shank, and a blade. The blade is the curved portion applied to the sides of the fetal head. The blades of most forceps (the Tucker-McLean is an exception) have a **fenestrum**, a large opening or window to enhance the grip on the fetal head. The blades usually consist of two curves, a cephalic curve, which conforms to the shape of the head, and a pelvic curve, to follow the curve of the birth canal. Axis-traction forceps, such as the Tarnier, have a mechanism attached below that permits the pulling to be done more directly in the axis of the birth canal. An axis-traction handle also is available for use on standard forceps. The two blades of the forceps are designated as right and left. The left blade is introduced into the vagina on the client's left side; the right blade goes in on the right side.

Types of Forceps Applications

Forceps applications have been classified according to the station and position of the presenting part at the time the forceps are applied (American College of Obstetricians and Gynecologists [ACOG], 1989):

- Outlet forceps—45-degree rotation or less required; applied when the scalp is visible at the introitus without spreading the labia. The skull has reached the pelvic floor, the sagittal suture is in the anteroposterior diameter or right or left anterior or posterior position, and the fetal head is at the perineum.
- Low forceps—subdivided into rotation requiring more than 45 degress or less than 45 degrees; ap-

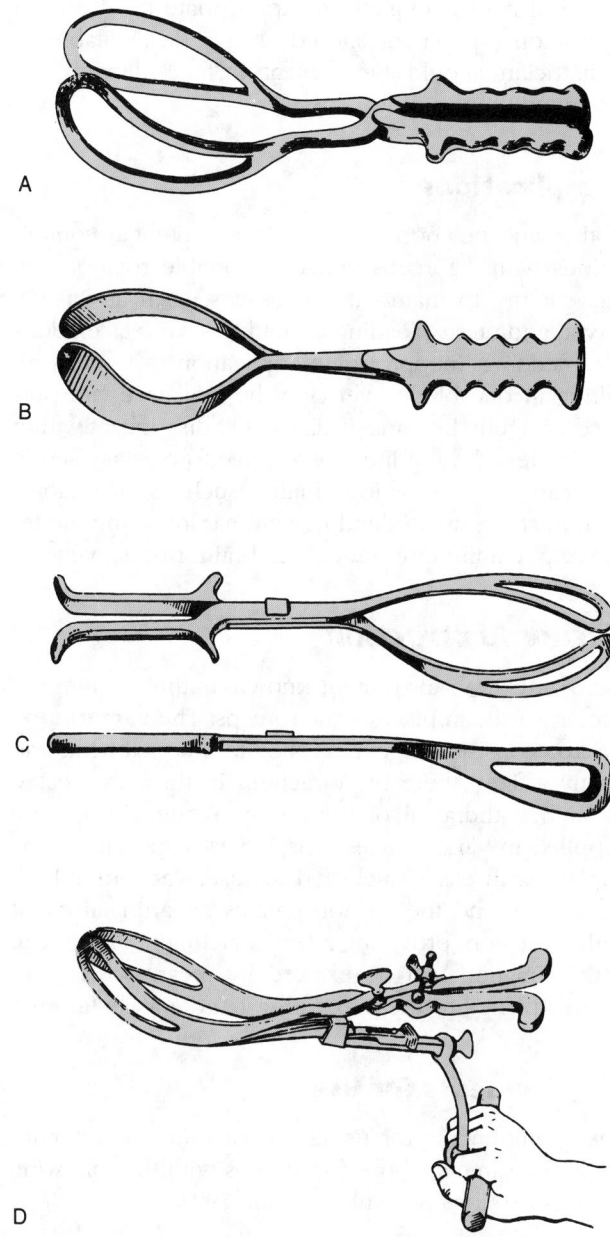

FIGURE 37–1 Types of forceps. **(A)** Simpson forceps. **(B)** Tucker-McLean forceps. **(C,** top) Kielland forceps, front view. **(C,** bottom) Kielland forceps, side view. **(D)** Tarnier axis-traction forceps.

plied when the leading point of the skull is at station +2 or more

■ Mid forceps—applied when the head is engaged but the leading point of the skull is less than +2. This is a controversial forceps application, because it has been associated with birth trauma. Today, most obstetricians perform a cesarean delivery if the head is arrested above +2 station to avoid any untoward maternal and fetal injury in the birthing process.

Under no circumstances should forceps be applied to an unengaged presenting part.

Procedure

After a decision is made to use forceps, the obstetrician selects the type of instrument to be used. Several pairs of the generally approved forceps, each encased in suitable wrappings, are autoclaved and kept in the delivery room for immediate use. The other instruments needed for a forceps delivery are the same as those required for a spontaneous vaginal delivery.

The client is placed in the lithotomy position and prepared and draped in the usual fashion. After checking the exact position of the fetal head by vaginal examination, the physician introduces two or more fingers of one hand into the left side of the vagina. These fingers guide the left blade into place and at the same time, protect the maternal soft parts (vagina and cervix) from injury. The other hand is used to introduce the left blade of the forceps into the left side of the vagina, gently placing it between the fetus' head and the fingers of the hand (Fig. 37-2).

The same procedure is carried out on the right side. Then the blades are articulated (attached together at the shank). Traction is applied intermittently, not continuously (see Fig. 37-2*B*). Between traction, the blades are partially disarticulated to release pressure on the fetal head. Episiotomy is routinely performed in these cases to allow adequate room for forcep maneuvering without tearing maternal tissues.

Piper Forceps for Breech Delivery. The Piper forceps have been designed to assist in the delivery of the aftercoming head in breech presentations. They are applied after the shoulders have been delivered and the head has been brought into the pelvis by gentle traction combined with suprapubic pressure. Suspension of the body and arms with a towel facilitates application of the blades (Fig. 37-3).

The left blade is introduced in an upward direction along the fetal head on the left side. The right blade is applied in a similar fashion. The forceps are locked in place, and their position on the head is confirmed by palpation. An episiotomy is made, and as traction is applied, the chin, mouth, and nose emerge over the perineum. The Piper forceps are often used electively as a substitute for the Mauriceau-Smellie-Veit maneuver, or when the Mauriceau-Smellie-Veit maneuver has failed to deliver the fetal head (see Chap. 36).

Nursing Management

When forceps delivery is anticipated, the nurse can briefly explain the procedure and its necessity to the woman and her partner. The woman feels pressure and pulling but does not feel pain with adequate regional or spinal anesthesia. Breathing techniques to prevent muscle tensing and pushing during application of the

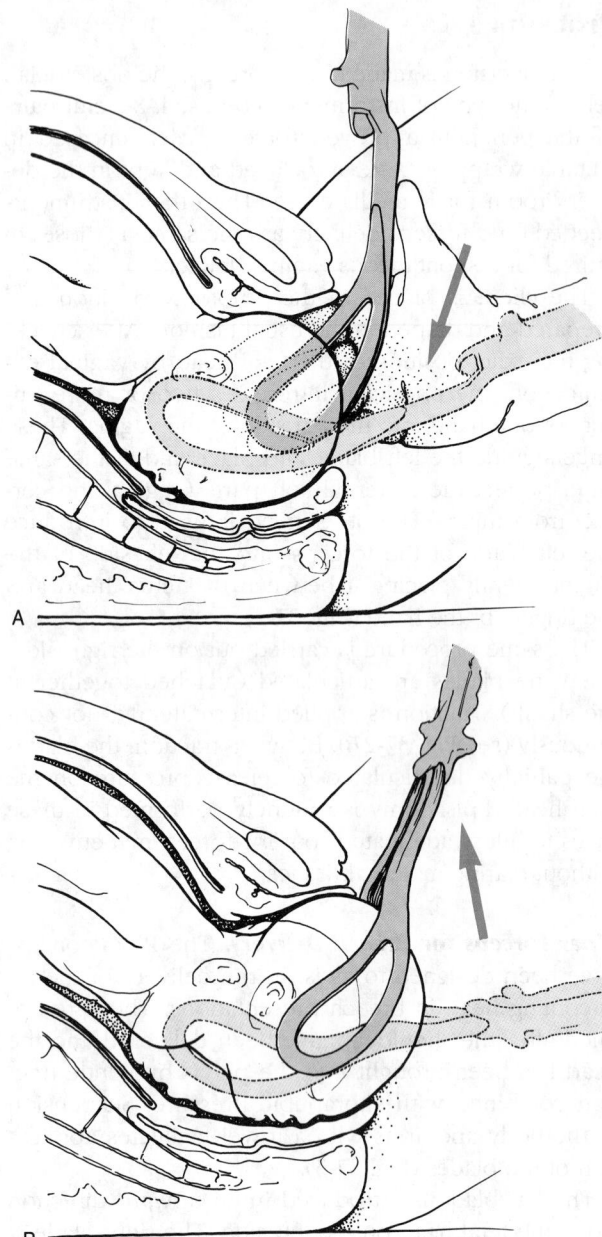

FIGURE 37–2 (A) Insertion of forceps blade and **(B)** applied forceps and direction of traction.

forceps and other techniques used by the woman and couple to cope with labor should be encouraged.

The nurse provides the physician with the required type of forceps. Often determined in advance, the forceps can be put on the delivery table. Once the forceps are applied, the nurse monitors contractions and advises the physician, so traction with the forceps can be coordinated with contractions. The mother also is encouraged to continue pushing as the physician applies traction.

Continuous fetal monitoring is important because fetal bradycardia is common with forceps delivery, due to the increased pressure on the fetal head or some

umbilical cord compression. Appropriate newborn resuscitation equipment should always be available. A pediatrician should be present if fetal distress has prompted the use of forceps.

Complications

Mother and newborn are at risk for potential complications with a forceps delivery. Forcible rotation can cause injury to maternal soft tissues, such as vagina, cervix, and uterus, leading to mild to severe lacerations and bleeding. Inappropriate application of forceps resulting in one blade overlying the fetal face can produce unsightly bruising. This usually disappears within the first few days of life. If excessive force was used, it can lead to more serious injury, such as lacerations, skull fracture, or subdural hematoma, involving the fetal scalp, cranium, or underlying brain, respectively.

Vacuum Extraction

Increasingly, an instrument known as the vacuum extractor is used in place of the forceps. The **vacuum extractor** consists of a cup applied to the fetal head and tightly affixed there by a vacuum in the cup created through withdrawal of the air by a pump. Cups are supplied in various sizes. The largest cup that can be applied with ease is selected for use. Vacuum is built up slowly, and the suction creates an artificial caput within the cup, providing a firm attachment to the fetal scalp. Traction can be exerted by means of a short chain attached to the cup with a handle at its far end.

Requirements for Use

The requirements for using the vacuum extractor include the same as those for forceps with the following three exceptions (Newnham et al., 1992):

1. In multiparous women with only a small rim of cervix that is easily stretched over the fetal head remaining, the vacuum can be used.
2. The vacuum extractor should never be used in preterm delivery, because the fetal head and scalp are prone to injury from the suction cup.
3. It should never be used for breech or face deliveries.

Nursing Management

The nurse should briefly explain the procedure and its necessity to the woman and her partner. The mother feels pressure and pulling sensations but does not feel pain with adequate regional or spinal anesthesia. Breathing techniques to prevent tensing and pushing are encouraged during application of the vacuum ex-

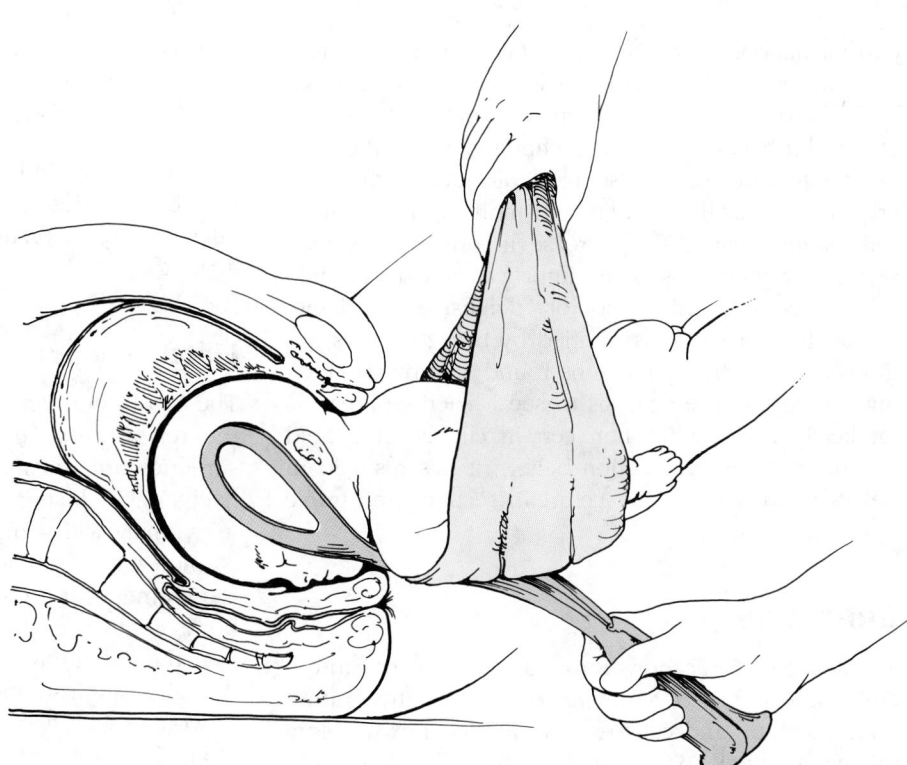

FIGURE 37–3 Piper forceps are used to deliver the aftercoming head in breech presentations, while the body and arms are suspended in a towel.

traction cup. The woman is kept informed by the nurse during the procedure.

The nurse provides the physician with the vacuum extraction equipment, including the size cup requested and sterile tubing. After the physician assembles the cup and tubing, the nurse attaches the distal end to suction. With the cup applied to the fetal head, the nurse activates the suction. To avoid damaging vaginal tissues, suction must be released if the cup slips off the fetal head. The nurse encourages the woman to push during contractions, while traction is applied by the physician.

The fetal heart rate should be monitored frequently by the nurse during the procedure. Newborn resuscitation equipment should be available, and the pediatrician should be called if complications are expected with the newborn. Parents should be informed that the newborn's head will have a caput (chignon) where the cup was applied, but that this disappears within a few days.

Complications

As with forceps, the use of the vacuum extractor can lead to maternal and fetal injuries. Vaginal lacerations can be prevented if a digital examination of the entire circumference of the suction cup is done after application but before initiation of vacuum. Fetal scalp injuries can be prevented by avoiding prolonged use. A general rule is that if traction on the suction cup during three contractions has not produced encouraging de-

scent of the fetal head, the trial of vaginal delivery by vacuum extraction should be abandoned (Newnham et al., 1992).

Cesarean Delivery

Cesarean delivery (also called cesarean section or C section) is the delivery of the fetus through incisions made in the abdominal wall and uterus. It is considered major abdominal surgery. The name is derived from the legend that Julius Caesar was born in this manner. Before the advent of safe surgery, abdominal birth was reserved for instances in which the mother was dying and the newborn was to be saved. It was not until the late 19th century that cesarean birth was safely accomplished.

Incidence

The incidence of cesarean birth has increased dramatically in the last several years, from about 5.5% in 1970 to 22.7% in 1985 and to 24% in 1988; the reported range currently is 10% to 40% of all births (Seiler, 1990; Newnham et al., 1992). The main indication for a cesarean delivery has been a repeat cesarean. Once the prevalance in primary cesarean sections increased, the total rate escalated primarily due to the greater number of women presenting with the history of cesearean section. The increase in cesarean deliveries has been controversial in healthcare, especially in light of the current national concern about the high cost of medical care. This increased rate has occurred in an environment of increased medical malpractice cases, declining birth rate, and new technologies like the fetal heart rate monitor. It also has coincided with a decreasing perinatal morbidity and mortality rate. Therefore, some believe the increase in primary cesarean sections was necessary to improve outcome, while others say it is only proof of "defensive" medicine, in which the therapy is justified by being the less litigious option. The truth can be found only by conducting a case by case analysis to see if each cesarean is medically indicated. When certain clients have held a generic, "anti-intervention belief," it has resulted in delays of truly necessary cesarean sections and tragic outcomes.

Indications

The accepted indications for cesarean delivery can occur singularly or in combination, are relative rather than absolute, and can be classified as shown below (Newnham et al., 1992; Cunningham et al., 1993):

- Maternal and fetal:
  Dystocia (abnormal progress of labor) is the second most common indication (30%), which usually presents as "failure to progress" in labor. It can be due to cephalopelvic disproportion, failed induction, or abnormal uterine action (see Chap. 36).
- Maternal:
  Severe maternal disease, such as severe heart disease, brittle diabetes, severe preeclampsia or eclampsia, cervical cancer, or severe infection (ie, herpes simplex virus type II or herpes genitalis in the active phase or within 2 weeks of active lesions). These conditions necessitate a cesarean for several reasons: to expeditie the delivery in a critical condition; because the woman and fetus are unable to tolerate labor; or the fetus would be exposed to increased risks passing through the birth canal.
  Previous uterine surgery, including myomectomy, previous cesarean delivery with a classic incision, or uterine reconstruction
  Obstruction of the birth canal by fibroids or ovarian tumors
- Fetal:
  Fetal distress, such as with cord prolapse, severe uteroplacental insufficiency
  Malpresentations, such as transverse lie, brow presentation
  Multiple gestation in which the presenting twin is breech transverse

- Placental:
  Placenta previa
  Premature separation of the placenta (abruption)

Controversial indications include unknown previous scar, breech presentation, post-term pregnancy, and fetal macrosomia (estimated fetal weight of more than 4,500 g).

Elective Repeat Cesareans

The most common indication for cesarean delivery is the repeat cesarean section (33%). Several of these surgeries are not medically required but done "electively," as a matter of physician or client preference in women with only one prior cesarean section. In women with multiple previous cesareans, the medical requirement for a cesarean section versus a trial of labor is controversial, because there are insufficient data to make a definitive recommendation (Scott, 1993). Although some institutions currently allow a trial of labor in women with two prior cesarean sections (Newnham et al., 1992), recent studies have shown that there is a threefold increased incidence of uterine rupture during labor in women with two or more previous cesareans compared with those with only one previous cesarean (Leung et al., 1993).

Because prematurity is the most common fetal complication of elective repeat cesarean birth, ACOG has recommended that one of the following criteria be used to confirm fetal age assessment prior to the elective delivery (ACOG, 1991):

- Ultrasound at 12 to 20 weeks, confirming estimated gestational age of more than 39 weeks as obtained by clinical history and physical examination
- Ultrasound measurement of crown to rump length at 5 to 11 weeks, which supports an estimated gestational age of more than 39 weeks
- Fetal heart tones documented for 20 weeks by nonelectronic fetoscope or 30 weeks by Doppler
- 36 weeks since a positive human chorionic gonadotropin pregnancy test
- Amniocentesis for fetal lung maturity if unsure of dating

Classification of Cesarean Sections

Classification of cesarean sections refers to the uterine incision used. Although there are three currently performed types, the transverse incision in the lower-segment of the uterus is usually the operation of choice. Other types of cesarean delivery include the classic cesarean section, in which a vertical incision is made in the upper segment of the uterus, or the low vertical cesarean, made in the lower segment. Only the two most common types are described below.

Transverse (Low-Segment) Cesarean Delivery

Transverse, or low-segment, cesarean delivery is usually the operation of choice for a number of reasons. Because the incision is made in the lower segment of the uterus, its thinnest portion with the least uterine activity, there is minimal blood loss. This area is easier to repair, and there is a decreased chance of rupture of the scar in a subsequent pregnancy. There also is a lower incidence of peritonitis, paralytic ileus, and bowel adhesions.

The initial incision (the abdominal cavity having been opened) is made transversely across the uterine peritoneum, where it is attached loosely just above the bladder. The lower peritoneal flap and the bladder are dissected from the uterus, and the uterine muscle is incised either vertically or transversely. The membranes are ruptured, and the fetus is delivered (Fig. 37-4). The placenta is extracted, and intravenous oxytocin is administered to contract the uterus. The uterine incision is sutured in two layers, with the second layer imbricat-

ing the first. This two-flap arrangement seals off the uterine incision and is believed to prevent the lochia from entering the peritoneal cavity. Then the visceral peritoneum is reapproximated with a continuous layer of absorbable suture. Packs are removed from the abdominal cavity. A normal saline lavage is done to reduce postoperative infection and the abdomen is closed in layers.

Classic Cesarean

A vertical incision is made directly into the wall of the body of the uterus. The fetus and the placenta are extracted, and the incision is closed by three layers of absorbable sutures. This approach requires going through the full thickness of the uterine corpus. It is particularly useful when the bladder and lower segment are involved in extensive adhesions resulting from a previous cesarean section. Occasionally, it is selected when the fetus is in a transverse lie or when there is an anterior placenta previa.

Because classic cesarean is more spacious, providing rapid access to the fetus, it is the method of choice when acute hemorrhage is occurring or in other emergency situations in which time is critical and the lives

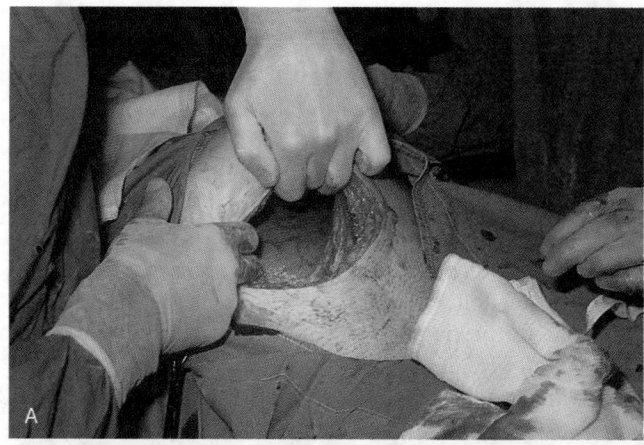
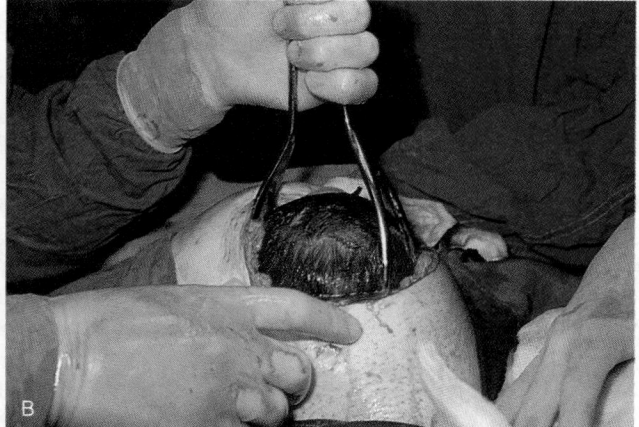
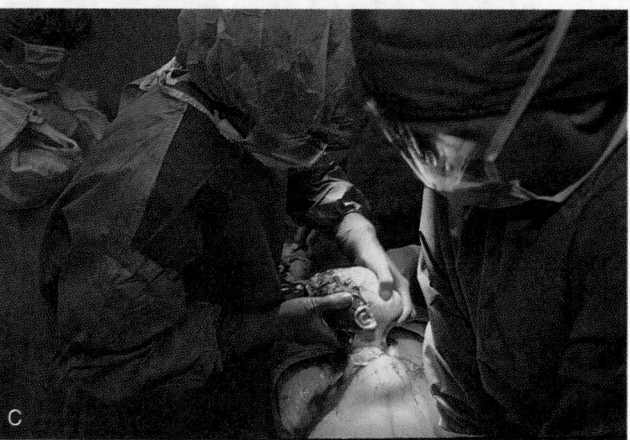

FIGURE 37–4 Cesarean birth. (**A**) The peritoneum has been opened, and the lower uterine segment is visible through the incision. (**B**) The head is gently delivered through the uterine and abdominal incisions using forceps. (**C**) The posterior shoulder is delivered first. Gentle upward traction is used to pull it through the uterine and abdominal incisions.

of the woman and fetus are threatened. Five other conditions also warrant classic incisions (Newnham et al., 1992):

- A preterm fetus less than 34 weeks who presents by breech, because the lower segment is still poorly formed and a transverse incision may be too narrow to allow an atraumatic delivery of the fetus
- Access to the lower segment restricted by fibroids
- Hysterectomy immediately following the cesarean section
- Postmortem cesarean section performed in an attempt to rescue a live fetus from a dead woman
- Invasive cervical cancer present

Preoperative Care

Assessment

Having an operative delivery is often anxiety producing for the client and her family, adding numerous factors that must be understood and accepted, making postdelivery recovery more difficult, placing additional strain on the developing mother–newborn relationship, and creating a need for processing and integrating the altered birth experience (See Nursing Care Plan: The Woman Experiencing Cesarean Birth).

Nursing assessment in the preoperative period includes evaluating the client's physical parameters and readiness for and understanding of the procedure and identifying possible risk factors. If the cesarean is an elective procedure, verification of gestational age is important and needs to be addressed with the physician if it has not been verified already. Information is gathered from the client's prenatal records (often transferred to the hospital before the delivery date), physical assessment (vital signs, laboratory data), and interview of the client and her support person at the time of admission.

Nursing Diagnosis

After completing the assessment, the nurse can identify possible nursing diagnoses. For a list of possible nursing diagnoses, see Box 37-1.

Planning and Intervention

Preparation for cesarean birth involves readying the woman for surgery and making the necessary preparations for care of the newborn. The usual laboratory tests, physical examination, typing and cross-matching blood, abdominal shaving, and other customary procedures are carried out. The physician discusses the type of operation and anesthesia with the woman and family, and informed consent is obtained. When the client is admitted for an elective cesarean section, nursing care includes checking fetal heart tones and being alert to signs of labor. Oral intake should be discontinued for at least 8 hours before surgery.

The lower abdomen is shaved, including the pubic hair. A retention catheter may be inserted and attached to a continuous drainage system to ensure that the bladder remains empty during the operation. The nurse should make certain that the catheter is draining properly before the procedure.

An intravenous infusion (commonly Ringer's lactate solution or 5% dextrose in water) 1,000 mL is started. Valuables are taken for safe keeping, and routine preoperative precautions are taken, such as removing fingernail polish, dentures, glasses, and contact lenses.

Preoperative medications are administered according to the physician's orders. In addition to the preparation of the operating room for the surgical procedure, the nurse makes the necessary preparations for care of the newborn. The nurse makes sure that the necessary equipment is present, including a warm crib and resuscitation equipment. A newborn resuscitator, equipped with heat, suction, oxygen (open mask and positive pressure), and an adjustable frame to permit proper positioning of the newborn, is most useful. Care Path: Cesarean Birth provides an example of care given to the client from the intrapartum period up to 72 hours after birth.

Childbirth Education Classes. If a cesarean delivery is planned, education is essential. Childbirth classes in preparation for cesarean birth are increasing in number. Some educators feel all childbirth classes should present information about cesarean delivery, even when vaginal delivery is anticipated. Considering that in some medical centers, the cesarean rate is nearly one in four deliveries, this approach has merit.

Cesarean prenatal classes usually cover content common to all prenatal classes, including onset of labor and the contact person, should labor begin at home. Special emphasis is given to prenatal testing, such as tests of fetal condition; preoperative tests; surgical procedures; analgesia and anesthesia; diagnostic procedures, including sonography; treatments, including intravenous fluids and urinary retention catheter; the operating room experience; and postoperative recovery.

Techniques for increasing comfort and relaxation also are taught. Although labor is not anticipated, the woman will find these techniques useful during tests and examinations and to help alleviate pain after surgery. Hospital policies are reviewed, including the partner's presence in the operating room and after surgery. The delivery and care of the newborn are detailed, including procedures in the operating and recovery rooms and normal variations in early mother–newborn relations. The course of postoperative recov-

Nursing Goals

1. Mother and family indicate readiness for cesarean birth.
2. Mother and family indicate understanding of the cesarean process.
3. Normal maternal–infant bonding occurs.
4. Mother's comfort and body functions are maintained or restored.
5. Mother and family indicate integration of the cesarean birth as a positive and satisfying birth experience.

Assessment	Potential Nursing Diagnoses	Intervention/ Rationale	Evaluation
Preparation for cesarean birth (unanticipated, elective)	Knowledge Deficit related to reasons for cesarean, procedures, relaxation, pain relief	Include cesarean birth in childbirth preparation classes *to provide information to prevent anxiety*	Parents recognize the potential for cesarean birth and feel prepared
	Fear related to condition of self or baby, pain, procedures, outcomes, aftermath	Provide information and explanation of reasons for cesarean, preparations for surgery, and processes to anticipate *to increase understanding*	Parents verbalize understanding, accept need and processes, cooperate in preparations
	Risk for injury, maternal–fetal	Assist parents to express their feelings of fear, disappointment, grief, powerlessness, and so forth *to allay their anxiety*	Parents express feelings freely and begin to accept and prepare for cesarean delivery
		Provide information and reassurance (as much as possible) about condition of mother and baby *to allay anxiety*	Parents feel reasonably reassured or able to cope with risks
		Remove prosthetic devices (eg, contacts, dentures) and jewelry *to prevent injury*	
		Placement of indwelling urinary catheter to deflate bladder *to prevent damage to bladder during surgery*	
		Shave abdomen "nipple to thigh" to remove hair around incisional area *to prevent infection*	
		Remove nail polish *to visualize nail beds perfusion*	
		Assist with positioning for anesthesia; *spine should be arched to increase access area to intervertabral spaces*	
		Continue fetal monitoring of heart rate patterns up until the removal of fetus from uterus if distress has been present (remove thigh leads & scalp electrode by reaching under leg drapes) *to maintain adequate fetal surveillance*	

(continued)

Assessment	Potential Nursing Diagnoses	Intervention/ Rationale	Evaluation
Postoperative condition: Fundal contraction Bleeding Vital signs Input and output Incision Respiratory function Comfort	Potential complications: hemorrhage, uterine atony, hematomas, shock, depressed respiratory function	Monitor postoperative progress, report early signs of problems, take emergency actions as needed *to prevent complications*	
	Alteration in Comfort: pain related to incision, after-pains, stretched abdominal muscles	Administer analgesics, change position, adjust bedding *to increase comfort*	Mother reports increased comfort or sleeps or rests
Early bonding with infant Mother Father	Risk for Altered Parenting related to lack of early contact, complications, pain, anesthesia, disappointment over birth, powerlessness	Provide opportunity for parents to see, hold, and explore infant in recovery area (if possible); or report on infant's condition and characteristics (sex, weight, normalcy, progress) *to enhance bonding*	Parents have satisfying early contact or have their questions about the baby answered and feel well informed
	Risk for Altered Parenting related to lack of early contact due to exclusion, condition of mother or infant, powerlessness, disappointment		Mother is awake and reasonably comfortable; can hold and interact with baby
		Discuss parents' feelings and reactions to cesarean birth; provide information and explanations	Parents express feelings freely, fit missing pieces together, begin to integrate the experience
Postpartum observations: Incision healing Pain Fluids and nutrition Bowel function Bladder function Respiratory function	For general postpartum care, see Nursing Care in the Postpartum Period, Chapter 27. Observations specific to cesarean sections are included here.	Monitor condition of incision, input and output, bowel and bladder function, respiratory function *to assess possibility of infection*	Mother takes fluids and food, moves bowels as expected, voids well after removal of catheter, and aerates lungs adequately
	Risk for Complications: infection, hematoma, incisional bleeding, wound dehiscence	Identify signs of complications early; report and take action *to decrease severity of complication*	Mother feels comfortable
	Altered Comfort related to incision, after-pains, stretched abdominal muscles, gas	Administer analgesics, assist in positioning, teach splinting and movement to minimize pain *to enhance recovery*	Mother reports increased comfort, holds and cares for infant, and interacts with partner satisfactorily
	Risk for Complications: persistent nausea and vomiting, continued intravenous therapy, lack of appetite, decreased gastrointestinal functioning		
	Altered Bowel Elimination: decreased functioning related to anesthesia and surgery (decreased peristalsis and activity), gas, constipation		
	Altered Urinary Elimination related to surgery, anesthesia, indwelling catheter; risk for urinary retention		
	Risk for Complications: decreased oxygenation due to limited ventilation, pneumonia, pulmonary embolus		

ery, both in the hospital and at home, is related to the pacing of caretaking responsibilities and need for assistance at home.

Interventions for Unanticipated Cesarean Delivery.

Emergency cesarean deliveries are performed when fetal or maternal complications pose serious risks. Complications may arise at any time. Often the decision for surgery arises after hours of nonprogressive labor or as a result of abnormal tracings on the fetal monitor. The woman may be discouraged, exhausted, worried about her own or the fetus' condition, and possibly dehydrated with low glycogen reserves. Preoperative preparations usually must be done rapidly, leaving little time for explanations.

The nurse should provide short, simple, and concise explanations of the surgery and procedures that must be done. The nurse must offer as much reassurance about the woman's and fetus' conditions as can reasonably be given. However, the client's and her partner's anxiety levels are high, and they may not recall much information. They also may misunderstand information given. After the operation, the nurse should spend time reviewing events leading up to the surgery, what occurred in the operating room, and the newborn's status to allow the parents to understand and integrate their experiences.

Care During Surgery

Nurses assist during cesarean delivery by scrubbing or circulating in the operating room. The surgical team consists of obstetrician, surgical assistant, anesthesiologist, pediatrician, and nurses. The nurse has a special role in keeping parents informed, providing calm reassurance, and interpreting events for the parents. Many cesarean deliveries are done under regional anesthesia, so the woman is aware of events. The father or support person, gowned appropriately, also may be in the room, sitting close to the woman's head. The surgical team must take the above into consideration in their communications with each other.

A trained professional should be present at the cesarean delivery to give the newborn initial care and to resuscitate if necessary. This person may be an experienced nurse with advanced training in newborn resuscitation, a nurse anesthetist, anesthesiologist, or perinatologist. Immediate transport to the neonatal intensive care unit must be available in case the newborn is compromised at birth. Depending on the newborn's condition and hospital policies, newborn care and evaluation may be done in the operating room. In many hospitals, it is customary to have a pediatrician available to take over the care of the newborn as soon as it is born. This frees the obstetrician to devote full attention to the mother. The support person may be given the newborn to hold and show to the mother, or they may be united in the recovery room.

The nurse should encourage and foster the parent–newborn bonding process by providing the mother and the partner the opportunity to touch and hold the newborn. When it is difficult for the mother to hold the newborn, the nurse can hold the newborn in an en face (face-to-face) position to facilitate the maternal–newborn bonding process.

Immediate Postoperative Postpartum Care

The woman who has had a cesarean delivery has undergone both abdominal surgery and birth. Postoperative care includes the same procedures as for any abdominal surgery with the added dimension of postpartum care.

Assessment

Assessment of the client postcesarean delivery involves close monitoring of all body systems. Two crucial areas to assess include the amount of blood loss and fluid balance.

Blood Loss. Bleeding is assessed in the same manner as for any delivery. The woman must be watched for hemorrhage by frequently inspecting the perineal pad and checking the fundus. Usually, the abdominal dressings are not bulky, and the nurse can palpate the fundus to see if the uterus is well contracted. Skin and uterine sutures are secure, and gentle but firm pressure can be used to assess uterine consistency. This may cause some discomfort, but it does not disturb the sutures. If a classic incision was used, gentle palpation along the side of the uterus will cause less discomfort. Oxytocics are usually ordered to contract the uterus and control bleeding.

The amount and character of lochia are noted, using the same guidelines as with vaginal deliveries (see

(text continues on page 1022)

Name _____

This care path is a guideline and is not intended to create a standard of care. This guideline may be modified based on individual client's needs.

Prob. #		Intrapartum	0-4 Hours/Date:	4-8 Hours/Date:	
3	ADL	Bedrest or ambulation as tolerated	Bedrest PRN	Dangle x 1 Ambulate with assist PRN Chair/rocker PRN	
1,3	Assessment Monitor	Perinatal Unit admission assessment Ongoing assessments PRN	Immediate postpartum assessments VS q 15 min x4, q 30 min, then q 4 hr VS are WNL	Immediate postpartum assessments-are WNL Assess mother/infant interaction VS q 4 hr while awake VS are WNL	
1,2,4	Consults	Perinatal CNS Anesthesia PRN House officer PRN Resolve PRN NICU staff PRN	⟶ ⟶ ⟶ ⟶ ⟶	⟶ ⟶ ⟶ ⟶ ⟶	
3	Procedures/ Tests	CBC Type and screen	Assess Rubella Titer status Assess need for Rhogam	⟶ ⟶	
1,3	Treatments	EFM IV Foley catheter Abdominal shave prep	Ice to incision Foley cath TCDB q 2 hr Peri care q 4 hr I&O q shift x 48 hr	⟶ ⟶ ⟶ ⟶ ⟶	
1,3,5	Meds/IVs	Epidural IVF-LR/D5LR	PCA/Epidural IV fluids Pitocin to IV Antiemetic PRN Antibiotics PRN Benadryl PRN	⟶ ⟶ ⟶ ⟶ ⟶ ⟶	
1,2	Nutrition	NPO (as ordered for scheduled sections)	Ice chips PRN (sips and chips)	⟶	
2,4	Client/Family Education	EFM Explain procedures	Mother/Baby booklet Safety issues Pharmacologic and non-pharmacologic pain control and comfort measures Initiate breast feeding/bottle feeding	Initiate infant care Normal involution, lochia, perineal care	
2,4	Discharge Planning	Mother/baby teaching form	Determine LOS	Begin discharge instructions	
2,4	Spiritual/Psycho/ Social/Emotional Needs	Support client/significant other Facilitate positive childbirth experience	Assess maternal role strenghts	Assist mother's transition through tasks of taking on maternal role	
	Multi-disciplinary Team Signatures	_____ _____	_____ _____	_____ _____	

Client Problems

1. Discomfort/pain
2. Learning needs
3. Potential for instability - postpartum involution
4. Potential alteration in coping related to childbirth
5. Potential for infection

CLIENT IDENTIFICATION

8-12 Hours/Date	12-24 Hours/Date:	24-48 Hours/Date:	48-72 Hours/Date:
———→ ———→	———→ ———→	**Encourage ambulation**	Up ad lib
Listen for bowel sounds ———→ ———→ **VS are WNL**	———→ ———→ ———→ **VS are WNL**	**Bowel sounds present** **Assessments BID are WNL** Assess mother/infant interaction VS q 4 hr while awake **VS are WNL**	VS QID
Lactation consultant PRN Social Service PRN WIC PRN	Lactation consultant Social Service, WIC, PRN	Lactation consultant Social Service, WIC PRN	Lactation consultant Social Service, WIC PRN
Rhogam screen PRN			H&H
———→ ———→ ———→ ———→ Dressing removed PRN	Foley cath PRN Peri care q 4 hr PRN ———→	Cath PRN I&O q shift x 48 hr Dressing removed PRN Supportive bra PRN	Staple removal PRN
———→ ———→ ———→ ———→ ———→ ———→	IV fluids PRN Pitocin PRN ———→ ———→ ———→	PO analgesics PRN Pitocin PRN Antiemetic PRN Antibiotics PRN Benadryl PRN IV fluids PRN Rhogam PRN Rubella vaccine PRN Mylicon PRN Stool softeners PRN	Mylicon PRN Stool softeners PRN PO analgesics PRN Suppositories/laxative PRN
Clear liquids	Advance as tolerated	Advance as tolerated	Regular diet
Initiate self care	Reinforce self care with demos Baby/cord care demo Breast pump if indicated	Breast pump if indicated	Self care and infant care return demos
———→	Assess parent interaction ———→	Discharge instructions Assess parent interaction Assess need for home health follow-up	Reinforce discharge instructions Assess parent interaction Assess need for home health follow-up
———→	———→	Assist mother's transition through tasks of taking on maternal role Encourage family and other support systems	Assist mother's transition through tasks of taking on maternal role

Chap. 27). Some women have less lochia after cesarean birth because of the operative techniques used in placenta removal and hemostasis. If the client has been on her back for a prolonged time, it is important to check under the buttocks for pooling of blood that may trickle down the perineum without getting trapped on the perineal pad. The skin incision is examined regularly for signs of hematoma, bleeding, or infection. Vital signs are taken every 4 hours for the first few postoperative days, or until stable. It is particularly important to watch for signs of shock or infection.

Fluid Balance. A retention catheter often remains in place for 12 to 24 hours. It should be monitored closely to see that it drains freely. The nurse should note the color, clarity, amount, and odor of the urine, notifying the physician of any abnormalities. Intravenous fluids are usually administered during the first 24 hours. Small amounts of fluids may be given by mouth after nausea has subsided. A record of the mother's intake and output is kept for the first 24 to 48 hours or until the need is no longer indicated.

Nursing Diagnoses

In the immediate postoperative period, the following nursing diagnoses are possible:

- Ineffective Breathing Pattern related to shallow breathing secondary to incisional pain
- Altered Tissue Perfusion related to blood loss from surgery and inadequate contraction of the uterus
- Alteration of fluid and electrolyte balance
- Alteration of comfort related to incisional pain and uterine involution

Planning and Intervention

Postoperatively, analgesic drugs should be used to keep the mother comfortable and encourage her to rest. Her position in bed during the early postoperative hours may be dictated by the type of anesthesia she received. She should be encouraged to turn from side to side every hour. Deep breathing, coughing, and incentive spirometry also should be encouraged to promote good lung ventilation. Most mothers who deliver by cesarean are allowed ambulation once fully recovered from anesthesia. Ambulation usually is usually encouraged 12 to 24 hours following delivery. This contributes considerably to maintaining good bladder and intestinal function, reducing thrombus formation, and preventing pneumonia.

Pain after cesarean birth most often involves the incisional site, gas pain as bowel function is restored, flank pain from stretching of abdominal muscles during surgery, muscle aches from immobility, afterpains, and sometimes discomfort from bladder distention. Analgesic medication should be timed to provide maximum relief during the times the mother spends feeding and caring for the newborn. Patient-controlled analgesia often is used to treat the pain and allow the client to have a sense of control over the situation. She can devote her energy to the newborn and avoid the distraction of postoperative pain.

Continued Postoperative Postpartum Care

After the immediate postoperative period, the mother receives routine postpartum care and continued post-surgery observations. Care includes vital sign assessment; lochia observation; fundal assessment; breast, perineal, and incisional care; attention to bladder and bowel elimination; nutrition; ambulation; hygiene; and pain management.

Assessment

Care related to the surgery includes observation of the incision, pain control, respiratory function, and increased need for rest and recovery. Showers may be taken by the second day if staples were used to close the incision.

Assessment and intervention in the development of mothering skills and family adaptations to cesarean birth are of central importance. The woman's and family's response to the birth process must be carefully observed and assessed. According to research conducted more than 15 years ago by investigators, such as Affonso and McClellan, women can have negative emotional reactions following cesareans. Levels of anxiety, anger, disappointment, and confusion may be high. This especially is true in unanticipated cesarean deliveries. Many women feel overwhelmed by an unexpected cesarean birth and are completely unprepared for their physical and emotional responses. They express feelings of anxiety for themselves or the newborn. They experience anger or depression because they expected a vaginal birth. They may feel a sense of loss about not experiencing vaginal delivery, not witnessing the birth, or not having their partner's or family's participation. There are often altered body perceptions and many concerns surrounding mothering the newborn during their recovery from surgery. The physical discomfort of the mother after the surgery, combined with her feelings of disappointment or guilt, can interfere with her ability to bond with her newborn.

However, mothers who were allowed early and continuous contact with their newborns after cesarean birth (with spinal anesthesia and delivery of a healthy, normal newborn) were found to have significantly more positive perceptions of their newborns in the early postpartum period. They also displayed more maternal behavior in caretaking at this time and when the newborn was 1 month old than cesarean mothers who only had brief contact in the first 12 hours after birth.

At this time, the woman finds herself burdened with an abdominal operative procedure. Her need for physical and emotional recovery may dominate her mothering interests initially. She may need to deal with her reduced ability to care for the newborn, separation from the newborn (especially with maternal or neonatal complications), discomfort in holding and feeding, and concern about the newborn's well-being. The father or support person likewise may need to review and integrate the experience and to learn the new processes involved in recovery and procedures after cesarean birth.

Nursing Diagnoses

After assessing the client, the nurse can identify possible postpartum nursing diagnoses, in addition to those appropriate for any client postoperatively. For a list of possible nursing diagnoses for the client with a cesarean delivery in the postpartum, postoperative period, see Box 37-2.

Planning and Intervention

In addition to caring for the mother's physical needs in the postpartum period, the nurse has a large responsibility for providing explanations of events and decisions and giving support through physical contact, calmness, comfort measures, verbal reassurances, and assisting the mother to gain mastery of her body and newborn care tasks.

BOX 37–2
Cesarean Postoperative Nursing Diagnoses

- Knowledge Deficit related to the cesarean birth
- Altered Parenting
- Body Image Disturbance
- Self Esteem Disturbance
- Grieving related to cesarean birth or fetal demise
- Altered Family Process

Nursing care must provide opportunity to review events, seek understanding of what happened and why, remember responses and work through these, clear up questions and misunderstandings, and alter self-concept and expectations to be congruent with reality. An interesting study done almost 20 years ago by Affonso revealed that 1 or 2 days after the birth, a visit from the labor and delivery nurse who assisted the couple during the childbirth was often beneficial for the integration of the event into their lives. It is important for all women to fill in missing pieces if they experience gaps in their memories of the labor and birth of their newborn.

This may be more important when the woman is attempting to understand the reasons for surgical intervention in what is often expected to be a natural process. These visits also provide the couple with the opportunity to discuss any feelings of failure, guilt, or anger that they may be experiencing. A sensitive and responsive nurse can effectively help the couple work through such feelings by remaining open to their comments and honestly addressing their concerns. If the family unit is to be strengthened through the childbearing process and childbirth is to be a family-centered event, the obstetric staff should make every attempt to help families incorporate this experience into their lives.

Issues of sexuality also can be addressed in the postpartum period. The mother may fear pain with intercourse or that the surgery will affect her partner's concept of her body. Reassurance and factual information usually assist the mother in resolving these issues. Involvement of the partner in this discussion often helps the couple in their adjustment.

Grief counseling should be available, especially in cases of fetal demise or when the newborn is seriously ill. Chapter 42 addresses the emotional, psychological, and spiritual care of the family in this instance.

Discharge Planning

Hospitalization after cesarean birth usually lasts 2 to 5 days but often only 48 to 72 hours. Discharge preparation includes that for any postpartum client (see Chap. 27), with added teaching specific to postoperative considerations. Mothers may be prescribed analgesics for use at home and should be reminded of their increased need for rest. The client should be instructed to begin limited exercises when abdominal pain has decreased. Lifting objects heavier than the newborn should be avoided for 2 to 3 weeks. Additional exercises should be avoided until after the client sees her physician for follow-up.

Instruction about complications is important. These should include signs of infection (fever, dysuria, flank pain), hemorrhage, thrombosis (severe chest or leg pain, leg swelling), and wound dehiscence. Guidelines for contacting the physician or clinic should be given. The client should be instructed that intercourse may be resumed when lochia has ceased and there is no undue abdominal or perineal discomfort. Contraceptive information should be provided as for any other postpartum client. A return visit is usually scheduled for 3 weeks after delivery and another at 6 weeks.

A referral for follow-up by the public health nurse or home care service is appropriate if the nurse observes the mother exhibiting undue difficulty in adapting to her newborn, with teenage mothers with no support system in the home, or when ongoing assistance may be desired.

Vaginal Birth After Cesarean

As previously stated, more women are electing to attempt labor and vaginal birth after a cesarean (VBAC). Safety and feasibility are being demonstrated repeatedly (Aylsworth, 1990). In 1980, the National Institutes of Health's Consensus Development Task Force on Cesarean Childbirth provided guidelines for attempting a VBAC. In 1988, ACOG (1988) elaborated on these guidelines, stressing the individual assessment of candidates and the development of institutional policies for VBAC (Boxes 37-3 and 37-4). In addition, studies have shown that the use of oxytocin augmentation and epidural anesthesia presents no greater risk to the VBAC client than to the client with no history of operative delivery if no other risk factors exist (Chazotte et al., 1990; Harlass et al., 1990).

Careful selection of clients and prudent monitoring of the pregnancy can enhance the chance for successful VBAC. Routine obstetric care provided by physicians or nurse-midwives is essential (Hangsleben et al., 1989). Concurrent medical conditions, such as gestational diabetes, must be successfully managed. In such cases, close observation of fetal weight gain using ultrasound can assist in the detection of a fetus who might be too large to deliver vaginally (Hangsleben et al., 1989).

The primary risk of VBAC is uterine rupture. The rate of dehiscensce of a low transverse scar according to some studies has been 2% to 4% overall (Scott, 1993). The rupture is usually only a small window, but in some cases, it can be a complete rupture, with catastrophic hemorrhage and extrusion of the fetus into the peritoneal cavity. Therefore, it is imperative that the nurse caring for a client uncergoing VBAC knows the symptoms of impending uterine rupture to allow for prompt emergency cesarean (see Chap. 36).

BOX 37–3
Report of the National Institutes of Health Consensus Development Task Force on Cesarean Childbirth

In 1979, the National Institutes of Health convened a Consensus Development Task Force to examine cesarean childbirth. A group of experts from medicine, research, law, social sciences, and the public examined all available evidence about cesareans and arrived at consensus recommendations for practice. In 1980, their report was published with these recommendations for lowering the cesarean birth rate:

1. Labor and vaginal delivery are a safe, relatively low-risk choice after a previous low-segment transverse uterine incision.
2. Trials of labor after previous cesareans should take place in facilities with the capability of a prompt emergency cesarean if necessary. Hospitals that lack such facilities should inform clients in advance and refer them to the nearest fully equipped hospital.
3. Prolonged labor (dystocia) should be treated with such measures as rest, hydration, sedation, ambulation, and oxytocin stimulation before resorting to cesarean.
4. Research should continue into means for evaluating the progress of labor, the effects of conservative treatment of dystocia, and the effects of emotional support and regional anesthesia.
5. Vaginal breech delivery should continue to be an accepted practice with a full-term newborn not expected to be over 8 lb, normal pelvis, frank breech presentation without hyperextended head, and an experienced obstetrician.
6. All clients should have the choice of regional anesthesia.
7. Fathers should be allowed to be present at cesarean births.
8. Parents and newborns should not be routinely separated after birth, unless indicated by the mother's or newborn's condition.
9. Parent education and information about cesareans should be provided during pregnancy by childbirth educators and health professionals.

Clients electing a trial of labor and VBAC should be encouraged to participate in childbirth education classes. Specialized classes for VBAC couples are becoming available across the country. These classes use information provided by the growing research on VBAC and can provide the couple with realistic expectations for the experience. Women experiencing VBAC have been shown to have similar labor patterns to those without a history of cesarean birth. In other words, prior cesarean birth does not affect the time required for the first full labor and vaginal birth (Chazotte et al., 1990).

BOX 37–4

Guidelines for Vaginal Delivery After a Previous Cesarean Birth

Each hospital should develop its own protocol for management of clients who are encouraged to deliver vaginally after a previous cesarean birth. Suggested guidelines include the following:

1. The concept of routine repeat cesarean birth should be replaced by a specific indication for a subsequent abdominal delivery, and in the absence of a contraindication, a woman with one previous cesarean delivery with a low transverse incision should be counseled and encouraged to attempt labor in her current pregnancy.
2. A woman with two or more previous cesarean deliveries with low transverse incisions who wishes to attempt vaginal birth should not be discouraged from doing so in the absence of contraindications.
3. In circumstances in which specific data on risks are lacking, the question of whether to allow a trial of labor must be assessed on an individual basis.
4. A previous classic uterine incision is a contraindication to labor.
5. Professional and institutional resources must have the capacity to respond to acute intrapartum obstetric emergencies, such as performing cesarean delivery within 30 minutes from the time the decision is made until the surgical procedure is begun, as is standard for any obstetric client in labor.
6. Normal activity should be encouraged during the latent phase of labor; there is no need for restriction to a labor bed before actual labor has begun.
7. A physician who is capable of evaluating labor and performing a cesarean delivery should be readily available.

(ACOG [1988]. Guidelines for vaginal delivery after a previous cesarean birth: ACOG Committee Opinion, 64. Washington, DC: ACOG)

Summary Points

✔ Operative obstetrics involves methods to expedite the delivery by using instruments to assist second stage expulsive efforts (forceps or vacuum extractor) or by abdominal surgical intervention (cesarean section).

✔ Indications for cesarean delivery are classified as maternal or fetal, such as dystocia; maternal, such as maternal disease; fetal, such as cord prolapse and fetal distress; or placental, such as placenta previa or abruptio placentae.

✔ Forceps application and use must be done carefully to avoid maternal and fetal complications, injury to maternal soft tissues, unsightly bruising of the fetal face, and more serious injury to the fetal scalp, cranium, or brain. When a vacuum extractor is used, a general rule is that if traction on the suction cup during three contractions has not produced encouraging descent of the fetal head, the trial of vaginal delivery by vacuum extraction should be abandoned.

✔ Low-segment cesarean delivery is usually the operation of choice because there is minimal blood loss, it is easier to repair, there is a decreased chance of rupture of the scar in a subsequent pregnancy, and there is a lower incidence of peritonitis, paralytic ileus, and bowel adhesions.

✔ The main risk of VBAC is uterine rupture. It is imperative that the nurse knows the symptoms of impending rupture so that an emergency cesarean delivery can be done if necessary.

REFERENCES

American College of Obstetrics and Gynecologists (1988). *Guidelines for vaginal delivery after a previous cesarean birth. Committee Opinion No. 64.* Washington, DC: Author.

American College of Obstetricians and Gynecologists (1989). *Obstetric forceps. Committee Opinion No. 71.* Washington, DC: Author.

American College of Obstetricians and Gynecologists (1991). *Elective repeat cesarean: Fetal maturity testing. Committee Opinion No. 71.* Washington, DC: Author.

Aylsworth, J. (1990). Vaginal birth after cesarean section: Where do we stand now? *OB/GYN Nursing and Patient Counseling, 1*(1), 6–8.

Chazotte, C., Madden, R., & Cohen, W. (1990). Labor Patterns in women with previous cesareans. *Obstetrics and Gynecology, 75,* 353–355.

Cunningham, F., Mac Donald, P., Gant, N., Leveno, K. et al. (1993). *Williams obstetrics.* Norwalk, CT: Appleton & Lange.

Hangsleben, K., Taylor, M., & Lynn, N. (1989). UBAC program in a nurse–midwifery service, five years experience. *Journal of Nurse Midwifery, 34*(4), 179–184.

Harlass, F., & Duff, F. (1990). The duration of labor in primiparas undergoing vaginal birth after cesarean delivery. *Obstetrics and Gynecology, 75,* 45–47.

Leung, A., Leung, E., & Paul, R. (1993). Uterine rupture after previous cesarean delivery: Maternal and fetal consequences. *American Journal of Obstetrics and Gynecology, 169,* 945–950.

Newnham, J., & Hobel, C. (1992). Operative delivery. In N. Hacker and J. G. Moore (Eds.), *Essentials of obstetrics and gynecology* (2nd ed.) (pp. 308–315). Philadelphia: W.B. Saunders.

Scott, J. (1993). Cesarean delivery. In J. Scott, P. Disaia, C. Hammond, & W. Spellacy (Eds.), *Danforth's obstetrics and gynecology* (7th ed.) (pp. 563–576). Philadelphia: J.B. Lippincott.

Seiler, J. (1990). The demise of vaginal operative obstetrics: A suggested plan for its revival. *Obstetrics and Gynecology, 75,* 710–712.

38

Postpartum Complications

Objectives

- Identify the common complications associated with the postpartum period.
- Discuss risk factors for postpartum infections.
- Discuss the nursing assessment and care for clients with an infection of the genital tract, postpartum hemorrhage, and a thromboembolic condition.
- Discuss the nursing assessment and care of the client with mastitis.
- Describe the nursing care for the client with urinary tract infection.
- Describe the nursing care for the client with postpartum depression.

Key Terms

Aerobic	Peritonitis
Affective (neurotic) depression	Postpartum hemorrhage
Anaerobic	Postpartum psychosis
Chorioamnionitis	Puerperal infection
Crepitus	Pulmonary embolism
Cystitis	Pyelonephritis
Endometritis	Salpingitis
Mastitis	Thrombophlebitis
Pelvic cellulitis (parametritis)	

The postpartum period is a time of increased physiologic stress and major psychological transition. Energy depletion and fatigue of late pregnancy and labor, soft-tissue trauma from delivery, and blood loss increase the woman's vulnerability to complications. Most women recover from the stresses of pregnancy and childbirth without significant complications. However postpartum complications can occur. The potential seriousness of many postpartum complications; associated pain, procedures, and medications; frequent need to be isolated or separated from the newborn; and emotionally disruptive effects of the physiologic malfunction can interfere with the maternal–newborn bonding process. Using a nursing process framework, this chapter discusses the most common postpartum complications, including infections involving the genital tract, breasts, and urinary system; hemorrhagic and thromboembolic disorders; and postpartum depression.

Infections of the Genital Tract

Puerperal infections, postpartum infections of the genital tract associated with childbirth, usually are the result of bacteria ascending from the genital tract. The bacteria may be commonly found within the genital tract or introduced from the outside. Puerperal infections often remain localized, but they may extend along vascular or lymphatic pathways to produce extensive pelvic or systemic infections. Fever is the principal sign. The course of the illness varies according to the size of the bacterial inoculum, the virulence of the organisms, the pelvic tissues affected, and the host's defense mechanisms, including general health and im-

munologic status. Puerperal infection is one of the most common causes of morbidity in the postpartum period. It is a leading cause of death associated with childbearing.

The postpartum woman is assumed to have an infection if she has an elevated temperature of 39°C (102.2°F) at any time, or 38.0°C (101.4°F) on two successive occasions 4 hours apart after the first 24 hours following delivery. Low-grade temperature elevations are not uncommon and have been attributed to such factors as dehydration, infusion of fetal protein, breast engorgement, and respiratory infection. With vaginal birth, the spontaneous clearance of necrotic decidua and blood from the uterine cavity usually is adequate to remove bacteria. The transient temperature elevation seen in the first 24 hours after delivery represents this process. With cesarean birth, a much higher risk of postpartum infection exists. The woman with a cesarean birth has a 5 to 30 times higher risk for infection than the woman who delivered vaginally (Creasy et al., 1994). Figures 38-1 and 38-2 show febrile patterns of transient temperature elevation in the first 24 hours compared with clinically significant postpartum infection.

Pathophysiology

The exact pathogenesis of postpartum infections is not completely understood. However, many factors are associated with an increased risk of postpartum genital

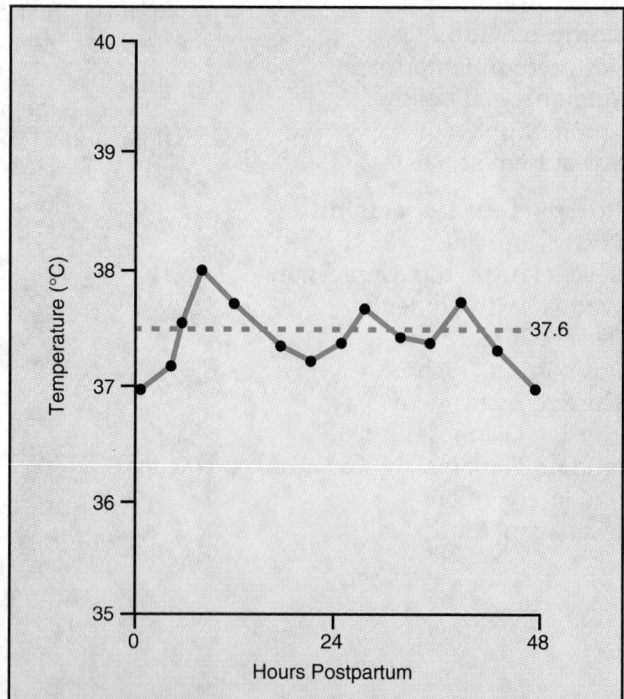

FIGURE 38–1 The pattern of resolving postpartum fever (single spike) after spontaneous vaginal delivery.

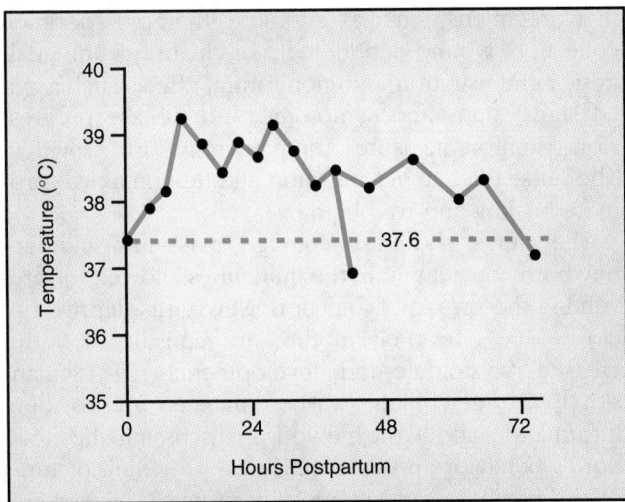

FIGURE 38-2 The pattern of fever (>38.4°C) in the first 3 days postpartum after either spontaneous vaginal delivery or cesarean birth. Fever may persist longer in more serious infections.

tract infection. Cesarean delivery is probably the single greatest risk factor for developing a postpartum infection. Prolonged labor and prolonged rupture of membranes, often associated with a greater number of vaginal examinations, are among the most important factors because they increase the size of the bacterial inoculum. Low socioeconomic status, with related suboptimal prenatal care and nutritional deficiencies, appears to be a key factor in host defense mechanisms (Creasy et al., 1994; Mead, 1990; Box 38-1). Postpartum genital tract infections involve **anaerobic** (not requiring oxygen for growth) and **aerobic** (requiring oxygen for growth) microorganisms, most of which are normal microflora of the vagina and cervix (Charles, 1993). The most common organisms are the aerobic gram-positive cocci (such as *Streptococcus* species) and anaerobic gram-negative bacilli (such as *Bacteroides* species; Gall, 1990; Sweet, 1990). Box 38-2 lists the

most common causative microorganisms. The reappearance of *Streptococcus*, a beta-hemolytic microorganism (Nathan et al., 1993), and the emergence of antibiotic-resistant bacteria are a concern in today's practice. The most frequent soft-tissue infections following vaginal birth include endometritis, salpingitis, tubo-ovarian abscess, pelvic abscess, pelvic cellulitis, and surgical site infection (Gall, 1990).

Nursing Assessment

Postpartum nursing assessment focuses on identifying the signs and symptoms of infections early; monitoring progress and physiologic functions, including uterine involution; noting needs for comfort and education; and identifying emotional reactions and needs.

Any signs and symptoms of infection are noted. Vital signs, condition of perineum and uterus, character of lochia, condition of extremities and breasts, and status of bladder and bowel function are evaluated. The mother's needs for physical comfort, including rest and sleep, nutrition and hydration, and pain relief, are assessed. Information about the client's relationship with the newborn, client and family responses to the complications, and relationship with the husband or partner are collected to complete the psychosocial component of the assessment.

Nursing Diagnoses

The nursing diagnoses identified based on the nursing assessment involve a maturational process (childbirth) and physiologic deficits, such as decreased resistance and tissue trauma. Contributing factors include tissue hypoxia and trauma, pain, fatigue, and altered immune function. Injury from postpartum infections can lead to delayed healing, abscess formation, and serious sequelae, such as septicemia, shock, or death. For a list of possible nursing diagnoses, see Box 38-3.

BOX 38-1
Risk Factors for Developing Postpartum Infections

Related to General Infection Risk	*Related to Labor Events*	*Related to Operative Risk Factors*
Anemia	Prolonged labor	Cesarean delivery
Poor nutrition	Prolonged rupture of membranes	General anesthesia
Lack of prenatal care	Chorioamnionitis	Urgency of operation
Obesity	Intrauterine fetal monitoring*	Breaks in operative technique
Low socioeconomic status	Number of examinations during labor*	Manual placental removal
Sexual intercourse after rupture of membranes	Hemorrhage	Forceps delivery
Immunosuppression		Episiotomy
		Lacerations

*Related to longer labors and high-risk maternal status.

BOX 38–2
Microorganisms Commonly Involved in Postpartum Genital Tract Infections

---

Aerobes	**Anaerobes**
Gram Positive	**Gram Positive**
Streptococcus	*Peptostreptococcus*
Group B	*Peptococcus*
Alpha hemolytic (A)	*Clostridium*
Streptococcus	
Staphylococcus	
Gram Negative	**Gram Negative**
Gardnerella vaginalis	*Bacteroides*
Escherichia coli	*B. bivius*
Klebsiella pneumoniae	*B. disiens*
Proteus mirabilis	*B. fragilis*
Enterobacter	*Fusobacterium*

Sexually Transmitted
Chlamydia trachomatis
Neisseria gonorrhoeae
Mycoplasma hominis
Ureaplasma urealyticum

Nursing Planning and Intervention

Prompt diagnosis and treatment of postpartum infections to minimize serious sequelae and reduce their effects on the client's ability to function are essential. The nurse plays a role in carrying out medical treat-

---

BOX 38–3
Nursing Diagnoses— Puerperal Infections

- Risk for Injury related to
  - Childbirth and physiologic stressors
  - Spread of infection
- Risk for Infection related to
  - Exposure to others or equipment
  - Lack of knowledge of infection transmission
- Pain related to infection site, procedures, or treatments
- Anxiety related to interference with recovery
- Risk for Altered Parenting related to limited contact, pain, or inability to focus attention on neonate
- Risk for Altered Parent/Infant Attachment related to client's inability to bond with neonate
- Situational Low Self Esteem related to infection and interference with caretaking responsibilities
- Knowledge Deficit related to infectious process, treatment regimen, and implications for care of self and neonate

---

ment regimens, such as antibiotic therapy, specimen collection, wound débridement or cleansing, and analgesic administration and monitoring, effects such as vital signs, signs and symptoms, and disease progression. Comfort measures for pain relief are provided. The nurse encourages nutrition and fluid intake to promote healing and well-being.

The nurse should encourage maximum mother–newborn contact within the guidelines allowed for preventing the spread of infection. Newborns deprived of close access to their mother are considered at increased physiologic and developmental risk (Symanski, 1992). Attachment can be enhanced by providing information about the newborn, discussing the newborn's behavior and characteristics, providing pictures of the newborn, and supporting visits to the nursery. As soon as the infection allows, the mother can be assisted to hold and care for her newborn as much as possible.

Teaching about the infectious process and its expected course and treatment is essential. The partner should be involved in these discussions when possible. The nurse can provide support and encouragement for the client or family and assist them to work through fears of the consequences or grief about the effects of the infection on the postpartum experience (see the Nursing Care Plan).

Prevention of Infection

The prevention of infection is important throughout the maternity cycle. Health teaching is emphasized. The client is advised to avoid possible sources of infection, especially upper respiratory tract and urinary tract infections (UTIs) and communicable diseases.

During labor and delivery, care is exercised to limit opportunity for ascending infection from the genital tract and to reduce exposure to exogenous bacteria. Each postpartum client should have her own equipment to reduce the chance of cross-contamination. Careful handwashing after contacts with each client also helps to prevent the transfer of infection from one client to another. Standard precautions are followed for all procedures.

Personnel with an infection of the skin or respiratory tract should not work in the maternity department. The nasopharynx of personnel is a common exogenous source of contamination. To be effective, clean, dry masks covering the nose and mouth are worn during delivery and procedures. They must be changed frequently and should not hang around the neck when not in use.

For many days following delivery, the surface of the birth canal is a vulnerable area for pathogenic bacteria. The nurse inspects the perineum and lochia at least every 8 hours for signs and symptoms of infection. Clients are taught proper principles of perineal care,

NURSING CARE PLAN
The Woman With Postpartum Complications

Nursing Goals

1. Client receives prompt diagnosis and treatment of postpartum complications to minimize risk of morbidity, mortality, and dysfunctional effects.
2. Client indicates comfort is increased by physical care measures and pain relief therapies.
3. Client and family indicate understanding of the complication and integration of the experience.
4. Separation of mother and newborn is minimized and mother–newborn relationship is enhanced through information and support.
5. Client and family indicate ability to deal with anxiety, anger, grief, and fear through self-expression and acceptance.

Assessment (for All Complications)	Potential Nursing Diagnoses	Intervention/ Rationale	Evaluation
Physiologic Assessment Vital signs Patterns of temperature elevation Condition of perineum and uterus Character of lochia Tenderness and pain Condition of legs Condition of breasts Status of bladder and voiding	Risk for complications, such as hemorrhage, urinary tract infection urinary retention, infection of the genital tract, embolism, subinvolution, vulvar hematoma, mastitis related to abnormal conditions of the puerperium Risk for Injury related to physiologic deficits	Monitor for signs and symptoms *to provide a database on the body's response to the insult and to the treatments.* Monitor vital signs *to establish baseline data and the deviation from baseline and from "normal."* Monitor fluids *to enhance hydration and circulation.* Collect specimens *to aid the process of identifying the causative agent(s).* Record and report findings *to enhance collaboration with the team.*	Mother's vital signs are stabilized. Mother voids completely. Mother becomes and remains symptom free.
Physical Comfort Rest and sleep Appetite, nutrition, and hydration Pain or discomfort	Pain related to spread of infection, procedures, incisions, uterine contractions	Provide physical care *to promote comfort (eg, cold–heat therapy, bath, backrub, clean and dry linens, positioning).* Enhance fluid and food intake (relaxed atmosphere, preferences) *to maintain hydration and provide body with its caloric needs.* Administer antibiotics, other medications, and treatments *to combat the infectious organisms and to correct the abnormal state with a return to "normalcy."*	Mother rests and sleeps well. Mother takes adequate fluids and food. Mother reports relief of pain and discomfort.
Psychosocial Assessment Relation to newborn Response to complication Response of partner	Knowledge Deficit related to cause, progress, and care of complication	Encourage maximum mother–newborn contact, and provide continuous information on newborn *to enhance the bonding or attachment process.*	Mother assumes as much caretaking of newborn as condition permits.

(continued)

NURSING CARE PLAN *(Continued)*
The Woman With Postpartum Complications

Assessment (for All Complications)	Potential Nursing Diagnosis	Intervention/ Rationale	Evaluation
Psychosocial Assessment	Altered Parenting related to physical or emotional effects of complication	*To enhance optimal individual and family functioning:* ■ Explain and discuss complication, expected course and treatment. ■ Involve partner in education about complication, relating to newborn, understanding mother's emotional needs, providing support. ■ Respond to needs for support and encouragement, working through grief and fear.	Mother maintains interest in newborn. Mother understands treatment and expected course of complication. Partner understands above and provides support. Mother expresses grief and fear.
Genital Tract Infection Fundal size, consistency, tenderness; lochia odor, character; temperature, condition of perineum, wound, legs	Pain related to progress of infection Knowledge Deficit of self-care related to particular infection	Obtain specimens, report findings, administer antibiotics or medications, monitor signs and symptoms. *Rationale as above. Isolate as needed to prevent the spread of infection.*	Mother is pain free. Mother performs self-care and newborn care.
Hemorrhage Fundal size, consistency, tenderness; amount of lochia, clots, character; pulse and blood pressure; blood loss	Risk for Injury: complications of hemorrhage (tissue damage, cerebral anoxia, death) Altered Tissue Perfusion	Massage uterus, facilitate voiding, report blood loss, prepare for IVs and transfusion, monitor for shock, administer medications and oxygen, keep family informed. *Rationale as stated above.*	Mother returns to stable condition. Mother and family understand events and treatment.
Pulmonary Embolism Respiratory distress and pain, hypotension, cyanosis, hemoptysis	Risk for Injury: complications of pulmonary embolism (cerebral anoxia, death)	Evaluate respiratory status, report signs and symptoms and frequent vital signs, administer medications and oxygen, note response to treatment, obtain specimens, and institute emergency cardiopulmonary resuscitation or therapy if needed. *Rationale as stated above.*	Mother breathes normally. Mother returns to symptom-free condition. Mother's vital signs and cardiopulmonary condition stabilize.
Mastitis Temperature and pulse; swelling, pain, redness of breasts; nipple soreness, fissures; axillary nodes, tenderness	Pain related to infection Knowledge Deficit related to care of breasts Self Esteem Disturbance related to inability to nurse	Obtain specimens for milk culture, report findings, assist at procedures (incision and drainage), change dressings, administer antibiotics or medi-	Mother's vital signs are stable. Mother returns to symptom-free condition. Mother continues nursing.

(continued)

NURSING CARE PLAN *(Continued)*
The Woman With Postpartum Complications

Assessment (for All Complications)	Potential Nursing Diagnosis	Intervention/ Rationale	Evaluation
Mastitis		cines, provide ice packs or hot compresses and comfort measures (support brassiere), and monitor vital signs and progress of healing. *Rationale as stated above.*	
Urinary Retention or Infections Frequency and amount of voiding, dysuria, hematuria, suprapubic or flank pain, temperature and pulse, height and consistency of uterine fundus	Risk for Injury: complications of urinary retention, cystitis, pyelonephritis related to trauma or decreased tonus Pain related to infection	Obtain specimens, report findings, administer antibiotics or medications, insert intermittent or indwelling catheter as needed, note response to treatment, isolate as needed, monitor signs and symptoms. *Rationale as stated above.*	Mother voids normally. Mother is pain free. Mother's vital signs are stabilized.
Thrombophlebitis Pain, swelling, stiffness in leg and calf, temperature, chills	Pain Risk for Injury from embolism	To reduce the risk of embolization, rest and elevate the leg; use bed cradle and handle leg with care; administer prescribed anticoagulants; heat and cold, antibiotics or analgesics, support, and teaching. *Rationale as above.*	Mother is comfortable. Signs of thrombophlebitis improve or resolve. Mother is able to provide self-care and newborn care.

with emphasis on not touching the labia or perineal pad with the fingers and not separating the labia because this permits the cleansing solution to enter the vagina (see Chap. 27). Breast-feeding mothers are taught to inspect their nipples for redness or cracks after each feeding and to report soreness early. Clients are taught to report signs of genital tract infection promptly to their physician or primary care provider.

Evaluation

Anticipated outcomes of nursing care include the following:

- The client's temperature returns to normal.
- Vital signs are within normal limits.
- The client states that appetite has returned.
- The client ambulates without difficulty.
- The client verbalizes no pain at the site of infection.
- The client's uterus and lochia are normal for the stage of involution.

- The client demonstrates self-care and newborn care-taking with minimal assistance. Additionally, the client's partner provides support, and the client resumes breast-feeding if she had been breast-feeding previously.

When alterations in self-esteem or parenting, anxiety, and knowledge deficits are present, nursing care is successful when the mother and partner have worked through their concerns and negative feelings, feel assured of normal functioning, have intergrated the disappointments of experiencing a complication, are ready to assume self- and newborn-care responsibilities, and feel knowledgeable about illness processes, treatment, and recovery.

Infections of the Perineum and Vulva

Infections of the perineum and vulva are localized infections commonly involving a repaired perineal laceration or episiotomy wound. These infections usually are not severe, involve moderate discomfort, and may only minimally affect functioning.

Nursing Assessment

The nurse assesses the client for the usual symptoms, including elevated temperature, pain, and a sensation of heat in the affected area. On inspection, the area involved is red and edematous, the skin edges separate, and seropurulent discharge is present. In some vulval infections, the entire vulva may become edematous, causing the client considerable pain.

Nursing Planning and Intervention

These localized infections seldom cause severe problems, provided that good drainage is established and the client's temperature remains below 38.4°C (101°F). To promote good drainage, the physician removes the sutures and opens the wound. Because the drainage is a source of contamination, care must be taken when handling items possibly contaminated with drainage to prevent the spread of infection. The wound must be kept clean and perineal pads changed frequently. Sitz baths provide pain relief and promote drainage. They also increase circulation to the area, which helps to increase healing. A perineal heat lamp also may be used to provide pain relief. Prescribed antibiotics are administered according to schedule.

The nurse continually observes the wound for healing, noting characteristics of any drainage and condition of the wound site. The presence of fever, malaise, and decreased appetite are recorded and reported. Additional fluid intake to 2,000 mL/d is encouraged. The client is instructed in proper perineal care, pad hygiene, and measures to prevent the spread of infection. She is encouraged to care for and feed her newborn. The client is reassured that the risk of infection to the newborn is minimal when preventive techniques are followed.

Endometritis

Endometritis is a localized infection of the inner uterine wall. It frequently begins at the placental site and may spread to involve the entire endometrium. Following vaginal delivery, about 2% to 3% of women develop endometritis. Prolonged labor and ruptured membranes, which lead to increased colonization of the lower uterine segment due to numerous vaginal examinations, are two important risk factors. Amniotic fluid infection develops in about one-third of women whose membranes are ruptured longer than 6 hours before birth. When risk factors are present, the incidence of vaginal birth endometritis increases to 6%, rising to 13% when **chorioamnionitis**, an inflammation

of the amniotic fluid, is present (Cunningham et al., 1993). Studies have shown that intrauterine fetal monitoring has minimal or no impact on the development of intrauterine infections (Creasy et al., 1994).

Nursing Assessment

When endometritis develops, it is usually manifested 48 to 72 hours after delivery. In the milder forms, the client may have no signs or symptoms other than a rise in temperature above 38°C (100.4°F). This elevated temperature persists for several days and then subsides. More typically, infections are accompanied by lower abdominal pain, uterine tenderness, foul-smelling discharge, higher fever, tachycardia, and leukocytosis (Fig. 38-3). The client often experiences chills, malaise, loss of appetite, headache, and backache. There may be severe and prolonged afterpains. The uterus is usually large and extremely tender when palpated. The lochial discharge may be decreased, red-brown, and foul smelling (see Fig. 38-3). If the infection is caused by hemolytic *Streptococcus*, the lochia usually is odorless.

Nursing Planning and Intervention

Nursing care includes emotional support, client teaching, and family interventions to assist with integrating the experience, working through feelings, and learning about the infection and its treatment. Assistance is provided with self-care and newborn care, and any modifications needed are identified. Medically, endometritis is treated with parenteral antibiotics, using broad-spectrum second- and third-generation cephalosporins or semisynthetic penicillins (Box 38-4). A trend toward using single-agent rather than combination therapy has emerged with the advantages of less toxicity and greater effectiveness. Treatment with antibiotics is continued for 36 to 48 hours after the woman becomes asymptomatic. At this time, she may be discharged home. Continued oral antibiotics are generally unnecessary (Creasy et al., 1994).

The nurse encourages the client to assume the Fowler's position to promote lochial drainage. Oxytocic medications may be ordered (ergonovine or methylergonovine) to promote uterine contractions and aid lochial flow. The nurse monitors the progress of involution, including fundal height and firmess, tenderness, and the amount and characteristics of lochia. The client is encouraged to increase fluids to 3,000 to 4,000 mL/d and eat a well-balanced diet. Temperature, pulse, and blood pressure are taken every 4 hours. The client may be isolated to prevent exposure to other clients and to offer the mother greater rest. The nurse needs to provide supportive understanding to help the client adjust with this separation. If it is necessary for the client to discontinue breast-feeding, such as when the client is

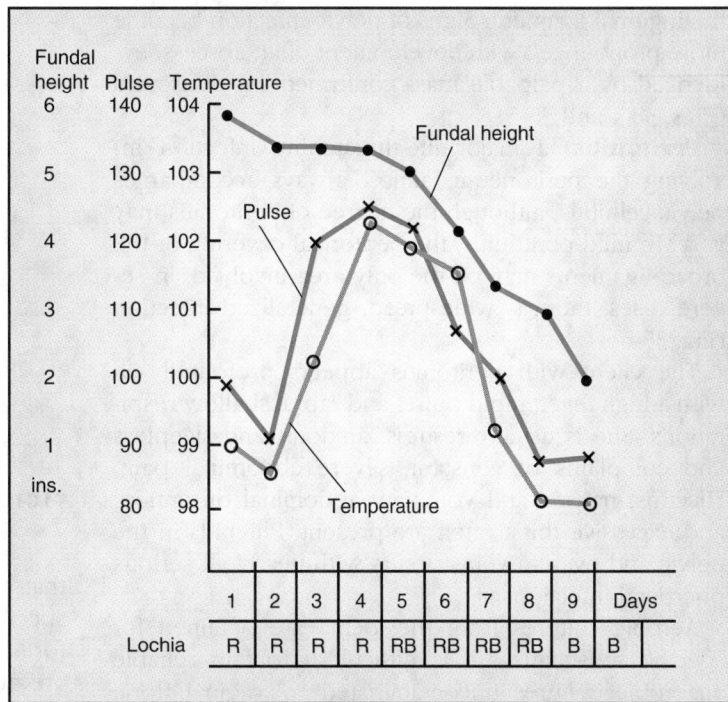

FIGURE 38–3 Febrile pattern in endometritis. The four classic signs of postpartum endometritis are temperature elevation to 38.4°C (101°F), increase in pulse rate (100–120), delayed involution with fundal height not decreasing, and lochia remaining red with foul odor. (R, red; B, brown.)

acutely ill or is receiving an antibiotic that is passed in breast milk and would be harmful to the newborn, the client needs reassurance that the newborn's needs can be met with formula feedings. If breast-feeding is to resume, the nurse instructs the client in manual expression of breast milk to ensure an adequate supply.

BOX 38–4
Antimicrobial Regimens for Treatment of Genital Tract Infections

Combination Regimens

Clindamycin and aminoglycoside

Metronidazole and aminoglycoside

Clindamycin and aztreonam

Clindamycin and gentamicin

Single-Agent Regimens

Cephalosporins and cephamycins
  Cefoxitin
  Cefotetan
  Cefmetazole
  Ceftizoxime
  Cefotaxime
  Moxalactam

Extended-spectrum penicillins
  Mezlocillin
  Piperacillin

Carbapenems
  Imipenem

Beta-lactams and enzyme blockers
  Ampicillin-sulbactam
  Ticarcillin-clavulanic acid

With prompt antibiotic treatment, the infection often resolves, and the client is discharged after 3 to 4 days. The nurse provides discharge teaching, which includes drinking 8 to 10 glasses of water daily, eating a diet high in proteins and vitamins, monitoring for signs of infection, and keeping follow-up appointments.

Pelvic Cellulitis and Peritonitis

Pelvic cellulitis (parametritis) is an infection that extends along the blood vessels and lymphatics to the loose connective tissue of the broad ligament or other pelvic structures. The source of infection may be cervical lacerations, which provide a direct pathway for organisms already found in the cervix to enter the pelvis or endometrium. Ascending organisms from the vaginal microflora are the most common pathogens; usually more than one organism is involved. Pelvic cellulitis usually is unilateral, but it may involve both broad ligaments.

Nursing Assessment

The client has persistent fever that may reach 39.5° to 40°C (103°–104°F), with chills, malaise, and lethargy. The pulse rate is elevated. On examination, the uterus is boggy and tender, limited in mobility, and may be displaced to one side. The client complains of marked abdominal pain on palpation. Laboratory analysis reveals an elevated white blood count, which may reach 30,000/mm³ or more. An abscess may develop in the center of the area of cellulitis, which may extend downward into the posterior cul-de-sac or upward to the inguinal ligament. Signs of pelvic infection become more pronounced with development of an abscess, evidenced by a palpable mass confirmed by ultrasound (Figs. 38-4 and 38-5).

Peritonitis, a major life-threatening infection involving the peritoneum, almost always accompanies pelvic cellutitis, although the degree of peritonitis may vary. In mild peritonitis, the peritoneal covering of the broad ligaments may be the only area involved; in severe cases, there is widespread, generalized infection (Fig. 38-6).

The client with peritonitis appears profoundly ill with a high fever, rapid pulse, and rapid, shallow respirations. She is usually restless, anxious, and sleepless and complains of constant, severe abdominal pain. Hiccups, nausea and vomiting, abdominal distention, and excessive thirst often are present. Phlebitis in the pelvic and ovarian veins occurs with nearly all serious puerperal infections.

Aerobic cultures from the lochia are obtained for specific sensitivities; it is difficult to obtain reliable anaerobic cultures uncontaminated by vaginal flora. Blood cultures may provide useful information, especially in clients who do not respond to standard therapy or who develop an abscess or peritonitis.

Nursing Planning and Intervention

Medically, pelvic cellulitis and peritonitis are treated with antibiotic therapy. If the infection is severe, parenteral antibiotics are used. It is especially important

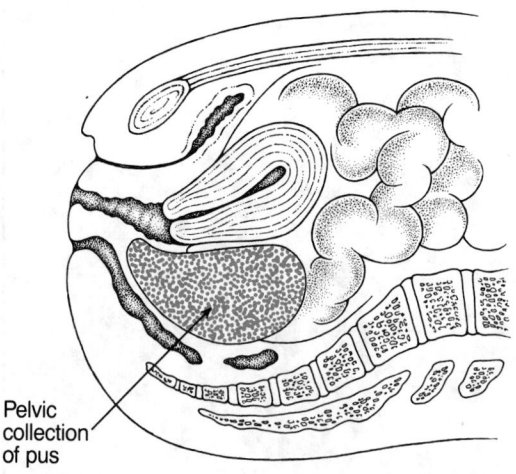

Pelvic collection of pus

FIGURE 38-5 Pelvic abscess.

that the antibiotic be effective against *Enterobacter* species, which commonly cause peritonitis, abscess formation, and sepsis (Sweet, 1990). Analgesic drugs are prescribed for discomfort. Mild sedatives are given to relieve the client's restlessness and apprehension. If there is intestinal involvement, oral feedings are withheld until normal intestinal function is restored. If a paralytic ileus occurs, nasogastric suctioning may be

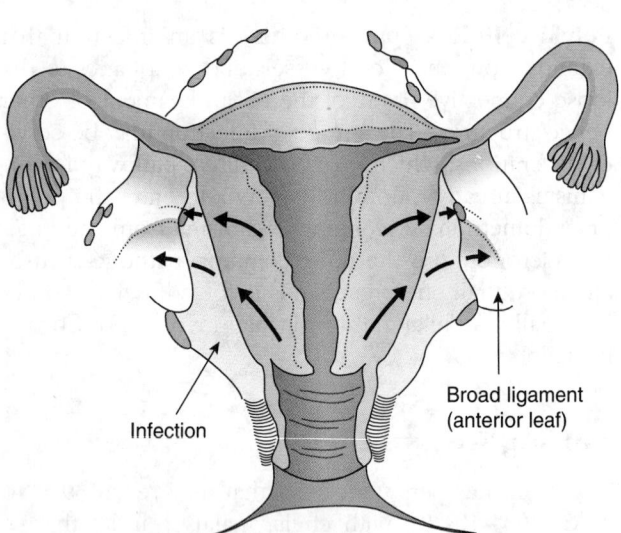

Infection

Broad ligament (anterior leaf)

FIGURE 38-4 Parametritis or pelvic cellulitis. Infection may spread from the uterus, a cervical laceration, or thrombophlebitis into the loose connective tissue. It may extend retroperitoneally in any direction, commonly between leaves of the broad ligament and around the vagina or rectum. Pelvic examination reveals a large, hard mass representing a pelvic abscess in some instances.

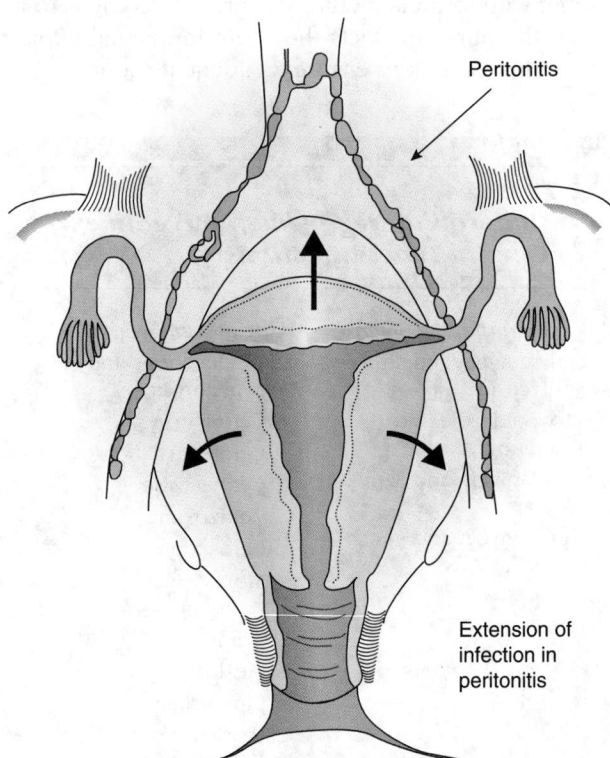

Peritonitis

Extension of infection in peritonitis

FIGURE 38-6 Postpartum peritonitis. The pelvic peritoneum may become involved in an infection in the same ways as the parametrium. Generalized peritonitis may occur with development of paralytic ileus. Although uncommon, peritonitis can be severe and life-threatening.

necessary. Incision and drainage are necessary if an abscess develops. After the abscess is drained, it may be packed with medicated gauze to enhance drainage and promote healing.

The nurse plays a key role in administering and monitoring intravenous fluids, electrolytes, and antibiotic therapy. Intake and output are measured and recorded frequently. Strict aseptic technique is required for wound care following incision and drainage of the abscess. If the client is acutely ill, she may be transferred to the intensive care unit.

Continuous emotional support and guidance are necessary. The client may be frightened by her condition, isolated from others, and unable to care for her newborn. The nurse needs to assist the client with adjusting to her illness and its treatment while helping her adjust to her new role.

Salpingitis

Salpingitis, an infection of the fallopian tubes, may occur following childbirth. Bacteria may ascend from the uterine cavity or spread venously to cause salpingitis. The fallopian tubes become hyperemic and edematous, and purulent discharge often fills the tubal lumina. Tubal abscesses may occur, causing tender adnexal masses (Fig. 38-7). Laparoscopy may be necessary to establish the correct diagnosis. Salpingitis usually is a multibacterial infection, involving *Neisseria gonorrhoeae* and many gram-positive and gram-negative aerobes and anaerobes. Cervical cultures are taken to detect *N. gonorrhoeae.*

Symptoms often resemble peritonitis and include high fever, rapid pulse, nausea and vomiting, and abdominal pain and rigidity. Although usually bilateral, unilateral right-sided salpingitis may occur and mimic

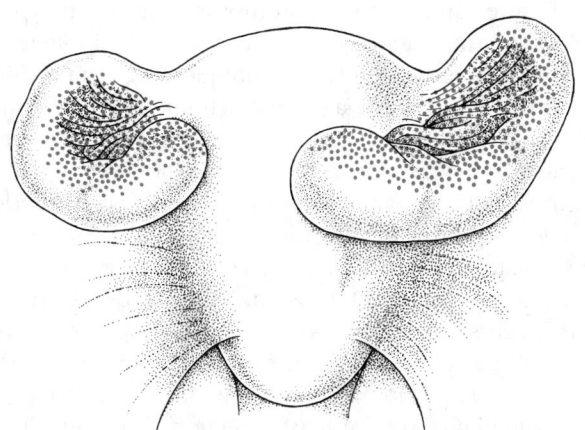

FIGURE 38–7 Postpartum salpingitis. Infection of the fallopian tubes leads to hyperemia, edema, and purulent discharge into the tubal lumina. The tubes are enlarged, swollen, and tender. Tubal abscesses may occur, creating tender adnexal masses.

appendicitis. Problems with tubal patency and subsequent infertility are frequent sequelae of salpingitis.

Infection Following Cesarean Delivery

Cesarean birth significantly increases the risk of genital tract infections, with endometritis occurring in 12% to 51% of these women (Creasy et al., 1994). Despite use of prophylactic antibiotics, 10% to 20% of women with cesarean births will experience endometritis (Stoval et al., 1993). Prolonged rupture of the membranes or prolonged labor contributes to the development of endometritis (Mead, 1990; Soper, 1993).

Bacterial vaginosis, a common vaginal infection in pregnant women associated with high concentrations of *Bacteroides, Peptostreptococcus,* and *Gardnerella vaginalis* organisms, is an important risk factor for postcesarean endometritis. Women with bacterial vaginosis were found to be six times more likely to develop endometritis after cesarean delivery, especially when associated with prolonged ruptured membranes and maternal age less than 20 years (Watt et al., 1990).

Operative trauma also increases the risk of infection. The resultant tissue ischemia and collection of blood and serum in the wound, myometrium, or endometrium play an important role in the development of postpartum endometritis, pelvic abscesses, and incisional wound infections and abscesses.

The incidence of wound infections following primary cesarean birth is 5% to 7% (Eschenbach, 1991). Risk factors for development of wound infections include obesity, diabetes, number of vaginal examinations, length of labor, emergency cesarean, and duration of operation. The organisms causing wound infections are endogenous and commonly include aerobic and anaerobic gram-positive cocci, predominately *Streptococcus, G. vaginalis, Staphylococcus epidermidis, Bacteroides, Escherichia coli,* and rarely *Clostridium.*

Nursing Assessment

The initial signs of wound infection usually begin within 48 hours after surgery with temperature elevation, pain, induration, and erythema of the incision. Areas of swelling often develop and may form into abscesses. Foul odor, the presence of gas in the tissue (**crepitus**), and necrosis of the wound area are present with anaerobic wound infections.

Nursing Planning and Intervention

Each client is evaluated individually for antibiotic prophylaxis when cesarean delivery occurs. Risk of postcesarean infection is increased with prolonged labor, membranes ruptured 6 to 12 hours before surgery, obesity, anemia, and low socioeconomic status. A 1-day, three-dose regimen or a single perioperative dose of cephamycins has been effective in providing prophylaxis (Galask, 1990; Sweet, 1990).

Medical treatment involves the use of broad-spectrum antimicrobial therapy, drainage of abscesses, and complete removal of crepitant and necrotic tissue. The wound may be packed several times daily to keep it open and draining. Intravenous fluids are usually administered. The nurse initiates intravenous infusions, administers antibiotics, performs dressing changes, and monitors physiologic signs, including wound characteristics and drainage, evidence of wound healing, vital signs, and involution progress.

Women undergoing cesarean birth may experience problems with self-esteem, self-concept, altered parenting, anxiety, fear, altered comfort, and altered family processes. They often must grieve the deviations in the childbearing experience caused by a cesarean birth and may feel inadequate as mothers or women. The additional pain, functional limitations, and separation from the newborn may affect mother–newborn bonding and development of caretaking skills. Nursing intervention provides an opportunity for the client and family to express and explore feelings, relive the birth experience, and grieve the loss of a vaginal birth. Emotional support, comfort measures, assistance with newborn caretaking, client teaching, and family counseling may be included in nursing care.

Other Infections

The postpartum client also is at risk for infections other than those of the genital tract. These infections include mastitis and UTIs. Mastitis is common in first-time mothers who are breast-feeding for the first time. UTIs are common because of bladder and urethral trauma and possible catheterization during or after labor.

Mastitis

Mastitis in the postpartum period is an acute infection of the glandular tissue of the breast. It occurs predominantly in breast-feeding mothers. The microorganism most frequently involved in mastitis is *Staphylococcus aureus.* Occasionally it may be caused by group A beta-hemolytic *Streptococcus.* The infection is usually preceded by fissures or erosions of the nipple or areola, providing an entry site for microorganisms into the ductal system. Occasionally, plugged lactiferous ducts are involved, providing a medium for microbial growth. The newborn may be a source of infection having acquired the pathogen orally from the mother's skin or from a healthcare provider. The client's hands

can be a source of infection, particularly when mastitis is caused by other organisms. On occasion, epidemics of mastitis occur when organisms are transmitted by nursery personnel to many newborns and then by newborns to their mothers.

Nursing Assessment

Puerperal mastitis may occur any time during lactation. Daily observation of breasts, including consistency, color, surface temperature, and nipple condition, is crucial to early identification. The nurse also observes the mother breast-feeding to ensure proper technique. Engorgement of the breast may precede mastitis, although engorgement does not cause the infection. The woman usually reports a tender area in one breast that is warm, firm, and red. The client experiences pain in the affected area of the breast and may have malaise, chills, and elevated temperature. The inflammation may be generalized or confined to a lobe or local area of the breast, with induration, tenderness, and erythema. Red streaks may occur along lymphatic channels, and tender, enlarged axillary nodes may be present. Cultures or Gram stains may be taken of breast milk to identify the causative organism. Mastitis is usually unilateral. Without effective treatment, local abscesses may form (Fig. 38-8).

Nursing Diagnoses

Based on the nursing assessment, appropriate nursing diagnoses are identified. For a list of possible nursing diagnoses, see Box 38-5.

Nursing Planning and Intervention

The client usually can prevent mastitis by avoiding nipple fissures and receiving prompt treatment if they develop. Client teaching about breast and nipple care and proper breast-feeding techniques is essential (see Chap. 30). The nurse also instructs the client in signs and symptoms of infection and need for prompt treatment. Nipples are inspected every 8 hours for cracks, fissures, blisters, and excoriated areas. Sore, tender nipples reported by the mother should be inspected immediately. There may be a very small break in the skin surface or slight erosion. Once a break in the skin occurs, the chances of infection are greatly increased. Early identification of mastitis is important to prevent complications and minimize its impact on breast-feeding. Many breast infections are caused by penicillin-resistant staphylococci; antibiotic treatment with oxacillin or cloxacillin, cephalosporins, or vancomycin, depending on microorganism sensitivity, is used. If areas of fluctuation or abscesses develop, these must be incised and drained. Cold and heat therapy also is used. The nurse administers antibiotics, per-

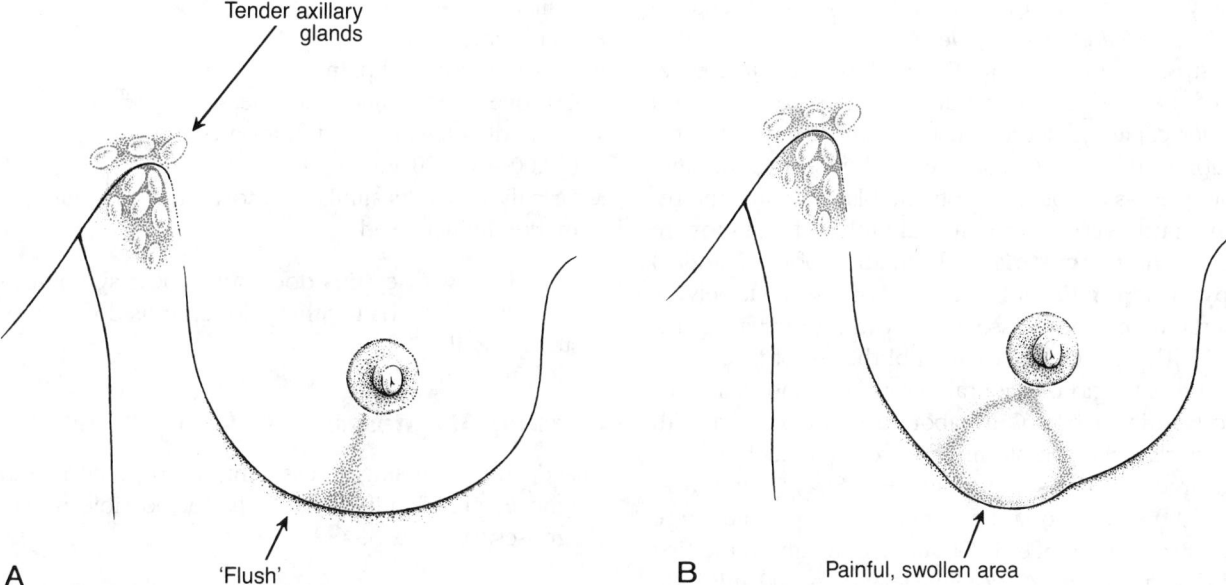

FIGURE 38–8 Mastitis. (**A**) Early mastitis. Fever is followed by a painful area on the breast and a "flush" that is red and tender but not fluctuant or swollen. (**B**) Overt inflammation in mastitis. A swollen, painful, red-to-brawny area develops. The purulent drainage gradually localizes into an abscess; when fluctuant, it must be incised and drained.

forms dressing changes following incision and drainage, and monitors the client's wound for signs of healing. With effective antibiotic therapy, the infection can often be controlled within 24 hours.

Opinions about whether or not to discontinue breast-feeding vary. When the client's fever is high or an abscess develops requiring incision and drainage, it is recommended that she temporarily stop breast-feeding. To maintain lactation, the client is encouraged to express milk from the affected breast every few hours once the pain has subsided. The client also is encouraged to wear a firm supportive brassiere for breast support.

If breast-feeding is discontinued, it should be resumed as soon as the temperature is normal and the signs of infection (pain, redness, edema) have decreased. If a decision has been made to discontinue breast-feeding, the woman's acceptance, adjustment to formula feeding, and alterations in role and self-concept are explored. Emotional support and guidance are provided to help the client cope with these changes.

Nursing Evaluation

Anticipated outcomes of nursing care for the client with mastitis include the following:

- The client demonstrates proper breast and nipple care and breast-feeding techniques.
- The client verbalizes the signs and symptoms of mastitis.
- The client verbalizes a decrease in pain in affected breast.
- The client demonstrates evidence of resolving infection.
- The client verbalizes acceptance of condition.
- The client demonstrates positive coping behaviors.

Urinary Tract Infections

The physiologic urinary stasis, dilatation of the ureters, and vesicoureteral reflux that occur during pregnancy persist for several months after delivery. Therefore, the client remains as vulnerable to UTIs postpartum as she was in the prenatal period (Stray-Pedersen et al., 1990). UTIs occur in about 5% of postpartum clients and are

---

BOX 38–5
Nursing Diagnoses—Mastitis

- Knowledge Deficit related to
  - Care of the breasts
  - Proper breast-feeding techniques
  - Prevention of infection
- Pain related to inflammation and infection
- Anxiety related to effect of infection on breast-feeding
- Interrupted breast-feeding related to infection and pain
- Altered Parenting related to client's inability to continue breast-feeding
- Risk for Altered Parent/Infant Attachment related to possible isolation from newborn
- Situational Low Self Esteem related to client's inability to continue breast-feeding

usually caused by coliform bacteria (*E. coli,* enterococci, *Klebsiella pneumoniae*).

Postpartum urinary retention and incomplete emptying of the bladder are common because of increased bladder capacity, decreased tone, and decreased perception of the urge to void caused by perineal trauma. If the client is unable to empty the bladder fully, the remaining urine is a culture medium for bacterial growth, often leading to **cystitis** (inflammation of the bladder) or **pyelonephritis** (inflammation of the renal pelvis).

Certain factors are associated with an increased risk of UTI. These include cesarean birth, use of forceps or vacuum extraction, epidural anesthesia, and catheterization during labor. Only about 20% of women with bacteriuria have symptoms of lower UTI, such as dysuria, urgency, and suprapubic pain (Stray-Pedersen et al., 1990). It is common for women to void large amounts of urine (500–1,000 mL) frequently in the first few days postpartum. Voiding less than 300 mL indicates urinary retention.

Nursing Assessment

A thorough history and physical examination are important to identify possible risk factors predisposing the client to UTIs. The nurse is alert to possible signs and symptoms of cystitis and pyelonephritis.

Postpartum screening for bacteriuria is routinely performed in many facilities. The diagnosis is by cultures of voided midstream urine specimens and confirmed by urine culture. Sensitivity studies usually are performed to identify the appropriate antibiotic to treat the causative organism.

Signs and symptoms of cystitis include the following:

- Burning or pain on urination
- Urgency
- Frequency
- Suprapubic tenderness
- Low-grade fever

Urinalysis examines the following:

- Leukocytosis
- Red blood cells
- Bacteria

Urine culture reveals the following:

- Positive results

Signs and symptoms of pyelonephritis include the following:

- Dysuria
- Urgency
- Frequency
- Temperature elevation to 40° to 41°C (104°–106°F), spiking then dropping

- Chills
- Flank pain
- Lower abdominal pain
- Costovertebral angle tenderness
- Markedly elevated white blood count (20,000–30,000/mm^3)
- Urinalysis results similar to those of cystitis but markedly increased

The client with cystitis does not appear systemically ill; however, the client with pyelonephritis does appear systemically ill.

Nursing Diagnoses

Based on the nursing assessment, appropriate nursing diagnoses are identified. For a list of possible nursing diagnoses, see Box 38-6.

Nursing Planning and Intervention

The nurse plays a key role in preventing UTIs and identifying the signs and symptoms of infection as soon as possible. Crucial to this role is client teaching. See Client Teaching Guidelines: Preventing Urinary Tract Infections for a list of topics to address.

The client should void within 6 hours after delivery (see Chap. 27). If she has not voided within 8 hours, depending on the degree of bladder distention, catheterization may be necessary. When the mother voids in small amounts (less than 300 mL) at frequent intervals, an overflow of residual urine is indicated, especially when there is some bladder fullness and suprapubic discomfort. The client usually is catheterized after each voiding until the residual urine becomes less than 30 mL. If necessary, intermittent catheterization may be indicated. Catheterization for residual urine, to be completely accurate, must be done within 5 minutes after the client voids. If 100 mL or more of urine still remains in the bladder, voiding is considered incomplete. Immediately after voiding, uterine assessment reveals

---

BOX 38–6
Nursing Diagnoses—Urinary
Tract Infections

- Pain related to dysuria from infection
- Altered Urinary Elimination related to postpartum urinary stasis and infection.
- Knowledge Deficit related to
  - Prevention of urinary tract infection
  - Infection, treatment, and possible sequelae
- Risk for Altered Parenting related to infection and interference with bonding

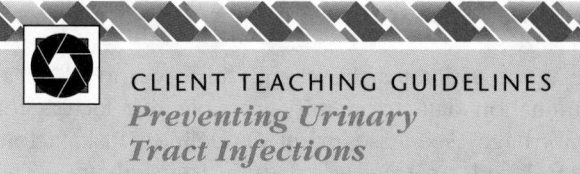

the uterus located higher in the abdomen and to the side of midline, indicating inadequate voiding.

The nurse can institute measures to improve bladder function, thereby decreasing residual urine. The client is encouraged to try to void every 2 to 4 hours and not to delay voiding when she feels the urge. To promote voiding, the client is helped to the bathroom or bedside commode or is assisted on the bedpan if she cannot ambulate. Running water in the sink, pouring warm water over the perineum, or helping her to sit in a sitz bath can help stimulate voiding.

The client is encouraged to rock back and forth slowly on the commode to promote complete bladder emptying. Increasing ambulation and instructing the client in Kegel exercises also can be helpful.

When symptoms of cystitis or pyelonephritis are present, nursing care includes collecting urine specimens, either by voided clean-catch midstream specimens or catheterization. Because catheterization increases the risk of infection, a clean-catch midstream voided specimen often is preferred. Uncontaminated specimens can be obtained if done carefully under the continued supervision of the nurse. In addition, the nurse initiates nonpharmacologic measures for comfort and promotes proper nutrition, hydration, and rest. Careful monitoring of intake and output also is necessary to prevent the possibility of hypovolemic shock.

Medical treatment centers on the use of antibiotic therapy. Commonly used antibiotics include amoxicillin or ampicillin; for penicillin allergy or resistant bacteria, cephalexin, sulfamethoxazole-nitrofurantion, or sulfamethoxazole-trimethoprim are used. Medication usually is administered orally, except in acute febrile pyelonephritis, in which intravenous antibiotics are often used. Antispasmodics and analgesics also may be ordered to relieve discomfort. Symptoms usually are relieved within 24 to 48 hours. Treatment is

continued for 10 days to 2 weeks. Repeat urine cultures are performed following the course of therapy to be certain the urine is free of organisms. The nurse is responsible for instituting medical treatment in a timely matter as prescribed to minimize the risk of ascending infection and the development of a systemic infection.

If the client is unable to void, an indwelling urinary catheter may be necessary. Clients with indwelling catheters for longer than 4 days have a significantly higher incidence of bacteriuria. Almost all such infections are caused by *E. coli*. Clients with indwelling catheters for longer than 24 hours usually are treated with prophylactic antibiotic therapy.

The necessity of treating asymptomatic bacteriuria in nonpregnant women is controversial. Among postpartum women, about 30% have persistent asymptomatic bacteriuria, predisposing them to pyelonephritis resulting from the physiologic changes occurring during pregnancy that are not yet resolved. Asymptomatic postpartum women with positive midstream voided urine specimens should have repeat evaluations. With confirmed bacteriuria, a 3-day course of antibiotic therapy should be sufficient to clear the urine of bacteria (Stray-Pedersen et al., 1990).

Anticipated outcomes of nursing care for the client with a postpartum UTI include the following:

- The client verbalizes understanding of the signs and symptoms of UTI.
- The client identifies measures to prevent UTI.
- The client verbalizes relief of pain on urination.
- The client reports that the bladder feels empty after voiding.
- The client resumes bonding with the neonate.

Hemorrhagic and Thromboembolic Complications

After delivery, the woman's cardiovascular system undergoes substantial changes back to prepregnant conditions. Reductions in cardiac output and blood volume occur after the first 48 hours, with most changes occurring by 2 weeks postpartum. The increase in coagulation factors associated with pregnancy continues postpartum. Fibrinogen and thromboplastin remain elevated for 3 weeks after delivery (see Chap. 25). Postpartum women are at increased risk for hemorrhage and thromboembolic problems.

Postpartum Hemorrhage

Postpartum hemorrhage, the blood loss of more than 500 mL, complicates 5% to 10% of vaginal deliveries and is a leading cause of maternal mortality (Veronikis et al., 1994). Immediate postpartum hemorrhage occurs during the first 24 hours after delivery. It most commonly is the result of uterine atony caused by overdistention during pregnancy or factors complicating labor and delivery. Hemorrhage also may be delayed, occurring more than 24 hours after delivery. Late hemorrhage most frequently occurs between the 5th and 15th postpartum day, but it can occur as long as 6 weeks after delivery. Delayed and late postpartum hemorrhage usually occur suddenly and may be so massive that they produce hypovolemia. Late postpartum hemorrhage is uncommon, occurring in less than 1% of deliveries (American College of Obstetricians and Gynecologists, 1990).

The most frequent causes of delayed and late postpartum hemorrhage are subinvolution of the placental site, retained placental tissue, and infection. Regeneration of the placental site takes longer (about 42 days) than the rest of the endometrium (about 21 days). Until the site is firmly epithelialized, sloughing of clots may cause bleeding. Certain factors are associated with clot sloughing and hemorrhage, including low-grade fever, a history of abortion, uterine bleeding during pregnancy, and not breast-feeding.

Placental fragments that have been retained may become necrosed. As fibrin is deposited and builds up, pseudopolyps can form. When pseudopolyps become detached, brisk bleeding may occur from the placental site, which has not accomplished adequate hemostasis. This leads to delayed or late postpartum hemorrhage.

Nursing Assessment

The nurse evaluates the client's history and physical examination data to identify possible risk factors for hemorrhage (see Assessment Guidelines: Risk factors for Delayed or Late Postpartum Hemorrhage). The condition of the fundus, amount of bleeding, and lochial flow are observed carefully in these clients during the postpartum period.

Hemorrhage may be signaled by a sudden, profuse outpouring of blood from the vagina or a very large pool of blood found under the mother's hips. Often hemorrhage is steady, heavier than usual vaginal bleeding that continues for hours. It may not be immediately recognized as hemorrhage, especially if the fundus is well contracted. A steady flow of blood from the vagina when the uterus is firmly contracted indicates bleeding from cervical or vaginal lacerations. The presence of clots in vaginal blood indicates heavy bleeding or pooling of blood in the vagina. Restlessness, anxiety, and thirst also can indicate excessive bleeding. As blood loss increases, signs and symptoms of hypovolemic shock become more pronounced (see Assessment Guidelines: Assessing Extent of Hemorrhage).

Because of compensatory cardiovascular mechanisms, changes in pulse rate and blood pressure may not occur until a large amount of blood has been lost (up to 1,500 mL). Cardiac output remains adequate until about 15% to 20% of the woman's total blood volume has been lost. After this, pulse and blood pressure may change suddenly as cardiac output and stroke vol-

ASSESSMENT GUIDELINES
Risk Factors for Delayed or Late Postpartum Hemorrhage

Prior History	*Related to Present Pregnancy and Labor*
High parity (grand multipara)	Overdistention of the uterus (multiple pregnancy, polyhydramnios, macrosomic newborn)
Prior postpartum hemorrhage	
Uterine fibroids	Bleeding problems (placenta previa, abruptio placentae)
Systemic diseases (leukemia, idiopathic thrombocytopenia, coagulation defects)	Labor or delivery trauma (midforceps, cesarean delivery, intrauterine manipulation)
	Hypertonic–hypotonic contractions (precipitate, dysfunctional, prolonged labor)
	Deep anesthesia
	Pregnancy-induced hypertension
	Chorioamnionitis
	Subinvolution

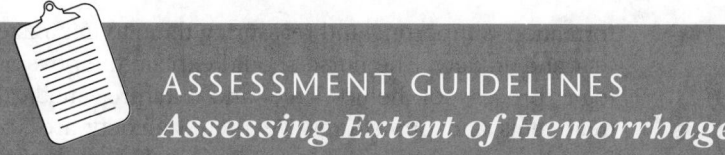

ASSESSMENT GUIDELINES
Assessing Extent of Hemorrhage

Signs and Symptoms	Blood Volume Loss
Uterus boggy	15%–20% reduction (750–1,250 mL)
Blood pressure normal or slightly decreased	
Pulse rate normal or slightly elevated	
Mild vasoconstriction (cool hands, feet)	
Normal urinary output	
Aware, alert, oriented, may have anxiety	
Atonic uterus	25%–35% reduction (1,250–1,750 mL)
Systolic blood pressure < 90 to 100 mm Hg	
Moderate tachycardia 100 to 120 beats/min	
Moderate vasoconstriction (skin pallor, cold, moist extremities)	
Decreased urinary output (oliguria)	
Increased restlessness, may become disoriented	
Atonic uterus	35%–50% reduction (1,800–2,500 mL)
Systolic blood pressure < 60 mm Hg, may be unobtainable by cuff	
Severe tachycardia > 120 beats/min	
Pronounced vasoconstriction (extreme pallor, cold, clammy, cyanotic lips and fingers)	
Urinary output ceases (anuria)	
Mental stupor, lethargy, semicomatose	

ume decrease. By the time significant tachycardia (100–120 beats/min) and hypotension occur (<90–100 mm Hg systolic), the woman has lost about 25% to 35% of her blood volume.

When hemorrhage is suspected, the nurse should monitor the pulse rate and blood pressure every 5 to 10 minutes. Because these signs may not change in early hypovolemic shock while the client is supine, the nurse can help the client sit up. This may produce dizziness, hypotension, and tachycardia, indicating substantial blood loss and shock. The nurse should be alert to women with pregnancy-induced hypertension (PIH) who may appear to have normal blood pressure in early hypovolemic shock. However, these women develop symptoms of shock earlier than women with normal blood pressure readings because PIH causes an interstitial fluid shift that rapidly produces hypovolemia.

Nursing Diagnoses

After completing the nursing assessment, the nurse can identify possible nursing diagnoses. For a list of possible nursing diagnoses, see Box 38-7. The nurse should be alert to the possible collaborative problem of hypovolemic shock and potential complications of it, such as brain and kidney damage, cardiac arrest, and possibly death.

Nursing Planning and Intervention

Identification and correction of the cause of bleeding are essential for treatment. Postpartum hemorrhage and shock are treated with immediate intravenous fluid administration to replace circulatory volume and to serve as a quick route for intravenous medications, particularly oxytocins to help contract the uterus. The nurse administers the intravenous fluids and anticipates medication orders. Oxygen may be administered in severe emergencies when a large blood volume has been lost. The client is often placed in Trendelenburg position to increase venous blood return to the heart and maximize cardiac output.

The nurse monitors vital signs every 5 to 10 minutes and observes the client's color, oxygen saturation by pulse oximetry, skin temperature, and sensorium. The fundus is palpated for firmness and massaged to restore tone when indicated. The amount of vaginal bleeding is evaluated, noting the extent of perineal pad saturation in a given period, color and consistency of bleeding, clots, and pooling on the underpad.

Intravenous or intramuscular medications are administered as ordered, and their effects are monitored. Blood transfusions are administered to replace blood loss. If bleeding is not controlled, surgery may be necessary to determine and halt the source of bleeding. Cervical or vaginal lacerations may need to be sutured. A curettage usually is the first procedure in which retained placental fragments are removed. Severe, uncontrolled bleeding from a uterine source may require a hysterectomy to save the woman's life. The nurse assists with preparations for these surgical procedures.

The nurse needs to use a calm, reassuring manner when caring for clients experiencing hemorrhage. The family or partner should be encouraged to remain with the client to the extent possible. Nursing care includes responding to the woman's and family's needs for in-

formation, supporting and reassuring them to minimize fear and anxiety. The nurse should explain the physiologic process of hemorrhage and interpret medical treatments and procedures. Fears and anxiety are acknowledged, and reassurance is given that all necessary measures are being taken. Once hemorrhage is controlled, the nurse assists the woman and family to understand what happened and why; to anticipate what impact this complication will have on the postpartum course, caretaking, and self-care activities; and to plan for special needs at home. Complications that may occur as an aftermath of hemorrhage, such as infection or persistent weakness, are discussed. The normal progression of lochia is reviewed, and the need to contact the physician if bleeding recurs or fever develops is emphasized.

In cases of delayed or late postpartum hemorrhage when the mother must return to the hospital, the beginning relationship with the newborn is upset. Much of the mother's anxiety or desire to return home as quickly as possible may arise from the often abrupt and temporary arrangements that she has had to make. Understanding and counseling the mother about these concerns and helping with planning can relieve much anxiety. Arrangements for the mother to get adequate rest after her return home also are helpful.

Evaluation

Intervention for postpartum hemorrhage is successful when the bleeding is controlled and blood is replaced as necessary to maintain the client's health and strength.

Possible anticipated outcomes of nursing care for the client with postpartum hemorrhage include the following:

- Client's vital signs and laboratory values will return to normal limits.
- The client and family express understanding of the complication and its treatment.
- The client and family demonstrate ability to integrate this experience psychologically and emotionally.
- The client resumes newborn care-taking and self-care activities.
- The client states that pain is relieved or minimized.
- The client verbalizes resolution of fears and anxiety.

Pulmonary Embolism

Pulmonary embolism is usually caused by a thrombus fragment (embolus) carried by venous circulation to the right side of the heart. It occurs once in every 2,500 to 3,000 deliveries. The thrombus usually originates in a uterine or a pelvic vein. When the embolus occludes the pulmonary artery, it obstructs the passage of blood into the lungs, and the client may die of asphyxia within a few minutes. If the clot is small, the initial episode may not be fatal, but recurrent emboli increase the mortality risk. Emboli may follow infection, thrombosis, severe hemorrhage, or shock.

Nursing Assessment

Prompt assessment of the client with a pulmonary embolus is crucial. Symptoms associated with smaller pulmonary emboli include sudden onset of chest pain, cough or the feeling of the need to clear the throat, and expectoration of blood-streaked mucus. Larger pulmonary emboli cause sudden, intense chest pain, severe dyspnea, air hunger, apprehension, syncope, hemoptysis, tachypnea, pallor, cyanosis, and irregular or faint pulse. Fever, tachycardia, disphoresis, and hypotension may occur. The client often reports headache or lethargy and may experience confusion, restlessness, and anxiety. Respiratory or cardiac arrest may occur. With severe pulmonary obstruction, death may result within a few minutes or hours.

Nursing Planning and Intervention

When embolism occurs, emergency measures to combat anoxia and shock must be carried out promptly. Cardiopulmonary resuscitation may be necessary. Diagnosic tests include chest x-ray, electrocardiogram, arterial blood gasses, lung scan, and pulmonary angiography. Shock and acid–base imbalances are treated, and anticoagulants are often administered. Intravenous morphine or meperidine (Demerol) may be given to help relieve the client's apprehension and pain.

During the acute, life-threatening phase, the nurse monitors blood pressure, pulse, and respirations every 5 minutes. An intravenous infusion is initiated; dextran is infused, and defibrinating agents, such as streptokinase, urokinase, and tissue plasminogen activator are administered. Skin color, breathing difficulty, and neck vein distention are assessed. The chest is auscultated for rales, friction rub, or atelectasis. The nurse prepares the client for diagnostic testing and assists with collection of specimens and performance of procedures. The client and family are kept informed about the client's progress, diagnosis, and treatment. Support, encouragement, and reassurance are provided as much as possible to allay anxiety and apprehension.

Once the crisis phase and need for hospitalization are over, anticogagulant therapy with heparin or warfarin is continued to prevent recurrent emboli. The length of treatment with anticoagulant therapy depends on the client's clinical response lasting from 6 weeks to 6 months. The mother–newborn relationship may be severely disrupted because of the mother's acute, life-threatening complication. Nursing measures are instituted to provide information, reduce knowledge deficits, allay anxiety, and minimize alterations in parenting.

Thrombophlebitis

Thrombophlebitis is an infection of the vascular endothelium with clot formation attached to the vessel wall. The veins of the leg, including the femoral, popliteal, and saphenous veins, are most often involved. Septic pelvic thrombophlebitis involving the ovarian and uterine veins may accompany severe pelvic infections (Fig. 38-9).

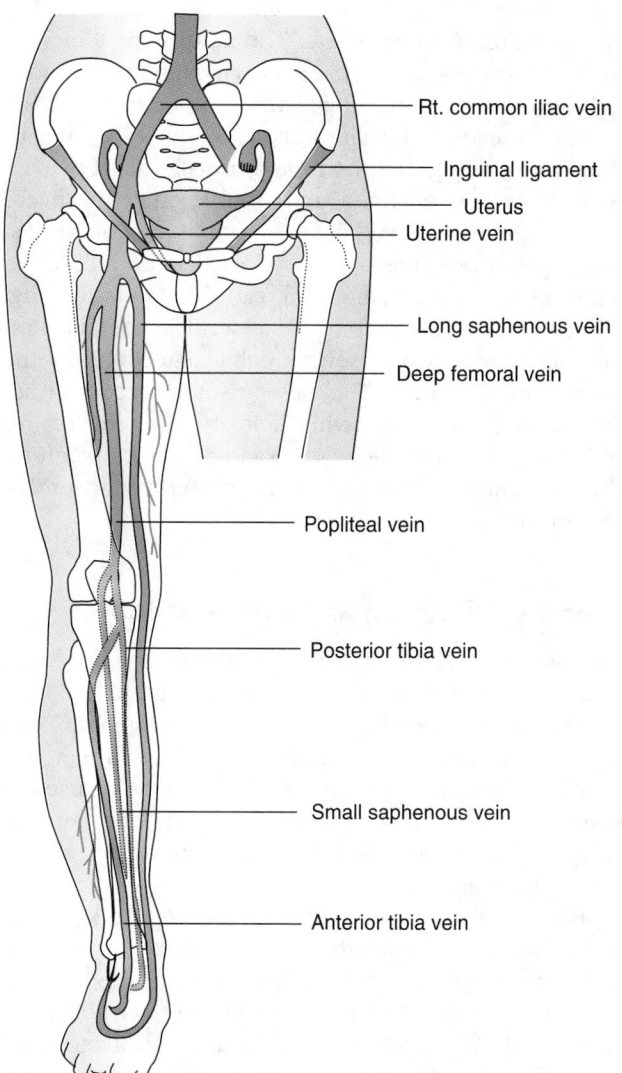

Rt. common iliac vein

Inguinal ligament

Uterus
Uterine vein

Long saphenous vein

Deep femoral vein

Popliteal vein

Posterior tibia vein

Small saphenous vein

Anterior tibia vein

FIGURE 38–9 Sites of postpartum thrombophlebitis. Pelvic thrombophlebitis involves the uterine and ovarian veins. Femoral thrombophlebitis involves the femoral, popliteal, and long saphenous veins. When the small saphenous vein is involved, the term is *phlebothrombosis*, because the thrombus is caused more by stasis than infection, although deep calf thrombi do become infected.

Nursing Assessment

Femoral thrombophlebitis usually appears about 10 days after delivery. However, it can occur as late as the 20th day postpartum. It is characterized by pain, stiffness, pale skin, and swelling of the calf or thigh. These symptoms result from the formation of a clot in the veins interfering with blood return. The woman often experiences malaise, chills, and fever. As with acute febrile diseases occurring after labor, the secretion of milk may cease.

The client usually complains of pain. Pain may begin in the groin or the hip and extend downward, or it may begin in the calf of the leg and extend upward. In about 24 hours after the onset of pain, the leg begins to swell, and the pain may decrease. Often pain is severe enough to prevent sleep. The skin over the swollen area is shiny white. The acute symptoms last from a few days to a week, after which the pain gradually subsides, and the client slowly improves.

The course of the illness is 4 to 6 weeks. The affected leg slowly returns to its normal size. However, it may remain enlarged and troublesome. In severe cases, abscesses may form. Possible complications, such as serious infections or clots that may dislodge causing pulmonary embolism, can be life-threatening.

Pelvic thrombophlebitis is a serious complication and may accompany severe pelvic infections in the postparturm period. The onset usually occurs about the second week following delivery with severe, repeated chills and dramatic swings in temperature. The infection is baterial, usually caused by anaerobic organisms.

Nursing Planning and Intervention

Treatment of femoral thrombophlebitis consists of rest, elevation of the affected leg, and analgesics as indicated for pain. Anticoagulants, such as heparin and dicumarol, may be prescribed to prevent further formation of thrombi. Antimicrobial drugs may be used to treat abscesses or generalized infection. The nurse is responsible for administering medications and monitoring their effects.

Bed rest with a bed cradle can be used to keep the pressure of the bedclothes off the affected part. Heat or cold therapy also may be applied along the affected vessels. The affected part should not be rubbed or massaged. When changing dressings, applying bandages, making the bed, or giving a bath, the leg is handled with care to avoid trauma and dislodgement of the clot.

Surgical treatment may be indicated in some cases that are severe or do not respond to treatment measures. Incision of the affected vessel, removal of the clot, and repair of the vessel is performed. Ligation of the major vessels may be necessary as a preventive measure for pulmonary embolism. Devices such as an umbrella filter or Greenfield filter can be inserted transvenously to catch the embolism.

Women with pelvic thrombophlebitis are often ill. Breast-feeding may be interrupted, and the significant emotional and physiologic changes following childbirth may be compounded by the illness. Antimicrobial therapy with broad-spectrum antibiotics and anticoagulant therapy are used.

Nursing care for the client with pelvic thrombophlebitis includes accurate observation, recording, and reporting of signs and symptoms. The nurse is responsible for monitoring progress of the illness and assessing to prevent and detect complications. Physical care focuses on comfort, fluid intake, and prevention of further complications. Supportive care to help the mother and family work through possible feelings of depression and discouragement is provided.

Vulvar Hematomas

Blood may escape into the connective tissue beneath the skin covering the external genitalia or beneath the vaginal mucosa to form vulvar or vaginal hematomas. Hematomas occur once in every 500 to 1,000 deliveries and are usually caused by rupture or trauma to blood vessels without laceration of the superficial tissues. Delayed hematoma formation can result from sloughing of a necrotic blood vessel that was damaged by prolonged pressure during childbirth. Smaller hematomas may reabsorb spontaneously. Large hematomas require immediate attention because they can produce tissue necrosis, rupture, and profuse bleeding.

Nursing Assessment

Vulvar hematomas cause severe perineal pain with a tense, fluctuant, and sensitive tumorlike swelling of varying size covered by bluish-black skin. Vaginal hematomas may temporarily escape detection, but the client's pain and difficulty voiding alert the nurse to this complication. The client often reports perineal, vagina, bladder, or rectal pressure that is not relieved by analgesia.

Nursing Planning and Intervention

Small hematomas are usually treated supportively and allowed to resolve on their own. Heat and cold therapy can be used for pain relief. If pain is severe or the hematoma enlarges, incision and evacuation of the blood with ligation of bleeding points is required. Because of possible cardiovascular instability, clients may receive general anesthesia for this procedure (Varner,

1991) rather than a regional anesthetic (ie, epidural or spinal), which may increase the hypotension. Following evacuation of deep hematomas, drains may be inserted. Large genital hematomas nearly always result in a blood loss that is more than the clinical estimate. Hypovolemia and anemia are prevented by using blood replacement as necessary.

Vulvar or vaginal hematomas, particularly those that are opened and drained, may become infected. Aseptic technique and teaching the client about proper perineal and bowel hygiene help to reduce the risk of infection. Dressings or perineal pads must be changed frequently. Client observation to detect early signs of infection, such as foul-smelling discharge or temperature elevation, is essential. Any signs must be reported at once. The use of broad-spectrum antibiotics may be necessary.

Postpartum Depression

During the postpartum period, women may experience a wide range of emotional responses, with depression being a central feature of these responses. Women may exhibit the mild, transitory "blues"; a deeper, often incapacitating depression; or a severe depression with psychotic aspects. The literature commonly refers to these mood disorders as "the blues," postpartum depression, and postpartum psychosis (Beck, 1992; Ugarriza, 1992). However, absent from the literature are clear and consistent definitions of these states. Landy et al. (1989) have described three such emotional responses and added a fourth description: depression in the woman with a borderline personality (Table 38-1).

Depression in the postpartum period transcends culture with no appreciable difference in incidence found between women in western developed countries and other developing countries (Unterman et al., 1990). The frequency of depression increases with time after birth; 8.5% of women exhibit signs of depression in the first several days. By 12 weeks, 14.2% exhibit signs of depression. The overall rate of depression in postpartum women is 10.4% (Unterman et al., 1990).

Postpartum Blues

The most common type of depression in the postpartum woman is postpartum blues, an adjustment disorder to a life event (childbirth). Women experience a depressed mood during this transitory condition, which lasts from 1 to 14 days, with symptoms peaking on day 5 (Beck et al., 1992). Women feel "down" and cry easily for no apparent reason. Many women have pronounced fatigue, poor concentration, and feelings of loss, sadness, and hostility toward their partners. Current research indicates a possible link between se-

vere postpartum blues and later postpartum depression (Hannah et al., 1992; Pop et al., 1993).

Severe Postpartum Depression

Affective (neurotic) depression is more severe depression that may occur shortly after birth but may not be recognized or diagnosed for several months postpartum. The woman experiences a deep, persistent sense of loss and sadness, accompanied by anxiety, irritability, sleep disturbances, lack of appetite, guilt, hypochondriasis, and at times, phobias. Most women do not have suicidal ideation or thoughts of harming the newborn. This type of depression generaly persists for about 1 year postpartum. In Beck's study of postpartum depression, women found life to be a "living nightmare" (Beck, 1992). Many such women do not seek professional help despite the misery and chaos of daily living (McIntosh, 1993).

Women With Borderline Personalities

Women with borderline personalities have many of the previous symptoms but additionally have feelings of helplessness, emptiness, nothingness, and loneliness following childbirth. These feelings may have been present before pregnancy but are accentuated by delivery. There may be transitory psychotic episodes with a sense of being out of control, fear of going crazy, and periods of depersonalization and disorientation (Landy et al., 1989).

Postpartum Psychosis

The woman with **postpartum psychosis** (psychotic depression) loses contact with reality and experiences delusions, hallucinations, and disorientation. Common themes for delusions and hallucinations are associated with childbirth, the newborn's health, and sexuality. There are often strong feelings of anger toward self and the newborn, accompanied by delusions in which the woman believes that she is being told to harm the newborn. Paranoia and strong aggressive feelings may be present. Postpartum psychosis can be unipolar with depression only or bipolar, swinging between mania and depression. The risk of suicide or harming the newborn is substantially increased (Guscott et al., 1991; Ugarriza, 1992).

Causative Factors in Postpartum Depression

Physiologic factors have long been suspected of playing an important role in postpartum depression, al-

TABLE 38-1
Types of Postpartum Depression

	Postpartum Blues	Postpartum (Neurotic) Depression	Depression in Women With Borderline Personality (Borderline Depression)	Postpartum Psychosis (Psychotic Depression)
ONSET	Transitory; usually strongest about 3–5 d after birth	May be up to 6 mo after birth	Could be up to 12 mo after birth	Usually within first month after birth; most common onset after 2 wk postpartum
SYMPTOMS	Mild depression; tears; some feelings of loss and being overwhelmed with responsibility; fatigue; rapid mood changes; poor concentration	May include anxiety states, phobias, fears of harming baby, hypochondriasis, loss of weight, insomnia, obsessive thoughts, irritability, feelings of guilt, apathy, lack of energy, feelings of loss of love and self-esteem	Could fluctuate from neurotic depression to periods of psychosis	Accompanied by delusions and hallucinations, disorientation, strong feelings of anger toward self and baby; may be paranoid, strong obsessive reaction; may be unipolar (only depression) or bipolar (swinging from mania to depression)
CONTACT WITH REALITY	Maintained throughout	May be accompanied by feelings of depersonalization and disorientation with reality testing maintained	May have transitory loss of contact with reality; depersonalization and acting out	Loss of contact with reality
RISK FACTORS	Minimal	Suicide	Suicide	Suicide, infanticide, or both
INCIDENCE	75% of mothers	One in 10 (10%–15%)	Not known	One in 500 to 700 births (2%)
DEFENSES	Usually get "primary maternal preoccupation" with newborn, some sublimation, rationalization, intellectualization, and altruism	Mainly characterized by repression and restriction of ego functioning; may try to control through thinking, detachment, isolation, reaction formation, somatization, and introjection	Restriction of ego functioning, splitting, depersonalization, and acting out	Severe regression, breakdown and splitting into primitive images; primary process and magical thinking, may get severe; acting out, including turning against self and infant
ORGANIC ETIOLOGY	Minimal, although loss of sleep and endocrine change may contribute	May be some hormonal imbalance, depressive disposition associated with psychogenic factors	Possible vulnerability; no clear causality	May be strong organic predisposition to schizophrenia, and so forth
CHILDHOOD HISTORY	No strong evidence of deprivation, loss, repression, or abuse in first 6 y of life	May be characterized by deprivation in early years and strong parental control from 3–6 y	Typically experienced problems with separation and individualization	Often characterized by deprivation, loss or abuse in first year or two of life; previous psychiatric illness common
TREATMENT	Opportunity to discuss feelings of loss and to ventilate feelings of anger; patience, support, and understanding	Insight-oriented psychotherapy; drug therapy and hospitalization if anxiety and suicidal feelings persist; infant–parent psychotherapy	Long-term intensive therapy	Hospitalization; supportive psychotherapy; drug therapy, ECT as a last resort

(continued)

TABLE 38-1 *(Continued)*
Types of Postpartum Depression

	Postpartum Blues	Postpartum (Neurotic) Depression	Depression in Women With Borderline Personality (Borderline Depression)	Postpartum Psychosis (Psychotic Depression)
PROGNOSIS	Excellent; difficulties and feelings usually integrated into personality for growth	Good depending on history and willingness to remain in psychotherapy; complete recovery common	Guarded without long-term intensive psychotherapy and help with parenting	Poor: may continue to need drug therapy
EFFECT ON INFANT	Minimal	May reduce orienting responses and cause delay of attachment and developmental milestones; may result in feeding or sleeping disorders	Abuse and neglect possible; difficulties most likely in second year postpartum	If extreme and no substitute caregiver available, could result in infant's withdrawal from animate and inanimate environment

ECT = electroconvulsive therapy.
(Landy, S., Montgomery, J., Walsh, S. [1989]. Postpartum depression: A clinical view. *Maternal Child Nursing Journal 18* (1), 1–29.)

though no evidence makes this link conclusively. Given the massive physiologic shifts during pregnancy and the postpartum period, the timing and transience of postpartum blues suggest a hormonal etiology. These physiologic changes could trigger depressive reaction in women with predisposition or risk factors. Postpartum affective disorders and psychosis appear much less related to physiologic events of pregnancy and childbirth (Unterman et al., 1990).

Psychosocial stressors are more important than physiologic factors in causation of affective depression. A principal feature seen through several generations is the mother–daughter relationship that may lead to rejection of the reproductive role. Postpartum depression is associated with a lack of early support, attention, and a dependable relationship with either parent; mothers who were not warm, nurturing, or dependable or who had negative attitudes toward their mothering roles; and fathers who were absent, preoccupied, or minimally available (Unterman et al., 1990).

Currently, life situation is an important factor in postpartum depression. Any stressful life event, such as death of a loved one, loss of job, or change of residence, occurring around the vulnerable postpartum period will have an impact on the woman's mood. An unstable relationship with the husband or partner has a strong association with depression. Other factors that increase the risk of depression include inadequate financial resources, housing difficulties, and dissatisfaction with education. In this last area, the critical factor is not the level of education, but the woman's satisfaction with that level and her disappointment in herself (Collins et al., 1993; O'Hara et al., 1991; Unterman et al., 1990).

Coping with psychosocial stress is more difficult when new adaptations are necessary, such as a taking care of a newborn and integrating him or her into the family. Sleep deprivation, discomfort, and fatigue often contribute to overwhelming the mother's coping abilities. Lack of feelings of competence also appear significant in postpartum depression. Obtaining satisfactory information, feeling in control of self and over events during the childbirth experience, and companionship in labor are positively related to postpartum psychological outcomes (Beck, 1993; Green et al., 1990; Wolman et al., 1993).

Nursing Assessment

Early identification of risk factors for postpartum depression will enable the nurse to take preventive steps so that depressive disorders can be avoided or minimized. A history of postpartum depression, familial affective disorders, or depression not related to pregnancy should alert the nurse to a potential problem. Other risk factors include low socioeconomic status, martial instability, single parent with limited support systems, ambivalence or negativity about parenthood, history of abuse or neglect as a child, self-disappointment and criticism, feeling incompetent to care for the newborn, and recent stressful life events. During the postpartum period, the nurse also should assess for early predictive signs in the mother's behavior and interaction with the newborn. Such signs may include a lack of warm and caring support people; ambivalence about the pregnancy or newborn; sleep disturbances, nightmares; crying episodes; extreme feelings of loss (personal routines, goals, body image), sadness, anxiety, or guilt; anger; lack of interest and warmth in new-born caregiving (see Assessment Guidelines: Early Predictive Signs of Postpartum Depression).

Nursing Diagnoses

After a thorough assessment, the nurse can identify possible nursing diagnoses. For a list of possible nursing diagnoses, see Box 38-8.

Nursing Planning and Intervention

Nursing care for women with postpartum blues is mainly supportive, because the condition usually resolves spontaneously in a few days. With early discharge, the woman will be at home when the full impact of "the blues" occurs. Hence, the nurse must take a proactive role to prepare the woman and her family for this condition (Beck et al., 1992). The nurse assists the mother and family to understand the temporary nature of this condition, the mother's need to express her feelings in an accepting environment, and the mother's need to explore options for her concerns. For milder affective depressions, emotional support and practical assistance, such as obtaining help with household tasks and newborn care so the mother can sleep adequately, often are sufficient to enhance coping abilities and decrease depression. The nurse assists the woman to problem solve constructively and teaches relaxation techniques. Strategies that rely on her personal strengths and experiences and help establish a supportive network of understanding people are encour-

aged. Self-help and support groups are excellent resources for help.

Women who experience more intense depression need mental health consultation and therapy. Counseling to deal with feelings and concerns may be behavioral, supportive, or insight oriented, depending on the mother's needs and capacity to integrate new perspectives into her functioning. Depending on resources available, the mother may obtain individual psychiatric or group therapy or participate in self-help or support groups. Parenting groups, hot lines, and mental health drop-in centers provide additional sources of assistance. Psychotherapy for the mother (with the newborn present), which focuses on confrontation and working through previously unresolved and unconscious conflicts related to her own experience of being parented, is often especially beneficial (Landy et al., 1989).

For women with severe affective depressions, borderline personalities, or psychotic depression, tranquilizers or antidepressant medications usually are necessary. Psychiatric referral and management should be instituted as soon as possible. Hospitalization may be needed if the depression is not controlled with medication or the woman is acting out, planning suicide, or posing a serious threat to the newborn.

The long-term prognosis for women with severe affective depression, borderline personalities, and psychotic depression varies. About 25% to 43% of women with postpartum depression still have some impairment 1 year after delivery. Services needed often are multifaceted, and not all communities have adequate

ASSESSMENT GUIDELINES
Early Predictive Signs of Postpartum Depression

In providing care during the postpartum period, the nurse assesses the mother's behavior and interaction with the infant for these signs:

Mother has no visitors and does not share news about birth with relatives or friends.
Spouse or partner is not warm, supportive, or caring toward mother.
Mother expresses rejection or ambivalence toward pregnancy, childbirth, or newborn.
Mother views newborn as rejecting her, or behaving badly or aggressively; she may call baby a "monster."
Mother experiences sleep disturbances or severe nightmares.
Mother demonstrates lack of warmth and interest in newborn during feeding and caretaking; may not want to hold newborn; does little verbalization; lacks eye-to-eye contact; exhibits little reciprocity.
Mother expresses intense feelings of loss involving body image, independence, personal routines, status, goals.
Mother shows extreme feelings of sadness, anxiety, guilt, and anger and cries frequently.

Adapted from Landy, S., Montgomery, J., & Walsh, S. [1989]. Postpartum depression: A clinical view.
Maternal Child Nursing Journal, 18(1), 1–29.)

BOX 38–8
Nursing Diagnoses—Postpartum Depression

- Ineffective Individual Coping related to
  - Stress of childbirth
  - Negative self-concept
  - Change in life pattern
  - Inadequate support systems
- Impaired Social Interaction related to severe depression
- Altered Parenting related to
  - Postpartum blues
  - Feelings of inadequacy
  - Delusions and hallucinations
- Altered Family Processes related to maternal depression
- Risk for Injury related to postpartum psychosis
- Ineffective Family Coping: Disabling related to maternal depression and effect on family unit

mental health facilities. The nurse's role includes assessing the client's behaviors, feelings, ideations, coping skills, support systems, and mother–newborn interactions. Such assessments help identify clients at risk for, suffering with, or recovering from a postpartum depression disorder. Nurses implement interventions, such as assisting clients to vent feelings, use effective problem solving and coping skills, obtain appropriate referrals for treatment and hospitalization. Obtaining and providing an appropriate and safe environment for the client and her newborn is an integral part of the nurse's role. Nurses teach clients and family members signs and symptoms of various postpartum depressive states and provide clients with acceptance and support through active listening and nonjudgmental approaches.

Evaluation

Anticipated outcomes for the client with postpartum blues and mild affective depression include the following:

- The client expresses feelings openly.
- The client identifies appropriate coping patterns and consequences.
- The client identifies her strengths and accepts support from others.
- The client participates in decision making, following through with action to accomplish goals or make desired changes.
- The client's depression resolves or significantly decreases.
- The client demonstrates a positive attitude and assumes caretaking and family responsibilities.

Summary Points

✔ Astute nursing assessments and interventions are important in preventing complications and reducing their impact on the woman and her family.

✔ Endometritis is a common postpartum infection, which usually responds promptly to antibiotic therapy.

✔ Women are as vulnerable to UTIs in the postpartum period as they are in the prenatal period.

✔ Late postpartum hemorrhage is due to retained products of conception, subinvolution of the placental site, or infection.

✔ Large hematomas require urgent interventions rather than a "wait and watch" approach to reduce maternal morbidity and mortality.

✔ Thromboembolic problems can be life-threatening if the clot attached to the vascular wall breaks free, causing a pulmonary embolism.

✔ Mastitis most often occurs in breast-feeding mothers and is usually caused by *S. aureus*.

✔ Depression in the postpartum period ranges from the mild, transient "blues" to a more significant, incapacitating depression to a severe depression with psychotic features.

REFERENCES

American College of Obstetricians and Gynecologists (1990). *Diagnosis and treatment of postpartum hemorrhage* (No. 143). ACOG Technical Bulletin. Washington, DC: Author.

Beck, C. T. (1993). Teetering on the edge: A substantive theory of postpartum depression. *Nursing Research, 42*(1), 42–48.

Beck, C. T. (1992). The lived experience of postpartum depression: A phenomenological study. *Nursing Research, 41–43*, 166–170.

Beck, C. T., Reynold, M. A., & Rutowiski, P. (1992). Maternity blues and postpartum depression. *Journal of Obstetric, Gynecologic, and Neonatal Nursing, 21*(4), 287–293.

Collins, N. L., Dunkel-Schetter, C., Lobel, M., & Scrimshaw, S. C. M. (1993). Social support in pregnancy: Pschosocial correlates of birth outcome and postpartum depression. *Journal of Personality and Social Psychology, 65*(6), 1243–1258.

Charles, D. (1993). *Obstetric and perinatal infections*. St. Louis: Mosby Year Book.

Creasy, R. K., & Resnik, R. (1994). *Maternal-fetal medicine: Principles and practice* (3rd ed.). Philadelphia: W.B. Saunders.

Cunningham, F. G., MacDonald, P. C., Leveno, K. J., Gant, N. F., & Gilstrp III, L. C. (1993). *Williams obstetrics* (19th ed.). Norwalk, CT: Appleton & Lange.

Eschenbach, D. A. (1991). Wound infections—more serious than acknowledged. *Contemporary Obstetrics and Gynecology, 36*(9), 21–36.

Green, J. M., Coupland, V. A., & Kitzinger, J. V. (1990). Expectations, experiences, and psychological outcomes of childbirth: A prospective study of 825 women. *Birth 17*(3), 15–24.

Galask, R. P. (1990). The challenge of prophylaxis in cesarean sections in the 1990s. *Journal of Reproductive Medicine, 53*(Suppl. 11), 1078–1081.

Gall, S. (1990). Therapeutic dilemnas in the treatment of pelvic infections. *Journal of Reproductive Medicine, 35* (Suppl. 11), 1091–1094.

Guscott, R. G., & Steiner, M. (1991). A multidisciplinary treatment approach to postpartum psychosis. *Canadian Journal of Psychiatry, 36*(8), 551–556.

Hannah, P., Adams, D., Lee, A., Glover, V., & Sandler, M. (1992). Links between early postpartum mood and post-natal depression. *British Journal of Psychiatry, 160*, 777–780.

Landy, S., Montgomery, J., & Walsh, S. (1989). Postpartum depression: A clinical view. *Maternal-Child Nursing Journal, 18*(1), 1–29.

McIntosh, J. (1993). Postpartum depression: Women's help seeking behaviours and perceptions of cause. *Journal of Advanced Nursing, 18*(2), 178–184.

Mead, P. B. (1990). Postpartum endometritis. *Contemporary Obstetrics and Gynecology, 35*(12), 29–34.

Nathan, L., Peters, M. T., Ahmed, A. M., & Leveno, K. J. (1993). The return of life threatening puerperal sepsis caused by group a streptococcus. *American Journal of Obstetrics and Gynecology, 169*(3), 571–572.

O'Hara, M. W., Schlechte, J. A., Lewis, D. A., & Wright, E. J. (1991). Prospective study of postpartum blues: biological and psychosocial factors. *Archives of General Psychiatry, 48*(9), 801–806.

Pop, V. J. M., Essed, G. G. M., Digeus, C. A., VanSon, M. M., & Komproe, I. H. (1993). Prevalence of postpartum depression—or is it post-puerperium depression? *Acta Obstetricia Et Gynecologica Scandinavica, 72*(5), 354–358.

Soper, D. E. (1993). Bacterial vaginosis and postoperative infection. *American Journal of Obstetrics and Gynecology, 169*(Part 2), 467–469.

Stovall, T. G., Thorpe, E. M., & Ling, F. W. (1993). Treatment of post cesarean endometritis with ampicillin and sulbactam or clindamycin and gentamicin. *Journal of Reproductive Medicine, 38*(11), 843–848.

Stray-Pedersen, G., Glakstad, M., & Bergan, T. (1990). Bacteriuria in the puerperium. *American Journal of Obstetrics and Gynecology, 162*(2), 792–797.

Sweet, R. L. (1990). Role of cephamycins in obstetrics and gynecology. *Journal of Reproductive Medicine, 35*(Suppl. 11), 1064–1069.

Symanski, M. E. (1992). Maternal-infant bonding: practice issues for the 1990s. *Journal of Nurse-Midwifery, 37*(Suppl. 2), 67–73.

Ugarriza, D. N. (1992). Postpartum affective disorders. *Journal of Psychosocial Nursing, 30*(5), 29–32.

Unterman, R. R., Posner, N. A., & Williams, K. N. (1990). Postpartum depressive disorders: changing trends. *Birth, 17*(3), 131–137.

Varner, M. (1991). Postpartum hemorrhage. *Critical Care Clinics, 7*(4), 883–897.

Veronikis, D. R., & O'Grady, J. P. (1994). What to do—or not to do—for postpartum hemorrhage. *Contemporary Obstetrics and Gynecology, 39*(8), 11–33.

Watts, D. H., Krohn, M. A., Hillier, S. L., & Eschenbach, D. A. (1990). Bacterial vaginosis as a risk factor for post-cesarean endometritis. *Obstetrics and Gynecology, 75*(1), 52–58.

Wolman, W. L., Chambers, B., Hofmeyr, J., & Nikodem, V. C. (1993). Postpartum depression and companionship in the critical birth environment: A randomized controlled study. *American Journal of Obstetrics and Gynecology, 186*(5), 1388–1393.

SUGGESTED READINGS

American College of Obstetricians and Gynecologists (1988, revised 1991). *Antimcrobial therapy for obstetric patients* (No. 117). ACOG Technical Bulletin. Washington, DC: Author.

Berkeley, A. B. (1992). Septic pelvic thrombophlebitis. *Contemporary Obstetrics and Gynecology, 37*(5), 109–113.

Cosico, J. N., & Rothlauf, E. B. (1992). Indications, management, and patient education: Anticoagulant therapy. *American Journal of Maternal Child Nursing, 17*(3), 130–135.

Dildy, G. A., & Clark, S. L. (1993). Postpartum hemorrhage. *Contemporary Obstetrics and Gynecology, 38*(8), 21–39.

Gerrard, J., Holden, J. M., Elliott, S. A., McKenzie, P., McKenzie, J., & Cox, J. L. (1993). Trainer's perspective of an innovative programme teaching health visitors about the detection, treatment, and prevention of postnatal depression. *Journal of Advanced Nursing, 18*(11), 1825–1832.

Jones, R. M. (1990). Role of a new cephamycins in the management of obstetric and gynecologic infections. *Journal of Reproductive Medicine, 35*(Suppl. 11), 1070–1077.

O'Hara, M. W., & Engeldinger, J. (1990). Postpartum depression. *Postgraduate Obstetrics and Gynecology, 10*(4), 1–6.

Silver, R., & Clark, S. L. (1994). Venous thromboembolism. *Contemporary Obstetrics and Gynecology, 39*(3), 11–23.

Steiner, M. (1990). Postpartum psychiatric disorders. *Canadian Journal of Psychology, 35*(1), 89–95.

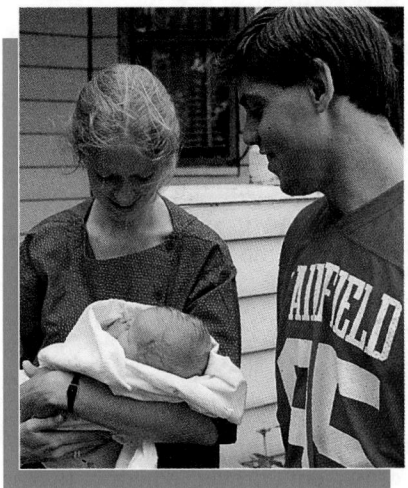

VII

Assessment and Management of High-Risk Maternal Conditions

Critical Thinking Questions

1. Dolores Collette, a 38-year-old gravida 5 client, developed preeclampsia during the last trimester of her pregnancy. Now, at term, she is admitted to the hospital because of suspected abruptio placentae. After consultation, she is informed of the need for an emergency cesarean delivery.

    After formulating appropriate nursing diagnoses and expected outcomes for this client, organize your proposed nursing care based on the client's priority needs prior to the cesarean delivery, and then postoperatively.

2. Jean Wolf is a 25-year-old multipara whose labor was complicated by prolonged early rupture of the membranes. There were no complications of delivery. On her second postpartum day, her temperature rises to 39° C, 102.2° F, and her pulse rate is 118. She complains of increased afterpains and headache. On examination, you note fundal tenderness and a foul smelling lochia which has decreased in amount from previous assessments and is red-brown in color. A diagnosis of endometritis is made. Cultures are taken and antibiotic therapy is started. Jean is breastfeeding her baby.

    Propose effective strategies for this client's care, integrating the client's needs related to the complication, breast-feeding, and discharge.

3. Patty Martin, 24 weeks pregnant, comes to the emergency department accompanied by her husband Tom. She appears anxious and frightened and has bruises on her arms and face. On further examination, she has contusions on her abdomen, breasts, and perineum. While questioning the client about what happened, you notice that her anxiety level increases and she looks to her husband before explaining, "I fell down the steps a few days ago." You suspect spousal abuse.

    After analyzing your feelings about spousal abuse, how would you approach this situation, tak-ing into consideration the priority needs of the client and fetus at this time?

4. As part of a community outreach program, you are asked to go into the local schools and provide primary pregnancy prevention to the adolescents, both male and female. You are assigned to go to one inner city school and one suburban private school.

    Devise an appropriate plan for teaching each group, comparing and contrasting any similarities and differences in your approach for each group.

5. Amy Gasparro, 26 weeks pregnant, is admitted for treatment of preterm labor. After treatment with tocolytic therapy, the client is to be discharged home. You are the home care nurse assigned to care for this client who is on terbutaline pump therapy.

    How would you approach your first visit with the client; include any predictions for possible priority needs based on your knowledge about preterm labor and tocolytic therapy.

Multiple Choice Questions

1. A pregnant client with Class 2 heart disease and a history of rheumatic fever as a child develops shortness of breath and chest discomfort with moderate exertion. The nurse would anticipate that the condition that would increase her risk for further complications of pregnancy is:

    A. Anemia
    B. Nocturia
    C. Heartburn
    D. Supine hypotension

2. A client with severe pre-eclampsia is receiving magnesium sulfate intravenously. During hourly assessments, the nurse obtains the following information: blood pressure remaining 136/90; urine output, 80 cc/hr; deep tendon reflexes 2+; and respirations, 11 breaths per minute. The nurse interprets this information and concludes that:

A. The medication isn't working because her blood pressure remains elevated.
B. The client is exhibiting signs of magnesium sulfate toxicity as evidenced by 2+ deep tendon reflexes.
C. The client's urine output is inadequate based on expected output during magnesium sulfate administration.
D. The client is exhibiting magnesium sulfate toxicity based on her respiratory rate.

3. After 14 hours of labor, vaginal examination of a primipara client reveals cervical dilation at 5 cm, an increase from 3 cm in the last hour. Fetal station has remained at -2 since admission 6 hours ago. The client is experiencing moderate contractions every 5 to 6 minutes, lasting for 50 seconds. The nurse interprets this labor pattern as:

A. Early transitional labor
B. Arrested fetal descent
C. Prolonged latent phase of labor
D. Hypertonic uterine contractions

4. Following spontaneous rupture of membranes, the nurse discovers umbilical cord prolapse. The nurse anticipates that the action that takes priority at this time is:

A. Relieving umbilical cord compression.
B. Preparing the client for cesarean birth.
C. Increasing client comfort.
D. Alleviating client anxiety.

5. An insulin-dependent diabetic client who is in her first trimester is experiencing persistent nausea and vomiting. Her blood glucose levels have been ranging from 60 to 78 mg/dl. When planning this client's care, the nurse anticipates that she is at risk for:

A. Hyperglycemia
B. Hypoglycemia
C. Glycosuria
D. Ketoacidosis

6. When assessing a client with abruptio placentae, which of the following would the nurse expect to find?

A. Soft nontender uterus
B. Elevated temperature
C. Bright red vaginal bleeding
D. Knifelike abdominal pain

7. Which of the following anomalies would the nurse anticipate as a problem in a client with dystocia?

A. Cephalhematoma
B. Caput succedaneum

C. Hydramnios
D. Hydrocephalus

8. The physician orders prostaglandin gel for a client prior to induction with oxytocin. The nurse understands that the rationale for the action is to:

A. Stimulate uterine contractions
B. Soften and efface the cervix
C. Prevent an episiotomy
D. Decrease the client's pain

9. A client is admitted to the labor and delivery area with a diagnosis of placenta previa. Which of the following procedures would be contraindicated?

A. Urine specimen for urinalysis
B. Baseline serum laboratory studies
C. Enema to prepare for delivery
D. Shave and prep of the perineal area

Study Questions

1. Name the predominant symptom associated with tubal rupture with an ectopic pregnancy.
2. Identify the most common cause of bleeding in late pregnancy.
3. List the four main medical strategies for managing DIC.
4. Name the triad of symptoms seen with PIH.
5. When is the diagnosis of GDM usually made?
6. Identify the major threat imposed by pregnancy for clients with heart disease.
7. What is the criteria on which the diagnosis of IDA is based?
8. List seven possible effects of smoking on the infant.
9. Explain the effect of alcohol on the fetus.
10. Identify five possible effects on the infant of a client who uses cocaine.
11. What drug is contraindicated in treating hypertonic uterine contractions?
12. Explain why the postterm fetus is at risk.
13. Name three causes of early postpartum hemorrhage, in order of frequency.
14. Name the microorganism most frequently involved in mastitis.
15. List the most frequent cause of delayed and late postpartum hemorrhage.

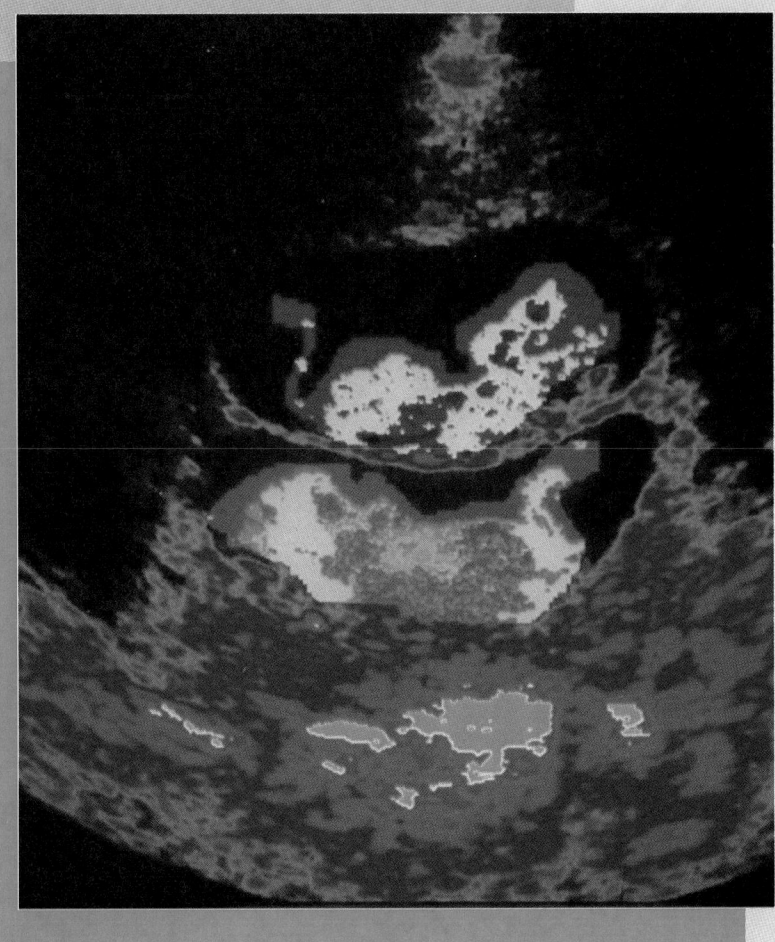

Assessment and Management of High-Risk Perinatal Conditions

VIII

39

Fetal Diagnosis and Treatment

Objectives

- Discuss clinical applications of ultrasound.
- List obstetric applications for MRI.
- Identify what is assessed during a biophysical assessment of the fetus.
- Discuss the role that maternal serum studies play in assessment of the fetus.
- Identify the types of fetal treatments that are available.
- Discuss the role of the nurse within the area of fetal diagnosis and treatment.

Key Terms

Abdominal circumference
Acoustic window
Amniocentesis
Amniotic fluid index
Biparietal diameter
Cephalic index
Contraction stress test
Crown to rump length
Femur length
Fetal biophysical profile

Fetal cell isolation
Magnetic resonance imaging
Nipple stimulation test
Nonstress test
Percutaneous umbilical blood sampling
Ultrasound
Vibroacoustic stimulation

The concept of the fetus as an individual client whose specific anatomic and physiologic problems are subject to diagnosis and treatment is relatively new to the practice of obstetrics. Prior to the 1960s, the diagnosis of fetal condition was limited to the assessment of fetal activity perceived by the mother, movement palpated by the physician, or simply auscultation of the fetal heart beat. Plain x-rays offered only a minimum of information, such as fetal position and major bony abnormalities, and were recognized as potentially harmful to the developing fetus. Amniograms (the introduction of radiopaque materials into the amniotic fluid) increased the risk of preterm labor or premature rupture of membranes without offering much more diagnostic data. In the last 3 decades, a series of rapidly evolving developments have opened the way to more accurate approaches to fetal diagnosis. These developments include ultrasound techniques, behavioral assessment, electronic fetal monitoring, biochemical sampling, and safer use of amniocentesis (which has allowed greater access to amniotic fluid for cytogenetic and biochemical assessment of the fetus).

Several circumstances exist in which the fetus might be in jeopardy that demand evaluation of fetal status. Such instances range from the first-trimester client with a threatened abortion to midtrimester pregnancy studies to determine congenital anatomic and chromosomal disorders. In the third trimester, serial evaluations are necessary in chronic maternal disorders, such as diabetes and hypertension, and in more acute problems, such as preeclampsia and the postdate pregnancy. The application of sophisticated tests to determine fetal condition is currently limited to women with a determined fetal risk; normal pregnancies are evaluated largely by clinical means. Some or all of these techniques may soon be routinely applied as a form of prenatal screening.

The period of gestation determines the action to be taken for the fetus in definite jeopardy. If the pregnancy is determined to be nonviable in the first trimester, the uterus can be evacuated. In the midtrimester, with a previable fetus, assessment of well-being is of variable moment. In some instances, in utero medical, surgical, and pharmacologic therapy can be directed toward the fetus, thereby allowing the pregnancy to continue. Many of these approaches, however, are investigative. If in utero fetal therapy is not initiated, there may be no recourse if serious fetal problems are uncovered during the second trimester of pregnancy, given the fact that delivery is unacceptable. Fetal evaluations performed in the third trimester can present the perinatal healthcare team with a choice between delivering a potentially viable premature newborn to begin neonatal therapy or prolonging intrauterine life with the risk of fetal death. When the indications of in utero jeopardy are severe, the decision to deliver often results in the birth of a seriously ill newborn and a potential neonatal death. More commonly, however, the studies are reassuring and permit prolongation of the pregnancy.

Advances in fetal assessment have led to advances in understanding that permit significant, albeit limited, treatment of the fetus beyond simply converting the fetus to a newborn. The proliferation of technology has been accompanied by a parallel rapid growth in the number and types of specialized professional and supportive personnel in the broad area of perinatology. Subspecialties have evolved for maternal–fetal medical specialists and neonatologists. Obstetric anesthesia has emerged as a growing and well-defined area of study. Training programs have been developed for perinatal nurse clinicians. Also, the concept of the perinatal team has become well established. Such a team includes the obstetrician, neonatologist, anesthesiologist, nurse specialist, nutritionist, genetics counselor, social worker, and other supporting consultants. The combined efforts of this team have resulted in a decrease of perinatal morbidity and mortality.

Noninvasive Methods of Fetal Diagnosis

Ultrasound in Pregnancy

Only with the development of ultrasound was a noninvasive, direct in utero visualization of the fetus possible. Ultrasound has provided obstetric healthcare providers a technique to delineate accurately normal and abnormal fetal anatomy with considerable detail. Fetal parts can be measured for growth and determination of gestational age. Heart motion can be seen and cardiac structure and function assessed. Fetal body and eye movements, breathing, sucking, swallowing, and urination are easily visualized with sonography. Ultrasound guidance may be used in invasive diagnostic procedures, such as amniocentesis, chorionic villus sampling, fetal blood sampling, and even tissue sampling (ie, biopsies).

Ultrasound is the transmission of low-energy, high-frequency sound waves through a medium, such as fluid or tissue. The intensity and delay time for reflected echoes are recorded. A transducer, containing crystals that vibrate in response to an electronic stimulus and produce an electric signal, generates sound waves. As sound is generated, it passes through various tissues at different speeds based on the density and elasticity of the tissue structure. In general, the denser the tissue, the higher the velocity of sound transmission. Sound travels through tissue until it comes to another tissue of a different density, a tissue interface (boundary). The change in density results in a small proportion of sound energy being reflected back toward the transducer. The echoes are received by the transducer crystals, converted into electric signals, and displayed on a monitor.

Ultrasonic information can be displayed in a variety of ways. Real-time B-scan is the mainstay of obstetric ultrasonic imaging. Dots on a monitor produced by electronic signals display motion picture-like, two-dimensional, sectional images. The brightness of the dots reflects the strength of the signal. The differences among these signals indicate anatomic structures:

- Black areas that are completely devoid of echoes frequently relate to fluid areas, such as amniotic fluid. These regions are called *anechoic*.
- Bright white areas are generated by strong reflectors, such as bone tissue.
- Gray areas are generated by small echoes arising from tissues of intermediate density, such as cardiac, renal, or brain tissue.

Currently, state-of-the-art equipment displays signal strengths in 128 shades of gray, and prototype methods are available for color conversion of these images. Real-time scanning also provides a method of visualizing fetal heart activity, fetal behavior, and fetal bladder and stomach filling and emptying.

Another display of information used in obstetric ultrasound is M-mode, which yields lines that depict movement of anatomic structures versus time. M-mode provides valuable information about cardiac structure and dynamic changes occurring in the fetal heart.

Finally, Doppler ultrasound analyzes data on the frequencies of returning echoes to determine the velocity of moving structures. The primary use of Doppler ultrasound in obstetrics has been to detect and measure blood flow in the uterine arteries and fetal umbilical, carotid, and intracranial vessels.

Three-Dimensional Ultrasound

Traditional two-dimensional (2D) real-time ultrasound provides easily visualized and accurate images of normal fetal anatomy and pathologic findings. 2D sonography, however, provides only a linear (length and width) observation of fetal structures. These images may be confusing and difficult to construe because they must be interpreted to form a three-dimensional impression of the anatomic structures represented (Hamper et al., 1994). For several years, clinicians have been investigating the use of three-dimensional (3D) sonography to visualize the fetus. With this recent development in ultrasound, three continual different planes, representing longitudinal, transverse, and horizontal sections, are displayed simultaneously. These three planes can be rotated and computer translated to obtain accurate anatomic sections needed for diagnosis and geometric measurements, such as distances, areas, and volume (Kuo et al., 1992; Steiner et al., 1994). Thus, 3D sonography may provide new fetal assessment parameters, such as surface views of fetal organs and the fetal face, fetal organ volumes, and weight-length correlations (Lee et al., 1994; Pretorius et al., 1995). While currently being used in tertiary centers only, 3D sonography has the potential to be used in primary care settings. In this situation, computerized images would be transferred by a computer modem for on-line assessment by specialists (Pretorius et al., 1995).

M-Mode Echocardiography

Real-time directed M-mode echocardiography supplies information about a single portion of the linear sector display and plots it over time. The result is a wavy pattern in the presence of movement. M-mode echocardiography is a useful supplement to cross-sectional (real-time B-scan) imaging for evaluating myocardial wall thickness, chamber dimension, and valve and wall motion (Fig. 39-1; DeVore, 1985; DeVore et al., 1984; DeVore et al., 1985). The detection of such conditions by M-mode echocardiography allows for pharmacologic intervention that averts in utero heart failure.

Doppler Ultrasound

Doppler ultrasound technology is based on the Doppler effect; when a sound wave of a defined frequency is reflected from moving matter, the shift in reflected frequency provides a measure of the speed of movement. The Doppler effect has applications in everyday life ranging from police radar detectors to home burglar alarms. In obstetrics, Doppler detects the movement of red blood cells in vessels and is used to measure blood velocity and flow.

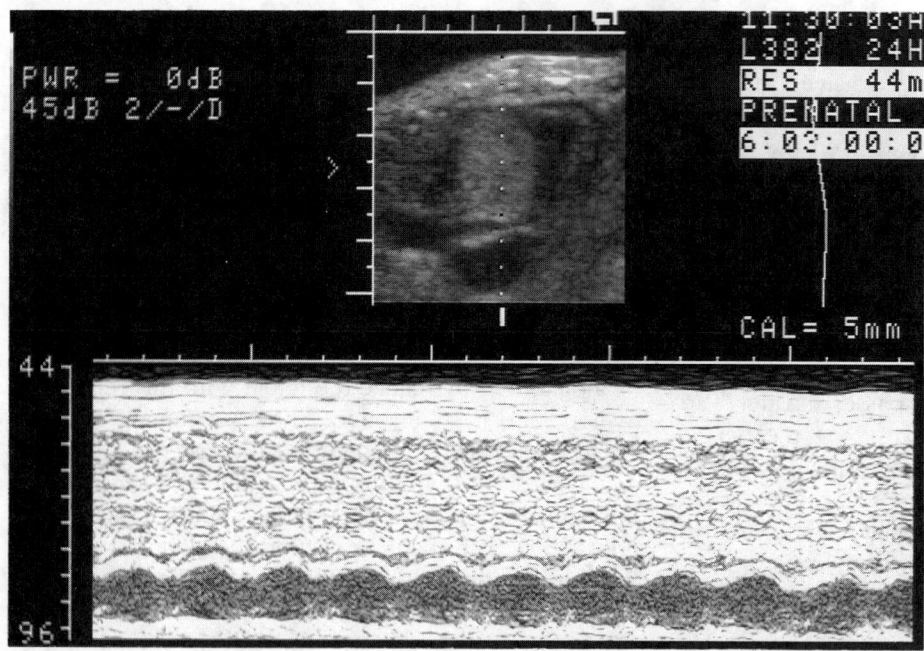

FIGURE 39–1 Movement of the cardiac valves and walls can be studied using M-mode ultrasound of the fetal heart. This case demonstrates a fetal cardiac tumor (rhabdomyoma).

Currently, the implementation of Doppler ultrasound is achieved in three modes:

1. Continuous-wave Doppler
2. Pulsed-wave Doppler
3. Two-dimensional Doppler color-flow imaging

In continuous-wave Doppler, the transducer contains two crystals, one for the transmission of sound and the other for reception of the echo. The frequency of the received echo is compared with the frequency of the transmitted echo to derive the Doppler shift. Any motion within the region of the overlapping beams is capable of producing the shift. Continuous-wave Doppler, therefore, is unable to measure the depth or range (ie, the source) of the shift (Maulik et al., 1990).

In pulsed-wave Doppler, the transducer contains a single crystal that emits short bursts of sound and receives the reflected signals after a variable time delay during the interpulse interval. In general, pulsed-wave Doppler transmits a signal 0.1% of the time while receiving returning signals 99.9% of the time. The location, range, or depth of the sound can be determined by adjusting the gate (the sending and receiving times for the crystal; Maulik et al., 1990). A duplex ultrasound system combines pulsed-wave Doppler with real-time imaging to visualize directly and sample vessels at specific anatomic locations.

Whereas pulsed-wave Doppler is based on a single range-gated signal, color-flow Doppler image uses multiple gates that measure mean frequency shifts at multiple points and at multiple ranges. The resulting information is represented as color-coded flow patterns superimposed on real-time images of fetal anatomy (Fig. 39-2; Maulik et al., 1990). The choice of color assignment for the received echo is determined by the direction of motion with respect to the transducer. Conventionally, a red color is assigned to designate flow toward the transducer and a blue color designates flow away from the transducer. Because color assignment depends only on flow direction, tortuous vessels will vary in color assignment as their flow changes.

A Doppler waveform of a vessel represents the velocity waveform, which in turn reflects the upstream and downstream circulatory condition (ie, systole and diastole). Doppler measurements relate maximum frequencies observed during end diastole (D) to those noted during peak systole (S). These include the simple S/D ratio and Pourcelot's resistance index:

$$RI = \frac{(S-D)}{S}$$

They also include the pulsatility index:

$$PI = \frac{(S-D)}{\text{Mean value of the maximum frequencies}}$$

Doppler waveform has been used to measure the velocity in several vessels in the maternal–fetal unit, including the intracerebral, renal, internal iliac, femoral, and umbilical arteries. The widest application of Doppler in obstetrics is umbilical artery Doppler studies, which measure the velocity of blood returning from the fetus to the placenta. Approximate values of normal S/D ratios are 4.0 at 20 weeks' gestation, 3.0 at 30 weeks, and 2.0 at 40 weeks.

Studies that compare values of normal fetuses with values from fetuses suspected of being growth retarded have found that elevated values for gestational

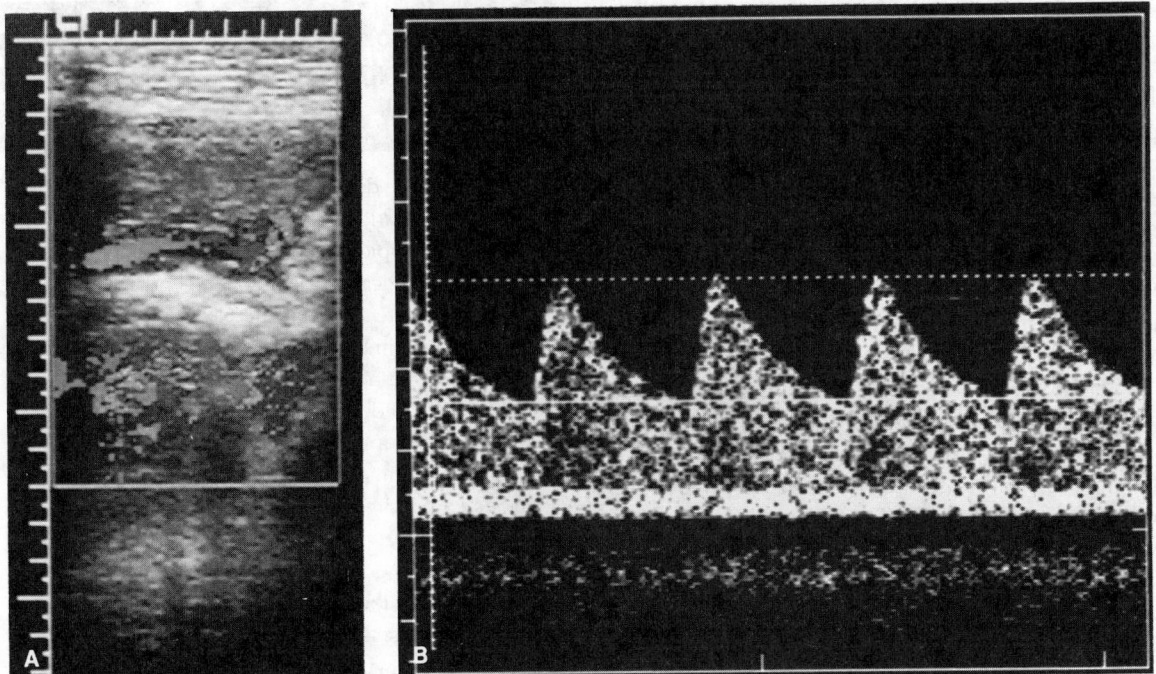

FIGURE 39–2 Doppler velocity waveforms. (**A**) Color flow Doppler imaging is used to detect a location for amniocentesis. When only real-time B-scan was used, the top colored area appeared black, seeming to contain only amniotic fluid. Color flow imaging demonstrates that this pocket is packed with umbilical cord. (**B**) Normal Doppler waveform of the umbilical artery.

age are associated with a higher risk for intrauterine growth retardation (IUGR; Fleischer et al., 1985). Doppler ultrasound is therefore a logical tool for the detection of IUGR. Although these reports are promising, the sensitivity of Doppler ultrasound in the prediction of IUGR ranges from 55% (Berkowitz et al., 1988) to 78.3% (Fleischer et al., 1985). In an effort to improve the sensitivity of Doppler as a test, other vessels in the fetal circulatory system have been investigated. Internal carotid artery velocities were chosen for study because fetuses with growth retardation are thought to have an increase of blood flow to the brain in asymmetrical growth retardation (Wladimiroff et al., 1987; Arduini et al., 1987). These studies demonstrated that the proportion of blood flowing during diastole in the cerebral vasculature increased with advancing gestation, whereas diastolic flow in the umbilical circulation declined in growth-retarded fetuses. Although Doppler ultrasound apparently has potential as a quick, noninvasive, and relatively easy diagnostic tool in predicting perinatal outcome, additional prospective studies are needed prior to the widespread clinical use.

Color flow imaging is the most recent of Doppler techniques to be used in obstetrics. This diagnostic modality has a number of established uses. Color Doppler can be used in the evaluation of placenta previa by better determining what portion of the placenta is in continuity with the cervix. Imaging of the placenta with color also can be used to trace out the fetal circu-

lation in multiple gestations in which a twin-to-twin transfusion is suspected. Color is valuable in umbilical cord identification as an adjunct to percutaneous umbilical blood sampling (PUBS) and amniocentesis. Several congenital anomalies can be detected with color flow imaging. These include intracranial anomalies, such as hydrocephalus; renal anomalies; and anomalies of the umbilical cord or vein. Doppler color flow imaging also is used in fetal echocardiography to detect intracardiac and great vessel flow disturbances and diagnose structural malformations of the heart.

Safety of Ultrasound

Obstetric ultrasound examinations are performed during the most sensitive periods of human growth and development. Diagnostic studies may be conducted during any or all three trimesters of pregnancy, including periods in which a disruption in normal embryonic process may have disastrous effects. Thus, since the inception of obstetric ultrasonography more than 25 years ago, the safety of ultrasound to the fetus and woman has been questioned. Extensive research has examined the possible unexpected harmful effects of ultrasound; however, conclusions regarding risk still remain relatively elusive (Sabbagha, 1994).

The American Institute of Ultrasound in Medicine issued a report concerning the safety of ultrasound delivered at diagnostic intensities and stated that there has been no independently confirmed evidence of bioeffect of ultrasound delivered at diagnostic intensities (AIUM Bioeffects Reports Subcommittee, 1988). Additionally, they state that "although the possibility exists that such biological effects may be identified in the future, current data indicate that the benefits to clients of the prudent use of diagnostic ultrasound outweigh the risks, if any, that may be present."

In 1984, the National Institutes of Health (NIH) and the U.S. Food and Drug Administration (FDA) convened a Consensus Development Conference of Diagnostic Ultrasound Imaging in Pregnancy (U.S. Department of Health and Human Services, 1984). They determined that ultrasound should be performed only when there are firm clinical indications. Table 39-1 lists the indications for obstetric ultrasound as recommended by the NIH panel. These recommendations, however, have been questioned by many authors who advocate routine screening of obstetric clients.

Although it is widely believed among medical practitioners that ultrasonagraphy is safe and beneficial, research continues to eliminate unwanted reactions and ensure the well-being of the woman and fetus. Additional research that increases awareness of potential risk factors or lack thereof and improved technology that lessens the frequency of exposure to ultrasound will be instrumental in this pursuit (Sabbagha, 1994).

The Ultrasound Examination

Ultrasound examinations may take one of three forms: the basic examination, the targeted examination, and the limited examination (American College of Obstetricians and Gynecologists, 1993). Every client who undergoes ultrasound assessment should have a basic examination that includes the following:

- Determination of fetal number
- Presentation
- Documentation of fetal life
- Placental localization
- Amniotic fluid volume
- Gestational dating
- Detection and evaluation of maternal pelvic masses
- Survey of fetal anatomy for gross malformations

This examination is adequate for most obstetric clients and takes an average of 20 minutes. However, a client who has a fetus with a known or suspected defect should be sent for a targeted examination (ie, an examination that is performed by a sonographer who has more expertise in sophisticated scanning techniques). An examination of this type may take up to 40 minutes to perform. The third type of ultrasound examination, the limited examination, is performed in situations in which only specific or limited urgent clinical information is required, but it is unnecessary or impos-

TABLE 39-1
Summary of the National Institutes of Health Guidelines for the Use of Diagnostic Ultrasound in Obstetrics

Ovarian follicle development surveillance
Suspected hydatidiform mole
Suspected ectopic pregnancy
Adjunct to cervical cerclage placement
Pelvic mass detected clinically
Suspected uterine abnormality
Intrauterine contraceptive device localization
Suspected fetal death
Suspected multiple gestation
Abnormal serum alpha-fetoprotein value
Suspected polyhydramnios or oligohydramnios
Follow-up observation of identified fetal anomaly
History of congenital anomaly
Adjunct to amniocentesis
Estimation of gestational age:
  1. In clients who are late registrants for prenatal care
  2. In clients who are to undergo elective termination of pregnancy
Evaluation of fetal growth
  1. In clients who have an identified etiology for uteroplacental insufficiency leading to intrauterine growth retardation
  2. In clients when macrosomia is suspected
Significant uterine size—clinical date discrepancy
Serial evaluation of fetal growth in multiple gestation
Estimation of fetal weight or presentation in premature rupture of membranes or premature labor
Vaginal bleeding of undetermined etiology
Suspected abruptio placentae
Biophysical profile for fetal well-being
Adjunct to special procedures
Adjunct to external version
Determination of fetal presentation in labor when the presenting part cannot be adequately assessed
Observation of intrapartum events

(Modified from Shearer, M. H. [1984]. Revelations: A summary and analysis of the NIH Consensus Development Conference on ultrasound imaging in pregnancy. *Birth, 11,* 23.)

sible to perform a complete fetal anatomic survey. A limited examination could include the fetal biophysical profile (FBP), amniotic fluid assessment, confirmation of fetal cardiac activity, fetal number and presentation, and placental localization.

Obstetric ultrasound may be performed by two techniques: transabdominal scanning or transvaginal scanning. Transabdominal ultrasound is the more traditional method and can be used throughout all trimesters of pregnancy regardless of the size of the pregnant uterus (Fig. 39-3).

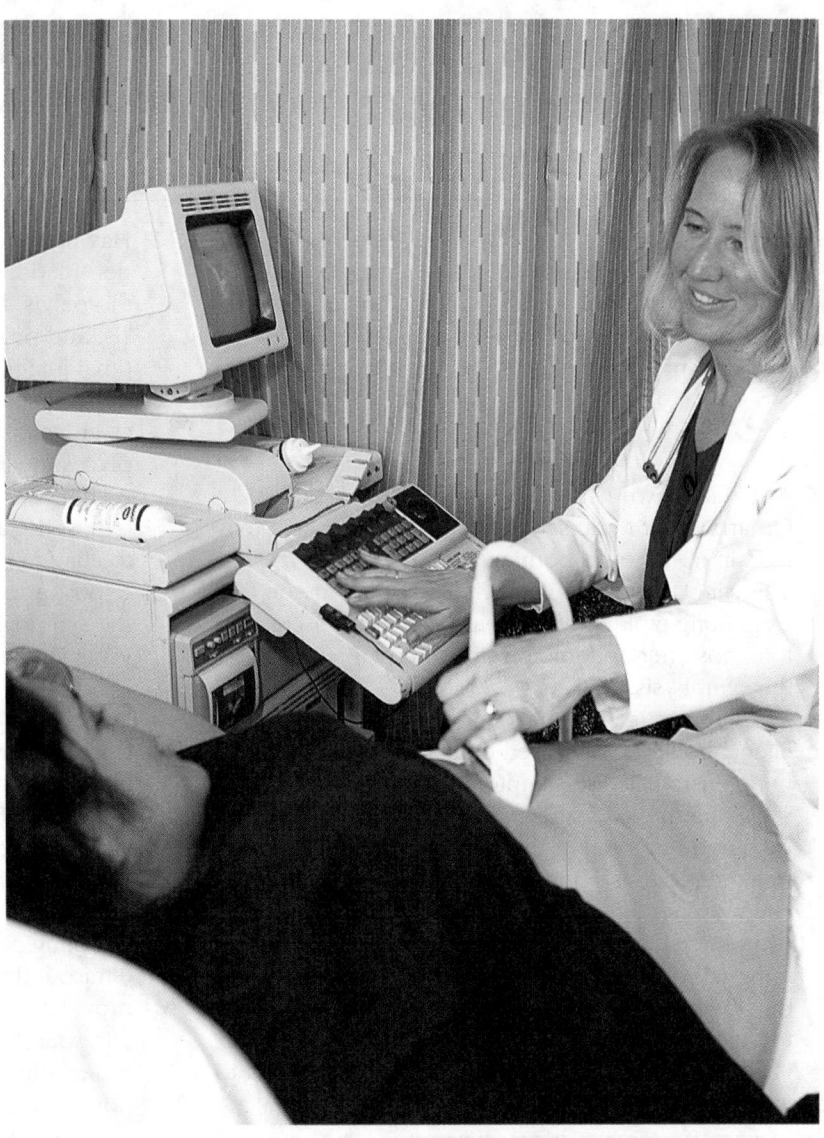

FIGURE 39–3 Transabdominal ultrasound can be used throughout the pregnancy.

For optimal imaging of the fetus with transabdominal ultrasound an "**acoustic window**" must be available. In a first-trimester pregnancy, a filled bladder is required for the examination because most pelvic structures are located behind gas-filled loops of bowel. An ultrasound beam is unable to penetrate gas; water, however, is an excellent transmission medium. Bladder distention displaces the bowel out of the pelvis, lifts the uterus from behind the symphysis, and provides an acoustic window to the pelvic structures (Jeanty et al., 1984). Bladder filling is usually unnecessary for the second and third trimester scans, because there normally is sufficient amniotic fluid to serve as an acoustic window, and the expanded uterus pushes the intestines out of the way. One of the exceptions to this is when a client is undergoing sonographic examination for placental localization (Procedure 39-1).

Transvaginal ultrasound scanning consists of placing an elongated ultrasound transducer within the vagina to visualize the pelvic structures. One of the advantages of transvaginal ultrasound over abdominal scanning is that no acoustic window is required for transvaginal scanning. Clients, therefore, do not have to fill their bladders and may find this technique more comfortable. A second advantage is that the transvaginal probe is closer to the pelvic structures than the abdominal transducer, allowing these structures to be visualized more clearly (Rebar, 1988). This technique is especially useful in obese women, women with abdominal wall scarring, or clients who display interfering bowel gas. Obstetric indications for transvaginal scanning include documentation of early intrauterine pregnancy, identification of early ectopic pregnancy, assessment of embryonic development and detection of anomalies, and cervical incompetence (Berman, 1991). Transvaginal ultrasound has limited use in fetal anatomic visualization and biometrics measurements after 16 weeks' postmenstrual age, being used primarily to evaluate

PROCEDURE 39–1
Preparing a Client for a Transabdominal Ultrasound Scan

Procedure	Rationale
1. In the first trimester of pregnancy, the woman should be instructed to drink four 8-oz glasses of water 2 hours prior to the examination and not to void. This is not necessary for second- and third-trimester pregnancies.	1. Having the client drink water will distend her bladder. Bladder distention displaces the bowel out of the pelvis, lifts the uterus from behind the symphysis, and provides an acoustic window, enabling optimal imaging of the fetus. During the second and third trimesters of pregnancy, amniotic fluid serves as an acoustic window, while the gravid uterus displaces the bowel.
2. A special gown is not needed for the procedure. On arrival for a transabdominal scan, the client may remain in her own clothing.	2. As long as the client's abdomen can be adequately exposed with her own clothing, she does not need to change into a gown.
3. The client should be instructed to lie supine on the examining table and either lift or lower her clothing to expose her abdomen from the costal margin to the symphysis.	3. Exposure of the abdomen from the costal margin to the symphysis will provide a complete area for fetal visualization.
4. From approximately 20 weeks' gestation on, the client should be observed for symptoms of supine hypotension. These symptoms include sudden onset of faintness, dizziness, nausea, ringing in the ears, and numbing of the extremities. Immediate treatment of this phenomenon involves turning the client on her left side.	4. Lying supine can result in hypotension resulting from compression of the vena cava by the enlarged uterus, which also reduces uteroplacental and renal perfusion. Turning the client to her left side will alleviate the compression and increase blood flow.
5. After the client is comfortably situated on the examining table, coupling gel is generously applied to the abdomen. A towel or sheet should be provided to the client to protect her clothing. Ultrasound gel is notoriously cold, and gel warmers can be used to ease client discomfort.	5. Coupling gel eliminates the air interface between the ultrasound transducer and the client's skin, thereby providing a better transmission and reception of the ultrasound waves. Even though the gel is usually water soluble and does not stain, it can leave a temporary mark on clothing until the gel dries.

the presenting fetal part in middle to late pregnancy (Procedure 39-2).

Important to any ultrasound examination is documentation of the study. A written report of the ultrasound findings should be included in the client's medical record. The report should contain any measurements made and the anatomic findings observed during the examination. A permanent record of ultrasound images obtained during the examination should be added to the client's record. Various recording devices can produce a record of an ultrasound examination. A multiformat camera uses x-ray film, which requires developing. Nine images can be recorded on a single sheet of film. Instant-film cameras, such as a Polaroid, are a common method of recording images. The major disadvantage of this method is the expense of the film; the cost per picture is often just under a dollar. A popular method of recording images is a video image recorder. This device records images on a sheet of thermal paper, resulting in a good-quality picture at

a relatively inexpensive cost (ie, less than 10 cents per picture). Dynamic imaging as obtained by real-time ultrasound can be saved on a video recorder. The value of this device is that complete ultrasound examinations can be recorded and referred to another physician for a second opinion. Lastly, ultrasound images can be saved on computer disks, allowing approximately 10 images per disk. The major disadvantage of this method is that it is time consuming. Whatever method is used for recording an ultrasound examination, the images should be labeled with the client's name and the date of the examination.

Clinical Applications of Ultrasound

Detection of Early Intrauterine Pregnancy. Ultrasound in the first 11 postmenstrual weeks can have a significant role in the diagnosis of early intrauterine pregnancy and embryonic life. In a normal pregnancy, the gestational sac can routinely be detected with

PROCEDURE 39-2
Preparing the Client for a Transvaginal Ultrasound

Procedure	Rationale
1. No pre-examination preparation is involved in transvaginal scanning.	1. No acoustic window is required for a transvaginal scan because the transducer is in direct contact with the pelvic organs.
2. Upon arrival for the examination, the client is asked to remove any clothing below the waist.	2. The sonographer must have access to the vagina.
3. The client should be placed in a lithotomy position, or a pillow may be placed under her buttocks to raise the pelvic area.	3. Elevating the client's hips will provide better imaging of higher pelvic structures.
4. A transducer sheath or a condom partially filled with coupling gel is placed over the vaginal transducer. A lubricant can be placed over the outside of the transducer sheath for ease of insertion.	4. Coupling gel will eliminate the air interface between the transducer and the client's skin. Lubricant applied to the transducer will facilitate gentle insertion of the transducer without client discomfort.
5. The transducer is then inserted through the introitus and into the midvagina. Although clinics follow varying practices, it is recommended that a female chaperon be present when the transvaginal scan is performed.	5. A female chaperon should be present as with any pelvic examination.
6. At the end of the examination, the condom is removed, and the transducer is cleaned with Cidex or some other disinfectant (Berman, 1991).	6. Disinfectant is used to eliminate the spread of any possible infection.

transvaginal ultrasound between 4 and 5 postmenstrual weeks (deCrespigny et al., 1988). The mean sac diameter should be measured; in a normally developing pregnancy, the sac should be 5 mm at 5 weeks (Nyberg et al., 1985). The accuracy of the mean sac diameter for dating purposes is ±2 weeks (DuBose, 1991). During the middle of the fifth postmenstrual week, the embryo measures between 2 and 5 mm. After 6 postmenstrual weeks, heart pulsations can be detected with vaginal ultrasound, whereas abdominal ultrasound may detect heart motion between 7 and 8 weeks. By the end of the ninth week of development, the embryonic head, body, and extremities can clearly be identified with either abdominal or vaginal ultrasound, and fetal movements are clearly recognizable. Deviation from normally identified sonographic signs could indicate complications of early pregnancy, such as blighted ovum, incomplete or complete abortion, or an embryonic pregnancy (Fleischer et al., 1991).

Fetal Measurements. Sonographic measurement of the fetus is important in determining the gestational age of the fetus, evaluating fetal growth to identify IUGR, and detecting congenital malformations. During the ultrasound examination, measurements are made with electronic calipers as the sonographer identifies the desired fetal part. Various tables and nomograms have been created to describe normal growth of various fetal pa-

rameters and can be located in any basic clinical ultrasound book.

Crown to Rump Length. The **crown to rump length** (CRL) is the longest demonstrable length of the embryo or fetus, excluding the limbs and yolk sac (Robinson et al., 1975). The CRL is considered one of the most accurate indicators of fetal age due to the excellent correlation between length and age in early pregnancy when growth is rapid and minimally affected by pathologic disorders. At about 9 weeks' gestation, extension and development of the head and regression of the tail occur. Coupled with the fetus assuming its natural curvature, this is an appropriate time to make an accurate CRL measurement (Goldstein et al., 1994). Therefore, it has been argued that CRL measurements may be inappropriate before 7 weeks' gestation (Harrington et al., 1993). The CRL can be used reliably until 12 weeks' gestation, after which a linear measurement of the fetus is difficult because of increasing flexion and extension of the fetal trunk. For purposes of dating, the accuracy of the CRL is ±3 days from 7 to 10 weeks' gestation and ±5 days between 10 and 14 weeks (Jeanty, 1991).

Measurements of the Fetal Head. The **biparietal diameter** (BPD) is the maximum distance between the two fetal parietal bones. It is one of the most widely used measurements in obstetric ultrasound because it is easy to obtain, has a distinctive appearance, and provides a relatively accurate measurement (Fleischer et al., 1991). The BPD is used in determining gestational age and fetal weight and diagnosing anomalies, such as microcephaly and hydrocephaly. The measurement is taken at the widest portion of the fetal skull with the thalamus positioned midline (Fig. 39-4; Hadlock et al., 1982). The BPD can be measured as early as 9 to 10 weeks' gestation when the head can be differentiated from the rump; however, at this time, the internal anatomy of the head is not consistently visualized. This measurement can be used most reliably from 12 to 20 weeks when internal structures of the head are routinely identified (Hearn-Stebbins, 1995). Accuracy of the BPD decreases with increasing gestational age due to shaping of the fetal head, growth disturbances, and individual variation. At 16 weeks' gestation, the BPD has an accuracy of ±5 to 7 days, whereas at more than 28 weeks' gestation, the accuracy is ±3 weeks.

Cephalic index (CI) is the ratio of the BPD to occipitofrontal diameter. The CI is used to determine if the shape of the fetal head is normal. During the course of pregnancy, pressure from the maternal parts, such as the ribs, pelvic bones, or tumors, can result in an abnormal shaping of the fetal head. The fetal head can become dolichocephalic (flattened and elongated) or brachycephalic (short and widened). If these conditions occur, the BPD should not be used to determine gestational age. In normal conditions, the CI ranges between 0.74 and 0.83 (±1 standard deviation) and should remain constant throughout pregnancy (Sabbagha, 1994).

Head circumference (HC) in the fetus can be computed from measurements of the BPD and the occipitofrontal diameter:

$$HC = (BPD + OFD) \times 1.57$$

They also can be directly measured with a digitizer, map reader, or the assistance of computer software installed in state-of-the-art ultrasound equipment. The HC is not affected by abnormal head shape as is the BPD; therefore, it can be used to determine gestational age. It is also used in the diagnosis of IUGR and various anomalies, such as microcephaly.

Measurements of the Fetal Body. **Abdominal circumference** (AC) is used as a parameter in the diagnosis of IUGR. It is an estimation of the size of the fetus at the level of the liver and the left portal vein. The measurement of the abdomen is taken at this location because the fetal liver will be most severely affected in growth-retarded fetuses (Jeanty et al., 1984). The AC also reflects subcutaneous fat, which has an influence on fetal weight. AC is also used in the determination of gestational age. The AC can be used from 16 weeks' gestation to term; however, optimal use is at 34 weeks (±1 week; Hearn-Stebbins, 1995). As in HC, the AC can be measured mechanically, electronically, or computationally:

$$AC = (\text{Transverse diameter of the abdomen} + \text{anteroposterior diameter}) \times 1.57$$

The AC measurement should be reinforced with other methods of measurement.

Measurement of the Fetal Extremities. Fetal long bones are good indicators of fetal growth because the bones are not subject to changes in shape due to pressure or position. Although all long bones of the fetus can be identified and measured with real-time ultrasound, the **femur length** (FL) is the most widely used parameter. The fetal femur is the largest, easiest to identify, and least movable of the long bones of the fetal body. It is also one of the most reproducibly measured structures obtained in obstetric ultrasound. FL is used as a parameter in determining gestational age and is considered to be as accurate as the BPD by some investigators (Jeanty et al., 1984; Wolfson et al., 1986). It is also used in the diagnosis of skeletal dysplasias. The femur is measured from the origin to the distal end of the shaft (Fig. 39-5) and can be obtained as early as 10 weeks' gestation.

Determination of Fetal Age. Although it is customary to use Nägele's rule to determine the period of gestation and estimated date of confinement from the first day of the last menstrual period, this method is fraught with error for various reasons. In at least 20% of women, menstrual age is not a reliable factor in determining gestational age because of a history of ab-

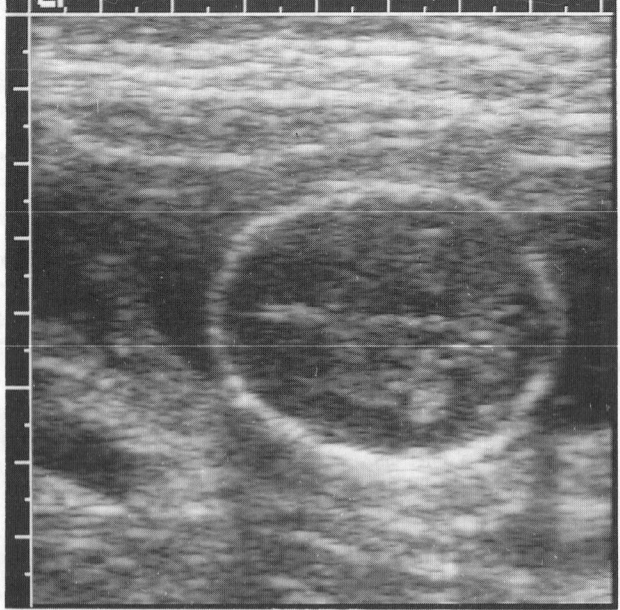

FIGURE 39-4 Normal fetal biparietal diameter.

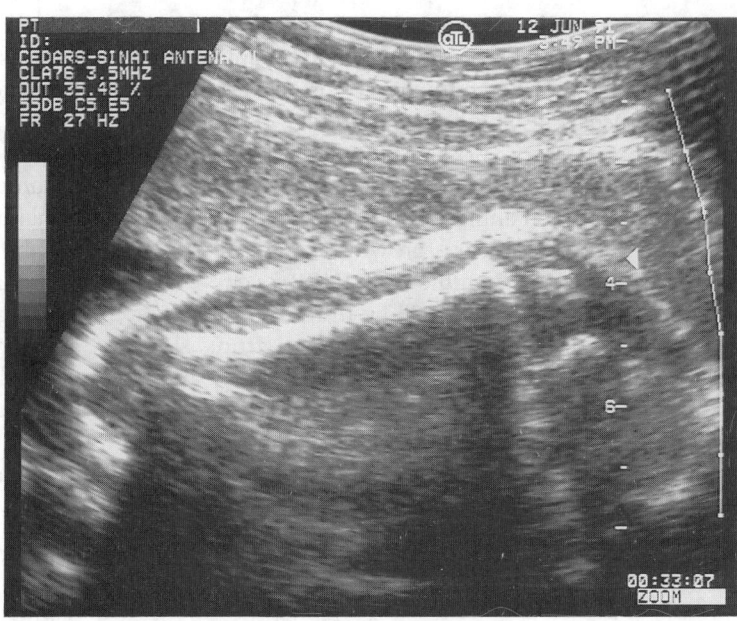

FIGURE 39–5 Normal fetal femur.

normally infrequent menstruation (oligomenorrhea), bleeding in the first trimester, or becoming pregnant after the use of oral contraceptives or during the postpartum period. In addition, a significant number of women fail to remember exact dates. In these women, only 70% delivered within ±2 weeks of their estimated date of confinement (Campbell et al., 1985). Physical measurements, such as fundal height, are increasingly inaccurate as the woman approaches term. In the first trimester, a physical examination may predict fetal age to ±2 weeks; by the third trimester, the fundal height may vary by as much as ±4 to 6 weeks (Kurtz et al., 1988). In the case of an uncomplicated pregnancy, not knowing the exact length of gestation may not represent a serious problem. In the high-risk woman for whom timing of the delivery is critical, however, the information is vital.

Real-time ultrasound has become the standard for determining gestational age. There are, however, some constraints on the use of ultrasound as a dating tool. As a rule, the most accurate sonographic measurements of gestational age are those made early in pregnancy before individual growth patterns have much effect on the fetus. These individual patterns emerge in the third trimester of pregnancy and account for the lack of precision in sonographic dating after 28 weeks' gestation. Although any published fetal size-age nomograms may be used for dating purposes, some differences in normal growth patterns may exist owing to environmental and genetic factors, such as altitude and race. Though these differences may be small in most instances, nomograms should be developed for each specific population being served. However, this is not always practical or possible. Therefore, the examiner should select nomograms that were generated from a population that most closely mirrors the population being examined.

Other than CRL, a single morphometric measurement is not accurate for dating purposes, especially during the third trimester of pregnancy. An average of sonographically determined ages of multiple fetal parameters (BPD, HC, AC, and FL) yields a more accurate estimation of fetal age throughout gestation than any single parameter (Hadlock et al., 1987). Using multiple parameters tends to minimize operator errors and limitations in instrumentation and averages out normal individual variations in fetal anatomy (DuBose, 1985).

Determination of Fetal Growth

Intrauterine Growth Retardation. One of the most commonly recognized abnormalities of the fetus is IUGR, in which the fetus fails to prosper in utero. Depending on the severity of the problem, death rates among IUGR fetuses and infants are significantly increased. Compared with normal pregnancies, the overall perinatal mortality of the IUGR infant is six to eight times higher (Scott et al., 1994). Many longitudal studies have indicated long-term neurologic deficits among IUGR children (Scott et al., 1994).

Many definitions have been provided for IUGR. Fetuses with an estimated weight below the 10th percentile are commonly classified as growth retarded; however, an estimated fetal weight below the third percentile has also been used to define IUGR. Streeter et al. (1980) demonstrated a progressive increase in the incidence of serious morbidity as birth weight percentile decreased. Their results ranged from a morbidity of less than 10% in the 5th to 10th percentile to as high as 36% below the 5th percentile. Thus, if third percentile is accepted as the cut-off for normal growth, a higher percentage of abnormal fetuses will be missed than if the cut-off is set at the 10th percentile. Conversely, if the 10th percentile cut-off is accepted, more normal fetuses will be followed with high-risk management than necessary. Most institutions follow the conservative definition of IUGR as estimated fetal weight below the 10th percentile.

Two types of abnormal growth patterns are commonly recognized. Asymmetrical IUGR occurs when the fetus grows normally until the third trimester. After 28 weeks' gestation, growth of the fetal trunk slows relative to head growth, a result of "brain sparing." Brain sparing results from a hypoxemic reflex redistribution of cardiac output. Preferential channeling of oxygen and nutrient-rich blood from the placenta to the brain results in an increased cerebral blood flow and a reduction in perfusion of the kidney and lung, resulting in diminished amniotic fluid production (Manning et al., 1991). The etiology of asymmetrical IUGR is uteroplacental insufficiency due to a variety of maternal disorders, including chronic hypertension, collagen vascular disease, chronic renal disease, preeclampsia, and classes F to R diabetes. Symmetrical IUGR is a growth lag of the fetal head and body (ie, the entire fetus is proportionately small for gestational age). The insult in this disorder occurs within the first trimester and is so severe that the brain is not spared as in asymmetrical IUGR. TORCH (toxoplasmosis, other infections, including hepatitis B, HIV, syphilis, Group B *Streptococcus, Chlamydia,* and varicella; rubella; CMV; and herpes simplex) infections, congenital malformations, drugs, and chromosomal abnormalities are causative factors of symmetrical IUGR.

Clinical diagnosis of IUGR includes measurement of fundal height, maternal weight gain assessment, and estimation of fetal weight (EFW) by palpation. These methods have been shown to be insufficiently accurate in identifying the growth-retarded fetus (Andersen et al., 1981; Beazley et al., 1970). IUGR is clinically undiagnosed in 50% of the cases prior to birth. Accurate diagnosis of IUGR depends on ultrasonic morphometric assessment. Sonographic parameters that are used in the evaluation of IUGR include BPD, HC, AC, and FL. Additionally, body proportionality indices (eg, the ratio of the HC to AC) are used to determine asymmetrical IUGR. Clearly measuring the HC alone is potentially insufficient and may cause a diagnosis of IUGR to be overlooked, because the brain of the asymmetrical IUGR continues to grow (Scott et al., 1994). Serial measurements of growth parameters are recommended for all fetuses with proven or suspected IUGR. The interval between examinations varies with gestational age, severity of growth retardation, fetal well-being, and maternal condition at the time of diagnosis. The usual interval between examinations, however, is 2 weeks to minimize biologic variation and measurement error.

EFW can be computed by a number of formulas using various sonographic measurements, but it has a ±15% estimate of error (Hadlock et al., 1983; Campbell et al., 1975). Therefore, EFW is not a reliable independent indicator of IUGR.

Large-for-Gestational Age Fetus. The large-for-gestational-age (LGA) fetus presents a number of problems for the obstetric team. Fetuses who are suspected of being LGA are at risk for intrapartum complications, including cephalopelvic disproportion, shoulder dystocia, and asphyxia. The detection of the LGA fetus provides the obstetric team with information for selecting the timing and route of delivery (Acker et al., 1985). Etiologic factors of macrosomia (LGA) include the following:

■ Diabetes
■ Postdatism
■ Maternal obesity
■ Previous delivery of a macrosomic newborn

Macrosomia, defined as birth weight in excess of 4,000 to 4,500 g, is present in 1% of all deliveries. Sonographic growth parameters used to diagnose LGA include BPD, AC, and EFW. EFW, however, has a tendency to underestimate the true weight in LGA fetuses. As in evaluation of growth retardation, fetuses with suspected LGA should have serial scans to assist in the obstetric management of these clients.

Detection of Congenital Anomalies. A congenital anomaly consists of a departure from the normal anatomic structure of an organ or system. Major structural anomalies are identified in 7% of newborns and account for 20% of perinatal deaths (Chung et al., 1987; Myrianthopoulos et al., 1974). Infants with nonlethal malformations may require major surgery and have neurologic abnormalities and psychiatric deficits that impose an economic burden on society and significant financial and emotional stresses on their families. For these reasons, the detection of congenital anomalies is considered an important goal of prenatal care.

Prenatal detection of fetal malformations is not performed for the purpose of termination of undesirable pregnancies. Although the recognition of fetal anomalies can provide parents with an opportunity to interrupt pregnancy if they desire, prenatal diagnosis enhances the obstetric management of the dysmorphic pregnancy in several ways. It allows a predelivery consideration of referral for prepared delivery at a perinatal center that can provide immediate care for neonatal medical and surgical problems. Prenatal diagnosis can result in further testing, such as chromosome analysis or magnetic resonance imaging (MRI), which can better define the anomaly. Parents can be offered prebirth counseling to prepare them for the appearance and care of their affected newborn. Heroic intrapartum interventions can be avoided if the anomaly is demonstrated to be lethal, as in the case of anencephaly and acardia. Lastly, early prenatal detection can result in the initiation of in utero fetal therapy if appropriate.

Ultrasound plays a key role in the management of developmental anomalies. All ultrasound examinations should include a detailed review of fetal anatomy. The sonographer focuses on the recognition of a departure from normal fetal anatomy, as in the following examples (Fig. 39-6):

- The absence of a normal structure
- The presence of an abnormal structure
- A disruption of the shape, size, or location of a normal structure
- Abnormal measurements
- Abnormal fetal motion (Romero et al., 1991).

Accuracy of diagnosis is based on the gestational age at the time of the examination. Many malformations are not apparent until 16 to 18 weeks' gestation, and others may not be expressed until much later. A scan in early pregnancy, therefore, does not exclude the presence of anomalies. On the other hand, first-trimester scans sometimes falsely indicate fetal anamolies, because the fetus is in an early stage of development (McGahan et al., 1994). Accuracy of the examination also is affected by the index of the sonographer's suspicion at the time of the examination. An examination of the fetal spine will be more detailed in a client with an elevated maternal serum alpha-fetoprotein than a routine scan for gestational age determination. Finally, the accuracy of detection varies with the expertise of the sonographer. Sonographer experience and recent advances in ultrasound technology have permitted the detailed prenatal diagnosis of multiple congenital anomalies. If the anomalies fit a pattern, chromosomal studies are warranted. Obstetric management and client counseling on the prognosis of morbidity and mortality may change with a diagnosis of a lethal aneuploidy, such as trisomy 18. Suggestive markers of the aneuploidic fetus include the following:

- Abnormalities of the hands, feet, and limbs (Fig. 39-7; Chervenak et al., 1985; Jeanty et al., 1985; Benacerraf et al., 1988a; Benacerraf et al., 1988b; Jeanty et al., 1990)
- Abnormalities of the face and head (Berry et al., 1990; Nicolaides et al., 1992)
- Diaphragmatic hernia (Benacerraf et al., 1988a)
- Thickened nuchal skin folds (Benacerraf et al., 1987)
- Congenital heart defects (Copel et al., 1988; Bundy et al., 1986)
- Fetal choroid plexus cysts (Platt et al., 1991)
- Renal pyelectasis (Benacerraf et al., 1990)

Assessment of the Fetal Environment

Amniotic Fluid Assessment. Ultrasound assessment of amniotic fluid plays a crucial role in pregnancy assessment. Several methods of amniotic fluid measurement have been documented since the 1980s. One of the most common methods is the single measurement of the vertical axis of the largest pocket of amniotic fluid (Manning et al., 1981; Chamberlain et al., 1984). In this method, decreased fluid (oligohydramnios) is defined as an amniotic fluid pocket measurement <2 cm (<3 cm in some institutions), whereas increased fluid, known either as hydramnios or polyhydramnios, is de-

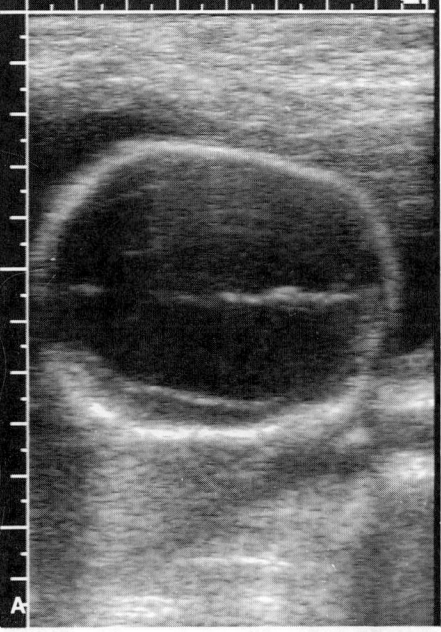
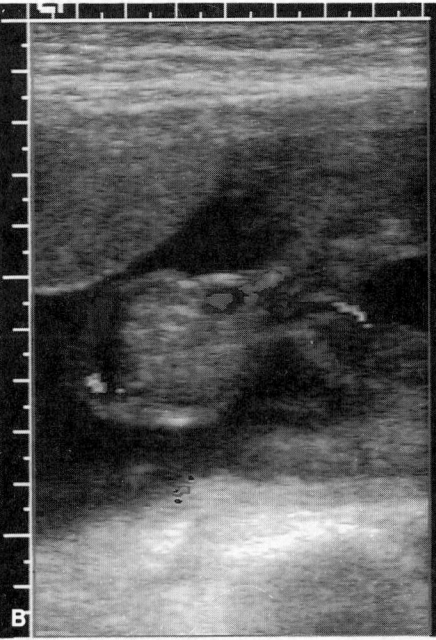

FIGURE 39–6 Ultrasound can be used to detect a number of congenital anomalies. (**A**) Severe hydrocephalus. Lack of visualization of the normal internal structures of the fetal brain in conjunction with ventricular dilatation and macrocephaly are indicative of this congenital disorder. (**B**) Anomalies also can be detected by the presence of an abnormal structure. Transverse scan of the fetal abdomen at the insertion of the umbilical cord illustrates an omphalocele. Fetal intestines can be seen within the umbilical cord. The umbilical vein, viewed with color flow Doppler imaging, surrounds the abnormally placed bowel.

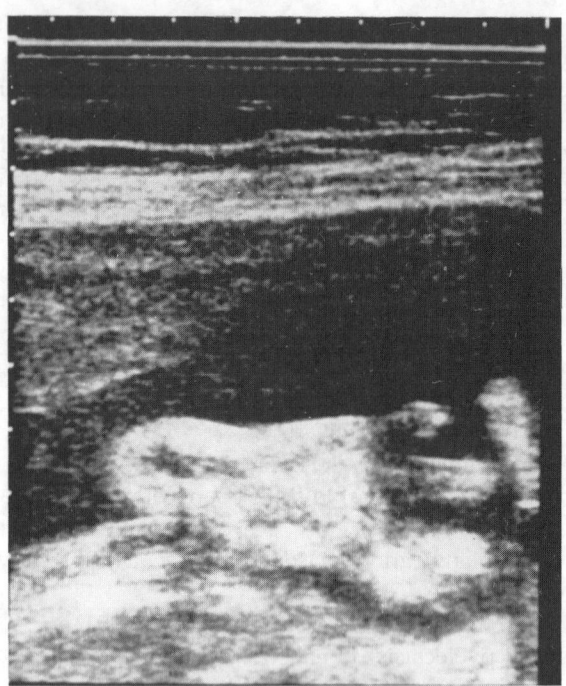

FIGURE 39-7 Wide spacing of the second toe on the foot of a fetus diagnosed with trisomy 18.

scribed as a single vertical amniotic fluid pocket ≥8 cm. A technique that has gained popularity is a four-quadrant approach called the **amniotic fluid index** (AFI; Phelan et al., 1987). The AFI involves dividing the maternal abdomen into four quadrants using the umbilicus and linea nigra as the horizontal and vertical

reference points of division. Holding the ultrasound transducer perpendicular to the floor, the vertical diameter of the largest pocket of amniotic fluid is identified and measured. The numbers from each quadrant are summed, the result of which is the AFI (Fig. 39-8). For clinical purposes, decreased amniotic fluid is defined by an AFI ≤5 cm, whereas increased amniotic fluid is an AFI ≥24 cm (Carlson et al., 1990). Studies have compared the AFI with the maximum vertical pocket techniques to detect oligohydramnios and hydramnios (Moore, 1990; Croom et al., 1992; Williams et al., 1992). These investigations suggest that the AFI may identify abnormal amniotic fluid volumes more efficiently than the single-pocket technique; however, the superiority of one technique over another has not been consistently demonstrated from one study to the next.

Oligohydramnios is associated with post-term gestation, IUGR, renal dysfunction, obstructive uropathy, and rupture of membranes. Oligohydramnios predisposes the fetus to cord compression, which can lead to fetal distress in labor or fetal demise. If prolonged, decreased fluid can result in fetal pulmonary hypoplasia. Hydramnios is associated with maternal illness, such as diabetes and anemia. It is also related to congenital anomalies of the central nervous system (anencephaly) and the gastrointestinal system (tracheoesophageal fistula, upper gastrointestinal tract obstruction), idiopathic macrosomia, hydrops fetalis, and aneuploidy. An increased volume of amniotic fluid can result in preterm labor, premature rupture of membranes, cord prolapse, and perinatal death.

AMNIOTIC FLUID INDEX
AFI   15.0 cm

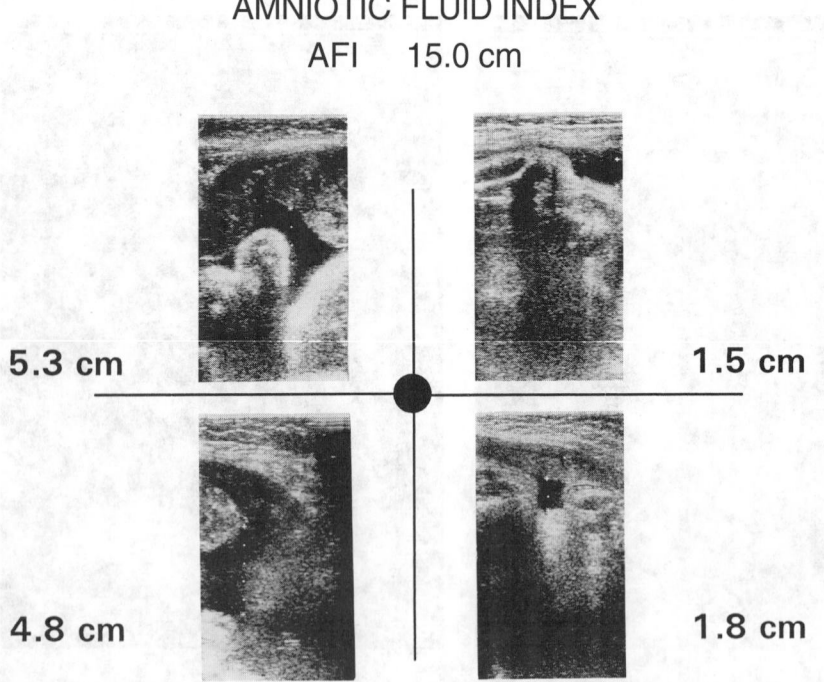

5.3 cm   1.5 cm

4.8 cm   1.8 cm

FIGURE 39-8 The four-quadrant method of evaluating amniotic fluid volume—the amniotic fluid index (AFI). Using the umbilicus as one reference, the uterus is divided into upper and lower halves. The linea nigra is used to divide the uterus into right and left halves. If the umbilical cord completely fills a quadrant, that quadrant is not measured. If the quadrant has a part of the umbilical cord visualized, amniotic fluid is measured only to the point where the cord can be detected. The AFI demonstrated in this figure is 13.4 cm.

Placenta. The placenta is easily assessed by ultrasound and is used in the diagnosis of placenta previa and abruptio placentae as discussed in Chapter 31.

The most common abnormality of the placenta assessed with ultrasound is variation in size in certain high-risk pregnancies. The placenta may be markedly enlarged in cases of hemolytic disease of the newborn, diabetes, and anemia due to edema of the chorionic villi (Perrin et al., 1984). Placentas from preeclamptic women tend to be smaller than the norm. The observations of the size of placentas may assist in diagnosing the presence and severity of these diseases.

Placental maturation changes can be evaluated during the sonographic examination. Placental calcium deposition is a normal physiologic process that occurs throughout pregnancy. The incidence of placental calcification increases exponentially with increasing gestational age, beginning around 29 weeks' gestation. Calcium is deposited in the basal and chorionic plate and in the perivillous and subchorionic spaces. A sonographic grading system (grade 0 to III) has been developed to describe the presence of echogenic areas within the placenta: Grade 0 is the least calcified placenta, and grade III demonstrates significant calcification (Grannum et al., 1979). Placental grading in conjunction with BPD and FL has been used as a noninvasive method to evaluate fetal lung maturity and determine the timing of elective deliveries.

Multiple Gestation. Assessment of the uterine environment includes the determination of the number of fetuses in utero. Of all twin gestations, 98% may be detected by routine ultrasound performed at 16 to 18 weeks (Fig. 39-9; Sabbagha, 1994). Studies have proven that early identification of twin gestation improves perinatal outcome, due to closer observations

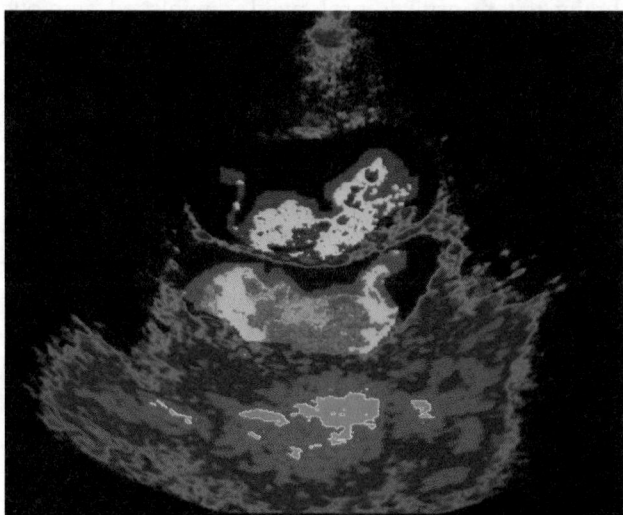

FIGURE 39–9 Routine ultrasound will detect 98% of all twin pregnancies.

and more timely interventions (Sabbagha, 1994). Ultrasound is also used to diagnose conjoined twins and assess characteristics of the placenta and membrane, providing information about zygosity and relative risks. Monoamniotic twins have an increased incidence of fetal wastage (Mahony et al., 1985). Twin-to-twin transfusions resulting from placental arteriovenous anastomoses may occur in monochorionic twins. The donor twin is usually growth retarded and has a marked reduction of amniotic fluid. The recipient twin may suffer from complications of overperfusion, such as cardiomegaly, fetal hydrops, and hydramnios.

Magnetic Resonance Imaging

Obstetric **MRI** is a noninvasive diagnostic tool that provides high-resolution cross-sectional images of fluid-filled soft tissues in the reproductive system, including the fetus, placenta, and uterus. Images are produced using an interaction between hydrogen nuclei, static magnetic fields, and radio waves (Lowe et al., 1985). When the magnetic field of the MRI is turned on, it causes the hydrogen nuclei in the body to align themselves. These nuclei emit signals that are converted into computer images (Fishbach, 1996). The images that are produced are often as precise as can be seen by direct visual examination.

The MRI is specifically suited for the detection of soft-tissue abnormalities that cannot be identified by ultrasound. Obstetric applications for MRI include the following:

■ Known or suspected hydatidiform mole (Powell et al., 1986a)
■ Placenta previa (Powell et al., 1986b)
■ Fetal anomalies, including hydrocephaly, cystic hygroma, urethral obstruction, hydronephrosis, and anencephaly (McCarthy et al., 1985; Thickman et al., 1984)
■ IUGR (Stark et al., 1985)

The advantage of MRI over ultrasound is that MRI can be used in adverse scanning conditions. These include maternal obesity, overlying bony structures, and gas-filled intestines, which may interfere with optimal sonographic imaging. MRI has a particular advantage over ultrasound in clients with oligohydramnios because ultrasound diagnosis is often difficult in clients with decreased amniotic fluid. Oligohydramnios is not a limiting factor in MRI diagnosis because amniotic fluid is not required for fetal visualization in this technique. In fact, decreased amniotic fluid may be a benefit because it can restrict fetal movement, which is a disadvantage in MRI. Other disadvantages of MRI are the expense and the length of the examination, which may be 1 to 2 hours (Lowe et al., 1985).

Biophysical Assessment of the Fetus

Fetal Behavior

More specific and direct examination of the fetus has been made possible with the development of high-resolution, real-time ultrasound. The ability to visualize the fetus directly and monitor fetal activities and responses to stimuli has provided insight into the functional maturation of the fetal central nervous system. Behavioral patterns (states) and fetal reactions to stimuli indicate that several stages of neurologic organization can be defined in relation to other parameters of intrauterine development. Associated with the direct observation of fetal behavior comes an increasing recognition of fetal disease and the opportunity to affect treatment.

Fetal Movement

There is a successive development of simple movement involving the entire fetal body to more complex movements of individual fetal parts. Movements can be discerned with ultrasound as early as 7 weeks' gestation. By 8 weeks, general movements of the limbs, trunk, and head can be appreciated. Hiccups are observed as early as 9 weeks, and fetal breathing is initiated at 10 weeks. By 12 weeks of pregnancy, sucking and swallowing are incorporated into the repertoire of fetal movement (deVries et al., 1984). All movements that can be identified in the term fetus are present by 15 weeks' gestational age.

The development of periodic individual movements, fixed combinations of individual movements, and the association of fetal heart rate (FHR) patterns and fetal motility occurs in the second and third trimesters of pregnancy. In general, movement normally decreases as gestational age increases. The maximum incidence of motor activity in the 20- to 22-week fetus is 21%. In the 30- to 40-week fetus, it is only 10%. The quality of movement patterns is also age dependent in that the frequency of rest-activity cycles decreases with gestational age. The younger fetus moves for an average of 10 minutes, then rests for 9 minutes, thus having three rest-activity periods within a 1-hour interval. The average term fetus, however, will move for 23 minutes, then rest for 40 minutes, having only one rest-activity pattern within 1 hour. Individual variations occur. Up to 90 minutes may elapse before movement can be detected in a normal fetus. A late night-early morning rhythm of movement develops during the second trimester of pregnancy, with the 24- to 28-week fetus moving more often between 11:00 PM and 8:00 AM. The third-trimester fetus, however, has a burst of activity between 9:00 PM to 1:00 AM. Correlations of fetal movements with FHR have been found as early as 20 to 22 weeks, with this interaction increasing with gestational age. The number and amplitude of FHR accelerations associated with movements increase as the fetus approaches 32 weeks (deVries et al., 1987; Patrick et al., 1982; deVries et al, 1982; Dierker et al, 1982).

Fetal Breathing Movements

Although fetal breathing movements are considered a preparatory exercise for extrauterine breathing, they are essential for fetal lung growth. Fetal respiratory activity enhances neuromuscular and skeletal development of the respiratory system and makes the appropriate respiratory epithelial development of the gas-exchanging surfaces of the fetal lung possible (Maloney et al., 1980). Fetal breathing is detected at 10 weeks' gestation and increases with gestational age. The frequency of breathing decreases, however, as early as 3 days prior to the initiation of labor and persists until delivery. A pattern of fetal breathing revolving around a 24-hour cycle appears at 24 weeks' gestation. At this stage, breathing occurs more frequently between 11:00 PM and 2:00 AM. The 30- to 39-week fetus has a higher incidence of breathing between 4:00 AM and 7:00 AM (Patrick et al., 1980; Natale et al., 1988; Carmichael et al., 1984).

Effects of Asphyxia on Fetal Biophysical Activities

As in the extrauterine client, asphyxia (insufficient intake of oxygen) produces effects on multiple organ systems in the fetus, including the lungs, kidneys, and central nervous system. Signs of fetal asphyxia depend on the extent, duration, and persistence of the asphyxial insult. Acute episodes of asphyxia result in a shunting of blood from the fetal lung and kidney to the brain. If the insult is prolonged, diminished amniotic fluid production occurs owing to decreased urine production and lung fluid flow. If an acute episode of total asphyxia (no oxygen is delivered to the fetus) or a prolonged partial asphyxia occurs, the fetal central nervous system can become affected. The results of asphyxia are then observed as alterations in the frequency and patterning of fetal behavior. In extreme cases, hypotonia, absent fetal breathing, absent fetal movements, and absent heart rate reactivity can progressively be observed. In the fetus, asphyxia commonly occurs as a result of a chronic reduction in uteroplacental perfusion.

Fetal Behavioral States

Behavioral states are stable periods of specific, fixed combinations of several physiologic variables that recur over time. Well-developed behavioral states are exhibited by the neonate born at or near term (Nijhuis et al., 1984). The assessment of neonatal behavioral states is important because these states influence the responsiveness of the newborn during a neurologic examination. Behavioral states are considered indicators of the functional condition of the central nervous system (Junge, 1979).

Behavioral states have been studied in the 32 weeks to term fetus, based on the criteria of body movements, breathing movements, eye movements, and heart rate patterns (Table 39-2). In general, the term fetus spends approximately 98% of the time in quiet or active sleep (state 1 or state 2), which is similar to the normal newborn. The fetus alternates between these two states over a 20- to 40-minute period. States 3 and 4 (quiet and active awake states) are recognized only 2% of the time (Arduini et al., 1986; Arduini et al., 1985).

The influence of behavioral states on fetal biophysical activities is of major importance in the interpretation of fetal behavior. The observation of normal biophysical activities indicates a functional and therefore nonasphyxiated fetal central nervous system. Therefore, consideration of fetal behavioral state is unnecessary. In contrast, failure to recognize the presence of normal biophysical activities requires consideration of fetal behavioral state. Differentiating between a normal sleep state and asphyxiation can be determined by extending the observation beyond the time for pattern shift or repeating the observation at a later point. In either instance, subsequent observation of normal activities confirms normality, whereas persistent absence of activities suggests asphyxia.

Fetal Biophysical Profile

Scoring of the FBP is a method of fetal surveillance based on a composite assessment of several markers of fetal disease (Manning et al., 1980; Platt et al., 1985; Manning et al., 1990). The basic premise of the FBP is that the perdictive accuracy of observing a number of biophysical variables is superior to that achieved by observing any one variable. Thus, the compromised fetus can be better identified by considering variables that reflect immediate fetal condition (heart rate reactivity [the nonstress test, NST], fetal movement, fetal breathing, and fetal tone) and a variable that reflects fetal condition over a long period (amniotic fluid volume). Except for FHR activity, all variables are measured by real-time ultrasound. For scoring purposes, each variable is assigned a score of 2 when normal and a score of 0 when abnormal. The variable is coded as normal whenever fixed criteria (Table 39-3) are reached, regardless of the duration of observation, up to a maximum of 30 minutes. The highest obtainable combined score possible is 10. The lowest score that can be observed when all the parameters are abnormal is 0. A combined score of 10 or 8 is regarded as normal. A combined score of 6 is equivocal and indicates that the profile should be repeated within 24 hours. A combined score of 4, 2, or 0 indicates fetal compromise, and delivery of the fetus should be considered. A deviation in this system is in the case of oligohydramnios. In any fetus with decreased amniotic fluid, intact membranes, and all other normal FBP variables, delivery is considered at many institutions (Chamberlain et al., 1984; Bastide et al., 1986).

Clinical experience with the FBP as a measure of fetal compromise has yielded encouraging results. Manning et al. (1990) have reported on FBP results of more than 26,000 high-risk clients and demonstrated that a significant exponential rise in perinatal morbidity and mortality occurs with decreasing profile scores. Other prospective studies have shown similar results (Platt et al., 1985; Baskett et al., 1987).

Maternal Perception of Fetal Movement

Although maternal perception of fetal movement is the oldest and least expensive means of monitoring fetal

---

TABLE 39–2
Fetal Behavioral State Criteria

State Criteria	State 1F	State 2F	State 3F	State 4F
Body movements	Incidental	Periodic	Absent	Continuous
Eye movements	Absent	Present	Present	Present
Heart rate pattern	Stable, little variability, isolated accelerations	Greater variability than 1F, frequent accelerations	Greater variability than 1F, no accelerations	Unstable, large, and long-lasting accelerations, often fused into sustained tachycardia
Breathing movements	Regular	Irregular	Irregular	Irregular

(Adapted from Nijhuis, J. G., Prechtl, H. F. R., Martin, C. B. Jr. et al. [1982]. Are there behavioral states in the human fetus. *Early Human Development, 6,* 177–195; Nijhuis, J. G., Martin, C. B. Jr., Gommers, S. et al. [1983]. The rhythmicity of fetal breathing varies with behavioral state in the human fetus. *Early Human Development, 9,* 1–7.)

TABLE 39–3
Characteristics of the Fetal Biophysical Profile

Parameter	Score 2 (Normal)	Score 0 (Abnormal)
Nonstress test	Reactive: two or more fetal heart rate accelerations of at least 15 beats/min in amplitude and at least 15-sec duration in 10 min within a 40-min testing period	Nonreactive: one or less fetal heart rate acceleration of at least 15 beats/min and 15-sec duration in 10 min within a 40-min testing period
Fetal breathing movements	At least one episode of fetal breathing of at least 30-sec duration in 30-min observational period	Absence of fetal breathing or less than 30 sec of breathing within a 30-min observation period
Fetal body movements	At least three discrete episodes of fetal movements in a 30-min period; episodes of active continuous movement counted as a single movement	Two or less discrete fetal movements in a 30-min observation period
Fetal tone	At least one episode of extension of extremities, hand, or trunk with return to position of flexion	Extremities in position of extension or partial flexion; spine in position in full extension; fetal movement not followed by return to flexion
Amniotic fluid volume	Amniotic fluid index greater than 5 cm	Amniotic fluid index less than or equal to 5 cm

(Modified from Walla, C. A., & Platt, L. D. [1991]. Observing fetal maturation through fetal movement and fetal behavior. In M. Berman (Ed.), *Diagnostic medical sonography, Vol. I. Obstetrics and gynecology.* Philadelphia: J.B. Lippincott.)

condition, only recently has it re-emerged as an effective screening tool in high- and low-risk pregnancies. Arguably, perceptions of fetal movement do not fully

RESEARCH HIGHLIGHT

Maternal Perception of Fetal Movement

Prenatal fetal surveillance in the high-risk pregnancy has been shown to significantly reduce fetal and perinatal mortality. Nearly half of all stillbirths, however, are associated with no identifiable maternal or fetal risk factors. Moore and Piacquadio conducted a prospective study evaluating the effectiveness of a fetal movement screening program in reducing fetal mortality.

From 28 weeks' gestation, 256 low-risk women were asked to record the time interval to appreciate 10 fetal movements between 7:00 PM to 11:00 PM. Subjects who failed to perceive 10 movements in 2 hours were instructed to report for further evaluation.

The mean time interval of monitoring was 30 minutes. During the study period, the number of prenatal tests performed increased 13%. Fetal mortality among clients with decreased movement dropped from 44 per 1,000 during the control period to 10 per 1,000 births during the study period.

Critique: The count-to-10 fetal movement screening program is a simple and effective method of reducing the rate of fetal demise. Nurses need to educate women on procedures of counting fetal movements and the importance of immediately reporting a decrease in fetal activity.

Moore, T. R., & Piacquadio, K. (1989). A prospective evaluation of fetal movement screening to reduce the incidence of antepartum fetal death. *American Journal of Obstetrics and Gynecology, 160,* 1075–1080.

indicate the type and quality of fetal movements, fetal maturity, or health; however, maternal perception of fetal movements do have a predictive value (Sabbagha, 1994). Several studies have reported that a reduced or total absence of fetal activity is associated with fetal compromise (Sadovsky et al., 1977; Liston et al., 1982; Rayburn, 1982).

Numerous protocols have been proposed to record maternal perception of fetal movement. They all involve either counting for a fixed time and recording the number of movements or recording the time taken to count a fixed number of movements. One frequently used method is the Cardiff "count-to-10" chart (Pearson et al., 1976), which involves having the mother note fetal movements up to a maximum of 10. When 10 movements are felt, she discontinues counting. Less than 10 movements within a 12-hour period are to be reported to her care provider. Variations on this technique involve a reduction in time defining the counting period to eliminate having abnormal results reported in the evening when further fetal evaluation is difficult to arrange (see Research Highlight).

The effectiveness of this assessment technique is based on several factors:

- An adequate explanation must be given to the client on how to keep a movement chart.
- The woman should be instructed to lie on her side in a quiet location, concentrate on the fetus' movements, and record the movements (Rayburn, 1995).
- She also must be instructed on the importance of reporting a reduction in fetal movements (Draper et al., 1986).

- Maternal compliance is more favorable when counting is for 1 hour or less each day and when her risk factors are specifically defined (Eggersen et al., 1987; Smith et al., 1992).

Prenatal Fetal Heart Rate Monitoring

Periodic electronic fetal monitoring during the third trimester has become a common method for evaluating the fetus in a high-risk pregnancy. As with many other forms of fetal assessment, a normal result is highly accurate in indicating fetal well-being. On the other hand, false-positive results occur with a relatively high frequency. For this reason, two or more different tests of fetal well-being are required before premature delivery or other remedial measures are instituted. Figure 39-10 shows a management scheme of prenatal fetal surveillance.

Contraction Stress Test

A **contraction stress test** (CST), or *oxytocin challenge test*, evaluates FHR in the presence of sponta-neous or oxytocin-induced contractions. The CST was developed with the premise that oxygenation of a marginally compromised fetus will transiently worsen with uterine contractions. The CST was widely applied clinically prior to the development of the Nonstress Test (Procedure 39-3).

Contraction Stress Test Interpretation. Results of the CST are classified as follows:

- Negative or passed test—No late decelerations of the FHR occur when an adequate frequency of three contractions in 10 minutes has been established, a "negative window."
- Positive—Late decelerations occur with three contractions in 10 minutes, a "positive window."
- Equivocal—No positive or negative window occurs, or late decelerations are associated with maternal hypotension or uterine hyperstimulation. In some areas of the country, any late decelerations are considered equivocal. Equivocal tests should be repeated within 24 hours.
- Hyperstimulation—Excessive uterine activity (more than three contractions in a 10-minute interval) is

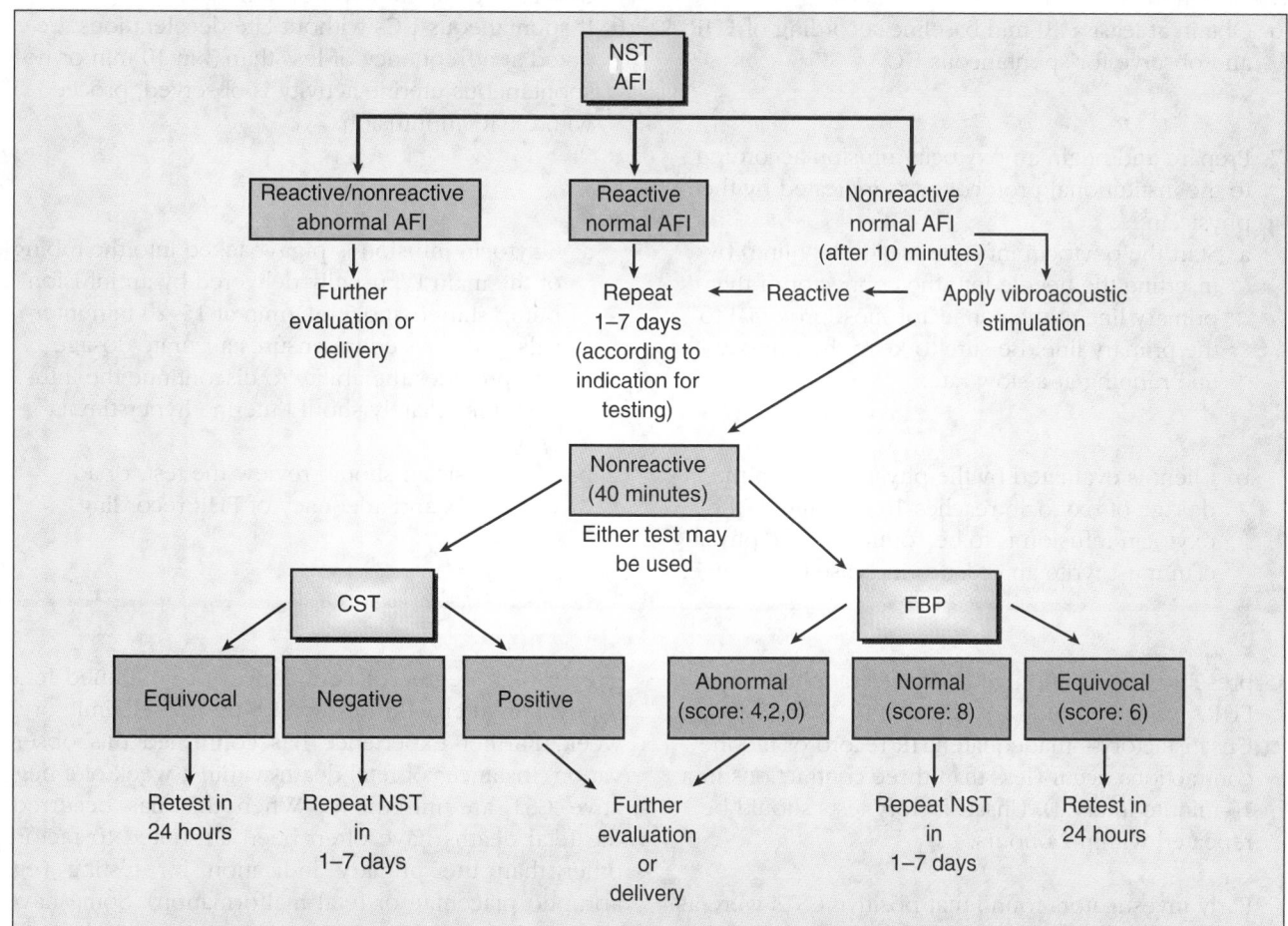

FIGURE 39-10 An example of a management scheme of prenatal fetal surveillance.

PROCEDURE 39–3
Performing the Contraction Stress Test

Procedure	Rationale
1. Take client to a labor or prenatal testing unit.	1. This ensures that qualified personnel will administer the test correctly.
2. Explain to client the testing procedure and the time involved. (The test requires an average of about 90 min, but it is not uncommon for the procedure to take 3 h.)	2. Giving a full explanation of the test and the average time of the test will help ease the client.
3. Place client in a semi-Fowler's position at a 30- to 45-degree angle with a slight left tilt.	3. This position will help eliminate supine hypotension resulting from compression of the vena cava by the enlarged uterus, which also reduces uteroplacental perfusion; this could result in late decelerations and a false-positive test. A semi-Fowler's position and turning the client to her left side will alleviate the compression and increase blood flow.
4. Place client on an external monitor. An ultrasound transducer is used to record the fetal heart rate (FHR), and a tocodynamometer is used to measure uterine contractions (UC).	
5. Record client's blood pressure initially and at 5- to 10-min intervals.	5. Blood pressure is taken to determine if the client is developing supine hypotension.
6. Obtain at least a 10-min baseline recording of FHR, and observe for spontaneous UC.	6. If spontaneous UCs without late decelerations are noted at a frequency of less than 3 in 10 min or no spontaneous uterine activity is observed, proceed with oxytocin infusion.
7. Prepare and begin an oxytocin infusion according to the institutional protocol or as indicated by the physician. a. Start the oxytocin infusion (secondary line) by inserting the needle into the connector of the primary line at the connector most proximal to the primary line. Be sure to keep the primary line running at a slow rate.	 a. Oxytocin infusion is piggybacked into the tubing of the main IV, usually delivered by an infusion pump started at 0.5 mU/min at 15–20-min intervals. This procedure ensures accurate dosage and provides the ability to discontinue the infusion immediately should uterine hyperstimulation occur.
b. Client is evaluated by the physician when the dosage of oxytocin reaches 10 mU/min. If the oxytocin infusion is to be continued, the physician must write an order to increase the dosage.	b. The physician should review the test for adequate UCs and adequacy of FHR recording.

present in association with a deceleration of the FHR.

■ Unsatisfactory—Inadequate FHR record or uterine contractions occur (less than three contractions in a 10-minute interval). Unsatisfactory tests should be repeated within 24 hours.

Early investigators found that positive CSTs were associated with a relatively high frequency of poor outcome, such as intrauterine fetal death, fetal distress, or poor condition of the newborn at birth. A normal CST gave a high degree of confidence for continued fetal survival in utero during an arbitrarily set limit of 1 week. Further experience has confirmed this observation. Instances of fetal death within 1 week of a negative CST are infrequent. When this has occurred, the fetal deaths have often been attributed to factors other than the primary indication for testing (eg, abruptio placentae or fetal malformation). Some have suggested performing CSTs more frequently when the maternal condition is deteriorating (eg, increasing severity of pregnancy-induced hypertension) or in certain very high-risk disorders (eg, diabetes with vascular disease).

Clinical studies in which clients were induced to labor and electronically monitored following a positive CST have demonstrated a high false-positive rate (25%–40%); that is, late decelerations did not recur in labor. Because of this, more than one test of fetal well-being should be carried out before a preterm delivery for fetal compromise is indicated. Clearly, the greatest benefit of the CST lies in the reassurance that allows continuation of a high-risk pregnancy when the test result is normal.

Nipple Stimulation Test

The **nipple stimulation test** is a noninvasive technique in prenatal testing that achieves a CST. This technique is based on the principle that nipple stimulation causes oxytocin to be released from the neurohypophysis, and if successful, the need for intravenous infusion of oxytocin (Pitocin) is eliminated. Several methods have been suggested to achieve an adequate test without effecting uterine hyperstimulation. The following protocol has been used successfully in a number of institutions.

- The client is instructed to roll both nipples between her fingers for 2 minutes.

- The client rests for 3 minutes, and then the procedure is repeated.
- Stimulation is continued for 20 minutes.
- If inadequate uterine contractions occur, the client increases stimulation to 3 minutes and rests for 2 minutes.
- Stimulation is discontinued if three contractions occur in 10 minutes, a positive CST is observed, a prolonged FHR deceleration occurs, or hyperstimulation is observed.
- If after 60 minutes, adequate contraction frequency is not achieved, an oxytocin challenge test is initiated.

The CST is an invasive and lengthy test. An average CST takes 90 minutes or more to achieve adequate contraction frequency. Because of the simplicity of nipple stimulation, the disadvantages of the CST can be avoided. Several reports have demonstrated that nipple stimulation is practical and has a predictive value similar to that of the CST (Huddleston et al., 1984; Oki et al., 1987; Rosenzweig et al, 1989; Fig. 39-11).

Nonstress Test

The **Nonstress Test (NST)** observes changes in FHR associated with spontaneous or evoked fetal movement. Studies have indicated that the heart rate of a nonacidotic fetus will temporarily accelerate with fetal move-

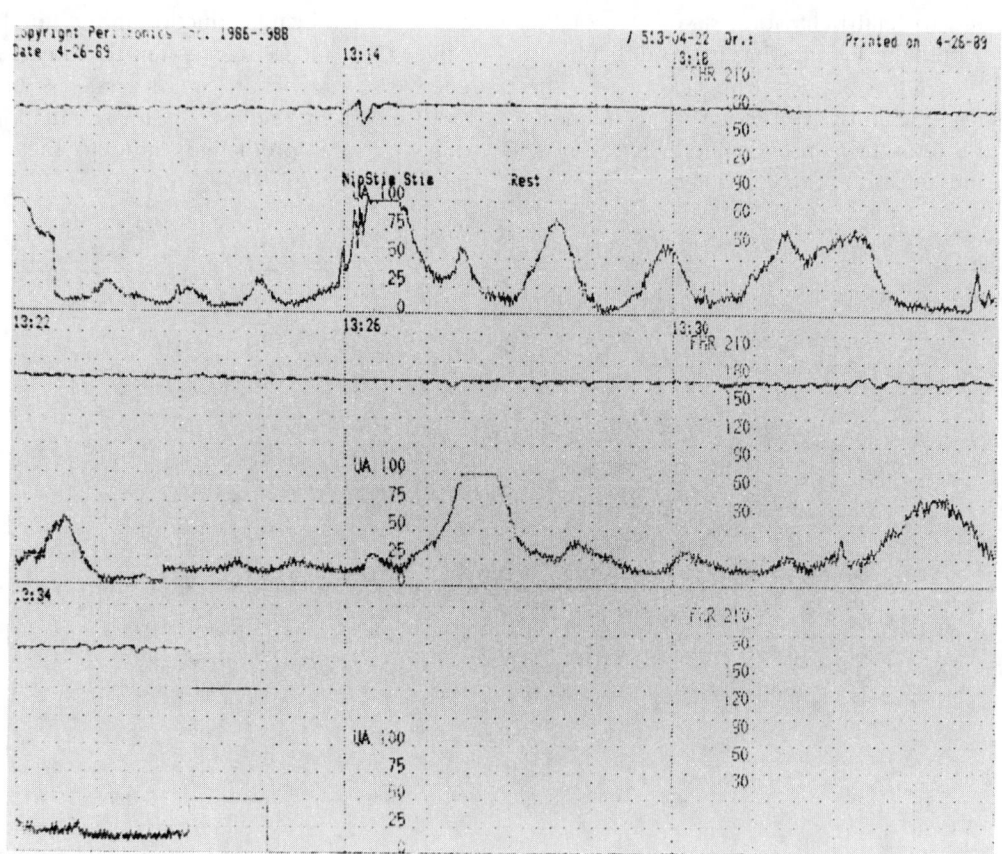

FIGURE 39–11 Computer printout of a negative CST performed with nipple stimulation.

ment. Because this form of testing does not require intravenous administration of drugs, it can be safely and more quickly performed in an outpatient area. These features, coupled with the apparent reliability of the NST as a screening test, have lessened the use of CSTs.

Various criteria have been applied for interpreting the NST. The occurrence of five accelerations of greater than 15 beats/min for more than 15 seconds in 20 minutes was initially required as a normal or reactive test. More recent studies have suggested that fewer accelerations of the same magnitude may be adequate. Many institutions define a reactive NST as the occurrence of two qualifying accelerations within a 10-minute period. Because the fetus has cyclic periods of rest, external stimulation has been used to elicit movement for the testing. Also, immature fetuses (fetuses less than 33 weeks' gestation), have fewer qualifying accelerations, leading to a higher incidence of nonreactive patterns (Smith et al., 1985; Baskett, 1988). Failure to demonstrate a reactive pattern because of lack of accelerations with movement or lack of fetal movement is taken as an indication for further evaluation of the fetus by a CST or FBP.

Vibroacoustic Stimulation

The reactive NST is a safe and reliable indicator of fetal well-being. Although a nonreactive NST may be a useful test of fetal compromise, episodes of nonreactivity are often related to fetal behavioral state. One of the problems with prenatal FHR testing is the difficulty in separating healthy fetuses at rest from sick fetuses who are not moving because of asphyxia. Various attempts to stimulate the fetus have proven ineffective. These include the administration of orange juice prior to test-

ing and manual manipulation of the maternal abdomen (Eglinton et al., 1984; Druzin et al., 1985). **Vibroacoustic stimulation** is used to reduce the number of falsely nonreactive tests presumably due to fetal sleep states. A state of reactivity is generated by an artificial larynx that provides acoustic and vibratory stimuli. This device emits fundamental tones of approximately 85 to 100 dB with a fundamental frequency of 850 Hz. When applied to the maternal abdomen, the fetus changes state and reacts with a startle response. The vibroacoustic stimulator has received FDA approval for prenatal use between 28 and 42 weeks' gestation. Use of the vibroacoustic stimulator prior to 28 weeks' gestation has been found to have little benefit because fetal hearing begins to develop at 24 to 25 weeks' gestation (Birnholz et al., 1983). Therefore, prior to 28 weeks, an inconsistent response to vibroacoustic stimulation occurs (Druzin et al., 1989).

Vibroacoustic stimulation is initiated in nonstress testing after 10 minutes of nonreactivity. The stimulator is applied to the maternal abdomen for 1 second, and FHR response is observed for 1 minute. If the criteria for adequate accelerations are not met, the fetus is stimulated for 2 seconds. If accelerations are not achieved after an additional 1 minute of observation, a third application of stimulation is performed for 3 seconds. The FHR is then observed until it becomes reactive or 40 minutes have elapsed. Several studies have reported that the use of vibroacoustic stimulation results in a significant reduction in the number of nonreactive NSTs and a decrease in the time required for a reactive test to occur (Smith et al., 1986; Clark et al., 1989). Reactivity achieved with stimulation was found to have equal predictive value to that of a spontaneously reactive NST (Fig. 39-12).

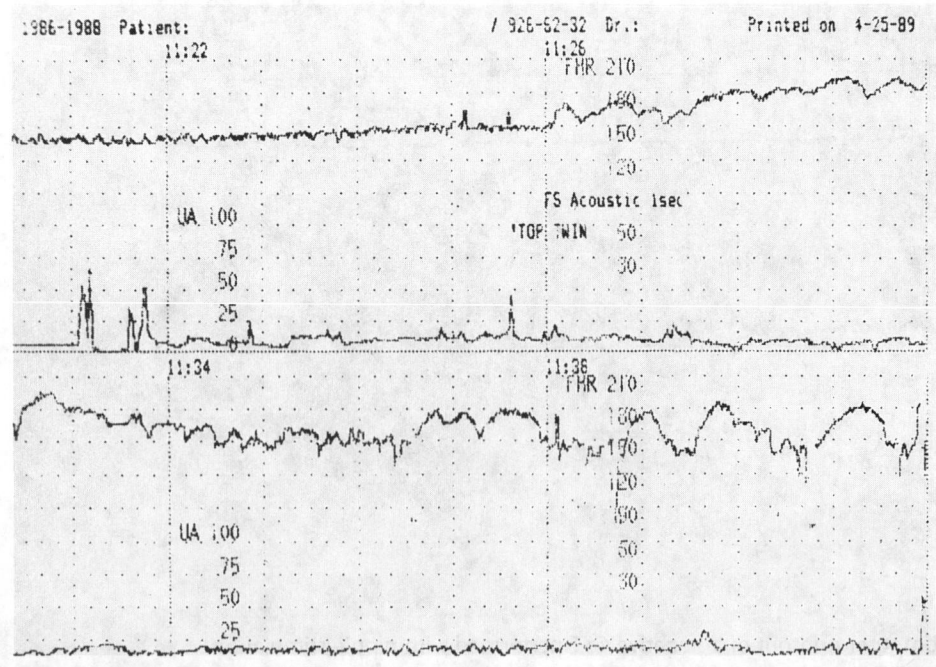

FIGURE 39–12 Computer printout of a reactive NST performed with vibroacoustic stimulation.

Modified Biophysical Profile

Many institutions advocate the use of a modified biophysical profile, the NST, and AFI as the primary testing mode of fetal surveillance (Clark et al., 1989; Nageotte et al., 1994). If nonreactivity is observed, the remaining three variables of the FBP can be performed to ensure fetal well-being. This method of testing is equal in predictive value to the CST and FBP.

Biochemical Assessment of the Fetus

Maternal Serum Studies

Alpha-fetoprotein

First introduced as a method to identify the fetus at risk for a neural tube defect, maternal serum alpha-fetoprotein screening now incorporates a whole new area of high-risk clients. This includes those at risk for fetal growth disturbances, stillbirth, preterm labor, low birth weight, and chromosomal disorders (Sabbagha, 1995; Wald et al., 1988; Burton, 1988). In the past, this was tested at 15 weeks' gestation. However, new technology has made it possible to analyze alpha-fetoprotein as early as 11 weeks' gestation, when alpha-fetoprotein begins to rise (Crandall et al., 1993). A detailed discussion of alpha-fetoprotein can be found in Chapter 14.

Human Chorionic Gonadotropin

Human chorionic gonadotropin (hCG), a glycoprotein hormone, is exclusively produced during pregnancy. Produced principally in syncytiotrophoblasts, hCG is detectable in maternal plasma soon after implantation. Plasma levels rise rapidly and double in concentration every 1.4 to 2.5 days, peaking at about 10 weeks' gestation; they fall off to relatively low levels in the second and third trimesters. The function of this hormone is to maintain corpus luteum function during early pregnancy (Martin et al., 1990). It is the basis for most pregnancy tests.

Values of hCG that deviate from the norm suggest an abnormally developing pregnancy. Abnormally slow production of hCG in early pregnancy is associated with threatened abortion or ectopic pregnancy (Kadar et al., 1981; Pittaway et al., 1985). However, 15% of normal intrauterine pregnancies demonstrate a slow production. Ultrasound in conjunction with hCG determinations can be used to differentiate normal from abortive or ectopic pregnancies (Coleman et al., 1988).

Elevated hCG levels are associated with hydatidiform mole. Values that remain elevated after 100 days of pregnancy strongly suggest a molar pregnancy. Values that are increased prior to this period are not necessarily due to a mole but may be due to multiple pregnancy. Evaluation with ultrasound is used to make a differential diagnosis (Coleman et al., 1988).

Recently it has been demonstrated that hCG levels in midtrimester pregnancies may be predictive of Down syndrome in conjunction with maternal age, maternal serum alpha-fetoprotein levels, and maternal serum estriol levels (see Chap. 14).

Estrogen and Estriol

Prior to maternal serum alpha-fetoprotein testing for gestational screening, serial plasma or urinary estriol (E3) determinations were the most widely used markers of fetoplacental well-being. Estrogen levels in maternal serum and urine rise progressively during the course of normal pregnancy. Although estrone and estradiol also increase during pregnancy, estriol is the predominant estrogen, increasing 1,000-fold and accounting for 90% of the total estrogen. At least 90% of the estrogen precursors are produced by the fetal adrenal cortex. The conversion of these precursors to estriol is a function of the placenta. If either the fetus or the placenta becomes compromised, decreased production of E3 is expected to occur (Martin et al., 1990; Ray, 1987). Therefore, abnormal estriol levels have been thought to predict poor perinatal outcome.

Serum and urine estriol levels have been used extensively in the past to determine fetal condition in a number of high-risk pregnancies, including diabetes, post-term pregnancies, hypertension, preeclampsia, and IUGR. Currently, however, estriol determinations are not used clinically in the obstetric management of these complicated pregnancies.

Maternal serum estriol levels in midtrimester pregnancies may predict Down syndrome in conjunction with maternal age, maternal serum alpha-fetoprotein levels, and hCG levels (see Chap. 14).

Progesterone

Progesterone, a steroid hormone, is produced by the placenta in progressively increasing quantities during pregnancy. It can be measured as serum progesterone or urinary pregnanediol; however, it has little value in evaluating fetal well-being, because progesterone does not require fetal precursors and can persist in significant quantities even after an intrauterine fetal death has occurred.

Human Placental Lactogen

Also known as human chorionic somatomammotropin, human placental lactogen is synthesized by the syncytiotrophoblast of the placenta in progressively increasing quantities throughout pregnancy. This hormone presently is not used in clinical management of high-risk pregnancies.

Maternal Blood Enzyme Measurement

A number of enzymes increase in concentration in maternal serum during pregnancy, including heat-stable alkaline phosphatase, diamine oxidase, and oxytocinase. The measurement of these enzymes is not used in the assessment of fetal well-being.

Fetal Cell Isolation

For some time it has been known that various fetal cell types (trophoblast, erythrocytes, and leukocytes) cross the placenta and circulate in the maternal blood in extremely small amounts (1 in 1 million in 1 cm³ of maternal blood; Senyei et al., 1993). Various techniques have been used to isolate assorted fetal cells based on the presence of specific fetal cell surface antigens. These cells are analyzed for fetal chromosomal abnormalities. Thus, **fetal cell isolation** is a noninvasive approach to identifying trisomic fetuses in utero. The fetal nucleated erythrocyte is the primary fetal cell used in isolation technology for a number of reasons. It is unlikely to be found in peripheral adult blood yet is abundant in the fetus early in gestation (Holzgreve et al., 1992). Further, because they have nuclei, these fetal erythrocytes contain a full complement of fetal genes.

To make a successful prenatal genetic diagnosis using fetal cells, it is vital to have a sensitive and specific technique to recover, identify, and analyze them. Fluorescence in situ hybridization (FISH) is a method by which probes (chemical compliments of the DNA of chromosomes) are synthetically created and used to hybridize (bind) their exact copy on the DNA. Hybridization is detected by a fluorescent signal placed on the probe. Isolated cells are examined on a microscope slide, and the signals are detected under a fluorescent microscope. Each chromosome is detected as a colored dot. The number of dots indicates the number of copies present of that specific chromosome. Thus, a cell from an individual with trisomy 21 (Down syndrome) will show three dots after hybridization to a chromosome 21 probe set, whereas a normal cell displays two dots (Geifman-Holtzman et al., 1994). Specific probes have been developed for the chromosomes most frequently involved in liveborn aneuploidies: 13, 18, 21, X, and Y (Ried et al., 1992). Only the chromosome number can be assessed by FISH; definitive chromosomal analysis must be achieved from specimens obtained by amniocentesis or chorionic villus sampling. Thus far, this technique is performed only on a research basis. While fetal cell isolation or FISH offers a potential promise for a noninvasive method of prenatal cytogenetic diagnosis, clinical evaluations are necessary to offer these techniques in place of amniocentesis, chorionic villus sampling, and triple marker studies.

Invasive Methods of Fetal Diagnosis

Amniocentesis

Amniocentesis, the oldest prenatal invasive procedure, has been in use for more than 100 years. Initial use of amniocentesis in the 19th century was the treatment of polyhydramnios (Romero et al., 1991). The most common indication for amniocentesis is prenatal diagnosis, followed by the evaluation of lung maturity in the third trimester of pregnancy. However, it is used in a number of procedures and diagnostic tests:

- Amniography
- Elective termination of pregnancy
- Management of isoimmunized pregnancies
- Diagnosis of chromosomal and metabolic disorders
- Detection of neural tube defects
- Evaluation of fetal lung maturity
- Detection of intra-amniotic infections

The technical aspects of amniocentesis and related nursing care are discussed in Chapter 14.

Amniotic Fluid Studies

Phospholipids: Assessment of Fetal Lung Maturity

Assessment of fetal lung maturity has evolved through extensive investigation of fetal pulmonary fluids. Because there are respiratory movements in utero, the composition of amniotic fluid reflects the content of pulmonary fluids. Analysis of amniotic fluid phospholipids is the most accurate method of determining the degree of fetal lung maturity. This analysis is recommended when elective preterm delivery is anticipated or required and when elective term delivery is planned, but gestational age is uncertain.

The stability of lung airway spaces depends on the presence of adequate amounts of surfactant. Synthesized by the type II pneumocytes in the lung, surfactant promotes lung airway space stability by reducing alveolar surface tension. Although it is present in small quantities from midpregnancy and increases slowly with advancing gestation, the mature pathway for surfactant synthesis is activated at 35 weeks in the normal pregnancy. In certain stressful circumstances, such as preeclampsia, class D and F diabetes, and IUGR, the process is accelerated. In others, such as class A, B, and C diabetes, it may be delayed.

There are several techniques for measuring this activity, including the "Shake" test, lecithin/sphingomyelin (L/S) ratio, latex agglutination of phosphatidylglycerol, and optical density at 650 nm. The Shake test determines the stability of foam on the surface of mixtures of ethyl alcohol and various dilutions of amniotic fluid. Maturity is indicated when the foam is stable in the presence of a 2:1 dilution. A kit (Lumadex-FSI Test) that uses these principles but varies the concentrations of ethanol and amniotic fluid has the advantage of being commercially available and prepackaged. Used carefully under controlled conditions, the Shake test has been quite accurate in predicting lung maturity.

The most widely used technique is the L/S ratio. Lecithin is a major constituent of surfactant. Because the concentration of sphingomyelin remains relatively constant, a rising L/S ratio indicates increasing surfactant production. The separation of lecithin and sphingomyelin is achieved by thin-layer chromatography. The ratio is determined either by visual inspection or by densitometry. Pulmonary maturity is established when the L/S ratio exceeds 2:1. The chances of encountering severe neonatal respiratory distress syndrome with an L/S ratio greater than 2:1 are extremely low.

A specific phospholipid in amniotic fluid, phosphatidylglycerol, has proven to be valuable in borderline instances of the L/S ratio and in women with class A, B, and C diabetes in whom fetal pulmonary maturity is often delayed to 37 weeks or later. The presence of phosphatidylglycerol in more than trace amounts, associated with an L/S ratio of more than 2:1, virtually ensures fetal pulmonary maturity.

Slide agglutination tests for the presence of phosphatidylglycerol are available. They appear to predict reliably the absence of respiratory distress syndrome when positive. When the slide test is negative, performance of a more definitive test (such as chromatography) is recommended.

Within recent years, two additional tests for fetal lung maturity have developed. The first of these, optical density measurement of amniotic fluid, has been used as a rapid screening test of lung maturity. The determination of the absorbance of light by amniotic fluid of 650 nm wavelength has been adopted by some institutions. The second test, which has developed since the early 1990s, is the evaluation of lamellar body number. Lamellar bodies consist almost entirely of surface-active phospholipids and are secreted by the pulmonary alveolar type II cells into the amniotic fluid (Oulton et al., 1980). Lamellar body concentration increases exponentially with gestation as does the L/S ratio. Lamellar body counts >30,000 to 55,000 particles/μL are associated with fetal pulmonary maturity (Lemuel et al., 1991; Ashwood et al., 1993; Fakhoury et al., 1994; Greenspoon et al., 1995). The appeal of this test is that lamellar bodies can be counted with a Coulter counter or any particle counter for automated platelet quantitation. Virtually all hospital-based laboratories in the United States are equipped with such counters. Thus, the test has 24-hour availability in any laboratory, with the procedure typically taking approximately less than 2 hours to perform. Furthermore, less amniotic fluid is required for this examination (0.4 mL versus 3 mL for an L/S ratio and phosphatidylglycerol), and it is much less expensive than the L/S ratio and phosphatidylglycerol tests (Ashwood et al., 1993; Fakhoury et al., 1994). Lamellar body counts appear to have potential as a sensitive and rapid test for determining fetal lung maturity; however, studies continue to evaluate how such factors as oligohydramnios, polyhydramnios, blood, and meconium in the amniotic fluid affect the results.

Bilirubin: Assessment of the Isoimmunized Pregnancy

Hemolytic disease is the excessive destruction of red blood cells in the newborn. It is caused by maternal antigens, usually in response to Rh or ABO blood incompatibilities. Hemolytic disease is one of the complications of pregnancy in which there may be devastating fetal effects with virtually no maternal risk. Although the fetal pathology of severe hemolytic disease had been described before the 1900s, the exact nature of the problem was not known until after the discovery of the Rh factor in 1940. Most of the attention has been focused on the Rh factor (D antigen) as a cause of hemolytic disease; however, the ABO blood groups and other blood factors, such as Kell, c, E, and C, also may cause a form of hemolytic disease.

For more than 20 years, this disease has been declining in the United States, due to the availabilty of Rh antibody prevention. In 1970, the incidence of hemolytic disease in newborns was approximately 45 in 10,000 births. By 1980, it had dropped to 13 in 10,000 births. The majority of new cases result from ABO incompatibility or the failure to prevent maternal sensitization by not administering or administering an inadequate dose of Rh immunoglobulin during the prenatal and postpartum periods.

All pregnant women should be tested for ABO and Rh types and screened for antibodies to these and other red blood cell antigens. Any red blood cell antibody present must be specifically identified, and appropriate titers must be obtained to determine whether there is a risk to the fetus. If an antibody is present that is known to cause fetal or newborn hemolytic disease, the father's blood type and zygosity for that antigen should be determined if possible.

Anti-D Globulin. The ability to prevent Rh sensitization has been an established fact since Rh (anti-D) globulin became commercially available in 1969. It prevents sensitization by clearing the fetal cells from the maternal circulation and perhaps also by depressing the client's immune response. A single dose (300 μg) is capable of clearing up to 15 mL of fetal erythrocytes. Microdoses (50 μg) have been made available for use in situations when only small fetomaternal hemorrhages are likely.

Candidates for Rh immunoglobulin are the following unsensitized Rh-negative clients:

- Have delivered Rh-positive newborns
- Have had untypeable pregnancies, such as stillborns, ectopic pregnancies, or spontaneous or induced abortions
- Have received ABO-compatible Rh-positive blood
- Have had an invasive diagnostic procedure, such as amniocentesis

It is of no value in the client who is already sensitized. It should be administered within 3 days of delivery.

Pathophysiology. Even though the maternal and fetal circulation are normally completely separated, breaks in this barrier permit the entry of fetal red blood cells into the maternal circulation. This happens during the second and third trimesters and at delivery in up to 50% of pregnancies. Such breaks also occur with abortions beyond 6 to 8 weeks of pregnancy. Isoimmune hemolytic disease of the fetus and newborn is caused by a fetal–maternal blood group incompatibility, with maternal immunization against a fetal blood group antigen. Maternal antibodies bind fetal circulation and trigger fetal reticuloendothelial system digestion of fetal red blood cells. Deformed cells are removed from circulation and disposed of by hemolysis and phagocytosis. With worsening anemia, the fetus compensates by maximizing red blood cell production. Hemolysis continues, so the anemia remains uncorrected and worsens. In the worst possible case, hydrops fetalis occurs, resulting in ascites, pericardial effusion, cardiac failure, impaired placental circulation, and finally fetal death (Harman, 1991).

Management. The severity of the hemolytic anemia in the fetus can be determined by the quantity of bilirubin in the amniotic fluid (ie, the higher the bilirubin level, the lower the fetal hemoglobin). Thus, amniocentesis with analysis of bilirubin in the fluid is used for making therapeutic decisions in sensitized women. Using spectrophotometry, bilirubin produces an optical density peak at 450 nm, and the height of this peak (or OD450) is used to evaluate fetal involvement. In most laboratories, a significant antibody titer below which fetal morbidity is unlikely can be determined. Although this varies from institution to institution, titers above 1:8 to 1:16 are generally considered significant. Amniocentesis can be instituted as early as 20 weeks' gestation. The frequency of repeated amniocentesis is determined by the level of the OD450; weekly taps are indicated if values are high.

The common method for evaluating OD450 is the Liley chart, which is illustrated in Figure 39-13. Values in the lower zone for the particular gestation indicate a mildly affected or even unaffected fetus, whereas those in the middle zone indicate an affected fetus but one not in immediate danger of death. Values in the upper zone suggest the fetus will not survive 10 to 14 days without intervention. Management decisions are not based on single values but rather on the trend. If the OD450 remains in the lower zone, no interference is indicated, and the pregnancy is allowed to proceed to term. If the values remain in the middle zone, the fetus is best delivered as soon as there is evidence of maturity. Upper-zone values indicate immediate intervention by delivery if beyond 33 to 34 weeks' gestation or by intrauterine transfusion if before that age.

Ultrasound is a vital element in the management of the isoimmunized fetus. The fetus is examined for signs of congenital abnormalities, edema, or ascites. Routine measurements are obtained to verify gestational age to ensure proper usage of the Liley chart. When measurements are made, any changes in the AC that may be due to hepatosplenomegaly are specifically noted. M-mode ultrasound is effective in identifying pericardial effusions (DeVore et al., 1982). Doppler ultrasound has several uses in the assessment of the isoimmunized fetus. For example, affected fetuses have higher than usual velocities in umbilical arteries when the fetus is anemic (Copel et al., 1988). Color flow imaging can be used to diagnose fetal anemia directly by visualizing the umbilical cord for purposes of fetal blood sampling.

Percutaneous Umbilical Blood Sampling

In utero blood sampling has been possible since 1972 when Valenti obtained samples under endoscopic visualization (Valenti, 1972). Prior to 1982, blood sampling was performed by fetoscopy, which is a difficult and invasive technique that has a significant associated fetal risk. In 1983, Daffos et al. (1983) were the first to report PUBS, also known as cordocentesis, under direct ultrasound guidance.

Indications for PUBS follow:

- Risk of fetal hemolytic disease
- Rapid karyotype
- Diagnosis of congenital infection
- Hemoglobinopathies
- Coagulopathies
- Immunodeficiency syndromes
- Fetal well-being (Romero et al., 1991).

Additionally, PUBS is performed to study the development of various fetal biologic parameters. Prior to PUBS, these factors could be studied only in products of abortion. Fetal blood can now be studied for hema-

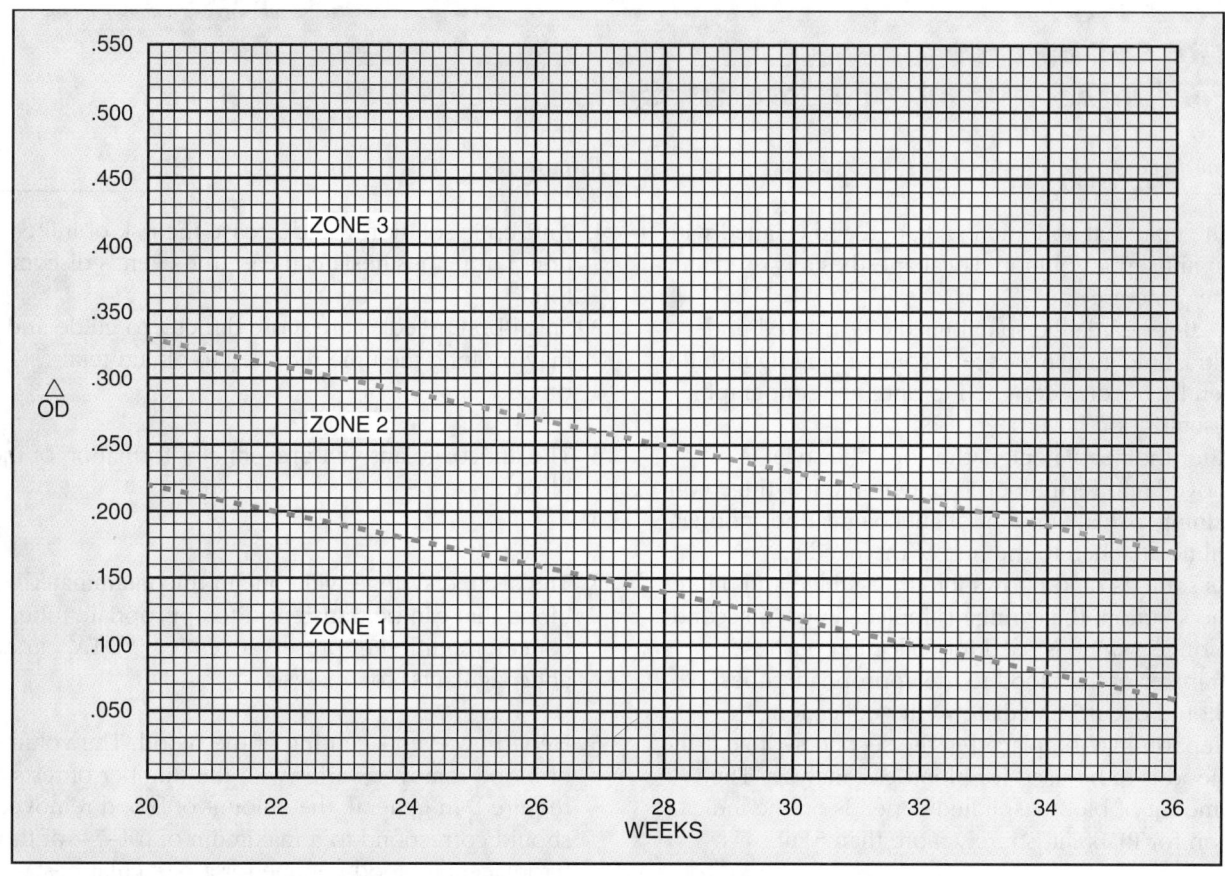

FIGURE 39-13 Modified Liley graph for relating OD450 to weeks of gestation in determining the severity of hemolytic disease. (Recreated from [1972]. *Management of erythroblastosis [Technical Bulletin, 17].* Chicago: ACOG.)

tologic, biochemical, hemostasis, endocrinologic, immunologic, and acid–base parameters (Daffos, 1990).

The PUBS can be performed as an inpatient or outpatient procedure. Immediately before the procedure, a complete ultrasound examination is performed. The insertion site of the umbilical cord in the placenta is then identified. This site is preferred for sampling because the cord is in its most fixed position and can be punctured more easily at this point. Free-floating cord is more difficult to penetrate because it slips away from the needle. Color flow Doppler is useful in determining the proper location. The site may be obstructed by the fetus, so it may be necessary to empty or fill the bladder or manipulate the fetus manually to gain access to the umbilical cord (Procedure 39-4).

The sampling procedure is relatively short, taking approximately 10 minutes to perform (Daffos, 1990). This technology is associated with a 2% risk of complication (Scott et al., 1995). Complications of PUBS include spontaneous abortion in 0.8% of the procedures and fetal demise in 1.1% of the procedures. Additional complications associated with the procedure are bleeding from the puncture site, fetal bradycardia, infection, thrombosis of the umbilical vein, and formation of um-

bilical cord hematoma (Daffos et al., 1985; Muller et al., 1988; Jauniaux et al., 1989).

Chorionic Villus Sampling

Chorionic villus sampling is an effective method for obtaining living trophoblastic tissue for genetic diagnosis in the first trimester of pregnancy. The tissue can be tested for a rapidly increasing number of biochemical and chromosomal disorders of the fetus. A detailed discussion of chorionic villus sampling is presented in Chapter 14.

Fetal Tissue Sampling

Several genetic disorders cannot be diagnosed by chromosomal analysis. In these cases, direct sampling of fetal tissue can be performed. Fetal skin sampling is performed if there is a suspicion of severe skin disorders associated with high rates of morbidity and mortality. In this procedure, biopsy forceps are inserted through an Angiocath. Under continuous ultrasound guidance, the biopsy forceps are used to take fetal skin samples (Shulman et al., 1990).

PROCEDURE 39-4
Percutaneous Umbilical Blood Sampling (PUBS)

Procedure	*Rationale*
1. The maternal abdomen is draped and cleaned with an antiseptic solution. Local anesthesia is used at the puncture site.	1. Antiseptic solution will decrease the risk of infection. Local anesthesia can ease the client's discomfort.
2. A 20- or 22-gauge spinal needle is inserted under ultrasonic guidance (see accompanying figure). Recently, needles designed to optimize sonographic visualization have been used.	2. Small-bore needles are more difficult to guide and may prolong the time required to obtain fetal blood.
3. After the needle enters the cord, the stylet is removed and fetal blood is drawn into a syringe containing a small amount of anticoagulant or normal saline attached to the hub of the needle.	3. The anticoagulant will prevent clot formation of the blood.
4. As soon as blood flows into the syringe and dilutes the solution, the syringe is replaced with a second syringe, which is used for collection purposes. Transfer of the blood to the appropriate tubes should occur immediately after collection.	4. The second syringe will contain uncontaminated blood that can be transferred to appropriate tubes containing different preservatives (eg, EDTA, citrate, anticoagulants) for analysis.
5. Heparin may be placed in the second syringe if the blood is to be used for blood gas analysis. The amount of blood aspirated depends on the indication for PUBS; it is rarely more than 5 mL.	5. Heparin prevents clotting of the blood. The volume of blood removed varies with the number of tests required. In general, the amount of blood removed should correspond to a maximum of 6%–7% of the fetoplacental blood volume for a particular gestational age.
6. On completion of sampling, the needle is withdrawn, and ultrasound is used to determine fetal status.	6. Fetal heart motion is confirmed with ultrasound.
7. The fetal heart rate is then monitored for 1 to 2 hours following the procedure (Ghidini et al., 1996).	7. Complications of PUBS include cord hematoma and fetal hemorrhage, which could result in a prolonged bradycardia and rapid deterioration of the fetus. Further, a vasospasm reflex of the umbilical artery can elicit a vasovagal response in the fetus, leading to a transient fetal bradycardia. The procedure also may stimulate the uterus, thereby resulting in uterine contractions. Monitoring of the fetus will alert the caretakers to possible complications resulting from the procedure.

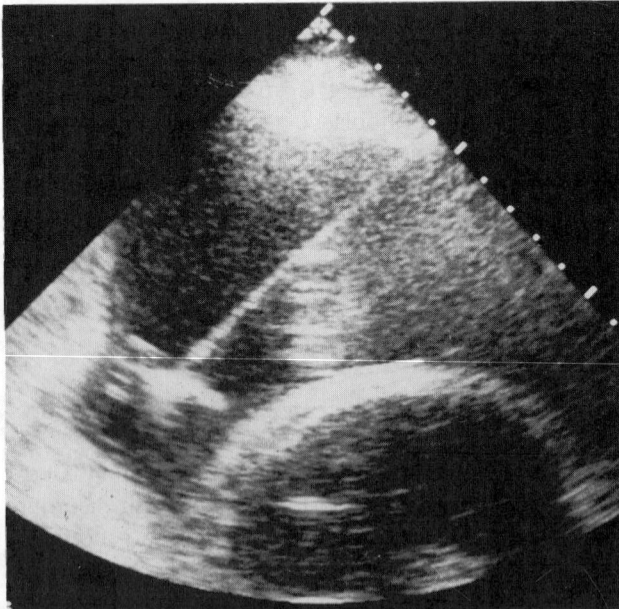

A needle penetrating the umbilical cord in percutaneous umbilical blood sampling.

Fetal liver biopsy is performed to diagnose inborn errors of metabolism limited to liver enzyme abnormalities. The biopsy is performed under continuous ultrasound guidance. A biopsy needle is inserted directly into the fetal liver, and fetal liver tissue is aspirated (Shulman et al., 1990). These tissue sampling techniques are investigational and not widely used.

Fetal Treatment

The art of fetal treatment is far less developed than that of fetal diagnosis. The most common approach to fetal treatment by the obstetrician is to select an appropriate time for delivery, convert the fetus to a newborn, and allow active treatment by the neonatologist. Perhaps the most important approach to fetal treatment is to provide appropriate support throughout the pregnancy. This includes adequate prenatal diet and sufficient glucose and oxygen during labor, especially if there is fetal distress.

Treatment in the case of a positive prenatal diagnosis of severe congenital disease is generally limited to therapeutic abortion. In some instances, however, in utero treatment may correct an increasing number of fetal defects and diseases.

Pharmacologic and Nutritional Therapy

Many drugs administered to the mother cross the placenta into the fetal circulation. Transplacental passage is generally a function of the molecular size of the drug. Substances with molecular weights less than 500 cross readily by simple diffusion. Although there should always be concern about the possible harmful effects of drugs, one can sometimes achieve a desirable therapeutic effect in the fetus by treating the mother. An example of this is the administration of digitalis to the mother when the fetus is suffering from supraventricular tachycardia. This cardiac arrhythmia is suspected when there is an elevated FHR and is confirmed by fetal echocardiography. Administering digitalis through the mother to the fetus is the treatment of choice.

Another example of fetal drug therapy is the administration of glucocorticoids to the mother to induce the production of surfactant by the type II cells of the fetal lung. There is evidence that if this is done between 26 to 28 and 32 to 34 weeks' gestation and delivery can be delayed for 24 to 48 hours, there will be a significant reduction in respiratory distress. The effect appears to be transient; the frequency of respiratory distress increases when delivery is delayed for more than 7 days following treatment. The effectiveness of this approach is still under investigation. There are risks, however,

associated with the use of glucocorticoids during pregnancy. For example, they may increase the risk of in utero infection. Additionally, long-term effects on the child exposed to glucocorticoids in utero include the following:

- Steroid-induced moon face
- Diabetes mellitus
- Psychosis
- Adrenocortical insufficiency
- Osteoporosis
- Aseptic necrosis (Scott et al., 1995)

Nutritional supplementation has been proposed as a method for treating IUGR. Supplemental nutrients can be provided to the growth-retarded fetus by three main routes: maternal administration, amniotic fluid, and direct administration to the fetus. These methods are experimental, and research is ongoing (Harding et al., 1990).

Transfusion

Intrauterine fetal transfusion in Rh disease is the most publicized form of fetal treatment. When the hematocrit determined by fetal blood sampling is low or hydrops is present, intrauterine transfusion is indicated. Prior to PUBS, intraperitoneal transfusion was the treatment of choice for the isoimmunized fetus. The direct intravascular route for fetal transfusions, however, is now favored over the intraperitoneal route because it yields direct information with regard to the severity of the disease, corrects fetal anemia more physiologically, and is associated with a lower risk of complications. The survival rate reaches 80% to 90% even in hydropic fetuses. Transfusions can be performed from 18 to 34 weeks' gestation by a technique similar to that for fetal blood sampling. Type O Rh-negative blood that is packed to a hematocrit of 65% to 85% is infused at a rate of 5 to 10 mL/min. The amount of transfused blood is calculated according to the estimated fetoplacental blood volume for gestational age and fetal pretransfusion hematocrit (Nicolaides et al., 1986). Intravascular transfusion has transformed the prognosis for immune hydrops, particularly if it is already present before 25 weeks.

Intrauterine intravascular transfusions also have been used to infuse platelets into the fetus diagnosed with severe thrombocytopenia. The fetus is transfused at 37 weeks to allow vaginal delivery. Cesarean section does not eliminate the risk of hemorrhage in the fetus and is unnecessary in most cases (Daffos et al., 1984).

Surgery and Needle Aspiration

Refinements in sonography have resulted in earlier and more accurate diagnosis of fetal abnormalities. Efforts to treat these have received substantial press coverage, captured public attention, and engendered substantial public and professional debate. Successful intrauterine treatment of lower urinary tract obstruction has been reported. Previously, this obstruction would have resulted in extensive fetal kidney damage. Particularly noteworthy is the intrauterine treatment of hydrocephalus. Efforts have been made to relieve the hydrocephalus by intermittent sonographically directed needle aspiration through the woman's abdomen or even by the surgical insertion of a shunt to provide continuous drainage into the amniotic sac (Cendron et al., 1994; Paidas et al., 1994). The risk-to-benefit ratio of these procedures is not established, and they must still be considered experimental. Clearly, there are substantial ethical issues, because such treatment could allow the survival of a severely retarded child who might otherwise have died in utero (Chervenak et al., 1991).

Future Therapy

The future undoubtedly holds many advances—from the prenatal correction of congenital defects to the unscrambling of genetic mishaps. There may well be treatments of maladies that are presently unknown in this rapidly developing area of fetal medicine.

Nursing Care of the Fetus and Family at Risk

Nursing Process

The nursing process is designed to accomplish the major client goals for care of the fetus and family at risk:

- The fetus maintains optimal health.
- The compromised fetus is detected and treated to permit appropriate delivery and neonatal care.
- The client and family indicate knowledge of fetal diagnostic and treatment procedures.
- The client and family psychologically adjust to the defective or compromised fetus.

Nursing care is planned in conjunction with the desires of the woman, family, and with various members of the perinatal team, including the perinatologist, sonographer, laboratory personnel, and neonatologist. Fetal diagnostic techniques are most often performed as outpatient procedures. Thus the nurse has minimal time and client contact to achieve effective and therapeutic care as proposed by the perinatal team. A wide knowledge base of diagnostic methodologies and fetal disease processes, communications skills, and an organized plan of care are essential in assisting the fetus and its family to accomplish desired goals in a timely manner.

Nursing Assessment

Assessment of the fetus is initiated by obtaining a complete medical and obstetric history on the client's arrival for testing. Factors that may alter fetal diagnosis and treatment can be identified at this time. Psychosocial factors are appraised to determine the level of anxiety and stress the woman and family are experiencing in relation to the possibility of having an abnormal fetus. The family may be grieving and experiencing a sense of loss of their anticipated "perfect" child. Capacity of learning should be assessed to ascertain the level of knowledge the family can absorb. When the family is faced with the possibility of having an impaired newborn, they are often unable to assimilate information relating to the diagnostic procedure or the prognosis of their fetus.

Potential Nursing Diagnoses

Nursing assessment can identify several potential diagnoses relating to the fetus in jeopardy and its family. These may include

- Risk for Injury to fetus related to diagnostic tests and/or treatment
- Ineffective Family Coping
- Knowledge Deficit of fetal diagnosis, treatment, and prognosis

Nursing Intervention

Several clinical evaluations of the fetus can be accomplished by the nurse. These include fundal height, determination of estimated date of delivery, and maternal weight. Education of fetal activity counting also is a vital nursing function. Most diagnostic techniques, however, are usually performed by sonographic and laboratory specialists and the perinatologist. It is often the nurse's responsibility to explain the indications, risks, accuracy, and methodology of the procedures and the rationale for their use. The family must be allowed to ask questions about the tests and express their fears and concerns about their fetus.

Many obstetric nurses across the country are now performing expanded roles as nurse specialists in the field of prenatal fetal surveillance. With specialized training, these nurses have the ability to perform not only prenatal FHR monitoring, but also various sonographic procedures. In 1993, the Association of Women's Health, Obstetric, and Neonatal Nurses (AWHONN) set forth nursing practice competencies and educational guidelines for nurses who perform limited ultrasound examinations. Limited ultrasound examinations, as discussed previously, include confirmation of fetal life or death, identification fetal number and presentation, amniotic

NURSING CARE PLAN
The Fetus and Family at Risk

Nursing Goals:
1. Fetus maintains optimal health throughout pregnancy.
2. Fetal compromise is detected early to allow for appropriate and timely intervention.
3. Client understands and complies with prenatal treatment.
4. Client and family accept and adapt to fetal compromise and injury.

Assessment	*Diagnoses*	*Intervention/Rationale*	*Evaluation*
Care of the fetus			
Gestational age Nägele's rule ultrasound	Risk for Injury to fetus related to lack of early prenatal care, diagnosis, and intervention	Obtain history from client *to assess baseline status.* Determine fetal gestational age *to provide basis for future assessments.* Perform serial fundal height measurements *to assess internal fetal growth.*	Gestational age of fetus is determined and confirmed early in the first trimester.
Fetal well-being Prenatal diagnosis using maternal serum alpha-fetoprotein (MSAFP) testing, ultrasound, and amniocentesis or chorionic villus sampling (CVS)		Explain purpose of MSAFP test and obtain consent *to promote informed client participation.* Prepare client and family for ultrasound, genetic counseling, and amniocentesis or CVS procedure as indicated *to alleviate concern about procedural techniques.*	Fetal compromise is identified as soon as possible, and options are discussed with the client and her family.
Fetal growth and development	Risk for Altered Nutrition related to disease process (ie, chronic hypertension, diabetes)	Check maternal weight at each prenatal visit *to measure weight gain.*	Fetus grows appropriately for gestational age.
	Risk for Impaired Gas Exchange related to disease process (ie, chronic hypertension, diabetes)	Provide nutritional counseling for the client *to provide optimal potential for fetal growth and development.*	Results of fetal testing continue to be reassuring for gestational age and condition.
		Arrange for serial ultrasounds as ordered *to monitor more closely fetal growth.* Arrange for serial nonstress testing and fetal biophysical profiles as indicated *to monitor fetal well-being.* Teach client to initiate fetal kick counts *to monitor fetal activity closely.* Report all test results to appropriate health-care provider *to promote coordinated client care.*	Developing fetal compromise is identified and treated as early as possible.

(continued)

NURSING CARE PLAN *(Continued)*
The Fetus and Family at Risk

Assessment	Diagnoses	Intervention/Rationale	Evaluation
Delivery of high-risk fetus	Risk for Birth Trauma related to compromised fetal condition	Facilitate transfer if indicated *to promote optimal care of high-risk neonate.* Prepare for high-risk delivery *to promote smooth resuscitation and treatment as needed.* Coordinate availability of qualified personnel at delivery *to maximize potential neonatal outcome.* Arrange for resuscitation and specialty equipment at delivery *to ensure readiness for delivery and treatment of newborn.*	High-risk newborn is delivered atraumatically at appropriate facility. Qualified personnel are present at delivery.

Care of the woman and her support system

Assessment	Diagnoses	Intervention/Rationale	Evaluation
Coping behaviors	Ineffective Individual and Family Coping related to perceived parental role failure	Promote communication and coping by asking open-ended questions and allowing client and family to vent. Explain all procedures prior to starting them *to alleviate anxiety.* Reinforce prior explanations *for consistency.* Facilitate meeting with multidisciplinary staff prior to delivery *to teach client and family what to expect at delivery.*	Client and family are able to communicate freely with staff. Client and family voice their concerns regarding the pregnancy. Client and family voice understanding of all procedures. Client and family demonstrate appropriate coping behaviors.
Learning capabilities Readiness modalities	Knowledge Deficit related to etiology and treatment of high-risk fetal condition	Assess client's and family's readiness to learn *enabling a successful session.* Assess client's and family's preferred learning methods *so that teaching style is appropriate.* Develop a personalized teaching plan that is appropriate to educational level and method of client and family *to ensure dissemination of information.*	Client and family demonstrate readiness to learn. Client and family achieve learning goals. Client and family are actively involved in the plan of care.
Capability for compliance	Risk for Noncompliance with plan of care related to lack of resources	Arrange for client and family transportation as needed *to promote compliance.* Contact social worker *to arrange for financial assistance as needed.*	Client and family arrive for all scheduled visits. Client is not denied necessary treatments or procedures due to financial constraints.

fluid assessment, FBP, and localization of the placenta. Each institution's policies and procedures should specifically identify which components of a limited examination its obstetric nurses can perform (AWHONN, 1993). AWHONN further suggests that the obstetric nurse performing limited examinations should have a minimum of 12 hours of didactic instruction relating to ultrasound physics and instrumentation, client education, and nursing accountability. Clinical experiences should include "hands on" practicums. When meeting the institution's requirements for performing these sonographic examinations, the obstetric nurse should then participate in continuing education sessions, such as reviews and clinical update sessions, to maintain competency in this area (AWHONN, 1993; see Nursing Care Plan).

Evaluation

The fetus and the family must be reevaluated in light of the results of the diagnostic procedures. It is anticipated that the fetus will maintain optimal health as a result of assessment and intervention. It is also desirable that the family understands the reasons for testing and the treatment that may ensue as a result of the diagnostic outcome. Finally, it is expected that the family members will have the ability to communicate freely among themselves and staff members about their fears and concerns.

Summary Points

✔ Early in pregnancy, ultrasound is used to confirm the presence of a viable intrauterine pregnancy. As the pregnancy progresses, many congenital abnormalities can be identified at an early gestational age. Throughout pregnancy, serial ultrasound examinations reflect fetal growth patterns. All of the information enables the healthcare team to provide early diagnosis and treatment of problems for the client and family.

✔ Maternal serum studies and amniotic fluid studies provide a variety of information regarding fetal well-being. The presence of hCG is a conclusive indicator of pregnancy, but deviations from the normal range can indicate impending threats to the viability of the pregnancy. Similarly, assessment of fetal pulmonary phospholipids found in the amniotic fluid reflect the degree of fetal lung maturity.

✔ The FBP, composed of fetal behaviors and physiologic markers, is a method of fetal surveillance that enables a composite assessment with a predictive accuracy that surpasses indiviual assessment of

these same factors. This collective picture of fetal behavior reflects either fetal well-being or progressive fetal compromise, enabling appropriate and timely intervention as needed.

✔ Prenatal FHR monitoring involves noninvasive assessment of FHR patterns. These patterns provide information about fetal oxygenation and central nervous system activity. Testing can involve observation of the heart rate during spontaneous or evoked fetal movement, natural or induced uterine contractions, or a combination of scenarios.

✔ The primary goal of fetal treatment is to prolong gestation safely until the appropriate time for delivery, which varies depending on the condition of the woman and fetus. Fetal treatment ranges from relatively noninvasive interventions, such as adequate maternal diet, to extremely invasive interventions, such as fetal transfusion or surgery. Fetal treatment is a developing technology with promising opportunities for the future.

REFERENCES

Acker, D. B., Sachs, B. P., & Friedman, E. A. (1985). Risk factors for shoulder dystocia. *Obstetrics and Gynecology, 66,* 762.

AIUM Bioeffects Reports Subcommittee (1988). Bioeffects considerations for the study of diagnostic ultrasound. *Journal of Ultrasound Medicine, 7,* S4.

American College of Obstetricians and Gynecologists (1993). *Ultrasound in pregnancy* (Technical Bulletin 187). Washington, DC: Author.

Andersen, H. F., Johnson T. R. B., Barclay, M. L. et al. (1981). Gestational age assessment: I. Analysis of individual clinical observations. *American Journal of Obstetrics and Gynecology, 139,* 173.

Arduini, D., Rizzo, G., Giorlandino, C. et al. (1985). The fetal behavioral states: An ultrasonic study. *Prenatal Diagnosis, 5,* 269–276.

Arduini, D., Rizzo, G., Giorlandino, C. et al. (1986). The development of fetal behavioral states: A longitudinal study. *Prenatal Diagnosis, 6,* 117–124.

Arduini, D., Rizzo, G., Romanni, C. et al. (1987). Fetal blood flow velocity waveforms as predictors of growth retardation. *Obstetrics and Gynecology, 70,* 7.

Ashwood, E. R., Plamer, S. E., Taylor, J. A., & Pingree, S. S. (1993). Lamellar body counts for rapid fetal lung maturity testing. *Obstetrics and Gynecology, 81,* 619–624.

Association of Women's Health, Obstetric and Neonatal Nurses (1993). *Nursing practice competencies and educational guidelines for limited ultrasound examinations in obstetric and gynecologic/infertility settings.* Washington, DC: Author.

Baskett T. F. (1988). Gestational age and fetal biophysical assessment. *American Journal of Obstetrics and Gynecology, 158,* 332–334.

Baskett, T. F., Allen, A. C., Gray, J. H. et al. (1987). Fetal biophysical profile and perinatal death. *Obstetrics and Gynecology, 70,* 357–360.

Bastide, A., Manning, F. A., Harman, C. R. et al. (1986). Ultrasound evaluation of amniotic fluid: Outcome of pregnancies with severe oligohydramnios. *American Journal of Obstetrics and Gynecology, 154*, 895.

Beazley, J. M., & Underhill, R. A. (1970). Fallacy of the fundal height. *British Medical Journal, 4*, 404.

Benacerraf, B., Gelman, R., & Frigoletto, F. D. (1987). Sonographic identification of second trimester fetuses with Down's syndrome. *New England Journal Medicine, 317*, 1371–1376.

Benacerraf, B. R., Mandell, J., Estroff, J. A., Harlow, B. L., & Frigoletto, F. D. (1990). Fetal pyelectasis: A possible association with Down syndrome. *Obstetrics and Gynecology, 76*, 58–60.

Benacerraf, B. R., Miller, W. A., & Frigoletto, F. D. (1988a). Sonographic detection of fetuses with trisomies 13 and 18: Accuracy and limitations. *American Journal of Obstetrics and Gynecology, 158*, 404–409.

Benacerraf, B. R., Osathanondh, R., & Frigoletto, F. D. (1988b). Sonographic demonstration of hypoplasia of the middle phalanx of the fifth digit: A finding associated with Down syndrome. *American Journal Obstetrical Gynecology, 159*, 181–183.

Berkowitz, G. S., Chitkara, U., Rosenberg, J. et al. (1988). Songraphic estimation of fetal weight and Doppler analysis of umbilical artery velocimetry in the prediction of intrauterine growth retardation: A prospective study. *American Journal of Obstetrics and Gynecology, 158*, 1149–1153.

Berman, M. C. (1991). Principles of scanning technique in obstetric and gynecologic ultrasound. In M. C. Berman (Ed.), *Diagnostic medical sonography: Vol I. Obstetrics and gynecology* (pp. 3–18). Philadelphia: J.B. Lippincott.

Berry, S. M., Gosden, C. M., Snijders, R. J. M., & Nicolaides, K. H. (1990). Fetal holoprosencephaly: associated malformations and chromosomal defects. *Fetal Diagnosis and Therapy, 5*, 92–9.

Birnholz, J. C., & Benacerraf, B. R. (1983). The development of human fetal hearing. *Science, 222*, 516.

Bundy, A. L., Saltzman, D. H., Pober, B. et al. (1986). Antenatal sonographic findings in Trisomy 18. *Journal of Ultrasound in Medicine, 5*, 361–364.

Burton, B. K. (1988). Elevated maternal serum alpha-fetoprotein (MSAFP): Interpretation and follow-up. *Clinical Obstetrics and Gynecology, 31*, 293–305.

Campbell, S., Warsof, S. L., Little, D. et al. (1985). Routine ultrasound screening for the prediction of gestational age. *Obstetrics and Gynecology, 65*, 613.

Campbell, S., & Wilkin, P. (1975). Ultrasonic measurement of fetal abdominal circumference in the estimation of fetal weight. *British Journal of Obstetrics and Gynaecology, 82*, 689–697.

Carlson, D. E., Platt, L. D., Medearis, A. L. et al. (1990). Quantifiable polyhydramnios: Diagnosis and management. *Obstetrics and Gynecology, 75*, 989–992.

Carmichael, L., Campbell, K., & Patrick, J. (1984). Fetal breathing, gross fetal body movements, and maternal fetal heart rates before spontaneous labor at term. *American Journal of Obstetrics and Gynecology, 148*, 675–679.

Cendron, M., D'Alton, M. E., & Crombleholme, T. M. (1994). Prenatal diagnosis and management of the fetus with hydronephrosis. *Seminars in Perinatology, 18*, 163–181.

Chamberlain, P. F., Manning, F. A., Morrison, I. et al. (1984). Ultrasound evaluation of amniotic fluid volume. I. The relationship of marginal and decreased amniotic fluid volumes to perinatal outcome. *American Journal of Obstetrics and Gynecology, 150*, 245–249.

Chervenak, F. A., & McCullough, L. B. (1991). An ethically based standard of care for fetal therapy. *Journal of Maternal-Fetal Investigation, 1*, 175–180.

Chervenak, F. A., Tortora, M., & Hobbins, J. C. (1985). Antenatal sonographic diagnosis of clubfoot. *Journal of Ultrasound Medicine, 4*, 49–50.

Chung, C. S., & Myrianthopoulos, N. C. (1987). Congenital anomalies: Mortality and morbidity, burden and classification. *American Journal of Medical Genetics, 27*, 508.

Clark, S. L., Sabey, P., & Jolley, K. (1989). Nonstress testing with acoustic stimulation and amniotic fluid volume assessment: 5973 tests without unexpected fetal death. *American Journal of Obstetrics and Gynecology, 160*, 694–697.

Coleman, B. G., & Arger, P. H. (1988). Ultrasound in early pregnancy complications. *Clinical Obstetrics and Gynecology, 31*, 3–18.

Copel, J. A., Grannum, P. A., Belanger, K. et al. (1988). Pulsed Doppler flow-velocity waveforms before and after intrauterine intravascular transfusion for severe erythroblastosis fetalis. *American Journal of Obstetrics and Gynecology, 158*, 768–774.

Copel, J. A., Cullen, M., Green, J. J. et al. (1988). The frequency of aneuploidy in prenatally diagnosed congenital heart disease: An indication for fetal karyotyping. *American Journal of Obstetrics and Gynecology, 158*, 409–413.

Crandall, B. F. et al. (1993). Maternal serum screening for alpha-fetoprotein, unconjugated estriol, and human chorionic gonadotropin between 11 and 15 weeks of pregnancy to detect fetal chromosomal abnormalities. *American Journal of Obstetrics and Gynecology, 168*, 1864.

Croom, C. S., Banias, B. B., Ramos-Santos, E., Devoe, L. D., Bezhadian, A., & Hiett, A. K., (1992). Do semiquantitative amniotic fluid indexes reflect actual volume? *American Journal of Obstetrics and Gynecology, 167*, 995–999.

Daffos, F., Capella-Pavlovsky, M., & Forestier, F. (1985). Fetal blood sampling during pregnancy with use of a needle guided by ultrasound: A study of 606 consecutive cases. *American Journal of Obstetrics and Gynecology, 153*, 655.

Daffos, F. (1990). Fetal blood sampling. In M. R. Harrison, M. S. Golbus, & R. A. Filly (Eds.), *The unborn patient* (pp. 75–81). Philadelphia: W.B. Saunders.

Daffos, F., Forestier, F., Muller, J. Y. et al. (1984). In utero platelet transfusion in alloimmune thrombocytopenia. *Lancet, 2*, 1103.

Daffos, F., Capella-Pavlovsky, M., & Forestier, F. (1983). A new procedure for fetal blood sampling in utero: Preliminary results of fifty-three cases. *American Journal of Obstetrics and Gynecology, 146*, 985–987.

deCrespigny, L., Cooper, D., & McKenna, M. (1988). Early detection of intrauterine pregnancy with ultrasound. *Journal of Ultrasound Medicine, 7*, 7–10.

DeVore, G. R. (1985). The prenatal diagnosis of congenital heart disease: A practical approach for the fetal sonographer. *Journal of Clinical Ultrasound, 13*, 29–245.

DeVore, G. R., Donnerstein, R. I., Kleinman, C. S. et al. (1982). Fetal echocardiography: II. The diagnosis and significance of a pericardial effusion in the fetus using real-time-directed M-mode ultrasound. *American Journal of Obstetrics and Gynecology, 144*, 693–701.

DeVore, G. R., Siassi, B., & Platt, L. D. (1984). Fetal echocardiography: IV. M-mode assessment of ventricular size and contractility during the second and third trimesters of pregnancy in the normal fetus. *American Journal of Obstetrics and Gynecology, 150*, 981–988.

DeVore, G. R., Siassi, B., & Platt, L. D. (1985). M-mode echocardiography of the aortic root and aortic valve in second and third trimester normal human fetuses. *American Journal of Obstetrics and Gynecology, 152,* 543–550.

deVries, J. I. P., Visser, G. H. A., Mulder, E. J. H. et al. (1987). Diurnal and other variations in fetal movement and heart rate patterns at 20–22 weeks. *Early Human Development, 15,* 333–348.

deVries, J. I. P., Visser, G. H. A., & Prechtl, H. F. R. (1982). The emergence of fetal behaviour: I. Qualitative aspects. *Early Human Development, 7,* 301–322.

deVries, J. I. P., Visser, G. H., & Prechtl, H. F. R. (1984). Fetal motility in the first half of pregnancy. *Clinics in Developmental Medicine, 94,* 46–64.

Dierker, L. J., Rosen, M. G., Pillay, S. et al. (1982). The correlation between gestational age and fetal activity periods. *Biology of the Neonate, 42,* 66–72.

Draper, J., Field, S., Thomas, H. et al. (1986). Womens' views on keeping fetal movement charts. *British Journal of Obstetrics and Gynaecology, 93,* 334–338.

Druzin, M. L., Edersheim, T. G., Hutson, J. M., & Bond, A. L. (1989). The effect of vibroacoustic stimulation on the non-stress test at gestational ages of thirty-two weeks or less. *American Journal of Obstetrics and Gynecology, 161,* 141–145.

Druzin, M. L., Gratacos, J., Paul, R. H. et al. (1985). Antepartum fetal heart rate testing: XII. The effect of manual manipulation of the fetus on the nonstress test. *American Journal of Obstetrics and Gynecology, 151,* 61.

DuBose, T. J. (1985). Fetal biometry: Vertical calvarial diameter and calvarial volume. *Journal of Diagnostic Medical Ultrasonography, 1,* 205–217.

DuBose, T. J. (1991). Assessment of fetal age and size: Techniques and criteria. In M. C. Berman (Ed.), *Diagnostic medical sonography: Vol I. Obstetrics and gynecology* (pp. 273–300). Philadelphia: J.B. Lippincott.

Eggertsen, S. C., & Benedetti, T. J. (1987). Maternal response to daily fetal movement counting in primary care settings. *Journal of Perinatology, 4,* 327–330.

Eglinton, G. S., Paul, R. H., Broussard, P. M., Walla C. A., & Platt, L. D. (1984). Antepartum fetal heart rate testing: XI. Stimulation with orange juice. *American Journal of Obstetrics and Gynecology, 150,* 97–99.

Fakhoury, G., Daikoku, N. H., Benser, J., & Dubin, N. H. (1994). Lamellar body concentrations and the prediction of fetal pulmonary maturity. *American Journal of Obstetrics and Gynecology, 170,* 72–76.

Fishbach, F. (1996). *A manual of laboratory and diagnostic tests* (p. 690) (4th ed.). Philadelphia: Lippincott-Raven Publishers.

Fleischer, A., Schulman, H., Farmakides, G. et al. (1985). Umbilical artery velocity waveforms and intrauterine growth retardation. *American Journal of Obstetrics and Gynecology, 151,* 502–505.

Fleischer, A. C., Pennell, R. G., Sacks, G. A. et al. (1991). Sonography in early intrauterine pregnancy emphasizing transvaginal scanning. In A. C. Fleischer, R. Romero, F. A. Manning et al. (Eds.), *The principles and practice of ultrasonography in obstetrics and gynecology* (pp. 39–56). Norwalk, CT: Appleton & Lange.

Geifman-Holtzman, O., Blatman, R. N., & Bianchi, D. W. (1994). Prenatal genetic diagnosis by isolation and analysis of fetal cells circulating in maternal blood. *Seminars in Perinatology, 18,* 366–375.

Ghidini, A., Munoz, H., & Romero, R. (1996). Fetal blood sampling. In A. C. Fleischer, F. A. Manning, P. Jeanty, R. Romero. (Eds.), *Sonography in obstetrics and gynecology* (pp. 659–691). Stamford, CT: Appleton & Lange.

Goldstein, S. R., & Wolfson, R. (1994). Endovaginal ultrasonic measurement of early embryonic size as a means of assessing gestational age. *Journal of Ultrasound Medicine, 13,* 27–31.

Grannum, P. A. T., Berkowitz, R. L., & Hobbins, J. C. (1979). The ultrasonic changes in the maturing placenta and their relation to fetal pulmonic maturity. *American Journal of Obstetrics and Gynecology, 133,* 915–922.

Greenspoon, J. S., Rosen, D. J. D., Roll, K., & Dubin, S. B. (1995). Evluation of lamellar body number density as the initial assessment in a fetal lung maturity test cascade. *Journal of Reproductive Medicine, 40,* 260–266.

Hadlock, F. P., Harrist, R. B., Shah, Y. P. et al. (1987). Estimating fetal age using multiple parameters: A prospective evaluation in a racially mixed population. *American Journal of Obstetrics and Gynecology, 156,* 955.

Hadlock, F. P., Deter, R., Harrist, R. et al. (1983). A date-independent predictor of intrauterine growth retardation: Femur length/abdominal circumference ratio. *American Journal of Roentgenology, 141,* 979.

Hadlock, F. P., Deter R. L., Carpenter, R. J. et al. (1981). Estimating fetal age: Effect of head shape on BPD. *American Journal of Roentgenology, 137,* 83–85.

Hadlock, F. P., Deter R. L., Harrist, R. B. et al. (1982). Fetal biparietal diameter: Rational choice of plane of section for sonographic measurement. *American Journal of Roentgenology, 138,* 871–874.

Hamper, U. M., Trapanotto, V., Sheth, S., DeJong, M. R., & Caskey, C.I. (1994). Three-dimensional US: preliminary clinical experience. *Radiology, 191,* 397–401.

Harding, J. E., & Charlton, V. (1990). Experimental nutritional supplementation for intrauterine growth retardation. In M. R. Harrison, M. S. Golbus, & R. A. Filly (Eds.), *The unborn patient* (pp. 598–610). Philadelphia: W.B. Saunders.

Harman, C. R. (1991). Ultrasound in the management of the alloimmunized pregnancy. In A. C. Fleischer, R. Romero, F. A. Manning et al. (Eds.), *The principles and practice of ultrasonography in obstetrics and gynecology* (pp. 393–416). Norwalk, CT: Appleton & Lange.

Harrington, K., & Campbell, S. (1993). Fetal size and growth. *Current Opinion in Obstetrics and Gynecology, 5,* 186–194.

Hearn-Stebbins, B. (1995). Fetal growth assessment: A literature review. *Journal of Diagnostic Medical Sonography, 11*(4), 176–187.

Holzgreve, W., Garritsen, H. S. P., & Ganshirt-Ahlert, D. (1992). Fetal cells in maternal circulation. *Journal of Reproductive Medicine, 37,* 410–418.

Huddleston, J. F., Sutliff, G., & Robinson, D. (1984). Contraction stress test by intermittent nipple stimulation. *Obstetrics and Gynecology, 63,* 669.

Jauniaux, E., Donner, C., Simon, P. et al. (1989). Pathologic aspects of the umbilical cord after percutaneous umbilical blood sampling. *Obstetrics and Gynecology, 73,* 215.

Jeanty, P., Rodesch, R., Delbekd, D. et al. (1984). Estimation of gestational age from measurement of fetal long bones. *Journal of Ultrasound Medicine, 3,* 75–79.

Jeanty, P. (1991). Fetal biometry. In A. C. Fleischer, R. Romero, F. A. Manning et al. (Eds.), *The principles and practice of ultrasonography in obstetrics and gynecology* (pp. 93–108). Norwalk, CT: Appleton & Lange.

Jeanty, P., & Romero, R. (1984). *Obstetrical ultrasound.* New York: McGraw-Hill.

Jeanty, P., Romero, R., d'Alton, M. et al. (1985). In utero sonographic detection of hand and foot deformities. *Journal of Ultrasound Medicine, 4,* 595–601.

Jeanty, P. (1990). Prenatal detection of simian crease. *Journal of Ultrasound Medicine, 9,* 131–136.

Junge, H. D. (1979). Behavioral states and state related fetal heart rate and motor activity patterns in the newborn infant and the fetus antepartum: A comparative study. *Journal of Perinatal Medicine, 7,* 85.

Kadar, N., Caldwell, B., & Romero, R. (1981). A method of screening for ectopic pregnancy and its indications. *Obstetrics and Gynecology, 58,* 162–166.

Kleinman, C. S., Copel, J. A., Weinstein, E. M. et al. (1985). Treatment of fetal supraventricular tachyarrhythmias. *Journal of Clinical Ultrasound, 13,* 265–273.

Kuo, H.-C., Chang, F.-M., Wu, C.-H., Yao, B.-L., & Liu, C.-H. (1992). The primary application of three-dimensional ultrasonography in obstetrics. *American Journal of Obstetrics and Gynecology, 166,* 880–886.

Kurtz, A. B., & Needleman, L. (1988). Ultrasound assessment of fetal age. In P. W. Callen (Ed.), *Ultrasonography in obstetrics and gynecology.* Philadelphia: W.B. Saunders.

Lee, A., Deutinger, J., & Bernaschek, G. (1994). "Voluvision": Three-dimensional ultrasonography of fetal malformations. *American Journal of Obstetrics and Gynecology, 170,* 1312–1314.

Lemuel, J., Bowie, P. H. D., Shammo, J., Dohnal, J. C., Farrell, E., & Vye, M. V. (1991). Lamellar body number density and the prediction of respiratory distress. *Clinical Chemistry, 95,* 781–786.

Liston, R. M., Cohen, A. W., Mennuti, M. T. et al. (1982). Antepartum fetal evaluation by maternal perception of fetal movement. *Obstetrics and Gynecology, 60,* 424–426.

Lowe, T. W., Weinreb, J., Santos-Ramos, R. et al. (1985). Magnetic resonance imaging in human pregnancy. *Obstetrics and Gynecology, 66,* 629–633.

Mahony, B. S., Filly, R. A., & Callen, P. W. (1985). Amnioticity and chorionicity in twin pregnancies: Prediction using ultrasound. *Radiology, 167,* 383–385.

Maloney, J. E., Alcorn, D., Bowes, G. et al. (1980). Development of the future respiratory system before birth. *Seminars in Perinatology, 4,* 251–260.

Manning, F. A., Platt, L. D., & Sipos, L. (1980). Antepartum fetal evaluation: Development of a fetal biophysical profile score. *American Journal of Obstetrics and Gynecology, 136,* 787–795.

Manning, F. A., Hill, L. M., & Platt, L. D. (1981). Qualitative amniotic fluid volume determination by ultrasound: Antepartum detection of intrauterine growth retardation. *American Journal of Obstetrics and Gynecology, 139,* 254–258.

Manning, F. A. (1989). Reflections on future directions of perinatal medicine. *Seminars in Perinatology, 13,* 342–351.

Manning, F. A., & Hohler, C. (1991). Intrauterine growth retardation: Diagnosis, prognostication, and management based on ultrasound methods. In A. C. Fleischer, R. Romero, F. A. Manning et al. (Eds.), *The principles and practice of ultrasonography in obstetrics and gynecology* (pp. 331–348). Norwalk, CT: Appleton & Lange.

Manning, F. A., Harman, C. R., Morrison, I. et al. (1990). Fetal assessment based on fetal biophysical profile scoring: IV. An analysis of perinatal morbidity and mortality. *American Journal of Obstetrics and Gynecology, 162,* 703–709.

Martin, J. N., & Cowan, B. D. (1990). Biochemical assessment and prediction of gestational well–being. *Obstetric and Gynecology Clinics of North America, 17,* 81–93.

Maulik, D., Yarlagadda, P., & Downing, G. (1990). Doppler velocimetry in obstetrics. *Obstetric and Gynecology Clinics of North America, 17,* 163–186.

McGahan, J., & Porto, M. (1994). *Diagnostic obstetrical ultrasound* (pp. 20–21). Philadelphia: J.B. Lippincott.

McCarthy, S., Filly, R., Stark, D. et al. (1985). Magnetic resonance imaging of fetal anomalies in utero: Early experience. *American Journal of Roentgenology, 145,* 677–682.

Moore, T. R. (1990). Superiority of the four-quadrant sum over the single-deepes-pocket technique in ultrasonographic identification of abnormal amniotic fluid volumes. *American Journal of Obstetrics and Gynecology, 163,* 762–767.

Morrison, I., & Olson, J. (1985). Weight specific stillbirths and associated causes of death: An analysis of 765 consecutive stillbirths. *American Journal of Obstetrics and Gynecology, 152,* 975.

Muller, J., Giovangrandi, Y., Parnet-Mathieu, F. et al. (1988). Acute fetal distress after blood sampling (case report). *European Journal of Obstetrics and Gynecology, 28,* 269.

Myrianthopoulos, N. C., & Chung, C. S. (1974). Congenital malformation in singleton: Epidemiologic survey. In D. Bergsma (Ed.), *Birth defects.* New York: Stratton Inter-Continental Medical Book.

Nageotte, M. P., Towers, C. V., Asrat, T., & Freeman, R. K. (1994). Perinatal outcome with the modified biophysical profile. *American Journal of Obstetrics and Gynecology, 170,* 1672–1676.

Natale, R., Nasell-Paterson, C., Connors, G. et al. (1988). Patterns of fetal breathing activity in the human fetus at 24–28 weeks of gestation. *American Journal of Obstetrics and Gynecology, 158,* 317–321.

Nicolaides, K. H., Soothill, P. W., Rodeck, C. H. et al. (1986). Rh disease: Intravascular fetal blood transfusion by cordocentesis. *Fetal Therapy, 1,* 185.

Nicolaides, K. H., Snijders, R. J. M., Gosden, C. M., Berry C., & Campbell, S. (1992). Ultrasonographically detected markers of fetal chromosomal abnormalities. *Lancet, 340,* 704–707.

Nijhuis, J. G., Martin, C. B. Jr, & Prechtl, H. F. R. (1984). Behavioral states of the human fetus. *Clinics in Developmental Medicine, 94,* 65–78.

Nyberg, D. A., Filly, R. A., Mahony, B. S. et al. (1985). Early gestation: Correlation of hCG levels and sonographic identification. *American Journal of Roentgenology, 144,* 451–454.

Oki, E. Y., Keegan, K. A., Freeman, R. K. et al. (1987). The breast stimulated contraction stress test. *Journal of Reproductive Medicine, 32,* 919.

Oulton, M., Martin, T. R., Faulkner, G. T., Stinson, D., & Johnson, J. P. (1980). Developmental study of a lamellar body fraction isolated from human amniotic fluid. *Pediatric Research, 14,* 722–728.

Paidas, M. J., & Cohen, A. (1994). Disorders of the central nervous system. *Seminars in Perinatology, 18,* 266–282.

Patrick, J., Campbell, K., Carmichael, L. et al. (1980). Patterns of human fetal breathing during the last 10 weeks of pregnancy. *Obstetrics and Gynecology, 56,* 24–30.

Patrick, J., Campbell, K., Carmichael, L. et al. (1982). Patterns of gross fetal body movements over 24-hours observation during the last 10 weeks of pregnancy. *American Journal of Obstetrics and Gynecology, 142,* 363–371.

Pearson, J. F., & Weaver, J. B. (1976). Fetal activity and fetal wellbeing: An evaluation. *British Medical Journal, 1,* 1305–1307.

Perrin EVDK, & Sander, C. H. (1984). How to examine the placenta and why. In Perrin EVDK (Ed), *Pathology of the Placenta*. New York: Churchill Livingstone.

Phelan, J. P., Smith, C. V., Broussard, P. et al. (1987). Amniotic fluid volume assessment with the four-quadrant technique at 36-42 weeks gestation. *Journal of Reproductive Medicine, 32*, 540–542.

Pielet, B. W., Socol, M. L., MacGregor, S. N. et al. (1988). Cordocentesis: An appraisal of risks. *American Journal of Obstetrics and Gynecology, 159*, 1497.

Pittaway, D. E., Reish, R. L., & Wentz, A. C. (1985). Doubling times of human chorionic gonadotropin increase in early viable intrauterine pregnancies. *American Journal of Obstetrics and Gynecology, 152*, 299.

Platt, L. D., Walla, C. A., Paul, R. H. et al. (1985). A prospective trial of the fetal biophysical profile versus the nonstress test in the management of high-risk pregnancies. *American Journal of Obstetrics and Gynecology, 153*, 624–633.

Platt, L. D., Carlson, D. E., Medearis, A. L., & Walla C.A. (1991). Fetal choroid plexus cysts in the second trimester of pregnancy: A cause for concern. *American Journal of Obstetrics and Gynecology, 164*, 1652–1656.

Powell, M. C., Buckley, J., Price, H. et al. (1986b). Magnetic resonance imaging and placenta previa. *American Journal of Obstetrics and Gynecology, 154*, 565–569.

Powell, M. C., Buckley, J., Worthington, B. S. et al. (1986a). Magnetic resonance imaging and hydatidiform mole. *British Journal of Radiology, 59*, 561.

Pretorius, D. H., & Nelson, T. R. (1995). Fetal face visualization using three-dimensional ultrasonography. *Journal of Ultrasound in Medicine, 14*, 349–356.

Ray, D. A. (1987). Biochemical fetal assessment. *Clinical Obstetrics and Gynecology, 30*, 887–898.

Rayburn, W. F. (1995). Fetal movement monitoring. *Clinical Obstetrics and Gynecology, 38*, 59–67.

Rayburn, W. F. (1982). Clinical implications from monitoring fetal activity. *American Journal of Obstetrics and Gynecology, 144*, 4967–4980.

Rebar, R. W. (1988). Transvaginal sonography. *Journal of Reproductive Medicine, 33*, 931–938.

Ried, T., Landes, G., Dackowski, W. et al. (1992). Multicolor fluorescence in situ hybridization for the simultaneous detection of probe sets for chromosomes 13, 18, 21, X and Y in uncultured amniotic fluid cells. *Human Molecular Genetics, 1*, 307–313.

Robinson H. P., & Fleming J. E. E. (1975). A critical evaluation of sonar crown-rump length measurements. *British Journal of Obstetrics and Gynaecology, 82*, 702–710.

Romero, R., Athanassiadis, A. P., & Inati, M. (1991). Fetal blood sampling. In A. C. Fleischer, R. Romero, F. A. Manning et al. (Eds.), *The principles and practice of ultrasonography in obstetrics and gynecology* (pp. 455–474). Norwalk, CT: Appleton & Lange.

Romero, R., Oyarzun, E., Sirtori, M. et al. (1991). Prenatal detection of anatomic congenital anomalies. In A. C. Fleischer, R. Romero, F. A. Manning et al. (Eds.), *The principles and practice of ultrasonography in obstetrics and gynecology* (pp. 193–210). Norwalk, CT: Appleton & Lange.

Romero, R., Pupkin, M., Oyarzun, E. et al. (1991). Amniocentesis. In A. C. Fleischer, R. Romero, F. A. Manning et al. (Eds.), *The principles and practice of ultrasonography in obstetrics and gynecology* (pp. 439–454). Norwalk, CT: Appleton & Lange.

Rosenzweig, B. A., Levy, J. S., Schipious, P. et al. (1989). Comparison of the nipple stimulation and exogenous oxytocin contraction stress tests. *Journal of Reproductive Medicine, 34*, 950–954.

Sabbagha, R. (1994). *Diagnostic ultrasound: Applied to obstetrics and gynecology* (pp. 72, 108–11, 177, 224–225, 255–268) (3rd ed.). Philadelphia: J.B. Lippincott.

Sadovsky, E., & Polishuk, W. Z. (1977). Fetal movements in utero: Nature, assessment, prognostic value, timing of delivery. *Obstetrics and Gynecology, 50*, 49–55.

Scott, J., DiSaia, P., Hammond, C. et al. (1994). *Danforth's obstetrics and gynecology* (pp. 284, 317–321, 409–411) (7th ed.). Philadelphia: J.B. Lippincott.

Senyei, A, E., & Wassman, E. R. (1993). Fetal cells in the maternal circulation. *Obstetrics and Gynecology Clinics of North America, 20*, 583–598.

Shulman, L. P., & Elias, S. (1990). Percutaneous umbilical blood sampling, fetal skin sampling, and fetal liver biopsy. *Seminars in Perinatology, 14*, 456–464.

Smith, C. V., Phelan, J. P., Platt, L. D. et al. (1986). Fetal acoustic stimulation test: II. A randomized clinical comparison with the nonstress test. *American Journal of Obstetrics and Gynecology, 155*, 131–134.

Smith C. V., Phelan, J. P., & Paul, R. H. (1985). A prospective analysis of the influence of gestational age on the baseline fetal heart rate and reactivity in a low risk population. *American Journal of Obstetrics and Gynecology, 153*, 780.

Smith C., Davis S., & Rayburn W. F. (1992). Patient acceptance of monitoring fetal activity: A randomized comparison of charting techniques. *Journal of Reproductive Medicine, 37*, 144–146.

Stark, D., McCarthy, S., Filly, R et al. (1985). Intrauterine growth retardation: Evaluation by magnetic resonance. *Radiology, 155*, 425–427.

Steiner, H., Staudach, A., Spitzer, D., & Schaffer, H. (1994). Three-dimensional ultrasound in obstetrics and gynaecology: technique, possibilities and limitations. *Human Reproduction, 9*, 1773–1778.

Streeter, H., & Manning, F. A. (1980). *Classification of neonatal morbidity and mortality by birth weight percentile in IUGR neonates (abstract)*. Proceedings of the Society of Obstetrics and Gynecology, Canada.

Thickman, D., Mintz, M., Mennuti, M. et al. (1984). MR imaging of cerebral abnormalities in utero. *Journal of Computer Assisted Tomography, 8*, 1058.

U.S. Department of Health and Human Services (1984). *Diagnostic ultrasound imaging in pregnancy* (Publication No. PHS, NIH 84-667). Washington, DC: NICHD consensus report.

Valenti, C. (1972). Endoamnioscopy and fetal biopsy: A new technique. *American Journal of Obstetrics and Gynecology, 114*, 561–564.

Wald, N., Cuckle, H., Densem, J. et al. (1988). Maternal serum screening for Down's syndrome in early pregnancy. *British Medical Journal, 297*, 883–887.

Williams, K. Wittmann, G. K., & Dansereau, J. (1992). Correlation of subjective assessment of amniotic fluid with amniotic fluid index. *European Journal of Obstetrics and Gynecology and Reproductive Biology, 46*, 1–5.

Wladimiroff, J. W., vdWijngaard, J. A., Degani, S. et al. (1987). Cerebral and umbilical arterial blood flow velocity waveforms in normal and growth retarded pregnancies. *Obstetrics and Gynecology, 69*, 705–709.

Wolfson, R. N., Peisner, D. B., Chik, L. L. et al. (1986). Comparison of biparietal diameter and femur length in the third trimester: Effects of gestational age and variation in fetal growth. *Journal of Ultrasound Medicine, 5*, 145.

40

Intrapartum Fetal Monitoring and Care

Objectives

- Describe the process of evaluating the information obtained from the external and internal uterine activity panel of the fetal monitor.
- Identify two methods of auscultating the fetal heart rate.
- Compare and contrast the external and internal methods of electronic fetal monitoring.
- Define fetal heart rate baseline, variability, and periodic and nonperiodic changes.
- Define fetal scalp stimulation and scalp blood sampling in the assessment of fetal status.
- Describe the nursing management associated with assessing and interpreting fetal heart rate patterns.

Key Terms

Acme
Amnioinfusion
Amplitude
Baseline bradycardia
Baseline tachycardia
Beat-to-beat variability
Calibration
Decrement
Doppler ultrasound
Dysrhythmia
Early deceleration
Fetal
  electrocardiogram
Fetal spiral electrode
Fetoscope
Increment
Late deceleration
Long-term variability

Nadir
Nonperiodic changes
Nonreassuring patterns
Periodic changes
Prolonged
  decelerations
Real-time
  ultrasonography
Reassuring patterns
Saltatory variability
Scalp electrode
Short-term variability
Sinusoidal pattern
Tetanic contraction
Tocodynamometer
Variable deceleration
Zeroing

Uterine Activity Assessment

Palpation and external or internal electronic methods are used to monitor uterine activity (UA). Palpation yields information about the frequency, duration, and relative intensity of contractions. Palpated contractions are felt as **mild** (ie, like the tip of the nose), **moderate** (ie, like the chin), or **strong** (ie, like the forehead; Association of Women's Health, Obstetric and Neonatal Nursing [AWHONN], 1993). This type of assessment of contractions is highly subjective and not always useful, especially in labor situations when contraction quality is questionable. External monitoring provides a recording of the frequency and duration of uterine contractions (UC). Internal monitoring, using a pressure catheter placed by physician, midwife, or registered nurse, provides an accurate measurement of intrauterine pressure for assessing baseline tone, frequency of contractions, and intensity of contractions.

Most labors that are monitored can be adequately assessed by the external method. The method used and any change of method should be noted directly on the fetal monitoring record and in the nursing notes, nursing flow sheet, or electronic medical record.

The primary goal of intrapartum fetal monitoring is to detect fetal stress and distress so that appropriate actions can be undertaken by the perinatal team. Timely actions are vital during the labor process for the delivery of a physically and neurologically intact newborn. For many years, the forces of labor and the well-being of the fetus were evaluated by palpation of the maternal abdomen and by periodic sampling of the fetal heart rate (FHR) through auscultation. These methods were the mainstay of fetal intrapartum surveillance until the advent of continuous electronic monitoring of the fetal heart rate and uterine activity (UA) 30 years ago.

Fetal monitoring, whether by auscultation or electronic means, has expanded the role of the nurse in caring for the family during labor and delivery. With this expanded role have come additional responsibilities in parent education, counseling, client care, and fetal and maternal surveillance.

This chapter describes the important elements of intrapartum fetal monitoring and care. It begins by describing the methods currently used to assess UA. It then presents information about the methods used for FHR auscultation. Next, it addresses electronic FHR monitoring and FHR patterns. The chapter concludes with a discussion of the psychological aspects of fetal monitoring. Nursing management, including evaluation of data, is integrated throughout the chapter.

External Monitoring

A pressure transducer called a **tocodynamometer** (toco) monitors UA. The device converts one form of energy (uterine pressure) to another (electrical signals). The tocodynamometer is a flat, rectangular disk with a flush button. It is placed over the fundus above the umbilicus and secured with an elastic belt. As the uterus contracts, the abdominal wall rises and presses against the transducer button. The subsequent movement of the pressure-sensitive button is converted into an electrical signal and recorded on the paper, giving a continuous record of the frequency and duration of the contractions. Intensity of the contractions is assessed by palpation (see Nursing Care Plan: The Woman Participating in External Fetal Monitoring).

The tocodynamometer must be placed correctly to gather interpretable data. The toco is placed over the area where the greatest displacement of the uterus occurs during a contraction (ie, the uterine fundus). Displacement of the abdominal wall by the uterus may not be adequate to record UC in a client with a small uterus (ie, less than 20 weeks' gestation) or in one who is extremely overweight. Movement of the maternal abdominal wall caused by respirations, coughing, vomiting, or position changes may be reflected on the monitoring record. Any such interfering factors should be noted on the monitor tracing.

NURSING CARE PLAN
The Woman Participating in External Fetal Monitoring

Nursing Goals
1. Mother and fetus maintain optimal health.
2. Mother indicates knowledge and acceptance of the benefits and limitations of fetal monitoring.
3. Intrapartum fetal stressors are detected early so that appropriate and timely interventions may occur.

Assessment	Potential Nursing Diagnoses	Intervention/ Rationale	Evaluation
Determination of need for EFM			
Assess current maternal status.	Risk for Injury (fetal distress) related to unexpected factors	Review maternal records and fetal data if available *to assess risk factors*.	Mother's data show risk factors for possible fetal distress in labor; monitor with electronic fetal monitor (EFM).
		Check maternal vital signs and observe or question regarding physical status *to record baseline information*.	Continue monitoring electronically if aberrations from the norm occur.
Assess labor progress.		Review chart and question mother regarding onset of labor, status of membranes, and other pertinent data; examine if indicated *to ensure admission status*.	Report and record data as indicated and ongoing.
		Observe for behavioral manifestations of normal or abnormal labor progress *to determine need for education, coaching, or intervention*.	
Assess FHR.		Auscultate or apply EFM per institution protocol and client's desire.	Policy dictates initial EFM; mother concurs.
Assess couple's knowledge of EFM			
Assess client's knowledge of EFM.	Knowledge Deficit of EFM related to lack of prenatal education	Discuss fully what EFM can and cannot be used for; allow for questions and concerns.	Mother and family verbalize knowledge and understanding of EFM process.
		Apply monitor so that it is comfortable but recording data appropriately.	Mother exhibits relaxed posture and verbalizes comfort and understanding of proper positioning.
		Position for comfort and maximal uteroplacental blood flow.	
		Place monitor in view of client; review tracing with mother and family *to educate, allay fears*.	Client and family ask appropriate questions and use monitor as tool for assisting controlled breathing techniques.
Problem Assessment			
Assess FHR.	Risk for Ineffective Fetal Oxygenation related to labor stressors, maternal position, or condition	Evaluate FHR for need for internal monitoring.	FHR baseline is 120–160 beats/min, +variability, +accelerations with fetal movement; no ominous decelerations are present.

(continued)

NURSING CARE PLAN *(Continued)*
The Woman Participating in External Fetal Monitoring

Assessment	Potential Nursing Diagnoses	Intervention/ Rationale	Evaluation

Problem Assessment
Determine baseline, variability, periodic or nonperiodic changes, uterine tone.
		Review tracing data per protocol *to ensure acceptable FHR parameters.*
		Review maternal drug or medication use *to assess potential fetal effects.*
		Institute remedial measures for stress or distress patterns *to maintain optimal fetal oxygenation:*
		  Position change
		  Oxytocin discontinuation if applicable
		  Oxygen by mask if indicated
		  Fluid bolus if indicated
		  Vaginal exam if indicated
		Assess vital signs.
		Give complete report to primary provider.
		Remain with client; explain all procedures.
		Document all interventions and fetal and maternal responses to interventions in a timely manner.
			Reassuring fetal data return: normal baseline rate, variability, deceleration patterns abated, +accelerations.

It may not be possible to obtain consistent data with this method from clients who are extremely restless. Occasionally, clients who are experiencing discomfort find that the firm elastic straps become uncomfortable or interfere with breathing techniques and effleurage. When this occurs, repositioning the toco and straps may be useful. If the fetus is also being monitored externally, it may sometimes be possible to secure both transducers with one belt, thereby eliminating one of the belts.

Evaluation of Data

As stated previously, only the frequency and duration of the UC may be determined with external monitoring. The onset of the contraction is determined by the upswing of the pen, which signals the **increment**. The highest level recorded on paper is the peak or **acme**, followed by the progressive relaxation of the contraction, or **decrement**. When the baseline is reached, uterine relaxation occurs, and the contraction is completed. The total duration of the contraction and the interval from the onset of one contraction to the onset of the next contraction may be calculated when the paper speed is known (3 cm/min). Maternal respiratory movement may be noted as fine "saw-tooth" deflections confirmed by comparing the rate with that observed clinically. Coughing, sneezing, and many fetal movements may appear as large spiking deflections. Bearing-down efforts, or pushing, cause multiple sharp spikes superimposed on the contractions. Changes of position cause sudden, sharp changes of the baseline. Documentation on the monitor paper of known events such as these assists in reconstructing the data when time permits and documentation is being completed.

Internal Monitoring

The use of an internal pressure catheter permits the most accurate assessment of UA. Thus, the internal method is particularly useful when evaluating clients receiving oxytocic drugs or when the timing of FHR changes in relation to UCs is unclear. Internal uterine monitoring also is helpful in documenting the adequacy of labor in clients who experience an arrest of cervical dilatation. A labor pattern of frequent contractions of low intensity may appear impressively strong when using either palpation or the external technique. The clinical impression of weak contractions perceived by an experienced nurse palpating contractions may be confirmed with internal pressure monitoring. In such cases, oxytocin augmentation may be used.

Internal monitoring of the UA is performed if the cervix is partially dilated and the membranes have ruptured. A physician or certified nurse passes a soft plastic catheter using a firm plastic introducer into the uterus beyond the presenting fetal part. The catheter, if it is fluid filled, is connected to a pressure transducer (strain gauge). The intrauterine pressure is transmitted from the amniotic fluid through the sterile water in the catheter to the pressure transducer. The transducer produces an electrical signal that is amplified by the recorder. Changes in intrauterine pressure that occur with contractions or increased intra-abdominal pressure from, for example, the Valsalva maneuver or coughing are recorded on the monitor.

The internal pressure catheter provides a means for sampling amniotic fluid for meconium or bacteria during labor if this becomes clinically useful. The catheter may become plugged by vernix, meconium, or blood. If this occurs, intrauterine pressure will not be transmitted to the transducer. Flushing with small amounts of sterile water usually corrects the problem. When this fails, the catheter should be withdrawn slightly and repositioned. This may relieve kinking of the catheter or entrapment between the lower uterine segment and fetus. The portion of the catheter in the vagina or outside the client should not be advanced into the uterus because it may result in bacterial contamination. Generally, advancing the catheter is ineffective because the flexible catheter may coil alongside the presenting fetal part. When excessive vaginal bleeding occurs after catheter placement and UA fails to be recorded, perforation of the uterus and placental injury should be suspected. Perforation into the broad ligament has been reported, in which case hemorrhage is concealed. The presence of maternal hypotension and tachycardia following catheter insertion might suggest this rare complication.

Several modifications of the traditional fluid-filled internal pressure catheters have been manufactured. A popular model is a catheter with a pressure sensor in its tip, which transmits measured uterine pressure directly to the fetal monitor through the transducer port. This type of catheter is disposable, easily calibrated, and does not require any water column or irrigation to transmit intrauterine pressure accurately (Freeman et al., 1991). Its disadvantages include the increased diameter of the tip and the increased stiffness of the catheter, which could promote greater client discomfort and increased risk of uterine perforation (Freeman et al., 1991). However, recent improvements to this device have increased its pliability and streamlined the transducer tip.

Another modification made on the pressure catheter is the addition of a second lumen. This device can be used to measure intrauterine pressure through one lumen and infuse fluids into the uterus through the second lumen for purposes such as amnioinfusion.

Evaluation of Data

Intrauterine pressure can be quantitated following proper **zeroing** and **calibration** (ie, establishing an accurate baseline) only when internal monitoring is used. The baseline uterine tone is measured as the height of the baseline during the interval between contractions. It usually ranges from 5 to 15 mm Hg. If a transducer-tipped catheter is used, the uterine baseline may read as high as 25 mm Hg in its resting state.

An elevated baseline may indicate any of the following:

- Misplacement of the pressure transducer in relation to the catheter tip
- Excessive oxytocin administration
- Abruptio placentae
- Hypertonic uterine dysfunction

The contraction strength or **amplitude** may range from 30 to 60 mm Hg or more. Although contraction amplitudes of less that 25 to 30 mm Hg may occur in normal active phase labor, they are most frequently associated with early labor or hypotonic uterine dysfunction.

Hypertonic labor occurs when UC amplitudes exceed normal, the frequency between onset of contractions is less than 2 minutes, or the resting interval between contractions is less than 1 minute. A contraction that lasts 2 minutes or greater is a **tetanic contraction**. Hypertonic labor or uterine tetany is observed with administration of an excessive amount of oxytocic drugs, abruptio placentae, or hypertonic uterine dysfunction. Hypertonic UA may have a deleterious effect on the fetus. Sustained increases in intramyometrial pressure will decrease blood flow to the placenta and delivery of oxygen to the fetus. The effects of hypertonicity are most immediately reflected in FHR, including late or prolonged decelerations. Efforts to abolish hypertonia include cessation of oxytocin administration, position changes, and occasionally, the administration of uterine relaxants.

Fetal Heart Rate Auscultation

Auscultating the FHR has long been a method for evaluating fetal well-being. However, conflicting research has sparked controversy about its use and effectiveness compared with continuous fetal monitoring. Recent analysis of 12 randomized control trials has demonstrated that intermittent auscultation is equivalent to routine electronic fetal monitoring regarding neonatal morbidity and mortality. The primary difference in modalities is that electronic fetal monitor use did correlate with a decrease in the incidence of neonatal seizures in the groups studied (Thacker et al., 1995). Long-term follow-up of these children was similar in both groups.

In 1992, the American Academy of Pediatrics (AAP) and the American College of Obstetricians and Gynecologists (ACOG) published new guidelines for FHR assessment during labor (AAP and ACOG, 1992). These guidelines state that continuous FHR monitoring and intermittent auscultation are acceptable methods of monitoring the fetus in low- and high-risk pregnancies. Furthermore, in 1995, ACOG reiterated its guidelines for assessment whether risk factors are present or not (ACOG, 1995). The guidelines established are based on protocols delineated in randomized clinical trials. In these investigations, however, usually one nurse was assigned to one client in the auscultation group, a situation that may not be available in many labor and delivery services. Because of economic constraints, many institutions can meet the AAP-ACOG guidelines only by providing their clients in labor with continuous electronic fetal monitoring (Table 40-1).

Techniques of Auscultation

Auscultation of the FHR can be performed with a **fetoscope** (De Lee stethoscope) or a **Doppler ultrasound** device. The fetoscope, first used in 1917, has changed little in appearance since that time. The fetoscope has a stethoscope attached to a metal headpiece that is placed on the examiner's head. Sound is conducted through the frontal bone of the examiner's head and is used to assist in amplifying the heart beat (Fig. 40-1). The Doppler device is a continuous-wave ultrasound that uses sound to detect cardiac wall or valve motion. Ultrasound waves bounce off the fetal heart, producing echoes that are transformed into machine-generated noises that reflect the FHR.

Leopold's maneuvers (described in Chap. 20) are performed to determine fetal presentation and position. Identifying fetal position and presentation aids in locating fetal heart sounds. In the cephalic presentation and left occiput anterior (LOA) or left occiput posterior (LOP) position (fetal head down and back to the mother's left side), fetal heart tones are best heard in the lower left quadrant of the maternal abdomen. In the breech presentation, the fetal heart sounds are heard at or above the level of the umbilicus.

After locating fetal heart sounds, a baseline FHR should be obtained, noting the rate, rhythm, and presence or absence of any **nonperiodic changes** (accelerations or decelerations not associated with UCs). These can be detected by auscultating between contractions (NAACOG, 1992). To determine the baseline FHR, the heart beat can be counted for 15 seconds and multiplied by 4, counted for 30 seconds and multiplied by 2 or counted for a full 60 seconds. The mother's pulse should always be determined to differentiate between it and the fetal rate. The minimal standard of practice is to evaluate and record the FHR during a contraction and for 30 seconds thereafter to determine the presence or absence of accelerations or decelerations in the FHR.

Reassuring patterns of the FHR include normal baseline rate, accelerations with fetal movement or stimulation, and absence of decelerations. **Nonreassuring patterns** observed during auscultation include a baseline FHR less than 100 beats/min between UCs, a rate less than 100 beats/min 30 seconds after a UC, or

TABLE 40-1
Guidelines for Intrapartum Fetal Heart Rate Monitoring

	Rate of Assessment	
	HIGH-RISK PREGNANCY	LOW-RISK PREGNANCY
INTERMITTENT AUSCULTATION		
First stage of labor		
Latent phase	Every 30 min	Every 60 min
Active phase	Every 15 min	Every 30 min
Second stage of labor	Every 5 min	Every 15 min
CONTINUOUS ELECTRONIC FETAL MONITORING		
First stage of labor	Every 15 min	Every 30 min
Second stage of labor	Every 5 min	Every 15 min
ACOG Technical bulletin 207. July 1995		

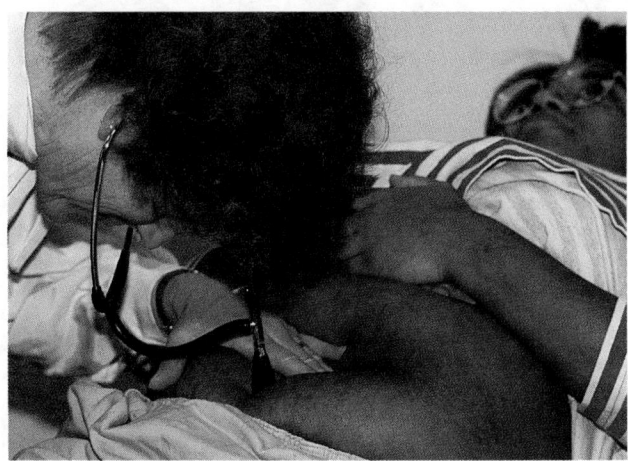

FIGURE 40–1 Auscultation of the fetal heart rate can be performed with a fetoscope.

an unexplained baseline tachycardia greater than 160 beats/min (ACOG, 1989). Continuous electronic monitoring can be initiated in clients exhibiting nonreassuring patterns.

Documentation of auscultated FHR monitoring should include FHR and UA data, maternal pulse, nursing interventions, and client and fetal responses to the interventions. Statements concerning the FHR, rhythm, and nature of identified FHR changes should be recorded in the client's chart (NAACOG, 1992). Documentation of FHR monitoring is discussed later in this chapter.

Electronic Fetal Heart Rate Monitoring

Prior to the development of electronic fetal monitoring, evaluation of FHR was restricted to periodic auscultation during the interval between contractions. FHR changes occurring with the contractions or during the first 30 seconds following the contraction generally were not easily detected. The ability to diagnose fetal distress was limited to sustained and extreme variation in FHR, such as severe bradycardia. With auscultation, the evaluation of periodic changes (ie, those occurring with contractions—decelerations or accelerations) and nonperiodic changes (ie, heart rate changes occurring in the absence of contractions) remains somewhat subjective, especially when they occur at a rate that is within the normal range.

Electronic FHR monitoring allows for continuous assessment, either externally or internally. In addition to monitoring FHR, UA also is assessed continuously externally or internally (see Procedure 40-1). With continuous electronic FHR monitoring, the interval between successive heart beats can be calculated as a rate and recorded graphically. For this calculation to be made,

the fetal signal obtained with a transducer is amplified and then counted by a cardiotachometer. This is converted to a rate between successive beats and recorded continuously during and between contractions.

External Method

The Doppler ultrasound method is the most commonly used method of external electronic FHR monitoring. With this technique, high-frequency sound waves are transmitted from a transducer into the fetus and are reflected from the moving fetal heart back to the Doppler for processing. The difference in frequencies of the transmitted and the reflected sound waves constitutes the signal. This is converted to an averaged rate between successive beats and recorded continuously during and between contractions. This signal is amplified, counted, and displayed by the cardiotachometer and is heard as an audible heart rate from the monitor. It should be stressed to the client that the sound emanating from the monitor is machine generated, not the actual fetal heart sounds.

When the Doppler transducer is used, the transducer is applied to an area directly over the fetal heart. This site is selected by auscultation and by palpation of the fetus. The position from which the sharpest (not necessarily the loudest) audible fetal signal can be heard is determined before securing the Doppler with the elastic belt. If the pregnant full-term client is in labor and the fetal head is engaged, the fetal heart sounds are usually midline between the umbilicus and pubic bone. Periodic maternal and fetal position change or movement may require readjustment of the transducer to maintain high-quality data (see Nursing Guidelines: Care During Fetal Heart Rate Monitoring).

Internal Method

In many centers, the **fetal spiral electrode** (FSE) is a widely used method for FHR monitoring in labor. A transducer, which is a small electrode, is attached to the scalp of the fetus and detects the direct **fetal electrocardiogram** (FECG). The most commonly used electrode is a small spiral wire that is advanced into the fetal scalp by clockwise rotation while gentle pressure is applied.

Application of the electrode requires that the membranes be ruptured and that the cervix be dilated at least 1 to 2 centimeters or more. The presenting part must be known and fixed in the pelvis. Attempts to apply the electrode when the fetus is floating are hazardous, possibly dislodging the fetus to an abnormal lie, and increasing the risk for umbilical cord prolapse. During application, the electrode should be rotated until mild resistance is met; it should never be forced. Additionally, the electrode should not be placed over the fetal face or fontanel. In a breech presentation, the

PROCEDURE 40-1
Application of the External Monitor

Equipment Needed

- Fetal monitor and paper
- Ultrasound transducer
- Tocodynamometer
- Two straps
- Conductive jelly

Preparation of Equipment

- Plug transducers into appropriate outlets on front of monitor.
- Turn monitor on.
- Test monitor by pushing test button.

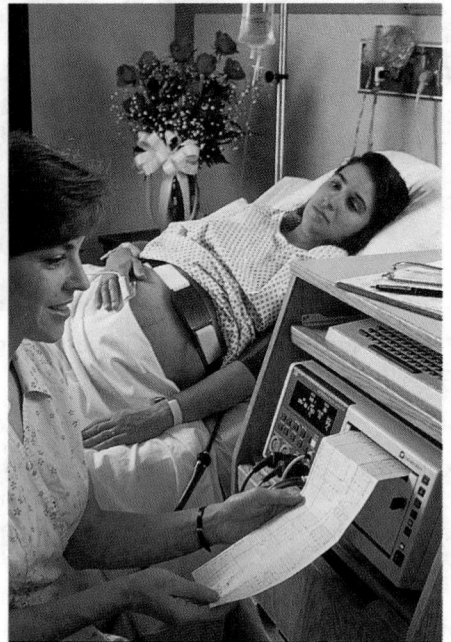

Client being monitored with external transducers secured to her abdomen. (Photo courtesy of Corometrics Medical Systems, Wallingford, CT.)

Nursing intervention	*Rationale*
1. Explain procedure to mother and support person.	Explanation allays fears, gains cooperation, and promotes compliance.
2. Elevate head of bed 15–30 degrees, or place client in lateral position.	Elevation and uterine displacement decrease aorta and vena caval compression.
3. Perform Leopold's maneuvers and place two straps under client.	This locates fetal position and best placement of Doppler.
4. Apply conductive jelly to Doppler, and place on client's abdomen until strong FHR is heard and consistent signal is obtained.	The jelly helps locate the area of maximum FHR signal.
5. Attach straps to Doppler and secure.	Straps should be snug but not tight.
6. Push recorder button if not already on.	Machine will not record data if off.
7. Place tocodynamometer on abdomen between umbilicus and top of fundus.	Fundus is the contractile portion of the uterus; care must be taken to avoid placing toco too high on fundus; respirations will record on monitor.
8. Attach straps to tocodynamometer and secure.	Straps should be snug but not tight; if too tight, pressure-sensitive button will not record data.
9. Adjust sound and equipment as needed, particularly when a procedure is performed or client's position is changed.	Monitor is sensitive to change or disturbance to equipment.
10. Review FHR and UA data with client and family. Use thorough descriptions of data.	This review promotes understanding of what client and family will be observing on the monitor.

genitalia should be avoided (see Nursing Guidelines: Application of a Fetal Spiral Electrode). Standard precautions must be used during application and care of the FECG. Use of the FECG is contraindicated in cases of infection, such as human immunodeficiency virus or hepatitis.

The FECG serves as the fetal signal for counting the heart rate. On occasion, the maternal signal may be obtained by this method and may produce an artificial tracing (eg, the maternal ECG may be conducted through a dead fetus). The use of **real-time ultrasonography** (ultrasound detection of echoes reflected from fetal structures in the path of the ultrasound pulse; Manning, 1994) to detect heart motion and assessment of the maternal pulse can usually resolve this question and avoid unnecessary cesarean delivery. With direct FECG recording, the true beat-to-beat variation in the FHR can be evaluated based on the principle that the FSE records each successive fetal R wave

in the QRS complex (signaling ventricular depolarization), thereby counting each beat of the heart. Filtering or editing of the direct FECG signal may sometimes result in inability of the monitor to detect certain fetal cardiac dysrhythmias. Spiral electrodes are easily removed before or after delivery by gentle counterclockwise rotation of the attached wires or by gently pulling the wires apart.

Nursing Management

In many institutions, continuous electronic fetal monitoring is used with all clients in labor. In other institutions, the responsibility for selection of clients to be monitored rests with the physician, nurse midwife, and nurse. The client's preferences should always be respected. The nurse's role in selection is particularly important when the number of clients in labor exceeds the number of available monitors. Priorities for monitoring must be established through institutional policy. The decision to monitor a client generally is made on the basis of one of the following primary indications:

- Prenatal risk factors, including maternal complications, such as diabetes, hypertension, and cardiac, renal, and hematologic diseases; fetal problems, such as suspected intrauterine growth retardation or postdate pregnancy

- Intrapartum risk factors, such as third-trimester bleeding, passage of meconium, or abnormalities of FHR determined by auscultation
- Other obstetric factors (eg, to evaluate abnormal progress of labor or the effects of drugs such as oxytocics and some anesthetic agents)

After the decision has been made to monitor a client, the method of monitoring is selected. This is contingent on status of the cervix and membranes, indication for monitoring, client acceptance, and availability. When the membranes are intact or the cervix is not dilated, external methods of monitoring must be used. If adequate data cannot be obtained with the available external systems, internal monitoring should be considered. In cases in which the most accurate data are required (eg, true beat-to-beat variation, temporal relationship of decelerations to contractions, or true intrauterine pressures), internal monitoring must be used (see Nursing Guidelines: Care During Fetal Heart Rate Monitoring).

Fetal Monitor Tracing

Fetal monitors are equipped to provide a continuous recording of FHR and UA. This information is recorded on perforated paper that folds "accordion style" (Fig 40-2). The UA is recorded on the lower channel. The

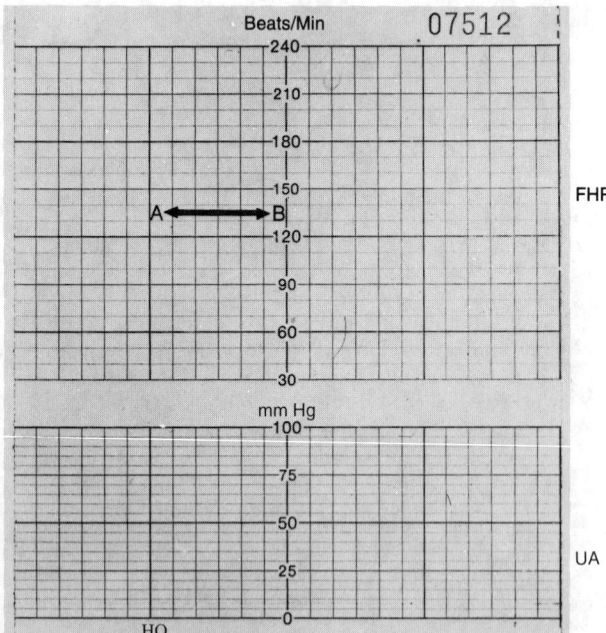

FIGURE 40–2 Recording paper for fetal monitor. Note fetal heart rate (beats per minute) recorded on upper channel, uterine activity (UA, mm Hg) recorded on lower channel, and panel number at top of sheet. Distance from A to B equals 1 minute when paper speed is 3 cm/min.

recording paper provides a vertical scale for measuring the intrauterine pressure, usually in millimeters of mercury (mm Hg). UA is also displayed numerically on the front of the monitor. Most monitors are equipped with a zeroing and calibration device to ensure that the record accurately reflects the true intrauterine pressure. The FHR in beats per minute is displayed on the upper channel of the paper and numerically on the front of the monitor.

In the United States, the paper speed is set at 3 cm/min. Other countries generally use the 1 or 2 cm/min paper speed. Divisions on the horizontal scale provide a measurement of the time elapsed. They are useful as markers to correlate events on both channels. Numbering on the individual sheets of the record provides a reference for rapid calculation of elapsed time for longer intervals, such as when trending of data is desired.

Centralized Fetal Heart Rate Monitoring

Advances in technology have permitted centralized fetal monitoring, that is, a monitoring system that allows a simultaneous display of every monitored bed in a labor and delivery unit. Real-time displays of several clients' FHR tracings and status screens that provide an overview of client data can be viewed. These displays can be placed at the nurses' station, allowing constant surveillance of the client even when a nurse is not physically present in the client's room. An additional advantage of such a system is that FHR tracings and related nursing notes can be saved on an optical computer disk and therefore are permanently archived. Care must be taken to ensure the archived fetal heart data correlate with the information recorded on the strip chart.

Interpretation of Data

Proper interpretation of the data obtained from electronic fetal monitoring requires a systematic approach to examine the tracings and correlate them with clinical events. The interpretation of monitor tracings can be learned from annotated atlases of monitor tracings and clinical experience. Expertise in this area often takes several years to acquire. To provide teaching in monitoring interpretation, many institutions have periodic in-service programs and conferences in which tracings are reviewed by members of the team caring for the clients.

Documentation of Fetal Heart Data

Because the data obtained become a part of the client's permanent record, a systematic method of identification must be used at the beginning of each new fetal

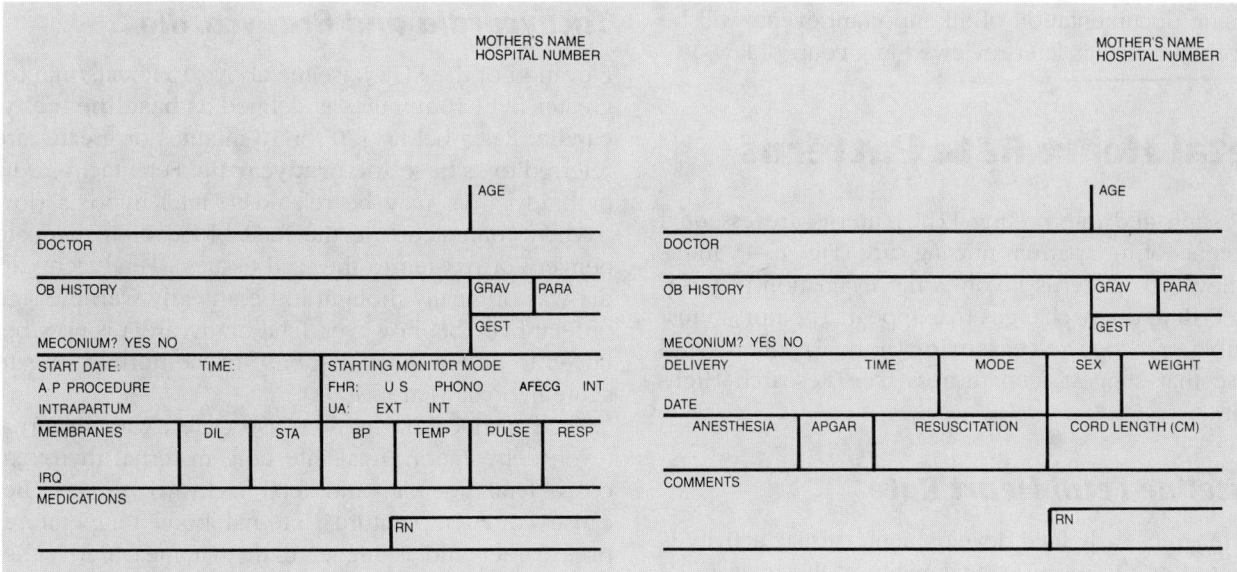

FIGURE 40-3 (Left) Label provides identification and clinical information for interpretation of tracing and is applied when monitoring is initiated and at the start of each new monitor strip. **(Right)** Label provides identification and clinical information for correlation of monitor data with neonatal condition and is applied following delivery.

monitor tracing paper and at delivery. A sample format for identification is shown in Figure 40-3.

The clock time and important clinical data should be identified on the strip and in the client record. These include vital signs, vaginal examinations, rupture of membranes, physician and nurse review of the tracing, medications (dose and route of administration), interventions, and client and fetal responses to interventions. Documentation should also include the starting number on the strip and strip number notations when the paper is changed or a break in the tracing occurs. This information is important for interpreting the record, retrospectively reviewing the tracing for teaching purposes, and defending against litigation (Eganhouse, 1991).

Nursing documentation of the FHR data also must be recorded on a flow sheet, in a nurse's narrative note, or in the electronic medical record if one is used. In 1992, AAP and ACOG stipulated that nurses use descriptive terms, such as early, variable, and late deceleration, for FHR patterns when documenting data (AAP and ACOG, 1992). The client's record should include nursing assessments of the FHR and UA. Identification of nonreassuring FHR patterns demands initiation of appropriate nursing interventions and physician notification. The attending physician is expected to respond. If the physician does not respond or is unfamiliar with monitoring, the nurse should follow hospital protocols for dealing with the situation (AWHONN, 1993). These actions must be documented factually in the client's chart. If they are not documented adequately, a retrospective review of the chart can assume that these nursing interventions were not performed. In charting,

the nurse's note should include appropriate terminology (Box 40-1).

These notes are an integral part of the client record. Any discrepancies or omissions concerning nursing and physician notes should be corrected at the time of labor and delivery. All notations should be dated and timed. With the advent of computerized documentation, it is essential that notations be made as close to the time in which the events occurred as possible because although the nurse may enter the event time into the electronic record, the computer will additionally enter real time into the data base. Careful and timely

---

BOX 40-1
Sample Charting

0930: IUPC and FECG in place. UA resting tone 20–25 mm Hg. Ctx q3min X 60 sec with peak 70–75 mm Hg. FHR BL 130–142 +LTV. O periodic changes noted. Oxytocin at 10 mU/min. H. Keller, RN

1000: UC q1–3min X 70–80 sec. Resting tone 25–30 mm Hg with peak 80–90 mm Hg. FHR BL 130–132. 0STV noted. Late decels noted with last 4 ctx. Client to L side, Oxytocin d/c'd. O₂ per face mask at 8 L/min. IV fluid bolus of 250 mL. Dr. Bond notified @ 1003 and in to review tracing at 1005. H. Keller, RN

1012: Ctx now q2–4min X 60 sec with resting tone 20–25 mm Hg and peak of 60–70 mm Hg. FHR BL 130–140. +STV noted. VE done. CX 4cm dil, 0.5 cm effaced with vertex at 0 station. + acceleration with scalp stimulation. H. Keller, RN

nursing documentation of all important events will be helpful if a case is later reviewed in a court of law.

Fetal Heart Rate Patterns

Assessing and interpreting FHR patterns are essential elements of intrapartum nursing care (Fig. 40-4). Interpreting FHR patterns involves the evaluation of baseline FHR and any changes that appear. The nurse must be able to recognize **reassuring** (normal) patterns and those that suggest fetal distress (see Research Highlight).

Baseline Fetal Heart Rate

During very early fetal development, cardiac activity is initiated by the intrinsic rhythmicity of the myocardial cells. Soon after, the sinoatrial node assumes the function of initiating the impulses, which are transmitted throughout the conduction system of the heart, resulting in the mechanical events known as the heart beat.

The baseline rate refers to the average FHR assessed between UCs, periodic changes, and periods of fetal movement or stimulation. It is generally counted for 10 minutes. The FHR decreases slightly as pregnancy advances and normally ranges between 120 and 160 beats/min. The baseline is affected by maternal or fetal factors, such as fever, infection, hypoxia, anemia, drugs, and catecholamine production; it also is affected by maternal and fetal physiologic problems, such as hyperthyroidism.

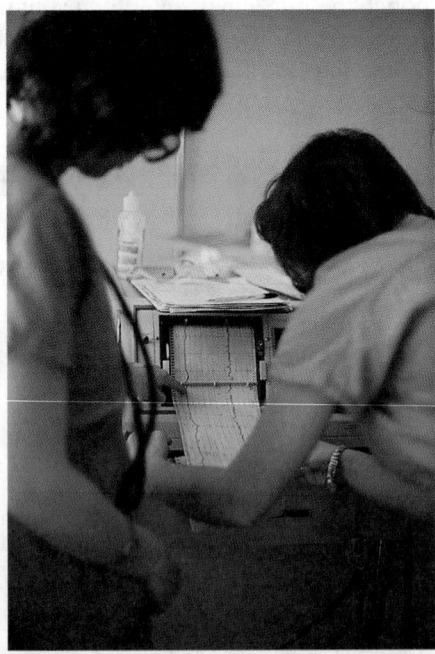

FIGURE 40–4 Intrapartum nursing care involves assessing, interpreting, and evaluating fetal heart rate patterns.

Tachycardia and Bradycardia

Elevation of the FHR baseline above 160 beats/min for greater than 10 minutes is defined as **baseline tachycardia**. Rates below 120 for 10 minutes or greater are referred to as **baseline bradycardia**. Fetal tachycardia or bradycardia may be related to fetal hypoxia (low oxygen content of the the fetal blood or inadequate delivery of oxygen to the fetal tissues). Fetal tachycardia was originally thought to be an early warning sign of fetal hypoxia; however, fetal bradycardia is now believed to be the initial response of the normal fetus to acute hypoxia (Parer, 1994).

Fetal tachycardia may be associated with maternal fever, dehydration, fetal infection, maternal thyrotoxicosis, fetal anemia, and fetal tachyarrhythmias. Because core temperature (internal body temperature) rises earlier and is higher than that measured either orally or rectally, fetal tachycardia may precede maternal fever by a short time.

Likewise, fetal bradycardia may be associated with maternal hypothermia, but this is unusual clinically. Fetal bradycardia also may be caused by drugs administered to the mother, such as beta-blockers. Fetal congenital heart block may produce a baseline bradycardia. This phenomenon has been observed in infants of mothers with systemic lupus erythematosus, who produce an antibody that crosses the placenta and destroys the fetal conduction system. Abnormalities in baseline FHR also may be attributed to **dysrhythmias** (abnormal discharge or transmission of impulses through the conduction system of the heart). These are usually benign and transient but may be associated with congenital heart defects or heart failure.

Variability

As fetal development advances, the autonomic nervous system assumes an increasingly important role in regulating FHR. Sympathetic nerve stimulation causes an increase in rate, whereas parasympathetic nerve stimulation causes a slowing of the heart rate. By 28 to 32 weeks' gestation, the fetus demonstrates the "push-pull" effect of the sympathetic and parasympathetic branches. The normal continuous opposition of these two stimuli results in beat-to beat variation, or variability, noted in the heart rate of the normal fetus. Variability is subdivided into two categories. **Long-term variability** is defined as the fluctuations or oscillations in the FHR for 1 minute. Long-term variability is expressed in amplitude (between 6 and 25 beats/min) and cycles per minute (between 3 and 6). The responsiveness of the fetus and its behavioral state and wake state account for this wide variation. **Beat-to-beat variability,** or **short-term variability**, is the rate counted from one R wave to the next in each cardiac

RESEARCH HIGHLIGHT

Using Fetal Pulse Oximetry to Monitor Fetal Heart Rate

Reassuring fetal heart rate patterns are predictive of a positive outcome; however, questionable patterns or patterns that indicate fetal stress or distress may not be as predictive of a negative outcome. To that end, the use of fetal scalp stimulation, vibroacoustic stimulation, and scalp sampling assists the clinician in the diagnosis of the fetus who exhibits nonreassuring patterns. Another technique currently under investigation is the measurement of fetal oxygen saturation by pulse oximetry. Pulse oximetry is used to assess arterial blood oxygen saturation in the neonatal, pediatric, and adult populations with much success.

The purpose of this study was to evaluate this technique in the assessment of the fetal pulse and fetal arterial oxygen saturation and tissue perfusion. The study group consisted of 73 term women in the active phase of labor. The pulse oximeter sensor was a noninvasive catheter set in the reflectance mode inserted intravaginally and alongside the surface of the fetal head. In this study, reliable data were defined as adequate signal quality (ie, physical contact between the oxisensor and the fetus as measured by the electrical impedance between the contact electrodes on the front surface of the sensor) at least 50% of the time; this was achieved in all of the subjects during the time the satu-

ration monitor was in use. The mean fetal SPO_2 in the monitored clients was 57.9 +/-10%, which correlates to other published values in animal experiments. In contrast, the adult values generally range between 95% and 100%.

The authors hope to conduct larger studies that will trend SPO_2 values during labor and expand on factors that affect values and correlation with umbilical cord blood samples.

The potential value of reflectance fetal pulse oximetry includes the ability to differentiate between nonreassuring fetal heart rate tracings that require immediate delivery and those that may only be false-positives. It also provides for direct assessment of fetal oxygen status and tissue perfusion.

Critique: If this investigational technique were used in obstetric practice, it would require additional education for nursing care providers to interpret appropriately but would add to the number of tools available to ensure fetal well-being during the intrapartum period. The limitations to this study include the relatively small sample size, the wide range of normal values, the lack of continuous information, and the intrinsic difficulty working with the medium (amniotic fluid) in which the sensor is placed. Because of the placement of the sensor alongside the fetal face, contamination from blood, amniotic fluid, and meconium occurs readily.

Dildy, G. A., Clark, S. L., & Loucks, C. A. (1993). Preliminary experience with intrapartum fetal pulse oximetry in humans. *Obstetrics and Gynecology, 81*(4), 630–635.

---

cycle. It is reflected by the fine, jittery irregularity seen on the normal FHR tracing (Fig. 40-5). Short-term variability is defined as being present or absent. When it is present, the tracing line of the fetal heart appears "rough." Absent short-term variability produces a "smooth" tracing line.

True beat-to-beat variability can be assessed only by internal fetal monitoring using the spiral electrode, although recent technological advances in Doppler ultrasound have created external transducers that closely rival the data obtained from the electrode. Normal beat-to-beat variability is probably the most reliable indication of fetal well-being. When variability is present, no matter what other FHR patterns are present, the fetus is thought to have an intact nervous system with normal regulatory influence over the FHR. Whereas several factors may be responsible for the loss of heart rate variability, a flat FHR baseline in the absence of an explainable cause is considered ominous and potentially indicative of hypoxia (Fig. 40-6). Increased (**saltatory**) **variability** (greater than 25 beats per minute) is thought to be a result of mild fetal hypoxemia and is seen with excessive uterine or fetal activity and postdate pregnancy as well as with certain medications (Cabaniss, 1993).

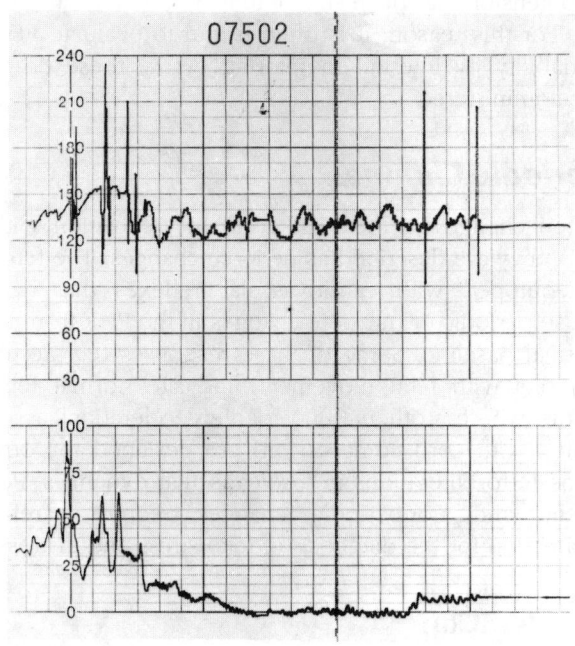

FIGURE 40-5 Fetal heart rate tracing. Note fine irregularity or beat-to-beat (short-term) variability.

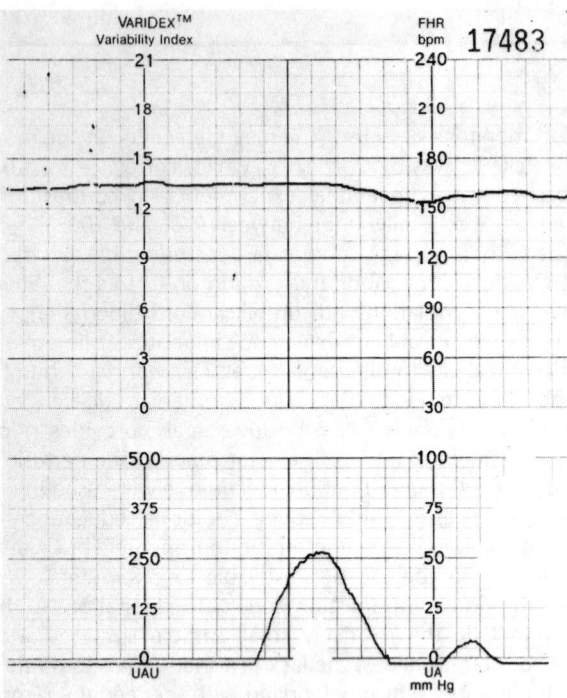

FIGURE 40–6 Fetal heart rate tracing with absent beat-to-beat variability. Note subtle late deceleration.

The influence of drugs is obvious in the assessment of FHR variability. It has become increasingly apparent that a large proportion of drugs administered to the woman will cause decreased or minimal FHR variability. Specific drugs that decrease variability include narcotics, barbiturates, phenothiazines, atropine, and tranquilizers. Ephedrine, used to treat anesthesia-related hypotension, has been shown to increase FHR variability. For this reason, it is often useful to evaluate FHR variability by internal monitoring before these drugs are administered.

Periodic Changes

When changes in the FHR occur in association with UCs, they are described as periodic changes. The fetus is equipped with cardiovascular reflexes that may cause periodic or transient changes in the FHR from its normal baseline. Some of these responses (eg, accelerations with fetal movement) indicate normal fetal status, whereas others (eg, variable decelerations associated with cord compression) are designed to compensate for alterations in cardiovascular dynamics. Periodic and nonperiodic changes require careful evaluation for the diagnosis of fetal stress and distress.

Accelerations

Transient increases of the FHR of more than 15 beats/min for more than 15 seconds have been noted

since fetal monitoring was first used (Fig. 40-7). They are, at times, associated with contractions but may be unrelated to UA. The outcome of fetuses demonstrating accelerations in labor has been uniformly good. It is believed that the increased FHR is due to transient discharges of the sympathetic nervous system. It also has been suggested that accelerations associated with contractions may be caused by partial compression of the cord, which results in selective occlusion of the umbilical vein, causing fetal hypotension and a transient increase in the FHR (Freeman et al., 1991; AWHONN, 1993; Cabaniss, 1993). The observation that accelerations are associated with fetal movement in the healthy fetus is the basis of the nonstress test for prenatal evaluation of the high-risk fetus. (See Chap. 39 for more information about the nonstress test.)

Early Decelerations

Transient slowing of the FHR in a pattern that is almost a mirror image of the contraction is known as an **early deceleration**. These decelerations are believed to be related to compression of the fetal head associated with the contraction, resulting in a para-

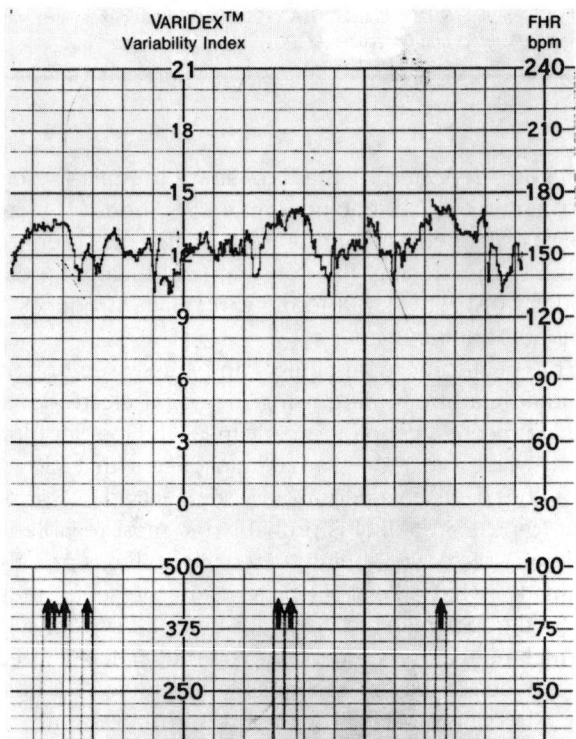

FIGURE 40–7 Transient accelerations of fetal heart rate noted during nonstress test. Arrows were made by the client to indicate when fetal movements were perceived.

sympathetic discharge mediated by the vagus nerve. Parasympathetic stimulation results in slowing of the FHR. This pattern represents a normal response of the fetus to this stimulus and in the absence of other periodic FHR changes is associated with a uniformly good outcome. Early decelerations, although not often seen, are more commonly observed in early active labor, usually between 4 and 6 cm dilatation (AWHONN, 1993).

Characteristically, these decelerations have a waveform that coincides with and resembles an inverted UC (Fig. 40-8). They are uniform in shape, of short duration, and of low amplitude. The FHR at the **nadir** (lowest point) of the deceleration is usually 100 beats/min or greater. When slower FHRs are observed with contractions, the decelerations are usually of the variable type (see below). Early decelerations do not respond to oxygen administered to the mother or to position change. Because of the benign nature of this pattern, however, remedial action is not necessary.

Late Decelerations

Like the term early decelerations, the designation **late deceleration** indicates a uniform shape and a consistent relationship of the deceleration to contractions. In contrast to early decelerations, the onset of the late deceleration, its nadir, and its recovery do not coincide with the onset, amplitude, and recovery of the UC. Rather, they are delayed (Fig. 40-9). Late decelerations may be subtle, entirely within the normal FHR range, yet ominous. This is particularly true if FHR variability is decreased. Several studies have demonstrated that subtle late decelerations accompanied by reduced heart rate variability are more likely to be associated with fetal acidosis than are more obvious late decelerations in which variability is preserved (reflex lates) (Cabaniss, 1993; Parer, 1994).

Late decelerations are thought to reflect the effects of intermittent hypoxia on the fetal autonomic nervous system, causing transient fetal hypertension and triggering a vagally mediated bradycardia. Prolonged tissue hypoxia leads to the accumulation of lactate and results in fetal acidosis. Such effects on acid–base balance may have a direct effect on the fetal myocardium and conduction system, causing slowing of the heart rate.

The hypoxia reflected by late decelerations results from the reduced oxygen delivered by the placenta as a result of the diminished intervillous blood flow that occurs with the UC. When the fetus is unable to extract sufficient oxygen during a UC, deceleration occurs. Hypoxia causing late decelerations may be elicited

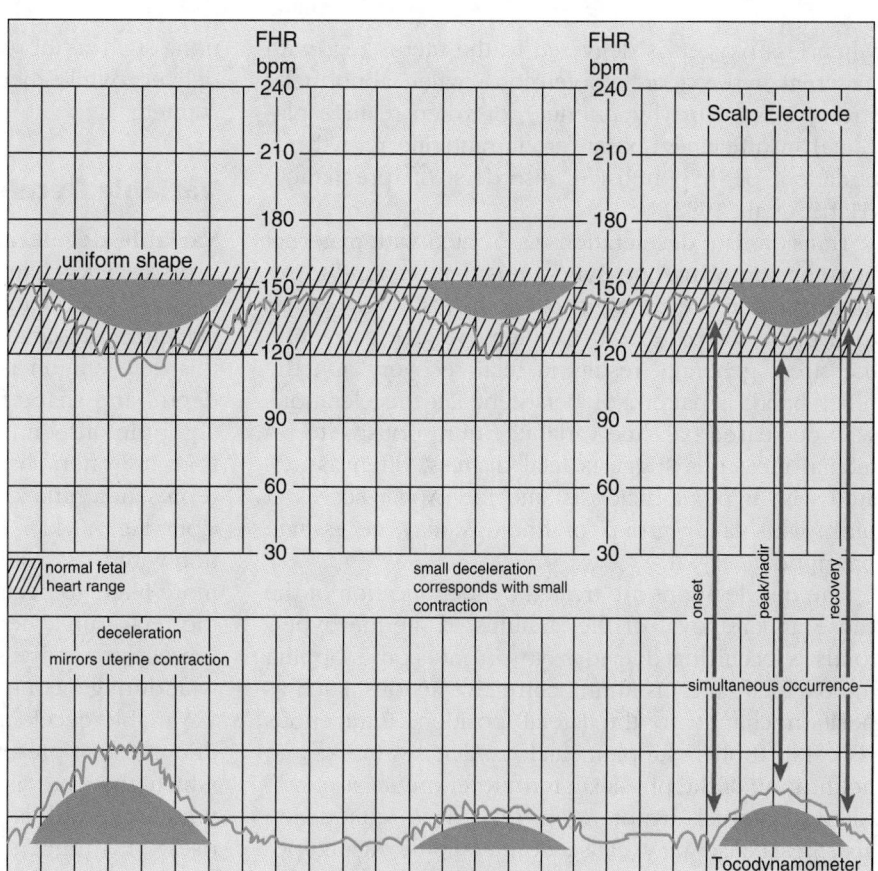

FIGURE 40–8 Early decelerations. Note how early decelerations appear to be "mirror images" of the contraction. (From Cabaniss, M. [1993]. *Fetal monitoring interpretation*. Philadelphia: J.B. Lippincott.)

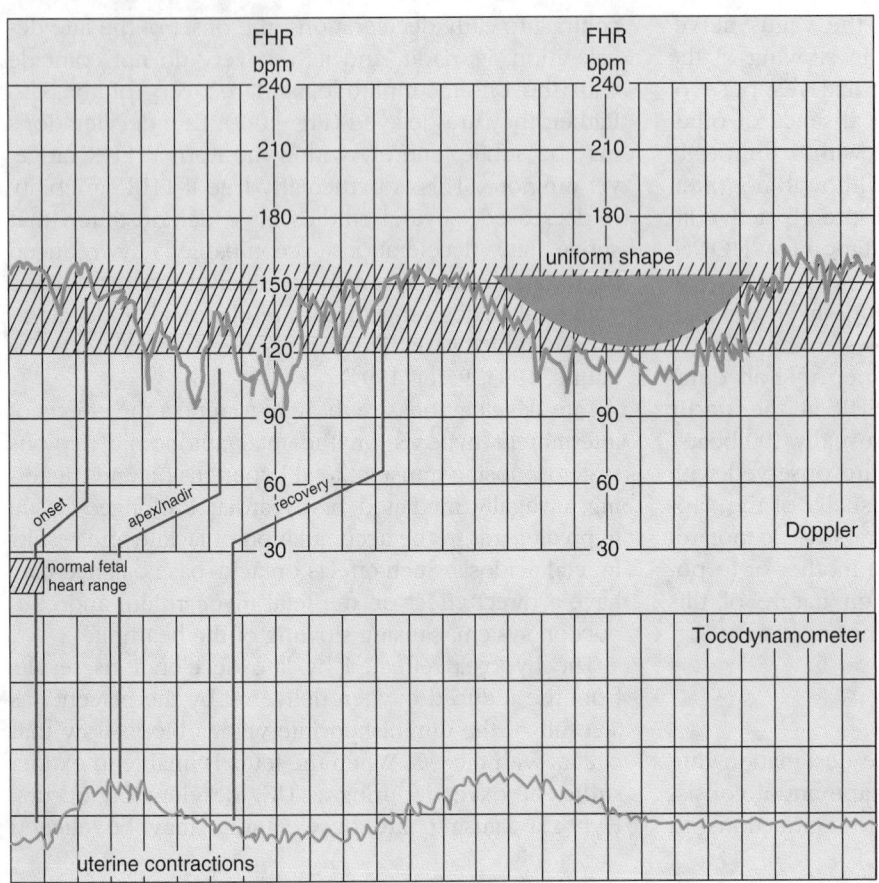

FIGURE 40-9 The timing of late deceleration. Note the presence of long-term variability. (From Cabaniss, M. [1993]. *Fetal monitoring interpretation.* Philadelphia: J.B. Lippincott.)

when less oxygen is delivered to the uterus (eg, with maternal hypoxia or hypotension), when abnormally strong UCs occur (hypertonus), or when relative placental insufficiency exists (eg, intrauterine growth retardation or hypertensive disorders of pregnancy) (Harris et al., 1982).

Transient late decelerations associated with maternal hypotension or uterine hypertonus that respond to remedial action are thought to signal fetal stress rather than distress (see Fig. 40-10). Removing or correcting the stress generally results in fetal recovery. On the other hand, a pattern of persistent late decelerations with decreased baseline variability unresponsive to remedial measures suggests fetal distress, often associated with hypoxia, acidosis, and low Apgar scores at birth. This latter group of findings may necessitate prompt delivery.

Late decelerations are treated by identification of the cause and removal of the stimulus. If uterine hypertonus is occurring due to oxytocin infusion, stopping the oxytocin and instituting corrective actions, such as position change to the lateral position, intravenous (IV) fluid bolus, supplemental oxygen by mask, and notification of the physician for further orders, are indicated. Maternal hypotension related to conduction anesthesia also may cause decelerations. Again, position change and IV fluid administration are primary interventions. Noncorrectable causes of late decelera-

tion, such as abruptio placentae, warrant immediate delivery while therapeutic interventions are being instituted.

Variable Decelerations

Variable decelerations are the most commonly observed FHR change during labor. The relationship of these decelerations to the contractions and the waveform is variable (Fig. 40-10). The appearance of this deceleration is described as variable in duration, depth, and shape from contraction to contraction and abrupt in onset and return to baseline. These decelerations are often characterized as V, W, or U shaped and represent a reflex response to umbilical cord compression (Fig. 40-11). They are often observed in association with UCs, a situation in which cord compression is more likely to occur. The cord can be wrapped around the fetal trunk, neck, or an extremity. They may also represent compression of the cord against the uterine wall during a contraction.

Variable decelerations often are seen when oligohydramnios is present. This is a circumstance during which the cord is particularly vulnerable. When the umbilical cord is compressed, fetal blood pressure rises. This triggers baroreceptors, which stimulate the vagus nerve and cause a drop in the FHR. The firing of the vagus nerve is erratic, resulting in the variable on-

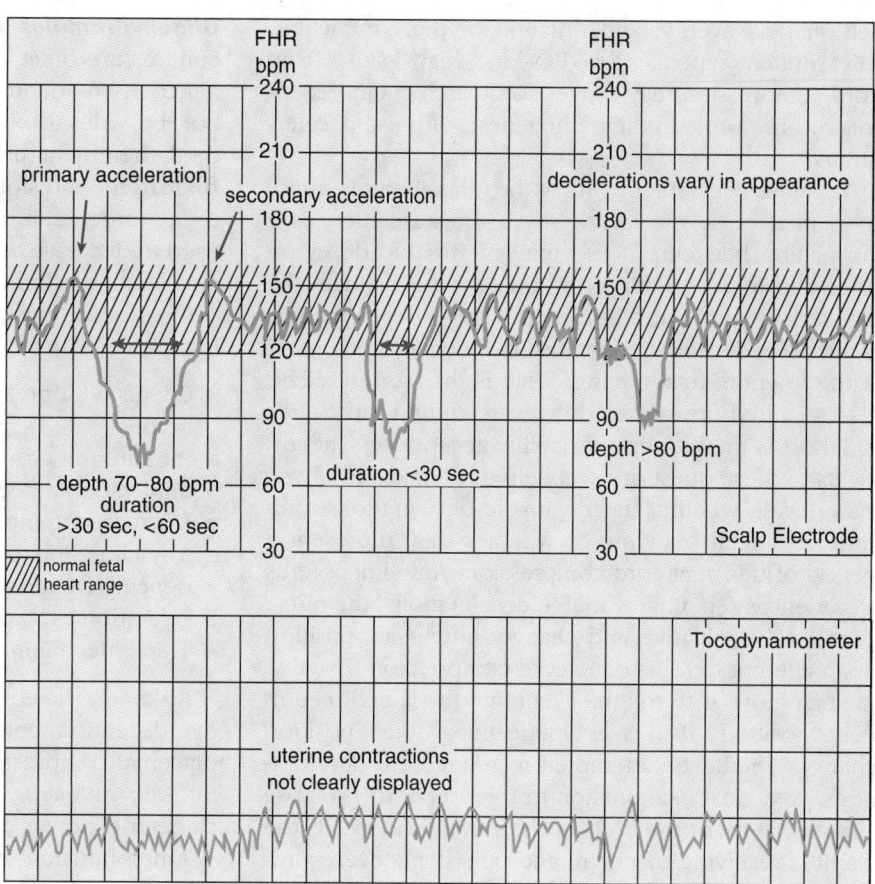

FIGURE 40–10 Classic mild variable decelerations. (From Cabaniss, M. [1993]. *Fetal monitoring interpretation.* Philadelphia: J.B. Lippincott.)

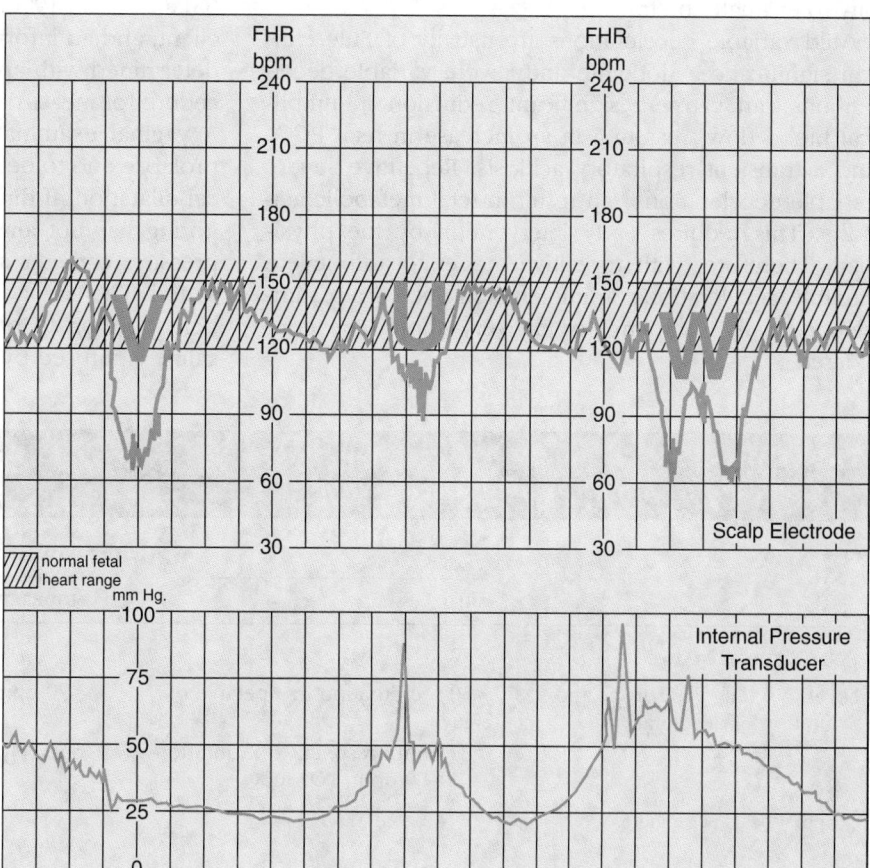

FIGURE 40–11 Variable decelerations. (From Cabaniss, M. [1993]. *Fetal monitoring interpretation.* Philadelphia: J.B. Lippincott.)

set, shape, severity, and duration of the contraction. The sudden hypoxia (low PO_2 and high PCO_2) from cord compression may trigger aortic arch chemoreceptors to play a role in the pathogenesis of these decelerations.

Variable decelerations may be classified as mild, moderate, or severe (Table 40-2). Because there is a correlation between the severity of variable decelerations and fetal condition, the nurse must evaluate the frequency, depth, and duration of these decelerations.

Variable decelerations must be judged in context with the entire fetal tracing. What is the baseline FHR? Has it shifted upward or downward during the course of labor? Is the baseline variability acceptable? The answers to these questions will help the nurse and physician decide whether these variable decelerations indicate poor fetal outcome or whether they represent a period of transient cord compression. Any time a fetus experiences repetitive variable decelerations, the nurse should take initiative and change the client's position in an attempt to relieve the cord compression. Usually, the first move is to roll the client into the lateral recumbent position. If this is ineffective, other position changes should be attempted to relieve the decelerations. A vaginal examination to rule out cord prolapse should be performed if not contraindicated. If the client is receiving oxytocin, and persistent severe variable decelerations are present, oxytocin infusion should be stopped until the physician has the opportunity to evaluate the tracing.

Mild variable decelerations are usually of little clinical significance. Moderate and severe variable decelerations can cause a significant reduction in umbilical blood flow, resulting in an increase in fetal PCO_2 and a transient respiratory acidosis. Repetitive severe variable decelerations can result in fetal metabolic acidosis. This requires early intervention by the physician. Therefore, with repetitive moderate and severe variable decelerations, amnioinfusion, fetal scalp stimulation, scalp sampling, or delivery should be considered.

Oligohydramnios and Amnioinfusion. Variable decelerations are often seen with oligohydramnios. Maintenance of an adequate amniotic fluid volume during labor provides protective cushioning of the umbilical cord, thereby minimizing cord compression. **Amnioinfusion**, the infusion of normal saline into the amniotic cavity through an intrauterine pressure catheter, can be used to decrease the frequency and severity of variable decelerations during labor (Strong et al., 1990; ACOG, 1995). Indications for amnioinfusion include the following:

- Clients with preterm premature rupture of membranes
- Intrauterine growth retarded fetuses experiencing mild variable deceleration
- Decreased amniotic fluid index (AFI) ≤ 5 cm
- Any client in labor with ruptured membranes experiencing frequent, prolonged, or severe variable deceleration
- Thick meconium staining

Risks associated with amnioinfusion include uterine overdistention, cord prolapse, amniotic fluid embolus, placental compression, electrolyte imbalances from the infusate, infection, and uterine perforation from the catheter (Thomas et al., 1993).

Amnioinfusion can be performed through a single- or dual-lumen pressure catheter. The use of an infusion pump and warming the solution are unnecessary (Glantz et al., 1996). The procedure is explained to the client, and an informed consent is obtained. The AFI is determined with an ultrasound examination. (The procedure for measuring the AFI is described in Chap. 39.) A vaginal examination is performed to rule out cord prolapse and to determine fetal presentation and cervical dilatation. If direct continuous electronic fetal monitoring has not already been initiated, an intrauterine pressure catheter and **scalp electrode** should be inserted. The client should be placed in a lateral recumbent position to prevent supine hypotension. Normal saline is infused by gravity at a rate of 10 mL/min. The

---

TABLE 40–2
Principles of Grading Variable Decelerations

	Criteria of Grading		
	MILD	**MODERATE**	**SEVERE**
VARIABLE DECELERATION			
Level to which FHR drops and duration of deceleration	<30-sec duration irrespective of level	<70 bpm, 30–60 sec	<70 bpm, >60 sec
	>80 bpm irrespective of duration 70–80 bpm, <60 sec	70–80 bpm, >60 sec	

bpm = beats per minute.

amount of saline infused is variable. Some physicians infuse saline at a rate of 10 mL/min for 1 hour, after which it is reduced to 3 mL/min until delivery (Nageotte et al., 1991; Thomas et al., 1993; ACOG, 1995). Amnioinfusion increases uterine tone significantly during and after the infusion (Posner et al., 1990). To decrease the risk of increased intrauterine pressure resulting in decreased uteroplacental perfusion, some practitioners prefer to limit the total volume of infusate. In women with oligohydramnios, an infusion of 250 mL saline has been found to increase the AFI by approximately 4 cm (Strong et al., 1990). A total of 500 mL amnioinfusate will achieve an AFI greater than or equal to 8 cm (Strong et al., 1990; Posner et al., 1990). Clients receiving amnioinfusion may undergo hourly AFI determination. Repeat amnioinfusion is performed whenever the AFI drops below 8 cm. Studies are ongoing to determine the optimal method of infusion and the amount of saline used during the procedure.

Prolonged Decelerations

When the FHR drops outside of the normal range (generally decreases of 30 beats/min below the fetus' normal baseline) for up to 10 minutes, they are defined as **prolonged decelerations** (AWHONN, 1993). There is some controversy in the literature about the duration of prolonged decelerations. Freeman et al. (1991) define the decelerations as lasting at least 60 to 90 seconds; AWHONN (1993) defines them as lasting at least 2 minutes; and Cabaniss (1993) defines them as lasting at least 2 to 3 minutes but less than 10 minutes. When the deceleration lasts 10 minutes, it is considered a baseline change (bradycardia).

Prolonged decelerations are defined only by their duration and not by their etiology. They can be caused by maternal hypotension, abruptio placentae, uterine hyperstimulation or rupture, cord compression or prolapse, rapid fetal descent, and occasionally, vagal stimulation from vaginal examination or Valsalva's maneuvers (Fig. 40-12). Prolonged fetal hypoxia is a factor in this type of deceleration with its resultant central ner-

vous system response to changes in the intrauterine or fetal environment.

Interventions for prolonged decelerations are similar to those used for the other types of decelerations. Position change, IV fluid bolus, vaginal examination to rule out cord prolapse, discontinuation of oxytocic medications, and supplemental oxygen by mask are all potentially useful in treating this type of deceleration. If the interventions for prolonged decelerations are ineffective, emergent delivery should be accomplished.

Nonperiodic Accelerations and Decelerations

Periodic changes in the FHR refer to accelerations and decelerations that occur during UCs. Nonperiodic changes occur in the absence of UCs. Examples of nonperiodic changes include accelerations of the FHR associated with fetal movement or stimulation and decelerations not related to UCs, as with cord prolapse or supine hypotension (Fig. 40-13). Treatment for nonperiodic decelerations is the same as for other classifications of decelerations.

Sinusoidal Pattern

An unusual abnormality in FHR in which there is a repetitive undulation of the baseline resembling a "sine wave" has been called a **sinusoidal pattern** (Fig. 40-14). Occasionally, tracings of a normal fetus appear to have a transient sinusoidal (pseudosinusoidal) pattern associated with maternal narcotic administration. This has not been correlated with any particular fetal abnormality. A persistent sinusoidal pattern sometimes indicates fetal hypoxia or severe fetal anemia. The latter is most frequently observed in fetuses suffering from hydrops fetalis due to Rh isoimmunization. Severe fetal anemia also can be seen in cases of fetomaternal hemorrhage. This can occur spontaneously from a chronic placental abruption or following transplacental amniocentesis.

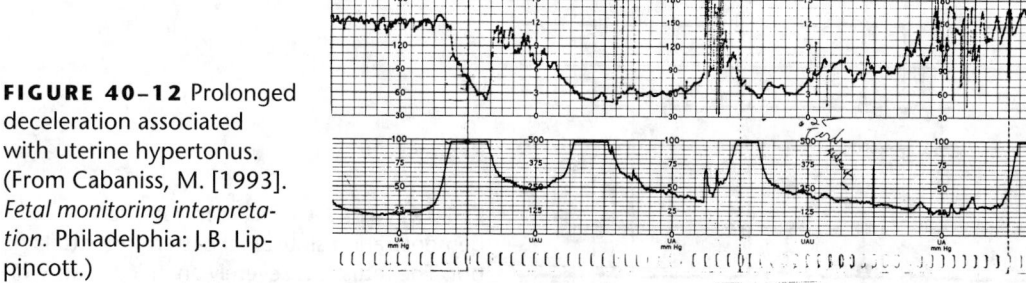

FIGURE 40–12 Prolonged deceleration associated with uterine hypertonus. (From Cabaniss, M. [1993]. *Fetal monitoring interpretation*. Philadelphia: J.B. Lippincott.)

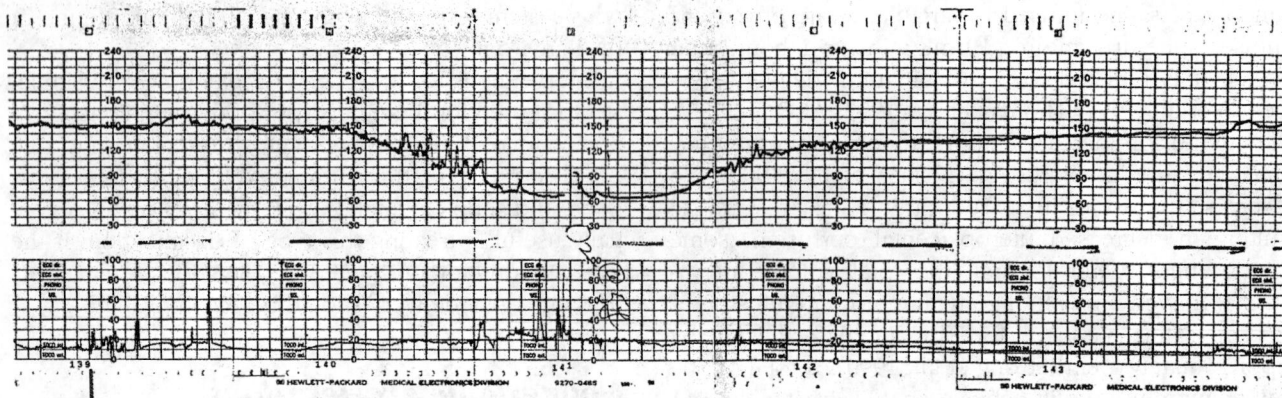

FIGURE 40–13 Nonperiodic prolonged deceleration associated with maternal hypotension. (From Cabaniss, M. [1993]. *Fetal monitoring interpretation.* Philadelphia: J.B. Lippincott.)

The pathophysiology of the development of a sinusoidal pattern is not well understood. This pattern may reflect an absence of autonomic nervous control over the FHR due to severe hypoxia. This pattern has been observed and is considered ominous in the hydropic (massively edematous) fetus.

Fetal Scalp Stimulation and Scalp Sampling

When confusing FHR patterns or patterns suggesting fetal distress occur, the clinician may determine the fetal scalp pH through a technique known as scalp blood sampling. Determination of the scalp pH is clinically useful in the diagnosis of fetal distress. For this measurement, a small volume of fetal blood may be obtained by puncturing the fetal scalp. Blood samples are obtained in glass capillary tubes, and the scalp's acid–base parameters are determined. Clinical studies have demonstrated a correlation between the pH of scalp blood and abnormalities in FHR, Apgar scores, and umbilical cord pH. This measurement may help when the fetal monitoring data are unclear. This procedure may be difficult to perform under the best of circumstances because it is usually performed when the client is actively laboring and often uncomfortable; many times, this must be repeated to ensure accurate information. Traditionally, a scalp blood pH of less than 7.20 is considered acidotic; values between 7.2 and 7.25 are equivocal and bear repeating. Values above 7.25 are considered normal for fetuses during labor. Although scalp sampling may be helpful in select cases, it is not commonly used in current practice (ACOG, 1995; Goodwin et al., 1994).

A newer technique to qualitatively assess fetal acid–base status is fetal scalp stimulation. This technique has been described as a viable alternative to scalp sampling (Clark et al., 1984). Fetal scalp stimulation can be performed using digital pressure during a vaginal ex-

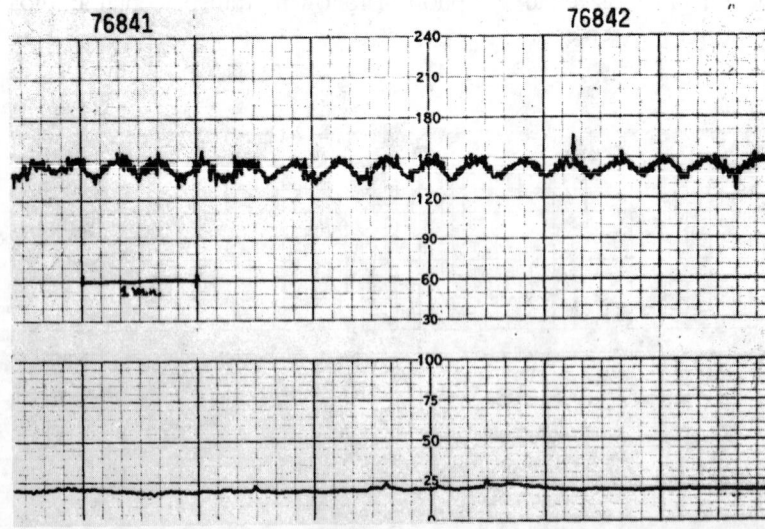

FIGURE 40–14 Fetal heart rate tracing demonstrating sinusoidal pattern prior to labor. The fetus was severely anemic because of Rhesus isoimmunization.

amination or by gentle pressure on the fetal scalp with an atraumatic Allis clamp. Fetal acoustic stimulation, described in Chapter 39, is another method to rule out fetal acidosis during labor. Regardless of the technique used, acceleration of the FHR of more than 15 beats/ min for more than 15 seconds indicates a normoxic fetus.

Nursing Management

Evaluation of the woman and fetus undergoing intra-partum monitoring is a continuous process until the delivery of the newborn. FHR and UA pattern recognition in light of maternal and fetal condition must be constantly reassessed.

The keys to excellent nursing care in the client with abnormalities in FHR patterns are careful attention to detail and fast, calm action. The goal of care is to maintain adequate fetal oxygenation by maintaining adequate uteroplacental blood flow and umbilical blood flow. Keeping these two objectives in mind will assist the nurse in achieving this goal.

As was stated previously, normal FHR variability almost always reflects a fetus who is adequately oxygenated. Abolishing those insults (decelerations) that can decrease the fetus' ability to maintain a normoxic state is the goal of nursing intervention. Early decelerations are not considered ominous and do not require intervention. Mild variable decelerations are thought to be reassuring by some authors and are therefore generally only treated with position change. Moderate and severe variables, late decelerations, and prolonged decelerations warrant nursing, and sometimes medical, intervention to abolish the patterns.

In the event of repetitive late decelerations, the cause should be ascertained. If oxytocin is in use, it should be discontinued. Oxygen by face mask at 8 to 10 L/min may be necessary. Maternal vital signs should be assessed. If the client is hypotensive, an attempt should be made physiologically to raise the blood pressure by changing maternal position to the far lateral and increasing the rate of intravenous crystalloid infusion. If the client has received regional anesthesia and this has caused hypotension, an anesthesiologist should be summoned to assess the need for vasopressive medication.

In the event of repetitive late decelerations that do not correct with the previous measures, fetal scalp stimulation or sampling may be indicated, or delivery should be considered.

Moderate and severe variable decelerations warrant similar interventions with the addition of a vaginal examination to rule out cord prolapse. If cord prolapse is found, the fetal head should be elevated vaginally and the client placed in the lateral Trendelenburg position or knee–chest position and taken to the surgical delivery room for immediate cesarean delivery. For a summary of interventions, see Nursing Guidelines: Intervention for Fetal Heart Rate Patterns.

Psychological Aspects of Fetal Monitoring

Fetal monitoring can occasionally have an important psychological impact on the client. The need for fetal monitoring should have been discussed with the client before the onset of labor. If it has not, this task may fall on the labor room nurse. It is important to stress to the parents that the purpose of monitoring is to detect any evidence of fetal distress before the fetus is compromised, not because the physician believes the fetus is already in danger. This will usually alleviate much of the client's fear. When counseling parents, the nurse should state the intended benefits of fetal monitoring without ignoring the infrequent complications. The nurse should never tell the family that intrapartum monitoring guarantees a healthy neonate.

The nurse must make the client aware that the FHR is consistently changing and that there is a wide range of normal variation. The nurse also must assure the client that with external FHR tracing, movement by the woman or fetus can cause a temporary loss of the FHR signal on the monitor. The client must know that this is a mechanical phenomenon and does not reflect a real loss of the FHR. Often the nurse also must explain to the client that internal monitoring is safe for the fetus.

Because most clients desire to observe the monitor tracing, the equipment should be placed in view of the woman, her partner, and the nurse. Couples often find that observing the onset and decrement (downslope) of the contractions is useful in assisting breathing techniques. This is particularly true for the partner. The reassurance obtained from observing or listening to the fetal heart beat during labor is often a secondary benefit to the couple.

Fetal monitoring requires a nurse who is professional, composed, and diplomatic. The nurse must be ready to take initiative. If an abnormal FHR pattern is noted, the nurse must take immediate action while allaying the client's anxiety and notifying the physician. Also, should scalp pH sampling or cesarean delivery become necessary, the nurse must exert a calming influence on the client while helping prepare her and the equipment for the appropriate procedure.

The responsibility of helping the mother cope with the psychological aspects of fetal monitoring usually rests with the labor nurse. This nurse must be a competent, compassionate, and secure person who can help the client understand the purpose of and procedures involved in fetal monitoring. This person also should be able to act swiftly in the event of an emergency and still maintain the client's confidence and allay her fears.

NURSING GUIDELINES

Intervention for Fetal Heart Rate Patterns

I. Periodic Changes—Uniform Decelerations
   A. Early decelerations
      Description: Fetal heart rate (FHR) begins to slow with the onset of the uterine contractions and returns to baseline when the contraction is over.
      Pathophysiology: Head compression

Nursing Intervention	*Rationale*
1. Be aware that the FHR may slow with a contraction. 2. Chart descriptive note or chart on flow sheet according to institutional practice.	Fetal head compression is associated with the contraction, resulting in a parasympathetic discharge mediated by the vagus nerve. Parasympathetic stimulation results in slowing of the FHR. This pattern represents normal response of the fetus to this stimulus and is associated with a good outcome.

   B. Late decelerations
      Description: FHR begins to fall after the onset of contraction and returns to baseline after the contraction has ceased. Usually the FHR remains within the normal range. Decelerations may be subtle but ominous.
      Pathophysiology: Uteroplacental insufficiency

Nursing Intervention	*Rationale*
1. Recognize the pattern on the tracing and be alert for audible changes in the rhythm of the FHR. 2. Follow institution policy: do you assess and wait for next deceleration to occur before notifying physician or proceed to intervention #3? 3. Turn client to her left side, and give oxygen 8–10 L/min by mask if indicated. 4. Chart a descriptive note or chart on flow sheet.	Nursing personnel must have knowledge and experience in FHR monitoring. Effective nursing and physician management provides for safe labor and delivery for mother with an uncompromised infant; compliance with institution policies is important. Changing position relieves aorta or vena cava pressure. Hypotension, hyperstimulation, or conduction anesthesia also may be the cause and need to be addressed by nurse and physician. Nursing management is dictated by institution policies.

II. Nonuniform Decelerations
   A. Variable decelerations
      Description: The FHR slows either with a contraction or between contractions. The pattern of the deceleration is often either a U, V, or W shape that drops suddenly from the baseline and returns abruptly to the baseline. FHR usually falls outside normal range.
      Pathophysiology: Cord compression

Nursing Intervention	*Rationale*
1. Recognize the pattern, and assess the frequency, depth, and duration of the deceleration. 2. Follow institution policy: Do you assess before notifying the physician and carrying out the interventions of #3? 3. Turn client to her left side or to lateral Trendelenburg position and give oxygen 8–10 L/min by mask if indicated.	There is correlation between the severity of the variable deceleration and fetal condition. Some institutions have 24-hour physician coverage on the unit; in other institutions, the nurse must inform the physician by phone, because they have standing orders. Changing position may help to remove the pressure on the cord. If this is not effective, physician or nurse may attempt upward displacement of presenting part.

   B. Prolonged decelerations
      Description: The FHR is at least 30 beats below the fetus' normal baseline for greater than 2 minutes and less than 10 minutes.
      Pathophysiology: Cord compression or uteroplacental insufficiency and rapid descent of the fetus through the birth canal

Nursing Intervention	*Rationale*
1. Recognize the pattern, and assess the depth and duration of the deceleration. Discontinue oxytocic medications. 2. Change client's position to the lateral and lateral Trendelenburg and knee–chest if indicated (if cord prolapse found). 3. Perform vaginal examination if indicated.	The nurse must act quickly to relieve stressors causing the deceleration and begin interventions. This may relieve pressure on cord or relieve aortacaval compression. Rule out cord prolapse and assess for rapid cervical progress and fetal descent.

(continued)

NURSING GUIDELINES (*Continued*)

Intervention for Fetal Heart Rate Patterns

Nursing Intervention	*Rationale*
4. Provide fluid bolus.	Hydrate client if hypotensive
5. Give oxygen by mask at 8–10 L.	Raising the PO_2 of the mother may have a positive impact on the oxygenation of the fetus.
6. Notify physician or nurse-midwife immediately, depending on cause and fetal response to interventions.	Delivery may be necessary.

III. Baseline Changes
  A. Tachycardia
    Description: A baseline FHR of more than 160 beats/min persists for more than 10 minutes.
    Pathophysiology: Fetal hypoxia, maternal fever, maternal dehydration, idiopathic maternal anxiety, prematurity, drug related, fetal arrhythmia or dysrhythmia

Nursing Intervention	*Rationale*
1. Confirm by auscultating FHR.	Confirm that monitor is operating properly and FHR has increased. Tachycardia may be in response to fetal movement.
2. Monitor maternal vital signs.	Tachycardia may be due to maternal fever or dehydration.
3. Monitor contractions.	FHR may increase in response to excessive contractions.
4. Change maternal position.	Aortoiliac compression is alleviated.
5. Continue to watch closely by reviewing tracings for changing patterns.	Etiologic factors might be identified. Tachycardia may be a sign of fetal distress; arrhythmias may be identified by fetal electrocardiogram.
6. Chart descriptive note on flow sheet or on electronic medical record.	Nursing management is dictated by institution policies.

  B. Bradycardia
    Description: An FHR of less than 120 beats/min persists for more than 10 minutes.

Nursing Intervention	*Rationale*
1. Change maternal position.	Changing position alleviates uterine pressure on the aorta and vena cava.
2. Give oxygen by mask at 8–10 L/min if indicated.	
3. Continue to watch closely for	
Bradycardia (<100 beats/min) with loss of variability and late decelerations	
Bradycardia (100–120 beats/min) with good FHR variability and absence of late decelerations	
Bradycardia due to heart block	Fetus may have congenital heart abnormality.
	Ominous signs indicate fetal distress, even impending death.
	This is a sign of fetal distress.
	This is generally not a sign of fetal distress.
4. Chart descriptive note on flow sheet or on electronic medical record.	Nursing management is dictated by institution policies.

  C. Variability
    Description: The normal variation in the fetal heart rate that reflects an intact autonomic nervous system
    Marked: >25 beats/min
    Average: 6–25 beats/min
    Minimal: <6 beats/min
    Pathophysiology: Maternal medication, fetal acidosis, fetal neurologic immaturity

Nursing Intervention	*Rationale*
1. Observe variability of the FHR.	Variability is an indication of normal neurologic control of heart rate and a measure of fetal reserve.
2. Increased variability may require nursing intervention.	This may be due to external uterine palpation, uterine hypertonus, mild fetal hypoxemia, fetal activity, or maternal activity.
3. Decreased variability: perform acoustic external or scalp stimulation; follow physician's orders based on cause.	Possible causes include prematurity, drugs, hypoxia and acidosis, fetal sleep, fetal cardiac arrhythmias, or anomalies.
4. Chart descriptive note, on flow sheet, or in electronic medical record.	Nursing management is dictated by institution policies.

Summary Points

✔ External UA monitoring provides a recording of the frequency and duration of UCs. Internal UA monitoring measures intrauterine pressure for assessing baseline tone, frequency, and intensity of contractions.

✔ Fetal heart rate auscultation can be performed using a fetoscope or a Doppler ultrasound device.

✔ The two methods of electronic fetal monitoring discussed in this chapter are the indirect, or external, mode, which uses a Doppler device and pressure-sensitive transducer for assessment, and the direct, or internal, mode, which uses a scalp electrode for heart rate assessment and intrauterine pressure catheter for uterine pressure readings.

✔ Fetal well-being is generally assured in the presence of a baseline FHR in the normal range, variability within the acceptable range, and accelerations with fetal movement or stimulation. The deceleration patterns that may be exhibited are a sign of the "insult" to the fetus.

✔ In addition to electronic fetal monitoring, other techniques have been identified as diagnostic adjuncts to ascertain fetal status. They include fetal scalp stimulation and scalp blood sampling.

✔ The role of the nurse caring for the intrapartum client has expanded during the last few decades. With the advent of electronic fetal monitoring, the nurse is expected not only to assess the client and fetus for abnormalities, but also to intervene appropriately. Knowledge of electronic fetal monitoring allows the nurse to provide more comprehensive care to the client. A thorough discussion with the client and her partner about the benefits and risks of monitoring techniques is essential.

REFERENCES

American Academy of Pediatrics and American College of Obstetricians and Gynecologists (1992). *Guidelines for perinatal care* (3rd ed.). Washington, DC: Author.

American College of Obstetricians and Gynecologists (1989). *ACOG technical bulletin 132—Intrapartum fetal heart rate monitoring*. Washington, DC: Author.

American College of Obstetricians and Gynecologists (1995). *ACOG technical bulletin 207—Fetal heart rate patterns: Monitoring, interpretation, and management*. Washington, DC: Author.

Association of Women's Health Obstetric and Neonatal Nursing (1993). *Fetal heart monitoring principles and practice*. Washington, DC: AWHONN.

Cabaniss, M. L. (1993). *Fetal monitoring interpretation*. Philadelphia: J.B. Lippincott.

Clark, S. L., Gimovsky, M. L., & Miller, F. C. (1984). The scalp stimulation test: A clinical alternative to fetal scalp blood sampling. *American Journal of Obstetrics and Gynecology, 148*, 274–277.

Eganhouse, D. J. (1991). Electronic fetal monitoring: Education and quality assurance. *Journal of Obstetric, Gynecologic, and Neonatal Nursing, 20*, 16–22.

Freeman, R. K., Garite, T. J., & Nageotte, M. P. (1991). *Fetal heart rate monitoring* (2nd ed.). Baltimore: Williams & Wilkins.

Glantz, J. C., & Letteney, D. L. (1996). Pumps and warmers during amnioinfusion: Is either necessary? *Obstetrics and Gynecology, 87*(1), 150–155.

Goodwin, T. M., Masterson, L. M., & Paul, R. H. (1994). Elimination of fetal scalp blood sampling on a large clinical service. *Obstetrics and Gynecology, 83*(6), 971–973.

Harris, J. L., Krueger, T. R., & Parer, J. T. (1982). Mechanisms of late decelerations of the fetal heart rate during hypoxia. *American Journal of Obstetrics and Gynecology, 144*, 491.

Manning, F. A. (1994). General principles and applications of ultrasonography. In Creasey & Resnick (Eds.), *Maternal-fetal medicine principles and practice* (3rd ed.). Philadelphia: W.B. Saunders.

Nurse's Association of the American College of Obstetricians and Gynecologists (1992). *NAACOG position statement. Nursing responsibilities in implementing intrapartum fetal heart rate monitoring*. Washington, DC: Author.

Nageotte, M. P. et al. (1991). Prophylactic amnioinfusion in pregnancies complicated by oligohydramnios: A prospective study. *Obstetrics and Gynecology, 77*, 677–680.

Parer, J. T. (1994). Fetal heart rate. In Creasey & Resnick (Eds.), *Maternal-fetal medicine principles and practice* (3rd ed.). Philadelphia: W.B. Saunders.

Posner, M. D., Ballage, S. A., & Paul, R. H. (1990). The effect of amnioinfusion on uterine pressure and activity: A preliminary report. *American Journal of Obstetrics and Gynecology, 163*, 813–818.

Strong, T. H., Hetzler, G., & Paul, R. H. (1990). Amniotic fluid volume increase after amnioinfusion of a fixed volume. *American Journal of Obstetrics and Gynecology, 162*, 746–748.

Thacker, S. B., Stroup, D. F., & Peterson, H. B. (1995). Efficacy and safety of intrapartum electronic fetal monitoring: An update. *Obstetrics and Gynecology, 86*(4), 613–620.

Thomas, S. J., & Nageotte, M. P. (1993). Amniotic fluid volume during labor and delivery. *Seminars in Perinatology, 17*(3), 210–219.

41

The High-Risk Newborn: Disorders of Gestational Age and Birth Weight

Objectives

- List risk factors implicated in alterations in gestational age and birth weight.
- Discuss the nursing process in high-risk neonatal care.
- Describe the neonatal intensive care environment.
- Describe the physiologic problems associated with the preterm newborn.
- Identify complications experienced by the preterm neonate.
- Compare and contrast problems associated with small-for-gestational age and large-for-gestational age newborns.

Key Terms

Appropriate for gestational age

Barotrauma

Bronchopulmonary dysplasia

Cephalopelvic disproportion

Extracorporeal membrane oxygenation

Fat emulsion

Gestational age

Intrauterine growth standards

Intrauterine growth retardation

Large for gestational age

Low birth weight

Necrotizing enterocolitis

Point of maximum impulse

Post-term

Preterm

Pulse oximetry

Respiratory distress syndrome

Retinopathy of prematurity

Small for gestational age

Surfactant

Term

Transcutaneous oxygen tension

Very low birth weight

All neonates are assessed as soon as possible after birth for specific needs necessary for adaptation to extrauterine life. These needs include respiratory initiation and maintenance, extrauterine circulatory patterns, body temperature control and maintenance, adequate nutrition and waste elimination, infection prevention, parent–newborn relationship development, and developmental requirements. These needs are especially important for the neonate with a disorder of gestational age or birth weight who is considered high risk, because the neonate's survival may be in jeopardy. Care focuses on supporting the newborn's basic functioning while also providing care to compensate for any inadequacies. The particular, precise, and highly specialized practice of neonatal nursing could cover an entire text. Because of the newborn's condition, the neonate and family are completely dependent on the skill of the primary caretaker, the neonatal nurse. This makes the nurse's task that much more demanding, challenging, rewarding, and stressful. From the time of birth, resuscitation, stabilization, possible transport, and continued care in the neonatal intensive care unit (NICU), the newborn is cared for by an ever-vigilant specialized team.

This chapter focuses on the nursing care of the neonate with a disorder of gestational age or birth weight. It begins by defining the terms commonly used for classifying gestational age and birth weight varia-

tions. Using the nursing process format, care of the high-risk newborn is discussed. Each variation is described, along with the common physiologic problems associated with each.

Gestational Age and Birth Weight Variations

Gestational age, the number of weeks the neonate remained in utero, and birth weight are important aspects to consider when assessing the newborn because they are associated with perinatal morbidity and mortality. Advances in modern technology have helped to improve the health and overall survival of neonates at risk because of gestational age or birth weight. However, coupled with these advances, conditions have resulted that may negatively affect the long-term quality of the newborn's life.

The size of a newborn is influenced by many factors affecting the maternal and fetal environments. The relationship between low birth weight and perinatal morbidity and mortality has long been recognized. In the past, however, different implications of birth weight relative to gestational age have been established. Newborns with low birth weight may be of appropriate size for their gestational age but immature because they are born before pregnancy has progressed to full term. Other low birth weight newborns may be undersized for the length of their gestation, whether delivered before or at term.

The associated problems and potential causes are different among the various types of alterations, requiring individualized assessment and management approaches. The particular causes of alterations in fetal growth also determine the newborn's immediate and long-term prognosis. The challenge for effective assessment and management of fetal growth disorders begins with an understanding of the intricate and complex mechanisms that control normal fetal growth.

Factors That Affect Fetal Growth

Fetal growth is influenced by a variety of factors of maternal, placental, and fetal origin (Box 41-1).

Classification of Newborns by Birth Weight and Gestational Age

The American Academy of Pediatrics Committee on Fetus and Newborn has recommended that all newborns be classified by birth weight and gestational age. Gestational age classifications are based on the age of the neonate calculated from the date of the onset of the

BOX 41-1

BOX 41-1
Factors Affecting Fetal Growth

Maternal

Low prepregnancy weight
Inadequate pregnancy weight gain
Malnutrition
History of low–birth-weight pregnancy
Adolescent
Short stature
Frequent pregnancies
Low socioeconomic status
Anemia
Chronic disease
Illicit and prescription medications
Smoking
High altitude
Race (African American)
Premature rupture of membranes

Placenta

Small size (decreased weight and volume)
Placental insufficiency
Decreased placental prostacyclin
Placenta or cord defects

Fetal

Genetic factors
Multiple gestation
Congenital malformations
Chromosomal disorders
Congenital infections
Male sex
Birth order

mother's last menstrual period until birth. These classifications include the following:

- **Preterm**—birth before completion of the 37th week of gestation regardless of birth weight; also called premature birth
- **Term**—birth occurring between 38 and 42 weeks' gestation
- **Post-term**—birth after completion of 42nd week of gestation

Birth weight varies normally for each gestational week. **Intrauterine growth standards**, graphic charts involving weight (in grams) and number of weeks' gestation, are used to compare a newborn's weight and gestational age with population averages. Although these standards have shortcomings when applied to particular situations, such as differences in weight due to race, parity, sex, and altitude, they are useful guides

in the assessment of high-risk newborns. The most widely used growth chart, developed in Colorado, gives percentiles of intrauterine growth for weight, length, and head circumference. However, the effects of altitude have made this estimate low for the rest of the country. A more recent fetal growth chart includes correction factors for parity, race, and sex and presents average fetal weights for the 10th, 25th, 50th, 75th, and 90th percentiles (Fig. 41-1).

Birth weight classifications include the following:

- **Large for gestational age**—Weight is above 90th percentile (or 2 or more standard deviations above the norm) at any week.
- **Appropriate for gestational age**—Weight falls between 10th and 90th percentile for neonate's age.
- **Small for gestational age** (SGA)—Weight falls below the 10th percentile (or 2 standard deviations below the norm).
- **Low birth weight**—Weight is 2,500 g or less at birth.
- **Very low birth weight**—Weight is 1,500 g or less at birth (Fig. 41-2).

Birth weight variations may occur in the preterm, term, and post-term neonate. For an illustration of how birth weight and gestational age classifications are related, see Figure 41-3.

Weight helps assess growth, and gestational age helps assess maturity. A newborn of 40 weeks' gestation who weighs less than 2,500 g (below the 10th percentile for weight or length) would be mature but undergrown. This disorder is called **intrauterine growth retardation,** in which the fetus' rate of growth does not meet expected norms; the newborn is classified as SGA. An newborn of 36 weeks' gestation who weighs 3,500 g (above the 90th percentile for weight) would be immature but overgrown. Such large-for-gestational age newborns are typical for diabetic mothers. Although this newborn has attained average term weight, it is actually premature, with incomplete maturation of organ systems. Because some newborns plot below the 10th or above the 90th percentiles and have normal growth patterns, a weight to length ratio or ponderal index may be calculated for a more accurate assessment. The formula may be calculated by multiplying the weight in grams by 100 and dividing by the length in centimeters cubed.

$$\frac{\text{Birth weight (g)} \times 100}{\text{length (cm}^3)}$$

$$\frac{2500 \text{ g} \times 100}{50 \text{ cm}^3} = \frac{250,000}{125,000} = 2$$

Newborns are at risk for various medical problems, depending on their gestational age.

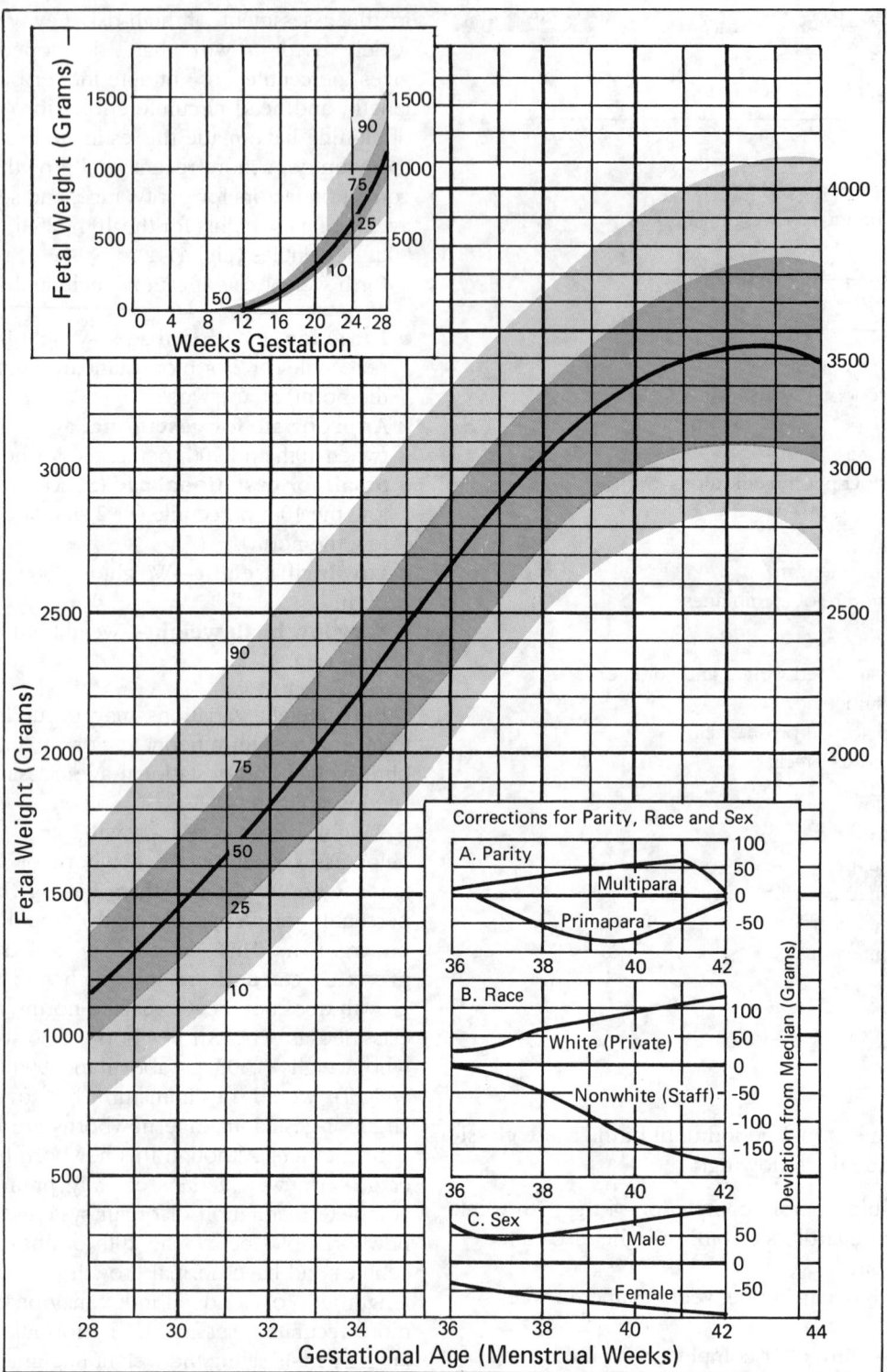

FIGURE 41–1 Fetal weight. The 10th, 25th, 50th, 75th, and 90th percentiles of fetal weight in grams throughout pregnancy and correction factors for parity, race (socioeconomic status), and sex are graphed. Data were obtained from 31,202 prostaglandin-induced abortions and spontaneous deliveries. (Brenner, W. E., Edelman, D. A., & Hendricks, C. H. [1976]. A standard of fetal growth for the United States of America. *American Journal of Obstetrics and Gynecology, 126,* 555–564.)

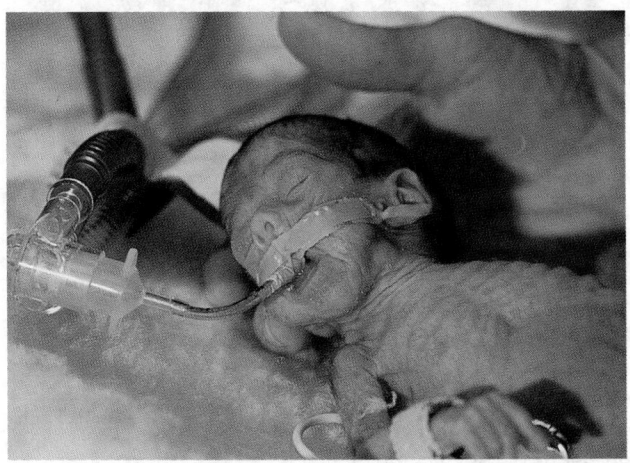

FIGURE 41–2 Born at 24 weeks gestation and weighing only 540 g, this infant is classified as a preterm/very low birth weight (VLBW).

Nursing Process in High-Risk Neonatal Care

When caring for the high-risk neonate, the nurse uses all the steps of the nursing process to achieve the most optimal outcome for the neonate and family. Essential to the care is information about the risk factors and the probable gestational age of the fetus about to be born. This section focuses on planning and intervention in high-risk neonatal care. Although the examples given are usually related to the preterm newborn, the term newborn also could receive similar interventions.

Nursing Assessment

During the first few days of life, the neonate undergoes more profound physiologic changes than at any other time in his or her life. In the neonate who is considered high risk, these changes may pose serious threats to survival. In many cases, the delivery of a high-risk newborn can be anticipated based on information from the mother's health history or prenatal or intrapartum course.

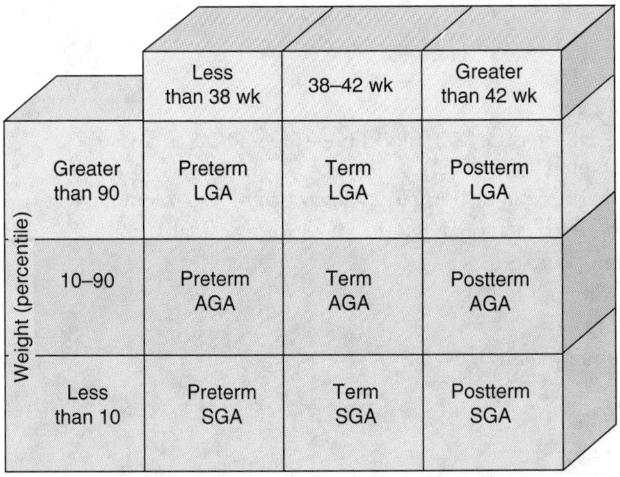

Assessment of the high-risk neonate is an ongoing process, beginning with the history. This history includes family and maternal history and information about the mother's labor and delivery. Factors that may have influenced the neonate's development in utero also are identified.

Although the causes of high-risk neonates are not completely understood, several associated factors have been identified that alert nurses and physicians to the possibility of these problems. Early recognition of mothers with high-risk pregnancies and careful prenatal care can often contribute to a better outcome for the neonate and the mother. Many of the factors contributing to the birth of a high-risk neonate are not specific for a particular problem or condition but are generally related to increased morbidity and mortality. Others are specifically associated with neonatal disorders or fetal abnormalities. Those related to preterm birth include diabetes, placental insufficiency, multiple pregnancy, preeclampsia and hypertensive disorders, and infection. Several of the same factors are associated with the increased incidence of SGA neonates, including preeclampsia and hypertensive disorders, placental insufficiency, infections, discordant twin, and altitude. Congenital anomalies are more highly correlated with term SGA neonates. Chapter 28 covers assessment of gestational age. Assessment considerations related to SGA and large-for-gestational age neonates may be found in the assessment sections of this chapter. Table 41-1 identifies some of the factors associated with high-risk neonates.

Immediately after birth, Apgar scoring and careful observations are correlated with information about the labor and delivery, including such areas as maternal anesthesia and analgesia and any complications that may have occurred. Continuing assessments using various monitoring techniques are made and evaluated in conjunction with the initial assessments made immediately after birth and the physical examination of the newborn (see Chap. 28).

Nursing Diagnoses

To intervene most successfully, the nurse needs to formulate appropriate nursing diagnoses. Examples of nursing diagnoses pertaining to the high-risk neonate are listed in Box 41-2.

Planning and Intervention

Nursing care of the high-risk neonate involves minute to minute observations and assessments with prompt intervention. Initial intervention focuses on supporting

	Less than 38 wk	38–42 wk	Greater than 42 wk
Greater than 90	Preterm LGA	Term LGA	Postterm LGA
10–90	Preterm AGA	Term AGA	Postterm AGA
Less than 10	Preterm SGA	Term SGA	Postterm SGA

Weight (percentile)

FIGURE 41–3 Birth weight and gestational age groups as defined by Lubchenko and coworkers.

TABLE 41–1
Identification of High-Risk Neonate: Associated Factors

PRENATAL FACTORS	Age <15 or >35
Maternal characteristics	Low socioeconomic status
	Unmarried
	Family or marital conflicts
	Emotional illness or family history of mental illness
	Persistent ambivalence or conflicts about the pregnancy
	Shorter than 5 ft
	20% underweight or overweight
	Malnutrition
Reproductive history	Parity ≥ three previous abortions
	Previous stillborn or neonatal death
	Previous premature labor or low birth weight newborn (<2,500 g)
	Previous excessively large newborn (>4,000 g)
	Newborn with isoimmunization or ABO incompatibility
	Newborn with congenital anomaly, genetic disorder, or birth trauma
	Prior preeclampsia or eclampsia
	Uterine fibroids >5 cm or submucous
	Abnormal Pap smear
	Infertility
	Prior cesarean section
	Prior fetal malpresentations
	Contracted pelvis
	Ovarian masses
	Genital tract abnormalities (incompetent cervix, subseptate or bicornate uterus)
	Pregnancy occurring 3 mo or less after last delivery
	Previous prolonged labor or significant dystocia
	Prior multiple birth
Substance abuse	Drugs
	Alcohol
	Smoking
Environmental hazards	Exposure to known teratogens
Medical problems	Anemias with hemoglobin <9 g and hematocrit <32%
	Pulmonary disease
	Endocrine disorders
	Gastrointestinal or liver disease
	Epilepsy
	Malignancy
	Chronic hypertension
	Renal disease
	Diabetes mellitus
	Heart disease
	Sickle cell trait or disease
Complications of present pregnancy	Low or excessive weight gain
	Hypertension (mean arterial pressure >90, blood pressure 140/90, increase >30 mm Hg systolic or >20 mm Hg diastolic)
	Recurrent glycosuria and abnormal fasting blood sugar or glucose tolerance test
	Uterine size inappropriate for gestational age (too large or too small)
Complications of present pregnancy	Recurrent urinary tract infections
	Severe varicosities or thrombophlebitis
	Recurrent vaginal bleeding
	Premature rupture of membranes
	Multiple pregnancy
	Hydramnios with a single fetus
	Rh-negative with a rising titer
	Late or no prenatal care

(continued)

Viral infections (rubella, cytomegalovirus, herpes, mumps, rubeola, chickenpox, shingles, smallpox, vaccinia, influenza, poliomyelitis, hepatitis, western equine encephalitis, coxsackievirus B)

Syphilis, especially late pregnancy

Bacterial infections (gonorrhea, tuberculosis, listeriosis, severe acute infection)

Protozoan infections (toxoplasmosis, malaria)

Postmaturity

Anemia with hemoglobin of 9 g or less

Severe pregnancy-induced hypertension

Abnormal fetal assessment tests

INTRAPARTUM FACTORS

Complications of labor and delivery

Labor longer than 24 h in primigravida

Labor longer than 12 h in multigravida

Second stage longer than 1 h

Ruptured membranes more than 24 h

Abnormal presentation or position

Heavy sedation or injudicious anesthesia

Maternal fever or infection

Placenta previa or abruptio placentae

Cesarean section

Meconium-stained amniotic fluid

Fetal distress demonstrated by monitoring or scalp blood sampling

Prolapsed cord

High forceps or midforceps delivery: difficult or operative delivery

Premature labor

Severe pregnancy-induced hypertension

Precipitous labor less than 3 h

Elective induction

Oxytocin (Pitocin) augmentation

Immediate problems of newborn

Malformation or other significant abnormality

Birth injury

Asphyxia (Apgar <6 at 5 min)

NEONATAL FACTORS

Characteristics of newborn

Clinical problems

Preterm

SGA or LGA

Birth weight <5½ lb or >9 lb

Low-set ears

Enlargement of one or both kidneys

Single palmar crease

Single umbilical artery

Small head size

Feeding problems

Anemia

Hyperbilirubinemia

Temperature instability

Respiratory distress

Hypoglycemia

Polycythemia

Sepsis

Rh or ABO incompatibilities

Hypocalcemia

Persistent cyanosis

Shock

Seizures

Heart murmur

SGA, small for gestational age; LGA, large for gestational age.

BOX 41-2
Nursing Diagnoses—High-Risk Neonate

- Risk for Fluid Volume Deficit related to insensible water loss
- Ineffective Airway Clearance related to amniotic fluid or mucus in airway
- Altered Cardiopulmonary Perfusion related to pulmonary compromise
- Ineffective Thermoregulation related to
  - Immaturity
  - Stress of illness or condition
- Activity Intolerance related to increased energy expenditures and lack of reserve capacity
- Altered Nutrition: Less than body requirements related to
  - Gastrointestinal immaturity
  - Increased energy expenditure
  - Problems with sucking
- Risk for Infection related to
  - Immaturity of immune system
  - Use of invasive procedures and treatments
- Inability to Sustain Spontaneous Ventilation related to asphyxia
- Anticipatory Grieving related to
  - Birth of "less than perfect" neonate
  - Neonate's serious conditions
- Risk for Altered Parent/Infant Attachment related to transfer of neonate to another facility
- Risk for Altered Parenting related interruption in bonding because of neonate's condition
- Impaired Gas Exchange related to
  - Surfactant deficiency
  - Alveolar compromise
- Altered Family Processes related to birth of high-risk neonate and adjustments necessitated by neonate's condition and hospitalization
- Altered Growth and Development related to
  - Functional immaturity
  - Prolonged environmental stress
  - Lack of stimulation appropriate for gestational age and physical condition
- Anxiety (parental) related to neonate's condition and uncertainty of outcome
- Knowledge Deficit (parental) related to hospital course and care and treatment of the high-risk neonate

---

vital functions and preventing complications. Throughout the course of care for the high-risk neonate, the parents play a crucial role. They must be kept informed of the neonate's conduction and progress, be allowed to participate in the neonate's care, be given opportunities to interact with the neonate, be allowed to voice their concern and fears, and be assisted in learning about the neonate and his or her care.

Resuscitation

Successful resuscitation includes anticipation, adequate preparation, and appropriate management. A NICU nurse, neonatologist, and respiratory therapist should be present at all high-risk deliveries. These personnel also should be available in the event that unanticipated problems occur with the neonate. Obstetric and neonatal nurses should be trained in resuscitation; delivery areas or labor rooms should be equipped appropriately. Equipment needs to be replaced as it is used, and the cart should be checked for inventory, expiration dates, and drugs every shift (Box 41-3). As part of preparation, personnel should be comfortable working with the equipment.

Chapter 24 discusses the universally known Apgar scoring system, which provides an assessment and guide for resuscitation required. Factors that can lower the Apgar are central nervous system disorders, maternal anesthetics, sedatives, other medications, fetal sepsis, and extreme prematurity. Although this score is a guideline, the caregiver should evaluate the neonate immediately and proceed with intervention (Phibbs, 1994).

Resuscitation encompasses the skills of maintaining an open airway, assisting with breathing, and maintaining circulation—the ABCs of cardiopulmonary resuscitation (Fig. 41-4). All procedures should be carried out under the open radiant warmer to allow easy access along with continuous temperature monitoring of the neonate. The neonate should be dried thoroughly to avoid evaporative heat loss.

Airway. As the head emerges at the time of birth, the nose and mouth are cleared of mucus with a bulb syringe. If further suctioning is required, the newborn should be placed in the radiant warmer. The mouth is suctioned again first, followed by the nose, to avoid reflex aspiration if the nose is stimulated first. Intermittent suction with a suction catheter for brief periods is recommended. The American Academy of Pediatrics recommends limiting suctioning to 3 to 5 seconds at one time. Continuous heart rate monitoring should be maintained by the use of electrocardiogram electrodes because suctioning can stimulate the vagus, resulting in bradycardia. Oxygen should be administered under intermittent positive pressure ventilation at 5 L/min. The neonate should be mechanically ventilated between suctioning if he or she is apneic.

Breathing. The newborn is placed in the "sniffing" position, without hyperextension of the neck; some neonates may require a towel roll under the shoulders to maintain this position. The mask is placed over the nose and mouth to create a seal. Various mask sizes should be available, because mask size must be appropriate for each newborn. The bag should have a one-way valve on the neck piece to allow for expiration. The bag also should have a collar and reservoir to permit 100% oxygen administration. Some bags have a pop-off valve to control maximum peak pressures, al-

BOX 41-3
Neonatal Resuscitation Equipment

1. Oxygen and air tanks with oxygen diluter, corrugated tubing
2. Infant warmer with suction machine, thermometer, two bottles of sterile water for suctioning, and stethoscope
3. Cardiac monitor with leads, strain gauge (to be brought to room when delivery expected)

Shelf Supplies

IV instrument tray

Catheter-assist tray (see next section)

Blood-culture tube, culturettes

Blood-collecting tubes

Dextrostix with heel stick equipment

Hematocrit tubes with sealing material

Extra syringes—eight each of tuberculin, 3 mL, 5 mL, and 10 mL

Safety pins

Feeding tubes–two No. 8

Suction supplies—one connecting tube; two each of numbers 5, 8, and 10 DeLee

Endotracheal suction tubes (two) and adapter

Sterile gloves—four of each size

Sterile drapes (two packs)

Sterile towels (four)

Ice basins for blood gases

Infant hood

Two continuous positive airway pressure (CPAP) setups— 1 always set up and 1 extra

Face masks—one each of three different infant sizes

Chart and pens on clipboard

Oxygen analyzer—brought in before delivery

Lab slips and white tape for identification labels

Stop watch

Stockinette and safety pins for restraints

1 hemoset

1 metriset

1 250-mL $D_{10}W$

1 150-mL $D_5/2$ NS

Betadine

Needle electrodes

Catheter-Assist Tray

One 20-mL syringe

Two 10-mL syringes

Two 5-mL syringes

Five 3-mL syringes

Five tuberculin syringes

Four packages 4-0 silk suture

Four No. 20 knife blades

Four disposable No. 16 blunt needles (Luer stub adapters)

Four disposable Tomac stopcocks

Four No. 5 arterial catheters

Four No. 3½ arterial catheters

One roll of 1-in pink tape

Cord clamp and cord tie

Disposable scalpels

Alcohol sponges

Corks

Extra 2 × 2 gauzes

Four steri-drapes

Two intraflo

Medicine Tray

Four heparin, 100 U/mL

One 20-mL vial of 1% lidocaine and 1% lidocaine for IV use

Two calcium gluceptate, 200 mg/mL

Two sodium bicarbonate

Two each normal saline and sterile water vials

One KCl vial; one NaCl vial

One salt-poor 25% albumin

Two adrenalin 1:1,000 (dilute 0.1 mL to total volume of 1 mL)

Neosporin ointment

Narcan 0.4 mg/mL, one vial

50% dextrose, 50-mL bottle

Intubation Tray

Laryngoscope with regular and premature size blades and batteries

Forregger tubes—1 each of sizes 2.5, 3.0, 3.5, 4.0, 8, 10, 12, 14, 16

Portex tubes—2 each of sizes 2.5, 3.0, 3.5, and 4.0

Benzoin and cotton swabs

Elastoplast, pink tape, precut tapes (preemie and regular)

Pneumothorax equipment

Needle holder, tweezers, and scissors

4-0 sutures and stylette

(Adapted from the Nursing Manual, *Nursery, Mt. Zion Hospital and Medical Center, San Francisco, CA.)*

though others have attached gauges to give this information (see the Research Highlight).

The usual rate for hand bagging is from 40 to 60 breaths per minute to simulate the usual respiratory rate. Most newborns require 100% oxygen during a re-

suscitation effort. Some newborns already receiving oxygen therapy may require only the percentage they are receiving. The majority of neonates who require ventilatory support may be adequately ventilated with a bag and mask. Positive pressure ventilation is indi-

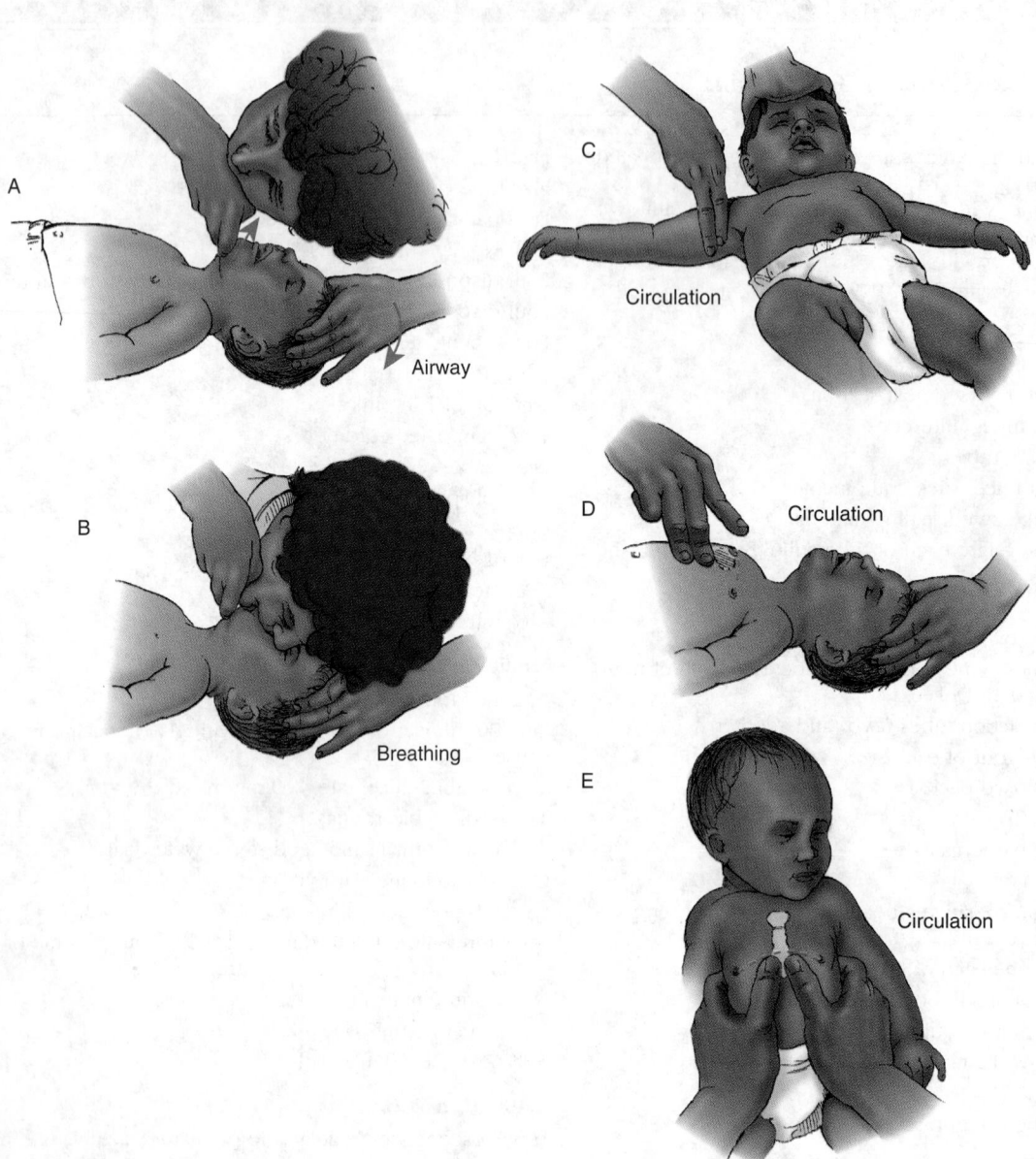

FIGURE 41–4 (**A**) Head tilt and chin lift. (**B**) Mouth-to-mouth rescue breathing and nose seal. (**C**) Locating and palpating the brachial pulse. (**D**) Locating the finger position for chest compressions in an infant. (**E**) Side-by-side thumb placement for chest compressions in small neonates. (From JAMA, Copyright, American Medical Association.)

cated when the neonate is apneic and bradycardic (heart rate less than 100 beats/min) and has persistent central cyanosis despite oxygen supplementation. Although pressure required for establishing air breathing is variable and unpredictable, initial lung inflation may require pressures of 30 to 40 cm H_2O or higher (JAMA, 1992). Less pressure is usually necessary for succeeding breaths (Table 41-2). A nasogastric tube should be placed to prevent gastric distension and aspiration of stomach contents for neonates requiring positive pressure ventilation for longer than 2 minutes (Jain et al., 1993). Chest movement should be observed with each mechanical breath, a more reliable indicator than any

specific pressure read from a manometer. Some respiratory effort and improvement of color should ensue. If spontaneous respirations do not occur quickly, endotracheal intubation should be accomplished by an experienced resuscitator.

Endotracheal Intubation. Endotracheal intubation is indicated when bag-mask ventilation is ineffective, when tracheal suctioning is required, and when prolonged positive pressure ventilation is necessary or anticipated. During chest compressions, endotracheal intubation may facilitate ventilation and minimize gastric distention.

RESEARCH HIGHLIGHT

The Use of Manometers to Control PIP

Variations exist in the techniques used to perform manual ventilation in neonates and in the proficiency levels of nurses in neonatal intensive care units (NICUs) who perform the procedure. Howard-Glenn and Koniak-Griffin investigated 1) whether significant differences exist in nurses' ability accurately to control prescribed peak inspiratory pressure (PIP) when using manometers compared with when they are not used during manual ventilation in NICU and 2) whether the number of years of NICU work experience is related to manometer use and success in controlling prescribed PIP.

A convenience sample of 60 professional nurses whose work experience ranged from 1 to 26 years participated in the study. Each nurse was observed performing one manual ventilation procedure. Pneumogards provided recordings of peak airway pressures during manual ventilation. Observation was made of the number of times the nurse looked at the manometer for insufflations during the ventilation procedure. Scores were given for successful PIP achievement while using the manometer and compared with successful PIP achievement without using the manometer.

Results revealed that 78% of the nurses using the manometers achieved successful PIP, whereas 41% of the nurses not using the manometers achieved successful PIP.

This difference was statistically significant and supports nurses' need to use manometers to control PIP successfully. Analysis also showed that the greater the nurses' NICU work experience, the less likely they were to use the manometer during manual ventilation; however, the correlation between the number of years' experience and success controlling PIP was insignificant.

Supplementary findings included the following: (1) 49% of the time, nurses used the manometer with 60% accuracy; (2) nurses used the manometer more during initiation of ventilation, with use declining in the middle and rising at the end of the procedure; (3) the successful control of PIP increased correspondingly to use of the manometer; and (4) as manometer use declined, accuracy was maintained for several insufflations, then declined until the manometer was used again.

Critique: The research was limited by the fact that the sample was a convenience sample with data collected by the principal investigator. Nurses' performances of the skills of manual ventilation and suctioning may have been affected by observation. Implications for nursing practice are the necessity to establish and use standards of care regarding the use of pressure-regulating devices during manual ventilation of neonates.

(Howard-Glenn, L., & Koniak-Griffin, D. [1990]. Evaluation of manometer use in manual ventilation of infants in neonatal intensive care units. *Heart Lung, 19*[6], 620–627.)

The newborn is again placed in the proper position to straighten the airway. Once positioning is accomplished, the laryngoscope is inserted, and the endotracheal tube of correct size is inserted on the right side of the mouth and advanced into the trachea. The tube size is determined by the neonate's weight. It is helpful to measure the distance from the mouth to the suprasternal notch before placing the tube. According to the American Academy of Pediatrics (1994), "Some prefer using the 'tip to lip' measurement for inserting the ET tube. Another quicker way to measure is to add 6 to the neonate's weight in kilograms" (Fig. 41-5). The presence of bilateral breath sounds when bagged with 100% oxygen indicates that placement is accurate. If one side has diminished breath sounds, the tube is probably inserted too far. An x-ray will confirm placement, which may be difficult during a delivery area resuscitation. After insertion is accomplished, the newborn is mechanically ventilated by rapid bagging with 100% oxygen. It is important to secure the tube some-

TABLE 41–2
Suggested Methods of Emergency Hand Ventilation

Condition of Neonate	Rate in Breaths per Minute	Concentration of Inspired Oxygen (FIO²)	Peak Pressure (cm H₂O pressure)
Depressed neonate in delivery room (state of lungs unknown)	40–60	90%–100%	Very first breath: 30–40 Other breaths: 16–25
Neonate with normal lungs (acute distress)	40–60	90%–100%	15–20
Neonate with known diseased lungs (as initial stabilization before transport)	40–60	90%–100%	20–40

(Adapted from American Academy of Pediatrics [1995]. *Textbook of neonatal resuscitation.*)

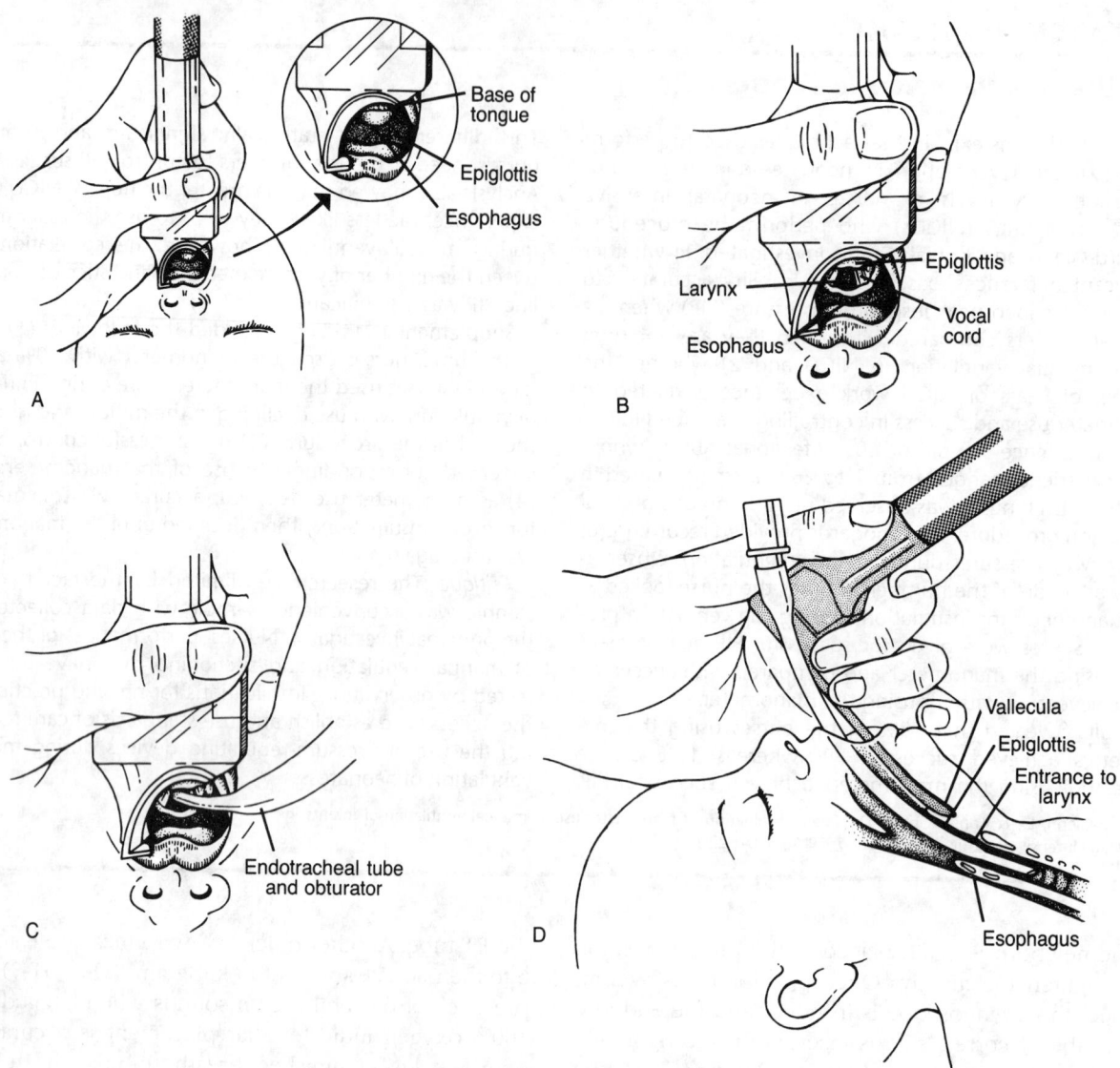

FIGURE 41–5 Technique of endotracheal intubation. (**A** and **B**) The Miller blade should be inserted near the midline and moved to the left side of the mouth, gently deflecting the tongue. As it is advanced, the base of the tongue and epiglottis are visualized. (**C** and **D**) The blade should be advanced in the same plane of movement into the vallecula (see **D**); as the blade is gently raised, the epiglottis swings anteriorly, revealing the opening of the larynx. If secretions or meconium is noted, gentle suctioning should be done before insertion of the endotracheal tube. On certain occasions when the epiglottis is not adequately raised, the blade tip may be placed posterior to the epiglottis, which can then be gently raised to expose the vocal cords. The endotracheal tube is advanced from the right corner of the mouth and inserted while maintaining direct visualization. The laryngoscope blade is then carefully withdrawn while the position of the tube is maintained by the right hand on the newborn's face. Note the tip of the blade in the vallecula.

what before transporting the newborn from the delivery area. Application of tincture of benzoin to the upper lip and cheeks followed by adhesive strips helps stabilize the tube until it can be more permanently secured for long-term care.

Circulation. While other resuscitative measures are being accomplished, the pulse should be monitored and

cardiac compression performed in the event of cardiac arrest or severe bradycardia.

Two techniques are appropriate for chest compressions in the neonate. With the preferred technique, two thumbs are placed on the middle third of the sternum with the fingers encircling the chest and supporting the back. The thumbs should be positioned on the sternum just below an imaginary line between the nipples. In the very small neonate, the thumbs may have to be superimposed. If the resuscitator's hands are too small to encircle the chest, two-finger compression with ring and middle fingers of one hand on the sternum just below the nipple line is used. The other hand should be used to support the neonate's back (JAMA, 1992).

The sternum is compressed ½ to ¾ in in a smooth, nonjerky fashion. Chest compression is interposed with ventilation in a 3:1 ratio. The rate of compression combined with ventilations should be 120 per minute, providing 90 compressions and 30 breaths each minute. Compressions should always be accompanied by positive pressure ventilation with 100% oxygen (JAMA, 1992).

If the procedure is effective, the femoral or brachial artery pulses are palpable in synchrony with depression of the sternum. The procedure is to be discontinued periodically to determine the presence of spontaneous cardiac activity. When this occurs, cardiac compression may be discontinued.

If the heart rate continues to be less than 80 beats/min in spite of adequate ventilation and chest compressions for 30 seconds, medications are indicated (Jain et al., 1993). An umbilical venous catheter can be placed to provide vascular access. Medications most commonly given are epinephrine, which can be given intravenously or endotracheally. The dosage for epinephrine is 0.1 mL/kg of a 1:10,000 solution. Naloxone hydrochloride (0.01 mg/kg) is a narcotic antagonist that may be given for a neonate of a drug-dependent mother or a mother who received narcotics in labor. Naloxone may be given intravenously or intramuscularly. Sodium bicarbonate may be used sparingly for documented metabolic acidosis. A summary of the resuscitation process is shown in Figure 41-6.

Once other resuscitative measures have been accomplished—airway, breathing, circulation, and drugs—the neonate's axillary temperature should be taken. Controlled heat and slow rewarming are recommended. Temperature is continuously monitored using a temperature probe taped to the abdomen. The newborn with cold stress may exhibit respiratory distress syndrome (RDS) symptoms of tachypnea, flaring, grunting, and retractions. These symptoms disappear as the temperature returns to normal. Once the newborn is supported and stabilized, immediate transport to the NICU is recommended, whether in-house or to a regional center. Parents should be informed of all events and should be permitted to see their newborn as soon as possible.

Transport of the Newborn at Risk

Recent advances and specialization in the care of the neonate have resulted in the regionalization of services for the high-risk newborn. Transport is accomplished when sick newborns are identified and admitted to a tertiary care center. In some cases, in utero transport can be carried out when the birth of a critically ill neonate is anticipated. Unfortunately, it is not always possible to transport the mother, so most centers have a transport team available to accompany the neonate from the referral hospital to the center. Transportation is accomplished by ground or air ambulance. The transport team usually consists of a registered nurse or physician and a registered respiratory therapist. General indications for neonatal transport and the equipment required are listed in Box 41-4. It is essential that the parents have the opportunity to see the newborn before the transport team departs. It is helpful for the parents to have a picture of the newborn to keep with them.

Neonatal Intensive Care Unit. Developed to provide highly skilled nursing and medical care to the high-risk neonate, NICUs require extensive sophisticated equipment. The first of such types of nurseries emerged in the mid-1960s in the United States. Nurses provide 24-hour care, with one nurse for every one or two critically ill neonates. With the emphasis now on the development of the whole neonate and family, sole physical care is obsolete. Nurseries are designed with newborn stimulation in mind and with a comfortable setting for the families involved.

Providing a Neutral Thermal Environment

A neutral thermal environment keeps the newborn's metabolic rate and oxygen consumption at a minimum and temperature within normal range. The neutral thermal environment is based on the neonate's weight and age. Skin temperature should be maintained between 36.1° and 36.7°C (96.8°–97.8°F). Axillary temperature should be kept in the range of 36.4° to 37.2°C (97.5°–99°F). Newborns of low birth weight have more difficulty maintaining a normal temperature because of a decrease in subcutaneous fat; a small body mass in relation to a larger surface area; thin, fragile skin; an extended-limbs posture; and underdeveloped central and peripheral temperature control mechanisms (Scanlon, 1994).

Temperature of the neonate may be assessed by one or several of the following means:

- Probe taped to an exposed section of skin
- Axillary temperature
- Anal (core) temperature
- Tympanic method

Environmental temperature should be assessed frequently in conjunction with the newborn's tempera-

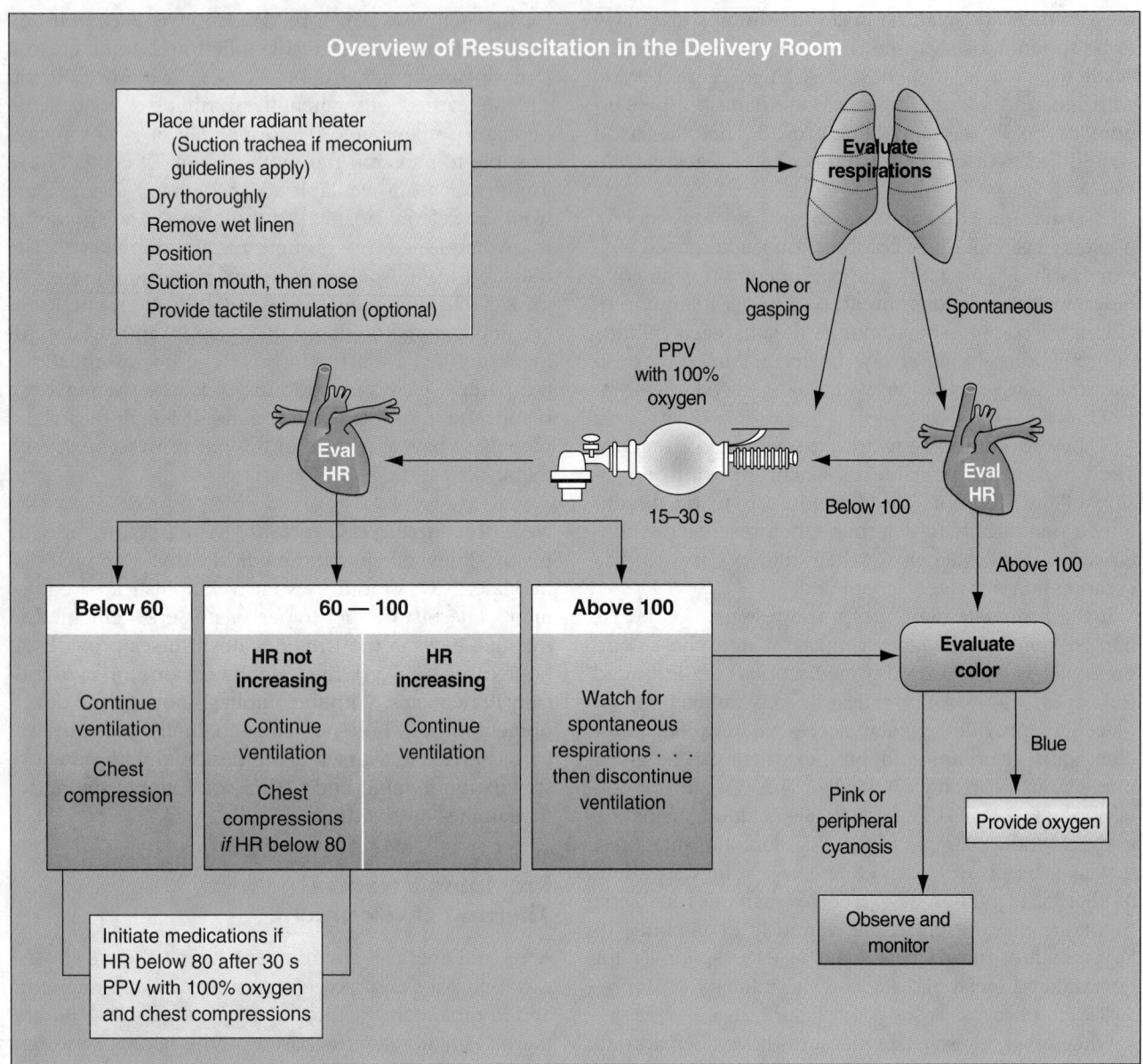

Overview of Resuscitation in the Delivery Room

Place under radiant heater
  (Suction trachea if meconium
  guidelines apply)
Dry thoroughly
Remove wet linen
Position
Suction mouth, then nose
Provide tactile stimulation (optional)

Evaluate respirations

None or gasping

Spontaneous

PPV with 100% oxygen

Eval HR

15–30 s

Eval HR

Below 100

Above 100

Below 60	**60 — 100**		**Above 100**
	HR not increasing	**HR increasing**	
Continue ventilation	Continue ventilation	Continue ventilation	Watch for spontaneous respirations . . . then discontinue ventilation
Chest compression	Chest compressions *if* HR below 80		

Initiate medications if HR below 80 after 30 s PPV with 100% oxygen and chest compressions

Evaluate color

Blue

Provide oxygen

Pink or peripheral cyanosis

Observe and monitor

FIGURE 41–6 Overview of resuscitation in the delivery room. (From American Academy of Pediatrics. [1994]. *Textbook of neonatal resuscitation.* Elk Grove Village, IL: Author; copyright American Heart Association.

ture. Several types of equipment may be used to warm the neonate. Isolettes can provide humidity and isolation. The isolette can be flooded with oxygen but only to a maximum of about 40%. The temperature of the isolette can be adapted by a servocontrol mechanism and a thermistor probe taped to an exposed section of the skin. Newborns in isolettes gain heat by convection but lose heat by evaporation, conduction, and radiation. When portholes are opened, cooler nursery air is sucked in and warm air escapes, resulting in heat loss by convection. Cuffs around the portholes can help with this problem. Dressing the newborn with caps and booties without interfering with assessment and the apparatus helps to protect the against heat loss (Scanlon, 1994).

The radiant overhead warmer provides improved visibility and accessibility to the neonate. A temperature probe unit adjusts the heat flow in accordance with the newborn's skin temperature. One significant disadvantage of the radiant warmer is insensible water loss, the water that is lost from the lungs and skin through the mechanisms of convection and evaporation. The use of plastic sheeting has been most effective in reducing insensible water loss. The use of heat shields may interfere with radiant heat transfer and impede the servocontrol function. The use of plastic wrap in addition to head and feet covers also help reduce heat loss (Scanlon, 1994).

All equipment used must be checked thoroughly and frequently for correct functioning. Temperature

BOX 41–4
Neonatal Transport

General neonatal indications for transport:

- Low birth weight or preterm
- Respiratory assistance needed
- High acuity level
- Life-threatening surgery
- Seizures
- Persistent fetal circulation

Equipment required:

- Battery-operated monitors for vital signs, blood pressure
- Transcutaneous oxygen monitor
- Suction equipment
- Intravenous pump, equipment
- Respirator
- Blood-drawing equipment
- Resuscitation equipment
- Transport equipment checked every shift

---

probes used must be taped on the skin. Units housing newborns should be kept away from drafts. All those caring for newborns should always have warm hands when handling the neonates, warm surfaces when placing neonates on them, and warmed oxygen. All procedures should be carried out in a warm area or under a radiant heat source.

Nurses should observe newborns for signs of cold stress, such as tachypnea, apneic spells, color changes, hypoglycemia, and metabolic acidosis. If newborns do become chilled, they should be warmed slowly over a period of hours to avoid apnea. The heating unit's desired temperature should be increased gradually until the newborn's temperature is stable. The newborn may require a calorie source to correct hypoglycemia or to stabilize blood gases. As the newborn's condition stabilizes, he or she can be weaned slowly from an isolette. Initially, the newborn is dressed in a shirt and diaper as the isolette's temperature is gradually lowered. If this is successful, the portholes are opened, the heat is turned off, and the newborn eventually is transferred to an open crib.

Maintaining Skin Integrity

The skin functions as a barrier against infection, helps regulate body temperature, stores fats, discharges electrolytes and water, and protects organs. The preterm neonate's skin is particularly fragile and susceptible to trauma and irritation. The outside layer of the epidermis, the stratum corneum, becomes thicker as maturation occurs. Skin permeability decreases with increasing gestational age. Finally, bonds between the layers of epidermis and dermis strengthen with increasing

gestational age (Lefrak-Okikawa et al., 1993). Current recommendations regarding skin in the NICU are as follows:

- Bathe two or three times a week with neutral pH soap. For neonates less than 28 weeks' gestation, avoid a soap bath for at least the first week of life.
- Use lubricants sparingly and only if the skin is excessively dry. Only use lubricants that are perfume and dye free.
- Change diapers to avoid heat loss from wetness and to avoid diaper dermatitis.
- Use povidone-iodine ointment before any invasive skin punctures, allow to dry for 60 seconds before a skin puncture, and remove with sterile water. Avoid using isopropyl alcohol in very low birth weight newborns because skin necrosis has been reported.
- Use pectin-based barriers, such as Hollihesive, between skin and tape, remove any adhesive with water-soaked cotton balls, and use gelled electrodes for electrocardiogram monitoring.
- Use transparent dressings, such as Opsite and Tegaderm, for intravenous (IV) sites to prevent skin excoriation over bony prominences and to prevent fluid losses in very low birth weight newborns.

Preventing Infection

The nurse is responsible for minimizing the neonate's exposure to invasive microorganisms. The high-risk newborn is at risk for infection. The preterm newborn also is vulnerable as a consequence of its immature immunologic state. Many neonates require invasive procedures and diagnostic tests that can be routes for organisms.

All caregivers, parents, and visitors who come into contact with the high-risk neonate must be instructed in and follow the handwashing procedure required by the NICU. In addition, the nursery dress codes, as described in detail in Chapter 29, must be followed. Refer to Chapter 29 for guidelines for staff members' health status. As with all clients, standard precautions are required.

Isolettes and radiant warmers should be changed weekly. IV tubing and solutions should be changed using aseptic technique according to agency policy. Other equipment used must be cleaned according to institutional policy.

Respiratory Care

Observation of the high-risk newborn provides numerous clues as to respiratory status. Respirations should be counted for 1 full minute because irregularity is common. Instances of periodic breathing are to be expected; however, apnea may be of a more pathologic nature. The usual respiratory rate ranges from 30 to 60 breaths per minute. The newborn's color should be generally pink. In the first few hours after birth, acrocyanosis may occur from vasomotor instability.

Respiratory movements should be symmetrical. The abdomen can be seen rising and falling as breaths are inspired and expired. Respiratory distress is indicated by tachypnea, retractions, grunting, nasal flaring, cyanosis, pallor, hypotonia, and bradycardia.

Additional data regarding respiratory status are provided by auscultation to ascertain abnormal breath sounds and indications of airway obstructions. Accurate identification of abnormal breath sounds requires considerable practice and skill on the part of the nurse. A stethoscope with a small diaphragm should be used so that it picks up more local sounds than those transmitted across the small chest. Breath sounds should be auscultated bilaterally, moving the stethoscope down the chest along the midaxillary line laterally and anteriorly. Breath sounds should be equal bilaterally. The presence of crackles (fine or coarse), wheezes, grunting, or other adventitious sounds should be assessed and documented (Koszarek, 1991).

During auscultation of the chest, the heart sounds are assessed by counting the rate and describing the quality and location of the **point of maximum impulse** (PMI), located in the fourth intercostal space to the left of the sternum in the midclavicular line. Murmurs and displacement of the PMI may be noted. A displacement of the PMI may indicate pneumothorax.

Chest physiotherapy may be necessary to assist in the mobilization of secretions. Chest physiotherapy is used with newborns who have pneumonia, meconium aspiration, or other respiratory diagnoses resulting in atelectasis and hypercapnea. Various devices, such as padded nipples and electric toothbrushes, may be used for percussion and vibration techniques (Turner, 1991). Procedure 41-1 provides guidelines for performing chest physiotherapy.

Invasive Monitoring. Newborns experiencing respiratory distress and requiring additional oxygen or ventilatory support must have frequent blood gas samples analyzed to titrate oxygen requirements and ventilatory settings. Arterial blood is sampled intermittently by arterial puncture or from an indwelling arterial catheter. Intermittent arterial sticks are painful, and test results are altered by crying and breath holding. The use of an umbilical arterial line provides ready access for withdrawing frequent and accurate blood gas samples.

Placement of the umbilical line is a sterile procedure; confirmation is made by radiograph. Complications of umbilical catheters include arterial emboli, aortic thrombosis, and infection (Guzzetta, 1994). The longer the umbilical catheter is in place, the greater the chance for infection. Signs of infection are temperature instability, drainage, redness or foul odor from cord,

lethargy, irritability, vomiting, poor feeding, and diminished muscle tone. In addition, the nurse must be alert to blanching or cyanosis of one or both extremities, necessitating removal of the catheter.

Percutaneous arterial placement is an alternative to the umbilical catheter. Preferred sites include the radial and posterior tibial arteries (Guzzetta, 1994). Extremities must be assessed for adequate circulation. Capillary blood samples have been found to correlate closely with arterial blood, especially in newborns older than 24 hours. The extremity must be warmed prior to collection of the sample for adequate capillary arterial flow. The site should be cleaned with alcohol and dried. Any alcohol residue can cause hemolysis. The first drop obtained after puncture should be discarded because it contains more interstitial fluid than subsequent blood flow.

Noninvasive Monitoring. **Transcutaneous oxygen tension** ($TcPO_2$) monitoring is a noninvasive method that provides continuous monitoring of PO_2 readings through measurement of skin oxygen tension. The monitoring of continuous status is helpful to observe the neonate's response to nursing interventions, such as weighing, nasogastric feedings, suctioning, and postural drainage.

The electrode is placed in an area with good capillary blood flow and little fat. The electrode should not be placed on a bony prominence. Commonly used sites include the upper chest, abdomen, and inner thigh. The site should be changed and the electrode recalibrated minimally every 4 hours (Turner, 1991). Some reports of skin erosion beneath the electrode make diligent assessment of skin a vital task.

Pulse oximetry is another noninvasive method of oxygen monitoring, using an infrared light source to determine the amount of saturated oxygen in tissues and read out the client's pulse rate. Oxygen saturation is measured by placing a probe emitting red spectrum light on one side of a pulsating vessel and a receptor on the opposite side of the vessel. The probe can be left in place indefinitely, because the sensor is wrapped around an extremity, such as a finger or toe. Significant complications have not been reported; however, oximeters are very sensitive to client movement and work optimally when the client is resting quietly or sleeping. Because pulse oximetry indicates hemoglobin saturation and not arterial oxygen tension, once the hemoglobin saturation reaches 90% to 95%, the arterial oxygen tension must be checked. Pulse oximetry enables the nurse to position the neonate and perform procedures with optimal oxygenation results. The oxygen saturation monitor is reliable, practical, and accurate for use in neonates with varying birth weights, gestational ages, and pulses (Turner, 1991).

PROCEDURE 41–1
Chest Physiotherapy

Overall Objective: To mobilize secretions and maintain patent airway

Nursing Action	*Rationale*
1. Check chart for orders; wash hands.	Chart will ascertain validity of order.
2. Auscultate lungs before and after procedure.	This establishes baseline and helps determine effectiveness of therapy.
3. Perform procedure prior to feeding and oral medications.	This timing prevents regurgitation and aspiration.
4. Perform percussion and vibration in position best for the particular client, depending on which part of lung is affected. Use padded toothbrush for vibration and soft percussor for percussion technique.	This position promotes most effective mobilization of secretions. Use of padded devices is less traumatic to chest.

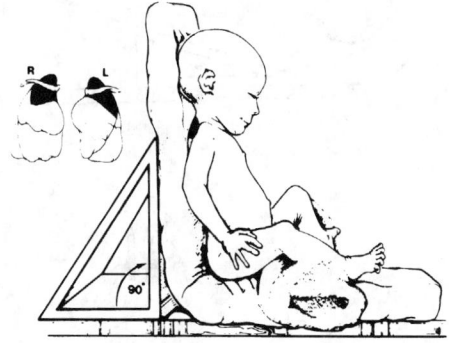

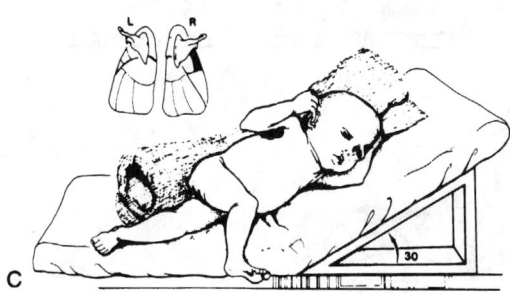

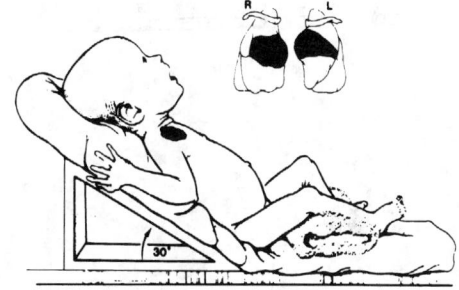

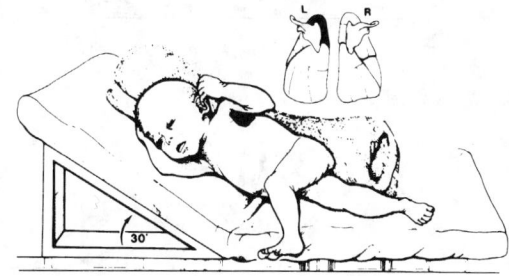

Postural drainage chest physiotherapy positions. Insets indicate the segments drained for each position. Shading on the newborn indicates the area for chest percussion and vibrations. The dependent-head position should be used with caution. (Fletcher, M. A., MacDonald, M., & Avery, G. [1983]. *Atlas of procedures in neonatology.* Philadelphia: J.B. Lippincott.)

(continued)

PROCEDURE 41-1 *(Continued)*
Chest Physiotherapy

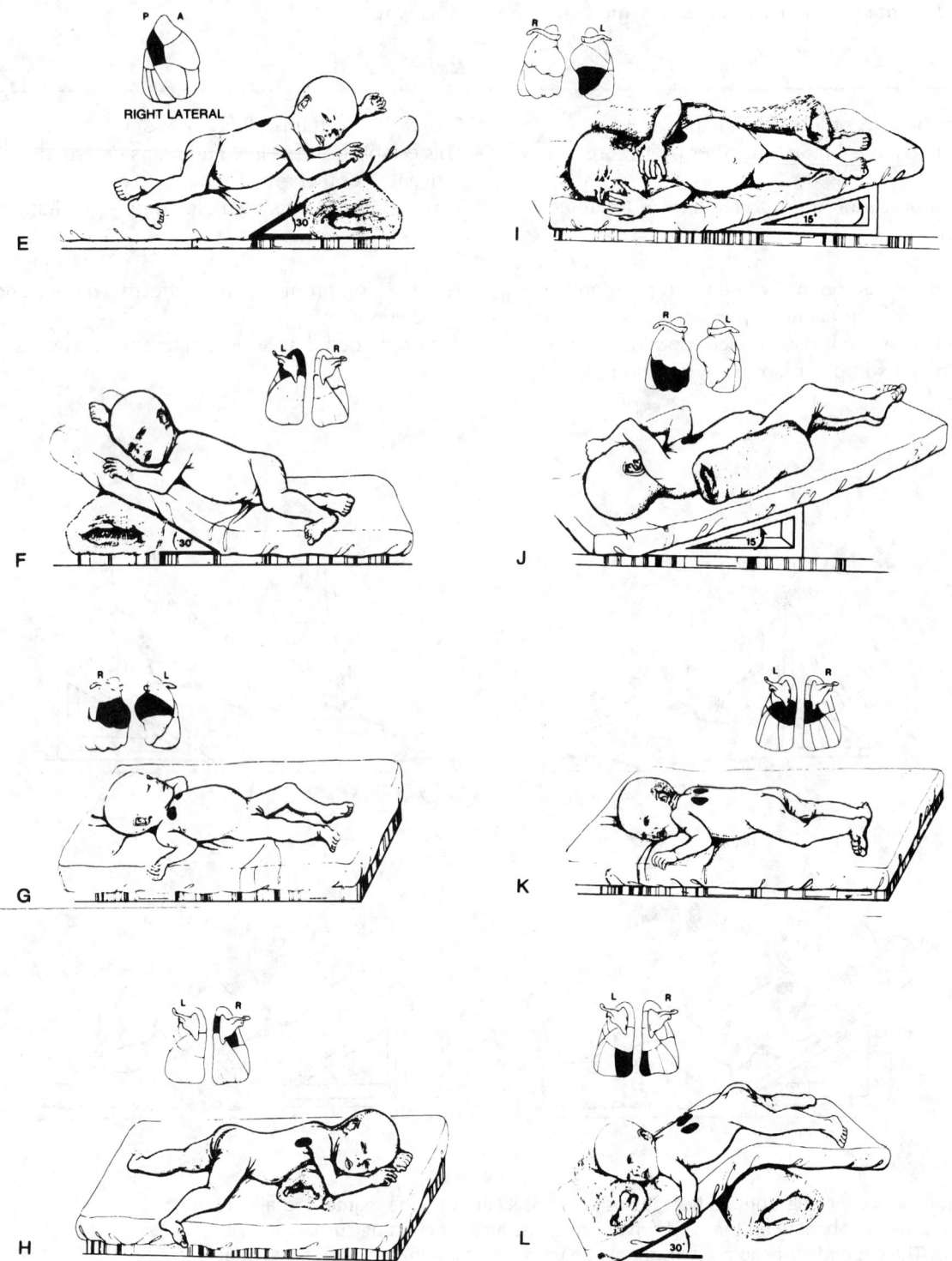

(continued)

PROCEDURE 41-1 *(Continued)*
Chest Physiotherapy

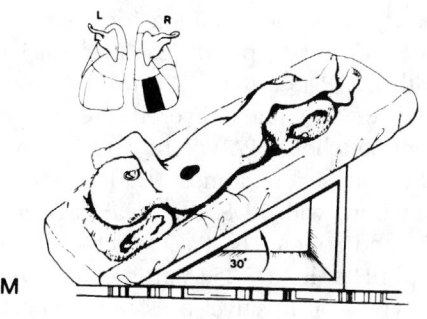

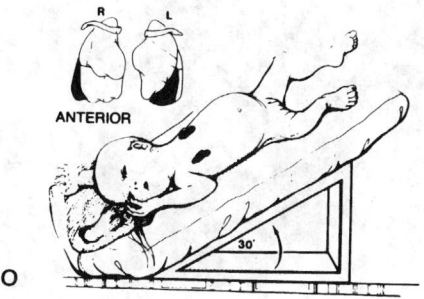

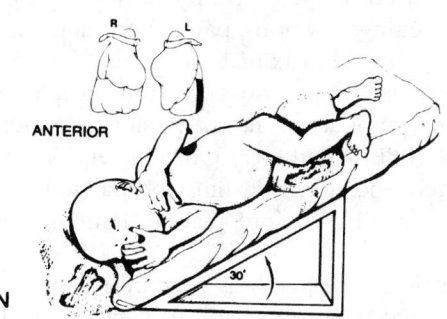

5. Monitor O$_2$ saturation throughout procedure, not to exceed 10 min.	Monitoring prevents fatigue and hypoxia.
6. Suction gently following percussion and vibration.	Suctioning removes secretions mobilized into the larger airways.
7. Place in position of comfort, and document character and amount of secretions and tolerance to treatment.	Documentation provides for continuity of care and notes effectiveness of treatment.

Oxygen Ventilatory Support. Flooding of the isolette with oxygen presents problems because the maximum concentration is probably no more than 30% to 40%. Frequent opening of the portholes makes maintaining a constant flow impossible. When other ventilator support is not necessary, administration of oxygen by hood is an option (Fig. 41-7). Oxygen delivered by the hood may be the optimal method of administration for neonates who have transient tachypnea of the newborn, RDS, or aspiration (Turner, 1991). The typical oxygen hood is made of plexiglass, with head and neck openings and doors or openings for cables and tubings. An oxygen analyzer must be kept in the hood to measure the percent of oxygen administered. Oxygen should be warm and kept at a stable temperature. The neonate should be suctioned periodically to main-

tain the open airway. Blood gases should be monitored every 4 hours and 10 to 20 minutes following each change in fraction of inspired oxygen (fIO$_2$). The use of TcPO$_2$ or pulse oximetry has significantly decreased the need for frequent blood gases.

Continuous positive airway pressure (CPAP) results from a machine applying pressure throughout the lungs of the neonate. This type of pressure helps to keep the alveoli open, thus decreasing the work of breathing and oxygen requirements. Newborns with RDS benefit the most from CPAP, because atelectasis is a common complication. CPAP is indicated for a PaO$_2$ of less than 50 mm Hg in the presence of 60% oxygen (Carlo, 1992). CPAP is measured in centimeters of H$_2$O. The initial amount delivered is usually 4 to 6 cm H$_2$O, depending on whether endotracheal (4) or nasal (6).

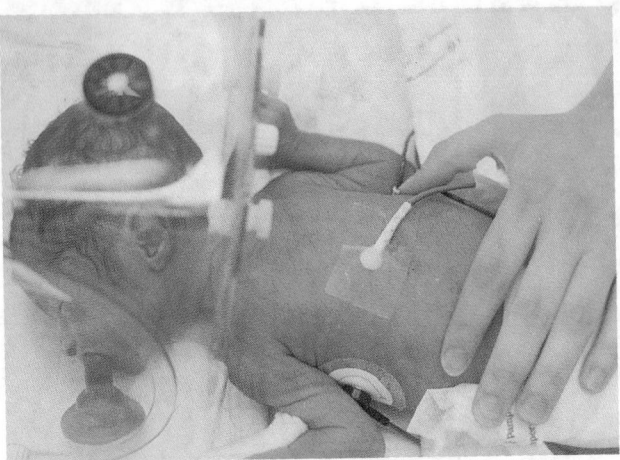

FIGURE 41–7 Oxygen can be administered to the newborn via an oxygen hood when there is no need for other ventilatory support.

This pressure is slowly increased until oxygenation is sufficient as measured by blood gas readings.

Nasal prongs or endotracheal intubation is usually the method of delivery of CPAP (Fig. 41-8). The neonate on nasal CPAP must have frequent nares care. Nasal prongs need to be removed periodically and cleaned with sterile water and cotton-tipped applicators. The nasopharynx and oropharynx should be suctioned with a bulb syringe. Nasal prongs must be anchored securely at all times. If the prongs are too loose, effective therapy will not be achieved. If they are too tight, erosion of the nasal membranes may occur (Turner, 1991).

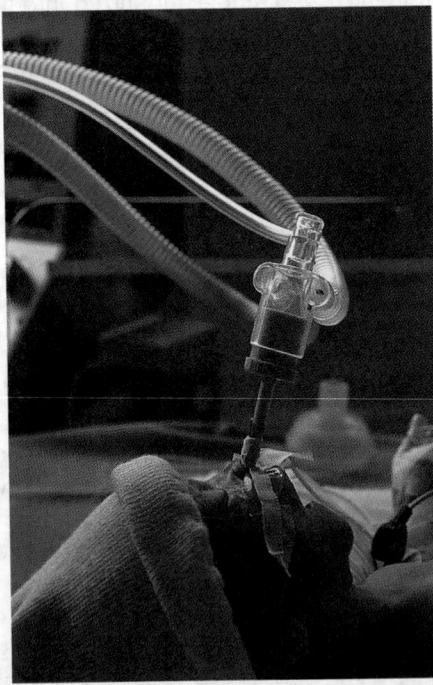

FIGURE 41–8 This newborn is receiving nasal continuous positive airway pressure (CPAP).

Conventional Mechanical Ventilation. In the event of apnea or inability to maintain adequate oxygenation with CPAP, endotracheal intubation (tubes size based on neonate's weight, gestational age, and unit protocol) and positive pressure ventilation may be essential for respiratory assistance. Criteria for assisted ventilation include pH of 6.0, pH of less than 7.25 in 100% oxygen with CPAP less than 7.20 to 7.25, hypoxemia on 100% oxygen flow rate delivered (FIO_2), hypoxemia while on endotracheal CPAP of 10 cm H_2O and 60% to 100% FIO_2, and severe apnea (Carlo, 1993). In the preterm newborn with RDS, the ideal PaO_2 should be between 50 and 80 mm Hg, $PaCO_2$ between 40 and 50 mm Hg, and pH at least 7.25 (Martin et al., 1993).

Various types of positive pressure ventilators are available. The nurse must become familiar with the machine used in the unit and the implications of the various settings. Various parameters that may be altered to provide maximal assistance for each client include peak inspiratory pressure, respiratory rate, inspiratory-expiratory ratio, positive end-expiratory pressure (PEEP), and FIO_2. Once the endotracheal tube is inserted, the newborn must be bagged to estimate ventilator settings before placing him or her on the ventilator.

Skeletal muscle paralysis may be required with the neonate receiving mechanical ventilation. Pancuronium (Pavulon) may be administered to block transmission of acetylcholine across the neuromuscular synapse. Because painful stimuli are still perceived, morphine sulfate may be required to promote comfort.

Condensation in the endotracheal tube will be evident if the tube is placed in the trachea (Turner, 1991). Securing the tube is essential for anticipated long-term therapy. Once the newborn is placed on the ventilator, the ventilator settings and alarms must be checked frequently. Blood gases must be checked at least every 4 hours and 10 to 20 minutes after a change in ventilator settings.

Suctioning is essential to keep the airway open. The suction catheter size can be estimated by multiplying the endotracheal tube size by two. The next size suction catheter above this size should pass into the tube. Negative effects of suctioning include hypoxemia; changes in heart rate, blood pressure, and intracranial pressure; and pneumothorax. Other possible long-term effects include mucosal trauma and sepsis. Negative effects can be minimized by preoxygenation with hyperventilation or continuous oxygen administration, limiting the depth of catheter insertion to just beyond the distance of the tube, using sedation, and minimizing the amount of newborn handling (Shorten, 1991). Procedure 41-2 provides guidelines for endotracheal tube suctioning.

High-Frequency Ventilation. To attempt to reduce the effects of **barotrauma** (injury due to high pressure) or the progression of injury in newborns with advanced

PROCEDURE 41–2
Endotracheal Tube Suctioning

Overall Objective: To promote patent airway by removing secretions and to promote optimal ventilation

Nursing Action	*Rationale*
Check chart, wash hands, and gather equipment: sterile gloves, suction catheter and machine, Ambu bag, stethoscope, oxygen, normal saline, and 1-mL syringe.	This promotes smooth procedure; minimizing possible interruptions, which could interfere with neonate's status.
Perform procedure after chest physiotherapy.	Suctioning is most effective when secretions are mobilized into the larger airways.
Auscultate breath sounds before and after procedure.	Auscultation establishes a baseline and determines effectiveness of suctioning; determines continued placement of ET tube.
Insert 0.2 to 0.5 mL of normal saline into endotracheal (ET) tube, and give three breaths with bag or ventilator.	This thins secretions and preoxygenates neonate.
With sterile glove on, pick up suction catheter. Measure distance from top of ET tube to earlobe to midsternum.	This is a sterile procedure. Measuring approximates distance to carina to ensure proper insertion.
Gently insert catheter to measured point, if resistance is felt withdraw 0.5–1 cm. Apply suction and withdraw catheter, rolling between fingers as it is removed.	This promotes correct placement and avoids trauma.
Do not suction longer than 10 seconds for entire procedure.	Airway is occluded and hypoxia can result.
Give three ventilations with bag or ventilator.	The ventilators promote reexpansion of lungs.
Place neonate on regular ventilator settings until vital signs stabilize.	These settings allow neonate to rest and stabilize.
Repeat procedure again with neonate's head turned and changing catheter angle.	Changes assist in clearing secretions effectively.
Do not suction if cyanosis, distress, or persistent bradycardia occurs. Bag neonate, notify physician, and attempt later.	Respiratory compromise will be avoided.

lung disease, a new method of high-frequency ventilation has been developed. Indications for high-frequency ventilation include RDS, pulmonary interstitial emphysema, meconium aspiration, diaphragmatic hernia, and thoracic surgery (Myrer, 1992).

Extracorporeal Membrane Oxygenation. **Extracorporeal membrane oxygenation** (ECMO) is a method of establishing a pulmonary bypass circuit, permitting the exchange of gases to occur outside of the lung in the machine. This therapy allows the lung to rest and has been used in newborns with severe RDS, meconium aspiration syndrome, and persistent pulmonary hypertension. During ECMO, blood is removed by gravity through a venous catheter that has been placed into the right atrium. The blood circulates from the catheter to the ECMO machine where it is reoxygenated and rewarmed. It then returns to the neonate's aortic arch by way of a catheter that has been inserted through the carotid artery. ECMO usually is used for 4 to 7 days. ECMO is associated with many complications, including intracranial hemorrhage (the most serious), which is believed to occur from the use of anticoagulant therapy necessary to prevent thromboembolism.

The neonate receiving ECMO requires constant diligent nursing care. Close monitoring of blood volume, oxygenation, and signs and symptoms of bleeding are essential components of care.

Liquid Ventilation. Liquid ventilation is a developing technology that uses oxygenated perfluorochemical liquids to reduce surface tension in pulmonary disease, such as RDS, aspiration syndromes, persistent pulmonary hypertension, and pneumonia (Greenspan, 1993).

Nutritional Support Fluid Therapy

Because high-risk newborns are particularly susceptible to water losses due to the high surface to body mass ratio, permeable skin, radiant warmers, phototherapy, and through urine and stool, they require adequate fluid intake at all times. Further, most preterm newborns initially are too critically ill to tolerate enteral feedings.

Parenteral fluid administration through a peripheral or central venous route may be used. Peripheral venous routes, such as in scalp veins or extremities, may be used when fluids are considered supplementary or temporary. Teflon angiocaths are preferred to steel scalp vein needles because the venous access can be maintained longer with less risk of infiltration.

The nurse inserts the device using aseptic technique and carefully secures it, allowing for the opportunity to observe the site for signs of infiltration. IV fluids should be administered at the prescribed rate using infusion pumps, microdrip tubing, and a fluid reservoir, such as a drip-controlled chamber or burette. If an extremity is used, it may need to be restrained to maintain the venous access. The site and extremity need to be assessed frequently for signs of infiltration and circulation.

If long-term therapy is anticipated, especially with total parenteral nutrition (TPN), a central line may be inserted into the internal and external jugular vein. From there, the catheter is threaded into the superior vena cava. This placement facilitates the use of hyperosmolar solutions and high-dextrose solutions, such as TPN.

Several factors determine fluid replacement. Factors determining fluid requirements include data collection of fluid intake and output, body weight changes, urine-specific gravity and osmolarity, serum electrolyte and creatinine concentration, and blood urea nitrogen (Bell et al., 1994). High fluid intake has been associated with patent ductus arteriosus, bronchopulmonary dysplasia (BPD), intraventricular hemorrhage (IVH), and necrotizing enterocolitis (NEC; Price et al., 1993). Fluid requirements of premature neonates vary widely, as do protocols regarding maintenance fluid intake. Ongoing clinical assessment of hydration status is a critical nursing intervention (Table 41-3). The prescribed amount of IV fluid must be administered per hour, using an infusion pump with a volumetric chamber or syringe to ensure a constant, precise amount of infusion. Alterations in the fluid rate could cause problems with blood glucose and overhydration or underhydration.

Formulas especially composed for the high-risk newborn, such as the preterm newborn, are available. Such formulas use the type of proteins similar to that of human milk. There is no agreement on the ideal formula for the preterm newborn. Preterm infant formulas have been modified to provide adequate calories, carbohydrate changes to give lower osmolarity, and fat modifications to promote absorption. Preterm breast

TABLE 41-3
Signs of Fluid Imbalance in the Neonate

Dehydration	Overhydration
EARLY SIGNS	
Lower urine volume (less than 1 mL/kg per hour)	Higher urine volume (more than 3 mL/kg per hour)
Higher urine osmolality (more than 400 mOsm)	Lower urine osmolality (less than 10 mOsm)
Higher urine-specific gravity (more than 1.012)	Lower urine-specific gravity (less than 1.008)
SIGNS OF DECOMPENSATION	
Weight loss (5%–15% a day)	Weight gain (5%–15% a day)
Higher serum sodium (more than 150 mEq/L)	Lower serum sodium (less than 130 mEq/L)
Higher serum osmolality (more than 300 mOsm)	Lower serum osmolality (less than 270 mOsm)
Dry mucous membranes	Subcutaneous edema
Sunken fontanels	
Poor skin turgor	
Higher hematocrit (10% or more)	Lower hematocrit (≤10%)
Higher serum protein (>6 g/dL)	Lower serum protein (less than 4 g/dL)
Lower blood volume	Higher blood volume
LATE SIGNS	
Shock	Pulmonary edema and rales
	Cardiac failure

milk, while adequate in its immunologic properties, is low in calcium and phosphorus. Several types of breast milk modifiers have been developed to boost any inadequacies of preterm breast milk, while still maintaining their valuable properties. These additives are available in powdered or liquid form and are mixed with breast milk. See Chapter 30 for details on pumping breast milk and breast-feeding. If the mother prefers to use breast milk, traditional methods of establishing breast-feeding in the preterm newborn have begun with the mother expressing milk until the newborn is at least 34 to 35 weeks' gestation. Mothers of preterm neonates may have difficulty expressing milk because the neonate has not been nursing, thus providing stimulation for the letdown reflex. Lactation consultants may be helpful with assistance in pumping breast milk and nursing the preterm neonate.

A significantly high failure rate has been documented in this population, because many mothers discontinue breast-feeding even before the neonate has been discharged from the NICU. Nurses have been identified as the caregivers most likely to determine the neonate's readiness to nipple feed. Often there are no established protocols for the initiation of nipple feeding in the preterm neonate. Factors that nurses have identified for readiness to nipple feed are non-nutritive sucking and postconception of 34 weeks or greater (Kinneer et al., 1994).

Three main categories of mothers' concerns about breast-feeding preterm neonates after discharge are whether the neonate has consumed enough milk during breast-feeding, the quality of the milk, and the mechanics of breast-feeding preterm newborns (Kavanaugh et al., 1995). Data suggest that preterm newborns' mothers share different concerns than term newborns' mothers about breast-feeding and that interventions need to be developed to assist in nutritional home care of the preterm newborn.

Feeding schedules vary depending on the neonate's status and nutritional needs. Very low birth weight newborns may require hourly or every 2-hour feedings. Volumes are begun with small amounts and increased gradually as tolerated.

Gavage Feeding. For the newborn whose gastrointestinal (GI) tract is intact but cannot tolerate oral feedings, gavage feeding, whether intermittent (bolus) or continuous, is commonly used. Newborns who may require gavage feeding include those younger than 32 weeks' gestation and those unable to coordinate their sucking, swallowing, and breathing. Appropriate-for-gestational-age newborns who tire easily may require gavage feeding to avoid needless energy expenditure and loss of calories. Procedure 41-3 explains how to perform gavage feeding.

According to the research, bolus-fed neonates grow faster than continuously fed neonates, and bolus feed-

ing is more physiologic than continuous feeding (Hill et al., 1993).

Neonates receiving tube feedings may be soothed by sucking on a pacifier. This kind of non-nutritive sucking has been studied extensively in relation to growth and development and various disease entities. While some studies suggest that non-nutritive sucking increases growth, more recent research has found that it did not affect growth (Hill et al., 1993; see Research Highlight).

Transpyloric Feedings. Continuous infusions by the transpyloric route represent alternative methods of nutritional support. Transpyloric feedings are infusions into the duodenum or jejunum. This method represents a small portion of all tube feedings. It may be the feeding of choice for preterm newborns at risk for aspiration, newborns with chronic lung disease, ventilator-dependent newborns, and preterm newborns who have repeated residuals following intragastric feedings (Hill et al., 1993). The tube is passed into the stomach, and placement is checked by x-ray when a gastric residual pH of 7 is obtained. The tube may be difficult to insert, and placement maintenance may be an ongoing problem.

As the neonate progresses, certain behaviors may indicate that the newborn may be ready to advance to oral feeding. These include a strong, vigorous suck; coordination of sucking and swallowing; sucking in response to the gavage tube; and wakefulness before feedings. The newborn may be challenged with oral feedings gradually, slowly increasing in frequency and amount. If the newborn is expending too much energy on the work of feeding, the result could be a weight loss instead of steady gain. Special "preemie" soft nipples are available to facilitate the sucking process. The nurse performs a thorough abdominal assessment of the newborn's tolerance to the feeding challenge and for development of complications, such as NEC. Feeding intolerance and NEC are identified by large gastric residuals, emesis, abdominal distension, and blood or reducing substances in the stool (Hill et al., 1993). See Chapter 30 for further details regarding oral nutrition for the neonate.

Total Parenteral Nutrition. Previously termed *hyperalimentation,* TPN is an aseptically prepared, nutritionally complete, hypertonic solution composed of protein, carbohydrates, electrolytes, vitamins, and minerals. When oral feedings must be delayed, even for only 2 to 3 days, TPN has been able to provide adequate nutrition to the neonate (Table 41-4). TPN is indicated for use in newborns with abdominal surgical defects, preterm or chronically ill newborns who are not tolerating other feedings, newborns with severe diarrhea, and newborns receiving ECMO (Fletcher, 1994).

(*text continues on page 1144*)

PROCEDURE 41–3
Gavage Feeding

Overall Objective: To provide adequate nutrition to neonates with inadequate feeding reflexes

Nursing Action	*Rationale*
Check chart for correct feeding type and amount. Wash hands.	Checking the chart confirms correct amount and type of feeding
Obtain equipment: 20 syringe and 5F or 8F feeding tube, depending on size of neonate.	Obtaining the equipment promotes smooth procedure minimizing possible interruptions that may interfere with neonates status.
Obtain formula or breast milk.	
Elevate head of bed 30 degrees. Place neonate on right side or prone. Bundle, hold, or have parents hold newborn after tube is inserted.	Elevation prevents reflux and promotes stomach emptying.
	This promotes neonate comfort, bonding, and parent confidence.
Measure catheter length for insertion from mouth to earlobe, then xiphoid process; mark the point with tape.	Measuring ensures accurate placement in stomach by approximating distance.

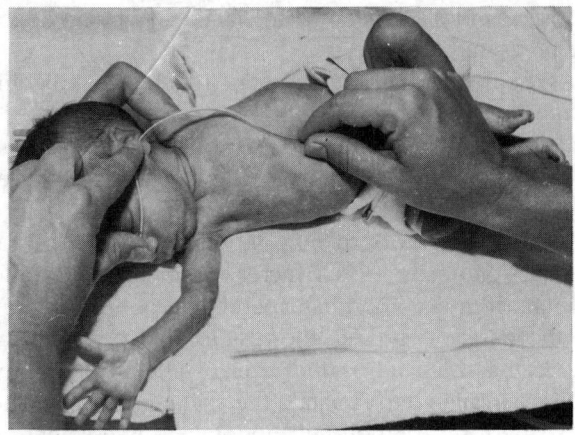

Measurement for gavage feeding.

Dip catheter in sterile water and insert through mouth to marked point. In some cases, the nose also may be used.	Water provides lubrication.
	Signs of distress indicate improper placement into trachea.
Remove catheter immediately if cyanosis, coughing, apnea, or bradycardia occur	Vagus nerve stimulation can cause bradycardia.
Determine accurate placement by attaching syringe and injecting 0.5 to 1 mL of air and auscultating over stomach area. Withdraw air.	Listening to air injection is one method to determine correct placement.
	Withdrawing air prevents regurgitation and abdominal distention.
Aspirate stomach contents, and note amount, color, and consistency. Report abnormalities.	This provides additional means for confirming placement; excess residuals indicate intolerance to feedings.
	Color abnormalities of brown-, red-, or green-tinged residuals may indicate gastrointestinal disease.

(continued)

PROCEDURE 41–3 (Continued)
Gavage Feeding

Nursing Action   *Rationale*

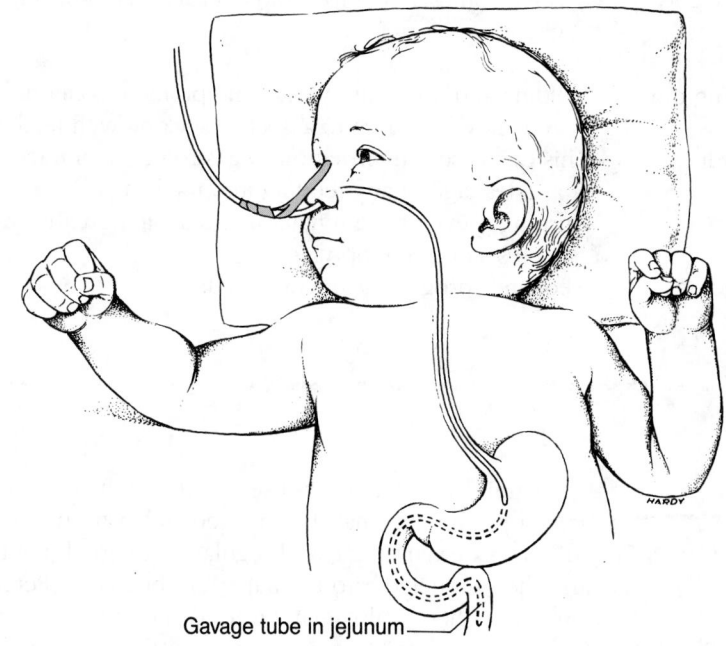

Gavage tube in jejunum

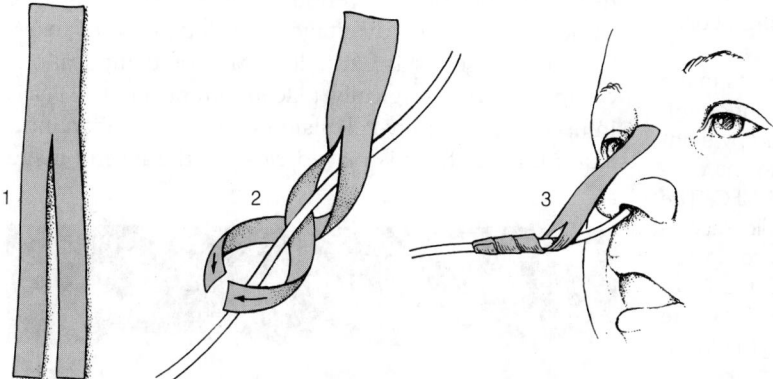

Gavage feeding.

Nursing Action	Rationale
Inject aspirate back into stomach. Subtract residual amount from total amount of feeding and feed the remaining amount.	Electrolyte imbalance and overdistension are prevented.
Tape tube in place.	Taping secures tube and reduces risky possible movement of tube into trachea.
Remove plunger from syringe, and pour feeding into syringe.	Trauma to stomach lining and overdistension are avoided.
Allow feeding to flow slowly into tube.	
If feeding does not flow, reinsert plunger to get it started, but do not push entire feeding into tube.	

(continued)

PROCEDURE 41–3 *(Continued)*
Gavage Feeding

Nursing Action	Rationale
Raise or lower the syringe to control the flow by gravity.	Syringe controls flow to avoid overdistension or regurgitation.
Give feeding over 15–30 min.	
Hold newborn, and provide non-nutritive sucking during feeding.	Holding and non-nutritive sucking promote comfort and allow newborn to associate sucking with feeding.
On completion of feeding, pinch tube and withdraw quickly.	This decreases any irritation to gastrointestinal tract and leakage of any feeding into trachea.
Burp neonate and place on right side or prone with head of bed up.	Burping prevents regurgitation and aspiration and promotes stomach emptying.
Document time, amount of feeding, type of feeding, characteristics and amount of residuals, tolerance to feeding.	Neonate's progress is documented.

RESEARCH HIGHLIGHT

Non-nutritive Sucking and Necrotizing Enterocolitis

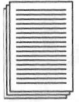

This study investigated the potential protective effect of non-nutritive sucking (NNS) against the development of necrotizing enterocolitis (NEC).

To conduct this study, a chart review was made of 12 preterm newborns who had been studied longitudinally on the effects of NNS on energy expenditure, weight gain, and feeding readiness. The six newborns in the control group who did not receive NNS developed NEC. The six newborns in the experimental group who did receive NNS did not develop NEC. The two groups were compared using clinical correlates that are linked to NEC. Clinical correlates used included race, gender, birth weight, 5-minute Apgar, maternal bleeding, maternal age, and length of ruptured membranes. For newborns who developed NEC, the number of clinical correlates ranged from one to four. For newborns who received NNS, the range of clinical correlates ranged from one to five. Because the sample size was so small, further research is necessary to examine the possible protective effect of NNS against NEC. Nursing implications include providing NNS during gavage feedings and during periods of stress for all neonates. NNS helps to promote gastric motility and the release of digestive enzymes and hormones. In addition, nurses need to minimize stress and carefully monitor newborns' physiologic responses to procedures.

Critique: Prospective studies are needed with larger sample sizes to investigate the effect of NNS on gastric motility and secretion of hormones and enzymes necessary for digestion.

(Pickler, R. H., & Terrell, B. V. [1994]. Non-nutritive sucking and necrotizing enterocolitis. *Neonatal Network, 13*[8], 15–17.)

Central venous catheters used for TPN infusion, such as a triple lumen, may be inserted into various sites, such as external or internal jugular or internal jugular and then tunneled into the superior vena cava. Percutaneous catheters also may be used (Fig. 41-9). Percutaneously inserted central venous catheters may be used for prolonged venous access. These Silastic catheters have the advantages of safety, ease of insertion, prolonged stay, and low rate of complications compared with surgically placed central lines. TPN is infused at a carefully calculated rate by way of an infusion pump. A filter is placed close to the insertion site

TABLE 41–4
Daily Requirements of Total Parenteral Nutrition

Protein	2.5–3.5 g/kg
Fat emulsion	2–4 g/kg
Calories	90–110 kcal/kg
H_2O	125–150 mL/kg or as needed
Na	3–4 mEq/kg
K	2–3 mEq/kg
Ca	50–100 mg/kg depending on size of newborn
P	1–1.5 mmol/kg
Mg	0.5–1 mEq/kg
Multivitamins* (MVI Pediatric)	10 mL (65% of dosage to newborns <3 kg; 30% to newborns <1 kg)

*Multivitamin preparations are undergoing scrutiny because of the preservatives in them. Practitioners must keep abreast of current recommendations.

(From Avery, G. B., & Fletcher, A. B. [1994]. Nutrition. In G. B. Avery (Ed.), *Neonatology* [3rd ed.]. Philadelphia: J.B. Lippincott.)

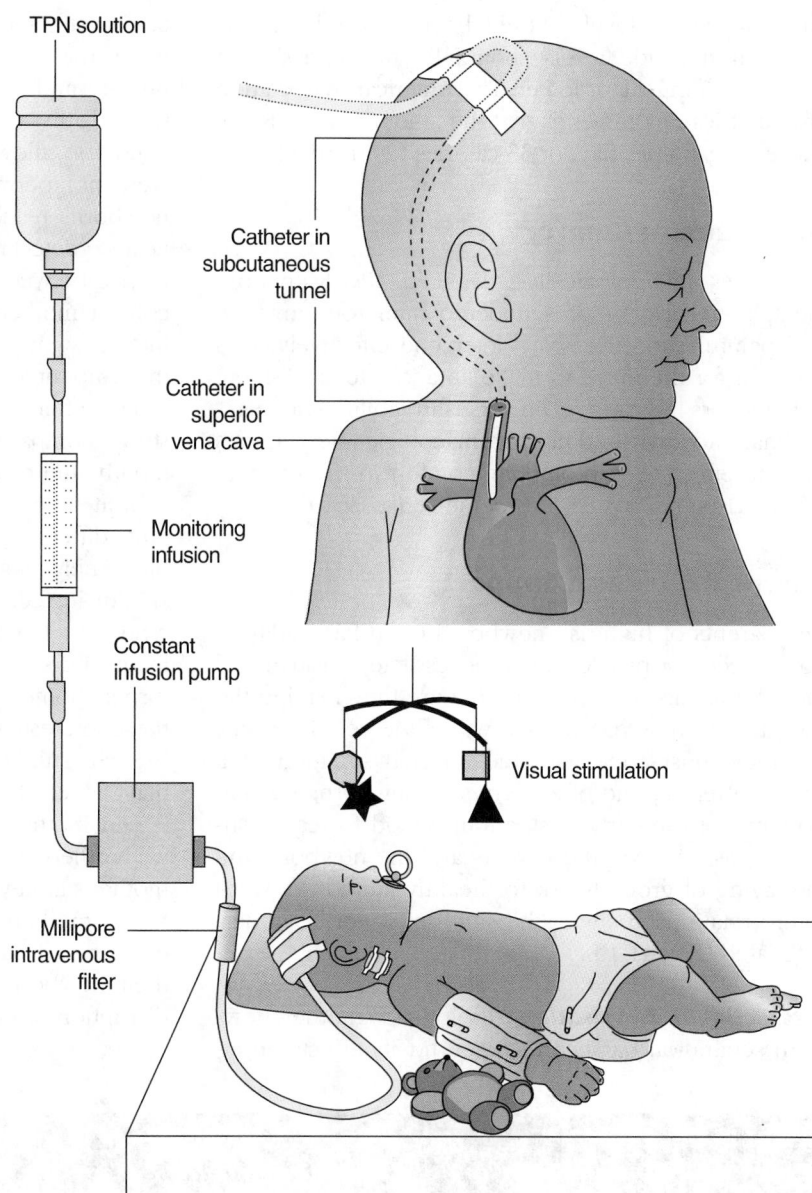

FIGURE 41–9 Total Parenteral Nutrition aseptically feeds the newborn through, in this case, the superior vena cava. The solution is infused at a carefully calculated rate by way of an infusion pump.

to help prevent infection. A sterile occlusive transparent dressing is placed securely over the insertion site. Neither medications nor blood should be given through the TPN line. If a triple-lumen catheter is used, the other parts can be accessed for administration of other IV fluids, medications, and blood.

Nursing care for the newborn receiving TPN involves monitoring the equipment, the infusion, and the newborn. The solution is prepared aseptically in the pharmacy and refrigerated until used. The solution container, tubing, and filter must be changed at least every 24 hours. The container label is carefully checked against the physician's order for correct ingredients and amounts. The insertion site is inspected carefully for any signs of infection. The insertion site dressing is changed at least three times a week using strict aseptic technique and following agency procedure. The infusion itself is maintained at the desired rate using an in-

fusion pump. Various parameters are measured, such as glucose levels, urine-specific gravity, sugar and acetone, intake and output, and daily weights. Blood studies, such as hemoglobin, hematocrit, electrolytes, and serum osmolarity, are done frequently to check electrolyte balance and needs. Numerous complications can occur, including catheter-related complications and metabolic complications. The newborn's non-nutritive sucking needs may be satisfied by a pacifier.

Newborns on TPN alone develop fatty acid deficiencies rapidly. Intralipid, a **fat emulsion,** is a Swedish soybean oil-egg emulsion designed to deliver extra calories and lower glucose concentration in addition to TPN. Intralipid should be infused slowly (preferably for 12–24 hours) in a line separate from other IV solutions but may be run in the same line through a Y connector or close to the insertion site. Serum is checked for turbidity daily to ensure fat clearance. Serum fatty acids and triglyceride levels should be monitored weekly. Serum triglyceride levels should be maintained at a level of 150 mg/dL or lower. The American Association of Pediatrics recommends that the amount of lipids not exceed 3 g/kg per day, or 33 calories (Sterk, 1983).

Alteration in Comfort

In today's technologically advanced NICU environment, preterm newborns undergo numerous invasive and painful procedures. To intervene effectively, it is essential for the nurse to make an accurate assessment of behaviors indicating pain versus irritability (Table 41-5). Pharmacologic and nonpharmacologic interventions may be effective in promoting comfort in the neonate (Table 41-6 and Box 41-5; Broome et al., 1990).

Parental Care and Support

The parents of high-risk newborns often have adaptational needs or problems that necessitate sensitive and thoughtful nursing care. Not only are they making the transition to new parenthood with all its requirements, but they must cope with the unusual situation of a small, different, and often very sick newborn. The importance of the early postpartum period for establishing bonds between the parents and the newborn and the laying of groundwork for healthy attitudes toward future relationships with the child must not be underestimated (Fig. 41-10).

Interactional Deprivation. Prolonged mother–newborn separation has been studied for its effects on attachment. As soon as possible after the birth, the mothers in the early contact group were admitted into the nursery and encouraged to touch their newborns and to perform such caretaking duties as the newborn's condition allowed. Mothers in the late contact group were not permitted into the nursery until after their newborns reached almost 1 month of age. Results revealed detectable differences in mothering performance between these two groups. In one study, high contact mothers had higher scores on an attachment interview, maternal performance, *en face* feeding, and the amount of fondling of newborns when tested 1 month after delivery (Klaus et al., 1972). In another study comparing late and early contact mothers 1 month after discharge of the infants and after 200 feedings at home, the late contact mothers held their infants differently and changed their positions less, bubbled their infants less frequently, and were not as skillful in feeding (Klaus et al., 1970). Some mothers who were barred from interaction with their newborns in the nursery resumed prior interests when they returned home. The infants then had to compete with these interests when they were discharged.

Such studies suggest that prolonged separation may adversely affect commitment or attachment between mother and newborn, may reduce confidence in mothering abilities, and may interfere with the mother's ability to develop an efficient routine of care. When mothers were allowed into the high-risk nursery for early and frequent contact and caretaking of their newborns, no increase in nursery infections or disruption of nursery routine was found (Barnett et al., 1970).

TABLE 41–5
Pain and Agitation Behaviors of Premature Neonates

Mode of Expression	Pain Behaviors	Irritable Behaviors
Verbal	Crying, often sudden and loud	Whining cry
Nonverbal	Decreased activity	Frown
	Grimace	Flailing of extremities
	Flexing extremities	Random movements of head and body
	Tensing muscles	Rigid posture
	Rigid posture	Altered feeding patterns
	Flushed face	
	Decreased period of alertness (withdrawal)	
Physiologic	Sudden heart rate increase, up to 40% (may follow temporary initial decrease)	Heart rate and blood pressure increase only with activity
	Blood pressure increase	No diaphoresis
	Duskiness	No color changes unless prolonged
	Oxygen saturation decrease	No oxygen saturation decrease unless prolonged

(Broome, M. E., & Tanzillo, H. [1990]. Differentiating between pain and agitation in premature neonates. *Journal of Perinatal and Neonatal Nursing, 4*[1], 55.)

TABLE 41–6
Pharmacologic Management of Neonatal Pain and Restlessness

Drug	Dose	Route	Frequency	Comments	Side Effects
ANALGESIC					
Morphine	15 µg/kg per hour	IV	Continuous infusion without loading dose	Inexpensive, well studied, very effective	Dose-related respiratory depression and sedation; decreased intestinal motility
Fentanyl	2–4 µg/kg	IV	Every 1–2 h, given over minimum of 2 min	Monitor plasma levels if given frequently; particularly useful for short procedures	
ANESTHETIC					
Lidocaine (for use during painful procedures)	0.2–0.8 mL	Intradermal	2–3 min prior to procedure		Hypotension, restlessness uncommon
SEDATION					
Chloral hydrate	6–8 mg/kg	po			Nausea, increased peristalsis, paradoxic excitement

IV = intravenous; po = per os (by mouth).
(Broome, M. E., & Tanzillo, H. [1990]. Differentiating between pain and agitation in premature neonates. *Journal of Perinatal and Neonatal Nursing, 4*[1], 57.)

BOX 41–5
Nonpharmacologic Management of Neonatal Pain and Irritability

Pain
Swaddling or containment during procedure
Alternative distraction: music, light, conversation
Pacifier during and after procedure
Calming before and after procedure
Tactile stimulation
Rocking

Irritability
Swaddling
Decreased light and noise
Decreased handling; increased rest periods between procedures
Rhythmic activities; stroking, patting
Vestibular stimulation: upright positioning

(Broome, M. E., & Tanzillo, H. [1990]. Differentiating between pain and agitation in premature neonates. Journal of Perinatal Neonatal Nursing, 4[1], 59.)

Modifying hospital routine to allow mothers early contact with their high-risk newborns appears to have a positive effect on later maternal behavior. This lends support to the concept of a sensitive time for bonding to occur between the mother and her newborn. This time is probably within the first several hours of delivery. Greater maternal attentiveness and better caretaking seem related to later exploratory behavior in infants; thus, removing barriers to maternal attachment during the sensitive period may have a potent influence on the later development of these newborns. It may be most helpful for the father to nurture the mother so that the mother may nuture the neonate (Weingarten et al., 1990).

Parental Reactions and Psychological Tasks. The birth of a high-risk newborn is often experienced as an acute emotional crisis by the family. This causes a certain amount of disorganization in the parents before they are able to master their feelings and accept the event. Because the newborn may be born before term, parents are often deprived of the last 6 to 8 weeks in which the final psychological (and sometimes material) preparation for the birth is made (Box 41-6).

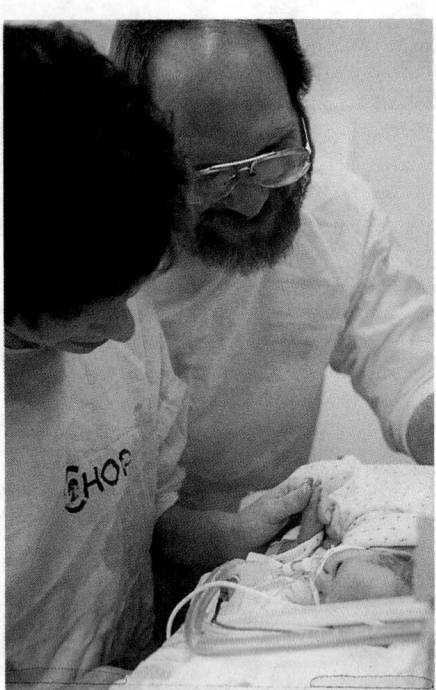

FIGURE 41–10 Parents should be encouraged to establish bonds with their high-risk newborn in the early postpartum period.

The nurse's first action is to assess the parents' reactions to the high-risk birth, based on the knowledge that certain behaviors may be anticipated. The nurse assists the parents to work through the grieving process by allowing expression of feelings, facilitating communication with healthcare team members, and providing support, information, and referrals as needed. Parents are encouraged to visit and telephone at any time, whether the newborn receives care at the birth medical center or transported to a tertiary care facility. If the the newborn is transported to a tertiary care center, the parents need to be informed of the circumstances and encouraged to see and touch the newborn before transport occurs. It is helpful for the parents to be given a snapshot of the newborn. Some nurseries have developed a pamphlet describing the unit. It is beneficial to try to transport both mother and newborn to the same medical center if possible (Fig. 41-11).

The father may often be the first parent to visit the neonatal unit and assume the role of communicator to the mother if the mother is not housed at the transport hospital or her physical condition does not permit her to visit immediately. The father's visit may be overwhelming at first, although the nurse may have tried to prepare him in advance. It is best simply to explain the equipment and its functions and then allow the father to ask questions. The nurse may encourage him to touch the newborn and begin the attachment process at a tolerable pace. The mother's first visit can be handled in a similar fashion. If she plans to breast-feed, she should be taught how to express and save her milk. This is a positive act that can definitely enhance the mother–newborn relationship.

As visits continue, parents may be encouraged to bring small objects from homes, such as toys and clothes. Siblings and other relatives may be allowed to visit, depending on unit policy. Given the proper guidelines and precautions, infection control should not be a problem. As time goes by, specific caretaking tasks may be assumed by the parents under the nurse's supervision. This will prepare the parents gradually for discharge, greatly enhance their self-confidence, and promote attachment. Any pamphlets that will help stress important information are always appreciated. If the tertiary care center is far from the parents' home, a return transport may be offered and may be acceptable to the parents (Klaus et al., 1992). A return transport sends the neonate back to the hospital of birth. Other interventions that may be explored are rooming in within the nursery, nesting in a private room with mother and newborn, referral to parent support groups, kangaroo care, and early discharge programs. Nesting occurs when the mother cares for the neonate by herself in a private room, with ongoing consultations with nurses. Kangaroo care is holding the neonate with skin-to-skin contact for periods of time. Ongoing community-based home care support is essential to provide assessment of the neonate's status and support the caregiver's positive interventions.

Evaluation

The nursing process in high-risk neonatal care is challenging, stressful, and rewarding. This highly specialized area seeks to intervene successfully for the critically ill neonate.

Possible anticipated outcomes include the following:

■ Then neonate maintains an adequate core temperature.

BOX 41–6
Psychological Processes of Parents After Birth of a High-Risk Newborn

Shock, disbelief, and denial
Anger and searching self and others for causes
Grieving over loss of fantasized perfect newborn
Grieving over own inability to produce perfect newborn
Anticipatory worrying over loss of newborn
Initiation of contact with newborn
Belief and desire that newborn will live
Readiness to establish caretaking relationship

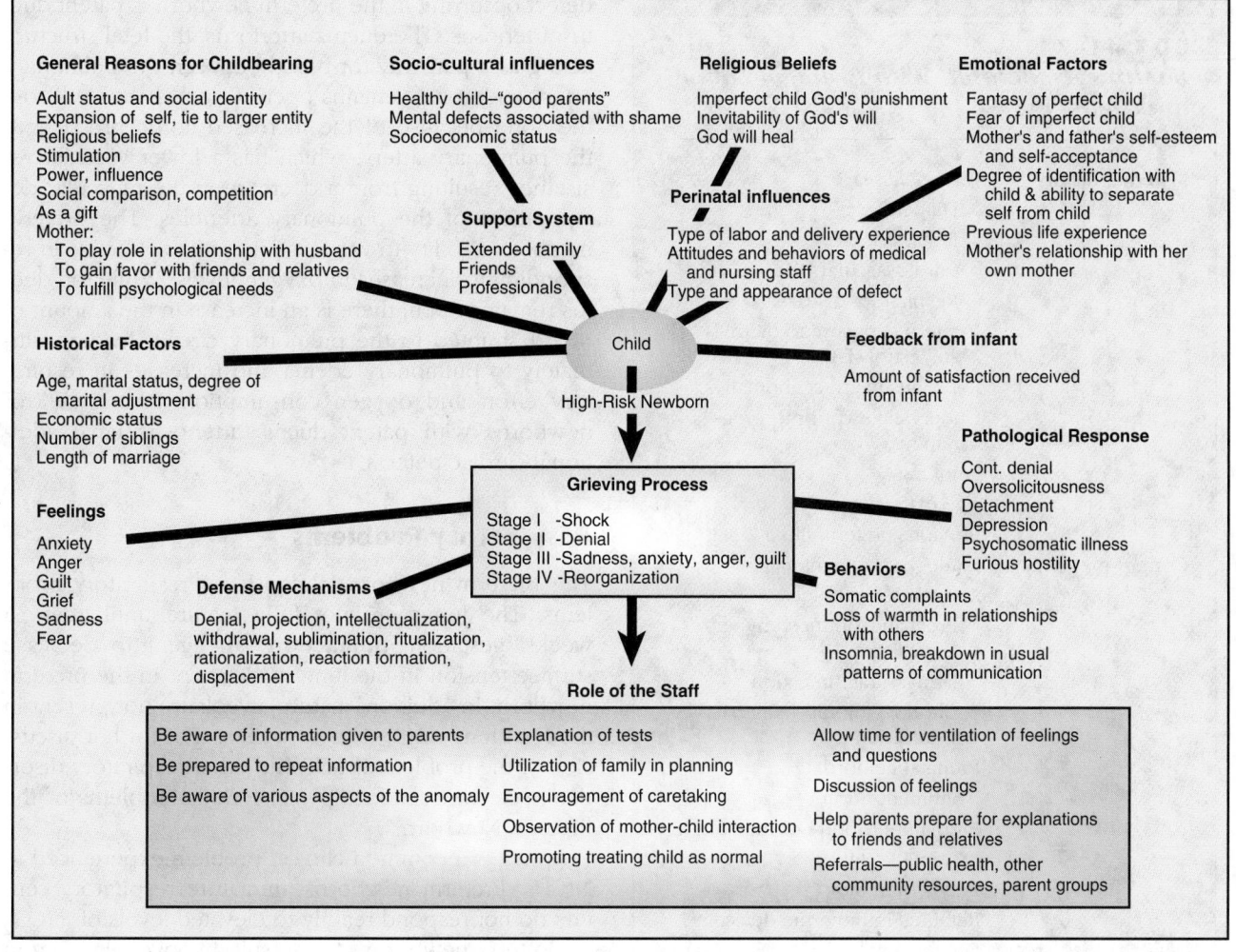

FIGURE 41-11 Parental response to the high-risk newborn.

- The neonate's cardiopulmonary status demonstrates improvement or remains within acceptable limits.
- The neonate tolerates feedings and gains adequate weight.
- The neonate remains free of skin breakdown.
- The neonate remains free of complications.
- The neonate remains free of apneic periods.
- The parents demonstrate positive coping abilities in response to the neonate's condition.
- The parents demonstrate adequate knowledge about the neonate's condition and necessary care activities.
- The parents demonstrate appropriate knowledge and skills to care for the neonate at home.
- The neonate is discharged home with little or no functional impairment.
- The neonate is assisted to a peaceful and dignified death.

The many technical aspects are beyond the scope of this text, and the reader is referred to one of the many texts on the subject of neonatal intensive care.

Preterm Newborns

Preterm newborns are born before the 37th week of gestation, regardless of birth weight. The main criterion is gestational age. Most babies who weigh less than 2,500 g at birth are premature, as are almost all those weighing less than 1,500 g. However, not all newborns weighing less than 2,500 g are necessarily premature. Most of these preterm newborns are appropriate for gestational age, but some are SGA. A number of factors are associated with preterm labor and delivery (Box 41-7). For a further discussion on preterm labor, see Chapter 36.

As neonatal technology advances, the survival of newborns of very low birth weight has improved yearly. Very low birth weight neonates weighing as little as 600 g commonly survive in the 1990s. The focus of care is moving toward intact survival for these neonates. More low birth weight neonates require ongoing multidisciplinary management and home care. Assessment and planning for discharge begin with the

BOX 41-7
Factors Associated With Preterm Labor and Delivery

Maternal history	Chronic disease
	Diabetes
	Renal disease
	Cardiovascular disease
	Respiratory disease
	In utero exposure to diethyl-stilbestrol (DES)
	Reproductive tract anomalies
	Underweight (prior to pregnancy)
	Smoking
	Age extremes (<18, >40)
	Previous preterm labor
Current pregnancy	Inadequate weight gain
	Acute maternal illness
	Pregnancy-induced hypertension
	Urinary tract infection
	Chorioamnionitis, vaginal infection
	Prenatal hemorrhage
	Isoimmunization
	Premature rupture of membranes
	Multiple gestation
	Polyhydramnios
	Retained intrauterine device
Fetal factors	Fetal anomalies
	Intrauterine fetal demise
	Infection

(Bartram, J., & Clewell, W. H. [1989]. Prenatal environment: Impact on neonatal outcome. In G. B. Merenstein & S. L. Gardner [Eds.], Handbook of neonatal intensive care [p. 42] [2nd ed.]. St. Louis: C.V. Mosby.)

parents' first bedside visit (see Nursing Care Plan: Preterm Infant and Family).

Physiologic Problems

The preterm newborn is at risk because of the immature organ systems and lack of adequate reserves. These newborns lack the adequate growth and development necessary for a smooth adaptation to extrauterine life, placing them at a distinct disadvantage for optimal health and survival. Various physiologic problems are a direct result.

Cardiovascular Problems

Changes in fetal circulation that occur at birth are covered in Chapter 7. The most common cardiovascular defect occurring in the preterm newborn is patent ductus arteriosus. The ductus arteriosus, the fetal structure acting as a pathway for blood between the pulmonary artery and aorta, remains open. Blood is shunted from the aorta because of the increased aortic pressure to the pulmonary artery, which has a lower vascular resistance resulting from a decrease in the muscular development of the pulmonary arterioles. The preterm newborn's ability to vasoconstrict is less effective in responding to increases in oxygen levels. While the ductus remains open, there is an increase in the amount of blood shunted to the pulmonary circuit, leading ultimately to pulmonary edema and increases in respiratory effort and oxygen consumption. About 15% of newborns with patent ductus arteriosus have additional cardiac defects.

Respiratory Problems

The preterm newborn is at risk for respiratory problems. The lungs are not fully mature until after 35 weeks' gestation. **Surfactant,** an agent to decrease surface tension in the lung, is deficient in the preterm newborn. In addition, mature alveoli are not present in the fetal lung until 34 to 36 weeks. (For further discussion of the problem of RDS and other respiratory disorders, see the section "Special Health Problems of the Preterm Newborn.")

Apnea is a common clinical problem experienced in NICUs. Preterm newborns' immature respiratory centers do not respond readily to elevated levels of $PaCO_2$ as do term newborns. As a result, hypoventilation and hypercapnia occur. Patterns of periodic breathing in the preterm newborn (pauses of 5–10 seconds) have been reported frequently. However, true apneic episodes last for 10 to 15 seconds and are accompanied by pallor, cyanosis, hypotonia, and bradycardia. Repeated apneic episodes occur most often in preterm newborns weighing less than 1,000 g. This problem represents immaturity of the respiratory control systems in the brain. Apneic episodes in the neonate, which must be treated promptly if possible, may be precipitated by the following disorders:

1. Temperature instability
2. Central nervous system problems
3. Drugs (maternal or fetal)
4. Infection
5. Metabolic disorders
6. Neonatal asphyxia
7. Abdominal distention

All newborns at risk should be placed on an apnea monitor for the first 2 weeks of life. The use of tactile stimulation and repositioning to avoid pharyngeal obstruction by hyperflexion of the neck has been helpful in managing and preventing apneic episodes. Other management techniques include low nasal CPAP at 3

NURSING CARE PLAN
Preterm Infant and Family

Nursing Goals

1. Infant breathes normally or at ease with ventilator assistance, without evidence of respiratory distress.
2. Noninvasive monitoring indicates adequate oxygenation.
3. Infant maintains normal fluid/electrolyte balance.
4. Infant loses minimal birth weight and gains steadily.
5. Infant adjusts to method of feeding.
6. Infant maintains normal bowel movements.
7. Infant maintains healthy, intact skin.
8. Infant does not experience cold stress.
9. Infant maintains stable temperature.
10. Infant remains or becomes infection free.
11. Infant demonstrates level of comfort.
12. Parents indicate knowledge and skill by performing caretaking tasks.
13. Parents voice confidence in caring for the infant.
14. Parents follow through on referrals.

Assessment	Potential Nursing Diagnoses	Intervention/ Rationale	Evaluation
Maternal Factors			
Placenta previa Abruptio placentae Hypertensive disease of pregnancy Cervical incompetence Premature rupture of membranes Uterine anomalies Infections Previous preterm delivery	Impaired Gas Exchange related to lack of surfactant	Observe, record, and report signs and symptoms of respiratory distress Tachypnea Cyanosis Retractions Grunting Nasal flaring Diminished breath sounds Suction *to maintain open airway* Administer oxygen along with appropriate monitoring of blood gases *to maintain adequate oxygenation* Monitor ventilator function and settings *to maintain adequate ventilation* Change position frequently; use chest physical therapy *to mobilize secretions* Maintain intravenous lines and monitor closely for any infiltration *to maintain fluid and electrolyte balance*	Infant breathes normally or at ease with ventilator without evidence of respiratory distress Infant maintains normal fluid and electrolyte balance
Fetal Factors			
Multiple gestation Infections	Fluid Volume Deficit related to insensible water loss and inadequate fluid intake	Administer correct fluid and correct amount per hour *to maintain fluid and electrolyte balance*	Infant loses minimal birth weight and gains steadily

(continued)

NURSING CARE PLAN *(Continued)*
Preterm Infant and Family

Assessment	Potential Nursing Diagnoses	Intervention/ Rationale	Evaluation
		Total intake per shift and daily *to monitor intake*	
		Observe for signs of dehydration *to maintain fluid balance*	
		Check skin turgor	
		Check urine output	
		Check mucous membranes	
		Check character of fontanel	
		Monitor color, odor, specific gravity, Clinitest, and amount of urine *to detect changes in output*	
		Weigh daily at approximately the same time *to detect fluid losses*	
		Use heat shields or plastic sheeting with radiant warmers *to maintain neutral thermal environment*	
	Altered Nutrition: Less than body requirements related to actual intake less than caloric requirements	Provide adequate calorie intake with most efficient method according to individual needs	Infant adjusts to method of feeding
		Nipple	Infant maintains normal bowel movements
		Breast	
		Gavage	
		Nasojejunal	
		Gastrostomy	
		Measure abdominal girth as needed *to monitor distention*	
		Measure residuals and replace *to maintain electrolyte balance*	
		Allow parents to participate in feeding plan *to provide caregiving time*	
		Observe stool patterns closely and report any abnormalities *to monitor output closely*	
	Impaired Skin Integrity related to tapes and other abrasive materials used with monitoring devices	Place as little tape as possible on skin *to maintain skin integrity*	Infant maintains healthy, intact skin
		Use OpSite for other skin devices *to avoid skin abrasion*	
		Keep any lotions having direct skin contact to a minimum *to avoid absorption of lotion*	

(continued)

NURSING CARE PLAN *(Continued)*
Preterm Infant and Family

Assessment	Potential Nursing Diagnoses	Intervention/ Rationale	Evaluation
		Place infant on water bed or sheepskin *to avoid pressure on skin*	
		Turn and reposition frequently *to avoid skin pressure*	
	Risk for Injury (cold stress) related to immature temperature-regulating mechanism	Maintain neutral thermal environment *to avoid cold stress*	Infant does not experience cold stress
		Monitor skin temperature by probe method	Infant maintains stable temperature
		Frequently check temperature of heating unit *to maintain neutral thermal environment*	
		Avoid subjecting infant to heat losses by evaporation, convection, conduction, and radiation *to avoid cold stress*	
	Risk for Infection related to immature immune system	See Care Plan for infection, Chap. 43	Infant remains or becomes infection free
	Anticipatory Grieving of parents related to loss of perfect infant	See Care Plan for grieving family, Chap. 42	
	Parental Knowledge Deficit related to care of the preterm infant	Give parents adequate and realistic information regarding infant's condition *to decrease anxiety*	Parents indicate knowledge and skill by performing caretaking tasks
		Encourage parents to perform many caretaking tasks *to promote confidence*	Parents voice confidence in caring for the infant
		Refer to home healthcare, social services, parental support group *as needed*	Parents follow through on referrals
Numerous invasive painful procedures Crying Grimace Rigid posture Heart rate and blood pressure increase Oxygen saturation decrease	Alteration in Comfort related to invasive, painful procedures	Administration of pain medications *to promote comfort* Swaddle Use of pacifier Tactile stimulation Rocking *to promote comfort and soothe*	Infant exhibits absence of painful behaviors and demonstrates comfort level

to 5 cm H_2O, water beds, and respiratory stimulants, such as theophylline or caffeine (Klaus et al., 1993).

Gastrointestinal Problems

Maturity of the GI tract is established by 36 to 38 weeks' gestation. Therefore, the preterm newborn's GI tract may not be as functional as the term newborn's GI tract.

The preterm newborn is subject to the following factors, which may interfere with mature GI functioning:

- Uncoordinated sucking and swallowing until 34 to 35 weeks
- Incompetent cardiac sphincter
- Delayed gastric emptying time
- Decreased absorption of fat
- Incomplete digestion of protein

■ Decreased or uncoordinated motility (Bucuvalas et al., 1992)

Central Nervous System Problems

The stage of development of the nervous system at birth depends on the degree of maturity. The fetus has a majority of neurons by 18 to 20 weeks' gestation. The basement membrane of brain capillaries is of minimum thickness compared with the adult brain. This phenomenon may be one factor predisposing the preterm newborn to subependymal hemorrhage and IVH. Reflexes, such as Moro and tonic neck, are present in the preterm newborn.

Sleep–wake cycles are difficult to evaluate in the preterm newborn. Preterm newborns experience more quiet sleep, less active sleep, and higher pO_2 levels in the prone position. More quiet sleep is experienced in a neutral thermal environment.

Additional problems are related to the degree of nervous system maturation based on the number of weeks' gestation. Little facial expression is noted before 30 to 32 weeks' gestation. Little spontaneous crying occurs before 30 to 32 weeks. From this time on, hunger is expressed by crying. Rhythmic, non-nutritive sucking is noted only after 33 weeks' gestation. The auditory system functions from 26 weeks' gestation. Consistent auditory responses are noted at 32 to 34 weeks. A gradual increase in muscle tone is noted with increasing gestational age. As muscle tone increases, the extremities gradually assume a flexed position. This posturing and flexible nature of the extremities represent a part of the gestational age assessment scoring. By 36 weeks, muscle movements become more coordinated (Hack, 1992).

Renal Problems

In the preterm newborn, the kidneys and related urinary structures have immature properties. The kidneys do not concentrate urine well or excrete large amounts of fluid. Further, drug excretion takes longer. Glomerular filtration rate efficiency parallels gestational age. The buffering capacity of the kidneys is low, with decreased excretion of bicarbonate and acid, predisposing the neonate to acidosis (Spitzer, 1992).

Hepatic Problems

The preterm newborn's immature liver presents serious problems during the immediate neonatal period. In the preterm newborn, bilirubin levels rise more rapidly than in the term newborn because of the liver's inability to process bilirubin. Hypoglycemia in the preterm neonate may be due to low liver glycogen stores. Lower serum protein levels, deficiency of blood-clotting factors, and deficient conjugation and detoxification of certain drugs are all attributed to liver immaturity.

Immunologic Problems

Of the five major immunoglobulins (Ig), only IgM is produced by the newborn. IgG does not cross the placenta in significant amounts until 34 weeks' gestation, thus putting the preterm newborn in jeopardy. IgA is found in breast milk (Fuller, 1992).

Integumentary Problems

The skin of the preterm newborn is thin, transparent, and covered with abundant vernix. There is a high rate of insensible water loss, especially with newborns of less than 30 weeks' gestation. Further, the preterm newborn's skin absorbs chemicals readily, so precautions must be taken with topical ointments and solutions covering the skin. Finally, the skin is extremely vulnerable to damage from adhesive materials, so care must be taken with the amount and kind of adhesive used with monitors and other items placed on the skin. The use of tape on the skin should be avoided whenever possible, because its removal can easily damage the vulnerable epidermis.

Bathing should be minimized because it destroys the acid pH mantle of the skin. Bony prominences should be protected by frequent turning, sheepskin, water beds, and semipermeable membrane dressings, such as Opsite or Tegaderm (Loisel et al., 1994).

Temperature Problems

The preterm newborn has difficulty regulating body temperature. The following factors foster temperature regulation problems in the preterm newborn:

■ Decreased fat insulation
■ Reduced brown fat stores
■ Large surface area to weight ratio
■ Inadequate calorie intake
■ Extended posture of extremities
■ Ineffective ability to increase oxygen consumption
■ Immature thermal regulatory abilities
■ Increased insensible fluid loss
■ Increased body water content (Thomas, 1994)

The American Academy of Pediatrics and the American College of Obstetrics and Gynecology recommend rectal and axillary temperatures to be 36.5° to 37.5°C (97.7°–99.5°F) and abdominal skin temperatures to be 36° to 36.5°C (96.8°–97.7°F; Thomas, 1994).

Special Health Problems of the Preterm Newborn

The preterm newborn is at risk for special health problems that are a direct result of the immaturity of body systems and lack of reserve. These health problems require prompt assessment and treatment to improve the newborn's possibility of survival. However, even with survival, economic, emotional, and long-term effects are associated with the treatments and care necessary.

Respiratory Distress Syndrome

Previously known as hyaline membrane disease, **respiratory distress syndrome** type I is a developmental disease of preterm newborns who are appropriate for gestational age. By estimate, 20,000 to 30,000 newborns develop RDS each year in the United States. RDS is the most common cause of respiratory distress in neonates, almost exclusively occurring in the preterm newborn. Although advances in neonatal care have improved the prognosis of these newborns, RDS is still a leading cause of neonatal mortality.

Pathophysiology. Respiratory distress syndrome is a partial persistence of the fetal cardiopulmonary state. The disease is primarily a developmental disorder involving underdevelopment of the lungs, because the synthesis of surfactant in utero must have taken place for lung maturation to be complete, which occurs at about 35 weeks' gestation. Surfactant, a complex biochemical substance composed of phospholipids and proteins, exerts a detergent-like action over the inner surface of the alveoli, decreasing their tendency to collapse. With low surfactant production (by the type II alveolar cells), alveolar collapse, atelectasis, and decreased lung compliance occur. The combination of atelectasis and pulmonary hypoperfusion from vasospasm leads to hypoxia and hypercapnia. Prolonged hypoxia and hypercapnia result in metabolic and respiratory aci-

dotic states. Hypoxic and acidotic states aggravate vasospasm, which increases pulmonary hypoperfusion. Hypoxia and acidosis also cause destruction of capillaries and alveoli. Capillary damage and destruction of alveoli lead to an increase in surfactant deficiency. Right-to-left shunting of blood may persist at the foramen ovale and ductus arteriosus as a result of increased blood pressure in the pulmonary circuit. Blood is thus diverted from the lungs, enhancing their hypoperfusion.

Perinatal complications that may increase the incidence or severity of RDS include asphyxia, maternal diabetes, and possibly cesarean birth. RDS occurs more often in boys than girls and in the second of twins. Factors enhancing the production of surfactant and lung maturation include the stress of intrauterine infections, premature rupture of membranes, maternal hypertensive disorders, and maternal administration of glucocorticoids.

Clinical Manifestations. The neonate exhibits respiratory distress, usually within 4 hours after birth. Distress results from diminished lung compliance and atelectasis, significantly increasing the work of breathing. The Silverman score is an index for measuring observations indicating respiratory distress. The index reflects other diseases and those that are the result of respiratory compromise in the neonate. The major signs exhibited are cyanosis, tachypnea, retractions, grunting, nasal flaring, and see-saw respirations. Breath sounds are diminished (Fig. 41-12). Hypotension also may be present.

Laboratory Data. Arterial blood gas analysis shows hypoxia, hypercapnia, and respiratory or metabolic

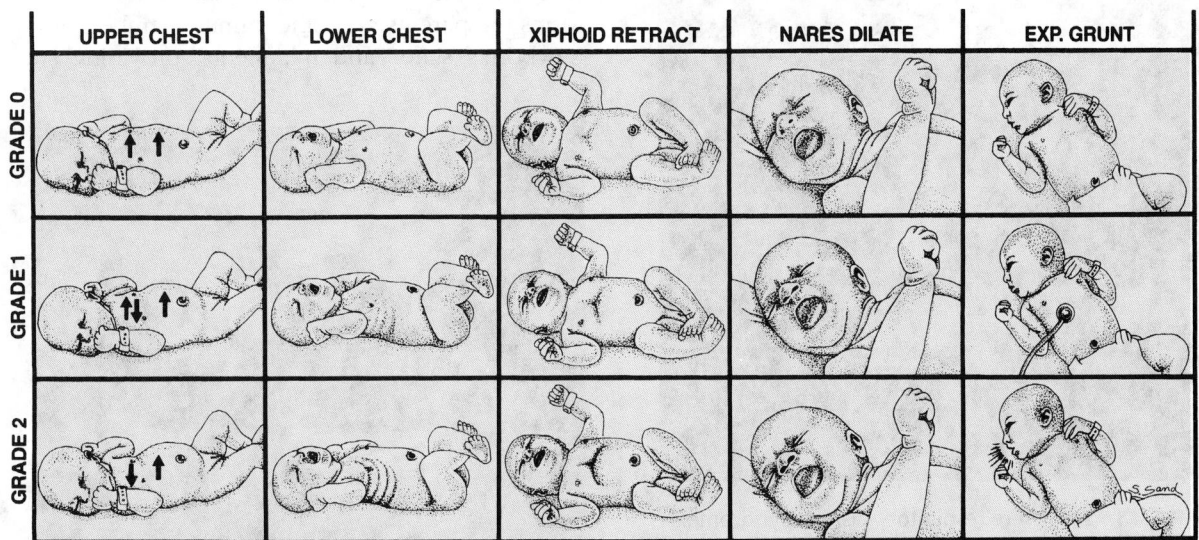

FIGURE 41–12 Observation of retractions using the Silverman score. An index of respiratory distress is determined by grading each of five arbitrary criteria. Grade 0 indicates no difficulty; grade 1 indicates moderate difficulty; and grade 2 indicates maximum respiratory difficulty. The retraction score is the sum of these values; a total score of 0 indicates no dyspnea, whereas a total score of 10 denotes maximal respiratory distress.

acidosis. The typical x-ray appearance shows a diffuse reticulogranular pattern over both lungs, peripheral air bronchograms, and loss of lung volume (Fig. 41-13).

Management and Prognosis.
Management is geared toward correcting hypoxia and acidosis, alleviating the work of breathing, and maintaining homeostasis. Measures include the administration of oxygen, assisted ventilation with continuous positive pressure, conventional mechanical ventilation, or high-frequency ventilation. The current use of synthetic surfactant as a treatment modality has been proven to decrease the morbidity and mortality in newborns with RDS.

Usually symptoms begin to lessen as surfactant production is established at about 48 to 72 hours of life. Gradual improvement is usually seen on day 3 of life. Preterm newborns with RDS may encounter complications of pneumothorax, pulmonary interstitial emphysema, BPD, retinopathy of prematurity, and IVH (Grobman et al., 1992).

Nursing Assessment.
By performing a gestational age assessment correctly, the nurse can ascertain quickly that the newborn is preterm and therefore at risk for RDS. Consequently, the nurse is alert for the clinical manifestation of respiratory distress, as previously described. The nurse also provides continuous respiratory assessment and observes for potential complications associated with RDS (Fig 41-14).

Nursing Diagnoses.
After completing the assessment, the nurse will be able to identify appropriate nursing diagnoses. For a list of possible nursing diagnoses, see Box 41-8.

Nursing Planning, Intervention, and Evaluation.
Nursing care goals for the neonate with RDS include recognizing and assessing the newborn at risk, stabilizing the critically ill newborn, preventing further complications, and providing support for the family in crisis. Nursing care priorities should focus primarily on the respiratory system and alleviation of the work of breathing. The nurse monitors the respiratory status of the newborn by physical assessment and the use of invasive and noninvasive measurements of oxygenation. The nurse administers oxygen and other respiratory medications as ordered, monitoring for therapeutic and adverse effects. Mechanical ventilation and associated care are important components of the plan. Nutritional status, fluids, and acid–base balance must be assessed frequently and corrected as needed. The nurse should be alert for potential complications associated with RDS and their clinical manifestations. The nurse informs the parents and other family members about the newborn's status and treatments, providing support,

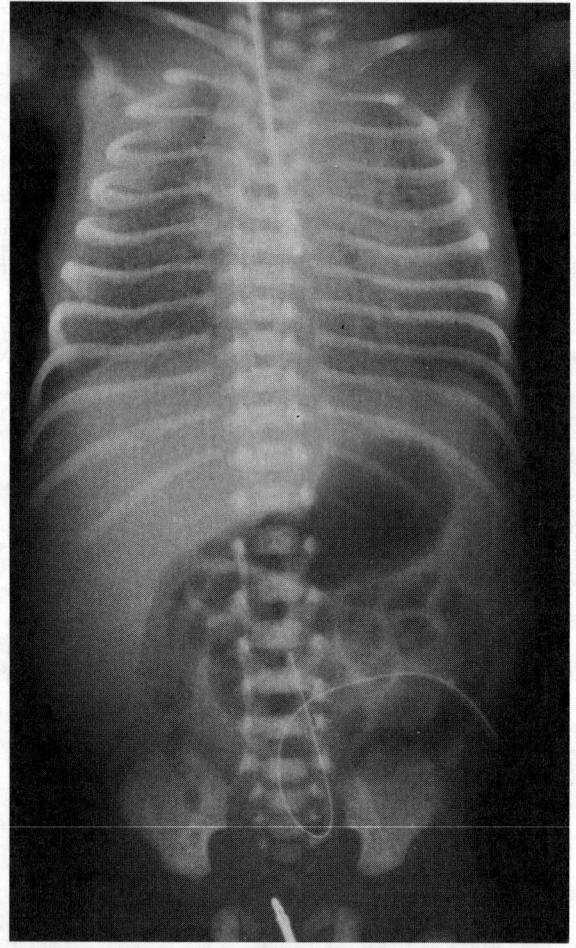

FIGURE 41–13 Severe respiratory distress syndrome. Note diffuse density of the lung fields compared with intestinal gas, with well-defined air brochograms. Both lungs are uniformly involved. An umbilical artery catheter lies at the aortic bifurcation (third lumbar vertebra). (Avery, G. B. [1987]. *Neonatology: Pathophysiology and management of the newborn* [3rd ed.]. Philadelphia: J.B. Lippincott.)

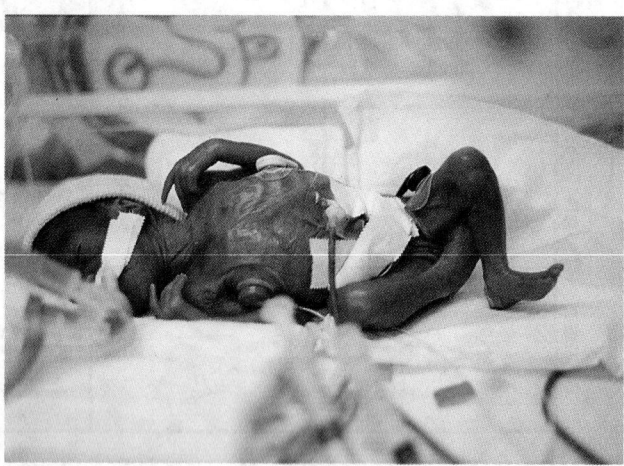

FIGURE 41–14 Note the substernal and intercostal retractions in this newborn with respiratory distress syndrome. Nasal continuous airway pressure is being used to treat the condition.

BOX 41-8
Nursing Diagnoses—
Respiratory Distress Syndrome

- Impaired Gas Exchange related to
  - Inadequate lung surfactant
  - Diminished alveolar perfusion
- Ineffective Airway Clearance related to increased secretions
- Altered Nutrition: Less than body requirements, related to
  - Caloric expenditure greater than intake
  - Treatments
- Activity Intolerance related to diminished pulmonary function
- Risk for Infection related to invasive treatment methods
- Risk for Altered Parent/Infant Attachment related to newborn's condition and treatments
- Knowledge Deficit related to newborn's condition, treatment, and possible complications
- Altered Family Processes related to interruption in parent–newborn attachment

and encouraging them to visit and provide caretaking. Further details regarding nursing interventions and evaluation are provided in the nursing care plan and in the section "Planning, Intervention, and Evaluation in High-Risk Neonatal Care."

Bronchopulmonary Dysplasia

Bronchopulmonary dysplasia is a significant chronic lung disorder in neonates. The etiology is multifactorial but most often is the result of pulmonary immaturity, surfactant deficiency, acute lung injury, oxygen toxicity, and barotrauma.

Current diagnostic criteria for BPD include the following:

- Requirement for intermittent positive pressure ventilation during the first week of life
- Respiratory distress continuing through 28 days of life
- Supplemental oxygen requirements for more than 28 days of life to keep $PaO_2 > 50$ mm Hg
- A characteristic chest x-ray finding of "persistent strands of increased density in both lungs, alternating with areas of unequal aeration" (Knoppert et al., 1994). Some researchers have proposed that changing the 28-day requirement to the expected date of delivery for the neonate may be more specific in terms of diagnosis.

Pathophysiology. With BPD, destructive inflammatory changes in the lung tissue are described as thickening and eventual destruction of alveolar walls, basement membrane, and bronchiolar epithelial lining layers. Fibrosis and atelectasis are present.

Clinical Manifestations. Clinical manifestations include respiratory distress, oxygen dependence, retractions, rales, CO_2 retention, respiratory acidosis, and potential congestive heart failure.

Prognosis. Although most newborns with BPD eventually achieve normal lung function, there is a high risk of mortality or complications during the first year of life. Complications include abnormal pulmonary function tests, reactive airway disease, and cardiac failure. Increased susceptibility to infection, especially respiratory syncytial virus, can lead to repeated hospitalizations and ventilator dependency. Newborns with BPD also are at risk for growth failure and developmental delays.

Nursing Assessment. The nurse performs a thorough respiratory assessment to determine the severity of respiratory distress. Ongoing invasive and noninvasive determinations of oxygen status are a priority because the newborn's status can change dramatically with the smallest change in oxygen therapy. The nurse assesses nutritional and fluid balance status on a regular basis. Evaluating the newborn's nutritional status is of primary concern, because malnutrition will delay development of new alveoli and predispose the newborn to infection. The nurse is alert for signs of sepsis and respiratory infection, which must be recognized as early as possible to initiate treatment.

Nursing Diagnosis. After completing the assessment, the nurse will be able to identify appropriate nursing diagnoses. For a list of possible nursing diagnoses, see Box 41-9.

Nursing Planning and Intervention. The goals of nursing care include maintaining oxygenation, maintaining fluid balance and optimal nutrition, and preventing infection. The nurse must diligently monitor respiratory status. Respiratory assessment, oxygen administration, ventilator care, and chest physiotherapy are integral components of this care. Weaning the newborn from oxygen with extreme caution is an ongoing intervention. Newborns may continue to require oxygen or ventilator assistance at home, necessitating parental involvement, education, and support. Adequate nutrition by parenteral and oral caloric intake is crucial to maintain optimal status. Because these newborns are subject to congestive heart failure, signs of fluid overload, such as increase in weight, rales, edema, and hepatomegaly, are noted and reported. Diuretics, bronchodilators, corticosteroids, vasodilators, and oxygen are administered as ordered.

(*text continues on page 1160*)

NURSING CARE PLAN
The Neonate With Respiratory Distress Syndrome

Nursing Goals
1. The neonate demonstrates adequate oxygenation as evidenced by adequate arterial blood gases and adequate oxygen saturation.
2. The neonate demonstrates effective breathing pattern without assistance.
3. The neonate has steady weight gain.
4. Parents verbalize understanding of home care instructions.

Assessment	*Potential Nursing Diagnoses*	*Intervention/ Rationale*	*Evaluation*
Preterm birth Tachypnea Retractions Grunting Flaring Cyanosis Pallor Low arterial paO₂ or low O₂ saturation Apnea Diminished breath sounds Crackles Rhonchi	Impaired Gas Exchange related to lack of lung surfactant	Auscultate breath sounds *to determine any change in status and if treatment is effective* Administer oxygen if ABGs decrease or O_2 saturation decreases *to improve oxygenation* Perform chest physiotherapy *to mobilize secretions* Suction as needed *to maintain patent airway* Monitor oxygen calibration *to ensure accurate oxygen delivery* Monitor blood gas levels every 4 to 6 hours or 20 to 30 minutes after fiO_2 levels *to ensure adequate oxygenation* Maintain linen roll under neck when in supine position *to maintain patent airway* Monitor and maintain stable body temperature *to avoid increase in respiratory rate and effort*	Arterial blood gases and oxygen within normal limits
	Ineffective Breathing Pattern related to disease process	Continuous positive airway pressure (CPAP) Auscultate breath sounds, note point of maximum impulse (PMI), chest symmetry *to check for bilateral expansion and monitor for pneumothorax* Check nasal prongs for patency *to prevent airway obstruction* Insert an orogastric tube *to prevent abdominal distention* Ventilator Monitor ventilator settings every hour *to maintain correct functioning*	Effective breathing pattern maintained

(continued)

NURSING CARE PLAN (Continued)
The Neonate With Respiratory Distress Syndrome

Assessment	Potential Nursing Diagnoses	Intervention/ Rationale	Evaluation
		Monitor for signs of extubation—crying, color change, diminished color change	
		Keep ambu bag at the bedside *to use in case of extubation*	
		Suction the endotracheal tube *to maintain patency*	
		Administer muscle relaxants *to promote pulmonary vascular relaxation, thereby promoting oxygenation*	
Low birth weight Preterm status NPO Respiratory distress	Altered Nutrition: Less than body requirements related to respiratory distress	Provide parenteral nutrition *to promote adequate nutrition until neonate can feed orally*	Neonate demonstrates steady weight gain
		Assess ability to suck, gag, and swallow when respiratory distress stabilized *to provide oral nutrition*	
		If reflexes inadequate, provide alternate routes—orogastric, nasogastric, nasojejunal as ordered *to promote adequate nutrition*	
		Provide adequate calories via preterm formula or breast milk fortified by supplements	
		Weigh daily *to assess nutritional status*	
Parental questions regarding home care Lack of parental experience with preterm neonate	Knowledge Deficit related to home care	Encourage intense caretaking sessions and rooming in while still in the hospital *to promote parental confidence*	Parents verbalize understanding of home care instructions
		Provide information regarding signs and symptoms of respiratory distress and infection *to promote prompt medical attention*	
		Encourage parental infant CPR certification and knowledge regarding any home devices, *ie,* IV pumps or apnea monitors *to promote safety in the home setting*	
		Provide referrals to appropriate support groups and other health professionals *to promote continuity of care and decrease parental anxiety*	
		Give instructions in medication administration *to promote parental confidence*	

BOX 41-9
Nursing Diagnoses—Bronchopulmonary Disease

- Impaired Gas Exchange related to inflammatory changes in the lung tissue
- Activity Intolerance related to diminished pulmonary function
- Inability to Sustain Spontaneous Ventilation related to diminished pulmonary function
- Dysfunctional Ventilatory Weaning Response related to interference with maintaining adequate oxygen saturation (dependence on ventilator)
- Ineffective Airway Clearance related to retained secretions
- Altered Nutrition: Less than body requirements related to
  - Increased caloric expenditure
  - Treatments
- Risk for Infection related to condition and invasive treatments
- Knowledge Deficit (parental) related to oxygen therapy and ventilator care at home
- Risk for Altered Parenting related to high-risk condition of newborn and need for treatments

Evaluation. The nursing process has been effective when the client outcomes have been met. Possible anticipated outcomes include the following:

- The newborn demonstrates adequate or stable oxygenation, with minimal assistance of oxygen or ventilator.
- The newborn is free of any clinical signs of sepsis.
- The newborn demonstrates signs of adequate hydration and nutritional status.

Pneumothorax

Pneumothorax is a potential complication of assisted ventilation and PEEP. Clinical signs indicate a sudden, rapid deterioration in condition, especially in a newborn with respiratory disease. Tachypnea, grunting, pallor, or cyanosis may occur. Breath sounds may be decreased. The cardiac apex may shift away from the affected side. Bradycardia and hypotension may occur.

Management. Diagnosis may be ascertained by transillumination of the chest followed by chest x-ray. High oxygen administration alone or further intervention may be necessary to reinflate the affected lung. Caution must be used with oxygen administration in preterm newborns due to their susceptibility for retinopathy of prematurity. The air leak can be decompressed by needle aspiration and subsequent placement of a chest tube with water-seal drainage and suction of 10 to 20 cm H_2O. When air movement in the tube and bubbling cease, the tube is clamped and re-moved in 24 hours if the newborn's condition remains stable.

Retinopathy of Prematurity

Retinopathy of prematurity (ROP) is an acquired disease resulting in eye injury and blindness in the low–birth-weight newborn. Although oxygen administration has been implicated in the past, evidence exists that other factors contribute to its development. The incidence is inversely proportional to birth weight. The disease progression ranges from dilation and tortuosity of retinal vessels to retinal detachment.

Management. Newborns who meet the following criteria are considered at risk for ROP and should receive routine ophthalmologic examinations in the NICU:

- Birth weight less than 1,500 g
- Mechanical ventilation administered more than 24 hours
- Oxygen requirement of more than 40% for 12 hours

Studies do not agree on the benefits of vitamin E therapy because side effects of sepsis and NEC exist. Recommendations are to maintain vitamin E levels within a physiologic range (1.5–2 mg/dL; Friendly, 1994). Vitamin E may reduce the incidence of ROP because it modifies the tissue response to oxygen. Newborns with advanced disease may benefit from transscleral cryotherapy, which freezes scarred retinal vessels. Cryotherapy has been shown to decrease the risk of blinding complications of ROP by 50%. Routine follow-up is essential to detect and treat vision problems as the newborn grows (Long, 1989).

Intraventricular Hemorrhage

A major disorder in preterm newborns is IVH. Incidence increases with decreasing gestational age. IVH is a leading cause of death. Impairment in survivors ranges from no impairment to severe impairment. IVH occurs more often among males, newborns who are growth retarded, and those with RDS (Dietch, 1993). The disorder is multifactorial in origin and can be related to various intravascular, vascular, and extravascular factors (Box 41-10).

Pathophysiology. The subependymal germinal matrix, a highly vascular area, is located at the level of the foramen of Monro and the head of the caudate nucleus. It is evident between 28 and 32 weeks' gestation; little of this structure is present at term. Bleeding is thought to originate from the capillaries of the germinal matrix. Because the sick preterm newborn does not regulate cerebral circulation well, several mechanisms can increase cerebral blood flow. Abrupt changes in blood pressure, complicated by hypoxia and hyper-

---

BOX 41–10
Factors Contributing to Intraventricular Hemorrhage in the Low–Birth-Weight Newborn

---

Intravascular
Fluctuating cerebral blood flow
Increase in cerebral blood flow
Increase in cerebral venous pressure
Decrease in cerebral blood flow
Abnormal platelet function and co-agulation

Vascular
Susceptibility of periventricular capillaries in germinal matrix to hypoxia

Extravascular
Physical stress
Adrenalin
Corticosteroids

---

capnea, result in increased cerebral blood flow and dilated cerebral blood vessels. Further, hypoxia and acidosis injure the endothelium of the vessels, making them rupture easily. In preterm newborns, the mechanism for keeping cerebral blood flow constant may be impaired. Arterioles dilate as stimulated by hypoxia or hypercarbia. A rise in blood pressure at this point may result in capillary rupture and hemorrhage. Bleeding may be isolated in the subependymal germinal matrix or extend into the neighboring ventricles (Dietch, 1993). The classification system shown in Box 41-10 can be used to isolate the severity of the hemorrhage.

Clinical Manifestations. Clinical signs may range from none to a dramatic change in condition. Observations of a deterioration may come about quickly. The nurse may notice apnea, bradycardia, hypotension, seizures, or decerebrate posturing. The anterior fontanel bulges, and the temperature becomes unstable, indicating increasing intracranial pressure.

Spinal fluid shows an increased number of red blood cells, elevated protein, and low glucose. Computed tomography and ultrasound techniques can pinpoint the timing, location, and size of the hemorrhage.

Treatment. Hemorrhage can be monitored by computed tomography and ultrasound. Small hemorrhages do not require any treatment and resolve spontaneously. Others require removal of the blood by spinal tap, direct ventricular puncture, or ventricular reservoir. Daily lumbar punctures may be required to decrease ventricular size. If posthemorrhagic hydrocephalus occurs, surgery is required to insert a ventriculoperitoneal shunt to drain the accumulated cerebrospinal fluid into the peritoneal cavity, where it is reabsorbed.

Nursing Assessment and Interventions. Prenatal prevention of preterm labor is crucial to eliminating a major risk factor of RDS. Elective intubation of very low–birth-weight newborns helps to eliminate hypoxia and hypercarbia and ensures adequate ventilation. Following the delivery, the nurse remembers to avoid

head compression by limiting the use of phototherapy masks, tight caps, excessive head rotation from one side to another, and rapid volume expansion. Avoiding rapid administration of hypertonic sodium bicarbonate or glucose also is helpful. These solutions can cause fluctuating cerebral arterial or verous pressures. During the first crucial week of life, the nurse intervenes to decrease risk in the environment while caring for neonates at risk. These interventions prevent stress, minimize heat loss, and maintain hemodynamic stability.

Continuing observation of the neonate at risk can alert the nurse to those subtle cues that indicate a change in status. Status of the fontanels (ie, flat, full, tense, or bulging) should be noted regularly. Signs of seizure activity, such as brief apneic periods, may be extremely subtle and difficult to identify. In an newborn diagnosed with IVH, the nurse must continue to be alert for signs of increasing intracranial pressure, such as apnea, bradycardia, hypotension, and temperature instability. Ongoing measurements of head circumferences and observation of fontanels are required. Assistance with treatment procedures and care of drains may be necessary. Depending on the severity of the hemorrhage, mild to severe neurologic deficits can result.

Patent Ductus Arteriosus

Patent ductus arteriosus is more common in the preterm newborn than in the term newborn. The ductus arteriosus in the fetus is a connection between the pulmonary artery and the aorta, functioning as a bypass for the lungs and possibly as a volume recipient from the left ventricle. In the term newborn, the ductus arteriosus closes in stages. Early or functional closure occurs in the first 24 hours. Later or anatomic closure of the tissue occurs in a few days. In the preterm newborn, these events occur but at a later time, when age and weight approach that of a term newborn.

Clinical Manifestations. The appearance of clinical signs of patent ductus arteriosus depends on the balance between the pulmonary and systemic vascular beds. If the pulmonary vascular resistance is low, there may be a left-to-right shunt, increasing the work of breathing for the neonate. If there is severe RDS, pulmonary vascular resistance is high, resulting in a right-to-left shunt.

Signs are more evident on the third or fourth day, when RDS would be resolving. Murmurs can be auscultated. Wide pulse pressures, tachycardia, and bounding pulses are noted. Signs and symptoms of pulmonary edema, such as tachypnea, grunting, retractions, and rales, occur. Elevation of $PaCO_2$, recurrent apnea, and increasing need for oxygen are noted. Chest x-ray, contrast echocardiography, and Doppler evaluation are used to confirm the diagnosis.

Treatment. Fluid restriction is necessary to decrease the workload of the heart. Adjustments are necessary when overhead radiant warmers are used to combat insensible water loss. Diuretics, such as furosemide (Lasix), may be used to control fluid volume. Controversy exists as to whether the use of digoxin in preterm newborns is therapeutic. Preterm newborns exhibit a high incidence of arrhythmias. Because anemia can increase the heart's workload, the hematocrit needs to be maintained as close to 40 as possible. Using prostaglandins to keep the ductus open and indomethacin to inhibit prostaglandin synthesis are medical advances in the treatment of patent ductus arteriosus. Overall, indomethacin has been successful, although in some neonates, the ductus has reopened. Because it affects the kidney, indomethacin should not be administered if the blood urea nitrogen is above 25 mg/dL or the creatinine is above 1.8 mg/dL. Renal function will be affected, with a decrease in urine output, decrease in serum sodium, and increase in potassium. These effects last only 72 hours. Three doses are given every 12 hours intravenously, orally, or rectally. If status does not improve, surgical intervention may be necessary. The timing of medical or surgical intervention and the choice of candidates remain open to debate and the individual situation.

Nursing Assessment and Interventions. Care of a newborn with a congenital heart defect is described in detail in Chapter 42.

Necrotizing Enterocolitis

Necrotizing enterocolitis, a disease of the neonate characterized by necrosis of the bowel, is a significant cause of death in the very low birth weight population; 80% of the clients with NEC are preterm low or very low birth weight newborns. The incidence of NEC increases with decreasing gestational age (MacKendrick et al., 1993).

Etiology. The development of the disease is multifactorial. Major factors that appear to be involved in the disease are toxins or infectious agents, enteral feeding, and tissue hypoxia and mesenteric ischemia. The role played by oxygen radicals, which may be produced by neutrophils or results of localized ischemia-reperfusion injury, is continuing to be investigated.

Clinical Manifestations. Clinical manifestations of NEC may be subtle and vary from neonate to neonate. Signs most often noted are lethargy, abdominal distension, temperature instability, and retention of feedings. Stool tests may indicate occult blood, and sugars may be noted prior to onset of NEC (Fanaroff et al., 1993). X-rays indicate pneumatosis intestinalis with bubbles or layers of gas in the intestinal wall.

Treatment. The neonate receives nothing by mouth, instead receiving IV fluids. Nasogastric suction is initiated and maintained. Broad-spectrum antibiotics are administered. Resection of necrotic segments of bowel and enterostomy are performed if intestinal perforation and peritonitis occur.

Nursing Assessment. The nurse plays a key role in identifying newborns at risk for NEC. The nurse's observations are crucial in establishing the correct diagnosis and subsequent management. During feedings, the preterm newborn is observed for how he or she tolerates the feedings.

Nursing Planning and Interventions. The goals of nursing care include preventing infection, promoting optimal hydration and nutrition, providing comfort, and maintaining a neutral thermal environment. Nurses must be aware of the risk factors that may contribute to gut ischemia. Once an at-risk newborn has been identified, the he or she should receive nothing by mouth, and IV fluids should be maintained; these measures permit the intestinal wall to rest and heal. Once feedings are initiated, fresh breast milk through nasogastric tube is the optimal choice. Breast milk is considered ideal because the organisms responsible for NEC grow more rapidly in cow's milk, and cow's milk lacks the antibodies breast milk provides. The nurse must check for gastric residuals while feeding through a nasogastric tube because increasing amounts of gastric residuals suggest intestinal malfunction. Nasojejunal tubes should be avoided because the introduction of formula into the bowel may cause mucosal damage and subsequent bowel perforation. A neutral thermal environment must be maintained because hypothermia leads to increased oxygen consumption and hypoxemia. All of these contribute to NEC by promoting bowel ischemia. Newborns with NEC usually are placed on long-term TPN therapy until the bowel is rested or re-anastomosed. Comfort may be promoted by careful positioning, stroking and tactile stimulation, and administering pain medications.

Post-term Newborns

Considering an accurate gestational age of greater than 42 weeks, the post-term newborn may experience the effects of the placental insufficiency from aging. This newborn is usually larger than the term neonate, so **cephalopelvic disproportion,** a condition in which the newborn's head is of such a shape, size, or position that it cannot pass through the mother's pelvis, may be a problem during the birth process. Resultant birth trauma also may present significant problems as a result of vaginal deliveries. With placental insufficiency occurring in the latter part of the gestation, physical characteristics may resemble those of the SGA newborn.

Physiologic Problems

Problems common to the post-term newborn include hypoxia, perinatal asphyxia, meconium aspiration, hypoglycemia, polycythemia, and ineffective thermal regulation.

Nursing Process

The nurse uses knowledge about the post-term newborn and possible problems and complications to plan and implement appropriate care. The nurse institutes a plan of care that is geared toward accurate assessments and measures to prevent complications and provide education and support to the parents.

Nursing Assessment

To aid in determining whether a newborn is post-term, it is essential to verify the date of the mother's last menstrual period and confirm the estimated date of delivery. The prenatal history also is received for findings that suggest a post-term newborn. These include maternal weight loss (3 lb or more per week) in the last weeks of pregnancy, reduction in fetal and uterine growth, palpation of a hard fetal head, meconium-stained amniotic fluid, or oligohydramnios.

A gestational assessment tool is used to ascertain that the pregnancy is at 42 weeks or longer and to verify the post-term status. The nurse assesses the newborn for characteristic physiologic abnormalities and potential physiologic complications. Physical characteristics of postmature newborns include decreased or absent vernix caseosa or lanugo; abundant scalp hair; dry, cracked, thin skin; little subcutaneous fat; yellow staining of skin, nails, and cord; and an alert, wide-eyed look.

Potential Nursing Diagnoses

Following assessment, appropriate nursing diagnoses that may apply to the post-term newborn can be developed. For a list of possible nursing diagnoses, see Box 41-11.

Planning and Intervention

When planning for the post-term newborn, the nurse prepares for injuries that may result from birth trauma or asphyxia. Using the Apgar score and immediate observations, the nurse in the delivery area may need to provide resuscitation and other immediate support measures for the neonate. Parenteral and other forms of nutrition are provided as soon as possible after birth. Heel stick glucose determinations are monitored frequently to detect hypoglycemia. The newborn's hematocrit is closely monitored, and any deviations from normal are reported. The temperature is assessed frequently, and measures to ensure appropriate environmental temperature are provided. The nurse informs the parents about the newborn's condition and provides support and resources as needed.

Evaluation

When caring for the post-term newborn, the nurse determines whether the care was effective. Possible anticipated outcomes include the following:

- The newborn experiences minimal or no birth trauma.
- The newborn maintains spontaneous, unassisted, and regular respirations.
- Arterial blood gases are within normal limits.

BOX 41–11
Nursing Diagnoses—
Post-term Newborn

- Impaired Gas Exchange related to meconium aspiration
- Ineffective Thermoregulation related to diminished subcutaneous fat stores
- Risk for Injury related to
  - Hypoglycemia
  - Vaginal delivery of a large newborn (birth trauma)
- Knowledge Deficit (parental) related to condition, treatment, and possible complications associated with post-term birth
- Risk for Altered Parenting related to newborn's condition

- Pulse oximeter readings demonstrate adequate oxygenation.
- The newborn tolerates adequate nutritional intake for the maintenance of homeostasis.
- The newborn's blood glucose determinations are within normal limits.
- The newborn remains free of cold stress.
- The newborn remains free of any complications associated with post-term birth.
- Parents demonstrate an understanding of the neonate's potential and actual needs.
- Parents demonstrate appropriate bonding behaviour with the newborn.

Small-for-Gestational Age Newborns

Newborns whose weights fall below the 10th percentile on an intrauterine growth chart for their gestational age have experienced some impairment of the normal intrauterine growth process during the prenatal period. These SGA newborns may be preterm, term, or post-term. However, most SGA newborns are born at or close to term and weigh less than 2,500 g. Under the old classification, these newborns would have been called *premature,* although their period of intrauterine life was not significantly shortened. Although small, these newborns are mature in comparison with newborns of similar weight but younger gestational age.

Growth-retarded newborns have an increased risk of perinatal morbidity and mortality. The newborn's condition results from intrauterine insult or deprivation. This insult or deprivation begins many weeks before birth. It is often related to abnormalities of the pregnancy or of the fetus.

The cause, severity, and gestational age at which the deprivation or insult occurs determines how the fetus is affected and what problems will be present. Fetal growth retardation may occur early or late in the pregnancy. Conditions occurring early in the pregnancy, such as the first trimester, which affects all aspects of fetal growth, result in symmetrical growth retardation. Newborns have proportional head circumference, weight, and length. Newborns affected by the maternal TORCH (Toxoplasmosis Other Rubella Cytomegalovirus Herpes) infections may experience early growth retardation. Growth retardation in later stages of pregnancy often results from impaired uteroplacental function or nutritional deficiency during the third trimester. These newborns experience asymmetrical growth retardation, with the head growing at a normal rate when compared with the growth of various other body organs (Kliegman, 1992). Often the weight will be less than the 10th percentile, while the head circumference and length will be greater than the 10th percentile.

Physiologic Problems

When adapting to extrauterine life, the problems encountered by the SGA newborn are different from those of the appropriate-for-gestational age preterm newborn. If the problem of poor growth in utero has been detected during pregnancy, nurses and physicians skilled in resuscitation should be present at delivery. Certain disorders tend to occur more frequently in the SGA newborn. These should be anticipated by the caregiver.

Asphyxia

Any neonate may be a victim of asphyxia during the labor and delivery process or immediately after birth. However, SGA newborns appear to be particularly vulnerable to this immediate neonatal complication. This may result from one of the following mechanisms:

- Lack of umbilical circulation
- Lack of placental exchange, as in abruptio placentae, or the SGA newborn's chronic hypoxia in utero
- Inadequate perfusion of the maternal side of the placenta

Neonatal asphyxia also may be the result of excess fluid in the lungs, airway obstruction, or ineffective respiratory effort. The failure to initiate or maintain normal respirations at birth is a severe, life-threatening emergency that requires immediate intervention to prevent anoxic cellular damage and to save the newborn's life.

Management. Nursing personnel need to be able to predict when a newborn may be born with asphyxia and require a resuscitative effort. Fetal monitoring during labor and delivery plays a significant role in that process. Indications of fetal distress on the monitor assist the staff to prepare for the birth of a depressed newborn. (See Chap. 40 for more details on monitoring and indications of fetal distress.) Other maternal indications include prolapsed cord, uterine rupture, abruptio placentae, placenta previa, chorioamnionitis, premature labor, malpresentation, maternal diabetes, polyhydramnios, and oligohydramnios. These conditions compromise fetal oxygenation status and promote fetal asphyxia. Neonates with asphyxia require immediate resuscitation at birth.

Meconium Aspiration Syndrome

Term, post-term, and SGA newborns are at risk for developing meconium aspiration syndrome. Meconium aspiration into the alveoli occurring in utero or at birth may result from fetal hypoxia. The etiology may be multifactorial because fetal distress and asphyxia do not always result in meconium aspiration syndrome. In addition to reflex gasping, the fetus responds to hypoxia with reflex relaxation of the anal sphincter and accelerated intestinal peristalsis, which draws the meconium into the tracheobronchial system. Meconium in the respiratory tract acts like a foreign body blocking the flow of air into the alveoli. Increasing inflation of the alveoli distal to the obstruction can lead to rupture and leakage of air into the interstitial tissue. This mechanism leads to hypoxemia, acidosis, and hypercapnea. Physiologically, these results lead to pulmonary vasoconstriction and ultimately, persistent pulmonary hypertension of the newborn (Wiswell et al., 1993).

Management. The syndrome may be prevented or minimized by prompt removal of meconium from the newborn's upper respiratory tract immediately after birth and through appropriate obstetric management of the mother when meconium-stained amniotic fluid is evident. Direct visualization and suctioning, essential preventive measures, are being reevaluated (Whitsett et al., 1994). In addition, the use of amnioinfusion during labor with women experiencing oligohydramnios may be helpful to relieve cord compression and dilute meconium. Despite preventive efforts, the newborn may require neonatal intensive care for stabilization and prevention of further complications.

Although few data exist on standardizing ventilator settings, management may include conventional assisted ventilation. ECMO has been effective when conventional ventilation is inadequate. High-frequency jet ventilation and surfactant therapy are still under investigation. Chest physiotherapy also may be helpful with neonates experiencing obstruction in the respiratory tract.

Nursing care primarily focuses on continuing observations, assessments, and interventions related to the neonate's respiratory system. In addition to ventilator care, assessment of respiratory status includes frequent monitoring and documentation of transcutaneous oxygen or pulse oximeter readings. The nurse's knowledge of potential complications, such as seizures, GI bleeding, and renal failure, requires frequent, comprehensive assessments (Turnage, 1989).

Hypoglycemia

Neonatal hypoglycemia is a frequent occurrence in SGA newborns and in newborns of diabetic mothers, stressed preterm newborns, and others (Klaus et al., 1993). Hypoglycemia is defined as a blood glucose of less than 40 mg/dL. Hypoglycemia in the SGA neonate is considered to be the result of a high metabolic rate along with low glycogen stores. Hypoglycemia usually occurs during the first 12 hours but can occur as late as 48 hours after birth (Klaus et al., 1993).

Management. The neonate should be screened according to agency protocol until tolerating oral feedings well. Parents need to be taught the signs and symptoms of hypoglycemia, because if stable, the neonate may be discharged early. The blood glucose concentration may be monitored by dipstick screening tests, such as Dextrostix or Chemstrips, or other screening devices. It is essential to follow the directions carefully to achieve the most accurate reading. Any low or questionable reading should be checked and confirmed by laboratory determination. Blood sugars must be carefully monitored and early feedings with 5% dextrose and water (D_5W) or formula given if necessary. Boluses of IV 10% dextrose and water ($D_{10}W$) solutions may be required for newborns who are symptomatic or do not tolerate feedings. Symptoms such as tremors, cyanosis, convulsions, apnea, abnormal cry, hypotonia, hypothermia, tachypnea, and cardiac arrest are often nonspecific. Continuous low blood sugar may increase the risk of cerebral damage. Finally, in newborns with hypoglycemia resulting from a specific medical problem, such as sepsis, the specific problem and the hypoglycemia must be treated (Di-Giacomo et al., 1989).

Ineffective Thermal Regulation

Newborns who are SGA have difficulty maintaining body temperature. They lack adequate muscle mass, brown fat (an internal fuel source), subcutaneous tissue, and ability to control skin capillaries. Additionally, basal metabolic rates differ from normal. Effects of asphyxia also are aggravated by cold stress. When sensing heat loss, the neonate attempts to produce heat by increasing physical work, such as by crying or becoming hyperactive. With cold stress, increased oxygen is necessary to increase metabolism. If the neonate has asphyxia, the increased work and need for increased oxygen further contribute to the asphyxia.

Management. Treatment and nursing care focus on maintaining a neutral thermal environment.

Polycythemia

On the average, SGA newborns have a higher plasma volume than appropriate-for-gestational age newborns. This polycythemic, hyperviscosity state may be due to intrauterine hypoxia, which stimulates erythropoiesis. In addition, a placental–fetal blood shift may occur during labor or as a result of fetal asphyxia. Polycythemia increases the cardiac workload because the neonate is less able to circulate blood effectively. The alteration in blood viscosity leads to hypoxia and hypoglycemia. If the polycythemia is severe, vessel blockage and thrombus formation may occur.

Management and Nursing Care. With a hematocrit greater than 65% and symptoms of hypoxia and hypoglycemia present, treatment is required. An exchange transfusion may be necessary to dilute the concentration of blood. Nursing care focuses on maintaining a well-controlled environment to maintain the neonate's body temperature and decrease the cardiac workload. The neonate is monitored closely for possible complications (Kliegman, 1992).

Nursing Process

The nurse uses knowledge about the SGA neonate and possible problems to plan and implement appropriate care. The nurse institutes a plan of care that addresses accurate assessments and measures to prevent complications and provide education and support to the parents.

Nursing Assessment

Most newborns with growth retardation resemble appropriate-for-gestational age preterm newborns. During assessment of the neonate, the nurse needs to be aware of common characteristics. Common physical characteristics of the SGA newborn with extreme growth retardation are listed in Box 41-12. However, assessment of gestational age according to physical characteristics may be altered or misleading for several reasons. Vernix is often decreased or absent. Consequently, the skin is more exposed to amniotic fluid. Sole creases appear more mature than they actually are. Breast tissue formation is reduced in SGA newborns. In girls, the adipose tissue covering the labia is decreased; thus, external genitalia appear less mature. Because the newborn's age is more advanced than the weight implies, the SGA newborn may have better developed neurologic responses. Thus, neurologic crite-

---

BOX 41–12
Common Physical Characteristics of Small-for-Gestational Age Newborn

- Decrease in subcutaneous tissue
- Loose, dry skin; poor skin turgor
- Decrease in normal chest and abdominal circumference
- Sunken abdomen
- Thin, slightly yellow, dull, dry umbilical cord
- Sparse scalp hair, dull and lusterless
- Wide-eyed look
- Skull sutures widely separated (from lack of normal bone growth)

BOX 41–13
Nursing Diagnoses— Small-for-Gestational Age Newborn

- Impaired Gas Exchange related to meconium aspiration
- Ineffective Thermoregulation related to inadequate muscle and fat stores
- Risk for Injury related to
  - Hypoglycemia
  - Effects of treatments and therapy
- Altered Cardiopulmonary Tissue Perfusion related to asphyxia
- Inability to Sustain Spontaneous Ventilation related to
  - Asphyxia
  - Hypoxia
- Risk for Altered Parenting related to
  - Neonate's appearance
  - High-risk condition

---

ria tend to be more accurate than physical criteria (Kliegman, 1992).

Nursing Diagnoses

Following assessment, appropriate nursing diagnoses can be developed. For a list of possible nursing diagnoses, see Box 41-13.

Nursing Interventions

The nurse uses information about maternal risk factors, gestational age, weight, length, head circumference, and other characteristic observations to anticipate interventions. Knowledge about various complications that may occur also is crucial. Any pertinent risk factors are identified, and the labor record is reviewed in preparation for possible resuscitation. If any meconium-stained amniotic fluid is detected, suctioning at the time of delivery is performed. Ongoing respiratory and neurologic assessments are essential when monitoring the neonate's status and adaptation to extrauterine life. Nutritional requirements need to be met from the time of delivery. Parenteral or oral nutrition is provided. It is imperative that the nurse screen the neonate's blood glucose according to the unit protocol; glucose is administered if necessary to prevent hypoglycemia. Because the SGA neonate is at risk for temperature instability, frequent temperature assessments are performed; measures to prevent infection and cold stress and provide a neutral thermal environment are instituted. The neonate's hematocrit is monitored for abnormal increases. Any deviations from the normal range are reported.

Evaluation

When caring for the SGA neonate, the nurse determines whether care was effective. Possible anticipated outcomes include the following:

- The neonate maintains spontaneous, unassisted, and regular respirations.
- Arterial blood gases are within normal limits.
- Pulse oximeter readings demonstrate adequate oxygenation.
- The neonate displays minimal or absent lung disease.
- The newborn tolerates adequate nutritional intake for maintenance of homeostasis.
- The neonate demonstrates appropriate weight gain.
- The neonate's glucose determinations are within normal limits.
- The neonate remains free of cold stress.
- The neonate remains free of any complications associated with gestational age.
- Parents demonstrate an understanding of the neonate's potential and actual needs.
- Parents demonstrate a beginning relationship with the neonate.

Large for Gestational Age Newborns

The large for gestational age (LGA) newborn fits into the 90th percentile or above on the intrauterine growth chart. Excessive birth weight often is the result of genetic influence. LGA newborns are susceptible to hypoglycemia and potential birth trauma as a result of their size. For further discussion of an example of an LGA newborn, see the section on the infant of a diabetic mother in Chapter 43.

Summary Points

✔ The environment in the NICU is a highly technical area in which critically ill newborns receive ongoing, competent, and compassionate nursing care. The NICU nurse is ever-diligent to assess the high-risk newborn for status changes and risk factors that will affect nursing diagnoses, outcomes, interventions, and subsequent outcome evaluations.

✔ The preterm newborn is potentially subject to numerous physiologic and psychosocial complications related to immaturity and family stressors. Many technologic advances have been accomplished, especially in the area of respiratory disease management, that have resulted in more positive outcomes.

✔ The post-term newborn may require vigorous resuscitation and frequent assessments for hypoglycemia, polycythemia, and temperature regulatory problems.

✔ The SGA newborn has characteristic physical features indicating possible impaired intrauterine growth. The nurse assesses and intervenes in the event of asphyxia, meconium aspiration, hypoglycemia, thermal regulation problems, and polycythemia.

✔ With a large-for-gestational age newborn, the nurse notes the potential complications of birth trauma and hypoglycemia and intervenes accordingly.

✔ Regardless of the factors requiring intensive care, the caregivers involve the family to the fullest extent possible in the care of the neonate so that family members will be comfortable with the neonate when he or she is discharged from the hospital. The family needs many resources to cope with problems that they may experience in the home care setting.

REFERENCES

Barnett, C., Leidermann, P., Grobstein, R. et al. (1970). Neonatal separation: The maternal side of interactional deprivation. *Pediatrics, 45,* 197.

Bell, E. F., & Oh, W. (1994). Principles of fluid and electrolyte therapy. In G. B. Avery, M. A. Fletcher, & M. G. Macdonald (Eds.), *Neonatology: Pathophysiology and management of the newborn* (pp. 312–327) (4th ed.). Philadelphia: J.B. Lippincott.

Broome, M. E., & Tanzillo, H. (1990). Differentiating between pain and agitation in premature neonates. *Journal of Perinatal and Neonatal Nursing, 4*(1), 53–62.

Bucuvalas, J. C., & Balistreri, W. F. (1992). The neonatal gastrointestinal tract development. In A. A. Fanaroff & R. S. Martin (Eds.), *Neonatal-perinatal medicine* (pp. 1019–1023) (5th ed.). St. Louis: C.V. Mosby.

Carlo, W. A. (1992). Assisted ventilation. In M. H. Klaus & A. A. Fanaroff (Eds.), *Care of the high risk neonate* (pp. 260–281) (4th ed.). Philadelphia: W.B. Saunders.

Dietch, J. (1993). Periventricular-intraventricular hemorrhage in the very low birth weight infant. *Neonatal Network, 12*(1), 7–12.

DiGiacomo, J. E., Hagedorn, M. I., & Hay, W. W. (1989). Glucose homeostasis. In G. B. Merenstein & S. L. Gardner (Eds.), *Handbook of neonatal care* (pp. 223). St. Louis: C.V Mosby.

Fanaroff, A. A., & Kleigman, R. M. (1993). Necrotizing enterocolitis. In M. H. Klaus & A. A. Fanaroff (Eds.), *Care of the high risk neonate* (pp. 260–281). (4th ed.). Philadelphia: W.B. Saunders.

Fletcher, A. (1994). Nutrition. In G. B. Avery, M. A. Fletcher, & M. G. Macdonald (Eds.), *Neonatology: Pathophysiology and management of the newborn* (pp. 330–356) (4th ed.). Philadelphia: J.B. Lippincott.

Friendly, D. (1994). Eye disorders. In G. B. Avery, M. A. Fletcher, & M. G. Macdonald (Eds.), *Neonatology: Pathophysiology and management of the newborn* (pp. 1195–1210) (4th ed.). Philadelphia: J.B. Lippincott.

Fuller, R. (1992). Group B streptococcal infection in the newborn. *Critical Care Nursing Clinics of North America, 4*(3), 487–492.

Gartner, L., & Lee, K. S. (1992). Jaundice and liver disease-unconjugated hyperbilirubinemia. In A. A. Fanaroff & R. S. Martin (Eds.), *Neonatal-perinatal medicine* (pp. 1093–1104) (5th ed.). St. Louis: C.V. Mosby.

Greenspan, J. (1993). Liquid ventilation: A developing technology. *Neonatal Network, 12*(4), 23–28.

Grobman, D. W., & Foley, M. M. (1992). Surfactant replacement therapy in newborns with hyaline membrane disease. *Critical Care Nursing Clinics of North America, 4*(3), 515–519.

Guzetta, P. C. et al. (1994). General surgery. In G. B. Avery, M. A. Fletcher, & M. G. Macdonald (Eds.), *Neonatology: Pathophysiology and management of the newborn* (pp. 914–951) (4th ed.). Philadelphia: J.B. Lippincott.

Hack, M. (1992). The sensorimotor development of the preterm infant. In A. A. Fanaroff & R. J. Martin (Eds.), *Neonatal-perinatal medicine* (pp. 759–782) (5th ed.). Philadelphia: W.B. Saunders.

Hill, A. S., & Rath, L. (1993). The care and feeding of the low-birth weight infant. *Journal of Perinatal and Neonatal Nursing, 6*(4), 56–58.

Jain, L., & Vidyasagar, D. (1993). Cardiopulmonary resuscitation of newborns. *Pediatric Clinics of North America, 40*(2), 287–300.

Kavanaugh, K., Mead, L., Meier, P., & Mangurten, H. (1995). Getting enough: Mothers' concerns about breastfeeding a preterm infant after discharge. *Journal of Obstetric, Gynecologic, and Neonatal Nursing, 24*(1), 23–32.

Kinneer, M. D., & Beachy, P. (1994). Nipple feeding premature infants in the neonatal intensive care unit: Factors and decisions. *Journal of Obstetric, Gynecologic, and Neonatal Nursing, 23*(2), 105–112.

Klaus, M. H., Jerauld, R., Kreger, N. et al. (1972). Maternal attachment: Importance of the first postpartum days. *New England Journal of Medicine, 286,* 460.

Klaus, M. H., & Kennell, J. H. (1970). Mothers separated from their newborn infants. *Pediatric Clinics of North America, 17,* 1015–1037.

Klaus, M. H., & Kennell, J. H. (1992). Care of the mother, father, and infant. In A. A. Fanaroff & R. S. Martin (Eds.), *Neonatal-perinatal medicine* (pp. 465–477) (5th ed.). St. Louis: C.V. Mosby.

Kliegman, R. M. (1992). Intrauterine growth retardation: Determinants of aberrant fetal growth. In A. A. Fanaroff & R. J. Martin (Eds.), *Neonatal-perinatal medicine* (pp. 149–185) (5th ed.). St. Louis: C.V. Mosby.

Knoppert, D. C., & MacKanjee, H. R. (1994). Current strategies in management of bronchopulmonary dysplasia: The role of corticosteroids. *Neonatal Network, 13*(3), 53–59.

Koszarek, K. (1991). Nursing assessment and care for the neonate in acute respiratory distress. In J. Nugent (Ed.), *Acute respiratory care of the neonate* (pp. 47–71). Petaluma, CA: NICU Link.

Lefrak-Okikawa, L., & Lund, C. H. (1993). Nursing practice in the neonatal intensive care unit. In M. H. Klaus & A. A. Fanaroff (Eds.), *Care of the high risk neonate* (pp. 212–227) (4th ed.). Philadelphia: W.B. Saunders.

Loisel, D. B., Korzelove, S., & Shatz, V. (1994). The intensive care nursery. In G. B. Avery, M. A. Fletcher, & M. G. Macdonald (Eds.), *Neonatology: Pathophysiology and management of the newborn* (pp. 54–67) (4th ed.). Philadelphia: J.B. Lippincott.

Long, C. (1989). Cryotherapy: A new treatment for retinopathy of prematurity. *Pediatric Nursing, 15*(3), 269–272.

MacKendrick, W., & Caplan, M. (1993). Necrotizing enterocolitis. *Pediatric Clinics of North America, 40*(5), 1047–1056.

Martin, R. J., Fanaroff, A. A., & Klaus, M. H. (1993). Respiratory problems. In M. H. Klaus & A. A. Fanaroff (Eds.), *Care of the high risk neonate* (pp. 228–259) (4th ed.). Philadelphia: W.B. Saunders.

Myer, M. L. (1992). New trends in neonatal mechanical ventilation. *Critical Care Nursing Clinics of North America, 4*(3), 507–512.

Phibbs, R. H. (1994). Delivery room management. In G. B. Avery, M. A. Fletcher, & M. G. Macdonald (Eds.), *Neonatology: Pathophysiology and management of the newborn* (pp. 248–268) (4th ed.). Philadelphia: J.B. Lippincott.

Pillitteri, A. (1995). *Maternal and child health nursing* (pp. 728–776). Philadelphia: J.B. Lippincott.

Price, P. T., & Kalhan, S. C. (1993). Nutrition and selected disorders of the GI tract. In M. H. Klaus & A. A. Fanaroff (Eds.), *Care of the high risk neonate* (pp. 130–175) (4th ed.). Philadelphia: W.B. Saunders.

Scanlon, J. W. (1994). The very low birth weight infant. In G. B. Avery, M. A. Fletcher, & M. G. Macdonald (Eds.), *Pathophysiology and management of the newborn* (pp. 399–416) (4th ed.). Philadelphia: J.B. Lippincott.

Spitzer, A., Bernstein, J., Boichis, H., & Edelmann, C. M. (1992). Kidney and urinary tract. In A. A. Fanaroff & R. J. Martin (Eds.), *Neonatal-perinatal medicine* (pp. 1293–1327) (5th ed.). St. Louis: C.V. Mosby.

Sterk, M. B. (1983). Understanding parenteral nutrition. *JOGNN, 12,* (3), 475.

Turnage, B..S. (1989). Meconium aspiration syndrome. *Journal of Perinatal and Neonatal Nursing, 3*(2), 69–80.

Turner, B. S. (1991). Nursing procedures. In J. Nugent (Ed.), *Acute respiratory care of the neonate* (pp. 75–96). Petaluma, CA: NICU Link.

Weingarten, C. T. et al. (1990). Married mothers' perceptions of their premature or term infants and the quality of their relationship with their husband. *Journal of Obstetric, Gynecologic, and Neonatal Nursing, 19*(1), 64.

Whitsett, J. A. et al. (1994). Acute respiratory disorders. In G. B. Avery, M. A. Fletcher, & M. G. Macdonald (Eds.), *Neonatology: Pathophysiology and management of the newborn* (pp. 429–452) (4th ed.). Philadelphia: J.B. Lippincott.

Wiswell, T. E., & Bent, R. C. (1993). Meconium staining and the meconium aspiration syndrome. *Pediatric Clinics of North America, 40*(5), 955–977.

SUGGESTED READINGS

Beachy, P., & Deacon J. (1992). *Core curriculum for neonatal intensive care nursing.* Philadelphia: W.B. Saunders.

Beckmann, C. A. (1990). Postterm pregnancy: Effects on temperature and glucose regulation. *Nursing Research, 39*(1), 21–14.

Bell, P. L., & Ellerbee, S. (1993). Impaired cerebral vascular blood flow in the premature infant. *Journal of Perinatal and Neonatal Nursing, 7*(1), 49–55.

Bell, S. G. (1994). The national pain management guideline: Implications for neonatal intensive care. *Neonatal Network, 13*(3), 9–15.

Bozzette, M. (1993). Observation of pain behavior in the NICU: An exploratory study. *Journal of Perinatal and Neonatal Nursing, 7*(1), 76–87.

Bruno, J. P. (1995). Systematic neonatal assessment and intervention. *MCN: American Journal of Maternal Child Nursing, 20*(1), 21–24.

Burchfield, D. J., Berkowitz, I. D., Berg, R. A., & Goldberg, R. N. (1993). Medications in neonatal resuscitation. *Annals of Emergency Medicine, 22*(pt. 2), 435–439.

Chally, P. S. (1992). Moral decision making in neonatal intensive care. *Journal of Obstetric, Gynecologic, and Neonatal Nursing, 21*(6), 475–482.

Clancy, G. T., Anand, K. J. S., & Lally, P. (1992). Neonatal pain management. *Critical Care Nursing Clinics of North America, 4*(3), 527–533.

Comer, D. (1992). Pulse oximetry-implications for practice. *Journal of Obstetric, Gynecologic, and Neonatal Nursing, 21*(1), 35–41.

Cusson, R. M. (1993). Instruments in neonatal research: Measuring attachment behavior. *Neonatal Network, 12*(4), 69–71.

Drosten-Brooks, F. (1993). Kangaroo care: Skin to skin contact in the NICU. *MCN: American Journal of Maternal Child Nursing, 18*(5), 250–253.

Gardner, S. L. (1994). Pain and pain relief in the neonate. *MCN: American Journal of Maternal Child Nursing, 19*(2), 85–89.

Gennaro, S., Brooten, D., & Bakewell-Sachs, S. (1991). Postdischarge services for low birth weight infants. *Journal of Obstetric, Gynecologic, and Neonatal Nursing, 20*(1), 29–35.

Georges, J. M. (1992). Glucose management and nutritional support of low birth weight neonates. *Journal of Perinatal and Neonatal Nursing, 6*(1), 71–77.

Gortner, L. (1992). Natural surfactant for neonatal respiratory distress syndrome in very premature infants: A 1992 update. *Journal of Perinatal Medicine, 20*(6), 409–419.

Graves, B. W. (1992). Newborn resuscitation revisited. *Journal of Nurse Midwifery, 32*(Suppl. 2), 36S–42S.

Haney, C., & Allingham, T. M. (1992). Nursing care of the neonate receiving high-frequency jet ventilation. *Journal of Obstetric, Gynecologic, and Neonatal Nursing, 21*(3), 187–198.

Kenner, C., Brueggemeyer, A., & Gunderson, L. P. (1993). *Comprehensive neonatal nursing, a physiologic perspective.* Philadelphia: W.B. Saunders.

Khan, N. S., & Luten, R. C. (1994). Neonatal resuscitation. *Emergency Medical Clinics of North America, 12*(1), 239–256.

Klaus, M. H., & Fanaroff, A. A. (1993). *Care of the high risk neonate* (4th ed.). Philadelphia: W.B. Saunders.

Kliegman, R. M., Walker, W. A., & Yolken, R. H. (1993). Necrotizing enterocolitis: Research agenda for a disease of unknown etiology and pathogenesis. *Pediatric Research, 34*(6), 701–708.

Krause, K. D., & Youngner, V. J. (1992). Nursing diagnoses as guidelines in the care of the neonatal ECMO patient. *Journal of Obstetric, Gynecologic, and Neonatal Nursing, 21*(3), 169–176.

Medoff-Cooper, B. (1994). Transition of the preterm infant to an open crib. *Journal of Obstetric, Gynecologic, and Neonatal Nursing, 23*(4), 321–328.

Meier, P. P. (1994). Transition of the preterm infant to an open crib: Process of the project group. *Journal of Obstetric, Gynecologic, and Neonatal Nursing, 23*(4), 329–335.

Merenstein, G. B., & Gardner, S. L. (1993). *Handbook of neonatal intensive care* (2nd ed.). St. Louis: C.V. Mosby.

Miles, M. S., Funk, S. G., & Carlson, J. (1993). Parental stressor scale:neonatal intensive care unit. *Nursing Research, 42*(3), 48–52.

Miller, H. D., & Anderson, G. C. (1993). Nonnutritive sucking: Effects on crying and heart rate in intubated infants requiring assisted mechanical. *Nursing Research, 42*(5), 305–307.

NAACOG (1991). Prevention, recognition, and management of neonatal pain. *OGN Nursing Practice Resource,*

NAACOG (1991). Physical assessment of the neonate. *OGN Nursing Practice Resource,*

NAACOG (1991). Facilitating breastfeeding. *OGN Nursing Practice Resource,*

NAACOG (1992). Neonatal skin care. *OGN Nursing Practice Resource,*

Oellrich, R. G., Murphy, M., Goldberg, L. A., & Aggarwal, R. (1991). The percutaneous central venous catheter for small or ill infants. *MCN: American Journal of Maternal Child Nursing, 16*(2), 92–96.

Phelps, D. L. (1993). Retinopathy of prematurity. *Pediatric Ophthalmology, 40*(4), 705–723.

Pickler, R. H., & Terrell, B. V. (1994). Nonnutritive sucking and necrotizing enterocolitis. *Neonatal Network, 13*(8), 15–17.

Pokela, M. L. (1994). Pain relief can reduce hypoxemia in distressed neonates during routine treatment procedures. *Pediatrics, 93*(3), 379–383.

Pramanik, A. K., Holtzman, R. B., & Merritt, T. A. (1993). Surfactant replacement therapy for pulmonary disease. *Pediatric Clinics of North America, 40*(5), 913–932.

Pridham, K. F., Sandel, S., Chang, A., & Green, C. (1993). Nipple feeding for preterm infants with bronchopulmonary dysplasia. *Journal of Obstetric, Gynecologic, and Neonatal Nursing, 22*(2), 147–155.

Shiao, S. Y. (1992). Fluid and electrolyte problems of infants of very low birth weight. *AACN Clinical Issues in Critical Care Nursing, 3*(3), 698–704.

Shogan, M. G., & Schumann, L. L. (1993). The effect of environmental lighting on the oxygen saturation of preterm infants in the NICU. *Neonatal Network, 12*(5), 7–13.

Stevens, B. J., & Johnston, C. C. (1994). Physiological responses of premature infants to a painful stimulus. *Nursing Research, 43*(4), 226–230.

Suddaby, E. C., & O'Brien, A. M. (1993). ECMO for cardiac support in children. *Heart and Lung, 22*(5), 401–407.

Thomas, K. (1994). Thermoregulation in neonates. *Neonatal Network, 13*(2), 15–21.

Urritia, N. L. (1991). Sorting the complexities of RDS. *MCN: American Journal of Maternal Child Nursing, 16*(6), 308–311.

Wung, J. T. (1993). Respiratory management for low birth weight infants. *Critical Care Medicine, Sept 21*(Suppl. 9), S364–S365.

Zahr, L. K., & Montijo, J. (1993). The benefit of home care for sick premature infants. *Neonatal Network, 12*(1), 93–97.

42

The High-Risk Newborn: Developmental Disorders

Objectives

- Describe the grieving process for parents whose neonates are born with congenital anomalies or developmental defects.
- Compare and contrast maladaptive and adaptive responses to a perinatal development crisis or loss.
- Discuss the common neonatal developmental disorders, including congenital and genetic abnormalities, musculoskeletal disorders, chromosomal anomalies, and inborn errors of metabolism.
- Identify potential nursing diagnoses applicable to the care of a newborn with a congenital or developmental disorder.
- Apply the nursing process to the care of the high-risk newborn with a selected developmental disorder.

Key Terms

Ambiguous genitalia	Grieving process
Aminoacidurias	Hydrocephalus
Anencephaly	Hypospadias
Cleft palate	Imperforate anus
Cleft lip	Meningocele
Congenital	Meningomyelocele
diaphragmatic hernia	Microcephaly
Congenital disorder	Omphalocele
Diaphragmatic hernia	Phenylketonuria
Epispadias	Polydactyly
Esophageal atresia	Spina bifida
Galactosemia	Spina bifida occulta
Gastroschisis	Talipes equinovarus
Genetic disorder	Tracheoesophageal
Grief	fistula

During labor, delivery, and the first several hours of newborn life, many changes occur in the fetus and newborn that allow physiologic adaptation to extrauterine life. Developmental characteristics of the newborn, such as genetic or congenital abnormalities, birth weight, and gestational age (see Chap. 41), may have significant influence on this process. Perinatal teams must be constantly alert to signs of possible complications in the newborn, identifying problems early, correcting disorders quickly or minimizing subsequent effects, preventing permanent disabilities, and promoting the parental bonding process.

This chapter describes the most common congenital and genetic abnormalities encountered in the perinatal setting. The psychosocial stresses experienced by the parents of a newborn with a congenital or genetic abnormality and their effect on family functioning and relationships are presented. Using a nursing process framework, nursing care of the newborn with various congenital or genetic abnormalities is described.

Parental and Staff Reactions to Defects and Disorders

The birth of a newborn with congenital anomalies or developmental defects presents significant psychosocial stresses for the family, precipitating an adaptive crisis. A variety of emotional difficulties may interfere with the parents' relationship with the newborn and disrupt family functioning. Parents often express feelings of anxiety, guilt, fear, inadequacy, helplessness, failure, and anger. The way parents cope with crisis

and work through their feelings will influence how realistically they perceive their newborn's medical condition and needs, how they are able to adapt to the newborn's hospital environment, their ability to assume the primary caretaking role, their ability to assume responsibility for the newborn's care after discharge, and for some, the ability to cope with the death of their newborn (Fig. 42-1).

Grief

Grief is the characteristic physiologic and psychological responses to the loss (anticipated or actual) of a valued object. A grief reaction may be precipitated by certain perinatal situations, such as abortion, stillbirth, preterm birth, newborn deformity or illness, neonatal death, or relinquishment of a newborn.

Stages of the Grieving Process

When a person experiences a loss, he or she goes through a **grieving process**, a means by which the person attempts to respond and adapt to the loss. The grieving process has been studied at length and in various settings. The various common behaviors noted during grief have been grouped into stages. Stages may be labeled differently but basically contain the same behaviors. Grieving parents may not exhibit all of the behaviors. In addition, they may repeat behaviors during the process. Bowlby et al. (1970) have described the grief process in the following manner.

Shock. Shock, denial, disbelief, and withdrawal behaviors characterize the first phase. Parents may experience a feeling of numbness. Physiologic reactions include loss of appetite, palpitations, fatigue, and shortness of breath. A tendency to withdraw from the situation may be observed in the case of a defective or critically ill newborn. This coping mechanism allows the potential loss to be less painful if attachment has not occurred.

Searching. The second stage involves seeking an answer or reason for the event. Behaviors of anger, guilt, hostility, and emptiness are commonly seen. Parents may feel that their actions are to blame for the loss. Healthcare professionals may be the target of their anger.

Disorientation. Disorientation is a bridge stage to reorganization. During this time, a gradual change to normal activities will occur. Parents may still be experiencing some depression. If a setback occurs, such as a complication in the health course of the preterm newborn, they may have little emotional energy to deal with it.

Reorganization. For a considerable time, parents adjust and accommodate to the loss. Minimal energy is

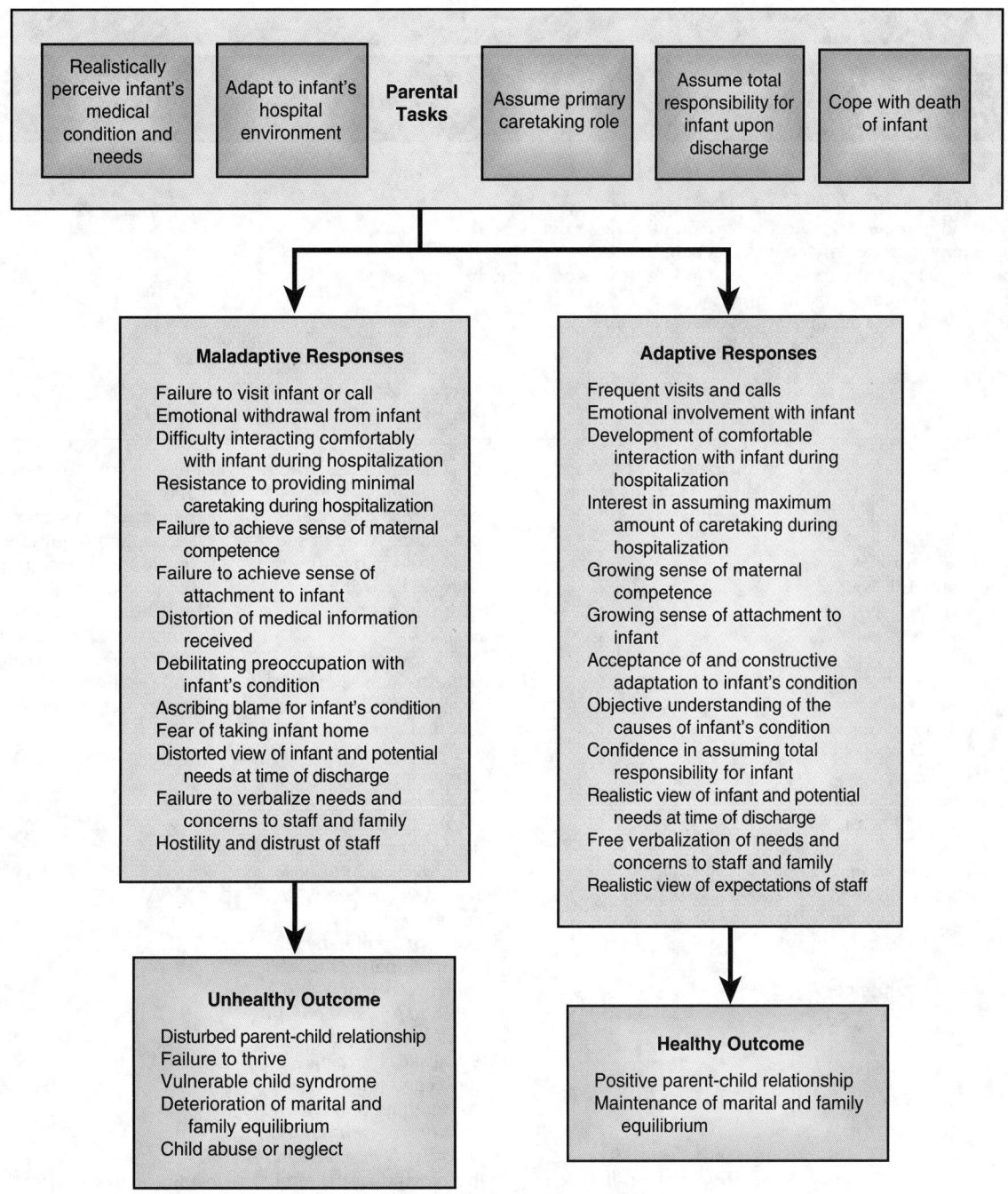

Parental Tasks

- Realistically perceive infant's medical condition and needs
- Adapt to infant's hospital environment
- Assume primary caretaking role
- Assume total responsibility for infant upon discharge
- Cope with death of infant

Maladaptive Responses

Failure to visit infant or call
Emotional withdrawal from infant
Difficulty interacting comfortably with infant during hospitalization
Resistance to providing minimal caretaking during hospitalization
Failure to achieve sense of maternal competence
Failure to achieve sense of attachment to infant
Distortion of medical information received
Debilitating preoccupation with infant's condition
Ascribing blame for infant's condition
Fear of taking infant home
Distorted view of infant and potential needs at time of discharge
Failure to verbalize needs and concerns to staff and family
Hostility and distrust of staff

Adaptive Responses

Frequent visits and calls
Emotional involvement with infant
Development of comfortable interaction with infant during hospitalization
Interest in assuming maximum amount of caretaking during hospitalization
Growing sense of maternal competence
Growing sense of attachment to infant
Acceptance of and constructive adaptation to infant's condition
Objective understanding of the causes of infant's condition
Confidence in assuming total responsibility for infant
Realistic view of infant and potential needs at time of discharge
Free verbalization of needs and concerns to staff and family
Realistic view of expectations of staff

Unhealthy Outcome

Disturbed parent-child relationship
Failure to thrive
Vulnerable child syndrome
Deterioration of marital and family equilibrium
Child abuse or neglect

Healthy Outcome

Positive parent-child relationship
Maintenance of marital and family equilibrium

FIGURE 42–1 Parental response during crisis period. (Grant, P. [1978]. Psychosocial needs of families of high-risk infants. *Family Community Health 1*(3),93 November)

devoted to the grief process, and most energy is directed toward normal living (Klaus et al., 1993).

Nursing Process

The nursing care of the family with a newborn who has a congenital or genetic anomaly is complex and demanding. Not only must the nurse care for the newborn, the nurse must also deal with parental disappointment and disillusionment and the parents' and the nurse's own possible negative feelings for the new-

born. An outline of the nursing process is found in the Nursing Care Plan: The Grieving Family.

Assessment

Not all congenital disorders can be predicted. Nursing assessment begins with establishing that an actual or potential perinatal loss has occurred. Variables to consider include the family's experiences and usual coping strategies in dealing with loss or crisis, support systems available, cultural and religious factors, and age and

NURSING CARE PLAN
The Grieving Family

Nursing Goals
1. The family members are supportive of one another.
2. The family applies its energy to working through grief.
3. The family uses healthy coping mechanisms.
5. The parents verbally repeat understanding of prognosis and resources.
6. Parents of ill infants visit the nursery.
7. Family is able to verbalize positive self-esteem.
8. Family verbalizes information related to loss.

Assessment	Potential Nursing Diagnoses	Intervention/ Rationale	Evaluation
Perinatal loss Abortion Stillbirth Neonatal death Intrauterine death Infant of low birth weight or preterm Infant with a congenital anomaly Infant with a life-threatening illness Family support systems available Past grief experiences Religious beliefs Age and maturity level of parents Cultural considerations Usual coping methods for crises Family expression of feelings Physical and emotional expressions	Anticipatory or Dysfunctional Grieving related to a perinatal loss	Allow family time to ventilate feelings *to provide supportive atmosphere* Allow family time to see and hold baby—describe how baby will look Ask if parents wish to name baby Provide photographs or other remembrances of baby if family wishes *to facilitate grieving* Seek parents' permission for an autopsy *to provide validation, if possible, of cause of death* Ask if parents wish baby baptized and notify clergy *to provide for religious needs* In case of an ill baby, encourage parents to visit nursery as much as possible *to promote bonding and subsequent grieving* Be realistic regarding prognosis and any long-term care required *to offer accurate information and avoid any misconceptions*	Family is supportive of one another Family applies its energy to working through grief Family applies healthy coping mechanisms Family adapts to crisis Parents verbally repeat understanding of prognosis and resources Parents of ill infants visit nursery Family seeks assistance as needed
Repeat abortions, fetal or neonatal Verbalization of guilt feelings Perinatal loss as result of trauma, teratogenic exposure, or genetic problem	Self Esteem Disturbance related to loss	Observe and assess family responses to loss, especially any expression of guilt *to validate grief response* Be available and listen to expression of feelings *to validate feelings using therapeutic communication* Assist with referrals as needed *to facilitate ongoing contact with caregivers of other disciplines and promote continuity of care*	Family is able to verbalize positive self-esteem Family identifies positive coping behaviors

(continued)

NURSING CARE PLAN *(Continued)*
The Grieving Family

Assessment	Potential Nursing Diagnoses	Intervention/ Rationale	Evaluation
Verbalization of concerns and questions	Knowledge Deficit related to perinatal loss	Provide information and review events as appropriate *to validate understanding* Provide information regarding the grief process, what to expect with siblings *to confirm understanding*	Family verbalizes correct information related to loss

maturity level of the parents. These variables guide the nurse in individualizing care for various family needs. The nurse considers these variables while communicating therapeutically and providing information to these families.

Nursing Diagnoses

Identifying potential nursing diagnoses is essential for appropriate planning and intervention. For a list of possible nursing diagnoses, see Box 42-1.

Planning and Intervention

The nurse plans to facilitate and support the family's grieving process. In addition, the nurse provides the family with information regarding the loss, including any implications for future childbearing. Nurses and caregivers in many settings and disciplines may interact with grieving family members. A comprehensive checklist may be used to ensure continuity of care throughout the grief process (see Assessment Guidelines: Comprehensive Checklist for Perinatal Loss and Research Highlight).

Evaluation

Adaptive responses to a crisis, such as a perinatal loss, are outlined in the nursing care plan and Figure 42-1. For more information about appropriate measures, see Chapter 41. Possible anticipated outcomes include the following:

- The parents demonstrate positive coping strategies to deal with the loss.
- The parents verbalize feelings and concerns openly and honestly.

- The parents demonstrate knowledge about care measures and adaptations necessary for the newborn.
- The parents demonstrate a beginning parent–newborn relationship.
- The parents choose a course of action in agreement with their family's goals and values.

Congenital and Genetic Abnormalities

A **congenital disorder** is present at birth and results from genetic or environmental factors or both. A **genetic disorder** is transmitted from generation to gen-

---

BOX 42–1
Nursing Diagnoses

- Anticipatory Grieving related to the uncertainty of outcome with newborn's condition
- Dysfunctional Grieving related to
  - Actual perinatal loss
  - Birth of newborn with a defect
- Self Esteem Disturbance related to
  - Loss of "perfect child"
  - Idea that parental action caused the defect.
- Knowledge Deficit related to
  - Treatment and care of newborn
  - Newborn needs, available resources, and necessary care after discharge
- Anxiety related to uncertainty of outcome or poor prognosis
- Risk for Altered Parenting related to negative feelings toward newborn
- Altered Family Processes related to difficulty coping with effects of newborn's condition
- Risk for Altered Parent/Infant Attachment related to negative feelings toward newborn

ASSESSMENT GUIDELINES
Comprehensive Checklist for Perinatal Loss

Parents' names _____

Address _____

Phone _____

Description of loss: _____

_____

Description of previous loss(es) _____

_____

L.M.P. _____ E.D.C. _____

Weeks of gestation _____

Sex of baby (if known) _____

Religious affiliation _____

	Office Staff	E.R. Staff	Labor/Delivery	Postpartum	Neonatal ICU	O.R. Staff	GYN/Postop	Community Health	Date(s)
Received pregnancy confirmation									
Lab/amnio results	☐	☐	☐			☐			___
Sonogram photo	☐		☐			☐			___
Acknowledgment of loss/impaired fertility	☐	☐	☐	☐	☐	☐	☐	☐	___
Bring up the subject									
Refer to the baby/expected child									
Call the baby by name									
Anticipatory guidance about normal grief									___
Mother	☐	☐	☐	☐	☐	☐	☐	☐	___
Father	☐	☐	☐	☐	☐	☐	☐	☐	___
Family members	☐	☐	☐	☐	☐	☐	☐	☐	___
Postloss options given									
To go home/maternity floor/alternate floor	☐	☐	☐			☐			___
Father to remain with mother/private room			☐	☐			☐		___
Saw/touched/held baby or products of conception	☐	☐	☐		☐	☐	☐		___
If refused, later offers made			☐	☐	☐		☐		___
Family members included in offer	☐	☐	☐	☐	☐	☐	☐		___
Received mementos									
Footprints			☐	☐	☐				___
Bracelet			☐	☐	☐				___
Lock of hair			☐	☐	☐				___
Crib card			☐	☐	☐				___
Blanket			☐	☐	☐				___
Tape measure			☐	☐	☐				___
Certificate of life/remembrance	☐	☐	☐	☐	☐	☐	☐	☐	___
Photographs taken									
Given to parents			☐		☐				___
Filed with chart			☐		☐				___
Bathed/dressed baby			☐		☐				___
Postdeath options discussed	☐	☐	☐	☐	☐		☐		___
Need/desire for funeral director									
Type/location/timing of service									
Burial/cremation/hospital disposal									
Parent involvement									
Choosing burial outfit/mementos									
Announcements—public/personal									
Religious options									
Baby baptized	☐	☐	☐		☐	☐	☐		___
Clergy notified	☐	☐	☐	☐	☐	☐	☐	☐	___
Received information about									
Birth/death certificates	☐	☐		☐	☐		☐	☐	___
Autopsy option discussed	☐	☐	☐	☐	☐		☐		___
Marked chart/room with identifying symbol (eg, butterfly, rainbow, rose)	☐	☐	☐	☐	☐	☐	☐	☐	___
Received literature/suggested readings	☐	☐	☐	☐	☐	☐	☐	☐	___
Hospital admitting office notified	☐	☐							___
SHARE/support group referral made	☐	☐	☐	☐	☐	☐	☐	☐	___

From Family Nursing Associates. JOGNN, Sept/Oct 1991

Nursing Interventions After Neonatal Loss

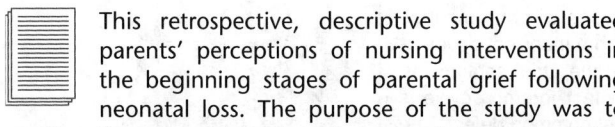

This retrospective, descriptive study evaluated parents' perceptions of nursing interventions in the beginning stages of parental grief following neonatal loss. The purpose of the study was to confirm the appropriateness of nursing interventions that are commonly accepted as beneficial to parents suffering the loss of a newborn. The researcher analyzed the data from Likert scale questionnaires administered to grieving parents. The sample population included parents who had experienced the loss of a viable newborn within the last calendar year. Parents were members of a national grief support group. Analysis of three major categories of acknowledgement of the newborn, education, information, or written materials; and general emotional support revealed that interventions acknowledging the newborn were the most beneficial to grieving parents.

The study's findings correlate with a study by Sexton and Stephen. Acknowledgement of the newborn included receiving photographs, footprints, hat, blanket, and lock of hair and ability to hold the newborn.

Critique: A replication of this study with a different sample group whose members were not in a support group might reveal different data. The interventions preferred reflect those most advocated in the event of a neonatal death.

Nursing implications of this study only emphasize the importance of the acknowledgement of the newborn, despite the primary impetus to provide emotional support in the event of a neonatal death.

Calhoun, L. K. (1994). Parents' perceptions of nursing support following neonatal loss. *Journal of Perinatal and Neonatal Nursing, 8*(2), 57–66.

eration. (See Chap. 14 for a detailed discussion of genetic disorders.)

Approximately 2% of newborns are born with abnormalities that significantly alter the structure and function of their bodies. Prevention, detection, and various treatment modalities are improving. As a result of the varied and complex nature of congenital and genetic disorders, an organized multidisciplinary approach is required, including medical, surgical, rehabilitation, financial, and community health resources. Enormous psychological and financial burdens can be overwhelming to the parents without competent resources at their disposal.

Congenital Heart Disease

For a review of the changes in the fetal circulation after birth see Chapter 7. Congenital heart disease has an incidence of about 7.5 per 1,000 births. Sick newborns requiring **cardiac catheterization** or cardiac surgery represent about 2.7 per 1,000 newborns (Flanagan et al., 1994). Most congenital heart disease is thought to be multifactorial in origin, implying both genetic and

environmental factors. Some congenital heart diseases are associated with syndromes, such as trisomy 21 and Turner's syndrome. Some defects are associated with maternal rubella exposure, maternal use of anticonvulsant medications, or maternal alcohol consumption.

Types of Congenital Cardiac Anomalies

Major types of congenital cardiac anomalies are illustrated and described in Figure 42-2. Although more than 100 different types of physiologic cardiac anomalies are known, ventricular septal defect is the most common congenital heart defect found in newborns. Others that are more common include transposition of the great arteries, coarctation of the aorta, and hypoplastic left heart (Heymann et al., 1993).

In the absence of respiratory disease, the presence of cyanosis is usually the result of a serious cardiac defect. Cyanotic defects include transposition of the great arteries, tetralogy of Fallot, pulmonary stenosis, tricuspid atresia, total anomalous pulmonary verous return, truncus arteriosus, and hypoplastic left heart syndrome.

Acyanotic cardiac defects include coarctation of the aorta, aortic stenosis, myocardial disease, tricuspid valve disease, ventricular septal defect, and endocardial cushion defects.

Assessment

The nurse reviews the history for evidence of familial congenital heart defects. The nurse assesses the newborn for possible signs, including cyanosis, respiratory distress, congestive heart failure, diminished peripheral pulses, abnormal cardiac rhythm, and abnormal heart sounds. The nurse also assesses the newborn for evidence of diminished cardiac output and decreased tissue perfusion. The newborn with congestive heart failure, which implies that the heart is unable to pump effectively enough to meet the body's circulatory requirements, may exhibit the following signs and symptoms:

- Tachycardia
- Tachypnea
- Cardiac enlargement
- Gallop rhythm
- Diminished peripheral pulses
- Decreased urine output
- Diaphoresis
- Edema
- Hepatomegaly
- Failure to thrive
- Feeding problems

Various diagnostic tests, including arterial blood gases, chest x-ray, electrocardiogram, echocardiogram, and cardiac catheterization, may be used. Whether cardiac catheterization is used in the neonatal period de-

Transposition of the great arteries

This anomaly is an embryologic defect caused by a straight division of the bulbar trunk without normal spiraling. As a result, the aorta originates from the right ventricle, and the pulmonary artery from the left ventricle. An abnormal communication between the two circulations must be present to sustain life.

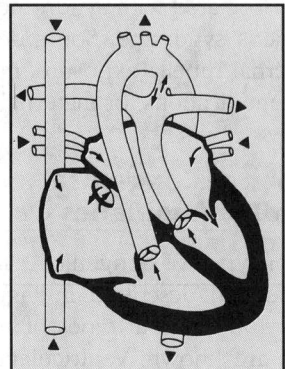

Atrial septal defect

An atrial septal defect is an abnormal opening between the right and left atria. Basically, three types of abnormalities result from incorrect development of the atrial septum. An incompetent foramen ovale is the most common defect. The high ostium secundum defect results from abnormal development of the septum secundum. Improper development of the septum primum produces a basal opening known as an ostium primum defect, frequently involving the atrioventricular valves. In general, left to right shunting of blood occurs in all atrial septal defects.

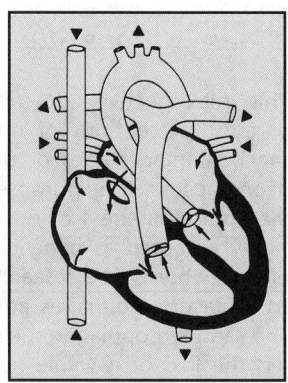

Patent ductus arteriosus

The patent ductus arteriosus is a vascular connection that, during fetal life, short circuits the pulmonary vascular bed and directs blood from the pulmonary artery to the aorta. Functional closure of the ductus normally occurs soon after birth. If the ductus remains patent after birth, the direction of blood flow in the ductus is reversed by the higher pressure in the aorta.

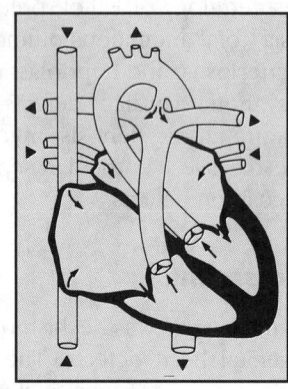

Ventricular septal defect

A ventricular septal defect is an abnormal opening between the right and left ventricle. Ventricular septal defects vary in size and may occur in either the membranous or muscular portion of the ventricular septum. Due to higher pressure in the left ventricle, a shunting of blood from the left to right ventricle occurs during systole. If pulmonary vascular resistance produces pulmonary hypertension, the shunt of blood is then reversed from the right to the left ventricle resulting in cyanosis.

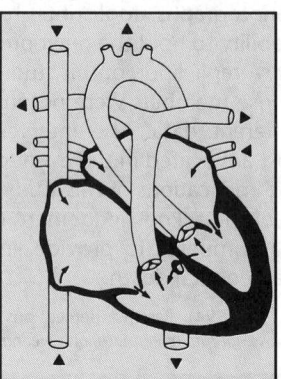

Coarctation of the aorta

Coarctation of the aorta is characterized by a narrowed aortic lumen. It exists as a preductal or postductal obstruction, depending on the position of the obstruction in relation to the ductus arteriosus. Coarctations exist with great variation in anatomical features. The lesion produces an obstruction to the flow of blood through the aorta causing an increased left ventricular pressure and work load.

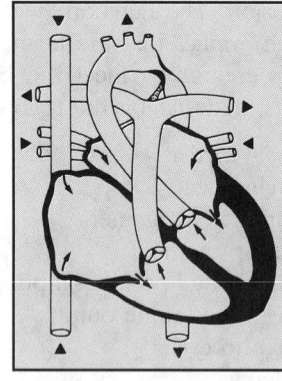

Tetralogy of Fallot

Tetralogy of Fallot is characterized by the combination of four defects—(1) pulmonary stenosis, (2) ventricular septal defect, (3) overriding aorta, and (4) hypertrophy of right ventricle. It is the most common defect causing cyanosis in patients surviving beyond two years of age. The severity of symptoms depends on the degree of pulmonary stenosis, the size of the ventricular septal defect, and the degree to which the aorta overrides the septal defect.

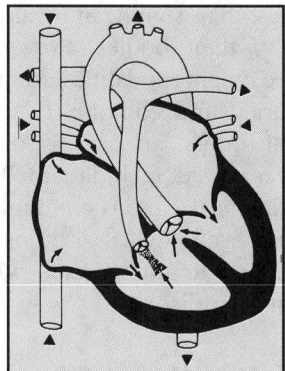

FIGURE 42–2 Six types of congenital heart anomalies. (Courtesy of Ross Laboratories.)

pends on the accuracy of other diagnostic tests and the type of defect suspected, whether cyanotic or acyanotic, and whether there is an increase or decrease in pulmonary blood flow.

The data obtained from a cardiac catheterization can indicate anatomic defects, pressure changes and oxygen saturation of blood in the chambers of the heart and great vessels, and changes in cardiac output or stroke volume. Complications of this procedure include hemorrhage, arrhythmias, infection, reactions to dye, and obstruction in the vessels. The data obtained from this procedure can assist the surgical team greatly if surgery is warranted. Once the lesion is definitely identified, the decision of whether medical or surgical intervention is the best approach can be made. Various surgical procedures may be used, depending on the type and extent of the defect. An example of the surgery used to repair pulmonary atresia or any other lesion requiring an increase in pulmonary blood flow is the Blalock-Taussig shunt. In this procedure, the subclavian artery is anastomosed to the pulmonary artery with or without a Gortex graft.

Nursing Diagnoses

Once assessment is completed, potential nursing diagnoses can be identified. For a list of possible nursing diagnoses, see Box 42-2.

Planning and Nursing Interventions

When the newborn is suspected of having congenital heart disease, the nurse gathers assessment data to plan ongoing care for the newborn. A cardiopulmonary monitor and pulse oximeter are used to assist in identifying bradycardia, tachycardia, arrhythmias, or any impairment in gas exchange. The newborn is observed for any indications of respiratory distress, and oxygen is administered as required. The newborn may be placed in an infant seat to facilitate respiratory effort. A neutral thermal environment is indicated to minimize energy expenditure and oxygen consumption. Fluid and electrolyte balance is maintained by monitoring intake and output and recording daily weights. Oral feedings may be tiring for the newborn as he or she attempts to coordinate sucking, swallowing, and breathing. Frequent rest periods are needed to avoid excess energy expenditure. Anticipating feedings is helpful to avoid excess crying and fatigue. Alternate feeding methods, such as gavage, may be needed (Merenstein et al., 1989).

Medications, such as antiarrhythmics, antihypertensives, diuretics, and sympathomimetics, may be administered. Prostaglandins, such as indomethacin, may be administered to maintain patency of the ductus arteriosus to promote oxygenation of major organs. Follow-

---

BOX 42-2
Nursing Diagnoses: Congenital Heart Defect

- Ineffective Breathing Patterns related to congestive heart failure
- Impaired Gas Exchange related to interference with blood flow resulting from cardiac defect
- Activity Intolerance related to limited energy expenditures and difficulty with ventilation
- Altered Nutrition: Less than body requirements related to
  - Difficulty breathing, sucking, and swallowing
  - Easy fatigability
- Fluid Volume Excess related to congestive heart failure and cardiac defect
- Risk for Injury related to physiologic effects of defect or treatment
- Altered Cardiopulmonary Tissue Perfusion related to diminished oxygen saturation resulting from congenital heart defect
- Knowledge Deficit (parental) related to cardiac defect, treatments, procedure, and care

---

ing cardiac catheterization, the equality of peripheral pulses and the temperature and color of the affected extremity are monitored. Following surgery, the newborn is observed closely in the intensive care unit. Monitors are used for constant recording of vital signs, including blood pressure. All readings should be compared with the baseline information. The nurse should be alert to possible environmental and anesthetic influences that may decrease the temperature initially. In addition, some temperature elevation due to the inflammatory process may be noted in the first 24 to 48 hours postoperatively. Any temperature elevation after this time may indicate infection.

All intravenous lines, sites, and dressings are observed and changed as needed. An intra-arterial line with heparinized saline is suggested. Central venous pressure readings are taken frequently. Respiratory status is monitored carefully. Turning, chest physiotherapy, and assessment of breath sounds are essential respiratory care measures. Suctioning accompanied by prebagging and postbagging with oxygen may be necessary to remove secretions. Chest tubes in place postoperatively are checked for adequate functioning. The color and amount of drainage are noted.

Fluid and electrolyte requirements are calculated according to the newborn's weight and laboratory reports. Initially, parenteral fluids are used until feedings are gradually resumed. Blood replacement may be necessary. Frequent monitoring of hematocrit, hemoglobin, and blood levels is essential.

Prior to discharge and community-based home care, parents need caregiving experience and detailed discharge instructions. Explanations of the heart defect medication's instructions, signs and symptoms to observe, and guidelines for care are provided. Parents should be instructed to phone the physician if the following signs or symptoms are noted.

- Poor feeding
- Diaphoresis
- Persistent vomiting
- Increased respiratory rate or distress
- Weight loss or failure to gain weight
- Frequent colds

Evaluation

Possible anticipated outcomes include the following:

- The newborn remains free of injury caused by the congenital cardiac defect.
- The newborn displays signs of adequate circulating oxygen.

- The newborn demonstrates adequate weight gain and growth.
- The newborn displays increasing tolerance of feedings and other activities.
- The parents demonstrate adequate knowledge of defect and treatment.
- The parents demonstrate ability to care for newborn following discharge.

Cleft Lip and Cleft Palate

Cleft lip and **cleft palate,** a congenital fissure or opening in the lip or palate that may occur separately or in combination, result from the failure of the soft or bony tissues of the palate and the upper jaw to unite during the fifth to 12th weeks of gestation. The defect commonly may be unilateral or bilateral. Rarely, the defect may be midline and incomplete or complete. Only the lip may be involved, or the disunion may extend into the upper jaw or the nasal cavity (Fig. 42-3).

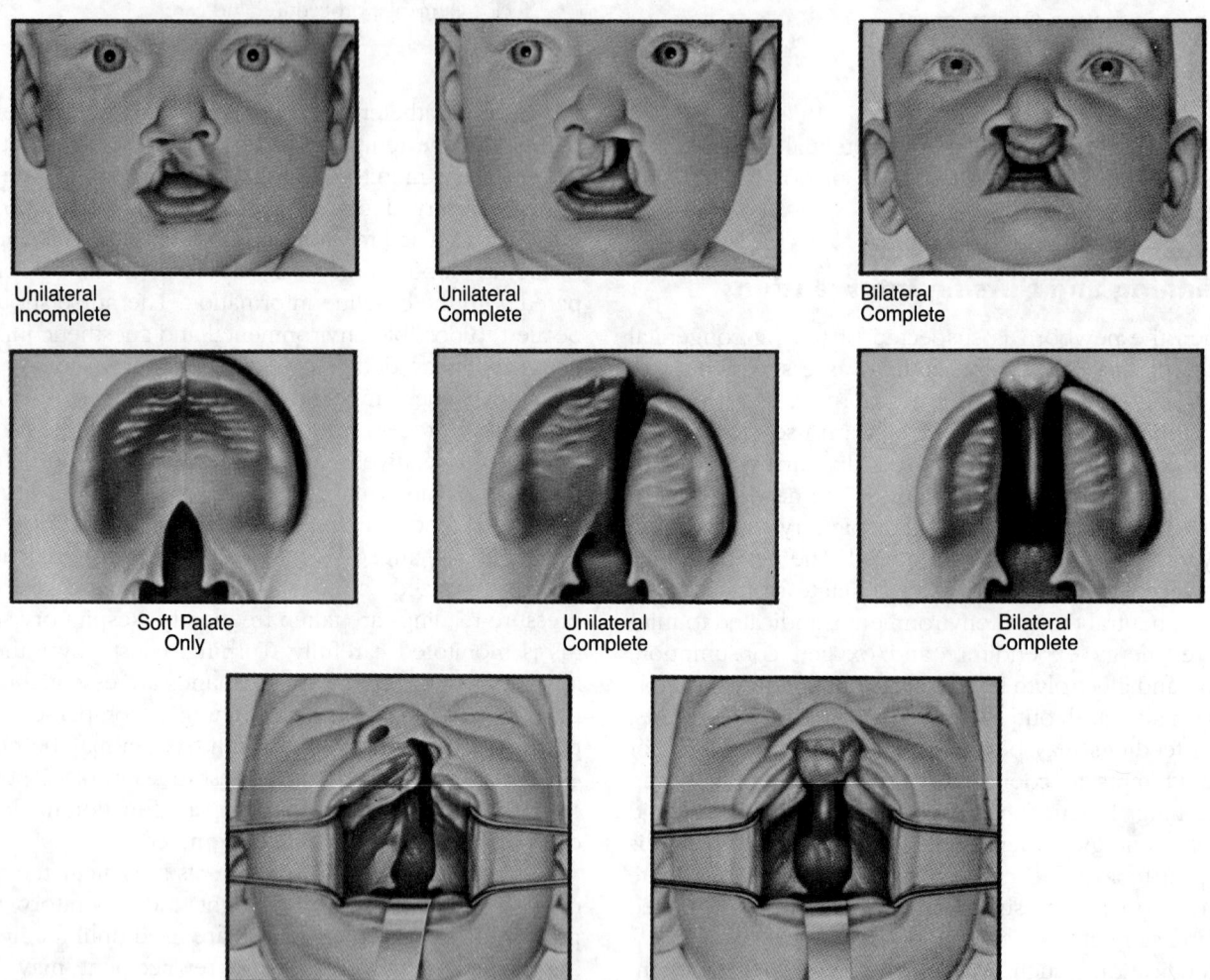

Unilateral
Incomplete

Unilateral
Complete

Bilateral
Complete

Soft Palate
Only

Unilateral
Complete

Bilateral
Complete

Unilateral
Complete

Bilateral
Complete

FIGURE 42-3 Illustrations of cleft lip and cleft palate. (Redrawn from drawing provided by Ross Laboratories.)

Each year, about 1 in 700 newborns are born with a cleft lip or cleft palate, making this condition one of the most common birth defects (Guzzetta et al., 1994). More boys than girls are affected by the combination cleft lip and cleft palate disorder. Cleft palate alone has an increased incidence in girls. These disorders may be associated with other syndromes. Multiple genetic influences may be involved.

Surgery for cleft lip repair is most often accomplished at approximately 3 months; for cleft palate, surgery occurs at 9 to 12 months. When surgery is performed later, a prosthetic speech device usually is fitted so that speech development is not hindered. Cleft palates usually involve other difficulties, such as recurrent ear infections and speech problems. Therefore, these children require coordinated, multidisciplinary care. Professionals from a craniofacial team may include a pediatrician, audiologist, otolaryngologist, speech pathologist, geneticist, dental specialists, plastic surgeon, pedodontist, orthodontist, nurses, and social workers (Guzzetta et al., 1994).

Nursing Assessment

Early assessment should be made by the craniofacial team. The newborn is assessed for the severity of the defect; he or she also is assessed thoroughly for any respiratory distress, airway obstruction, and feeding ability and tolerance.

Nursing Diagnoses

Once assessment is completed, potential nursing diagnoses can be identified. For a list of possible nursing diagnoses, see Box 42-3.

Planning and Intervention

The nurse provides the family with clear explanations and addresses questions as needed. The family should see the newborn immediately after birth, emphasizing the positive aspects of the newborn's appearance. The nurse should demonstrate acceptance of the newborn in the same manner as with all the other newborns in the nursery. Nurses can expect that parents will display grief behaviors and need to ventilate. The nurse should encourage parental involvement with caretaking because bonding may be initially delayed. Providing assistance with feeding may help to decrease any parental anxieties.

Feeding. Potential feeding problems may include ineffective sucking and difficulty swallowing properly. Secretions pool in the nasopharynx and predispose the newborn to aspiration.

The newborn also can have difficulty creating an effective seal for sucking, so nutritional intake could be compromised. The nurse needs to consider the variables affecting the situation, such as the severity of the defect, and promote the most natural feeding method possible.

Newborns with less severe defects may be able to breast-feed successfully. The mother can be instructed to stimulate the let-down reflex with the use of a breast pump. The nurse may refer the mother to a lactation specialist or home health agency for further assistance after discharge.

For bottle-fed newborns, special types of long nipples and soft bottles are available (Fig. 42-4). The parents should be instructed to hold the newborn as upright as possible during the feeding and to aim the nipple toward the intact part of the palate. The caregiver may need to squeeze the bottle to assist the newborn. An acrylic prosthetic device may be used to create a seal over the defect. Occasionally, other feeding methods, such as gavage feeding or rubber-tipped asepto syringe feeders, may be necessary.

Preoperative and Postoperative Interventions. Prior to surgery, parents require information concerning the surgery, such as the type of anesthesia, extent of parental involvement and participation permitted, and special types of restraints and other apparatus to be expected postoperatively. Postoperatively, elbow restraints to prevent flexion may be required. Lip care as prescribed is carried out. The use of a **Logan's bow** (a wire bow taped to both cheeks) is optional to prevent tension on the suture line.

Most centers resume feedings 24 hours after lip surgery and 48 hours after palate surgery (Curtin, 1990). During the first 24 hours, children with palate repairs may have a suture passed through the tip of the tongue and secured to the cheek to maximize airway management. A mist tent may be used to treat upper airway congestion.

BOX 42-3
Nursing Diagnoses: Cleft Lip and Palate

- Altered Nutrition: Less than body requirements related to inability to suck adequately or create an effective seal
- Risk for Aspiration related to difficulty clearing airway
- Risk for Injury related to special devices for feeding
- Risk for Infection related to retained secretions
- Knowledge Deficit (parental) related to cleft lip and palate, treatments, procedures, possible surgery, and care

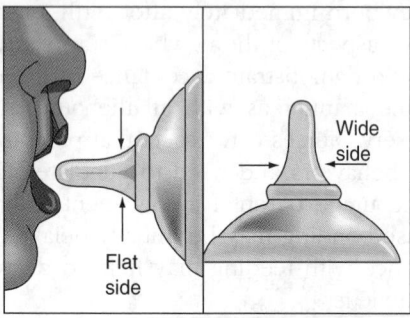

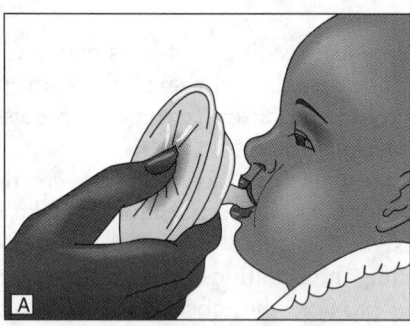

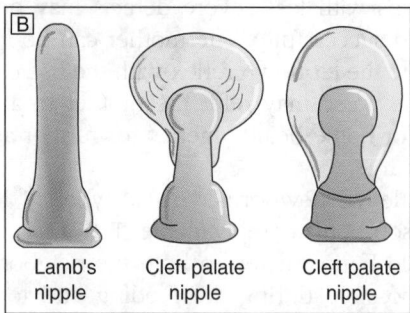

FIGURE 42–4 Nipples used for feeding newborns with cleft lip and palate. (**A**) Beniflex Nurser. (**B**) Other types of nipples. (Beniflex Nurser courtesy of Mead Johnson.)

Evaluation

As a result of appropriate nursing interventions, possible anticipated outcomes may include the following:

- The family demonstrates an adequate knowledge base to care for the newborn.
- The family verbalizes feelings and concerns related to grief.
- The newborn is free of signs of respiratory distress and infection.
- The newborn demonstrates adequate growth and weight gain.
- The newborn demonstrates increased nutritional intake for body requirements.

Hypospadias

Hypospadias is a disorder in which the urethral meatus lies somewhere proximal to the tip of the glans penis, either on the ventral surface of the glans or penile

shaft or in severe cases, on the perineum. In contrast, **epispadias** is a congenital anomaly in which the urethral meatus is located on the dorsal surface of the penis (Fig. 42-5). Epispadias is usually associated with exstrophy of the bladder, but it also may be a solitary defect.

Hypospadias is the second most common genital abnormality (after cryptorchidism) in the male newborn (Danish, 1992). Newborns with hypospadias have familial histories. Severe hypospadias may be associated with other genital abnormalities, such as endocrine, intersex, or chromosomal abnormalities.

Management

Management includes obtaining a maternal history for evidence of possible maternal progestin or estrogen exposure and family history of hypospadias, endocrine, or other intersex problems. Maternal progestin exposure may have occurred at 8 to 14 weeks' gestation.

The newborn is assessed for the extent of hypospadias and for any urinary tract abnormalities. Sexual organs are evaluated to rule out the possibility of intersex problems. Circumcision is withheld, selection of sex is accomplished, and the newborn is evaluated for any rare associated syndromes. Ideally, surgical repair is carried out during the first year of life. A severe form of hypospadias may require staged surgeries (Danish, 1992).

Intersex Problems

Any discrepancy in the genetic, gonadal, or genital makeup of a person is defined as an intersex problem.

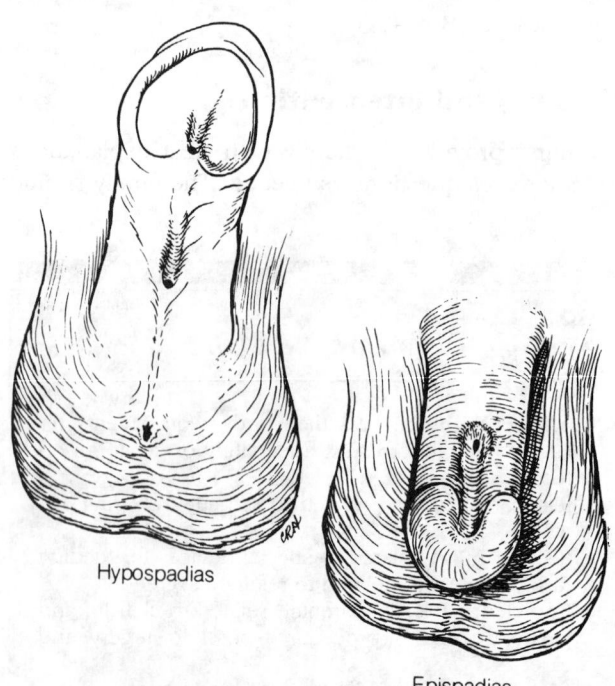

FIGURE 42–5 Hypospadias and epispadias.

Ambiguous genitalia is one sign that the newborn has an intersex problem. Most intersex newborns have some abnormality of the external genitalia (Fig. 42-6). (See Chap. 7 for normal fetal differentiation and Chap. 14 for genetic defects in sex chromosomes.) It is essential to identify and diagnose intersex problems quickly to provide sex assignment, identify any associated anomalies requiring treatment, provide genetic counseling, and correct problems early so that the client will have a strong sense of gender identity. The complexity and number of intersex problems are beyond the scope of this text; the reader is referred to the suggested reading list.

Management

If an intersex problem is suspected, such as ambiguous genitalia, the parents should be told that sexual assignment (whether the newborn will be designated male or female) is delayed until definitive diagnostic evaluation is made. This should require only 2 to 3 days. Diagnostic evaluation begins with a history, physical examination, and chromosomal analysis. Various biochemical studies and hormonal assays are completed. Internal genital structures are assessed using endoscopy. Based on complex selection criteria, sex is selected. Subsequent management of the client may involve hormonal treatment and reconstructive surgery.

Surgery for the client to be reared as a girl should be completed in the first year. Surgery for the client to be reared as a boy should be done in infancy so that he can stand to urinate and have a normal genital appearance (Danish, 1992). The family is provided with genetic counseling once the specific diagnosis is known.

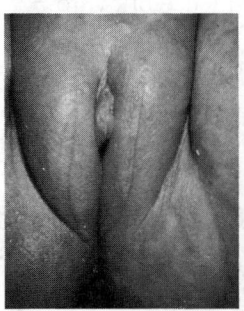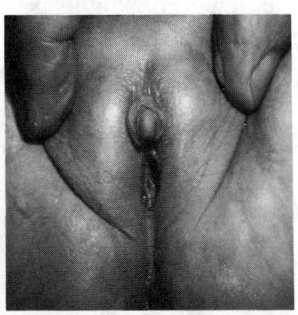

FIGURE 42-6 Ambiguous genitalia. This newborn was considered a normal girl at birth. At 6 months, a nurse practitioner questioned the nature of the symmetrical masses in the labia majora (*left*). Spreading the labia (*right*) discloses the obvious enlargement of the phallus and foreshortened introitus. Throughout the diagnostic procedures and following surgical procedures, every effort was made to support the parents by assuring them that the gender role assigned at birth remained correct. This case underscores the importance of careful examination of neonatal genitalia. (Source: Oski, F. A., DeAngelis, C. D., Feigin, R. D., & Warshaw, J. B. [1994]. *Principles and practice of pediatrics*. Philadelphia: J.B. Lippincott.)

Spina Bifida

Spina bifida, a common malformation (1 in 500 live births) involving the closure of the spinal cord, is the result of the congenital lack of one or more vertebral arches, usually at the lumbar site. When the membranes covering the spinal cord bulge through the opening, the condition is known as **meningocele.** It forms a soft, fluctuating tumor filled with cerebrospinal fluid. The extrusion of the cord along with the meninges is known as **meningomyelocele. Spina bifida occulta** is the failure of the vertebrae to close without any herniation of the membranes or spinal cord (Fig. 42-7*A–D*). The degree of neurologic deficit associated with the malformation is determined by the level of lesion.

The decision to intervene surgically is made by the physician and family, bearing in mind the associated complications and long-term follow-up required. Surgical closure should take place within the first few hours of life to prevent infection and further deterioration of the spinal cord and roots. Depending on the site of the lesion, hydrocephalus may develop, requiring serial shunting procedures. Computed tomography or magnetic resonance imaging scans can define the type and severity of hydrocephalus. The bowel and bladder frequently are involved. Orthopedic devices and surgery may be required, depending on the site of the lesion.

Assessment

The family's level of understanding, strengths, coping strategies, and grief is evaluated. The degree of neurologic impairment is determined. The newborn is assessed for associated bowel and bladder complications and motor and sensory functions of the lower extremities. Because there is a strong association with hydrocephalus, the newborn is assessed for possible signs and symptoms.

Nursing Diagnoses

After completing the assessment, potential nursing diagnoses can be identified. For a list of possible nursing diagnoses, see Box 42-4. Nursing diagnoses also are highlighted in the Nursing Care Plan: Family of the Neonate With Meningomyelocele and the nursing care plan regarding grief found earlier in this chapter.

Planning and Intervention

Immediately after identification, the sac is covered with sterile saline gauge. The nurse positions the newborn comfortably and protects the sac from trauma and infection.

Preoperatively, the nurse provides parental support and referral to the appropriate healthcare profession-

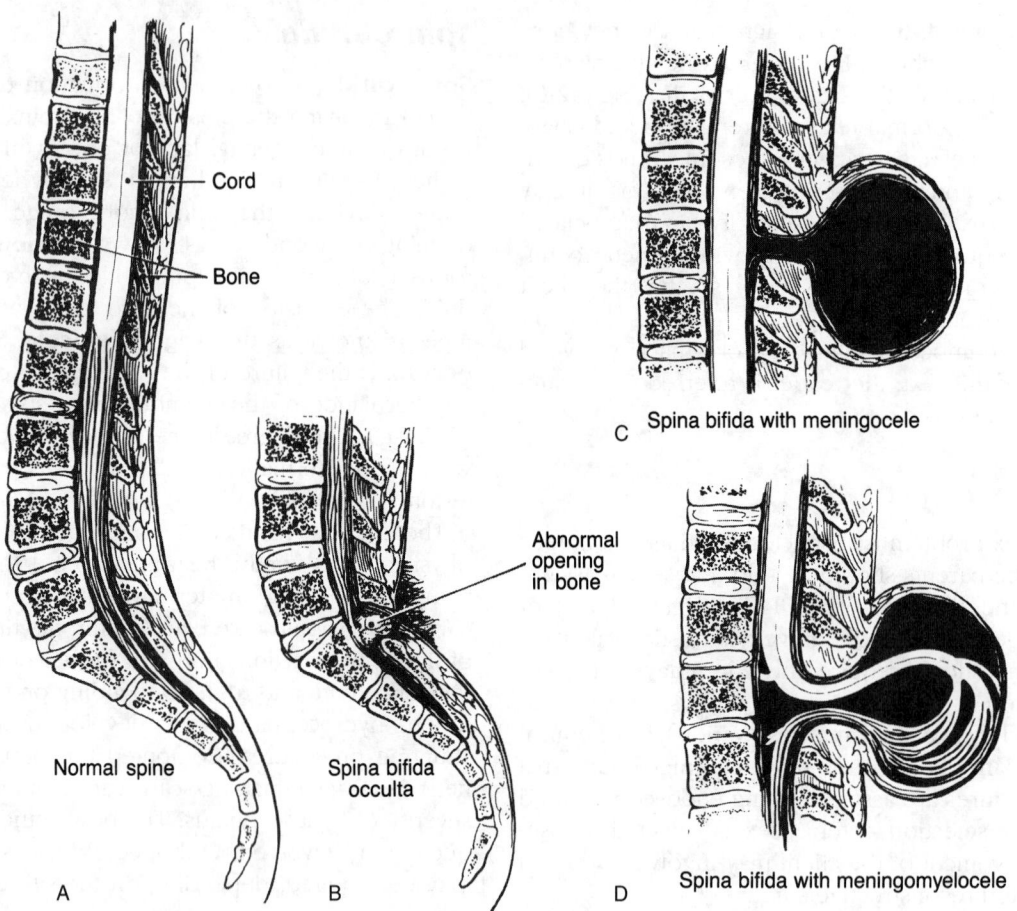

Cord

Bone

Normal spine

A

Spina bifida occulta

B

Abnormal opening in bone

C Spina bifida with meningocele

D Spina bifida with meningomyelocele

FIGURE 42-7 Spina bifida.

als, especially physicians and spina bifida specialist, social service, home healthcare, and parental support groups. The nurse provides information to the parents and promotes caretaking and bonding activities.

Postoperatively, the nurse positions the newborn, usually in the prone or the lateral positions to keep the incisional site free from infection. Meticulous skin care and ongoing assessments are crucial. The nurse evaluates the newborn's bowel and bladder function, noting patterns and assisting with elimination measures as necessary. The bladder may need to be emptied by **Credé's method** (manual bladder compression used to stimulate urination).

Passive range of motion exercises are performed to the lower extremities. Physical therapists may be helpful in providing appropriate exercises.

Evaluation

As a result of interventions, possible anticipated outcomes may include the following:

■ The newborn exhibits stable vital signs.
■ The newborn maintains optimal motor and sensory function.

■ The newborn remains free of discomfort.
■ The newborn exhibits no decrease in bowel and bladder function.
■ The newborn exhibits no evidence of hydrocephalus.
■ Parents demonstrate positive adaptation to newborn's condition.

BOX 42-4
Nursing Diagnoses: Spina Bifida

■ Impaired Skin Integrity related to protruding sac
■ Risk for Impaired Skin Integrity related to immobility and surgery
■ Bowel Incontinence related to level of spinal cord involvement
■ Altered Urinary Elimination related to level of spinal cord involvement
■ Altered Cerebral Tissue Perfusion related to hydrocephalus
■ Risk for Infection related to protruding sac
■ Risk for Injury related to degree of neurologic impairment

NURSING CARE PLAN
The Family of the Neonate with Meningomyelocele

Nursing Goals
1. The neonate's lesion site is identified early, and spinal cord involvement is established.
2. The neonate remains sepsis free.
3. The neonate does not experience trauma to the lower extremities.
4. Any developing hydrocephalus or increased intracranial pressure is identified.
5. The neonate's bowel and bladder functions are maintained.
6. The parents are knowledgeable regarding long-term care and prognosis.
7. The parents exhibit caretaking skills.
8. The parents use referrals and multidisciplinary care as necessary.

Assessment	*Potential Nursing Diagnoses*	*Intervention/ Rationale*	*Evaluation*
Neural tube dysfunction detected by alpha-feto-protein levels prenatally Herniated sac noted at delivery Increased head circumference Bulging fontanels Urinary retention Urinary dribbling Constipation Diminished sensation and movement below the level of the defect	Impaired Skin Integrity related to sac and surgical site	Place neonate in prone position with buttocks higher than head *to decrease pressure on sac and avoid rupture of sac* Cover sac with moist sterile dressing *to maintain sac integrity* Observe sac for fluid leakage *to detect and prevent meningitis* Use transparent occlusive dressing on buttocks *to prevent contamination of sac or surgical incision* Observe neonate frequently for signs and symptoms of infection *to permit prompt treatment*	Neonate remains free of sepsis
	Potential for Impaired Skin Integrity related to altered mobility	Maintain clean, dry, supportive bed *to avoid skin irritation* Change position at least every 2 hours and massage pressure points *to avoid skin breakdown* Provide passive ROM to extremities as prescribed by physical therapy *to prevent contractures* Observe for signs of skin breakdown *to provide early treatment*	Neonate's skin remains intact, without pressure areas Extremities are free of contractures
	Altered Bowel and Urinary Elimination related to level of spinal cord involvement	Observe, record, and report bowel movement pattern *to recognize early bowel dysfunction* Assess anal sphincter functioning by stimulation *to note any abnormalities* Note frequency, amount, and urine stream patterns *to assess bladder function*	Neonate exhibits normal bowel pattern Neonate exhibits normal elimination pattern without signs and symptoms of infection

(continued)

NURSING CARE PLAN *(Continued)*
The Family of the Neonate with Meningomyelocele

Assessment	Potential Nursing Diagnoses	Intervention/ Rationale	Evaluation
		Maintain intake and output records *to detect adequate output*	
		Use intermittent catheterization *to assure complete bladder emptying and decreasing potential for infection*	
	Altered Tissue Perfusion, cerebral, related to hydrocephalus	Daily head circumference measures *to detect possible increase in intracranial pressure*	Neonate exhibits no sign of increased intracranial pressure
		Assess neurologic status q 2–4 hours, noting irritability, bulging fontanels, seizures, *to obtain a baseline and detect any changes indicative of hydrocephalus*	
	Parental Anxiety related to uncertainty of long-term prognosis	Allow parents to discuss feelings, prognosis, and ask questions *to acknowledge feelings and obtain information*	Parents are knowledgeable regarding long-term care and prognosis
		Provide teaching sessions and written materials on caregiving skills *to reinforce learning and diminish anxiety when questions arise.* Refer to support groups or other appropriate resources *to assure ongoing follow-up and support.*	Parents exhibit caretaking skills
			Parents use referrals and multidisciplinary care as necessary

- Parents discuss their feelings and concerns openly, asking pertinent questions.
- Parents demonstrate appropriate caretaking skills, using support services as needed.

Hydrocephalus

Hydrocephalus results from an excess accumulation of cerebrospinal fluid in the ventricles of the brain. Normal cerebrospinal fluid circulation is impaired. The abnormal accumulation of fluid may occur between the brain and dura mater (external) or in the ventricular system of the brain (internal). As a result of the enlarged head, the fetus is often breech, necessitating cesarean delivery as a result of cephalopelvic disproportion.

Assessment

The newborn's head is enlarged as a result of increased intraventricular cerebrospinal fluid pressure. Additional signs include "setting sun" appearance of the eyes, separated sutures, tense fontanels, and prominence of the forehead (Fig. 42-8). Neurologic deficits may result, despite surgical shunting.

Nursing Interventions

The nurse provides skin care to prevent pressure areas and infection of the skin. The head must be supported with care, especially during handling and feeding, to prevent trauma to the area. Documentation of possible signs of increased intracranial pressure, including tense, enlarged fontanels and suture separation, is essential. In

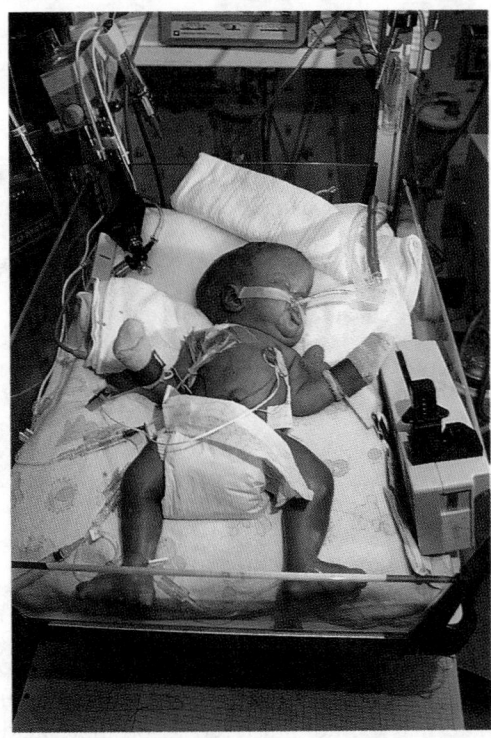

FIGURE 42-8 Hydrocephalus. Note the enlargement of the head and the prominent veins in the skin.

addition, the head circumference is serially assessed. If a shunt procedure is performed, the newborn's shunt site is assessed for signs and symptoms of infection. Initially, the newborn is positioned off the shunt site and in a flat plane to avoid sudden decompression and evacuation of the shunt. Parents are taught to assess the newborn for signs of increasing intracranial pressure and infection. Instructions about shunt care are provided.

Anencephaly

In **anencephaly,** there is complete or partial absence of the newborn's brain and of the skull overlying the brain. The cause is not known. Although there is a familial tendency, multiple environmental factors seem to be involved. Fifty percent of pregnancies involve polyhydramnios. If newborns survive labor and delivery, their life expectancy is short.

Nursing interventions

Supportive care is provided because the newborns seldom live more than a few days. The parents need much support in grieving and adjusting to this traumatic situation.

Microcephaly

In **microcephaly,** the head is generally well formed but small. The microcephalic newborn has an occipital frontal head circumference that is greater than three standard deviations below the mean on the growth chart or less than the third percentile on a growth chart. Microcephaly may be congenital or acquired. Congenital microcephaly may be associated with a maternal virus, or it may be the result of a chromosomal abnormality. Acquired microcephaly may occur as a result of maternal herpes, ischemic insults, hypothyroidism, or **aminoacidurias** (an excess of amino acids in the urine). Diagnostic evaluation includes a **TORCH** (T—Toxoplasmosis, O—Other, R—Rubella, C—Cytomegalovirus, H—Genital herpes) titer, skull x-rays, and amino acid screenings. No treatment is carried out.

Nursing interventions

The nurse is responsible for carefully assessing for any neurologic deficit, measuring head circumference on a daily basis, and assisting with diagnostic studies.

Congenital Diaphragmatic Hernia

Congenital diaphragmatic hernia is a condition involving incomplete embryonic development of the diaphragm, allowing the abdominal viscera to herniate into the thoracic cavity (Fig. 42-9).

This defect is caused by failure of the pleuroperitoneal cavity to fuse at 7 to 8 weeks' gestation. It is the most urgent neonatal emergency. Despite advances in

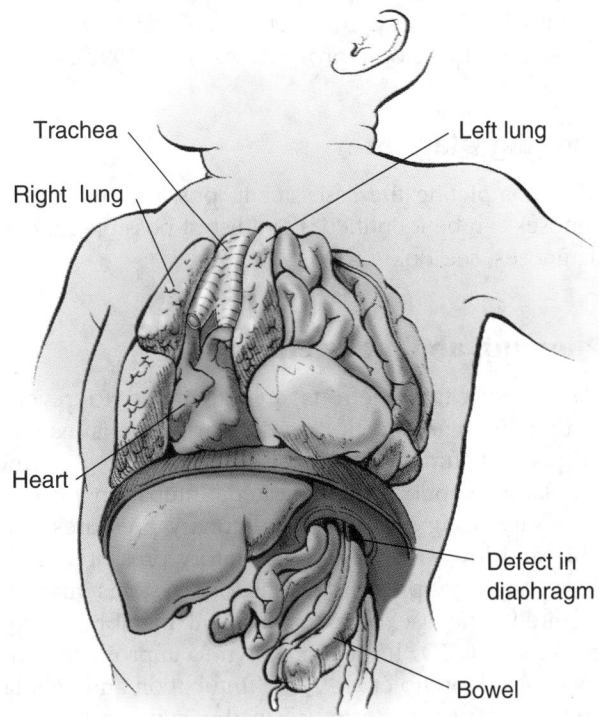

FIGURE 42-9 Diaphragmatic hernia showing abdominal contents within the thoracic cavity. This is considered a true pediatric emergency.

care, the mortality rate remains 50% to 80% (Moreno et al., 1993). The left side is affected in 80% to 85% of the cases because closure of the left posterolateral pleuroperitoneal membrane occurs later, and the right posterolateral pleuroperitoneal membrane is protected by the liver. Herniation of the small intestine with intestinal malrotation occurs in most cases, and about half involve herniation of the liver.

Lung maturity is arrested because varying degrees of pulmonary hypoplasia result. Other related lung disorders develop, including abnormalities of pulmonary arteries, decreased number of pulmonary vessels, and predisposition for persistent pulmonary hypertension (Theorell, 1990).

If prenatal diagnosis has already been confirmed, delivery should be arranged at a tertiary care center for optimum care. (See Chap. 39 for more information on fetal diagnosis and treatment.) The defect is surgically correctable by removing the herniated viscera from the thorax and repairing the diaphragm.

Assessment

The newborn is noted to be in varying degrees of respiratory distress, depending on the extent of lung hypoplasia. Because of the mediastinal shift, venous return is decreased, compromising cardiac output. The newborn may be cyanotic and in a shocky state. The most common defect is in the left diaphragm. Breath sounds may be decreased on the left side; a barrel or asymmetric chest may be observed. The abdomen is scaphoid and empty. In severe cases, the Apgar score is low and does not improve (Kent et al., 1992).

Nursing Diagnoses

After completing the assessment, possible nursing diagnoses can be identified. For a list of possible nursing diagnoses, see Box 42-5.

Planning and Intervention

Major resuscitation efforts are attempted to reverse cardiopulmonary shock. A nasogastric tube is inserted to prevent further bowel distension. Oxygen and ventilatory support are indicated. Intubation may be necessary using the lowest pulmonary pressures possible and low positive end-expiratory pressure. High-frequency, low-pressure ventilatory systems may be required. The use of extracorporeal membrane oxygenation (ECMO) has been shown to improve the survival rate (Moreno et al., 1993). Intubation and ventilation could promote rupture in the hypoplastic lung. The newborn requires close monitoring in case emergency surgery, such as a thoracotomy, is required.

BOX 42-5
Nursing Diagnoses: Congenital Diaphragmatic Hernia

- Impaired Gas Exchange related to hypoplastic lung syndrome
- Altered Cardiopulmonary Tissue Perfusion related to increased thoracic cavity pressure
- Ineffective Breathing Pattern related to pulmonary hypoplasia
- Inability to Sustain Spontaneous Ventilation related to pulmonary hypoplasia and increased thoracic cavity pressure
- Risk for Infection related to surgery

An intravenous line is inserted to administer vasopressors and volume expanders as ordered. Dopamine or tolazoline drips may be administered. Pulse oximetry and arterial blood gases are required for monitoring respiratory status. Medications such as sodium bicarbonate may be administered to promote acid–base balance.

Once the newborn is medically stable, surgical repair is performed. The transabdominal approach remains the method of choice; however, a transthoracic approach also may be used.

Postoperatively, the priority is the promotion of effective neonatal breathing patterns. Administration of oxygen and maintenance of assisted ventilation are essential. Other modes of ventilatory therapy, such as ECMO, have been used with some success (Roberts et al., 1990; Moreno et al., 1993). Prevention of respiratory complications, such as pneumothorax and acid–base imbalances, is a crucial element in care. Vasodilators and vasopressors may be necessary to promote adequate circulation. Some research has indicated that fentanyl and pancuronium may be useful in managing persistent pulmonary hypertension in the immediate postoperative period (Moreno et al., 1993).

Evaluation

The prognosis for the newborn with this severe respiratory involvement depends on the speed and efficiency of the management effort.

Possible anticipated outcomes may include the following:

- The newborn demonstrates respiratory parameters within normal limits.
- The newborn's vital signs and cardiopulmonary status are within normal limits.
- The newborn remains free of infection and complications.

Esophageal Atresia and Tracheoesophageal Fistula

Esophageal atresia and **tracheoesophageal fistula** (TEF) are common anomalies involving some interference that does not allow the esophagus and trachea to separate normally.

Esophageal atresia refers to an abnormal closure of the esophagus, resulting in a blind pouch. It may or may not be accompanied by an abnormal opening between the trachea and esophagus (TEF). The four types of esophageal atresia that occur are as follows:

- The esophagus ends in a blind pouch or is severely narrowed with no opening or connection to the trachea.
- The esophagus ends in a blind pouch with a fistula between the distal part of the esophagus and the trachea.
- The esophagus ends in a blind pouch with a fistula between the proximal part of the esophagus and the trachea.
- The esophagus ends in a blind pouch with numerous fistulas present between both widely spaced segments of the esophagus and trachea.

The most common type is esophageal atresia with a distal fistula to the trachea (occurrence rate of 85%–90%). Pure esophageal atresia with no connection to the trachea accounts for only a small portion of these defects. See Figure 42-10 for an illustration of the types of atresia.

Assessment

A history of polyhydramnios is common with newborn with esophageal atresia. Newborns with TEF have symptoms of esophageal obstruction or other respiratory complications. They appear to be "mucousy" and frequently cough or have choking episodes. Intermittent cyanosis may be noted. When the trachea and distal esophagus communicate anatomically, abdominal distension occurs. Crying and coughing lead to increasing air in the gastrointestinal tract and subsequent gastroesophageal reflux.

The diagnosis is confirmed by placing a nasogastric suction catheter tube. With esophageal atresia, the tube cannot be advanced beyond 10 cm. Radiographs also confirm placement of this catheter in the esophageal pouch and identify the TEF and air-filled esophagus. If the diagnosis is unclear at this point, small amounts of barium may be used to identify the blind pouch and fistula and then quickly suctioned to prevent aspiration.

Treatment

Various types of surgical options are available. Primary repair is best used for newborns who have no life-threatening abnormalities, have a stable respiratory

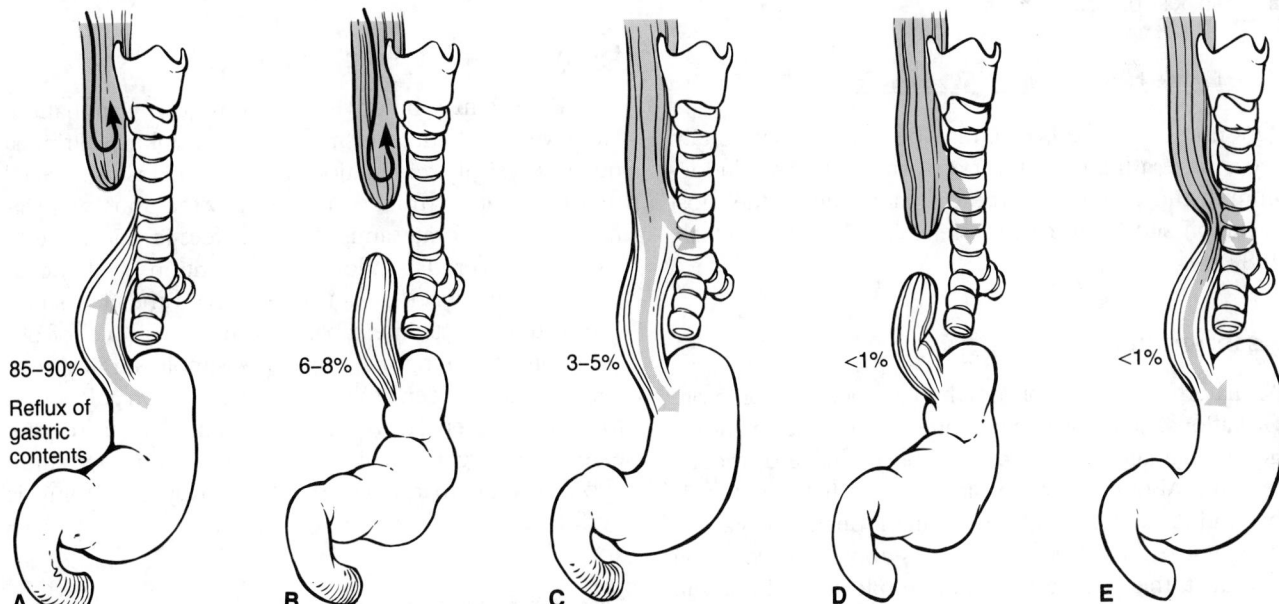

FIGURE 42-10 Tracheoesophageal abnormalities. Colored areas and arrows indicate path of feedings or oral secretions. (**A**) Blind pouch of upper esophageal segment with a fistula between lower segment and trachea. (**B**) Blind pouches of upper and lower segments. (**C**) Intact esophagus with tracheoesophageal fistula. (**D**) Blind pouches of both esophageal segments with fistula between upper segment and trachea. (**E**) Esophageal atresia with fistulas between both segments.

status, and weigh more than 2,000 g. Delayed surgical repair is chosen for full-term newborns who have pneumonia or other physiologic problems requiring diagnostic workup before surgery. Staged surgery is best used for preterm newborns, newborns with pneumonia or life-threatening anomalies, and complicated surgical cases (Ryckman et al., 1992).

Nursing interventions

When diagnosis is made and prior to surgery, the newborn is positioned in a 30-degree upright position. The administration of oxygen and positioning of a suction catheter are crucial interventions. Other anomalies must be recognized because treatment decisions might be affected. Significant coexisting anomalies occur in 30% to 40% of newborns with esophageal atresia. Newborns with TEF need close assessment of cardiac, renal, and skeletal systems. Postoperatively, a gastrostomy tube is in place for decompression and future feeding purposes. Nasotracheal intubation and low pressure ventilation are maintained until the respiratory status is stabilized. Total parenteral nutrition is maintained to provide nutritional support. Chest tube care is maintained. Ongoing assessment is essential. Nurses need to be alert for the following potential complications:

- Anastomotic leak
- Recurrent fistula
- Atelectasis and pneumonia
- Stricture
- Gastroesophageal reflux

Bowel Atresia and Stenosis

Any portion of the bowel may be narrow, but certain areas have a higher risk for abnormalities. The duodenum at the entrance of the common duct is the most common site for atresia or stenosis (Merenstein et al., 1989).

Assessment

A maternal history of polyhydramnios is common. Gestational age assessment often reveals a small-for-gestational-age newborn. Newborns have difficulty feeding. Abdominal distension occurs. If the defect is beyond the entrance of the common duct, bile-stained vomiting occurs. If the stenosis is above the common bile duct, the vomiting will not be bile stained but will contain saliva or undigested milk.

Treatment

Diagnosis is made by x-ray. A classic "double bubble" is seen on an abdominal upright film in duodenal atresia. Surgical repair may be accomplished by end-to-end anastomosis; if this is not possible, various types of ostomies are used.

Nursing

Preoperatively, an orogastric tube is inserted. This tube is maintained postoperatively to prevent abdominal distension. Fluids are administered intravenously. A central venous catheter, such as a Broviac catheter, may be inserted during surgery for administering total parenteral nutrition.

If an ostomy is created, the site is covered with a saline gauze dressing until the stoma begins to function. An appliance can then be applied. Accurate gastric output is monitored, because fluid and electrolyte balance depends on intravenous replacement of fluid losses.

Imperforate Anus

Imperforate anus consists of atresia of the anus. The defect may be low, stenosis of the anal opening or a membrane covering the normal anal opening, or high, termination of the rectum in a blind pouch or no communication between the normal anus and the rectum (Fig. 42-11). The defect may be accompanied by a fistula to the vagina, bladder, or urethra. Various anomalies are associated with imperforate anus, including urogenital, cardiac, and spinal cord anomalies; esophageal atresia; and TEF.

Diagnosis and Treatment

Low defects may be obvious on physical examination. However, high defects may be overlooked during a quick physical examination. Inability to insert a rectal thermometer or rubber catheter into the anus will signify an imperforate anus. If the defect is not immediately discovered, abdominal distention will occur when the newborn is not able to pass the first stool. Ultrasound assists in establishing the exact level of obstruction and ruling out a fistula. A simple surgical procedure may be performed during the neonatal period for low defects. However, most high defects require extensive surgery, which is usually postponed until about 1 year. In this case, a temporary colostomy is performed.

Omphalocele

Omphalocele is a congenital abdominal wall defect, in which a portion of the abdominal contents protrudes at the base of the umbilicus (Fig. 42-12). It occurs in 1 in 5,000 births.

Omphaloceles develop between the 10th and 12th weeks of fetal life. The mass is covered with a layer

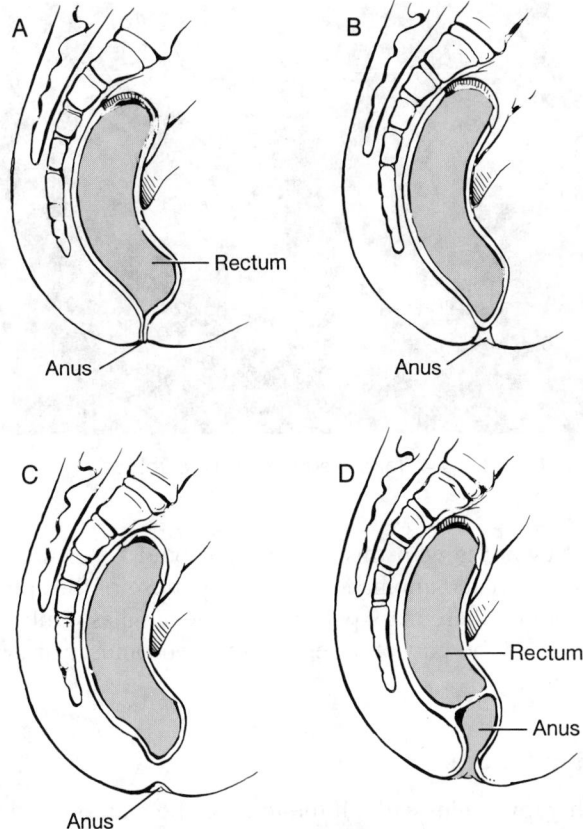

FIGURE 42–11 Types of imperforate anus. (**A**) Anal stenosis—Anal opening is present but constricted. (**B**) Membranous atresia—Anal and rectal structures appear normal except for a shiny, translucent membrane. (**C**) Anal agenesis—Rectum terminates in a blind pouch (80% of all anorectal abnormalities). (**D**) Rectal atresia—Anal canal is developed but does not communicate with the rectum.

of peritoneum and amnion and may rupture at delivery. Omphaloceles often are seen in conjunction with other cardiac, genitourinary, neurologic, or chromosomal anomalies.

Treatment

Surgery is indicated, and the repair should be prompt. A staged repair may be necessary. Various factors are considered when determining the individual surgical management for each client. Factors include the presence of an intact sac, size of eviscerated contents relative to the abdominal cavity, the nature of the herniated viscera, and the possibility of associated anomalies (Flake et al., 1992).

Nursing Interventions

Before surgery, the bowel should be cleansed gently and covered with a plastic sac, layer of plastic food wrap, or saline-soaked sponge covered with a dressing. This covering assists in maintaining thermoregulation by decreasing evaporative loss. It also prevents possible contamination and trauma to the defect. An orogastric tube is placed. The newborn should be positioned in the lateral position and the bowel supported to prevent injury to the mesenteric blood supply. Antibiotics are administered. Maintenance and replacement fluids are administered intravenously. Volume expanders, such as normal saline, albumin, or plasma protein fraction (Plasmanate), assist in maintaining intravascular integrity.

Postoperatively, the newborn may require a central venous catheter for long-term total parenteral nutrition. The nurse should be alert to several postoperative complications. Respiratory distress could occur as a result of the increase in abdominal pressure. Ventilatory assistance may be needed. The abdominal vessels may be compressed following surgical replacement of abdominal contents. The result can be a decrease in cardiac return. Edema of the lower extremities results from third spacing of fluid into tissue and an increase in extravascular volume. Elevation of the extremities may alleviate swelling.

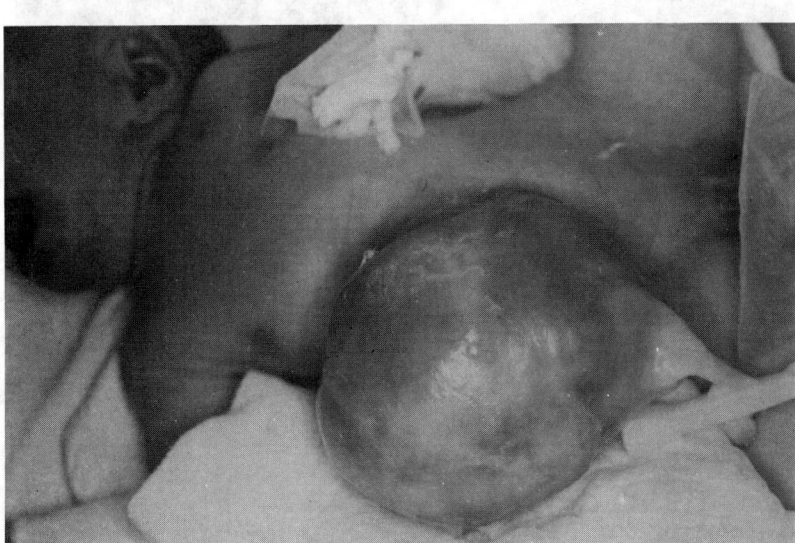

FIGURE 42–12 Large omphalocele. Note covering of the sac and its relationship to the umbilicus, which protrudes from the lower portion. (Avery, G. B. [1987]. *Neonatology: Pathophysiology and management of the newborn* [3rd ed.]. Philadelphia: J.B. Lippincott.)

Infection is a major potential postoperative problem, so broad-spectrum intravenous antibiotic therapy is continued, and the newborn is assessed for signs of sepsis. For newborns experiencing a staged repair, antimicrobial solutions are used to care for the silastic "pouch."

Thorough gastrointestinal system assessment and interventions remain a priority. The nurse monitors the newborn for signs and symptoms of complications, including vomiting, diarrhea, guaiac-positive stools, irritability, lethargy, and abdominal distension.

Gastroschisis

Gastroschisis is a condition similar to omphalocele, except that the abdominal wall defect is a distance from the umbilicus, and the abdominal organs are not contained by peritoneal membrane but rather spill from the abdomen freely. Newborns with gastroschisis are often small for gestational age and preterm. Unlike omphalocele, gastroschisis has few associated anomalies. The lesion is not covered with membrane, and the umbilical cord protrudes lateral to the defect in the abdominal wall. The herniated viscera is usually limited to the small intestine. Treatment is similar to that for omphalocele (Fig. 42-13).

Talipes Equinovarus (Clubfoot)

Talipes equinovarus (clubfoot), a musculoskeletal disorder, occurs twice as often in boys as in girls, with an overall incidence of 1 in 1,000 births (Cooperman, 1992). The three elements of this deformity are equinus or plantar flexion of the foot at the ankle, varus or inversion deformity of the heel, and forefoot adduction (Fig. 42-14). All three are present in classic talipes equinovarus.

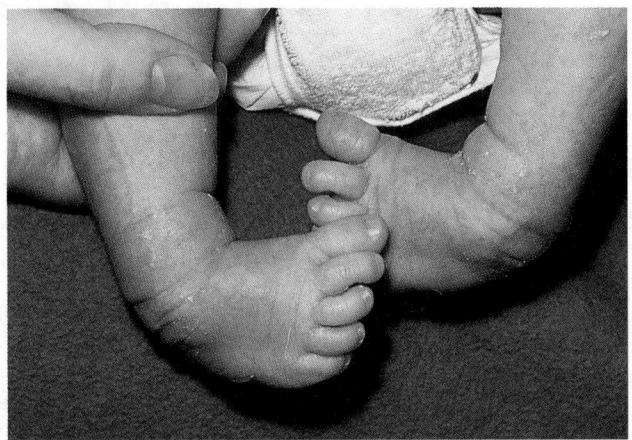

FIGURE 42–14 Talipes equinovarus (clubfoot).

Newborns with this deformity should be examined for associated anomalies, especially those of the spine. There is a hereditary pattern in some families. Clubfoot also may be part of a generalized neuromuscular syndrome.

Treatment

Therapy begins early. If the foot can be manipulated to the other direction, simple exercise may correct the abnormality. Plaster casts may be applied after the affected foot structures have been stretched and manipulated. Casts are applied sequentially, correcting first the forefoot adduction, then the heel inversion, and finally, the equinus flexion at the ankle. Serial casting is needed as the newborn grows.

After correction is obtained, braces are usually needed for months to years to prevent recurrences of the deformities. Surgery is rarely required (Griffin, 1994).

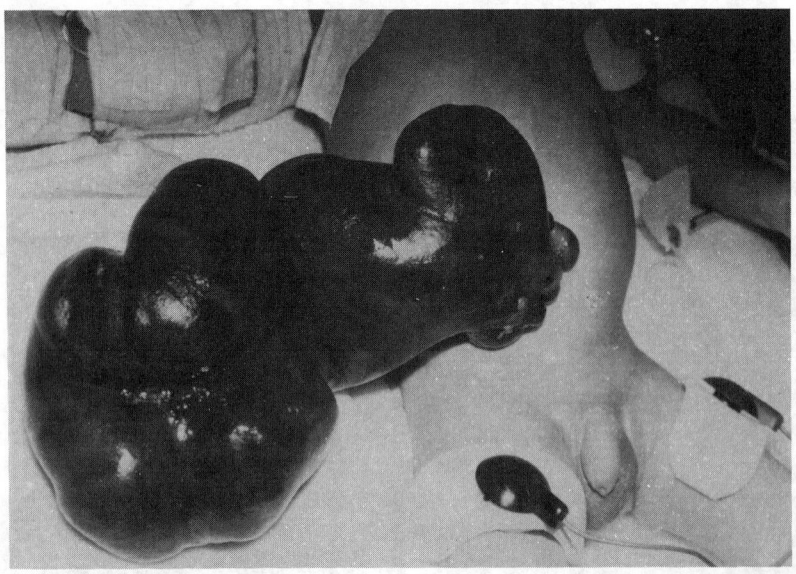

FIGURE 42–13 Client with gastroschisis. Note edematous, matted bowel, the result of the intestines floating freely in the amniotic fluid. Remarkably, these distorted viscera will ultimately fit back into the abdominal cavity and will finally assume a normal appearance and function. (Avery, G. B. [1987]. *Neonatology: Pathophysiology and management of the newborn* [3rd ed.]. Philadelphia: J.B. Lippincott.)

Congenital Hip Dysplasia

Congenital hip dysplasia refers to malformations of the hip involving various degrees of deformity that are present at birth. Congenital hip dysplasia occurs more frequently in girls than in boys. One-fourth of the cases are bilateral. If unilateral, the left hip more often is involved than the right. There is a significantly higher incidence of congenital hip disorders and breech presentation.

The hip may be dislocated or subluxated. Dislocation (luxation) refers to the femoral head lying outside the acetabulum but still within the stretched and elongated capsule. Subluxation of the femoral head refers to the head riding on the edge of the acetabulum.

When dislocation or subluxation occurs, acetabular dysplasia results.

Assessment

Ortolani's maneuver is carried out when the newborn is supine with the knees bent and hips flexed to 90 degrees and fully abducted (Fig. 42-15). When the hip is reduced by abduction, a click is felt as the femoral head slides across the posterior aspect of the acetabulum and enters the socket. With hip adduction, the femoral head redislocates out of the acetabulum with a click. The Ortolani test is positive in the dislocated hip until 6 to 8 weeks of age or longer (Griffin, 1994). Ultrasound also assists with physical assessment and diagnosis.

Treatment

Early diagnosis and intervention are essential for the prevention of this chronic deformity. No matter what type of deformity, the hip needs to be maintained in a position of flexion and abduction. Methods used include triple diapering and orthopedic splints, such as the Pavlik harness or Frejka pillow splint (Fig. 42-16).

If these methods are ineffective, a hip spica cast may be applied, followed by a brace. Successful treatment is usually accomplished in 3 to 4 months (Cooperman, 1992).

Nursing Interventions

Parents need education and support in applying corrective measures or appliances, using adaptive feeding and holding techniques, and understanding the course of treatment and expected results. If the client is identified and treated early, the long-term prognosis for correction is good.

Polydactyly

Polydactyly, a hereditary condition, consists of extra digits on the hands and feet. If the digits do not include bones, ligation with a silk suture during the neonatal period is often adequate to cause sloughing of the tissue, leaving only a small scar after a few days. Surgery is required if bones are present in the extra digits. Surgery should wait until the function of each of the duplicated digits is certain. Surgery is usually performed sometime between 6 and 18 months (Cooperman, 1992).

Trisomy 13

Trisomy 13 is a chromosomal anomaly characterized by an extra chromosome in the D group, which includes pairs 13 through 15. Newborns with this abnormality frequently have difficulty establishing and maintaining respiration.

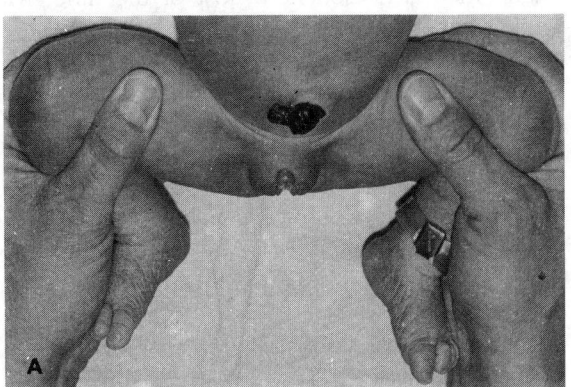 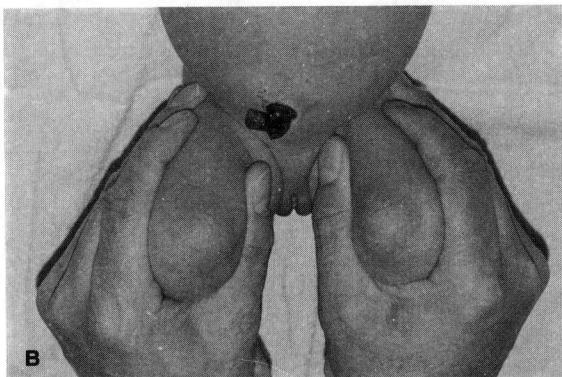

FIGURE 42–15 (**A**) Ortolani's sign. The fingers are on the trochanter, and the thumb grips the femur as shown. The femur is lifted forward as the thighs are abducted. If the head was dislocated, it can be felt to reduce. (**B**) The thighs are abducted, and if the head dislocates, it will be felt and seen as it suddenly jerks over the acetabulum. (Avery, G. B. [1994]. *Neonatology: Pathophysiology and management of the newborn* [4th ed.]. Philadelphia: J.B. Lippincott.)

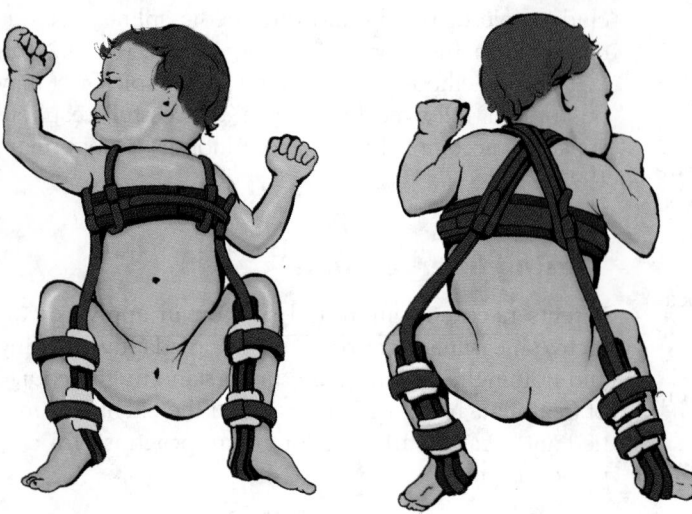

FIGURE 42–16 Application of the Pavlik harness.

Assessment

One of the most striking features is the abnormal cranial development. The cranium is usually small, with a sloping forehead. The ears may be malformed and low set, and the eyes usually have some defect, such as cataracts, iris defects, or unusual smallness, often bilaterally. Cleft palate and lip are commonly present. In addition, the hands and feet are often grossly deformed. Extra digits are common on hands and feet. The thumbs may be retroflexible (double jointed). The foot frequently has a posterior prominence of the heel sometimes accompanied by a convex sole, known as "rocker-bottom" foot. Other defects may include a bulbous nose, umbilical and diaphragmatic hernias, abnormal genitalia, scalp defects, and extensive capillary hemangiomatas far in excess of what is usually found in the normal newborn.

Neurologic examination reveals these newborns to have a weak or absent Moro reflex and little or no response to loud noises; hence, they appear to be deaf. They are prone to develop myoclonic seizures. All suffer from apneic spells of unknown origin. Autopsy often reveals the complete lack of olfactory nerves and tracts. All of these newborns are mentally retarded, and most have severe cardiac defects, such as dextroposition of the heart and ventricular septal defect, which are the major contributors to death. The average life span is less than 1 year, although several have lived to 5 years (Dickerman et al., 1992).

Nursing Interventions

The nurse performs ongoing physical assessment, maintains fluid balance, and positions for comfort. The family benefits from emotional support and referrals for care and support.

Trisomy 18

Trisomy 18 is a genetic anomaly characterized by an extra chromosome in the E group, which includes pairs 17 and 18 (see Chap. 14). These newborns are usually born at term but are small, averaging about 2 kg (5 lb). Their placentas are often very small.

Assessment

The head is small with an occiput that is prominent but proportionate to body size. The eyes are usually normal, but the ears are generally malformed and low set. The mouth appears small because of the short upper lip. The mandible is small, giving the appearance of a receding chin. The hands of these newborns are always malformed but in a different way from those in trisomy 13 newborns. The hands give the best diagnostic clue to the condition. These newborns keep their fists clenched most of the time, with the index finger overlying the third finger. Profuse lanugo covers the forehead, back, and extremities, and the skin usually has a mottled appearance. The sternum is very short; thus, the abdomen appears long. The pelvis is small, with limited abduction of the hips. There also may be abnormal genitalia. Inguinal and umbilical hernias are frequent; **diaphragmatic eventration** (elevation of a thinned portion of the diaphragm) occurs more often than frank hernia in these clients.

Neurologic examination reveals abnormal muscle tone. These newborns progress from a hypertonic state to frank **opisthotonos,** a dorsal arched position of the body in which the feet and head touch the floor or bed. Unlike trisomy 13, trisomy 18 babies demonstrate no gross brain abnormalities. Cardiac abnormalities are common, and either these or aspiration accounts for death in these newborns. The life span of these new-borns is less than 6 months on the average. During this time, they become progressively undernourished and present a failure-to-thrive syndrome. As with trisomy 13, some newborns have survived to childhood, so death in infancy cannot be predicted.

Nursing Interventions

Because the sucking reflex is poor, gavage feeding is often instituted. The nurse provides gavage feedings with care, because the risk of aspiration is high. Parents require teaching for home care and feeding and multidisciplinary referral and support.

Trisomy 21, or Down Syndrome

In Down syndrome, an extra chromosome belonging to pair 21 or pair 22 or a translocation of 15/21 is found (see Chap. 14). Although these newborns are apt to have congenital defects and are more susceptible to infection, they can be expected to live much longer and have less severe mental retardation (although it can be very severe) than the other trisomy newborns.

The incidence of Down syndrome is 1 in 150 new-borns in women older than 45 years, compared with 1 in 2,500 newborns in women younger than 20 years (Tunnessen, 1994). The usual causes of death in these newborns are heart defects and infectious illnesses. The survival rate is variable.

Types

The most common chromosomal defect of the ovum in Down syndrome is trisomy of chromosome 21 or 22. This results in a total chromosomal count of 47 instead of the normal number of 46. This type, commonly called standard trisomy, usually occurs in newborns of older women and is rarely familial. The incidence of standard trisomy is 1 in 600 births.

The second type of abnormality results from a 15/21 translocation. In this type, the actual chromosomal count is 46. The translocation type of Down syndrome is rare, of the familial type, and usually occurs in new-borns of younger parents. The third type of the disorder, **mosaicism,** is very rare. A unique factor in mosaicism is that one person may have cells with different chromosomal counts. Laboratory tests may demonstrate that the affected person's blood cells, for example, have 47 chromosomes, whereas the skin cells may show 46 chromosomes. This is not a familial type of Down syndrome, and the abnormalities may be less severe.

Assessment

The eyes are set close together and are slanting, have narrow palpebral fissures, and contain **Brushfield's spots** (white spots on the iris). The nose is flat. The tongue is large and fissured and usually is obvious because it protrudes from the open mouth. The head is small, and posteriorly, the occiput appears flat above the broad, pudgy neck (Fig. 42-17). The hands are short and thick, especially the fingers (the little finger is curved), with simian creases apparent on the palmar surfaces. In addition to having mental defects and the deformities mentioned previously, these newborns have underdeveloped muscles, loose joints, and heart and alimentary tract abnormalities.

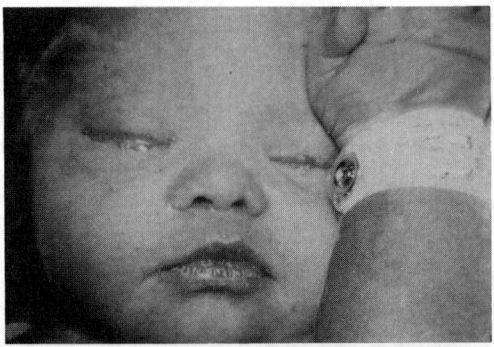
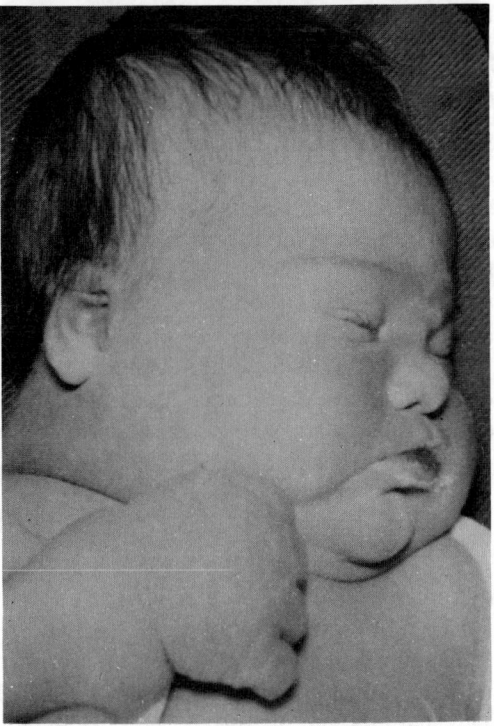

FIGURE 42–17 Newborn with Down syndrome. (Avery, G. B. [1987]. *Neonatology: Pathophysiology and management of the newborn* [3rd ed.]. Philadelphia: J.B. Lippincott.)

Planning and Intervention

Immediate care is supportive for the newborn. Warmth, prevention of infection, maintenance of fluid and electrolyte balance, and often oxygen therapy are provided. Because the immune system is often compromised, protection from infection by using good handwashing and medical asepsis is important. The nurse prioritizes the assessment to focus on the affected systems, for example cardiovascular. Nursing interventions are aimed primarily at supporting the parents in helping them to work through their grief. The supportive aspect is particularly important because of the grave prognosis for these newborns. It is often helpful to institute home healthcare for long-term referrals.

Inborn Errors of Metabolism

Numerous metabolic disorders, called inborn errors of metabolism, originate from mutations in the genes that alter the genetic constitution of a person to the extent that normal function is disrupted. These biochemical disorders arise because of the mutation in a molecule of the gene itself. They do not stem from some mishap or alteration during the embryonic development of tissue or organs. The mode of transmission of these inborn errors usually is recessive; for example, to be affected, a newborn must receive a pair of defective genes, one from the mother and one from the father. The mother and father, in these cases, would be carriers of the defective genes and would not be affected by the resulting disorder.

Fortunately, defective genes are found infrequently in the general population, and the chance of their joining is rare. Hence, the diseases they produce are rare. Newborns who have positive screening tests or are symptomatic need immediate diagnostic confirmation and treatment.

Screening for inborn errors of metabolism varies among states and countries. Testing for phenylketonuria is universal. Tests for other disorders available on a statewide basis are (in order of incidence) congenital hypothyroidism, galactosemia, maple syrup urine disease, homocystinuria, and biotinidase deficiency.

Phenylketonuria

Phenylketonuria (PKU), the result of an inborn error of metabolism, reflects the absence of the liver enzyme phenylalanine hydroxylase. Without this enzyme, phenylalanine cannot be converted to tyrosine. Toxic levels of phenylalanine and its metabolites, phenylpyruvic acid and phenylacetic acid, accumulate in blood, urine, and the central nervous system. The affected child has a musty odor, decreased pigmentation of skin and hair, and progressive mental retardation.

Several genetic disorders produce hyperphenylalaninemia: classical PKU, persistent non-PKU hyperphenylalaninemia, and hyperphenylalaninemia caused by one of several defects in tetrahydrobiopterin (BH4) metabolism. Nongenetic causes of hyperphenylalaninemia in the newborn are transient and disappear in the first year of life (Zinn, 1992).

The incidence is about 1 in 10,000 to 15,000 live births. Minimal central nervous system damage will occur if early diagnosis is made and treatment is begun before 1 month of age.

Screening. Newborn screening programs diagnose clients with genetic and nongenetic causes. The most commonly used screening method is the Guthrie method, which uses small amounts of blood placed on filter paper. Accuracy of the test depends on adequate ingestion of protein for 24 to 48 hours. With current short hospital stays, a repeat test may be necessary in 5 days. Phenylalanine levels of about 4 to 8 mg/dL are a presumptive positive.

Treatment. Treatment is begun as soon as possible after birth to prevent mental retardation. The treatment is dietary restriction to keep phenylalanine levels between 2 and 8 mg/dL. Diet needs to be low in phenylalanine yet with sufficient blood phenylalanine levels to allow for growth. The newborn may receive Lofenalac (low phenylalanine) or PKU-1. Total or partial breast-feeding may be possible with close monitoring because breast milk is low in phenylalanine. Frequent monitoring of phenylalanine levels is essential. Parents require multidisciplinary support. Transient hyperphenylalaninemia and non-PKU hyperphenylalaninemia do not require treatment.

Galactosemia

Galactosemia is an autosomal recessive disease and an inborn error of carbohydrate metabolism. The body is unable to metabolize galactose and lactose because of a lack of complex enzyme structures. Levels of galactose in the blood lead to cataract formation, renal disease, liver dysfunction, and some degree of mental retardation.

Treatment. Formulas such as Nutramigen or ProSobee may be used as treatment because they are lactose free. Soy protein is a formula of choice. Other treatment may be necessary for concomitant clinical problems.

Congenital Hypothyroidism

Congenital hypothyroidism results from inadequate production of thyroid hormone. Signs and symptoms develop gradually (ie, temperature instability, mottling, poor tone, jaundice, poor feeding, lethargy, and respiratory distress). If not treated promptly, the newborn will suffer growth failure, deafness, neurologic abnormalities, and mental retardation.

Maple Syrup Urine Disease

In **maple syrup urine disease,** three branched-chain amino acids are unable to be metabolized. The result is a rapidly progressing disease characterized by severe depression of the central nervous system and ultimately death from respiratory failure. Some degree of success is reported in a diet low in leucine, isoleucine, and valine. Frequent monitoring of these amino acids is essential to provide for adequate growth but not excess amino acids.

Homocystinuria

Homocystinuria is an inborn error of metabolism inherited in an autosomal recessive pattern with progressive clinical symptoms. There is a reduction in the activity of cystathionine synthetase, an enzyme that leads to the building of homocystine in the blood and urine and methionine in the blood. As a result, the body is unable to metabolize methionine for protein synthesis.

Clinical presentation in the newborn includes lethargy, poor feeding, and (rarely) thromboembolic disorders. If untreated, the disorder leads to musculoskeletal anomalies, dislocated optic lens, an increased bleeding tendency, thromboembolic vascular disease, and mental retardation. Administration of pyridoxine or a diet low in methionine and high in cystine is used (Zinn, 1992).

Summary Points

✔ The nursing care for the high-risk newborn experiencing various developmental disorders presents a challenge and an opportunity for the nurse to care for the family experiencing a situational crisis.

✔ The nurse must be confident and experienced in therapeutic communication skills, because many of the family's needs at this time may be psychosocial (ie, grief, denial and sorrow over the loss of the perfect expected newborn). The family requires information and ongoing teaching for community-based home care.

✔ Some developmental disorders, such as congenital heart disease, diaphragmatic hernia, spina bifida, and TEF may require immediate intervention to achieve the optimal outcome for the newborn and family.

✔ Other disorders may require a more staged approach and care, such as cleft lip and palate, imperforate anus, omphalocele, and gastroschisis.

✔ The nurse's unique assessment skills provide crucial data to the healthcare team and are an integral part in multidisciplinary care.

REFERENCES

Bowlby, J., & Parkes, C. M. (1970). Separation and loss within the family. In E. J. Anthony & C. Koupernik (Eds.), *The child and his family.* New York: Wiley.

Cooperman. D. R. (1992). Congenital deformities of the upper and lower extremities. In A. A. Fanaroff & R. J. Martin (Eds.), *Neonatal-perinatal medicine* (5th ed.) (pp. 1409–1420). St. Louis: C.V. Mosby.

Curtin, G. (1990). The infant with lip or palate: More than a surgical problem. *Journal of Perinatal and Neonatal Nursing, 3*(3), 80–80.

Danish, R. K. (1992). Abnormalities of sexual differentiation. In A. A. Fanaroff & R. J. Martin (Eds.), *Neonatal-perinatal medicine* (5th ed.) (pp. 1222–1292). St. Louis: C.V. Mosby.

Dickerman, L. H., & Park, V. M. (1992). Cytogenic and molecular aspects of genetic disease and prenatal diagnosis. In A. A. Fanaroff & R. J. Martin (Eds.), *Neonatal-perinatal medicine* (5th ed.) (pp. 57–79). St. Louis: C.V. Mosby.

Flake, A. W., & Ryckman, F. C. (1992). Selected anomalies and intestinal obstruction. In A. A. Fanaroff & R. J. Martin (Eds.), *Neonatal-perinatal medicine* (5th ed.) (pp. 1038–1065). St. Louis: C.V. Mosby.

Flanagan, M. F., & Fyler, D. C. (1994). Cardiac disease. In G. B. Avery, M. A. Fletcher, & M. G. Macdonald (Eds.), *Neonatology* (4th ed.) (pp. 914–951). Philadelphia: J.B. Lippincott.

Griffin, P. G. (1994), Orthopedics. In G. B. Avery, M. A. Fletcher, & M. G. Macdonald (Eds.), *Neonatology* (4th ed.) (pp. 1179–1194). Philadelphia: J.B. Lippincott.

Guzzetta, P. C., Anderson, K. D., Eichelberger, M. R., Newman, K. D., Rouse, T. M., Schnitzer, J. J., Boyajian, M., & Tomaski, S. M. (1994). General surgery. In G. B. Avery, M. A. Fletcher, & M. G. Macdonald (Eds.), *Neonatology* (4th ed.) (pp. 914–951). Philadelphia: J.B. Lippincott.

Heymann, M. A., Teital, D. F., & Leibman, J. (1993). The heart. In M. H. Klaus & A. A. Fanaroff (Eds.), *Care of the high risk neonate* (4th ed.). Philadelphia: W.B. Saunders.

Kent, P. A., & Curley, M. A. Q. (1992). Challenges in nursing: infants with congenital diaphragmatic hernia. *Heart and Lung, 21*(4), 381–388.

Klaus, M. H., & Kennell, J. H. (1993). Care of the parents. In M. H. Klaus & A. A. Fanaroff (Eds.), *Care of the high risk neonate* (4th ed.). Philadelphia: W.B. Saunders.

Kurcynski, T. W. (1992). Congenital malformations. In Fanaroff, A. A. & Martin, R. J. (Eds.), Neonatal-perinatal medicine (5th ed.) (pp. 372–398). St. Louis: C. V. Mosby.

Merenstein, G. B., & Gardner, S. L. (1989). *Handbook of neonatal intensive care* (2nd ed.) (pp. 539–547, 593–595). St. Louis: C.V. Mosby.

Moreno, M. C. N., & Iovanne, B. A. (1993). Congenital diaphragmatic hernia. Part II. *Neonatal Network, 12*(2), 21–26.

Roberts, P. M., & Jones, M. B. (1990). Extracorporeal membrane oxygenation and indications for cardiopulmonary bypass in the neonate. *Journal of Obstetric, Gynecologic, and Neonatal Nursing, 19*(5), 391–400.

Ryckmann, F. C., Flake, A. W., & Balistreri, W. F. (1992). Upper gastrointestinal disorders. In A. A. Fanaroff & R. J. Martin (Eds.), *Neonatal-perinatal medicine* (5th ed.) (pp. 1024–1029). St. Louis: C.V. Mosby.

Speers, A. T., & Speers, M. (1992). Care of the infant in a Pavlik harness. *Pediatric Nursing, 18*(3), 229–232.

Strobel, S. E., & Keller, C. S. (1993). Metabolics screening in the Nicu population: A proposal for change. *Pediatric Nursing, 19*(2), 113–117.

Theorell, C. J. (1990). Congenital diaphragmatic hernia: A physiological approach to management. *Journal of Perinatal and Neonatal Nursing, 3*(3), 66–79.

Tunnessen, W. W. (1994). Common syndromes with morphologic abnormalities. in F. A. Oski et al. (Eds.), *Principles and practice of pediatrics.* Philadelphia: J.B. Lippincott.

Zinn, A. B. (1992). Inborn errors of metabolism. In A. A. Fanaroff & R. J. Martin (Eds.), *Neonatal-perinatal medicine* (5th ed.) (pp. 1118–1151). St. Louis: C.V. Mosby.

SUGGESTED READING

Avery, G. B. (Ed.) (1993). *Neonatology: Pathophysiology and management of the newborn* (4th ed.). Philadelphia: J.B. Lippincott.

Beachy, P., & Deacon, J. (1992). *Core curriculum for neonatal intensive care nursing.* Philadelphia: W.B. Saunders.

Behrman, R. E. (1992). *Nelson textbook of pediatrics* (14th ed.). Philadelphia: W.B. Saunders.

Brentner, S. (1987). Abdominal defects: Omphalocele and gastroschisis. *Neonatal Network, 6*(3), 29–41.

Composto, R., & Eichelberger, C. (1992). Congenital diaphragmatic hernia: Pathophysiology and nursing care. *Neonatal Network, 11*(6), 57–61.

Daberkow, K., & Washington, R. L. (1993). Cardiovascular diseases and surgical interventions. In G. B. Merenstein & S. L. Gardner (Eds.), *Handbook of neonatal intensive care* (2nd ed.). St. Louis: C.V. Mosby.

Gomella, T. L. (Ed.) (1992). *Neonatology: Management, procedures, on-call problems, diseases, drugs* (2nd ed.). Norwalk, CT: Appleton-Lange.

Kenner, C., Brueggemeyer, A., & Gunderson, L. P. (Eds.), *Comprehensive neonatal nursing, a physiological perspective.* Philadelphia: W.B. Saunders.

Krause, K. D., & Youngner, V. J. (1992). Nursing diagnoses as guidelines in the care of the neonatal ECMO patient. *Journal of Obstetric, Gynecological, and Neonatal Nursing, 21*(3), 169–176.

Mattson, S., & Smith, J. E. (Eds.) (1992). *NAACOG core curriculum for maternal-newborn nursing.* Philadelphia: W.B. Saunders.

43

The High-Risk Newborn: Acquired Disorders

Objectives

- Describe common neonatal injuries resulting from birth trauma.
- List various perinatal risk factors for neonatal infections.
- Explain the nursing process in the care of the newborn experiencing an infectious process.
- Discuss the care of the infant of a diabetic mother.
- Describe risk factors for pathologic neonatal hyperbilirubinemia and the nursing care of a newborn experiencing pathologic jaundice.
- Explain the challenges facing the nurses caring for a newborn of a substance-abusing mother.

Most newborns make the transition to extrauterine life smoothly. For those who do not, the professional's skills in the delivery room and the nursery are important to future development. Certain factors have been identified as having an impact on the newborn's transition to extrauterine life. One group, **acquired disorders,** are those that result from environmental factors rather than genetic or congenital circumstances. These groups may include birth trauma, postnatal infections, physiologic processes affected by the newborn's environmental system, and maternal disorders and conditions. Newborns with acquired disorders may be only mildly affected, or they may be confined to an intensive care unit for months. Parents of these newborns need teaching from nurses to be able to cope with any unexpected illness. Parents also need assistance in dealing with guilt associated with this traumatic experience.

This chapter describes the most common acquired disorders seen in the newborn. Each disorder is presented using the nursing process as a framework.

Birth Trauma

Birth trauma refers to the physical injury that occurs during labor and delivery. Theoretically, most birth injuries may be avoidable by careful assessment and planning. However, some injuries may be unavoidable even with this careful assessment and planning because some injuries cannot be anticipated until a particular event occurs during labor and delivery.

Assessment

Immediate observation of the newborn in the delivery room usually permits the nurse to identify injuries or anoxia resulting from the birth process. A thorough neonatal assessment (discussed in Chap. 28), alertness to subtle changes in the newborn's behavior and condition, and careful recording of observations are important in the ongoing care.

Nursing Diagnoses

Nursing diagnoses will help to determine interventions in physical problems of the newborn and psychosocial problems concerning the family. For a list of possible nursing diagnoses, see Box 43-1.

Planning and Intervention

Some kinds of birth trauma require emergency intervention to save the newborn's life. Others can be treated later or will resolve spontaneously in several days. Ease in working with emergency techniques enables the nurse to promote the well-being of the high-risk newborn with an acquired disorder.

After managing the emergency situation, the nurse is responsible for providing overall care to the newborn, while adapting that care to his or her special needs. If the newborn is experiencing pain, the nurse must use judgment in using procedures that will alleviate pain or lessen it as much as possible. Gentle handling of the newborn is important. Positioning also aids in pain relief. The newborn's vital functions must be supported. If immobilization of a fracture is necessary, the nurse must take steps to avoid skin breakdown. Observations and management with general cast care are adapted to the newborn.

Communicating with parents by providing information and support is a major nursing responsibility. The nurse should share with the parents the description of the condition and possible outcomes. They should be shown how to handle the baby and be given time for touching and stroking if the newborn's movements must be kept to a minimum. Parent education and skill training in measures necessary for home care will give the family confidence in its ability to care for the newborn when he or she is released. Follow-up appointments should be made and a telephone number provided that the parents may call for additional help. Specific interventions are included in the discussion of each condition.

Evaluation

As mentioned previously, some injuries will resolve spontaneously. Others will go home with the newborns, while other newborns may be moved to a neonatal intensive care unit. Evaluations will differ in each case. Possible anticipated outcomes may include the following:

- The newborn demonstrates little or no pain.
- The newborn's vital signs remain within normal limits.

BOX 43-1
Nursing Diagnoses: Birth Trauma

- Pain related to injury and tissue trauma
- Risk for Impaired Skin Integrity related to immobility and casting of fractures
- Risk for Injury related to
  - Birth trauma
  - Procedures and treatments for the birth trauma
- Risk for Infection related to
  - Environmental influences
  - Procedures and treatments
- Altered Cerebral Tissue Perfusion related to intracranial hemorrhage
- Anxiety (parental) related to lack of knowledge about birth trauma and related treatments
- Knowledge Deficit related to trauma, prognosis, and care
- Anticipatory Grieving related to
  - Uncertainty of outcome and possible sequelae
  - Loss of "perfect newborn"
- Risk for Altered Parent/Infant Attachment related to
  - Guilt about birth trauma
  - Negative feelings toward newborn and appearance
  - Separation from newborn in intensive care unit

- The newborn remains free of further injury or infection.
- The newborn demonstrates no signs or symptoms of skin breakdown.
- The parents verbalize feelings and concerns openly.
- The parents demonstrate a beginning parent–newborn relationship.
- The parents demonstrate knowledge about their newborn's condition. The parents demonstrate confidence in their ability to care for the newborn at home.

Head Trauma

The newborn's head is large in proportion to the rest of the body. It also is soft with pliable skull bones. As a result, various types of head trauma may occur.

Caput Succedaneum and Cephalhematoma

Caput succedaneum refers to swelling or edema in or under the fetal scalp. This soft, edematous swelling of the scalp frequently occurs over a portion of the presenting part. Pressure from the uterus or birth canal can precipitate the accumulation of serum or blood above the periosteum. Vacuum extraction also may cause a caput. The caput may vary from a small area to a severely elongated head. Swelling may cross suture lines. No treatment is indicated. A caput succedaneum

usually resolves spontaneously within 12 hours or in a few days after birth (Margileth, 1994).

Cephalhematoma is a collection of blood caused by ruptured blood vessels between the bone and periosteum that does not cross the suture lines. Cephalhematoma is not as common as caput succedaneum. The incidence is 0.4% to 2.5% of all live births (Mangurten, 1992).

Cephalhematoma occurs during labor and delivery from the rupture of blood vessels crossing the skull to the periosteum. It may be precipitated by prolonged labor or the use of forceps. Because the bleeding is a slow process, it may take hours or days for the swelling to be noticeable. Usually it is unilateral, but it may be bilateral. It may be obvious by the second or third day. Most cephalhematomas resolve in 2 weeks to 3 months, with the majority resolving by 6 weeks Mangurten, 1992; Fig. 43-1). A skull fracture is present in 10% to 25% of affected newborns.

Interventions. The nurse's role in caring for newborns with caput succedaneum and cephalhematoma is supportive. The nurse needs to reassure the parents that both conditions will resolve without treatment.

Intracranial Hemorrhage

Intracranial hemorrhage is a result of birth trauma, more likely to occur in the full vein, large newborn. In the newborn, more than one type of hemorrhage can occur. The two most common types include subdural hemorrhage and subarachnoid hemorrhage.

Subdural Hemorrhage. **Subdural hemorrhage** refers to a collection of blood in the subdural space. It is a life-threatening condition most commonly the result of stretching and tearing of the large veins in the cerebellar tentorium. Subdural hemorrhage occurs less frequently today because of advances and improvements in obstetric monitoring and care.

Subarachnoid Hemorrhage. **Subarachnoid hemorrhage**, bleeding into the subarachnoid space, is the most common type of neonatal intracranial hemorrhage. Trauma is the most common cause in term newborns; hypoxia is the most common cause in preterm newborns. The bleeding is usually venous bleeding, possibly accompanied by a contusion.

Assessment. The clinical picture can vary; some newborns are asymptomatic. Irritability, decreased level of consciousness, seizures, and apnea may occur in subarachnoid hemorrhage. Subdural hemorrhage can cause definitive neurologic abnormalities, such as apnea, coma, unequal pupils, nuchal rigidity, and **opisthotonos,** a tetanic spasm resulting in an arched, hyperextended body position. Lumbar punctures and

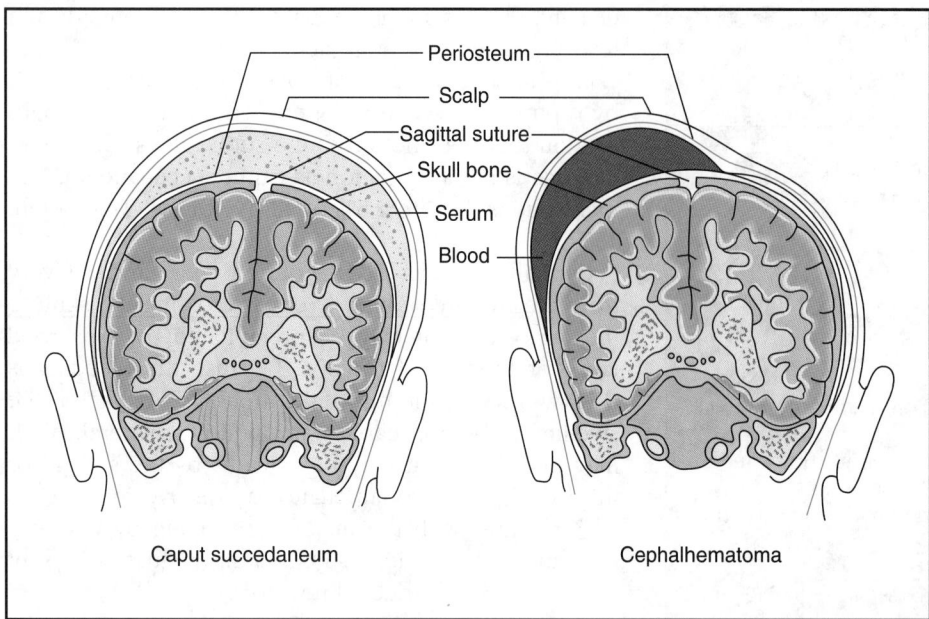

Periosteum

Scalp

Sagittal suture

Skull bone

Serum

Blood

Caput succedaneum

Cephalhematoma

FIGURE 43-1 Comparative diagram of the underlying pathophysiology in caput succedaneum and cephalhematoma.

computed tomography scans assist in and confirm the diagnosis.

Interventions. The nursing care of the newborn with intracranial hemorrhage is generally supportive. Ventilatory status is monitored closely for changes. The newborn is assessed for the possibility of seizures. Seizure precautions are instituted and maintained. Measures to prevent increased intracranial pressure are instituted. Intravenous therapy is used to maintain hydration and fluid and electrolyte balance. The newborn should be handled minimally to promote rest and reduce stressors.

Parent teaching and referral to support groups are essential, gearing information to the newborn's prognosis. The nurse should be alert for possible complications; complications of subdural hemorrhage may range from none to permanent neurologic deficits. The major potential complication of subarachnoid hemorrhage is hydrocephalus (Hill et al., 1994).

Perinatal Hemorrhage and Shock

Blood loss from hemorrhage can occur at any time in the perinatal period. If significant blood loss occurs, the result may be shock. Anemia occurring early in neonatal life also may be due to some form of perinatal hemorrhage.

Major blood loss can occur from various obstetric problems (Blanchette et al., 1994). Fetal–maternal transfusion is common but not usually severe enough to cause anemia in the newborn. Fetal–fetal transfusion occurs only in identical twins. Significant anemia occurs in only 15% of the cases (Table 43-1).

TABLE 43-1
Sources of Blood Loss

Prenatal	Perinatal	Neonatal
Placenta previa	Ruptured umbilical cord	Intracranial hemorrhage
Abruptio placentae	Hematoma of umbilical cord	Ruptured internal organs
Following external cephalic version	Placenta previa	Intraventricular hemorrhage
Traumatic amniocentesis	Abruptio placentae	Cephalhematoma
Twin to twin transfusion	Incision of placenta during cesarean birth	Iatrogenic anemias
	Rupture of anomalous placental vessels	

(Blanchette, V., Doyle, J., Schmidt, B. & Zipursky, A. [1994]. Hematology. In G. B. Avery, M. A. Fletcher, M. G. Macdonald (Eds.), *Neonatology: Pathophysiology and management of the newborn* [4th ed.] [pp. 952–999]. Philadelphia: J.B. Lippincott.)

Assessment

A neonate in hypovolemic shock has cool, clammy skin; mottled or gray extremities; diminished pulses; and decreased capillary refill. Low blood pressure and central venous pressure (CVP) will be evident along with compensatory tachycardia. Because renal blood flow depends on cardiac output, any decrease leads to decreased urine output. Dry mucous membranes, poor skin turgor, and sunken fontanels indicate dehydration. Laboratory values may indicate electrolyte imbalances, metabolic acidosis, hypoglycemia, and abnormal coagulation patterns (Table 43-2).

Interventions

Immediate resuscitative treatment is essential. Central and peripheral intravenous lines are inserted for fluid replacement using volume expanders. Blood and blood products are administered as needed (Rimar, 1989). The nurse must be alert to possible risks during transfusion therapy and intervene appropriately (Table 43-3).

Critical care monitoring is used, including electrocardiogram, CVP, pulmonary artery pressure, pulse oximetry, or transcutaneous oxygen saturation. Pharmacologic interventions also may be necessary (Table 43-4).

Nervous System Problems

Injury to the nervous system may result from birth trauma. Common injuries include facial paralysis, arm paralysis, and phrenic nerve injury.

Facial Paralysis. Facial paralysis due to pressure on cranial nerve VII may occur as a result of a difficult vaginal delivery or the pressure of forceps on the facial nerve. Temporary paralysis of the muscles of one side of the face occurs so that the mouth is drawn to the other side. This is particularly noticeable when the newborn cries. Other signs include the inability to close the eye on the affected side and absence of wrinkling of the forehead. The condition is usually transitory and disappears in a few days, often in a few hours. No medical treatment is necessary.

Interventions. Because the newborn can look disfigured, the parents will need an explanation about the temporary nature of this affliction (Fig. 43-2). If the mother is allowed to feed the newborn, the nurse should be with her consistently during the first feedings to help her as necessary. Sucking may be difficult for the newborn, and the mother needs to develop patience and skill in feeding.

If one eye remains open because of the affected muscles, the physician prescribes appropriate treatment. Artificial tears instilled daily to prevent drying or a protective eye patch may be used. Any necessary instructions regarding continuing care after discharge should be given to the mother before she leaves the hospital. Often when disorders occur, parents are afraid to handle their newborn for fear of hurting him or her. Thus, parents should be encouraged to hold and cuddle their newborn whenever the condition permits.

Arm Paralysis. Brachial plexus injury is the most common nerve injury of the newborn. Damage to the upper plexus (**Erb's palsy**) is more common than damage to the entire plexus. Isolated damage to the lower plexus (**Klumpke's palsy**) is rare. The prognosis for recovery of function varies with the severity of the injury.

Erb's palsy usually occurs as a result of pulling or stretching the shoulder away from the head, a result of vertex or breech delivery. Symptoms include a limp arm with elbow extended, wrist pronated, and arms internally rotated. The grasp reflex is present, but the deep tendon reflex is absent. The Moro reflex is lessened or absent on the affected side.

Symptoms of lower plexus injury are limited to the forearm and hand. There may be edema and cyanosis of the affected part. The wrist and hand are limp,

---

TABLE 43-2
Normal Erythrocyte Values During Gestation*

Weeks of Gestation	Erythrocytes ($\times 10^{12}$/L)	Hemoglobin (g/dL)	Hematocrit (%)	Mean Corpuscular Volume (fl)
18–21	2.85 ± 0.36	11.7 ± 1.3	37.3 ± 4.3	131.11 ± 10.97
22–25	3.09 ± 0.34	12.2 ± 1.6	38.6 ± 3.9	125.1 ± 7.84
26–29	3.46 ± 0.41	12.9 ± 1.4	40.9 ± 4.4	118.5 ± 7.96
>36	4.7 ± 0.4	16.5 ± 1.5	51.0 ± 4.5	108 ± 5

*Values are given ±1 standard deviation.
(Blanchette V., Doyle J., Schmidt, B., & Zipursky A. [1994]. Hematology. In G. B. Avery, M. A. Fletcher, & M. G. MacDonald (Eds.), *Neonatology: Pathophysiology and management of the newborn* [4th ed.] [p. 953] Philadelphia: J.B. Lippincott.)

TABLE 43-3
Guidelines for Safe Transfusions

Risk	Nursing Interventions
Volume overload	Adjust fluid intake as prescribed; report excessive weight gains and symptoms of congestive heart failure. Monitor fluid intake and output. Except in emergencies, give routine transfusions slowly over 3–4 h.
Thromboemboli	Avoid using regional arterial lines; use venous lines when possible. Use saline flushes before and after transfusion. (Glucose flushes will cause clotting when in contact with blood for transfusion.)
Infection	
Cytomegalovirus (CMV)	Use CMV-negative blood. Use blood screened for hepatitis and AIDS.
Hepatitis	
Acquired immunodeficiency syndrome (AIDS)	
Hemolytic transfusion reactions	Type and cross-match blood, then identify correct recipient of the blood product by double-checking client's ID number and name with another qualified staff member.
Graft-versus-host disease (GVHD)	Use irradiated blood components for clients susceptible to GVHD.
Metabolic derangements	
Hypothermia	Warm blood before giving.
Acidosis/alkalosis*	Monitor blood pH values as indicated, especially with exchange transfusion.
Hyperkalemia*	Usually only with exchange transfusion: monitor serum potassium levels, and report abnormal values.
Hypocalcemia*	Usually only with exchange transfusion: monitor calcium levels; watch for cardiac arrhythmias.
Hypoglycemia	Monitor blood sugar levels according to established unit policy. Maintain levels at 45 mg/dl or above.

*These problems can be minimized if fresh blood (stored no longer than 5–6 days) is used for exchange transfusions. (Kelting, S., Johnson, C. [1987]. Erythropoiesis and neonatal blood transfusions. *MCN: American Journal of Maternal Child Nursing, 12*(3), 176.)

and the deep tendon reflex is present, but the grasp is absent.

Interventions. Initially, the area is immobilized while the affected extremity is maintained in a functional position. An intense program of physical therapy follows this initial period of approximately 7 to 10 days. Surgery may be indicated if recovery does not occur after a year or two (Brann et al., 1992).

Phrenic Nerve Injury

Phrenic nerve injuries occur most often in conjunction with brachial palsy, which is usually the result of a difficult breech delivery. Because the phrenic nerve is the only nerve innervating the diaphragm, paralysis of the diaphragm occurs, usually unilaterally. Symptoms are those of respiratory distress. Respiratory effort of the involved side of the diaphragm is ineffective. The abdomen does not bulge during inspiration because breathing is almost completely thoracic. The diaphragm cannot be felt under the costal margin on the affected side.

Interventions. The newborn should be positioned on the affected side and given intravenous fluids and oxygen if necessary. More severe respiratory distress may require mechanical ventilation. Surgical intervention to move the diaphragm down may be necessary if spontaneous recovery does not occur with time. Most newborns recover spontaneously in weeks or months with supportive treatment. Pneumonia in the atelectatic lung is a potential complication (Mangurten, 1992).

Fractures

Fractures also may result from birth trauma. Common sites of fractures include the clavicle, long bones of the arms or legs, and skull.

Clavicle

The clavicle is the bone most commonly fractured during delivery. It usually is a result of dystocia, such as shoulder delivery in vertex delivery or extended arms in breech delivery. The newborn may be asymptomatic. Symptoms that might be observed are decreased or absent mobility of the affected arm, discoloration of the site, crepitus along the clavicle, and absence of the Moro reflex on the affected side.

TABLE 43-4
Cardiovascular Drugs Used in the Treatment of Pediatric Shock

Drug	Usual Intravenous Dose	Comments
Isoproterenol	0.1–0.5 µg/kg per minute	Increases strength and rate of cardiac contraction. Dilates peripheral vessels. May increase myocardial work and oxygen consumption. May include arrhythmias.
Epinephrine	0.05–0.1 µg/kg per minute	At low doses, increases strength and rate of cardiac contraction to moderate degree and causes systemic vascular resistance (SVR) to decrease slightly at low doses. At high doses, causes marked increase in strength and rate of cardiac contraction and severe vasoconstriction of peripheral vasculature (increased SVR). Because epinephrine may decrease renal blood flow significantly, monitor urine output.
Dopamine	2–20 µg/kg per minute (higher doses may be used)	Effects vary with dose: low dose response primarily dopaminergic; midrange causes moderate increase in heart rate and contractility; high doses (10–20 µg/kg per minute) vasoconstriction predominates. May cause arrhythmias.
Dobutamine	2–15 µg/kg per minute (higher doses may be used)	Increases strength of cardiac contraction but causes minimal change in heart rate. On occasion, causes tachycardia and hypertension.
Amrinone	3 mg/kg initially; over 20–30 min 5–10 µg/kg per minute	Increases strength of cardiac contraction and relaxes vascular smooth muscle, causing decreased afterload and preload. Clinical studies regarding use in children are ongoing.
Nitroprusside	0.5–10 µg/kg per minute	Dilates peripheral arteries and veins. May produce severe hypotension. Do not use in boluses. Immediate onset and short duration (2–4 sec) of action. Protect from light.
Tolazoline	1–2 mg/kg initially; 1–5 mg/kg per hour	Decreases peripheral resistance and increases venous capacitance. Causes cardiac stimulation. Reduces pulmonary arterial pressure and resistance.

(Adapted from Gregory, G. [1994]. *Pediatric anesthesia.* [3rd ed.]. New York: Churchill Livingstone, and Karch, A. [1996]. *1996 Lippincott's nursing drug guide.* Philadelphia: J.B. Lippincott.)

Interventions. No treatment or interventions are necessary except proper alignment and gentle handling to minimize pain. The affected arm and shoulder should be immobilized with the arm abducted above 60 degrees and the elbow flexed above 90 degrees (Mangurten, 1992). The prognosis is very good for complete recovery.

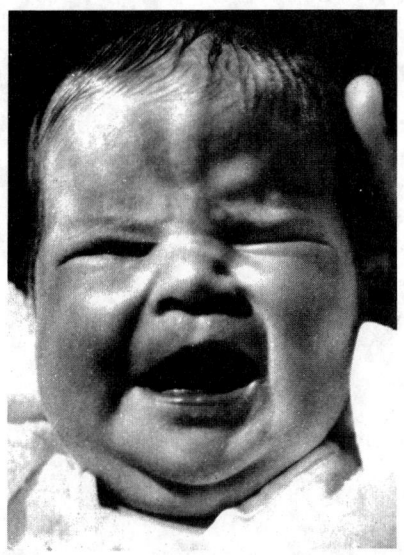

FIGURE 43-2 Facial nerve paralysis. Note the asymmetry of the mouth during crying.

Long Bones

The humerus is the second most often fractured bone. Fracture of the humerus occurs with difficult delivery of the arms or shoulders in a vertex delivery. Immobility of the affected arm is the presenting sign. The Moro reflex is absent on the affected side. The affected arm must be immobilized in the adducted position for 2 to 4 weeks for healing to occur. Immobilization may be carried out by splints or a cast.

Fracture of the femur is the most common fracture of the lower extremities. Fracture of the femur may occur during a breech delivery. Deformity of the thigh, swelling, or immobility may be noted. Treatment involves traction, suspension, and casting for about 3 to 4 weeks (Mangurten, 1992).

Skull

Because of the flexibility and molding of the newborn's head, skull fractures are uncommon. They occur as a result of prolonged, difficult labor or forceps delivery. Fractures may be linear or depressed. Most skull fractures are linear. The newborn will be asymptomatic with a linear fracture unless blood vessels become involved, which leads to a subdural hematoma. Depressed fractures may require surgery if brain tissue is involved (Minarcik et al., 1989).

Neonatal Infections

Sepsis, the presence of microorganisms or their toxins in the blood or other tissues, is one of the most significant causes of neonatal morbidity and mortality. The newborn is particularly vulnerable to infection for two reasons. The protective environment of the uterus is no longer available, and the newborn has not acquired defenses against disease (see Chap. 28).

The fetus may have become infected in utero, or the newborn may become infected during passage through the birth canal or from ascending infection following rupture of the membranes. These perinatal influences cause a vertical transmission of infection. Examples of vertical transmission include the TORCH (Toxoplasmosis, Other, Rubella, Cytomegalovirus, Congenital Herpes) infections and hepatitis. Serious defects in the fetus and newborn may result from the vertical transmission of infection.

An example of horizontal transmission is a newborn who acquires an infection, such as a staphylococcal infection, from the mother, caregivers, equipment, or environment.

Assessment

Nurses play a crucial role in assessing the newborn for signs of infection. The behaviors, signs, and symptoms of sepsis in the newborn are often subtle and are noticed only by experienced caregivers. Neonatal nurses have the responsibility to note such behaviors so that diagnosis and treatment can begin early. The nurses' observations also may prevent an epidemic of infection within the newborn nursery (see Assessment Guidelines: Clinical Signs of Sepsis in the Newborn).

Newborns at Risk

Certain maternal factors have been identified as influencing neonatal sepsis. These include symptomatic bacteriuria during pregnancy, low socioeconomic sta-

ASSESSMENT GUIDELINES
Clinical Signs of Sepsis in the Newborn

Central Nervous System

- Full or bulging fontanels
- Lethargy
- Jitteriness
- Temperature instability
- Irritability
- Hypotonia
- Tremors, seizures

Gastrointestinal System

- Diminished interest in feeding
- Decreased oral intake
- Vomiting
- Diarrhea
- Abdominal distension
- Increased gastric residuals

Integumentary System

- Jaundice
- Lesions
- Rashes

Respiratory System

- Apnea
- Cyanosis

- Tachypnea
- Decreased oxygenation saturation
- Nasal flaring, grunting, retractions
- Mottling

Cardiovascular System

- Tachycardia
- Diminished peripheral pulses
- Pallor, mottling
- Hypotension

Laboratory Tests

- Positive cultures of blood, cerebrospinal fluid, urine, gastric aspirate
- Leukocytosis
- Decreased neutrophils
- Increased bands
- Decreased platelets
- Hypoglycemia or hyperglycemia
- Chest x-ray changes

tus, lack of prenatal care, substance abuse, rupture of membranes for more than 18 hours, peripartal infections, use of invasive procedures in the antepartal and intrapartal periods, amnionitis, and colonization of the genital organs. Risk factors for the newborn include preterm birth, low birth weight, multiple gestations, male sex, hypoxia, maternal infections, and intrauterine growth retardation. Other factors relate to the environment, nosocomial transmission, and neonatal invasive procedures (Lott et al., 1994).

Nursing Diagnoses

Following assessment, appropriate nursing diagnoses can be identified. For a list of possible nursing diagnoses, see Box 43-2.

Planning and Intervention

An important aspect of infection control is prevention (see Chap. 29). Once an infection is identified in a newborn, steps must be taken to prevent further spread. Antibiotics used in infection management are listed in Table 43-5. Further interventions and a summary of common neonatal infections are found in Table 43-6 and in the Nursing Care Plan: Neonates with Infections.

BOX 43-2
Nursing Diagnoses: Neonatal Infections

- Risk for Infection related to
  - Resuscitative measures
  - Invasive procedures and treatments
  - Immaturity and lack of body reserves
- Ineffective Thermoregulation related to infection
- Impaired Tissue Integrity related to invasive procedures and treatments
- Diarrhea related to infection and effects of treatment
- Fluid Volume Deficit related to diarrhea, vomiting, or feeding problems
- Ineffective Airway Clearance related to increased mucous from respiratory infection
- Pain related to infection or invasive procedures and treatments
- Knowledge Deficit related to
  - Infectious process, treatments, and prognosis
  - Care of newborn after discharge
- Altered Protection related to infection and newborn's immature immune system
- Impaired Gas Exchange related to physiologic effects of sepsis
- Risk for Fluid Volume Deficit related to physiologic effects of sepsis

---

Infant of a Diabetic Mother

The successful control of diabetes with insulin has led to increased survival and fertility of a greater number of women. Better control of the diabetic state during pregnancy has increased the newborn's chances for a healthy birth. The infant of a diabetic mother (IDM), however, still presents with a number of clinical problems that are best treated in the intensive care nursery setting. IDMs may be large for gestational age, but most are appropriate for gestational age. Typically, the IDM has a round face, soft skin, an abundance of subcutaneous fat tissue, and a **plethoric appearance**, a condition marked by an excess of blood and fullness of pulse, accompanied by a feeling of tension in the head, florid complexion, and a tendency for nosebleeds.

Clinical Problems and Related Management

The IDM is at risk for various clinical problems. These include hypoglycemia, hypocalcemia, hyperbilirubinemia, respiratory disease, and birth defects.

Hypoglycemia

Newborns of class A to C or type I diabetic mothers are at risk for hypoglycemia. Maternal hyperglycemia is accompanied by fetal hyperglycemia. The fetal pancreas is thus stimulated, leading to hypertrophy of islet cells and hyperplasia of beta cells with subsequent increase in insulin content. On delivery, the newborn is no longer dependent on maternal glucose. Thus, a hypoglycemic state ensues. Because insulin stimulates fetal organ growth, a hyperinsulin state produces an increase in organ size and macrosomia (large for gestational age). There is an impetus for increased deposition of fat in the third trimester. Potential birth injuries may occur with attempted vaginal delivery of very large newborns. These potential birth injuries include cephalhematoma, subdural hemorrhage, facial palsy, ocular hemorrhage, clavicular fracture, and brachial plexus injury.

Hypoglycemia is defined as a blood glucose level of less than 40 mg/dL (Samson, 1992). Any random samples using test strips or glucose monitors should be verified by a laboratory blood glucose determination. Blood glucose levels usually drop within the first 30 to 60 minutes of life. Most IDMs are asymptomatic. Signs or symptoms that do occur include tremors, respiratory difficulty, or central nervous system dysfunction. The kind or severity of the symptoms does not

(*text continues on page 1212*)

TABLE 43-5

*Antibiotics That may be used for Treatment of Neonatal Sepsis or Meningitis**

Agent	First Week of Life or Premature			Full-Term Newborn Older Than 1 Week			Comment
	DOSAGE	ROUTE	SCHEDULE	DOSAGE	ROUTE	SCHEDULE	
Amikacin	15 mg/kg per day	IM, IV	q12h	30 mg/kg per day	IM, IV	q8h	When using IV, infuse over 30 min.
Ampicillin	100–150 mg/kg per day	IM, IV	q8h or q12h	150–300 mg/kg per day	IM, IV	q6h or q8h	Use highest dosage in meningitis. Use 100 mg/kg per day in premature newborns between 1 and 4 weeks old with sepsis.
Aztreonam	60 mg/kg per day	IV, IM	q8h or q12h	90–120 mg/kg per day	IM, IV	q8h or q6h	Not approved to date by FDA.
Carbenicillin	225 mg/kg per day	IM, IV	q8h	300 mg/kg per day	IM, IV	q6h	Give loading dose of 100 mg/kg to all clients. Full-term newborns may be given 300 mg/kg per day even during first week of life.
Cefotaxime	100–150 mg/kg per day	IV	q12h	150–200 mg/kg per day	IV	q6h or q8h	Use highest dosage in meningitis.
Ceftazidime	100 mg/kg per day	IV	q12h	150 mg/kg per day	IV	q12h	
Ceftriaxone	50 mg/kg per day	IM, IV	q day	50–100 mg/kg per day	IV	q day or q12h	May displace bilirubin from albumin-binding sites.
Cephalothin	50 mg/kg per day	IM, IV	q8h	50–100 mg/kg per day	IM, IV	q6h	
Chloramphenicol	25 mg/kg per day	IV	q8h	50 mg/kg per day	IV	q6h	If used, serum concentrations should be monitored.
Clindamycin	20 mg/kg per day	IV	q8h	30 mg/kg per day	IV	q6h	Do not use in clients with meningitis.
Colistimethate	5 mg/kg per day	IM	q12h	8 mg/kg per day	IM	q8h	
Erythromycin	Not established			40 mg/kg per day	PO	q6h	Use only for treatment of *Chlamydia trachomatis* pneumonia.
Gentamicin	5 mg/kg per day	IM, IV	q12h	7.5 mg/kg per day	IM, IV	q8h	When used IV, infuse over 30 min. Intraventricular therapy also may be required in clients with meningitis.

Drug	Dosage	Route	Interval	Dosage	Route	Interval	Comments
Kanamycin	15 mg/kg per day	IM, IV	q12h	25 mg/kg per day	IM, IV	q8h or q12h	When used IV, infuse over 30 min. Recent pharmacologic studies suggest that these dosage recommendations may require revision upward, but clinical studies to support lack of toxicity at increased dosages not available.
Methicillin	100 mg/kg per day	IM, IV	q8h	200 mg/kg per day	IM, IV	q6h	Give q12h on first day of life.
Metronidazole	15 mg/kg per day	IM	q12h	15–30 mg/kg per day	IM, PO	q12h	
Mezlocillin	150 mg/kg per day	IM, IV	q12h	300 mg/kg per day	IM, IV	q6h	Premature newborns older than 1 week may be given 225 mg/kg per day on an q8h schedule.
Nafcillin	100 mg/kg per day	IM, IV	q12h	200 mg/kg per day	IM, IV	q6h	
Neomycin	50–100 mg/kg per day	PO	q6h	50–100 mg/kg per day	PO	q6h	Use only if lack of systemic absorption can be ensured.
Nystatin	200,000–400,000 U	PO	q6h	200,000–400,000 U	PO	q6h	Do not use for systemic infections.
Oxacillin	100 mg/kg per day	IM, IV	q12h	200 mg/kg per day	IM, IV	q6h	
Penicillin	100,000–150,000 units/kg per day	IM, IV	q8h or q12h	100,000–300,000 units/kg per day	IM, IV	q6h or q8h	Use highest dosage in meningitis.
Polymyxin B	3 mg/kg per day	IM, IV	q12h	4 mg/kg per day	IM, IV	q8h	If used IV, infuse over 30 min. Intrathecal administration also required if used in treatment of meningitis.
Ticarcillin	150–225 mg/kg per day	IM, IV	q8-12h	225–300 mg/kg per day	IM, IV	q6h or q8h	Use lower dosage and longer interval for premature newborns.
Tobramycin	4–5 mg/kg per day	IM, IV	q12h	5–7.5 mg/kg per day	IM, IV	q6h or q8h	If used IV, infuse over 30 min; use higher dosage for meningitis.
Vancomycin	20–40 mg/kg per day	IV	q12h	30–60 mg/kg per day	IV	q6h or q8h	Use highest dosage in meningitis; infuse over 60 min to avoid histamine-like reactions; serum concentrations should be monitored.

(from Feigin R, Adcock LM, Edwards MS. The Immune system Part 2 Postnatal bacterial infections. Fanaroff, A.A. & Martin, R.S. (Eds) [1992]. Neonatal–perinatal medicine [5th ed.]. St. Louis, C.V. Mosby [pp.626–627].)

TABLE 43–6
Common Neonatal Infections

Infection	Transmission or Risk Factors	Clinical Picture	Diagnostic Tests	Treatment
Group Beta *Streptococcus*	Perinatal Positive maternal vaginal cultures in labor Premature or prolonged rupture of membranes Preterm birth Fetal distress 5-minute Apgar score less than 5	Early onset Respiratory distress Acidosis Hypovolemia Late onset Meningitis at 2 to 4 weeks of age	Chest x-ray with local infiltrates, "wet lung" or reticulogranular pattern Leukocytosis Thrombocytopenia Urine positive for GBS latex agglutination	Supportive Ampicillin Gentamycin
Hepatitis B virus	Positive Hepatitis B Surface Antigen (HBSAG) transplacental and perinatal transmission	Asymptomatic Risk for chronic carrier state Preterm birth	Positive HBSAG Positive HBeAG	Supportive Hepatitis B vaccine Hepatitis B immune globulin
Toxoplasmosis	Transplacental parasitic transmission	Asymptomatic Preterm or low birth weight Intrauterine growth retardation (IUGR) Chorioretinitis Microcephaly Neurologic defects Hepatosplenomegaly	Postive antitoxoplasmic IGM antibodies	Pyrimethamine Sulfadiazine therapy Supportive
Rubella	Transplacental	Deafness Cataracts IUGR Cardiovascular defects Microcephaly Hepatosplenomegaly	Positive serum antibody tests	Supportive Multidisciplinary referral Isolate from pregnant women
Cytomegalovirus	Transplacental Perinatal	Hepatosplenomegaly Jaundice Hearing Loss Microcephaly Chorioretinitis	Positive viral cultures	Supportive
Herpes Simplex Virus (HSV)	Transplacental Ascending cervical infection	Lesions Jaundice Hepatosplenomegaly	Positive viral cultures	Supportive Acyclovir

Disease	Etiology/Transmission	Clinical manifestations	Diagnosis	Treatment
Syphilis	Transplacental Maternal infection	Purpura Respiratory distress Shock Central nervous system defects IUGR Chorioretinitis ? Asymptomatic	Positive cultures: Rapid Plasma reagin/venereal disease research laboratory (RPR/VDRL) Serum Umbilical cord serum Long bone x-rays Nontreponemal antibody titers	Supportive Parenteral Penicillin
Human immunodeficiency virus (HIV)	Positive maternal HIV titer Transplacental Perinatal Breast-feeding	Failure to thrive Lymphadenopathy Recurrent bacterial infections Neurologic involvement	Rising HIV Antibody tests	Retrovir Prophylactic therapy for *pneumocystitis carinii* pneumonia and opportunistic bacterial infections
Chlamydia	Positive maternal culture Transplacental Perinatal	Conjunctivitis Interstitial pneumonia	Tissue culture of conjunctiva, oropharyngeal, genital, or rectal	Ophthalmic or systemic erythromycin
Listeria	Transplacental Premature rupture of the membranes Maternal infection	Preterm Meconium stained amniotic fluid Respiratory distress Hepatic dysfunction	Perinatal Positive blood, cerebrospinal fluid Urine cultures	Ampicillin, Aminoglycoside Respiratory support Total parenteral nutrition
Respiratory syncytial virus	Preterm Congenital heart disease Immunosuppression	Bronchiolitis Pneumonia Coughing Wheezing Cyanosis Respiratory failure Clear nasal discharge Fever Otitis media	Chest x-ray infiltrates Positive nasal swab	Supportive Ribavarin for serious illness

(Feigin, Adcock, Miller, 1992) (Baley and Goldfarb, 1992) (Feigin, Adcock, Edwards, 1992) (Lott and Kenner, 1994) (Fuller, 1994) (Benson, 1994)

NURSING CARE PLAN
Neonates With Infections (Prevention and Management)

Nursing Goals
1. Infected infants are identified and managed immediately.
2. Infants at risk for infection are assessed.
3. The infant is isolated, and spread of infection is curtailed.
4. Bowel patterns are adequate.
5. Fluid balance is present.
6. Infant demonstrates adequate weight gain.
7. Infant's respiratory status is stable.
8. Infant's vital signs remain stable.
9. Infant exhibits comfort behaviors.
10. Other infants in the nursery remain symptom free.

Assessment	Potential Nursing Diagnoses	Intervention/ Rationale	Evaluation
Maternal factors		Continue to observe newborn for signs and symptoms *to prevent further complication*	Infected infants are identified and managed immediately
Smoking	Risk for Infection related to immature immune system, environmental factors, maternal exposure or actual infectious disease process, sharing of nursery	Skin: rashes, lesions, jaundice	Infants at risk for infection are assessed
Low socioeconomic status		Central nervous system: hypotonia, temperature instability, irritability, lethargy, full or bulging fontanel	The infant is isolated, and the spread of infection is curtailed
Bacterial or viral infections of the urinary tract, vagina, or cervix			
Rupture of membranes more than 24 h	Altered Bowel Elimination, diarrhea related to infection		Bowel patterns are adequate
Amnionitis			
Maternal bleeding			
Neonatal factors			Fluid balance is present
Male sex	Fluid Volume Deficit related to vomiting, diarrhea, or feeding problems	Respiratory: tachypnea, apnea, cyanosis, grunting, retractions, nasal flaring	Infant demonstrates adequate weight gain
Preterm			Infant's respiratory status is stable
Invasive procedures (surgery, diagnostic)		Gastrointestinal: vomiting and diarrhea, feeding problems	Infant's vital signs remain stable
Certain congenital malformations (ie, meningomyelocele, gastroschisis)	Altered Respiratory Functions, inefficient airway clearance related to specific infection	Circulatory: hypotension; cool skin, mottling	Infant exhibits comfort behaviors
		Frequently monitor vital signs and intake and output *to insure adequate hydration*	Other infants in the nursery remain symptom free
		Pay careful attention to environmental temperature *to provide optimal temperature*	
		Administer antibiotics as ordered *to maximize resistance*	

necessarily reflect the degree of potential damage from unrecognized or undertreated hypoglycemia (Samson, 1992). Glucose screening procedures should continue frequently until the newborn stabilizes. Treatment includes the administration of intravenous glucose by continuous infusion, calculated according to the weight of the newborn. In lieu of intravenous administration, early feedings may begin within the first 30 minutes after delivery if bowel sounds are present.

Hypocalcemia

Hypocalcemia is defined as a calcium level below 7 mg/dL. It is one of the most common clinical problems for the IDM. About 50% of newborns of insulin-dependent women experience hypocalcemia during the first 3 days of life. During pregnancy, a maternal hyperparathyroid state exists that seeks to increase maternal calcium that has been diverted to the fetus. After delivery, neonatal serum calcium falls because of the levels of parathyroid hormone, vitamin D, and calcitonin. Subsequently, parathyroid hormone and vitamin D levels rise to correct this deficiency.

Symptoms of hypocalcemia include jitteriness, convulsions, and twitching. This type of early-onset hypocalcemia usually resolves spontaneously in a few days. Normal calcium levels can be restored with the assistance of early feedings, intravenous calcium gluconate, or calcium supplements.

Hyperbilirubinemia

The etiology of hyperbilirubinemia in IDMs is not clear, although several theories have been postulated. The rate of erythrocyte breakdown appears to be increased as a result of changes in erythrocyte membrane composition from changes in maternal glucose availability (Ogata, 1994). Of these, polycythemia, commonly seen in IDMs, emerges as a significant factor associated with hyperbilirubinemia. Bruising in macrosomic newborns at birth also may be a factor resulting in hyperbilirubinemia. Treatment is the same as for jaundice due to other factors.

Respiratory Disease

The IDM is more likely to develop respiratory distress than other newborns in term pregnancies. In diabetic pregnancies, there exists a fetal hyperinsulinemia due to excess stimulation of the fetal pancreas. When a fetal hyperinsulinemic state exists, surfactant synthesis is inhibited because the elevated levels of insulin change the movement of surfactant-associated proteins (SAPs) from type two alveolar cells. In addition to the traditional components of lecithin and sphingomyelin needed for surfactant, SAPs also are needed for the production of mature surfactant. SAP-35, a critical element in surfactant production, has been noted to be reduced in IDMs. Even term infants of diabetic mothers may experience respiratory distress syndrome as a result of changes in lung maturation. Acceptable lecithin-sphingomyelin ratios of 3.5 to 4.1 are considered acceptable in maternal diabetic pregnancies, because adequate amounts of lecithin may be present despite limited surfactant quantities.

The clinical picture of respiratory distress syndrome and interventions are the same as those discussed in Chapter 41. Current studies do not support the administration of exogenous surfactant supplementation for term infants of diabetic mothers experiencing respiratory distress syndrome. Exogenous surfactant seems to have the greatest benefit prior to 34 weeks' gestation (Samson, 1992).

Birth Defects

An increase in congenital defects has been noted in IDMs, specifically neural tube defects, caudal regression syndrome, and cardiac defects. For further discussion of the fetus of a diabetic mother, see Chapter 32.

Jaundice in the Newborn

Hyperbilirubinemia may occur as a result of physiologic or pathologic factors. **Physiologic jaundice** is common in the newborn and is typically mild and self-limiting (see Chap. 28). Pathologic jaundice may result from hemolytic disease of the newborn, related to either Rh incompatibility or ABO incompatibility. It also can result from excess production or decreased excretion of bilirubin.

Hemolytic disease of the newborn is significant but decreasing in severity because of screening and detection. The administration of anti-D globulin (RhoGAM) to eligible women has been important in combating Rh incompatibility and erythroblastosis fetalis. For extensive discussion of the pathophysiology of these entities, see Chapter 39.

Examples of increased bilirubin load are hemolytic disease of the newborn; hereditary hemolytic anemias; glucose-6-phosphate dehydrogenase deficiency; polycythemia; enclosed hemorrhage, such as cephalhematoma and extensive bruising; swallowed maternal blood; increased enterhepatic circulation of bilirubin; neonatal sepsis; and IDMs (Maisels, 1994). Decreased clearance of bilirubin can occur as a result of inborn errors of metabolism, hypothyroidism, breast milk jaundice, and prematurity.

Pathologic forms of jaundice may pose a serious threat to the newborn because of the possible complication of kernicterus. **Kernicterus** results from the accumulation of unconjugated and unbound bilirubin in brain cells. Neurologic signs occur, and ultimately, intellectual function is impaired. The exact bilirubin level at which kernicterus occurs varies with each newborn, occurring sooner in the preterm newborn.

Assessment

Chapter 28 discusses the physical assessment of a newborn suspected of being jaundiced. The following newborns requiring further evaluation for hyperbilirubinemia include:

■ Those born to Rh-negative mothers

- Those who exhibit jaundice during the first 24 hours of life
- Those who exhibit jaundice below the umbilicus between 24 and 48 hours of life or jaundice below the knees or on the hands and feet
- Jaundice that persists after 2 weeks of age

Diagnostic tests may include direct and total serum bilirubin concentration. Additional laboratory studies should be performed if serum bilirubin results are as follows:

- Cord blood: 4 mg/dL or more
- Rising by 0.5 mg/dL per hour or more over a 4- to 8-hour period
- Rising by a rate of 5 mg/dL or more per day
- Full-term newborns: 13 to 15 mg/dL or more at any time
- Preterm newborns: 10 mg/dL or greater at any time
- Jaundice persisting beyond 10 days of life in a term newborn or 21 days in a preterm newborn, except in breast-fed newborns (Gartner et al., 1992)

Additional diagnostic tests include maternal group and Rh type, neonatal group and Rh type, direct Coombs' test, hematocrit and hemoglobin, and total serum protein. A noninvasive screening tool that may be used to correlate skin color with a total serum bilirubin value is **transcutaneous bilirubinometry,** a hand-held fiberoptic instrument that illuminates the skin and measures the intensity of the yellow color (see Research Highlight: Percutaneous Bilirubinometer).

RESEARCH HIGHLIGHT

Transcutaneous Bilirubinometer

This article, by way of a descriptive review of the literature, presents the technical aspects of the operation of the transcutaneous bilirubinometer, potential problems that may be encountered by the user, and research concerning the instrument's validity and reliability.

The transcutaneous bilirubinometer can be a useful tool for nursing research and to evaluate neonatal jaundice in the home setting. The instrument can identify newborns requiring serum bilirubin determination and prevent other newborns from being subjected to unnecessary blood sampling. Responses to treatment, such as home phototherapy, can be evaluated by the nurse, using the instrument as a guide. Recommendations are made that each institution establish its own criteria for the interpretation of the data and related interventions.

Critique: The study is a basic beginning to other potential research, which could compare various interventions based on the data obtained by the instrument.

Brown, L. et al. (1990). Transcutaneous bilirubinometer: An instrument for clinical research. *Nursing Research, 39*(4), 241–243.

Because early discharge for newborns is becoming the norm, it is imperative that the newborn be evaluated in the home or in a follow-up visit by a healthcare professional. Parents must be taught to recognize the initial and progressive signs of jaundice and to notify the healthcare provider of any progression of jaundice or changes in the newborn's feeding, activity, or elimination patterns.

Nursing Diagnoses

After assessment is completed, appropriate nursing diagnoses can be identified. For a list of possible nursing diagnoses, see Box 43-3.

Planning and Intervention

In the event of a positive Coombs' test or a very low birth weight, phototherapy often may be initiated without waiting for bilirubin results. The decision to initiate phototherapy is somewhat individualized, with criteria varying from center to center. The use of phototherapy, generally considered a benign treatment, has almost eliminated the onset of kernicterus and significantly lowered the use of exchange transfusion as a treatment modality. Benefits need to be weighed against risks when making the decision to initiate phototherapy. The potential negative effects on the family, including possible interruption of breast-feeding and bonding, are factors to be considered.

Phototherapy

Phototherapy, the use of intense fluorescent light to reduce serum bilirubin, has gained acceptance in the treatment of hyperbilirubinemia. Phototherapy, by the

---

BOX 43–3
Nursing Diagnoses: Hyperbilirubenemia

- Risk for Injury related to elevated bilirubin levels
- Risk for Fluid Volume Deficit related to phototherapy and its effects
- Diarrhea related to effects of phototherapy
- Risk for Impaired Skin Integrity related to phototherapy
- Ineffective Thermoregulation related to phototherapy
- Knowledge Deficit related condition, treatments, and required care
- Risk for Altered Parent/Infant Attachment related to confinement during phototherapy
- Altered Family Processes related to needed phototherapy care at home

processes of photoisomerization and photo-oxidation, results in more water-soluble bilirubin end-products, which are rapidly excreted in urine and bile. Phototherapy generally consists of a single quartz halogen lamp or a bank of four to eight cool-white, daybright, or special blue fluorescent bulbs covered by a Plexiglas shield and positioned 12 to 30 in from the newborn. The energy output from the lights must be checked periodically to confirm the desired output. The success of phototherapy depends on the energy output in the blue spectrum of the lights and on the surface area of the newborn exposed to the treatment (Fig. 43-3).

Once phototherapy has been initiated, serum bilirubin levels must be monitored frequently, because visual assessment of any jaundice is no longer valid. Ongoing studies continue to investigate the possibility of any long-term or permanent side effects of phototherapy. So far, none are known. The nurse focuses on the care of the newborn receiving phototherapy and any subsequent short-term side effects (see Procedure 43-1). Fiberoptic light systems have been developed that emit light from a high-intensity lamp to a fiberoptic pad or blanket. Advantages of these systems are that the newborn can be held or nursed while still receiving treatment and that eye patches will probably be unnecessary. These systems appear to be as effective as conventional phototherapy.

Home Phototherapy. Home phototherapy may be a viable alternative when used carefully with families meeting the program's criteria. With the trend toward early discharge, home phototherapy can prevent readmission should hyperbilirubinemia occur. Parental education regarding newborn care and home visits by a home healthcare nurse are essential components of a home phototherapy program. Risks of home therapy programs are reported to be minimal. Benefits include financial savings, uninterrupted maternal–newborn bonding, and increased parental satisfaction.

Exchange Transfusion

Treatment could involve immediate exchange transfusion, as in the event of a **hydropic** newborn. A hydropic newborn is severely affected by hemolytic disease, exhibiting pallor, edema, ascites, congestive heart failure, and pleural effusion. Exchange transfusions may be performed in newborns subjected to hemolytic disease (eg, Rh incompatibility or ABO incompatibility). The exchange transfusion will decrease levels of bilirubin and correct any anemia. The donor blood used must be compatible with newborn's and mother's serum.

An exchange transfusion alternately removes a small amount of blood from the newborn and replaces it with the same amount of donor blood. An umbilical catheter is used to perform the exchange, usually a double-volume type. In a double-volume exchange, the amount of donor blood is twice that of the newborn volume. Small amounts up to 20 mL are exchanged at a time. An infusion of albumin can be given several hours prior to the procedure to increase the number of bilirubin binding sites, thereby making the exchange more efficient.

Pre-exchange. The nurse is the primary caregiver who assesses the newborn's color, observing for any increased jaundice. The newborn's behavior is assessed for increasing lethargy, necessitating more diagnostic workup. The nurse checks to see that all pre-exchange blood samples have been collected. An informed consent must be signed by the parents. Donor blood ordered must be checked for the type, unit number, and expiration date. Usually a hematocrit of donor blood is obtained. The desirable donor hematocrit is between 45 and 55.

Blood must be warmed slowly. Blood-warming units keep blood at an even temperature during the procedure. The newborn must be placed on monitors and restrained. The nurse prepares the newborn for umbilical artery catheterization, if needed, by restraining him or her and setting up the sterile tray, solutions, and surgical gloves.

Procedural Tasks. The newborn's temperature and other vital signs are taken and recorded at frequent intervals during the procedure. Ideally, the newborn is placed on a continuous cardiopulmonary monitor. Vital signs are recorded on the newborn's flow sheet and on the exchange record itself. The amount of blood placed in and out and any drugs given are recorded on the exchange transfer sheet. For example, a dose of calcium may be given for every 100 mL exchanged. To-

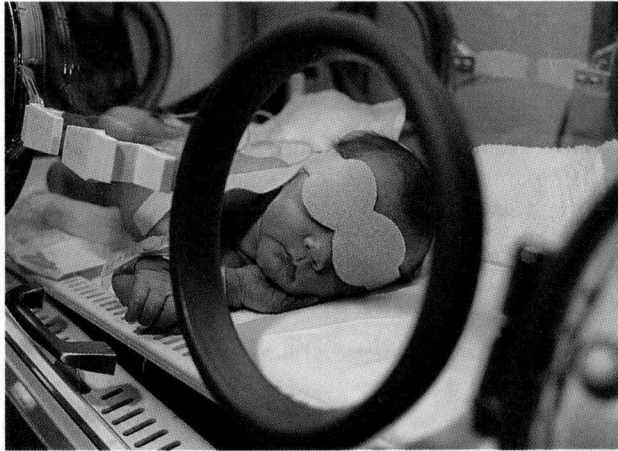

FIGURE 43–3 An infant receives phototherapy wearing eye patches to prevent any potential retinal damage.

PROCEDURE 43-1
Phototherapy

Overall Objective: To initiate and maintain phototherapy safely while promoting the psychosocial needs of the newborn and family unit

Nursing Actions	*Rationale*
Preparation	
1. Explain procedure to parents.	1. This alleviates anxiety concerning light therapy.
Procedure	
1. Place newborn in isolette with phototherapy bank of lights about 12–30 in from newborn.	1. Close lights promote more effective therapy. Distance is determined by type of bulb used.
2. Use fiberoptic blanket if available.	2. Newborn can be held and nursed and still receive treatment.
3. Shield newborn's eyes using a soft eyeshield. Take care to avoid obstructing nares. Remove eyeshields frequently and inspect for any eye discharge from reaction to routine prophylaxis or infection (conjunctivitis) from exposure to organisms in the birth canal.	3. Any potential damage to eyes and airway obstruction are avoided. Assessment and family eye contact can occur.
4. Keep newborn nude except diaper, and change position frequently.	4. This promotes maximal use of light working on subcutaneous tissue and shields external genitalia from light.
5. Monitor skin condition, and change diapers frequently.	5. Loose stools can cause skin breakdown.
6. Monitor intake and output, and observe for evidence of dehydration.	6. Potential for dehydration related to loose stools and body temperature increase from isolette and lights.
7. Monitor temperature, and maintain neutral thermal environment.	7. This avoids hyperthermia and prevents excessive stress.
8. Monitor light intensity with bilimeter.	8. Effectiveness of therapy is maintained.
9. Remove newborn from therapy for holding and feeding, unless contraindicated.	9. Family bonding is promoted and lactation is maintained if appropriate.

tal amounts of blood infused and withdrawn also are recorded. Postexchange blood samples are drawn at the end of the procedure.

Post-transfusion. Frequent monitoring of vital signs continues following the procedure. Ongoing assessments are crucial to identify potential complications. Some complications to anticipate include rebound hyperbilirubinemia, electrolyte imbalances, hypoglycemia, hypervolemia or hypovolemia, cardiac arrhythmias, air embolism, and infection.

Evaluation

Possible anticipated outcomes may include the following:

■ The newborn receives as much tactile stimulation and care as possible.

■ The newborn's fluid and electrolyte balances remain within normal limits.
■ The newborn's vital signs remain within normal limits.
■ The newborn remains free of complications.
■ The parents demonstrate knowledge of the newborn's condition and required care.
■ The parents demonstrate a beginning parent–newborn relationship.

Breast Milk Jaundice

The incidence of increased bilirubin at about the fourth to seventh day, with a peak at 2 weeks, has been reported in 1% to 2% of breast-fed babies (Wilkerson, 1988). The exact etiology of true breast milk jaundice is unknown. Theories have focused on the roles of pregnanediol, increased enzyme activity, and increased free fatty acids in breast milk. A recent hypothesis proposes that true breast milk jaundice occurs as a result of increased amounts of β-glucuronidase in breast milk, which leads to increased intestinal absorption of bilirubin. Jaundice associated with breast-feeding, a different phenomenon, appears to correlate with the newborn's success at breast-feeding. Research indicates that newborns who do not nurse well tend to have higher average bilirubin levels than those who nurse often and well (Wilkerson, 1988).

Treatment for elevated bilirubin levels varies depending on the type. Rising levels of bilirubin associated with true breast-feeding jaundice may necessitate phototherapy and temporary cessation of breast-feeding. Jaundice associated with breast-feeding is usually temporary and resolves with frequent nursing. The mother may need help in learning to pump her breasts if cessation of breast-feeding is recommended.

Newborn of Substance-Addicted Mother

The lifestyle of addicted women during the childbearing years promotes other health problems affecting the fetus and subsequently the newborn. Chapter 34 discusses the typical effects of smoking, drugs, and alcohol on the fetus and newborn. This section focuses on the nursing process used in the care of newborns of addicted mothers.

Nursing Assessment

Newborns exposed to toxic substances in utero exhibit characteristic appearances and behaviors described in detail in Chapter 34. If there is a known positive maternal history for drug or alcohol abuse, assessment priority focuses on any obvious congenital anomalies.

Prominent behavior alterations are demonstrated in the gastrointestinal and central nervous systems, in addition to vasomotor disturbances. Newborns may display vomiting, diarrhea, excessive sucking, and ineffective feeding patterns as a result of uncoordinated sucking and swallowing. Numerous central nervous system abnormalities can be noted with varying developmental implications. Newborn behaviors range from highly irritable to passive, with most displaying irritability and difficulty sleeping. Tremors of hands, arms, legs, chin, and tongue are common, increasing as the newborn fatigues. Increased muscle tone interferes with normal motor development; the ability to be pulled to a sitting position is delayed, and arms are typically widespread in "W" position. Resistance is exhib-

ited when bringing arms to the midline. This increased muscle tone inhibits development of fine motor skills. Lifelong developmental disabilities, such as short- and long-term learning problems, slower intellectual development, emotional and behavioral differences, and delayed language development, become increasingly evident as the infant grows and matures (Lewis, 1989).

Nursing Diagnoses

Various physiologic and psychosocial nursing diagnoses are possible for newborns exposed prenatally to drugs and alcohol. For a list of possible nursing diagnoses see Box 43-4.

Interventions

The nurse assists with nutritional deficits by providing small, frequent feedings; rest periods; and gavage feedings if necessary. The newborn is fed in an upright position, with the chin supported by a hand to facilitate sucking. To help diminish the newborn's irritability and tremors, the nurse adjusts the environment by decreasing noise and dimming lights. Soft music or background noise may have a calming effect. Swaddling, holding, and rocking the newborn; carrying the newborn in a front-pouch carrier; and offering the newborn a pacifier may be soothing. Newborns may be swaddled, carried, or held in positions that facilitate arm placement at midline rather than in "W" position.

BOX 43-4
Nursing Diagnoses: Newborn of Drug-Abusing Mother

- Altered Nutrition: Less than body requirements related to uncoordinated and ineffective sucking and swallowing reflexes
- Altered Growth and Development related to prenatal exposure to toxic substances
- Risk for Fluid Volume Deficit related to vomiting or diarrhea
- Altered Protection related to physiologic effects of drug abuse in the newborn
- Risk for Injury related to effects of drug abuse in the newborn
- Risk for Impaired Skin Integrity related to hyperactivity and diarrhea
- Risk for Altered Parenting related to newborn's behavioral problems
- Knowledge Deficit (parental) related to
  - Condition, treatment, and care
  - Effects of substance abuse on fetus and newborn
- Risk for Altered Parent/Infant Attachment related to
  - Continued maternal substance abuse
  - Newborn's behavioral problems

Sedatives may be administered as ordered to assist in promoting less irritability and tremors (Lewis, 1989).

Several drugs may be used in the treatment of neonatal abstinence syndrome for newborns of an opiate-using mother. The two most often used are tincture of opium and phenobarbital (Jorgensen, 1992). Other medications may include paregoric, diazepam (Valium), and chlorpromazine (Thorazine).

Separation between mother and newborn should be minimized, and the mother's active participation in caregiving should be encouraged (see Research Highlight: Maternal Perception and Parent-Newborn Interaction of Vulnerable Cocaine-Exposed Couples). Complications that may be encountered with newborns of drug-abusing women are infection, developmental delays, and special discharge planning considerations (Jorgensen, 1992). Multidisciplinary referrals are essential to attempt to establish a safe home environment for the newborn. Follow-up care and ongoing assessment of the home are vital in light of the evidence that these newborns are at high risk for abuse and neglect (see Nursing Care Plan: Infants Born to Drug Abusers).

Evaluation

As a result of effective nursing interventions, possible anticipated outcomes may include the following:

- The newborn demonstrates adequate nutrition and fluid balance by appropriate weight gain.
- The newborn demonstrates decreasing episodes of irritability and muscle rigidity.
- The newborn remains free of injury.
- The parents interact positively with the newborn on frequent occasions.
- The mother (or parents) participates in caretaking activities.
- The newborn returns to a safe environment.

Summary Points

✔ Various birth injuries may be immediately apparent in the moments following birth and after a thorough physical assessment.

✔ The most common birth injuries include head trauma, such as caput succedaneum, cephalhematoma, and intracranial hemorrhage; perinatal hemorrhage; and shock. Nervous system problems also occur, such as facial paralysis, Erb's palsy, and fractures of the clavicle, long bones of the extremities, and the skull.

✔ Nurses must be aware of maternal risk factors impacting the newborn who is at risk for various infections. Some septic newborns may be treated immediately with a positive outcome, while others may require long-term multidisciplinary referral, community-based assistance, and home care.

✔ Although advances have been made in the care of pregnant diabetic women, newborns remain vulnerable to various metabolic alterations, such as hypoglycemia, hypocalcemia, hyperbilirubinemia, respiratory disease, and birth defects.

✔ Numerous perinatal factors may impact the possibility of a newborn experiencing pathologic jaundice. Nursing assessment of jaundice patterns will impact treatment options.

✔ Nurses face the challenge of caring for newborns of maternal drug abusers. These mothers require teaching concerning the various neonatal physiologic and behavioral alterations that they may anticipate to achieve the most positive outcome.

RESEARCH HIGHLIGHT

Maternal Perception and Parent–Newborn Interaction of Vulnerable Cocaine-Exposed Couples

The purpose of this pilot study was to compare maternal perceptions of the newborn and parent–newborn interaction between mothers with positive urine drug screens for cocaine use and mothers with negative urine drug screens for cocaine use. The researchers designed the study to answer two questions: Will mothers with positive urine drug screens for cocaine have more negative perceptions of their newborns than mothers with negative urine drug screens? Will mothers with positive urine drug screens for cocaine have lower scores on parent–newborn interactions than mothers with negative urine drug screens for cocaine? The sample was composed of 30 low-risk women who delivered vaginally and were bottle feeding. Mothers' perceptions of their newborns were measured by the Neonatal Perception Inventory, and parent–newborn interaction was measured by the Nursing Child Assessment Scale. The data suggest that mothers with positive urine drug screens perceived their newborns in the same way as mothers with negative drug screens. However, the newborns exposed to cocaine sent poor cues to their mothers, while the mothers were less sensitive and responsive to the cues.

Critique: Study limitations were the small sample size and mothers' knowledge that they were being observed, with possible behavioral alterations. As a result of this study, nursing interventions should include the provision of information to mothers regarding neonatal withdrawal symptoms and other neurobehavioral alterations and assistance with parenting skills.

Barabach, L. M., Glazer, G., & Norris, S. C. (1992). Maternal perception and parent-infant interaction of vulnerable cocaine-exposed couplets. *Journal of Perinatal and Neonatal Nursing, 6*(3), 76–84.

NURSING CARE PLAN
Infants Born to Drug Abusers

Nursing Goals
1. Infant receives adequate nutrition.
2. Infant maintains fluid-volume balance.
3. Irritability and muscle rigidity are lessened.
4. Maternal–infant interactions are ongoing and positive.
5. Maternal caretaking is competent and ongoing.
6. A safe home environment is established prior to discharge.
7. Follow-up care is planned.

Assessment	Potential Nursing Diagnoses	Intervention/ Rationale	Evaluation
Known history of maternal drug abuse Amount, type of drug, and type of last dosage Positive maternal and neonatal drug screens Noted associated congenital anomalies Characteristic behaviors observed and documented Lack of quiet sleep Nonnutritive sucking patterns Tremors Irritability Vomiting Diarrhea Constipation	Altered Nutrition: Less than body requirements, related to uncoordinated and ineffective sucking and swallowing reflexes Risk for Fluid Volume Deficit related to inadequate fluid intake, vomiting, diarrhea Altered Growth and Development related to exposure to toxic substances prenatally Risk for Altered Parenting	Provide small, frequent feedings *to provide adequate nutrition* Gavage feed if necessary *to provide adequate nutrition* Feed in upright position *to provide adequate nutrition* Begin intravenous fluid administration *to assure fluid balance* Monitor intake and output *to ensure balance* Assess mucous membranes, skin turgor *for hydration status* Reduce stimuli in environment *to provide appropriate tactile stimulation* Position to avoid arms in "W" posture Promote maternal–infant interaction and caretaking *to promote bonding*	Infant receives adequate nutrition Infant maintains fluid-volume balance Irritability and muscle rigidity are lessened Maternal–infant interactions are ongoing and positive Maternal caretaking is competent and ongoing A safe home environment is established prior to discharge Follow-up care is planned

REFERENCES

Baley, J. E., & Goldfarb, J. (1992). Viral infections. In A. A. Fanaroff & R. S. Martin (Eds.), *Neonatal-perinatal medicine* (5th ed.) (pp. 662–682). St. Louis: C.V. Mosby.

Benson, M. S. (1994). Management of infants born to women infected with human immunodeficiency virus. *Journal of Perinatal and Neonatal Nursing, 7*(4), 79–89.

Blanchette, V., Doyk, J., Schmidt, B., and Zipursky, A. (1994). Hematology. In G. B. Avery, M. A. Fletcher, M. G. Macdonald (Eds.), Neonatology: Pathophysiology and management of the newborn (4th edition) pp. 952–999. Philadelphia: J.B. Lippincott.

Brann, A., & Schwartz, J. (1992). Central nervous disturbances-birth injury (part 3). In A. A. Fanaroff & R. S. Martin (Eds.), *Neonatal-perinatal medicine* (5th ed.) (pp. 703–718). St. Louis: C.V. Mosby.

Braune, K. W., & Lacey, L. (1983). Common hematologic problems of the immediate newborn period. *Journal of Obstetric, Gynecologic, and Neonatal Nursing, 12*(Suppl. 3), 19s–26s.

Feigin, R., Adcock, L. M., & Edwards, M. S. (1992). Fungal and protozoal infections. In A. A. Fanaroff & R. S. Martin (Eds.), *Neonatal-perinatal medicine* (5th ed.) (pp. 683–689). St. Louis: C.V. Mosby.

Feigin, R., Adcock, L. M., & Miller, D. J. (1992). Postnatal bacterial infections. In A. A. Fanaroff & R. S. Martin (Eds.), *Neonatal-perinatal medicine* (5th ed.) (pp. 619–659). St. Louis: C.V. Mosby.

Freij, B. J., & McCracken, G. H. (1994). Acute infections. IN G. B. Avery, M. A. Fletcher, & M. G. MacDonald (Eds.), *Neonatology: Pathophysiology and management of the newborn* (4th ed.) (pp. 1082–1116). Philadelphia: J.B. Lippincott.

Fuller, R. (1992). Group B streptococcal infection in the newborn. *Critical Care Nursing, 4*(3), 487–492.

Gartner, L., & Lee, K. S. (1992). Jaundice and liver disease-unconjugated hyperbilirubinemia. In A. A. Fanaroff & R. S. Martin (Eds.), Neonatal-perinatal medicine (5th ed.) (pp. 1093–1104). St. Louis: C.V. Mosby.

Hill, A., & Volpe, J. (1994). Neurological disorders. In G. B. Avery, M. A. Fletcher, & M. G. Macdonald (Eds.), *Neona-*

tology: Pathophysiology and management of the newborn (4th ed.) (pp. 1082–1116). Philadelphia: J.B. Lippincott.

Jorgenson, K. M. (1992). The drug-exposed infant. *Critical Care Nursing, 4*(3), 481–485.

Lewis, K. D., Bennett, B., Schmeder, N. H. (1989). The care of infants menaced by cocaine abuse. *MCN* 14(5), 324–329.

Lott, J. W., & Kenner, C. (1994). Keeping up with neonatal infections: Designer bugs. Part I. *MCN: American Journal of Maternal Child Nursing, 19*(4), 207–213.

Lott, J. W., & Kenner, C. (1994). Keeping up with neonatal infections: Designer bugs. Part II. *MCN: American Journal of Maternal Child Nursing, 19*(5), 264–271.

Maisels, M. J. (1994), Jaundice. In G. B. Avery, M. A. Fletcher, & M. G. Macdonald (Eds.), *Neonatology: Pathophysiology and management of the newborn* (4th ed.) (pp. 630–725). Philadelphia: J.B. Lippincott.

Mangurten, H. (1992). Birth injuries. In A. A. Fanaroff & R. S. Martin (Eds.), *Neonatal-perinatal medicine* (5th ed.) (pp. 346–371). St. Louis: C.V. Mosby.

Margileth, A. (1994). Dermatologic conditions. In G. B. Avery, M. A. Fletcher, & M. G. Macdonald (Eds.), *Neonatology: Pathophysiology and management of the newborn* (4th ed.) (pp. 1229–1268). Philadelphia: J.B. Lippincott.

Minarcik, C. J. and Beachy, P. (1989). Neurologic disorders. In G. B. Merenstein and S. L. Gardner (Eds.) *Handbook of Neonatal Intensive Care* (pp. 501–530). St. Louis: C. V. Mosby.

Ogata, E. S. (1994). Carbohydrate homeostasis. In G. B. Avery, M. A. Fletcher, & M. G. Macdonald (Eds.), *Neonatology: Pathophysiology and management of the newborn* (4th ed.) (pp. 1229–1268). Philadelphia: J.B. Lippincott.

Rimar, J. M. (1988). Shock in infants and children: Assessment and treatment. *MCN* 13(2), 98–105.

Samson, L. F. (1992). Infants of diabetic mother: Current perspectives. *Journal of Perinatal and Neonatal Nursing, 6*(1), 61–70.

Wilkerson, N. N. (1988). A comprehensive look at hyperbilirubinemia. *MCN: American Journal of Maternal Child Nursing, 13*(5), 360–364.

SUGGESTED READING

Barbach, L. M., Glazer, G., & Norris, S. C. (1992). Maternal perception and parent-infant interaction of vulnerable cocaine-exposed couplets. *Journal of Perinatal and Neonatal Nursing, 6*(3), 76–84.

Barbour, B. G. (1989). Is fetal alcohol syndrome completely irreversible? *MCN: American Journal of Maternal Child Nursing, 14*(1), 44–46.

Beachy, P., & Deacon, J. (1992). *Core curriculum for neonatal intensive care nursing*. Philadelphia: W.B. Saunders.

Chavez, G. F., Mulinara, J., & Edmonds, L. D. (1991). Epidemiology of Rh hemolytic disease of the newborn in the United States. *Journal of the American Medical Association, 265*(24), 3270–3274.

Flandermeyer, A. A. (1993). The drug-exposed neonate. In C. Kenner, A. Brueggemeyer, & L. P. Gunderson (Eds.), *Comprehensive neonatal nursing, a physiologic perspective.* Philadelphia: W.B. Saunders.

Free, T., Russell, F., Mills, B., & Hathaway, D. (1990). A descriptive study of infants and toddlers exposed prenatally to substance abuse. *MCN: American Journal of Maternal Child Nursing, 15*(4), 245–249.

Giacoia, G. P. (1993). New approaches for the treatment of neonatal sepsis. *Journal of Perinatology, 13*(3), 223–237.

Hoskins, S. K. (1990). Nursing care of the infant of a diabetic mother: An antenatal, intrapartal and neonatal challenge. *Neonatal Network, 9*(4), 39–46.

Klaus, M. H., & Fanaroff, A. A. (1993). *Care of the high-risk neonate* (4th ed.). Philadelphia: W.B. Saunders.

Klein, J. M. (1992). Neonatal morbidity and mortality secondary to premature rupture of the membranes. *Obstetrics and Gynecology Clinics of North America, 19*(2), 265–280.

Lassiter, H. A. (1992). Intravenous immunoglobulins in the prevention and treatment of neonatal bacterial sepsis. *Advances in Pediatrics, 39*, 71–99.

Ludwig, M. A. (1990). Phototherapy in the home setting. *Journal of Pediatric Health Care, 4*(6), 304–308.

Mattson, S., & Smith, J. E. (Eds.) (1992). *NAACOG core curriculum for maternal newborn nursing.* Philadelphia: W.B. Saunders.

Norris, M. K., & Hill, C. S. (1992). Assessing congenital heart defects in the cocaine-exposed neonate. *Dimensions of Critical Care Nursing, 11*(1), 6–12.

Payne, N. R., Schilling, C. G., & Steinberg, S. (1994). Selecting antibiotics for nosocomial bacterial infections in patients requiring neonatal intensive care. *Neonatal Network, 13*(3), 41–51.

Platt, M. W., & Gilson, G. J. (1994). Group B streptococcal disease in the perinatal period. *American Family Physician, 49*(2), 434–442.

Polin, R. A., & St. Geme, J. W. (1992). Neonatal sepsis. *Advances in Pediatric Infectious Diseases, 7*, 25–61.

Schuman, A. J., & Karush, G. (1992). Fiberoptic versus conventional home phototherapy for neonatal hyperbilirubinemia. *Clinical Pediatrics, 31*(6), 345–352.

Van Maldergem, L., Jauniaux, E., Fourneau, C., & Gillerot, Y. (1992). Genetic cause of hydrops fetalis. *Pediatrics, 89*(1), 81–86.

Weisman, L. E. (1993). Standard versus hyperimmune intravenous immunoglobin in preventing or treating neonatal bacterial infections. *Clinics in Perinatology, 20*(1), 211–224.

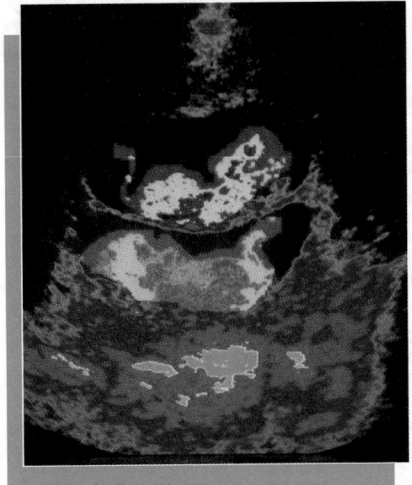

Assessment and Management of High-Risk Perinatal Conditions

Critical Thinking Exercises

1. Andrea Gasparro gave birth prematurely. Her daughter weighed only 2000 grams at 30 weeks' gestation. Her newborn had respiratory problems at birth that resulted in the need for mechanical ventilation. She was admitted to the NICU. Andrea is going to visit her daughter for the first time since giving birth. She appears anxious and fearful, stating, "How can I hold my baby? What if I do something wrong? I don't know what to do."

    Propose appropriate strategies based on your understanding of this newborn's needs that will assist the client with initiating the maternal-neonatal relationship.

2. A male neonate is born with a cleft lip and palate and polydactyly. Further examination reveals no other problems. The parents are distraught, upset and crying. They state, "Our son is deformed. How did this happen?" The mother then begins to blame herself for this "tragedy" because she did not follow all of her physician's instructions during her pregnancy, particularly about good nutrition.

    Outline the phases of the grieving process and recommend appropriate interventions to assist this couple in working through the grieving process.

3. John and Annie Lopez are planning to take their newborn daughter home today. Their daughter was diagnosed with hyperbilirubinemia and is to be treated with home phototherapy.

    Develop an appropriate teaching plan for John and Annie that addresses their needs prior to discharge and then once they take their baby home.

Multiple Choice Questions

1. When preparing a teaching plan for a group of students about possible disorders affecting an infant, the nurse is correct in identifying which of the following as an inborn error of metabolism?

    A. Phenylketonuria
    B. Kernicterus
    C. Down syndrome
    D. Sepsis

2. A client is scheduled for an amniocentesis to determine the lung maturity of the fetus. Which of the following is used for this purpose?

    A. Indirect and direct bilirubin
    B. Cytology smears
    C. Creatinine clearance
    D. Lecithin/sphingomyelin ratio

3. A client in her first trimester is scheduled for a transabdominal ultrasound. The nurse instructs the client to:

    A. Take nothing by mouth for 8 hours before the test
    B. Drink 6 to 8 glasses of water before the test
    C. Void frequently before the test
    D. Lie down in the lithotomy position

4. The nurse is preparing to auscultate the fetal heart tones of a client in labor. The fetus is in a cephalic presentation, LOA position. The nurse anticipates that the fetal heart sounds would be heard best:

    A. At or above the level of the umbilicus
    B. Midline between the umbilicus and the pubis
    C. In the left lower quadrant of the abdomen
    D. In the right lower quadrant of the abdomen

5. The nurse documents early decelerations for a client receiving electronic fetal monitoring is in place for a client. The pattern that the nurse is observing on the fetal heart tracing is one that is:

    A. U-shaped curve
    B. Mirror image of the uterine contraction
    C. W-shaped curve
    D. Occurring after the onset of the uterine contraction

6. Approximately 1 hour after birth, a neonate is diagnosed with a diaphragmatic hernia. He is cyanotic and close to going into shock. The nurse's priority when caring for this infant is:

A. Assisting with an umbilical catheter insertion
B. Obtaining footprints and bracelet for identification
C. Establishing adequate ventilation and oxygenation
D. Placing neonate prone to enhance lung expansion

7. While assessing a neonate of 38 weeks' gestation, the nurse notes that the neonate's skin is loose and dry, with sparse scalp hair, sunken abdomen, and minimal subcutaneous fat. The nurse determines that the neonate is:

A. Appropriate for gestational age
B. Large for gestational age
C. Small for gestational age
D. Postterm

8. A fetal monitoring strip shows FHR deceleration beginning about 30 seconds after the onset of each contraction and returning to baseline after the contraction is over. The nurse is correct in identifying that the cause of this pattern is:

A. Umbilical cord compression
B. Uteroplacental insufficiency
C. Cardiac anomalies
D. Fetal head compression

9. A neonate, transferred to the NICU because of respiratory distress, is receiving mechanical ventilation. The neonate's father is waiting to see his baby. The nurse should:

A. Tell the father to return when the baby is stable
B. Contact the facility's pastoral care department to wait with the father outside the unit
C. Allow the father to visit after explaining the baby's condition and what he will see
D. Take a photograph of the baby and give it to the father outside in the waiting area.

10. A neonate develops asphyxia shortly after birth and the neonatal team begins resuscitative measures. The nurse correctly maintains the neonate's head:

A. Fully hyperextended
B. In the sniff position
C. In a neutral position
D. Turned to the left side

11. A neonate is diagnosed with hydrocephalus. During assessment, the nurse would expect to find:

A. Closely approximated suture lines
B. Upward eye slanting
C. Bulging fontanels
D. Small forehead

12. At 34 weeks, a client delivers a neonate who dies shortly after birth. To assist this client, the nurse should:

A. Limit contact with the client to allow her to grieve
B. Allow the client to see and touch the neonate's body
C. Allow the client's partner to decide what the client should do
D. Avoid giving any information to the client or partner

13. Which of the following outcome criteria should receive the highest priority following percutaneous umbilical blood sampling?

A. Demonstrates increased knowledge about the procedure
B. Displays no signs of infection
C. Demonstrates fetal heart rate within normal limits
D. Reports relief of pain

Study Questions

1. Name the more traditional technique for performing an ultrasound.

2. Identify the fetal measurements that can be obtained with an ultrasound.

3. Name the most widely used method of external electronic FHR monitoring.

4. Identify the technique used to qualitatively assess fetal acid base status.

5. List four placental factors that may affect fetal growth.

6. Identify three complications of using an umbilical cord catheter.

7. Name the most common cardiovascular defect in the preterm neonate.

8. Define myelomeningocele.

9. How long does it take for a cephalhematoma to resolve?

10. State the most common nerve injury in the newborn.

11. List four life-long developmental disabilities associated with neonates born to substance-addicted mothers.

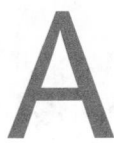

The Pregnant Patient's Bill of Rights

American parents are becoming increasingly aware that health professionals do not always have scientific data to support common American obstetric practices and that many of these practices are carried out primarily because they are part of medical and hospital tradition. In the last 40 years, many artificial practices have been introduced that have changed childbirth from a physiological event to a very complicated medical procedure in which all kinds of drugs are used and procedures carried out, sometimes unnecessarily, and many of them potentially damaging for the baby and even for the mother. A growing body of research makes it alarmingly clear that every aspect of traditional American hospital care during labor and delivery must now be questioned as to its possible effect on the future well-being of both the obstetric patient and her unborn child.

One in every 35 children born in the United States today will eventually be diagnosed as retarded; one in every 10 to 17 children has been found to have some form of brain dysfunction or learning disability requiring special treatment. Such statistics are not confined to the lower socioeconomic group but cut across all segments of American society.

New concerns are being raised by childbearing women because no one knows what degree of oxygen depletion, head compression, or traction by forceps the unborn or newborn infant can tolerate before that child sustains permanent brain damage or dysfunction. The recent findings regarding the cancer-related drug diethylstilbestrol have alerted the public to the fact that neither the approval of a drug by the U.S. Food and Drug Administration nor the fact that a drug is prescribed by a physician guarantees that a drug or medication is safe for the mother or her unborn child. In fact, the American Academy of Pediatrics Committee on Drugs has recently stated that no drug, whether prescription or over-the-counter, has been proven safe for the unborn child.

The pregnant patient has the right to participate in decisions involving her well-being and that of her unborn child, unless there is a clear-cut medical emergency that prevents her participation. In addition to the rights set forth in the American Hospital Association's "Patient's Bill of Rights" (which has also been adopted by the New York City Department of Health) the pregnant patient, because she represents *two* patients rather than one, should be recognized as having the additional rights listed below.

1. *The pregnant patient has the right,* prior to the administration of any drug or procedure, to be informed by the health professional caring for her of any potential direct or indirect effects, risks, or hazards to herself or her unborn or newborn infant which may result from the use of a drug or procedure prescribed for or administered to her during pregnancy, labor, birth, or lactation.

2. *The pregnant patient has the right,* prior to the proposed therapy, to be informed, not only of the benefits, risks, and hazards of the proposed therapy but also of known alternative therapy, such as available childbirth education classes, which could help to prepare the pregnant patient physically and mentally to cope with the discomfort or stress of pregnancy and the experience of childbirth, thereby reducing or eliminating her need for drugs and obstetric intervention. She should be offered such information early in her pregnancy in order that she may make a reasoned decision.

3. *The pregnant patient has the right,* prior to the administration of any drug, to be informed by the health professional who is prescribing or administering the drug to her that any drug she receives during pregnancy, labor, and birth, no matter how or when the drug is taken or administered, may adversely affect her unborn baby, directly or indirectly, and that there is no drug or chemical that has been proven safe for the unborn child.

4. *The pregnant patient has the right,* if cesarean section is anticipated, to be informed prior to the administration of any drug, and preferably prior to the hospitalization, that minimizing her and, in turn, her baby's intake of nonessential preoperative medicine will benefit her baby.

5. *The pregnant patient has the right,* prior to the administration of a drug or procedure, to be informed if there is NO properly controlled follow-up research that has established the

safety of the drug or procedure with regard to its direct or indirect effects on the physiological, mental, and neurological development of the child exposed, via the mother, to the drug or procedure during pregnancy, labor, birth, or lactation (this would apply to virtually all drugs and the vast majority of obstetric procedures).

6. *The pregnant patient has the right,* prior to the administration of any drug, to be informed of the brand name and generic name of the drug in order that she may advise the health professional of any past adverse reaction to the drug.

7. *The pregnant patient has the right* to determine for herself, without pressure from her attendant, whether she will accept the risks inherent in the proposed therapy or refuse a drug or procedure.

8. *The pregnant patient has the right* to know the name and qualifications of the individual administering a medication or procedure to her during labor or birth.

9. *The pregnant patient has the right* to be informed, prior to the administration of any procedure, whether that procedure is being administered to her for her or her baby's benefit (medically indicated) or as an elective procedure (for convenience or teaching purposes).

10. *The pregnant patient has the right* to be accompanied during the stress of labor and birth by someone she cares for, and to whom she looks for emotional comfort and encouragement.

11. *The pregnant patient has the right* after appropriate medical consultation to choose a position for labor and for birth which is least stressful to her baby and to herself.

12. *The obstetric patient has the right* to have her baby cared for at her bedside if her baby is normal and to feed her baby according to her baby's needs rather than according to the hospital regimen.

13. *The obstetric patient has the right* to be informed in writing of the name of the person who actually delivered her baby and the professional qualifications of that person. This information should also be on the birth certificate.

14. *The obstetric patient has the right* to be informed if there is any known or indicated aspect of her or her baby's care or condition that may cause her or her baby later difficulty or problems.

15. *The obstetric patient has the right* to have her and her baby's hospital medical records complete, accurate, and legible and to have their records, including Nurses' Notes, retained by the hospital until the child reaches at least the age of majority, or, alternatively, to have the records offered to her before they are destroyed.

16. *The obstetric patient,* both during and after her hospital stay, *has the right* to have access to her complete hospital medical records, including Nurses' Notes, and to receive a copy upon payment of a reasonable fee and without incurring the expense of retaining an attorney.

It is the obstetric patient and her baby, not the health professional, who must sustain any trauma or injury resulting from the use of a drug or obstetric procedure. The observation of the rights listed above will not only permit the obstetric patient to participate in the decisions involving her and her baby's health care, but will help to protect the health professional and the hospital against litigation arising from resentment or misunderstanding on the part of the mother.

(Reprinted by permission of the Committee on Patient's Rights, Box 1900, New York, N.Y. 10001.)

B

Standard Precautions

Use Standard Precautions, or the equivalent, for the care of all patients. *Category IB**

A. Handwashing
  (1) Wash hands after touching blood, body fluids, secretions, excretions, and contaminated items, whether or not gloves are worn. Wash hands immediately after gloves are removed, between patient contacts, and when otherwise indicated to avoid transfer of microorganisms to other patients or environments. It may be necessary to wash hands between tasks and procedures on the same patient to prevent cross-contamination of different body sites. *Category IB*
  (2) Use a plain (nonantimicrobial) soap for routine handwashing. *Category IB*
  (3) Use an antimicrobial agent or a waterless antiseptic agent for specific circumstances (eg, control of outbreaks or hyperendemic infections), as defined by the infection control program. *Category IB* (See Contact Precautions for additional recommendations on using antimicrobial and antiseptic agents.)
B. Gloves
  Wear gloves (clean, nonsterile gloves are adequate) when touching blood, body fluids, secretions, excretions, and contaminated items. Put on clean gloves just before touching mucous membranes and nonintact skin. Change gloves between tasks and procedures on the same patient after contact with material that may contain a high concentration of microorganisms. Remove gloves promptly after use, before touching noncontaminated items and environmental surfaces, and before going to another patient, and wash hands immediately to avoid transfer of microorganisms to other patients or environments. *Category IB*
C. Mask, Eye Protection, Face Shield
  Wear a mask and eye protection or a face shield to protect mucous membranes of the eyes, nose, and mouth during procedures and patient-care activities that are likely to generate splashes or sprays of blood, body fluids, secretions, and excretions. *Category IB*

D. Gown
  Wear a gown (a clean, nonsterile gown is adequate) to protect skin and to prevent soiling of clothing during procedures and patient-care activities that are likely to generate splashes or sprays of blood, body fluids, secretions, or excretions. Select a gown that is appropriate for the activity and amount of fluid likely to be encountered. Remove a soiled gown as promptly as possible, and wash hands to avoid transfer of microorganisms to other patients or environments. *Category IB*
E. Patient-Care Equipment
  Handle used patient-care equipment soiled with blood, body fluids, secretions, and excretions in a manner that prevents skin and mucous membrane exposures, contamination of clothing, and transfer of microorganisms to other patients and environments. Ensure that reusable equipment is not used for the care of another patient until it has been cleaned and reprocessed appropriately. Ensure that single-use items are discarded properly. *Category IB*
F. Environmental Control
  Ensure that the hospital has adequate procedures for the routine care, cleaning, and disinfection of environmental surfaces, beds, bedrails, bedside equipment, and other frequently touched surfaces, and ensure that these procedures are being followed. *Category IB*
G. Linen
  Handle, transport, and process used linen soiled with blood, body fluids, secretions, and excretions in a manner that prevents skin and mucous membrane exposures and contamination of clothing, and that avoids transfer of microorganisms to other patients and environments. *Category IB*
H. Occupational Health and Bloodborne Pathogens
  (1) Take care to prevent injuries when using needles, scalpels, and other sharp instruments or devices; when handling sharp instruments after procedures; when cleaning used instruments; and when disposing of used needles. Never recap used needles, or otherwise manipulate them using both hands,

or use any other technique that involves directing the point of a needle toward any part of the body; rather, use either a one-handed "scoop" technique or a mechanical device designed for holding the needle sheath. Do not remove used needles from disposable syringes by hand, and do not bend, break, or otherwise manipulate used needles by hand. Place used disposable syringes and needles, scalpel blades, and other sharp items in appropriate puncture-resistant containers, which are located as close as practical to the area in which the items were used, and place reusable syringes and needles in a puncture-resistant container for transport to the reprocessing area. *Category IB*

(2) Use mouthpieces, resuscitation bags, or other ventilation devices as an alternative to mouth-to-mouth resuscitation methods in areas where the need for resuscitation is predictable. *Category IB*

I. Patient Placement

Place a patient who contaminates the environment or who does not (or cannot be expected to) assist in maintaining appropriate hygiene or environmental control in a private room. If a private room is not available, consult with infection control professionals regarding patient placement or other alternatives. *Category IB*

---

*Category IB. Strongly recommended for all hospitals and reviewed as effective by experts in the field and a consensus of HICPAC based on strong rationale and suggestive evidence, even though definitive scientific studies have not been done.

(From Guideline for isolation precautions in hospitals developed by the Centers for Disease Control and Prevention and the Hospital Infection Control Practices Advisory Committee (HICPAC), January 1996.)

C

Prenatal and Postpartum Exercises

Conditioned Relaxation

Directions: Lie or sit in a comfortable position with pillows for support. Someone may read this to you while you learn to relax or this may be read while recording on an audio cassette. Pause in the reading 3 seconds at each . . . and 6 seconds between paragraphs. Practice 3 to 5 times per week.

Take a few slow, deep breaths . . . Inhale . . . Exhale . . . Inhale . . . Exhale . . .

Focus your attention on your breathing throughout this exercise, and recognize how easily slow, deep breathing alone can help to produce relaxation. Let your body breathe itself, according to its own natural rhythm . . . Slowly and deeply . . .

Now let's begin the exercise with what we call a "cleansing breath," a special message that tells the body we are ready to enter a state of deep relaxation. The cleansing breath is taken as follows . . . Exhale . . . Take a deep breath in through your nose . . . Then blow it out through your mouth.

You may notice a kind of "tingling" sensation when you take the cleansing breath. Whatever you feel is a signal or message to your body that will become associated with relaxation, so that as you practice this exercise over and over again, simply taking the cleansing breath alone will produce the same degree of relaxation that you'll be able to get by completing the entire exercise.

Breathe slowly and deeply . . . As you concentrate your attention on your breathing, focus your eyes on an imaginary spot in the center of your forehead . . . Look at the spot as if you are trying to see it from the inside of your head . . . Raise your eyes way up so as to stare at that spot from the inside of your head. Concentrate your attention on it . . . The more you are able to concentrate on the spot, the better your relaxation response will be . . .

As you continue to focus your attention on the spot, you might notice that your eyelids have become quite tense . . . That's fine, because what we want to do is to teach your body the difference between tension and relaxation. Your eyelids are controlled by some of the smallest muscles in your body, and they become easily tired and fatigued as they become more and more tense. When I count to three, we'll demonstrate the difference between tension and relaxation by allowing your eyelids to close gently, allowing the feelings of tension to melt away quickly.

One . . . Two . . . Three . . . Close your eyelids firmly but not too tightly, and as they close, sense a soothing feeling or relaxation radiate all around your eyes . . . the top of your eyes . . . the bottom . . . the sides . . . the front and back . . .

Breathe slowly and deeply . . . Feel the relaxation in your eyes and how nice it feels . . . Let these feelings of gentle relaxation radiate all around your eyes and out to your forehead . . . to your scalp . . . all around the back of your head . . . to your ears and temples . . . to your cheeks and nose . . . to your mouth and chin . . . and around to your jaw . . . As you feel all the tension flow out of your face and the area around your mouth, relax your jaw muscles . . . As you do so, let your jaw gently open slightly so that all the tension can smoothly flow away . . .

Remember your breathing, slowly and deeply . . . Relax the muscles in your neck . . . As you do so, feel all the tension flow away from the muscles in the back of your neck . . . Let this nice, gentle feeling of relaxation now radiate down into your shoulders . . . Feel the heaviness of your shoulders as the shoulder muscles gently relax . . . This is one of the most important areas of the body to relax because we all tend to store a lot of tension in our necks and shoulders . . . Feel all the tension flow away, and sense the nice, gentle feeling of deep relaxation . . .

Remember your breathing, slowly and deeply . . . Let this feeling of relaxation now radiate down your arms . . . to your elbows . . . forearms . . . wrists . . . and hands . . . Spend a moment to relax each of your fingers . . . your thumb, index finger, middle finger, ring finger, little finger . . . As your hands and arms completely and gently relax, you may notice feelings of warmth and heaviness . . . Some people report pulsations or tingly sensations . . . Some can even sense their heartbeat in their fingertips . . . Others report even magnetic or pulling sensations . . . Whatever you experience is your own body's way of expressing relaxation . . . Remember, you cannot *force* yourself to relax, you can only *allow* yourself to relax . . . Trust your body . . . It knows what to do . . .

Remember your breathing, slowly and deeply . . . Relax your chest . . . and abdomen . . . and let this feeling of relaxation radiate around your sides and ribs, as waves of relaxation cross your shoulder blades to meet at your upper back . . . middle back . . . and lower back . . . Feel all the muscles on either side of your spine softly relax . . . Let this feeling of gentle relaxation now radiate down into your pelvic area . . . to your buttocks . . . sphincter muscle . . . genitals . . . Feel your whole pelvic area open up and gently relax . . . Relax your thighs . . . knees . . . calves . . . ankles . . . and feet . . . Spend a moment to relax each toe . . . your big toe, second toe, third toe, fourth toe, and little toe . . . Breathe slowly and deeply . . . Relax and enjoy it . . .

Now that your body is gently relaxed and quiet, take a moment, starting from the top of your head working down, to check lightly to see how much relaxation you have obtained . . .

If there is any part of your body that is not yet fully relaxed and comfortable, simply inhale a deep breath and send it into that area, bringing soothing, relaxing, nourishing, healing oxygen into every cell of that area, comforting and relaxing it . . . As you exhale, imagine blowing out, right through your skin, any tension, tightness, pain, or discomfort in that area. Again, as you inhale, bring relaxing, healing oxygen into every cell of that area, and as you exhale, blow away, right through the skin, any tension or discomfort.

In this way you can send your breath to relax any part of your body which is not yet as fully relaxed and comfortable as it can be . . . Breathe slowly and deeply, and with each breath, allow yourself to become twice as relaxed as you were before . . . Inhale . . . Exhale . . . Twice as relaxed . . . Inhale . . . Exhale . . . Twice as relaxed . . .

When you find yourself quiet and fully relaxed, take a moment to enjoy it . . . Sense the gentle warmth and feeling of well-being all through your body . . . If any extraneous thoughts try to interfere, simply allow them to pass through and out of you . . . Ignore them and go back to your breathing, slowly and deeply . . . Slowly and deeply . . . Enjoy this nice state of gentle relaxation . . .

Remember your breathing, slowly and deeply . . . When you end this exercise, you may be surprised to notice that you feel not only relaxed and comfortable, but energized with such a powerful sense of well-being that you will easily be able to meet any demands that arise . . . To end the exercise, tell yourself that you can reach this nice gentle state of Conditioned Relaxation any time you wish by simply taking the cleansing breath . . . Reinforce that cleansing breath by concluding the exercise with it . . . Exhale . . . Inhale deeply through your nose . . . Blow out through the mouth . . . And be well . . .

(Adapted from Bresler DE: Free Yourself from Pain, pp 261–263. New York, Simon & Schuster, 1979.)

Tense–Release Relaxation

Assume a comfortable position, making sure that all your limbs are supported and slightly bent. Start to become aware of your breathing, slowing down and relaxing more on each exhaled breath. Allow your eyes to close . . .

Wrinkle your forehead, lifting your eyebrows as high as you can, and hold for a few seconds. Release and feel the tension flowing from your forehead and scalp . . . Now close your eyes tightly and wrinkle your nose. Hold it for a few seconds, and let go. Feel the tension flowing out of your face . . . Purse your lips and clench your teeth together. Hold for a few seconds. Now release the tension, and feel your jaw drop and your tongue rest loosely in your mouth . . . Push your head down toward your chest and hold for a few seconds. Relax . . .

Now shrug your shoulders up toward your ears, and hold for a few seconds. As you release, feel the tension leaving your neck and upper back . . .

Clench your fists tightly, and feel the tension in your hands. Hold. Now release the tension, and allow your hands to relax . . . Now tense your arms all the way to the shoulders. Hold for a few seconds and relax . . . Hold. Now release the tension and allow your hands to relax . . . Now tense your arms all the way to the shoulders. Hold for a few seconds and relax . . .

Arch your back for a few seconds. Now release . . . Tighten your adominal muscles and hold for a few seconds. Let go . . . Now tense your buttocks, Hold, and release . . . Tighten your feet, pulling your toes up toward your knees. Hold for a moment. Relax your feet . . . Tense your legs all the way up from your feet to your hips. Hold for a few seconds. Now relax, and feel the tension flowing out of your feet . . .

Breathe slowly, releasing any residual tension on each exhaled breath. Bring your attention to any part of your body that feels tight or uncomfortable, and release it, tensing first if necessary . . . Take time to enjoy this relaxed state, noting the relaxation in your muscles now that you have let go of all tension. Your muscles feel limp and heavy, warm and comfortable . . . Enjoy this good feeling for a few minutes. When you are ready to get up, stretch your arms and legs, take a deep breath, and open your eyes. Always get up slowly so you don't become "dizzy."

From Lieberman A: Easing Labor Pain. Garden City, NY, Doubleday and Co., 1992.)

Imagery Exercises

- Imagine that you are lying on a billowy cloud, moving gently through space. Feel the texture of the cloud as it buoys you up and its slow rocking motion. If colors come into your mind, let yourself be surrounded by them. Be held aloft and carried, or simply rest weightless, as you choose. Let yourself be lulled, as if you were in a hammock. Continue to breathe deeply, as your breath becomes one with the breath of the cloud.

- Imagine that you are floating on your back in water, staring up at the immense, harmonious blue of a cloudless sky. You may be in a lake, or on the ocean, or lying on a lily pad in a pond. You choose the place. Imagine how it feels to be held and gently moved by the natural flow of water. Let your breath be one with the motion of the water, and fill your eyes with the blue of the sky. See nothing else. If sounds come to you, let them flood your ears. Continue to breathe deeply as you float suspended.

- Imagine that you are lying in the cool, high grasses of a fresh green meadow, with a lilting spring breeze rushing over you. In your own hollowed-out hiding place the grass bends down and brushes you, caressing you with long blades that are almost like cool water. Feel the motion of the meadow as it ripples with the wind, a rhythm that is one with the long, peaceful motion of your own relaxed breath.

Let yourself be calmed by the sparkling sound of the nearby brook, running full with the first rains of spring.

(Bogin M: The Path to Pain Control, pp 214–215. Boston, Houghton-Mifflin, 1982.)

The Opening Flower

The "Opening Flower" is probably the single most effective guided imagery exercise for labor. Many laboring women find this exercise very effective for coping with contractions and hastening labor's progress.

The "Opening Flower" is an ideal metaphor for the dilating cervix during first stage and for the opening birth canal during second stage. No image better captures the qualities of warmth, beauty, softness, moisture, fragrance, and opening.

* * * * *

During contractions, imagine a blossoming flower. Choose any flower at all—a rose, lily, water lily—as long as it is beautiful. Then imagine the flower open-

Verbal Cue by Partner	Action by Woman	Partner's Role
1. Contract your right leg	Tense right thigh and calf; flex ankle Focus gaze on one spot to enhance concentration Think about the feeling of tension in the right leg and of relaxation in the rest of the body	Look over rest of body for obvious signs of tension; lift leg gently under knee to check relaxation; check both arms; turn head gently side to side to check relaxation of neck Where tension is detected, stroke and give cue, "Relax" or "Release"
Relax your right leg	Relax completely	Stroke right leg; lift gently under right knee to detect tension
2. Contract your left leg	As above	As above
Relax your left leg	As above	As above
3. Contract your left arm	Make a fist; tense entire arm and lift slightly off the floor Focus gaze on one spot to enhance concentration Think about the feeling of tension in the left arm and of relaxation in the rest of the body	Check rest of body for signs of tension; lift right arm gently by hand, swing freely from shoulder; lift knees slightly; observe face; turn head gently side to side to detect neck tension; stroke to signal its release
Relax your left arm	Relax completely	Stroke left arm and shoulder Lift left arm gently by hand; swing from shoulder
4. Contract your right arm	As above	As above
Relax your right arm	As above	As above
5. Contract your left arm and right leg	As above	As above
Relax only your left arm	Relax arm	As above
	Keep leg tense	As above
Relax your right leg	Relax completely	As above

(The previous chart is a combination of two sources—Birth Guide. West Los Angeles ASPO Certified Childbirth Educators, 1990; and Hassid P: Textbook for Childbirth Educators, 3rd ed. Philadelphia, JB Lippincott, 1987.)

ing petal by petal, opening, opening, opening, until it is fully in bloom.

You can add as many details to this exercise as you want, such as the shape of the petals, their delicate or bold shading, dewdrops on the flower, fragrance, the sun's rays coaxing the flower to open, and so on.

You can also vary the exercise by imagining that you are in a beautiful garden or in a field surrounded by hundreds of flowers. You can take a mental journey of the garden or field and choose the most beautiful flower of all. Then imagine that flower blossoming and opening, petal by petal.

Neuromuscular Control—"Partner Feedback Relaxation"

Directions: Choose a comfortable position with pillows for support. The emphasis is always on the relaxation, not on the tensing or how quickly the woman can respond. Relax to touch as well as to verbal instructions so these can be conditioned for labor. Breathe comfortably throughout the exercise. The woman learns what relaxation really feels like by partner feedback. She practices how to relax muscles while others are tense like it will be in labor. Practice together for 5 minutes daily.

Continue on with contracting: left arm and left leg, right arm and left leg, buttocks, neck—make up your own!

Prenatal Exercises

Do each exercise twice at first, progressing at your own pace to five times. The sequence can be repeated in reverse order. Relax and breathe deeply between each exercise.

1. Abdominal-Tightening on Outward Breath

Position: Lying on back or side, knees bent. Place hands on abdominal area below ribs (for the learning process; they can be removed later).

Action: Take a deep complete breath in through the nose, feeling the nostrils widen slightly. Breathing through the nose warms and filters the air. Keep the ribs as still as you can, and let the abdominal wall expand upward. Then, lips slightly parted, blow the air out through the mouth slowly but forcibly, pulling in your abdominal muscles all the while until you feel you have completely emptied your lungs. It's like sustaining a note while blowing a trumpet or singing.

Progression: Other positions, such as sitting or standing. Avoid taking too many deep breaths in succes-

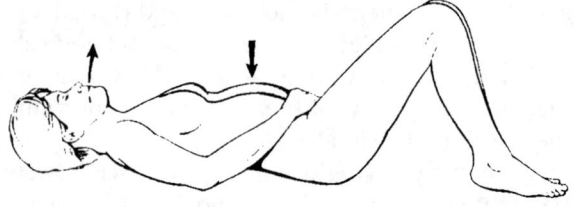

sion—you may get dizzy. Deep breathing is very important in pregnancy and the early postpartum phase, but at other times this exercise can be done as simple abdominal muscle contractions on normal outward breath in standing, sitting, or other positions. A rocking chair is ideal!

2. Pelvic Floor Exercise

Position: Lying down on back, side, or front. (On the front is the most comfortable position postpartum if you have had stitches.) Legs apart and chest relaxed for normal breathing.

Action: Draw up the pelvic floor, feel the additional squeeze from the sides as the sphincters are tightened and the inside passages become tense. Concentrate particularly on the front portion of the pelvic floor—the master sphincter surrounding the vagina and urethra. Place one hand over the pubic bones and think about tightening the birth canal as high as the level of your hand.

Hold for 2 to 3 seconds and then completely relax. Note the sensation as the pelvic floor lets down loosely. Try to slacken it a little more, releasing any residual tension. (This is what you must be able to do during delivery.) Release your jaw, too.

Do only two or three in succession before resting for a couple of minutes, and always end with a contraction to return the muscle floor to its supportive resting state. You can provide effective exercise of the muscle by doing this frequently, 50 times or more a day, in a series of five, holding each contraction for 5 seconds.

3. Foot-Bending and Foot-Stretching

The movement of frequent foot-bending and -stretching and ankle-rotating provides a venous pump to assist the return of blood from the lower legs, and will minimize varicosities and swelling of the ankles. Cramps, which often occur from lack of exercise, may be relieved.

Position: Sitting or lying. In either position, legs can be relaxed over a pillow or the feet can be elevated. At other times, rest foot on the opposite knee. (This makes it easier to see your feet late in pregnancy!)

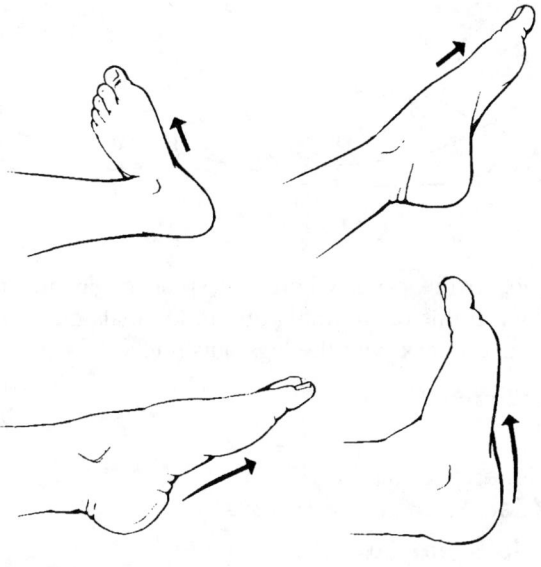

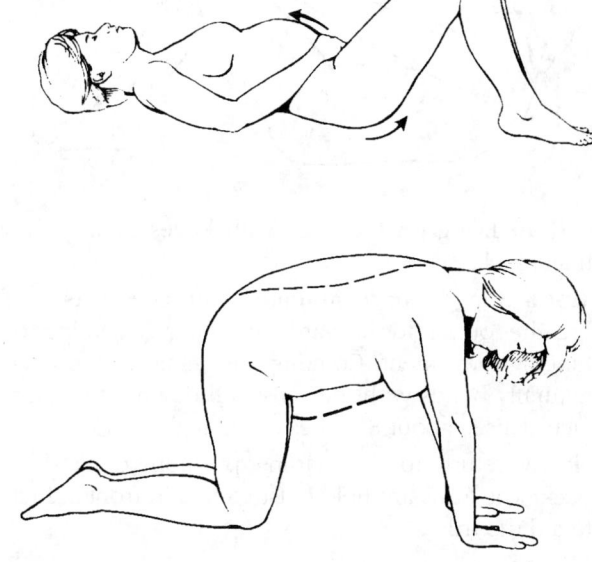

It's also a good way to put on socks or pantyhose. Sitting with the legs out straight provides additional stretch of the calf muscles.

Action: Bend the ankle as far as you can, pulling your toes up toward you, thus stretching the calf muscles; then point the foot downward, making an arch. Do this several times and take a short rest before repeating. If pointing the foot results in cramps, just stretch up . . . relax . . . stretch up.

4. Ankle-Rotating

Position: As for above Exercise and any time you're off your feet.

Action: Make large slow circles with each foot, first in a clockwise, then in a counterclockwise direction.

5. Pelvic-Tilting

Position: Lying on the back with the knees bent is the easiest starting position for learning the basic front-to-back action, which is important in the childbearing year. In late pregnancy, however, the weight of the uterus compresses the major blood vessels in this position, so if you experience discomfort or feel faint, practice this in one of the other recommended positions.

Action: Roll the pelvis back by flattening the lower back down on the floor. Then make an extra effort. Contract the abdominal muscles on outward breath and tighten the buttock muscles, too. Additional strong contraction of the muscles is necessary to make this an active strengthening exercise, not just a semipassive movement. To encourage more action in the lower abdominal muscles, place a hand just above the pubic bones so you can feel the muscles working. Hold the position for 3 seconds and then relax. Keep breathing! Make sure that you do not raise your buttocks at all or shift your shoulders. Do not rock the pelvis upward as this will force the curve in the lower back. *Always emphasize the flattening of the hollow* and add as much additional abdominal wall retraction as you can. Postpartum, think about "making yourself thin" from front to back.

Progression: When you feel that you understand the correct movement, try it standing, side-lying, sitting or on all-fours.

6. Straight Curl-Up

If you are well into the last trimester and have not been exercising the abdominal muscles, save the curl-ups for your postpartum program. If you cannot readily perform a movement, then you must not exert undue strain. In any case, during the last few weeks of pregnancy the size of the baby gets in the way. The other exercises will maintain existing strength at this time and can be done with ease and comfort.

Prenatal: This exercise is for early starters. If you are well into the last trimester and cannot readily perform these movements, then do not try. If the recti muscles have parted, from this pregnancy or a previous one, postpone this exercise and concentrate on supporting the muscles and raising just the head at first (see Chapter 19).

Postpartum: Always check the midline of your abdominal wall before doing this exercise. If the recti muscles have separated more than three fingers' width, support them as described in Chapter 19; this is actually a progression of the same exercise.

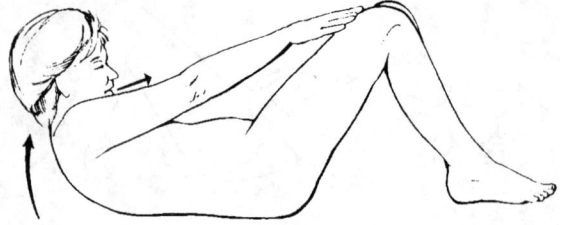
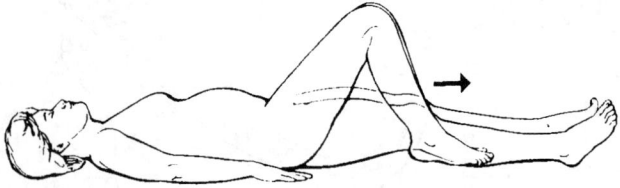

Position: Lying on the back with knees bent, pelvis tilted back.

Action: Bring your chin onto your chest. As you breathe out, fold forward without any jerking or hinging movement. Come up just as far as the back naturally bends with the waist still down on the surface. This is about 8 inches or an angle of 45°.

Slowly return to the starting position; don't drop back. The arms are held outstretched in front at first, to aid the trunk.

Postpartum Exercises

Commence within 24 hours; repeat each exercise twice to start, progressing at your own pace through the phases. Relax and breathe deeply between each exercise. The sequence can be repeated in reverse order. Do the exercises at least twice daily.

Phase I

1. Abdominal-Tightening on Outward Breath (See prenatal exercises)
2. Pelvic Floor Exercise (See prenatal exercises)
3. Foot-Bending and Foot-Stretching (See prenatal exercises)
4. Ankle-Rotating (See prenatal exercises)
5. Pelvic-Tilting (See prenatal exercises)

Add Phase II

7. Leg-Sliding

Position: Lying on back, knees bent, pelvis tilted backward, and lumbar spine flattened. Keep breathing normally throughout.

Action: Hold the position of corrected pelvic tilt as, sliding the heels, you slowly stretch the legs out straight. If the abdominals are unable to keep the back flat, draw the knees back up again, one at a time, to the point where the spine began to arch. Work in this range until your abdominals maintain a flattened back with the legs outstretched.

Add Phase III

8. Straight Curl-Up (See Prenatal Exercises)

9. Diagonal Curl-Up

If there is a separation of the recti muscles (see pages 346 and 347), postpone this exercise until the condition has been corrected.

Prenatal: This exercise is also for early starters, although it is a little easier than the straight curl-up since you move obliquely and have more help from other muscles in the corset. If you are in the last trimester and cannot perform this movement with ease and comfort, then do not try.

Position: Lying on the back with knees bent.

Action: Bring your chin onto your chest. As you breathe out, fold forward reaching with your outstretched arms to the outside of the left knee. Slowly return back to the starting position. Repeat the movement to the right knee.

(All exercises and illustrations are from Noble E: Essential Exercises for the Childbearing Year. Boston, Houghton-Mifflin, 1988.)

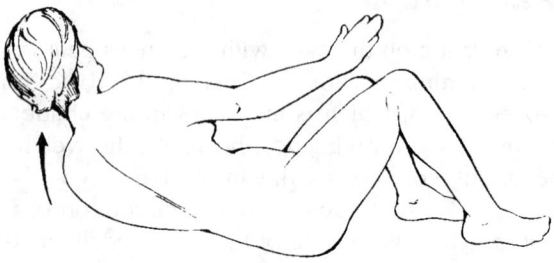

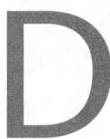

Standards for Maternity Care and Employment (U.S. Children's Bureau)

1. Facilities for adequate prenatal medical care should be readily available for all employed pregnant women, and arrangements should be made by those responsible for providing prenatal care, so that every woman has access to such care. Local health departments should make the services of prenatal clinics available to industrial plants, and the personnel management or physicians and nurses within the plant should make available to employees information about the importance of such services and where they can be obtained.

2. Pregnant women should not be employed on a shift including the hours between 12 midnight and 6 AM. Pregnant women should not be employed more than 48 hours per week, and it is desirable that their hours of work be limited to not more than 40 hours per week.

3. Every woman, especially a pregnant woman, should have at least two 10-minute rest periods during her work shift, for which adequate facilities for resting and an opportunity for securing nourishing food should be provided.

4. It is not considered desirable for pregnant women to be employed in the following types of occupations, and they should, if possible, be transferred to lighter and more sedentary work:
   a. Occupations that involve heavy lifting or other heavy work
   b. Occupations that involve continuous standing and moving about

5. Pregnant women should not be employed in the following types of work during any period of pregnancy
   a. Occupations that require a good sense of bodily balance, such as work performed on scaffolds or stepladders and occupations in which the accident risk is characterized by accidents causing severe injury, such as operation of punch presses, power-driven woodworking machines, or other machines having a point-of-operation hazard
   b. Occupations involving exposure to toxic substances considered to be extra hazardous during pregnancy, including the following:
      Aniline
      Benzene and toluene
      Carbon disulfide
         Carbon monoxide
      Chlorinated hydrocarbons
      Lead and its compounds
      Mercury and its compounds
      Nitrobenzol and other nitro compounds of benzol and its homologues
      Phosphorus
      Radioactive substances and x-rays
      Turpentine
      Other toxic substances that exert an injurious effect upon the blood-forming organs, the liver, or the kidneys

   Because these substances may exert a harmful influence upon the course of pregnancy, may lead to premature termination, or may injure the fetus, the maintenance of air concentrations within the so-called maximum permissible limits of state codes is not, in itself, sufficient assurance of a safe working condition for the pregnant woman. Pregnant women should be transferred from workrooms in which any of these substances are used or produced in any significant quantity.

6. A minimum of 6 weeks' leave *before* delivery should be granted with the presentation of a medical certificate of the expected date of confinement.

7. At any time during pregnancy, a woman should be granted a reasonable amount of additional leave with the presentation of a certificate from the attending physician to the effect that complications of pregnancy have made continuing employment prejudicial to her health or to the health of the child.

   To safeguard the mother's health she should be granted sufficient time off after delivery to return to normal and to regain her strength. The infant needs her care, especially during the first year of life. If it is essential that she return to work, the following recommendations are made:
   a. All women should be granted an extension of at least 2 months leave of absence after delivery.
   b. Should complications of delivery or of the postpartum period develop, a woman should be granted a reasonable amount of additional leave beyond 2 months following delivery with presentation of a certificate to this effect from the attending physician.

E

Drug Use During Breast-Feeding*

Drug or Agent	Contra-indicated	R_x With Caution	No Apparent Harm	Insufficient Information	Comment
ANALGESICS					
Acetaminophen			X		
Aspirin			X		
Propoxyphene (Darvon)			X		
ANTICOAGULANTS					
Ethyl biscoumacetate	X				Bleeding infant
Phenindione	X				Bleeding infant
Heparin			X		No passage into milk
Warfarin Na (Coumadin)			X		
Bishydroxycoumarin (Dicumarol)		X			
ANTICONVULSANTS					
Phenobarbital			X		Low levels in infant
Primadone (Mysoline)			X		? Drowsiness
Carbamazepine				X	Significant infant levels; no reported effects
Diphenylhydantoin (Phenytoin, Dilantin)			X		Low levels in infant, methemoglobin, one case
ANTIHISTAMINES					
Diphenhydramine (Benadryl)			X		Small amounts excreted
Trimeprazine (Temaril)			X		Small amounts excreted
Tripelennamine (Pyribenzamine)			X		Small amounts excreted
ANTI-INFECTIVE AGENTS					
Aminoglycosides (Kanamycin, gentamicin)			X		Significant excretion in milk; not absorbed
Chloramphenicol	X				Bone marrow depression; gastrointestinal and behavioral effects
Penicillins			X		Possible sensitization
Sulfonamides		X			Hemolysis, G-6-PD deficiency, bilirubin displacement
Tetracyclines			X		Limited absorption by infant
Nalidixic acid		X			Hemolysis
Nitrofurantoin		X			Possible G-6-PD hemolysis
Metronidazole (Flagyl)		X			Low absorption but potentially toxic
Isoniazid		X			High levels in milk, possible toxicity
Pyramethamine	X				Vomiting, marrow suppression, convulsions
Chloraquine			X		Not excreted
Quinine		X			Thrombocytopenia

(continued)

Drug or Agent	Contra-indicated	R$_x$ With Caution	No Apparent Harm	Insufficient Information	Comment
ANTI-INFLAMMATORY					
Aspirin			X		
Indomethacin		X			Seizures, one case
Phenylbutazone		X			Low levels, ? blood dyscrasia
Gold	X				Found in baby; nephritis, hepatitis, hematologic changes
Steroids				X	Low levels with prednisone and prednisolone
ANTINEOPLASTIC					
Cyclophosphamide	X				Neutropenia
Methotrexate	X				Very small excretion
ANTITHYROID					
Radioactive iodine	X				Thyroid suppression
Propylthiouracil	X				Thyroid suppression
BRONCHODILATORS					
Aminophylline			X		Irritability, one case
Iodides	X				Thyroid suppression
Sympathomimetics				X	Inhalers probably safe
CARDIOVASCULAR AGENTS					
Digoxin			X		Insignificant levels
Propanolol			X		Insignificant levels
Reserpine	X				Nasal stuffiness, lethargy
Guanethidine (Ismelin)			X		Insignificant levels
Methyldopa (Aldomet)				X	
CATHARTICS					
Anthroquinones (Cascara, danthron)	X				Diarrhea, cramps
Aloe, senna		X			Safe in moderate dosage
Bulk agents, softeners			X		
CONTRACEPTIVES, ORAL[†]					
Diethylstilbestrol	X				Possible vaginal cancer
Depo-provera		X			May affect lactation
Norethisterone		X			May affect lactation
Ethinyl estradiol		X			May affect lactation
DIURETICS					
Chlorthalidone				X	Low levels, but may accumulate
Thiazides		X			May affect lactation; low levels in milk
Spironolactone			X		Insignificant levels
ERGOT ALKALOIDS					
Bromocriptine	X				Lactation suppressed
Ergot	X				Vomiting, diarrhea, seizures
Ergotamine				X	
Ergonovine	X				Brief postpartum course may be safe
Methylergonovine	X				Brief postpartum course may be safe

(*continued*)

Drug or Agent	Contra-indicated	R$_x$ With Caution	No Apparent Harm	Insufficient Information	Comment
HORMONES					
Corticosteroids				X	Low levels with short-term prednisone or prednisolone
Sex hormones (see above, Contraceptives, Oral)					
Thyroid (T$_3$ or T$_4$)			X		Excreted in milk; may mask hypothyroid infant
Insulin			X		Not absorbed
ACTH			X		Not absorbed
Epinephrine			X		Not absorbed
NARCOTICS					
Codeine			X		
Meperidine (Demerol)				X	In usual doses
Morphine			X		Low infant levels on usual dosage
Heroin	X				Addiction withdrawal in infants
Methadone		X			Minimal levels
PSYCHOTHERAPEUTIC DRUGS					
Lithium	X				High levels in milk
Phenothiazines		X			Drowsiness; chronic effects uncertain
Tricyclic antidepressants				X	Low levels; effects uncertain
Diazepam (Valium)	X				Lethargy, weight loss, EEG changes
Meprobamate (Equanil)	X				High levels in milk
Chlordiazepoxide (Librium)			X		Low levels in milk
RADIOPHARMACEUTICALS					
^{131}I	X				72 hr, no breast-feeding
Technetium (99M Tc)	X				48 hr, no breast-feeding
^{131}I albumin	X				10 days, no breast-feeding
SEDATIVES-HYPNOTICS					
Barbiturates		X			Short-acting, less depressant
Chloral hydrate		X			Drowsiness
Bromides	X				Depression, rash
Diazepam (Valium)	X				Depression, weight loss
Flurazepam				X	Chemically related to diazepam
Nitrazepam				X	
SOCIAL-RECREATIONAL DRUGS					
Alcohol			X		Milk levels equal plasma, moderate consumption apparently safe, high levels inhibit lactation
Caffeine			X		Jitteriness with very high intakes
Nicotine			X		Low levels in milk
Marijuana			X		Minimal passage in milk
MISCELLANEOUS					
Atropine		X			May cause constipation or inhibit lactation
Dihydrotachysterol		X			Renal calcification in animals

*Drug use during breast-feeding remains controversial.
†Controversy in literature; long-term effects uncertain; one case of gynecomastia.
(Avery GB [ed]: Neonatology, 3rd ed. Philadelphia, JB Lippincott, 1987.)

Glossary

abdominal pregnancy. Ectopic pregnancy occurring in the cavity of the abdomen.

abdominal circumference. A parameter used in the diagnosis of IUGR, in which the size of the fetus is estimated based on the measurement of the abdomen at the level of the liver and the left portal vein.

abortifacients. Agents that induce abortions.

abortion. The termination of pregnancy by any means before the fetus has attained a stage of viability (ie, before it is capable of extrauterine existence). See also *elective a., incomplete a., induced a., missed a., recurrent a.,* and *spontaneous a.*.

abruptio placentae. Premature separation of a normally implanted placenta. The separation may be complete or partial and very often is considered a medical emergency. See also *covert a.p., marginal sinus rupture,* and *overt a.p.*.

acculturation. The adaptation of cultural traits and social patterns of another group.

acme. The time of greatest intensity. In obstetrics, the period when the intensity of a contraction is at its height.

acoustic window. The space through which an ultrasound beam is able to penetrate, such as water.

acquired disorders. Disorders that result from environmental factors rather than genetic or congenital circumstances.

acrocyanosis. Cyanosis of the extremities, especially of the hands and feet, seen in the newborn for the first few hours after birth.

acupressure. An ancient oriental technique of applying pressure to specific points to promote relaxation, increase energy, relieve pain, and aid homeostasis.

adolescence. The period of life beginning at puberty, when the secondary sex characteristics begin to develop and the capacity for reproduction is reached, and ending with adulthood.

aflatoxins. Cancer-causing toxins produced by a wide variety of foodstuffs.

afterbirth. The structures cast off after the expulsion of the fetus, including the membranes and the placenta with the attached umbilical cord.

afterpains. Uterine contractions, which are similar to menstrual cramps, that result from the contractile efforts of the uterus to return to its normal condition. Afterpains often occur 2 days after delivery.

allele. One of two or more alternate genes that occur at a particular locus of a chromosome, which decide alternate inherited characteristics.

alternate birth center (ABC). A hospital organization or a free-standing labor and delivery area that provides a homelike, family-centered atmosphere with liberal policies regarding labor, delivery, and postpartum care.

ambiguous genitalia. External genitals that are not clearly masculine or feminine.

amenorrhea. Absence or suppression of the menstrual discharge.

aminoaciduria. An excess of amino acids in the urine.

amniocentesis. The perforation, by use of a needle, through the abdominal wall into the uterus to obtain a sample of amniotic fluid for the purpose of fetal genetic or fetal maturity diagnosis.

amnioinfusion. Injection of a solution into the uterus, usually to induce abortion or increase in utero fluid levels.

amnion. The most internal of the fetal membranes, containing the waters that surround the fetus in utero.

amniotic fluid. The clear fluid that is 98% water contained in the amnion. This fluid provides protection to the fetus, keeps the temperature constant, and provides some nourishment to the fetus.

amniotic fluid embolism. The blocking of a maternal artery with amniotic fluid forced into it by strong uterine contractions.

amniotic fluid index. The sum of the vertical diameters of the largest amniotic fluid pocket in each of the four quadrants of the maternal abdomen. This index is used as an amniotic assessment tool.

amniotomy. The artificial rupture of the amniotic sac to induce labor.

amplitude. Strength, extent, fullness, size.

analgesia. A mild to moderate lessening or dulling of central nervous system function, thereby rendering the client conscious, but sedated, and experiencing a decreased level of pain.

androgenesis. A phenomenon in which chromosomes are completely of paternal origin.

android pelvis. One of the four main types of female pelvis, generally characterized as resembling the pelvis of a male and having a wedge-shaped inlet and narrow anterior segment.

anemia. A condition of the blood in which there is a deficiency in the red blood cells per unit volume, in the quantity of hemoglobin, or in the total volume. See also *megoblastic a.* and *microangiopathic hemolytic a.*

anencephaly. A congenital deformity characterized by complete or partial absence of the newborn's brain and the skull overlying the brain.

anesthesia. The loss of sensation or feeling, especially the feeling of pain.

aneuploidy. A condition of numeric chromosome errors, which result in major developmental defects of the fetus.

anovulation. Failure of the ovaries to release or produce mature eggs.

anterior fontanel. The diamond-shaped space between the frontal and two parietal bones in very young infants. Also known as the *soft spot* just above a baby's forehead

antepartal. The period from conception to the onset of labor; prenatal.

anthropoid pelvis. One of the four main types of female pelvis, generally characterized by a long anteroposterior diameter of the inlet.

anthropometric measurements. Various objective, noninvasive measurements of body size and composition.

antithrombin. A glycoprotein and major in vivo inhibitor of thrombin generation, which is used as a laboratory parameter for the diagnosis of disseminated intravascular coagulation (DIC).

Apgar scoring system. A system for appraising the condition of a newborn on the basis of heart rate, respiratory effort, muscle tone, reflex irritability, and color. The maximum score is 10. The evaluation is done at 60 seconds after birth, then again at 5 minutes and at 10 minutes if the neonate is unstable.

apnea. Cessation of aspirations for more than 20 seconds.

areola. The ring of pigment surrounding the nipple. See also *secondary areola.*

arrest of descent. Failure of the fetal head to descend for more than 1 hour in a nullipara and more than .5 hours for a multipara.

artificial insemination. The introduction of semen into the cervical os or uterus by mechanical means.

assisted reproductive technologies (ART). Procedures that aid in childbearing for couples unable to conceive and carry their own biologic child. These procedures include in vitro fertilization, GIFT or ZIFT, artificial insemination, surrogate parenting, and adoption.

asynclitism. An oblique presentation of the fetal head in labor.

atrial septal defect. A congenital cardiac anomaly in which there is an abnormal opening between the right and left atria of the heart.

attachment. The long process of staying in love with and affectionate toward another person.

attitude. A posture or position of the body. In obstetrics, the relation of the fetal parts to each other in the uterus. The basic attitude is either flexion or extension.

autosomal recessive disorder. A condition in which both members of a gene pair are abnormal.

autosome. Any of the 22 ordinary paired chromosomes as distinguished from the two sex chromosomes.

azoospermia. The absence of spermatozoa in the ejaculate.

bacterial endocarditis. Inflammation of the inner lining of the heart, usually involving the heart valves.

bagging. A resuscitative procedure in which oxygen is administered by bag and mask ventilation at a rate of 40 to 60 breaths per minute to deliver oxygen into the newborn's bronchi.

ballottement. Literally means tossing. A term used in examination when the fetus can be pushed about in the pregnant uterus.

Bandl's ring. See *pathologic retraction ring.*

Bartholin's glands. Glands situated one on each side of the vaginal canal opening into the groove between the hymen and the labia minora.

basal body temperature (BBT). The resting temperature taken in the morning before arising or performing any activity. Characteristic changes in BBT that usually occur in fertile women are used to identify the time ovulation has occurred.

battledore placenta. A placenta characterized by a cord inserted at the placental margin rather than in the center of the placenta as with normal insertion.

bearing down. Reflex effort by the mother to help with the uterine contractions.

bifidus factor. A growth enhancer of lactobacilli found in the milk of women but not in other mammalian species.

bilirubinometer. A hand-held, fiber optic noninvasive screening tool that illuminates the skin, measures the intensity of the yellow color, and correlates skin color with a total bilirubin value. This tool is useful in monitoring for jaundice.

bimanual palpation. Examination of the pelvic organs of a woman by placing one hand on the abdomen and the fingers of the other in the vagina.

biparietal diameter. The maximum distance between the two fetal parietal bones.

birth trauma. The physical injury that occurs during labor and delivery.

blastocyst. The inner solid mass of cells within the fertilized ovum that develop into the embryo and embryonic membranes.

body mechanics. The efficient use of the body to distribute weight and stress evenly among several muscle groups, rather than overtaxing a particular muscle group with undue strain.

bonding. The initial attraction and desire to get to know another person.

bradycardia. FHR below 120 beats/min for 10 minutes or greater.

Braxton Hicks contractions. Uterine contractions, occurring periodically during pregnancy, that enlarge the uterus to accommodate the growing fetus. During the third trimester, they are felt as a painless hardening or tightening of the uterus. They can become painful and are often difficult to differentiate from labor.

breech presentation. Fetal position in which the feet or buttocks are the presenting part.

broad ligament. Fibrous sheath covered by peritoneum extending from each side of the uterus to the lateral wall of the pelvis.

bronchopulmonary dysplasia. A significant chronic lung disorder in neonates that is most often the result of pulmonary immaturity, surfactant deficiency, acute lung injury, oxygen toxicity, and barotrauma.

brow presentation. Fetal position in which the largest diameter of the fetal head, the occipitomental, presents at the pelvic inlet.

brown fat. Fat cells that contain many small fat vacuoles and have a rich blood supply, which aid in the distribution of heat. Brown fat develops between the 17th and 20th weeks of gestation and usually is not found in adults.

Brushfield's spots. White spots on the iris.

burr cells. See *echinocytes*.

calendar method. The use of a menstrual calendar based on calculations of an 8-month menstruation pattern to determine periods of fertility.

Candida albicans. A yeastlike fungus that causes infections, commonly involving the mucous membranes of the mouth and vagina. During pregnancy, women are more susceptible to candidal infections due to the changed pH of the vagina and increased glycogen in vaginal cells.

capacitation. The process by which a spermatozoon is conditioned to fertilize an ovum after it is exposed to the female reproductive tract.

caput succedaneum. An edematous swelling that sometimes appears on the presenting part of the fetal head during labor.

cardinal movements. Positional changes that help the fetus meet minimal resistance as it passes through the birth canal. These movements include descent, flexion, internal rotation, extension, external rotation, and expulsion.

cephalhematoma. A collection of blood caused by ruptured blood vessels crossing the skull to the periosteum.

cephalic index. The ratio of the biparietal diameter to the occipitofrontal diameter used to determine if the shape of the fetal head is normal.

cephalic presentation. Presentation of any part of the fetal head in labor. Cephalic presentations are categorized into groups according to the relation of the fetus' head to its body.

cephalopelvic disproportion (CPD). A condition in which the fetal head is disproportionately large for passage through the maternal pelvis.

cervical cap. A barrier method of contraception having a 1¼ to 1½ soft rubber dome with a flexible rim, which fits snugly over the cervix and is held in place by suction between its rim and the base of the cervix.

cervical dilatation. Enlargement of the cervical os from an orifice of a few millimeters in size to an aperture large enough to permit the passage of the fetus (ie, a diameter of about 10 cm).

cervical ripening. The maturational process of softening and effacement of the cervix.

cervix. Neckline part; the lower, constricted, cylindrical portion of the uterus, between the os and the body of the organ.

cesarean delivery. Delivery of the fetus by an incision through the abdominal and uterine walls.

Chadwick's sign. The blue-purple color on the mucous membrane of the vagina just below the urethral orifice, caused by increased vascularity.

Chlamydia trachomatis. A sexually transmitted organism responsible for a spectrum of diseases, including cervicitis, urethritis, and acute salpingitis (PID).

chorioamnionitis. An intrauterine infection of the fetal membranes and amniotic fluid.

choriocarcinoma. A malignant sequel of a hydatidiform mole.

chorion. The outermost membrane of the growing zygote, or fertilized ovum, that serves as a protective and nutritive covering.

chorionic villus. Pl. villi. One of the fingerlike projections growing in tufts on the external surface of the chorion.

chorionic villus sampling. A method of fetal cell analysis during the first trimester, in which placental and chorionic tissue are collected, processed, and reviewed.

chromosome. A small, dark-staining and more or less rod-shaped body that contains DNA and proteins and appears in the nucleus of every body cell. See also *sex chromosome*.

chronic hypertension. A hypertensive vascular disorder that is unrelated to pregnancy and is evident prior to gestation or persists postpartum.

circumcision. The surgical excision of the end of the prepuce, or foreskin, of the penis.

circumvallate placenta. A condition in which the membranes of the placenta are folded back on the fetal surface, exposing a ring of the fetal surface around the umbilical cord.

cleavage. The process of rapid miotic cell division during the development of a fertilized ovum, in which male and female chromosomes mingle and split forming two sets of 46 chromosomes.

cleft lip. Congenital incomplete closure of the lip.

cleft palate. Congenital fissure of the palate and roof of the mouth.

clitoris. A small, elongated, erectile body situated at the anterior part of the vulva. It is the female organ that is homologous with the male penis.

clonus. Rapid, alternating contraction and relaxation of muscles occurring involuntarily in response to stretching of the muscle.

clubfoot. See *talipes equinovarus*.

coitus. Sexual intercourse, copulation.

coitus interruptus. The practice of withdrawal as a means of contraception. The penis is withdrawn from the vagina before ejaculation.

colostrum. The thin yellow fluid, high in protein and in-organic salts, that is secreted from the breasts before milk is produced (most often during the 3 days after delivery).

colposcope. An instrument designed for close examination of the cervical tissues, similar to a low-magnification microscope with binocular vision.

compound presentation. Presentation of an extremity that prolapses alongside and enters the pelvis at the same time as the presenting part.

conception. The impregnation of the female ovum by the spermatozoon of the male.

condom. See *male c., female c.*.

congenital anomaly. Abnormality present at birth.

congenital heart disease. Any pathologic condition of the heart present at birth.

contracted pelvis. A pelvis in which any important diameter is reduced significantly enough to interfere with the progress of labor.

contraction. The intermittent shortening of a muscle, especially the uterus during labor in order to expel the contents. See also *tetanic c.*

contraction stress test. A method of evaluating FHR in the presence of spontaneous or oxytocin-induced contractions. The premise is that oxygenation of a marginally compromised fetus will transiently worsen with uterine contractions.

corpus albicans. The white fibrous tissue that replaces the corpus luteum in the ovary as it regresses.

corpus luteum. The yellow matter found within the ruptured follicle after the ovum has been discharged.

couplet care. See *mother-newborn couple care.*

Couvade syndrome. A phenomenon whereby the father or partner manifests pregnancy-related symptoms, such as nausea, vomiting, alterations in appetite, weight gain, abdominal pain, backache, leg cramps, elusive toothaches, and other aches and pains in different parts of the body.

Couvelaire uterus. A severe uterine condition seen in some cases of placental separation, when coagulation is impaired and there is extensive bleeding into the uterine muscle, causing a blue discoloration.

covert abruptio placentae. Abruptio placentae whereby central separation entraps lost blood between the uterine wall and the placenta.

Cowper's glands. Two glands located at the base of the prostate gland and on either side of the membranous urethra. These glands produce a mucinous substance that lubricates the urethra and coats its surface.

crack. A derivative of cocaine that can be smoked.

Crede's method. Manual bladder compression used to stimulate urination.

critical thinking. A method of problem analysis that includes the examination of assumptions, beliefs, prospective and the meaning and uses of words, statements, and arguments related to a problem.

crowning. The phase in the second stage of labor when the largest diameter of the fetal head is visible and circled by the vulva. The anus is open, and the perineum is distended.

crown to rump length. The longest demonstrable length of the embryo or fetus, excluding the limbs and yolk sac.

cryptorchidism. Undescended testes.

Cullen's sign. A blue-tinge to the umbilicus that indicates bleeding in the peritoneal.

curettage. (Fr.) The removal of substances from the wall of a cavity, especially the uterine cavity, with a spoon-shaped instrument called a curet.

cystitis. An infection or inflammation of the urinary bladder.

cystocele. The descent or pouching downward of a portion of the posterior bladder wall and trigone into the vagina.

cytomegalovirus. A herpes virus that produces unique large cells bearing intranuclear inclusions.

dancing reflex. See *stepping reflex.*

deceleration. decrease in velocity of the fetal heart rate. See also *early d., late d., prolonged d.,* and *variable d.*

decidua. The structure of thickened endometrium that develops after conception and, except for the deepest layer, sheds during childbirth.

decidua basalis. The part lying directly under the embedded ovum that forms the maternal component of the placenta.

decidua capsularis. The portion that overlies the ovum, separating it from the rest of the uterine cavity.

decidua vera. The remaining portion that is not in immediate contact with the ovum. Sometimes called the *d. parietalis*

decrement. Decrease; in obstetrics, a period when the intensity of a contraction decreases.

dependent edema. edema of the lower body parts.

descent. Passage of the presenting part of the fetus into and through the birth canal; it begins at the onset of labor and proceeds during effacement and dilatation of the cervix.

developmental stressors. Extrafamilial stressors that are a result of developmental events, such as pregnancy, parenthood, and other family life changes.

developmental tasks. Physical or cognitive skills that a person must accomplish during a particular age to continue developing.

diabetes or **diabetes mellitus.** An endocrine disorder that involves disruption of normal carbohydrate metabolism caused by a deficiency of insulin. Because pregnancy causes a significant change in the course of diabetes, closely supervised prenatal care of a diabetic gravida is required. See also *gestational diabetes.*

diagonal conjugate measurement. The chief internal pelvic measurement made to determine the actual diameter of the pelvic passage. It is the distance between the sacral promontory and the lower margin of the symphysis pubis.

diaphoresis. Profuse sweating. In obstetrics, it is part of the reversal of water metabolism, in which excess fluid accumulated during pregnancy is eliminated.

diaphragm. A dome-shaped rubber contraceptive device that is inserted into the vagina and covers the anterior wall and cervix to act like a cap. To be effective, the device is used with spermicidal cream or jelly.

diaphragmatic hernia. A defect in the development of the diaphragm, which allows the abdominal viscera to herniate into the thoracic cavity.

diastasis. Separation of the abdominal recti muscles, which may occur during pregnancy, due to stretching of the abdominal wall.

Dick-Read approach to childbirth. The approach that is based on the understanding that fear of pain produces muscular tension, which produces pain and greater fear. This approach includes an educational program to teach physiological processes of labor, exercise to improve muscle tone, and techniques to assist in relaxation and prevent the fear-tension-pain mechanism.

differentiation. Maturation of physiologic processes, resulting in the organs being able to perform specialized functions.

disseminated intravascular coagulation. An acquired disorder in which there is acceleration of thrombi formation and also increasing fibrinolytic activity resulting in hemorrhage. The disorder can be either chronic or acute. In obstetrics it is usually acute and considered a medical emergency.

Doppler ultrasound. Ultrasound that measures the speed of movement by comparing the shift of frequency among transmitted sound waves and reflected sound waves.

doula. An experienced woman in childcare who provides continuous physical, emotional, and informational support to the woman in labor.

Down syndrome. A chromosomal abnormality characterized by slanting eyes set close together; narrow palpebral fissures, flat nose; protruding large fissured tongue; small head and flat occiput; broad pudgy neck; short, thick hands with simian creases on the palms; defective mentality; underdeveloped muscles loose joints, and heart and alimentary tract abnormalities. The syndrome may be inherited, although its incidence increases with maternal age. Also called *trisomy 21* and, formerly, *mongolism.*

duration. The time during which something lasts. In obstetrics, the length of a contraction from increment to decrement.

dysfunctional labor. Abnormal uterine contractions that interfere with the normal progress of labor.

dysfunctional uterine bleeding. Abnormally heavy, light or irregular menstrual bleeding

dysmenorrhea. Painful menstruation.

dyspareunia. Painful intercourse, which can result from penetration, frictional movement, and deep thrusting.

dysphoria. Exaggerated feeling of depression or anxiety.

dysplasia. Abnormal cellular growth.

dyspnea. Rapid respirations exceeding 50 breaths per minute.

dysrhythmia. Abnormal discharge or transmission of impulses through the conduction system of the heart.

dystocia. Difficult, slow, or painful birth or delivery. It is distinguished as maternal or fetal (ie, the difficulty is due to some deformity on the part of the mother or on the part of the child).

early deceleration. Transient slowing of the FHR in a pattern that is almost a mirror image of the contraction.

echinocytes. Contracted red blood cells with spiny projections; also known as *burr cells.*

eclampsia. A severe complication occurring in pregnancy or the early puerperium, characterized by hypertension, edema, proteinuria, seizures, and coma.

ectopic pregnancy. Gestation in which the fetus is implanted outside uterine cavity. It includes gestations in the interstitial portion of the tube or in a rudimentary horn of the uterus (cornual pregnancy) and cervical pregnancy, as well as tubal, abdominal, and ovarian pregnancies. Also known as *extrauterine pregnancy.*

edema. Abnormal swelling due to large amounts of fluid in the tissues. See also *dependent e..*

effacement. Obliteration. In obstetrics, refers to thinning and shortening of the cervical canal.

effleurage. (Fr.) A rubbing movement, as in a massage. In obstetrics, an abdominal massage to aid in the pain management of labor.

elective abortion. Deliberate termination of a pregnancy.

electronic fetal monitor. A system for monitoring fetal heart rate and uterine activity by electrically operated instruments.

embryo. The product of conception in utero from the second through the eighth week of gestation.

embryotoxins. Substances that kill or alter the embryo.

endometriosis. Pathologic condition in which endometrial tissue is present on the pelvic peritoneum, contributing to infertility.

endometrium. The mucous membrane that lines the uterus.

endorphin. An opiatelike substance naturally produced by the body.

en face. (Fr.) The position in which the mother's face is rotated so that her eyes and those of her infant meet fully.

engagement. 1. In clinical obstetrics, applies to the entrance of the presenting part into the superior pelvic strait and the beginning of the descent through the pelvic canal. 2. Also relating to parent-infant interaction; behaviors designed to induce and sustain social interchanges.

engorgement. Hyperemia; local congestion; excessive fullness of any organ or passage. In obstetrics, refers to an exaggeration of normal venous and lymph stasis of the breasts, which is caused by increased amounts of milk in the lobules and ducts and circulating blood and lymph in the mammary glands.

enterocele. Herniation of the rectouterine pouch into the rectovaginal septum.

epidural anesthesia. Anesthesia produced by injecting a volume of anesthetic between the vertebral spines and beneath the ligamentum flavum into the epidural space. It is used in obstetric anesthesia to alleviate maternal pain with minimal danger to the infant. It requires the expertise that is afforded a surgical patient.

epidural space. The outer covering of the dura, spinal fluid and cord. It is filled with segments of nerve roots from the spinal cord, fatty tissue and an intricate networking of blood vessels. It is surrounded by a series of protective and supportive ligaments and the bony vertebral column.

episiotomy. Surgical incision of the vulvar orifice for obstetric purposes.

epispadias. A congenital anomaly in which the urethral meatus is located on the dorsal surface of the penis.

Erb's palsy. The upper-arm type of brachial birth palsy, due to damage to the upper plexus.

Escherichia coli. A short, rod-shaped genus of gram-negative bacteria found in the large intestines of humans and warm-blooded animals, which often causes urinary tract infections, diarrhea and other infections. Commonly referred to as *E. coli.*

esophageal atresia. A congenital defect in which the esophagus closes abnormally and ends in a blind pouch rather than a continuous tube to the stomach. It is characterized by excessive drooling, gagging, coughing, vomiting when fed, cyanosis, and dyspnea.

estradiol. An estrogen produced in ovarian follicles. It inhibits the release of follicle-stimulating hormones prior to ovulation.

estrogen. A steroid hormone produced primarily by the ovaries but also by the adrenal cortex. It is responsible for the development of secondary sex characteristics and the cyclic nature of female reproductive physiology.

estrogenic phase. See *proliferative phase.*

ethical dilemma. An ethical situation where there is no satisfactory decision, or there are satisfactory decisions but they are in opposition of one another.

ethnocentrism. The practice of judging different cultural beliefs or practices by standards from one's own culture.

euglycemia. Blood glucose levels as near the normal range as possible.

exophthalmos. Abnormal protrusion of the eye.

expected date of delivery (EDD). The calculated date for the birth of the fetus, which is usually based on the last menstrual period.

extension. Movement of the fetal head as it approaches the pelvic floor to allow for delivery of the head, face, and chin.

external cephalic version. Manipulation to turn the fetus from a breech presentation to a vertex.

external rotation. In childbirth, a change in the position of the fetus following the birth of the head during which the shoulders are born.

extracorporeal membrane oxygenation (ECMO) A method of establishing a pulmonary bypass circuit that permits the exchange of gas to occur outside the lung in a machine. This therapy has been used in newborns with respiratory distress syndrome, meconium aspiration syndrome, and persistent pulmonary hypertension.

extraction vacuum. In assisted childbirth, the use of a cup affixed to the fetal head by creating a vacuum between it and the head to assist in the delivery of a fetus. Traction is exerted by means of a short chain attached to the cup, with a handle at its far end.

extrauterine pregnancy. See *ectopic pregnancy.*

eye prophylaxis. Administration of anti-infective agents to prevent infectious conjunctivitis in newborns.

face presentation. A less common head presentation in which the fetal face (chin) enters the pelvic inlet first.

failure of descent. Absence of descent during the first stage, deceleration phase, or second stage of labor.

failure to progress. The cessation of labor due to the inability of the cervix to dilate normally. This occurs when the rate of progress in active labor falls below the Friedman curve, but there is normal uterine activity and no CPD.

fallopian tubes. Two trumpet shaped, thin flexible tubes about 12 cm long extending from the uterine cornua along the upper margin of the broad ligaments to the ovaries.

false labor A condition in the latter weeks of some pregnancies in which irregular uterine contractions are felt but the cervix is not affected.

false pelvis. The part of the pelvis superior to a plane passing through the linea terminalis, which supports the uterus during late pregnancy and directs the fetus into the true pelvis at the proper time.

family function. The actions of the family that produce competent persons who can survive in a complex ever-changing world. These functions include generating affection, ensuring continuity of companionship, providing personal security and acceptance, giving satisfaction and a sense of purpose, providing social placement and socialization, and instilling controls and a sense of what is right.

female condom. A prelubricated, polyurethane condom for vaginal use, which has a closed end covering the cervix and an open end fitting in the introitus.

female reproductive cycle (FRC). The combination of the menstrual and ovarian cycles which makes childbearing possible and influences the unique qualities and lives of women.

femur length. A diagnostic parameter used in determining gestational age and skeletal dysplasia, whereby the femur is measured from the origin to the distal end of the shaft.

fenestrum. A large opening or window on obstetric forceps to enhance the grip on the fetal head.

fertility. The ability to produce offspring; power of reproduction.

fertility awareness. The development of familiarity with the bodily signs of impending ovulation and bodily signs after ovulation, which enables a woman to anticipate her fertile period and its ending.

fertility rate. The number of births per 1000 women aged 15 through 44 years.

fertilization. The fusion of the spermatozoon with the ovum; it marks the beginning of pregnancy.

fetal. Pertaining to a fetus.

fetal alcohol syndrome. Birth defects caused by excessive intake of alcohol by the mother during pregnancy. Symptoms include prenatal and infant growth deficiencies, developmental delay or mental retardation, microcephaly, fine motor dysfunction, and facial dysmorphology in infants.

fetal biophysical profile. A method of fetal surveillance based on a composite assessment of several immediate and long-term markers of fetal disease. These markers include heart rate reactivity, fetal movement, fetal breathing, fetal tone, and amniotic fluid volume.

fetal cell isolation. A method of detecting fetal chromosomal abnormalities by evaluating various fetal cells that cross the placenta and circulate in the maternal blood.

fetal death. Death of the fetus that occurs in the uterus prior to birth.

fetal distress. A condition of fetal difficulty in utero that can occur during either the antenatal or the intrapartum period. Signs are fetal tachycardia, decrease in variability, and repetitive late or severe variable decelerations.

fetal heart rate (FHR). The heart rate of the fetus. Normally, it can be heard about the middle of pregnancy and usually ranges between 120 to 160 beats per minute.

fetal lie. The relationship of the long axis (spine) of the fetus to the long axis of the mother.

fetoscope. 1. A head stethoscope designed especially for listening to fetal heart tones. 2. An endoscope for viewing a fetus.

fetus. The baby in utero from the end of the 8th week of gestation until birth.

first stage of labor. The dilating stage that begins with the onset of regular labor contractions and ends with the complete dilatation of the cervix.

folic acid. One of the vitamins of the B complex that is essential for growth and necessary to the proper formation of blood in the body. Folic acid is particularly important to the development of the fetus.

follicle-stimulating hormone (FSH). A gonadotropic hormone secreted by the anterior pituitary, which stimulates the development of graafian follicles.

follicular phase. See *proliferative stage*.

fontanels. Intersections of sutures found on the upper part of the cranium. See also *anterior f.* and *posterior f.*.

fornix of the vagina. The arched or vaulted surface of the vaginal mucous membrane onto the cervix uteri.

fourth stage of labor. The recovery stage that begins with the delivery of the placenta and extends to the first 1 to 4 hours postpartum.

frequency. The number of times a process repeats within a certain period of time. In labor and delivery, the time between the beginning of one contraction to the beginning of the next.

fundal height. The measurement of the fundal position in relation to the umbilicus in order to determine the length of the fetus or uterine status.

fundus. The upper rounded portion of the uterus between the insertion points of the fallopian tubes.

funic souffle. A soft blowing sound, occurring simultaneously with the fetal heart sounds, that is supposed to be produced in the umbilical cord.

galactorrhea. Lactation after cessation of breast-feeding.

galactosemia. An inherited autosomal recessive disease and an inborn error of galactose metabolism caused by a lack of the enzyme necessary for proper metabolism of galactose.

gamete. A sexual cell; a mature germ cell, as an unfertilized egg or mature sperm cell.

gamete intrafallopian transfer (GIFT). An assisted reproductive procedure in which eggs are retrieved from the woman, mixed with sperm, then immediately introduced into the tubal segment known to be patent, usually through laparoscopy.

gametogenesis. The process of formation and development of the specialized male (spermatozoon) and female (ovum) gametes for fertilization.

gastroschisis. An abdominal wall defect in which abdominal organs are not contained by peritoneal membranes but spill from the abdomen freely.

gene. A functional unit of heredity in the chromosome that carries on a hereditary transmissible character.

genetic anomaly. A marked deviation from the expected standard as a result of an inherited defect.

genetics. The science of heredity.

genital herpes. A viral skin disease of the genitals marked by groups of vesicles 3 mm to 6 mm in diameter.

genotype. An individual's entire genetic composition.

gestational age. The number of weeks the neonate remains in utero.

gestational diabetes. Diabetes initially diagnosed during pregnancy, due to glucose intolerance.

gestational hypertension. A relatively benign condition of elevated BP during pregnancy without signs of proteinuria and edema.

glycosuria. The presence of glucose (sugar) in the urine.

glycosylated hemoglobin (HbA1c). Hemoglobin A with a glucose group attached to the terminal amino acid of the beta chains. Levels of glycosylated hemoglobin are measured to evaluate overall glycemic control.

gonadotropin. A substance produced by the anterior pituitary and placenta that has an affinity for or a stimulating effect on the gonads.

gonorrhea. A disease that is caused by *Neisseria gonorrhea*, spread by sexual contact, and affects the mucosa of the genital tract. The disease may be asymptomatic in women, except for a vaginal discharge. It can produce puerperal infection if present in the cervix at the time of delivery. The infection can infect the infant's eyes at birth.

Goodell's sign. Softening of the cervix, a probable sign of pregnancy.

graafian follicles or vesicles. Small spherical bodies in the ovaries, each containing an ovum.

grasp reflex. The reflex present at birth in an infant's hands and feet causing the fingers and toes to curl around an object touching them.

gravida. A pregnant woman.

growth. Increase in size, involving cell division and elaboration of cell products.

gynecoid pelvis. The most prevalent of the four main types of female pelvis, having a rounded oval shape.

gynecologic age. Number of years past onset of menarche.

gynecology. The branch of medicine that studies and treats women's diseases, especially of the genital tract.

habituation. The decreased response to a repeated stimulus.

Hegar' sign. An extreme softening of the lower uterine segment; a sign of pregnancy.

HELLP syndrome. Hypertension during pregnancy characterized by symptoms of hemolysis, elevated liver enzymes, and low platelet count.

hepatitis. Inflammation of the liver.

heterozygous. Having dissimilar genes at a specific locus.

hip dysplasia. A hereditary condition involving dislocation with partial or complete loss of contact between the femoral head and the cup-shaped cavity on the lateral surface of the hip bone.

histoplasmosis. A systemic respiratory disease caused by *Histoplasma Capsulatum*, a genus of parasitic fungi.

homocystinuria. Inborn error of metabolism inherited in an autosomal recessive pattern with progressive clinical symptoms.

homologous. Corresponding in structure or origin but not necessarily in function; derived from the same source.

hormone replacement therapy. Therapy of estrogen alone (ERT) or a combination of estrogen and progestogen (HRT) used to treat changes associated with menopause, such as hot flashes, vaginal and urinary tract atrophy, skin changes, and mood changes.

human chorionic gonadotropin (HCG). A hormone secreted by the placenta that prolongs the life of the corpus luteum. It is excreted in the mother's urine and makes possible the standards for pregnancy testing.

human immunodeficiency virus (HIV). A virus that causes a gradual decline of immune system function, resulting in AIDS when specific opportunistic infections develop. HIV substitutes its own RNA and DNA for a portion of the T4 cell's DNA, continues to destroy healthy T4 cells, and replicates infected ones.

human placental lactogen (HPL). An insulin antagonist produced by the placenta that promotes lipolysis to increase the amount of free circulating fatty acids for maternal metabolic use. HPL influences somatic growth and facilitates preparation of the breasts for lactation.

hydatidiform mole. Transformation and proliferation of the chorionic villi into grapelike cysts, characterized by poorly vascularized and edematous villi.

hydramnios. An excessive amount of amniotic fluid.

hydrocephalus. An excessive accumulation of cerebrospinal fluid in the ventricles of the brain with subsequent enlargement of the cranium.

hydropic. swollen; edemic

hyperemesis gravidarum. Excessive nausea and vomiting that results in fluid and electrolyte imbalance, marked weight loss, acetonuria, and nutritional deficits. Also called *pernicious vomiting.*

hyperglycemia. A condition characterized by an increase in or excess of blood glucose.

hypertension. Persistent high blood pressure, especially arterial blood pressure. See also *chronic h., gestational h., late or transient h.,* and *pregnancy-induced h..*

hypertonic. 1. Having high osmotic pressure. 2. A state of great tension.

hypertonic uterine dysfunction. An abnormality in the functioning of the uterus to propel the fetus through the birth canal. Uterine action is incoordinate; although there is constant tension in the muscle, the force of the contractions is distorted.

hypochromic. Insufficient hemoglobin in the erythrocyte.

hypofibrinogenemia. Deficiency of fibrinogen in the blood.

hypomenorrhea. Short, scant menstrual flow.

hypospadias. A developmental anomaly in which the urethra lies somewhere proximal to the tip of the glans penis, either on the ventral surface of the glans or penile shaft or in severe cases, on the perineum.

hysterectomy. The abdominal or vaginal surgical removal of all or a portion of the uterus.

hysterosalpingography. A x-ray procedure in which dye is passed through the fallopian tubes to test for tubal blockage.

ilium. Pl. ilia. The upper and largest portion of the hip bone.

imagery. A conscious, temporary shift from the here and now, which has a physiologic, pain-reducing effect on the body. Also called *visualization.*

imperforate anus. An abnormal closing of the anus.

implementation. The action stage of the nursing process in which the plan is initiated, the response to the plan is evaluated, and the nursing activities and client's responses to these activities are recorded. Implementation requires the use of intellectual, interpersonal, and technical skills.

inborn errors of metabolism. Hereditary deficiency of specific enzymes needed for normal metabolism of specific chemicals.

incompetent cervix. A mechanical defect in the cervix, which causes the cervical os to dilate prematurely during the midtrimester of pregnancy resulting in late habitual recurrent abortion or preterm labor.

incomplete abortion. An abortion in which some but not all the products of conception are passed.

increment. That by which anything is increased. In obstetrics, a period when the intensity of a contraction increases.

induced abortion. An abortion that is produced artificially and intentionally.

induction. Artificial initiation of labor after the fetus is viable.

infertility. The condition of being unfruitful or barren; sterility. The general criteria for a diagnosis of fertility is 1 year of coitus without conception.

inlet. The upper limit of the pelvic cavity (brim).

insulinase. An enzyme that accelerates insulin degradation.

insulin resistance. A glucose sparing mechanism that allows for an abundant supply of glucose for fetal use.

intermenstrual bleeding. Any bleeding or spotting between menses.

internal rotation. The process in the delivery of a baby in which the fetal head is rotated so that it enters the pelvis in the transverse position and exits in the anteroposterior position.

interstitial pregnancy. An ectopic pregnancy that develops in the portion of the tube that passes through the uterine wall.

intensity. The degree of strength. In obstetrics, the strength of a contraction during acme.

internal podalic version. A maneuver designed to change any fetal presentation to a breech presentation to facilitate delivery.

intrauterine growth retardation (IUGR). The condition of an infant born at 40 weeks' gestation and weighing less than 2500 g (or below the tenth percentile for weight or length). IUGR may be the result of a congenital anomaly, poor nutritional intake of the mother, or any other condition that significantly alters maternal, fetal, or placental health.

intrauterine growth standards. Graphic charts that are used to compare a newborn's weight (in grams) and gestational age with population averages.

inversion of the uterus. The state of the womb being turned inside out, associated with a placenta that has fundal implantation.

inverted nipple. A nipple that recedes rather than becoming erect when gentle pressure is used to compress the area behind the nipple.

in vitro fertilization. A system of impregnation in which ova are extracted from a woman, fertilized in a test tube, and implanted in the uterus.

involution. 1. A rolling or pushing inward. 2. A retrograde process of change that is the reverse of evolution; particularly applied to the return of the uterus to its normal size and condition after parturition.

ischium. The posterior and inferior bone of the pelvis, distinct and separate in the fetus and the infant, or the corresponding part of the hip bone in the adult.

jaundice. A condition characterized by hyperbilirubinemia and yellowness of the skin, eyes, mucous membranes, and body fluids. Jaundice is considered physiologic in the absence of disease or specific causes.

karyotype. The chromosome makeup of the nucleus of a human cell; the photomicrograph of chromosomes arranged in an organized way.

Kegel's exercise. The tightening and relaxing of the pubococcygeal muscle. It aids in toning the vagina, strengthening the perineum, preventing hemorrhoids, and controlling stress incontinence of urine.

kernicterus. The accumulation of unbound bilirubin in brain cells resulting in neurologic impairment.

Ketonemia. Ketone bodies in the blood.

Klumpke's palsy. Paralysis due to isolated damage to the lower plexus.

labia. The nominative plural of labium. Lips or liplike structures.

labia majora. The folds of skin containing fat and covered with hair that form each side of the vulva.

labia minora. The nymphae, or folds of delicate skin inside the labia majora.

labor. Parturition; the physiologic process by which regularly occurring uterine contractions result in progressive effacement and dilation of the cervix. See also *dysfunctional l., false l.,* and the *first stage of l., fourth stage of l., second stage of l., third stage of l.*

LaLeche League. An organization that holds classes about breast-feeding for women either before or after the baby is born.

Lamaze method of delivery. A widely practiced method of prepared childbirth that uses an individualized approach with classes for both parents or partners in the anatomy and neuromuscular activity of the reproductive system, breathing techniques in labor, and exercises. Sometimes other subjects such as nutrition, hygiene, and child care are taught. Also called *psychoprophylactic method of prepared childbirth.*

laminaria. A genus of seaweeds. Also, a small stick of hygroscopic material that absorbs moisture rapidly and expands. It is used to begin initial dilation of the cervix prior to abortion.

lanugo. The fine, downy hair found on nearly all parts of the fetus' body except the palms of the hands and the soles of the feet.

laparoscopy. The introduction of a slender, long surgical instrument (the laparoscope) into the abdominal cavity through very small incisions, not involving actual opening of the abdominal cavity. This procedure is often used for female sterilization. It is also used for direct visualization into the pelvic area in an effort to diagnose intrauterine adhesions, fibroid tumors, and other uterine anomalies.

large for gestational age (LGA). Pertaining to an neonate weighing above the 90th percentile for the gestational age. LGA infants are immature but overgrown and are typical of diabetic mothers.

late deceleration. A change in the FHR in which the onset, nadir, and recovery of the deceleration does not coincide with the onset, amplitude, and recovery of the uterine contraction.

late or transient hypertension. Hypertension that develops without edema or proteinuria during labor or the early postpartum period and then returns to normal after 10 days following delivery.

Leopold's maneuver. Maneuvers for diagnosing the fetal position by external palpation of the mother's abdomen.

let-down reflex. The activation of a process by which contractions of the myoepithelial cells in a mother's breast propel milk along the duct into the lactiferous sinuses. Also called *milk ejection reflex.*

lightening. Descent of the uterus into the pelvic cavity, which occurs from 2 to 3 weeks before the onset of labor, most often in primigravidas.

linea alba. The central tendinous line extending from the pubic bone to the ensiform cartilage.

linea nigra. A dark line appearing on the abdomen and extending from the pubis toward the umbilicus—considered one of the signs of pregnancy.

linea terminalis. The oblique ridge on the inner surface of the ilium, continued on the pubis, which separates the tube from the false pelvis. Formerly called the *iliopectineal line.*

lochia. The discharge from the genital canal during the first or second week following delivery.

lochia rubra. A bright red discharge consisting primarily of blood with small amounts of mucus, particles of decidua and cellular debris from the placental site; lasts for 3 days.

lochia serosa. A pinkish watery discharge consisting of old blood, serum, leukocytes and tissue debris; occurs as bleeding from the endometrium diminishes and lasts until 10 days after birth.

lochia alba. A thin, scant, whitish-tan discharge consisting of leukocytes, epithelial cells, mucus, serum and decidua; occurs after the 10th day of birth and disappears by the end of the 3rd week, although a brownish mucoid discharge may persist for 6 weeks.

Logan's bow. A wire bow taped to the cheeks after cleft surgery to prevent tension on suture lines around the lips.

long-term variability of FHR. The fluctuations or oscilations in the FHR for 1 minute, expressed in amplitude (between 6 and 25 beats/min) and cycles per minute (between 3 and 6).

low birth weight. A birth weight of 2,500 g or less.

luteal phase. See *secretory phase.*

luteinizing hormone (LH). A hormone released by the pituitary gland to bring about the final ripening of the graafian follicle and ovulation.

macrosomia. Excessive fetal growth.

magnetic resonance imaging. A noninvasive diagnostic tool that provides high-resolution cross-sectional images of fluid-filled soft tissue.

male condom. A thin sheath of latex rubber or processed collagenous tissue placed over the penis that acts as a mechanical barrier prohibiting sperm and bodily fluids from entering the vagina, thus preventing pregnancy and STDs.

marginal sinus rupture. A disorder of placental attachment; a mild type of abruptio placentae in which slight separation occurs at the edge of the placenta in the region of the marginal sinus of the mother.

mastitis. An acute infection in the glandular tissue of the breasts.

maternal mortality. Refers to the rate of maternal deaths that result from complications of pregnancy, childbirth, or the puerperium.

maternal role attainment. A process, which occurs over 3 to 10 months, in which the mother gains gratification and competence in mothering behaviors and mother-infant interactions through identifying, claiming, and interacting with the child.

maternity-perinatal nursing. The delivery of professional quality healthcare that recognizes, focuses on, and adapts to the physical and psychosocial needs of the childbearing woman, family, and newborn.

maximal effectiveness. A method's effectiveness in preventing pregnancy under ideal conditions.

McDonald's measurement. Measurement of the height of the uterine fundus with a tape measure; the distance from the symphysis pubis to the fundus.

meconium. The dark green or black substance found in the large intestine of the fetus or newborn.

megoblastic anemia. Anemia characterized by immature red blood cells that fail to divide, then become enlarged and fewer in number.

meiosis. The method for cell division that male and female germ cells undergo through which they mature and their genetic material, or chromosomes, are halved in preparation for fertilization; the creation of gametes.

menarche. The establishment or beginning of menstrual function.

meningocele. A congenital hernia in which the membranes covering the spinal cord bulge through an opening.

meningomyelocele. An extrusion of the spinal cord and meninges that forms a soft fluctuating tumor filled with cerebrospinal fluid.

menopause. The period at which menstruation ceases; the "change of life," usually between 48 and 52 years.

menorrhagia. Excessive uterine bleeding occurring at the regular time of menstrual flow, usually lasting 7-8 days with blood loss of more than 80–100 ml.

menstrual cycle. The recurring cycle of physiologic changes in the endometrium and sex organs that includes the menstrual, proliferative, and secretory phases.

menstrual phase. Approximately the 1st to the 5th day of the menstrual cycle, during which the endometrium, blood, glandular secretions and unfertilized egg are expelled.

menstruation. The periodic discharge of blood, mucus, and epithelial cells from the uterus that normally recurs at approximately 4-week intervals, in the absence of pregnancy, during the reproductive period.

metaplastic process. The replacement of one adult cell in a tissue by another adult cell that is not normal for that tissue.

microangioplastic hemolytic anemia. A reduction in the number of circulating blood cells in the small blood vessels.

microcephaly. Abnormal smallness of the head, which may be congenital or acquired.

microcytic. Small or immature red blood cells.

Mifepristone (RU486). A progesterone antagonist that has been investigated as an early abortifacient and a mid-cycle contraceptive.

milk ejection reflex. See *let-down reflex.*

missed abortion. The condition in which the embryo has died and subsequently the products of conception are retained in the uterus, and often expelled within 4-5 weeks of fetal death.

mitosis. The process by which body (somatic) cells replicate to produce two new identical cells with the same genetic makeup.

mitral valve prolapse. Prolapse of the mitral valve leaflets into the left atrium during ventricular systole, causing some backflow of blood.

mittelschmerz. Painful discomfort sometimes experienced during ovulation or in the middle of the menstrual cycle.

molding. The skull bones overlapping major sutures in order to adjust the fetal head to the size and shape of the birth canal.

mongolian spots. Gray-blue pigmented areas seen on some infants, especially those with dark skins. These have no relationship to mongolism and disappear spontaneously later.

monoclonal antibodies. Specific antibodies used to identify antigens on viruses and bacteria.

monosomy. The condition of a missing chromosome from a pair.

mons veneris. A firm cushionlike formation of subcutaneous fatty tissue and loose connective tissue over the symphysis pubis.

morning sickness. A symptom of pregnancy in some women, characterized by waves of nausea and sometimes vomiting. It usually occurs in the early part of the day and subsides after a few hours. It is common between 6–16 weeks of pregnancy.

Moro reflex. The reflex that is present from birth to age 3 months that indicates an awareness of equilibrium by a lateral extension of the upper extremities, and opening of the hands with the thumb and forefingers forming a characteristic "C."

morphogenesis. Development of form, including mass cell movement that allows cells to interact with each other during the formation of tissues and organs.

morula. The fertilized ovum at the 16-cell stage 3 days after conception. It travels from the fallopian tube into the uterine cavity prior to implantation.

mosaicism. The presence of two or more sets of cells that differ in their genetic makeup but arise from a single cell.

mother-newborn couple care. Care of the mother and newborn by the same nurse to help facilitate more flexible routines and increased opportunities for parenting education. Also called *couplet care.*

multipara. A woman who has given one or more prior births.

multiple pregnancy. The condition in which two or more embryos develop in the uterus at the same time.

mutagen. A chemical or substance that causes a change in inherited chromosomal structure or alteration of genetic information

mycobacteria tuberculosis. An acid-fast organism of the genus *Mycobacterium*, which is the causative agent of tuberculosis.

Nagele's rule. A method of calculating the expected date of confinement. The date is calculated by subtracting 3 calendar months from the 1st day of the last menstrual period and adding 7 days.

natural chilldbirth. See *prepared childbirth.*

Neonatal Behavioral Assessment Scale. A tool developed by Brazelton (1973) to evaluate newborn behavior by measuring 27 specific behavioral items that fall into one of the six designated categories—habituation, orientation, motor maturity, variation, self-quieting abilities, and social behavior.

neonatal death. Death of a neonate occurring shortly after birth.

neonate. The infant from birth through the first 28 days of life.

neoplasia. New and abnormal tissue growth. Also, called *tumors*.

nipple stimulation test. A noninvasive technique in prenatal testing based on the principle that nipple stimulation causes oxytocin to be released from the neurohypophysis, thus leading to the same results of a contraction stress test but eliminating the need for intravenous infusion of oxytocin.

nondisjunction. The unequal disturbance of chromosomes to the daughter cells during mitosis or meiosis.

nonperiodic changes of FHR. Accelerations or decelerations in the fetal heart rate that are not associated with uterine contractions.

nonreassuring patterns of FHR. Patterns of the FHR, observed during auscultation, that include a baseline FHR less than 100 beats/min 30 seconds after a uterine contraction, or an unexplained baseline tachycardia greater than 160 beats/min.

nonstress test. A test providing information about fetal well-being, by using the external fetal monitor and evaluating the fetal heart rate for accelerations from the baseline rate.

Norplant. A long-acting subdermal hormonal contraceptive, whereby six Silastic membrane capsules containing 35 mg of levonorgestrel (a type of progestin) are inserted into the woman's upper arm.

nullipara. A woman who has not borne children.

nurse-midwife. A registered nurse who has completed a recognized program of study and clinical experience leading to a certificate in nurse-midwifery.

obstetrics. The branch of medicine that is concerned with the management of women during parturition, its antecedents, and its sequelae.

oligomenorrhea. Irregular menses with long cycles.

omphalocele. Congenital abdominal wall defect in which portions of the abdominal content protrude at the base of the umbilicus.

oogenesis. The maturation process of the ovum.

operative obstetrics. Methods to expedite a complicated delivery and prevent harm to the newborn and mother, such as cesarean delivery or assisted delivery with forceps or a vacuum extractor.

ophthalmia neonatorum. Infectious conjunctivitis of the newborn, usually due to gonorrheal or chlamydial infection.

opisthotonos. A tetanic spasm resulting in an arched, hyperextended body position.

oral contraceptive. Hormonal agents consisting of a combination of estrogen and progestin or progestin alone that act on the central nervous system to inhibit ovulation.

Ortolani's maneuver. A diagnostic procedure performed on the newborn to determine congenital hip dysplasia.

osteopenia. A condition in which bone mass is substantially lower than the mean level of peak bone mass.

osteoporosis. An absolute decrease in the amount of bone to a level below that required for mechanical support function of the bone.

ovary. The almond-shaped glandular organs of the female in which the ova are developed. There are two ovaries located in the upper portion of the pelvic cavity on either side of the uterus.

overt abruptio placentae. Abruptio placentae whereby a separation occurs at the margin allowing blood to pass between the uterine wall and fetal membranes, creating an external hemorrhage. Also called *revealed abruptio placentae*.

ovulation. The growth and discharge of an unimpregnated ovum, usually coincident with the menstrual period.

ovum. The female reproductive cell developed in the ovary. The human ovum is a round cell about 1/120 of an inch in diameter.

oxytocic. 1. Accelerating parturition. 2. A drug that stimulates uterine contraction and controls bleeding.

oxytocin challenge/contraction stress test. A test providing information about uteroplacental function by using the external fetal monitor and evaluating the fetal heart rate in response to either spontaneous or induced uterine contractions.

pain. A localized sensation of hurt. In clinical practice, it can be defined as whatever the experiencing person says it is, existing whenever he or she says it does.

pain experience. All of the sensations, feelings, and behavioral responses, including physiologic activities and actions that impact others, experienced by a client.

pain intensity. The severity of the pain sensation.

pain tolerance. The intensity or duration of pain that the client is willing to endure without making further efforts to relieve it.

Papanicolaou smear. Cytology test of cervical cells used as a screening for cervical cancer.

para. The term referring to past pregnancies that have produced a viable infant, whether the infant was alive at birth or not.

paracervical block. The blocking of neuropathways of pain through a submucosal injection of local anesthetics near uterine nerve fibers at the vaginal fornix lateral to the cervix.

parametritis. An infection that extends along the blood vessels and lymphatics to the loose connective tissue of the broad ligaments or other pelvic structures.

partogram. A graph used to asses the normal progress of labor.

parturition. See *labor*.

passageway. The birth canal through which the fetus travels.

passenger. A term referring to the fetus during labor and delivery.

pathologic retraction ring. An exaggeration of the normal physiologic retraction ring that occurs at the junction of the upper and lower uterine segments. Bandl's ring is a pathologic constriction of the retraction ring.

patient-controlled analgesia. A method of pain relief in which the patient controls low-intensity stimulation emitted from a transcutaneous electric nerve stimulation unit.

pelvic. Pertaining to the pelvis.

pelvic cavity. The space between the inlet above, the outlet below, and the anterior, posterior, and lateral walls of the pelvis.

pelvic contractures. Disorders of pelvic muscles or fibrosis of supporting muscle tissue that cause an abnormal shortening of muscle tissue and make it difficult for the pelvic muscles to stretch.

Pelvic exenteration. Removal of the rectum, vagina, bladder, uterus, and cervix.

pelvic inflammatory disease (PID). Infection of the pelvic organs often caused by sexually transmitted disease or the presence of an IUD.

pelvic inlet. The entryway between the sacral promontory and symphysis pubis through which the fetal head must pass to the true pelvis.

pelvis. The lower part of the body bounded by the two hip bones, the sacrum, and the coccyx. See also *android p., anthropoid p., contracted p., false p., gynecoid p., platypelloid p.,* and *true p.*

percutaneous umbilical blood sampling (PUBS). A method of obtaining a sample of blood from the umbilical cord inside the placenta to study developments of various fetal biologic parameters.

perimenopause. The period beginning from irregular fertility and menses through at least 1 year after permanent cessation.

perinatal. Pertaining to the time before and after birth; defined as beginning at conception through the 28th day of life.

perinatal mortality. Refers to the rate of both fetal and neonatal deaths.

perineum. The muscle and fascia between the vagina and the rectum.

periodic breathing. Normal pauses, lasting up to 20 seconds, in the newborn's respiration.

period of reactivity. A phase in which the newborn exhibits outbursts of diffuse, purposeless movements that alternate with periods of relative immobility in a quiet alert state.

peritoneum. A strong serous membrane investing the inner surface of the abdominal walls and the viscera of the abdomen.

peritonitis. A major life-threatening infection of the peritoneum.

pernicious vomiting. See *hyperemesis gravidarum.*

persistent occiput posterior. Rotation of the fetal head through a 45-degree arc to the direct occiput posterior position.

phenotype. Observable characteristics.

phenylketonuria (PKU). An inborn error of metabolism that reflects the absence of the liver enzyme phenylalanine hydroxylase. It may be detected by blood or urine tests. Early treatment prevents mental retardation.

phimosis. A condition in which the opening of the foreskin is so small it cannot be pulled back at all.

phototherapy. The use of intense fluorescent light to treat a disease, especially to reduce serum bilirubin in the treatment of hyperbilirubinemia.

pica. An eating disorder characterized by the abnormal intake of specific substances such as clay dirt, cornstarch, or plaster. It may characterize the behavior of malnourished children or pregnant women.

placenta. The circular, flat, vascular structure in the impregnated uterus, which is formed through the union of the chorionic villa and the decidua basil. The placenta serves as the principal medium of communication between the mother and the fetus. See also *abruptio p., battledore p., circumvallate p.,p. accreta, p. previa, succenturiate p., velamentous p.*

placenta accreta. Implantation of the placenta in which an abnormally firm adherence to the uterine wall exists and makes separation of the placenta difficult or impossible.

placenta previa. A placenta that is implanted in the lower uterine segment so that it wholly or partially covers the internal os of the cervix.

placental expulsion. Delivery of the placenta in the third stage of labor, after the placenta has separated from the uterine wall.

platypelloid pelvis. One of the four main types of female pelvis, having a flattened pelvic inlet.

plethoric appearance. A condition marked by an excess of blood and fullness of pulse, accompanied by a feeling of tension in the head, florid complexion, and a tendency for nosebleeds.

Pneumocystis carnii. The causative organism of interstitial plasma cell pneumonia.

polydactyly. A hereditary condition characterized by extra digits on the hands or feet.

positive signs of pregnancy. Signs that undoubtedly confirm pregnancy, such as the detection of fetal heart sounds, fetal movements felt by the examiner, and visualization of the fetus.

posterior fontanel. A small, triangular fontanel between the occipital and parietal bones.

postpartum. After delivery or childbirth, referring to the mother.

postpartum hemorrhage. Loss of 500 ml or more of blood from the uterus after completion of the third stage of labor.

postpartum psychosis. Psychotic depression after childbirth, characterized by the loss of contact with reality, delusions, hallucinations, disorientation, sometimes anger, and possibly paranoia and strong aggressive feelings.

post-term pregnancy. A common complication of pregnancy when labor fails to start spontaneously in a pregnancy of 42 weeks or more.

powers. The combined force from involuntary uterine contractions (primary powers) and maternal pushing efforts (secondary powers), which allow for expulsion of the fetus and placenta.

precipitate delivery. A delivery that occurs with undue rapidity (less than 3 hours) and usually without the benefit of asepsis.

preeclampsia. A disorder encountered during pregnancy or early in the puerperium, characterized by hypertension, pathologic edema, and proteinuria.

pregnancy-induced hypertension (PIH). A diagnostic label used to describe the syndrome of hypertension, edema, and proteinuria evident in certain pregnant women. Preeclampsia and eclampsia are two categories of PIH.

premenstrual magnification pattern (PMM). High severity symptoms of PMS, such as medical, psychiatric or other affective disorders, that occur during the postmenses phase and become worse during premenses.

premenstrual phase. See *secretory phase.*

premenstrual syndrome (PMS). A complex set of recurrent, cyclic physical behavioral and emotional symptoms experienced during the 10 days preceding menstruation, which vary in severity. It is characterized by irritability, insomnia, headache, pain in the breasts, abdominal distention, nausea, anorexia, constipation, emotional instability, and urinary frequency.

premonitory signs. Symptoms experienced before the onset of labor that warn of the forthcoming event.

prepared childbirth. The methods by which parents or partners actively participate in childbirth. Some approaches include the concepts and techniques of Dick-Read, Lamaze, and Bradley. Also called *natural childbirth.*

presentation. Term used to designate that part of the fetus nearest the internal os, or that part that is felt by the examiner's hand when doing a vaginal examination. See also *breech p., brow p., cephalic p., compound p., face p.,* and *shoulder p.*

presumptive signs of pregnancy. Signs that suggest but do not prove that a healthy woman is pregnant. These include menstrual suppression, nausea, vomiting, frequent urination, tenderness and other changes of breasts, "quickening," Chadwick's sign, and fatigue.

preterm birth. The termination of pregnancy, spontaneously or therapeutically, after the fetus is viable but before it has attained full term, that is before the end of 37 weeks' gestation.

prickly heat. A closely grouped, pinhead size rash of papules and vesicles most often on the face and neck caused by the blockage of sweat pores.

primary prevention. Prevention of disease or high-risk situations through health promotion efforts, such as education and immunization.

primigravida. Pl. primigravidas. A woman who is pregnant for the first time.

primordial follicle. The whole structure of the ovum and surrounding cells in its underdeveloped state at birth.

probable signs of pregnancy. Signs strongly suggesting that the likelihood of pregnancy is great. These include enlargement of the abdomen, changes in the size, shape, and consistency of the uterus, fetal outline felt by palpation, ballottement, changes in the cervix, Braxton Hicks contractions, and a positive pregnancy test.

progestational phase. See *secretory phase.*

progesterone. The pure hormone contained in the corpus luteum whose function is to prepare the endometrium for the reception and development of the fertilized ovum.

prolactin. A proteohormone from the anterior pituitary that stimulates lactation in the mammary glands.

prolapse of umbilical cord. Delivery of the umbilical cord in labor prior to the delivery of the fetus.

proliferative phase. The phase of the menstrual cycle that occurs just after menstruation when the endometrium is growing or proliferating. Also called the *follicular* or *estrogenic phase.*

prolonged deceleration. A drop in the FHR that is outside the normal range, generally a decrease of 30 beats/min below the fetus' normal baseline, for up to 10 minutes.

prostate gland. A gland in the male that surrounds the neck of the bladder and urethra.

protracted active phase dilation. A slower than normal rate of cervical dilation.

protracted descent. Delayed descent of the fetal head in the active phase of labor.

protraction disorders. Disorders of labor and delivery characterized by protracted active phase dilation and protracted descent.

psychoprophylactic method of prepared childbirth. See also *Lamaze Method of delivery.*

puberty. The entire transitional period between childhood and sexual maturity.

pubis. The os pubis or public bone forming the front of the pelvis.

pudendal block. The blocking of neuropathways of pain by injecting a local anesthetic into the pudendal nerve. It abolishes pain in the vagina, perineum, and rectum.

puerperal infection. A wound infection of the birth canal after childbirth, which sometimes extends to cause phlebitis or peritonitis.

puerperium. The period elapsing between the termination of labor and the return of the reproductive organs to their prepregnant condition, about 6 weeks.

pulmonary embolism. Obstruction of the pulmonary artery. This is caused by a thrombus fragment that usually originates in the uterine or pelvic vein and is carried by venous circulation to the right side of the heart.

pulse oximeter. A noninvasive method of oxygen monitoring in the newborn that uses an infrared light source to determine the amount of saturated oxygen in tissues and read out the client's pulse rate.

pyelonephritis. Inflammation of the kidney and renal pelvis due to bacterial infection. In pregnancy, hormonal and anatomic changes cause narrowing of the lower ureter and dilation of the upper ureter and renal pelvis, thus increasing the risk of infection.

quickening. Perception of fetal movements.

rape. Sexual contact in the absence of consent.

rape trauma syndrome. Psychological crisis experienced by most victims of sexual assault, characterized by initial symptoms of confusion and disorganization of reactions, proceeding through an intermediate adjustment phase, and concluding with a long-term reorganization process.

reassuring patterns of FHR. Patterns of FHR that include a normal baseline rate, accelerations with fetal movement or stimulation, and the absence of decelerations.

real-time ultrasonography. B-mode ultrasonography that relies on several detectors to reflect echoes from the fetal structures and quickly provide multiple images in the form of motion.

recommended dietary allowances. Standards for the daily dietary intake of calories and nutrients for the people of the United States set by the Food and Nutrition Board of the National Research Council.

rectocele. The protrusion by hernia of a part of the rectum into the vagina, caused by disruption of the recto-vaginal fascia during childbirth.

recurrent abortion. Three or more consecutive first-trimester sponta-neous losses.

red reflex. A reflex of the eye that causes the pupil to appear as a small red-orange circular spot when light is directed at it.

regional blockade. The use of a local anesthetic to interfere with a group of sensory nerve fibers.

reproductive wastage. Loss of the products of conception.

research utilization. A complex ac-tivity involving planned change, the transfer of specific research-based knowledge into practice, and the activity of client problem-solving.

respiratory acidosis. A condition secondary to pulmonary insuffi-ciency in which an increase in hy-drogen ion concentration lowers blood pH below 7.35 and results in retention of carbon dioxide.

respiratory distress syndrome. A disease of premature infants charac-terized by the formation of a translucent membrane in the respi-ratory passages and the incapacity of the lungs to expand adequately.

retinopathy of prematurity (ROP). An acquired disease of the retina re-sulting in eye injury and blindness in the low-birth-weight newborn.

retraction ring. A ridge on the uterus marking the physiologic boundary between the upper, or contracting, segment and the lower, or dilating, segment of the uterus. See also *pathologic r.r.*

revealed abruptio placentae. See *overt abruptio placentae.*

rheumatic heart disease. Any patho-logic condition of the heart resulting from consequences of rheumatic fever, such as recurrent inflamma-tion and valvular scarring.

Rh factor. A term applied to an inher-ited antigen in the human blood.

RhoGAM. A preparation of anti-Rh an-tibodies administered by injection to unsensitized Rh-negative women following childbirth or abortion, to prevent the development of en-dogenous antibodies that could later lead to erythroblastosis fetalis (Rh disease of the fetus) in a subsequent pregnancy.

rhythm method. A birth control method relying on abstinence from sexual intercourse before, during, and after the period of time the ovum is capable of being fertilized.

role. Behavior that reflects the goals, values, and sentiments operating in a certain situation.

role allocation. The assignment of roles to family members based on the role structure of the family.

role conflict. Tension or interruption in role relations; Also referred to as *role strain.*

role differentiation. Structuring and delineating a role; the association of certain behaviors with each role.

role modeling. The act of giving spe-cific instructions regarding a certain facet of behavior and providing ex-amples of desired behavior to assist with the socialization of an indi-vidual.

role strain. See *role conflict.*

role structure. The way a family is organized based on each member's values, goals, and ability to perceive and attach meaning to events.

rooming-in. A family-centered, hos-pital practice in which newborns remain in the mother's room with the family all the time, except for necessary examinations or proce-dures.

rooting reflex. The tendency of in-fants to open their mouths and turn toward an object that is gently stroking their cheeks or the corner of their mouths.

salpingitis. Inflammation of the fal-lopian tubes.

scalp blood sampling. A technique of evaluating fetal scalp pH by puncturing the fetal scalp and ob-taining a small volume of blood.

scarf sign. A test to assess infant ma-turity. The infant's arms are drawn across the neck and as far across the opposite shoulder as possible. In the premature infant there is less re-sistance and greater draping (or scarf) effect; the elbow will reach near or across the midline. In the full-term infant, the elbow will not reach the midline.

schistocytes. Red blood cell frag-ments or portions of disrupted cells.

secondary areola. A circle of faint color sometimes seen just outside the original areola at about the 5th month of pregnancy.

secondary arrest of dilation. The lack of progress in cervical dilation during active labor for more than 2 hours.

secondary prevention. Early diagno-sis of disease or high-risk situations with prompt therapy to maximize outcomes.

second stage of labor. The pelvic stage that begins with the complete dilatation of the cervix and ends with the delivery or birth of the newborn.

secretory phase. The last 14 +/- 2 days of the menstrual cycle, during which progesterone is released in addition to estrogen. Also called the *progestational, luteal,* or *premen-strual phase.*

semen. 1. A seed. 2. The fluid se-creted by the male reproductive or-gans that contains the spermatozoa and nutrients.

semi-Fowler's position. A position of labor whereby the client's knees are flexed on the abdomen, hands grasped just below the knees during the onset of a contraction, and the head and shoulders possibly raised in a 45-degree angle.

seminiferous tubules. Coiled ducts, located within the lobules of the testes, where spermatogenesis occurs.

sepsis. The presence of microorgan-isms or their toxins in the blood or other tissues.

sex chromosome. One of two chro-mosomes in human cells that are as-sociated with the determination of the sex of the individual. A male cell normally contains one X and one Y chromosome, and a female cell contains two X chromosomes.

sexual abuse. Sexual contact and mis-treatment without consent, usually with the intent to harm

sexuality. The complex feelings, atti-tudes, preferences, and behaviors related to the individual's expres-sion of the sexual self and eroticism that are influenced biologically and culturally.

sexually transmitted diseases (STD). A variety of diseases usually trans-mitted by direct sexual contact with an infected individual.

short-term variability of FHR. The rate of FHR counted from one R wave to the next in each cardiac cycle.

shoulder dystocia. A serious compli-cation in the birth of an oversized infant whose unusually large shoulders arrest at either the pelvic brim or the outlet.

shoulder presentation. A serious complication of birth in which the infant lies crosswise in the uterus instead of longitudinally, thus the shoulder is usually the fetal part in the brim of the inlet.

show. The blood-tinged mucus discharged from the cervix after the mucus plug has become dislodged.

Sim's position. A position of labor in which the woman lies on her left side with her left leg extended and her right knee flexed at her side and up against the abdomen or with both knees flexed.

sinusoidal pattern. An unusual abnormality in FHR in which there is a repetitive undulation of the baseline resembling a "sine wave."

situational stressors. Extrafamilial stressors that are a result of situational events, such as illness, loss of a job, destruction of property through natural catastrophes, divorce, and separation of families because of job obligations or financial needs.

sitz bath. A treatment for perineal or perianal discomfort in which the client sits for 20 minutes three to four times per day in very warm water that may have astringents or solutions added.

Skene's gland. One of two glands just within the meatus of the female urethra; regarded as the homologue of the prostate gland in the male.

small for gestational age (SGA). Pertaining to a neonate weighing below the 10th percentile or standard deviations below the norm for the gestational age.

socialization. The process by which an individual learns society's expectations for behavior.

socioeconomic status. A theoretical formulation of relationships between societal subgroups, in which populations are subdivided into descriptive categories that differ in a variety of social and economic characteristics, backgrounds, and behaviors.

sound. An instrument introduced into the body passages or cavities for dilation or detection of foreign bodies.

spermatogenesis. The production and release of spermatozoa from the testes.

spermatozoon. Pl. spermatozoa. A mature male germ cell; the mobile microscopic sexual element that resembles in shape an elongated tadpole.

spina bifida. A common malformation involving closure of the spinal cord due to the congenital absence of one or more vertebral arches, usually at the lower part of the spine.

spina bifida occulta. The failure of the vertebrae to close without any herniation of the membranes or spinal cord.

spinal anesthesia. See *subarachnoid blockade.*

spiral electrode. A widely used method for FHR monitoring in which a spiral wire electrode is advanced into the fetal scalp in a clockwise rotation while gentle pressure is applied.

spontaneous abortion. An abortion that starts of its own accord through natural causes; commonly called a *miscarriage.*

startle reflex. A protective reflex in the newborn up until the 4th month characterized by a symmetrical drawing up of legs and grasping of arms in response to a sudden jarring.

stepping reflex. The reflex, which is present at birth but disappears within 2 months, that causes infants to make little stepping or prancing movements when they are held upright with their feet touching a surface. Also known as *dancing reflex.*

sterilization. 1. A process of eliminating microbial viability. 2. A permanent method of contraception; a surgical procedure by which an individual is made incapable of reproduction.

stressor. Something that produces stress. See also *developmental s.* and *situational s.*

striae gravidarum. Elongated streaks of red or pink often found on the abdomen and breasts of a pregnant woman; stretch marks.

stripping the membranes. The manual separation of chorioamniotic membranes from the lower uterine segment.

stroma. Tissue forming the framework of an organ.

subarachnoid blockade. Injection of a local anesthetic into the subarachnoid space where the medicine mixes with cerebrospinal fluid. Also called *spinal anesthesia.*

subarachnoid hemorrhage. A common type of intracranial hemorrhage in which bleeding into the subarachnoid space results.

subarachnoid space. The area between the pia mater and the arachnoid membrane.

subdural hematoma. A collection of blood between the arachnoid and dura mater (subdural space).

succenturiate placenta. An anomaly in which one or more small accessory lobes of the placenta develop in the membranes at a distance from the main placenta.

sucking reflex. The reflex in infants to suck anything that comes in contact with their lips. It seems to be a great need for the first 2 months of life, is present while sleeping, and need not be nutritive.

suffering. The state of anguish that might accompany pain.

surfactant. Secretions of the lungs and air passages that reduce the surface tension in the lungs; deficient in the preterm infant.

surrogate motherhood. The contractual hiring of a woman to bear another couple's child. Either the father's sperm impregnates the surrogate or the surrogate is implanted with the genetic parent's embryo.

sutures. Membranous interspaces between the four bones of the upper part of the cranium—the frontal, occipital, and two partial bones.

symptothermal method. Combination of the cervical mucus and ovulation symptom method with the BBT method to determine fertility. This approach tends to improve effectiveness of the fertility awareness approach to birth control. It also decreases the number of days on which a couple is permitted to have sexual intercourse.

tachycardia. Elevation of the FHR above 160 beats/min for greater than 10 minutes.

talipes equinovarus. The typical clubfoot. Its elements are equinus or plantar flexion of the foot at the ankle, varus or inversion deformity of the heel, and forefoot adduction.

Tay-Sachs disease. A hereditary metabolic disorder characterized by a degeneration of brain cells and a red spot on each retina, and eventually dementia, blindness, paralysis, and death.

teratogen. A chemical substance that interferes with fetal development after conception, producing a congenital malformation.

term. Birth occurring between 38 and 42 weeks gestation.

testosterone. The principal male sex hormone produced in the testes in response to the luteinizing hormone. It is believed to be responsible for regulating spermatogenesis, male characteristics, and maintaining muscle mass and bone tissue in the adult.

tetanic contraction. A contraction that lasts 2 minutes or greater.

tetralogy of Fallot. A combination of four congenital cardiac anomalies including ventricular septal defect, pulmonary stenosis, overriding aorta, and hypertrophy of the right ventricle.

therapeutic touch. A method of pain relief based on the folk-healing practice known as *laying on of hands*, whereby healers place themselves in a meditative state, hold their hands just above the client, and transfer their energy to the client to relieve pain or other problems.

third stage of labor. The placental stage that begins with the birth of the newborn and terminates with the delivery of the placenta.

thrombocytopenia. A decrease of clotting factors and the number of platelets in circulating blood.

thrombophlebitis. A condition in which inflammation of the vessel wall accompanies thrombosis.

thrombosis. The formation of blood clots.

tocodynamometer. An instrument that measures the expulsive force of uterine contractions in childbirth.

tocolytic drug. A drug used to inhibit uterine contractions primarily in an effort to suppress preterm labor.

tonic neck reflex. The tendency of infants while lying on their backs to turn their heads to one side and extend the arm and leg on that side, flexing the arm and leg on the other side.

toxemia. A condition cause by toxins circulating in the body.

toxic shock. Multisymptom infectious disease caused by toxin-producing strains of *Staphylococcus aureus*.

toxoplasmosis. A congenital disease characterized by lesions of the central nervous system. It is caused by the protoan *Toxoplasma gondii*, which is transmitted to the infant via maternal ingestion of raw meat, unpasteurized goat milk, or cat feces.

transabdominal ultrasound. Ultrasound in which a transducer transmits sound waves through the abdomen; for this procedure to be successful an acoustic window must be present.

transcutaneous electric nerve stimulation. The use of a mild electric current through the skin to relieve pain.

transvaginal ultrasound. Ultrasound in which an elongated transducer is placed within the vagina to visualize the pelvic structure.

transverse arrest. An abnormal fetal position in which rotation of the head is incomplete and the head is stopped in the transverse position.

tracheoesophageal fistula. An abnormal, tubelike opening between the trachea and esophagus.

traditional family. A mainstream form of the family that may be one of the following; single adult, nuclear family, nuclear dyad, single-parent family, or extended family/kin network.

transcutaneous oxygen tension (TcPO2). A noninvasive method of oxygen monitoring in the newborn that provides continuous monitoring of PO2 readings through measurement of skin oxygen tension.

transient circulation. The period during which anatomic changes of the circulatory system occur.

transitional stool. Stool after the first few days of life that is yellowish brown, less sticky than meconium, and contains some milk curds.

translocation. A structural chromosomal error that results from breakage and restructuring of the chromosomes.

trial of labor. An attempted labor to determine whether the fetal head can pass through the pelvis with adequate contractions.

Trichomonas vaginalis. A genus of parasitic flagellate protozoa sometimes found in the vagina and skene's ducts.

trichomonas vaginitis. A vaginal infection caused by *Trichomonas vaginalis* with characteristic increased discharge and pruritus, or itching.

trisomy. A chromosomal abnormality in which a particular chromosome is in triplicate rather than the usual pair.

trisomy 21. See *Down syndrome*.

trophoblast. The outer layers of the fertilized ovum, which attach the fertilized ovum to the uterine wall, secure food for the embryo, and develop into the chorion.

true pelvis. The part of the pelvis inferior to a plane passing through the linea terminalis that forms the bony canal through which the fetus must pass during parturition.

tubal ligation. A contraceptive surgical procedure designed to block the tubal conduit through which spermatozoa and ova pass, by binding or tying a the vessel with a substance such as string or catgut .

tubal pregnancy. An ectopic pregnancy in which the fertilized ovum is embedded in one of the fallopian tubes rather than the wall of the uterus.

Turner's syndrome. A genetic defect characterized by undifferentiated gonads, short stature, and other abnormalities, which may include webbing of the neck, low posterior hairline, and cardiac defects.

typical effectiveness. A method's effectiveness in preventing pregnancy under actual use, in which some people use the method correctly and others use it carelessly or incorrectly.

ultrasound. The use of high-frequency sound waves to detect the differences in tissue density and visualize outlines of structures within the body. Used for fetal assessment because it poses a minimal risk. See also *Doppler u.*, *transabdominal u.*, and *transvaginal u.*

umbilical cord. (Latin, funis umbilicalis.) The cord connecting the placenta with the umbilicus of the fetus that provides nutrition to the fetus and in turn removes the fetus' waste. At the close of gestation, it is principally made up of the two umbilical arteries and the umbilical vein, encased in a mass of gelatinous tissue called Wharton's jelly.

ureter. The tube through which urine passes from the kidney to the bladder.

uterine atony. Lack of uterine tone or strength due to stretching of the uterus.

uterus. The hollow, thick-walled, muscular organ in the female designed for the lodgement and nourishment of the fetus during its development until birth.

vagina. (Latin, a sheath.) The dilatable, mucus membrane-lined passage between the bladder and the rectum.

vaginal spermicide. A physical barrier to sperm penetration that also exerts a chemical action on the sperm.

vaginosis. An infection of the vagina caused by *Gardnerella vaginalis.* Vaginosis is characterized by an increase of vaginal discharge that is typically thin, gray white, homogeneous and has a fishy odor particularly after intercourse and during menstruation.

Valsalva's maneuver. Bearing down efforts accompanied by long and sustained pushes without audible sounds.

variable deceleration. A change in the FHR in which the relationship of the deceleration to the contraction and the waveform is variable in duration, depth, and shape from contraction to contraction and abrupt in onset and recovery.

varicocele. Varicose veins of the scrotum.

vasectomy. The surgical interruption and ligation of the vas deferens, the spermatic duct, to prevent sperm from being in the ejaculate. It is the method of male sterilization.

vegan. A pure vegetarian who abstains from all meats and animal by-products.

vegetarianism. A dietary pattern of abstaining from the consumption of meats or animal by-products for religious, health, or social reasons. Vegetarian diets vary in the extent to which animal proteins are excluded.

velamentous placenta. Abnormality of the umbilical cord in which blood vessels course unprotected for long distances through the membranes to insert into the margin of the placenta.

ventricular septal defect. A congenital cardiac anomaly in which there is an abnormal opening between the right and left ventricles.

vernix caseosa. "Cheesy varnish." The layer of fatty matter that covers the skin of the fetus.

vestibule of the vagina. A triangular space between the attachment lines of the labia minora; the urinary meatus and the vagina open into it.

viability. The capacity of the fetus to live outside the uterus at the earliest gestational age.

vibroacoustic stimulation. A method of stimulating reactivity in a presumably resting fetus during a nonstress test. An artificial larynx provides acoustic and vibratory stimulation.

villus. Pl. villi. A small vascular process or protrusion growing on a mucous surface, such as the chorionic villi seen in tufts on the chorion of the early embryo.

visualization. See *imagery*.

vulva. The external genitals of the female.

Wharton's jelly. (Thomas Wharton, English anatomist, died 1673.) The jellylike mucous tissue composing the bulk of the umbilical cord.

witches' milk. A milky fluid secreted from the breast of the newborn.

withdrawal. The practice of retracting the penis from the vagina in intercourse prior to ejaculation, used as a method of contraception.

X-linked recessive disorder. A condition resulting from abnormal genes located on the X chromosome.

zygote. A cell resulting from the fusion of two gametes that contains the characteristics of the woman and man.

zygote intrafallopian transfer (ZIFT). An assisted reproductive procedure in which eggs are retrieved, fertilized in vitro, and transferred to the fallopian tube at the pronuclear stage prior to cell division. ZIFT is used when proof of fertilization is essential in situations such as severe male factor infertility or immunologic infertility.

Photo Credit List

Figure 1-1B: ©Simon Fraser/Department of Child Health, RVI, Newcastle/Science Photo Library/Photo Researchers

Figure 1-2: ©Kathy Sloane

Figure 3-1: ©Seth Resnick/Stock, Boston

Figure 3-4: Photo by C. Shea

Figure 4-2: ©Kathy Sloane

Figure 4-5: ©B. Proud

Figure 7-6: ©P. Motta/Dept. Of Anatomy/University "La Sapienza," Rome/Science Photo Library/Photo Researchers

Figure 7-7: ©P. Motta/Dept. Of Anatomy/University "La Sapienze," Rome/Science Photo Library/Photo Researchers

Figure 7-12A: ©SIU/Photo Researchers

Figure 7-12B: ©Martin M. Rotker/Photo Researchers

Figure 7-15 A-D: ©Petit Format/Nestle/Science Source/Photo Researchers

Figure 8-1: Reprinted from Craven R. (1996) Fundamentals of Nursing—Human Health and Function. (2nd ed.). Philadelphia: Lippincott-Raven.

Figure 9-1: Photo by D. DiPalma

Figure 11-2: Reprinted from Allen, K. (1997) Women's Health Across the Lifespan. Philadelphia: Lippincott-Raven.

Figure 13-2: ©Science Photo Library/Photo Researchers

Figure 14-9: ©P. Saada/Eurelios/Science Photo Library/Photo Researchers

Figure 16-1: ©B. Proud

Figure 16-2 A&B: Photo by D. DiPalma

Figure 17-5: ©B. Proud

Figure 17-6 A&B: Photo by D. DiPalma

Figure 18-1: ©B. Proud

Figure 18-2: Photo by D. DiPalma

Figure 19-3: ©Kathy Sloane

Figure 19-4: Photo by D. DiPalma

Figure 22-2: ©Kathy Sloane

Figure 22-3: ©Kathy Sloane

Figure 22-8: ©Kathy Sloane

Figure 22-10: ©Kathy Sloane

Figure 22-12: ©Fred McConnaughey/Photo Researchers

Figure 23-2: Reprinted from Taylor, C. (1997) Fundamentals of Nursing: The Art and Science of Nursing Care. (3rd ed.). Philadelphia: Lippincott-Raven.

Figure 23-3: Reprinted from Taylor, C. (1997) Fundamentals of Nursing: The Art and Science of Nursing Care. (3rd ed.). Philadelphia: Lippincott-Raven.

Figure 24-1: ©SIU/Photo Researchers.

Figure 24-4: ©David J. Sams/Stock, Boston

Figure 26-2: ©Kathy Sloane

Figure 26-3: ©Kathy Sloane

Figure 28-2: ©Kathy Sloane

Figure 28-4: ©Kathy Sloane

Figure 28-5: ©Kathy Sloane

Table 28-5, Unnumbered Figure 1: ©Biophoto Associates/Photo Researchers

Table 28-5, Unnumbered Figure 2: ©Science Photo Library/Photo Researchers

Table 28-5, Unnumbered Figure 3: Reprinted from Scherer J. (1995) Introductory Medical-Surgical Nursing. (6th ed.). Philadelphia: J.B. Lippincott Co.

Figure 29-3: ©Kathy Sloane

Figure 29-8: ©Gates/Rhodes

Unnumbered Figure 29-1: photo courtesy S. Ludington

Figure 30-1: ©Kathy Sloane

Figure 30-3: ©Kathy Sloane

Figure 30-8: ©Dorothy Littell Greco/Stock, Boston

Figure 30-9: ©Sue Klemens/Stock, Boston

Procedure 32-1, Unnumbered Figure 32-1: Reprinted from Smeltzer S. (1996) Brunner and Suddarth's Textbook of Medical-Surgical Nursing. (8th ed.). Philadelphia: Lippincott-Raven.

Figure 34-2: Photo by D. DiPalma

Figure 35-2: ©Bob Daemmrich/Stock, Boston

Figure 35-3: Reprinted from Craven R. (1996) Fundamentals of Nursing—Human Health and Function. (2nd ed.). Philadelphia: Lippincott-Raven.

Figure 35-4: ©Kathy Sloane

Figure 37-4A: ©Biophoto Assoc./Photo Researchers

Figure 37-4B: ©Biophoto Assoc/Photo Researchers

Figure 37-4C: ©Bob Daemrich/Stock, Boston

Figure 39-3: ©Kathy Sloane

Figure 39-9: Reprinted from Craven R. (1996) Fundamentals of Nursing—Human Health and Function. (2nd ed.). Philadelphia: Lippincott-Raven.

Unnumbered Figure 40-1: ©Kathy Sloane

Figure 40-1: ©B.A. Rupert

Figure 40-5: ©Kathy Sloane

Figure 41-2: ©Susan Leavines/Photo Researchers

Figure 41-7: ©Gates/Rhodes

Figure 41-8: ©John Watney/Photo Researchers

Figure 41-10: ©Gates/Rhodes

Figure 41-14: ©Gates/Rhodes

Figure 42-8: ©Susan Leavines/Photo Researchers

Figure 42-15: ©Jim Stevenson/Science Photo Library/Photo Researchers

Figure 43-3: ©Photo Researchers

Unit Openers

Unit I: Photo by C. Shea

Unit II: ©P. Motta/Dept. Of Anatomy/University "La Sapienze," Rome/Science Photo Library/Photo Researchers

Unit III: Reprinted from Craven R. (1996) Fundamentals of Nursing—Human Health and Function. (2nd ed.). Philadelphia: Lippincott-Raven.

Unit IV: ©B. Proud

Unit V: Reprinted from Craven R. (1996) Fundamentals of Nursing—Human Health and Function. (2nd ed.). Philadelphia: Lippincott-Raven.

Unit VI: ©Kathy Sloane

Unit VII: Reprinted from Craven R. (1996) Fundamentals of Nursing—Human Health and Function (2nd ed.). Philadelphia: Lippincott-Raven.

Unit VIII: Reprinted from Craven R. (1996) Fundamentals of Nursing—Human Health and Function (2nd ed.). Philadelphia: Lippincott-Raven.

Index

Page numbers followed by f indicate figures; those followed by t indicate tables; those followed by box indicate boxed material.

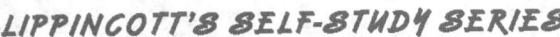
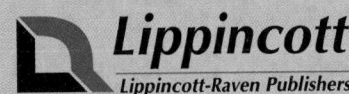

Maternity Nursing *Self-Study Disk Instructions*

SYSTEM REQUIREMENTS

A PC-compatible computer with an Intel 386 or better processor.

Windows 3.1 or later.

4 Megabytes of RAM (minimum); but recommend 8 MB RAM on Windows 3.1

8 Megabytes of RAM (minimum); but recommend 12 MB RAM minimum on Windows 95

3 Megabytes of available hard disk space.

INSTALLATION

Installing *Maternity Nursing* for Windows

1. Start up Windows.
2. Insert the *Maternity Nursing* disk into the floppy disk drive.
3. From the Program Manager's File Menu, choose the Run command.
4. When the Run dialog box appears, type a:\setup (or b:\setup if you're using the B drive) in the Command Line box. Click OK or press the Enter button.
5. The *Maternity Nursing* installation process will begin. A dialog proposing the directory "MATNSG" on the drive containing Windows will appear. If the name and location are correct, click OK. If you want to change this information, type over the existing data, then click OK.
6. When the *Maternity Nursing* setup routine is complete, a new group called "*Maternity Nursing*" will appear on your desktop.
7. Start the *Maternity Nursing* self-study program by double-clicking on its icon.

MATERNITY NURSING *SELF-STUDY PROGRAM*

Maternity Nursing contains approximately 250 questions that review the content covered in *Maternity Nursing*, Eighteenth Edition.

This is not a timed test. Take your time, consider the questions and the possible answers carefully.

The Main Menu screen allows you to select which unit you would like to review. To begin a unit test, choose Start Test for that unit. To continue a test that you have already begun, choose Resume Test. To restart the test and erase your results from a previous test, choose Restart Test. To review the answers you have given and compare them with the correct answers, choose Answers.

When you choose Start Test, Resume Test, Restart Test, or Answers the test and the program's Toolbar will appear.

MATERNITY NURSING'S *TOOLBAR*

The Toolbar contains a series of buttons that provide direct access to all test program functions. When you move the cursor over a button, an explanation of its function displays in the Status Bar, which is immediately above the Toolbar.

To get help at any time during the test, choose the Program Help button. Program Help reviews basic functions of the program.

Answer each question by clicking on the oval to the left of an answer selection or by selecting the appropriate letter on the keyboard (e.g. A, B, C, D, etc.). When an answer is selected, its oval will darken. If you change your mind about an answer, simply select that choice, by mouse or keyboard, again.

To register your answer selection and proceed to the next question, click on the Right Arrow button or press Return.

After taking the test and receiving your score you may review your answers by clicking on the Answers button on the Main Menu screen.

If you are unsure about an answer to a particular question, the program allows you to mark it for later review. Flag the question by clicking on the Mark button. To review all marked questions for a test, click on the Table of Contents button, which is immediately to the right of the Mark button.

The Table of Contents window lists every question included on the test and summarizes whether it has been answered, left unanswered, or marked for later review. Click on an item in the Table of Contents window, and the program will move to that test question.

Use the Arrow buttons to move to the first, previous, next, or last question.

At any time during the test or when you are finished taking the test, click on the Stop button. If you wish, you may return to the session at a later time without erasing your existing answers by clicking on the Resume Test button on the Main Menu.

After taking a test, view the correct answer for each test question by using the Answers button on the Main Menu. This will take you back to the test, but you will not be able to modify the answers you have given. Click on the Q/A button (to the right of the Stop button) and a window will pop up explaining the correct answer to the question. (The Q/A button will only appear when you are in the "Answers" section of the test.) You may also wish to use the Table of Contents button to show you which questions you marked for review.

To exit the *Maternity Nursing* program, click the Quit button on the Main Menu.